ROTHMAN–SIMEONE

THE SPINE

ROTHMAN–SIMEONE

THE SPINE *Fourth Edition*

VOLUME II

Harry N. Herkowitz, M.D.

Chairman, Department of Orthopaedic Surgery,
Willliam Beaumont Hospital;
Director, Section of Spine Surgery,
Department of Orthopaedic Surgery,
William Beaumont Hospital,
Royal Oak, Michigan

Steven R. Garfin, M.D.

Professor and Chair, Department of Orthopaedics,
University of California, San Diego;
Chief, Section of Spine Surgery,
UCSD Medical Center,
San Diego, California

Richard A. Balderston, M.D.

Professor, Orthopaedic Surgery, and Associate
  Professor, Neurosurgery;
Vice-Chair, Department of Orthopaedics;
Chief, Spine and Scoliosis Service,
Allegheny University Hospitals,
Philadelphia, Pennsylvania

Frank J. Eismont, M.D.

Professor, Department of Orthopedics, and
Clinical Professor of Neurologic Surgery,
University of Miami School of Medicine;
Co-Director of Spinal Cord Injury Service,
Jackson Memorial Hospital,
Miami, Florida

Gordon R. Bell, M.D.

Vice Chairman, Department of Orthopaedic
  Surgery;
Head, Section of Spinal Surgery;
Cleveland Clinic Foundation,
Cleveland, Ohio

Sam W. Wiesel, M.D.

Professor and Chairman, Department of
  Orthopaedic Surgery,
Georgetown University School of Medicine and
  Medical Center,
Washington, D.C.

W.B. SAUNDERS COMPANY
A Harcourt Health Sciences Company

Philadelphia   London   New York   St. Louis   Sydney   Toronto

W. B. SAUNDERS COMPANY
A *Harcourt Health Sciences Company*
The Curtis Center
Independence Square West
Philadelphia, PA 19106

Library of Congress Cataloging-in-Publication Data

Rothman-Simeone, the spine.—4th ed. / Harry N. Herkowitz . . . [et al.]

p.   cm.

Rev. ed. of: The spine / founding editors, Richard H. Rothman and Frederick A. Simeone. 3rd ed. © 1992.

Includes bibliographical references and index.

ISBN 0–7216–7176–4

1. Spine—Surgery.   2. Spine—Diseases.   3. Spine—Wounds and injuries.
   4. Spine—Abnormalities.   I. Herkowitz, Harry N.   II. Rothman, Richard H.
   III. Simeone, Frederick A.
[DNLM: 1. Spinal Diseases.   2. Spinal Injuries.
3. Spine—surgery.   WE 725 R846 1999]

RD533.S68   1999   617.5′6—dc21

DNLM/DLC   97-2672

Volume I ISBN 0–7216–7807–6
Volume II ISBN 0–7216–7808–4
Set ISBN 0–7216–7176–4

ROTHMAN-SIMEONE THE SPINE

Printed in the United States of America.

Last digit is the print number: 9   8   7   6   5   4   3   2

The fourth edition of The Spine *is based on the principles taught to us, the Editorial Board, by Drs. Rothman and Simeone as Fellows or practice partners. These are (1) thorough knowledge of the basic science as it relates to the clinical picture, (2) understanding of the natural history of spinal disease, (3) knowledge and interpretive skills of imaging modalities and laboratory studies, (4) treatment decisions based on sound scientific principles, and (5) commitment to education and research to further the knowledge base of spinal disorders.*

These principles continue to guide our daily practices and our educational responsibilities. As with the previous edition, this fourth edition remains dedicated to Drs. Rothman and Simeone, teachers and friends.

Each member of the Editorial Board has special dedications, which are listed below.

Harry N. Herkowitz, M.D.

To my wife, Jan, and my children, Seth Adam and Rachael Helene, for their love, understanding, and support. To the residents and fellows whose enthusiasm for knowledge and "all the answers" inspires me to continue academic pursuits.

Steven R. Garfin, M.D.

Susan, Jessica, and Cory. Textbooks may change by 20–30% every three to five years. My love and respect for my wonderful family, however, continues to grow regularly. They understand and accept my commitment to patients and education.

Richard A. Balderston, M.D.

To my wife Claudia, for her constant love and support, and my children Philip and Jessica, who make it all worthwhile.

Frank J. Eismont, M.D.

To my wife Emily and my children Adam, April, Allison, and Andrew, whose love and encouragement and tolerance have allowed me to avidly pursue my medical interest, and to Drs. Charles Herndon, Henry Bohlman, Fred Simeone, and Richard Rothman, who have been excellent role models for me to try to emulate regarding medical education and patient care.

Gordon R. Bell, M.D.

To my wife Kathy, for her patience and understanding.
To my children Gordie, Michael, and Megan, for making efforts such as this worthwhile.
To my parents, Gordon and Ann, for their support in making this possible.

Sam W. Wiesel, M.D.

To Vicki and Phil Bowie, who have provided unwavering support over the years.

List of Contributors

Jean-Jacques Abitbol, M.D.
Clinical Instructor, Department of Orthopaedic
Surgery, State University of New York, Health Science
Center at Syracuse, Syracuse, New York; Attending
Orthopaedic Surgeon, St. John's Episcopal Hospital,
Smithtown, New York; Attending Orthopaedic
Surgeon, Huntington Hospital, Huntington, New York
Adult Scoliosis

Todd J. Albert, M.D.
Associate Professor, Department of Orthopaedics,
Thomas Jefferson University; Co-Director,
Reconstructive Spine Service and Spinal Fellowship
Program, Thomas Jefferson University Hospital and
Rothman Institute, Philadelphia, Pennsylvania
Spinal Instrumentation

Marshall B. Allen, M.D.
Professor Emeritus, Medical College of Georgia,
Augusta, Georgia
Intraspinal Infections

Michael J. Aminoff, M.D., F.R.C.P.
Professor of Neurology, School of Medicine,
University of California, San Francisco; Attending
Physician, Director of Clinical Neurophysiology
Laboratories, University of California Medical Center,
San Francisco, California
*Electrodiagnosis: Somatosensory and Motor Evoked
Potentials*

Glenn Amundson, M.D.
Assistant Professor of Orthopedics, University of
Kansas Medical Center, Kansas City, Kansas
Spondylolisthesis

Howard S. An, M.D.
The Morton International Professor of Orthopaedic
Surgery, Rush Medical College; Director of Spine
Fellowship Program, Department of Orthopaedic
Surgery, Rush–Presbyterian–St Luke's Medical Center,
Chicago, Illinois
*Juvenile Kyphosis; Surgical Management of Cervical
Disc Disease*

David F. Apple, Jr., M.D.
Associate Clinical Professor of Orthopaedic Surgery,
Clinical Associate Professor in Rehabilitation
Medicine, Emory University; Medical Director,
Shepherd Center; Piedmont Hospital, Atlanta, Georgia
Spinal Cord Injury Rehabilitation

Richard A. Balderston, M.D.
Professor, Orthopaedic Surgery, and Associate
Professor, Neurosurgery; Vice-Chair, Department of
Orthopaedics; Chief, Spine and Scoliosis Service,
Allegheny University Hospitals, Philadelphia,
Pennsylvania
Juvenile Kyphosis; Spinal Instrumentation

Gordon R. Bell, M.D.
Vice Chairman, Department of Orthopaedic Surgery;
Head, Section of Spinal Surgery; Cleveland Clinic
Foundation, Cleveland, Ohio
*Differential Diagnosis of Sciatica; Radiology of the
Lumbar Spine*

Robert J. Benz, M.D.
Clinical Instructor, Department of Orthopaedics,
University of California, San Diego, San Diego,
California
Adult Scoliosis

Joseph R. Berger, M.D.
Professor and Chairman, Department of Neurology;
Professor, Department of Internal Medicine,
University of Kentucky College of Medicine,
Lexington, Kentucky
Medical Myelopathies

Kel Bergmann, C.P.O.
Vice President and Board Member, California
Orthotics and Prosthetics Association; Board Member,
National Multiple Sclerosis Society; Member,
American Orthotics and Prosthetics Association and
American Academy of Orthotics and Prosthetics;
Southern California Orthotics and Prosthetics
(SCOPE), San Diego, California
Spinal Orthoses for Traumatic and Degenerative Disease

Mark Bernhardt, M.D.
Clinical Associate Professor, Department of
Orthopaedic Surgery, University of Missouri–Kansas
City School of Medicine; Dickson-Diveley Midwest
Orthopaedic Clinic, St. Luke's Hospital of Kansas
City, The Children's Mercy Hospital, Kansas City,
Missouri
Biomechanical Considerations of Spinal Stability

Joseph Bernstein, M.D.
Assistant Professor, Orthopedic Surgery, University of
Pennsylvania School of Medicine; Attending
Orthopedic Surgeon, Hospital of the University of
Pennsylvania, Philadelphia, Pennsylvania
Metabolic Bone Disorders of the Spine

Scott D. Boden, M.D.
Associate Professor of Orthopaedics, Emory
University School of Medicine; Director, The Emory
Spine Center, Atlanta, Georgia
*Spinal Fusion; The Multiply Operated Low Back: An
Algorithmic Approach; Workers' Compensation As It
Affects the Spine*

Henry H. Bohlman, M.D.
Professor, Department of Orthopedic Surgery;
Director, The University Hospitals Spine Institute;
Chief, The Acute Spinal Cord Injury Service–Veterans
Administration Medical Center; Case Western Reserve
University, School of Medicine, Cleveland, Ohio
Spine Trauma in Adults: Spine and Spinal Cord Injuries

Robert E. Booth, Jr., M.D.
Professor of Orthopaedic Surgery at Allegheny
University of the Health Sciences; Chair of the
Orthopaedic Hospital at Allegheny University
Hospitals–Graduate, Philadelphia, Pennsylvania
Arthritis of the Spine

Michael J. Botte, M.D.
Head, Section of Neuromuscular Reconstructive
Surgery and Rehabilitation, Division of Orthopaedic
Surgery, Scripps Clinic and Research Foundation, La
Jolla, California; Orthopaedic Surgery Service,
Veterans Affairs Medical Center, San Diego,
California; Clinical Professor, Department of
Orthopaedic Surgery, University of California, San
Diego, School of Medicine, San Diego, California
Spinal Ortheses for Traumatic and Degenerative Disease

Brian C. Bowen, M.D., Ph.D.
Associate Professor of Radiology and Neurological
Surgery, University of Miami School of Medicine;
Attending Physician, Jackson Memorial Medical
Center, Miami, Florida
Syringomyelia

David S. Bradford, M.D.
Professor and Chairman, Department of Orthopaedic
Surgery, University of California, San Francisco, San
Francisco, California
Lumbar Pseudarthrosis: Diagnosis and Treatment

Richard S. Brower, M.D.
Assistant Professor of Orthopaedic Surgery,
Northeastern Ohio Universities College of Medicine,
Rootstown, Ohio; Active Staff, Summa Health System,
Akron, Ohio
*Cervical Disc Disease: Clinical Syndromes and
Differential Diagnosis of Cervical Disc Disease*

H. Ulrich Bueff, M.D.
Formerly Department of Orthopaedic Surgery,
University of California, San Francisco, San Francisco,
California
Lumbar Pseudarthrosis: Diagnosis and Treatment

Richard P. Bunge, M.D.
Late Professor of Neurological Surgery and Cell
Biology and Anatomy, University of Miami School of
Medicine, Miami, Florida
*Experimental Spinal Cord Injury: Pathophysiology and
Treatment*

James C. Butler, M.D.
Associate Professor, Tulane University School of
Medicine; Full Time Orthopaedic Staff Member,
Tulane University Medical Center, New Orleans,
Louisiana
*Complications of Spinal Surgery: Postlaminectomy
Kyphosis of the Cervical Spine*

Thomas P. Byrne, O.T.C.
University of California, San Diego, Medical Center,
San Diego, California
Spinal Orthoses for Traumatic and Degenerative Disease

Charles R. Clark, M.D.
Professor of Orthopaedic Surgery, Professor of
Biomedical Engineering, University of Iowa; Staff
Physician, University of Iowa Hospitals and Clinics,
Iowa City, Iowa
Rheumatoid Arthritis: Surgical Considerations

Mark S. Cohen, M.D.
Assistant Professor, Director, Orthopaedic Education,
Director, Hand and Elbow Program, Department of
Orthopaedic Surgery, Rush–Presbyterian–St. Luke's
Medical Center, Chicago, Illinois
*Anatomy of the Spinal Nerve Roots in the Lumbar and
Lower Thoracic Spine*

Patrick J. Connolly, M.D.
Associate Professor/Orthopedic Surgery, SUNY
Health Science Center at Syracuse, Syracuse, New
York
*Complications of Spinal Surgery: Complications
Associated With Posterior Spinal Instrumentation*

Bryan W. Cunningham, M.Sc., Ph.D.
Director of Spinal Research, Orthopaedic
Biomechanics Laboratory, Union Memorial Hospital,
Baltimore, Maryland
*Spine Trauma in Adults: Spinal Instrumentation for
Thoracic and Lumbar Fractures*

Bradford L. Currier, M.D.
Assistant Professor, Orthopaedic Surgery, Mayo
Medical School; Consultant, Department of
Orthopaedics, Joint Appointment, Department of
Neurosurgery, Mayo Clinic; Head, Mayo Clinic Spine
Group; Director, Mayo Clinic Spine Fellowship, Mayo
Medical Center, Rochester, Minnesota
Thoracic Disc Disease; Infections of the Spine

George Cybulski, M.D.
Associate Professor, Division of Neurological Surgery,
Northwestern University Medical School; Chief,
Section of Neurosurgery, Lakeside VA Hospital,
Chicago, Illinois
*Spinal Stenosis: Clinical Evaluation and Differential
Diagnosis*

Rick B. Delamarter, M.D.
Associate Clinical Professor, UCLA School of
Medicine; Co-Director, UCLA Comprehensive Spine
Center, UCLA Medical Center, Los Angeles, California
Surgical Management of Cervical Disc Disease

Richard A. Deyo, M.D., M.P.H.
Professor, Department of Medicine, Professor,
Department of Health Services, University of
Washington; Head, Section of General Internal
Medicine, University of Washington Medical Center,
Seattle, Washington
Outcomes Research for Spinal Disorders

William H. Dillin, M.D.
Spinal Surgery Consultant, Kerlan-Jobe Clinic, Los
Angeles and Anaheim, California
*Back Pain in Children and Adolescents; Cervical Disc
Disease: Clinical Syndromes in Cervical Myelopathy;
Surgical Management of Cervical Disc Disease*

Thomas J. Dowling, M.D.
Attending Orthopaedic Surgeon, St. John's Episcopal
Hospital, Smithtown, New York; Attending
Orthopaedic Surgeon, Huntington Hospital,
Huntington, New York
Adult Scoliosis

Thomas B. Ducker, M.D.
Professor of Surgery, Department of Neurosurgery;
Clinical Professor, Division of Neurosurgery, Johns
Hopkins University, Baltimore, Maryland; Johns
Hopkins Hospital, Baltimore, Maryland; Anne
Arundel Medical Center, Annapolis, Maryland
Spine Trauma in Adults: Spine and Spinal Cord Injuries

Joseph Dunn, M.D.
Assistant Clinical Professor, Anesthesiology,
University of California, San Diego, San Diego,
California; Pain Consultants of Oregon, Eugene,
Oregon
*Chronic Pain Management: Nonsurgical Management of
Chronic Back Pain*

Charles C. Edwards, M.D.
Professor of Orthopedic Surgery, University of
Maryland; Director, Section of Spinal Surgery,
University of Maryland Hospital, Baltimore, Maryland
Spondylolisthesis

Frank J. Eismont, M.D.
Professor, Department of Orthopedics, and Clinical
Professor of Neurologic Surgery, University of Miami
School of Medicine; Co-Director of Spinal Cord Injury
Service, Jackson Memorial Hospital, Miami, Florida
Thoracic Disc Disease; Infections of the Spine

Ronney L. Ferguson, M.D.
Chief of Staff, Shriners Hospitals for
Children—Spokane, Spokane, Washington
*Thoracic and Lumbar Spinal Trauma of the Immature
Spine*

Jeffrey S. Fischgrund, M.D.
Attending Spinal Surgeon, William Beaumont
Hospital, Royal Oak, Michigan
*Cervical Disc Disease: Cervical Spondylotic
Radiculopathy: Natural History and Pathophysiology*

Ann Marie Flannery, M.D.
Associate Professor, Service Chief, Pediatric
Neurosurgery, Medical College of Georgia, Augusta,
Georgia
Intraspinal Infections

Bruce E. Fredrickson, M.D.
Professor of Orthopedic and Neurologic Surgery,
SUNY Health Science Center at Syracuse; Crouse
Irving Memorial Hospital—Active; Veterans
Administration—Active; St. Joseph's
Hospital—Courtesy; Harrison Center Out-Patient
Surgery Center—Attending, Syracuse, New York
*Complications of Spinal Surgery: Complications
Associated With Posterior Spinal Instrumentation*

Trey Fulp, D.O.
Associate Clinical Professor of Orthopaedics,
University of North Texas Health Science Center, Fort
Worth, Texas; Spine Surgeon, Texas Back Institute,
Plano, Texas
*Surgical Management of Cervical Disc Disease:
Complications of Cervical Spine Surgery*

Steven R. Garfin, M.D.
Professor and Chair, Department of Orthopaedics,
University of California, San Diego; Chief, Section of
Spine Surgery, UCSD Medical Center, San Diego,
California
*Anatomy of the Spinal Nerve Roots in the Lumbar and
Lower Thoracic Spine; Lumbar Disc Disease; Spinal
Stenosis; Spondylolisthesis; Spinal Orthoses for Traumatic
and Degenerative Disease*

Timothy A. Garvey, M.D.
Assistant Professor of Orthopaedic Surgery,
University of Minnesota Medical School; Fairview-
University Medical Center; Twin Cities Spine Center/
Abbott Northwestern Hospital, Minneapolis,
Minnesota
Redo Disc Surgery—Techniques and Results

Eric B. Geller, M.D.
Head, Intraoperative Monitoring and Evoked
Potentials, Department of Neurology, The Cleveland
Clinic Foundation, Cleveland, Ohio
*Intraoperative Neurophysiologic Monitoring of the
Spinal Cord*

P. Langham Gleason, M.D.
Assistant Professor of Clinical Neurosurgery, Eastern
Virginia Medical School; Staff Neurosurgeon,
Children's Hospital of the King's Daughters, Norfolk,
Virginia
*Alternate Forms of Disc Excision: Automated
Percutaneous Lumbar Discectomy (APLD)*

Jeffrey A. Goldstein, M.D.
Clinical Instructor, Department of Orthopaedic
Surgery, New York University School of Medicine;
Director of Spine Services, NYU Downtown Hospital;
Attending Surgeon, Hospital for Joint Diseases
Orthopaedic Institute, New York, New York
*Spine Trauma in Adults: Spinal Instrumentation for
Thoracic and Lumbar Fractures*

Barth A. Green, M.D.
Professor of Neurological Surgery, University of
Miami School of Medicine; Chief of Service, Jackson
Memorial Hospital, Miami, Florida
*Thoracic Disc Disease; Experimental Spinal Cord Injury:
Pathophysiology and Treatment; Syringomyelia*

Anthony F. Guanciale, M.D.
Assistant Professor and Director, Division of Spine
Surgery at the University of Cincinnati College of
Medicine, Department of Orthopaedic Surgery,
Cincinnati, Ohio
Back Pain in Children and Adolescents

Richard D. Guyer, M.D.
Associate Clinical Professor, Department of
Orthopaedics, Southwestern School of Medicine,
Dallas, Texas; Director, Texas Back Institute Spine
Fellowship, Plano, Texas
Surgical Management of Cervical Disc Disease

Edward N. Hanley, Jr., M.D.
Clinical Professor, Department of Surgery, School of
Medicine, University of North Carolina at Chapel
Hill, Chapel Hill, North Carolina; Chairman and
Program Director, Department of Orthopaedic
Surgery; Vice-President, Clinical Activities, Carolinas
Healthcare System, Carolinas Medical Center,
Charlotte, North Carolina
*Spinal Stenosis (Surgical Management of Lumbar Spinal
Stenosis); Spinal Fusion*

John G. Heller, M.D.
Associate Professor of Orthopaedic Surgery, Emory
University School of Medicine; Director of Education,
Emory Spine Center, Atlanta, Georgia
*Complications of Spinal Surgery: Postoperative
Infections of the Spine*

Robert N. Hensinger, M.D.
Professor and Section Head, Orthopaedic Surgery,
University of Michigan Medical School; University of
Michigan Hospitals and Health System, Ann Arbor,
Michigan
Congenital Anomalies of the Cervical Spine

Harry N. Herkowitz, M.D.
Chairman, Department of Orthopaedic Surgery,
William Beaumont Hospital; Director, Section of Spine
Surgery, Department of Orthopaedic Surgery, William
Beaumont Hospital, Royal Oak, Michigan
*Arthritis of the Spine; Cervical Disc Disease: Cervical
Spondylotic Radiculopathy: Natural History and
Pathophysiology; Surgical Management of Cervical Disc
Disease; Spinal Stenosis; Spinal Fusion: Techniques and
Complications of Bone Graft Harvesting*

Kiyoshi Hirabayashi, M.D., Ph.D.
Professor, Department of Orthopaedic Surgery, Keio
University School of Medicine; Dean, Keio Hunior
College of Nursing, Tokyo, Japan
Ossification of the Posterior Longitudinal Ligament

Steven C. Humphreys, M.D.
Spine Surgeon, Memorial Hospital, Chattanooga,
Tennessee
Juvenile Kyphosis

Gordon Irving, M.B., B.S., M.Sc., M.Med.
Associate Professor, Department of Anesthesiology,
University of Texas Health Science Center at Houston;
Medical Director, University Center for Pain Medicine
and Rehabilitation at Hermann, Houston, Texas
*Chronic Pain Management: Nonsurgical Management of
Chronic Back Pain*

Kenneth L. Jarolem, M.D.
Spinal Surgeon, Orthopaedic Center of South Florida,
Plantation, Florida
Thoracoscopy of the Spine

Rollin M. Johnson, M.D.
Associate Clinical Professor of Orthopaedics and
Rehabilitation, Yale School of Medicine, New Haven,
Connecticut; Attending Surgeon, Cooley Dickinson
Hospital, Northampton, Massachusetts
Surgical Approaches to the Spine

Alexander M. Jones, M.D.
Orthopedic Surgeon, Denver Orthopedic Specialists,
Denver, Colorado
Spinal Instrumentation

Neil Kahanovitz, M.D.
Anderson Orthopedic Clinic, Arlington, Virginia
Spinal Fusion

Parviz Kambin, M.D.
Professor of Orthopaedic Surgery, Hahnemann School
of Medicine; Director of Spine Diagnostic and
Treatment Center, Allegheny University Hospitals
MCP, Philadelphia, Pennsylvania
*Alternative Forms of Disc Excision: Minimally Invasive
Spine Surgery*

John P. Kostuik, M.D.
Professor of Orthopaedics, Johns Hopkins University,
Baltimore, Maryland
Adult Scoliosis

Lawrence T. Kurz, M.D.
Attending Staff, Section of Spinal Surgery,
Department of Orthopaedic Surgery, William
Beaumont Hospital, Royal Oak, Michigan
*Cervical Disc Disease: Nonoperative Treatment; Spinal
Fusion*

Myron M. LaBan, M.D.
Clinical Professor, Wayne State University, Detroit,
Michigan; Director, Department of Physical Medicine
and Rehabilitation, William Beaumont Hospital, Royal
Oak, Michigan
*Spinal Stenosis: Conservative Management of Lumbar
Spinal Stenosis*

Joseph M. Lane, M.D.
Professor of Surgery (Orthopaedics), Assistant Dean,
Medical School, Cornell University Medical College;
Chief, Metabolic Bone Disease Service, Hospital for
Special Surgery, New York, New York
Metabolic Bone Disorders of the Spine; Spinal Fusion

William C. Lauerman, M.D.
Associate Professor of Orthopaedic Surgery, Chief of
Spine Division, Georgetown University Medical
Center, Washington, D.C.
*The Multiply Operated Low Back: An Algorithmic
Approach*

Alan M. Levine, M.D.
Professor, Orthopaedic Surgery and Oncology,
Consultant in Spinal Injury, Maryland Shock Trauma
Center, University of Maryland; Director, The Cancer
Institute of Sinai Hospital, Baltimore, Maryland
*Spine Trauma in Adults: Surgical Techniques for the
Treatment of Thoracic, Thoracolumbar, Lumbar, and Sacral
Trauma*

Marc J. Levine, M.D.
Central Jersey Spine Associates, Lawrenceville, New
Jersey
*Complications of Spinal Surgery: Postoperative
Infections of the Spine*

Stephen J. Lipson, M.D.
Associate Professor of Orthopaedic Surgery, Harvard
Medical School; Chairman, Department of
Orthopaedic Surgery, Beth Israel Deaconess Medical
Center, Boston, Massachusetts
Spinal Stenosis: Pathophysiology

John E. Lonstein, M.D.
Clinical Associate Professor of Orthopedic Surgery,
University of Minnesota, Minneapolis, Minnesota;
Chief, Spine and CP Spine Service, Gillette Children's
Specialty Healthcare, St. Paul, Minnesota
Juvenile and Adolescent Scoliosis

Gregory E. Lutz, M.D.
Assistant Professor of Rehabilitation Medicine,
Cornell University Medical Center; Chief, Physical
Medicine and Rehabilitation, the Hospital for Special
Surgery, New York, New York
Lumbar Disc Disease

Parley W. Madsen, III, M.D., Ph.D.
Assistant Clinical Professor of Anatomy and
Neurobiology, St. Louis University School of
Medicine; Member, Board of Directors, Practical
Anatomy and Surgical Technique Workshop of St.
Louis, St. Louis, Missouri
Syringomyelia

Joseph C. Maroon, M.D.
Professor of Surgery (Neurosurgery), Allegheny
University of the Health Sciences, Allegheny Campus;
Chairman, Department of Surgery and Neurosurgery,
A.U. H.S./Allegheny General Hospital, Pittsburgh,
Pennsylvania
*Alternate Forms of Disc Excision: Automated
Percutaneous Lumbar Discectomy (APLD)*

Lawrence F. Marshall, M.D.
Professor and Chair, Division of Neurosurgery,
University of California at San Diego, San Diego,
California
*Complications of Spinal Surgery: Cerebrospinal Fluid
Leaks: Etiology and Treatment*

Alberto Martinez-Arizala, M.D.
Associate Professor, Department of Neurology,
University of Miami School of Medicine, Miami,
Florida
*Experimental Spinal Cord Injury: Pathophysiology and
Treatment*

Thomas J. Masaryk, M.D.
Professor of Radiology, Ohio State University,
Columbus, Ohio; Section Head, Neuroradiology,
Cleveland Clinic Foundation, Cleveland, Ohio
Interventional Neuroradiology of the Spine

Tom G. Mayer, M.D.
Clinical Professor of Orthopedic Surgery, University of Texas Southwestern Medical Center; Medical Director, Productive Rehabilitation Institute of Dallas for Ergonomics (PRIDE), Dallas, Texas
Lumbar Musculature: Anatomy and Function; Spinal Functional Restoration: Tertiary Nonoperative Care

Paul C. McAfee, M.D.
Associate Professor of Orthopedic Surgery Johns Hopkins Hospital, The Johns Hopkins University School of Medicine; Chief of Spinal Surgery, St. Joseph's Hospital, Baltimore, Maryland
Spine Trauma in Adults: Spinal Instrumentation for Thoracic and Lumbar Fractures

Paul C. McCormick, M.D.
Associate Professor of Clinical Neurosurgery, Columbia University College of Physicians and Surgeons; Associate Attending Medical Director, Columbia-Presbyterian Spine Center, Columbia-Presbyterian Medical Center, New York, New York
Arteriovenous Malformations of the Spinal Cord

John A. McCulloch, M.D., F.R.C.S.C.
Professor, Department of Orthopaedic Surgery, Northeastern Ohio Universities College of Medicine, Rootstown, Ohio; Chief of Spine Surgery, Department of Spinal Surgery, Summa Health System, St. Thomas Hospital, Akron, Ohio
Alternative Forms of Disc Excision: Microdiscectomy; Chemonucleolysis

Robert F. McLain, M.D.
Staff Surgeon, Director of Spine Research, Department of Orthopaedic Surgery, The Cleveland Clinic Foundation, Cleveland, Ohio
Tumors of the Spine

Arnold H. Menezes, M.D.
Professor of Neurosurgery, University of Iowa; Staff Physician, University of Iowa Hospitals and Clinics, Iowa City, Iowa
Rheumatoid Arthritis: Surgical Considerations

Luis A. Mignucci, M.D.
Clinical Assistant Professor of Neurological Surgery, University of Texas Southwestern Medical School, Dallas, Texas; Neurosurgeon, Spine Surgeon, Medical Center of Plano, Plano, Texas; Medical City Hospital at Dallas, VA Medical Center at Dallas, Dallas, Texas
Differential Diagnosis of Sciatica

Srdjan Mirkovic, M.D.
Assistant Clinical Professor of Orthopaedics, Northwestern University School of Medicine; Attending, Northwestern Memorial Hospital, Chicago, Illinois
Spinal Stenosis: Clinical Evaluation and Differential Diagnosis

Michael T. Modic, M.D.
Professor, Department of Radiology, Ohio State University, Columbus, Ohio; Chairman, Division of Radiology, Cleveland Clinic Foundation, Cleveland, Ohio
Radiology of the Lumbar Spine

David M. Montgomery, M.D.
Clinical Assistant Professor, Wayne State University School of Medicine, Detroit, Michigan; Orthopedic Spine Surgeon, William Beaumont Hospital, Royal Oak, Michigan
Spinal Stenosis: Clinical Evaluation and Differential Diagnosis

Vert Mooney, M.D.
Professor of Orthopaedic Surgery, University of California, San Diego (UCSD), La Jolla, California
Sacroiliac Joint Dysfunction

Gabrielle F. Morris, M.D.
Senior Resident, Division of Neurosurgery, University of California, San Diego, San Diego, California
Complications of Spinal Surgery: Adhesive Arachnoiditis; Cerebrospinal Fluid Leaks: Etiology and Treatment

Scott J. Mubarak, M.D.
Clinical Professor, Department of Orthopedics, University of California, San Diego; University of California Medical Center; Director of Orthopedic Program at Children's Hospital, San Diego, California
Neuromuscular Scoliosis

Michael J. Murphy, M.D.
Assistant Clinical Professor of Orthopaedic Surgery, Yale University School of Medicine; Attending Surgeon, Yale–New Haven Hospital, New Haven, Connecticut
Surgical Approaches to the Spine

George F. Muschler, M.D.
Full Staff, Department of Orthopaedic Surgery; Director, Bone Biology Laboratory, Learner Research Institute; The Cleveland Clinic Foundation, Cleveland, Ohio
Spinal Fusion

Imad M. Najm, M.D.
Associate Staff, Cleveland Clinic Foundation, Cleveland, Ohio
Intraoperative Neurophysiologic Monitoring of the Spinal Cord

Peter O. Newton, M.D.
Assistant Clinical Professor, Department of Orthopedic Surgery, University of California, San Diego, Medical Center; Staff Pediatric Orthopedic Surgeon, Children's Hospital and Health Center, San Diego, California
Neuromuscular Scoliosis

Kjell Olmarker, M.D., Ph.D.
Associate Professor, Department of Orthopedics, Gothenburg University, Gothenburg, Sweden
Anatomy of the Spinal Nerve Roots in the Lumbar and Lower Thoracic Spine; Pathophysiology of Spinal Nerve Roots as Related to Sciatica and Disc Herniation

Manohar M. Panjabi, Ph.D., D. Tech.
Professor of Biomechanics in Surgery, Yale University School of Medicine; Director of Bioengineering Research, Department of Orthopaedics and Rehabilitation, Yale University School of Medicine, New Haven, Connecticut
Biomechanical Considerations of Spinal Stability

Wesley W. Parke, Ph.D.
Professor and Chairman, Emeritus, Department of Anatomy and Structural Biology, University of South Dakota School of Medicine, Vermillion, South Dakota
Development of the Spine; Applied Anatomy of the Spine

Eric Phillips, M.D.
Immanuel Medical Center, Bergan Mercy Hospital, Methodist Hospital, Clarkson Hospital, Omaha, Nebraska
Spinal Fusion

Matthew Quigley, M.D.
Associate Professor of Surgery (Neurosurgery), Allegheny University of the Health Sciences; Associate Professor of Surgery (Neurosurgery), Department of Neurosurgery, A.U.H.S./Allegheny General Hospital, Pittsburgh, Pennsylvania
Alternate Forms of Disc Excision: Automated Percutaneous Lumbar Discectomy (APLD)

John J. Regan, M.D.
Associate Clinical Professor, University of Texas–Southwestern Medical School; Texas Back Institute, Dallas, Texas; Presbyterian Hospital of Plano, Plano, Texas
Thoracoscopy of the Spine

Richard H. Rothman, M.D.
Professor and Chairman, Department of Orthopaedic Surgery, Thomas Jefferson University; Director, the Rothman Institute, Philadelphia, Pennsylvania
Lumbar Disc Disease

Michael E. Russell, II, M.D.
Azalea Orthopedic and Sports Medicine Clinic, East Texas Medical Center, and Mother Francis Hospital, Tyler, Texas
Spinal Stenosis (Surgical Management of Lumbar Spinal Stenosis)

Stephen J. Ryan, M.D., M.A.
Assistant Professor, Department of Neurology, University of Kentucky College of Medicine, Lexington, Kentucky
Medical Myelopathies

Björn L. Rydevik, M.D., Ph.D.
Professor and Chairman, Department of Orthopaedics, University of Gothenburg, Gothenburg, Sweden
Anatomy of the Spinal Nerve Roots in the Lumbar and Lower Thoracic Spine; Pathophysiology of Spinal Nerve Roots as Related to Sciatica and Disc Herniation; Spinal Stenosis: Pathophysiology

L. Carl Samberg, M.D.
Clinical Assistant Professor of Orthopaedic Surgery, Wayne State University School of Medicine, Detroit, Michigan; Director of Orthopaedic Education, William Beaumont Hospital, Royal Oak, Michigan
Spinal Fusion

Kazuhiko Satomi, M.D., Ph.D.
Associate Professor, Department of Orthopaedic Surgery, Kyorin University School of Medicine; Chief of Spine Group, Kyorin University Hospital, Tokyo, Japan
Ossification of the Posterior Longitudinal Ligament

Jonathan L. Schaffer, M.D.
Assistant Professor, Department of Orthopedic Surgery, Harvard Medical School; Associate Orthopedic Surgeon, Associate Director, Decision Systems Group, Brigham and Women's Hospital, Boston, Massachusetts
Alternative Forms of Disc Excision: Minimally Invasive Spine Surgery

Jeffrey H. Schimandle, M.D.
Department of Surgery, Orthopedic and Reconstructive Spine Surgery, St. Anthony Hospital, Oklahoma City, Oklahoma
Spinal Fusion

Daniel M. Schwartz, Ph.D.
Surgical Monitoring Associates, Bala Cynwyd, Pennsylvania
Congenital Anomalies of the Spinal Cord

Kanwaldeep S. Sidhu, M.D.
Attending Surgeon, St. Clair Orthopaedics, Orthopaedic Spine Surgery, St. John's Hospital and Medical Center, Detroit, Michigan
Surgical Management of Cervical Disc Disease

Frederick A. Simeone, M.D.
Chairman of Neurosurgery, Jefferson Medical College; Chairman of Neurosurgery, Thomas Jefferson University Hospital, Philadelphia, Pennsylvania
Surgical Management of Cervical Disc Disease; Intradural Tumors; Complications of Spinal Surgery

Edward H. Simmons, M.D., B.Sc.(Med), F.R.C.S.(C), M.S.(Tor), F.A.C.S.
Professor of Orthopaedic Surgery, State University of New York at Buffalo; Emeritus Chief, Department of Orthopaedic Surgery, Buffalo General Hospital, Buffalo, New York
Ankylosing Spondylitis: Surgical Considerations

J. Michael Simpson, M.D.
Assistant Professor, Medical College of Virginia;
Director of Spinal Surgery, Tuckahoe Orthopaedics,
Richmond, Virginia
Arthritis of the Spine

Andrew V. Slucky, M.D.
Assistant Professor, University of California, San
Francisco, Department of Orthopaedic Surgery, San
Francisco, California
Thoracic Disc Disease

John M. Small, M.D.
Spine Surgeon, Florida Orthopaedic Institute, Tampa,
Florida
*Cervical Disc Disease: Clinical Syndromes in Cervical
Myelopathy*

Samuel D. Small, D.O.
Clinical Instructor, Department of Orthopaedic
Surgery, UCLA School of Medicine, Los Angeles,
California; Orthopaedic Spine Surgeon, Ventura
Orthopaedic Group, Community Memorial Hospital,
Ventura, California
Surgical Management of Cervical Disc Disease

Wayne O. Southwick, M.D.
Professor Emeritus, Department of Orthopaedics and
Rehabilitation, Yale University School of Medicine,
New Haven, Connecticut
Surgical Approaches to the Spine

Dan M. Spengler, M.D.
Professor and Chairman, Vanderbilt Orthopaedics and
Rehabilitation, Nashville, Tennessee
*Workers' Compensation As It Affects the Spine:
Management of the Workers' Compensation Patient With
Low Back Pain*

Gray C. Stahlman, M.D.
Tennessee Orthopaedic Associates, Nashville,
Tennessee
Spinal Fusion

Jeffery L. Stambough, M.D., M.B.A.
Co-Director of the Musculoskeletal Research Center,
Associated with the University of Cincinnati, College
of Engineering, and Consultant to the Back Treatment
Center, Deaconess Hospital, Cincinnati, Ohio
*Discitis; Complications of Spinal Surgery: Vascular
Complications in Spine Surgery; Neurologic Complications
in Spine Surgery*

Bennett M. Stein, M.D.
Professor Emeritus of Clinical Neurosurgery,
Columbia University College of Physicians and
Surgeons; Professor Emeritus, Columbia-Presbyterian
Medical Center, New York, New York
Arteriovenous Malformations of the Spinal Cord

Leslie N. Sutton, M.D.
Professor of Neurosurgery, University of
Pennsylvania; Director of Neurosurgery, Children's
Hospital of Philadelphia, Philadelphia, Pennsylvania
Congenital Anomalies of the Spinal Cord

Ronald S. Taylor, M.D.
Clinical Assistant Professor, Wayne State University
School of Medicine, Detroit, Michigan; Director,
Rehabilitation Services, William Beaumont Hospital,
Royal Oak, Michigan
*Spinal Stenosis: Conservative Management of Lumbar
Spinal Stenosis*

Vernon Tolo, M.D.
John C. Wilson, Jr., Professor of Orthopaedics,
University of Southern California School of Medicine;
Head, Division of Orthopaedics, Childrens Hospital
Los Angeles, Los Angeles, California
*Spinal Disorders Associated With Skeletal Dysplasias
and Metabolic Diseases*

Ensor E. Transfeldt, M.D.
Associate Professor of Orthopaedic Surgery,
University of Minnesota Medical School; Fairview-
University Medical Center, Twin Cities Spine Center,
Abbott-Northwestern Hospital, Minneapolis,
Minnesota
Redo Disc Surgery—Techniques and Results

Alexander R. Vaccaro, M.D.
Associate Professor of Orthopaedic Surgery, Thomas
Jefferson University and the Rothman Institute,
Philadelphia, Pennsylvania
*Spinal Ortheses for Traumatic and Degenerative Disease;
Spinal Instrumentation*

Eric J. Wall, M.D.
Director, Sports Medicine at Children's Hospital;
Assistant Professor of Clinical Orthopaedic
Surgery—Affiliate, Children's Hospital, Cincinnati,
Ohio
*Anatomy of the Spinal Nerve Roots in the Lumbar and
Lower Thoracic Spine*

Mark S. Wallace, M.D.
Assistant Clinical Professor of Anesthesiology;
Director, Pain Management Medical Group and
Clinical Pain Research, University of California, San
Diego, Medical Center, San Diego, California
*Chronic Pain Management: Nonsurgical Management of
Chronic Back Pain*

Robert C. Wallace, M.D.
Director of Neuroangiography, Department of
Neuroradiology, Barrow Neurological Institute and St.
Joseph's Hospital, Phoenix, Arizona
Interventional Neuroradiology of the Spine

Ay-Ming Wang, M.D.
Co-Chief, Neuroradiology Division, Department of
Diagnostic Radiology, William Beaumont Hospital,
Royal Oak, Michigan
*Cervical Disc Disease: Radiologic Evaluation; Spinal
Stenosis: Clinical Evaluation and Differential Diagnosis*

Robert G. Watkins, M.D.
Professor of Clinical Orthopedic Surgery, University
of Southern California; Director, Center for
Orthopedic Spinal Surgery, University of Southern
California, Los Angeles, California
*Back Pain in Children and Adolescents; Cervical Disc
Disease: Clinical Syndromes in Cervical Myelopathy*

James N. Weinstein, D.O., M.S.
Professor, Dartmouth School of Medicine, Dartmouth
College, Hanover, New Hampshire; Orthopaedic
Surgeon, Dartmouth-Hitchcock Medical Center,
Lebanon, New Hampshire
*Outcomes Research for Spinal Disorders; Tumors of the
Spine*

Dennis R. Wenger, M.D.
Director, Pediatric Orthopedics, Children's Hospital,
San Diego; Clinical Professor of Orthopedic Surgery,
University of California, San Diego, San Diego,
California
Neuromuscular Scoliosis

David P. Wesolowski, M.D.
Director of Neuroradiology Fellowship, Co-Chief,
Division of Neuroradiology, William Beaumont
Hospital, Royal Oak, Michigan
*Cervical Disc Disease: Radiologic Evaluation; Spinal
Stenosis: Clinical Evaluation and Differential Diagnosis*

F. Todd Wetzel, M.D.
Associate Professor, Department of Surgery, Section of
Orthopaedic Surgery and Rehabilitation, and
Anesthesia and Critical Care, University of Chicago;
Chief, Section of Orthopaedic Surgery, Director,
University of Chicago Spine Center, Louis A. Weiss
Memorial Hospital (University of Chicago–North
Campus), Chicago, Illinois
*Chronic Pain Management: Surgical Procedures for the
Control of Chronic Pain*

Augustus A. White III, M.D., D. Med. Sci.
Professor of Orthopaedic Surgery, Harvard Medical
School; Orthopaedic Surgeon-in-Chief, Emeritus, Beth
Israel Deaconess Medical Center, Boston,
Massachusetts
Biomechanical Considerations of Spinal Stability

Thomas S. Whitecloud III, M.D.
Ray J. Haddad Professor and Chairman, Tulane
University School of Medicine; Chief, Division of
Spinal Surgery, Tulane University Medical Center,
New Orleans, Louisiana
*Complications of Spinal Surgery: Postlaminectomy
Kyphosis of the Cervical Spine*

Sam W. Wiesel, M.D.
Professor and Chairman, Department of Orthopaedic
Surgery, Georgetown University School of Medicine
and Medical Center, Washington, DC
*The Multiply Operated Low Back: An Algorithmic
Approach; Workers' Compensation As It Affects the Spine:
Compensation Low Back and Neck Pain*

Asa J. Wilbourn, M.D.
Associate Clinical Professor (Neurology), Case
Western Reserve School of Medicine; Director, EMG
Laboratory, Department of Neurology, Cleveland
Clinic, Cleveland, Ohio
Electrodiagnosis: The Electrodiagnostic Examination

Robert B. Winter, M.D.
Clinical Professor, Orthopedic Surgery, University of
Minnesota; Medical Director of Research, Minnesota
Spine Foundation, Minneapolis, Minnesota
Juvenile and Adolescent Scoliosis

Ronald J. Wisneski, M.D.
Associate Professor of Surgery (Orthopaedics), Cornell
University Medical Center, The Hospital for Special
Surgery, New York, New York; Attending
Orthopaedic Surgeon, The Medical Center at
Princeton, Princeton, New Jersey
Lumbar Disc Disease

Tony Yaksh, Ph.D.
Professor and Vice Chairman for Research,
Department of Anesthesiology; Adjunct Professor of
Pharmacology, University of California, San Diego,
San Diego, California
*Chronic Pain Management: Nonsurgical Management of
Chronic Back Pain*

Kazuo Yonenobu, M.D.
Associate Professor, Department of Orthopaedic
Surgery, Osaka University Medical School, Osaka,
Japan
Surgical Management of Cervical Disc Disease

Hansen A. Yuan, M.D.
Professor of Neurologic and Orthopedic Surgery,
SUNY Health Science Center at Syracuse, Syracuse,
New York
*Complications of Spinal Surgery: Complications
Associated With Posterior Spinal Instrumentation*

Thomas A. Zdeblick, M.D.
Professor, Division of Orthopedic Surgery,
Department of Surgery, University of Wisconsin;
Director, University of Wisconsin Spine Center,
Madison, Wisconsin
Laparoscopic Spinal Fusion; Discogenic Back Pain

Preface

Fourth Edition The Spine

This edition of *The Spine*, the fourth, has been assembled under the direction of the same Editorial Board that was responsible for the third edition (1992). The guiding principles taught to us by our mentors, Richard H. Rothman, M.D., Ph.D., and Frederick A. Simeone, M.D., permeate throughout the chapters of this fourth edition. They include (1) understanding of the basic science behind the clinical aspects of spinal disorders, (2) knowledge of natural history and the clinical course, and (3) treatment based on the scientific literature and available outcomes research.

This fourth edition of *The Spine* continues the tradition of providing a comprehensive textbook of spinal disease affecting children and adults. It is dedicated to students of spinal disease regardless of specialty and rank. It is also dedicated to the patients whose care may be influenced by the words contained within its 59 chapters. Because history plays such an important role in furthering scientific knowledge, a review of the previous prefaces will help put this new edition in proper perspective.

The forerunner to *The Spine* was *The Intervertebral Disc* by Rothman and DePalma. In their preface written in 1970, the authors wrote: "The role of the intervertebral disc in the production of neck and back pain, with or without radiation into one of the extremities, has been the subject of much investigation for many decades. . . . The disc has been attacked from every conceivable angle, the most important of which is its biochemical nature and its response to physiologic aging and trauma. In spite of the exhaustive studies recorded in the literature, it is alarming to find how little of this knowledge has been acquired by those concerned with neck and back disorders. . . . This monograph deals with the modern concepts of the biochemical structure of the disc, its functional role, and how different phases of alterations in the disc are related to the presenting clinical syndrome. . . . We are sure that much that is recorded in this book is still very controversial. Yet, we believe that our approach to this complex problem will be helpful and rewarding to others." This comprehensive monograph on the disc totaled 373 pages. A sig- nificant portion of the information it contained was based on the authors' own work and rigorous analysis of their results. The sections on the chemistry and physiology of the disc, though the crux of the book, were limited and reflected the state of knowledge at the time. However, it did crystallize concepts of the disc for spine physicians of the day and served as the forerunner of the texts that were to follow.

In the preface to the first edition, Rothman and Simeone stated: "*The Spine* had as its genesis a strong feeling on the part of its editors that a need existed for a comprehensive textbook to include all aspects of diagnosis and treatment of spinal disease. Our goals were to lower the traditional disciplinary barriers and biases and to present a uniform guideline to problem solving in this area . . . this book has been designed to include all facets of disease related to the spine, whether orthopedic, neurosurgical, or medical in nature. . . . An attempt has been made to achieve completeness without exhaustive and burdensome details. The contributing authors have not merely recorded the possibilities in diagnosis and treatment of spinal disorders but have relied on their personal experience to offer concrete recommendations." The success of that effort is legend. The first edition of *The Spine* followed the dictates of the editors, covered the full range of knowledge of spinal disorders known at the time, and became an essential component of the libraries of all medical personnel who dealt with spinal disorders. The authors, one a neurosurgeon (F.A.S.) and one an orthopaedic surgeon (R.H.R.), combined their efforts to teach the world not only diseases of the spine, but also the importance of working together in an attempt to understand and treat the disease processes. Their spinal fellowship, as well as personal fellowship, was (is) based on this team, multidisciplinary, yet regimented approach to the spine, and has been the model that we have sought to achieve in our own clinical and teaching environments. In fact, it may be required that successful spine fellowships in the future be a coordinated effort between multispecialties, as envisioned and taught by Drs. Rothman and

Simeone, so that the spine is not broken up into multiple segments (bone, nerves, discs, etc.).

The preface to the second edition of *The Spine* stated: "Advancements in medicine generally follow broader scientific and even social trends. The treatment of spine diseases is no exception. Consequently, increments of new information have been added to the general body of knowledge in spotty, but predictable areas. These new developments constitute the raison d'etre for this second edition. The dramatic progress in radiologic imaging stands out as the most useful innovation. . . . Logic indicates that the next generation of (CT) scanners will delineate all thoracic and cervical disc lesions. Spinal trauma is managed better since the advent of computed tomography. Infections, tumor infiltration, and congenital malformations are being better understood as experience grows. . . . Each contributor has demonstrated his commitment to summarizing the most recent information in a manner useful to students and clinicians alike, and for this the editors are proud and appreciative."

The preface to the third edition included the following: "The current edition has new editorial leadership. Those of us involved in the direction of this project have tried to follow the model previously established by Drs. Rothman and Simeone in finding the best authors for each chapter. We, hopefully, have emphasized, as in past editions, the importance of understanding the basic science in a concise manner, which leads to the ability to make appropriate decisions and manage patients with simple or complex spinal problems. We have attempted to update each section, have eliminated those areas that are not current, and have separated some components of the basic science from the clinical to aid readers in locating pertinent information in the ever-increasing body of knowledge related to the spine."

The current editors have been involved with Dick Rothman and Fred Simeone in various ways. Some have been fellows, some residents, and some partners. Each of us has developed special feelings and interactions with them. Each of us has carried the messages they teach and actively practice to our own clinical and research environments. They have taught us the importance of combining scientific queries with active clinical practices and have fostered in us the desire to clinically and academically succeed in an open and honest fashion.

As stated, the fourth edition has been assembled under the direction of the Editorial Board responsible for the third edition. This fourth edition, the largest both in number of pages and length and width, has undergone considerable updating. This includes chapters on outcomes research, management of disc degeneration, laparoscopic and endoscopic surgery, and ossification of the posterior longitudinal ligament as it relates to myelopathy. Magnetic resonance imaging, which was introduced in the third edition, has an expanded presence in this edition, since it is now the imaging modality of choice for most spinal disorders.

The Editorial Board has maintained the broad-based appeal of this textbook by including basic scientists, neurologists, radiologists, physiatrists, and orthopaedic and neurosurgeons as chapter authors. In addition, this textbook remains unique in providing a comprehensive section on pediatric disorders as well as adult disease.

We, the Editorial Board, feel confident that readers of this fourth edition will find the information needed to understand the causes of and diagnose and care for patients afflicted with spinal disease.

HARRY N. HERKOWITZ, M.D.
STEVEN R. GARFIN, M.D.
RICHARD A. BALDERSTON, M.D.
FRANK J. EISMONT, M.D.
GORDON R. BELL, M.D.
SAM W. WIESEL, M.D.

Contents

SECTION 5

Trauma

Spine Trauma in Adults

Henry H. Bohlman, M.D.   *Alan M. Levine, M.D.*   *Jeffrey A. Goldstein, M.D.*

Thomas B. Ducker, M.D.   *Bryan W. Cunningham, M.Sc., Ph.D.*

                                                               Paul C. McAfee, M.D.

Spine and Spinal Cord Injuries

Henry H. Bohlman, M.D.

Thomas B. Ducker, M.D.

Acute injuries of the spine and spinal cord are among the most common causes of severe disability and death following trauma. The diagnosis of these injuries is often delayed, and the treatment is frequently unstandardized or inadequate, producing increasing problems with rehabilitation of the patient.[32, 34, 43, 46, 52, 54]

Five thousand years ago, the Edwin Smith Surgical Papyrus of Egypt described spinal cord injuries in case reports as ailments not to be treated. Unfortunately, this pessimistic attitude survived many hundreds of years. Over the past two decades, there has been a renewed interest in treatment and research in relation to patients with spine and spinal cord injuries. With the advent of trauma and spinal cord injury centers in this country, great strides have been made toward improving emergency care and initial medical and surgical treatment, as well as toward rehabilitation of the person sustaining a spinal cord injury.

Specifically, one of the great treatment advances has been the application of the anterior and anterolateral operative approaches to spinal injuries, as well as improved internal fixation devices used with this surgery.[11, 27, 28, 36, 39, 40, 42, 49, 50, 55, 65, 82, 84, 87, 119, 165, 219, 234]

There has been a major thrust toward research of these injuries to define electrical, pathophysiologic, biochemical, and mechanical events that occur with the acute spine and spinal cord injury.[25, 47, 48, 70, 71, 85, 86, 107, 114, 124, 126, 127, 151, 215, 225, 227, 360, 373]

The biomechanics of the normal spine, as well as the spinal injury, have been studied in the laboratory and have resulted in a more precise definition of instability.[209, 360] Various internal fixation devices for the spine have been analyzed for their effectiveness with

the combined efforts of the surgeon and engineer.[230, 282, 361] Recent studies by various investigators have classified spine and spinal cord injuries so that clinical analysis of various treatment modalities is more accurate.[7, 29, 46, 78, 93, 116, 138, 154, 168, 169, 249]

Studies of acute and chronic spinal cord compression and the effect of initial spine stabilization have added to our knowledge of these effects on recovery from spinal cord injury.[38, 44, 47, 72, 73, 130, 184, 227, 344-346]

The authors of this chapter have reviewed the literature, attempted to apply their experience from two large spinal cord injury centers, and have developed an approach to diagnosis and treatment based on clinical, experimental, and pathologic studies. The first part of this chapter covers mechanisms of injury, pathophysiology, and clinical assessment of spine and spinal cord injury. General principles of emergency management as well as treatment of spinal injuries are discussed. Past and present classifications of spinal cord injury are redefined.

The latter part of the chapter relates to general principles of diagnosis, pathology, and treatment of injuries at specific levels of the spine. Various complications are addressed, including instability, deformity, pain, and late paralysis.

MECHANISMS OF SPINE AND SPINAL CORD INJURY

Upper Cervical Injuries (Occiput, Atlas, and Axis)

The forces and mechanisms that produce spine and spinal cord injury relate very closely to the anatomic structures at the various levels of the spine and spinal cord. At the occipito-cervical joints, 40 per cent of the normal motion of the cervical spine occurs in flexion and extension. Any abnormal force or motion produced that is a major injury vector at this level may disrupt the strong ligamentous integrity of the atlanto-occipital joints, which includes the tectorial membrane, posterior atlanto-occipital membrane, and the apical and alar ligaments.

Dvorak et al.[137] tested seven human specimens of the cervical spine and found that the alar ligaments had an in vitro strength of 200 newtons and the transverse ligaments had an in vitro strength of 350 newtons. Therefore, the alar ligament had lower strength and might be more easily damaged, especially when rotational forces are applied.

Anderson and Montesano[9] reported six cases of occipital condyle fractures, which are quite rare. They classified these injuries into Type I, an impaction fracture; Type II, which included a basilar skull fracture; and Type III, avulsion fractures. All healed with rigid immobilization.

Approximately 40 per cent of rotation in the cervical spine occurs at the atlantoaxial joint, which is restricted by the alar ligaments extending from the odontoid process to the inner border of the occipital condyles. The apical ligament centrally attaches the odontoid to the anterior foramen magnum. The integrity of the atlantoaxial articulation is maintained by the very strong transverse ligament, as well as lateral joint capsules. A portion of structural support is also given by the anterior and posterior longitudinal ligaments, as well as the vertical odontoid process held against the atlas ring by the transverse ligament. Fielding et al.[157] and Spence et al.[335] studied in fresh cadavers the force required to stretch and completely disrupt these ligaments. A mean force of 84 kg is necessary to tear the transverse ligament by forced dislocation of the atlas on the axis. A force of 54 kg is necessary to disrupt the transverse ligament by lateral forces.

Approximately 80 per cent of cervical spine injuries occur by the accelerating head and body striking a stationary object.[44, 46, 107] Therefore, sites of head trauma, such as lacerations, contusions, or facial fractures, can be instructive in correlation of spinal fracture types with mechanisms of injury in both the upper and lower cervical spine. The most common mechanism of injury at the atlantoaxial level is flexion, which may produce a fractured odontoid process or, more rarely, may tear the transverse ligament and result in a dislocation of these vertebrae. Extension injury may fracture the odontoid with posterior displacement, but this is unusual. Rotatory forces play a role at the biconvex first and second cervical joints, but the traumatic unilateral rotary dislocation or subluxation that results is rare. Direct axial loading or a blow on the vertex of the skull produces centrifugal force against the lateral masses of the atlas, which fractures through its thinner parts of the ring posteriorly and anteriorly. A spread of the lateral masses greater than 7 mm indicates tearing of the transverse ligament.[192, 214, 327, 335]

A further injury produced by extension of the occiput on the cervical spine is bilateral pedicle fractures of the axis, and in rare instances there may be a flexion component with subluxation of the second or third cervical vertebrae.[156] Only 16 per cent of injuries at the atlantoaxial level produce neurologic deficit because of the anatomically wide spinal canal at these levels allowing for more osseous displacement, as opposed to the narrower lower levels of the cervical spine. Occasionally, the vertebral artery can be damaged.[286]

Effendi et al.[138] classified 131 patients with fractures of the ring of the axis[138] into three types. Type 1 fractures, the most common (65 per cent), are stable fractures and undisplaced and probably occur with extension. Type 2 fractures (28 per cent) are unstable, with displacement of the anterior fragment and abnormal disc between C2 and C3. In Type 3 fractures (7 per cent), facets are dislocated and displacement of the anterior fragment of the body is in the flexed position. Type 3 was the most unstable and required surgical intervention. Starr and Eismont[336] reported 19 cases of traumatic spondylolisthesis of the axis of which six were the atypical class II Effendi type of fractures, which are more commonly associated with significant neurologic dysfunction because of spinal canal compromise from fractures of the posterior aspect of the vertebral body of the axis or continuity of the pedicle.

Francis et al.[168] reported 123 patients with traumatic spondylolisthesis of the axis. They describe the lesion associated with extension and axial loading with a high incidence of injuries to the face and scalp and a low incidence of neurologic injury. They believed that operation was necessary only for chronic instability, and that most fractures heal with nonoperative stabilization. They also identified an anterior angulation of greater than 11 degrees seen in patients who developed nonunion.

Levine and Edwards[242] described the management of spondylolisthesis of the axis in 52 patients, in whom associated neurologic deficits were found in only four. They classified the fractures into four types, but essentially used Effendi's classification and added an additional subtype. Type 1 injuries had a fracture through the neural arch with no angulation, Type 2 had significant angulation and displacement, and Type 2A fractures showed minimal displacement but severe angulation. Type 3 fractures combined a bilateral facet dislocation with a fracture of the neural arch and displacement. The authors believe the mechanism of injury for Type 1 is hyperextension and axial loading. For Type 2, it is hyperextension and axial loading, with a second force, anterior flexion and compression. In addition, they believe that Type 2A and Type 3 injuries occur by a flexion as well as posterior distraction force. They also thought Types 1 and 2 injuries were stable and that Type 3 injuries were unstable and best treated by immediate skeletal traction and reduction and posterior fixation.

Fielding et al.[155, 157, 160] demonstrated instability of the atlantoaxial complex if greater than 3 mm of space in adults or 4 mm of space in children is present at the anterior atlantodental interval. Both indicate alteration or tearing of the transverse ligament.[155, 157, 160] Further development occurs with stretching of the accessory or alar ligaments. Instability may also occur if the odontoid fractures or is dysplastic, and atlantoaxial dislocation results.

Lower Cervical Fractures (C3–C7 and T1)

Between the third and seventh cervical segments, the spinal canal is less spacious, and the facet joints are oriented at a 45-degree angle to the vertical and limit rotational forces but allow for relatively more cervical flexion. The stabilizing influences of soft tissue and osseous structures at these levels of the spine may be divided into anterior and posterior complexes. The anterior portion comprises the vertebral body, disc, and annular ligament, as well as the anterior and posterior longitudinal ligaments. The posterior complex comprises the pedicles, facet joints, and their capsules, laminae, spinous processes, interspinous ligaments, and the ligamentum flavum in the cervical spine. There is a strong pattern of coupling, such that axial rotation is associated with lateral bending.

Instability may occur following acute cervical spine injury if the normal structures, either bone or ligament, are stressed beyond normal physiologic loads.[362] White and Panjabi[360] have defined clinical instability as "the loss of the ability of the spine under physiologic loads to maintain relationships between vertebrae in such a way that there is neither damage nor subsequent irritation to the spinal cord or nerve roots, and in addition, there is no development of incapacitating deformity or pain due to structural changes."

At the lower cervical segments, instability has been defined biomechanically by White et al.,[362] who tested fresh cadaver specimens, measuring abnormal motion of the adjacent vertebrae after serially sectioning posterior and anterior ligaments. Instability of the lower cervical spine was thus defined as "translatory displacement of two adjacent vertebrae greater than 3.5 mm, angulation of greater than 11 degrees between adjacent vertebrae, indicating a significant ligament disruption."[209, 360]

Fractures of the osseous structures may produce instability acutely; that is, severe compression fracture of the vertebral body anteriorly or fractures of the facet joints posteriorly, both of which may allow abnormal angulation or dislocation of the cervical spine.

Mechanisms of injury to the lower cervical spine are usually defined as specific forces applied individually; however, in reality multiple forces are probably involved with most severe cervical spine trauma.[27, 29, 31, 107] The most frequent injuries that occur are secondary to the following forces: flexion, extension, lateral rotation, axial loading, or a combination of these. Injuries of the cervical spine may be caused by a direct blow, such as a weight falling on the person's head, a missile, or a gunshot wound.

Allen et al.[7] developed a classification of cervical spine fractures based on mechanism of injury by studying 165 cases. He divided the cases into groups involving (1) compressive flexion, (2) vertical compression, (3) distractive flexion, (4) compressive extension, (5) distractive extension, and (6) lateral flexion. The probability of an associated neurologic lesion was related directly to the type and severity of cervical injury. The groups were then subdivided into other stages of varying degrees of fractures or vertebral displacement, which correlated with the severity of neurologic damage.

The syndrome of subacute instability was described by Herkowitz,[199] in which initial roentgenograms appear to be normal but ligament disruption later allows vertebral displacement and neurologic deficit.[199]

Torg and others surveyed 503 schools in the 1984 football season and reported neurapraxia of the cervical spinal cord with transient quadriplegia in 1.3 per cent of 10,000 athletes with a suggestive history.[349, 354, 379] They identified developmental spinal stenosis in 17 patients, congenital fusion in five, cervical instability in four, and intervertebral disc disease in six patients. Using a ratio method of measuring the spinal canal in relationship to the vertebral body width, they developed a ratio in which a measurement of less than 0.80 indicates significant spinal stenosis in a group of 24 patients for whom roentgenograms were available. This was compared to a ratio of approximately 1.00 or more in the control group. They found no evidence of occurrence of neurapraxia producing permanent neurologic injury. However, in patients who have the syndrome in association with instability of the cervical spine or acute or chronic degenerative changes, they recommended these people be prevented from further participation in contact sports.[353]

Similarly, Ladd and Scranton[231] described two patients in whom complete but transient quadriplegia developed after an injury incurred playing football. Severe congenital stenosis was found after an injury to the cervical disc. These authors advise that patients who have stenosis of the cervical spine should discontinue participation in contact sports.

Eismont and others[140] investigated the relationship between cervical spine sagittal canal diameter and neurologic injury in cases of cervical fracture dislocations. They analyzed 98 patients, of whom 45 had no neurologic deficits, 39 had incomplete quadriparesis, and 14 had complete quadriplegia. Their conclusions were that small diameter canals were correlated significantly with neurologic injury, whereas large diameter canals allowed protection from neurologic injury in cervical fractures. Torg identified the C3-C4 level as the most common dislocation in football injuries resulting in quadriplegia.[221, 352]

Pang and Wilberger[280] described spinal cord injury without radiologic abnormalities in children. They believe the inherent elasticity of vertebral columns in infants and young children renders the pediatric spine exceedingly vulnerable to the deforming forces and neurologic lesions, including a high incidence of complete and severe partial cord lesions.[88] Children under 8 years of age sustain more serious neurologic damage and suffer a larger number of upper cervical cord lesions than those over 8 years of age. It is of interest that in 52 per cent of the cases there was delayed onset of paralysis up to 4 days after injury. Delayed dynamic films were essential to exclude late instability, which, at present, should be managed with a halo fixation or surgical fusion. They found the long-term prognosis for recovery was grim with a complete cord lesion, and only those with mild neurologic injuries make satisfactory neurologic recovery. Other authors have identified specific cervical fractures in children with and without neurologic deficit.[108, 149, 195, 235, 291]

Kang et al.[221] studied the sagittal measurements of the cervical spine in subaxial fractures and dislocations and analyzed 288 patients with and without neurologic deficits. They found that the mean space available for the spinal cord at the level of injury was 10.5 mm for the patients who had complete injury of the spinal cord, 13.1 mm for those who had incomplete injury of the spinal cord, 15.9 mm for those who had an isolated nerve root injury, and 16.7 mm for those who had no neurologic deficit. When measuring the mean Pavlov ratio at the uninjured levels, they found no significant difference between the complete and incomplete spinal cord–injured patients and no difference between those with isolated nerve root injury and those without neurologic deficit. However, there was a significant difference between those with a spinal cord injury versus those with a nerve root or no neurologic injury.

Finally, they demonstrated that the severity of injury of the spinal cord was in part associated with space available for the spinal cord after the injury, as measured on the plain lateral radiographs. Also, patients who sustained a permanent injury of the spinal cord had a narrow sagittal diameter of the spinal canal before injury. They concluded that patients who have a large sagittal diameter of the canal may be more likely to be spared a permanent injury of the spinal cord following cervical trauma, compared with those individuals who have a narrow canal.

McGrory et al.[267] reported on a series of 143 acute fractures and dislocations of the cervical spine in children and adolescents. They studied patients between 2 months and 15 years of age. They described children less than 11 years of age having fewer injuries as a group, and the cervical spine trauma was predominantly ligamentous in nature in the cephalic portion of the cervical spine. These injuries were associated with a high rate of mortality. As a group, children 12 through 15 years of age had more injuries related to sports and recreational activities and were more frequently injured in the caudal portion of the cervical spine. The risk of death due to injury was 5.1 times higher in the younger age group.

Huelke et al.[208] described a new mechanism of cervical spine injury secondary to shoulder belt restraints by which injuries to the cervical spine occurred without head or torso impacts against the interior car structures. They state that the cervical spine injuries were due to neck flexion over the shoulder portion of the restraint.

Upper Thoracic Fractures (T2–T10)

By nature of the different anatomy and surrounding structures in the thoracic spine between the first and tenth thoracic vertebrae, other mechanisms of injury may occur to produce damage to the spine at these levels. Specifically, the thoracic rib cage, the costovertebral ligaments, intervertebral discs, and annulus fibrosus produce relatively more normal stability in this area as opposed to the cervical spine or thoracolumbar junction. In addition, the thoracic spinal canal is quite small and offers less room for fracture fragment and disc protrusion into the spinal canal without causing spinal cord injury, which is an important consideration. In the thoracic spine, more severe injuries are required to produce fractures and dislocations in this region. Anatomically, the facet joints of the thoracic spine are placed in a more sagittal plane than in the cervical spine, and with the rib cage offering greater support, rotational injuries are less common. Mechanisms of injury in the thoracic spine include flexion, most often axial loading, rotation, extension, or a combination of these. As in the cervical spine, direct blows, such as falling objects or missiles, may cause thoracic spine and cord injuries. Instability following injury is not as great a concern in the thoracic spine as it is in the more mobile cervical or thoracolumbar areas of the spine.[39, 40, 363]

Lower Thoracic and Lumbar Fractures (T11–L5)

At the thoracolumbar junction and distally, the spinal canal is relatively large, and the facet joints become sagitally placed so that rotational forces are strongly resisted. The thoracolumbar junction is a fulcrum for spine motion placed just below the rigid upper thoracic spine and chest cage, and it is here that abnormal forces frequently produce fractures and dislocations of the spine. As in other areas of the spine, the intervertebral disc, annular, interspinous, and longitudinal ligaments, and facet joint capsules aid in providing stability of the spine. Mechanisms of injury to the thoracolumbar and lumbar spine include flexion, lateral rotation, axial loading, extension, or a combination of these forces.[154, 272]

Acute instability of the thoracolumbar spine following injury is more commonly a problem requiring external or internal stabilization than in the upper thoracic region. The anatomy of the upper thoracic and thoracolumbar spine differs, from a neurologic as well as an osseous standpoint. With reference to traumatic upper thoracic spine and spinal cord injuries, of major concern is the spinal cord and, to a lesser extent, the nerve roots in this region. There is no major functional significance to loss of upper thoracic nerve root function at a few levels. At the thoracic lumbar junction, however, the spinal cord ends in the conus with the lumbar and sacral cord segments, and the lumbar nerve roots pass by this junction, which is a very important anatomic consideration in injuries at this level of the spine. Here nerve root function is quite important.[205, 206]

Instability may occur in the thoracolumbar spine following major disruption of the osseous or ligamentous structures, either in isolation or as combined injuries. Originally, when Holdsworth described his series of thoracolumbar fractures, he believed the unstable types included severe flexion injuries with posterior ligament complex tearing as well as flexion-rotation fractures that fractured the facets and end plate of the adjacent vertebra. When severe osseous displacement occurred, he recommended open reduction and internal fixation. Flexion injuries with compression fractures of the vertebral body were considered stable if the posterior ligaments were intact.[206] Little emphasis was placed on retropulsion of bone or disc fragments into the spinal canal or neural compression following attempts at reduction and alignment.[293] Ferguson and Allen[154] described a mechanistic classification of thoracolumbar spine fractures in a review of 54 patients. Of these, 34 had bone protrusion from the posterior vertebral body encroaching on the neural canal. They divided the three parts of the vertebrae into anterior, middle, and posterior elements, and classified injuries as (1) compressive flexion, (2) distractive flexion, (3) lateral flexion, (4) translational, (5) torsional flexion, (6) vertical compression, and (7) distractive extension. McAfee[265] described patients with "unstable" burst fractures of the thoracolumbar junction treated by posterolateral decompression and Harrington rod instrumentation. He noted that preoperative computed tomography (CT) could assess the mid-sagittal diameter of the spinal canal, and identified a large portion of cases having posterior element fractures as well as bone protrusion into the spinal canal. In 1983, McAfee et al. studied 100 consecutive patients with potentially unstable fractures and fracture dislocations with CT in the thoracolumbar spine. The mechanism of failure of the middle osteoligamentous complex of the spine was determined by three-dimensional analysis. Three modes of middle column failure were used to classify the injuries: axial compression (73 patients), axial traction (15 patients), and translation within the transverse plane (12 patients). Compression and distraction injuries of the middle complex could be appropriately treated by Harrington distraction and compression instrumentation, respectively. However, in translational injuries, routine Harrington instrumentation was contraindicated owing to the risk of overdistraction; these injuries were therefore treated with segmental spinal instrumentation.

Denis[116] additionally described the three-column concept of the thoracolumbar spine and its significance in the classification of acute thoracolumbar spinal injuries.

Other authors have stressed the demonstration and significance of neural compression after spinal injury.[194, 216, 293] Jelsma et al. indicate that continued neural compression following spinal injury is an important decision factor in making a case for anterior decompression

of the spinal cord, because this results in improved neurologic recovery.[182, 217, 262, 350, 351]

Gertzbein et al.[181] reclassified flexion and distraction injuries of the lumbar spine, which were previously described as seat-belt injuries.[181] They include three types of posterior fracture, with anterior fracture created with flexion and distraction as the mechanism of injury. This fracture was originally described by Kauffer and Hayes in 1966, in which the predominant fracture line occurs through the osseous elements of the vertebrae.[223] Reid et al. have described similar fractures in children.[296]

Rumball and Jarvis[309] reported on seat-belt injuries of the spine in young children, describing 10 patients, three of whom had neurologic deficit. Four of these had intra-abdominal injuries requiring laparotomy, and there was a delay in diagnosis of either the spinal or intra-abdominal injury in five cases. All of these children had contusion of the abdominal wall, the so-called "seat-belt sign." All of these injuries were treated conservatively.

Ching et al.[91] carried out a biomechanical study comparing the residual stability in thoracolumbar spine fractures using neutral zone measurements. They found that burst fractures retain the least residual stability, compression fractures the greatest, and flexion-distraction injuries were similar to burst fractures in flexion and extension.

Fractures of the fifth lumbar vertebra are quite unusual and have been reported by Court-Brown and Gertzbein.[100] They reported three cases, two of which were treated nonsurgically. In a third patient, posterior decompression with instrumentation was performed, which produced loss of lordosis. None of these patients had persistent neurologic deficit. Frederickson et al. reported an additional four cases in which the major mechanism of injury was vertical compression; all of the patients had some neurologic deficit. These authors and others[83, 274] described laceration and crushing of the nerve roots as well as dural tears. They recommended a decompression and a fusion from L4 to the sacrum without internal fixation.[170] Mick and others described a series of 11 patients sustaining burst fractures of the fifth lumbar vertebrae, five of whom had neurologic injury. Nonsurgical treatment yielded excellent results in young patients with minimal canal compromise; however, neurologic deficits responded more predictably to surgical decompression.[273]

Sacral Fractures

Sacral fractures are uncommon and usually occur by shear forces with or without neurologic involvement. These fractures are reasonably stable acutely with external support.

Recently, sacral fractures were reclassified by Sabiston and Wing, who describe the high association with pelvic fractures.[310] They identified a vertical fracture associated with pelvic fracture occurring through the sacral foramen, a lower segmental sacral fracture that was transversed through the lower sacral area, and an upper segmental transverse fracture through the S1 foramen. All patients were treated without surgery. Only one, with complete cauda equina injury, had no significant improvement neurologically. There were three associated nerve root injuries. Denis et al.[117] reported on a retrospective analysis of 236 patients with sacral fractures and classified them into three zones. Zone 1, the region of the ala, was occasionally associated with fifth nerve root injury. Zone 2, the region of the sacral foramen, was a vertical fracture frequently associated with sciatica but rarely with bladder dysfunction. Zone 3, the region of the central sacral canal, was frequently associated with saddle anesthesia and loss of sphincter function. Gibbons et al. reviewed 253 patients with pelvic fractures, of whom 44 were found to have sacral fractures in association. They classified their zones similarly to Denis and found similar neurologic impairment in the different zones. They and others believe that operative decompression has a place in useful recovery of neurologic function.[183, 283]

Pathophysiology of Spinal Cord Trauma: Experimental

The pathophysiology of spinal cord trauma has been reviewed by Saul and Ducker.[312, 313] Many mechanisms are operative once the spinal cord has been damaged, and, to a certain degree, they are progressive. Spinal cord tissue injury can be related to the mechanical insult, biochemical derangements, hemodynamic changes and, in certain cases, to ancillary problems as they relate to other systemic conditions of the patient.[294, 295, 346]

The mechanical insult to the spinal cord includes direct tissue disruption, motion stresses to a damaged cord, which may accentuate the pathology, and persistent compression of the neural tissue.[72, 73] The physical injury to the cord and the neuromembranes is responsible for the initial dysfunction.[225, 226] Anatomically, over a period of hours, the cord may become edematous, soft, and necrotic. The meningeal vessels change caliber, and the axons and their surrounding myelin may become fragmented. In the area of trauma, there is ischemia and diminished axoplasmic flow in the transverse axons. Histologically, progressive gray matter necrosis occurs with fragmentation in the white matter.[13, 58, 59, 124, 127, 358] The amount of tissue disruption is proportional to the injuring force, and progresses as a function of time. Within five minutes following injury, the venules in the gray matter of the spinal cord distend and red cells may appear in the perivascular spaces. Hemorrhages can be seen both in the gray matter and occasionally in the dorsal white matter. Vacuolation and swelling of capillary endothelium undergo occlusion with progressive gray matter necrosis.[224, 355]

Histologic changes in the white matter are not as prominent in the first few hours after injury as in gray matter; however, in the experimental animal, the central gray matter changes occur rapidly, as they do after three to four hours in the peripheral white matter. Initial edema leads to distortion of small vessels with altered perfusion and, after the maximum swelling, which is about 24 to 48 hours in the experimental animal, there may be progressive demyelinization and axonal loss with total tissue destruction. This process may last as long as five days in the human spinal cord injury.

Therapy may also be directed to the mechanical aspects of the injury. Although the direct tissue disruption cannot be altered by the physician once it has occurred, movement of the injured spinal cord or persistent compression of the neural structures by bone or disc fragments may be altered to preserve the remaining neural integrity. Immediate immobilization protects the spinal cord,[130] and any significant cord compression that can be readily corrected by a surgical procedure should be planned.

The electrophysiologic changes can be measured in an injured spinal cord and may reflect neuronal activity that is not readily assessable by a clinical examination.[190, 244] Griffiths[187, 188] and Bohlman et al.[45, 47, 48] studied both acute and chronic anterior cord compression in animals and showed that evoked cortical potentials transmitted in the dorsal columns are readily stopped with significant injury.[3] Gooding et al.[184] demonstrated the additive detrimental effect of compression and ischemia. Kobrine and coworkers[202, 225, 226] clearly demonstrated that initial weight drop on the cord causes disruption of the neural conduction mechanisms, and recovery depends on the rapidity, duration, and force of the inflicting injury. After the initial injury in the clinical setting, the spinal cord probably recovers to a certain degree, only to have a secondary pathologic process occur that may be related to the hemodynamic events that take over and lead to final cessation of cord function.[128]

Biochemical derangements have been demonstrated by many authors. On a cellular and organelle level, there is massive assimilation of lysosomes and a release of hydrolases,[222] as well as mitochondrial alterations with a decrease in cytochrome oxidase activity.[210] Clendenon et al. in 1978[94] demonstrated decreased sodium, potassium, and adenosine triphosphatase activity in the injured area of spinal cord. The importance of accumulation of lactic acid and changes in the overall glucose metabolic pathways was demonstrated by Locke et al.[246] The release of lipid peroxidase and the subsequent hydrolysis at the injury site with the substance breakdown of neuromembranes and neurofilaments occurs within six to eight hours, according to Bracken, and is extremely important in some of the delayed necrosis seen pathologically.[62, 63] If this secondary effect of lipid peroxidation can be inhibited, then the vasoactive byproducts of arachidonic metabolism might be reduced, which in turn would improve the blood supply at the injury site. There is some research evidence that high-dose steroids given in experimental spinal cord injury do affect this peroxidase activity and subsequent loss of blood flow. This may be an explanation for some of the experimental and clinical evidence that steroids may be effective in diminishing the damage to the spinal cord after injury. However, these basic metabolic derangements provide us with some pathophysiologic information that would influence our treatment. For example, high-energy consumption states secondary to fever, sepsis, or agitation should be avoided. We should try to minimize endogenous and exogenous toxins, which could further poison or interfere with the normal metabolic processes. It may be advisable to reduce the metabolic rate with cooling, as advocated in experiments by Albin et al.[5] Hydrocortisone therapy has resulted experimentally in stabilization of cell membranes, reducing the mechanical defects, and has recently been proved to have some beneficial effect in the clinical situation.[62, 63, 67, 69–71]

The hemodynamic changes that occur after cord trauma include response of the vasomotor system and alterations in blood flow, oxygen tension, and autoregulation. Vasomotor activity is almost completely lost immediately after the injury, in addition to changes in the responsiveness to carbon dioxide.[125, 224, 330] After three to four hours, blood flow in the injured spinal cord tends to diminish over time. There is diminished flow in the severely injured cord, which can be either primary or secondary to the ischemic process. Oxygen tension also falls in the contused spinal cord, but whether this is a primary or secondary effect has not been determined. Therapy aimed at trying to diminish the hemodynamic changes is possible in the clinical situation if normal systemic blood pressure is maintained for optimal cord perfusion and adequate oxygenation.

Regeneration of the spinal cord is not possible at the present time. Elaborate studies by Windle[369, 370] demonstrated no real functional value of the regeneration, which may in part be promoted by changes in temperature or using various enzyme preparations. Experiments in 1960 confirmed the earlier studies by Windle, although some regenerating bulbs were noted, but functional recovery was not possible. Russian experiments provided histologic evidence of nerve fiber regeneration and some electrophysiologic evidence of conduction between the sciatic nerve and the cerebral cortex; however, when these experimental studies were reproduced by Guth et al.,[192, 193] actual regeneration could not be shown and no functional recovery occurred.

To date, there is no inherent regeneration process that allows functional recovery of an anatomically disrupted spinal cord. Therefore, treatments have to be aimed at those pathophysiologic processes in which cord tissue that was not totally disrupted is preserved for future use and recovery.

Pathology of Spine and Spinal Cord Trauma: Clinical

It is difficult to assess the degree of spinal cord pathology from clinical evaluation of neurologic deficit.[215] There is no easy and direct correlation of findings at autopsy in spinal cord–injured patients with the clinical situation. As Bohlman[46] has pointed out in his review of 300 cervical spine injuries, the autopsy findings in 48 cases indicated that only three patients had total cord tissue disruption, and many of the patients with clinical evidence of total cord lesions had incomplete contusions and parenchymal hemorrhages. Conversely, some patients with anterior cord syndromes had normal cords microscopically without evidence of gross cord disruption (Fig. 33–1). This absence of cord dis-

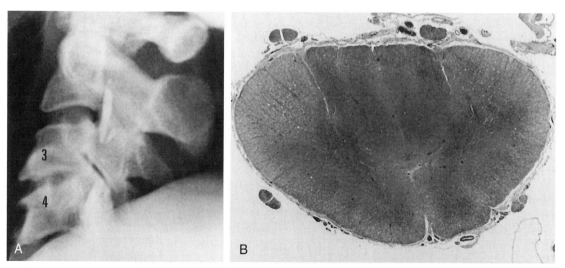

Figure 33–1. *A,* A 53-year-old man had a central cord quadriparesis at the third cervical level after he fell while intoxicated. A preoperative myelogram showed protrusion of disc material between the third and fourth vertebrae. After Robinson anterior cervical discectomy and fusion carried out 10 days after injury, there was a rapid recovery of function, but the patient died of a pulmonary embolus 10 months after injury. *B,* This histologic section of the spinal cord at the level of the third and fourth vertebrae shows little more than peripheral vacuolization (H & E × 10). (From Bohlman, H. H.: Acute fractures and dislocations of the cervical spine. J. Bone Joint Surg. *61A:*1119–1142, 1979.)

ruption supports the concept that ischemia and mechanical compression are the basis of the anterior cord syndrome. In addition, four cases with unilateral facet dislocations and impairment of major radicular feeder vessels to the cord demonstrated central cord necrosis, which would lend support to advocates of early reduction of spinal fractures. Bohlman et al.[47, 48] demonstrated in a chronic anterior cord compression model, as well as in an anterior weight drop contusion animal model, that central necrosis of the gray matter is the most common pathologic finding. Magnetic resonance imaging (MRI) carried out on acutely injured spinal cord patients may reveal similar pathology (see Fig. 33–78). The formerly described anterior and central cord syndromes may represent different degrees of the same pathologic process; that is, contusion of the cord initially followed by microvascular oligemia, edema, and subsequent necrosis of the cervical spinal cord. It would therefore seem appropriate, based on these findings, to reduce fractures and dislocations immediately with skeletal traction and to remove any offending anterior compressive pathologic condition that may interfere with normal recovery of the spinal cord.

Massive epidural hemorrhage is rare,[290] occurring in only four of the eight patients with ankylosing spondylitis in Bohlman's review series of 300 cases,[46] and not occurring to any great extent in the series by Davis, Bohlman and coworkers[107] of 50 fatal craniospinal injuries; therefore, compressive pathology of the spinal cord in cervical spine injuries is operable anteriorly with reference to the spinal cord, and any decompressive operative procedures should be approached in that direction (Fig. 33–2). Also, in the fatal craniospinal injury study, it was apparent that the spinal cord was injured predominantly in the upper cervical segments, whereas disc injuries occurred most commonly in the lower cervical segments. The vertebral artery was involved in only one case. The longitudinal ligaments were damaged very often with the disc, together indicating multiple forces involved in these severe injuries. The transverse ligament of the odontoid was spared.

Bucholz analyzed 170 multiple trauma victims brought to the Dallas County medical examiner's office, of whom 38 were discovered to have cervical spine injuries.[78] He too found a more commonly associated higher level of atlanto-occipital and atlantoaxial injuries. Eight bilateral pedicle fractures of the axis were analyzed. There was combined ligament disruption producing a very unstable situation, with a major dislocation of C2 on C3. The cord was transected in three of the patients.

Treatment of the osseous and ligamentous injuries depends on the degree of damage that has occurred with the original injury. A mild axial loading or compressive fracture of the lower cervical vertebral bodies may be treated with a rigid brace or halo apparatus and will heal uneventfully; however, more severe compression fractures of the vertebrae may produce osseous fragment protrusion into the spinal canal and necessitate skeletal traction for reduction and possible anterior arthrodesis. A compression fracture of the cer-

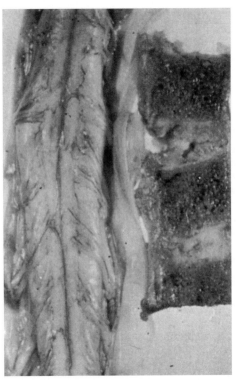

Figure 33–2. This specimen shows a large extruded disc fragment lying anterior to the posterior longitudinal ligament, and narrowing of the anteroposterior diameter of the spinal canal. Most herniated discs caused by cervical trauma remain anterior to the posterior longitudinal ligament and can be excised through the anterior approach. In this specimen, there was no gross evidence of necrosis of the spinal cord. (From Bohlman, H. H.: Acute fractures and dislocations of the cervical spine. J. Bone Joint Surg. *61A:*1119–1142, 1979.)

vical vertebrae may produce anterior cord or nerve root compression. If skeletal traction cannot reduce the fracture appropriately, thereby decompressing the spinal canal, anterior decompression and fusion are indicated to relieve neural compression. By the same reasoning, post-traumatic cervical disc herniations, if they are compressing the neural structures, should be decompressed anteriorly and fusion carried out, provided that posterior stability has been established. MRI and cervical myelography with CT scanning may be very useful in determining whether neural compression persists after attempted closed reduction of the fracture. The preferred technique that we recommend for anterior decompression of an axial loading vertebral body fracture and fusion is removal of the discs above and below the compression fracture and grafting with iliac bone. The Cloward dowel graft is not a stable graft for traumatic injuries of the cervical spine,[34] and although a strong fibular graft can be used, the latter does not incorporate very rapidly.[337] It is our policy to use a rigid, two-poster orthosis or halo-vest until the iliac crest graft is well incorporated, usually in two months. A further problem may arise in the case of combined anterior and posterior instability, where two procedures may have to be done.

The most common severe cervical spine injury involving the posterior elements is a subluxation or dislocation in which the posterior ligament complex is completely torn. This may be associated with anterior disc or ligament disruption. Displacement of disc material posteriorly into the spinal canal at the time of a unilateral or bilateral fracture dislocation has been demonstrated by Bohlman[34] and by Eismont as well as Zidman and Ducker (Fig. 33–3). Use of MRI in the evaluation of an acutely injured patient is becoming more common. Although it is difficult to do these studies, newer nonmagnetic halos and tongs make it possible. A traction device has been developed that is MRI compatible and allows for spinal stability and traction to be maintained during the study. It has been pointed out by Bohlman[46] that late instability is more common than previously realized, because ligamentous structures do not reconstitute normally, even with prolonged external rigid fixation (Fig. 33–4). Subluxations of the cervical vertebrae as a result of bilaterally perched facets in a flexion injury can be reduced with skeletal traction; however, they usually require posterior stabilization with wire and iliac crest graft for ultimate stability. In the case of severe posterior or ligament tearing, which fits White's criteria for instability, we would prefer to perform an early arthrodesis so

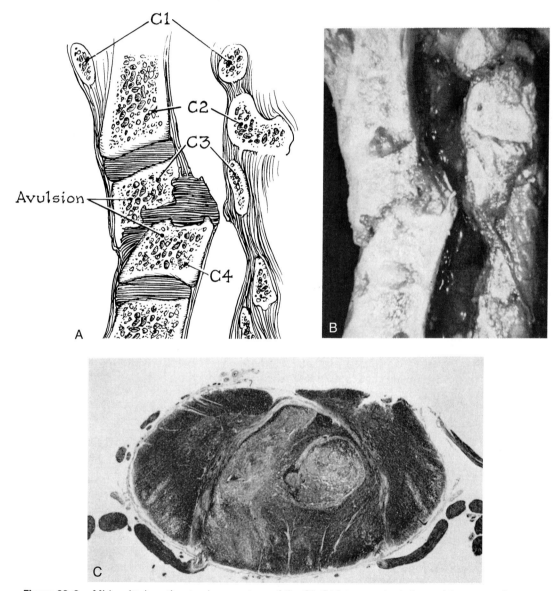

Figure 33–3. Midsagittal section to show rupture of the C3–C4 intervertebral disc and fractures of adjacent bodies with extravasation of intervertebral disc material compromising the neural canal and preventing reduction of the displacement. *A,* Sketch. *B,* Photograph. *C,* Photomicrograph of a section of the cervical spinal cord at C3–C4 showing the pulped central white and gray matter. (Loyez for myelin × 6.) (From Davis, D., Bohlman, H., Walker, A. E., et al.: The pathological findings in fatal craniospinal injuries. J. Neurosurg. *34:*612, 1971.)

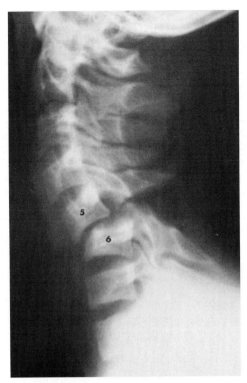

Figure 33–4. A 15-year-old male who fell on the ice, striking his occiput and sustaining a flexion-type injury with dislocation of C5 on C6. He was reduced in long traction and then placed in a Minerva jacket for 15 weeks and redislocated. Note spreading of the interspinous ligament between C5 and C6 on the lateral roentgenogram. Posterior fusion was required. (From Bohlman, H. H.: Complications of treatment of fractures and dislocations of the cervical spine. In Epps, C. H., Jr. [ed.]: Complications of Orthopedic Surgery. Philadelphia, J. B. Lippincott Co., 1985.)

that the patient may be mobilized in a rigid orthosis quickly, rather than waiting a three-month period after maintaining the patient in a halo brace and then finding on stress views that there is continued chronic instability and having to do the fusion at a later date. Patients with less severe ligamentous tearing and subluxations of the cervical spine may be treated conservatively and have the option of a late arthrodesis if necessary. Unilateral cervical facet dislocations usually impinge on the individual nerve root of that foramen and are extremely difficult to reduce nonoperatively with skeletal traction unless a manipulation is performed. It is our approach to attempt closed reduction without general anesthesia in skeletal traction and, if reduction is not obtained easily, then posterior reduction by operative intervention is carried out and arthrodesis with iliac graft and triple wiring is performed. However, if diagnostic studies such as MRI reveal a large disc herniation anterior to the cord, then the patient will need both an anterior and posterior operation carried out in skeletal traction or an anterior decompression with stabilization by bone graft and plate fixation. In the review series of cervical spine injuries, the only root lesions that did not recover were

those left untreated without adequate reduction or decompression. Unilateral facet fractures may allow subluxation of one vertebra on another and impinge against a nerve root dorsally; therefore, if they cannot be reduced adequately by skeletal traction so that the foramen is clear, open reduction and a limited posterior decompression should be performed by means of foraminotomy followed by a posterior arthrodesis. Fractures of the individual spinous processes or laminae will heal quite well with rigid immobilization and do not require operative treatment. Bilateral facet dislocations, which are usually associated with complete quadriplegia, frequently require open reduction to preserve one nerve root level above the cord injury and should be treated by posterior triple wiring and arthrodesis, so that early mobilization can be carried out and stabilization is assured.[139] The preceding indications for operative intervention are, of course, based on stabilization of the general medical status of the patient and other associated injuries.

A problem may arise in the case of the patient who presents with posterior instability and an incomplete cord injury with evident compressive pathology against the anterior cervical cord. This is usually a combination of an axial loading compression fracture with osseous protrusion into the spinal canal and a torn posterior ligament complex. In this instance, we believe that the patient should be immediately treated in the skeletal traction for attempted reduction and alignment, which is then followed by myelography to assess the canal and posterior arthrodesis and wiring for stabilization, and then a staged anterior decompression and arthrodesis if necessary. The patients who we have treated by this method have recovered significant neurologic function and are able to be ambulated in a rigid cervical brace immediately following the second surgical procedure. The timing of surgical decompression and stabilization is a matter of the surgeon's judgment; however, in the high-risk patient, such as a complete quadriplegic at the fifth cervical level, we have found that it is safe to do an early posterior reduction and fusion using local anesthesia. However, general anesthesia is required for anterior decompression and fusion.

Chronic Spinal Cord and Cauda Equina Compression: Experimental and Clinical

Bohlman et al.[47, 48] demonstrated experimentally that incomplete spinal cord injuries have the potential to recover to varying degrees, depending on the amount of initial cord contusion, as well as mechanical factors producing compression of neural tissue. If the spinal cord is incompletely damaged or contused during injury, varying amounts of functional cord tissue remain. Mechanical factors that subject this remaining viable cord tissue to anterior compression may prevent optimal recovery of spinal cord function. Compressive elements may physiologically block spinal cord function and recovery for extended periods of time without totally destroying neural tissue.[344-346] The spinal cord remains ischemic and deformed as long as compression is present.[122] When clinical neurologic recovery has reached a plateau, the spinal cord may still recover if compression is removed. Therefore, anterior decompression of the spinal cord aids in recovery of spinal cord function.[121] Important questions are how severely the spinal cord may be contused, and how low the spinal cord may be compressed anteriorly and still allow for recovery of neurologic function.[56]

How does one measure the degree of spinal cord damage noninvasively and predict the extent of eventual recovery? Bohlman et al. developed an experimental animal model of incomplete spinal cord injury by individually producing compression (pressure transducer) and contusion (weight drop) in animals through an anterior cervical spinal approach.[46, 48] To develop the incomplete spinal cord contusion model, beagle hounds were subjected to 250 to 1000 g/cm² of energy by the weight-drop method. Variable levels of quadriparesis occurred in all animals, and in order to consistently reproduce an incomplete paralysis that did not resolve, 800 g/cm² to 1000 g/cm² of energy was required. This is considerably greater than the 400 g/cm² of energy required to produce an incomplete paraplegia from the standard thoracodorsal approach.[126, 127] The increased energy required in the anterior cervical weight-drop experiments may be related to the larger spinal cord at the midcervical level, as well as an increased blood supply in this region of the spinal cord. The animal model of incomplete spinal cord injury secondary to compression was produced by inserting a pressure transducer through the anterior cervical approach at the fifth and sixth cervical interspace (Fig. 33–5). Immediate spinal cord compression was produced with approximately 5 to 20 pounds per square inch of pressure applied externally through a remote, spring-loaded fluid reservoir. Immediate paralysis occurred, which was then maintained by chronic compression for three to eight weeks until no further neurologic recovery occurred. The spinal cord was then decompressed by removing the pressure transducer, so that late recovery from paralysis could be studied.

It was demonstrated in this study that recovery from chronic paralysis could occur even though decompression was performed late after paralysis had been well established. Most of the dogs studied developed central cord syndromes, with forepaw paralysis greater than hindpaw, regardless of whether the animal model was produced by compression or contusion of the spinal cord. The spinal cords of the dogs were subjected to gross and histologic examination, which revealed varying degrees of central gray matter damage as the most common finding. The latter correlated well with the clinical syndromes of paralysis. Other animals demonstrated wallerian degeneration of the ascending sensory posterior columns, indicating a reason for loss of cortical evoked potentials (CEPs). Anterior and lateral corticospinal tracts were damaged, indicating descending wallerian degeneration. A number of animals had normal histologic examination, indicating that ischemia, or decreased vascular supply of the spinal cord,

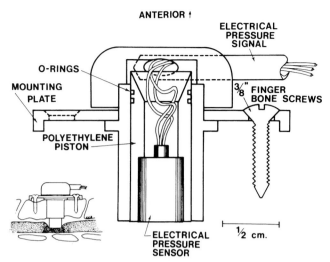

Figure 33–5. Newer design of pressure transducer with solid polyethylene piston and incorporated electrical pressure sensor to measure pressure directly applied to the spinal cord. The transducer piston is remotely controlled and monitored after insertion into the anterior cervical spine (inset). (From Bohlman, H. H., et al.: Mechanical factors affecting recovery of incomplete cervical spinal cord injury: A preliminary report. Johns Hopkins Med. J. *145:*115–125, 1979.)

may have played a role in the resultant clinical paralysis that later recovered.

With either mechanism of injury, that is, compression or contusion, complete neurologic recovery is possible, although histologic damage persists. In the acute contusion model progressively greater contusion forces cause proportionately increased neurologic damage and recovery time. Compression models demonstrate that neurologic recovery is possible with sustained cord compression; but recovery was much faster and more complete when anterior decompression was performed. Spinal cord monitoring was performed by measuring the computer-averaged CEP induced by peripheral nerve stimulation. As in other studies, the CEP paralleled the degree of recovery from both the contusive and compressive lesions.[47, 48, 129, 244] From this study, it is apparent that late recovery of spinal cord function can occur if mechanical factors such as protruding discs and bone fragments are removed from the spinal canal by the anterior surgical approach.

Delamarter, Bohlman, and others have developed an animal model of graded compression of the cauda equina in which the cortical evoked potentials, microvasculature, and histopathology were studied.[110, 111, 114] Animals with cauda equina constricted 25 per cent had no neurologic deficits, mild changes in cortical evoked potentials, and slight histologic change. Those with constriction of 50 per cent had mild initial motor weakness, major changes in cortical evoked potentials, edema and loss of myelin in the root of the seventh lumbar nerve, and moderate or severe venous congestion of the root or dorsal root ganglion of the seventh lumbar nerve. Constriction of 75 per cent produced

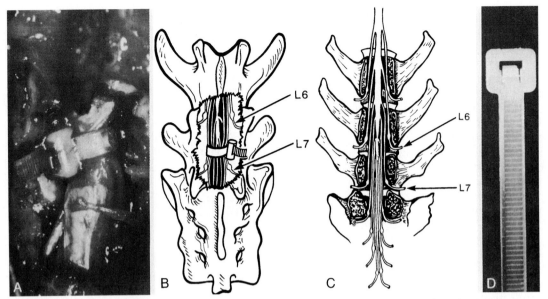

Figure 33–6. *A,* Intraoperative photograph of the site of the laminectomy of the sixth and seventh lumbar vertebrae, showing the constriction band with 50 per cent constriction of the cauda equina. *B,* Illustration of the photograph shown in *A.* The constriction band was always applied at the seventh lumbar level, and the roots of the seventh lumbar nerve were included in the constriction. *C,* Illustration of the canine cauda equina (dura removed). Note that the conus medullaris extends to the level of the fifth and sixth lumbar vertebrae, and the cauda equina begins at the sixth lumbar vertebra. *D,* Nylon constricting band. Each catch-ratchet is 0.35 mm apart, allowing precise measurements of constriction. (From Delamarter, R. B., Bohlman, H. H., Dodge, L. D., and Biro, C.: Experimental spinal stenosis. J. Bone Joint Surg. *72A:*111, 1990.)

significant paralysis and urinary incontinence, with marked change in CEPs. There was blockage of axoplasmic flow and wallerian degeneration of the motor nerve roots distal to the constriction and to the sensory roots proximal to the constriction, as well as degeneration of the posterior columns. Severe arterial narrowing at the level of constriction and venous congestion of the roots and dorsal root ganglia of the seventh lumbar and first sacral nerves were also present. CEPs revealed neurologic abnormalities before the appearance of neurologic signs and symptoms (Figs. 33–6, 33–7, and 33–8). Carlson et al.[86] developed an animal model of spinal cord compression and decompression to study the viscoelastic relaxation and regional blood flow response in spinal cord injuries. The first group of six animals that were decompressed five minutes after maximum compression was compared with six animals that had spinal cord compression maintained for three hours and were not decompressed; the authors found that five minutes after compression was stopped, the spinal cord interface pressure had dissipated 51 per cent and the somatosensory evoked amplitudes continued to decrease to 16 per cent of baseline. In contrast, in the sustained compression group, cord interface pressure relaxed to 13 per cent of maximum within 90 minutes; however, no recovery of somatosensory evoked potential occurred, and the regional spinal cord blood flow remained significantly lower than baseline. In those animals who were decompressed within 5 minutes, spinal cord blood flow recovered to baseline within 30 minutes. This study is the first to quantify and correlate the mechanical interface loads observed with precision loading and indicated that early electrical conduction effects of spinal cord compression are associated with a combination of mechanical and ischemic factors.

In addition, in another article by Carlson et al.,[85] they demonstrated early time-dependent decompression for

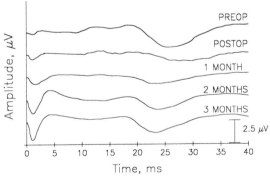

Figure 33–7. Cortical evoked potentials after bilateral stimulation of the posterior tibial nerve in a dog that had 50 per cent constriction. There were increased latency and decreased amplitude immediately after operation and one month postoperatively, with substantial recovery by the second postoperative month (amplitude axis, 2.5 μV per division). (From Delamarter, R. B., Bohlman, H. H., Dodge, L. D., and Biro, C.: Experimental spinal stenosis. J. Bone Joint Surg. *72A:*113, 1990.)

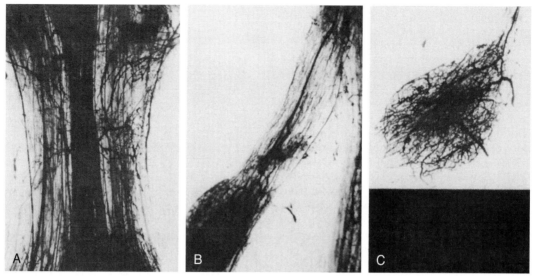

Figure 33–8. A dog that had 50 per cent constriction. *A,* Note the hourglass appearance, with excellent filling of the vessels, except for the peripheral radicular vessels. *B,* The root of the seventh lumbar nerve, just caudal to the constriction band, shows venous distention and a curlicued pattern. The large central radicular artery is normal. *C,* The dorsal root ganglion of the seventh lumbar nerve shows vascular congestion and leakage of dye. (From Delamarter, R. B., Bohlman, H. H., Dodge, L. D., and Biro, C.: Experimental spinal stenosis. J. Bone Joint Surg. *72A:*114, 1990.)

spinal cord injury and vascular mechanisms of recovery. They noted that electrophysiologic recovery was very significant if the decompression was performed within one hour of initial compression. In addition, these authors describe the degree of early reperfusion hyperemia after decompression as being proportional to the duration of the spinal cord compression and inversely proportional to the electrophysiologic recovery. Residual blood flow during the sustained compression period was significantly higher in those dogs that did not recover evoked potential function after decompression, suggesting a reperfusion injury. Their results indicate that a critical time period exists in which intervention by early spinal cord decompression can lead to electrophysiologic recovery if it is within one hour.

In addition to the animal experimentations, Bohlman and colleagues carried out late anterior decompression of severe spinal cord injuries with long-term follow-up.[11, 36] Between 1973 and 1983, late anterior decompressions were carried out on 60 patients with complete motor quadriplegia secondary to cervical injuries. Decompressions were carried out to gain further root recovery of the upper extremities and were performed an average time from injury to surgery of 14.3 months. Of 52 patients followed with re-examination from two to 15 years, neurologic recovery of at least two functional motor root levels was documented in eight and of one nerve root level in 18. Increased motor strength by two grades of muscle function was seen six times. Therefore, anterior decompression resulted in neurologic recovery with improvement in upper extremity function in 73 per cent of the patients. During the same period, 58 patients with incomplete cervical spinal cord injury were decompressed anteriorly;

the average time from injury to surgery was 12.8 months. Of 56 patients who were evaluated from two to 16 years after surgery, recovery of distal cord motor function in the legs occurred in 36, and 28 patients became functional ambulators or improved their ambulatory status. Only six were able to stand with aid preoperatively. Also, 39 patients made root recovery of one or more levels in the upper extremities. A delay of longer than 12 months from injury to surgical decompression adversely affected neurologic recovery. We therefore believe that anterior decompression and fusion, even late after injury, can result in further neurologic recovery of both upper extremity root and distal cord leg function in approximately 82 per cent of patients with incomplete motor paralysis.

Bohlman and others reported on the treatment of acute injuries of the upper thoracic spine with paralysis in 218 patients.[40] Of these, 184 had complete and 34 had incomplete lesions of the spinal cord. Thirty of the patients with an incomplete lesion of the spinal cord were followed for two to 20 years. Five patients with an incomplete lesion were treated without surgery (two having gunshot wounds and one a stab wound). Three of these recovered the ability to walk, while two were nonambulatory. Seventeen patients with an incomplete lesion of the spinal cord were treated by laminectomy. None of these recovered completely but more importantly, eight lost neurologic function or became completely paraplegic after surgery and did not recover. Of the eight patients with an incomplete lesion treated by anterior transthoracic decompression and fusion, three had had a previous laminectomy that did not improve their status. Five of these eight recovered the ability to walk without aid, two walked with braces, and one recovered some motor function but was nonambulatory. It was concluded that laminectomy is contraindicated for incomplete lesions of the upper region of the thoracic spinal cord and that anterior transthoracic decompression and fusion offers the best chance of recovery of neurologic function. No surgical procedure aided recovery of the 184 complete cord injuries.

McAfee, Bohlman, and Yuan reported on anterior decompression of traumatic thoracolumbar fractures with incomplete neurologic deficit using a retroperitoneal approach.[266] Between 1973 and 1981, 70 patients were reviewed, 48 of whom had been followed from two to 8.6 years. All surgery was done within one year of the injury. No patient lost any neurologic function. Thirty-seven of 42 patients with major motor deficit improved at least one class in motor strength. Fourteen of the 30 patients whose quadriceps and hamstrings were too weak to permit walking regained full independent ambulation. Surprisingly, of 32 patients who had conus medullaris injury with neurogenic bowel and bladder, 12 recovered bladder function. From this study, it was apparent that the degree of neurologic recovery of spinal cord injury after anterior decompression for thoracolumbar fractures appears to be more favorable than other reported series in which the spinal canal is not decompressed.[65, 104, 106, 119, 169, 205] Larson and Jelsma have separately reported similar findings with decompression of the spinal canal and stabilization.[21, 217, 234]

Patients with incomplete spinal cord injuries may have continued bone and disc fragments compressing the spinal cord, which prevent optimal recovery of neurologic function. Once the mechanical compressive pathology is recognized, then anterior surgical decompression and fusion are indicated. In principle, therefore, it appears necessary to evaluate patients with spinal cord injury for both acute and chronic cord compression that can be relieved by anterior decompression and fusion.[22, 28, 36, 46]

PATIENT EVALUATION

General Assessment

Recognition of the patient with a spine and spinal cord injury is the first step toward appropriate treatment. In a detailed review of 300 cervical spine injuries by Bohlman,[46] 100 were initially missed in the emergency room situation. Ideally, these injuries should be diagnosed at the scene of the accident, and at least visible paralysis should be assessed and recorded. Delay in diagnosis ranged from one day to over one year, and the most common causes for lack of recognition of cervical spine injuries are head injuries, acute alcoholic intoxication, and multiple injuries.[37] All of those factors distract from the cervical spine problem. Patients with a decreased level of consciousness or in coma do not complain of neck pain; therefore, a lateral roentgenogram must be obtained (Figs. 33–9 and 33–10). Severe scalp lacerations bleed profusely and are evidence of

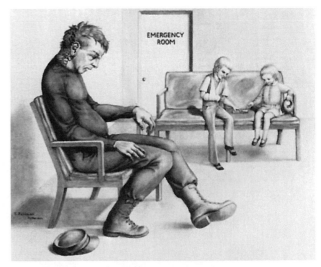

Figure 33–9. Patient sitting in the emergency room with head and neck injury and an associated lethargic level of consciousness. (From Bohlman, H. H.: The neck. *In* D'Ambrosia, R. [ed.]: Musculoskeletal Disorders. 2nd ed. Philadelphia, J. B. Lippincott Co., 1986.)

head trauma, but may lead the examining physician away from evaluation of the spine (Fig. 33–11). The acutely intoxicated patient usually falls down the stairs, striking his head, and may fracture the spine and not complain of neck pain (Fig. 33–12). The polytrauma patient may present in cardiovascular shock and not describe neck pain. Gentle palpation of the posterior cervical spine will reveal reaction to pain by the patient with cervical spine injury (Fig. 33–13). Finally, a small number of patients with traumatic injuries of the cervi-

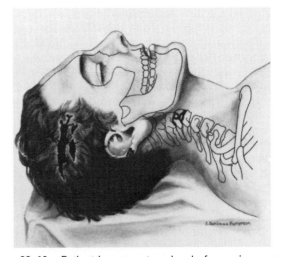

Figure 33–10. Patient in a comatose level of consciousness with a cervical fracture and scalp laceration. Since this patient will not complain of pain, cervical spine roentgenograms must be taken for diagnosis of neck injury. (From Bohlman, H. H.: The neck. *In* D'Ambrosia, R. [ed.]: Musculoskeletal Disorders. 2nd ed. Philadelphia, J. B. Lippincott Co., 1986.)

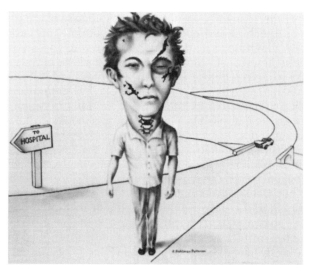

Figure 33–11. Patient with severe scalp lacerations that distract attention from a cervical fracture. (From Bohlman, H. H.: The neck. *In* D'Ambrosia, R. [ed.]: Musculoskeletal Disorders. 2nd ed. Philadelphia, J. B. Lippincott Co., 1986.)

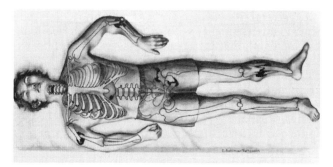

Figure 33–13. A patient with multiple trauma is frequently in shock and will not complain of neck pain. Incomplete paralysis may also be difficult to evaluate. (From Bohlman, H. H.: The neck. *In* D'Ambrosia, R. [ed.]: Musculoskeletal Disorders. 2nd ed. Philadelphia, J. B. Lippincott Co., 1986.)

cal spine may develop Brown-Séquard syndrome and appear to have a hemiparesis that mimics a cerebrovascular accident (Fig. 33–14).[37]

A high correlation of head and neck injury pathology has been demonstrated by Davis et al.[107] in fatal craniospinal injuries. Any patient with a head injury should be suspected of having a traumatic cervical spine injury and vice versa.

A detailed history of the mechanisms of injury should be taken from the patient if he or she is conscious, or from witnesses. Scalp lacerations or abrasions will offer some clue as to the sites of the forces applied to the head and, therefore, to the neck. An inquiry should be made as to the patient's consciousness and limb function immediately following the injury. Occasionally, a patient may have had a transient paralysis secondary to concussion of the spinal cord that resolves partially or completely prior to the patient's arrival at the emergency room. Pre-existing conditions such as cervical spondylosis or congenital anomalies may produce a narrow cervical spinal canal, thus predisposing the patient to spinal cord injury.[44, 140, 231, 348, 353, 354] Patients with mild motor weakness and relative sensory sparing may be mistakenly thought of as hysterical when in fact a spinal cord injury has occurred.

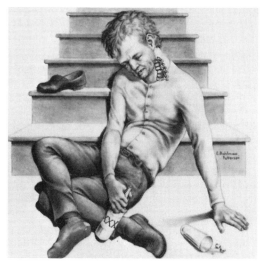

Figure 33–12. An acutely intoxicated patient usually sustains a cervical spine fracture by falling down the stairs. The obtunded patient will not complain of pain. Cervical spine roentgenograms must be taken for diagnosis. (From Bohlman, H. H.: The neck. *In* D'Ambrosia, R. [ed.]: Musculoskeletal Disorders. 2nd ed. Philadelphia, J. B. Lippincott Co., 1986.)

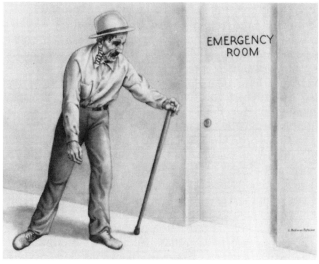

Figure 33–14. An elderly patient with scalp laceration and unilateral facet dislocation may consequently have hemiparesis. This clinical pattern may be mistaken for a cerebrovascular episode. (From Bohlman, H. H.: The neck. *In* D'Ambrosia, R. [ed.]: Musculoskeletal Disorders. 2nd ed. Philadelphia, J. B. Lippincott Co., 1986.)

A general physical examination should be performed on all patients with spinal trauma to evaluate associated injuries in other organ systems or the extremities.

Fractures and dislocations of the thoracic and lumbar spines occur with severe trauma and are often associated with cardiothoracic, abdominal, and cervical injuries. In a study by Bohlman et al.[40] of 218 upper thoracic spine fractures with paralysis, one third of these injuries were associated with intrathoracic trauma; that is, a hemopneumothorax or major vessel injury and ruptured diaphragm. Head and cervical injuries were found in many of the patients. Extremity fractures and soft tissue trauma also occur with upper thoracic fractures. Lumbar fractures, especially seatbelt fracture, are associated with abdominal trauma, including ruptured bowel and major vessel, liver, spleen, and urologic injury.[223, 296] The usual priorities for the multiple-injured patient should be observed, and the spinal fractures take on lesser importance in the face of life-threatening hypovolemic shock and major cardiothoracic trauma. This is not to say, however, that the spine should not be evaluated and stabilized during diagnosis and treatment of other injuries.

On physical examination of the patient with thoracolumbar spine fracture, there may be external clues to the type of fracture and particular force applied. Abrasions and contusions of the skin, gibbous deformity, and displaced or separated spinous processes may be observed and should be recorded to aid in reconstruction of the mechanism of injury.

Roentgenographic Assessment

Following general patient evaluation and external spine and neurologic assessment, the next step in identifying specific spine injuries is the roentgenographic examination in the emergency room. The surgeon diagnosing and treating spine and spinal cord injuries must be aware of the normal as well as abnormal roentgenographic findings with reference to the spine. Care must be taken not to misdiagnose normal variations in anatomy for pathologic situations, especially in children, as well as identifying spinal pathology when it really exists.[27, 29, 31] In a very young child, the head is proportionately larger than the neck and torso, so routine lateral cervical spine radiographs taken with the patient lying on a stretcher may actually be unintentionally flexing the neck. The back and shoulders should therefore be padded. Herzenberg et al.[200] studied emergency transport and positioning of young children with injuries of the cervical spine. Ten children who were less than seven years of age were found to have anterior angulation or translation or both on lateral roentgenograms taken with the child on a standard flat backboard that forces the child's neck into flexion. They therefore recommend a double mattress to raise the chest or a recess of the occiput to lower the head.

As mentioned before, cervical spine pathology is most easily missed in the emergency room situation, whereas severe injuries to the thoracic and lumbar spine are frequently associated with other severe injuries of the chest and abdomen and, therefore, are more easily diagnosed. In the emergency room, the lateral roentgenogram should initiate the diagnosis of severe cervical spine injury. Once the suspicion of cervical spine injury arises, the spine should be immobilized with sandbags or, in the case of obvious neurologic deficit, skeletal traction should be applied. Even head halter traction can be applied until appropriate roentgenograms are taken.

It is extremely uncommon not to recognize cervical spine pathology, that is, fractures or dislocations, on the initial lateral roentgenogram.[46, 59, 199] This roentgenogram should be taken with the patient in supine position, protected in cervical traction, and the superimposed shoulders should be pulled down by the physician who stands at the base of the table so that a good view of the lower cervical spine is obtained.[112] The cassette for the lateral roentgenograms is placed below the shoulder and above the cervical spine region, so that the atlanto-occipital area as well as the cervicothoracic areas of the spine are well visualized. If the patient is obese or extremely muscular, a swimmer's view may be obtained by extending one shoulder in the abducted position 180 degrees and directing the x-ray beam perpendicular to the lower cervical spine. The patient must be instructed to relax the shoulder muscles so that the shoulders may be pulled distally and completely free of the spine for the lateral roentgenogram. Once the lateral roentgenogram is obtained, it should be examined for soft tissue swelling anterior to the spine, which occurs in fractures of the anterior elements; that is, odontoid and vertebral body fractures.[287] Generally, flexion injuries of the cervical spine with torn posterior ligaments do not create soft tissue swelling. T2-weighted MRI can verify posterior interspinous ligament disruption.[146] Following the lateral roentgenogram, the anteroposterior view should be obtained of the cervical spine by angling the x-ray beam in the midline 20 degrees cephalically to visualize the joints of Luschka, disc spaces, and vertebral body end plates, which are often injured in compression fractures. The x-ray cassette may be placed under the patient by the physician, gently lifting the shoulders with both hands while clasping the head between the forearms so as to maintain stability of the cervical spine. In addition, alignment and rotation of the spinous processes may be visualized on this view. Chang et al.[89] published a biomechanical study of the geometric changes in the cervical spinal canal during impact. These authors believe that two potentially injurious geometric changes occur: occlusion of the cross-sectional diameter of the spinal canal, which can constrict the spinal cord, and changes in the length of the spinal canal. The authors believe that the radiographic measurements significantly underestimate the actual transient injury that occurs during impact.

The next important step in diagnosing cervical spine injuries is to obtain oblique views with the patient in the supine position. It is important to assess the pathology of the posterior elements, including the facet joints, to proceed with treatment of cervical spine injuries. Therefore, oblique roentgenograms must be taken in the emergency room prior to any closed or open reduction of a fracture dislocation. Distorted but very useful oblique roentgenograms may be obtained by the following method: once again the head, neck, and shoulders are lifted as a unit and the x-ray cassette is placed under the cervical spine more to the side where the facets are to be visualized; that is, further to the left if the left facets are to be seen on the oblique view, and more to the right if the right facets are to be visualized. The x-ray beam is then directed toward the midcervical spine 45 degrees from vertical and angled 10 degrees cephalically. This allows visualization of the foramina, articular facets, pedicles, and portions of the vertebral bodies. An alternate approach is to have the x-ray cassette placed in a holder under a translucent table, on which the patient lies supine. The cassette holder is at an angle 45 degrees from horizontal, and the oblique x-ray beam is therefore directed perpendicular to the cassette.

Following the oblique views, an open-mouth odontoid view may be taken, and occasionally it is necessary to prop a patient's mouth open by using a roll of gauze or cotton, which is usually available in the emergency room. Most odontoid fractures can be visualized initially on the lateral view; however, additional information should be gained by the anteroposterior view through the mouth.

Fractures of the laminae are frequently missed because they are not visualized on routine roentgenograms of the cervical spine. The view using the x-ray beam directed 30 degrees caudad is difficult to obtain in the acute injury situation, especially when one has to overextend the head on the neck to visualize the cervical spine. In addition, fractures of the laminae rarely cause compression of the spinal cord and, therefore, are not as important as far as treatment is concerned.

CT reconstruction may be helpful in defining greater details of cervical fractures, especially bone fragment protrusion into the spinal canal, as well as lateral mass fractures and fractures of the articular facets, but this special study should be performed only after routine roentgenograms of the cervical spine have been completed and evaluated. MRI is probably the best method of assessing intrinsic cord damage, but it may be difficult to differentiate acute hematomyelia from a syrinx.

In suspected upper thoracic spine fractures, routine anteroposterior and lateral views should be obtained with the patient in the supine position. It is extremely difficult to visualize the upper thoracic spine, especially in stocky individuals, on the lateral roentgenogram; therefore, CT reconstruction may be necessary to define the pathology. Certainly, if a patient presents with paraplegia, great effort should be exerted to define the osseous pathology in the upper thoracic region, because fractures are easily missed in this area because of poor-quality roentgenograms. Once again, as in cervical spine trauma, adequate roentgenograms should be obtained to determine what type of fracture dislocation has occurred, so that appropriate treatment can

be instituted. Frequently, soft tissue swelling of the paraspinous area may be a clue to significant thoracic spine trauma, as well as intrathoracic vascular injury or mediastinal pathology.[53] Routine chest roentgenograms should be obtained, and vascular contrast studies may be required to rule out intrathoracic trauma.

Thoracolumbar junction injuries as well as lumbar spine fractures can be initially evaluated with anteroposterior and lateral roentgenograms, as in the thoracic area. It is more important to obtain oblique films in the lumbar region than in the upper thoracic area of the spine. It is difficult to visualize the posterior elements at the thoracolumbar junction on lateral roentgenograms because of the usual overpenetration of that area in relation to the vertebral bodies in the supine position. Less penetrated views or CT reconstruction should be required to assess tearing of the interspinous ligaments; also, T2-weighted MRI can clearly demonstrate ligament disruption (Fig. 33–15).[146] As in the cervical area, oblique films should be obtained in the lumbar region to assess the osteoarticular pathology, to proceed with appropriate treatment.

Fractures of the sacral spine are uncommon. Anteroposterior and lateral roentgenograms should be obtained if fractures in this region are suspected, especially in association with fractures of the pelvis. However, as Denis has pointed out, the sacrum is poorly visualized on plain anteroposterior roentgenograms of the pelvis.[117] An anteroposterior view angled 20 to 25 degrees cephalically enables one to visualize the sacral foramen much better. Anteroposterior and lateral tomograms and CT scans should be used to further define the type and extent of fracture. Myelography is of limited value because the dural sac usually ends at S2 or above. MRI offers useful information with regard to the foramen and the nerve roots.

Following analysis of the preceding routine roentgenographic views of the spine, one should now determine whether special studies are indicated to further delineate specific fractures or intraspinal pathology. Bohlman[46] and Jelsma[216] have determined that early myelography can be extremely useful in acute spinal cord injuries without any major untoward side effects. Cervical myelography with CT scan or MRI may rule out spinal cord compressive pathology, such as anteriorly displaced bone and disc fragments that could be impairing spinal cord function. The same principles are true in relation to the thoracolumbar spine when one wishes to rule out herniated discs or bone intrusion into the spinal canal, compressing the neural elements. Myelography is therefore important in decision making with reference to early anterior decompressive surgery for spinal cord injuries.

The CT scan should be used in conjunction with myelography to assess bone and disc protrusion into the spinal canal and other spinal cord lesions such as a central cyst, although MRI is best for the latter.[144, 185, 279, 303, 314]

Neurologic Assessment

Evaluation of the spinal cord–injured patient should begin at the scene of the accident with trained para-

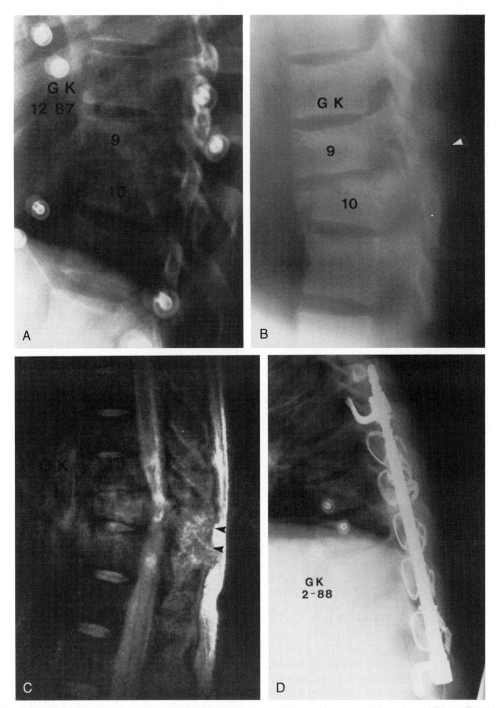

Figure 33–15. *A,* Lateral roentgenogram of a patient sustaining a fracture-dislocation of T9 on T10 in a motorcycle accident with complete paraplegia. Note the subluxation of T9 on T10 and the difficulty of visualizing the posterior elements or appreciating ligamentous disruption. *B,* Tomograms are helpful in delineating the osseous and ligamentous pathology. There is a fracture and dislocation of the facet as well as spread of the interspinous ligaments. *C,* T2-weighted MRI demonstrating ligament disruption posteriorly visualized by the hemorrhagic response of the disrupted interspinous ligaments. *D,* The patient was treated with posterior Harrington instrumentation and sublaminar wires, with reduction of the dislocation and fusion.

medics, where initial meaningful information can be gathered. The first question in obtaining a history has to deal with pain in the region of the neck or spine. If there is pain in the cervical region, the patient's neck should be placed in a collar on a spine board or, if the pain is in the lower spine, the patient should be placed on a transportation board in a neutral supine position. There should be no further movement of the spine until the patient has been completely evaluated by a physician with roentgenograms in the emergency room.[312, 313] Paramedics should be trained to ask patients to perform five movements as tests of motor function. It is not important initially to do a sensory examination or reflex evaluation. The first motor examination in the field simply tests the level of cord function. By asking the patient to move first the arms, then the hands, followed by the legs and toes, one can determine whether there is a true functional abnormality. On rare occasions, a hysterical patient will be transported by helicopter to the hospital, but we would rather err on the side of safety. The initial questions deal with extremity function, and the final question asks the patient to voluntarily "clamp down" with the anal sphincter during rectal examination. Clothing does not have to be totally removed from the patient when this assessment is carried out in the field, but in the emergency room, the full evaluation, including rectal tone and sacral sensation, requires that the patient be uncovered. All comatose patients need to be stabilized with a cervical collar because associated cervical spine injuries occur in 3 to 5 per cent of these patients and approximately 25 per cent have cord damage as well.

With regard to early assessment of vital signs and basic resuscitative measures, it is also important to maintain adequate oxygenation. Patients with cervical fractures may have paralyzed intercostal muscles of the chest, and the tidal volume may be severely reduced to 200 ml or, in certain thoracic injuries, the chest may be immobile because of fractured ribs or a hemopneumothorax. In the lower lumbar spine–injured patient, respiratory problems usually do not occur and abdominal injuries become more common.

In higher cervical spinal cord injuries, changes in vital signs readily occur, because the sympathectomy caused by cord damage may reduce blood pressure, pulse, and cardiac contractility and output. Low to normal pulse rate and low blood pressure in this situation should not be treated as hypovolemic or septic shock, in which the pulse rate is elevated. In spinal cord injury, the pulse is usually depressed and may be as low as 40 in a healthy young person. Low blood pressure as an isolated entity does not require treatment in the majority of cord-injured patients if renal perfusion is maintained and there is usually adequate urinary output. Fluid overload can be extremely dangerous in these patients, because cardiac output is often suppressed and the additional intravascular volume is tolerated poorly. Cardiac outputs measured in these patients with complete cord lesions can be 40 per cent of normal. Additional injuries or fluid overload is toler-

ated poorly and, in Viet Nam, many such patients developed pulmonary edema before the poor cardiac output problem was fully appreciated. Impaired sympathetic outflow changes not only the vital signs but also the myocardial tone and output, leaving these severely injured patients in a very dangerous state.[133]

Although spinal injury can occur without neurologic deficit when there is damage to the nervous system, the complexity of the problem increases considerably. At the scene of the accident and in the emergency room, the initial assessment should be primarily a motor examination, and any weakness, even if it is hysterical, should dictate that the patient be treated as seriously cord-damaged until there has been a full radiologic, orthopedic, and neurologic assessment.[27, 37] The hysterical patient will have a profound motor weakness, usually in the lower extremities, with normal reflexes and anal tone. The true cord-injured patient will be initially areflexic, but the patient under the influence of alcohol or other drugs can complicate and confuse the initial evaluation. In our current medicolegal environment, if intoxication is suspected, then it should be recorded because this may affect subsequent medical care.

Although the more detailed neurologic grading will be discussed later, the initial neurologic assessment should begin by having the patient take a deep breath. Both intercostal and diaphragmatic breathing should be assessed because the typical patient with mid- to low cervical and thoracic cord injury will have diaphragmatic breathing with paralyzed intercostal musculature and a decreased respiratory exchange. After respiratory assessment, the patient should be asked to move the arms and lift them high over the head. Many cervical cord-injured patients can do this if the paralysis is in lower cervical segments and, in this case, will be unable to use their hands. Therefore, the next test is to have the patient open and close the hands tightly and snap the fingers. Most cervical cord injuries, either partial or complete, initially result in paralysis of hand function.

If there is no evidence of cervical cord injury, again the patient is asked to take a deep breath to assess thoracic function, then the patient is instructed to elevate his or her head from the examining table to evaluate abdominal muscle tone. Contraction of the upper abdominal without the lower abdominal muscles produces cephalad movement of the umbilicus, referred to as Beevor's sign, indicating paralysis below the tenth thoracic level. If all abdominal muscles contract with equal strength, then the umbilicus will maintain its position, indicating intact thoracic levels.

Next, the patient should be asked to lift and extend the legs from the examining table, requiring upper lumbar cord function. After this, the patient should be instructed to move the toes and dig the heels into the examining table, requiring toe and knee flexion. Nerve root function related to hip flexion involves L1–L2, knee extension involves L3–L4, and dorsiflexion and plantar ankle flexion involve L5–S1 roots. If these segments are intact along with anal tone, then it is unlikely that there is serious cord damage.

This initial neurologic assessment can be done very quickly. Our teaching is that the motor examination should be performed in the field and by the emergency room physicians. A more detailed motor examination with evaluation of sensory function and reflexes is the responsibility of a trained surgeon who will care for spinal cord–injured patients, and this should include recording of posterior column function and any sacral sensory sparing. We now recommend the American Spinal Injury Association Motor Scale but with the inclusion of documentation of bladder function or dysfunction (Table 33–1).

Neurophysiologic tests can be of value with initial assessment. The most commonly used test is somatosensory evoked potentials (SSEP) in which a stimulus is delivered to peripheral nerves of the extremities and the electrical responses carried up the posterior columns to the sensory cortex can be evaluated by summation and computer averaging. Delays in conduction or depression of the spinal response may indicate cord damage or physiologic block of function. Absence of any conduction is associated with severe cord damage that is usually irreversible.[74, 103, 114, 190, 244, 289]

Recently, Li et al.[244] demonstrated clinically in 36 spinal cord–injured patients that the mean SSEP had the strongest individual relationship with outcome of improvement in Motor Index Score at six months. Joint position sense was the best clinical predictor of outcome.

Table 33–1. SUGGESTED SPINAL CORD INJURY MOTOR INDEX SCORE

Grade on Right	Muscle	Grade on Left
5	C5	5
5	C6	5
5	C7	5
5	C8	5
5	T1	5
5	L2	5
5	L3	5
5	L4	5
5	L5	5
5		5
50		50

This motor index score, when used accurately, provides a numerical grading system to document improvement or deterioration of motor function.

Motor grading system:
0—absent: total paralysis
1—trace: palpable or visible contraction
2—poor: active movement through range of motion (ROM) with gravity eliminated
3—fair: active movement through ROM against gravity
4—good: active movement through ROM against resistance
5—normal

	Present	Absent
Bladder function—		
Bowel function—		

Adapted from scoring system by Lucas and Ducker.

GENERAL TREATMENT PRINCIPLES: SPRAINS, SUBLUXATIONS, DISLOCATIONS, AND FRACTURES OF THE SPINE

Cervical Sprain

The most common traumatic spinal injury the practicing physician sees in the office following a vehicular accident is a sprain of the cervical spine. Usually, this is a combination of flexion and extension forces with or without rotation applied, and may involve the individual striking the skull on a stationary object. A sprain is ordinarily defined as an injury of the soft tissue-supporting ligaments in which the individual fibers of the ligament or ligaments are torn but the major ligament remains intact. The soft tissue injuries of the cervical region include articular facet capsular sprains, tearing of the interspinous ligaments, disruption of the individual cervical disc, or stretching of the longitudinal ligaments.[37, 135, 251] Ordinarily, roentgenographic examination of the cervical spine does not give any additional information unless there is a major disruption of ligament structures as in more severe injuries.[204] In the latter instance, vertebral bodies and osseous structures are separated posteriorly. Cervical sprain is a common cause of disability in this country and can usually be treated conservatively without operative intervention.

Neck pain is the usual complaint following a sprain of the cervical spine and soft tissue structures. The pathophysiologic mechanisms by which neck pain is produced are direct external neural compression of the cervical nerve roots or spinal cord, central or intrinsic spinal cord pressure, degenerative disc and joint disease, intrinsic osseous or ligamentous lesions, and abnormal motion or instability.[35, 37, 41] Cervical spine pain may radiate to distal sites because of direct neural compression or by stimulation of deep somatic nerve endings found in the joints, bone, and outer layers of the disc itself. For many years, there has been a misconception that all neck pain originates from neural compression. However, injuries to disc and ligamentous structures as well as joints of the cervical spine may produce pain by stimulating somatic nerve endings. Anatomically, the facet joint capsules, the outer layers of the annulus fibrosus, and the anterior and posterior longitudinal ligaments have all been shown to be innervated by c-nerve fibers with simple terminations in these structures. Also, bone itself has innervations that travel with the vascular supply. Therefore, it can be assumed that with abnormal motion or distortion of soft tissue structures such as the disc, longitudinal ligaments, and joint capsules, stimulation of the c-nerve fibers will occur and a pain syndrome is produced.

It seems likely after an acute cervical sprain that immobilization of the cervical spine and soft tissue structures would help alleviate and heal the original injury. Cervical traction and any type of manipulation of the spine following an acute sprain will only aggravate the situation, and for that reason a soft collar or cervical orthosis by means of a rigid brace is indicated. It is important to prevent hyperextension of the cervical spine in patients with pre-existing cervical spondylosis, which may aggravate the nerve roots or soft tissue structures. A period of three to six weeks of soft collar immobilization of the cervical spine usually resolves mild sprains of the cervical spine. A chronic cervical pain may be related to cervical disc disruption from an injury, and eventually may result in narrowing of the disc and cervical spondylosis, as documented by Hohl.[204] Unfortunately, these changes are seen late, usually years after a legal settlement of the particular accident.

Cervical Subluxation

Subluxation of the cervical spine indicates greater disruption of the ligamentous structures than a sprain, and complete tearing of the ligaments allows abnormal motion and the possibility of instability. In this instance, the decision has to be made whether skeletal traction is instituted initially to reduce the subluxation and whether the use of a rigid orthosis or a halo device is indicated. If the subluxation falls into the category of instability according to White's criteria mentioned before, then a rigid orthosis would be indicated for a period of eight to 12 weeks. At that time, flexion and extension views should be obtained to determine the extent of any progressive subluxation that occurs in the cervical spine, such as that of the bilaterally perched facets, which appear tip-to-tip on the lateral and oblique roentgenograms. This indicates severe posterior ligamentous tearing, which should be reduced with skeletal traction or a halo device. In many instances, as documented by Bohlman,[46] this amount of ligamentous tearing will not reconstitute adequately with long rigid immobilization unless spontaneous intervertebral body fusion occurs anteriorly. If late instability of this type is present, then usually a posterior arthrodesis is indicated.

Cervical Dislocation

Dislocation of the cervical vertebrae implies complete disruption of the ligamentous structures so that the facet joints are no longer in continuity. As mentioned before, initial oblique roentgenograms must be obtained in the emergency room to determine whether a dislocation is unilateral or bilateral and whether there are any fractures associated with the dislocation.[46] Initial treatment of unilateral or bilateral dislocations of the spine is by skeletal traction to attempt a closed reduction. It is now believed by the authors that immediate or certainly early reduction of dislocations should be carried out, especially in conjunction with those patients having a neurologic deficit. This may require general anesthesia or open reduction, which will be discussed later. The authors believe it is unwise to attempt closed reduction with greater than 50 pounds of skeletal traction, because excessive weight applied through skeletal traction to a dislocated or fractured

spine with severe ligament disruption may cause over-distraction at the injured level and stretch the spinal cord, thus producing ascending and cord edema and paralysis. It is safer to carry out an open reduction under controlled circumstances, followed by operative stabilization, than to increase the weight on skeletal traction in an inordinate uncontrolled manner over an extended period of time.

Using body build and weight, emergency skeletal immobilization and traction can be initiated. In distraction injuries, the head is placed in a horseshoe-shaped, nonenclosed halo ring. In compression injuries, with vertebral body burst fractures, traction is initiated at 10 per cent of body weight and incrementally increased to 40 per cent of body weight to achieve alignment. To maintain alignment, 25 to 35 per cent traction weight to body weight (TW/BW) is used. In flexion injuries, 10 per cent of TW/BW is increased to 30 to 55 per cent to achieve alignment, but only 15 per cent TW/BW is needed to maintain spinal alignment. Compression and flexion injuries in combination are present in two thirds of the patients. In extension injuries of the osteoarthritic spine with retrolisthesis, 10 per cent TW/BW is the initial traction, and alignment is maintained with 15 per cent TW/BW.

As one might expect, injuries of the third and fourth cervical levels usually respond to a lower TW/BW, as opposed to lower cervical injuries. Strong, muscular males may require higher weights, while elderly females may need less. Serial lateral radiographs are taken every 10 to 15 minutes, and alignment is accomplished rapidly in most patients. C-arm image intensifiers can be used and, once the spine is aligned and stabilized, the patient may be transferred for MRI, myelography, and CT scanning.

Although spinal manipulation is used in other countries, specifically England and Australia, for unilateral facet dislocations, it has not gained wide acceptance in the United States because of the medicolegal implications of such a maneuver. However, a high rate of success has been reported by manipulating unilateral facet dislocations of the cervical spine under controlled circumstances with skeletal traction and general anesthesia.[80] Initial decompression of the spinal canal and cord occurs by obtaining an anatomically reduced fracture dislocation, and this is the initial goal of skeletal traction and treatment.[77] Surgical intervention is not contemplated unless closed reduction fails.

Cervical Compression Fractures

Compression fractures or axial loading injuries of the cervical spine, if not severe and without paralysis, are treated with a rigid brace for eight to 12 weeks until healing has occurred. The more severe compression fracture of the cervical spine may be quite unstable and, if there is a bone fragment protruding posteriorly into the spinal canal, skeletal traction is immediately instituted and closed reduction is attempted. If bone protrusion into the spinal canal remains after traction for seven to 10 days, or if the compression fracture is so severe that potential kyphosis may result at a later date, surgical intervention may be indicated from the anterior approach. Once again, as pointed out previously, unless spontaneous fusion occurs anteriorly between the adjacent vertebrae, late instability and kyphosis can occur.[92] Occasionally, a cervical spine–injured patient presents with major tearing of the posterior ligament complex and anterior compression fracture of the vertebral body, as in a severe flexion and axial loading injury. This then presents a problem of posterior as well as anterior instability. Initially, skeletal traction is instituted and realignment is attempted in a nonsurgical fashion. Once the spine is stable, a halo brace or a rigid cervical orthosis is used, provided that late instability is not anticipated.

If the patient is to be treated in skeletal traction for a cervical spine injury, the nature of the injury will determine which type of bed is to be used during the period of skeletal traction. If a dislocation is to be reduced, then a turning frame should be used in conjunction with the skeletal traction; otherwise, a regular bed can be used with cervical traction attached to the head of the bed. The CircOlectric bed is contraindicated for all spine and spinal cord injuries. The reasons are that in a vertical position, the spine is loaded because the patient actually stands on a foot piece, and respiratory arrest occurs when the CircOlectric bed compresses the abdomen from distally to proximally, applying the anterior frame prior to turning. The abdominal contents are compressed in a wedge-shaped pattern, pushing up against the diaphragm and resulting in difficult breathing for patients with paralysis. In addition, asensory patients develop severe heel pressure sores because of the foot plate. For these reasons, we have abandoned the use of the CircOlectric bed in spine and spinal cord injuries.[34]

Upper Thoracic Spine Injuries (T2–T10)

Upper thoracic spine fractures are reasonably stable in the acute injury situation because of the surrounding chest cage and the strong costovertebral ligaments. For these reasons, patients with upper thoracic spine fractures may be treated in a regular bed. Patients with mild compression fractures and those with gunshot wounds are very stable and can be treated with brief recumbency and then ambulated with an appropriate orthosis. More severe fractures and dislocations of the upper thoracic spine require one to three weeks of recumbency, and then ambulation can be carried out with a molded orthosis, provided the medical condition of the patient is stable and there are no other associated injuries preventing ambulation.

Thoracolumbar Injuries (T11–L5)

The thoracolumbar spine junction and the lumbar spine itself are much more unstable and require a longer recumbency unless internal fixation is carried out by means of operative intervention.[205] A patient with a mild wedge compression fracture (less than 40

per cent) at the thoracolumbar junction and no neurologic deficit can be ambulated in a molded orthosis, when comfortable, within days. However, appropriate roentgenography or even myelography should be carried out to make sure that there is no fracture protrusion into the spinal canal. Mild compression fractures of the lumbar spine may be treated in the same fashion with a lumbosacral orthosis. More severe fractures or dislocations of the thoracolumbar junction or lumbar spine require a longer recumbency for stabilization. Fracture dislocations, severe compressions, or burst fractures are frequently associated with neural compression and deficit, and therefore should be treated recumbent until a decision is made regarding surgical decompression and stabilization. A common mistake in treating fractures of the thoracolumbar spine is in not recognizing osseous protrusion into the spinal canal in the hidden zone behind the pedicle, as viewed on the lateral roentgenogram. In most instances, the degree of neurologic deficit will parallel the degree of osseous injury. When there is significant neurologic deficit in the face of very little osseous injury, then a massive herniated disc or bone fragment intrusion into the spinal canal should be suspected. In these instances, a CT scan and lumbar myelography or MRI may be performed to define the situation. Principles for management of thoracolumbar vertebral injuries are similar to those for cervical spine fractures; that is, restoration of spinal alignment should be achieved first by a closed or nonsurgical manipulation on a turning frame or, if necessary, by surgery.[169, 272] In the case of patients with thoracolumbar fractures and neurologic deficit, restoration and alignment of the spinal canal is the first step in decompression of the neural structures.

GENERAL TREATMENT PRINCIPLES: SPINAL CORD INJURY

History

Treatment of spinal cord–injured patients began in the 17th century B.C., when Egyptian physicians recognized such syndromes with the patient "unaware of hands, penis is erect and urine escaping unknowingly." They recognized that it was secondary to dislocation of vertebrae, and noted that it varied in severity and classified the syndrome into "a disease I will fight, a disease I will support and a disease which cannot be treated." Galen, in 150 B.C., reportedly performed the first experimental laminectomy and distinguished signs for different levels of vertebral trauma. This was later supplemented in 1895 by Roentgen's discovery, which allowed the correlation of vertebral trauma to the clinical signs of neuronal dysfunction by cord segment level. Since that time, the major impetus has been that of further subdivision of the partial cord lesions (Brown-Séquard, anterior cord, and central cord) and the response to various treatment regimens. Subsequently, many authors have tried to develop varying methods of classification to delineate similar groups for study. Probably the best attempt was that of Sir

Table 33–2. CLASSIFICATION OF SPINAL CORD INJURIES

Complete lesions
Posterior cord syndrome (crude sensation only)
Anterior cord syndrome
Central cord syndrome
Partial cord lesion, including Brown-Séquard type
Root syndrome

These are the known and recognized spinal cord injury syndromes, including the syndrome of isolated nerve root compression.

Ludwig Guttmann, who used a motor grading system. In Guttmann's classification, however, a patient with a complete spinal cord lesion (group A) can recover to a functional level (group D), which leads to some confusion as to exactly what is complete with the initial injury, because most authors describe only rare episodes of patients with total spinal cord injuries recovering function. Probably, recovery from group A in this classification relates to return of nerve root function in the upper extremities and not of spinal cord function.

Table 33–2 lists the various classifications of spinal cord injury syndromes as they appeared in the literature in the 1950s and 1960s.[316-321, 323] Complete lesions were not subdivided initially, except in terms of quadriplegia and paraplegia, but partial lesions were divided into various syndromes. Quadriparesis and paraparesis have been and still are acceptable terms to indicate incomplete motor paralysis. Names for syndromes of incomplete cord injury were selected to designate the area of the spinal cord that had been the most severely damaged.

In the anterior cord syndrome, the damage is primarily in the anterior two thirds of the spinal cord, leaving the posterior columns intact. In these patients, there is a motor paralysis and a sensory deficit that spares posterior column tracts that carry position sense, proprioception, and vibratory sensation. Evaluation of the anterior cord syndrome by the initial roentgenograms may reveal bone or disc compressing the anterior aspects of the spinal cord (Fig. 33–16).

The central cord syndrome is more commonly associated with patients who have pre-existing cervical spondylosis and who then sustain a hyperextension injury with compression of the cord by anterior osteophytes and posteriorly by the bulging ligamentum flavum (Fig. 33–17).[255] Most of the damage to the spinal cord lies within the central gray matter, which is more susceptible to injury, and there is a partial neurologic deficit involving the central gray and white matter, resulting in loss of motor function in the arms and hands with sparing of function to some degree of the musculature in the lower extremities. These patients have proportionately greater paralysis in their hands and arms but are able to move their legs and feet. Central cord syndrome occurs distally in the thoracic and lumbar cord, where the patient has more marked proximal trunk weakness in the upper lumbar cord segments and is unable to lift the legs off the examining table but is able to move the toes and may have a certain amount of anal tone.[40]

Another less common partial cord syndrome is referred to as the cord hemisection or the Brown-Séquard syndrome, in which one half of the cord is damaged while the opposite half is spared. In this case, there is ipsilateral paralysis of motor function as well as loss of position sense and contralateral loss of pain and temperature sensation.

Finally, certain patients will present with only a nerve root syndrome at the level of spinal fracture. Any root in the cervical area, lumbar area, or both may be so involved. Single-root lesions are rare in the thoracic levels of the spine. The cervical area usually involves the fifth or sixth roots with an isolated paralysis of the deltoid or biceps musculature, respectively, or seventh root with associated triceps weakness. Rarely, we have seen bilateral deltoid paralysis secondary to a fourth or fifth cervical dislocation without cord damage; however, more typically a unilateral deficit occurs.

Classifications of Spinal Cord Injury Syndromes

The older descriptive terms of spinal cord injury are useful in understanding the pathophysiology and will

Figure 33–16. *A* and *B,* Diagram of the anterior cord syndrome. A herniated disc or bone fragment compresses the anterior spinal artery and cord. This may produce ischemia of the anterior two thirds of the cord and sparing of posterior column function (touch, position, and vibratory senses). (From Bohlman, H. H.: The neck. *In* D'Ambrosia, R. [ed.]: Musculoskeletal Disorders. 2nd ed. Philadelphia, J. B. Lippincott Co., 1986.)

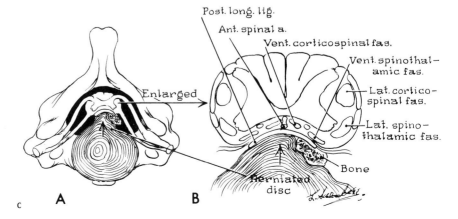

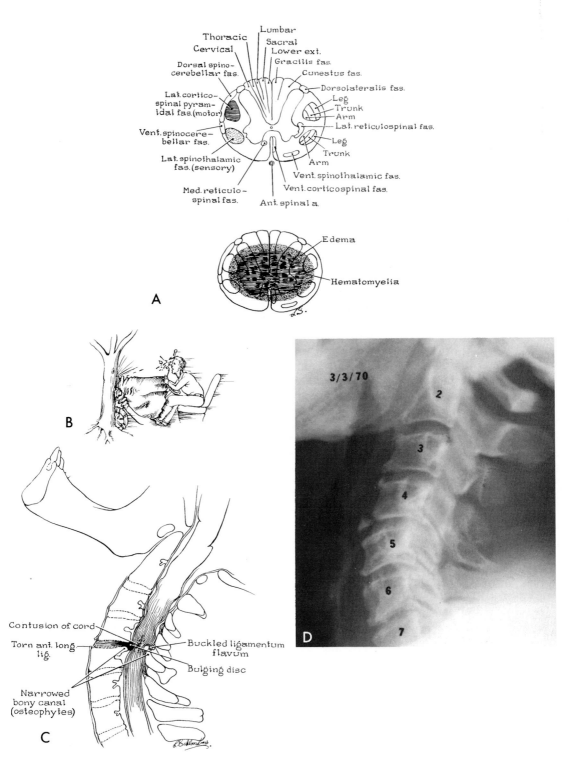

Figure 33–17. *A,* Diagram of the central cord syndrome. Centrally placed tracts are affected by central edema or necrosis. Note that the most medial portion of the pyramidal tract is for arm function. The upper extremity paralysis is therefore greater than the lower extremity. *B,* Frontal head injury producing hyperextension with cervical spondylosis. *C,* Note that the ligamentum flavum buckles inwardly against the posterior spinal cord, while the bulging disc compresses the cord anteriorly. The combined forces contuse the cord. The disc is also disrupted. *D,* Lateral cervical spine roentgenogram at the C5 level in a totally quadriplegic patient. Note the slight posterior subluxation of C4 on C5. Avulsion fracture of the anterior inferior body of C4 indicates a hyperextension injury. (From Bohlman, H.H.: The neck. *In* D'Ambrosia, R. [ed.]: Musculoskeletal Disorders. 2nd ed. Philadelphia, J. B. Lippincott Co., 1986.)

give some hint as to the major compressive force affecting the cord and can be used as information in guiding therapy. The more incomplete the spinal cord lesion is, the better the prognosis, and, conversely, in the patient with complete cord injury with persistent neurologic deficit for 48 hours, the prognosis is guarded and neurologic recovery of the spinal cord is unlikely to occur.

Previously, standard neurologic terms were used in the American literature, but in European literature, especially the British, various letters and numbers were used to grade the spinal cord injury and to assess recovery. The 0 or A lesion was a complete lesion with no neurologic function below the level of trauma to the cord, and the 1 or B lesion had no motor function but some sensory sparing. The remaining grades were subdivided by motor function, whereby the patient was listed as motor useless, motor useful, motor functional, or normal motor neurologic examination. This motor evaluation was used in reports in the British literature to evaluate surgical intervention in the early course of the spinal cord–injured patient. Laminectomy proved to be of little benefit and led to a nonoperative approach in the majority of patients treated.[17, 81, 92, 98, 169, 275] A 1970 registry was created by Ducker for the evaluation of acutely injured patients, primarily on the basis of motor function. Although the sensory and reflex evaluation is important for the patient's initial assessment, those parameters could not be used in a meaningful way to carry out calculated recovery rates to make some definitive statements on the best therapeutic modalities. Our registry included over 500 patients with acute injuries who had medically audited follow-up examinations.[249, 250] The patients were classified into two groups with complete lesions, three groups with partial lesions, and a subdivision with isolated root damage. A complete transverse cord lesion is defined as a one-segment cord injury in a patient without any function below the damaged area. A graded complete lesion is one in which the osseous damage may be at the C5–C6 level, while there is still some motor function at lower seventh and eighth cord levels. If meticulous neurologic examinations are performed, graded complete lesions are more common than initially appreciated. Many anterior cord syndromes, according to older definitions, fit into this group because of some spared touch sensation but no distal motor function.

Partial cord lesions are divided into those in which the caudal segments of the cord are either very weak, very strong, or the same as where the cord segment is injured. A partial lesion with caudal loss (anterior cord syndrome) is usually found in a severely cord-damaged patient with the only evidence of incompleteness being minimal movement of the toes. A partial lesion with proportionately better caudal motor strength is the same as the central cord lesion. The neurologic deficit is greater in the cervical areas of the spinal cord with caudal sparing, so that the legs have greater motor function than the arms. The uniform partial cord lesion, although not common, can occur with loss below the osseous lesion but predominantly on one side.

Many of these patients were previously classified as the Brown-Séquard type, where there seemed to be more of a loss on one side of the spinal cord, while there was uniform strength on the preserved side.

Patients with isolated nerve root lesions are uncommon and are classified as having neurologic loss without cord damage.

Our registry data reveal that complete cord lesions are more common than partial cord lesions. The complete lesions occurred in 60 per cent of the cervical injuries and in over 70 per cent of the thoracic and upper lumbar cord segment injuries. Partial lesions of the cervical levels were typically central cord syndromes, in our classification referred to as partial cord injuries with caudal gain or caudal sparing.

A single level of fracture or dislocation occurred in 87 per cent of the patients and multiple levels in 7 per cent, and no fracture could be identified in 5 per cent of the patients. Roentgenograms were too poor in quality in 1 per cent of the patients for proper analysis. These statistics are very similar to Bohlman's 300 cervical spine injury review series.[46] This classification of cervical cord injuries includes a definition of total (complete) cord syndrome, as well as grading of incomplete cord syndromes. The total cord lesion is defined as quadriplegia with complete loss of all motor and sensory functions below the level of injury present more than 48 hours after injury. The incomplete cord syndromes are graded from 1+ to 4+ with increasing severity of the lesion. One plus (1+) means the patient can move limbs and feet with good sparing of position and vibratory sense; 2+ means slight distal motor function (toe wiggle) and good position and vibration sense; 3+ indicates no distal motor function, touch sensation present, and good position and vibration sense; and 4+ indicates no distal motor function, touch sensation present, but little or no position or vibratory sense. This is basically a motor grading system with an indication of gross sensory sparing. No patient in this series recovered leg function after a complete quadriplegia occurred.

Classification of Spinal Cord Injury by Neurologic Examination

If one accepts the motor classification of patients with spinal cord injury as a means of predicting recovery rates, then a standard of motor grading has to be applied. The most universally accepted scale is the motor function scale, listed as 0; 1, trace; 2, poor; 3, fair; 4, good; and 5, normal. Recovery from individual or multiple muscles can be documented over a period of time.

Our first attempt to develop a standardized examination form included osseous level of injury documented radiologically and the neurologic examination based on reflex, sensory, and motor findings. The examination was documented at the time of injury and one year later. A standard motor examination was studied by linear regression technique to determine the major prognostic indicators; that is, initial examination, treatment, and the neurologic outcome one year after injury. The major prognostic indicator one year following injury was determined to be most related to the initial neurologic examination findings. This enabled us to establish controls for further evaluation of the varying treatment regimens of cervical spinal cord injuries.[248]

Our initial examination form tested 14 different muscle groups and four sensory functions in quadriplegic patients. Important information was included, such as time of injury, level of osseous disruption, and associated medical problems. The motor examination at follow-up was sampled by two methods: (1) individual muscle groups, and (2) the examiner's judgment of the patient's gait. The individual groups of muscles were tested for motor strength on a 0 to 5 system, as described earlier. There was a positive correlation between the gait and individual motor groups, with the latter being more sensitive. Sensory examination was listed as the lowest intact dermatome for a specific modality or lowest joint position sense. Reflexes were also listed. These modalities were studied by linear regression as to degree of prognostic correlation, with the final examination carried out one year following injury. The motor examination was found to be the most accurate prognostic indicator. Therefore, we relied on the motor examination primarily to draw conclusions on the best possible treatment. However, it must be noted that the muscles chosen for the examination form were a compromise with various levels of cord segment sampling.

Specific muscles that can be assessed only as strong, abnormal, or paralyzed are simply graded 2, 1, or 0. Respiration is included with intercostals, upper abdominals, lower abdominals, and anal tone. By selecting five muscle groups in the upper extremities, and a few others, a 100-point grading system can be applied to the spinal cord. The recovery rate was based on averaging all the muscles available on 0 to 5 rating, establishing a motor index, as listed in Table 33-1, from 0 to 100. One can then assess the recovery rate based on the patient's initial and follow-up examination. In patients with complete neurologic deficit, the recovery rate is minimal, usually in the upper extremities less than 20 per cent of that anticipated for a full recovery. Conversely, in partial lesions in which the neurologic deficit is minimal initially, the remaining neurologic loss can often be made up so that recovery is greater than 80 per cent. Recovery rates must be distinctly different from what would be expected to provide efficacy of a particular treatment.

The osseous level of injury is documented by radiologic examination and further subdivided into single and multiple levels. In the analytic data to follow, we will only deal with those osseous injuries considered to be single, defined as the subluxation of two adjacent vertebrae, numbering the caudal level, or a fracture without subluxation. For example, fractures of C6 or subluxation of C5 on C6 would be considered as one level. Although such restriction reduces the number of

patients studied, it allows for more accurate conclusions.

Various motor patterns are present in spinal cord–injured patients and can be subdivided. Motor complete or complete transverse traumatic myelitis is defined as zero motor function in the root exiting two levels below the site of osseous injury. Graded complete patients are defined as remaining at zero motor function between two and four segments below the level of osseous trauma. Partial lesions can be subdivided into three groups: (A) partial loss at the site of osseous lesion with a secondary loss of motor function (partial cord lesion [PCL] greater than four roots below the level of the osseous lesion); (B) partial loss at the site of osseous trauma with a secondary caudal (distal) gain in motor function (PCS—central cord syndrome); and (C) partial loss at site of osseous injury with uniform loss distally (PLC). When we discuss the influence of blood pressure, steroids, laminectomy, and anterior decompression and fusion operations, it is possible to subdivide the patients into neurologically similar groups. The mean recovery rate of each group has its own clinical characteristics and, as expected, the less the original neurologic injury, the greater the recovery. Also, the subgroups have certain characteristics that suggest different causes of cord dysfunction. Complete motor loss is primarily a result of physiologic or anatomic disruption of cord function occurring at the time of injury, but five per cent of patients in this group suffer from secondary neural tissue compression from a herniated cervical disc or dislocation; if decompression is performed within 48 to 72 hours, significant recovery may occur in those with secondary compression. In the graded complete lesions, there appears to be a perfusion or blood pressure problem secondary to ruptured viscera, and these patients may have poorer recovery rates. In the subdivision titled partial loss with caudal sparing or central cord syndrome lesions, our data indicate that those patients with congenital or degenerative spinal stenosis and continuous cord compression have significantly better recovery if a decompression is performed one or two weeks following injury.[132] In summary, the motor classifications are subdivisions involving multiple causes and clinical factors affecting recovery of spinal cord function.

SPECIFIC TREATMENT OF THE PATIENT WITH SPINAL CORD INJURY

There are five important steps in the treatment of a neurologic deficit associated with spinal cord injury: (1) immobilization, (2) medical stabilization, (3) spinal alignment, (4) surgical decompression if there is proved cord compression, and (5) spinal stabilization. Each of these five steps must be carefully planned and instituted. Each phase of treatment may influence the final neurologic function.[10, 36, 46, 298, 299]

Immobilization

Immobilization should be carried out as soon as possible, preferably at the scene of the accident. For cervical spine injuries, a soft collar or sandbags with a spine board are used to immobilize the head and neck. Continuous movement of an injured spinal cord will accentuate the pathologic damage within the spinal cord.[38, 130] Immobilization and splinting of an injured spinal cord are just as important as immobilization and splinting of the fractured vertebrae. There are isolated episodes reported of patients with partial deficits who, during transfer to or within a hospital, have lost neural function because of continuous movement of the damaged spine and spinal cord.[34, 46] Training of emergency medical technicians should stress initial immobilization and assessment of the clothed or unclothed patient and should include assessment of the following motor functions: The emergency medical technician needs to ask the patient about movement of the arms, hands, legs, and feet, and to check clamp-down anal tone by rectal examination. All personnel should be educated to test for various patterns of arm and hand function associated with cervical spine and cord injuries. If the patient has not been splinted in the field, then this is the first order of business on the arrival at an emergency room where treatment is carried out by physicians.

Medical Stabilization

Medical stabilization follows the same principles of any emergency resuscitation process; that is, to establish an airway and maintain circulation and perfusion. Patients with both cervical and thoracic cord injuries and intercostal muscle paralysis may have mechanical difficulties in exchanging adequate amounts of air for oxygenation of the blood. Although immediate intubation and respiratory support are rarely indicated, facilities to do this via nasal endotracheal intubation should be available. We try to avoid early tracheostomies because certain patients may require anterior operations, in which case incision will be near the tracheostomy site. Conversely, if respiratory embarrassment is a significant problem, then either nonmanipulative fiberoptic intubation or tracheostomy has to be carried out. Certain obese patients with very short necks will require airway support.

The influence of perfusion pressure in the spinal cord can be measured in relationship to spinal cord injury recovery.[127–129] When the diastolic pressure is 69 mm Hg or less, there is a possibility of inadequate cord perfusion, and when it is 70 mm Hg or greater, there is adequate systemic perfusion pressure. Poor perfusion pressure does not influence the complete transverse cord lesion. However, in the rare graded complete lesion and in certain partial lesions, there may be significant vascular compromise to the cord, and the low blood pressure is deleterious to the overall recovery rate.[152, 187] The older patient with a central cord lesion (partial cord lesion with caudal sparing) and shock may have cord recovery completely obliterated. Adequate blood pressure and volume support are mandatory, but may not always be possible because of cardiovascular instability.

In a high thoracic or cervical cord lesion, the sympathetic influence on the cardiac function and cardiovascular reflexes may be adversely affected, but the parasympathetic control to the heart through the vagus nerve is usually maintained. Typically, these patients have both low blood pressure and decreased pulse. This is to be differentiated from hypovolemic shock, in which low blood pressure is accompanied by a high pulse rate. The presence of low blood pressure alone is not reason for massive fluid replacement. A central venous catheter and even possibly a pulmonary wedge pressure catheter are required to monitor the blood pressure in these patients. The lack of sympathetic influence on the heart adversely affects myocardial contractility as well as cardiac rate and may cause a precipitous drop in cardiac output, but we more commonly see marked fluctuations in cardiac output with cardiac instability. It is not always possible to achieve adequate perfusion pressure, even with proper fluid volume replacement with cardiac support. Skilled anesthesiologists or critical care specialists are helpful in achieving the desired success in maintaining adequate perfusion pressure.

Spinal Alignment

The next most important step in the initial treatment of spinal cord injuries is spinal alignment. Vertebral dislocations produce compression of the central nervous system. Carrying out myelography, MRI, or other specific studies in a malaligned spine is not necessary prior to realignment unless a herniated disc is suspected. Spinal alignment of cervical fractures is usually accomplished with skeletal traction. Each part of the spine will be discussed separately later in this chapter, and there is no one specific rule that will apply to the entire spine. In high cervical injuries at the atlanto-occipital junction, positioning of the head on the spine is more important than any kind of traction or manipulation; however, with lower cervical spine injuries, axial traction with varying weights may be indicated.

Decompression of the Spinal Canal

Decompressive surgical procedures should be carried out only if there is proven compression of neural elements following spinal alignment. In certain injuries, there may be bone fragments or foreign bodies (such as a bullet) in the spinal canal, which require surgical removal in order to achieve the normal space for the injured cord. After spinal alignment, diagnostic procedures such as myelography or MRI should be carried out to make sure that there is no further compression of the neural elements. In the cervical area with the patient in traction and turned supine with the head elevated, a myelogram may be taken by insertion of dye through the C1–C2 lateral interspace. The patient can then be turned prone for the remaining radiographs and CT scan to rule out the presence of isolated herniated disc in the canal that would require surgical removal. MRI also may be used. In the thoracic and lumbar areas, myelography and CT scan should be used as well as MRI, where indicated, to plan a decompressive procedure. In our hands, fewer than one in four patients require a decompressive operation after there is satisfactory spinal alignment, and, if satisfactory spinal alignment cannot be achieved, then surgical reduction and decompression are indicated.

Spinal Stability

Spinal stabilization has to be individualized to the vertebral segment involved. An unstable spine can allow continuous subluxation, which may be reinjuring a recovering spinal cord or adjacent spinal nerve roots with resultant loss of motor function. It is important, therefore, to establish and maintain spinal stability until osseous healing occurs.[92]

CONTROVERSIES OF TREATMENT OF SPINAL CORD INJURIES

Although there is general agreement on the preceding statements on treating patients with spine and spinal cord injury,[347] controversy remains about the influence of specific treatments. The four most discussed controversies in acute care are (1) use of steroids, (2) laminectomy, (3) anterior spinal cord decompression and fusion, and (4) gunshot wounds. These have been statistically analyzed using the motor neurologic syndromes described.

Corticosteroids

The anti-inflammatory properties of glucocorticosteroids were well recognized by the early 1960s, and numerous studies had demonstrated the clinical benefits of their use in the treatment of various neurologic disorders, including brain tumors. The initial rationale for their use was grounded in the hypothesis that glucocorticosteroids might prevent post-traumatic spinal cord edema by the same mechanism as the reduction of peritumoral cerebral edema. Initial experiments compared placebo, hypothermia, and glucocorticosteroids for the treatment of spinal cord injury in dogs.[124] In that study, both hypothermia- and steroid-treated animals had a modified anti-inflammatory response and improved neurologic recovery when the treatment modality was delivered immediately after injury. Although the benefits were modest, the use of steroids for acute spinal cord injury rapidly gained widespread acceptance.[7a, 376a]

Over the past 30-year period the efficacy of glucocorticosteroids has been examined in preclinical and clinical spinal cord injury studies. Despite extensive experience, the role of glucocorticosteroids in the treatment of traumatic spinal cord injury remains poorly defined. Several groups have reported enhanced neurologic recovery with different drug treatments after spinal cord trauma in laboratory animals,[196b, 302a] but until very recently, no medical treatment was conclusively demonstrated to improve neurologic recovery and reverse the initial neurologic deficit.[60, 61, 61b, 61c]

Historically, steroids were thought to be minimally beneficial in the treatment of a few, selected cord-damaged patients, but improvement is difficult to document on a clinical basis.[63, 67, 127, 130] Our initial dose was 20 mg of dexamethasone or 125 mg of methylprednisolone. The dosage was repeated every six hours for the first three days. However, after three days, we again assessed the patient carefully, and if the patient had a partial lesion and was responding to our overall treatment with improvement, we continued the steroids for one week, then tapered for one week. In complete lesions, either transverse myelitis or graded traumatic myelitis, the recovery rate ranges from 11 to 15 per cent with or without steroids and therefore is not affected. In the partial lesions with caudal sparing (central cord syndrome), the recovery rate was slightly higher in the steroid-treated group. Also, it is in this group of patients that we have seen the rare steroid-dependent patient; when the drug was abruptly stopped after four or five days, neurologic deterioration occurred, but motor strength was reinstated within 24 hours with continuation of the steroids. The groups of patients with a partial caudal loss (anterior cord syndrome) and a uniform partial loss had different recovery rates that reflect a difference in the initial motor index, and we could not prove that steroids were helpful. Bohlman demonstrated no improvement in recovery rates in those spinal cord–injured patients treated with steroids as opposed to those treated without the drug.[46] In addition, there was a high incidence of gastrointestinal hemorrhage resulting in death in 12 per cent of the quadriplegic patients on steroids.

Brankman and others[67] performed a prospective, double-blind clinical trial on 161 patients with high-dose steroid therapy admitted with coma and blunt head injury. There was no significant difference found in the one-month survival rate or in the outcome after six months, regardless of severity of brain injury. In addition, there was no significant effect on morbidity and mortality. In 1985, Bracken and others[63] published a multicenter, double-blind, randomized clinical trial using high-dose and standard-dose steroids following acute spinal cord injury. There was no significant difference observed in neurologic recovery of motor function, pinprick response, or touch sensation one year after injury between the two treatment groups. Interestingly, the fatality rate was 10.7 per cent.

In 1990, Bracken et al.[62] evaluated the efficacy and safety of methylprednisolone and naloxone in a multicenter, randomized, double-blind, placebo-controlled trial. Steroids were given to 162 patients, naloxone was given to 154 patients, and placebos were given to 171 patients.[163] A dose of methylprednisolone given was a bolus of 30 mg/kg of body weight, followed by infusion at 5.4 mg/kg/hr for 23 hours. The patients were evaluated at six weeks and at six months after treatment. A motor scale of evaluation was rated from 0 to 70. Of the patients with complete motor and sensory spinal cord injuries, those treated with methylprednisolone had a gain of 10.5 in muscle power, those treated with naloxone 7.5, and those treated with placebo 4.2. Therefore, there was a difference of only three points gain between the steroid and the other groups. Of the patients with motor-complete and sensory-spared cord injuries, those treated with steroids had a motor score of 23, those with naloxone 28.9, and those treated with placebo 26.5 at six-month follow-up. Therefore, the patients treated without steroids improved from 3.5 to 5.9 motor points greater than the steroid-treated group. Among the patients with paresis and incomplete spinal cord lesions, the improvements in motor score were 24.3 in the steroid group, 14.5 in the naloxone group, and 12.9 in the placebo group at six-month follow-up. Therefore, there did seem to be a significant improvement in patients with incomplete cord injury.[374]

Unfortunately, many of the patients had various operative procedures on the spine for decompression and stabilization, and those data were not included in the report.[134] In addition, there was no discussion as to the true functional, that is ambulatory, status of any of the incompletely injured patients. The treatment with steroids was not beneficial if given longer than eight hours after injury. Wound infections occurred in 7.1 per cent of the steroid group, and 3.3 per cent and 3.6 per cent of the patients given naloxone and placebo, respectively. Gastrointestinal bleeding rates were 4.5, 2.0, and 3.0 per cent in the steroid, naloxone, and placebo groups, respectively.[180]

In the paretic patients, those treated with steroids had a lesser neurologic deficit on arrival to the emergency than did the control subjects. The end result of total motor recovery is approximately the same, whereas in the quadriplegic patients, there was slightly better improvement of motor function, that is, nerve root recovery, in the steroid-treated group.[131] It would, therefore, be of great importance to determine what the ambulatory status of the paretic patients was more than two years from initial treatment. In addition, an analysis of the various surgical procedures in relationship to recovery of neural function more than two years after treatment would be of great benefit to this study. Finally, if steroids are to be used in the acutely spinal cord–injured patients, they must be administered within the first eight hours according to the above protocol, taking into consideration the possibility of a 7 per cent wound infection rate in those patients on whom surgery is to be performed.[34, 46, 115, 147, 203, 239]

NASCIS I, which began in 1979, compared the efficacy of "low-dose" (100 mg bolus/day for 10 days) and "high-dose" (1000 mg bolus/day for 10 days) intravenous methylprednisolone.[61a] Researchers involved in NASCIS I decided on a Clinical Phase II study to determine the proper dosage of methylprednisolone. The study did not include a placebo arm. Clinical Phase I study with a placebo arm would have been preferable. Resulting data failed to demonstrate any difference between the low-dose and high-dose groups. The majority of clinicians concluded that steroids were not beneficial in the short-term management of spinal cord trauma, but basic research continued in the role for secondary injury processes potentially responsive

to pharmacologic therapy. Demopoulos et al.[11a] proposed that the principal molecular mechanism of post-traumatic neuronal degeneration was lipid peroxidation (LP). Braughler and Hall[69] demonstrated that an initial intravenous bolus of methylprednisolone protected the spinal cord from LP. Large intravenous doses of methylprednisolone were required to achieve a therapeutic effect, and a biphasic dose-response curve existed for many of the beneficial effects of methylprednisolone (i.e., an intravenous dose of 30 mg/kg inhibited LP, but doubling the dose negated that action). Treatment had to be initiated soon after injury to achieve a therapeutic effect. The half-life of methylprednisolone in spinal tissue is two to six hours, and frequent dosing is necessary to maintain blood flow, improve tissue conservation, and maximize recovery.

The ability to inhibit LP of central nervous system (CNS) tissue was correlated with positive effects on other pathophysiologic processes, including neurologic recovery. An effort to define the neuroprotective pharmacology of methylprednisolone in experimental spinal cord injury was initiated. Hall et al.[196a] found that an intravenous dose (30 mg/kg) given immediately after blunt spinal cord injury attenuated post-traumatic LP as well as supporting energy metabolism and preventing post-traumatic ischemia, neurofilament degradation in cats, and significantly higher recovery scores within two weeks of injury.[196a] A reduction in post-traumatic spinal-tissue loss was observed, the degree of which was inversely correlated with the neurologic recovery score. High-dose methylprednisolone increased blood flow, extracellular ionic shifts, and evoked potentials in cat spinal cords and increased locomotory recovery.[375a] Studies by others have shown that high-dose methylprednisolone facilitates neurologic recovery of spinal cord–injured cats,[203a, 269a] monkeys,[198a] and rats.[206a] The beneficial effects of antioxidant doses of methylprednisolone support the contention that post-traumatic LP is a critical mechanism that can be interrupted with an antioxidant agent. The postulated mechanisms of glucocorticosteroids in attenuating spinal cord injury include not only inhibition of CNS tissue LP, but also protection of energy metabolic function, reduction of post-traumatic ischemia, maintenance of neurofilament structure, and slowing of traumatic ionic shifts.[11a]

Results of preclinical trials are often difficult to extrapolate to humans, however, because of controversy regarding the applicability of the animal model to human injury, the reproducibility of the model, and differing responses of animals and humans to different drugs. Whereas more than 85 per cent of preclinical studies demonstrated some benefit with steroid therapy, until 1990 no unequivocal, clearly defining study in humans had yet been performed. Consequently, the National Institutes of Health (NIH) funded a second multicenter clinical trial to define the role of glucocorticosteroid therapy in spinal cord injury in a meaningful manner.

The second NIH study (NASCIS II) had an elaborate protocol consisting of the randomized, blinded use of methylprednisolone, naloxone, or placebo in 487 patients within 12 hours for spinal cord injury.[26a, 61b] Analysis of the entire population did not show a significant clinical difference among treatments, although data stratifications revealed a significant change in patients with a complete loss of function who received a high-dose methylprednisolone (a bolus of 30 mg/kg body weight as a loading dose, followed by an infusion of 5.4 mg/kg/h for 23 h) within 8 hours of the injury. NASCIS II was the first randomized, double-blind, placebo-controlled trial that demonstrated that a pharmacologic agent can beneficially modify the course of events after severe central nervous system injury. The dosage level and regimen were derived from pharmacologic investigations that focused on the mechanism of action, dose-response and time-action studies, and pharmacokinetics.

NASCIS II represents a positive first step in realizing the goal of successful neuroprotection; however, certain key issues remain unresolved.

There is a potential for serious steroidal side effects related to the dose and duration of treatment. Both NASCIS I and NASCIS II had a predictable trend toward complications with prolonged steroidal therapy. In NASCIS II, the administration of methylprednisolone was associated with a 7.1 per cent incidence of wound infection. Bohlman and Ducker[26a] reported a significant increase in the incidence of complications in patients given 10 days of high-dose methylprednisolone therapy. Galandiuk et al.[176a] suspected that pneumonia was more frequent and severe in steroid-treated patients and initiated prospective and retrospective studies evaluating the effect of high-dose methylprednisolone in 32 patients with cervical or upper thoracic spinal injuries. Complete spinal cord injury was present in 22 of 32 patients; 14 patients received steroids after injury. The hospital stay was longer in steroid-treated patients than in patients not treated with steroids (44.4 vs. 27.7 days, respectively). Seventy-nine per cent of steroid-treated patients had pneumonia, compared with 50% of patients not so treated. In steroid-treated patients, vital immune responses were adversely affected, pneumonia was more prevalent, and hospitalization was prolonged, and hospital costs increased by an average of $51,504 per admission.[176a] Additionally, the anti-inflammatory actions of methylprednisolone may impede the normal intraspinal clean-up process while inhibiting LP.

The results of NASCIS II were released to the press before publication in a peer-reviewed professional journal. The rationale for this early press release was the need for rapid dissemination of knowledge and therapy. Early disclosure to the press unfortunately resulted in data misinterpretation and oversimplification, failure to recognize exclusion criteria or appropriate legal ramifications, and lack of communication to appropriate physicians.[197a] Initial press reports overinflated the effectiveness of methylprednisolone in the treatment of spinal cord injury, and subsequent studies have provided a promising but less dramatic outlook for the pharmacologic therapy of acute spinal cord injury. Patients with incomplete spinal cord lesions treated with methylprednisolone beyond eight hours after injury had significantly worse neurologic recovery than patients with incomplete spinal cord lesions treated with placebo beyond eight hours after injury.

Whereas NASCIS II suggested a clinical benefit for high-dose intravenous methylprednisolone therapy, incomplete data and statistical descriptions reduced assertions. Discrepancies in the report included lack of radiologic data or descriptions of time-dependent surgical manipulations and extent of rehabilitative therapy. Justification for the broad eight-hour stratum and multiple hypothesis testing was unclear; incomplete design details included level of statistical significance, study power, stopping rules, trial duration, and odds ratio data.[197a]

In complete injuries, with complete loss of both caudal motor and sensory function, the adjacent spinal cord function was not enhanced by methylprednisolone. The placebo groups of patients showed improvements from 1.3 to 3.1 motor levels, and improvement in the glucocorticosteroid group was nearly the same. In the pinprick sensory levels, the placebo-treated groups improved 9 to 12.2 levels, and patients receiving methylprednisolone within the first eight hours improved 14.6. The latter number represents a positive trend. For touch, the placebo-treated groups improved 7.9 to 11.6 levels, and the patients receiving methylprednisolone within the first eight hours were on the high end of the spectrum at 10.4. When the drug was administered beyond eight hours, there was no appreciable benefit.

The true benefit of methylprednisolone is also questionable because of the difference in outcome of the two placebo groups who entered the protocol before and after eight hours. Patients with incomplete spinal cord injury treated with placebo within eight hours and patients with incomplete spinal cord injury treated with placebo beyond eight hours are significantly different from one another, with the latter group showing greater recovery. This goes against clinical observations that patients admitted earlier typically have a better outcome than those admitted later.

One interpretation of the data is that we could treat the patient with placebo after eight hours and obtain the same results as treatment with methylprednisolone within eight hours, which does not make intuitive sense. When compared with the control group, the treatment group needs to improve, and the placebo group should not have to become worse to demonstrate a positive drug effect. Therefore the initial promising results may indeed be negated by the better recovery of the delayed treatment or untreated group of patients or both, which would be listed in the placebo group beyond eight hours. The two placebo groups (or the patients studied before and after eight hours of entry into the protocol treatments) do not differ enough that firm conclusions are possible. We urge clinicians to perform their own independent analyses.

The current status of glucocorticosteroids, using our standardized mechanism for assessing drug development, is shown in Table 33–3.[186b] With that background information, the Third National Acute Spinal Cord Injury Randomized Clinical Controlled Trial was completed and reported in May of 1997 in JAMA.[269a] This study again used 16 acute spinal cord injury centers in North America and evaluated 499 patients who could be treated within eight hours. All patients received the standard intravenous bolus dose of methylprednisolone (30 mg/kg) as part of their initial treatment. They were then randomized into a 24-hour treatment group, a 48-hour treatment of steroids (methylprednisolone), and a third group treated with trilazad mesylate which was given for 48 hours. The motor function between the initial presentation, at six weeks, and at six months was the primary clinical outcome measure. In addition, a functional, independent measure was done at six weeks and six months.

If the large methylprednisolone dose was initiated within three hours of injury, there was no evidence that extending that for an additional 24 hours was of any benefit to the patient. However, if the treatment was initiated three to eight hours after injury, maintaining the high dose of steroids for 48 hours gave some modest additional benefit to the patient. The usage of trilazad mesylate (a potent lipid peroxidation inhibitor), which was developed to treat central nervous system trauma with the potential of fewer complications than anticipated from a 48-hour steroid regimen, failed to benefit the patients as much as the methylprednisolone. In this study, there were no patients entered for full evaluation who had no treatment (controls) or who were treated after the initial eight hours, which would have been important data for comparison.

Again, there is a price to be paid for using steroids. Although there is no statistical difference between the complication rate in the patients with just 24 hours of methylprednisolone treatment compared with those with 48 hours, the collective complication rate at 48 hours is slightly higher. Also, in analyzing survival probability, the shorter 24-hour course of steroid patients did slightly better.

Within three months of the NASCIS III study publication, there was an analysis of steroids used in patients with gunshot wounds in the spinal cord injury centers in Philadelphia and New Jersey, reviewing 254 consecutive patients treated between 1979 and 1994

Table 33–3. GLUCOCORTICOID STEROIDS IN SPINAL CORD INJURY

Laboratory Phase I:	1969, Ducker, Goodkin
Laboratory Phase II:	1970s–1990s, Demopoulos, Braughlen, Hall, Means, Hoerlein, Green, Holtz, Ross, Young
Laboratory Phase III:	Toxicology, related use
Clinical Phase I:	1984, Bracken et al. (NASCIS I)
Clinical Phase II:	1990, 1992, (NASCIS II)
Clinical Phase III:	1997 (NASCIS III)
Clinical Phase IV:	No FDA approval

with gunshot wounds to the spine and spinal cord injuries between the first cervical and the first lumbar vertebra. The patients were divided into three groups, those receiving the high-dose methylprednisolone, a second group receiving dexamethasone, and a third group receiving no steroids. There was no statistical difference in the neurologic recoveries from any of the three groups. Instead, infection complications were increased in both groups receiving steroids, whether dexamethasone or methylprednisolone. That report concluded that patients who sustained spinal cord injuries secondary to gunshot wounds to the spine should not be treated with steroids.[198a]

In conclusion, there is fairly good evidence to believe that, on an experimental basis, a very high dose of glucocorticosteroids given very soon after a blunt spinal cord injury would be beneficial to the patient if there is no contraindication to giving the medication. The sooner it is given for a shorter duration, the better; therefore, if it can be initiated within eight hours, it is acceptable to carry the dosage regimen for 48 hours. While this seems to apply to cases of the contusion injury, it does not apply to the open destructive injury secondary to gunshot wounds. In using high-dose steroids, one has to be cognizant that there may be an increase in problems with infection and gastrointestinal hemorrhage. At the time of this writing, use of methylprednisolone has not received Federal Drug Administration approval.[376a] Currently there are no further large-scale clinical trials planned to expand our information on this subject.[123]

Laminectomy

This procedure initially advocated to "decompress" a swollen cord has been found not to benefit many patients and to cause harm.[46, 205, 206, 299, 316, 338, 372] As a result, the treatment of cord-damaged patients by laminectomy in Great Britain and centers in this country is an abandoned procedure. Laminectomy may be indicated in very selected cord-damaged patients if there is proved posterior cord compression by laminar fractures or the rare large epidural hematoma.

In complete injuries, we could not improve recovery by a laminectomy; the recovery rate remained between 11 and 15 per cent for all patients studied. In partially cord-damaged patients, in whom the neurologic loss was quite severe but there was minimal function of the toes, the results of laminectomy simply reflect the biologic curve of recovery of the patients who were better before the operation. In the patients with a uniform partial loss, typically with high cervical cord injuries between the first and fourth cervical levels, the extra manipulation of the cord by a laminectomy was not helpful and on occasion was even harmful. The group of patients with the central cord syndrome and a narrow spinal canal received slight benefit from laminectomy. The patients with partial lesions and caudal sparing (central cord syndrome) without laminectomy had higher initial motor indices, but those treated with surgery had a slightly higher (6 per cent) recovery rate.

Both groups of patients had recovery rates from 65 to 71 per cent. The fact that the patients with a lower motor index initially (2.45 on a scale from 0 to 5) did better made us re-examine those patients who benefited from an operation. If the patient has continuous compression after cord injury, specifically patients with cervical spondylosis and stenosis whose clinical condition quickly plateaus, then anterior decompression or laminectomy may be indicated. Laminoplasty in these patients is done with the patient in skeletal traction on a frame and with high-speed air drills, so that no instrument is placed underneath the lamina at the time that the bone is removed. Many of these patients improve initially, but after the operation, which is performed in the first three weeks, there may be an additional 35 per cent improvement in recovery compared with 22 per cent in the groups who had very early surgery or nonsurgical groups, but these results will have to be analyzed with much longer than a one-year follow-up.

In Bohlman's series of patients, laminectomy produced a loss of function and high mortality rate in those with central cord syndromes as well as other partial and complete cord lesions. There was no apparent benefit from the operation at long-term follow-up. In those few patients with ankylosing spondylitis and massive epidural hemorrhage, however, laminectomy may be the only way to evacuate the hematoma.[23, 46, 186, 189]

Anterior Spinal Decompression and Fusion

Anterior spinal decompressive operations are indicated if there is proved compression of the spinal cord.[10, 14, 20, 22, 36, 96]

In Bohlman's series of 300 patients, anterior decompression and fusion appeared to be beneficial in patients with incomplete cord syndromes in relation to nonsurgical treatment or laminectomy.

There is strong evidence in the literature now that anterior decompression for spinal cord and cauda equina injuries benefits the ultimate neurologic recovery.[21, 28, 33, 40, 46, 65, 66, 75, 111, 141]

As previously documented in this chapter, Bohlman reported the long-term follow-up results of anterior decompression for cervical motor complete as well as incomplete injuries. We can now expect a 60 per cent improvement in nerve root function in complete quadriplegics with anterior decompression and fusion, and a significant number of the motor incomplete cord-injured patients can become ambulators following anterior decompression. The exact timing of anterior operative procedures in the very acute phase of the spinal cord injury is not clear; however, Bohlman has pointed out that it is statistically significant to decompress the cervical spinal cord–injured patients within the first few weeks or months rather than very late, such as one or two years after injury. A major question is whether more acute decompressions will be beneficial; that is, within hours of injury. However, the exact neurologic status of the patient may not be clear within the first 48 hours if the patient is in spinal cord shock.

Anterior decompression of upper thoracic incomplete spinal cord injuries is definitely beneficial in the ultimate neurologic recovery and is far superior to laminectomy and nonsurgical treatment.[40] To date, no one has proved whether timing of these decompressions is beneficial. However, based on experimental evidence as well as clinical observations, it would appear that earlier decompression would be more beneficial to the injured spinal cord. However, no early surgery should be done until the patient's medical status and other injuries have stabilized. More recently, Delamarter et al.[109] suggested in an experimental study that decompression within one hour of upper thoracic spinal cord injury might allow recovery, whereas those animals who sustained compression of the thoracic spinal cord for greater periods of time did not recover. Therefore, one may theorize that in the clinical situation, an anterior transthoracic decompression should be attempted if the patient is received within the first hour following injury and the bony fracture is not a severe one in which there is demonstrable spinal cord compression, even though the patient may present as a complete paraplegic.

Anterior decompression for thoracolumbar injuries has been shown to improve the ultimate neurologic outcome;[219, 253, 262, 356] but again, the timing of the operative procedure within the first year after injury has not been proved to be statistically significant.

Benzel and others[21] also demonstrated the significant benefits of anterior decompressive procedures in cervical and thoracolumbar spinal cord injuries. These authors carried out their decompressions within the first two to six weeks following the injury.

In summary, the anterior decompressive operation is indicated when there is proven compression of the spinal cord. The selection of a stabilization procedure is dependent on the associated osseous and ligamentous pathology, whereas a decompression procedure is dependent on the site of spinal cord compression.

Gunshot Wounds

Indications for decompressive procedures following gunshot wounds of the spine are based on the presence or absence of compressive pathology.[378] If a missile traverses the spinal canal, leaving behind no bullet or bone fragments, then surgical decompression as a general rule has little to offer and may cause harm.[338, 372] On rare occasions, a cerebrospinal fluid leak out of the wound or into the pleural cavity will require surgical dural closure. If the bullet or shell fragment lies near or in the spinal canal with bone compressing the neural structures, it is probably best to remove it. But a laminectomy is not always the proper operation. The fragment should be localized roentgenographically.[36] When a bullet has lodged in the vertebral body, causing anterior dural compression, an anterior cervical approach, costotransversectomy, or transthoracic anterior approach is used to decompress the spinal cord. If there is no compression or if the cord is completely injured, a surgical procedure may be more destructive than constructive. In gunshot wounds and war missile wounds more than in any other clinical setting, pulmonary and cardiovascular stability must be achieved. First, intrathoracic chest tubes must be placed if needed, intraperitoneal bleeding must be identified, and intravascular volume replacement must be completed. Once the patient is stable, which may be 24 to 48 hours following injury, any necessary decompressive procedure is carried out.

SPECIFIC LESIONS OF UPPER CERVICAL SPINE INJURIES: PATHOLOGY AND CURRENT TREATMENT CONCEPTS

Atlanto-Occipital Lesions

In a previous study of fatal craniospinal injuries by Davis et al., it was evident that injuries to the occipitocervical junction were very common; however, in the clinical situation, atlanto-occipital dislocations have rarely been reported with survival.[107, 145, 150] Fortunately, those patients who survive severe atlanto-occipital dislocations can have incomplete cord injuries, and recovery can occur with stabilization of the fracture by posterior cervico-occipital arthrodesis. When the spinal cord is completely transected at the first cervical level, survival is rare for more than two years because of pulmonary complications. The spinal pathology that is involved in these devastating injuries includes total disruption of all ligamentous structures between the

occiput and the atlantoaxial complex with sparing but distortion of the vertebral arteries.[322] This is a severely unstable dislocation that may occur in association with fractures of the atlas. Dislocation of the occiput on the atlas may be either anterior or posterior. In Bohlman's series of 300 cervical spine injuries, there were two patients with anterior atlanto-occipital dislocations associated with brain injury who were comatose on admission to the hospital. Both of these patients died within a short period of time secondary to their injuries.[46] Roentgenograms in both patients revealed the skull separated from the axis and displaced anteriorly to a significant degree. At autopsy, both patients were found to have transection of the spinal cord at the atlanto-occipital level (Fig. 33–18). Anderson and Montesano[9] have described and classified the rare occipital condylar fractures.

Atlantoaxial Lesions

Atlantoaxial injuries generally occur without neurologic deficit because of the relatively larger diameter of the spinal canal at this level. Of 69 patients with atlantoaxial lesions in Bohlman's review series of 300 injuries, 58 occurred without and 11 with neural deficit. The fractures at this region of the spine may occur singly or in combination. Isolated fractures of the atlas may occur in the posterior arch, anterior arch, or as a combination, producing the Jefferson fracture, in which four fractures occur in the ring of the atlas, producing lateral displacement of the lateral masses of the atlas.[214] Single lateral mass compression fracture may occur without interruption of the entire ring of the atlas (Fig.

Figure 33–18. *A,* Arteriogram of a pedestrian who was struck by an automobile, sustaining an anterior dislocation of the occiput on the atlas. Arteriography was performed because the patient was comatose. Note the forward displacement of the occipital condyles on the C1–C2 complex. The patient died 48 hours after injury. (From Bohlman, H.H.: The neck. *In* D'Ambrosia, R. [ed.]: Musculoskeletal Disorders. Chap. 6. Philadelphia, J. B. Lippincott Co., 1977.) *B,* This sagittal section of a specimen taken from the cervical spine, leaving the foramen magnum intact, shows complete transection of the spinal cord at the first cervical vertebra with complete disruption of all ligaments between the foramen magnum and the atlantoaxial complex. (From Bohlman, H. H.: Acute fractures and dislocations of the cervical spine. J. Bone Joint Surg. *61A:*1119–1142, 1979.)

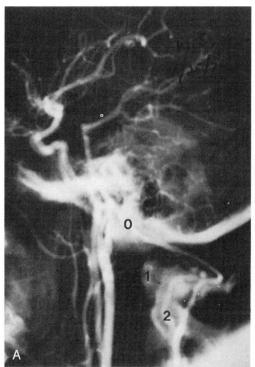
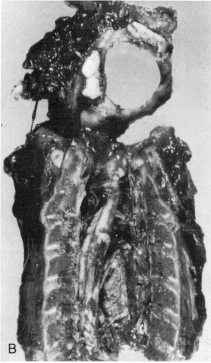

33–19). Fractures of the anterior arch of the atlas are usually associated with axial loading as well as flexion forces; however, posterior arch fractures require an extension force applied to the head that extends the head on the neck and therefore impinges on the posterior ring in the atlas. A direct blow to the head, as in falling or being struck on the head by a heavy falling object, may produce axial loading that is transmitted through both occipital condyles to the articulation of the lateral masses of the atlas, creating a "blowout fracture" or the so-called Jefferson fracture. This fracture occurs secondary to a centrifugal force applied to the wedge-shaped lateral masses, and the atlas fractures posteriorly at the two weaker points near the grooves of the vertebral arteries and anteriorly at its thinnest aspect. Ordinarily, there is no neurologic deficit in association with fractures of the atlas because there is enough room for the spinal cord, and the displacement usually occurs laterally. Levine and Edwards[240] reported on the treatment of 34 patients with fractures of the atlas with an average follow-up of 4.5 years. Of these 34, 17 had bilateral fractures of the posterior arch, six had fractures in the area of the lateral mass, and 11 sustained Jefferson blowout fractures. The majority of these patients were treated nonsurgically with either a rigid brace or a halo vest, and only patients who had an associated odontoid fracture or tear of the transverse ligament with instability required arthrodesis. The Jefferson fractures were treated with skeletal traction, but complete reduction was not always possible. Asymmetry of the atlantoaxial joint was not associated with long-term degenerative arthritis, but a significant number of patients had long-term neck pain that was not disabling.

Roentgenographically, these fractures may be diagnosed by visualization on the anteroposterior and lat-

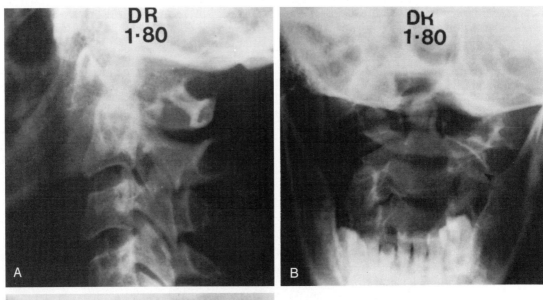

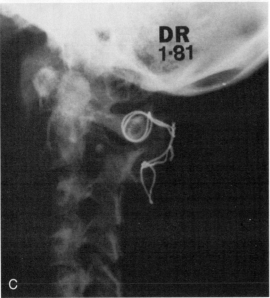

Figure 33–19. *A,* Lateral roentgenogram of a patient who was initially unconscious after sustaining a head injury in a vehicular accident. Upon awakening the patient was noted to have a torticollis, and the C1–C2 complex appears to show increased space at the anterior atlantodental interval with an oblique view of the posterior arch of the atlas in relationship to the body and posterior element of the axis. *B,* Open-mouth odontoid view of the same patient reveals a unilateral lateral mass fracture of the atlas and disruption of the atlantoaxial joint, resulting in a fixed torticollis. *C,* One year after injury the patient had persistent pain, which required posterior atlantoaxial arthrodesis. Lateral roentgenogram demonstrates the arthrodesis and wire in place. Fusion relieved the symptoms, and the torticollis was ultimately corrected by adaptation of the head and neck position.

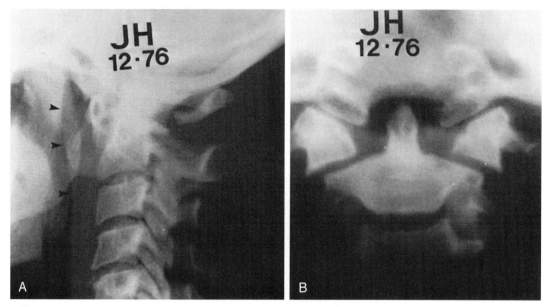

Figure 33–20. *A*, Lateral roentgenogram of a patient after a vehicular accident reveals a posterior arch fracture of the atlas. There is some widening of the soft tissue space anterior to the atlas and axis, indicating swelling of the soft tissues in the retropharyngeal area. *B*, Anteroposterior tomography of the upper cervical spine reveals bilateral spreading of the lateral masses of the atlas on the axis and on the occipital condyles, indicating total disruption of the ring of the atlas anteriorly and posteriorly with tearing of the transverse ligament.

eral views of the atlantoaxial region. On the open-mouth odontoid view, the lateral masses of the atlas are each displaced laterally beyond the upper articular surfaces of the axis (Fig. 33–20).[327] Anterior and posterior tomography may be necessary to confirm the diagnosis of the Jefferson fracture. The CT scan is very useful in judging the type of fracture as well as healing.

Not all of these fractures heal by osseous union; some heal instead by fibrous union and are stable.[326] Ordinarily, surgical intervention is not necessary for fractures of the atlas unless they are associated with odontoid fractures or rupture of the transverse ligament.[335] The treatment is by rigid cervical orthosis or halo vest for approximately two to three months. Isolated fractures of the lateral mass of the atlas may usually be treated conservatively with a rigid orthosis, and later problems, if they occur, are usually a result of incongruity of the joint surfaces, which produces pain with or without a spastic torticollis. In the latter instance, a posterior atlantoaxial arthrodesis may be indicated and the torticollis will resolve.

Atlantoaxial dislocations may occur with or without fractures. Anterior dislocation of the atlas on the axis without fracture is very rare, occurring in only three of 300 patients reviewed by Bohlman[46] (Fig. 33–21). This indicates complete disruption of the transverse ligament, which is a very unstable situation and requires posterior atlantoaxial arthrodesis following reduction.[153, 170] Posterior atlantoaxial dislocation is extremely rare and indicates disruption of the apical and alar ligaments with maintenance of the transverse ligament.

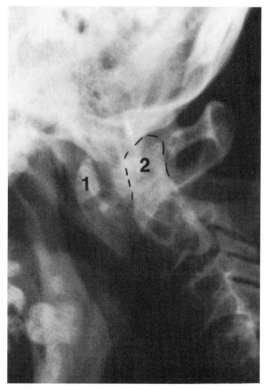

Figure 33–21. Roentgenogram of the driver of a milk truck that was struck by a train shows anterior dislocation of the axis on the atlas without fracture. This is evidence of a ruptured transverse ligament. (From Bohlman, H. H.: The neck. *In* D'Ambrosia, R. [ed.]: Musculoskeletal Disorders. 2nd ed. Philadelphia, J. B. Lippincott Co., 1986.)

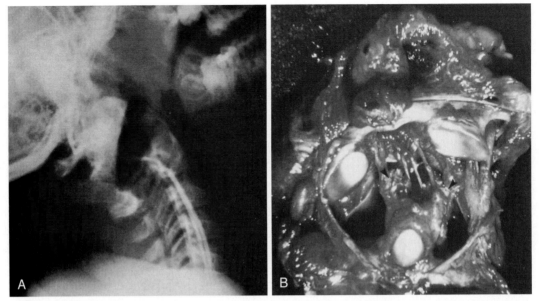

Figure 33–22. *A,* Autopsy roentgenogram of a child struck by a car, resulting in a secondary posterior atlantoaxial dislocation. (From Bohlman, H. H.: The neck. *In* D'Ambrosia, R. [ed.]: Musculoskeletal Disorders. Chap. 6. Philadelphia, J. B. Lippincott Co., 1977.) *B,* Photograph of a specimen with posterior atlantoaxial dislocation. Note that the odontoid process has been pulled through the ring in the atlas, whose inferior articular facets are shown in the picture. The alar ligaments are still attached to the odontoid process inferiorly and have been avulsed from the occipital condyles. The vertebral arteries remain intact, although there has been major ligamentous tearing between C1 and C2. (From Davis, D. D., Bohlman, H. H., Walker, A. E., et al.: Pathologic findings in fatal craniospinal injuries. J. Neurosurg. *34:*603–613, 1971.)

This injury has been reported in fatal craniospinal injuries and also with survival (Fig. 33–22).[107, 284, 311] Because of severe ligamentous disruption with posterior atlantoaxial dislocation, reduction should be obtained by axial skeletal traction, and posterior arthrodesis should be performed from the atlas to the axis following reduction. Anterior atlantoaxial dislocation may occur in association with an aplastic or dysplastic odontoid in adults or children (Fig. 33–23).[158, 160] The most common type of dysplastic odontoid found in children is in the Morquio dwarf.[24, 105, 158, 162, 269] This is frequently recognized after a traumatic episode and may be potentially fatal; therefore, posterior atlantoaxial arthrodesis should be performed when this entity is

Figure 33–23. Atlantoaxial dislocation diagnosed by a roentgenogram taken after an auto accident. Note the hypoplastic odontoid process on the lateral roentgenogram. (From Bohlman, H. H.: The neck. *In* D'Ambrosia, R. [ed.]: Musculoskeletal Disorders. 2nd ed. Philadelphia, J. B. Lippincott Co., 1986.)

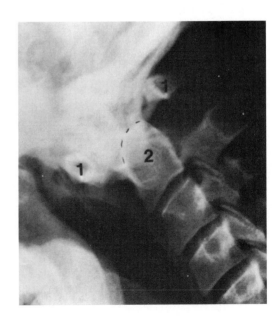

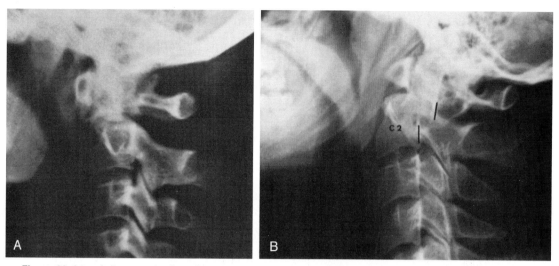

Figure 33–24. *A,* Fractured odontoid process with anterior displacement. The transverse ligament remains intact and carries the odontoid forward with the atlas. *B,* Fractured odontoid process with posterior displacement. The transverse ligament remains intact. (From Bohlman, H. H.: The neck. *In* D'Ambrosia, R. [ed.]: Musculoskeletal Disorders. 2nd ed. Philadelphia, J. B. Lippincott Co., 1986.)

recognized. Progressive myelopathy may develop if atlantoaxial dislocation is left untreated.[341, 357] Laminectomy in this instance is contraindicated because of its resultant high mortality.[105]

Fractures of the odontoid process may occur with or without dislocation or displacement of the atlas. Displacement may be anterior or posterior (Fig. 33–24). These fractures have been classified by Anderson et al. and Schatzker et al. with reference to their healing ability and necessity for arthrodesis.[8, 315] Basically, fractures may occur in adults through the upper aspect of the odontoid (Type I), through the base of the odontoid process without extending into the body of the axis (Type II), and by extension into the body of the axis (Type III). Fractures through the waist of the odontoid process have a poor prognosis for healing and may result in nonunion, especially if they are overdistracted in a halo-fixation apparatus (Fig. 33–25). Fractures into the vertebral body of the axis usually will heal uneventfully with rigid fixation by the use of a rigid orthosis or halo-fixation device.[276, 298] However, Clark and White[93] reported in a multicenter study that Type III

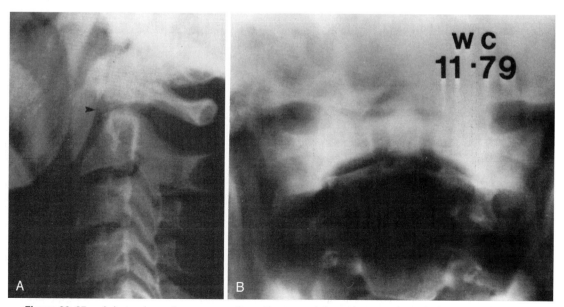

Figure 33–25. *A,* Lateral roentgenogram of a patient sustaining a fracture through the waist of the odontoid process in a vehicular accident. *B,* Anteroposterior view of the fractured odontoid through its poorly vascularized waist, indicating a high incidence of nonunion.

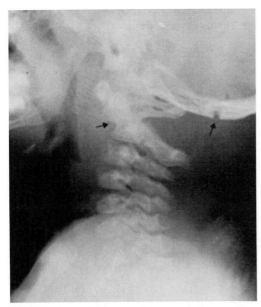

Figure 33–26. An epiphyseal fracture of the odontoid process and a fracture of the occiput are seen in this 2½-year-old child whose level of consciousness was decreased. The diagnosis was not determined for two days. (From Bohlman, H. H.: Acute fractures and dislocations of the cervical spine. J. Bone Joint Surg. *61A*:1119–1142, 1979.)

fractures may heal in a malunited position. More rarely in young children, a fracture may occur through the epiphyseal line, and displacement may occur (Fig. 33–26).[46, 108, 149, 195, 235, 291] These fractures heal quite nicely with rigid immobilization for two to three months. A major problem may occur with spinal cord compression if a fracture of the axis is either unrecognized or left to heal in malposition. The treatment of these fractures will be discussed later in this chapter in the sections on late deformity. Displaced fractures of the odontoid should be treated initially with skeletal traction to restore normal alignment, and at that time a decision should be made as to whether posterior arthrodesis is indicated with wire or transarticular screw fixation.[212]

Rarely, rotary atlantoaxial dislocation may be a result of trauma, in which case the patient presents with a painful torticollis.[161] On the lateral roentgenogram, the atlas appears to be subluxed forward with the lateral mass visible anterior to the odontoid process. On the anteroposterior open-mouth view, the atlantoaxial joint on the subluxed side is obliterated or overlapped.[37] In this instance, the capsule of the atlantoaxial joint has been torn or stretched to a significant degree, and usually skeletal traction is necessary to reduce the subluxation. These subluxations may be treated conservatively with rigid immobilization for six to eight weeks or by posterior atlantoaxial arthrodesis if the subluxation is severe or chronic and irreducible. In the case of the chronic rotatory subluxation of the atlas on the axis, reduction is not possible and manipulation should not be performed under anesthesia. Ordi-

narily, posterior arthrodesis results in adaptation of the head and neck to a straighter configuration once the arthrodesis is solid (see Fig. 33–19).[332]

Pedicle Fractures of the Axis

Pedicle fractures of the axis are not uncommon and ordinarily occur by hyperextension injury in which the occiput is forced into extension against the atlas, which in turn compresses the axis pedicles and produces a fracture (Fig. 33–27). If a flexion injury component is added, there may be disruption of the disc and ligaments between the second and third cervical vertebrae with forward subluxation at this segment of the spine. At the second and third level there is a relatively large amount of room for the spinal cord, and these injuries rarely result in a neurologic deficit.[46, 68] If these fractures are displaced, then skeletal traction is warranted to obtain reduction and maintain the pedicle fractures in alignment for healing.[194, 196] It has been our policy to treat nondisplaced pedicle fractures of the axis with a rigid brace or halo for three months. If the fractures are displaced, skeletal traction is instituted until reduction is obtained, which is then maintained for three weeks until early callus formation has occurred. At this point, a halo-cast is applied and the patient is ambulated. The patient who sustains bilateral pedicle fractures of the axis with disruption of the discs and ligaments between the second and third cervical vertebrae is in an extremely unstable situation and may require anterior cervical fusion at C2–C3 at a later date

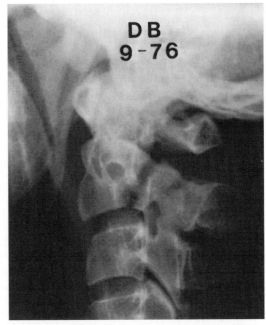

Figure 33–27. Lateral roentgenogram of a patient sustaining a bilateral pedicle fracture of the axis. Note the slight anterior subluxation of the axis on the third cervical vertebra. These fractures heal quite nicely with rigid immobilization and do not usually require arthrodesis.

if spontaneous arthrodesis does not occur. Francis et al.,[168] as well as Levine and Edwards,[242] documented this severe Type III displacement with facet dislocations in association with a high incidence of instability and nonunion.

Upper Cervical Spinal Cord Syndromes

When there is spinal injury between the occiput and the axis with damage to the central nervous system, survival of the patient is in great danger. High spinal cord lesions that are neurologically complete are, for the most part, fatal.[107] There is a loss of all respiratory function, with paralysis of the phrenic nerve innervating the diaphragm as well as all of the intercostal musculature. The phrenic nerve, arising from motor neurons in the third and fourth cervical cord segments, needs to have integrated central nervous system function for the patient to breathe. On occasion, the physician is confronted with such a patient who has received immediate cardiopulmonary resuscitation and is brought to a medical center with ventilatory support. Even after emergency resuscitation has allowed the patient to be alive for initial treatment, the prognosis is very poor and death usually occurs secondary to pulmonary complications.[18] Medical centers with great expertise in high spinal cord–injured patients may selectively try to stabilize such a severely damaged patient. Survival and rehabilitation of the C1–C2 complete cord-injured patients require tremendous nursing, family, and medical support. Independence can be achieved by diaphragmatic or phrenic nerve pacers and portable respirators with a spare machine. In addition, an electrical wheelchair with chin control is necessary for mobilization.

Fortunately, most of the patients we see with cord damage high in the cervical area have partial neurologic lesions where there is a larger amount of white than of gray matter.[145] The usual neurologic lesion is a partial cord syndrome with a uniform loss of arm and leg function with a Brown-Séquard type of pattern. If the spine is stabilized and the cord is protected, the prognosis for recovery is fairly good. Calculated recovery rates in these patients if 50 per cent of the total motor function was retained at the time of presentation range from 55 to 70 per cent. If the uniform neurologic loss is greater than 50 per cent, then the return of function may be only 35 per cent of the initially lost motor function.

The most important aspect of treatment of patients with upper cervical cord injury is immobilization and stabilization of the spine, because anterior decompression is not beneficial to the recovery. A cervical collar is required initially for immobilization, and traction is often applied; the weights added to the patient's traction apparatus should be kept to a minimum because, as previously mentioned, atlanto-occipital injuries tear major ligaments and create severe instability. The halo apparatus may be used to align the skull with the cervical spine. Because there is a considerable amount of ligamentous disruption, an occipitocervical ar-

throdesis is required, which can be performed in the halo device. Delaying the procedure until there is soft tissue healing may risk late instability and death (Fig. 33–28). We prefer the technique of fusion described by Wertheim and Bohlman.[359]

Generally speaking, cervical traction is started at approximately three to five pounds per vertebra in high cervical injuries. Jefferson fractures of the atlas will realign. Third and fourth cervical levels may be treated initially with nine to 10 pounds of traction, going to as high as 15 to 20 with caution. Because most of these lesions are partial cord injuries, the use of the halo-vest apparatus early in the treatment provides immobilization and stabilization of the spine, preventing any compression of the spinal cord and allowing the patient the shortest possible hospitalization.

SPECIFIC LESIONS BETWEEN THE THIRD CERVICAL AND FIRST THORACIC VERTEBRAE: PATHOLOGY AND CURRENT TREATMENT CONCEPTS

Osteoarticular Pathology

Fractures occurring in the lower cervical spine may be divided pathologically into injuries of the posterior, anterior, or lateral elements, or a combination.[7, 37, 46] As mentioned previously, most fractures or dislocations of the lower cervical spine may be initially diagnosed by a single lateral roentgenogram. If the series of roentgenograms is obtained in a methodical fashion as described, then an accurate assessment of the stability and fracture type may be obtained, and one can proceed with appropriate treatment as indicated.

It is rare that no vertebral fractures or displacements are seen on lateral roentgenograms so that stress views are necessary. Stress roentgenograms in flexion and extension should only be obtained in protected head halter or skeletal traction when there is no indication of cervical trauma on previous roentgenograms and the clinical situation indicates that there has been severe cervical injury.

Soft tissue and ligament injuries of the cervical region may occur posteriorly, in the anterior region, or as a combination of both. In the previously mentioned fatal craniospinal injury series, 38 per cent of these individuals had cervical disc disruption that could not be recognized on routine roentgenograms.[107] Distraction of the disc space in skeletal traction occurred only if there was major ligamentous disruption; that is, of the longitudinal ligaments and associated disc. Ligamentous injuries occurred in combinations, attesting to the fact that mechanisms of injury may occur in groups rather than individually as pure flexion or extension. Soft tissue swelling anterior to the cervical spine may occur by hemorrhage or edema, and in the fatal injury study, retroesophageal hemorrhage of as much as 700 mg was seen secondary to tearing of the radicular

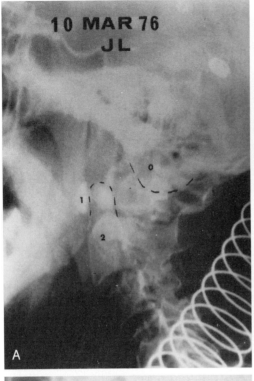

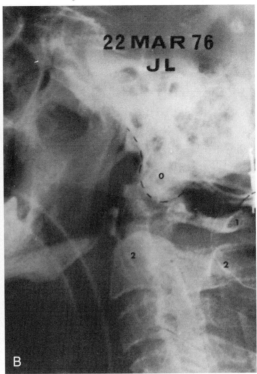

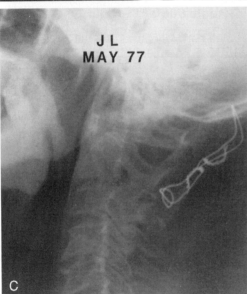

Figure 33–28. *A,* Lateral cervical roentgenogram demonstrating a posterior atlanto-occipital dislocation, as well as a fracture of the posterior arch of the atlas. Note that the basion is grossly posterior to the odontoid process. The lateral mass of the atlas also appears to be slightly posteriorly dislocated in relationship to the odontoid process, but this is due to the rotation of the head as shown by the asymmetric position of the mandibular rami. *B,* True lateral roentgenogram of the cervical spine centered at the level of the atlas, demonstrating reduction of the atlanto-occipital dislocation. *C,* Postoperative lateral radiograph revealing a completely solid cervical occipital arthrodesis. The patient was initially quadriparetic and recovered completely after stabilization. (From Eismont, F. J., and Bohlman, H. H.: Posterior atlanto-occipital dislocation with fractures of the atlas and odontoid process. Report of a case with survival. J. Bone Joint Surg. *60A:*397–399, 1978.)

vessels and not as a result of tearing of the vertebral artery.

Atlanto-occipital and atlantoaxial injuries are much more common in a fatal series than lower cervical spine disruption. Injury to the vertebral body was rare, and vertebral artery thrombosis and tearing was seen in only one case in the 50 injuries studied by Davis et al.[107] and Simeone and Goldberg.[329] Other authors have reported vertebral artery injury with upper as well as midcervical fractures.[57, 197, 213, 368]

Now that cervical myelography and MRI are used routinely in acute spinal injuries, it is apparent that extrusion of cervical disc material posteriorly into the spinal canal is much more common than previously realized.[27, 42, 258, 343] Cervical osteoarthritis may be a pre-existing condition in patients with cervical spine injuries and may play a role in the injury to the spinal cord.[16, 46, 79, 80, 255] Pathologic rupture of the posterior ligamentous structures usually occurs as a group with disruption of the interspinous ligament, the ligamentum flavum, and joint capsules, as in the usual flexion injury. This may be recognized by separation of the spinous processes at the injured segment of the spine with or without the vertebral body subluxation.

Fractures or dislocation of the posterior elements may include unilateral or bilateral facet dislocations, bilaterally perched facets, fractured facets or spinous processes, and laminar fractures. Injuries to the anterior elements include axial loading or compression fractures of the vertebral body with or without displacement, avulsion fractures, and fractures through the spondylitic disc space; in addition, there may be an isolated lateral mass fracture. Most of these injuries of the osseous structures are associated with ligamentous injury and disruption.

As mentioned previously, the lateral roentgenogram should initiate the diagnosis of cervical spine injury.[37, 46] One of the following conditions will usually be evident on the lateral roentgenogram: (1) slight posterior subluxation of the upper on the lower vertebra (Fig. 33–29), (2) moderate anterior subluxation of the upper vertebra on the lower one (Fig. 33–30), or (3) maximal anterior dislocation of the upper vertebra on the lower one (Fig. 33–31). Slight posterior subluxation usually occurs with hyperextension injuries in the patient with pre-existing cervical spondylosis where there is disruption of the disc space. This may be very subtle on lateral roetgenograms but usually indicates disruption of the disc and tearing of the longitudinal ligaments, which is an unstable subluxation. This reverse subluxation may be associated with an avulsion fracture of the anterior vertebral bodies, indicating the anterior ligament torn from the bone. Moderate anterior sublux-

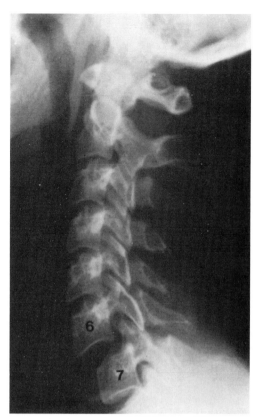

Figure 33–30. Lateral roentgenogram of a patient sustaining moderate anterior subluxation of C6 on C7. Note that the vertebral displacement is approximately one third of the width of the vertebral body. In this situation, oblique roentgenograms must be obtained to determine the specific pathology involving the posterior elements.

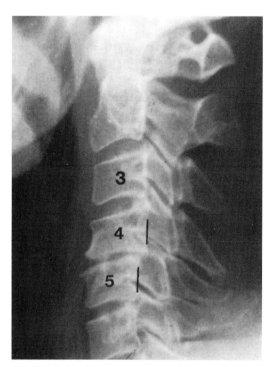

Figure 33–29. Lateral roentgenogram of the cervical spine of a patient who sustained a central cord quadriparesis in a surfing accident, being struck by a wave. Note the slight reverse subluxation of C4 on C5 and the relatively narrow cervical spinal canal at that level.

ation as seen on the lateral roentgenogram may indicate either a unilateral facet dislocation, a unilateral facet fracture, or bilaterally "perched facets" (Fig. 33–32). Moderate anterior subluxation may be associated with either incomplete cord or nerve root lesions, and maximal anterior dislocation usually indicates completely dislocated facets bilaterally and is usually associated with complete quadriplegia.[139] Oblique roentgenograms are obtained in the supine position. The preceding roentgenographic assessment and the classification by Allen et al.[7] are very helpful in determining the pathology involved and in planning a well-organized approach to treatment.

Neurologic Assessment of Lower Cervical Cord Injuries

Spinal cord injuries occurring between the third cervical and first thoracic levels result in either quadriplegia (complete motor paralysis) or quadriparesis (incomplete motor paralysis). These terms imply that there is weakness or paralysis in four extremities. Inadequate testing of upper extremity function in the emergency room or the use of wording such as "paraplegia with paralysis of the hand" has led only to misinterpretation

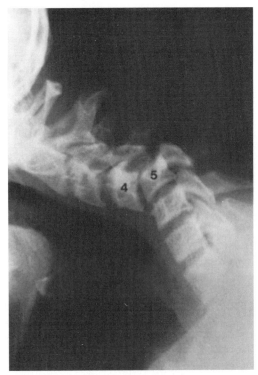

Figure 33–31. Anterior dislocation of C4 and C5 with bilateral dislocation of the articular processes is seen in a patient who was quadriplegic. (From Bohlman, H. H.: Acute fractures and dislocations of the cervical spine. J. Bone Joint Surg. *61A*:1119–1142, 1979.)

cian does have the added advantage of an immediate parameter on which to test the efficacy of the medical care rendered. Immediate immobilization is achieved by a cervical collar or sandbags, but skeletal traction needs to be applied as rapidly as possible. Skeletal traction can be used in any emergency situation.

Traction weight used initially is equivalent to body build and weight as previously described, and progressively increasing poundage up to 50 pounds with roentgenographic control is acceptable. One can either use a C-arm image intensifier or rapidly repeated lateral cervical spine films to measure the success of the traction by achieving spinal alignment. During this phase of treatment, it is advised to carefully supervise the patient. The traction weight necessary for each patient will vary; the exact poundage applied for every patient should be just sufficient to achieve alignment without overdistraction, and maintenance of alignment can usually be accomplished with roughly one third of the weight used in the reduction. Extension injuries sustained in osteoarthritic patients usually require less weight than flexion-dislocation injuries in younger patients, which in turn require less weight than flexion-compression injuries. In the flexion-compression injury with a burst fracture of the vertebral body, it is more important to maintain overall alignment than to use a maximal amount of weight to achieve reduction of the crushed vertebra, which may be quite difficult. Once the spinal canal seems to be decompressed by having provided spinal alignment, the patient can be turned on the frame from a supine to a prone position, and

of diagnosis or medicolegal problems. Although no spinal cord myotome segment is pure, as a general rule the fifth cervical nerve root exits between the fourth and fifth cervical vertebrae and supplies the deltoid and some of the biceps musculature; the sixth root supplies innervation to the biceps, supinator, and the radial wrist extensors; the seventh root supplies the triceps and much of the extensors of the forearm; the eighth root supplies the flexors in the forearm and some grip; and the first thoracic root function adds strength to the grip, as well as to the intrinsic hand muscle function. These general concepts can easily be applied to most patients with lower cervical cord injuries. The neurologic function for spinal cord–injured patients is assessed as described earlier by testing five upper extremity and four lower extremity muscle functions with diaphragmatic, abdominal, and anal function testing, which results in the muscle grading system totaling 100 points (see Table 33–1). The spinal cord injury muscle function sheet, which records the progress of all patients, is used for application of the mathematics defined in this chapter.

Treatment Methods

The treatment of patients with lower cervical spinal cord injuries is initially the same for complete and partial lesions. In partial neurologic lesions, the physi-

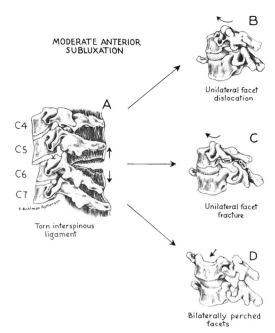

Figure 33–32. Various types of fractures and dislocations (*B, C,* and *D*) of the articular processes that may cause moderate anterior subluxation. (From Bohlman, H. H.: Acute fractures and dislocations of the cervical spine. J. Bone Joint Surg. *61A*:1119–1142, 1979.)

roentgenograms are taken again to check the alignment. If proper alignment is maintained, the further therapy can be planned, including MRI and myelographic studies. If there is continued compression of the spinal cord, which occurs in only the minority of cases, then a decompressive procedure may be indicated.

In patients with lower cervical cord injuries, medical stabilization is usually not a difficult problem, because the patient usually has strong diaphragmatic function, and a precipitous drop in blood pressure is not as commonly seen. Spinal alignment is often a more difficult problem, because it takes more weight to achieve a reduction of dislocations. It is in these cases that we have used as much as 50 pounds with roentgenographic or fluoroscopic control to try to achieve reduction of a bilaterally dislocated facet; however, use of high-weight traction is ill-advised for long periods of time because of over-distraction and the danger of ascending paralysis. If spinal alignment cannot be achieved in traction, the patient has to be taken to the operating room, where a posterior surgical reduction is performed. Once reduction is achieved, posterior arthrodesis is performed with the triple wire technique or plate fixation and iliac bone.[14, 16, 166, 342, 342]

An additional anterior decompressive operation of the cervical spine is occasionally indicated after posterior reduction, but before the operation can be carried out, there has to be proved external cord compression by bone or disc that is present in the spinal canal.[45, 50, 277] (Fig. 33–33). Roentgenographic evidence of spinal cord compression is necessary to make this decision. For example, we have been rewarded on rare occasion when a patient has sustained a severe spinal cord injury with no visible fracture in the midcervical area, where diagnostic studies have shown a large disc fragment within the spinal canal (see Fig. 33–33).[318, 319, 321]

A patient with an anterior cord syndrome treated with an anterior decompression and fusion may have significant return of motor function. Patients with a partial lesion of the central cord type (partial loss with caudal sparing) where there is spinal stenosis, either acquired or congenital, in whom diagnostic studies show continued cord compression anteriorly may benefit from multiple-level anterior discectomy or corpectomy and fusion (Fig. 33–34).

The timing of surgical treatment of spinal cord–injured patients will vary, but generally speaking, the same principles that apply to a tumor that compresses the spinal cord, causing a neurologic deficit, apply to a traumatic disc herniation that compresses the cord.[11, 36, 55] Even though the initial cord contusion may have caused most and, in many cases, all of the neurologic damage, it is the obligation of the treating physician to free the patient of any pathologic process that may continue to contribute to malfunction of the cord. Currently, we try to achieve immobilization at the scene of the accident and medical stabilization within two to three hours after injury, making sure there is no cord compression that would require a further decompressive procedure within the first six to 12 hours following injury. In cases of partial cord lesions in which the patient is improving and there is in addition compression of the spinal cord, decompression can be postponed until the patient's medical and neurologic condition stabilizes some 10 to 14 days after the initial insult. The final treatment of the neurologic deficit may require decompression combined with spinal stabilization by the techniques to be described.[45, 300, 308, 334]

Surgical Techniques

If a patient sustains a cervical dislocation with either unilaterally or bilaterally displaced facets and closed reduction is unsuccessful with skeletal traction, open reduction and arthrodesis are performed in the following manner. In the patient with fourth or fifth cervical complete quadriplegia, local anesthesia may be used because these patients are at high risk under general anesthesia and have a high incidence of subsequent pulmonary problems.[377] Otherwise, the patient is given general anesthesia, intubated in the supine position, then turned prone while protected in skeletal traction. Roentgenograms are taken to ascertain the status of the spine because occasionally spontaneous reduction will have occurred at this point with relaxation of the musculature. Open reduction and arthrodesis are performed with the aid of infiltration of saline and epinephrine solution (1:500,000) down to the laminae and periosteum. A midline incision is made posteriorly, with extreme care taken to dissect sharply in the midline between the muscle fascia. Sharp scalpel dissection is used to avoid harsh motions of the acutely injured spine. Once the laminae are exposed, a subperiosteal elevator is used with the assistant stabilizing the fractured spine with a clamp. When the laminae and facet joints are adequately exposed, lateral identifying roentgenograms are performed. Dislocated facets are reduced by burring off their edges with a power burr and gently levering the vertebrae into reduced position. If a fractured facet compresses the nerve root posteriorly, then a foraminotomy is performed, removing all compressing elements. The arthrodesis is performed with thick corticocancellous iliac grafts, one for each side of the spine. Drill holes are placed through the base of the affected spinous processes of the dislocated vertebrae. If two vertebral segments are involved, then these are the only levels arthrodesed. Multiple levels of laminar fractures may be encountered, in which case the fusion length may be extended. Overzealous arthrodeses only limit useful neck motion, which may be very important for the patient with complete quadriplegia. No decortication is necessary for lower posterior cervical arthrodeses. All posterior fusions reported in Bohlman's series of 300 cervical spine injuries healed without decortication.[46] Enlargement of the drill holes at the base of the spinous processes is carried out with the aid of a large towel clip; then a 20-gauge wire is passed through the cephalic vertebra, looped around the spinous process, passed back through the same hole, and is passed down through and around the caudal spinous process. The 20-gauge wire is pulled

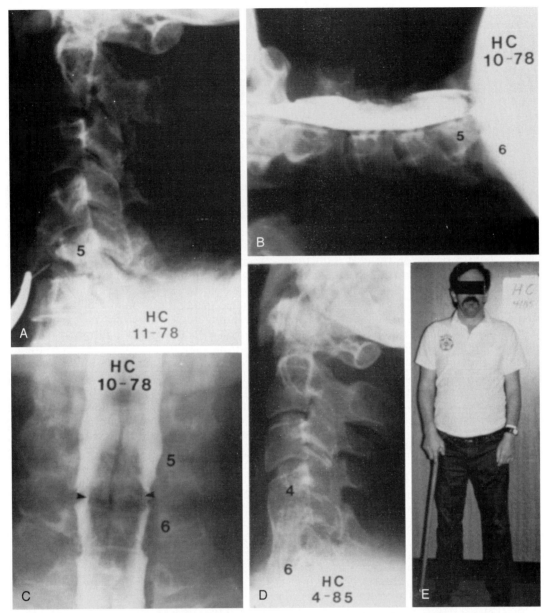

Figure 33–33. *A,* Lateral intraoperative roentgenogram of a male patient who sustained an axial loading compression fracture of C5 with bone protrusion into the spinal canal. Initially he had an anterior cord syndrome with sparing only of perianal-sacral sensation and a one-sided toe wiggle. In addition he had spared position and vibratory sense. He was treated conservatively for 18 months and recovered only minimal function in one leg. *B,* Lateral myelogram demonstrating anterior compression of the dural sac at C5–C6. *C,* Anteroposterior myelographic view demonstrating marked central compression of the spinal cord in the dye column. *D,* Lateral roentgenogram of the patient six years and five months after surgery. Note the incorporation of the anterior iliac bone graft at the level of decompression. *E,* The patient recovered almost completely with slight residual left arm weakness. He was able to walk with a cane and had normal bladder, bowel, and sexual function. This case demonstrates the feasibility of late anterior decompression for an incomplete spinal cord injury and potential neurologic recovery.

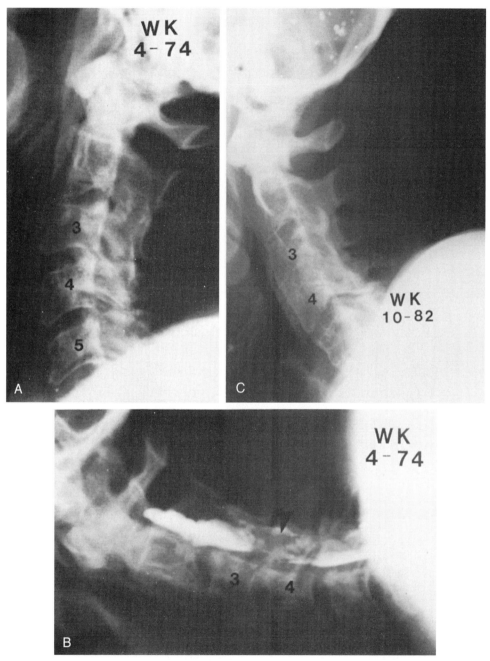

Figure 33–34. *A,* Lateral roentgenogram of a patient sustaining a central cord quadriparesis with no evident fracture or dislocations. The motor level of paralysis was at C4. Six weeks after injury, motor recovery was not occurring. *B,* Lateral view of the cervical myelogram demonstrating a large soft disc herniation between C3 and C4. (*B* from Bohlman, H. H.: Indications for late anterior decompression and fusion for cervical spinal cord injuries. *In* Tator, C. [ed.]: Early Management of Acute Spinal Cord Injury. New York, Raven Press, 1981.) *C,* Seven years after surgical decompression and fusion, a lateral roentgenogram shows the spine to be fused, and the patient has recovered to ambulatory status.

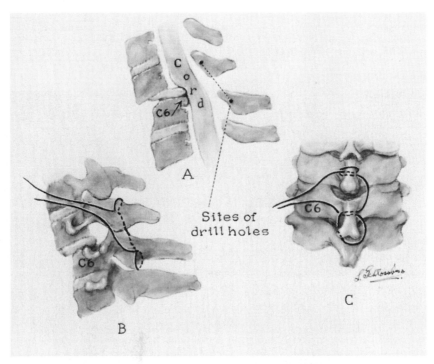

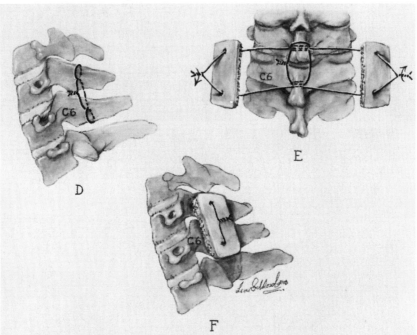

Figure 33–35. *A* to *C,* A posterior midline tethering wire (20 gauge) is passed through and around the base of the subluxed spinous processes in initial stabilization of a distraction-flexion Stage 3 injury. *D* to *F,* Two lateral wires are used to compress two large cortical cancellous iliac strut grafts against the individual lamina. Note that the illustrations demonstrate the fixation methods for a C5–C6 injury. No decortication is necessary. (From Sutterlin, C. E., 3d., McAfee, P. C., Warden, K. E., et al.: A biomechanical evaluation of cervical spine stabilization methods in a bovine model. Static and cyclical loading. Spine *13:*795–802, 1988.)

taut and is twisted on itself in a snug position. The first wire is used to stabilize the spinal reduction until osseous union has occurred. A second, 22-gauge wire is then passed through and around the upper spinous process, and both free ends are tagged with clamps. The same procedure is performed at the lower vertebra. Drill holes are then placed through either end of the one-half-inch–thick corticocancellous iliac grafts.

Each of these grafts is attached to the vertebrae individually with the free ends of the 22-gauge wire, which is passed through the holes in each end of the graft and pulled taut, with the assistant holding the cancellous parts of the graft in place against the laminae and spinous processes. The 22-gauge wire is then twisted down over the iliac graft on each side of the spine (Fig. 33–35). A drain is placed in the wound and removed within 48 hours following the operation. It has been our experience that patients stabilized in this matter may be immediately ambulated to sitting or standing position in a rigid two-poster orthosis (Fig. 33–36).

An additional surgical technique that can be used is posterior cervical fusion using AO reconstruction plates described by Anderson. The size of the plates is either 2.7 mm or 3.5 mm. In general, the smaller size is more malleable and adaptable. Drill holes are placed 1 mm medial to the center of the four boundaries of the

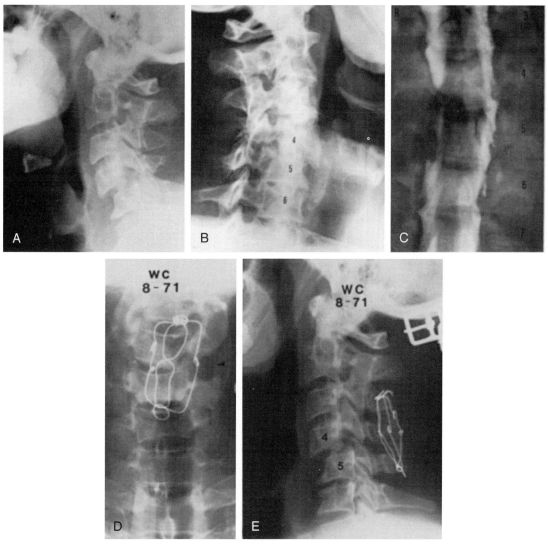

Figure 33–36. *A,* Roentgenogram of a patient with anterior dislocation of C4 on C5. Marked deltoid and mild biceps weakness was present on the right. Dislocation was missed for six weeks because the patient was initially intoxicated and did not complain of neck pain. *B,* Right oblique roentgenogram demonstrates a dislocated C4 facet and a fractured facet occluding the C4–C5 foramina. The latter pathology caused compression of the right fifth nerve root. *C,* Anteroposterior view of the cervical myelogram demonstrating a significant extradural filling defect at C4–C5 on the right, indicating severe fifth nerve root compression. *D,* Anteroposterior roentgenogram of postoperative foraminotomy and posterior arthrodesis. Note the two-wire technique. The first wire is placed through and around the spinous processes of the involved vertebra, locking the unstable vertebra in place, and then an additional wire is placed through the separate iliac bone grafts on either side, through and around the spinous processes, holding the bone grafts against the vertebra involved. *E,* Lateral roentgenogram showing postoperative arthrodesis with the double wiring and iliac bone graft. (*A* and *B* from Bohlman, H. H.: The neck. *In* D'Ambrosia, R. [ed.]: Musculoskeletal Disorders. 2nd ed. Philadelphia, J. B. Lippincott Co., 1986.)

lateral mass, which usually coincides with the highest elevation of the facet. A drill guide is used to allow a Kirschner wire to be used as a drill with advancement of no more than 15 mm. The wire is directed 30 to 40 degrees cranially, parallel to the facet joint, and 10 degrees laterally. The length of screw selected is 1 to 2 mm longer than the length needed to penetrate the far cortex of the lateral mass. The dorsal cortex tap uses a 3.5 mm AO bone tap. The facet joint is decorticated and packed with autogenous bone prior to insertion of the plate. The cancellous bone is added to the re-maining exposed bone. Postoperative immobilization includes a cervicothoracic orthosis for six to eight weeks.

When an anterior cervical vertebrectomy (corpec-tomy) is required to remove crushed bone protruding into the spinal canal, the following technique is used (Fig. 33–37A).[46, 49, 50] The patient is given a general anes-thetic and intubated in the supine position while being protected in skeletal traction. Patient positioning and the anterior cervical approach are performed as pre-viously described. Once the fractured level is identified

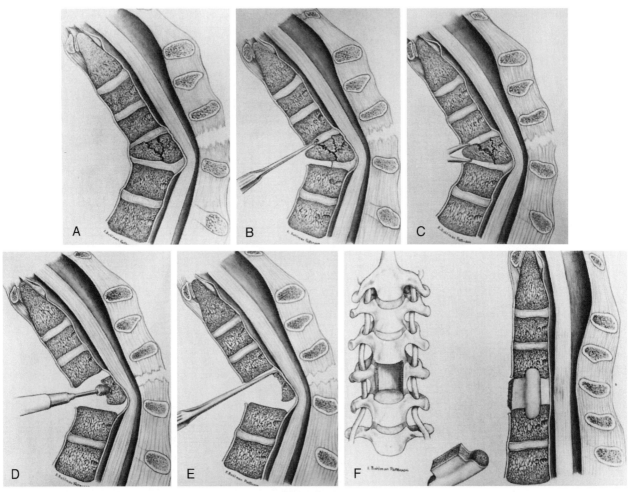

Figure 33–37. *A,* A typical compression fracture with protrusion of disc material, bone fragments, and a kyphotic deformity causing compression of the anterior aspect of the cord. *B,* Lateral view of the cervical spine showing initial removal of disc material on either side of the crushed vertebral body, which is used as a guide to identify the extent of the crushed bone superiorly and inferiorly, as well as posteriorly. *C,* After initial disc removal on either side of the crushed body, hand rongeurs are used to remove the first portion of the crushed vertebral body. *D,* The portion of the remaining crushed vertebral body is removed with a power burr. All of the disc is removed back to the posterior longitudinal ligament to identify the extent of bony protrusion. *E,* The remaining posterior vertebral cortex is removed using a curet to peel the bone from the longitudinal ligament. *F (left),* Anterior view of the cervical spine showing the extent of vertebral body resection to the posterior longitudinal ligament, sparing the lateral cortices to protect the vertebral arteries. The posterior longitudinal ligament is not violated, and no instruments enter the spinal canal. *Right,* A full-thickness iliac crest graft is inserted to replace the resected vertebra. The cortical surface of the crest is placed posteriorly. This procedure corrects the kyphotic deformity and relieves the spinal cord compression. (*A* and *F* from Bohlman, H. H.: Acute fractures and dislocations of the cervical spine. J. Bone Joint Surg. *61A:*1119–1142, 1979. *D* and *E* from Bohlman, H. H., and Eismont, F. J.: Surgical techniques of anterior decompression and fusion for spinal cord injuries. Clin. Orthop. *54:*57–67, 1981.)

by a lateral roentgenogram, the discs above and below the fractured vertebra are partially removed by incision of the anterior longitudinal ligament and curettage of the disc material (Fig. 33–37B); using a hand rongeur, the anterior aspect of the fractured vertebra is removed (Fig. 33–37C). High-intensity headlights and magnifying loops are very helpful at this stage of the procedure. The remaining disc material is cleaned out until the posterior longitudinal ligament is identified above and below the fractured vertebra. A diamond power burr is used at this point to remove more of the vertebral body (Fig. 33–37D) and, finally, the most posterior shell of bone is carefully elevated away from the posterior longitudinal ligament with small curets (Fig. 33–37E). No attempt is made to enter the spinal canal merely to inspect the spinal cord. In most cases, the protruding bone and disc fragments lie anterior to the posterior longitudinal ligament. The latter structure offers protection and strength to the construct. Once the major portion of the crushed vertebra is removed, the surgeons will usually be able to visualize the posterior ligament bulging anteriorly and becoming more convex. The cervical traction is now increased, and the osseous end plates of the vertebra above and below are removed centrally to accept and lock in the iliac graft.

A full-thickness corticocancellous iliac graft is taken with a power saw, shaped to fit the defect created by decompression, and tamped into place with the three-sided cortical portion directed posteriorly. The anterior cancellous bone is smoothed off with rongeurs to protect the esophagus (Fig. 33–37F). The wound is then drained and closed in the usual fashion. The patient is then ambulated in a rigid two-poster cervical orthosis unless posterior ligament tearing has occurred and posterior instability is present, in which case the patient is kept recumbent in skeletal traction until an additional posterior arthrodesis is performed.

Occasionally, a patient will present with a compression fracture producing an anterior cord syndrome and also will have had a severe flexion-distraction injury that has torn the posterior ligament complex. In this instance, it has become our policy to perform posterior stabilization first and then at the same time on a turning frame an anterior decompression and fusion is performed, or at a later date when the patient's medical status permits. Utilization of an anterior vertebral plate could be considered in this situation but biomechanically is not strong in flexion (Fig. 33–38).[178, 361] The patient may then be ambulated in a rigid orthosis (Fig. 33–39).[178]

SPECIFIC LESIONS OF UPPER THORACIC SPINE INJURIES (T2–T10)

Anatomic Considerations

Fractures of the upper thoracic spine differ from the cervical or thoracolumbar spine regions both from an osseous as well as a neurologic standpoint. These fractures are reasonably stable because of the surrounding ribcage and strong costovertebral ligaments that attach the ribs to the vertebral bodies. The ribcage, therefore, acts as a splint, and the relative motion at these levels of the upper thoracic spine is not as great in comparison with the thoracolumbar junction or cervical region, where motion is allowed to a greater extent by virtue of the basic anatomy of the osseous structures.[360] The articular facet joints are more horizontally oriented, which limits rotation around the axial plane; however, they allow for some flexion and extension. Because of the rigid chest cage, severe fracture dislocations of the upper thoracic spine occur only with great force. The thoracic spinal canal is quite narrow between the first and tenth vertebrae and, therefore, the risk of spinal cord damage is also very great with any displacement of the vertebrae. Although herniated discs are quite rare in the upper thoracic region with or without trauma, they can occur by protruding through or beneath the very thin posterior longitudinal ligament and can produce neural compression. The blood supply of the upper thoracic spinal cord may be sparse between the fourth and eighth thoracic vertebrae, where there is the so-called "critical zone"; however, Crock, in his monograph on blood supply of the spine and spinal cord, disputes this and states that the blood supply is quite good in this region.[101] The anterior spinal artery supplies the anterior two thirds of the cord substance, and double posterior spinal arteries supply the posterior third of the spinal cord.[236, 237, 375] The segmental arteries, which branch from the thoracic aorta, supply the anterior spinal and sulcal vessels of the spinal cord. Each segmental artery is located at the midportion of each vertebra under a thin layer of fascia. Inside the spinal canal is an epidural venous plexus that may bleed profusely with trauma of the spinal column. In addition, the segmental arteries send small radicular vessels into the foramina, which are the distribution points of the segmental arteries to the medullary vessels of the spinal cord.

Pathologic Considerations

Bohlman has reviewed and reported 218 upper thoracic spine fractures (T1–T10) with paralysis and analyzed this patient group in detail.[40] The causes of the injuries included missile wounds, both from Viet Nam and civilian injuries, as well as vehicular accidents and falls. Some of these patients were struck by heavy falling objects during industrial injuries. As mentioned previously, associated injuries of the chest, head, and cervical spine were common. Frequently, life-threatening emergencies are present, and cardiovascular, pulmonary, or head trauma takes precedent initially over the spine and spinal cord injury. On analysis of the types of vertebral fractures that occurred, these appeared to be somewhat different from those in the thoracolumbar region. Axial loading or compression fractures occurred most commonly, in which there was either a mild or moderately severe wedge compression fracture and a purely osseous injury (Figs. 33–40 and 33–41). These fractures included retropulsion of bone into the spinal canal to varying degrees. Burst fractures oc-

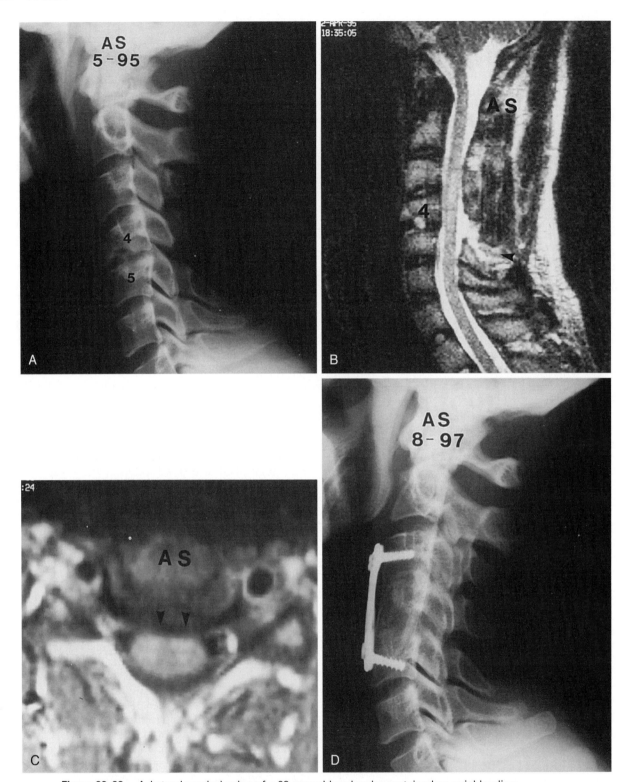

Figure 33–38. *A,* Lateral cervical spine of a 23-year-old male who sustained an axial loading compression fracture of C4 and posterior distraction injury in a motor vehicle accident. He has no paralysis, but persistent neck pain with ligamentous instability. *B,* Sagittal MR image demonstrating the torn posterior ligament complex as well as effacement of the spinal cord at C4. *C,* Axial MR image demonstrating effacement of the spinal cord by bone and disc protrusion. *D,* The patient underwent an anterior cervical corpectomy of C4 and an iliac strut graft with an anterior plate fixation because of the torn posterior ligament complex. Lateral cervical roentgenogram demonstrating complete healing two years following the surgery; the patient was relieved of his pain.

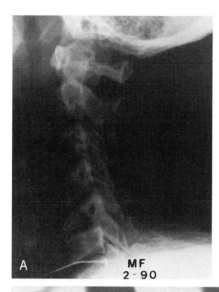

Figure 33–39. *A,* Lateral roentgenogram of an 18-year-old male who sustained an axial loading compression fracture of C5 with quadriparesis and an anterior cord syndrome. Note the posterior ligament disruption between C5 and C6 and the bone protrusion into the spinal canal. *B,* Sagittal reconstruction of the CT scan demonstrates bone protrusion into the spinal canal. *C,* Unenhanced cross-sectional CT scan reveals disc and bone protrusion into the spinal canal. *D,* The patient underwent a microscopic anterior decompression with an autologous rib graft placement at the referring hospital. At this stage he had marked quadriparesis with very little leg or foot function. The kyphotic deformity increased in the halovest and he was referred for further treatment. *E,* Cross-sectional image of the enhanced CT scan reveals the protruding rib graft and continued bone compression of the anterior spinal cord with inadequate decompression of the fracture.

Illustration continued on following page

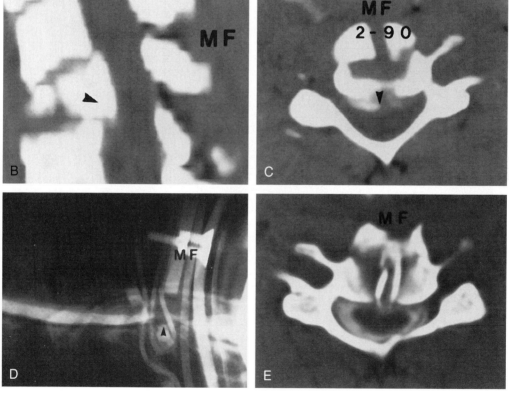

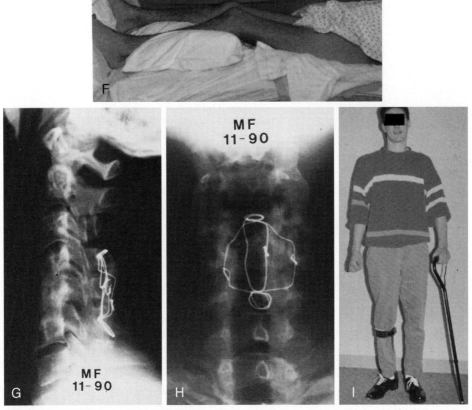

Figure 33–39 *Continued. F,* Photograph of the patient's lower extremities demonstrating no antigravity function; at this point he had only a trace of motor function in multiple muscle groups. *G,* Lateral roentgenogram. Six months after the second operation he underwent an anterior corpectomy, decompression of the spinal cord, and insertion of an iliac graft with intraoperative spinal cord monitoring followed by a posterior arthrodesis at the same operation. *H,* Anteroposterior view of the cervical spine demonstrating the triple-wire technique six months after surgery. *I,* Ambulatory function six months after the second operation: the patient uses a right short leg brace and one cane to walk short distances.

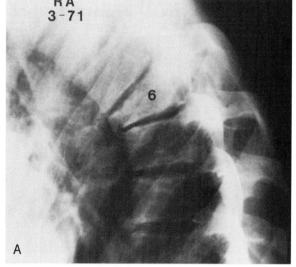

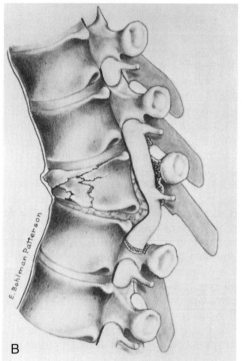

Figure 33–40. *A,* Lateral roentgenogram of a patient with complete paraplegia sustained after a fracture of T6. Note the mild wedge compression with narrowing of the disc spaces, as well as a small anterior fragment. *B,* Drawing of the lateral aspect of the mild wedge compression fracture indicating that bone and disc protrusion may occur against the anterior spinal cord. It is in this type of injury that there is most likely to be incomplete spinal cord injury, less devastating to the spinal cord and therefore more amenable to anterior transthoracic decompression.

Figure 33–41. *A,* Major wedge compression fracture of T3 with protrusion of bone into the spinal canal. The patient was paraplegic with sparing of posterior column functions. *B,* Major wedge compression fracture of the thoracic vertebra with severe disc and bone displacement anteriorly as well as into the spinal canal. Interspinous ligamentous tearing occurs posteriorly with separation of the spinous processes. Usually this type of fracture is associated with a complete cord injury.

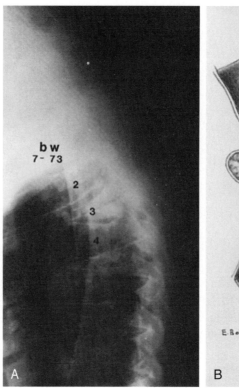

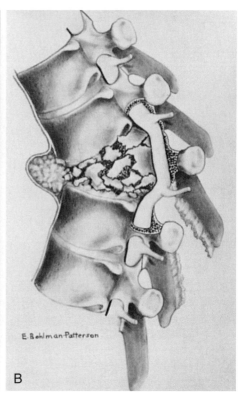

curred, which predominantly are osseous injuries in which an entire vertebra is retropulsed into the spinal canal and laterally to either side so that roentgenographically there appears to be no vertebra left on the anteroposterior or lateral view. On counting individual ribs, it is apparent that the vertebra has burst into the surrounding tissues. This fracture is ordinarily associated with a complete spinal cord injury (Fig. 33–42). Because of very little rotational ability of the upper thoracic spine, most of the osseous injuries occur in flexion or extension or gradations of each. One particular fracture that appeared to be dissimilar from thoracolumbar regional injuries was what we termed a sagittal slice fracture. This additionally is most purely osseous, in which the vertebra above slices down in a sagittal plane through the vertebra below, displacing half of the vertebra below laterally. Roentgenographically, this appears as a telescoped vertebra above overlapping the one below on an anteroposterior view. The more cephalic vertebral column is displaced to the side of the shear fracture. On the lateral roentgenogram, there appears to be a complete overlap of one vertebra on another (Fig. 33–43). The latter are severe injuries and ordinarily are associated with complete spinal cord damage. Predominantly ligamentous injuries may occur with varying degrees of anterior dislocation in which the posterior ligament complex is torn (Fig. 33–44) or, more rarely, posterior dislocation of the upper vertebra on the lower segment occurs (Fig. 33–45). Anterior or posterior dislocations may be associated with varying degrees of ligamentous tearing and occa-

sionally with wedging of the vertebra involved. On rare occasions in the upper thoracic spine, complete or near complete dislocation of the osseous elements may occur. This is a total ligamentous disruption occurring with severe violence, and bilateral facet dislocations result, in which case the upper vertebra is 100 per cent displaced on the one below and is telescoped anterior to the distal segment. This situation creates an overlap of two vertebral bodies on the anteroposterior roentgenogram, and a total displacement of the cephalic vertebra in front of the caudal one on the lateral roentgenogram (Fig. 33–46). These injuries are, of course, associated with total disruption of the spinal cord and complete paraplegia.

In rare instances, a massive thoracic intervertebral disc herniation occurs with paraparesis or complete paraplegia. This is difficult to diagnose unless on roentgenograms the intervertebral disc space is narrowed or myelography and CT scan or MRI are carried out to delineate the soft disc herniation. In the instance of the herniated disc with incomplete cord lesion, this patient should be decompressed anteriorly either by costotransversectomy or the transthoracic technique (Fig. 33–47).[35]

Instability

Although a gross instability in an acute injury of the upper thoracic spine is unusual because of the supporting chest cage, this can occur, and the patient has to have spinal instrumentation and posterior fusion.

Text continued on page 947

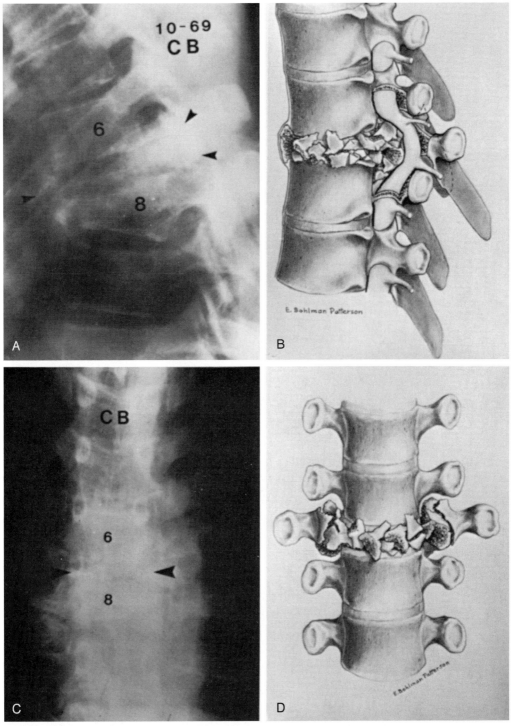

Figure 33–42. *A,* Lateral roentgenogram of a patient sustaining a severe burst fracture of T7 with retropulsion of a major portion of the vertebral body into the spinal canal. Note that there is only a thin wafer of bone left in the original vertebral space occupied by T7. There also is anterior bone expulsion. The patient was completely paraplegic. *B,* Drawing of a massive burst fracture from the lateral aspect. Note the telescoping of the upper vertebrae on the distal ones and massive bone protrusion into the spinal canal. This is ordinarily associated with a complete spinal cord injury. *C,* Anteroposterior roentgenogram demonstrating the burst fracture occurring at T7. Note that the vertebral body is exploded out to the side and there is very little space left for the original vertebra between the sixth and eighth levels. *D,* Anteroposterior view of a burst fracture with telescoping of the vertebrae above and below. Note that the lateral masses and transverse processes are displaced laterally to either side.

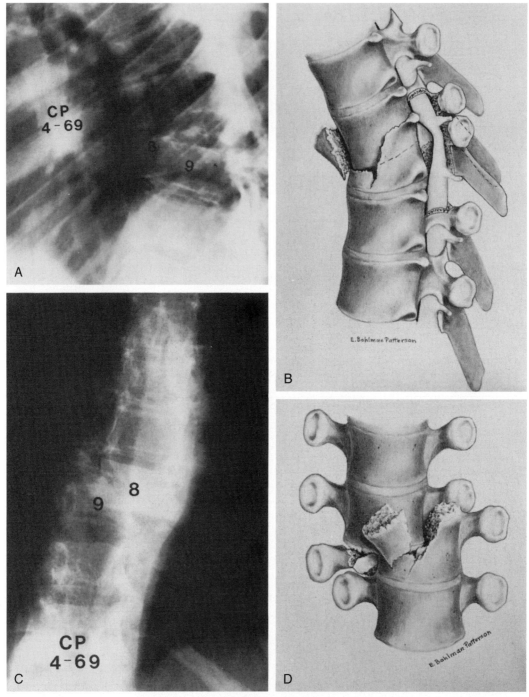

Figure 33–43. *A,* Lateral roentgenogram of a patient sustaining a sagittal slice fracture with dislocation of T8 on T9. Note the overlap of the vertebral bodies on the lateral view. The patient was completely paraplegic. *B,* Drawing of the sagittal slice fracture from the lateral view indicating that the more cephalic vertebra compresses the lower vertebra, producing a slice fracture in the sagittal plane. On lateral view this produces telescoping of the cephalic vertebra on the more caudal one. This type of fracture is almost always associated with a complete spinal cord injury. *C,* Anteroposterior roentgenogram of the patient revealing the sagittal slice fracture through the ninth vertebral body with telescoping of the eighth on the ninth vertebral bodies. There is also lateral shift of the individual vertebra. *D,* Drawing of the anteroposterior view of a sagittal slice fracture indicating the sagittal plane of the fracture and the lateral displacement of one vertebra on another.

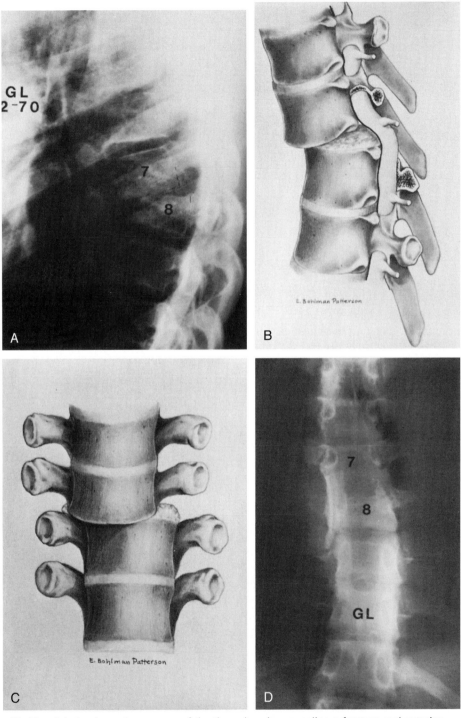

Figure 33–44. *A,* Lateral roentgenogram of the thoracic spine revealing a fracture and anterior subluxation of T7 on T8 secondary to a vehicular accident. *B,* Drawing of the lateral view of an anterior subluxation of the upper thoracic vertebrae. The disc space and longitudinal ligaments are disrupted, and this may result in incomplete spinal cord injury. *C,* Anteroposterior drawing of the anterior subluxation of the thoracic vertebrae indicating disc disruption and some lateral displacement of the vertebral bodies. *D,* Anteroposterior view of the patient after laminectomy. Note the slight lateral displacement of the upper seventh vertebra on the lower eighth vertebra.

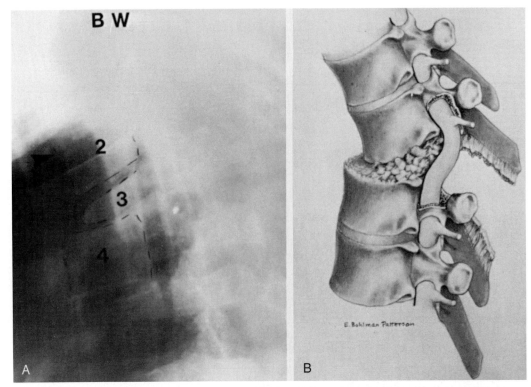

Figure 33–45. *A,* Lateral roentgenogram of a patient sustaining a fracture of the third vertebral body with posterior displacement of T2 and T3 in relationship to T4. The patient was completely paraplegic. *B,* Drawing of the lateral view of a posterior subluxation of upper thoracic vertebrae that includes posterior ligamentous as well as disc disruption.

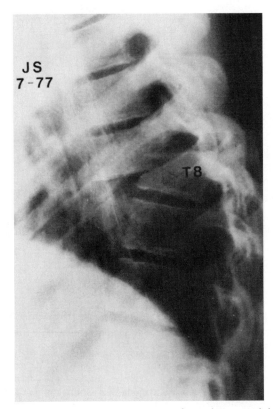

Figure 33–46. Lateral roentgenogram of a patient sustaining a complete dislocation of T7 on T8 after a vehicular accident. The patient was completely paraplegic. This represents marked ligamentous tearing and instability in the upper thoracic spine.

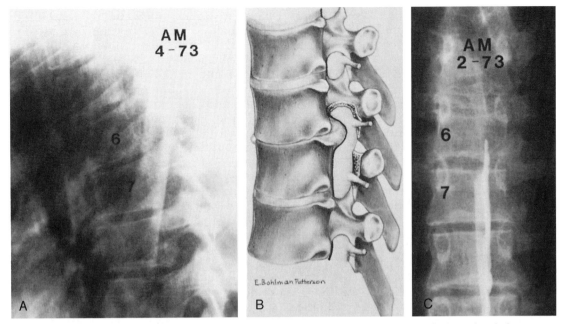

Figure 33–47. *A,* Lateral roentgenogram of a patient sustaining a complete paraplegia at the sixth thoracic level after a vehicular accident. Note the slight narrowing of the disc space between T6 and T7. No fractures could be discerned on the film. *B,* Drawing of the lateral view of a herniated disc protrusion in the upper thoracic spine, producing anterior cord compression. Usually the disc space is narrowed on the lateral roentgenogram, and this may be associated with either incomplete or complete cord lesions. *C,* Anteroposterior myelogram of a patient demonstrating complete block of the dye column at the interspace between the sixth and seventh thoracic vertebrae, indicating a large disc protrusion.

Instability in the upper thoracic area includes complete dislocation or abnormal motion of the vertebral segments with or without pain or increasing neurologic deficit. The latter problem is extremely uncommon in upper thoracic spine and cord injuries. Severe kyphosis may occur in those rare instances of complete dislocations of the vertebral bodies or in patients who have had laminectomies with removal of the posterior elements, in whom greater than 40 degrees of kyphosis exists secondary to a compression fracture anteriorly

(Fig. 33–48).[247, 299] Sagittal slice fractures may progress to some degree and telescope; however, this is usually not a major problem and the fractures heal with massive callus. Progressive dislocation as well as increasing kyphotic deformity may occur following laminectomy. Ducker has pointed out experimentally that immediate stability of the spine is important for recovery of spinal cord function.[130] The types of fractures that are generally stable in the thoracic spine are simple compression fractures in which major ligament tearing has not oc-

Figure 33–48. This lateral roentgenogram of a thoracolumbar fracture-dislocation was taken after a laminectomy and attempted posterior fusion in a patient who sustained complete paraplegia secondary to a vehicular accident. Removal of the posterior elements in this severe injury resulted in further dislocation of the vertebrae postoperatively and severe kyphosis.

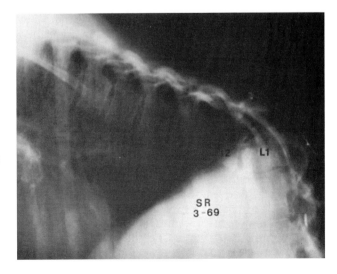

curred, burst fractures, mild subluxations, and gunshot wounds of the spine. Patients with the latter types of injuries may be ambulated in a molded orthosis when comfortable.

Spinal Cord Lesions

In Bohlman's[40] review of upper thoracic spine fractures with paralysis, approximately five sixths of the patients sustained a complete cord lesion with resultant complete paraplegia, and one sixth of the injuries resulted in some type of incomplete cord syndrome. The most common type of incomplete cord syndrome resembled the anterior cord syndrome described by Schneider[317] for the cervical region; that is, an incomplete paraparesis or complete paraplegia with sparing of posterior column modalities (position and vibratory sense with varying degrees of sacral sensation sparing). Usually, the incomplete paraparetic patient has an associated anterior wedge compression fracture with bone protrusion into the spinal canal to varying degrees or a mild anterior subluxation of the upper vertebral body on the lower segment. A less common spinal cord syndrome occurring in upper thoracic spine injuries is the Brown-Séquard syndrome with motor paralysis on one side of the body distal to the level lesion and sensory disassociation on the opposite side. This, of course, may occur with either fractures or stab wounds of the spinal canal and cord. A type of central cord syndrome occurred in a few patients with incomplete lesions in which the proximal trunk musculature was weaker than the distal muscles around the ankles and feet, with varying degrees of sensory loss. Finally, a few patients with incomplete cord lesions have a mixed type of injury with a paraparesis and an additional component of Brown-Séquard syndrome; that is, predominantly greater motor loss on one side as well as an element of sensory disassociation.

The diagnosis of spinal cord injury in the upper thoracic region is not as easily missed as it is in the cervical area; however, a number of patients can be mistaken for being hysterical if they have predominantly a motor loss with very little sensory loss, as occurred in a few of the patients reviewed. Ordinarily, these patients have sustained severe trauma and have other associated injuries that bring the attention to the spine and the paralysis that exists.

Treatment Methods

In principle, the treatment of upper thoracic spine fractures depends on the osseous as well as neurologic lesion. The treating physician must decide whether the osseous injury is stable or unstable, as reviewed before. Generally, mild wedge compression fractures, gunshot wounds, or mild subluxations of vertebrae are reasonably stable, and these patients may be ambulated within seven days in a molded orthosis. Patients with more severe osseous fractures, such as the sagittal slice fracture, the burst fracture, and the severe wedge compression fracture, should be treated with recumbency

for seven days or until surgically stabilized and then be ambulated to a wheelchair in a molded orthosis. These types of fractures do not usually require a surgical stabilization of any type. Patients with paralysis are divided into the complete and the incomplete cord-injured. In the patient with a complete cord injury lasting more than 48 hours, there should be no consideration for performing any decompressive procedure. In the review of these injuries by Bohlman, no surgical or nonsurgical treatment made any difference in complete cord injuries as far as recovery of neurologic function was concerned. That is, patients treated without surgery and appropriate recumbency until the osseous lesion was healed did just as well as patients treated with any type of decompression or stabilization procedure. As mentioned previously, these are very stable injuries from an osseous standpoint, and following a week of recumbency, most of these lesions will be healed enough to ambulate the patient in a molded orthosis. We do not recommend any stabilization procedure in the complete paraplegic patient with upper thoracic spine fractures unless a total dislocation exists, in which case severe gibbous deformity may result; in this instance, posterior open reduction and fusion with distraction rod fixation is indicated. Mild wedge compression fractures or minimal dislocations may be associated with incomplete spinal cord injury, and the approach to treatment in this instance is different. Almost all of these individuals will have anterior spinal cord compression by bone or disc fragments, in which case myelography with CT scan and MRI is used to demonstrate the cord compression. An early anterior transthoracic decompression and fusion are indicated to remove fragments of bone and disc that may be compressing the cord.[40, 285] This is carried out as soon as the medical status of the patient permits general anesthesia. The results of neurologic recovery for incomplete lesions are far superior with anterior decompression. Of the eight cases reported, six became ambulators and two recovered partially; of 17 treated by laminectomy, eight became completely paralyzed. The technique of anterior decompression may be by the transthoracic approach, which is our preference,[285] or by costotransversectomy,[84, 234] but the latter operation does not allow good visualization of the spinal cord or spinal column. The technique of transthoracic decompression that we prefer is described next (Fig. 33–49). Krengel et al.[229] reported on early stabilization and decompression for incomplete paraplegia in 14 patients with upper thoracic fractures. They found that early surgical reduction, stabilization, and decompression are safe and improved neurologic recovery in comparison to historic control subjects treated by postural reduction or late surgical intervention.

Operative Techniques

The patient who is to have anterior transthoracic decompression at the third through tenth thoracic levels is placed in the lateral decubitus position for a standard thoracotomy with the table slightly flexed (Fig. 33–

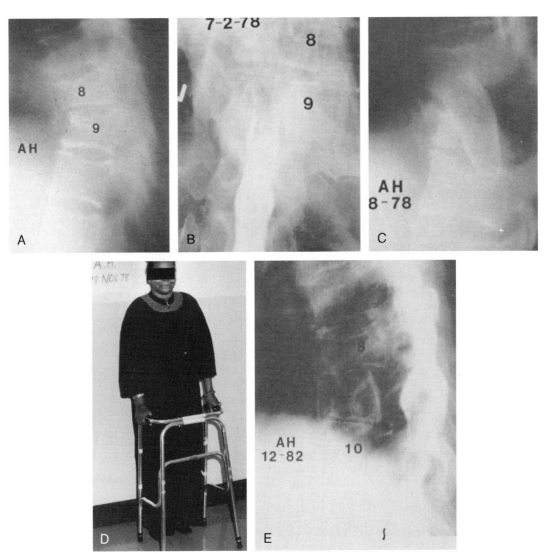

Figure 33–49. *A,* Lateral tomogram of a patient who sustained a fracture and anterior subluxation of the eighth and ninth thoracic vertebrae when a large steel beam fell on her back. This resulted in anterior spinal cord quadriparesis, with Grade B neurologic loss. *B,* Anteroposterior myelogram of the thoracic vertebrae, demonstrating total obstruction at the ninth thoracic level. *C,* Lateral tomogram of the spine six weeks after transthoracic anterior decompression and arthrodesis with an iliac graft. The patient recovered and was fully able to walk without braces six months after the operation. Note the early incorporation of the bone and area of decompression. *D,* The patient standing and walking with a walker four months after surgery. *E,* Lateral roentgenogram four years after thoracic decompression and fusion. The iliac graft is well incorporated. The patient recovered to normal Grade D neurologic function and walked without aid.

50*A*). We prefer to approach the spine through the right side to avoid the great vessels and the heart, and the exposure is made as a standard thoracotomy at the rib level corresponding to the vertebral fracture level. This allows exposure of one vertebra above and several vertebrae below the fracture. Once the thoracotomy has been performed and the self-retaining retractors are placed, the surgeon can visualize the vertebral bodies, and usually the fractured vertebra bulges out laterally to a certain extent. The thin layer of parietal pleura is seen, under which the segmental arteries and veins can be visualized. The segmental vessels lie in a small amount of fatty tissue between the periosteum and parietal pleura. The parietal pleura is then split longitudinally and is reflected gently to expose the segmental vessels. The segmental vessels over the fractured vertebra are then ligated with heavy silk sutures, transected, and mobilized dorsally and ventrally to expose the periosteum (Fig. 33–50*B*). The periosteum is then reflected from the vertebral bodies, exposing the crushed vertebra that is to be decompressed (Fig. 33–50*C*). At this point, the base of the rib is dissected free subperiosteally, and approximately four inches of the proximal rib are removed by transecting the costovertebral ligaments. This exposes the rib bed and the neurovascular bundle. The intercostal nerve is identified and followed

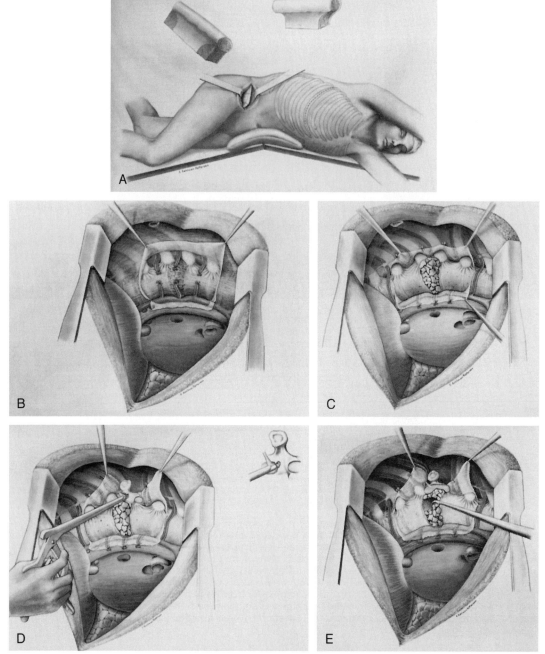

Figure 33–50. *A,* Artist's drawing of positioning of the patient for transthoracic anterior decompression and fusion. A standard thoracotomy is used through the rib associated with the specific fractured vertebra. The iliac crest is exposed and a full-thickness, three-sided corticocancellous graft is used. *B,* Transthoracic view of the crushed thoracic vertebra as seen through the periosteum. The parietal pleura has been reflected and the segmental vessels have been ligated. The diaphragm is shown to the left and the lung has been excluded on the right side. *C,* View of the transthoracic approach with the periosteum, segmental vessels, and parietal pleura reflected from the crushed vertebra. At this point the intercostal nerve is identified under the rib to be removed to lead the surgeon into the foramina, and therefore the spinal canal. *D,* Once the base of the rib has been removed, the intercostal nerve is followed into the foraminal area to identify the pedicle of the crushed vertebra. The pedicle is then delineated with a periosteal elevator and removed with a 40-degree Kerrison punch, exposing the dura and spinal cord. *E,* The decompression of the crushed vertebra is begun by removing the disc cephalically as well as caudally and the midportion of the vertebral body with a curet. Note that once the pedicle is removed, the crushed vertebra can be seen compressing the cord from the anterior aspect.

Illustration continued on opposite page

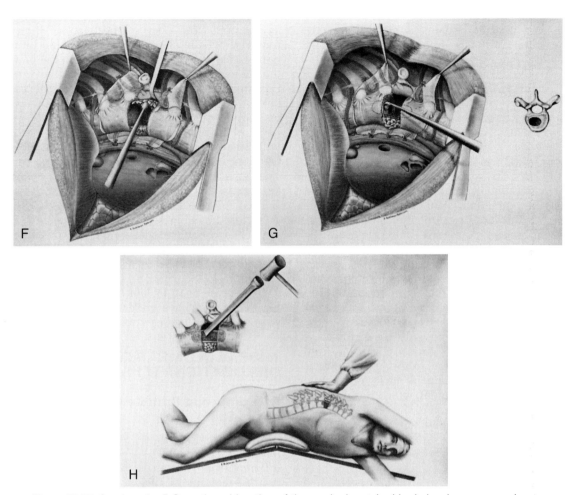

Figure 33–50 *Continued. F,* Once the midportion of the crushed vertebral body has been removed, attention is drawn to the posteriorly protruding fracture fragments that compress the spinal cord. Care is used to dissect the dura away from the fractured bone with a Penfield elevator, and once this has been freed the final bone and fracture fragments are pulled away from the spinal cord with a long-handled curet, care being taken to protect the spinal cord from trauma. *G,* After decompression of the crushed vertebral body, the spinal cord and dura are seen to expand into a more normal, round configuration. A bed for the bone graft is prepared by undermining the vertebral body above and the one below with a large curet. *H,* With an assistant placing a hand on the gibbus deformity posteriorly, the full-thickness iliac graft is inserted in the undermined area above and below and is tamped into place. The three-sided cortical portion of the graft is placed within the vertebral bodies for additional axial-loading strength in the erect position. (*E* from Bohlman, H. H., and Eismont, F. J.: Surgical techniques of anterior decompression and fusion for spinal cord injuries. Clin. Orthop. *154:*54–67, 1981.)

toward the pedicle of the crushed vertebra, identifying the foramina and the spinal canal, which is not easily seen but can be palpated gently. At this point, the pedicle that is to be removed is delineated with a periosteal elevator at its lateral, superior, and inferior aspects. The dura should then be identified where the nerve root exists. A high-intensity headlight and magnifying loupes are useful to visualize the structures. At this point, using an angled Kerrison punch, the pedicle is removed, exposing the underlying dura that is compressed from the anterior aspect by the crushed vertebra (Fig. 33–50D). The surgeon should be able to easily visualize the compressive pathology and, using a Penfield elevator, a plane of dissection is developed between the dura and the posterior longitudinal liga-

ment, so there is no scarring against the dura that will allow tearing of the dura during the decompression. Epidural bleeding is controlled with gelatin sponges and patties and with the use of bipolar coagulation. The adjacent intervertebral discs are then removed by incising the lateral annulus and curetting free the disc material. This identifies the upper and lower boundaries of the fractured vertebra that is to be removed. With the use of long-handled curets and gouges, the midportion of the vertebral body is removed (Fig. 33–50E) and bone wax is used for excessive bony bleeders. When the entire midportion of the vertebral body has been removed toward the opposite cortex, this then leaves a shell of posteriorly protruding bone (Fig. 33–50F). After the entire decompression has been performed, one can usually visualize a marked enlargement of the spinal cord and dural sac with resumption of pulsation of the dura. Care must be taken to decompress the spinal cord completely across the entire spinal canal, so that no shell of bone is left on the opposite side. At this point, a bed for the bone graft is prepared by removing the midportion of the superior end plate of the vertebra most cephalad and the inferior end plate of the vertebra caudad (Fig. 33–50G). The iliac graft is taken in the usual fashion, and the three-sided cortex of the superior aspect of the iliac crest is used for placement within the troughs formed in the end plate of the vertebral body above and below. This forms an internal strut of iliac bone that is quite strong, and additional bone chips may be placed beneath the periosteum, if necessary. Pressure is placed on the gibbous deformity posteriorly while the graft is tamped into place and countersunk. The graft is fashioned in a T-shape so that either end of the T can be locked into place in the hollows of the vertebra above and below (Fig. 33–50H). The parietal pleura is closed over the vertebral bodies to the extent possible. Gelatin foam is placed over the exposed dura to arrest any epidural bleeders that may still be present. In the upper thoracic spine decompressions, no attempt is made to preserve the posterior longitudinal ligament, which is quite thin, as opposed to the decompression of the cervical region. A chest tube is placed, and the wound is closed in the usual fashion. The chest tube is connected to underwater suction drainage and removed when drainage has ceased, usually on the third day. The patient is kept recumbent in a regular bed and turned every two hours for approximately four days. At this point, the patient is ambulated in a total contact thoracic orthosis. The iliac graft usually has healed to a great extent by eight weeks, and by three months osseous union has occurred, which can be assessed by anteroposterior and lateral roentgenograms.

A costotransversectomy approach can be used in those patients in whom small bone fragments are compressing the cord and a large bone graft is not necessary, or in the rare patient with a thoracic disc herniation in which a small bone graft is to be used or less exposure is necessary. We have found the transthoracic approach much easier, however, and there is much better visualization for placement of a large graft, especially if a complete vertebrectomy is to be performed. The costotransversectomy approach is as follows: The patient is placed in the lateral decubitus position and is rolled toward the operating surgeon, who stands on the ventral side of the patient. The patient's arms are extended above on the operating table. A curved incision is made, centering over the gibbous and fractured vertebra. The dissection is carried down through the latissimus dorsi fascia, and this is incised along the line of the incision. The erector spinae muscle is identified and dissected away from at least one rib above and one rib below the fractured vertebra. Perforating vessels are clamped and cauterized. The transverse processes of the three ribs exposed are removed, exposing the base of the ribs and the costovertebral

ligamentous attachments. The bases of three ribs are removed by subperiosteal dissection, and blunt dissection is carried out laterally external to the pleura along the lateral surface of the vertebral body. As in the transthoracic approach, the intercostal nerve existing below the pedicle of the fractured vertebra is exposed by subperiosteal dissection and delineated at its superior and inferior borders. The pedicle is then removed with an angled Kerrison punch, exposing the dura and the compressive pathology anterior to the spinal cord. The bone or disc protrusion is removed in the same fashion as in the transthoracic approach. An iliac graft is used if bone grafting is necessary. This wound is then closed over a drain in the usual fashion. Postoperative chest roentgenograms are taken to be certain there is no pneumothorax. The patient is treated following surgery in the same way as for transthoracic decompression.

In the case of an isolated herniated disc with incomplete cord injury, we prefer the transthoracic technique published by Zdeblick and Bohlman.[35, 376]

THORACOLUMBAR FRACTURES AND DISLOCATIONS (T11–L5)

Anatomic and Pathologic Considerations of the Spine

As previously mentioned, the thoracolumbar junction injuries of the spine and spinal cord are completely different from an osseous as well as a neurologic standpoint. Fractures at this level of the spine are much more unstable following the acute injury than are the upper spine fractures.[47, 119, 164, 165, 205, 206]

Various authors have classified thoracolumbar spinal fractures in relation to the mechanism of injury and resultant stability or instability.[205, 299] Ferguson and Allen[154] as well as McAfee[265] and Denis[116] have contributed greatly to the mechanistic classification of thoracolumbar fractures. Out of their writings have come the three-column concept, dividing the vertebrae into the anterior, middle, and posterior columns. White and Panjabi used a biomechanical analysis of motion of the contiguous spinal segments as a basis for a classification of injuries.[360] They presupposed six degrees of freedom in spinal motion, with compression-distraction and rotation occurring in the Y axis, flexion-extension and lateral translation in the X axis, and lateral flexion and anterior posterior translation in the Z axis. The three-dimensional description of forces is then translated into anatomic variations visualized by multiplanar CT. Panjabi and others[281] more recently tested the validity of the three-column theory of thoracolumbar fractures in a biomechanical investigation. Their results from this study supported the three-column theory and the concept of the middle column being the primary determinant of mechanical stability of this region of the spine. McAfee combined the classifications of other authors into a more simplified system based on three forces as they act to injure the middle column: axial compression, axial distraction, and trans-

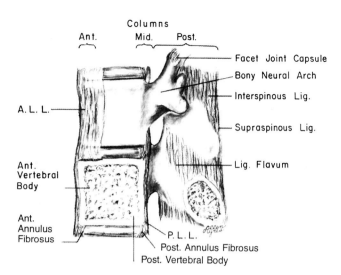

Figure 33–51. The anatomic structures making up the three longitudinal columns of stability in the thoracolumbar spine. Anterior column: anterior two thirds of the vertebral body, anterior part of the annulus fibrosus, and anterior longitudinal ligament. Middle column: posterior one third of the vertebral body, posterior part of the annulus fibrosus, and posterior longitudinal ligament. Posterior column: facet joint capsules, ligamentum flavum, osseous neural arch, supraspinous ligament, interspinous ligament, and articular processes. (From McAfee, P. C., Yuan, H. A., Fredrickson, B. E., and Lubicky, J. P.: The value of computed tomography in thoracolumbar fractures. J. Bone Joint Surg. *65A*:462, 1983.)

lation within the transverse plane (Figs. 33–51, 33–52, and 33–53). There are, therefore, basically six kinds of injury: (1) a wedge compression fracture, which is an injury resulting from forward flexion causing isolated failure of the anterior column. This is rarely associated with neural loss (Fig. 33–54). (2) A stable burst fracture is one in which the anterior and middle columns fail because of a compressive load without loss of integrity of the posterior elements (Fig. 33–55). (3) An unstable burst fracture is one in which anterior and middle columns fail in compression and the posterior column is disrupted, but does not fail in distraction because of the anterior and middle columns failing in compression (Fig. 33–56). (4) Chance fracture is a horizontal avulsion injury of the intervertebral body as a result of flexion about an axis, anterior to the anterior longitudinal ligament. The entire vertebra is pulled apart by a strong tensile force. This is the so-called seat-belt injury (Fig. 33–57).[208, 296, 331] Rumball and Jarvis reported, in 1992, 10 seat-belt injuries to the spine in young children. Paraplegia occurred in 3 of the patients; 4 individuals

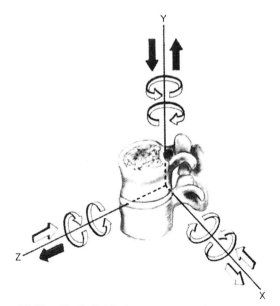

Figure 33–52. The individual components of a complex spinal injury can be analyzed with reference to the X, Y, and Z axes. In the X axis there are three mechanisms of injury: flexion, extension, and left and right lateral translation. In the Y axis there are axial compression, axial distraction, and clockwise and counterclockwise rotation. In the Z axis there are lateral flexion to either side and anterior or posterior translation. Axial compression, axial distraction, and translation are of prognostic significance and correlate with specific patterns of injury. (Adapted from White, A. A., and Panjabi, M. M.: Clinical Biomechanics of the Spine. Philadelphia, J. B. Lippincott Co., 1978, p. 38.)

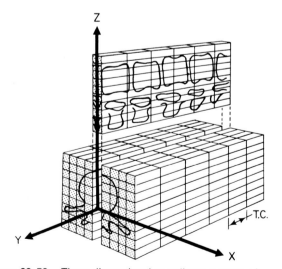

Figure 33–53. Three-dimensional coordinate system of multiplane computed tomography. A sagittal reconstructed image through the middle column has been derived from a series of transaxial cuts (T.C.). (From McAfee, P. C., Yuan, H. A., Fredrickson, B. E., and Lubicky, J. P.: The value of computed tomography in thoracolumbar fractures. J. Bone Joint Surg. *65A*:463, 1983.)

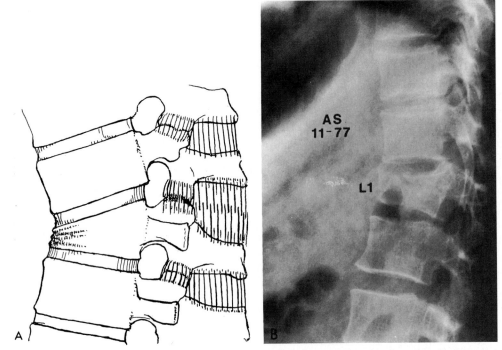

Figure 33–54. *A,* Axial loading compression fracture of the lumbar spine with the posterior ligamentous structures intact, producing a stable fracture. (From Holdsworth, F. W., and Hardy, A.: Early treatment of paraplegia from fractures of the thoracolumbar spine. J. Bone Joint Surg. *35B:*540–550, 1953.) *B,* Lateral roentgenogram of a patient sustaining a compression fracture of L1 having fallen from a second-story window, landing on his buttocks. He had a mild paraparesis with protrusion of bone into the spinal canal, necessitating anterolateral decompression at a later date because of increasing claudication.

sustained intra-abdominal injuries requiring laparotomy, and all had contusion of the abdominal wall as a "seat-belt sign." All 10 patients were treated conservatively with bed rest and then hyperextension casts.[309] (5) A flexion-distraction injury is one in which the flexion axis is posterior to the anterior longitudinal ligament and there is compressive failure of the anterior column, while the middle and posterior columns fail in tension. The posterior longitudinal ligament is torn, and if the facet joint capsules are disrupted, there may be subluxation or dislocation or fracture of the facets. This is similar to the flexion-type injury described by Holdsworth (Fig. 33–58; see Figs. 33–15 and 33–63). (6) Translational injuries occur when the alignment of the neural canal has been disrupted and the spinal column, therefore, has been displaced in the transverse plane. Usually all three columns have failed due to shear forces. This type of injury includes Holdsworth's so-called slice fracture as well as rotational fracture-dislocation and pure dislocation (Fig. 33–59).

A very uncommon injury is a pure extension injury of the lumbar spine, described by Ferguson and Allen as distractive extension, in which the anterior and middle columns are disrupted in extension and the upper vertebra is displaced posteriorly on the one below (Fig. 33–60).

All acute thoracolumbar fractures should be considered unstable initially and, therefore, immobilization and splinting should be provided. Ultimate stability after surgical or nonsurgical treatment is a matter of individual judgment.[198] Ching et al.[91] reported a biomechanical study comparing residual stability in thoracolumbar spine fractures using neutral zone measurements. They stated that burst fractures retained the least residual stability, and compression fractures the greatest, with flexion-distraction injuries having similar biomechanical characteristics to those of burst fractures.

McLain et al.[268] pointed out that pedicle screw rod fixation utilized in thoracolumbar fractures will commonly fail if the anterior column is unstable; therefore, the system is contraindicated in anterior column fractures.

Although a simple wedge compression fracture secondary to axial loading and flexion forces may not tear the posterior ligament complex, this may be associated with posterior osseous protrusion into the spinal canal with or without obvious neural compression and paralysis. If this situation exists, the patient cannot be immediately ambulated and may have to be treated surgically. It must be determined whether there is osseous protrusion into the spinal canal that is significant and may produce late neural compression and paralysis or whether the immediate bony compression is of significance with its associated paralysis. Spinal canal myelography with CT scanning or MRI may be very beneficial in aiding the surgeon in a decision as to whether a decompressive operation should be performed.[258] If a

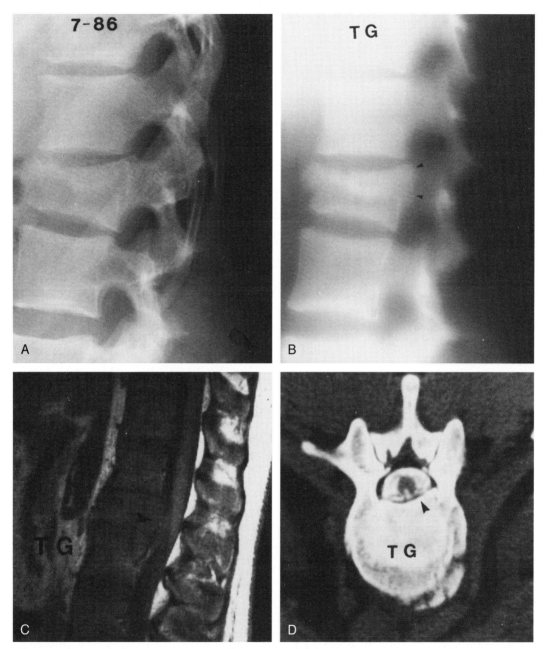

Figure 33–55. *A,* Lateral roentgenogram of a young male who sustained a purely axial loading injury of L1 with approximately 30 per cent compression of the vertebral body in both the anterior and middle columns. *B,* Lateral tomogram reveals a small bony protrusion into the spinal canal, and the posterior elements are intact. *C,* Lateral view of MRI scan demonstrating a small bone protrusion into the spinal canal and a small hematoma at the level of the conus. Note that there is no posterior ligament disruption. *D,* Enhanced CT scan reveals only a small amount of unilateral bone protrusion against the dural sac without deformation of the conus. There are no fractures of the posterior elements. The patient was treated conservatively with a molded thoracolumbar orthosis for three months.

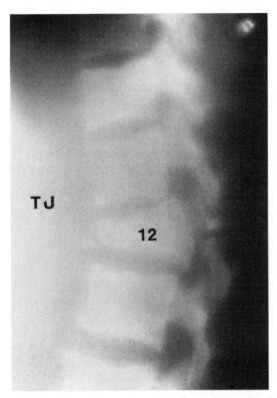

Figure 33–56. Lateral roentgenogram of an axial loading injury that has disrupted the anterior, middle, and posterior columns. The patient was paraparetic. Note the anterior column failure, the protrusion of bone into the spinal canal from the middle column, and the posterior column osseous disruption.

compression fracture is wedged greater than 40 per cent, then it usually requires a stabilization procedure posteriorly, if it is not associated with a neural deficit. Frequently, these fractures compress further even after they have consolidated at three months following the injury; therefore, a posterior fusion with instrumentation may be indicated. More severe wedge compression fractures in association with subluxations or dislocations usually indicate a disruption of the posterior ligament complex, which is a more unstable situation. The indications for doing a surgical stabilization in this case are much greater.[2, 19, 39, 65, 66, 176, 339, 367] Once again, posterior instrumentation in conjunction with a fusion can be carried out to gain stabilization. Subluxations and dislocations of the thoracolumbar spine may occur by total disruption of the posterior ligament complex, as well as the anterior disc and longitudinal ligaments. This may be an unstable situation and may endanger the neural structures if further subluxation occurs. The decision then has to be made whether posterior stabilization is indicated.[119, 181, 241]

We agree with McAfee that compression and distraction injuries of the middle complex should be appropriately treated by posterior distraction and compression instrumentation, respectively.[265] In translational injuries, routine distraction instrumentation is contraindicated because of the risk of overdistraction. Therefore, pedicle screw and rod fixation would be appropriate.

In treating patients with thoracolumbar fractures and a neurologic deficit, consideration must be taken of whether there is persistent neural compression by middle column bone fragments protruding into the spinal canal. In general, 75 per cent of thoracolumbar junction fractures will be some variation of burst or wedge compression fracture with bone protrusion into the spinal canal, especially in those patients with neurologic deficit. An additional important fact is that approximately 75 per cent of patients with thoracolumbar spine injuries and neurologic deficit will be incompletely injured neurologically, with some sparing of cauda equina or conus function. Both of these are important facts when considering anterior decompression and fusion primarily.[33, 39, 262, 297]

Patients with a complete cord and cauda equinal injury with grossly unstable translational fractures will require posterior reduction and internal fixation with arthrodesis. Primary anterior decompression is preferred for patients who have incomplete neurologic injury with a compression or burst fracture, if the posterior ligament complex has not been disrupted. This, of course, can be proved by MRI. In this situation, a retroperitoneal anterior decompression and fusion with iliac bone graft can accomplish a total decompression of the middle column and anterior spinal canal and stabilization without the necessity of internal fixation. If, however, as in the cervical spine, a flexion and distraction injury has occurred with total disruption of the posterior ligament complex, then it is appropriate to carry out posterior stabilization with distraction instrumentation and arthrodesis first and then reassess the spinal canal to see if there is any remaining bone fragment compression of the neural structures. If the latter is present, then an anterior retroperitoneal decompression is done at a later date. An alternative to the combined procedure would be a primary anterior retroperitoneal decompression and fixation with an anterior vertebral body device, such as described by Kaneda. More bulky anterior fixation devices have been associated with erosion and rupture of the aorta.[76] Shono and others[328] have demonstrated in an experimental study of thoracolumbar burst fractures that an anterior reconstruction method permits effective decompression of the spinal canal and offers superior mechanical stability compared with indirect decompression and stabilization with posterior instrumentation.

The question arises as to how much bone protrusion into the spinal canal warrants an anterior decompression. Delamarter and Bohlman have carried out an experimental study of lumbar spinal stenosis with graded compression of the cauda equina in the canine animal model.[111, 114] It is apparent from these studies that constriction of 60 per cent or greater of the spinal canal diameter produces consistent alteration in the electrophysiologic function, the blood supply, and the histopathology of the cauda equina, and neural deficit appears. Furthermore, 75 per cent constriction produces universal neurologic deficit and permanent damage to the cauda equina. Finally, surgical decompres-

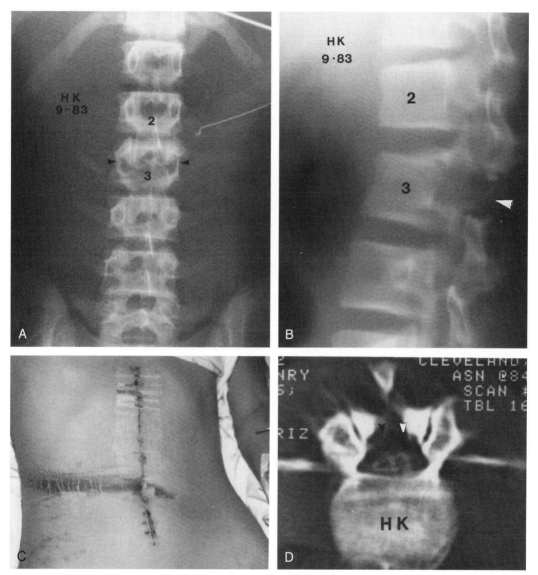

Figure 33–57. *A,* Anteroposterior roentgenogram of a 16-year-old male who was belted into the back seat of a car. After a vehicular accident he was paraparetic with loss of bladder function. Note the transverse fracture through the pedicles and disruption of the lamina. *B,* Lateral roentgenogram demonstrating total posterior and middle column disruption of the osseous structures, a typical chance fracture. *C,* Note the abrasion and seatbelt burn across the abdomen. The patient also had an exploratory laparotomy for internal bleeding. *D,* An enhanced CT scan and myelogram were performed and demonstrated dorsal compression of the cauda equina secondary to an infolded ligamentum flavum.

Illustration continued on following page

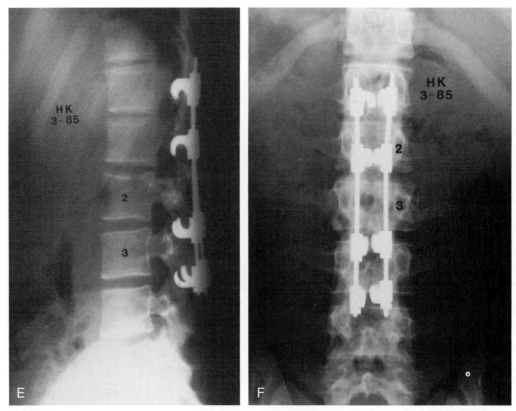

Figure 33–57 *Continued.* *E,* He underwent a posterior laminotomy; decompression of the thecal sac, followed by insertion of two Harrington compression rods, reducing the fracture; and a posterolateral fusion. *F,* Anteroposterior roentgenogram of the healed spine 18 months after the surgery. The patient had completely recovered from the paraparesis and regained bladder function.

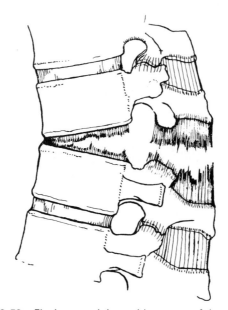

Figure 33–58. Flexion-type injury with rupture of the posterior ligaments and disc in which a pure dislocation can be produced. (From Holdsworth, F. W., and Hardy, A.: Early treatment of paraplegia from fractures of the thoracolumbar spine. J. Bone Joint Surg. *35B:*540–550, 1953.)

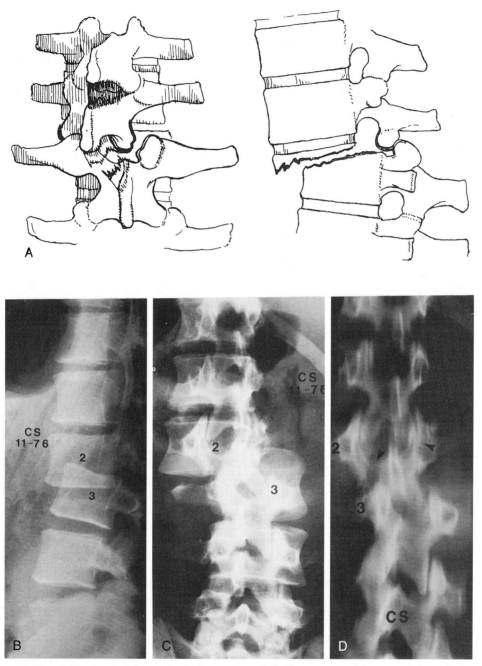

Figure 33–59. *A,* Torsional violence producing rupture of the ligaments and fracture of the articular processes, resulting in rotation and the typical horizontal slice fracture of the vertebral body. This fracture is unstable. (From Holdsworth, F. W., and Hardy, A.: Early treatment of paraplegia from fractures of the thoracolumbar spine. J. Bone Joint Surg. *35B:*540–550, 1953.) *B,* Lateral roentgenogram demonstrating a rotatory fracture-dislocation of L2 on L3 sustained in a vehicular accident. Note the overlap of the two vertebrae on the lateral view, as well as anterior displacement of L2 on L3. The patient was incompletely paraparetic. *C,* Anteroposterior roentgenogram of the rotatory fracture-dislocation of L2 on L3. The lower aspect of the lumbar spine appears to be a true anteroposterior view, whereas the upper lumbar spine is shown in oblique view because of the rotational deformity. The fracture of the pedicle of L2 can be noted on this view. A shear fracture of the upper end plate of L3 cannot be seen on this particular view. *D,* Anteroposterior tomogram of the fracture-dislocation of L2 on L3. Arrows are pointing to the pedicle fracture of L2 and facet fracture of the articular process on the right side. This injury requires rotational as well as flexion forces involving both major osseous and ligamentous injury.

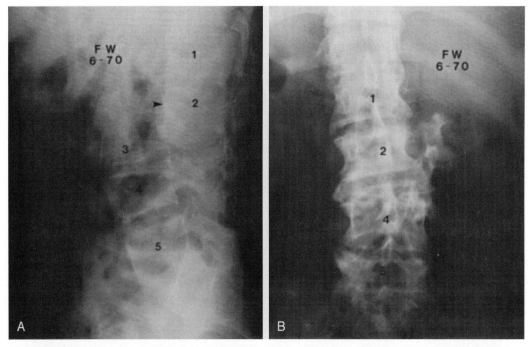

Figure 33–60. *A,* Lateral roentgenogram of a severe extension injury of the lumbar spine involving posterior dislocation of L2 on L3 with a fracture of the latter structure. The patient was completely paralyzed at the second lumbar level. *B,* Anteroposterior roentgenogram of the extension injury demonstrating loss of the third lumbar vertebral height with fracture fragments displaced laterally.

sion has resulted in axonal regeneration. Bolesta has carried out a similar study of graded compression at the conus level of the spinal cord and has found fairly consistent neurologic deficit and alteration of blood supply in 50 per cent or greater compression of the spinal canal. In addition, decompression resulted in significant neurologic recovery. Based on our clinical experience of anterior decompression of thoracolumbar fractures as well as the experimental data, we believe that when the spinal canal is compromised 60 per cent or greater, especially in association with a neurologic deficit, anterior decompression of the spinal canal is in order. The risk of this type of surgery in experienced hands is very slight, and we have not had any increase in neurologic deficit secondary to anterior decompression surgery in over 200 cases. Clohisy et al.[95] demonstrated in a small series of 20 patients that early anterior decompression of thoracolumbar-junction spine fractures within 48 hours of injury resulted in improved neurologic recovery in comparison with decompression carried out an average of 61 days after injury; however, the series is too small to make an absolute statement about timing of decompression and functional recovery. Similarly, Hu et al.[207] reported in a series of 69 patients with lumbar fractures and incomplete paraparesis that the 30 who underwent anterior vertebrectomy and decompression had superior neurologic recovery to those who were treated with posterior instrumentation without decompression.

Another concern of surgeons is the kyphotic deformity that occurs at the thoracolumbar junction. By and large, it is our belief that a 20- to 30-degree kyphotic deformity without associated posterior ligament disruption should be of no concern and does not have to be corrected as long as the spinal canal is decompressed and an anterior fusion is performed. It has been our experience, over 20 years and in more than 200 patients with anterior thoracolumbar decompression, that the kyphotic deformity will not progress unless there is posterior column ligament disruption and instability or a laminectomy has been performed without posterior instrumentation.[43, 51, 52]

Lower lumbar fractures are not common but can occur with severe axial loading and flexion forces. Previous reports of fifth lumbar fractures have indicated the difficulties of attempted instrumentation.[228, 271, 339] Ordinarily, an axial loading injury of the fifth lumbar vertebra produces a superior fracture fragment from the middle column, which protrudes into the spinal canal and which may or may not produce a neurologic deficit. If the canal is occluded at least 60 per cent and there is a neurologic deficit, we prefer to carry out a laminectomy and L4 to L5 discectomy, retrieving the posteriorly protruding fragment, which is usually split in a sagittal plane, and removing it from the spinal canal. This is then followed by a posterolateral fusion from L4 to the sacrum with or without pedicle screw and plate fixation (Fig. 33–61).[32, 39] Mick et al.[273] more recently reported on 11 patients who sustained burst fractures of the fifth lumbar vertebra. They documented a better response in terms of resolution of neurologic deficits with surgical decompression and

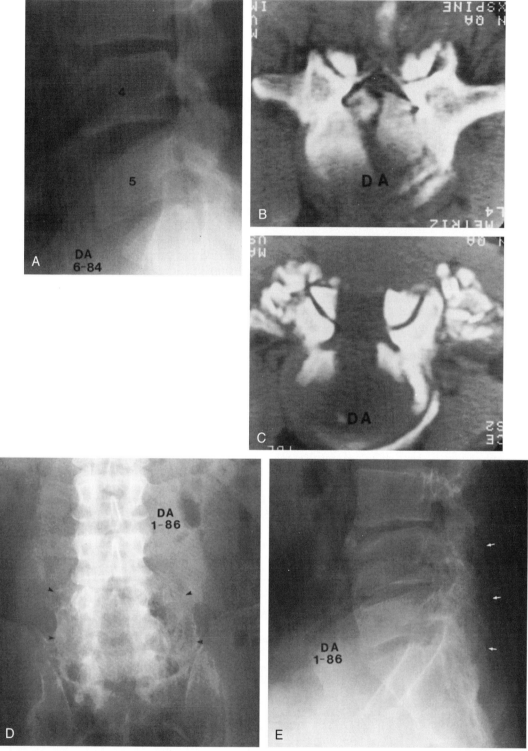

Figure 33–61. *A,* Lateral roentgenogram and myelogram of a 35-year-old dentist who crashed in his home-built aircraft, sustaining severe head and multiple extremity injuries and chest injuries. He was initially paraparetic. The x-ray film demonstrates an axial loading compression fracture of L5 and an anterior column failure of L4. *B,* CT scan reveals severe compromise of the spinal canal with cauda equina compression secondary to bone fragment protrusion at the superior aspect of L5. *C,* The patient underwent a lumbar laminectomy excision of bone fragments and posterolateral fusion, and the postoperative CT scan reveals complete decompression of the spinal canal. *D,* Anteroposterior roentgenogram 20 months after decompression and posterolateral fusion. Note the completely solid fusion from L4 to the sacrum and the laminectomy at L4–L5. *E,* Lateral roentgenogram demonstrating totally solid fusion from L4 to the sacrum and spontaneous anterior fusion at L4–L5. The patient totally recovered from the cauda equina deficit and was fully ambulatory without bracing.

stabilization by pedicle screw fixation in six patients who had neural compression of bone fragments. Fracture-dislocation of the fifth lumbar vertebra on the sacrum is rare and requires open reduction and fusion, usually with plate fixation. If the injury is discovered late, an interbody fusion, as described by Bohlman and Cook, can be done.[30]

Neurologic Assessment

With reference to those patients who have thoracolumbar spine fractures with neural deficit, one must first determine which type of neurologic injury has occurred. Holdsworth classified these neurologic injuries as (1) complete division of the sacral cord and lumbar roots, (2) complete division of the sacral cord with escape of nerve roots on one or both sides, and (3) incomplete division of the sacral cord with escape of nerve roots (Fig. 33–62).[205, 206] As mentioned previously, there may be various gradations of the incomplete cord and root lesions at the thoracolumbar junction, and one must determine this on initial neurologic evaluations. Only then can the treating physician proceed with a rational plan of appropriate care, whether surgical or nonsurgical. Initial evaluation in the field should include (1) motion in the patient's legs, (2) motion of the toes, and (3) estimation of anal tone by rectal examination. These should be reassessed in the emergency room, and in addition, at that point a complete neurologic examination is performed, including perianal sensory examination, anal reflexes (anal wink and bulbocavernosus reflexes), and distal extremity reflexes. Occasionally, one will be confused with a hysterical patient who has some injury or sprain of the lumbar spinal area and refuses to move the legs. Sensory function may be impaired by psychologic mechanisms; however, in the hysterical patient, reflexes are usually present. Typically, in the patient with acute spinal cord injury, reflexes are depressed or absent. The importance of assessing spinal cord as well as nerve root function cannot be overestimated. If the spinal cord is divided at or above the first sacral segment, there will be complete loss of voluntary power and loss of sensation of all parts supplied by the sacral segments. There may be isolated reflex activity as indicated by reflex bladder and bowel function, presence of bulbocavernosus and anal skin reflexes, and occasionally extensor plantar responses. The latter reflexes may return within hours or within a few days after this injury, but if complete paralysis and anesthesia of sacral segmental neurologic supply persists, then this indicates complete transection of the spinal cord at or above the first sacral level. The lumbar roots control flexion and adduction of the hips and extension of the knees and contribute to control of extension and abduction of the hips, flexion of the knees, and dorsiflexion of the foot. They are responsible for some sensation of the legs anteriorly and medially. Complete damage of the lumbar nerve roots causes loss of the movements and sensation. If there is complete damage of the spinal cord and nerve roots at the thoracolumbar junction, then no function or sensation will be present below the level of the first lumbar segment. Isolated reflexes will return when the spinal cord is out of shock, which may occur 48 hours following the injury. The lumbar reflexes will not return.

Lumbar root sparing is demonstrated by flexion and adduction movement of the hips with weak extension and abduction movement and weak flexion of the knees. There may be weak dorsiflexion in the ankles, but no plantar flexion of the foot or movement of the toes. Some sensation in the lumbar dermatomes may be present, and knee jerks may be present. The presence of voluntary activity in the lumbar segments is not evidence of an incomplete cord lesion but of lumbar nerve root escape, and there may be complete bladder and

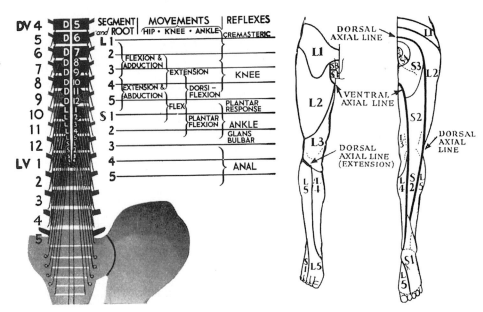

Figure 33–62. Diagram showing the relation of the vertebrae to the segments of the spinal cord. Opposite T12 lie the upper sacral segments in all the lumbar roots. Injury at this level divides the cord and all the lumbar roots and is therefore a mixed cord and root injury. The segmental control of leg movements and reflexes is also shown. The lumbar and sacral dermatomes are indicated. (From Holdsworth, F. W., and Hardy, A.: Early treatment of paraplegia from fractures of the thoracolumbar spine. J. Bone Joint Surg. *35B*:540–550, 1953.)

bowel paralysis as well as sacral motor function paralysis of the extremities, which remains permanent. It is only in the presence of voluntary activity of the sacral segments that an incomplete cord lesion can be diagnosed. The most common type of incomplete injury that we have seen is complete cord damage with sparing of lumbar roots to varying degrees. It is extremely important prognostically, for the patient's functional recovery, to make sure that everything possible is done to reduce dislocations, stabilize the spine, and clear the spinal canal of any protruding bone or disc fragments, which may compress these functioning lumbar nerve roots and the conus if the spinal cord is spared. Ultimate ability to walk with or without bracing may depend on the early diagnosis of the particular injury and its initial care.

On rare occasions, there may be a vascular syndrome associated with fractures of the upper lumbar vertebrae. A radicular artery (artery of the conus) traveling along the second and third lumbar roots may be a major supplier of the spinal cord.[101] Patients sustaining fractures of the second or third lumbar vertebra may present with a central cord syndrome involving the spinal cord segments of the eleventh thoracic through second lumbar regions. A large radicular (medullary) artery typically enters at the eighth or ninth thoracic level, supplying the cord in a cephalad direction, and a lower radicular (or medullary) artery supplies the cord segments between the eleventh thoracic and the lumbar vertebrae. If the lower artery is injured, the patient may present with a thoracolumbar central cord syndrome with greater weakness and hip flexion and moderately good foot and ankle function. The basic principles of treatment, including restoration of alignment, and decompression and stabilization, are the same. The importance of maintaining perfusion pressure and regulating hypovolemic shock obviously should be considered in this type of syndrome.

Treatment Methods

Once restoration of alignment has been achieved and medical stabilization of these patients has been accomplished, then the consideration of decompressive procedures should be entertained. Intra-abdominal injury must be ruled out. It is standard procedure now to perform intraperitoneal lavage or minilaparotomy to make sure there is no bleeding within the abdominal cavity. If there is no serious abdominal pathology and urine is clear on catheterization, then we proceed with ultimate treatment of the spinal condition. If proper spinal alignment cannot be obtained by closed nonsurgical methods and neural deficit is present, evaluation of bone or disc fragments protruding into the spinal canal must be carried out. MRI or myelography with CT scan is the most accurate means of determining bony protrusion into the spinal canal against the neural structures.

Surgical Techniques

If necessary, the next step in spinal alignment may be by surgical means with distraction instrumentation in association with posterior arthrodesis. Assessment of the ligamentous as well as osseous damage is carried out. If the articular facets are dislocated, these are reduced by partial removal of the facet and gentle manipulation of the spine. Once distraction instrument is placed to help realign the spine, reassessment postoperatively is then carried out by myelography and CT scan, as well as by anteroposterior and lateral roentgenograms. This will determine whether there is any remaining bone or disc protrusion in the spinal canal compressing the neural structures. It is our belief that all neural structures should be decompressed at the time of realignment and arthrodesis. If neural compression is still present, then anterior retroperitoneal decompression is performed at a later date. It is generally believed that distraction rods are placed two levels above and two levels below the fractured vertebra. We do not normally fuse the entire length of the rods that are inserted (Fig. 33–63). The decision to approach the injured spine and neural structures posteriorly or anteriorly is up to the individual surgeons and their particular expertise and depends also on the type of spinal injury. In the case of the flexion-distraction or translational injuries of the spine, the posterior approach appears to be best to restore alignment and perform a decompression; however, in the patient who has sustained a burst or compression fracture with protrusion of bone into the spinal canal, the anterolateral decompressive approach with stabilization may be superior. The advantages of the latter approach are that the anterior dura can be more easily visualized. The anterior compressive pathology can be more easily removed, and the spine stabilization is carried out by iliac grafting above and below the level of the fracture with or without internal fixation. Long segments of the spine are therefore not immobilized, and there is a more direct attack on the anterior compressive pathology. In addition, we have seen many patients over the past 18 years who have had internal fixation with Harrington instrumentation in whom the fracture was not reduced, the spinal canal was therefore not decompressed, and neural compression remained, which necessitated late anterior decompression if the patient was not recovering (Fig. 33–64). Also, a significant percentage of Harrington rods may become loose shortly after this insertion, and the stabilization effect is lost.[263] We have demonstrated in the biomechanics laboratory that Harrington distraction rods do not always stabilize forces applied to the spine, especially in rotatory fracture dislocations.[191, 230, 270] Overdistraction may occur with posterior instrumentation, and neurologic loss can occur from ascending paralysis or stretching of the neural structures. This is particularly true in the ankylosed spine, in which there is no ligamentous stability.[263] For most anterolateral decompressions we prefer the sympathetic retroperitoneal anterior approach to the vertebral bodies if the fracture involved is between T12 and L4 as reported by McAfee, Bohlman, and Yuan.[262] Good visualization of the anterior vertebral bodies and dura can be obtained. This sympathetic approach is much the same as described by Southwick

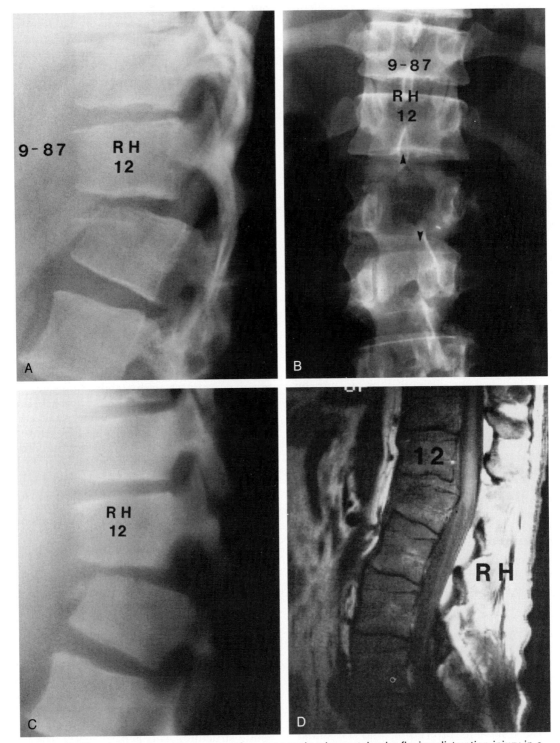

Figure 33–63. *A,* Lateral roentgenogram of a young male who sustained a flexion-distraction injury in a vehicular accident without neurologic deficit. Note the distraction of the posterior elements and slight anterior subluxation of T12 on L1, as well as failure of the anterior column. *B,* Note the marked spread of the spinous processes of T12–L1, indicating complete disruption of the posterior ligaments. *C,* Lateral tomogram reveals perched facets secondary to the disrupted posterior ligaments. *D,* Lateral view of MRI scan reveals only slight conus compression and ligament disruption posteriorly.

Illustration continued on opposite page

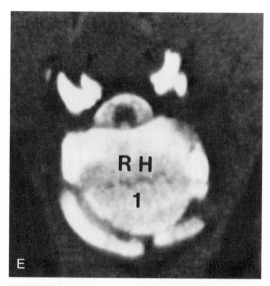

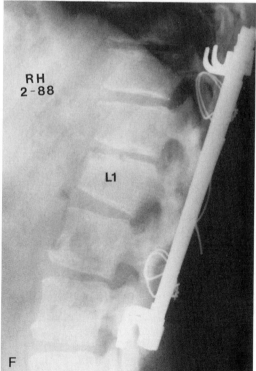

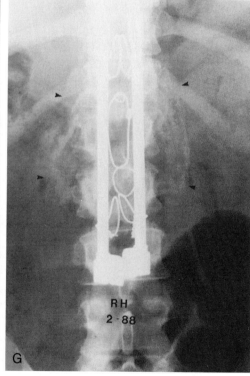

Figure 33–63 *Continued. E,* Enhanced CT scan reveals the naked facet sign and very slight thecal sac compression. *F,* Lateral roentgenogram five months after posterior open reduction and fusion with Harrington distraction and sublaminar wires. *G,* Anteroposterior roentgenogram demonstrating the solid posterolateral fusion from T12 to L2.

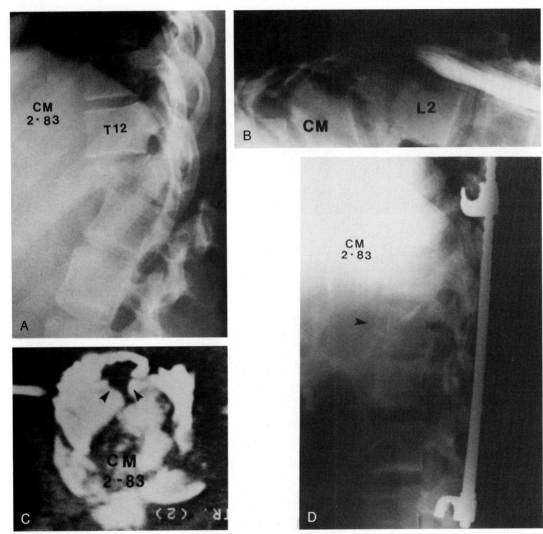

Figure 33–64. *A,* Lateral roentgenogram of a 25-year-old woman who sustained a severe fracture dislocation of T12–L1 in a vehicular accident. On arrival at the emergency room she was completely paraplegic with bladder and bowel paralysis, and the only sensory sparing was in the left L1, L2, and L3 dermatomes. An emergency laparotomy was performed for intraperitoneal blood. Note the complete disruption of the posterior ligament complex and the severe bursting injury of L1. This demonstrates major instability of the anterior, middle, and posterior columns with minimal sparing of neurologic function. *B,* Lumbar myelogram the day after injury reveals a complete block with severe bone protrusion into the spinal canal against the dural sac. *C,* CT scan reveals major protrusion of bone fragments into the spinal canal. *D,* Because of the posterior disruption and severe instability, a posterior open reduction and Harrington instrumentation was carried out with distraction rods. The postoperative lateral roentgenogram reveals what appears to be an adequate reduction of the L1 compression fracture.

Illustration continued on opposite page

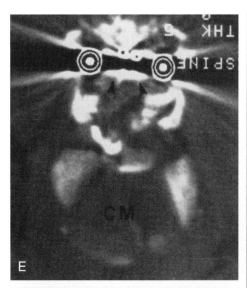

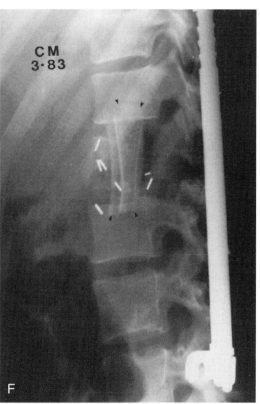

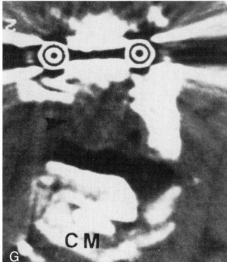

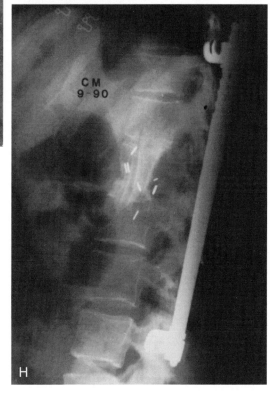

Figure 33–64 *Continued.* *E,* Postoperative CT scan reveals inadequate decompression of the spinal canal with continued severe bone protrusion. *F,* Lateral roentgenogram four weeks after retroperitoneal anterior decompression and iliac fusion. Note the extent of débridement of the protruding bone fragments and the placement of the grafts. *G,* Postoperative CT scan after anterior decompression reveals adequate débridement of the spinal canal across to the opposite pedicle, with the iliac graft in place ventrally. *H,* Lateral roentgenogram six years and seven months after the injury demonstrates total incorporation of the iliac grafts and a stable spine. At this point the patient had regained ambulatory status as a household walker, using one long leg and one short leg brace. Bladder function did not recover.

and Robinson.[334] The patient is placed in the lateral decubitus position and rolled slightly toward the surgeon, who stands on the abdominal side. An incision is made over the left twelfth rib from just lateral to the midline toward the region of the anterior abdomen just a few inches above the iliac crest, which is used for grafting. Dissection is carried subperiosteally around the twelfth rib, and the rib is then removed subperiosteally. Following this, the twelfth intercostal nerve is identified in the neurovascular bundle and followed into the foramen to identify the foramen between the twelfth thoracic and first lumbar vertebra. Blunt dissection is carried out in the retrorenal space to expose the vertebrae. At this point, if the first lumbar vertebra is the fractured one, then the pedicle that lies inferior of the twelfth intercostal nerve is removed. This is carried out in the same fashion as described before. The first lumbar nerve root sheath will be identified inferiorly in relation to the excised first lumbar pedicle. Following removal of the pedicle, it is possible to visualize the dura and osseous protrusion into the spinal canal. De-compression and fusion are carried out in the same fashion as described in the transthoracic approach. Internal stabilization may be performed with a plate or anterior fixation device, as deemed necessary. Patients who have not had a previous laminectomy can be ambulated at about four days following surgery (Fig. 33–65). Ambulation is carried out in a molded orthosis designed for three-point fixation of the spine. The orthosis is worn for three months following the surgery or until there is roentgenographic proof of osseous fusion. If the patient presents with three-column injury including tearing of posterior ligaments, then an option would be to carry out a retroperitoneal anterior decompression utilizing internal fixation, which then obviates the need for a posterior stabilization procedure in that situation (Fig. 33–66).[76] This anterior approach as described is most useful and probably is the only way to adequately decompress a spine and spinal cord injury at the thoracolumbar junction longer than three weeks following the injury. Of the 42 severely but incompletely paralyzed patients reported by McAfee and

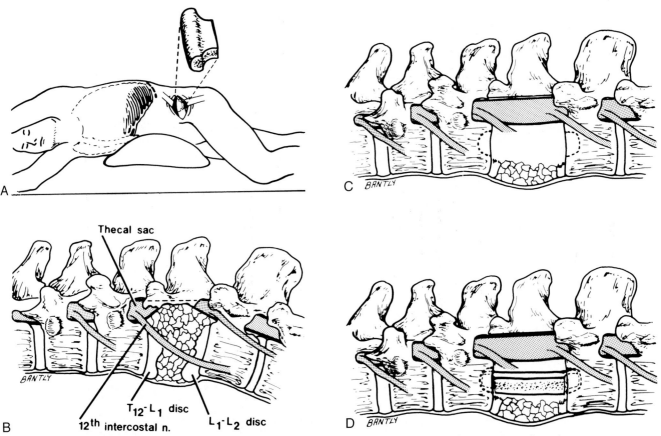

Figure 33–65. *A* to *G,* Technique for anterior retroperitoneal decompression of the lumbar spine. *A,* Retroperitoneal approach to the first lumbar vertebra from the left through an incision overlying the twelfth rib. *B,* Orientation to the spinal canal is facilitated by tracing the course of the twelfth intercostal nerve. After removal of the left pedicle of the first lumbar vertebra, the retropulsed vertebral body fragments of a burst fracture of the first lumbar vertebra are seen compressing the thecal sac. *C,* The fragments are removed with a high-speed burr until the base of the opposite pedicle is visualized. *D,* An iliac crest tricortical strut graft is locked into place with bone tamps. Each end is countersunk into the vertebral body above and below.

Illustration continued on opposite page

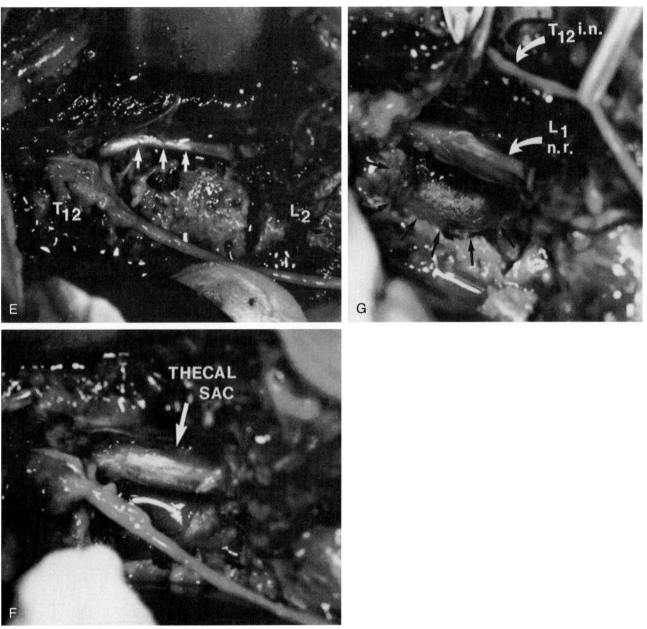

Figure 33–65 *Continued.* *E* to *G,* Intraoperative photographs demonstrate, from the operating surgeon's perspective, the appearance of the anterior aspect of the thecal sac before and after decompression. *E,* Burst fracture of the first lumbar vertebra compressing the thecal sac *(arrows).* For orientation, cephalad is to the left and anterior is toward the bottom of the picture. The left pedicle of the first lumbar vertebra and the discs between the twelfth thoracic and first lumbar and between the first and second lumbar vertebrae have been removed. *F,* After corpectomy of the first lumbar vertebra, the thecal sac expands anteriorly into the space occupied by retropulsed fragments of the vertebral body. The left twelfth thoracic intercostal nerve diagonally traverses the operative field. *G,* The area of decompression of the first lumbar vertebra is designated by the black arrows. The thecal sac is better visualized with the left twelfth thoracic intercostal nerve retracted posteriorly (T_{12}i.n.). This nerve is an important landmark in locating the twelfth thoracic–first lumbar neural foramina and the thecal sac during the initial operative exposure. The first lumbar–nerve root sleeve (L_1n.r.) is also visible. An iliac bone graft is ready to be inserted after locking holes are made in the twelfth thoracic and second lumbar vertebral bodies. (From McAfee, P. C., Bohlman, H. H., and Yuan, H. A.: Anterior decompression of traumatic thoracolumbar fractures with incomplete neurological deficit using a retroperitoneal approach. J. Bone Joint Surg. *67A:*92–95, 1985.)

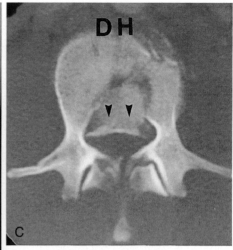

Figure 33–66. *A,* Lateral lumbar roentgenogram of a 17-year-old male who sustained an L2 burst fracture without paralysis secondary to a motor vehicle accident. He was a restrained right front seat passenger. Note the bony protrusion into the spinal canal at the middle column. *B,* Anteroposterior roentgenogram of the lumbar spine demonstrating the L2 burst fracture and fractured laminae. *C,* CT scan demonstrates approximately 70 per cent occlusion of the spinal canal by the posterior of the middle column fragment. *D,* The patient underwent an anterior retroperitoneal L2 decompression and iliac fusion with Z-plate fixation. This lateral roentgenogram demonstrates the healed fracture and solid fusion two years and four months postoperatively. *E,* Anteroposterior roentgenogram of the lumbar spine demonstrating a complete fusion and maintenance of the fixation device.

Bohlman,38 recovered one grade or more of neurologic function, 14 became ambulators, and one third recovered bladder function, which is far better statistically than the results with no decompression or with posterior instrumentation alone (Fig. 33–67). In addition, we have seen a number of patients develop neurologic symptoms years after a decompression fracture injury in which no decompression was performed.10, 43, 52 The anterior approach is then the one of choice. In those patients who have had posterior rod instrumentation with inadequate decompression or reduction of the spine, the anterior approach is also indicated.

SACRAL SPINE INJURIES

Injuries of the sacral spine and nerve roots are very unusual and, in most reports in the literature, account for less than 1 per cent of all spinal fractures.167 Frequently, the diagnosis is delayed in the polytrauma patient. As previously mentioned, Denis et al.,117 Sabiston and Wing,310 and more recently Gibbons et al.183 described large series of sacral fractures. The Denis classification is very useful (Fig. 33–68). If a catheter has been placed in the bladder to monitor the clinical condition of the multiple-injured patient, paralysis of

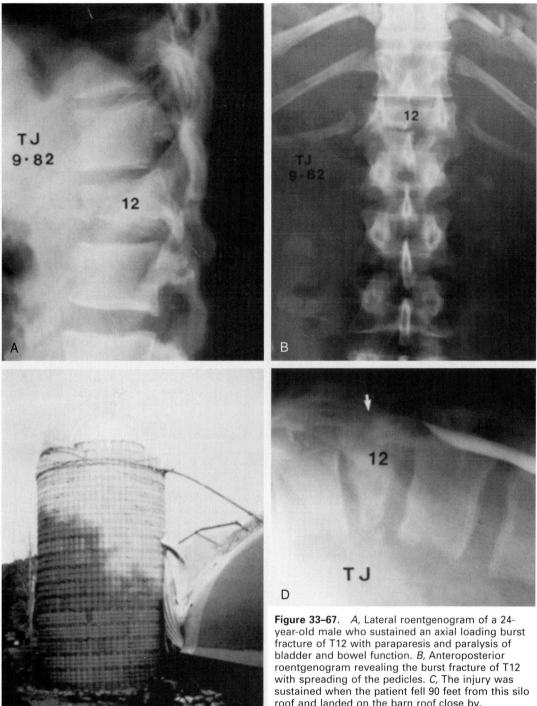

Figure 33–67. *A,* Lateral roentgenogram of a 24-year-old male who sustained an axial loading burst fracture of T12 with paraparesis and paralysis of bladder and bowel function. *B,* Anteroposterior roentgenogram revealing the burst fracture of T12 with spreading of the pedicles. *C,* The injury was sustained when the patient fell 90 feet from this silo roof and landed on the barn roof close by, whereupon he rolled onto the ground. *D,* Lateral view lumbar myelogram taken six weeks after injury, revealing a complete block and marked bone protrusion into the spinal canal into the thecal sac.

Illustration continued on following page

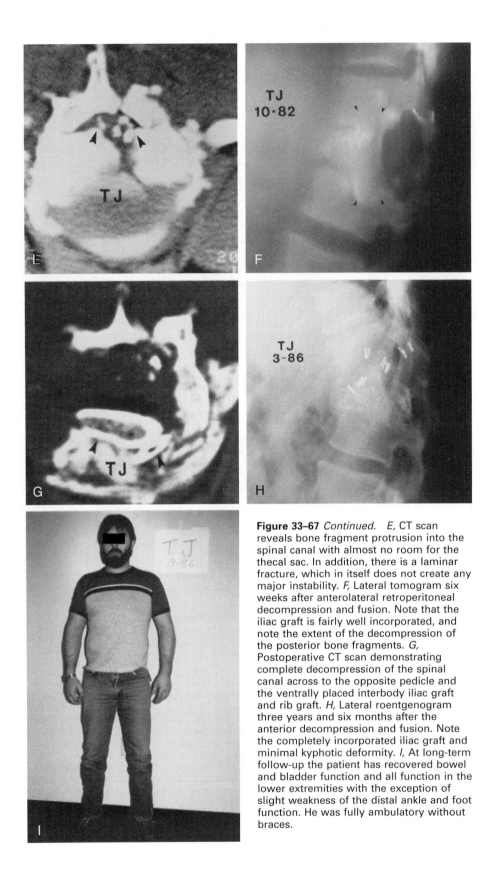

Figure 33–67 *Continued.* *E,* CT scan reveals bone fragment protrusion into the spinal canal with almost no room for the thecal sac. In addition, there is a laminar fracture, which in itself does not create any major instability. *F,* Lateral tomogram six weeks after anterolateral retroperitoneal decompression and fusion. Note that the iliac graft is fairly well incorporated, and note the extent of the decompression of the posterior bone fragments. *G,* Postoperative CT scan demonstrating complete decompression of the spinal canal across to the opposite pedicle and the ventrally placed interbody iliac graft and rib graft. *H,* Lateral roentgenogram three years and six months after the anterior decompression and fusion. Note the completely incorporated iliac graft and minimal kyphotic deformity. *I,* At long-term follow-up the patient has recovered bowel and bladder function and all function in the lower extremities with the exception of slight weakness of the distal ankle and foot function. He was fully ambulatory without braces.

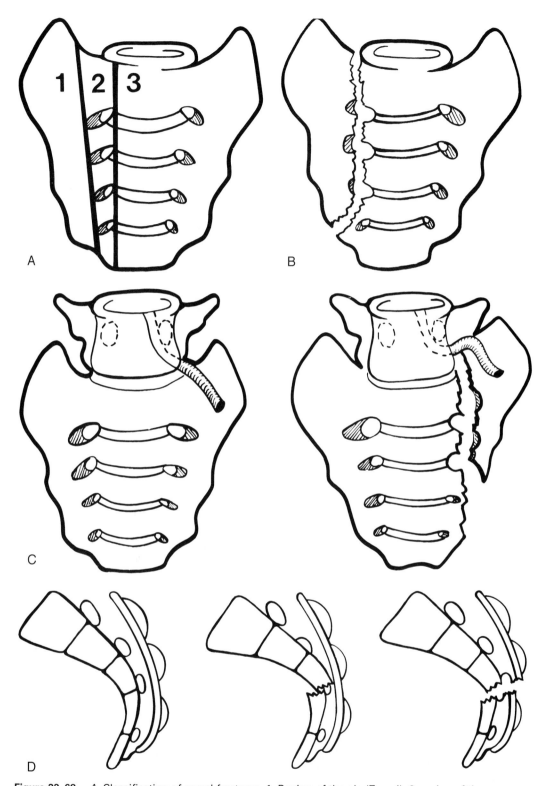

Figure 33–68. *A,* Classification of sacral fractures. 1, Region of the ala (Zone I); 2, region of the foramina (Zone II); 3, region of the central sacral canal (Zone III). *B,* Foraminal fracture (Zone II). *C,* Mechanism of L5 root damage and/or entrapment in the traumatic "far-out" syndrome. The L5 root is caught between the sacral ala and the transverse process of L5 as the alar fragment migrates superiorly and posteriorly. *D,* Zone III injuries: *left,* a normal sacrum for comparison; *middle,* sacral burst fracture with higher potential for sacral root compression; *right,* sacral fracture-dislocation with higher potential for sacral root disruption. (From Denis, F., Davis, S., and Comfort, T.: Sacral fractures: An important problem. Retrospective analysis of 236 cases. Clin. Orthop. *227*:67–81, 1988.)

the bladder and perianal sensory loss from injury to the lower sacral roots (S2 through S5) may not be appreciated initially. In addition, on the admitting examination, rectal tone is often overlooked. Fractures of the sacrum are frequently associated with fractures of the pelvis in the severely injured patient. The fractures of the sacrum without paralysis ordinarily do not need any surgical intervention and will heal quite nicely with proper immobilization. Analysis of fractures with neurologic deficit should include CT, laminography, and MRI to assess whether there is continued compression of the sacral nerve roots in the sacral spinal canal and foramen. There may be a place for sacral laminectomy and foraminotomy if bone protrusion into the sacral canal is observed to be compressing the nerve roots.[333] Fractures in Zone I of Denis' classification produce L5 root and in Zone II S1 root compression,[148] whereas transverse fractures through the body of the sacrum in Zone III may produce a cauda equina syndrome. The results of recovery of these lesions, however, remain variable and not totally predictable as far as bowel and bladder function recovery are concerned

(Figs. 33–69 and 33–70).[90] Complete fracture-dislocation of the sacrum has been reported also.[256] Hilibrand and others[202] recently reported five patients with acute spondylitic spondylolisthesis secondary to major trauma. Four of the patients had dislocations of the fifth lumbar or the first sacral vertebra. The deformity progressed in two adolescents who had been managed nonsurgically, and in one a cauda equina syndrome developed. These authors remarked that these deformities are very unstable with a propensity to progress and that surgical stabilization may be necessary to prevent progression and neurologic compromise (Fig. 33–71).

COMPLICATIONS OF TREATMENT OF CERVICAL SPINE AND SPINAL CORD INJURY

Gastrointestinal System

A common problem associated with the treatment of cervical spinal cord injuries is gastrointestinal hemorrhage, which occurs on or about the tenth to the four-

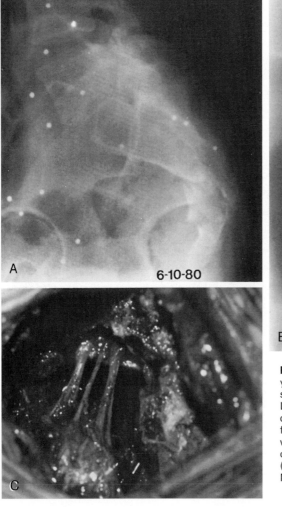

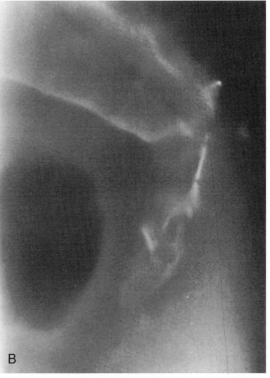

Figure 33–69. *A,* Lateral roentgenogram of a 32-year-old male who sustained an open fractured sacrum in a fall. The white dots are artifacts. *B,* Lateral tomogram of the sacral fracture. Note the comminution and bone protrusion into the sacral fracture. *C,* Operative photograph of the open wound and exposed sacral nerve roots in the canal. This was débrided and closed primarily. (Courtesy of Paul R. Meyer, Jr., M.D., Northwest Memorial Hospital, Chicago.)

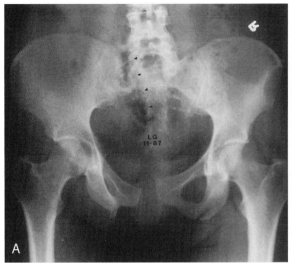

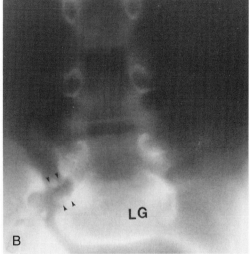

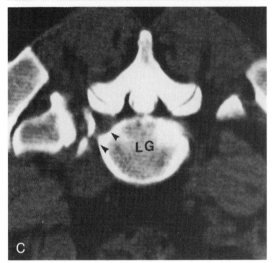

Figure 33–70. *A,* Anteroposterior view of the pelvis and sacrum in a 36-year-old woman involved in a vehicular accident. Note the left-sided Denis Zone 2 complete disruption as well as the diastasis of the pubic symphysis. After recovery, she presented with severe persistent left L5 and S1 radiculopathy lasting two years. *B,* Anteroposterior tomogram reveals the fracture fragment protrusion into the L5–S1 foramen. *C,* CT scan demonstrates fracture fragment protrusion into the L5 and S1 foraminal areas. The patient was treated with a posterior laminectomy of L5, and foraminotomies were performed for the L5 and S1 nerve roots. This was followed by a posterior fusion from L5 to the sacrum. At long-term follow-up the patient has had complete relief of leg pain as well as correction of the L5 root deficit.

teenth day following injury.[239] There is a high correlation with administration of steroids.[34, 46, 47] In Bohlman's review of 300 cervical spine injuries, 37 spinal cord–injured patients received steroids within 72 hours of injury, and 15 developed gastrointestinal hemorrhage (40 per cent), whereas of 97 patients with cord injuries who did not receive steroids, only 9 per cent had gastrointestinal hemorrhage.[46] There was no difference in recovery of neurologic function between the steroid and nonsteroid groups of patients. Twelve per cent of the quadriplegics died of massive gastrointestinal hemorrhage proved at autopsy, and all were treated with steroids. More recently, Bracken et al.[62] studied the effects of large-dose steroids within 24 hours of spinal cord injury and found no significant difference in gastrointestinal hemorrhage, although the steroid-treated group had 4.5 per cent, versus 2.0 per cent in naloxone-treated patients. There are certainly other factors associated with the increased incidences of gastrointestinal hemorrhage, such as gastric stasis, excessive gastric secretions, which may be as much as 3000 ml per day, and immobilization of the patient.[203] Na-

sogastric suction and appropriate medical prophylaxis should be instituted immediately following acute spinal cord injury. The major problem is gastrointestinal hemorrhage, and even perforation of an ulcer through the intestinal wall may occur silently in the asensory patient and may be manifested only by a precipitous hypovolemic episode with ileus and even death. Immediate surgical intervention may be necessary (Fig. 33–72).

If the quadriplegic patient is placed in a halo-cast and kept immobile, on rare occasions a superior mesenteric artery syndrome may occur with duodenal obstruction and persistent vomiting after taking food. This may merely require repositioning of the patient or, in some instances, surgical intervention. The duodenal obstruction occurs between the superior mesenteric artery and the second lumbar vertebra.

Pulmonary System

Pulmonary problems are most common in the cervical spinal cord injury and become more complicated with higher levels of paralysis. Initial hypoventilation is

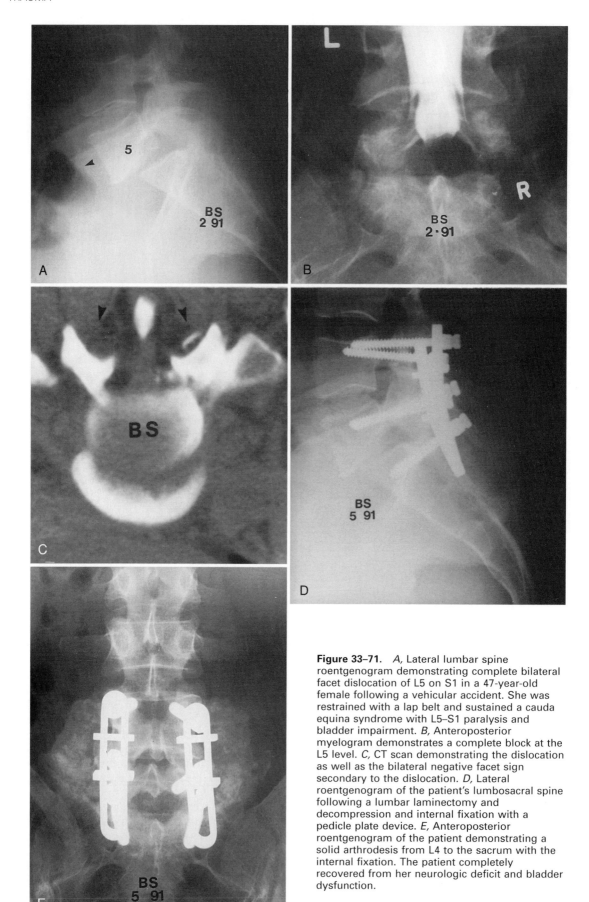

Figure 33–71. *A,* Lateral lumbar spine roentgenogram demonstrating complete bilateral facet dislocation of L5 on S1 in a 47-year-old female following a vehicular accident. She was restrained with a lap belt and sustained a cauda equina syndrome with L5–S1 paralysis and bladder impairment. *B,* Anteroposterior myelogram demonstrates a complete block at the L5 level. *C,* CT scan demonstrating the dislocation as well as the bilateral negative facet sign secondary to the dislocation. *D,* Lateral roentgenogram of the patient's lumbosacral spine following a lumbar laminectomy and decompression and internal fixation with a pedicle plate device. *E,* Anteroposterior roentgenogram of the patient demonstrating a solid arthrodesis from L4 to the sacrum with the internal fixation. The patient completely recovered from her neurologic deficit and bladder dysfunction.

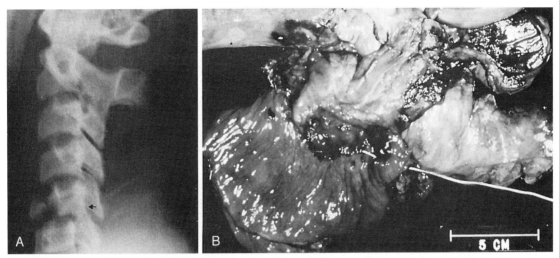

Figure 33–72. *A,* This compression fracture of C5 resulted in complete quadriplegia. The patient was treated by immediate laminectomy and steroids. Note the continuing bone protrusion *(arrow)* into the spinal canal after laminectomy. The patient died from massive gastrointestinal hemorrhage 10 days postoperatively. *B,* The autopsy assessment shows the stomach with a probe in one of the many perforated ulcers. (From Bohlman, H. H.: Complications of treatment of fractures and dislocations of the cervical spine. *In* Epps, C. H., Jr. [ed.]: Complications of Orthopedic Surgery. Philadelphia, J. B. Lippincott Co., 1985.)

caused by paralysis of the intercostal muscles and, of course, in the patient with a fourth cervical level quadriplegia, diaphragmatic paralysis occurs; in both instances, a hypoxic state may be produced that is complicated by atelectasis and pneumonia. Respiratory assistance and tracheostomy may be necessary.[18, 254] Frequent monitoring of blood gas levels is essential during the treatment of the acute quadriplegic patient.

Lieberman and Webb[245] recently reported on 41 patients over the age of 65 years who suffered cervical spine injuries, 12 with neurologic deficit. Eleven of these patients died during treatment, predominantly from respiratory disease. They point out that bed rest and traction are poorly tolerated by older people. Similarly, Alander et al.[4] described 44 patients sustaining cervical spinal cord injuries who were older than 50 years of age. Patients with complete cervical cord injuries who were over 65 years of age had a poor prognosis for survival. A major cause of death in patients was respiratory failure and pulmonary embolus, occurring in eight patients.[4]

Lemons and Wagner[238] described a group of 65 consecutive patients with cervical spinal cord injury and their respiratory complications. They found that the severity of spinal cord injury correlated strongly with the development of respiratory complications but not necessarily with the level of spinal cord injury. They recommend aggressive measures of pulmonary hygiene, an effort to clear pulmonary secretions accounting for a dramatic decrease in respiratory mortality in these individuals over the last 20 years, from 20 per cent to 5 per cent.

Central Nervous System and Spine

Ascending paralysis in spinal cord-injured patients can occur early or late after cervical spine trauma.[34, 257, 306,] [307, 320] The cause is ordinarily ascending central necrosis of the gray matter with an enlarging central syrinx (Fig. 33–73). In the acute stage of the disease, this is usually a fatal complication; however, many years after injury this may occur with formation of an expanding syrinx, which can be treated surgically and drained by means of a shunt. MRI is the most useful diagnostic tool in identifying a post-traumatic syrinx or hematomyelia.[179]

Massive epidural hemorrhage has been previously mentioned in the literature in relationship to certain hematologic diseases; however, it is quite rare in patients with traumatic spine and spinal cord injury. Davis et al.[107] studied 50 fatal craniospinal injuries in which no massive epidural hemorrhage was found, and of the 300 cervical spine injuries reviewed,[46] with 48 autopsy recoveries, four patients developed large epidural hemorrhages, all in association with ankylosing spondylitis. It is apparent that when the rigid ankylosed spine fractures, the bone bleeds profusely, and there is scarring in the epidural space, fixing the paravertebral veins, which then tear and result in profuse bleeding. Immediate immobilization of the fractured ankylosed spine helps to prevent this serious complication, which may require laminectomy to evacuate the hematoma (Fig. 33–74).[118] Respiratory arrest has been reported in association with posteriorly displaced odontoid fractures secondary to spinal cord compression.[243]

Traction and Immobilization Devices

Complications may occur in relationship to the use of immobilization or traction devices.[136] In previous years, the Minerva plaster jacket was used extensively prior to the era of the halo-cast or vest. The Minerva jacket,

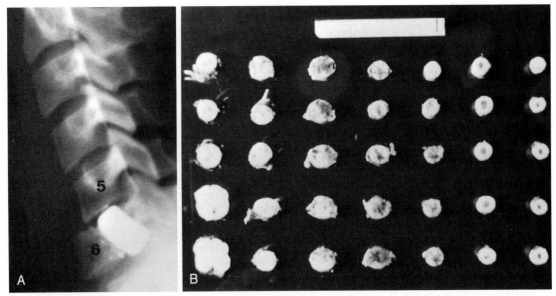

Figure 33–73. *A,* A lateral roentgenogram of a patient rendered quadriplegic by a gunshot wound of C6. The patient initially was quadriplegic at the C6 level but developed ascending paralysis with eventual respiratory paralysis and death. *B,* Multiple sections of the cervical spinal cord depict a pattern of ascending necrosis from the lower cervical cord to the pons. (From Bohlman H. H.: Complications of treatment of fractures and dislocations of the cervical spine. *In* Epps, C. H., Jr. [ed.]: Complications of Orthopedic Surgery. Philadelphia, J. B. Lippincott Co., 1985.)

even when properly applied, does not immobilize the cervical spine adequately, and progressive deformity may occur, especially in those patients with flexion injuries and torn posterior ligament complexes.[46] The halo-vest, therefore, is the preferred treatment for cervical fractures in those patients without neurologic deficit. Conversely, the halo-vest may produce overdistrac-

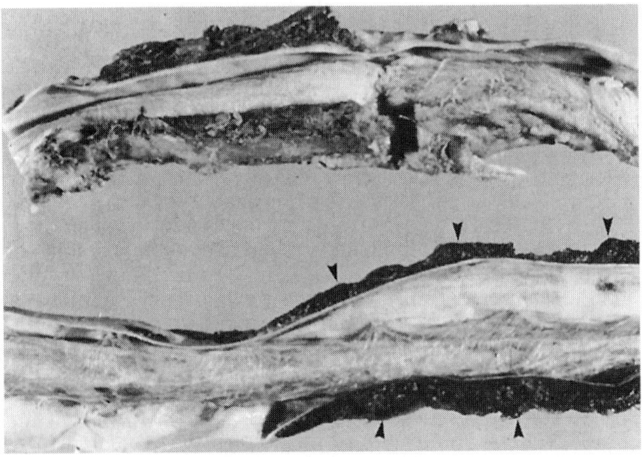

Figure 33–74. A 60-year-old man with ankylosing spondylitis fell and sustained a fracture of C7 without neural involvement. His facial lacerations were sutured on the day of injury and he was discharged. One week after injury he returned with progressive quadriparesis. Laminectomy revealed a massive epidural hemorrhage, which was confirmed at autopsy 18 days later. (From Bohlman, H. H.: Acute fractures and dislocations of the cervical spine. J. Bone Joint Surg. *61A:*1119–1142, 1979.)

tion of odontoid fractures and result in a nonunion, so care must be taken not to place the patient with upper cervical spine injuries in traction.

Skeletal traction by the use of tongs has been used since the 1930s, when Crutchfield described this method of immobilizing cervical fractures. These tongs are no longer used because of bone resorption around the tongs, which results in loosening and the tongs' falling out at two or three weeks following insertion. More appropriately, the Gardener-Wells tongs are less apt to loosen, or the halo-ring can be used for immediate traction, since it does not allow motion or produce bone resorption and can later be attached to a vest or cast. Careful daily pin care is necessary to prevent sepsis and osteomyelitis of the skull.[177] Unfortunately, pressure sores may develop under the halo-vest in asensory patients; therefore, it is probably wiser to continue with cervical tong traction and to stabilize asensory patients by means of an appropriate arthrodesis to achieve early ambulation in a cervical orthosis. In the obese patient, the halo-vest offers poor fixation around the pelvis and may allow excessive motion of the cervical spine.[365] In addition, dorsal pads should not be used in patients without sensation, because pressure sores will result.

Overdistraction may occur if all ligaments and discs are disrupted and too much weight is used during traction (Fig. 33–75).[175] It is rare for the patient with acute spinal cord injury to develop increased paralysis if properly immobilized. Early instability must be recognized, or subluxations and dislocations may further displace, compressing the neural structures; however, it is dangerous to test for acute instability with flexion-

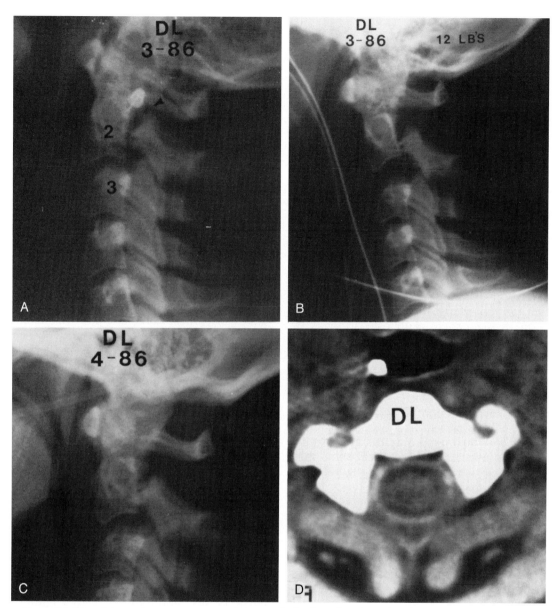

Figure 33–75. *A,* Lateral roentgenogram of the cervical spine of a young female who sustained a bilateral pedicle fracture of C2 in a vehicular accident. No paralysis was present on arrival at the emergency room, but there were distal extremity fractures. *B,* The patient was placed in 12 pounds of skeletal traction and taken to the operating room, where the distal long-bone fractures were openly reduced and fixed internally. Another cervical spine film was not taken until the following day (shown here). Note the overdistraction of the C2–C3 disc space, indicating total disruption of the osseous and ligamentous structures. The patient had developed an ascending paralysis with only slight sparing of distal motor function at approximately the C3 level. *C,* Traction was reduced and she was ultimately placed in a halo-vest for stabilization. *D,* A CT scan performed at a later date reveals what appears to be myelomalacia of the central spinal cord. The patient recovered only partial neurologic function and has remained quadriparetic.

extension roentgenograms prior to applying protective skeletal traction or the halo apparatus. As previously mentioned, one can usually assess the integrity of the posterior ligament complex by initial evaluation of the lateral roentgenogram, which demonstrates widening of the interspinous space or subluxation of vertebrae. Bohlman documented, in his review series, the hazards of manipulating odontoid fractures in roentgenographic studies as well as in the operating room.[46]

Mahale and others[252] documented neurologic complications of the reduction of cervical spine dislocations. They describe 16 patients in whom four had immediate onset of increased neurologic deficit, and 11 a delayed increase in deficit with either traction, manual manipulation, or open reduction of dislocations. The various causes included direct cord injury, spinal cord edema, herniated disk, and spondylosis producing further compromise of the spinal canal.

Early Deformity

In patients with complete quadriplegia from cervical fractures, failure to reduce dislocations or fractures may ultimately result in inability of the spinal cord or nerve roots to recover expected neurologic function.[49, 278, 340] Unreduced osteoarticular facets may continue to compress nerve roots and not allow recovery, or major radicular artery feeders may be compressed, resulting in central cord necrosis.[46] In the complete cord lesion, an unreduced dislocation may further compress the good spared nerve roots above the level of the cord lesion and, therefore, reduction should be carried out as soon as feasible, taking into account the associated medical problems. Severe kyphotic deformities with wedge-compression fractures may continue to produce anterior cervical cord compression and prevent ultimate total recovery from an incomplete cord lesion.[363, 364, 376]

Overdistraction in skeletal traction can occur with cervical fractures or dislocations if all the ligamentous structures are torn anteriorly and posteriorly.[15] This is most common in the patient with osteoarthrosis or ankylosing spondylitis. Ascending neurologic deficit has been reported secondary to overdistraction with cervical traction.[175] Generally, we do not apply more than 40 or 50 pounds of traction to cervical fractures below the third cervical level. Once again, careful analysis of the osteoarticular lesion will aid in predicting the degree of instability present (see Fig. 33–75).

Patients with ankylosing spondylitis and pre-existing kyphotic deformities of the cervical spine may sustain fractures and then be placed in a neutral position in tong traction that is abnormal for them.[118] This may result in severe pain and loss of nerve root or cord function until recognition of the previous deformity, when the patient is actually placed in a flexed position in skeletal traction. This may require use of a conventional hospital bed with the head elevated 45 to 50 degrees and traction applied vertically in the original deformed position.[34]

Sepsis

Sepsis occurring with fractures and dislocations of the spine usually results from an invasive injury such as a gunshot wound in which the associated soft tissue structures or the esophagus has been penetrated, thereby releasing bacteria into the surrounding tissues.[141] The same is true of gunshot wounds of the abdomen and lumbar spine in which the bullet traverses the bowel, spreading organisms to the spine and spinal canal.[302] In addition, sepsis following surgical procedures is more common in patients treated with steroids.[62]

Complications of Surgery

As one might expect, complications of surgical treatment are varied and common. Sepsis by direct introduction of bacteria during surgical procedures is rare but can occur. Contamination of posterior sites in oper-

ations of the upper cervical spine may result in meningitis and death. Iatrogenic perforation of the esophagus with sharp retractors may occur during an anterior cervical operation and result in esophagocutaneous fistulas and consequent osteomyelitis of the cervical vertebrae. The use of wires for tying an anterior bone graft has been abandoned by us because of two known cases of a resultant perforated esophagus. When bone remodeling occurs with healing, the anterior wire loop may be left to compress the esophageal wall and produce a perforation.[34] We do not recommend the use of foreign materials in cervical spine surgery for traumatic injuries, excluding wire for posterior fusions. Recently plates and screws have been used for anterior cervical spine surgery, but they are weak biomechanically in flexion and the screws loosen and may back out, causing esophageal perforation.[97] Methylmethacrylate has been used and reported in the literature; however, we have seen patients who have developed massive sepsis as a result of the implants. Bone cement does not attach to cortical bone, and the wire fixation used in conjunction with this technique soon loosens, and loss of reduction occurs.[142, 250] If one is to carry out a major surgical procedure for stabilization, then we believe it is very reasonable to use the patient's iliac bone, which will immediately stabilize the spine and result in arthrodesis. In Bohlman's review series, not one posterior cervical fusion between the third and seventh cervical levels failed to unite when autogenous bone and wire fixation were used.

Respiratory problems may occur intraoperatively, especially if patients have a high paralysis at the fourth or fifth cervical level. Ventilation is poor, and postoperatively there is a higher risk of pulmonary complications. Respiratory arrest may occur in patients with unreduced atlantoaxial dislocations when instruments are passed under the posterior arch of the atlas, where there is very little room for the spinal cord.[34, 46] Surgery for upper cervical spine injuries may produce Ondine's curse, or sleep-induced respiratory failure, as a result of damage to the respiratory pathway and the reticulospinal tract.[159] In addition, patients within the first few weeks following spinal cord injury may develop hyperkalemia as a result of loss of potassium from the paralyzed muscle cells. In these patients, succinylcholine has been reported to cause cardiorespiratory arrest and should not be used in conjunction with general anesthesia.

Central nervous system complications may be a result of surgical intervention, especially if the dura has been violated or left open, which was a previous technique that should no longer be used. It is our policy at the present time not to inspect the dura just for the sake of looking at it when an anterior cervical decompression is performed. Ordinarily, the posterior longitudinal ligament is not violated, and one can dissect the bone fragments away from it prior to grafting. Cutaneous spinal fluid fistulas are almost always a result of surgical intervention with poor closure of the dura and can usually be treated successfully with antibiotics, recumbency, and lumbar subarachnoid drainage.

The most common cause of increased neural deficit in cervical fractures is secondary to direct cord injury during laminectomy. In Bohlman's review of 300 cervical spine injuries, 22 per cent of the 55 patients who were treated by laminectomy had increased permanent loss of neural function immediately postoperatively.[46] Permanent loss of neural function did not occur after anterior or posterior fusion or adequate nonsurgical treatment. Laminectomy was particularly devastating in those patients with incomplete cord injuries. Also, there was a higher death rate in the patients with quadriplegia treated by laminectomy. It should be evident to most surgeons that laminectomy cannot decompress a spinal cord or retrieve bone and disc fragments that anteriorly compress the spinal cord. In addition, laminectomy causes increased instability and may allow subluxation or dislocation.[275]

An additional cause of increased neurologic deficit and spinal cord trauma may occur following reduction of dislocations of the cervical vertebrae.[34, 42, 54] In this instance, an anteriorly ruptured disc may be pulled back against the spinal cord and may produce further cord compression and increase neural deficit. This should be recognized immediately and followed by anterior discectomy and fusion for decompression. After preoperative visualization by MRI or myelogram and CT scan, the anterior procedure should be done first. The cervical spinal cord–injured patient must be carefully monitored following reduction of dislocations for this devastating complication.

Complications may occur as a result of anterior or posterior arthrodesis techniques. It has been reported that retinal artery thrombosis may occur because of headrests that apply circumferential pressure about the eye.[34] Presently we use the Gardner or Mayfield headrest, which attaches to the outer layer of the skull and rigidly fixes the head and neck in the prone position without any pressure on the face or eyes. One can adjust this to exert longitudinal traction and flexion or extension as necessary through the universal joints and then finally fix the entire head and neck rigidly prior to the surgery.

Vertebral artery damage has been reported with anterior cervical fusions; therefore, it is important to leave the lateral cortices of the vertebral body when performing an anterior corpectomy or vertebrectomy, to avoid this complication.

The type of bone graft used for arthrodesis of the cervical spine should have inherent strength as well as good osteogenic properties; therefore, we prefer the block-type iliac graft rather than the Cloward dowel or fibular graft.[96] Any type of anterior graft may collapse or extrude if the patient has posterior cervical ligamentous tearing and, therefore, instability. Protective skeletal traction or a halo-cast maintains alignment until healing takes place.

One must obtain intraoperative roentgenograms to ascertain the level of the fusion. Mistakes can be made

by fusing the wrong level if identifying roentgenograms are not taken.

Open reduction of cervical dislocations and posterior wiring or plating without fusion are to be condemned. This procedure only allows redislocation of the fracture because of the assumption that the fixation is sufficient until spontaneous anterior fusion occurs, which is an erroneous concept.[34] Not all injuries fuse spontaneously after cervical fractures.

Late Spinal Deformity and Paralysis

Late complications may occur with cervical spine injuries, specifically late instability or deformity. This may be associated with pain or with progressive neurologic deficit. Of the 229 patients studied by Bohlman with cervical injuries between the third and seventh cervical levels, 33 developed late instability following nonsurgical management.[46] This is a much higher incidence of instability than previously reported in the literature. Most of these injuries were flexion-distraction type injuries with posterior ligament tearing, and the remainder were hyperextension injuries in osteoarthritic spines with longitudinal ligament and disc disruption. Ligaments do not always adequately heal even with rigid fixation for three months, nor does spontaneous fusion always occur as mentioned. Arthrodesis may be required in these instances (Fig. 33–76).

Odontoid fractures that do not heal allow chronic atlantoaxial instability.[325] Wertheim, Bohlman and others have documented the high pseudarthrosis rate of onlay occipitocervical fusion, probably as a result of distraction or tension forces in this area of a bone graft.[359] Occipitocervical fusion grafts should be firmly fixed to the occiput as well as the cervical spine with wires. The technique that we have used for this level of fusion has been to pass a wire loop through a drill hole under the outer cortex of the skull along the nuchal ridge and to pass this wire through corticocancellous iliac grafts. An additional wire is used through a drill hole in the spinous process of the cervical vertebra to further stabilize the graft. Wertheim and Bohlman have published their results of this technique on 13 patients, with fusion in all cases. An alternative technique is to use atlantoaxial lateral mass screw fixation for a more rigid arthrodesis.

Crockard and others[102] reported on progressive myelopathy secondary to remote odontoid fractures and described 16 patients who presented from four months to 45 years after the initial injury, 10 of whom had myelopathy. In seven of these patients, the transverse ligament was found interposed in the fracture at the time of transoral surgery.[12]

Late pain and paralysis can occur secondary to fractures of the cervical spine if bone and disc fragments are not decompressed initially and stability is not achieved.[11, 36] Additional problems occur if dislocations of the vertebrae are not initially reduced and are allowed to heal in malposition.[376] Of particular importance is the patient with an atlantoaxial dislocation that has been allowed to heal in malposition secondary to

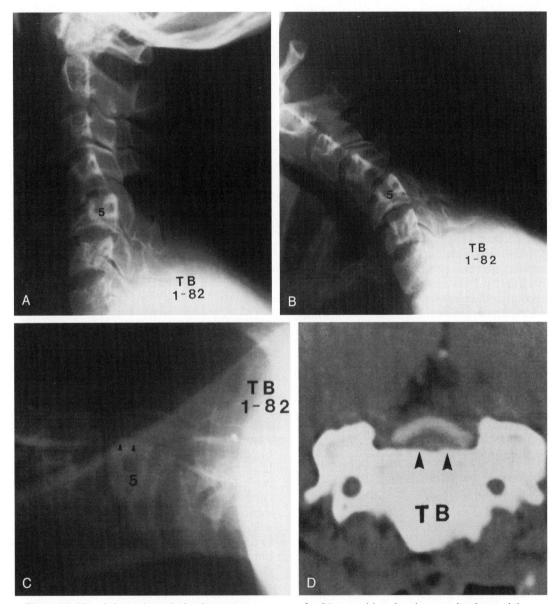

Figure 33–76. *A,* Lateral cervical spine roentgenogram of a 24-year-old male who sustained an axial loading injury of C5 with flexion and distraction of the posterior elements, tearing the interspinous ligaments, two years previously in a diving accident. He was an incomplete anterior cord quadriparetic barely able to stand and walk short distances. *B,* Lateral roentgenogram revealing the kyphotic deformity of the cervical spine in flexion. *C,* Lateral myelogram demonstrating anterior spinal cord compression even with the patient in neutral position. *D,* Enhanced CT scan at the fracture site demonstrating no posterior elements and severe flattening of the spinal cord over the kyphosis.

Illustration continued on opposite page

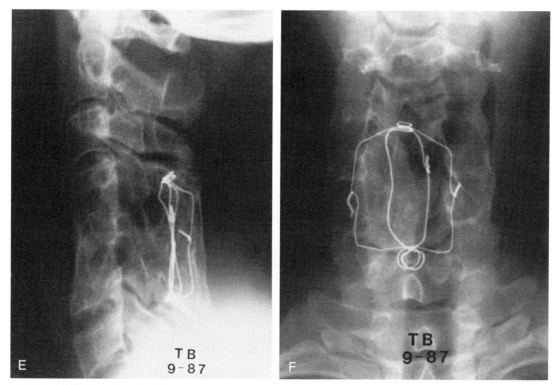

Figure 33-76 *Continued.* *E,* Lateral roentgenogram five years and eight months after surgery. The patient underwent an anterior corpectomy of C5, correction of the kyphosis in skeletal traction, and insertion of an iliac graft, immediately followed by a posterior stabilization with the triple wire technique and iliac grafting. *F,* Anteroposterior x-ray film at long-term follow-up demonstrating the triple wire technique and solid fusion. The patient had regained ambulatory status with the aid of one cane, and recovered bladder and sexual function.

a fracture of the odontoid that was not reduced (Fig. 33-77).[264] This produces chronic spinal compression and paralysis as well as pain.[105, 155, 233, 357] In this instance, if the posterior atlantodental interval is less than 13 mm, it may be hazardous to pass instruments under the arch of the atlas to establish an arthrodesis. Such patients have developed respiratory arrest and further paralysis with this maneuver.[34] In these instances, it is probably best to carry out a laminectomy of the arch of the atlas and then perform a posterior cervico-occipital arthrodesis, keeping the patient in a halo-cast postoperatively.

Spinal cord monitoring with CEPs is most useful if a general anesthetic is to be used during surgery.[289] This allows intraoperative monitoring of the patient's spinal cord to determine whether any decrease in neurologic function occurs during the procedure. One may also perform this operation with the patient in a halo-cast under local anesthesia, which we have done many times. The malunited atlantoaxial fracture dislocation may require additional transoral decompression of the odontoid;[11] however, there are significant complications with this procedure, and it is our belief now that the anterior extrapharyngeal approach to resect the body of the axis and odontoid with C1 to C3 fusion is best.[260] This procedure may have to be combined with a laminectomy of the atlas and posterior fusion.

LATE SURGICAL PROCEDURES

Late Anterior Decompression for Cervical Spinal Cord Injury

Fractures of the lower cervical spine that are unreduced may heal in a dislocated position, or compression fractures of the vertebrae may leave bone protrusion into the spinal canal, compressing the anterior surface of the spinal cord. It is in these patients that we believe ultimate recovery of neurologic function will not occur unless decompression and stabilization are carried out.[27, 29, 43, 321] Patients with incomplete spinal cord injuries have potential for recovery, depending on the amount of initial cord contusion as well as existing spinal cord compression.[344-346, 356] Many of these patients will recover neurologic function to a significant degree but then plateau in their neural recovery, and late anterior decompression may be indicated. Bohlman has had experience with over 300 late anterior decompressions of the cervical, thoracic, and lumbar spine with significant recovery in many of these patients, even up to two years following injury.[11, 22, 28, 36] The indications for late anterior decompression are in those patients who have stopped recovering neurologic functions, those who still have incomplete cord lesions, or those in whom there are demonstrable bone and disc frag-

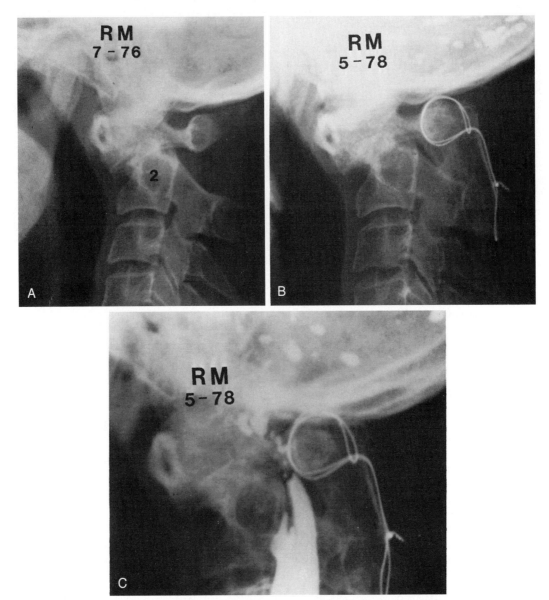

Figure 33–77. *A,* Lateral roentgenogram of an old C1–C2 dislocation secondary to an odontoid fracture. The patient had developed syncopal episodes and drop attacks. *B,* Posterior fusion and wiring were carried out. However, in the recovery room it was noted that the patient was quadriparetic with a central cord syndrome. The subluxation had recurred, and the fusion was allowed to heal in the displaced position. *C,* Two years after the original procedure the patient had recovered to ambulatory status but remained with a Brown-Séquard syndrome and left hemiparesis. A cervical myelogram revealed severe compromise of the spinal cord at the C1–C2 level. This necessitated a transoral anterior decompression, as well as a posterior decompression by removal of the arch of the atlas and a portion of the posterior fusion as separate procedures. The patient eventually regained some motor function.

Illustration continued on opposite page

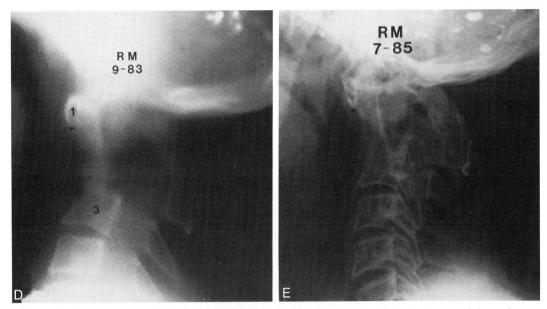

Figure 33–77 *Continued. D,* The transoral microscopic decompression was inadequate and the patient continued to have pain without major recovery of neurologic function. This necessitated a retropharyngeal anterior resection of the vertebral body of C2 and iliac fusion from C1 to C3. This lateral tomogram after surgery demonstrates the adequacy of anterior decompression and the incorporated iliac strut graft. *E,* Lateral roentgenogram two years after retropharyngeal decompression demonstrating the totally incorporated iliac graft. The patient had recovered further neurologic function and most of his pain was relieved.

Illustration continued on following page

ments compressing the anterior spinal cord. On occasion, the complete quadriplegic patient may have an unreduced dislocation or bony protrusion into the spinal canal that is compressing the good nerve roots coming from the spinal cord above the level of the cord injury itself and can obtain arm function recovery with late anterior decompression. Of 58 patients with incomplete neurologic injury so treated with long-term follow-up, 30 of the 52 who could not walk before surgery became functional ambulators with significant postoperative recovery (Fig. 33–78). Other authors have reported similar results in small series.[20] Even sensory recovery in the quadriplegic patient is beneficial to prevent pressure sores, and arm functional recovery of one to two nerve root levels may be quite beneficial in terms of the patient becoming an independent ambulator. Of more than 300 patients operated on to date, we have had one patient lose motor root function as a result of the surgical procedure. Other complications have occurred in the following types of high-risk patients: patients with complete high cervical injuries (fifth cervical cord segment or above), patients with chronic obstructive pulmonary disease, the older patient (more than 60 years of age), and the severely depressed patient without a will to live.[50] The simultaneous presence of more than one of the preceding factors may be a contraindication to surgery. The late deformity after cervical spine injury may produce a severe disabling pain as well as paralysis. MRI is used to visualize the cord compression.[99] Decompression may have to be carried out to relieve pain that is a result of either spinal cord or nerve root compression. In addition, it is our clinical impression that spasticity is much worse in those quadriplegic patients in whom there is major osseous compression of the spinal cord remaining, although this is not absolute. In our late decompression patients, we have seen improvement in spasticity following surgery, and patients may be able to discontinue the use of antispasticity medication.

Delayed Syrinx Formation

Another cause of delayed neurologic loss other than mechanical compressive pathology is that of the previously mentioned central syrinx.[305, 306, 324, 364] The pathophysiologic events following spinal cord trauma introduce central necrosis of the gray matter, which can progress at a later date.[120, 121, 125, 215, 313] Once necrosis has occurred, the central area, the gray matter, becomes liquified. On rare occasions, the central syrinx enlarges and becomes a symptomatic internal expansile lesion of the cord with progressive neurologic deficit and severe pain. MRI is the most accurate method of viewing the syrinx.[292] Ordinarily intractable dysesthetic pain prevents rehabilitation of the patient, and because of these problems, surgical intervention is necessary to decompress the central syrinx. It is preferable to carry out a laminectomy for this procedure after the spine is stabilized. In these patients, the cord is exposed above the damaged area, a bilateral cordotomy is performed to transect the anterior lateral spinal thalamic tracts for pain, and below this procedure a midline myelotomy

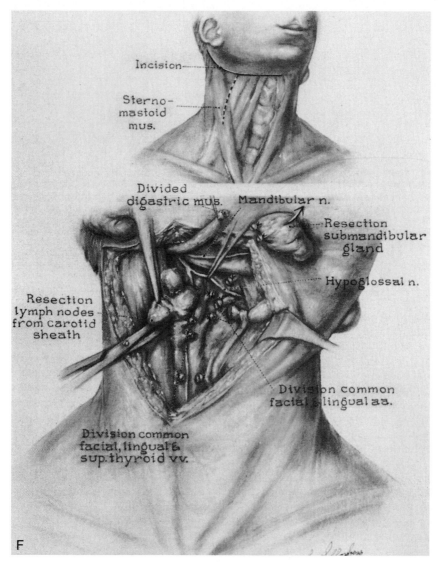

Figure 33–77 *Continued.* *F,* Key features of the extramucosal anterior approach to the atlas and axis. Through a submandibular incision on the right side, the submandibular gland is resected and the digastric tendon divided. It should be noted that the lower limb of the incision is not used unless concomitant exposure to the midcervical levels is required.

Illustration continued on opposite page

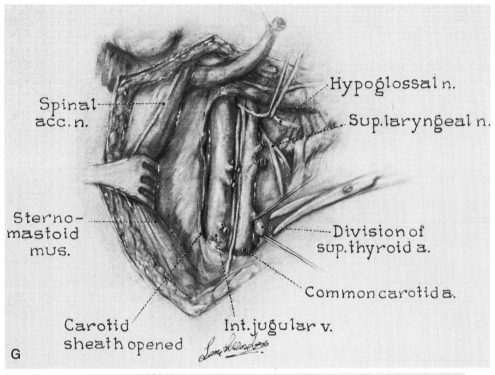

Spinal acc. n.

Hypoglossal n.

Sup. laryngeal n.

Sterno-mastoid mus.

Division of sup. thyroid a.

Common carotid a.

Carotid sheath opened

Int. jugular v.

G

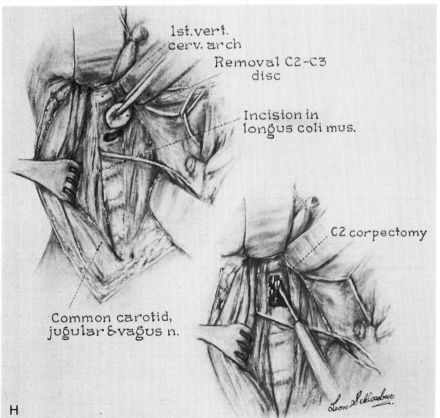

1st. vert. cerv. arch

Removal C2-C3 disc

Incision in longus coli mus.

C2 corpectomy

Common carotid, jugular & vagus n.

H

Figure 33–77 *Continued.* *G,* After the superficial layer of the deep cervical fascia is incised along the anterior border of the sternocleidomastoid muscle, the superior thyroid artery and vein are divided. The hypoglossal and superior laryngeal nerves are mobilized. Additional branches of the carotid artery and internal jugular vein are ligated to allow mobilization of the contents of the carotid sheath laterally as the hypopharynx is mobilized medially. *H,* The first step of the anterior spinal decompression is a meticulous removal of the disc between the second and third cervical vertebrae. The longus colli muscle is dissected in a lateral direction, exposing the second cervical vertebral body and the anterior arch of the atlas. Removal of the body of the second cervical vertebra can then be performed with a high-speed burr.

Illustration continued on following page

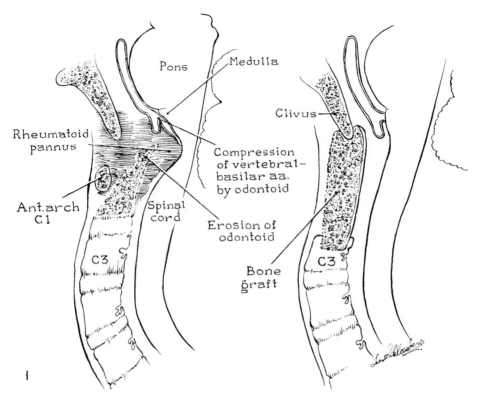

Figure 33–77 *Continued. I,* The most frequent non-neoplastic cause of compression at the level of the second cervical vertebra is rheumatoid pannus, associated with atlantoaxial subluxation and basilar invagination of the odontoid process. The goal of the anterior decompression and stabilization is to provide an arthrodesis from the clivus to the subaxial spine. (*F* to *I* from McAfee, P. C., Bohlman, H. H., Riley, L. H., Jr., et al.: The anterior retropharyngeal approach to the upper part of the cervical spine. J. Bone Joint Surg. *69A*:1374–1379, 1987.)

may be carried out, using the operating microscope.[1, 211] There may be associated severe arachnoiditis and scarring above the site of injury, especially after gunshot wounds, in which case drainage of the central cyst results in relief of pain.[304] Over a period of time after these procedures, pain can recur; however, if rehabilitation has been completed, the patient is more tolerant of this discomfort and does not usually require a second procedure. The central syrinx is normally drained with a plastic tube to bypass the damaged lesion, as in the case of syringomyelia (Fig. 33–79).

Hida and others[201] reported on 14 patients with post-traumatic syringomyelia and described MRI findings as well as surgical management. The onset of the syrinx occurred from three to 33 years, with a mean of 14 years. Eleven of the symptomatic patients underwent surgical treatment, including a syringosubarachnoid shunt in six, a syringoperitoneal shunt in four, and a ventricular peritoneal shunt in one. Motor improvement occurred in eight of nine patients, and relief of local pain in four of four patients. Also, Schurch and others[324] carried out a prospective study of 449 patients with spinal cord injury, of whom 20 displayed symptoms of post-traumatic syrinx. Neurologic deterioration was closely related to the enlargement of the cyst, and in the surgical patients, neurologic improvement or

stabilization correlated with collapse of the cyst. Cord compression, tense syrinx at the fracture site, and kyphosis seem to be closely linked to cyst enlargement.

Spasticity

Spasticity may be a severe problem in spinal cord–injured patients, affecting the lower abdominal wall, extremities, or the bladder. The spinal cord is isolated below the level of injury because it has lost its upper motor neuron influence to control muscle contractions. The exact mechanism of spasticity is not clear; however, this condition may be uncontrolled by medication and may prevent adequate rehabilitation. Many surgical procedures have been proposed to control spasticity, but no one procedure is universally satisfactory.[1, 211] At this time, the most common operation used is a T-shaped myelotomy through the dorsal spinal approach carried out between the two dorsal columns to interrupt the reflex arc between the entering sensory axon as it traverses to the motor neuron. The procedure can be selectively carried out to control lower abdominal spasms, upper leg spasms, and the uncontrolled spastic bladder. Some surgeons prefer a percutaneous dorsal rhizotomy. However, it is important for patients undergoing the operation for correction of the latter problem

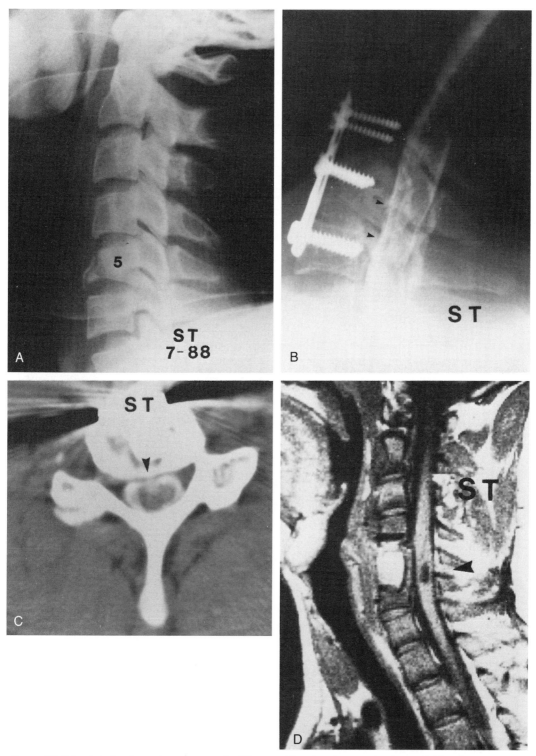

Figure 33–78. *A,* Lateral roentgenogram of a 16-year-old male who sustained an axial loading compression fracture of C5 in a diving injury. He initially had a severe anterior cord syndrome with very poor motor function. *B,* The patient underwent an anterior fusion using Caspar plates without decompression. He recovered some motor function but by six months was unable to ambulate. This lateral cervical myelogram demonstrates continued compression of the cervical spinal cord. In addition he was extremely spastic. *C,* Enhanced CT scan demonstrates continued bone compression of the spinal cord and some dye in the central portion of the spinal cord. *D,* The patient underwent removal of the Caspar plates and corpectomy of C5 with iliac fusion from C4 to C6. Immediately postoperatively a cervical MRI reveals a central contusion or myelomalacia of the spinal cord.

Illustration continued on following page

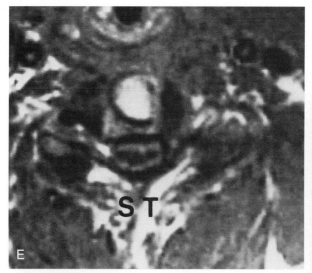

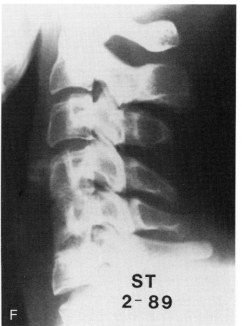

Figure 33–78 *Continued. E,* Axial MRI view reveals central myelomalacia with a surrounding shell of the spinal cord. *F,* Postoperative lateral x-ray film shows incorporation of the iliac graft. The patient has become fully ambulatory with the aid of crutches.

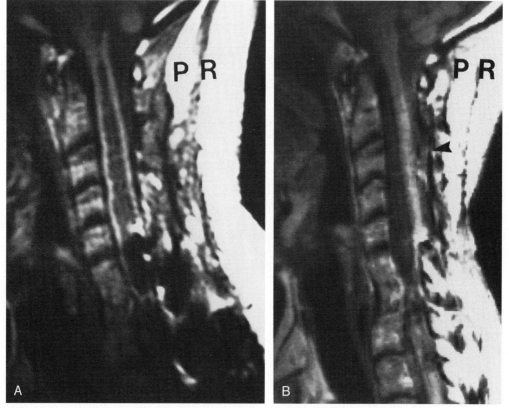

Figure 33–79. A patient sustained a remote spinal cord injury, motor complete C6. He underwent an anterior corpectomy and fusion and two years later developed ascending paralysis with loss of arm function, increased pain, and episodes of sweating. *A,* MRI demonstrates a very large syrinx ascending from the spinal cord injury level to C1. The patient underwent a cervical laminectomy, microscopic myelotomy, and a shunt procedure. This relieved his pain and restored the lost motor function to a preoperative state. *B,* The postoperative lateral MRI demonstrates complete resolution of the syrinx. (From Bolesta, M. J., and Bohlman, H. H.: Late complications of cervical fractures and dislocations and their management. *In* Frymoyer, J. [ed.]: The Adult Spine: Principles and Practice. New York, Raven Press, 1991, pp. 1107–1126.)

to have preoperative urologic evaluation. The potential for loss of erection or reflex bladder emptying is present following these procedures, which is quite disturbing to the patient. The spastic bladder may be controlled by sectioning the second, third, and fourth sacral segments selectively. In some patients, selective rhizotomies of the second and third sacral nerve roots have been carried out to control the spastic bladder condition. In addition, sphincterotomy of the bladder prior to the neurosurgical procedure may relieve the bladder symptoms. In all of the procedures to control spasticity, one is confronted with an isolated motor neuron for the so-called upper motor neuronal denervation syndrome, in which the cell acts independently of the brain and other higher centers. These motor cells react to the only input available to them, which is primarily segmental sensory responses. Once there is loss of central inhibition, this must be balanced by reducing the amount of local spinal cord input.

COMPLICATIONS OF TREATMENT OF THORACOLUMBAR SPINE INJURIES

Although the majority of complications occur with cervical spine and cord injuries, there may also be problems with upper thoracic spine fractures. As mentioned before, these are associated with intrathoracic injuries, which must be dealt with when they arise. As far as the upper thoracic spine is concerned, these fractures are generally stable if treated with recumbency for three weeks. It is rare to have progressive deformity of the upper thoracic spine unless a laminectomy has been performed previously, in which case all posterior stabilizing influences have been removed.[275, 299] In addition, laminectomy may increase paralysis in the complete cord lesion. In Bohlman's series of 17 patients so treated, eight became completely paralyzed permanently.[40] We believe laminectomy is therefore contraindicated in upper thoracic fractures with paralysis. The use of Harrington distraction rods in the upper thoracic spine is usually not necessary. Difficulties arise when the fractures are between the first and fifth thoracic vertebrae and there is no technical way of anchoring the hooks unless they are placed in the cervical spine, which is contraindicated. Overdistraction may occur, particularly in the ankylosed spine in which the ossified longitudinal ligaments are disrupted, and may produce ascending paralysis and cord necrosis.[263] Anterior osseous union occurs most readily in nearly all of the upper thoracic spine fractures, provided laminectomy has not been performed. As in the cervical spine, when approaching the upper thoracic area transthoracically or otherwise, care must be taken to be accurate in identification of the level of the vertebra. Preoperative assessment of the roentgenograms and counting ribs will avoid operating on the wrong level of the spine.

Fractures of the thoracolumbar spine present more difficulties than in the upper thoracic levels from both the osseous and neurologic standpoints. These fractures are considerably more unstable in the acute situation and result in late deformity if reduction and stabi-

lization are not carried out.[43, 366, 367] As Roberts and Curtis[299] have pointed out, these fractures are quite unstable if they are the translatory or flexion-distraction type, which require internal fixation. Progressive deformity and neurologic deficit most frequently occur following laminectomy if a stabilization has not been performed. We believe that laminectomy in this area is contraindicated without stabilization. Currently, distraction rod fixation with sublaminar wires is being used widely for reduction and stabilization of thoracolumbar fractures. This is a definite improvement in treatment of these fractures compared to the old approach, with laminectomy alone, because in most instances immediate stabilization can be carried out with reduction of the spine fracture; however, we have seen significant difficulties with the Harrington instrumentation system without sublaminar wires. The most common problems that we have experienced in our spinal cord injury units are (1) Harrington distraction rods may become loose in the immediate postoperative period and fixation is lost (Fig. 33–80); (2) long segments of the spine have to be fixed to reduce the fracture, and this may not be the best method ultimately in treating these injuries; (3) overdistraction may occur in patients with seat-belt injury or chance fractures and, therefore, a compression device should be used in the latter instance; and (4) in addition, overdistraction occurs in the ankylosed spine in which

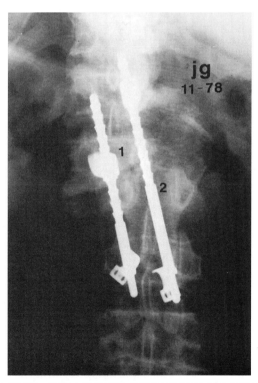

Figure 33–80. Anteroposterior roentgenogram of a patient who sustained a rotatory fracture-dislocation of L1 on L2 with complete paraplegia. Harrington rod instrumentation and fusion were carried out, but rotatory instability resulted in redislocation and extrusion of the rods.

the ossified ligaments are disrupted and there is no stability. Fracture-dislocations may not be reduced adequately by distraction rods. This is of particular concern in those patients with incomplete neurologic lesions in whom the osseous structures are still compressing the neurologic elements that are functioning.[6] This then necessitates anterior decompression and vertebral body fusion to alleviate the situation.[143, 287] We do not as a policy carry out decompressions on patients with complete neurologic lesions; however, stabilization may be required in the case of translatory fracture-dislocations to ambulate the patient. As an invasive procedure, any instrument and fusion may become infected, resulting in spinal osteomyelitis and meningitis, which necessitates removal of the device. If the rods loosen and the spinal deformity increases, they may protrude through the skin and have to be removed. In addition, Harrington rods alone do not offer significant rotatory or torsional stability of the spine. This is especially true in the case of rotatory fracture-dislocations; therefore, sublaminar wires or transpedicular fixation should be used and patients must be protected with a molded orthosis for three months or until arthrodesis occurs. Ultimately, it may be better initially to carry out anterolateral decompression and arthrodesis with or without internal fixation for compression fractures with neurologic deficit and to reserve rotatory fracture-dislocations for posterior reduction and internal fixation. Experimentally, the facet joints are affected by internal fixation.[218] Caution should be used if Edwards sleeves are inserted with distraction rods, especially if laminar fractures are present, because they can be pushed into the spinal canal, causing increased or new neurologic dysfunction. These injuries are quite variable, and it is up to the judgment of the surgeons involved to carry out the most optimal surgical procedure.

In children and adolescents with spinal cord injury, late paralytic spinal deformity is common and may require stabilization for sitting posture.[232, 259] We have seen and treated approximately 60 patients with late pain and paralysis following fractures of the thoracolumbar spine.[43] In most of these instances, patients have mild (20-degree) kyphotic deformity of the spine with bone protrusion into the spinal canal, compressing neural structures originating with the injury. They may have initially recovered a mild neurologic deficit and then have gone on to develop neurogenic deficit claudication or progressive paralysis, and have become functionally disabled. All of these patients have had demonstrable neural compression by myelography and CT scan or MRI, and have required anterolateral decompression and fusion. In most instances, decompression will relieve pain, and in some patients, recovery of function can occur late after injury, as described before.

In the asensory complete paraplegic patient, laminectomy without stabilization may result in a totally unstable Charcot spine, requiring internal fixation and fusion (Fig. 33–81).[333]

Patients with ankylosing spondylitis may have "silent" fractures of the spine, particularly of the thoraco-

lumbar junction after minor trauma. As Kanefield et al.[220] pointed out, these fractures are overlooked, and a nonunion occurs with a resultant build-up of fibrous pseudarthrosis tissue. This progressively compresses the spinal cord and nerve roots, producing a central neurogenic type of pain that may radiate to the legs and may or may not be associated with paralysis of the bladder and the extremities. These patients also require anterolateral decompression and fusion to recover function, gain stability, and relieve pain. We believe that pain is quite unusual after spinal fractures that have been treated appropriately with reduction and stabilization and adequate decompression. In those patients who present with pain later after injury, investigations are done to rule out mechanical compressive pathology against neural structures, which is most commonly the etiology of the problem. Arachnoiditis secondary to the original injury is rarely a cause of chronic pain and can be diagnosed with the MRI or myelography and CT scan.[113]

Bohlman and others[26] documented in a group of 45 patients the onset of late pain and paralysis following thoracolumbar fractures. These patients were treated with anterior decompression and fusion, with 41 having satisfactory relief of pain. Of 25 with neural deficit, 21 experienced an improvement in their neurologic deficit even years after injury.[26, 64]

Long-bone fractures occur in chronically paralyzed patients because of osteopenia. These can be treated with pillow splints.[172] Freehafer[171] reported on the treatment of a total of 133 patients with spinal cord injury and long-bone fractures. The majority of these fractures in the lower extremity were just above or below the knee and could be treated with pillow splints. None of the fractures of the femoral neck healed in patients with total paralysis, and these were treated symptomatically. Intertrochanteric and subtrochanteric fractures of the femur were treated with a pillow splint between the patient's knees and hips, and the patients were ambulated to their wheelchair.

REHABILITATION

The goal of rehabilitation of the spinal cord–injured patient is to treat all systems of the body that are affected and return the patient to social functioning in a lifestyle as independent and as close to normalcy as possible. The ultimate level of rehabilitation is determined by many factors, including the type of spinal cord injury (complete or incomplete), psychologic readjustment, the neurologic level of the injury, and appropriate care of associated organ systems; that is, pulmonary, genitourinary, gastrointestinal, and the integument. The pulmonary function problems usually stabilize within the first few weeks after injury unless of course the level of the injury is above the fourth cervical level, in which case a respirator may be required. Lower cervical injuries gradually adapt to intercostal muscle paralysis. In the less common instance of survival of a patient with a complete first cervical level quadriplegia, this necessitates a ventilatory sup-

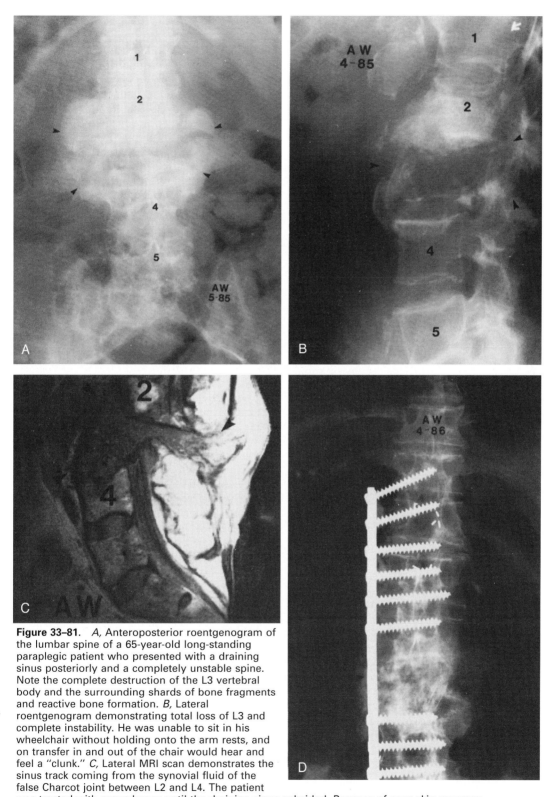

Figure 33–81. *A,* Anteroposterior roentgenogram of the lumbar spine of a 65-year-old long-standing paraplegic patient who presented with a draining sinus posteriorly and a completely unstable spine. Note the complete destruction of the L3 vertebral body and the surrounding shards of bone fragments and reactive bone formation. *B,* Lateral roentgenogram demonstrating total loss of L3 and complete instability. He was unable to sit in his wheelchair without holding onto the arm rests, and on transfer in and out of the chair would hear and feel a "clunk." *C,* Lateral MRI scan demonstrates the sinus track coming from the synovial fluid of the false Charcot joint between L2 and L4. The patient was treated with recumbency until the draining sinus subsided. Because of poor skin coverage posteriorly, it was elected to carry out a retroperitoneal anterior resection of the Charcot joint bone grafting with femoral head bank bone and use of an AO plate and cancellous screws for internal fixation. *D,* Anteroposterior roentgenogram reveals a solid fusion one year postoperatively. The patient was able to sit upright in his wheelchair and did not need to use his arms for a sitting posture.

port system. Phrenic nerve or diaphragmatic stimulators and pacers may be inserted to free the patient from a mechanical respirator. The mortality rate in these patients is very high in the first two years.

The care of the integument of the asensory patient is by frequent turning every two hours until the patient is ambulated in a wheelchair, in which case pressure on the buttocks and sacral region is relieved by frequent push-ups in the wheelchair or change of position. Pressure sores are treated by recumbency, débridement, and, occasionally, rotational flaps. The most important treatment is prevention.

Urinary tract care is begun by intermittent catheterization every four to six hours to provide reflex emptying of the bladder without a high residual capacity. Approximately 85 per cent of the patients should become catheter-free by using the intermittent catheterization program prior to their discharge from a rehabilitation program.[288] The treating physician and nursing staff should be aware of the problem of autonomic dysreflexia and how to treat it. If a severe hypertensive crisis occurs, one should check the catheter drainage of the bladder first. Nifedipine 10 mg is given sublingually stat, then Dibenzyline, 10 mg every day prophylactically. The bowel may be trained in similar fashion to empty with the use of suppositories and stool softeners. This may be by reflex emptying or by manual evacuation.

The expected functional levels of the quadriplegic patients are described subsequently. Above the fourth cervical level the patient is frequently dependent on a respirator but may drive an electric wheelchair equipped with a portable respirator and chin controls.

At the fifth cervical level there is no muscle power below the elbow flexion, and patients can drive an electric wheelchair or push a wheelchair without electrical control, dress themselves, and drive an automobile with hand controls. A flexor hinge splint may aid in function of the extremities provided extensor power is adequate at the wrist. Tendon transfers may improve hand and wrist functional ability.[173, 174]

At the seventh cervical level there is no finger muscle power; however, the patient can be independent in wheelchair transfers, drive an automobile with hand controls, and live independently.

Between the first and twelfth thoracic cord levels with complete paralysis, the patient may be totally independent in a wheelchair and may drive a car with hand controls but usually will be unable to walk even with the aid of bracing. The energy expenditure required to walk with long leg braces in paralysis above the T12 neurologic level is usually prohibitive, and the patient finds life much easier living in a wheelchair and being able to transfer in and out of it and drive a car.

Neurologic function at the thoracolumbar junction depends on the degree of lumbar root sparing; patients may be ambulatory to varying degrees with or without bracing. Patients with quadriceps function, flexor power at the hips, and control of the pelvis and trunk can learn to walk with crutches and short leg braces and will discard the wheelchair. However, when quadriceps function is absent but the patient has some hip flexion power and control of the pelvis, long leg braces and crutches will be required to walk. Without hip control, patients can learn to walk with long leg braces, crutches, and a swing-through gait, but functional walking is less likely to occur, and patients will usually prefer a wheelchair existence.

Other factors play a major role in whether a patient will ambulate functionally, including age, weight, associated medical problems, psychologic factors, and socioeconomic and family situations.[4]

Woolsey described the rehabilitation outcome of 100 consecutive patients with a recent spinal cord injury.[371] On admission, 80 per cent were predicted to become functionally independent and 70 per cent achieved this goal at discharge. Factors related to success or failure of rehabilitation effort were identified. Appropriate intervention neutralized negative influences and may increase the number of successfully rehabilitated patients with spinal cord injuries. The average length of stay for all quadriplegic patients was 5.5 months, and for paraplegic patients, 3.3 months. Average follow-up after discharge was 45 months. The functional goals to be achieved are to eat, drink, dress, and groom independently, to manage bladder and bowel care, to transfer to and from and operate a wheelchair, to provide for pressure relief, and to drive a car. Achievement of these goals may be affected by the level of paralysis, age, the status of pressure sores on admission, the degree of paralysis, and associated medical problems. Achievement of rehabilitation goals results in functional independence. No patient with a C5 or higher level injury was able to achieve functional independence. Patients with a C6 level injury required assistance and occasionally needed help transferring to and from a wheelchair. Almost all patients with C7 or lower level injuries were able to achieve functional independence. Three patient characteristics correlated highly with ultimate nursing home placement: (1) age older than 50 years, (2) absence of spouse or parent, and (3) injury to spinal level of C6 or above.

Prior to the patient's discharge, sexual activities should be discussed. The majority of male patients, especially those with incomplete cord injuries (85 per cent), will be able to have an erection; however, a much smaller per cent will have ejaculation. This varies from the upper motor neuron to lower motor neuron lesions. Female patients are capable of having pleasurable sexual experiences, becoming pregnant, and bearing children. Although sexual experiences are different after spinal cord injuries, with adjustment patients may achieve satisfaction. Counseling is extremely important to help the patient adapt to the injury. Long-term care of the spinal cord–injured patient includes follow-up examination, repeat neurologic documentation, examination for pressure sores, and genitourinary evaluation at appropriate times.

References

1. Adams, J. E., Lippert, R. G., and Hosobucki, Y.: Commissural myelotomy. Curr. Tech. Operative Neurosurg. 29:427–434, 1977.

2. Akbarnia, B. A., Fogarty, J. P., and Tayob, A. A.: Contoured Harrington instrumentation in the treatment of unstable spinal fractures: Effect of supplemental sublaminar wires. Clin. Orthop. *189*:186–194, 1984.
3. Aki, T., and Toya, S.: Experimental study on changes of the spinal evoked potential and circulatory dynamics following spinal cord compression and decompression. Spine *9*:800–809, 1984.
4. Alander, D. H., Andreychik, D. A., and Stauffer, E. S.: Early outcome in cervical spinal cord injured patients older than 50 years of age. Spine *19*:2299–2301, 1994.
5. Albin, M. S., White, R. J., Locke, G. S., et al.: Localized spinal cord hypothermia. Anesth. Analg. *46*:8–16, 1967.
6. Allen, B. L., Jr., Tencer, A. F., and Ferguson, R. L.: The biomechanics of decompressive laminectomy. Spine *12*:803–808, 1987.
7. Allen, B. L., Jr., Ferguson, R. L., Lehmann, T. R., and O'Brien, R. P.: A mechanistic classification of closed, indirect fractures and dislocations of the lower cervical spine. Spine *7*:1–27, 1982.
7a. Anderson D. K., Hall E. D., Braughler, J. M., McCall, J. M., Means E. D.: Effect of delayed administration of U74006F (trilazad mesylate) on recovery of locomotor function after experimental spinal cord injury. J. Neurotrauma *8*:187–192, 1991.
8. Anderson, L. D., and D'Alonzo, R. T.: Fractures of the odontoid process of the axis. J. Bone Joint Surg. *56A*:1663–1674, 1974.
9. Anderson, P. A., and Montesano, P. X.: Morphology and treatment of occipital condyle fractures. Spine *13*:731–736, 1988.
10. Anderson, P. A., and Bohlman, H. H.: Late anterior decompression of thoracolumbar spine fractures. Seminars in Spine Surgery *2*:54–62, 1990.
11. Anderson, P. A., and Bohlman, H. H.: Anterior decompression and arthrodesis of the cervical spine: Long-term motor improvement. Part II: Improvement in complete traumatic quadriplegia. J. Bone Joint Surg. *74A*:683–692, 1992.
11a. Arias M. J.: Effect of naloxone on functional recovery after experimental spinal cord injury in the rat. Surg. Neurol. *23*:440–442, 1985.
12. Ashraf, J., and Crockard, H. A.: Transoral fusion for high cervical fractures. J. Bone Joint Surg. *72B*:76–79, 1990.
13. Assenmacher, D. R., and Ducker, T. B.: Experimental traumatic paraplegia: The vascular and pathological changes seen in reversible and irreversible spinal cord lesions. J. Bone Joint Surg. *53A*:671–680, 1971.
14. Bailey, R. W., and Badgley, C. E.: Stabilization of the cervical spine by anterior fusion. J. Bone Joint Surg. *42A*:565–594, 1960.
15. Barros, T. E., and Fielding, J. W.: Traumatic spondylolisthesis of the axis with unusual distraction. A case report [published erratum appears in J. Bone Joint Surg. 72A:473, 1990]. J. Bone Joint Surg. *72A*:124–125, 1990.
16. Beatson, T. R.: Fractures and dislocations of the cervical spine. J. Bone Joint Surg. *45B*:21–35, 1963.
17. Bedbrook, G. M.: Spinal injuries with tetraplegia and paraplegia. J. Bone Joint Surg. *61B*:267–284, 1979.
18. Bellamy, R., Pitts, F. W., and Stauffer, E. S.: Respiratory complications in traumatic quadriplegia. J. Neurosurg. *39*:596–600, 1973.
19. Benson, D. R., and Keenen, T. L.: Evaluation and treatment of trauma to the vertebral column. A.A.O.S. Instructional Course Lectures *39*:577–589, 1990.
20. Benzel, E. C., and Larson, S. J.: Recovery of nerve root function after complete quadriplegia from cervical spine fractures. Neurosurgery *19*:809–812, 1986.
21. Benzel, E. C., and Larson, S. J.: Functional recovery after decompressive operation for thoracic and lumbar spine fractures. Neurosurgery *19*:772–778, 1986.
22. Benzel, E. C., and Larson, S. J.: Functional recovery after decompressive spine operation for cervical spine fractures. Neurosurgery *20*:742–746, 1987.
23. Bergmann, E. W.: Fractures of the ankylosed spine. J. Bone Joint Surg. *31A*:669–674, 1979.
24. Blaw, M. E., and Langer, L. O.: Spinal cord compression in Morquio-Brailsbord's disease. J. Pediatr. *74*:593–600, 1969.
25. Bodner, D. R., Delamarter, R. B., Bohlman, H. H., et al.: Neurologic changes after cauda equina compression in dogs. J. Urol. *143*:186–190, 1990.
26. Bohlman, H. H., Kirkpatrick, J. S., Delamarter, R. B., and Leventhal, M.: Anterior decompression for late pain and paralysis after fractures of the thoracolumbar spine. Clin. Orthop. *300*:24–29, 1994.
26a. Bohlman, H., Ducker, T.: Therapy for spinal cord injury. In Rothman, R. H., and Simeone, F. A. (eds.): The Spine. Philadelphia, W. B. Saunders, 1992, pp. 973–1104.
27. Bohlman, H. H.: Surgical management of cervical spine fractures and dislocations. A.A.O.S. Instructional Course Lectures *34*:163–187, 1985.
28. Bohlman, H. H.: Late anterior decompression and fusion for spinal cord injuries: Review of 100 cases with long term results. Orthop. Trans. *4*:42–43, 1980.
29. Bohlman, H. H.: Trauma of the cervical spine and cord. American Academy of Orthopaedic Surgeons Update II, pp. 267–280, 1987.
30. Bohlman, H. H., and Cook, S. S.: One stage decompression, posterolateral and interbody fusion for lumbosacral spondyloptosis. Description of a new technique using the posterior approach. J. Bone Joint Surg. *64A*:415–418, 1982.
31. Bohlman, H. H., Rekate, H., and Thompson, G. H.: Problem fractures of the cervical spine in children. In Haughton, G., and Thompson, G. (eds.): Problem Fractures in Children. Boston, Butterworth, 1983, pp. 101–125.
32. Bohlman, H. H.: Post-traumatic lesions of the spine and sacrum. In Laurin, C. A., Riley, L. H., and Roy-Camille, R. (eds.): Atlas of Orthopedic Surgery. Paris, Masson, 1989, pp. 393–410.
33. Bohlman, H. H., Stauffer, E. S., Ferguson, R., and Apple, D. F.: Paraplegia secondary to thoracolumbar spinal trauma. Contemporary Orthopaedics *16*:57–86, 1988.
34. Bohlman, H. H.: Complications of treatment of fractures and dislocations of the cervical spine. In Epps, C. (ed.): Complications of Orthopaedic Surgery. Philadelphia, J. B. Lippincott Co., 1985, pp. 897–918.
35. Bohlman, H. H., and Zdeblick, T. A.: Anterior excision of herniated thoracic disks. J. Bone Joint Surg. *70A*:1038–1047, 1988.
36. Bohlman, H. H., and Anderson, P. A.: Anterior decompression and arthrodesis of the cervical spine: Long-term motor improvement. Part I: Improvement in incomplete traumatic quadriparesis. J. Bone Joint Surg. *74A*:671–682, 1992.
37. Bohlman, H. H.: The neck. In D'Ambrosia, R. D. (ed.): Musculoskeletal Disorders, Regional Examination Differential Diagnosis. 2nd ed. Philadelphia, J. B. Lippincott Co., 1985, pp. 219–286.
38. Bohlman, H. H., and Emery, S. E.: The pathophysiology of cervical spondylosis and myelopathy. Spine *13*:843–846, 1988.
39. Bohlman, H. H.: Treatment of thoracic and lumbar fractures and dislocations. Current concepts review. J. Bone Joint Surg. *67A*:192–200, 1985.
40. Bohlman, H. H., Freehafer, A., and Dejak, J.: The results of treatment of acute injuries of the upper thoracic spine with paralysis. J. Bone Joint Surg. *67A*:360–369, 1985.
41. Bohlman, H. H.: Degenerative arthritis of the lower cervical spine. In Evarts, C. M. (ed.): Surgery of the Musculoskeletal System. 2nd ed. Vol. 2. New York, Churchill Livingston, 1989, pp. 2211–2231.
42. Bohlman, H. H., and Boada, E.: Fractures and dislocations of the lower cervical spine. In Cervical Research Society (ed.): The Cervical Spine. 2nd ed. Philadelphia, J. B. Lippincott Co., 1988, pp. 487–514.
43. Bohlman, H. H.: Late progressive paralysis and pain following fractures of the thoracolumbar spine: A report of 10 patients. J. Bone Joint Surg. *58A*:723, 1976.
44. Bohlman, H. H.: Cervical spondylosis with moderate to severe myelopathy: A report of 17 cases treated by Robinson anterior cervical discectomy and fusion. Spine *2*:151–162, 1977.
45. Bohlman, H. H., Riley, L. Jr., and Robinson, R. A.: Anterolateral approaches to the cervical spine. In Rugi, D., and Wiltse, L. L. (eds.): Spinal Disorders. Philadelphia, Lea & Febiger, 1977, p. 125.
46. Bohlman, H. H.: Acute fractures and dislocations of the cervical spine: An analysis of 300 hospitalized patients and review of the literature. J. Bone Joint Surg. *61A*:1119–1142, 1979.
47. Bohlman, H. H., Bahniuk, E., Raskulinecz, G., and Field, G.: Mechanical factors affecting recovery from incomplete cervical

spinal cord injury: A preliminary report. Johns Hopkins Med. J. *145*:115–125, 1979.

48. Bohlman, H. H., Bahniuk, E., Field, G., and Raskulinecz, G.: Spinal cord monitoring of experimental incomplete cervical spinal cord injury. Spine *6*:428–436, 1981.

49. Bohlman, H. H.: Indications for late anterior decompression and fusion for cervical spinal cord injuries. *In* Tator, C. H. (ed.): Early Management of Acute Cervical Spinal Cord Injury. New York, Raven Press, 1982, pp. 315–333.

50. Bohlman, H. H., and Eismont, F. J.: Surgical techniques of anterior decompression and fusion for spinal cord injuries. Clin. Orthop. *154*:57–67, 1981.

51. Bolesta, M. J., and Bohlman, H. H.: Surgical management of injuries to the thoracic and lumbar spine. *In* Findlay, G., and Owen, R. (eds.): Surgery of the Spine: A Combined Orthopedic and Neurosurgical Approach. Oxford, Blackwell Scientific Publications, 1992, pp. 1115–1129.

52. Bolesta, M. J., and Bohlman, H. H.: Late sequelae of fractures and fracture-dislocations of the thoracolumbar spine: Surgical treatment. *In* Frymoyer, J. (ed.): The Adult Spine—Principles and Practice. New York, Raven Press, 1991, pp. 1331–1352.

53. Bolesta, M. J., and Bohlman, H. H.: Mediastinal widening associated with fractures of the upper thoracic spine. J. Bone Joint Surg. *73A*:447–450, 1991.

54. Bolesta, M. J., and Bohlman, H. H.: Late complications of cervical fractures and dislocations and their surgical treatment. *In* Frymoyer, J. (ed.): The Adult Spine—Principles and Practice. New York, Raven Press, 1991, pp. 1107–1126.

55. Boling, D., Taxdal, D., and Robinson, R. A.: Six case histories demonstrating the feasibility of partial or total replacement of vertebral bodies by bone grafts. Am. Surg. *26*:236–247, 1960.

56. Bosch, A., Stauffer, E. S., and Nickel, V. L.: Incomplete traumatic quadriplegia—a ten-year review. JAMA *216*:473–478, 1971.

57. Bose, B., Northrup, B. E., and Osterholm, J. L.: Delayed vertebrobasilar insufficiency following cervical spine injury. Spine *10*:108–110, 1985.

58. Braakman, R., and Penning, L.: Injuries of the Cervical Spine. Amsterdam, Excerpta Medica, 1971, p. 262.

59. Braakman, R., and Penning, L.: Injuries of the cervical spine. *In* Vinken, P. J., and Bruyn, G. W. (eds.): Handbook of Clinical Neurology. Vol. 25. Amsterdam, Elsevier-North Holland, 1976, pp. 227–380.

60. Bracken, M. B., and Holford, T. R.: Effects of timing of methylprednisolone or naloxone administration on recovery of segmental and long tract neurological function in NASCIS 2. J. Neurosurg. *79*:500–507, 1993.

61. Bracken, M. B., Shepard, M. J., Collins, W. F. Jr., et al: Methylprednisolone or naloxone treatment after acute spinal cord injury: 1-year follow-up data. J. Neurosurg. *76*:23–31, 1992.

61a. Bracken, M. B.: Pharmacological treatment of acute spinal cord injury: Current status and future projects. J. Emerg. Med. *1*:43–48, 1993.

61b. Bracken, M., Collins, W., Freeman, D., et al.: Efficacy of methylprednisolone in acute spinal cord injury. JAMA *251*:45–52, 1984.

61c. Bracken, M., Shepard, M. J., Holford, T. R., et al.: Administration of methylprednisolone for 24 or 48 hours or Tirilazad Mesylate for 48 hours in the treatment of acute spinal cord injury. JAMA *277*:1597–1604, 1997.

62. Bracken, M. B., Shepard, M. J., Collins, W. F., et al.: A randomized, controlled trial of methylprednisolone or naloxone in the treatment of acute spinal cord injury: Results of the second National Acute Spinal Cord Injury study. N. Engl. J. Med. *322*:1405–1411, 1990.

63. Bracken, M. B., Shepard, M. J., Hellenbrand, K. G., et al.: Methylprednisolone and neurological function one year after spinal cord injury. Results of the National Acute Spinal Cord Injury Study. J. Neurosurg. *63*:704–713, 1985.

64. Bradford, D. S., Winter, R. B., Lonstein, J. E., and Moe, J. H.: Techniques of anterior spinal surgery for the management of kyphosis. Clin. Orthop. *128*:129, 1977.

65. Bradford, D. S., Akbarnia, B. A., Winter, R. B., and Seljeskog, E. L.: Surgical stabilization of fracture and fracture dislocation of the thoracic spine. Spine *2*:185–196, 1977.

66. Bradford, D. S., and McBride, G. G.: Surgical management of

67. Brankman, R., Schouten, H. J., Blaauw-van Dishoeck, M., and Minderhoud, J. M.: Megadose steroids in severe head injury: Results of prospective double-blind clinical trial. J. Neurosurg. *58*:326–330, 1983.

68. Brashear, H. R. Jr., Venters, G. D., and Preston, E. T.: Fractures of the neural arch of the axis. A report of twenty-nine cases. J. Bone Joint Surg. *57A*:789–887, 1975.

69. Braughler, J. M., and Hall, E. D.: Correlation of methylprednisolone levels in cat spinal cord with its effects on (Na+ = K+)-ATPase, lipid peroxidation and alpha motor neuron function. J. Neurosurg. *56*:838–844, 1983.

70. Braughler, J. M., and Hall, E. D.: Effects of multi-dose methylprednisolone sodium succinate administration on injured cat spinal cord neurofilament degradation and energy metabolism. J. Neurosurg. *61*:290–295, 1984.

71. Braughler, J. M., Hall, E. D., Means, E. D., et al.: Evaluation of an intensive methylprednisolone sodium succinate dosing regimen in experimental spinal cord injury. J. Neurosurg. *67*:102–105, 1987.

72. Brieg, A. H.: Adverse Mechanical Tension in the Central Nervous System. 2nd ed. New York, John Wiley & Sons, 1978.

73. Brieg, A., Turnbull, I., and Hassler, O.: Effects of mechanical stresses on the spinal cord in cervical spondylosis. A study of fresh cadaver material. J. Neurosurg. *25*:45–46, 1966.

74. Brodkey, J. S., Richards, E. E., Blasingame, J. P., and Nulsen, F. E.: Reversible spinal cord trauma in cats: Additive effects of direct pressure and ischemia. J. Neurosurg. *37*:591–593, 1972.

75. Brodkey, J. S., Miller, C. F. Jr., and Harmody, R. M.: The syndrome of acute central cervical spinal cord injury revisited. Surg. Neurol. *14*:251–257, 1980.

76. Brown, L. P., Bridwell, K. H., Holt, R. T., et al.: Aortic erosions and lacerations associated with the Dunn anterior spinal instrumentation. Orthop. Trans. *10*:16, 1986.

77. Brunette, D. D., and Rockswold, G. L.: Neurologic recovery following rapid spinal realignment for complete cervical spinal cord injury. J. Trauma *27*:445–447, 1987.

78. Bucholz, R. W.: Unstable hangman's fractures. Clin. Orthop. *154*:119–124, 1981.

79. Burke, D. C.: Hyperextension injuries of the spine. J. Bone Joint Surg. *53B*:3–12, 1971.

80. Burke, D. C., and Berryman, D.: The place of closed manipulation in the management of flexion-rotation dislocations of the cervical spine. J. Bone Joint Surg. *53B*:165–182, 1971.

81. Burke, D. C., and Murray, D. C.: The management of thoracic and thoracolumbar injuries of the spine with neurological involvement. J. Bone Joint Surg. *58B*:72–78, 1976.

82. Burrington, J. D., Brown, C., Wayne, E. R., and Odom, J.: Anterior approach to the thoracolumbar spine. Arch. Surg. *11*:456, 1976.

83. Cammisa, F. P. Jr., Eismont, F. J., and Green, B. A.: Dural laceration occurring with burst fractures and associated laminar fractures. J. Bone Joint Surg. *71A*:1044–1052, 1989.

84. Capener, N.: The evaluation of lateral rhachotomy. J. Bone Joint Surg. *36B*:173, 1954.

85. Carlson, G. D., Minato, Y., Okada, A., et al.: Early time-dependent decompression for spinal cord injury: vascular mechanisms of recovery. J. Neurotrauma *14*:951–962, 1997.

86. Carlson, G. D., Warden, K. E., Barbeau, J. M., et al.: Viscoelastic relaxation and regional blood flow response to spinal cord compression and decompression. Spine *22*:1285–1291, 1997.

87. Caspar, W., Barbier, D. D., and Klara, P. M.: Anterior cervical fusion and Caspar plate stabilization for cervical trauma. Neurosurgery *25*:491–502, 1989.

88. Cattell, H. S., and Filtzer, D. L.: Pseudosubluxation and other normal variations in the cervical spine in children: A study of one hundred and sixty children. J. Bone Joint Surg. *47A*:1295–1309, 1964.

89. Chang, D. G., Tencer, A. F., Ching, R. P., et al.: Geometric changes in the cervical spinal canal during impact. Spine *19*:973–980, 1994.

90. Chiaruttini, M.: Transverse sacral fracture with transient neurologic complications. Ann. Emerg. Med. *16*:111–113, 1987.

91. Ching, R. P., Tencer, A. F., Anderson, P. A., and Daly, C. H.: Comparison of residual stability in thoracolumbar spine fractures using neutral zone measurements. J. Orthop. Res. *13*:533–541, 1995.

92. Cheshire, D. J. E.: The stability of the cervical spine following the conservative treatment of fractures and fracture-dislocations. Paraplegia *7*:193–203, 1969.

93. Clark, C. R., and White, A. A. III: Fractures of the dens. A multicenter study. J. Bone Joint Surg. *67A*:1340–1348, 1985.

94. Clendenon, N. R., Allen, N., Gordon, W. A., et al.: Inhibition of Na$^+$-K$^+$ activated ATPase activity following experimental spinal cord trauma. J. Neurosurg. *49*:563–568, 1978.

95. Clohisy, J. C., Akbarnia, B. A., Bucholz, R. D., et al.: Neurologic recovery associated with anterior decompression of spine fractures at the thoracolumbar junction (T12-L1). Spine *17*:S325–S330, 1992.

96. Cloward, R. B.: Treatment of acute fractures and fracture-dislocations of the cervical spine by vertebral-body fusion: Report of eleven cases. J. Neurosurg. *18*:201–209, 1961.

97. Coe, J. D., Wharton, K. E., Sutterlin, C. E., and McAfee, P. C.: Biomechanical evaluation of cervical spinal stabilization methods in a human cadaveric model. Spine *14*:1122–1131, 1989.

98. Comarr, A. E., and Kaufman, A. A.: A survey of the neurological results of 858 spinal cord injuries. A comparison of patients treated with and without laminectomy. J. Neurosurg. *13*:95–106, 1956.

99. Condon, B. R., and Hadley, D. M.: Quantification of cord deformation and dynamics during flexion and extension of the cervical spine using MR imaging. J. Comput. Assist. Tomogr. *12*:947–955, 1988.

100. Court-Brown, C. M., and Gertzbein, S. D.: The management of burst fractures of the fifth lumbar vertebra. Spine *12*:308–312, 1987.

101. Crock, H. V., and Yoshizawa, H.: The Blood Supply of the Vertebral Column and Spinal Cord in Man. New York, Springer-Verlag, 1977.

102. Crockard, H. A., Heilman, A. E., and Stevens, J. M.: Progressive myelopathy secondary to odontoid fractures: clinical, radiological, and surgical features. J. Neurosurg. *78*:579–586, 1993.

103. Croft, T. J., Brodkey, J. S., and Nulsen, F. E.: Reversible spinal cord trauma: A model for electrical monitoring of spinal cord function. J. Neurosurg. *36*:402–406, 1972.

104. Dall, B. E., and Stauffer, E. S.: Neurologic injury and recovery patterns in burst fractures at the T12 or L1 motion segment. Clin. Orthop. *233*:171–176, 1988.

105. Dastur, D. K., Wadia, N. H., Desai, A. D., and Sing, G.: Medullispinal compression due to atlanto-axial dislocation and sudden haematomyelia during decompression. Pathology, pathogenesis and clinical correlations. Brain *88*:897–924, 1964.

106. Davies, W. E., Morris, J. H., Hill, V., and Phty, B.: An analysis of conservative (non-surgical) management of thoracolumbar fractures and fracture dislocations with neural damage. J. Bone Joint Surg. *62A*:1324–1328, 1980.

107. Davis, D., Bohlman, H. H., Walker, A. E., et al.: The pathological findings in fatal craniospinal injuries. J. Neurosurg. *34*:603–613, 1971.

108. deBeer, J. D., Hoffman, E. B., and Kieck, C. F.: Traumatic atlantoaxial subluxation in children. J. Pediatr. Orthop. *10*:397–400, 1990.

109. Delamarter R. B., Sherman, J., and Carr, J. B.: Pathophysiology of spinal cord injury: Recovery after immediate and delayed decompression. J. Bone Joint Surg. *77A*:1042–1049, 1995.

110. Delamarter, R. B., Bohlman, H. H., Bodner, D., and Biro, C.: Urological function after experimental cauda equina compression: Cystometrograms vs. cortical-evoked potentials. Spine *15*:864–870, 1990.

111. Delamarter, R. B., Bohlman, H. H., and Biro, C.: Decompression of experimental spinal stenosis: Analysis of cortical evoked potentials, vasculature, and histopathology. International Society for the Study of the Lumbar Spine Annual Meeting, Kyoto, Japan, May 1989. Orthop. Trans. *4*:34–35, 1990.

112. Delamarter, R. B., Batzdorf, U., and Bohlman, H. H.: The C7-T1 junction: Problems with diagnosis, visualization, instability and decompression. Orthop. Trans. *13*(2):218, 1989.

113. Delamarter, R. B., Ross, J. S., Masaryk, T. J., et al.: Diagnosis of lumbar arachnoiditis by magnetic resonance imaging. Spine *15*:304–310, 1990.

114. Delamarter, R. B., Bohlman, H. H., Dodge, L. D., and Biro, C.: Experimental lumbar stenosis, analysis of the vasculature, histology, and cortical evoked potentials following chronic compression of the dog cauda equina. J. Bone Joint Surg. *72A*:111–120, 1990.

115. DeMaria, E. J., Reichman, W., Kenney, P. R., et al.: Septic complications of corticosteroid administration after central nervous system trauma. Ann. Surg. *202*:248–252, 1985.

116. Denis, F.: The three column spine and its significance in the classification of acute thoracolumbar spinal injuries. Spine *8*:817–831, 1983.

117. Denis, F., Davis, S., and Comfort, T.: Sacral fractures: An important problem. Retrospective analysis of 236 cases. Clin. Orthop. *227*:67–81, 1988.

118. Detwiler, K. N., Loftus, C. M., Godersky, J. C., and Menezes, A. H.: Management of cervical spine injuries in patients with ankylosing spondylitis. J. Neurosurg. *72*:210–215, 1990.

119. Dickson, H. H., Harrington, P. R., and Erwin, W. D.: Results of reduction and stabilization of the severely fractured thoracic and lumbar spine. J. Bone Joint Surg. *60A*:799–805, 1978.

120. Drohrmann, G. L., Wagner, F. C., Jr., and Bucy, P. C.: The microvasculature in transitory traumatic paraplegia: An electron microscopic study in the monkey. J. Neurosurg. *35*:263–271, 1971.

121. Dolan, E. J., Tator, C. H., and Endrenyi, L.: The value of decompression for acute experimental spinal cord compression injury. J. Neurosurg. *53*:749–755, 1980.

122. Doppman, J. L., and Girton, M.: Angiographic study of the effect of laminectomy in the presence of acute anterior epidural masses. J. Neurosurg. *45*:195–202, 1976.

123. Ducker, T. B., and Zeidman, S. M.: Spinal cord injury. Role of steroid therapy. Spine *19*:2281–2287, 1994.

124. Ducker, T. B., and Hamit, H. F.: Experimental treatments of acute spinal cord injury. J. Neurosurg. *30*:693–697, 1969.

125. Ducker, T. B., and Kindt, G. W.: The effect of trauma on the vasomotor control of spinal cord blood flow. Curr. Top. Surg. Res. *3*:163–171, 1971.

126. Ducker, T. B., Kindt, G. W., and Kempe, L. G.: Pathological findings in acute experimental spinal cord trauma. J. Neurosurg. *35*:700–708, 1971.

127. Ducker, T. B.: Experimental injury of the spinal cord. *In* Vinken, P. J., and Bruyn, G. W. (eds.): Handbook of Clinical Neurology. Vol. 25. Amsterdam, Elsevier-North Holland, 1976, pp. 9–26.

128. Ducker, T. B., Salcman, M., Perot, P. L., et al.: Experimental spinal cord trauma. I: Correlations of blood flow, tissue oxygen and neurologic status in the dog. Surg. Neurol. *10*:60–63, 1978.

129. Ducker, T. B., Salcman, M., Lucas, J. T., et al.: Experimental spinal cord trauma. II: Blood flow, tissue oxygen, evoked potentials in both paretic and plegic monkeys. Surg. Neurol. *10*:64–70, 1978.

130. Ducker, T. B., Salcman, M., and Daniel, H. B.: Experimental spinal cord trauma. III: Therapeutic effect of immobilization and pharmacologic agents. Surg. Neurol. *10*:71–76, 1978.

131. Ducker, T. B.: Treatment of spinal cord injury [editorial]. N. Engl. J. Med. *322*:1459–1461, 1990.

132. Ducker, T. B., Lucas, J. T., and Wallace, C. A.: Recovery from spinal cord injury. Clin. Neurosurg. *30*:495–513, 1983.

133. Ducker, T. B., Bellegarrique, R., Salomon, M., and Walleck, C.: Timing of operative care in cervical spinal cord injury. Spine *9*:525–531, 1984.

134. Duh, M. S., Shepard, M. J., Wilberger, J. E., and Bracken, M. B.: The effectiveness of surgery on the treatment of acute spinal cord injury and its relation to pharmacological treatment. Neurosurgery *35*:240–249, 1994.

135. Dunn, E. J., and Blazar, S.: Soft-tissue injuries of the lower cervical spine. A.A.O.S. Instructional Course Lectures *36*:499–512, 1987.

136. Dunn, E. J., and LeClair, W. E.: How to reduce complications in treatment of cervical spine trauma. A.A.O.S. Instructional Course Lectures *34*:155–162, 1985.

137. Dvorak, J., Schneider, E., Saldinger, P., and Rahn, B.: Biomecha-

nics of the craniocervical region: The alar and transverse ligaments. J. Orthop. Res. *6*:452–461, 1988.

138. Effendi, B., Roy, D., Cornish, B., et al.: Fractures of the ring of the axis. A classification based on the analysis of 131 cases. J. Bone Joint Surg. *63B*:319–327, 1981.

139. Eismont, F. J., Borja, F., and Bohlman, H. H.: Complete dislocations at two adjacent levels of the cervical spine. A case report. Spine *9*:319–322, 1984.

140. Eismont, F. J., Clifford, S., Goldberg, M., and Green B.: Cervical sagittal spinal canal size in spine injury. Spine *9*:663–666, 1984.

141. Eismont, F. J., Bohlman, H. H., Soni, P. L., et al.: Pyogenic and fungal osteomyelitis of the spine with paralysis. J. Bone Joint Surg. *65A*:19–29, 1983.

142. Eismont, F. J., and Bohlman, H. H.: Posterior methylmethacrylate fixation for cervical trauma: A review of six cases with emphasis on complications. Spine *6*:21–27, 1981.

143. Eismont, F. J., Green, B. A., Berkowitz, B. M., et al.: The role of intraoperative ultrasonography in the treatment of thoracic and lumbar spine fractures. Spine *9*:782–787, 1984.

144. Eismont, F. J., Green, B. A., and Quencer, R. M.: Post-traumatic spinal cord cyst. A case report. J. Bone Joint Surg. *66A*:614–618, 1984.

145. Eismont, F. J., and Bohlman, H. H.: Posterior atlanto-occipital dislocation with fractures of the atlas and odontoid process: Report of a case with survival. J. Bone Joint Surg. *60A*:387–399, 1978.

146. Emery, S. E., Pathria, M. N., Wilber, R. G., et al.: Magnetic resonance imaging of post-traumatic spinal ligament injury. J. Spinal Disord. *2*:229–233, 1989.

147. Epstein, N., Hood, D. C., and Ransohoff, J.: Gastrointestinal bleeding in patients with spinal cord trauma. Effects of steroids, cimetidine, and mini-dose heparin. J. Neurosurg. *54*:16–20, 1981.

148. Epstein, N. E., Epstein, J. A., and Carras, R.: Unilateral S-1 root compression syndrome caused by fracture of the sacrum. Neurosurgery *19*:1025–1027, 1986.

149. Evans, D. L., and Bethem, D.: Cervical spine injuries in children. J. Pediatr. Orthop. *9*:563–568, 1989.

150. Evarts, C. M.: Traumatic occipito-atlantal dislocation. Report of a case with survival. J. Bone Joint Surg. *52A*:1653–1660, 1970.

151. Faden, A. I., Jacobs, T. P., Patrick, D. H., and Smith, M. T.: Megadose corticosteroid therapy following experimental traumatic spinal cord injury. J. Neurosurg. *60*:712–717, 1984.

152. Fairholm, D. J., and Turnbull, I. M.: Microangiographic study of experimental spinal cord injuries. J. Neurosurg. *35*:277–286, 1971.

153. Fang, H. S. Y., and Ogn, G. B.: Direct anterior approach to upper cervical spine. J. Bone Joint Surg. *44A*:1588–1604, 1962.

154. Ferguson, R. L., and Allen, B. L. Jr.: A mechanistic classification of thoracolumbar spine fractures. Clin. Orthop. *189*:77–88, 1984.

155. Fielding, J. W.: Injuries to the upper cervical spine. A.A.O.S. Instructional Course Lectures *36*:483–494, 1987.

156. Fielding, J. W., Francis, W. R. Jr., Hawkins, R. J., et al.: Traumatic spondylolisthesis of the axis. Clin. Orthop. *239*:47–52, 1989.

157. Fielding, J. W., Cochran, G. V. B., Lawsing, J. F. III, and Hohl, M.: Tears of the transverse ligament of the atlas: A clinical and biomechanical study. J. Bone Joint Surg. *56A*:1683–1691, 1974.

158. Fielding, J. W., and Griffin, P. P.: Os odonotoideum: An acquired lesion. J. Bone Joint Surg. *56A*:187–190, 1974.

159. Fielding, J. W., Tuul, A., and Hawkins, R. J.: "Ondine's curse": A complication of upper cervical spine surgery. J. Bone Joint Surg. *57A*:1000–1001, 1975.

160. Fielding, J. W., Hawkins, R. J., and Ratzan, S. A.: Spine fusion for atlanto-axial instability. J. Bone Joint Surg. *58A*:400–407, 1976.

161. Fielding, J. W., and Hawkins, R. J.: Atlanto-axial rotatory fixation. J. Bone Joint Surg. *59A*:37–44, 1977.

162. Finerman, G. A. M., Sakai, D., and Weingarten, S.: Atlanto-axial dislocation with spinal cord compression in a mongoloid child. J. Bone Joint Surg. *58A*:408–409, 1976.

163. Flamm, E. S., Young, W., Collins, W. F., et al.: A Phase I trial of naloxone treatment in acute spinal cord injury. J. Neurosurg. *63*:3990–3997, 1985.

164. Flesch, J. R., Leider, L. L. Jr., and Bradford, D. S.: Harrington instrumentation of thoracic and lumbar spinal injuries. J. Bone Joint Surg. *57A*:1025, 1975.

165. Flesch, J. R., Leider, L. L. Jr., Erickson, D. D., et al.: Harrington instrumentation and spine fusion for unstable fractures and fracture dislocations of the thoracic and lumbar spine. J. Bone Joint Surg. *57A*:143–153, 1977.

166. Forsyth, H. F., Alexander, E. Jr., Davis, C. R., and Underal, R.: The advantages of early spine fusion in the treatment of fracture-dislocation of the cervical spine. J. Bone Joint Surg. *41A*:17–36, 1959.

167. Fountain, S. S., Hamilton, R. D., and Jameson, R. M.: Transverse fractures of the sacrum. J. Bone Joint Surg. *59A*:486–489, 1977.

168. Francis, W. R., Fielding, J. W., Hawkins, R. J., et al.: Traumatic spondylolisthesis of the axis. J. Bone Joint Surg. *63B*:313–318, 1981.

169. Frankel, H. L., Hancock, D. O., Hyslop, G., et al.: The value of postural reduction in the initial management of closed injuries of the spine with paraplegia and tetraplegia. Paraplegia *7*:179, 1969.

170. Frederickson, B. E., Yaun, H. A., and Miller, H.: Burst fractures of the fifth lumbar vertebra. A report of four cases. J. Bone Joint Surg. *64A*:1088–1094, 1982.

171. Freehafer, A. A.: Limb fractures in patients with spinal cord injury. Arch. Phys. Med. Rehabil. *76*:823–827, 1995.

172. Freehafer, A. A., and Mast, W. A.: Lower extremity fractures in patients with spinal cord injury. J. Bone Joint Surg. *47A*:683–694, 1965.

173. Freehafer, A. A., and Mast, W. A.: Transfer to the brachioradialis to improve wrist extension in high cervical spinal cord injury. J. Bone Joint Surg. *49A*:648–652, 1967.

174. Freehafer, A. A., Von Haam, E., and Allen, V.: Tendon transfers to improve grasp after injuries of the cervical spinal cord. J. Bone Joint Surg. *56A*:951–959, 1974.

175. Fried, L. C.: Cervical spine cord injury during skeletal traction. JAMA *229*:181–183, 1974.

176. Gaines, R. W., Breedlove, R. F., and Munson, G.: Stabilization of thoracic and thoracolumbar fracture-dislocations with Harrington rods and sublaminar wires. Clin. Orthop. *189*:195, 1984.

176a. Galandiuk, S., Racque, G., Appel, S., Polk, H. J.: The two-edged sword of large-dose steroids for spinal cord trauma. Ann. Surg. *218*:419–425, 1993.

177. Garfin, S. R., Botte, M. J., Waters, R. L., and Nickel, V. L.: Complications in the use of the halo fixation device. J. Bone Joint Surg. *68A*:320–325, 1986.

178. Garvey, T. A., Eismont, F. J., and Roberti, L. J.: Anterior decompression, structural bone grafting, and Caspar plate stabilization for unstable cervical spine fractures and/or dislocations. Spine *17*:S431–S435, 1992.

179. Geisler, F. H., Mirvis, S. E., Zrebeet, H., and Joslyn, J. N.: Titanium wire internal fixation for stabilization of injury of the cervical spine: Clinical results and postoperative magnetic resonance imaging of the spinal cord. Neurosurgery *25*:356–362, 1989.

180. Gerndt, S. J., Rodriguez, J. L., Pawlik, J. W., et al.: Consequences of high dose steroid therapy for acute spinal cord injury. J. Trauma *42*:279–284, 1997.

181. Gertzbein, S. D., and Court-Brown, C. M.: Flexion-distraction injuries of the lumbar spine. Mechanisms of injury and classification. Clin. Orthop. *227*:52–60, 1988.

182. Gertzbein, D. S., Court-Brown, C. M., Jacobs, R. R., et al.: Decompression and circumferential stabilization of unstable spinal fractures. Spine *13*:892–895, 1988.

183. Gibbons, K. J., Soloniuk, D. S., and Razack, N.: Neurological injury and patterns of sacral fractures. J. Neurosurg. *72*:889–893, 1990.

184. Gooding, M. R., Wilson, C. B., and Hoff, J. T.: Experimental cervical myelopathy. Effects of ischemia and compression of the canine cervical spine cord. J. Neurosurg. *43*:9–17, 1975.

185. Grabb, P. A., and Pang, D.: Magnetic resonance imaging in the evaluation of spinal cord injury without radiographic abnormality in children. Neurosurgery *35*:406–414, 1994.

186. Graham, B., and Van Peteghem, P. K.: Fractures of the spine in ankylosing spondylitis. Diagnosis, treatment, and complications. Spine *14*:803–807, 1989.

186a. Green, B., Kahn, T., Klose, K.: A comparative study of steroid therapy in acute experimental spinal cord injury. Surg. Neurol. *13*:91–97, 1980.

186b. Greene, K. A., Marciano, F. F., Sonntag, V. K.: Pharmacological management of spinal cord injury: Current status of drugs designed to augment functional recovery of the injured human spinal cord. J. Spinal Disord. *9(5)*:355–366, 1996.

187. Griffiths, I. R.: Spinal cord blood flow in dogs: The effect of blood pressure. J. Neurosurg. Psychiatr. *36*:914–920, 1973.

188. Griffiths, I. R.: Vasogenic edema following acute and chronic spinal cord compression in the dog. J. Neurosurg. *42*:155–165, 1975.

189. Grisolia, A., Bell, R. L., and Peltier, L. F.· Fractures and dislocations of the spine complicating ankylosing spondylitis. A report of six cases. J. Bone Joint Surg. *49A*:339–344, 1967.

190. Grundy, B. L., and Frindman, W.: Electrophysiological evaluation of the patient with acute spinal cord injury. Crit. Care Clin. *3*:519–548, 1987.

191. Gurr, K. R., McAfee, P. C., and Shih, C. M.: Biomechanical analysis of anterior and posterior instrumentation systems after corpectomy. A calf-spine model. J. Bone Joint Surg. *70*:1182–1191, 1988.

192. Guth, L.: History of CNS regeneration research. Exp. Neurol. *48*:3–15, 1975.

193. Guth, L., Bright, D., and Donati, E. J.: Functional deficits and anatomical alterations after high cervical spinal hemisection in the rat. Exp. Neurol. *58*:511–520, 1978.

194. Hadley, M. N., Dickman, C. A., Browner, C. M., and Sonntag, V. K.: Acute axis fractures: A review of 229 cases. J. Neurosurg. *71*:642–647, 1989.

195. Hadley, M. N., Zabramski, J. M., Browner, C. M., et al.: Pediatric spinal trauma. Review of 122 cases of spinal cord and vertebral column injuries. J. Neurosurg. *68*:18–24, 1988.

196. Hadley, M. N., Browner, C., and Sonntag, V. K.: Axis fractures: A comprehensive review of management and treatment in 107 cases. Neurosurgery *17*:281–290, 1985.

196a. Hall, E. D.: The neuroprotective pharmacology of methylprednisolone. J. Neurosurg. *76*:13–22, 1992.

196b. Hall, E. D.: The effects of glucocorticoid and nonglucocorticoid steroids on acute neuronal degeneration. Adv. Neurol. *59*:241–248, 1993.

197. Handa, Y., Hayashi, M., Kawano, H., et al.: Vertebral artery thrombosis accompanied by burst fracture of the lower cervical spine: case report. Neurosurgery *17*:955–957, 1985.

197a. Hanigan, W. C., Anderson, R. J.: Commentary on NASCIS-2. J. Spinal Disord. *5*:125–131, 1992.

198. Hazel, W. A. Jr., Jones, R. A., Morrey, B. F., and Stauffer, R. N.: Vertebral fractures without neurological deficit. A long-term follow-up study. J. Bone Joint Surg. *70A*:1319–1321, 1988.

198a. Heary, R. F., Vaccaro, A. R., Mesa, J. J., et al.: Steroids and gunshot wounds to the spine. Neurosurg. *41(3)*:576–584, 1997.

199. Herkowitz, H. N., and Rothman, R. H.: Subacute instability of the cervical spine. Spine *9*:348–357, 1984.

200. Herzenberg, J. E., Hensinger, R. N., Dedrick, D. K., and Phillips, W. A.: Emergency transport and positioning of young children who have an injury of the cervical spine. The standard backboard may be hazardous. J. Bone Joint Surg. *71A*:15–22, 1989.

201. Hida, K., Iwasaki, Y., Imamura, H., and Abe, H.: Posttraumatic syringomyelia: Its characteristic magnetic resonance imaging findings in surgical management. Neurosurgery *35*:886–891, 1994.

202. Hilibrand, A. S., Urquhart, A. G., Graziano, G. P., and Hensinger, R. N.: Acute spondylotic spondylolisthesis. Risk of progression and neurological complications. J. Bone Joint Surg. *77A*:190–196, 1995.

203. Hinchey, J. E., Hreno, A., Benoit, P. R., et al.: The stress ulcer syndrome. *In* Welch, C. (ed.): Advances in Surgery, Vol. 4. Chicago, Yearbook Medical, 1970, pp. 325–393.

203a. Hoerlein, B., Redding, R., Hoff, E., Ja, M.: Evaluation of naloxone, crocetin, thyrotropin releasing hormone, methylprednisolone, partial myelotomy, and hemilaminectomy in the treatment of acute spinal cord trauma. J. Am. Anim. Hosp. Assoc. *21*:67–77, 1984.

204. Hohl, M.: Soft tissue injuries of the neck in automobile accidents. J. Bone Joint Surg. *46A*:1777–1779, 1964.

205. Holdsworth, F. W., and Hardy, A.: Early treatment of paraplegia from fractures of the thoracolumbar spine. J. Bone Joint Surg. *35B*:540–550, 1953.

206. Holdsworth, F. W.: Fractures, dislocations and fracture-dislocations of the spine. J. Bone Joint Surg. *52A*:1534–1551, 1970.

206a. Holtz, A., Gerdin, B.: Blocking weight-induced spinal cord injury in rats. Neurol. Res. *14*:49–52, 1992.

207. Hu, S. S., Capen, D. A., Rimoldi, R. L., and Ziegler, J. E.: The effect of surgical decompression on neurologic outcome after lumbar fractures. Clin. Orthop. *288*:166–173, 1993.

208. Huelke, D. F., Mackay, G. M., and Morris, A.: Vertebral column injuries and lap shoulder belts. J. Trauma *38*:547–556, 1995.

209. Huelke, D. F., and Nusholtz, G. S.: Cervical spine biomechanics. A review of the literature. J. Orthop. Res. *4*:232, 1986.

210. Ito, T., Allen, M., and Yashon, D.: A mitochondrial lesion in experimental spinal cord trauma. J. Neurosurg. *48*:434–442, 1978.

211. Ivan, L. P.: Longitudinal (Bishof's) myelotomy. Curr. Tech. Operative Neurosurg. *30*:435–447, 1977.

212. Jeanneret, B., and Magerl, F.: Primary posterior fusion of C1-2 in odontoid fractures: Indications, technique, and results of transarticular screw fixation. J. Spinal Disord. *5*:464–475, 1992.

213. Jeanneret, B., Magerl, F., and Stanisic, M.: Thrombosis of the vertebral artery. A rare complication following traumatic spondylolisthesis of the second cervical vertebra. Spine *11*:179–182, 1986.

214. Jefferson, G.: Fractures of the atlas vertebra. Report of four cases and a review of those previously recorded. Br. J. Surg. *7*:407–422, 1920.

215. Jelinger, K.: Neuropathology of cord injuries. *In* Vinken, P. J., and Bruyn, G. W. (eds.): Handbook of Clinical Neurology. Vol. 25. Amsterdam, Elsevier-North Holland, 1976, pp. 43–121.

216. Jelsma, R. K., Rice, J. F., Jelsma, L. F., and Kirsch, P. T.: The demonstration and significance of neural compression after spinal injury. Surg. Neurol. *18*:79–92, 1982.

217. Jelsma, R. K., Kirsch, P. T., Jelsma, L. F., et al.: Surgical treatment of thoracolumbar fractures. Surg. Neurol. *18*:156–166, 1982.

218. Kahanovitz, N., Bullough, P., and Jacobs, R. R.: The effect of internal fixation without arthrodesis on human facet joint cartilage. Clin. Orthop. *189*:204–208, 1984.

219. Kaneda, K., Abumi, K., and Fujiya, M.: Burst fractures with neurologic deficits of the thoraco-lumbar-lumbar spine. Results of anterior decompression and stabilization with anterior instrumentation. Spine *9*:788–795, 1984.

220. Kanefield, D. G., Mullins, B. P., Freehafer, A. A., et al.: Destructive lesions of the spine in rheumatoid spondylitis. J. Bone Joint Surg. *51A*:1369–1375, 1969.

221. Kang, J. D., Figgie, M. P., and Bohlman, H. H.: Sagittal measurements of the cervical spine in subaxial fractures and dislocations. An analysis of 288 patients with and without neurologic deficits. J. Bone Joint Surg. *76A*:1617–1627, 1994.

222. Kao, C. C., and Chang, L. W.: The mechanism of spinal cord cavitation following spinal cord transection. Part I: A correlated histochemical study. J. Neurosurg. *46*:197–209, 1977.

223. Kauffer, H., and Hayes, J. T.: Lumbar fracture-dislocations: A study of twenty-one cases. J. Bone Joint Surg. *48A*:712–730, 1966.

224. Kindt, G. W., Ducker, T. B., and Huddlestone, J.: Regulation of spinal cord blood flow. *In* Ross, R. W. (ed.): Brain and Blood Flow. London, Russell Pitman Medical and Scientific, 1971, pp. 401–405.

225. Kobrine, A. I., Doyle, T. F., and Martins, A. N.: Local spinal cord blood flow in experimental traumatic myelopathy. J. Neurosurg. *42*:144–149, 1975.

226. Kobrine, A. I., Doyle, T. F., and Rizzoli, H. V.: Spinal cord blood flow as affected by changes in systemic arterial blood pressure. J. Neurosurg. *44*:12–15, 1976.

227. Kobrine, A. I., Evans, D. E., and Rizzoli, H. V.: Experimental acute balloon compression of the spinal cord. J. Neurosurg. *51*:841–845, 1979.

228. Kramer, K. M., and Levine, A. M.: Unilateral facet dislocation of the lumbosacral junction. A case report and review of the literature. J. Bone Joint Surg. *71A*:1258–1261, 1989.

229. Krengel, W. F. 3rd, Anderson, P. A., and Henley, M. B.: Early stabilization and decompression for incomplete paraplegia due to a thoracic level spinal cord injury. Spine *18*:2080–2087, 1993.

230. Laborde, M. T., Bahniuk, E., Bohlman, H. H., and Samson, B.: Comparison of fixation of spinal fractures. Clin. Orthop. *152*:303–310, 1980.

231. Ladd, A. L., and Scranton, P. E.: Congenital cervical stenosis presenting as transient quadriplegia in athletes. A report of two cases. J. Bone Joint Surg. *68A*:1371–1374, 1986.

232. Lancourt, J. E., Dickson, J. H., and Carter, R. E.: Paralytic spinal deformity following traumatic spinal-cord injury in children and adolescents. J. Bone Joint Surg. *63A*:45–53, 1981.

233. Lansen, T. A., Kasoff, S. S., and Tenner, M. S.: Occipital-cervical fusion for reduction of traumatic periodontoid hypertrophic cicatrix. J. Neurosurg. *73*:466–470, 1990.

234. Larson, S. J., Holst, R. A., Hemmy, D. C., and Sances, A.: Lateral extracavitary approach to traumatic lesions of the thoracic and lumbar spine. J. Neurosurg. *45*:628–637, 1976.

235. Lawson, J. P., Ogden, J. A., Bucholz, R. M., and Hughes, S. A.: Physeal injuries of the cervical spine. J. Pediatr. Orthop. *7*:428–435, 1987.

236. Lazorthes, G., Gouaze, A., Bastide, G., et al.: La vascularisation arterielle du renflement lombaire. Etude des variations et des suppléances. Rev. Neurol. *114*:109–122, 1966.

237. Lazorthes, G., Gouaze, A., Zadeh, J. O., et al.: Arterial vascularization of the spine cord. Recent studies of the anastomotic substitution pathways. J. Neurosurg. *5*:253–262, 1971.

238. Lemons, V. R., and Wagner, F. C. Jr.: Respiratory complications after cervical spinal cord injury. Spine *19*:2315–2320, 1994.

239. Leramo, O. B., Tator, C. H., and Hudson, A. R.: Massive gastroduodenal hemorrhage and perforation in acute spinal cord injury. Surg. Neurol. *17*:186–190, 1982.

240. Levine, A. M., and Edwards, C. C.: Fractures of the atlas. J. Bone Joint Surg. *73A*:680–691, 1991.

241. Levine, A. M., Bosse, M., and Edwards, C. C.: Bilateral facet dislocations in the thoracolumbar spine. Spine *13*:630–640, 1988.

242. Levine, A. M., and Edwards, C. C.: The management of traumatic spondylolisthesis of the axis. J. Bone Joint Surg. *67A*:217–226, 1985.

243. Lewallen, R. P., Morrey, B. F., and Cabanela, M. E.: Respiratory arrest following posteriorly displaced odontoid fractures. Case reports and review of the literature. Clin. Orthop. *188*:187–190, 1984.

244. Li, C., Houlden, D. A., and Rowed, D. W.: Somatosensory-evoked potentials and neurologic grades as predictors of outcomes in acute spinal cord injury. J. Neurosurg. *72*:600–609, 1990.

245. Lieberman, I. H., and Webb, J. K.: Cervical spine injuries in the elderly. J. Bone Joint Surg. *76B*:877–881, 1994.

246. Locke, G. E., Yashon, D., Feldman, A., et al.: Ischemia in primate spinal cord injury. J. Neurosurg. *34*:614–617, 1971.

247. Lonstein, J. E.: Post-laminectomy kyphosis. Clin. Orthop. *128*:93–100, 1977.

248. Lucas, J. T., and Ducker, T. B.: Morbidity, mortality and recovery rates of spinal cord injuries undergoing anterior decompression and/or fusion procedures. Surg. Forum *27*:451–453, 1977.

249. Lucas, J. T., and Ducker, T. B.: Motor classification of spinal cord injuries with mobility, morbidity and recovery indices. Am. Surg. *45*:151–158, 1979.

250. Lucas, J. T., and Ducker, T. B.: Recovery in spinal cord injuries. Adv. Neurosurg. *7*:281–294, 1979.

251. Macnab, I.: Acceleration injuries of the cervical spine. J. Bone Joint Surg. *46A*:1797–1799, 1964.

252. Mahale, Y. J., Silver, J. R., and Henderson, N. J.: Neurological complications of the reduction of cervical spine dislocations. J. Bone Joint Surg. *75B*:403–409, 1993.

253. Maiman, D. J., Larson, S. J., and Benzel, E. C.: Neurological improvement associated with late decompression of the thoracolumbar spinal cord. Neurosurgery *15*:302–307, 1984.

254. Mansel, J. K., and Norman, J. R.: Respiratory complications and management of spinal cord injuries. Chest *97*:1446–1452, 1990.

255. Marar, B. C.: Hyperextension injuries of the cervical spine: The pathogenesis of damage to the spinal cord. J. Bone Joint Surg. *56A*:1655–1662, 1974.

256. Marcus, R. E., and Hansen, S. T. Jr.: Bilateral fracture-dislocation of the sacrum. A case report. J. Bone Joint Surg. *66A*:1297–1299, 1984.

257. Marshall, L. F., Knowlton, S., Garfin, S. R., et al.: Deterioration following spinal cord injury. A multicenter study. J. Neurosurg. *66*:400–404, 1987.

258. Masaryk, T. J., Ross, J. S., Modic, M. T., et al.: High resolution MR imaging of sequestered lumbar intervertebral disks. AJNR *9*:351–358, 1988.

259. Mayfield, J. K., Erkkila, J. C., and Winter, R. B.: Spine deformity subsequent to acquired childhood spinal cord injury. J. Bone Joint Surg. *63A*:1401–1411, 1981.

260. McAfee, P. C., Bohlman, H. H., Riley, L., et al.: Anterior extraoral approach to the atlas and axis. J. Bone Joint Surg. *69A*:1371–1383, 1987.

261. McAfee, P. C., Bohlman, H. H., Ducker, T., and Eismont, F. G.: Failure of stabilization of the spine with methylmethacrylate. A retrospective analysis of 24 cases. J. Bone Joint Surg. *68A*:1145–1157, 1986.

262. McAfee, P. C., Bohlman, H. H., and Yuan, H. A.: Anterior decompression of traumatic thoracolumbar fractures with incomplete neurological deficit using a retroperitoneal approach. J. Bone Joint Surg. *67A*:89–104, 1985.

263. McAfee, P. C., and Bohlman, H. H.: Complications following Harrington instrumentation for fractures of the thoracolumbar spine. J. Bone Joint Surg. *67A*:672–686, 1985.

264. McAfee, P. C., Bohlman, H. H., Han, J. S., and Salvagno, R. T.: Comparison of nuclear magnetic resonance imaging and computed tomography in the diagnosis of upper cervical spinal cord compression. Spine *11*:295–304, 1986.

265. McAfee, P. C., Yuan, H. A., Fredrickson, B. E., and Lubicky, J. P.: The value of computed tomography in thoracolumbar fractures. An analysis of one hundred consecutive cases and a new classification. J. Bone Joint Surg *65A*:461–473, 1983.

266. McAfee, P. C., and Bohlman, H. H.: One-stage anterior cervical decompression and posterior stabilization with circumferential arthrodesis. An analysis of twenty-four cases. J. Bone Joint Surg. *71A*:78–88, 1989.

267. McGrory, B. J., Klassen, R. A., Chao, E. Y. S., et al.: Acute fractures and dislocations of the cervical spine in children and adolescents. J. Bone Joint Surg. *75A*:988–995, 1993.

268. McLain, R. F., Sparling, E., and Benson, D. R.: Early failure of short-segment pedicle instrumentation for thoracolumbar fractures. A preliminary report. J. Bone Joint Surg. *75A*:162–167, 1993.

269. McRae, D. L.: The significance of abnormalities of the cervical spine. AJR *84*:3–25, 1960.

269a. Means, E., Anderson, D., Waters, T., Kalaf, L.: Effect of methylprednisolone in compression trauma to the feline spinal cord. J. Neurosurg *55*:200–208, 1981.

270. Meyer, F. R.: Complications of treatment of fractures and dislocations of the dorsolumbar spine. *In* Epps, C. H. Jr. (ed.): Complications in Orthopaedic Surgery. 2nd ed. 1986, pp. 713–789.

271. Meyer, P. R.: Posterior stabilization of thoracic, lumbar and sacral injuries. A.A.O.S. Instructional Course Lectures *35*:401–419, 1986.

272. Meyer, P. R.: Surgery of Spine Trauma. New York, Churchill Livingston, 1989.

273. Mick, C. A., Carl, A., Sachs, B., et al.: Burst fractures of the fifth lumbar vertebra. Spine *18*:1878–1884, 1993.

274. Miller, C. A., Dewy, R. C., and Hunt, W. E.: Impaction fracture of the lumbar vertebrae with dural tear. J. Neurosurg. *53*:765–771, 1980.

275. Morgan, T. H., Wharton, G. W., and Austin, G. N.: The results of laminectomy in patients with incomplete spinal cord injuries. Paraplegia *9*:14–23, 1971.

276. Nickel, V. L., Perry, J., Garrett, A., and Heppenstall, M.: The halo. J. Bone Joint Surg. *50A*:1400–1409, 1968.

277. Norrell, H., and Wilson, C. B.: Early anterior fusion for injuries of the cervical portion of the spine. JAMA *214*:525–530, 1970.

278. Osti, O. L., Fraser, R. D., and Griffiths, E. R.: Reduction and stabilisation of cervical dislocations. An analysis of 167 cases. J. Bone Joint Surg. *71B*:275–282, 1989.

279. Pan, G., Kulkarni, M., MacDougall, D. J., and Miner, M. E.: Traumatic epidural hematoma of the cervical spine: Diagnosis with magnetic resonance imaging. Case report. J. Neurosurg. *68*:798–801, 1988.

280. Pang, D., and Wilberger, J. E. Jr.: Spinal cord injury without radiographic abnormalities in children. J. Neurosurg. *57*:114, 1982.

281. Panjabi, M. M., Oxland, T. R., Kifune, M., et al.: Validity of the three-column theory of thoracolumbar fractures. A biomechanic investigation. Spine 20:1122–1127, 1995.

282. Panjabi, M. M., and Wrathal, J. R.: Biochemical analysis of spinal cord injury and functional loss. Spine 13:1365–1370, 1988.

283. Pattee, G. A., Bohlman, H. H., and McAfee, P. C.: Sacral nerve root compression as a complication of internal fixation of the sacroiliac joint. A case report. J. Bone Joint Surg. 68:764–771, 1986.

284. Patzakis, M. J.: Posterior dislocation of the atlas on the axis: A case report. J. Bone Joint Surg. 56A:1260, 1974.

285. Paul, R. L., Michael, R. H., Dunn, J. E., and Williams, J. P.: Anterior transthoracic surgical decompression of acute spinal cord injuries. J. Neurosurg. 43:299–307, 1975.

286. Pelker, R. R., and Dorfman, G. S.: Fracture of the axis associated with vertebral artery injury. A case report. Spine 11:621–623, 1986.

287. Penning, L.: Prevertebral hematoma in cervical spine injury: Incidence and etiologic significance. AJR 136:533–561, 1981.

288. Perkash, I.: Intermittent catheterization and bladder rehabilitation in spinal cord injury patients. J. Urol. 114:230–233, 1975.

289. Perot, P. L.: The clinical use of somatosensory evoked potentials in spinal cord injury. Clin. Neurosurg. 20:367–381, 1973.

290. Pierson, R. M.: Spinal and cranial injuries of the baby in breech deliveries. A clinical and pathological study of thirty-eight cases. Surg. Gynecol. Obstet. 37:802–815, 1923.

291. Pizzutillo, P. D., Rocha, E. F., D'Astous, J., et al.: Bilateral fracture of the pedicle of the second cervical vertebra in the young child. J. Bone Joint Surg. 68A:892–896, 1986.

292. Quencer, R. M., Sheldon, J. J., Post, M. J., et al.: MRI of the chronically injured cervical spinal cord. AJR 147:125–132, 1986.

293. Quencer, R. M., Montalvo, B. M., Eismont, F. J., and Green, B. A.: Intraoperative spinal sonography in thoracic and lumbar fractures: Evaluation of Harrington rod instrumentation. AJR 145:343–349, 1985.

294. Rawe, S. E., Roth, R. H., Boadle-Biber, M., et al.: Norepinephrine levels in experimental spinal cord trauma. I: Biochemical study of hemorrhagic necrosis. J. Neurosurg. 46:342–349, 1977.

295. Rawe, S. E., Roth, R. H., and Collins, W. F.: Norepinephrine levels in experimental spinal cord trauma. II: Histopathological study of hemorrhagic necrosis. J. Neurosurg. 46:350–356, 1977.

296. Reid, A. B., Letts, R. M., and Black, G. B.: Pediatric chance fractures: Association with intraabdominal injuries and seatbelt use. Trauma 30:384–391, 1990.

297. Riska, E. B., Myllynen, P., and Bostman, O.: Anterolateral decompression for neural involvement in thoracolumbar fractures. A review of 78 cases. J. Bone Joint Surg. 685B:704–708, 1987.

298. Roberts, A., and Wickstrom, J.: Prognosis of odontoid fractures. J. Bone Joint Surg. 54A:1353, 1973.

299. Roberts, J. B., and Curtis, P. H.: Stability of the thoracic and lumbar spine in traumatic paraplegia following fracture or fracture-dislocation. J. Bone Joint Surg. 52A:1115–1130, 1970.

300. Robinson, R. A., and Southwick, W. O.: Surgical approaches to the cervical spine. A.A.O.S. Instructional Course Lectures 17:299–330, 1960.

301. Rogers, W. A.: Fractures and dislocation of the cervical spine: An end result study. J. Bone Joint Surg. 39A:341–376, 1957.

302. Romanick, T. C., Smith, T. K., Kopaniky, D. R., and Oldfield, D.: Infection about the spine associated with low velocity missile injury to the abdomen. J. Bone Joint Surg. 67A:1195–1201, 1985.

302a. Ross, I. B., Tator, C. H.: Spinal cord blood flow and evoked potential responses after treatment with nimodipine or methylprednisolone in spinal cord injured rats. Neurosurgery 33:470–476, 1993.

303. Ross, J. S., Perez-Reyes, N., Masaryk, T. J., et al.: Thoracic disc herniation and magnetic resonance imaging. Radiology 165:511–515, 1987.

304. Ross, J. S., Masaryk, T. J., Modic, M. T., et al.: MR imaging of lumbar arachnoiditis. AJNR 8:885–892, 1987.

305. Rossier, A. B., Berney, J., Rosenbaum, A. E., and Hachen, J.: Value of gas myelography in early management of acute cervical spine injuries. J. Neurosurg. 42:330–337, 1975.

306. Rossier, A. B., Werner, A., Wildi, E., and Berney, J.: Contribution to the study of late cervical syringomyelic syndromes after dorsal or lumbar traumatic paraplegia. J. Neurol. Neurosurg. Psychiatry 31:99–105, 1968.

307. Rossier, A. B., Hussey, R. W., and Kenzora, J. E.: Anterior fibular interbody fusion in the treatment of cervical spinal cord injuries. Surg. Neurol. 7:55–60, 1977.

308. Ruge, D., and Wiltse, L. L. Jr.: Spinal Disorders: Diagnosis and Treatment. Philadelphia, Lea & Febiger, 1977.

309. Rumball, K., and Jarvis, J.: Seat-belt injuries of the spine in young children. J. Bone Joint Surg. 74B:571–574, 1992.

310. Sabiston, C. P., and Wing, P. C.: Sacral fractures: Classification and neurologic implications. J. Trauma 26:1113–1115, 1986.

311. Sassard, W. R., Heinig, C. F., and Pitts, W. R.: Posterior atlanto-axial dislocation without fracture. J. Bone Joint Surg. 56A:625–628, 1974.

312. Saul, T. G., and Ducker, T. B.: The spine and spinal cord. In Watt, J., et al. (eds.): American College of Surgeons: Early Care of the Injured Patient, 3rd ed. Philadelphia, W. B. Saunders Co., 1982, pp. 196–205.

313. Saul, T. B., and Ducker, T. B.: Treatment of spinal cord injury. In Cowley, R. A., and Trump, B. (eds.): Cellular Injury in Shock, Anoxia and Ischemia: Pathophysiology, Prevention and Treatment. Baltimore, Williams & Wilkins, 1981.

314. Schaefer, D. M., Flanders, A., Northrup, B. E., et al.: Magnetic resonance imaging of acute cervical spine trauma. Correlation with severity of neurologic injury. Spine 14:1090–1095, 1989.

315. Schatzker, J., Rorabeck, C. H., and Waddell, J. P.: Fractures of the dens (odontoid process): An analysis of thirty-seven cases. J. Bone Joint Surg. 53B:392–405, 1971.

316. Schneider, R. C., Cherry, G., and Pantek, H.: The syndrome of acute central cervical spinal cord injury: Special reference to the mechanisms involved in hypertension injuries of cervical spine. J. Neurosurg. 11:546–577, 1954.

317. Schneider, R. C.: The syndrome of acute anterior spinal cord injury. J. Neurosurg. 12:95–122, 1955.

318. Schneider, R. C., and Kahn, E. A.: Chronic neurological sequelae of acute trauma to the spine and spinal cord. I: The significance of the acute flexion or "tear drop" fracture dislocation of the cervical spine. J. Bone Joint Surg. 38A:958–997, 1956.

319. Schneider, R. C.: Chronic neurological sequelae of acute trauma to the spine and spinal cord. II: The syndrome of chronic anterior spinal cord injury or compression. Herniated intervertebral discs. J. Bone Joint Surg. 41A:449–456, 1959.

320. Schneider, R. C., and Knighton, R.: Chronic neurological sequelae of acute trauma to the spine and spinal cord. III: The syndrome of chronic injury to the cervical spinal cord in the region of the central canal. J. Bone Joint Surg. 41A:905–919, 1959.

321. Schneider, R. C.: Chronic neurological sequelae of acute trauma to the spine and spinal cord. V: The syndrome of acute cervical spinal cord injury followed by chronic anterior cervical cord (or compression syndrome). J. Bone Joint Surg. 42A:253–360, 1960.

322. Schneider, R. C., Gosch, H. H., Norrell, H., et al.: Vascular insufficiency and differential distortion of brain and cord caused by cervicomedullary football injuries. J. Neurosurg. 33:363–375, 1970.

323. Schneider, R. C., Crosby, E. C., Russo, R. H., and Gosh, H. H.: Traumatic spinal cord syndromes and their management. Clin. Neurosurg. 30:367–381, 1973.

324. Schurch, B., Wichmann, W., and Rossier, A. B.: Post-traumatic syringomyelia (cystic myelopathy): A prospective study of 449 patients with spinal cord injury. J. Neurol. Neurosurg. Psychiatry 60:61–67, 1996.

325. Scott, E. W., Regis, W. H., and Peace, D.: Type 1 fractures of the odontoid process. Implications for atlanto-occipital instability. J. Neurosurg. 78:488–492, 1990.

326. Segal, L. S., Grimm, J. O., and Stauffer, E. S.: Non-union of fractures of the atlas. J. Bone Joint Surg. 69A:1423–1434, 1987.

327. Sherk, H. H., and Nicholson, J. T.: Fractures of the atlas. J. Bone Joint Surg. 52A:1017–1024, 1970.

328. Shono, Y., McAfee, P. C., and Cunningham, B. W.: Experimental study of thoracolumbar burst fractures. A radiographic and biomechanical analysis of anterior and posterior instrumentation systems. Spine 19:1711–1722, 1994.

329. Simeone, F. A., and Goldberg, H. I.: Thrombosis of the vertebral artery from hyperextension injury to the neck. Case report. J. Neurosurg. 39:540–544, 1968.

330. Smith, A. J., McCreery, C. G., Bloedel, J. R., and Chou, S. N.: Hyperemia, CO_2 responsiveness and autoregulation in the white matter following experimental spinal cord injury. J. Neurosurg. 48:239–251, 1978.

331. Smith, W. S., and Kaufer, H.: Patterns and mechanisms of lumbar injuries associated with lap seat belts. J. Bone Joint Surg. 51A:239–254, 1969.

332. Smith, M. D., Kotzar, G., Yoo, J., and Bohlman, H. H.: A biomechanical analysis of atlantoaxial stabilization methods using a bovine model. Clin. Orthop. 260:285–295, 1993.

333. Sobel, J. W., Bohlman, H. H., and Freehafer, A. A.: Charcot's arthropathy of the spine following spinal cord injury. A report of five cases. J. Bone Joint Surg. 67A:771–776, 1985.

334. Southwick, W. O., and Robinson, R. A.: Surgical approaches to the vertebral bodies in the cervical and lumbar regions. J. Bone Joint Surg. 39A:631–644, 1957.

335. Spence, K. F. Jr., Decker, S., and Sell, K. W.: Bursting atlantal fracture associated with rupture of the transverse ligament. J. Bone Joint Surg. 52A:543–549, 1970.

336. Starr, J. K., and Eismont, F. J.: Atypical hangman's fractures. Spine 18:1954–1957, 1993.

337. Stauffer, E. S., and Kelly, E. J.: Fracture-dislocations of cervical spine. Instability and recurrent deformities following treatment by anterior interbody fusion. J. Bone Joint Surg. 59A:45–48, 1977.

338. Stauffer, E. S., Wood, W., and Kelly, E. G.: Gunshot wounds of the spine: The effects of laminectomy. J. Bone Joint Surg. 61A:389–392, 1979.

339. Stauffer, E. S.: Current concepts review: Internal fixation of fractures of the thoracolumbar spine. J. Bone Joint Surg. 66A:1136–1138, 1984.

340. Stauffer, E. S.: Neurologic recovery following injuries to the cervical spinal cord and nerve roots. Spine 9:532–534, 1984.

341. Stratford, J.: Myelopathy caused by atlanto-axial dislocation. J. Neurosurg. 14:97–104, 1957.

342. Sutterlin, C. E., McAfee, P. C., Warden, K. E., et al.: A biomechanical evaluation of cervical spinal stabilization methods in a bovine model. Static and cyclical loading. Spine 13:795–802, 1988.

343. Takahashi, M., Yamashita, Y., Sakamoto, Y., and Kojima, R.: Chronic cervical cord compression: Clinical significance of increased signal intensity on MR images. Radiology 173:219–224, 1989.

344. Tarlov, I. M., Klinger, H. A., and Vitale, S.: Spinal cord compression studies. I: Experimental techniques to produce acute and gradual compression. Arch. Neurol. Psychiatr. 70:813–819, 1953.

345. Tarlov, I. M.: Spinal cord compression studies. II. Tarlov, I. M., and Klinger, H.: Time limits for recovery after acute compression in dogs. Arch. Neurol. Psychiatr. 71:271–290, 1954; III. Time limits for recovery after gradual compression in dogs. Arch. Neurol. Psychiatr. 71:588–597, 1954.

346. Tarlov, I. M.: Acute spinal cord compression paralysis. J. Neurosurg. 36:10–20, 1972.

347. Tator, C. H.: Acute management of spinal cord injury. Br. J. Surg. 77:485–486, 1990.

348. Tator, C. H.: Spine-spinal cord relationships in spinal cord trauma. Clin. Neurosurg. 30:479–494, 1983.

349. Taylor, A. R.: The mechanism of injury to the spinal cord in the neck without damage to the vertebral column. J. Bone Joint Surg. 33B:543–547, 1951.

350. Tencer, A. F., Ferguson, R. L., and Allen, B. L. Jr.: A biomechanical study of thoracolumbar spinal fractures with bone in the canal. II: The effect of flexion angulation, distraction, and shortening of the motion segment. Spine 10:586–589, 1985.

351. Tencer, A. F., Allen, B. L. Jr., and Ferguson, R. L.: A biomechanical study of thoracolumbar spinal fractures with bone in the canal. I: The effect of laminectomy. Spine 10:580–585, 1985.

352. Torg, J. R., Truex, R. C., Marshall, J., et al.: Spinal injury at the level of the third and fourth cervical vertebrae from football. J. Bone Joint Surg. 59A:1015–1019, 1977.

353. Torg, J. S., Pavlov, H., Genuario, S. E., et al.: Neuropraxia of the cervical spinal cord with transient quadriplegia. J. Bone Joint Surg. 68A:1354–1370, 1986.

354. Torg, J. S., Vegso, J. J., Sennett, B., and Das, M.: The National Football Head and Neck Injury Registry: 14-year report on cervical quadriplegia, 1971 through 1984. JAMA 254:3439–3443, 1985.

355. Turnbull, I. M.: Microvasculature of the human spinal cord. J. Neurosurg. 35:141–147, 1971.

356. Verbiest, H.: Anterolateral operations for fractures and dislocations in the middle and lower parts of the cervical spine. Report of a series of forty-seven cases. J. Bone Joint Surg. 51A:1489–1530, 1969.

357. Wadia, N. H.: Myelopathy complicating congenital atlanto-axial dislocation (a study of 28 cases). Brain 90:449–472, 1967.

358. Wagner, F. C. Jr., Dohrmann, G. H., and Bucy, P. C.: Histopathology of transitory traumatic paraplegia in the monkey. J. Neurosurg. 35:272–276, 1971.

359. Wertheim, S. B., and Bohlman, H. H.: Occipito-cervical fusion, indications, technique and results in thirteen patients. J. Bone Joint Surg. 69A:833–836, 1987.

360. White, A. A., and Panjabi, M. M.: Clinical Biomechanics of the Spine. 2nd ed. Philadelphia, J. B. Lippincott Co., 1990.

361. White, A. A.: Clinical biomechanics of cervical spine implants. Spine 14:1040–1045, 1989.

362. White, A. A., Southwick, W. O., and Panjabi, M. M.: Clinical instability in the lower cervical spine. Spine I:15–27, 1976.

363. White, A. A., Panjabi, M. M., and Thomas C. L.: The clinical biomechanics of kyphotic deformities. Clin. Orthop. 128:8–17, 1977.

364. White, J. B., Kneisley, L. W., and Rossier, A. B.: Delayed paralysis after cervical fracture dislocation. Case report. J. Neurosurg. 46:512–516, 1977.

365. Whitehill, R., Richman, J. A., and Glaser, J. A.: Failure of immobilization of the cervical spine by the halo vest. A report of five cases. J. Bone Joint Surg. 68A:326–332, 1986.

366. Whitesides, T. E. Jr., and Shah, S. G. A.: On the management of unstable fractures of the thoraco-lumbar spine. Spine I:99–107, 1976.

367. Whitesides, T. E. Jr.: Traumatic kyphosis of the thoracolumbar spine. Clin. Orthop. 128:78–92, 1977.

368. Willis, B. K., Greiner, F., Orrison, W. W., and Benzel, E. C.: The incidence of vertebral artery injury after midcervical spine fracture or subluxation. Neurosurgery 34:435–442, 1994.

369. Windle, W. F., Clemente, C. D., and Chambers, W. W.: Inhibition of formation of a glial barrier as a means of permitting a peripheral nerve to grow into the brain. J. Comp. Neurol. 96:359–370, 1952.

370. Windle, W. F.: Regeneration of axons in the vertebrate CNS. Physiol. Res. 36:427–440, 1956.

371. Woolsey, R. M.: Rehabilitation outcome following spinal cord injury. Arch. Neurol. 42:116–119, 1985.

372. Yashon, D., Jane, J. A., and White, R. J.: Prognosis and management of spinal cord and cauda equina bullet injuries in sixty-five civilians. J. Neurosurg. 32:163–170, 1970.

373. Yoganandan, N., Sances, A., Maiman, D. J., et al.: Experimental spinal injuries with vertical impact. Spine 11:855–860, 1986.

374. Young, W., and Bracken, M. B.: The Second National Acute Spinal Cord Injury Study. J. Neurotrauma 9:S397–S405, 1992.

375. Young, W.: Blood flow, metabolic and neurophysiological mechanisms in spinal cord injury. In Becker, D., Povlishock, J. T. (eds.): Central Nervous System Trauma Status Report. Rockville, MD, National Institutes of Health, 1985, pp. 463–473.

375a. Young, W.: Methylprednisolone treatment of acute spinal cord injury: an introduction. J. Neurotrauma 8:S43–S46, 1991.

376. Zdeblick, T. A., and Bohlman, H. H.: Cervical kyphosis and myelopathy. Treatment by anterior carpectomy and strut-grafting. J. Bone Joint Surg. 71A:170–182, 1989.

376a. Zeidman, S. M., Ling, G. S. F., Ducker, T. B., Ellenbogen, R. G.: Clinical applications of pharmacologic therapies for spinal cord injury. J. Spinal Disord. 9(5):367–380, 1996.

377. Zigler, J., Rockowitz, N., Capen, D., et al.: Posterior cervical fusion with local anesthesia. The awake patient as the ultimate spinal cord monitor. Spine 12:206–208, 1987.

378. Zigler, J., Bahniuk, E., VanDyke, C., and Bohlman, H. H.: Localization of foreign bodies in the spinal canal by the computer-assisted biplaner digitizer. Spine 11:892–894, 1986.

379. Zwimpfer, T. J., and Bernstein, M.: Spinal cord concussion. J. Neurosurg. 72:894–900, 1990.

Surgical Techniques for the Treatment of Thoracic, Thoracolumbar, Lumbar, and Sacral Trauma

Alan M. Levine, M.D.

The goals of surgical intervention for thoracolumbar spine trauma are (1) anatomic reduction of the deformity, (2) rigid fixation, and (3) neural decompression when appropriate indications exist. The method used to achieve these goals for a specific patient is moderated by a number of different variables. It is difficult if not impossible to apply a single surgical technique that will fit all combinations of variables. Once the decision for surgical intervention has been made, the selection of approach (anterior versus posterior) and type of instrumentation must be made. Based on the fracture pattern, the condition of the patient, and the specific limitations and advantages of individual instrumentation systems, a rational decision-making process can be used to maximize the benefits and diminish the risks for an individual patient.[15]

The initial goal for most patients undergoing surgical intervention is that of anatomic reduction of the presenting deformity. The ability of any individual instrumentation system (whether posterior or anterior) to achieve this goal is based on the extent to which it can effectively oppose the directions of the forces that have caused the deformity and counteract the resultant instability. The selection of an appropriate instrumentation construct for a particular patient is based on understanding the mechanism by which the injury has occurred and, consequently, the forces that have caused the deformity. Once that initial information is understood, selection of the approach can be based on the knowledge of which instrumentation construct will best allow appropriate forces to be applied to the spine to achieve reduction.[42, 50, 71, 91, 97, 106]

Spinal injury can be classified using systems that are based on radiologic description, assessment of spinal instability,[53] prognosis for neural recovery, systematic assessment of structural impairment,[82] prediction of failure of specific fixation modalities, or mechanisms of injury. Although a number of types of classification systems have been used to categorize spinal injuries,[12, 27, 38] for this particular facet of decision making for surgical intervention, a classification subdivided into major mechanistic categories is necessary.[34, 65] The major forces the spine is subjected to during trauma are flexion, extension, axial loading, distraction shear, and lateral bending. The majority of injuries occur as a result of combinations of flexion and axial compression, with this group encompassing approximately 80 per cent of all patients with spinal injury who undergo surgical stabilization. The combination of flexion and axial compression forms a continuum of injuries, ranging from those resulting predominantly from a flexion moment (compression fracture) to those resulting predominantly from an axial compression moment (Denis type A burst fracture). In the middle are the large

majority of injuries, which result from a combination of the two. This continuum encompasses five major types of injuries: the compression fracture with less than 50 per cent loss of height, the compression fracture with more than 50 per cent loss of height, the Denis type A (posterior element involvement and significant body involvement), and the Denis B and C types (intact posterior elements with lesser degrees of body comminution). A compression fracture in the thoracic and lumbar spine generally results predominantly from a flexion force causing crushing and disruption of the anterior portion of the vertebral body, but leaving the posterior aspect of the vertebral body intact. The posterior ligamentous complex is generally not disrupted unless more than 50 per cent of the height of the vertebral body is lost; under these circumstances, posterior instability may result.

Injuries that combine flexion and compression generally result in disruption of the anterior portion of the vertebral body and comminution of the posterior vertebral wall, with the posterior superior fragment of the wall retropulsed into the neural canal. This will occur in varying degrees of severity, depending on the direction and magnitude of the forces causing the injury.[97] However, because the flexion component of the injury is the major force, the posterior elements are rarely disrupted and the neural arch, including the pedicles, remains attached to the lateral wall of the vertebral body. This pattern has a very distinctive appearance on computed tomography (CT) scan and comprises approximately 40 per cent of all patients with burst fractures undergoing treatment. In an uncommon variant of this type of injury, the fracture is inverted and the posterior inferior corner is retropulsed into the canal. The third type of injury in this continuum is the "true" burst fracture. This is predominantly an axial loading injury, although it may also have some lesser component of flexion. There is loss of height of the entire vertebra (both anterior and posterior walls of the vertebral body), as well as the posterior elements. The neural arch and pedicles are comminuted and frequently are detached from the vertebral body. Compression of the neural canal results from retropulsion of the posterior wall of the vertebral body and occasionally from displacement of laminar fractures into the canal. The combination of the flexion-axial load mechanism (Denis type B) and the predominantly axial load type burst fractures (Denis type A) constitute approximately 80 per cent of all injuries requiring surgical intervention.

The next group of injuries are those resulting from flexion and distraction.[7, 46, 83, 103] These constitute approximately 15 per cent of all injuries for which surgical intervention is undertaken. They are composed of several major groups, the first of which is the bilateral facet dislocation.[64] This is a pure ligamentous injury that disrupts the interspinous ligament, the facet capsules, ligamentum flavum, and the posterior aspect of the annulus of the intervertebral disc. Bilateral facet disruption most frequently occurs at the thoracolumbar junction and results in a very high frequency of complete paraplegia. Although its mechanism of injury is reasonably straightforward, surgical intervention for this particular type of injury can be somewhat confusing. Its predominant injury is not bony but ligamentous, and results in disruption of the posterior ligamentous complex and the intervertebral disc. Although it is logical that extension and compression should be used to reduce the deformity resulting from flexion and distraction, in the case of a bilateral facet dislocation a note of caution should be introduced. Although compression and extension applied through posterior instrumentation will in fact restore the normal sagittal alignment of the bony elements of the spine, they can potentiate disc extravasation of a severely injured disc.[64] This phenomenon is seen with reduction of cervical bilateral facet dislocations as well. In the patient who is initially neurologically intact or incomplete, care should be taken that extravasation of the disc causing neural deficit does not occur with the application of forces to reduce the bony spinal deformity.

The remainder of the flexion distraction injuries can be classified as either bony type injuries (Chance) or combinations of bony and ligamentous injuries. The majority of flexion distraction fractures transverse the spinous process, the pedicles, and the body, hinging off the anterior longitudinal ligament and the anterior portion of the body. However, instead of penetration through the spinous processes, occasionally the injury will propagate through the interspinous ligament and the facet joints into the pedicle and body. It is important to differentiate the latter group, which will continue to have posterior ligamentous instability in spite of healing of the bony vertebral fracture. When surgical intervention is necessary, extension and compression can be applied locally to this injured segment of the spine to reduce the deformity caused by flexion and distraction. The final group of deformities, which constitute approximately 3 to 5 per cent of all injuries, are those which are mixed deformities, usually having an element of shear. This group may be extremely difficult to differentiate initially, but is most important because of the gross instability related to the shear component of the injury.[54] The surgical reconstruction may require a complex configuration to achieve reduction of all deformities, counteracting the resultant shear instability to achieve a stable construct.

The second goal of surgical intervention is long-term postoperative maintenance of the reduction achieved intraoperatively. This requires that the instrumentation applied to the spine be stable and able to counteract all elements of instability. A common reason for postoperative loss of correction is that the device selected cannot possibly prevent subsequent recurrence of the deformity.[11, 26, 32, 52, 67, 75, 84] For example, even though

vertebral height may be restored on the operating room table, segmental spinal instrumentation does not have the ability to maintain distraction in axial burst fractures and therefore cannot be expected to maintain the vertical height. Smooth rods and sublaminar or spinous process wires have no intrinsic resistance to axial compression.[52, 69] Therefore, although reduction may be achieved initially with a variety of distraction devices, the height is lost when the patient becomes erect postoperatively. Similarly, if a significant flexion deformity is reduced on the operating table by postural reduction in the prone position but not maintained by some component of the instrumentation, the deformity recurs. The use of very short unilaminar hook fixation or pedicle fixation will result in such high forces (in the presence of severe anterior column disruption) that failure occurs. Similarly in multiple hook fixation systems,[11, 75] failure to impart an extension force at the apex of the construct may result in recurrence of deformity.

The final goal of surgical intervention is decompression of the dural sac. The type of injury and the timing of surgical intervention dictate in part the type of decompression that will be most effective. Those patients with compression of the dural sac based on sagittal alignment, rather than on comminution of the vertebral wall and retropulsion of bone, will obtain adequate decompression simply from spinal realignment (i.e., bilateral facet dislocations). Conversely, those patients with retropulsion of bone without significant sagittal plane deformity will be less likely to achieve decompression indirectly (by spine reduction) and more likely to need direct decompression. Three basic methods of decompression of the dural sac exist: direct anterior decompression,[10, 13, 22, 55, 73] posterolateral or transpedicular decompression,[10, 45, 49, 98] and indirect decompression achieved by spinal realignment.[25, 31, 33, 50, 66, 90, 99] Indirect decompression by anatomic restoration of spinal alignment has been shown to be an effective modality in achieving decompression of the dural sac in those patients who undergo surgical intervention acutely. After 48 hours, however, success with indirect decompression is more limited; after 10 days, it is generally not effective.[33] Advocates of posterior instrumentation as the preferred method of stabilization of spinal injuries may sometimes combine posterolateral decompression with stabilization in patients with neurologic deficit in whom indirect decompression has not been effective.[49, 98] The final method for neural decompression is anterior corpectomy with direct decompression. This is clearly the treatment of choice for those patients in whom decompression is indicated and surgical intervention is delayed more than 10 days from the time of injury. Additionally, in an incomplete spinal cord injury with significant canal compromise (bone or disc), primary anterior decompression and fusion should be considered because it allows direct and complete decompression of the neural canal from pedicle to pedicle.[31] Its major disadvantage is that reduction of deformity and stabilization are less reliable and more difficult from the anterior approach than from the posterior approach. Recent advances in anterior instrumentation now allow reasonable success in stabilization of injuries with significant deformity and instability.[6, 44, 55, 58, 60, 104] Overall there are no studies that clearly show a significant difference in neurologic recovery based on the method of decompression.[21, 34, 51, 63, 78, 100] The strength of the anterior approach is more certainly its ability to achieve "safe" decompression. In complex fractures with gross deformity and instability, posterior stabilization in conjunction with anterior decompression may prove the optimal treatment for the patient.

With a multitude of options from which to choose, delineation of a clear treatment protocol for spinal injury becomes increasingly difficult. Once the basic decision between surgical and nonsurgical treatment has been made,[4, 5, 17, 20, 40, 59, 96, 102] realistically organizing the various treatment modalities must be based on defining the goals of that particular surgery as well as considering the patient condition. Rather than dogmatically and sometimes irrationally espousing a single approach to surgery for spinal injury, it is more appropriate to consider the various indications for different approaches. Thus, if we consider the posterior approach to the treatment of spinal injuries, we may define the absolute indications for the use of the posterior approach, the absolute contraindications for that approach, and the relative indications.

There are certain combinations of clinical parameters when the use of the posterior approach for the reduction, stabilization, and decompression of spinal injury makes overwhelming sense. In polytraumatized patients, especially those with a spinal fracture and multiple extremity injuries, the posterior approach has overwhelming advantages. Irrespective of the neurologic status, the use of a posterior surgical approach will expedite the treatment of the other injuries. It may be necessary to first stabilize the thoracolumbar injury to allow positioning on the table for fixation of femoral, tibial, or humeral fractures. Likewise initial laparotomy or fixateur application for a pelvic injury may strongly influence the choice of a posterior approach to the spine. The use of the posterior approach in these acutely injured patients can achieve all the necessary surgical goals of reduction, decompression, and stabilization with relative efficiency and with minimal surgical time and blood loss. A subgroup of polytraumatized patients has been demonstrated to benefit from immediate stabilization, and the procedure should be performed from the posterior.[85] Patients with complete neurologic injury as a result of a major thoracic spine fracture will frequently also have significant chest contusions, which are a manifestation of the extreme force needed to create that spinal injury. Early stabilization has been shown to shorten the hospital course and decrease morbidity. Posterior spinal instrumentation is the most reasonable approach, as thoracotomy will only further compromise the patient's respiratory function. In those patients with shear injuries, both the nature of the canal compromise and the gross instability of their spines again make the posterior approach

optimal. It is difficult to achieve both reduction and sufficient stability from an anterior approach. Both patients with stiff spines (diffuse idiopathic skeletal hyperostosis or ankylosing spondylitis) and those with normal morbidity prior to injury must have multiple attachment points to the spine and sufficient lever arms to accomplish a stable anatomic reduction and fixation in these highly unstable injuries. Finally, for low lumbar fractures, the posterior approach is most often the most reasonable. For injuries to L4 and L5, anterior stabilization to L5 and S1 is more risky and difficult because of the position of the vessels. In addition, approximately 20 per cent of men undergoing an anterior approach at that level will have retrograde ejaculation after the procedure, clearly an unwanted complication in this relatively young population. In 25 to 40 per cent of patients with severe low lumbar burst fractures, a laminar split and a traumatic dural laceration accompany the fracture.[16, 29] These are always located on the posterior or posterolateral surface of the dural tube and thus must be approached from the posterior to free the entrapped nerve roots and repair the laceration. Patients with a flexion-distraction injury resulting in a true bilateral facet dislocation of the thoracolumbar spine must have a reduction of the dislocation from a posterior approach. Finally, in those rare patients in whom a depressed laminar fragment exists and causes any dural compression, the posterior approach allows the ability to both decompress and stabilize. Thus, in patients in whom the overwhelming goal of surgery is reduction of deformity and stabilization of the injury, the posterior approach continues to have many advantages over the anterior approach.

There are, however, absolute contraindications to the use of the posterior approach for the treatment of spinal injuries. In the majority of these situations, the predominant goal of surgery is neural decompression rather than correction of deformity. It has been well demonstrated that indirect reduction by ligamentataxis is most effective within the first 48 to 72 hours from the time of injury. By 10 days from the time of injury, it is not effective at all for reduction of fragments. Thus, for the patient who presents at 10 days or later with incomplete neurologic injury and requires decompression of the neural elements, it is more effectively done from an anterior approach. Additionally, certain fracture patterns are more effectively treated from the anterior approach when spinal decompression is the overwhelming concern. When a portion or the entire retropulsed fragment causing the neural compression is inverted, then indirect decompression is usually not terribly effective. In those circumstances, if neural decompression is a major consideration, then initial anterior decompression should be the primary approach. The inversion of the retropulsed fragment signifies the fact that either the posterior longitudinal ligament is disrupted or the fragment is no longer attached to the ligament. Indirect reduction of the fragment by ligamentataxis therefore cannot be effective in that circumstance. Additionally, if the patient has significant retropulsion of a fragment but minimal compression and kyphosis, indirect decompression is less effective. Both of these circumstances are rare, however, and occur in less than 5 per cent of thoracolumbar spine injuries requiring surgical treatment.

Finally, there is a group of patients with relative indications for posterior surgery who could also be managed using an alternate approach. In the neurologically intact patient, in whom the goals of treatment are correction of deformity and spinal stabilization, posterior instrumentation can be accomplished with the least risk and the most satisfactory results. The anterior approach requires more extensive dissection and has less efficient application of reduction forces than current methods of posterior stabilization. Thus the use of a multiple rod-hook system in the thoracic spine, the rod sleeve for the thoracolumbar junction, and pedicle screw systems for the lower lumbar spine requires less operative time and can achieve more effective reduction with less morbidity than the respective anterior approach. In addition, in those patients with neurologic deficit requiring neural decompression as well as reduction and stabilization in the acute injury setting (less than 48 hours), the posterior approach with indirect decompression by ligamentataxis has been shown to be as effective as direct anterior decompression. If the compression is focal to one side, then adjunctive posterolateral decompression could be added. Although either approach could be used for these patients, the operative risk, duration of surgery, and the length of the recovery period have to be considered.

POSTERIOR SURGICAL TECHNIQUE

Thoracic Injuries

There is little controversy concerning the requirements for instrumentation for optimal reduction and stabilization for injuries between T2 and T11. A rod-and-hook system is relatively simple, is low risk, and provides adequate reduction and stabilization of most fractures in the thoracic spine, because the majority are flexion-compression or axial-compression injuries.[23] Flexion-distraction injuries are extremely rare in this area. Reduction is achieved by distraction with some extension, and overall stability is aided by the intrinsic mechanical restraints of the chest wall. In patients with complete neurologic deficit and severe shear injury in the thoracic spine, augmentation with sublaminar wiring is helpful in achieving and maintaining rigid stability, thereby facilitating early rehabilitation[85] and minimizing brace wear.[95]

The most difficult area of the thoracic spine to achieve a reduction and adequate stabilization is the cervicothoracic junction. Fractures occurring at the T2 and T3 levels are difficult to manage both because of positioning and reduction problems and instrumentation problems. Both longitudinal as well as transverse rolls as well as most spinal frames tend to place the upper thoracic spine into significant kyphosis as a result of the positioning necessary for the head. This is accentuated by attempting to raise the position of the head and increasing the cervical lordosis. These high thoracic fractures can in fact both be positioned and posturally reduced by modified positioning technique. Gardner-Wells tongs are first applied to the head. The patient is then positioned on a regular operating table with longitudinal rolls and the head is placed on a Mayfield horseshoe headrest with 10 to 15 pounds of traction. The height of the headrest is adjusted to decrease the cervical lordosis. The combination of the longitudinal traction and the flattening of the cervical lordosis will significantly reduce the kyphosis inherent in most high thoracic fractures. It also improves the access to the posterior elements of the lower cervical spine that are necessary attachment points for the proximal end of the instrumentation for high thoracic fractures. As described subsequently, the instrumentation can be modified by using a plating technique to modify the hook pattern in a rod-hook configuration.

Surgical Technique

The surgical technique for the initial preparation and exposure of the spine is similar for most types of rod instrumentation. After appropriate radiographic studies, the patient is positioned in the prone position (Fig. 33–82). For most injuries in the thoracic spine, extension on the table is helpful in achieving partial fracture reduction. Therefore, transverse rolls placed at the levels of the clavicle and of the pubic symphysis tend to hyperextend the patient, thereby reducing the deformity. This position is easily achieved on a Stryker frame or on an operating table; however, a Stryker frame is convenient, especially in the patient with an unstable spine, because it allows easier turning from supine to prone position. The use of an operating table is possible, especially with the advent of radiolucent operating tables; however, care must be taken with transferring and turning patients to avoid further neurologic damage. To reduce this risk, one can either use awake intubation or delay the general anesthetic until positioning is complete and the neurologic status is reassessed. Similar results can be achieved with a Judet fracture table or a spinal frame. Care must be taken in positioning so that the abdomen is not compressed, because this may impede venous return and increase intraoperative bleeding.

The patient is prepped from the nape of the neck down to the iliac crest, with care being taken to allow preparation for an iliac crest bone graft. A midline incision is made, beginning approximately three levels above the level of injury and proceeding approximately three levels below the injury. The incision is carried directly down to the tips of the spinous processes, using a cautery to keep bleeding to a minimum. Frequently, in thoracic burst fractures there is tremendous soft tissue destruction from the force of the injury. Devascularized muscle in the thoracic spine should be débrided. Then, using a cautery, the paraspinous musculature is stripped subperiosteally from the spinous processes. Once the spinous processes are ex-

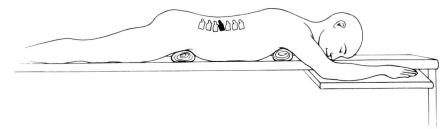

Figure 33–82. There are a variety of methods for positioning patients for surgical intervention from a posterior approach for thoracolumbar fractures. The precise positioning depends in part on the level of the injury: thoracic, thoracolumbar, or lumbar. For most types of posterior surgical intervention, passive or positional reduction of the deformity is helpful in achieving an optimal operative reduction. Therefore, since most injuries have a significant flexion component, it is helpful to apply extension. In addition, positioning is based on whether fluoroscopic control is necessary using an image intensifier. However, for most thoracolumbar level injuries, placing a transverse roll at the level of the clavicles and a second transverse roll at the level of the pubis allows the thoracolumbar junction to sag between the two rolls, both decompressing the abdomen, so that there is no pressure on the vena cava, and also allowing optimal postural reduction. This method can be used on a regular operating room table, a radiolucent table, or on a Stryker frame, which allows ease in turning and positioning. (Modified from Eismont, F. J., Garfin, S. R., and Abitbol, J-J.: Thoracic and thoracolumbar injuries. In Browner, B. D., Levine, A. M., Jupiter, J. B., and Trafton, P. G. [eds.]: Skeletal Trauma. Philadelphia, W. B. Saunders Co., 1992.)

posed, a towel clip is placed on the suspected level of injury and a roentgenogram taken to verify the position. This step is important because there may not be accurate landmarks to assess location. The majority of instrumentation systems for the thoracic spine require exposure of at least six segments, three above the level of injury and two below the level of injury. Again using a cautery to avoid causing excessive motion of the spine with subperiosteal stripping, all soft tissue is removed from the posterior elements, from the spinous processes, across the lamina, and out to the tips of the transverse processes. Care must be taken to expose the transverse process that is proximal to the superior hook site. This is easily overlooked because the inferior edge of the lamina of the superior vertebral segment may be exposed for preparation of the hook-seating site but the transverse process that lies approximately 1 cm proximal to it may not be exposed. Therefore, the most superior vertebral segment may not end up being grafted or fused. Fractures of the posterior elements should be carefully exposed. Loose pieces of spinous process can be excised and used for graft. After exposure of the posterior aspect of the spine and localization, the appropriate technique of hook insertion can be completed.

Harrington Distraction Rod Technique

Preparation of hook sites for Harrington distraction rodding[3, 26, 43, 52, 84] in the thoracic spine is most commonly at three levels above and two levels below the injury, irrespective of the type of injury (Fig. 33–83). A Harrington 1253 hook is seated in a sublaminar position under the most cephalad lamina; this is done by using a Penfield elevator to subperiosteally dissect the ligamentum flavum from the undersurface of the lamina. A Kerrison punch then can be used to square the

inferomedial edge of the lamina for symmetrical contact of the hook to the lamina. Because of the shoe width, the hooks may impinge on the medial aspect of the facet joint; using a curette, a small portion of the cartilage within the facet joint can be removed to allow proper seating of the hook. These hooks are meant, however, to seat in the sublaminar position, rather than in the facet joint. Once both sides of the spine are prepared, the two hooks should be placed before any rod is inserted to ascertain that they can be positioned symmetrically. Preparation of the inferior hook site is then undertaken (Fig. 33–83B). The hooks should be placed on the superior laminar edge of the vertebra two levels below the fractured vertebral body. A laminotomy is done after removing the facet joint capsules at the appropriate interspace. A portion of the inferior edge of the lamina and the facet joint of the vertebra proximal to the level of seating is removed, allowing exposure of the ligamentum flavum. This is often difficult to expose initially, and may require substantial resection of the inferior edge of the lamina above. A Kerrison punch can then be used to remove the ligamentum flavum and a portion of the superior facet of the level below. This portion of the laminotomy should be resected back until the line of the lamina is clearly evident and the laminotomy is wide enough to accept a hook. Care must be taken at this point to attempt to insert both of the distal hooks simultaneously to ensure that they do not overlap in the midline. Overlapping may cause significant impingement on the neural canal. If they do impinge medially, then additional bone should be resected laterally, up to and including the entire inferior facet of the level above. Care should be taken, however, not to remove or damage the pars interarticularis of the level on which the hooks are seated, which could result in an iatrogenic spondylolysis. After the hooks are seated appropri-

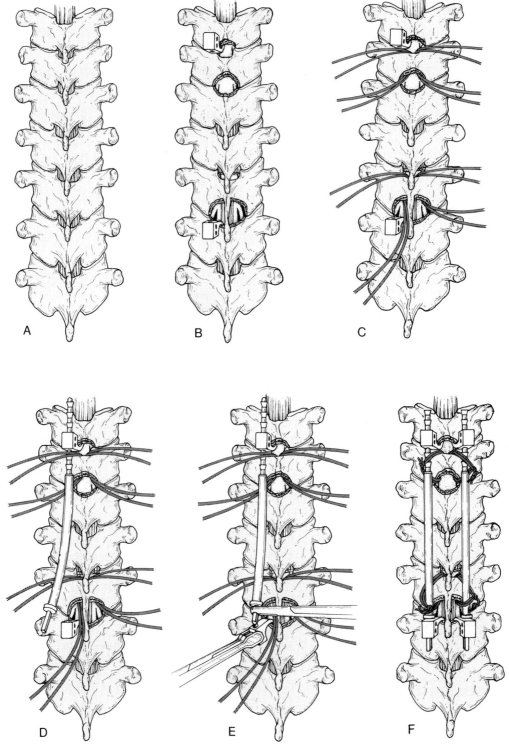

Figure 33–83 *See legend on opposite page*

ately, laminotomies can be made for passing sublaminar wires, if necessary (Fig. 33–83C). Frequently, augmentation with sublaminar wires will be necessary with straight or contoured Harrington or Moe rod instrumentation. Laminotomies should not be done at the level of injury, because passing a wire at the injury level may cause further deficit. In addition, care should be taken in passing the wires so that a dural leak is not propagated. The laminotomies for augmentation with sublaminar wires should not be placed in the interspaces above and below the construct for wiring of the proximal and distal level. This necessitates removal of the interspinous ligament and ligamentum flavum above and below what will be a rigid segment, and may result in postfusion kyphosis at those levels. The wires are then passed at the level proximal and distal to the injury site. Double 18-gauge wires are generally sufficient for this purpose.

There are two options available for rod selection. To accommodate the kyphosis of the thoracic spine, square-ended Moe rods or standard Harrington rods can be selected. The rods should be contoured slightly to accommodate the thoracic kyphosis. This tends to place less stress at the upper thoracic hook purchase

site and, with distraction, will minimize the tendency for the upper hooks to rotate out from under the lamina. Straight rods should be avoided in the upper thoracic spine. For the lower thoracic spine, minimal rod contouring is necessary; however, care must be taken to avoid placement of the upper hook sites at the apex of the thoracic kyphosis. This may make the hooks extremely prominent and also may increase the difficulty of obtaining satisfactory rod contour. The construct should be lengthened or shortened to avoid the apex. The rod length should be selected to have the minimum number of ratchets distal to the cephalad hook. However, approximately two to three ratchets are necessary proximal to the hook to prevent hook dislodgement. A hook holder is then placed on the cephalad hook and a rod holder on the appropriate rod. The rod is advanced up through the proximal hook until the nipple of the distal end of the rod clears the distal hook (Fig. 33–83D). This may necessitate sliding the smooth portion of the rod into the hook with the shorter ratcheted (seven ratchets) rods. The hook holder is then used to place downward pressure on the distal end of the rod, reducing the kyphosis caused by the fracture (Fig. 33–83E). Distraction is then

Figure 33–83. Technique for distraction instrumentation augmented with sublaminar wires. *A,* The spine is stripped of all soft tissue posteriorly across either five or six segments. With more standard Harrington technique, this is three above the injury to two below the injury. If sublaminar wiring is used, a minimum of six levels must be exposed to avoid passage of wires at the level of injury. The soft tissue should be completely and carefully stripped out to the tips of the transverse processes. If possible the interspinous ligaments should be left intact for subsequent reconstruction of the lumbodorsal fascia. Posterior elements should be carefully inspected for fractures. *B,* Hook placement is done initially at three levels above the fractured level and two levels below. Care should be taken in dissecting the proximal level to remove the ligamentum flavum from the undersurface of the superior lamina. The hook is then slipped up beneath the lamina and not in the facet joint. Occasionally the cartilage in the medial aspect of the facet joint must be removed to allow the hook to seat. This is done on both the right and left sides, and both hooks are placed together to make sure they seat symmetrically and do not overlap. Attention is then turned to the superior edge of the lamina at two levels below the fracture. Again, the interspinous ligament should be left intact, but a laminotomy is accomplished removing the inferior portion of the level above the edge on which the hooks must seat. The laminotomy is often carried laterally into the medial aspect of the facet joint. Since this facet is being fused, that is of little consequence. Laminotomy should be carried laterally enough out to the edge of the pedicle. Care must be taken not to resect bone from the superior edge of the lamina on which the hook is to be seated, as this may cause weakening of the lamina and subsequent fracture through the pars. Hooks are seated on both the right and left sides, and then both hooks are seated simultaneously to ensure that they are seated symmetrically and that (most important at this level) they do not overlap. *C,* A laminotomy is then accomplished by removing a portion of the spinous process and ligamentum flavum at the level just caudal to the proximal hooks and just proximal to the distal hooks. No attempt is made to prepare and pass wires at the two levels adjacent to the fracture. *D,* The rods are contoured in the standard fashion to maintain lordosis at the thoracolumbar junction or kyphosis in the thoracic region. Contouring is especially important in the thoracic spine to prevent prominence of the rod tips. The rod is then passed up through the proximal hook and distracted down into the distal hook. Constant downward force is necessary to reduce the kyphosis with the contouring of the rod so that the tip of the rod can be inserted in the distal hook. *E,* The distal hook is grasped with a hook holder and the end of the rod with a rod holder, allowing downward pressure to be achieved. The tip of the rod is inserted into the distal hook while the assistant uses a spreader to distract the rod into appropriate position. Constant downward pressure must be maintained on the distal end of the rod until the nipple of the rod is fully inserted into the hook. *F,* At this point the bone graft should be harvested and the spine should undergo viscoelastic relaxation before final distraction of the rod and tightening of the sublaminar wires. Sublaminar wires should not be tightened before full achievement of the reduction of the spine, as demonstrated on anteroposterior and lateral roentgenograms. An additional one to two ratchets of distraction will be achieved after viscoelastic relaxation. Two C-washers are placed below the proximal hooks and then the two sublaminar wires at either end are tightened. (Redrawn from Leona Allison.)

done at the upper end, engaging the appropriate nipple into the caudal hook. Pressure should be kept on the lower end of the rod until the nipple is fully engaged. The second side is similarly engaged. A lateral roentgenogram is then taken to check the reduction. If insufficient distraction has been applied, additional distraction can be used until appropriate height is restored. Kyphosis at the injury level in the thoracic spine should be reduced by the application of the rod against the posterior elements of the midthoracic spine. Corticocancellous graft can then be harvested, allowing time for stress relaxation. Additional ratchet distraction can usually be obtained after completion of harvesting the graft. After the reduction has been completed, C-washers are crimped below the Harrington 1253 hooks to prevent loss of distraction. If the construct is to be augmented with sublaminar wires, these are now twisted down into position (Fig. 33–83F). The conclusion of the procedure is the same for all types of instrumentation and will be described at the end of this techniques section.

Rod-Sleeve Techniques

The rod-sleeve method for thoracic and thoracolumbar injuries currently uses standard, straight Harrington rods, modified anatomic hooks, and rod-sleeves in four different sizes (Fig. 33–84). Its advantages include the application of an anteriorly directed extension force to counteract the flexion moment of most spinal injuries. In addition, the application of the sleeves wedged between the facets and spinous processes on either side gives more rotational stability than is obtained with straight or even contoured Harrington rods. It also allows flexibility in the application of forces, based on the fracture pattern. For flexion-compression injuries in which the posterior elements, especially the body-pedicle junction, are intact, the rod-sleeves can be applied directly over the pedicles of the fractured body (Fig. 33–85). This allows a three-point bending moment and extension applied directly at the level of injury, thereby reducing the flexion component. The rods are used to apply the distraction to counteract the axial compression force of the injury. Stability of this particular construct is not based as much on the number of levels instrumented (as with straight Harrington instrumentation) as on the relative length of the lever arm at either end of the rod. A minimum of 3 cm of space is required between the sleeve and hook, both proximally and distally. Therefore, because of the relatively small size of the lamina of the thoracic spine, a single rod-sleeve construct for a flexion-compression injury in most cases may require instrumentation of five vertebrae and four interspaces (two above and two below) (see Fig. 33–85). Occasionally, with very small laminar size, this may take six interspaces and five levels. Its advantage, however, is that as we progress caudally into the thoracolumbar junction and high lumbar spine, the size of the lamina increases, and, therefore, the number of instrumented levels decreases

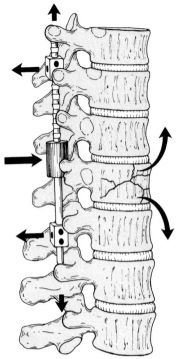

Figure 33–84. Rod sleeve construct for a flexion-compression–type burst fracture (Denis B). This construct has the rod-sleeve over the apical facets and pedicle of the injured body. This is because the pedicles remain connected to the lateral sides of the body, and therefore correction of kyphosis can actively be achieved by positioning of the rod-sleeve in that location. The rod-sleeve produces a three-point bending moment to both correct the kyphotic portion of the deformity and allow distraction with the rods to correct the axial compression of the deformity. The corrective forces are noted in this figure. The length of the construct is determined by the size of the vertebra at any particular level. With a smaller length of lamina, this will require a total of five vertebrae and four interspaces to achieve a minimum of 3 cm from the sleeve to the hooks on either end, with the sleeve roughly centered in the middle of the construct. However, in the high lumbar spine or thoracolumbar junction, this same application of forces may be achieved with only three interspaces and four segments, thus saving a distal and/or proximal interspace because of the increased size of the lamina in this region. (Modified from Eismont, F. J., Garfin, S. R., and Abitbol, J-J.: Thoracic and thoracolumbar injuries. *In* Browner, B. D., Levine, A. M., Jupiter, J. B., and Trafton, P. G. [eds.]: Skeletal Trauma. Philadelphia, W. B. Saunders Co., 1992.)

while the same stability of instrumentation is maintained. In the case of a true burst fracture with severe comminution of the posterior elements and pedicles, direct, three-point bending cannot be applied to the injured level. In that instance, a bridging construct can be used (Fig. 33–86). This places a set of sleeves at the intact pedicles, below the level of injury, thus avoiding the comminuted apical level. It still allows three-point bending to be applied to the spine as a whole, effectively reducing the kyphosis and augmenting stability. In the thoracic spine, this will generally require six levels of instrumentation over five interspaces.

The surgical technique for insertion of the rod-sleeve construct varies slightly from the standard Harrington

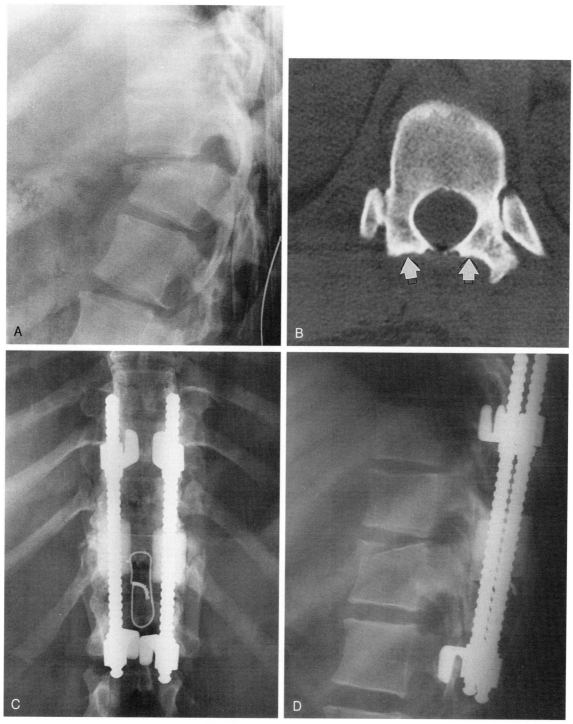

Figure 33–85. This 26-year-old female fell through the floor of a building, landing on her buttocks and sustaining complete and immediate paraplegia. The lateral roentgenogram *(A)* shows intact posterior walls of both bodies but comminution of the anterior column. The axial CT scan *(B)* shows the facet dislocation *(arrows)* and an intact canal. She underwent open reduction of the dislocation with preservation of the facet joints and rod-sleeve stabilization. An interspinous wire was used to complete the reduction before application of the rod-sleeve construct *(C)* and *(D)*. This injury requires the same five level four interspace configuration as the Denis B burst fracture.

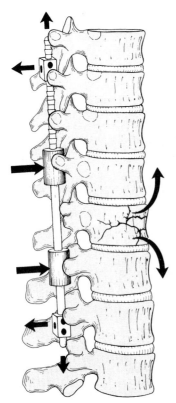

Figure 33–86. This diagram demonstrates the same principles as shown in Figure 33–85 but applied in a true burst fracture with predominantly axial loading force (Denis A) and with severe comminution of both the body pedicles and the posterior elements. A fracture pattern of this sort precludes the use of direct application of the corrective force over the apical segment because of the comminution of the neural arch. (Modified from Eismont, F. J., Garfin, S. R., and Abitbol, J-J.: Thoracic and thoracolumbar injuries. *In* Browner, B. D., Levine, A. M., Jupiter, J. B., and Trafton, P. G. [eds.]: Skeletal Trauma. Philadelphia, W. B. Saunders Co., 1992.)

instrumentation (Fig. 33–87). The exposure and preparation of the spine are the same as previously noted. However, once localization of the appropriate levels has occurred, insertion of the hooks is significantly different because of the variations in shape between anatomic hooks and Harrington hooks. For a standard rod-sleeve construct, a point approximately 3 cm proximal from the sleeve is chosen, with insertion of a hook on the inferior edge of that lamina. Anatomic hooks come in three standard sizes; the larger two, the medium and high-profile, are used most frequently in cases of trauma. The insertion of the anatomic hook in the middle to upper thoracic spine is done by first removing the ligamentum flavum from the undersurface of the lamina on which the hook is to be seated, as well as its attachments from the superior edge of the lamina below. Because the hook replicates the shape of the undersurface of the lamina and is not round, as the Harrington hook is, it must be seated directly and cannot be "rolled into position." Therefore, the superior edge of the lamina just below the insertion site will need to be burred flat so that the angle of entry

beneath the surface of the lamina is in line with the undersurface of the lamina (see Fig. 33–87A). This requires flattening of the level below. A curette can be used to ascertain that the ligamentum flavum is thoroughly detached. The facet joint should not be disrupted, because the width of the hook is narrower than that of a Harrington hook and will easily slide in the sublaminar position. These are not placed in the facet joints. Intact facet joints and capsules prevent lateral migration of the hooks with distraction. It is frequently necessary to remove a small portion of the medial corner of the spinous process to have the hook seated flush and not angled on the edge of the lamina. Care should be taken not to notch the lamina, because the force applied to the lamina with reduction is sufficient with this system to precipitate a laminar fracture if a stress riser is created. Using the pusher, the hook should slide easily into the sublaminar position. In the upper thoracic spine, a medium anatomic hook is most often used. This is done on both sides, and the two hooks should be checked to make sure they seat at the same angles and to the same depth. After insertion of the upper hooks, the lower hook sites are selected. These are generally two levels below the injured level for a standard rod-sleeve construct in the thoracic spine. A laminotomy involving resection of the inferior edge of the lamina above the one on which the hook is to be seated is performed. A rectangular laminotomy is necessary, because seating of these hooks requires a larger laminotomy than that for a Harrington hook and because, again, these anatomic hooks cannot be "rotated into position." The ligamentum flavum is then resected once it is visualized, and a portion of the superior facet is resected so that the hook seats directly on the edge of the lamina and not on the edge of the facet. Care must be taken not to resect the pars interarticularis, because iatrogenic spondylolysis can occur.[39] Minimal to none of the lamina should be resected at this lower level. Both hooks should be placed into the canal simultaneously to ensure that there is no overlapping of the hooks. Care is taken to leave the interspinous ligament intact with this technique. If there is medial impingement or difficulty seating the two hooks, resection of bone should be carried out to the pedicle. When the pedicle is palpable with the toe of the Kerrison punch, generally the size of the laminotomy is sufficient to accommodate the two hooks. All intervening facet capsules are removed and the cartilage is curetted. The appropriate standard Harrington or universal rods are then selected (square-ended rods should not be used). High-profile hooks are generally used distally, although in the middle and upper thoracic spine, medium-profile hooks are sometimes sufficient in size to clear the thickness of the lamina. Hooks with the small holes to accommodate the distal end of the Harrington rod are only available in a high-profile hook design, however. Therefore, the most common configurations are medium-profile hooks proximally with standard holes and high-profile hooks distally with small holes. If a modified universal rod is used, then standard hole hooks are used at both ends. The rod length is selected to leave approximately three ratchets proximal to the cephalad hooks. This prevents hook dislodgment. The amount of distraction with this system is somewhat less than with the Harrington system; therefore, rod length, except in cases of severe axial collapse, can be reasonably assessed by using a rod that has approximately six to seven ratchets proximal to the upper hook in the unreduced state (see Fig. 33–87B). The appropriate sleeve size is then selected from the four sizes. The small sleeve (thoracic) is most commonly used in the mid-thoracic spine. In the lower thoracic spine, the medium sleeve will be used in some individuals. When a bridging construct is used in the thoracic spine, generally four sleeves of similar size are used. The sleeves may not be of similar size at the lumbar junction and thoracolumbar spine. The sleeve is slid over the rod with a rod spreader, which can be used to move the sleeve. A special four-prong hook holder is placed on the proximal hook. The rod and sleeve combination is advanced up through the proximal hook until the nipple clears the distal hook. A hook holder is placed on the distal hook. With the surgeon on a standing stool so as to have appropriate visualization and adequate application of force through a rod holder, the distal end of the rod is firmly and continuously pushed down toward the depth of the distal hook. The greater the kyphosis at the fracture site, the more difficult this reduction will be. The placement of the sleeve should at this point be either at the level of the fracture or just distal to it (see Fig. 33–87C). If difficulty in engaging the hook is encountered, then the sleeve can be slid slightly more distally so as to diminish the force initially. This will allow engagement of the rod and hook with a less completely reduced sagittal alignment. However, moving the sleeve proximally at that point will complete the reduction. The application of force downward to reduce the kyphosis should be through continuous, rather than sporadic, applications. The spine will tend to relax, and the nipple can be inserted into the hook. Once the nipple is at the level of the hole in the hook, the assistant takes a rod spreader and distracts the rod down into the distal hook. Care needs to be taken not to cant the distal hook to engage the tip of the nipple into it; this can cause improper seating or dislodgment of the distal hook. Downward pressure should be kept on the rod until the nipple is fully engaged. At this point, before any distraction is applied, the sleeve should be slid directly over the pedicle of the fracture level or, in the bridging construct, over the pedicles proximal and distal to it. Minimal distraction should be applied to the single rod at this point. The amount of distraction should only be sufficient to begin to tighten the system. The second rod is inserted in a similar fashion. Once both sides are engaged, the system can be symmetrically distracted. The force placed on the spreader is "two-finger pressure." Once the limit of the distraction appears to be reached, the bone graft can be taken. After a 10- to 15-minute interval, an additional ratchet or two of distraction can be obtained and the system

further tightened. A lateral roentgenogram should be taken to verify sleeve position and completeness of reduction. Once the reduction has been completed and confirmed, C-washers are placed beneath the proximal hooks to block loss of distraction. The fusion is completed as detailed subsequently.

Multiple Hook-Rod Systems

The use of multiple hook-rod systems such as C-D, TSRH, Isola, and AO has now been extended to cases of trauma.[2, 24, 72, 74, 93] In the lumbar spine, to minimize construct length, combinations of hooks and screws can be considered[47, 48, 79, 96]; however, in the thoracic spine, the instrumentation is generally limited to the use of multiple-hook constructs. The experience with these systems for thoracolumbar spine trauma has increased exponentially in the last 10 years. Early experience with the use of short constructs, especially at the thoracolumbar junction and high lumbar spine, has been less than satisfactory. However, the use of multiple-hook, standard-length (six segments) constructs in the thoracic spine seems to offer satisfactory early results. The key to success appears to be a sufficient number of purchase sites and the length of the construct. The major disadvantages of the system are the time it takes to learn and the additional time required to assemble a construct. Although early data suggested that fracture reduction could be maintained without postoperative bracing, more recent results suggest that postoperative bracing may be required, depending on the number of hook sites utilized, the instability of the fracture, and the stiffness of the rod.[9]

The general plan of assembling any multiple system is based on combinations of unilaminar and bilaminar claw configurations above and below the level of injury (Fig. 33–88). A minimum of two unilaminar claws or an augmented claw (unilaminar plus a pedicle hook at the adjacent level) per side above the level of injury, and at least one bilaminar claw placed below the level of injury, are necessary. Additional hooks can be placed as required and varying amounts of compression and distraction can be applied between the claws. Placement technique for hooks is different than with Harrington instrumentation. The plan for a standard thoracic Denis type A or B burst fracture without significant posterior element comminution includes a unilaminar claw three levels above the level of injury. This is composed of a lumbar laminar hook over the transverse process and a pedicle hook in the facet joint and around the pedicle of the uppermost level. At the level above the injury, another unilaminar claw is inserted with a lumbar laminar hook over the transverse process and a pedicle hook placed facing cephalad in the facet and around the pedicle. If posterior element comminution exists at the hook placement level or if it is necessary to shorten the construct, a pedicle hook alone can be utilized at the level just distal to the cephalad-most claw. Below the level of injury, a thoracic laminar hook forms the upper end of

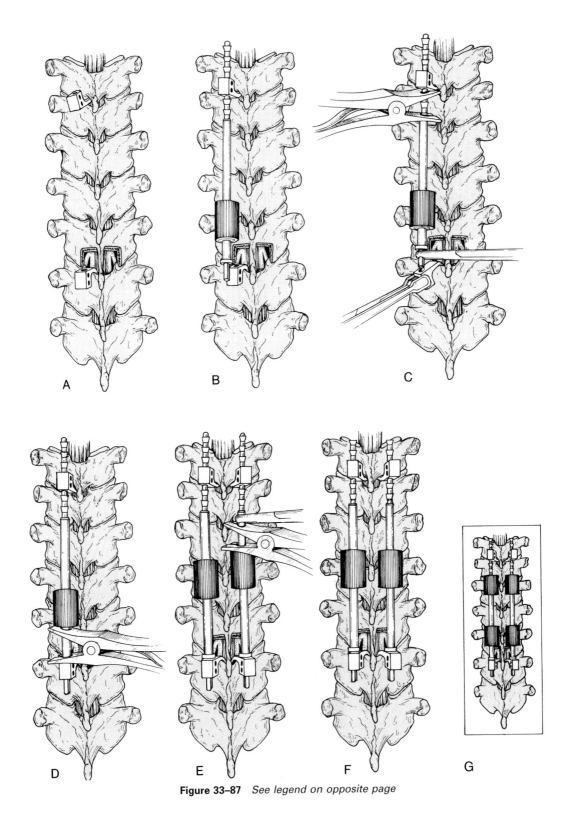

Figure 33–87 *See legend on opposite page*

the bilaminar claw, and a pedicle or laminar hook at the next level down forms the distal end of the claw.

Beginning at the proximal end, a laminar elevator is used to subperiosteally strip the soft tissue around the superior end of the transverse process of the uppermost level. A lumbar laminar hook is then placed over the top of that process, checking that the size is sufficient to allow seating around and not into the transverse process. At the upper thoracic levels, offset hooks may be necessary to engage the construct. On the undersurface of the proximal lamina, an osteotome is used to osteotomize the inferior edge of the facet joint. A high-speed burr can then be used to level the superior edge of the lamina and the medial aspect of the transverse process below that facet. A curette is used to remove the cartilage within the facet joint. A pedicle hook can then be inserted into the joint, engaging the inferior edge of the pedicle. The height of the shoe (standard versus increased) may need to be adjusted

so that the rod seats evenly in the claw configuration. The next level is not instrumented unless comminution exists at the level below; if so, a single pedicle hook is placed on either side, in the manner previously described. Under normal circumstances at the level directly above the fracture, a transverse process hook and a pedicle hook are inserted as described to assemble the second claw. At the superior end of the lamina, at the level below the injury, a laminotomy is performed. The laminotomy is different than those required for Harrington hooks in that it is directed in a medial-lateral direction. After completing the laminotomy, removing predominantly the inferior edge of the lamina above, the hook is inserted in a medial-lateral direction and rotated into position beneath the upper edge of the lamina. The shape of the laminotomy should prevent the hook from being forced into the canal. A thoracic laminar hook is preferred, both because of the size and the depth of the hook. Care

Figure 33–87. This technique demonstrates application of a rod sleeve for the thoracic spine. *A,* The determination of the placement of the hooks is based on the fracture pattern and the length of the lever arms. Generally in the thoracic spine this encompasses five segments and four interspaces for the standard flexion-compression type of injury. The rod-sleeve should be placed in its proper location over the apical segment, and then a distance of at least 3 cm should be determined from the rod-sleeve to the hook site. Because of the smaller size of the lamina, this will generally be two segments above the fractured level and two segments below, but on many occasions there will be three segments proximally as well. At the inferior edge of the selected level, the ligamentum flavum is removed. Because of the difference in the hook configuration from that of a Harrington hook, the insertion technique is slightly different for the anatomic hook. In the thoracic spine it is critical to burr down the superior edge of the lamina below so that the hook can slide directly under the lamina and does not lever on the lamina below. The hook is seated beneath the lamina and not in the facet joint. Care must be taken to dissect proximal to the hook site to achieve exposure of the proximal transverse processes for subsequent grafting. The interspinous ligament is left in position. Care is taken after inserting both hooks that they seat symmetrically. On the distal hook site, the laminotomy is achieved by removing only bone from the more proximal level, and no bone from the surface of the lamina on which the hook is to be seated. This is to prevent subsequent fracture of the pars at that location by weakening of the pars. The other critical feature is to widen the laminotomy out into the facet joints at the level of the pedicles so that the hooks do not overlap on seating. *B,* The proper size of sleeve, which in the upper thoracic spine is generally small and in the lower thoracic spine is medium, is placed over the rod on one side. The rod is then advanced through the proximal hook proximally enough so that the end of the nipple is rostral to the distal hook for ease of insertion. *C,* At this point, the surgeon grasps the distal hook with a hook holder and the nipple with a rod holder while the assistant readies a spreader at the proximal end of the construct. With a surgeon on a standing stool applying continuous pressure downward to reduce the kyphosis, the fracture kyphotic deformity is reduced before distracting the nipple into the distal hook. If reduction of deformity cannot be achieved, the sleeve size should be reassessed. If it is correct, the sleeve should be placed slightly distally on the rod engaged in the hook. The rod should be distracted only sufficiently to engage the distal hook. *D,* Once the rod is engaged in the distal hook and sufficient distraction is achieved to simply lock the construct in place, a rod spreader is used distally to move the sleeve to its proper location over the apical facet joints and pedicle. This completes the reduction. *E,* After the second rod is placed, that sleeve is also placed in the appropriate location so that the entire construct is symmetric. The construct should be checked to ensure that both hooks on the proximal and distal ends seat symmetrically and do not overlap in the canal. If the sleeves are not in an appropriate position, they can be moved up and down the rod. This should not be possible using finger pressure, as the impingement of the sleeve on the spine should be sufficient that it cannot easily be moved. This will generally require the use of the spreader. On the nonratcheted portion of the rod, a rod holder can be used to provide the second point so that the spreader can be placed between the rod holder and the sleeve, to allow enough force to be applied to move the sleeve to its appropriate position over the apical facet and pedicle. If the sleeves are loose and move easily with a finger, they are not effective and should be removed by disengaging the rods, and replaced with the next larger size. *F,* The entire construct is checked for symmetry and redistracted after harvesting of the bone graft. Generally one to two more ratchets can be achieved once a sufficient time interval (10 to 15 minutes) has elapsed. The washers are then placed below the upper hooks to prevent loosening of a construct subsequently. *G* demonstrates a correct position for the sleeves in a bridging construct in the thoracic spine. (Redrawn from Leona Allison.)

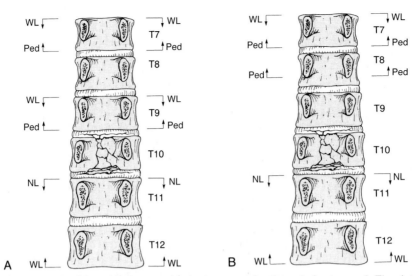

Figure 33–88. Patterns of Cotrel-Dubousset hook placement for thoracic fractures. *A*, The determination of the placement of the hooks for Cotrel-Dubousset instrumentation for fractures in the thoracic spine is critical and based on a combination of the length of the construct necessary to achieve the reduction of both the kyphosis and axial compression, and on the comminution of the posterior elements. The instrumentation must be configured to decrease the kyphosis of the injury. This generally requires at least one claw configuration proximally and distally. The proximal claw or claws are indirect claws. They are composed of a wide lumbar laminar hook placed over the transverse process of the uppermost level and a pedicle hook placed in the facet joint, capturing the pedicle at the same level. Generally, two sets of direct claws are necessary to achieve adequate strength of laminar fixation to counteract the kyphotic portion of the deformity without resulting in subsequent fracture of the lamina. This generally requires one direct claw three levels above the fractured level and a second one at the level above the fracture, with no instrumentation possible at the intervening level. Distal to the fracture, one indirect claw is generally sufficient to achieve adequate fixation. A single direct claw is not suggested, as this has frequently resulted in fracturing of the entire posterior elements at that level because of the amount of stress concentrated on a single lamina. The indirect claw distally can be composed of an narrow laminar hook at the level adjacent to the fracture level with a wide lumbar laminar hook or pedicle hook over the inferior edge of the next most distal level. An alternate, although less optimal, configuration in the higher thoracic spine is an indirect claw composed of a wide lumbar hook placed over the transverse processes at the proximal level and pedicle hooks placed at the distal level but not on the same lamina. *B*, An alternative construct for the same fracture pattern where the lamina of T9 is comminuted and does not allow placement of the second claw at that level. In that instance, a single open pedicle hook placed proximally can substitute for the claw at the next level distally. WL, wide lamina; Ped, pedicle; NL, narrow lamina. (Modified from Eismont, F. J., Garfin, S. R., and Abitbol, J-J.: Thoracic and thoracolumbar injuries. *In* Browner, B. D., Levine, A. M., Jupiter, J. B., and Trafton, P. G. [eds.]: Skeletal Trauma. Philadelphia, W. B. Saunders Co., 1992.)

should be taken to have the hook impinge on the dural sac. If this is a very proximal thoracic construct, a laminar hook over the transverse process can be substituted. The inferior portion of the bilaminar claw (encompassing two consecutive levels) in the upper thoracic spine can be a pedicle hook, whereas in the lower thoracic spine it should be a laminar hook on the inferior edge of the most distal lamina. After the rod is contoured to physiologic norms of the thoracic spine, it is inserted into the open bodies of the inserted hooks. If the fracture reduction is relatively complete simply by positioning on the table, then the rod shown fits easily into the majority of the hooks. This will allow insertion of the locking caps into the tops of the hooks with minimal application of force. The caps are not tightened at this point but are merely engaged in the hook. If significant kyphosis remains across the fracture site after positioning on the table, the rods and hooks can be used to achieve fracture reduction. The rods

should in that case be inserted bilaterally into the upper three (augmented claw) or four (two unilaminar claw) hooks and the locking caps inserted. The claws should be set by being compressed on the laminae and the caps tightened on both sides. If the reduction of the kyphosis is incomplete at this time, then the distal ends of the rods will be posterior to the hooks. Rod reduction tools can be placed on both sides and reduction of both rods into the hooks achieved. This will correct the kyphosis and the caps can then be inserted and tightened. If the rod can be inserted without use of a rod reduction tool, then the tightening pattern is as follows: Beginning at the proximal end of the construct, the cap on the most proximal hook is tightened. A hook approximator is used to tighten the upper claw. The hook at the level above the fracture is then advanced proximally using a spreader, and its cap is then tightened into place. Theoretically, the kyphosis should have been reduced by insertion of the appropriately contoured rod. Therefore, only slight distraction is now necessary between the hook above the level of the injury and the one below the level of the injury to further reduce it. Appropriate distraction is done and the cap is tightened. The distal claw can then be approximated, compressing the distal to the proximal hook that has just been tightened. A symmetric construct is placed on the contralateral side. Care must be taken with this particular construct to prepare all of the facet joints prior to insertion of the hardware. Appropriate roentgenograms are taken. The transverse connectors are placed at the proximal and distal ends of the construct, and all caps are broken off in the hooks (Fig. 33–89).

This technique is slightly modified for use with high thoracic fractures. Most of these fractures have some laminar comminution at the adjacent levels, thus instrumentation into the cervical spine is almost always necessary. The proximal hook in the cephalad claw is a small, offset, angled hook that is placed in the midline on the superior edge of the lamina. Care must be taken in preparing the seating site for these hooks so that the interspinous ligament and the facet capsules are not disturbed. A small bit of the inferior portion of the overlying lamina may need to be removed with a Kerrison punch to allow seating of the hook. This hook is inserted toward the midline and then rotated into

position. As a result of the small size of the cervical lamina, unilaminar claws are not applicable. Therefore for a T2 fracture, an offset hook would be inserted in the cephalad portion of the C6 lamina, a small laminar hook on the inferior portion of the C7 lamina, and a laminar or pedicle hook on the inferior portion of the T1 lamina. The distal end of the construct is the same as for other fracture patterns.

Plate-Screw Constructs

Under some circumstances, application of a hook-rod construct may not be appropriate for upper thoracic spine fractures. Both in Europe and in the United States, there have been reports of the use of plate-screw combinations for the fixation of thoracic fractures.[88] Although their potential for reduction of fracture deformity is relatively limited, they will satisfactorily hold a fracture reduction if sufficient number of points of fixation are selected. For upper thoracic fractures that can be reduced by postural reduction, stabilization with a plate-screw combination of reasonable thickness can be considered. Fixation in the lower cervical spine is attained with screws in the lateral masses. Fixation should not begin at C7 but rather at C6 because of the relatively poor fixation into the thin bone of the C7 lateral mass. Fixation in the upper thoracic spine can

Figure 33–89. These anteroposterior and lateral roentgenograms demonstrate a Cotrel-Dubousset construct for a fracture with severe laminar comminution at the central levels requiring an augmented claw proximally and a bilaminar claw distally.

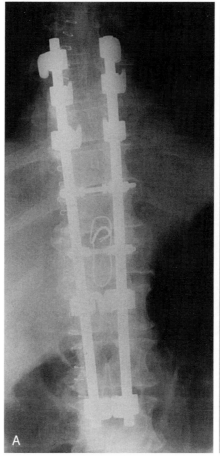
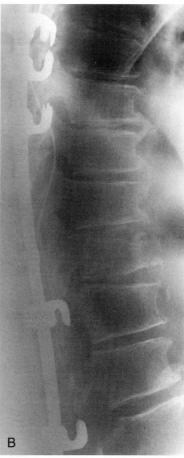

either be accomplished by fixation into the pedicles or four-cortex fixation through the transverse process and ribs with 3.5-mm or 4.0-mm screws. A minimum of three screws on each side of the fracture in each plate is necessary (Fig. 33–90).

Completion of Surgical Stabilization of the Thoracic Spine

Bone graft harvesting can be done for all of these constructs through a separate incision. A vertical inci-

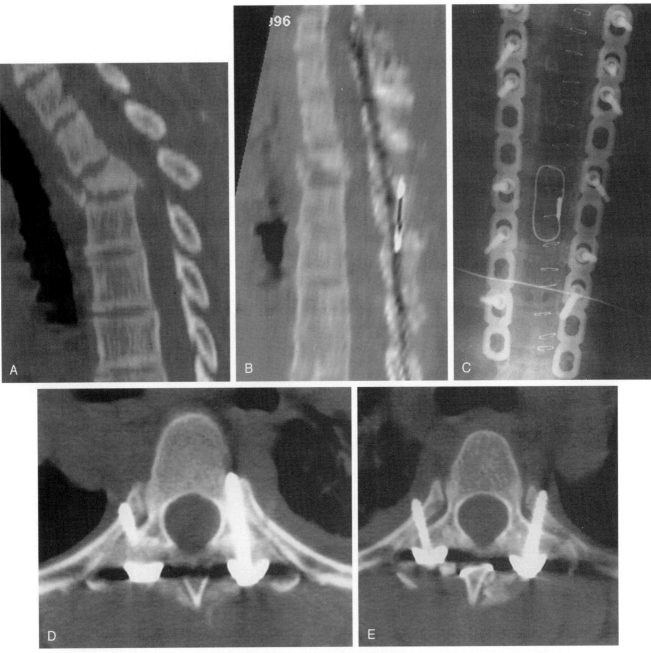

Figure 33–90. This midsagittal reconstruction (A) demonstrates a fracture of T2 in a patient with incomplete paraplegia. There is significant kyphosis and displacement. To reduce the fracture, the patient was placed in cervical traction in the prone position over a Mayfield headrest. The postoperative midsagittal reconstruction (B) shows the restoration of alignment and height achieved by this technique. As a result of the severe laminar comminution there were not enough purchase points to use a multiple hook-rod system, and therefore thoracic plating was done (C). Due to the relatively small size of the pedicles, it was difficult to obtain purchase in that structure (D) and therefore the majority of the screws were placed through the transverse processes and ribs, which gave secure purchase (E).

sion placed directly lateral to the posterior superior iliac crest allows exposure of the largest area of cancellous bone without significant disruption of the lumbodorsal fascia or interruption of the cluneal nerves. Graft harvested during the course of the procedure allows an interval for viscoelastic relaxation to occur. After completion of all the hardware insertion, the transverse processes are thoroughly decorticated. These should be exposed at the beginning of the procedure and can be decorticated with a high-speed burr or a rat-tooth rongeur, a curette, or a gouge. The lateral edges of the facet joints are similarly decorticated. Care must be taken in the Harrington and rod-sleeve methods to decorticate the transverse process proximal to the proximal hook. In the C-D construct, that transverse process is used for fixation; therefore, it is often difficult to obtain sufficient decorticated bone for fusion at that level. Care must be taken to apply bone to decorticated lamina throughout the length of the fusion. The paraspinous muscles should be sutured back in the midline. Suction drains are placed in both the spine and iliac crest hip wounds. In all constructs, the patient should be immobilized in a total-contact orthosis. Immobilization of the upper thoracic spine is difficult. With hooks placed at T3 or higher, a cervicothoracic orthosis is necessary. With the upper hooks placed at T4 or below, a standard thoracolumbar orthosis carried high in the front and in the back is sufficient.

Thoracolumbar and High Lumbar Trauma

The considerations for instrumentation of the region from T11 to L2 are somewhat different from those in the thoracic spine. First, the majority of injuries occur at the thoracolumbar junction as a result of the transition from the rigid thoracic spine (rib cage) to the more mobile lumbar spine. Second, there is the change in sagittal alignment from thoracic kyphosis to lumbar lordosis. Third, the injury patterns are somewhat different at the thoracolumbar junction as opposed to the thoracic spine, because injuries such as flexion distraction rarely occur in the thoracic spine but are most frequent at the thoracolumbar junction and in the high lumbar spine. This group of flexion injuries includes both Chance fractures and other flexion-distraction variants, as well as bilateral facet dislocations. The fourth consideration in treatment of thoracolumbar injuries is the necessity to preserve the overall sagittal alignment and, as important, minimize the length of fixation and fusion into the lumbar spine. Thus, instrumentation that requires significant length of fixation distal to the fracture site is less advantageous at the thoracolumbar junction or the high lumbar spine than it would be in the thoracic spine. Several of the techniques described in detail for the thoracic spine must be modified when applied to the thoracolumbar and high lumbar spine.[36]

Surgical Technique

Modifications in positioning for surgical intervention at the thoracolumbar junction are mainly related to the extreme flexibility of the lumbar spine and thoracolumbar junction. It has been well demonstrated that accentuating the lumbar lordosis in the prone position can significantly reduce the fracture deformity. Therefore, positioning for fractures at the thoracolumbar junction and high lumbar spine is extremely critical in that sufficient lordosis must be imparted to the fracture to augment the reduction. The use of transverse rolls or a spinal frame that allows extension is one extremely helpful technique. Care should again be taken to leave the abdomen unimpeded to prevent delay of venous return.

Several elements must be given meticulous attention in the surgical exposure of the thoracolumbar and lumbar spine in two areas. First, the lumbodorsal fascia must be preserved (see Fig. 33–91A) and, if possible, reattached to the spinous processes at closure. This means that care should be taken not to disrupt the supraspinous and interspinous ligaments. This is especially critical in exposure at the distal ends of the construct. Precise localization must be established for the levels being exposed to preserve the interspinous ligament and the facet capsules at the level just caudal to the planned end of the instrumentation. An error of one level of distal exposure can result in sufficient instability at the end of a rigid segment to cause marked late degenerative changes. Exposure is similar to the thoracic spine, with the exception that once localization has been verified by the use of a roentgenogram, exposure of the lumbar transverse processes should be done. This includes the stripping of all capsules from the facet joints. Care must be taken in the exposure of the distal hook site on the superior edge of the caudal end of the construct so that the facet and its capsule below are not damaged. At the proximal end of the construct, the transverse process that lies cephalad to the proximal hook purchase site must also be well visualized and prepared.

Harrington Distraction Instrumentation

Few modifications of Harrington distraction instrumentation are possible for use at the thoracolumbar junction and high lumbar spine. The length of instrumentation is fixed by the necessity to maintain sufficient lever arms to achieve stability. Therefore, the length of instrumentation at the thoracolumbar junction remains three above and two below. When necessary, augmentation with sublaminar wires may help prevent the unacceptably high hook dislodgement rate that accompanies distal hooks in the lumbar spine. In addition, contouring of the rods and the use of square-ended hooks can help maintain lumbar lordosis when the construct extends to the mid and lower lumbar spine (L2, L3, L4).[1, 28] The technique is not significantly modified from the thoracic technique, with the previously noted exceptions.

Rod-Sleeve Technique

As mentioned previously, the rod-sleeve technique is adaptable with certain fracture patterns to a short con-

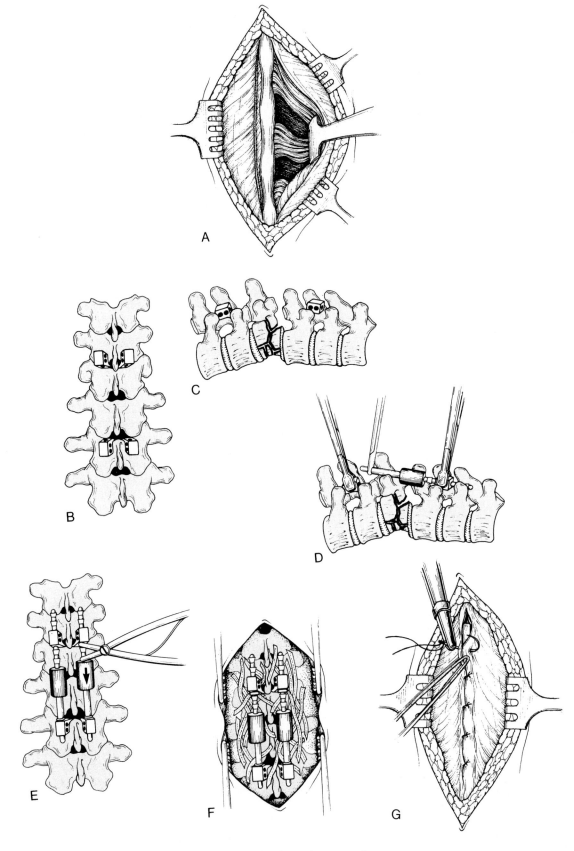

Figure 33–91 *See legend on opposite page*

struct (four levels/three interspaces) for the high lumbar spine and thoracolumbar junction. This is because there is an increase in the overall size of the individual lamina, and thus the necessity of a 3-cm lever arm between the rod-sleeve and hooks can be satisfied with fewer segments. For example, in the patient with an L2 fracture who has an intact posterior arch and body–pedicle junction but a large retropulsed fragment and severe kyphosis, a short rod-sleeve technique can be used (see Fig. 33–91B). For this injury, the sleeves are placed over the L1–L2 facets and centered over the L2 pedicle. The distal hooks are placed over the superior edge of the L3 lamina, and the superior hooks under the inferior edge of the T12 lamina. For an L3 fracture, the distal hooks can usually be placed at L4 and the proximal hooks at L1, thus immobilizing only four levels and three interspaces. This requires no further fusion or immobilization of segments caudally than either a direct anterior approach or a pedicle screw construct from posterior necessitates. It is, however,

---

Figure 33–91. Technique for short rod-sleeve construct. *A,* Exposure of the thoracolumbar junction and lumbar spine is critical because it is necessary to leave the interspinous and supraspinous ligament intact for reconstitution of the lumbodorsal fascia after the procedure. Therefore the incision is made down to the tips of the spinous processes, and then two separate straight incisions are made parallel to the outer bony edge of the spinous processes across the four segments to be instrumented. This is done on both sides without weaving into the interspinous area. Then, using a cautery and Cobb elevator for retraction, all soft tissue is removed from the spinous process and the lamina, but the facet joints are left intact until a roentgenogram is taken to ascertain the correct localization of levels. At that point, the dissection is carried out through the facet capsules, in which the ones to be fused are removed, and out to the tips to the transverse processes. *B,* For the L2 fracture illustrated, with the posterior arch intact but a large retropulsed fragment and significant kyphosis, the hook placement selection is based on the critical lever arm length. Generally at the thoracolumbar junction this can be accomplished with a single level below the injured vertebra; thus, for an L2 fracture the distal hooks can be placed at L3, still achieving a 3-cm lever arm, and proximal hooks two segments above. Thus, for an L2 fracture a T12 proximal hook site is sufficient. Occasionally, this may have to be increased one hook site proximally to T11, but rarely distally. Placement of the hooks as in the thoracic spine is critical because of the high forces placed on, especially, the proximal hooks. Care should be taken that no bone is removed from the edge of the lamina at the superior level on which the upper hooks are seated. Simply removing the ligamentum flavum from the undersurface of the lamina will allow easy seating of a medium profile hook. Care should be taken that the hooks are seated symmetrically and beneath the lamina. The facet capsules can be removed, but destruction of the joint should not take place, although the fusion mass will be proximal to the transverse processes at that level. At the caudal level, a laminotomy is done, removing simply the bone at the inferior edge of the lamina of the fractured level. This is sufficiently distal to the area of canal impingement that the hook placement in this location will not be a problem. The ligamentum flavum is removed through the laminotomy on both sides, and the resection of the facet joint is carried far enough laterally to be able to feel the pedicle with the tip of a Kerrison punch. The two high-profile hooks are then seated in the canal and checked to make sure there is no overlapping of the hooks and that they seat symmetrically. If there is a problem with seating, the laminotomy should be carried wider into the facet joints. Care should be taken, however, not to remove any bone of the superior aspect of the lamina of L3, as this will significantly weaken the lamina and may cause subsequent fracture. *C,* The appropriate position of the hooks in reference to the fractured vertebral body. Note the kyphosis at this level. *D,* The appropriate rod length is selected. This is determined by placing a rod over the construct and then estimating approximately three ratchets of distraction in the normal flexion compression (Denis type B) fracture. The appropriate size of sleeve is selected by making certain that the sleeve fits at the apical lamina and its medial-lateral width is appropriate. Generally, for a small woman, at the thoracolumbar junction or higher lumbar spine, a medium sleeve can be used; for a larger male a large sleeve will be necessary. The sleeve is placed on the rod, and the rod-sleeve combination is advanced through the proximal hook. With a surgeon now standing on a stool above, pressure is applied in a downward direction over the apical kyphosis to reduce the kyphosis before engaging the tip of the rod in the distal hook. Once the tip of the rod is at the level of the hook, downward pressure is maintained as the assistant distracts the rod to completely seat the rod in the distal hook before relieving the downward pressure. This is repeated on the contralateral side. *E,* A distractor can then be used to tension the rods initially so that they are just snug but not too tight. The sleeves are then positioned over the apical facet joints and pedicle, and the final rod tension is achieved. A roentgenogram is taken to ascertain the efficacy of reduction. A bone graft is then obtained and additional tension is applied to the construct after viscoelastic relaxation has occurred. *F,* Washers are placed beneath the upper rods after final tensioning to keep the correct amount of distraction. Decortication of the transverse processes and the lateral side of the facets is performed with bone grafting, including the upper transverse process, which is approximately 1.5 cm proximal to the upper end of the upper hooks. Care must be taken to graft that site carefully, as it is a frequent site of nonunions. *G,* In closure of the wound over a suction drain, care is taken to reapproximate the lumbodorsal fascia to the remaining supraspinous and interspinous ligament. For this technique, even when the ligament is disrupted at its central portion, the peripheral portions can be easily reapproximated, giving a satisfactory closure. (Modified from Eismont, F. J., Garfin, S. R., and Abitbol, J-J.: Thoracic and thoracolumbar injuries. *In* Browner, B. D., Levine, A. M., Jupiter, J. B., and Trafton, P. G. [eds.]: Skeletal Trauma. Philadelphia, W. B. Saunders Co., 1992.)

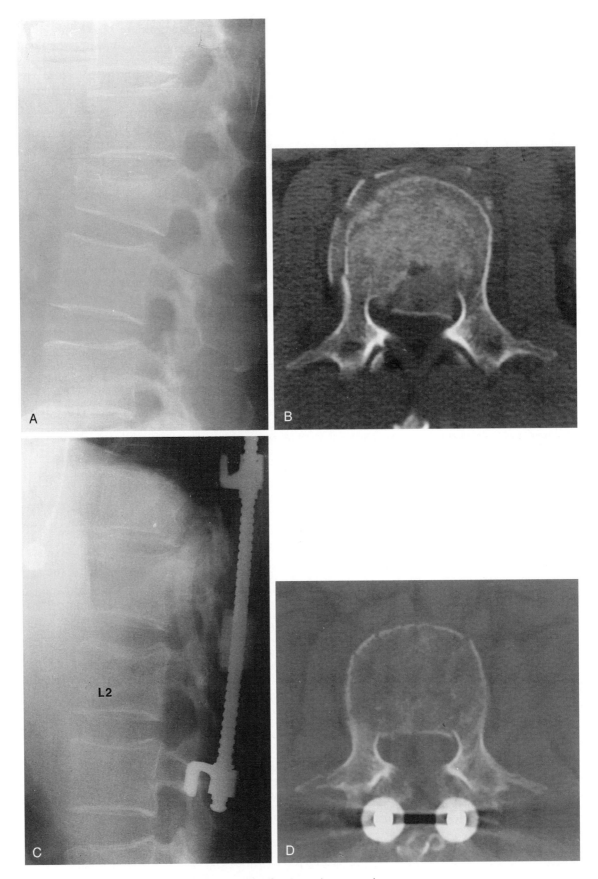

Figure 33–92 *See legend on opposite page*

limited to that group of patients in whom three-point fixation can be applied directly over the fractured level. This constitutes approximately 40 per cent of all patients with burst-type injuries. Those patients with burst injuries with comminution of the posterior elements and the body–pedicle junction require a bridging sleeve construct. In the lumbar spine, this can be accomplished over five levels and four interspaces. The sleeves are placed at the level proximal and distal to the fractured level. For an L1 fracture, the distal hooks are at L3; for an L2 fracture, the distal hooks are at L4 (see Fig. 33–91C). The major advantage of a rod-sleeve at this particular level is that the amount of lumbar lordosis can be controlled and maintained by the use of appropriate size sleeves. The short rod-sleeve construct for an L2 fracture will be detailed (see Fig. 33–91). The approach is similar to that previously described. Care in exposure is necessary because only one level below the level of injury is to be instrumented. Thus, maintenance of the L3–L4 facet joints and L3–L4 interspinous ligament is important. In addition, for an L2 fracture, when preparing the undersurface of the T12 lamina, care must be taken not to notch the lamina in any way. Simple detachment of the ligamentum flavum from the undersurface of the lamina is sufficient. The shape of the lamina will generally allow seating of a medium-profile hook without modification to the shape of the lamina. Occasionally, in a male with a very thick T12 lamina, a high-profile hook will be needed to accommodate the thickness of the lamina at this proximal hook site. At the L2–L3 interspace, the ligamentum flavum is easily exposed. As a result of the lordosis imparted to reduce the fracture, occasionally the interspace will be somewhat closed. In that case, additional excision of the inferior end of the L2 lamina is necessary to expose the interspace. The ligamentum flavum is then excised, but the superior edge of the L3 lamina is not modified in any way. It is extremely critical in the lumbar spine not to damage the pars interarticularis in the preparation of the hook site.[39] The laminotomy is completed and a high-profile hook is placed in position. Most frequently, the width of the laminotomy must be extended out to the pedicle. This may require partial excision of the inferior facet of L2. Once both laminotomies have been made, the two distal hooks are placed simultaneously to ascertain that they do not overlap in the canal.

After the spine and the hook sites are prepared, the appropriate length of rod is selected. Sleeve selection is based on patient size. For a small woman with a high lumbar fracture and a short construct, medium sleeves are adequate. Medium sleeves may be sufficient in some males; however, in a larger male in whom high-profile hooks are used proximally, a large sleeve will be necessary. Occasionally, the distance between the facets laterally and spinous process medially will not allow complete seating of a large sleeve, even though the depth of the sleeve is needed to maintain lordosis and reduce kyphosis. The sleeve can be narrowed in its medial-lateral direction at the operating table with the use of a high-speed burr or scalpel. Once the appropriate sleeve has been selected and prepared, the rod is advanced up through the proximal hook. Significant downward pressure is applied to reduce the kyphosis and allow engagement of the distal nipple of the rod into the distal high-profile hooks (see Fig. 33–91D). The downward pressure must be maintained until the rod is fully seated. If difficulty is encountered in engaging the rod into the distal hook, there are several alternatives. First, the sleeve can be pushed distally a slight distance to make engagement easier. Secondly, a smaller sleeve can be used initially to achieve a partial reduction, and then a larger sleeve can be reapplied in an alternating fashion after completing the reduction on the contralateral side. Finally, the assistant may engage a longer rod through the proximal hook on the contralateral side and apply gentle pressure with the longer rod over the apical segment, thus achieving partial reduction and aiding the surgeon with the reduction on his or her side. With the short rod-sleeve technique, very little distraction will be achieved, because kyphosis is the predominant deformity in these patients. Once the construct has been engaged, generally not more than two complete ratchets of distraction will be further obtained. Completion of the procedure is similar to that detailed for the thoracic spine (Fig. 33–92).

Multiple Hook-Rod Instrumentation

The use of a short construct for multiple hook-rod instrumentation at the thoracolumbar junction has met with less success[24] than the use of the same instrumentation for thoracic fractures[8] (see Fig. 33–87C). The use

Figure 33–92. This 43-year-old male was riding his bicycle and was struck by a motor vehicle, sustaining this L2 burst fracture. On the initial lateral roentgenogram *(A)* he had comminution of the upper 60 per cent of the vertebral body and 29 degrees of kyphosis and was neurologically intact with the exception of the inability to void. Preoperative CT scan *(B)* showed 60 per cent canal compromise. This fracture was felt to be a Denis type B burst fracture with intact body pedicle junction and posterior elements. Thus a single sleeve construct could be utilized with the point of lordosis centered directly over the L2 pedicle with the distal extent of the instrumentation only going to L3. On the postoperative lateral roentgenogram *(C),* restoration of vertebral height and sagittal alignment were achieved. Postoperative CT scan *(D)* at exactly the same level as the preoperative scan shows restoration of canal area as well as the placement of the sleeves. (From Browner, B. D., Jupiter, J. B., Levine, A. M., Trafton, P. G. [eds.]: Skeletal Trauma. 2nd ed. Philadelphia, W. B. Saunders, 1997.)

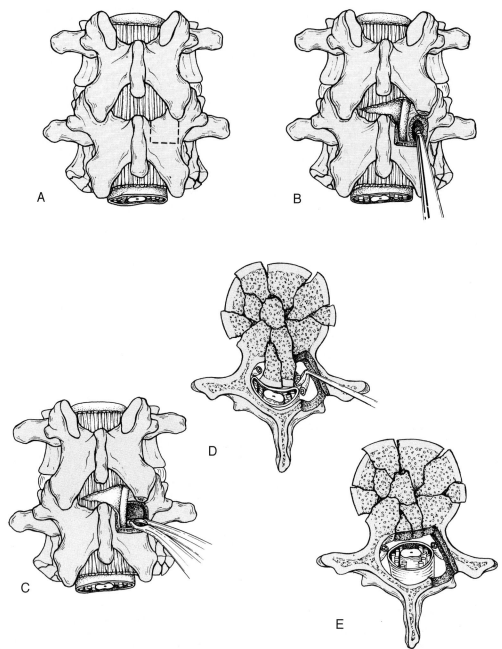

Figure 33–93. Technique for posterolateral decompression of a spinal fracture. *A,* On the basis of the preoperative CT scan, the area of maximal compression and the side of maximal compression are determined. This technique is most effective for unilateral compression, as only one side of the canal can be clearly visualized. A laminotomy is then performed, removing the lamina adjacent to the pedicle, which is generally the superior aspect of the lamina at the interspace, out to and including a significant portion of the facet joint. Fracture of the pars or division of the pars may occur from its thinning. Once the pedicle is located, the nerve root coming around the inferomedial portion of the pedicle is visualized and protected and the pedicle is inspected. *B,* After the nerve root is carefully protected, a high-speed burr is used to drill out the central portion of the pedicle down to the level of the vertebral body. The pedicle is thinned so that all that remains is the medial wall. Significant bleeding may be encountered as the fractured body is entered. *C,* Again the root is protected and the medial wall of the pedicle is removed using a pituitary rongeur and Kerrison punch down to the level of the canal. At this point, with appropriate retraction of the nerve root and the dural sac, it should be possible to visualize the retropulsed fragments *(D).* Generally a headlight is helpful in achieving this visualization. A reverse-angled curet can be used either to tamp the fragments back into the body or to gently tease the fragments out and remove them through the defect in the pedicle and lateral portion of the body. Care must be taken in separating the large fragments from the intact posterior longitudinal ligament. The extent of decompression can be checked with ultrasonography. *E,* The final result of the posterior lateral decompression. (Modified from Eismont, F. J., Garfin, S. R., and Abitbol, J-J.: Thoracic and thoracolumbar injuries. *In* Browner, B. D., Levine, A. M., Jupiter, J. B., and Trafton, P. G. [eds.]: Skeletal Trauma. Philadelphia, W. B. Saunders Co., 1992.)

of a four segment/three interspace construct with a unilaminar claw above and a unilaminar claw below results in frequent fracture of the claw purchase site proximally or distally. Thus, for an L2 fracture, the use of a claw on the upper and lower edge of the lamina of L3 and at T12 has met with a loss of correction and an unacceptable complication rate. Two solutions have been applied to make this a satisfactory technique for the thoracolumbar junction and still restrict the overall length of the construct. The first is the use of an anterior graft with the posterior instrumentation. The use of direct anterior decompression and tricortical graft from L1 to L3 with instrumentation from T12 to L3 has been a satisfactory alternative for patients requiring both anterior decompression and posterior stabilization. The second alternative, which at this point is investigational (not FDA approved), is the use of combined pedicle screw–hook fixation[47] at the same level distally to augment the distal purchase site and thus shorten the overall construct without compromise of the purchase strength. Further details of surgical technique for pedicle screws are in the following section.

Posterolateral Decompression

An adjunctive technique frequently applied at the thoracolumbar junction for many of these injuries is that of posterolateral decompression.[10, 43, 49, 98] The adequacy of decompression can be assessed by intraoperative ultrasonography. It must be stressed, however, that the use of a posterolateral approach may jeopardize the stability of fixation by removing important posterior elements, neural arch, and pedicles, which lend stability to the posterior stabilization techniques. Posterolateral decompression is also a one-sided technique. Exposure of one side will not lend exposure to the contralateral side and, if a symmetrical block is present, it may require bilateral transpedicular exposure. Generally, the instrumentation is inserted on one side first, leaving the other side available for decompression. A hemilaminectomy is performed and the ligamentum flavum removed (Fig. 33–93A). A small ultrasound probe can be used to verify the position of the fragment relative to the posterior and posterolateral structures. This can be correlated with the preoperative CT scan (Fig. 33–94). Once this has been done, the laminectomy is extended using a high-speed burr. The laminectomy is extended out to the medial border of the pedicle (Fig. 33–93B). A nerve root retractor is then used to retract the nerve root away from the site of excision of the pedicle, and the pedicle or its medial wall is excised (Fig. 33–93C). The body is then undercut, and fragments of bone are withdrawn through this hemilaminectomy and pediculectomy or are tapped back into the vertebral body if they are too large to remove (Fig. 33–93D). Intraoperative reduction can be verified by the use of ultrasonography. Direct inspection of the entire canal is difficult, but unilateral inspection is possible (Fig. 33–93D). The use of a headlight for visualization is necessary. Care must be taken in completion of the stabilization that no direct three-point bending

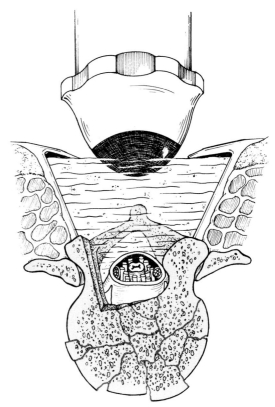

Figure 33–94. In this illustration after decompression of the area of maximal canal compromise by posterolateral decompression, the configuration of the canal can be checked with ultrasonography. Using a sterile barrier over the tip, the wound is filled with saline, and the orientation of the tip of the ultrasound probe can be used to visualize this transverse section of the canal at the level of the pedicles. For visualization of a posterolateral decompression, the laminotomy needs to be extended across the midline, with a window approximately 1.5 by 2 cm in dimension available for introducing the probe. (Modified from Eismont, F. J., Garfin, S. R., and Abitbol, J-J.: Thoracic and thoracolumbar injuries. *In* Browner, B. D., Levine, A. M., Jupiter, J. B., and Trafton, P. G. [eds.]: Skeletal Trauma. Philadelphia, W. B. Saunders Co., 1992.)

forces are placed over the level where the pedicle has been excised.

Low Lumbar Fractures

Surgical Technique

The region of L3 to L5 has been an area of considerable difficulty.[41, 76, 94] Fractures infrequently occur at this location. As a result of the multiple complexities involving the configuration of the vertebrae, the high shear stresses, and the necessity for maintenance of lordosis, instrumentation of low lumbar fractures has been fraught with many complications.[34, 65] The use of most rod-hook configurations in the low lumbar spine has required fusion to the sacrum, complicated by iatrogenic flatback and unacceptable instrumentation dislodgment and pseudarthrosis rates. Until 1985, surgical intervention consisted predominantly of direct decompression and uninstrumented posterolateral fusion. The advent of the investigational use of pedicle screw fixation changed the outlook for low lumbar fractures.[48, 105] Although pedicle screw fixation has been applied to fractures above L3,[18, 67, 68, 72, 75, 89] its use in that setting is even more controversial. The relative risks of the procedure as compared with the benefits imparted to the patient must be assessed,[19, 37, 80] and the outcome remains controversial.

Pedicle screw fixation in the lumbar spine can be divided into several different system types. These are predominantly (1) rod-based,[24, 34, 65, 75] (2) plate-based,[32, 86, 87, 106] and (3) internal fixateurs.[30, 35, 56, 57, 62, 68, 70, 72, 81] Although the technical details of placement of pedicle fixation vary from system to system, the overall concepts of placement of pedicle screws in the lumbar spine are reasonably constant. Rod-based systems allow combinations of both pedicle screws and hooks and may, because of their versatility, allow placement of screws at both the adjacent levels to the fracture and the fracture level itself.[34, 65] Plate-based systems frequently allow fixation at the adjacent levels as well as at the fracture level but lack the versatility in screw placement angle and are limited if significant displacement exists and reduction is necessary. The fixateur systems all depend on placement of screws only at the levels proximal and distal to the fracture.[35, 68, 72] Reduction of the fracture is based on cantilever bending. The ability to regain lordosis when there is marked deformity and comminution is therefore limited.

The relative advantages of the use of pedicle fixation are greater in the lumbar spine than in the thoracic spine. This is because in the former region there is the need for shorter constructs and less immobilization. Additionally, the larger diameter of the pedicles increases the ease of insertion and outweighs the relative disadvantages. At the thoracolumbar junction, the pedicle anatomy becomes less constant, the pedicles often being elliptical, with sufficient length but insufficient width to accommodate the necessary diameter of the pedicle screws. The difficulty with placement of screws at T12 has been well documented. At the thoracolumbar junction, the necessity for shorter constructs offered by pedicle-based systems over the length of a rod-hook construct is not as significant as in the low lumbar spine. Finally, the overall alignment of the thoracolumbar junction is at best neutral and, in many patients, slightly kyphotic. This allows the weight-bearing line of the axis of the body to fall anterior to the device after fracture reduction and applies significant cantilever-bending forces to the screws. This force may cause earlier failure than in the lumbar spine. With restoration of sagittal alignment of the lumbar spine, the relative lordosis causes the weight-bearing axis to fall posteriorly along the line of the body of the instrumentation, thus diminishing the bending stresses on the screws and imparting axial loading stresses on the device itself.[61, 92]

There are multiple screw configurations currently in use, but with two major variables. These are the core diameter and the thread size and pitch. Because of size restrictions imposed by the pedicle, a conflict in design exists. The larger the core diameter of the screw, the greater the resistance to bending strength. However, there is a finite limit to the size of the thread, because as thread size diminishes, pull-out strength similarly diminishes. Thus, in assessing a pedicle screw system, the relative stresses to which the screws are subjected must dictate the design of the screw. Those screws requiring significant pull-out strength will, by necessity, have a smaller core diameter and a larger thread size, whereas those subjected more to cantilever bending and less to pull-out will tend to have larger core diameter and smaller thread width. As screws have been introduced, the relative experience is that screw sizes under 6 mm that are rigidly fixed to the device generally fail by breakage. The range of screws currently in use is between 6 and 7 mm, a compromise between the maximum size that can be inserted in the lumbar pedicles and the relative strength of the screw. Smaller screws can be used, however, if the screw–plate junction is not extremely rigid. A slight bit of toggle built into that junction protects the screws, allowing screws as small as 3.5 mm to be used with some applications. Screw design is, by definition, flawed, with natural stress risers at junctions between screw threads and shank, and so on. The majority of resistance to pull-out is found in the pedicle, as opposed to the cancellous bone of the vertebral body. The depth of insertion is important only in that penetration of the anterior body can add approximately 20 per cent to the pull-out strength.

Surgical Technique for Pedicle Screw Insertion

The surgical technique for pedicle screw insertion in most cases includes radiologic control for placement of the screws. Several different techniques are available, and these are outlined here. Radiologic control can either be with plain roentgenograms taken in the anteroposterior and lateral positions, or with image intensification. In those cases in which anteroposterior and lateral roentgenograms are taken, a standard operating room table with a cassette holder can be used. This has the advantage of allowing flexion and extension of the patient during screw fixation. This flexibility in positioning may be offset by the cumbersome nature of time delays in obtaining plain roentgenograms. Conversely, the use of a radiolucent table without the ability to obtain flexion-extension is somewhat more difficult. The advent of radiolucent operating tables with the inherent ability to flex and extend the table makes the use of image intensification at this time slightly superior to the use of plain roentgenograms. In addition, the positioning of the image intensifier allows visualization of the pedicle in both direct and accurate anteroposterior and lateral planes as well as along the axis of the pedicle. The patient can be positioned in the prone position on longitudinal rolls. Care should be taken not to hyperextend the lumbar spine, because placement of pedicle screws with overextension of the spine will be more difficult. For exposure and initial placement, the table can be slightly flexed; once fracture reduction is begun, extension of the table for aid in reduction can be achieved. Positioning of the image intensifier can be beneath a radiolucent platform table to allow maximum convenience as well as radiographic control.

Surgical exposure for most pedicle screw systems is limited to one level above and one level below the level of injury. In the initial dissection, care must be taken to preserve the interspinous ligaments and the facet capsules at levels that are not to be instrumented. For an L4 fracture, exposure should be L3–L5 without destruction of the L2–L3 facet capsules, but with exposure of the transverse process of L3, which is lateral to the L2–L3 facet. Exposure for sacral screw placement requires exposure to S2 and laterally out to the sacral ala.

A midline posterior incision is used. Dissection is carefully done with a cautery to avoid excessive motion to the spine and to preserve the interspinous ligaments, so that restoration of the lumbodorsal fascia can be done on closure. The soft tissue is stripped off the appropriate levels of the spinous processes, laminae, facets, and transverse processes (Fig. 33–95A). As previously mentioned, the proximal transverse process lies opposite a level that is not to be instrumented, and the facet capsule at that level should not be damaged. The distal level is somewhat easier, because the transverse process lies lateral to the most distally fused facet joint. Care must be taken to clear all soft tissue from the junction of the transverse process and the inferior edge of the adjacent facet joint. Exposure of transverse processes can reveal fractures of these processes, as well as fractures of the posterior elements.

There are a number of methods for orientation of the screws. We will deal only with L3–S1. After the patient is positioned on the table, the orientation of the vertebrals with reference to vertical axis must be determined. After the spine is exposed, roentgenograms or fluoroscopic images should be obtained in the lateral position to verify the angles of the pedicles with reference to the vertical axis. For most low lumbar fractures, the most proximal level pedicle will be oriented slightly cephalad, and at the level of injury almost vertical. L5 is oriented approximately 15 degrees caudally, and S1 approximately 25 degrees caudally. In addition, the orientation of the screws in a medial lateral direction is critical. The orientation of the pedicles beginning at T12 is approximately 0 to −4 degrees from the sagittal. L1–L2 are approximately 5 degrees oriented medially, and L4 and L5 are oriented as much as 15 to 20 degrees medially (Fig. 33–95B). This can be determined preoperatively from assessment of the CT scans for individual patients. In addition, the pedicle diameters can be determined. The range is significant. Most patients have sufficient pedicle diameter in the medial-lateral direction to accommodate screws at L3–S1. Orientation of screw placement at S1[77] can be either medially into the pedicle (Fig. 33–95C) and through the anterior portion of the body, or laterally into the sacral

ala (Fig. 33–95D). In either case, the screw should parallel the end plate of S1 at an angle of approximately 25 degrees from the vertical. Medial orientation requires approximately 30 degrees of inward orientation from the sagittal, and lateral orientation of approximately 35 degrees to arrive in the sacral ala.

The most common entry position for lumbar pedicles is that described by Roy-Camille (Fig. 33–95E, F). For L3, L4, and L5, the entry point is at the intersection of lines drawn through the transverse processes in a medial-lateral direction and through the inferior-lateral edge of the proximal facet in a vertical direction. The screw holes are begun by entering through the posterior cortical bone using an awl or a high-speed burr. The burr should be angled to make the entry hole approximately in the same direction as previously described for orientation of the screw. The only exception is the most proximal level, where care must be taken to avoid the facet joint. Depending on the flexibility of the system, orientation of the screw can begin somewhat more inferior and lateral in this pedicle, to avoid impingement on the unfused proximal facet joint. In the sacrum, penetration of the posterior cortex with a high-speed burr is not necessary because most bone purchase is achieved at the posterior cortex and it should not be weakened. For L3–L5, once the posterior cortex is removed, entry into the pedicle can be done with power or by hand. A slowly rotating power drill can be used to feel the cancellous bone of the pedicle. Alternatively, a 3-0 or 4-0 curette can be gently worked down the pedicle in the proper orientation. It should go with minimal resistance. Once the depth of the pedicle has been probed, a 2.0-mm drill bit or Kirschner wire can be placed down the hole. It should not initially be inserted deeper than the depth of the pedicle (see Fig. 33–95G). At this point, anteroposterior and lateral roentgenograms can be taken, if that method is used. Two drill bits at the same level can be reversed so that one is shank down and the other is bit down, so that they can be differentiated on the lateral image. If image intensification is used, then the image intensifier should be orientated parallel to the orientation of the pedicles. This requires more angulation with more caudal pedicles. Visualization of the drill bit or Kirschner wire on the anteroposterior image should then be simply a round dot in the center of the pedicle, which on the oblique or lateral view should course centrally in the pedicle. Once the orientation of the drill bits within the pedicles has been ascertained, the holes are then deepened into the body. This can be done with any appropriate instrument, such as a larger drill bit, on a tap, curette, or probe. The depth of the hole is measured. With any technique, the integrity of the pedicles should be checked by feeling all four quadrants of the pedicle. This is easily accomplished with a depth gauge or blunt, bent-end Kirschner wire, using the small hook portion to run along the medial, lateral, superior, and inferior walls of the pedicles to ascertain that there is no penetration. This is necessary prior to inserting a screw.

For lateral placement in the sacrum, a small drill bit

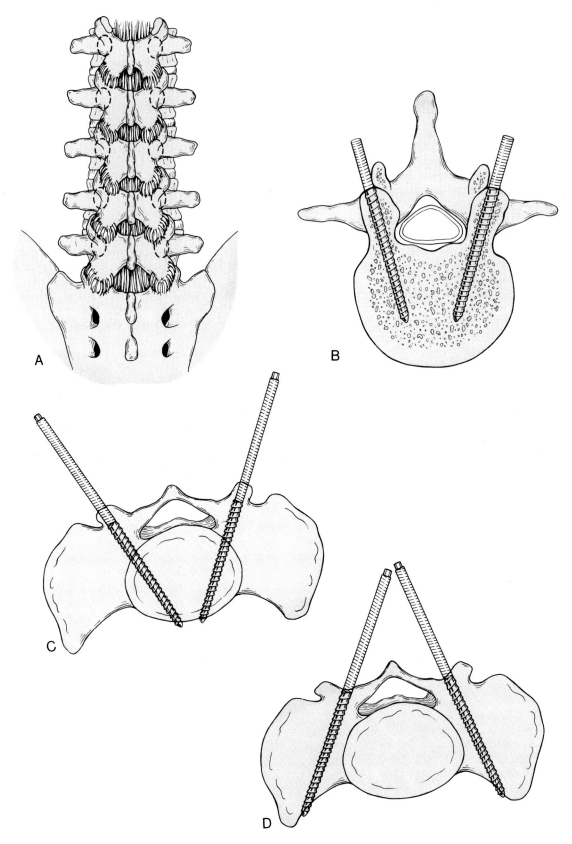

Figure 33–95 *See legend on opposite page*

is placed in the dimple that lies midway between the inferior edge of the L5–S1 facet joint take-off from the sacrum and the superior edge of the S1 dorsal foramen (Fig. 33–95*H*). The bit should be oriented approximately 35 degrees laterally and 25 degrees inferiorly, but this may be adjusted, especially in the superior-inferior direction, based on the position of the patient on the table. The posterior cortex of the sacrum is drilled in that orientation and the bit advanced through the cancellous bone to the anterior cortex simply by pushing it until the dense anterior cortical bone is encountered. The anterior cortical bone is not drilled at this time. Roentgenograms or image intensification should now be employed to view the position of the screws on both anteroposterior and lateral projections. Care should be taken in visualizing the lateral projection to remember that the marker is in the sacral ala and therefore will appear markedly anterior to the body of the sacrum. It should, however, parallel the superior end plate of the body of the sacrum, approximately 1 cm below it. For placement in a medial direction, a hand drill should be used and the starting point should be somewhat more lateral than described previously to stay within the pedicle. In either case, when drilling of the anterior cortex is done, care should be taken not to plunge but to control the drill carefully so that only the anterior cortex is penetrated. Careful depth gauging is necessary to obtain the optimal screw length. Screws are then placed and sufficient purchase (resistance) should be felt. For internal fixateur insertion, the screw insertion should be obtained only at the level proximal and distal to the fracture, whereas for rod-screw and plate-screw combinations, generally three or more levels should have fixation.

Care must be taken once screw insertion is completed to obtain a significant quantity of corticocancellous graft. Decortication of the appropriate transverse processes and lateral aspects of the facets should be accomplished prior to reduction of the fracture and insertion of the hardware. Often, the mass and location of the hardware make appropriate preparation of the transverse processes difficult if performed after instrumentation assembly. With careful preparation of the transverse processes under direct visualization, minimal additional bleeding should be encountered and adequate preparation and grafting accomplished prior to hardware insertion (Fig. 33–96).

ANTEROLATERAL DECOMPRESSION

Anterolateral decompression of the thoracic, thoracolumbar, and lumbar spine is a technique that can be employed in several different circumstances. As previously mentioned, it is extremely useful in patients requiring direct decompression of the dural sac whose presentation is delayed more than 10 days after the injury. It is also useful in patients in whom indirect decompression has not proved successful.[10, 14] This technique can be used alone for decompression or may be combined with either anterior or posterior stabilization techniques.[101]

There are three different approaches for the three predominant regions of the spine: the thoracic spine from approximately T3 to T10, the thoracolumbar spine from T11 to L1, and the lumbar spine from L2 to L4. There are differences in the surgical technique for the three areas; however, the basic positioning and preparation are similar. The only difference in initial preparation of the patient is that in those undergoing a thoracotomy, intubation should be done with a double-lumen tube so that the lung on the side of the approach can be selectively deflated, making exposure easier. The patient is placed in the lateral decubitus position. The side of the approach is more frequently left for the

Figure 33–95. Technique of pedicle screw insertion for low lumbar fractures. *A,* Exposure of the lumbar spine for pedicle screw instrumentation of a lumbar burst fracture requires very limited exposure. The appropriate levels of the spine should be localized using roentgenographic control, and then the spinous process lamina and transverse processes of those levels should be totally stripped of soft tissue. Care is taken to obtain excellent exposure of the transverse processes for subsequent grafting. Because of the bulk of the instrumentation, it is often difficult to apply adequate bone graft posteriorly. The lamina should be checked carefully for fractures and correlated with the preoperative CT scans. A note of caution in exposing the area of insertion of the uppermost pedicle: this may impinge on the intact facet joint just proximal to it that will not be fused. The location of the proximal pedicle is at the base of the intact unfused facet joint. Care must be taken to leave the interspinous ligament at that level intact as well as the facet capsule, although it is necessary to strip lateral to it to localize the transverse process. *B,* One technique requires that pedicle screws be placed perpendicular to the posterior elements in a transverse plane, as advocated by Roy-Camille. This requires a more medial starting hole. A second alternative, as noted in this illustration, is along the orientation of the pedicle, which in the lumbar spine generally is canted approximately 5 to 15 degrees medially, depending on the level. The screws are placed in a more lateral starting hole and oriented along the axis of the pedicle. *C,* One of the two safe areas and positions for screw placement in S1. These screws are oriented along the S1 pedicles parallel to the end plate and can penetrate the anterior portion of the body near its midline. This is a relatively safe zone with few large neurovascular structures. *D,* A second orientation of the screws in the sacrum directed laterally into the sacral ala. This should place the screws at an approximately 25- to 30-degree angle laterally from the midline, thus hitting another free zone lateral to the vessels and nerve roots.

Illustration continued on following page

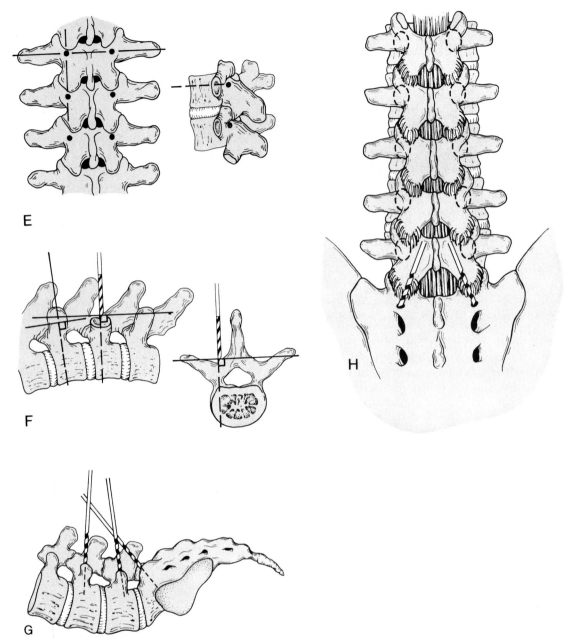

Figure 33–95 *Continued.* *E,* The orientation of the starting hole, as advocated by Roy-Camille. The starting hole should be at the intersection of a line drawn transversely through the midportion of the transverse process and vertically through the facet joints. This gives a slightly medial starting hole and is most effective for screws placed directly anteriorly, and with a slightly smaller screw diameter, a starting hole placed 1 to 2 mm more laterally along the same transverse line will allow orientation of the screw down the axis of the pedicle. *F,* The relative orientation in a caudal rostral direction of the screws with the changes and configuration in the lumbar spine. These screws should be placed roughly parallel to the end plate and down the axis of the pedicle. *G,* The insertion of drill bits for an L5 fracture requiring three points of fixation. The superior bit should be started somewhat more inferiorly and laterally and aimed slightly up toward the end plate of L4 to avoid impingement on the unfused L3–L4 facet joint just rostral to the starting point. The L5 screw can usually be perpendicular to the floor or slightly inclined inferiorly again to follow the axis of the end plate of L5. The S1 screw should be roughly parallel to the S1 end plate approximately 1 cm distal to it, oriented approximately 20 degrees caudally to achieve this angulation. The drill bits are placed only down to the depth of the pedicle so that in the anteroposterior roentgenogram or image they will not appear to cross, but give a true visualization of the orientation within the pedicle. *H,* The starting point and the medial-lateral orientation for the screws placed laterally out into the sacral ala. They should be started at a point midway from the inferior edge of the L5–S1 facet and the S1 dorsal foramen. (Modified from Eismont, F. J., Garfin, S. R., and Abitbol, J-J.: Thoracic and thoracolumbar injuries. *In* Browner, B. D., Levine, A. M., Jupiter, J. B., and Trafton, P. G. [eds.]: Skeletal Trauma. Philadelphia, W. B. Saunders Co., 1992.)

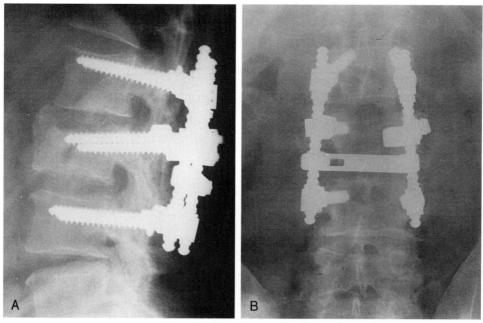

Figure 33–96. This patient sustained a burst fracture of L3 and was treated nonsurgically, with severe and incapacitating pain. The use of pedicle screw instrumentation allowed restoration of alignment with immediate relief of pain. Note that the central screw into the fractured body is angled inferiorly to purchase in the noncomminuted portion of the body.

lumbar spine, but can be done on either side if there is an asymmetric bone fragment that dictates the approach. The side of approach should also be modified depending on the prominence of the instrumentation. The more prominent instrumentation should be placed from the right side to avoid contact with the pulsatile aorta. An axillary roll is placed under the down side axilla, approximately six inches from the apex of the axilla. Hip supports are used to maintain the relative position of the patient on the table. The arm on the side of the approach is placed on a Mayo stand and well padded, especially around bony prominences. Especially when instrumentation is to be placed, the patient should be in a true decubitus position to allow adequate roentgenographic evaluation in both an anteroposterior and lateral position. However, the table can then be rolled back into a 45-degree oblique position to allow a more directly anterior view of the spine. Surgical preparation is made from the midline of the anterior chest wall beyond the midline of the posterior spine. Should posterior instrumentation need to be placed simultaneously, it can be placed through a simultaneous midline posterior incision. Approach to the upper thoracic spine requires elevation of the scapula on the central and lateral border. This will allow evaluation of the scapula for exposure of the third through sixth thoracic ribs. Elevation of the scapula generally requires division of the rhomboids and part of the trapezius. The spine should be approached through the rib lying one level above the fractured vertebra (Fig. 33–97A,B). The rib is stripped subperiosteally from its anterior tip as far posteriorly as possible, and then cut posteriorly and anteriorly at the costochondral junc-

tion, and the rib is removed and preserved for grafting. A chest retractor is then placed and slowly cranked open. Time for relaxation of the chest wall is necessary to prevent fractures of adjacent ribs. Once the chest is fully exposed, the lung can then be deflated to provide adequate exposure.

Generally, the fractured vertebra is readily evident as it bulges laterally and can be palpated easily. A spinal needle is then placed in an adjacent disc and a lateral roentgenogram is taken for verification. Using the cutting cautery, the parietal pleura is cut on the lateral surface of the vertebral body from the midportion of the body below to the midportion of the body above. Should instrumentation be necessary, the incision of the pleura can go to the disc space one level below the injury and the disc space above, thus exposing the lateral aspects of the three vertebra. In doing this, the segmental vessels are identified, ligated, and divided. The parietal pleura can be taken back in a flap fashion, with additional cuts parallel to the disc space at the body above and below the fracture level. Then, using a cutting cautery, the bodies can be stripped subperiosteally. At this point, the terminal end of the rib at the costal vertebral junction, once exposed, can be transected and removed with an osteotome. Additional subperiosteal dissection may be necessary anteriorly for final exposure of the affected body. At this point, the discs above and below the fractured body are entered. The disc material is removed using a pituitary rongeur and a curet; this isolates the fractured body (Fig. 33–97C). If it is a relatively acute fracture, the fractured fragments of the body can be removed using a combination of a rongeur and burr. This tech-

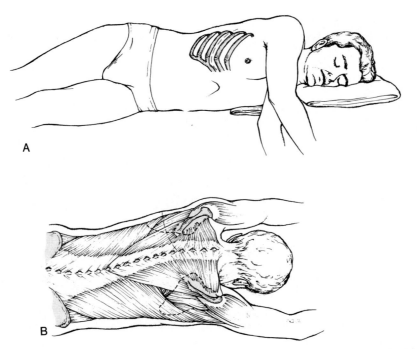

Figure 33–97. Technique of anterolateral decompression of a thoracic burst fracture. *A,* Positioning of the patient is critical in the true lateral position, especially if instrumentation is to be used. Subsequent screw placement is important, and thus orientation on the table becomes significant. An axillary roll is placed just below the axilla, and prepping and draping is done down to and including the iliac crest for subsequent grafting. The incision line *(B)* should parallel the course of the rib one level proximal to the fracture. The incision should begin approximately 3 to 4 cm from the posterior midline and carry on to the rib just anterior to it. *B,* Once the level is exposed, the disc on either end should be removed, isolating the fracture body. A triangular-shaped resection of the body, allowing optimal visualization of the dural sac, should be accomplished. Unfractured bone on the contralateral side should not be removed.

Illustration continued on opposite page

nique is continued until the bulk of the vertebral body is removed. The retropulsed posterior wall must be removed in a more delicate fashion. If the fracture is older and consolidation of the body has occurred, then removal of the vertebral body will be more difficult. A planned, triangular-shaped resection of the body should be done using the high-speed burr. This should allow adequate exposure of the retropulsed posterior wall. In either circumstance, the posterior wall should be thinned using a high-speed burr at an area where the compression of the dural sac is least significant (Fig. 33–97D). This is generally at the inferior end of the vertebra, because the predominant compression is usually at the more superior end, at the level of the pedicles. A small, angled curet can be used to tease the fragments loose away from the dural sac and back into the defect that has been made in the vertebral body (Fig. 33–97F). The decompression should continue from one disc space at the upper end to the lower disc space that had been previously evacuated, and from pedicle to pedicle. Irrespective of the type of fixation (anterior or posterior), after the decompression is completed, a slot should be made from the side of the exposed body toward the opposite side at the level above and below the fracture to allow firm seating of a tricortical iliac strut (Fig. 33–97G). If a significant kyphotic deformity

exists, it should be corrected using appropriate instrumentation prior to measuring and inserting the iliac graft. Appropriate instrumentation can then be adjusted or applied.

The technique will need to be modified for a thoracolumbar or lumbar fracture. In the thoracolumbar area, two possibilities exist for approaching fractures at the T11, T12, and L1 areas. At the upper end, a thoracoabdominal approach with splitting of the diaphragm can be done that allows excellent exposure. This, however, is not always necessary, and exposure of T12 and L1 can frequently be accomplished through a retroperitoneal approach, dissecting from caudal to rostral, elevating the crus of the diaphragm, with the entire approach staying extrapleural. In the lumbar spine for L2 to L4, a retroperitoneal approach provides excellent exposure. An anterior approach for L4 and L5 is infrequently necessary because fixation anteriorly is difficult and neural decompression, especially of root lesions, can be accomplished more easily from the posterior (laminectomy approach). In addition, in the low lumbar spine, more frequently the dural tears in patients with neurologic deficit are on the posterior surface[16, 29] as opposed to the anterior surface, and for those reasons an anterior approach to low lumbar lesions is not recommended.

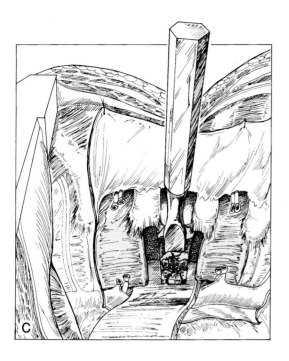
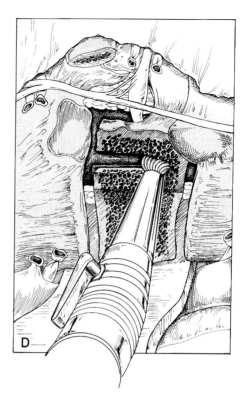
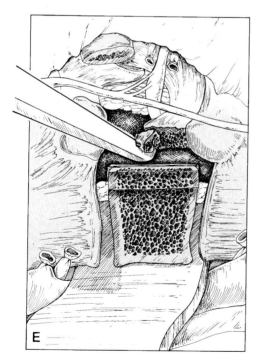
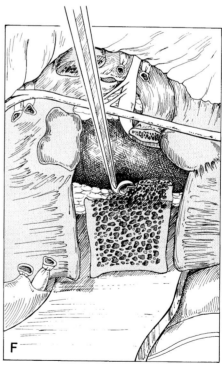

Figure 33–97 *Continued.* Loose fragments *(C)* can be removed with a gouge or osteotome and a curet. In older fractures in which the bone is consolidated, a high-speed burr *(D)* is often necessary to thin the remaining bone and fashion the triangular resection of the vertebral body. Care should be taken that the burr does not penetrate the posterior longitudinal ligament. *E,* Once the posterior cortex is thinned, the dissection should begin at the inferior edge of the vertebral body, working proximally toward the area of the pedicles, which is generally the area of maximal compression. A Kerrison punch can be used to remove the thinned area of bone. *F,* Finally, a small-angle curet can be used to gently ease the remaining fibers away from the posterior longitudinal ligament or dura, or both, in extremely stenotic areas adjacent to the pedicle.

Illustration continued on following page

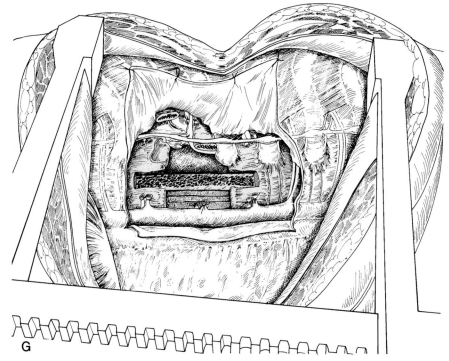

G

Figure 33–97 *Continued.* *G,* Once the decompression is complete, a slot should be cut encompassing the level above and the level below for insertion of an iliac crest graft. In areas where significant kyphosis exists, instrumentation may be considered. Current instrumentation can achieve limited correction of deformity and, most important, maintenance of correction subsequently. Care should be taken, however, that the instrumentation is placed extremely posterior away from the great vessels. In the thoracic spine, a right-sided approach should be used when instrumentation is considered. This requires that the slot cut for grafting be placed somewhat more anterior to allow a solid screw fixation of the device. Subsequent grafting of the vertebral body and slot should be done with a corticocancellous graft, and may be supplemented with available rib. (Modified from Eismont, F. J., Garfin, S. R., and Abitbol, J-J.: Thoracic and thoracolumbar injuries. *In* Browner, B. D., Levine, A. M., Jupiter, J. B., and Trafton, P. G. [eds.]: Skeletal Trauma. Philadelphia, W. B. Saunders Co., 1992.)

References

1. Akbarnia, B. A., Fogarty, J. P., and Tayob, A. A.: Contoured Harrington instrumentation in the treatment of unstable spinal fractures: The effect of supplementary sublaminar wires. Clin. Orthop. *189:*186–194, 1984.
2. Akbarnia, B. A., Moskowicz, A., Merenda, J. T., et al.: Surgical treatment of thoracic spine fractures with Cotrel Dubousset instrumentation. Poster exhibit presented at the Scoliosis Research Society, Amsterdam, September, 1989.
3. Akbarnia, B. A., Crandall, D. G., Burkus, K., et al.: Use of long rods and a short arthrodesis for burst fractures of the thoracolumbar spine. J. Bone Joint Surg. *76A(11):*1629–1635, 1994.
4. An, H. S., Vaccaro, A., Cotler, J. M., et al.: Low lumbar burst fractures. Comparison among body cast, Harrington rod, Luque rod, and Steffee plate. Spine *16(8)Supp:*S440–S444, 1991.
5. An, H. S., Simpson, J. M., Ebraheim, N. A., et al.: Low lumbar burst fractures: Comparison between conservative and surgical treatments. Orthopedics *15(3):*367–373, 1992.
6. An, H. S., Tae-Hong, L., Jae-Won, Y., et al.: Biomechanical evaluation of anterior thoracolumbar spinal instrumentation. Spine *20(18):*1979–1983, 1995.
7. Anderson, P. A., Rivara, F. P., Maier, R. V., et al.: The epidemiology of seatbelt-associated injuries. J. Trauma *31(1):*60–67, 1991.
8. Argenson, C., Lovet, L., De Peretti, F., et al.: Treatment of spinal fractures with Cotrel Dubousset instrumentation. Results of the first 85 cases. Poster exhibit presented at the Scoliosis Research Society, Amsterdam, September, 1989.
9. Baynham, G. C., Stahl, E. J., Odom, J. A., Jr., et al.: Treatment of acute spine fractures with Cotrel Dubousset instrumentation. Poster exhibit presented at the Scoliosis Research Society, Amsterdam, September, 1989.
10. Benson, D. R.: Unstable thoracolumbar fractures, with emphasis on the burst fracture. Clin. Orthop. *230:*14–29, 1988.
11. Benson, D. R., Burkus, J. K., Montesano, P. X., et al.: Unstable thoracolumbar and lumbar burst fractures treated with an AO fixateur interne. J. Spinal Disord. *5(3):*335–343, 1992.
12. Bohlman, H. H.: Current concepts review: Treatment of fractures and dislocations of the thoracic and lumbar spine. J. Bone Joint Surg. *67A:*165–169, 1985.
13. Bohlman, H. H., and Eismont, F. J.: Surgical techniques on anterior decompressions and fusion for spinal cord injuries. Clin. Orthop. *154:*57, 1981.
14. Bradford, D. S., and McBride, G. G.: Surgical management of thoracolumbar spine fractures with incomplete neurologic deficits. Clin. Orthop. *218:*201–216, 1987.
15. Cain, J. E., DeJong, J. T., Dinenberg, A. S., et al.: Pathomechanical analysis of thoracolumbar burst fracture reduction. Spine *18(12):*1647–1654, 1993.
16. Cammisa, F. P., Eismont, F. J., and Green, A. B.: Dural laceration occurring with burst fractures and associated laminar fractures. J. Bone Joint Surg. *71A:*1044–1052, 1989.
17. Cantor, J. B., Lebwohl, N. H., Garvey, T., et al.: Nonoperative management of stable thoracolumbar burst fractures with early ambulation and bracing. Spine *18(8):*971–976, 1993.
18. Carl, A. L., Tromanhauser, S. C., Roger, D. J.: Pedicle screw instrumentation for thoracolumbar burst fractures and fracture-dislocations. Spine *17(8S):*S317–S324, 1992.
19. Carragee, E. J., Khan, N., O'Sullivan: Complications in spinal

surgery with associated pedicle-screw fixation. Comps. Orthoped. Winter: 88–96, 1995.

20. Chan, D. P. K., Seng, N. K., Kaan, K. T.: Nonoperative treatment in burst fractures of the lumbar spine (L2–L5) with neurologic deficits. Spine *18(3):*320–325, 1993.

21. Chapman, J. R., Anderson, P. A.: Thoracolumbar spine fractures with neurologic deficit. Orthop. Clin. North Am. *25(4):*595–612, 1994.

22. Clohisy, J. C., Akbarnia, B. A., Bucholz, R. D., et al.: Neurologic recovery associated with anterior decompression of spine fractures at the thoracolumbar junction (T12–L1). Spine *17(8S):*S325–S330, 1992.

23. Cotler, J. M., Vernace, J. V., and Michalski, J. A.: The use of Harrington rods in thoracolumbar fractures. Orthop. Clin. North Am. *17:*87–103, 1986.

24. Cotrel, Y., Dubousset, J., and Guillaumat, M.: New universal instrumentation in spinal surgery. Clin. Orthop. *227:*10–23, 1988.

25. Crutcher, J. P., Anderson, P. A., King, H. A., et al.: Indirect spinal canal decompression in patients with thoracolumbar burst fractures treated by posterior distraction rods. J. Spinal Disord. *4(1):*39–48, 1991.

26. Dekutoski, M. B., Conlan, S., Salciccioli, G. G.: Spinal mobility and deformity after Harrington rod stabilization and limited arthrodesis of thoracolumbar fractures. J. Bone Joint Surg. *75(2):*168–176, 1993.

27. Denis, F.: The three column spine and its significance in the classification of acute thoracolumbar spinal injuries. Spine *8:*817–831, 1983.

28. Denis, F., Ruiz, H., and Searls, K.: Comparison between square-ended distraction rods and standard round-ended distraction rods in the treatment of thoracolumbar spinal injuries: A statistical analysis. Clin. Orthop. *189:*162–167, 1984.

29. Denis, F., Burkus, J. K.: Diagnosis and treatment of cauda equina entrapment in the vertebral lamina fracture of lumbar burst fractures. Spine *16(8)Supp:*S433–S439, 1991.

30. Dick, W., Kluger, P., Magerl, F., et al.: A new device for internal fixation of thoracolumbar and lumbar spine fractures: The 'fixateur interne.' Paraplegia *23:*225–232, 1985.

31. Doerr, T. E., Montesano, P. X., Burkus, J. K., et al.: Spinal canal decompression in traumatic thoracolumbar burst fractures: Posterior distraction rods versus transpedicular screw fixation. J. Orthop. Trauma *5(9):*403–411, 1991.

32. Ebelke, D. K., Asher, M. A., Neff, J. R., et al.: Survivorship analysis of VSP spine instrumentation in the treatment of thoracolumbar and lumbar burst fracture. Spine *16(8)Supp:*S428–S432, 1991.

33. Edwards, C. C., and Levine, A. M.: Early rod-sleeve stabilization of the injured thoracic and lumbar spine. Orthop. Clin. North Am. *17:*121–145, 1986.

34. Edwards, C. C., and Levine, A. M.: Fractures of the lumbar spine. *In* Evarts, C. M. (ed.): Surgery of the Musculoskeletal System. New York, Churchill Livingstone, 1990, pp. 2237–2275.

35. Esses, S. I., Botsford, D. J., Wright, T., et al.: Operative treatment of spinal fractures with the AO internal fixator. Spine *16(3) Supp:*S146–S150, 1991.

36. Esses, S. I., Botsford, D. J., Kostiuk, J. P.: Evaluation of surgical treatment for burst fractures. Spine *15(7):*667–673, 1990.

37. Farber, G. L., Place, H. M., Mazur, R. A., et al.: Accuracy of pedicle screw placement in lumbar fusions by plain radiographs and computed tomography. Spine *20(13):*1494–1499, 1995.

38. Ferguson, R. L., and Allen, B. L.: A mechanistic classification of thoracolumbar spine fractures. Clin. Orthop. *189:*77–88, 1984.

39. Fernyhough, J. C., Schimandle, J. H., Levine, A. M.: Iatrogenic spondylolysis complicating distal laminar hook placement: A report of two cases. Spine *16:*849–850, 1991.

40. Findlay, J. M., Grace, M. G. A., Saboe, L. A., et al.: A survey of vertebral burst-fracture management in Canada. Can. J. Surg. *35(4):*407–413, 1991.

41. Finn, C. A., Stauffer, E. S.: Burst fracture of the fifth lumbar vertebra. J. Bone Joint Surg. *74A(3):*398–403, 1992.

42. Fredrickson, B. E., Edwards, W. T., Rauschning, W., et al.: Vertebral burst fractures: An experimental, morphologic, and radiographic study. Spine *17(9):*1012–1021, 1992.

43. Gardner, V. O., Armstrong, G. W. D.: Long-term lumbar facet

joint changes in spinal fracture patients treated with Harrington rods. Spine *15(6):*479–484, 1990.

44. Gardner, V. O., Thalgott, J. S., White, J. I.: The contoured anterior spinal plate system (CASP): Indications, techniques, and results. Spine *19(5):*550–555, 1994.

45. Garfin, S. R., Mowery, C. A., Guerra, J., and Marshall, L. F.: Confirmation of the posterolateral technique to decompress and fuse thoracolumbar spine burst fractures. Spine *10:*218–228, 1985.

46. Gertzbein, S. D., and Court-Brown, C. M.: Flexion-distraction injuries of the lumbar spine. Mechanisms of injury and classification. Clin. Orthop. *227:*52–60, 1988.

47. Graziano, G. P.: Cotrel-Dubousset hook and screw combination for spine fractures. J. Spinal Disord. *6(5):*380–385, 1993.

48. Gurwitz, G. S., Dawson, J. M., McNamera, M. J., et al.: Biomechanical analysis of three surgical approaches for lumbar burst fractures using short-segment instrumentation. Spine *18(8):*977–982, 1993.

49. Hardaker, W. T., Cook, W. A., Freidman, A. H., et al.: Bilateral transpedicular decompression and Harrington rod stabilization in the management of severe thoracolumbar burst fractures. Spine *17(2):*162–171, 1992.

50. Harrington, R. M., Budorick, T., Hoyt, J., et al.: Biomechanics of indirect reduction of bone retropulsed into the spinal canal in vertebral fracture. Spine *18(6):*692–699, 1993.

51. Hu, S. S., Capen, D. A., Rimolda, R. L., et al.: The effect of surgical decompression on neurologic outcome after lumbar fractures. Clin. Orthop. Rel. Res. *288:*166–173, 1993.

52. Huckell, C. B., Powell, J., Eggli, S., et al.: A comparative analysis of distraction rods versus Luque rods in thoracic spine fractures. Eur. Spine J. *3:*270–275, 1994

53. James, K. S., Wagner, K. H., Schlegel, J. D., et al.: Biomechanical evaluation of the stability of thoracolumbar burst fractures. Spine *19(15):*1731–1740, 1994.

54. Jeanneret, B., Ho, P. K., Magerl, F.: Burst-shear flexion-distraction injuries of the lumbar spine. J. Spinal Disord. *6:*473–481, 1993.

55. Kaneda, K., Kuniyoshi, A., and Fujiya, M.: Burst fractures with neurologic deficits of the thoracolumbar-lumbar spine: Results of anterior decompression and stabilization with anterior instrumentation. Spine *9:*789–795, 1984.

56. Karlstrom, G., Olerud, S., and Sjostrom, L.: Transpedicular segmental fixation: Description of a new procedure. Orthopedics *11:*689–700, 1988.

57. Kinnard, P., Ghibely, A., Gordon, D., et al.: Roy-Camille plates in unstable spinal conditions: A preliminary report. Spine *11:*131–135, 1986.

58. Kirkpatrick, J. S., Wilber, R. G., Likavec, M., et al.: Anterior stabilization of thoraco-lumbar burst fractures using the Kaneda device: A preliminary report. Orthopedics *18:*673–678, 1995.

59. Knight, R. Q., Stornelli, D. P., Chan, D. P. K., et al.: Comparison of operative versus non-operative treatment of lumbar burst fractures. CORR *293:*112–121, 1993.

60. Kostuik, J. P.: Anterior fixation for fractures of the thoracic and lumbar spine with or without neurologic involvement. Clin. Orthop. *189:*103–115, 1984.

61. Kostuik, J. P., Munting, E., Valdevit, A.: Biomechanical analysis of screw load sharing in pedicle fixation of the lumbar spine. J. Spinal Disord. *7(5):*394–401, 1994.

62. Krag, M. H., Beynnon, B. D., Pope, M. H., et al.: An internal fixator for posterior application to short segments of the thoracic, lumbar or lumbosacral spine. Clin. Orthop. *203:*75–78, 1986.

63. Lemons, V. R., Wagner, F. C., Montesane, P. X.: Management of thoracolumbar fractures with accompanying neurological injury. Neurosurg. *30(5):*667–671, 1992.

64. Levine, A., Bosse, M., and Edwards, C. C.: Bilateral facet dislocations in the thoracolumbar spine. Spine *13:*630–640, 1988.

65. Levine, A. M., and Edwards, C. C.: Lumbar spine trauma. *In* Camins, M., and O'Leary, P. (eds.): The Lumbar Spine. New York, Raven Press, 1987, pp. 183–212.

66. Lindahl, S., Willen, J., and Irstam, L.: Unstable thoracolumbar fractures: A comparative radiologic study of conservative treatment and Harrington instrumentation. Acta Radiol. *I:*67, 1985.

67. Lindsey, R. W., Dick, W.: The fixateur interne in the reduction and stabilization of thoracolumbar spine fractures in patients with neurologic deficit. Spine *16(3)Supp*:S140–S145, 1991.

68. Lindsey, R. W., Dick, W., Nunchuck, S., et al.: Residual intersegmental spinal mobility following limited pedicle fixation of thoracolumbar spine fractures with the fixateur interne. Spine *18(4)*:474–478, 1993.

69. Luque, E. R., and Cassis, N.: Segmental spinal instrumentation in the treatment of fractures of the thoracolumbar spine. Spine *7*:312, 1982.

70. Magerl, F. P.: Stabilization of the lower thoracic and lumbar spine with external skeletal fixation. Clin. Orthop. *189*:125–141, 1984.

71. Mann, K. A., McGowan, D. P., Fredrickson, B. E., et al.: A biomechanical investigation of short segment spinal fixation for burst fractures with varying degrees of posterior disruption. Spine *15(6)*:470–478, 1990.

72. Markel, D. C., Graziano, G. P.: A comparison study of treatment of thoracolumbar fractures using the ACE posterior segmental fixator and Cotrel-Dubousset instrumentation. Orthopedics *18(7)*:679–686, 1995.

73. McAfee, P. C., Bohlman, H. H., and Yuan, H. A.: Anterior decompression of traumatic thoracolumbar fractures with incomplete neurological deficit using a retroperitoneal approach. J. Bone Joint Surg. *67A*89–104, 1985.

74. McBride, G. G.: Cotrel-Dubousset rods in surgical stabilization of spinal fractures. Spine *18(4)*:466–473, 1993.

75. McLain, R. F., Sparling, E., Benson, D.: Early failure of short-segment pedicle instrumentation for thoracolumbar fractures. J. Bone Joint Surg. *75A(2)*:162–167, 1993.

76. Mick, C. A., Carl, A., Sachs, B., et al.: Burst fractures of the fifth lumbar vertebra. Spine *18(13)*:1878–1884, 1993.

77. Mirkovic, S., Abitbol, J. J., Steinman, J., et al.: Anatomic consideration for sacral screw placement. Spine *16(6)Suppl*:S289–S294, 1991.

78. Mumford, J., Weinstein, J. N., Spratt, K. F., et al.: Thoracolumbar burst fractures. Spine *18(8)*:955–970, 1993.

79. Neumann, A., Nordwall, A., Osvalder, A-L.: Traumatic instability of the lumbar spine. Spine *20(10)*:1111–1121, 1995.

80. Nolte, L-P., Zamorano, L. J., Jiang, Z., et al.: Image-guided insertion of transpedicular screws: A laboratory set-up. Spine *20(4)*:497–500, 1995.

81. Olerud, S., Karltom, G., and Sjostrom, L.: Transpedicular fixation of thoracolumbar vertebral fractures. Clin. Orthop. *227*:44–51, 1988.

82. Panjabi, M., Oxland, T. R., Kifune, M., et al.: Validity of the three-column theory of thoracolumbar fractures: A biomechanic investigation. Spine *20(10)*:1122–1127, 1995.

83. Reid, A. B., Letts, R. M., Black, G. B.: Pediatric Chance fractures: Association with intra-abdominal injuries and seatbelt use. J. Trauma *30(4)*:384–391, 1990.

84. Riebel, G. D., Yoo, J. U., Fredrickson, B. E., et al.: Review of Harrington rod treatment of spinal trauma. Spine *18(4)*:479–491, 1993.

85. Rimoldi, R. L., Zigler, J. E., Capen, D. A., et al.: The effect of surgical intervention on rehabilitation time in patients with thoracolumbar and lumbar spinal cord injuries. Spine *17(12)*:1443–1449, 1991.

86. Roy-Camille, R., Saillant, G., Berteaux, D., and Salgado, V.: Osteosynthesis of thoraco-lumbar spine fractures with metal plates screwed through the vertebral pedicles. Reconstr. Surg. Traumatol. *15*:2–15, 1976.

87. Roy-Camille, R., Saillant, G., and Mazel, C.: Plating of thoracic, thoracolumbar, and lumbar injuries with pedicle screw plates. Orthop. Clin. North Am. *17*:147–159, 1986

88. Sasso, R. C., Cotler, H. B., Reuben, J. D.: Posterior fixation of thoracic and lumbar spine fractures using DC plates and pedicle screws. Spine *16(3)Suppl*:S134–S139, 1991.

89. Shiba, K., Katsuki, M., Ueta, T., et al.: Transpedicular fixation with Zielke instrumentation in the treatment of thoracolumbar and lumbar injuries. Spine *19(17)*:1940–1949, 1994.

90. Sjostrom, L., Jacobsson, O., Karlstrom, G., et al.: Spinal canal remodeling after stabilization of thoracolumbar burst fractures. Eur. Spine J. *3*:312–317, 1994.

91. Skalli, W., Robin, S., Lavaste, F., et al.: A biomechanical analysis of short segment spinal fixation using a three-dimensional geometric and mechanical model. Spine *18(5)*:536–545, 1993.

92. Slosar, P. J., Patwardhan, A. G., Lorenz, M., et al.: Instability of the lumbar burst fracture and limitations of transpedicular instrumentation. Spine *20(13)*:1452–1461, 1995.

93. Stambough, J. L.: Cotrel-Dubousset instrumentation and thoracolumbar spine trauma: A review of 55 cases. J. Spinal Disord. *7(6)*:461–469, 1994.

94. Stephens, G. C., Devito, D. P., McNamara, M. J.: Segmental fixation of lumbar burst fractures with Cotrel-Dubousset instrumentation. J. Spinal Disord. *3*:344–348, 1992.

95. Sullivan, J. A.: Sublaminar wiring of Harrington distraction rods for unstable thoracolumbar spine fractures. Clin. Orthop. *189*:178–185, 1984.

96. Tasdemiroglu, E., Tibbs, P. A.: Long-term follow-up results of thoracolumbar fractures after posterior instrumentation. Spine *20(15)*:1704–1708, 1995.

97. Tran, N. T., Watson, N. A., Tencer, A. F., et al.: Mechanism of the burst fracture in the thoracolumbar spine: The effect of loading rate. Spine *20(18)*:1984–1988, 1995.

98. Viale G. L., Silvestro, C., Francaviglia, N., et al.: Transpedicular decompression and stabilization of burst fractures of the lumbar spine. Surg. Neurol. *40*:104–111, 1993.

99. Vornanen, M. J., Bostman, O. M., Myllynen, P. J.: Reduction of bone retropulsed into the spinal canal in thoracolumbar vertebral body compression burst fractures. Spine *20(15)*:1699–1703, 1995.

100. Weyns, F., Rommens, P. M., Van Calenbergh, F., et al.: Neurological outcome after surgery for thoracolumbar fractures: A retrospective study of 93 consecutive cases, treated with dorsal instrumentation. Eur. Spine J. *3*:276–281, 1994.

101. Whitesides, T. E., and Ali Shan, S. G.: On the management of unstable fractures of the thoracolumbar spine: Rationale for use of anterior decompression and fusion and posterior stabilization. Spine *1*:99, 1976.

102. Willen, J., Anderson, J., Toomoka, K., et al.: The natural history of burst fractures at the thoracolumbar junction. J. Spinal Disord. *3(1)*:39–46, 1990.

103. Wiliams, N., Ratliff, D. A.: Gastrointestinal disruption and vertebral fracture associated with the use of seat belts. Ann. Royal Coll. Surg. *75*:129–132, 1993.

104. Yuan, H. A., Mann, K. A., Found, E. M., et al.: Early clinical experience with the Syracuse I-plate: An anterior spinal fixation device. Spine *13*:278–285, 1988.

105. Yuan, H. A., Garfin, S. R., Dickman, C. A., et al.: A historical cohort study of pedicle screw fixation in thoracic, lumbar, and sacral spinal fusions. Spine *19(205)*:2279S–2296S, 1994.

106. Zou, D., Yoo, J. U., Edwards, T., et al.: Mechanics of anatomic reduction of thoracolumbar burst fractures. Spine *18(2)*:195–203, 1993.

Spinal Instrumentation for Thoracic and Lumbar Fractures

Jeffrey A. Goldstein, M.D.

Bryan W. Cunningham, M.Sc., Ph.D.

Paul C. McAfee, M.D.

ASSESSMENT OF SPINAL STABILITY

An important conceptual advance in the determination and management of spinal stability after traumatic fractures is the development of the "three-column theory." Francis Denis defined three longitudinal columns of stability in the thoracolumbar spine (Fig. 33–98).[25] The anterior column comprises three structures: the anterior longitudinal ligament, the anterior portion of the vertebral body, and the anterior portion of the annulus fibrosus. The middle osteoligamentous column comprises the posterior longitudinal ligament, the posterior aspect of the vertebral body, and the posterior aspect of the annulus fibrosus. The third longitudinal column of spinal stability comprises the posterior elements such as the posterior facet joints and facet joint capsules, the ligamentum flavum, the interspinous ligaments, and the posterior aspect of the neural arch.

McAfee et al.[85] applied this anatomic three-column concept to evaluate 100 consecutive patients with potentially unstable thoracolumbar fractures and fracture-

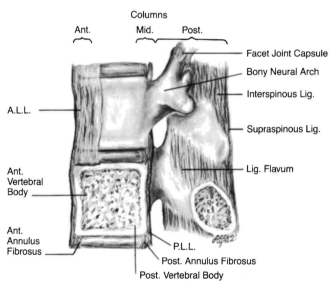

Figure 33–98. Three longitudinal columns of the spine contribute to stability. The anterior column consists of the anterior longitudinal ligament, the anterior two thirds of the vertebral body, and the anterior two thirds of the annulus fibrosus. The middle osteoligamentous column consists of the posterior longitudinal ligament, the posterior one third of the vertebral body, and the posterior one third of the annulus fibrosus. The posterior column consists of the posterior bony elements, the ligamentum flavum, and the supraspinous and interspinous ligaments. Key management decisions regarding anterior or posterior surgery, the types of instrumentation, and whether the surgery is indicated center around the mechanism of injury of the middle osteoligamentous column.

dislocations studied by multiplanar computed tomography (CT).[85] There are six main categories of injury based on the mechanism of injury of the middle osteoligamentous column.

1. **The wedge compression fracture.** This is defined as compressive failure of the anterior column secondary to an axial load. There is no posterior ligamentous injury and no failure of the middle osteoligamentous column, except by plastic deformation over an extended time period. The wedge compression fracture is therefore a stable injury and requires internal fixation only if it occurs high in the thoracic spine (T1–T4). Wedge compression fractures occurring at two or more vertebral levels in the upper thoracic spine can cause progressive cervicothoracic kyphosis and can therefore cause secondary spinal cord compression. Multiple adjacent wedge compression fractures should be observed carefully, because there is currently no adequate orthotic device for correcting upper thoracic kyphosis once it starts to develop. If kyphosis progresses in the early post-injury period, multiple adjacent wedge compression fractures should be stabilized with compression rods (Harrington compression rods, Cotrel-Dubousset compression rods, Texas Scottish Rite Hospital [TSRH] compression rods) extending at least two vertebral levels superior and two levels inferior to the injury.

2. **The stable burst fracture.** This is defined as failure of the anterior and middle longitudinal columns, secondary to an axial load. Because by definition there is no disruption of the posterior elements, these are stable injuries and do not normally require internal fixation. These fractures can be managed successfully with a thoracolumbar sacral orthosis (TLSO) or a body cast. Most stable burst fractures heal without subsequent deformity, without causing progressive pain, and are not associated with progressive neurologic deficit, provided the patient is maintained in a TLSO for a three- to six-month period. The duration of immobilization for a TLSO is determined by the radiographic appearance.

3. **The unstable burst fracture.** This is an injury with compressive axial failure of the anterior and middle columns that also involves complete disruption of the posterior elements. These are extremely unstable injuries and require internal fixation to prevent further compression of the spine. As the vertebral bodies compress, owing to axial loading, the bone fragments from the vertebral bodies are retropulsed against the neural structures. Denis and colleagues described five patterns of unstable burst fractures: type A (23.7 per cent), rupture of both inferior and

superior end plates; type B (49.2 percent), rupture of the superior end plate; type C (6.8 per cent), rupture of the inferior end plate; type D (15.2 per cent), burst rotation; and type E (5.1 per cent), burst lateral flexion.[24] It is extremely important to note that type B is the most common fracture pattern, so that while performing an anterior vertebral corpectomy, the surgeon should pay particular attention to extracting the posterosuperior aspect of the vertebral body from the spinal canal, because this is usually the site of the most severe neurologic compression.

4. **The flexion-distraction injury.** This is a potentially serious injury involving ligamentous disruption of the middle column and posterior elements. A flexion force applied to the thoracic spine usually results in a facet subluxation or dislocation. The anterior aspect of the vertebral bodies is crushed, whereas the posterior aspect of the thoracolumbar elements is spread apart. This injury requires posterior internal fixation with compression-type instrumentation. This injury is also associated with more severe neurologic deficits than the Chance fracture.

5. **The translation injury.** This is defined as any injury of the thoracolumbar spine that results from a shearing failure of the middle osteoligamentous middle column. Holdsworth originally described this injury and termed it a "slice" fracture. This is the most unstable of all thoracolumbar spinal injuries and is associated with the highest incidence of paraplegia and complete neurologic deficits. There is basically a complete loss in continuity of the patient's spinal canal, and ligamentous discontinuity from one vertebral level to the next. The treatment of these injuries is directed toward more rapid mobilization and earlier rehabilitation of the paraplegic patient. Therefore, these injuries are usually treated with a segmental type of instrumentation. In the generic sense, segmental instrumentation increases the biomechanical rigidity of a fixation system by spreading the load out among the intervening vertebral levels rather than concentrating the reduction forces to the "end vertebrae." For purposes of this chapter, all of the following are considered types of segmental instrumentation: Luque (SSI), L-rods, or Luque rectangular rods fixed to the spine by sublaminar wires; Wisconsin (ISSI) instrumentation, Harrington or Luque rods attached via Drummond buttons to the base of the spinous processes; Cotrel-Dubousset compression rods; Steffee (VSP) instrumentation, Roy-Camille transpedicular instrumentation, and TSRH instrumentation. Aside from having the highest incidence of neurologic injury, the translational injuries have the highest incidence of instrumentation failure. In a review of 45 Harrington instrumentation procedures referred from elsewhere owing to complications, McAfee and Bohlman found that seven of 16 patients with failed fixation had a translation injury of the middle column.[78] This is particularly significant because translation (flexion-rotation,

shear injuries) constitutes less than 10 per cent of all unstable thoracolumbar injuries.

OPERATIVE RATIONALE

The goals of operative treatment for thoracolumbar injury are: anatomic reduction of the fracture; rigid fixation; neural decompression when necessary; and, in the long term, a functional, painless spinal column. For each patient, the goals must be clearly defined and the appropriate treatment methods employed. Thus, the trauma patient who has a marked sagittal or coronal deformity of his or her spine (e.g., traumatic kyphosis, axial compression, and/or translation) but no neurologic deficit will need only to have correction of alignment and rigid fixation without the necessity for any canal decompression. However, the patient who has kyphosis and displacement of bone fragments into the neural tissues and an incomplete neurologic deficit will need to have spinal realignment, canal decompression, and stabilization.

The most important biomechanical consideration for the use of implants in spinal trauma is that the strengths of the system must be matched to the instabilities of the injury.[42, 67] Thus, for any injury with axial compression, the implant must have the ability to apply axial distraction to correct the deformity, maintain alignment, and resist axial compression in the erect position. Similarly, for the flexion component of an injury there must be a component of the instrumentation that can apply extension centered at the level of injury and it must be able to resist subsequent loss of reduction in flexion. For those injuries due to axial distraction, the implant must be able to apply axial compressive forces and resist further axial distraction. In some cases the applied construct may not be able to directly counteract a deforming force but, if it is part of a coupled motion, the correct applications of the hardware may be able to resist a coupled motion by resisting its force partner. Finally, for injuries that have a significant shear injury and have bidirectional instability, it must be within the capability of the hardware system to progressively reduce the deformity and then lock it into position, resisting displacement in all three planes of motion.

Controversies persist regarding the indications for the anterior approach versus the posterior approach for management of thoracolumbar injuries. This controversy has centered around the ability to achieve neural decompression and limit the length of fixation.

Posterior Instrumentation

Indications

The indications for the posterior approach may be divided into absolute indications, relative indications, and contraindications. An absolute indication is the patient with a complete neurologic deficit and an upper thoracic injury. These patients need rapid stabilization so that they can be mobilized to diminish the chance of pulmonary complications. In patients with complete neurologic deficits, posterior instrumentation is the most reasonable approach, as it can achieve axial realignment and rigid stabilization and allow rapid patient mobilization. In the multiply injured patient with chest trauma, the goals of the surgery are to stabilize and realign the spine but not necessarily to decompress the neural tissues. A second indication for posterior instrumentation is the patient with low lumbar burst fracture and dural lacerations. The traumatic dural lacerations are posterior and frequently have extravasation of the roots into the laminar fracture. An anterior approach would not provide access for dural repair nor is fixation to the fifth lumbar vertebra or sacrum ideal through an anterior approach.[12, 71] The third group of patients who should have a posterior reduction and stabilization are patients with segmental deformity without neural deficit at the thoracolumbar junction (either early or late). This procedure is more easily accomplished and maintained by the posterior approach.

The relative indications for posterior instrumentation are broad, including neurologically intact patients who have unstable fractures. If the surgical goal is the reduction of the deformity and rigid stabilization, it is best accomplished by posterior surgery and instrumentation up to four to six weeks from the time of initial injury. Other patients with relative indications for posterior instrumentation are patients with neural deficit and canal compromise who are less than 48 hours from injury. Indirect decompression by ligamentataxis and reduction of deformity is most effective in that time frame.[15, 19, 27, 30, 119] In these patients, the goal of the surgery is realignment, rigid fixation to protect the cord, and indirect neural decompression. In approximately 85 per cent of patients, posterior stabilization and reduction are sufficient to give adequate canal decompression in the neurologically compromised patient. Should the patient not attain satisfactory decompression, then a second-stage anterior decompression is indicated. Patients with low lumbar fractures are also more easily decompressed and stabilized from a posterior approach. Patients with unstable flexion-distraction injuries and Chance-type fractures who have significant ligamentous injuries are best treated surgically with posterior instrumentation. Finally, patients with shear injuries require segmental posterior instrumentation.

Contraindications to posterior instrumentation are patients who are more than 10 days from the time of injury with an incomplete neurologic deficit and canal compromise. These patients are best treated by direct canal decompression using an anterior approach.[33] Also, indirect decompression is not as satisfactory for patients whose CT scan demonstrates minimal axial compression or sagittal plane deformity but significant canal retropulsion, or in whom the posterior fragment of the wall is turned around so that the cancellous portion is facing posteriorly into the canal, indicating disruption of the posterior longitudinal ligament. In that case, anterior decompression can yield more opti-

mal results than posterior instrumentation. In patients with retropulsion localized to one side, a posterior decompression through a transpedicular route can be effective, but indirect decompression is generally not effective.[44, 114]

Posterior Instrumentation Systems

Harrington rod instrumentation was the first effective system for treatment of thoracolumbar fractures.[26, 45, 59, 99, 100] It applies a progressive reduction force in a single plane, either axial distraction or axial compression. With additional distraction, increased kyphosis is produced owing to lengthening of the posterior column. Harrington rods provide no rotational correction nor ability to correct or stabilize the flexion component of the deformity. To be effective, Harrington rods require intact longitudinal ligaments and instrumentation of two to three levels above and below the injury. In shear injuries, these ligaments have usually failed and therefore distraction instrumentation may result in iatrogenic overlengthening of the spinal column.[78]

Contouring of square-ended Harrington rods allows application of both a distraction force and extension moment to correct the traumatic kyphosis. The amount of lordosis in the rod is difficult to control and maintain. Also, they provide little or no rotational stability. The relatively loose fit between the proximal hook and rod tends to create kyphosis at the upper end of the construct. Segmental fixation with sublaminar wires applied to Luque rods or Harrington instrumentation poorly controls axial height and therefore has little role in management of spinal fractures.

The rod-sleeve method based on either Harrington distraction rods or Universal rods allows the application of a distractive force by the rod and a lordotic force by sleeves placed at the appropriate level.[29–31, 70] Lordosing forces are applied directly to the pedicles at the apex of the kyphosis in compression and burst-type fractures when the pedicles and posterior elements are intact. The sleeves can be placed in a bridging fashion at the pedicle above and below the injury, creating a three-point fixation for patients requiring a laminectomy, with comminution of the posterior elements, or with fracturing of the pedicles (Denis type A fractures). The rod-sleeve method also allows application of the lordotic force without compromising the proximal hook site. If the angle of the lamina is such that application of a straight rod will create excessive kyphosis at the proximal segment, slight contouring can be achieved at that level without sacrificing the overall lordotic force applied by the rod. In addition, because the sleeves wedge between the facets and spinous processes, a degree of rotational stability is imparted. Thus, they provide axial distraction and lordosis for use in compression fractures and burst-type fractures. For bilateral facet dislocations, a special application of the construct is required. Once the facets have been reduced, an interspinous wire is placed across the facet dislocation as a tension band posteriorly to hold reduction. A lordotic force is imparted at the apex and distraction is used to restore the disc height with the rod sleeve. In bony flexion-distraction injuries, a compression construct can be used with the same system, again using sleeves to impart lordosis. This rod-sleeve technique as a pure hook-rod-sleeve system does not provide adequate stabilization for shear injuries.

Segmental hook-rod methods are useful in many spinal injury patterns.[86] Distraction forces can be applied to the rods after seating of all of the hooks to restore axial compression failure. The rods can be prebent or bent in situ to reduce kyphosis. The rotational stability of segmental hook-rod methods is excellent, especially with the use of cross-locking devices. They are useful in patients with high thoracic injuries in whom segmental fixation precludes the use of external mobilization. For increased correction of kyphotic deformities, stiffer rods are available in most systems that will better resist the flexion forces. The disadvantage of segmental fixation is the increased length of instrumentation. Attempts to shorten the instrumentation by applying two hooks at the same lamina (either proximally or distally) result in a higher failure rate.

The use of pedicle screw constructs remains controversial. Difficulty in accurately placing pedicle screws increases above L1.[107, 109] In younger individuals, the pedicles at T10, T11, T12, and L1 are elliptical with too narrow a width to accommodate pedicle screws.[110] Smaller screws have been shown to have inadequate strength to withstand the loads and are subject to fatigue failure. Short segment pedicle screw constructs a single level above and below the fracture at the thoracolumbar junction may be inadequate to correct and withstand the applied forces.[89] Some systems have a coupled mechanism requiring both axial distraction and lordosis to be secured at the same time, which will lead to incomplete reductions. In addition, because the normal alignment at the thoracolumbar junction is slight kyphosis (0 to 5 degrees), the weight-bearing axis lies anterior to the linkage of the device. This creates excessive bending forces applied to the screws, which has resulted in frequent screw fracture and bending, and device loosening.[6, 89] Anterior fracture comminution increases bending and is more likely to result in failure of the plate-screw system. Cantilever (fixation) systems similarly have a high rate of loss of fixation and screw failure when applied at the thoracolumbar junction.[13, 32, 73, 89] Because of the higher complication rate and the difficulty of inserting large enough screws within the pedicles at the thoracolumbar junction, the use of screws at that level is less advantageous and carries a higher risk than the use of a rod-sleeve or a segmental rod-hook system. In the lower lumbar spine, the importance of saving levels and preserving open motion segments is critical. Also, distal hook fixation is tenuous and therefore pedicle screw systems are more advantageous. Here larger screws are able to be inserted in the pedicles and the weight-bearing axis falls posterior to the vertebral body. Depending on the screw rod linkage, pedicle screws can be used for the distal end of constructs with hooks used at the proximal end. Multiple pedicle screws may also be used to reduce and stabilize shear injuries.

Length of Arthrodesis

The length of the fixation and number of fused segments remain controversial. Two predominant theories are "rod long, fuse short" and arthrodesing over the entire length of instrumentation while attempting to minimize the number of levels instrumented, especially in the lumbar spine.[11, 49] Disadvantages of the rod long, fuse short technique are: (1) requirement for two surgical procedures; (2) insufficient data determining the optimal time for removal of the hardware, which is long enough for the fusion mass to mature and short enough to prevent damage to the joints that have been immobilized; (3) difficulty with hook placement without disruption of facet capsules and the ligamentous structures at adjacent levels; (4) temporary immobilization of facet joints may lead to degenerative changes.[53] Although recent studies show adequate functional outcome,[23, 50] this technique must be distinguished from reduction of the fracture without arthrodesis. This technique is associated with frequent collapse of the injury segment following hardware removal. The more common approach is to limit the number of levels of posterior stabilization and arthrodesis of the entire length of fixation. The number of segments instrumented are determined by the lever arms necessary to reduce the fracture. With straight Harrington rods, the forces were poorly concentrated and could not be applied specifically to the injured areas of the spine, and thus, two to three levels of instrumentation above and two levels below the fracture were necessary. Improved instrumentation systems such as pedicle screw systems and the rod-sleeve system allow specific application of forces directed in concentrated areas, enabling shortening of the construct. With the rod-sleeve system, this can be shortened to one level below and one to two interspaces above the injury. The segmental hook-rod systems generally instrument two normal levels above and below the fractured level. In the thoracic spine, this may be an appropriate exchange for the increased rigidity.

Outcomes of Posterior Instrumentation

Comparison of the results of Harrington instrumentation,[16, 19, 27, 33, 44, 88, 99, 100] rod-sleeve,[29–31, 36, 70, 72] and pedicle screw systems[1, 7, 8, 14, 15, 22, 28, 32, 40, 60, 61, 69, 73, 89, 101, 102, 103, 107, 110, 118] is given in Table 33–6 (see page 1067). The factors compared include the preoperative angular deformity and translation, the adequacy of correction, the maintenance of correction, and the rate of fusion. Harrington rod and Luque rod systems lost the correction achieved intraoperatively at long-term follow-up. This is less true with rod sleeves and segmental hook-rod systems. With the pedicle screw systems, similarly, there is a high rate of early failure of the systems when used at the thoracolumbar junction. In the lower lumbar spine,

Table 33–4. COMPLICATIONS OF ANTERIOR THORACOLUMBAR DECOMPRESSION, INSTRUMENTATION, AND FUSION*

Complication	Number
Iatrogenic spinal neurologic deficits	0
Lumbar plexus neuropraxia	3
Retraction of psoas muscle against transverse processes of L4 and L5	
Deep wound infections	0
Meningitis, resolved with 6 weeks of antibiotics	1
Pseudarthrosis	5
Graft displacement	1
Requiring additional posterior surgery	
Pulmonary complications	
Postoperative pneumothorax	2
Pneumonia	2
Tension hemopneumothorax	1
Pleural effusion requiring thoracentesis	1
Inadvertent detachment of the diaphragm off chest wall requiring intraoperative repair	1
Instrumentation failures	
Dwyer-Hall rod bending (275-pound patient) 10 days postoperatively	1
Axial slipping of Dwyer-Hall rod requiring posterior Cotrel-Dubousset instrumentation	1
Dwyer-Hall rod breaking, requiring revision of anterior stabilization using Kaneda system	1
Breakage of Kaneda screws, requiring posterior Cotrel-Dubousset instrumentation	2
L2 vertebral body screw in spinal canal, neurologically intact	1
Death	1
41 units postoperative blood loss following L3 corpectomy for *Mycobacterium tuberculosis* and *Escherichia coli* infection secondary to abdominal gunshot wound and pancreatitis; patient developed diffuse intravascular coagulation	
Residual kyphosis over 20 degrees (none with Kaneda device)	13

*Total procedures = 185.
Data from McAfee, P.C.: Complications of anterior approaches to the thoracolumbar spine: Emphasis on Kaneda instrumentation. Clin. Orthop. Rel. Res. *306*:110–119, 1994.

the degree of correction and fusion as well as maintenance of correction was satisfactory.[3]

Adjunctive Decompression
Decompression of the spinal canal is an important goal in the surgical treatment of thoracolumbar fractures. Previously it was recommended that patients who are neurologically intact with 30 per cent canal compromise should have anterior decompression to prevent symptoms related to spinal stenosis; however, there are no reported cases of spinal stenosis in patients who have reduction and stabilization of their fracture. In most cases in which late secondary decompressions were performed, patents had residual kyphosis deformities at the time of initial reduction. Long-term follow-up studies in patients treated both surgically and nonsurgically demonstrate that significant remodeling of the residual bone occurs.[70, 90]

Adjunctive posterior decompression at the time of initial surgery is occasionally recommended. Indirect canal depression is less effective in patients with low lumbar burst fractures. Because restoration of lordosis decreases the tension in the posterior longitudinal ligament, there is a decreased effect of ligamentataxis.[46] In addition, the larger spinal canals in the low lumbar spine afford easier access to the retropulsed fragments from the posterior approach. Therefore, in patients with a specific root deficit and a large retropulsed fragment on preoperative CT scan, a posterior decompression is easily accomplished. At the thoracolumbar junction, a transpedicular posterolateral decompression is an accepted technique if there is significant deformity and a unilateral retropulsion of either a free fragment or a large contained fragment.[36, 44, 79] The use of intraoperative ultrasonography has been an effective tool in gauging the adequacy of reduction. The alternative method is to postoperatively obtain a CT scan and determine whether neural compression is present. If the patient does not show adequate recovery, then a second-stage anterior decompression is indicated.

Patients with bilateral facet dislocations as a result of flexion-distraction injury may have associated intravertebral disc disruption.[37] If compression forces are applied, extravasation of the disc material into the spinal cord may occur with resultant neurologic injury.[72] Several treatment strategies are possible to avoid this complication. First, the fracture could be stabilized by a neutralization construct (after reduction) to prevent further axial compression of the disc space. Second, placement of a rod-sleeve system converts the deformity into a coupled force.[72] Once the facet dislocation is reduced, an intraspinous wire is placed and a rod-sleeve system is located directly over the dislocated facets, creating local lordosis. The rods can then be used to apply distraction and restore the height of the disc. Further dislocation is prevented, since both the wire and the rod-sleeve will prevent flexion. Finally, prophylactic discectomy could be performed and then a compression construct applied. In the low lumbar spine, to preserve levels, a pedicle screw construct is recommended.

Postoperative Orthosis

Postoperatively, a brace should be used in the majority of patients. The type of brace depends on fracture pattern, level of injury, and instrumentation system. The use of a total contact brace for fractures between T6 and L4 or the use of a total contact brace with a leg extension for those with fixation extending to the sacrum is recommended. Patients are rapidly mobilized out of bed but are maintained in braces for four to six months. The use of orthoses results in lower rates of instrumentation failure, pseudarthrosis, and loss of correction. In segmental hook-rod systems, especially in upper thoracic fractures, an orthosis is not required. The use of a total contact brace even in paraplegic patients is well tolerated with few complications. Patients are able to learn transfers, self-catheterization, and, eventually, driving.

Anterior Decompression and Arthrodesis

Rationale for Anterior Decompression

The goal of anterior spinal decompression is to provide an optimal environment for the recovery of incomplete neural deficits by achieving better reduction and decompression of the spinal canal.[54, 55, 79] In 90 per cent of unstable burst fractures, the offending agent is often the posterosuperior corner of the comminuted vertebral body. Some investigators attempt ligamentataxis or indirect closed reduction of the spinal canal by distracting the posterior longitudinal ligament. Often, if the surgery is performed more than 48 hours after injury, posterior distraction rods do not alleviate continued compression from displaced fragments of bone or disc within the spinal canal.[19, 30, 119] The rationale for anterior surgery is to perform an open reduction of the spinal canal under direct vision either through a retroperitoneal (L1 to L4) anterior approach or a thoracotomy (T2 to T12).

Alternatively, we are currently evaluating the use of the minimally invasive endoscopic approach to the spine for decompression and stabilization. The indications for minimally invasive decompression are the same as those for traditional open procedures.[38, 39, 76, 82, 83] In a prospective multicenter study, McAfee et al.[82] evaluated 15 patients who underwent video-assisted thoracic corpectomy for pathologic tumors, traumatic fractures, fracture-dislocations, or osteomyelitis. Fourteen of these patients presented with incomplete neurologic deficits and magnetic resonance (MR) or CT evidences of anterior spinal cord compression. After completion of VATS corpectomy, all patients had MR documentation of successful anterior spinal canal decompression. Twelve of the 14 patients with incomplete neurologic deficits demonstrated improvement of the Fränkel level of neurologic function. Stabilization was provided by a variety of techniques.[82] McAfee and others are also evaluating the use of endoscopically inserted fusion cages, anterior plates, and rods.

Anterior Instrumentation

It is beyond the scope of this text to describe in great detail the technique of anterior instrumentation. Currently marketed devices include the Kaneda device, Z-plate, CASP plate, and Thoracolumbar Locking Plate.[54, 55] Several principles are common to all of these devices, so their similarities will be emphasized. First and foremost, anterior instrumentation is a much more exacting procedure than posterior spinal instrumentation. All metal should be kept away from the great vessels to avoid vascular erosion and leaving a screw in juxtaposition to the iliac vein, aorta, or vena cava. Anterior instrumentation devices are load-sharing implants. Meticulous attention to detail is required in sizing and shaping a tricortical iliac strut graft so that its parallel surfaces are press-fit against the adjacent vertebral bodies.[41] In the transverse plane, the vertebral screws need to be directed in a triangular configuration to provide maximum resistance to pull-out. Finally, when the Kaneda paravertebral rods or others are attached to the vertebral screws, they need to apply a compressive force across the long axis of the iliac strut graft (preload). Once both rods are inserted properly, the graft is compressed. The importance of this maneuver cannot be overemphasized. Anterior instrumentation devices rely directly on load transmission through a healthy, strong tricortical graft for secure fixation and for long-term healing. If firm compression of the graft is not provided during instrumentation, the construct will fail (Fig. 33–99).

Outcome of Anterior Decompression and Arthrodesis

McAfee, Bohlman, and Yuan[79] reported the neurologic recovery of 70 patients undergoing anterior decompression for thoracolumbar fractures. At a minimum follow up of two years, no patient lost further cord or cauda equina function. Thirty-seven of 42 patients who had a motor deficit improved by at least one class (Eismont grading system) in motor strength. Fourteen of the 30 patients whose quadriceps and hamstrings were too weak to permit walking regained full independent walking ability. Twelve of the 32 patients who had a conus medullaris injury demonstrated recovery from neurogenic bowel and bladder dysfunction.

Kaneda documented the most comprehensive outcome study evaluating thoracolumbar spinal injuries treated by anterior decompression.[54] One hundred ten consecutive patients were followed for a minimum of four years postoperatively. The recovery of motor function was as follows: 11 patients improved two or more Fränkel levels; 46 patients improved one Fränkel level; 17 patients were unchanged. Using the McBride modified evaluation, 12 patients in this group improved from D1 to D2 or from D2 to D3.[86] Thirty-six patients who were intact remained normal at follow-up.

Using the Motor Index Scale (maximum total 50 points), the average preoperative score was 26.[75] After the anterior decompression and Kaneda instrumentation, the motor index was 49.4. Twenty-eight of 42 patients in the series with neurogenic bladder injury (lesion of the conus medullaris) demonstrated recovery of bladder function. The restoration of anterior spinal stability was also achieved at a high rate. In 106 of 110 procedures (96.4 per cent) a stable fusion was achieved by the primary procedure. Four failures of anterior instrumentation occurred and will be discussed in the complication section.

Kaneda recently compiled a series of 30 consecutive patients (average age, 41 years 6 months, with a range of 18 to 62 years) who had thoracolumbar spinal injuries treated by an anterior approach using the Kaneda SR (smooth rod) system (personal communication). The median follow-up was 23 months (minimum, 18

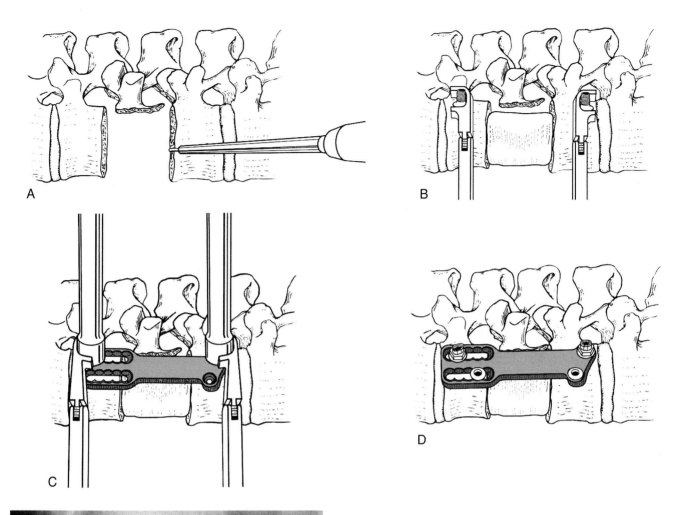

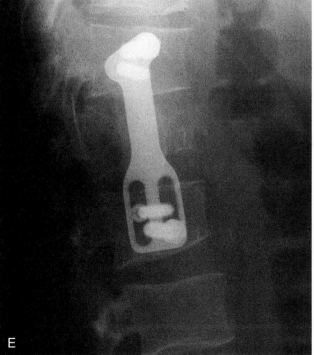

Figure 33–99. Anterior decompression and fusion of the spine using iliac crest strut graft and a Z-plate. (Illustrations and photographs courtesy of Thomas A. Zdeblick, M.D.) *A,* Anterior decompression of the spine and the resultant corpectomy defect. *B,* Placement of a tricortical iliac crest strut graft. *C,* Application of a compressive force across the strut graft. *D,* The Z-plate fixed to the spine with the compressed tricortical graft. *E,* Postoperative lateral radiograph demonstrates placement of the compressed tricortical strut graft and Z-plate.

months). Burst fractures occurred in 26 patients and four patients suffered a flexion-distraction injury with a burst component. Bowel or bladder dysfunction occurred in 12 (40%) of the patients.

At follow-up, four patients improved two or more Fränkel grades, 17 patients improved one Fränkel grade, and nine patients were unchanged. The average preoperative and postoperative Motor Index Scales were 46 and 49 points, respectively. Bladder function was recovered in nine of 12 (75%) of the patients. A stable fusion was achieved in 100% of the patients after the index procedure. The average preoperative kyphosis was corrected from 22.3 degrees to 7.5 degrees. At follow-up, the average loss of correction was 1.1 degree. There were no failures of instrumentation. The Kaneda SR system is illustrated in Figure 33–100. Preoperative and postoperative studies of one of Dr. Kaneda's patients are presented in Figure 33–101.

Currently we believe that anterior decompression and fusion can be performed as a primary procedure for patients with neurologic defects and burst-type fractures from T11 to L4. Alternatively, anterior decompression and fusion can follow a posterior instrumentation when there is residual cord or root compression and persistent neurologic deficits.

Complications of Instrumentation

Complications of treatment of patients with thoracolumbar trauma have been frequently reported. Many are due to lack of understanding of the patients' altered spinal mechanics, while others are due to poor technique or choice of instrumentation. In this section, complications of instrumentation are discussed.

McAfee reviewed 40 patients with failure of Harrington instrumentation for fractures of the thoracolumbar spine.[78] This series currently includes 120 cases of failure of posterior instrumentation in trauma patients. Forty-two patients had dislodgment or disengagement of the instrumentation with loss of fixation. Harrington distraction instrumentation requires intact ligaments for stability, and overdistraction is a complication more likely in translational injuries. The use of a claw-type configuration of pointing hooks placed in a segmental fashion toward each other decreases the incidence of loss of fixation. Twenty patients were referred with iatrogenic neurologic deficits. Nine patients had inadequate reduction of translational injuries. Twenty patients had persistent unrecognized neurologic compression. If primary posterior "indirect" reduction techniques are attempted for incomplete neurologic deficits, it is mandatory to obtain a CT myelogram postoperatively to determine whether a second-stage anterior corpectomy is indicated.

Steffee and Brantigan[112] performed a prospective multicentered study of 250 patients under an FDA-approved protocol. Overall fusion success was achieved in 186 of 200 (93 per cent) with no statistical difference when comparing the numbers of levels fused. There were 21 device-related complications (8.4 per cent). These included 10 wound infections; three

hematomas; three cases of leg pain; three cases of loss of bowel or bladder control; and one case of spinal cord infarction. The spinal cord infarction occurred in an 85-year-old patient who remained paraplegic postoperatively. Non–device related complications were reported on 16 occasions for 15 patients (6.4 per cent). These included ileus (n = 6); atelectasis (n = 3); chronic obstructive pulmonary disease (n = 1); myocardial infarction (n = 1); deep venous thrombosis (n = 2); pulmonary embolism (n = 1); urinary tract infection (n = 1); and idiopathic neuritis (n = 1). Screw breakage occurred in 33 of 1314 screws implanted in 31 patients.

West reported 124 consecutive cases of vertebral spinal plating (VSP) instrumentation and described complications in 33 patients (27 per cent).[116] Unfortunately, this study (and others on pedicle instrumentation) combined the medical postoperative complications with the complications specific to the pedicle screws. Neurologic deficit developed in seven patients (6 per cent). In five of them, the deficit was due to manipulation and reduction of the neural elements.

McAfee performed a survivorship analysis of pedicle instrumentation in 120 consecutive pedicle instrumentation cases (78 VSP procedures and 42 procedures utilizing Cotrel-Dubousset instrumentation).[84] Survivorship analysis was used to calculate a predicted cumulative rate of success for this series of patients over 10 years' postoperative follow-up. Out of 526 pedicle screws, there were 22 problem screws (4.18 per cent). In most patients, the hardware failure was an incidental radiographic finding. There were only five patients with screw breakage in association with a pseudoarthrosis. Actuarial analysis predicted the survivorship of solid posterolateral fusion at 90 per cent at 10 years' follow-up. This survivorship rate is similar to those predicted at 10 years for other more widely used orthopaedic surgical implants, such as total hip arthroplasty components.[51]

To reduce the incidence of complications in this series, the technique of "probing" rather than "drilling" the pedicle was utilized. McLain[89] demonstrated an increased risk of failure of short-segment Cotrel-Dubousset instrumentation when the anterior column was not properly addressed.

Pedicle screws are the instrumentation of choice in the posterior stabilization of lower lumbar (L4 or L5) unstable burst fractures. If pedicle instrumentation is applied in fractures across the thoracolumbar junction, it is important to supplement the pedicle screws with anterior structural bone grafting, placed via either an anterior or a posterolateral approach. Akbarnia reported a multicenter study of over 100 VSP used in thoracolumbar fractures.[2] Anterior load-sharing was necessary with pedicle instrumentation to prevent an unacceptably high rate of screw breakage and failure.

McAfee studied the incidence of complications occurring from 1984 to 1990 in 185 anterior thoracolumbar procedures (thoracotomies, transthoracic-retroperitoneal, and retroperitoneal approaches).[77] A complete listing of the complications encountered is shown in Table 33–4 (see page 1041). There were no cases of

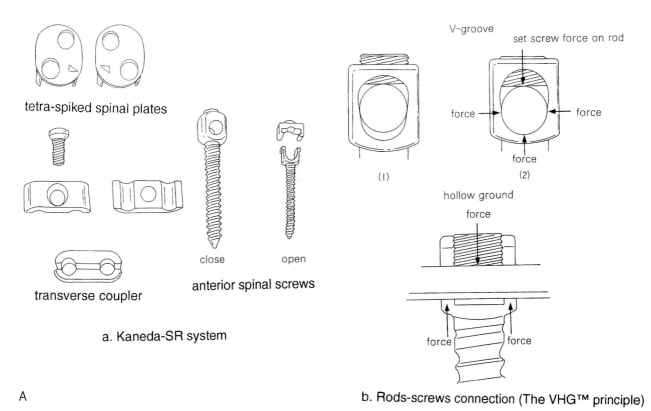

tetra-spiked spinal plates

transverse coupler

anterior spinal screws

close   open

a. Kaneda-SR system

V-groove

set screw force on rod

force   force

force

(1)   (2)

hollow ground

force

force   force

b. Rods-screws connection (The VHG™ principle)

A

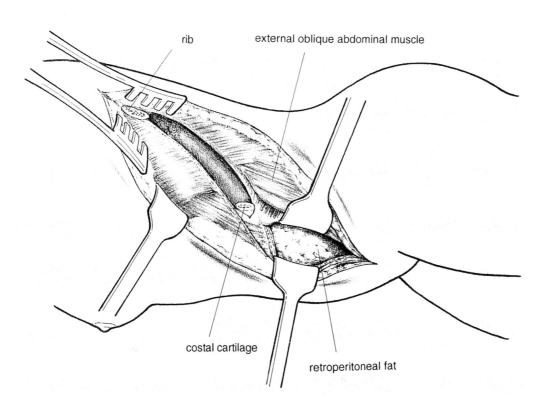

rib   external oblique abdominal muscle

costal cartilage

retroperitoneal fat

B

Figure 33–100. The Kaneda SR (smooth rod) system is available to treat thoracolumbar spinal injuries approached by the anterior approach. *A,* Depiction of the Kaneda SR (smooth rod). *B,* Extrapleural-retroperitoneal approach. The thoracolumbar junction is commonly approached through an incision over the tenth or eleventh rib. The costal cartilage is split longitudinally following resection of the corresponding rib, and blunt dissection separates the retroperitoneal fat and retroperitoneal structures from the iliopsoas muscle and spine.

Illustration continued on following page

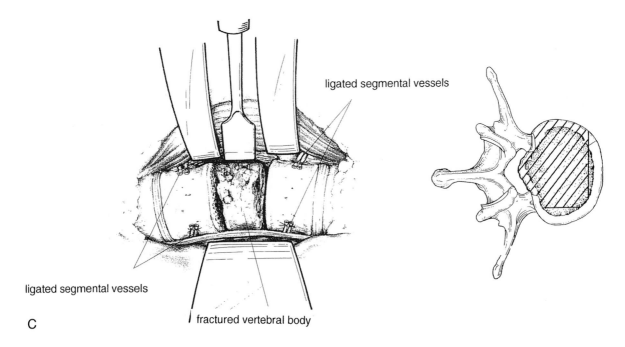

ligated segmental vessels

ligated segmental vessels

C

fractured vertebral body

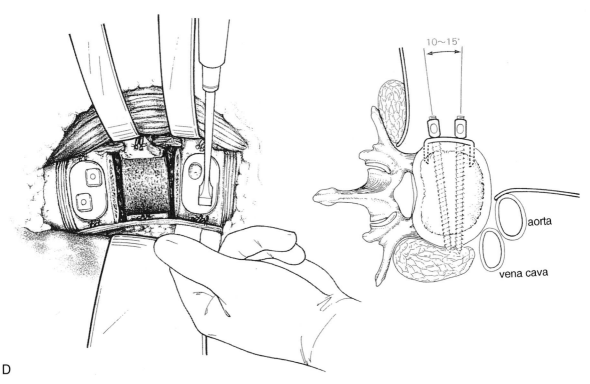

10~15°

aorta

vena cava

D

Figure 33–100 *Continued. C,* Decompression of the spinal canal. *Left,* A corpectomy is performed using chisels following resection of the discs above and below the damaged segment. Then, a decompression is carried out by removal of the retropulsed bony fragment into the spinal canal using chisels, curets, and rotatable Kerrison rongeur. *Right,* Extent of bone resection for anterior decompression is illustrated (axial plane). *D,* Placing spinal plates and screws. *Left,* Tetra-spiked spinal plates are correctly placed on lateral aspect of the vertebral body. Neither spike must be inserted into the intervertebral disc. *Right,* Two posterior screws are inserted with 10 degrees to 15 degrees anterior inclination to avoid the screw's penetration into the spinal canal. Each blunt-tipped screw is allowed to extend beyond the contralateral cortex by 2 to 3 mm to ensure secure bicortical purchase. Confirmation of each screw's placement through direct palpation is recommended to confirm bicortical purchase.

Illustration continued on opposite page

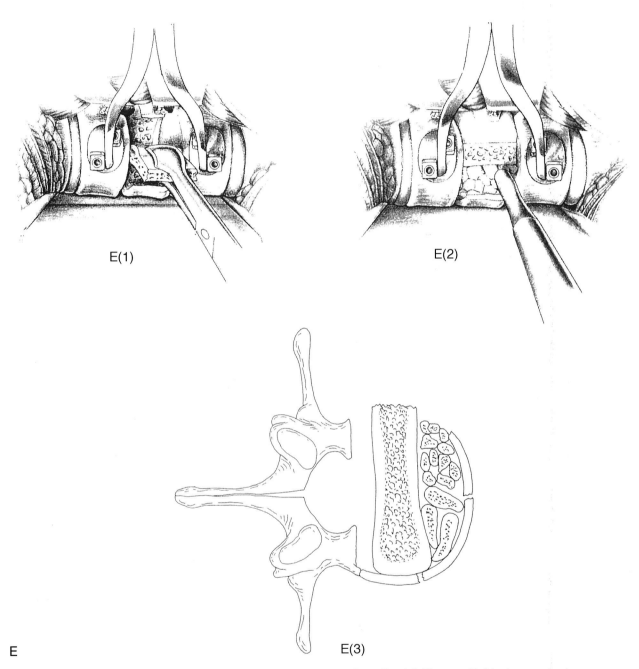

E(1)

E(2)

E(3)

E

Figure 33–100 *Continued.* *E,* Deformity correction and grafting. *Top left,* The vertebral body spreader is placed between the head of the rostral and caudal screws. Distraction is applied until the bodies have been returned to their anatomically correct location. The tricortical iliac crest graft is placed into the distracted vertebral resection defect. *Top right,* Additional morselized bone and rib strut are packed into the remaining anterior defect. *Bottom,* The tricortical portion of the iliac crest was inserted opposite the Kaneda plate near the contralateral pedicles.

Illustration continued on following page

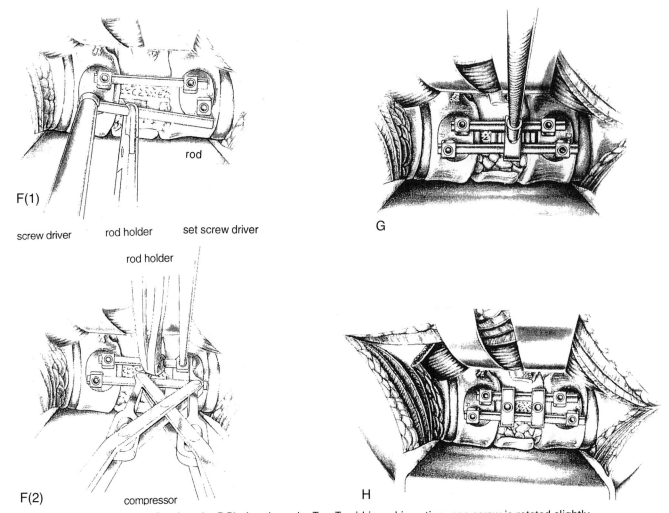

F(1)

screw driver   rod holder   set screw driver

rod holder

F(2)   compressor

G

H

Figure 33–100 *Continued.* *F,* Placing the rods. *Top,* To aid in rod insertion, one screw is rotated slightly away from the longitudinal axis of the construct, the rod is inserted, then the screw is rotated back onto the correct orientation. *Bottom,* A compressor is placed across the loose screw and the rod holder. Firm compression is applied, and the set screw is tightened. *G,* Placing the transverse couplers. *H,* Construct assembly is complete.

iatrogenic neurologic deficit. There were also no deep wound infections. One patient died one week postoperatively due to disseminated intravascular coagulopathy. None of the five patients with pseudarthrosis of the anterior corpectomy graft required repeat anterior surgery. All five cases were successfully revised with posterior Cotrel-Dubousset instrumentation and posterior spinal fusion.

In a similar finding, Kaneda did not have to remove any of the 110 anterior instrumentation devices.[54] The four patients with anterior pseudarthrosis or anterior implant failures were successfully stabilized by posterior spinal fusion and instrumentation (Kaneda paravertebral rod breakage, one patient; Kaneda vertebral screw breakage, one patient) (Fig. 33–102). One patient had rupture of the inferior vena cava that occurred during exposure of an untreated burst fracture with severe kyphosis. One postoperative death occurred at two weeks from pneumonia in a diabetic patient, two

patients had superficial wound infections, and five patients had postoperative atelectasis. It is our experience that there are more postoperative pulmonary problems with the contralateral lung than the lung on the side of the anterior approach, probably owing to dependency during surgery.

BASIC SCIENTIFIC CONSIDERATIONS OF THORACOLUMBAR SPINAL INSTRUMENTATION

Basic scientific evaluation of spinal instrumentation systems utilizes both in vitro and in vivo experimental methods. In vitro methods rely on bench-top modeling performed in a laboratory setting and typically provide information related to the stability of spinal reconstruction techniques using cadaveric or synthetic models. In many of these studies, intact ligamentous spine speci-

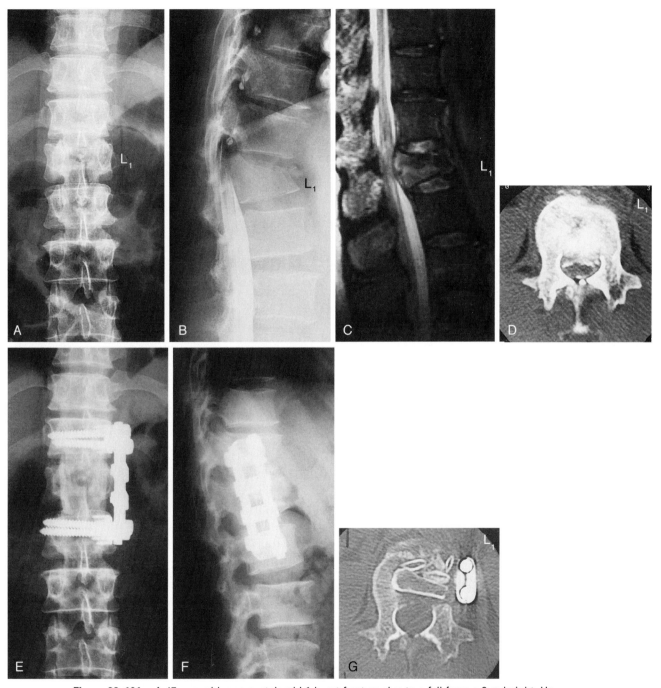

Figure 33–101.   A 47-year-old man sustained L1 burst fracture due to a fall from a 2 m height. He showed severe bowel and bladder dysfunction and mild motor weakness in bilateral lower extremities (modified Fränkel grade D1). Compression of the conus medullaris and the cauda equina was demonstrated by neuroradiologic studies. *A through D,* Preoperative plain film *(A),* myelogram *(B),* MRI (T2-weighted image) *(C),* and CT-myelogram *(D). E through G,* Anterior decompression and anterior reconstruction using the Kaneda SR and autologous iliac crest graft were carried out two days after injury. Motor function of the lower extremities and bowel-bladder function were fully recovered at follow-up (one year after surgery).

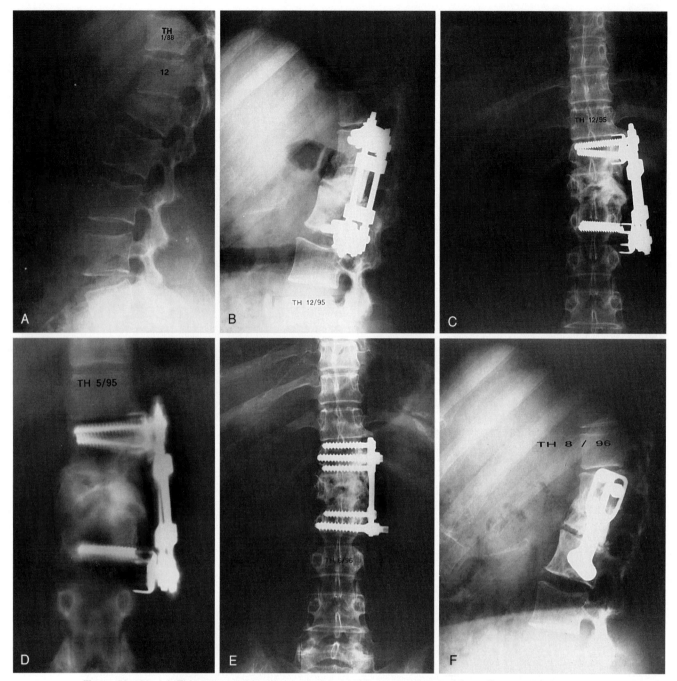

Figure 33–102. *A,* This 32-year-old woman was involved in a toboggan accident. She sustained an axial loading injury to her spine when the toboggan went off a jump, and she developed an L1 unstable burst fracture. Neurologically, she had weakness in both legs with dysesthetic pain in the L5 nerve root distribution on her right leg. *B,* The patient was initially treated with an anterior L1 corpectomy with iliac crest bone graft and anterior threaded rod Kaneda instrumentation from T12 to L2. The patient had a full neurologic recovery within the two months following surgery. However, by the time of this radiograph, six years postoperatively, she had developed mechanical back pain. *C,* An anteroposterior radiograph shows a fracture of the Kaneda screws within the L2 vertebral body. *D,* A tomogram demonstrates that the failure occurred between the screw head and the first thread. It is our experience that with anterior instrumentation, the most important factor is not the choice of instrumentation or the particular type of implant; the most important factor is a good result in obtaining load-sharing with the anterior tricortical iliac strut graft. Anteroposterior *(E)* and lateral *(F)* radiographs show revision through an anterior thoracotomy, resection of the Kaneda instrumentation, resection of the anterior pseudarthrosis, and use of iliac bone graft. In addition, an anterior Z-plate was utilized. The key was to compress the bone graft within the radiolucent pseudarthrosis defect at L1–L2. The patient had relief of mechanical back pain and she remained neurologically intact. In our experience, the biomechanical differences between anterior instrumentation constructs are very minor compared with several extremely important aspects of surgical technique common to all anterior implants:

1. The vertebral body screws need to have bicortical purchase.
2. The anterior implant needs to load-share with a tricortical iliac strut graft.
3. The implant must compress the iliac bone graft against the vertebral bodies.
4. A thoracolumbar sacral orthosis is used in all patients until there is radiographic evidence of fusion (usually by three or four months postoperatively).

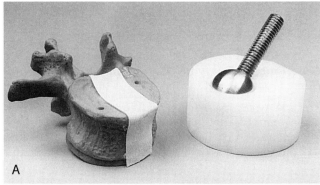

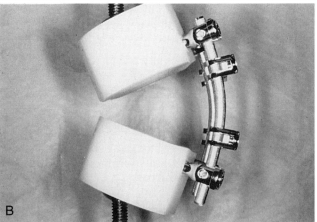

A

B

Figure 33–103. Cunningham et al.[21] developed a synthetic vertebral motion segment model composed of ultra-high molecular weight polyethylene (UHMWP) to better evaluate the intrinsic biomechanical properties of anterior and posterior spinal instrumentation systems. A total corpectomy defect was simulated using two independent fixation cylinders instrumented with the spinal system, and the bilateral posterior pedicle screw spinal constructs were tested in anterior compressive flexion utilizing a universal mechanism. The rods and plates served as the only connection between the cylinders, thus representing a "worst-case scenario" for the implant system with an entire vertebral body missing. The use of a synthetic fixation model addresses the limitations of biologic tissue deterioration, inherent strength, and tissue variability and also provides an invariable fixation medium for the destructive static and fatigue testing of spinal devices. *A,* The synthetic vertebral body motion segment *(right)* is composed of UHMWP and stainless steel rods. This is a biomechanical testing model used to simulate cyclical loading of a vertebral motion segment following spinal instrumentation. *B,* A lateral projection of the Texas Scottish Rite Hospital spinal implant system instrumented to the UHMWP fixation cylinders. This bilateral, bilevel posterior pedicle screw spinal device is undergoing a compressive bending test to quantify construct stiffness and bending strength.

In Vitro Biomechanical Studies of Spinal Instrumentation

The use of in vitro cadaveric models for comparative biomechanical testing of spinal instrumentation systems is well characterized.[43, 63, 87, 105, 106] However, the problems of biologic deterioration,[74] inherent tissue strength, and variability limit the use. To better evaluate the biomechanical properties of anterior and posterior spinal instrumentation systems, Cunningham et al.[21] developed a motion segment model (Fig. 33–103*A*). The experimental model allows for destructive static and fatigue testing.

Posterior and Anterior Thoracolumbar Spinal Implant Systems

Posterolateral pedicle screw spinal constructs have been evaluated in spinal flexion by Cunningham et al.[21] A total corpectomy defect was simulated and instrumented (Fig. 33–103*B*). Thirteen posterior pedicle screw spinal implant systems have been tested for stiffness, bending strength, and fatigue life (cycles at failure). Stiffness and bending strength differences as high as 500 percent were demonstrated (Figs. 33–104 and 33–105). Fatigue testing demonstrated the greatest differences between the systems (Fig. 33–106). Pedicle screw failure patterns were identical to those seen in in vivo canine and clinical studies.[4, 80, 116] Most of the screws fractured within the shank (Fig. 33–107*A*). The Dyna-Lok and VSP systems, however, fractured in the machine thread portion of the screw adjacent to the integral nut (Fig. 33–107*B*). The Compact Cotrel-Dubousset system was the only construct to demonstrate fracture within the spinal rod. The point of fracture in all cases was adjacent to the screw–rod junction and located between the screws (Fig. 33–107*C*). The

mens are first evaluated biomechanically and then injured to mimic a clinically relevant condition, followed by stabilization with instrumentation and retesting. The results of such studies compare the ability of different systems to restore stability to the injured spine.[41, 56, 63, 105, 106] In contrast, in vivo models allow for the characterization of the biologic response to destabilization and to spinal arthrodesis.[20, 57, 64, 80, 81, 104]

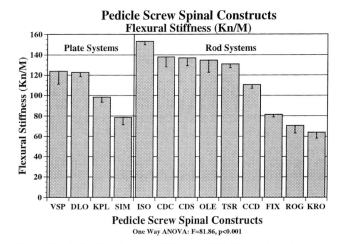

Figure 33–104. The flexural stiffness of 13 different posterior pedicle screw spinal constructs. A one-way analysis of variance yielded highly statistical differences between the systems. The ISOLA, Cotrel-Dubousset, Olerud, and TSRH were the stiffest systems evaluated, while the Fixateur Interne, Rogozinski, and Kirschner Rod were among the least stiff or most flexible.

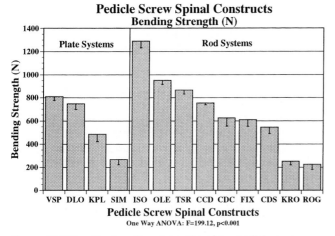

Figure 33–105. The bending strengths of the pedicle screw spinal constructs highlighted a 500 per cent difference when comparing the highest and lowest construct strengths. The ISOLA, Olerud, and TSRH rod constructs exhibited the highest bending strengths in a comparison of the 13 systems.

Plate Systems	Rod Systems	Rod Systems
VSP = Variable Screw Placement	ISO = ISOLA	FIX = Fixateur Interne
DLO = Dyna-Lok	OLE = Olerud	CDS = Cotrel-Dubousset Standard
Kirschner Plate	TSR = TSRH	KRO = Kirschner Rod
SIM = Simmons Plate	CCD = Compact Cotrel-Dubousset	CD ROG = Rogozinski
		CDC = Cotrel-Dubousset Cold Rolled

fatigue failure modes of the ISOLA implant system, the strongest system evaluated in the current study, were identical to those observed in the clinical setting (Fig. 33–108).

A similar study by Kotani et al.[65] evaluated the intrinsic mechanical properties of anterior thoracolumbar systems. Anterior spinal devices were evaluated for stiffness, bending strength, and fatigue life (Figs. 33–109 and 33–110). Most of the plate systems fractured at the screw–plate junction. The Z-plate, however, fractured within the plate at the screw nest (Fig. 33–111).

In all constructs, bending strengths were less than 1300 N. The compressive strength of nonosteoporotic lumbar vertebrae has been shown to range between 5000 and 6000 N.[5, 97] Nachemson's work on intradiscal pressures demonstrated the L3–L4 disc to undergo compressive loads as high as 3400 N when lifting 20 kg with bent back and knees straight.[91] This is approximately 400 per cent higher than the mean bending strengths afforded by these implant systems. Under axial loading conditions, the force-bearing capacity of the posterior and anterior lumbar columns has been shown to be 20 per cent and 80 per cent, respectively.[92]

All implants evaluated demonstrated bending strengths below the normal load distribution through the anterior column. This indicates that without adequate anterior column support, normal physiologic loads exceed the bending strengths of the implant sys-

tems. To maximize the endurance of posterior and anterior implants, an optimal anterior-posterior column load-sharing environment is necessary.

Experimental Study of Thoracolumbar Burst Fractures

The goals of surgery for thoracolumbar burst fractures are to provide anatomic reduction, obtain adequate decompression of the spinal canal, and maintain stable fixation. To date, studies have primarily focused on reduction mechanisms of intracanal fragments via a distraction force applied to the osteoligamentous tissue.[17, 34, 35] We developed an in vitro technique for creating clinically realistic burst fractures at a desired vertebral level. Using this model, Shono et al.[106] addressed three questions:

1. Can indirect posterior decompression and stabilization adequately restore spinal alignment and reduce fracture fragments?
2. What factors influence the degree of reduction of intracanal bone fragments?
3. Are there mechanical differences between anterior and posterior stabilization techniques for treating thoracolumbar burst fractures?

Reproducible burst fractures were created at the L1 level (Fig. 33–112). Fractures were classified using Denis' classification,[24] and reductions were evaluated (Table 33–5). Shono and coworkers[111] developed a model to reproducibly recreate clinically realistic burst fractures at a desired vertebral level. Using this technique, a biomechanical study was performed investigating the axial stability of unstable burst fractures and the relative contribution of load-sharing with bone graft alone, the anterior Kaneda device, and the poste-

Text continued on page 1057

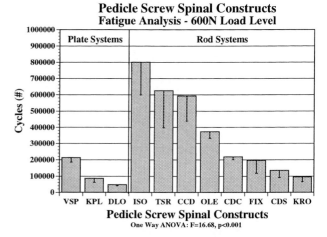

Figure 33–106. Comparison of the cyclical fatigue properties of 11 spinal implant systems. This load level highlighted the greatest differences among the spinal constructs, with the ISOLA, TSRH, and Compact Cotrel-Dubousset systems exhibiting the highest fatigue properties. There is an indicated statistical difference among the systems.

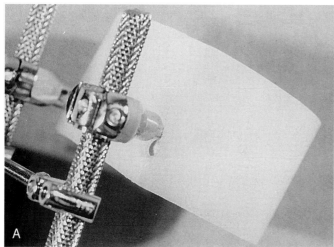

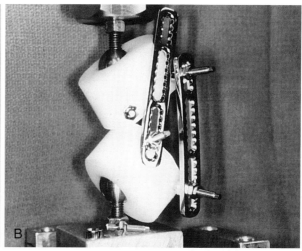

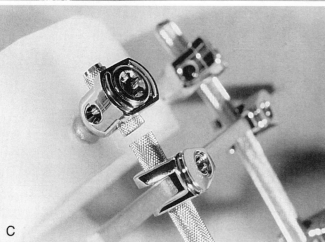

Figure 33–107. Simulated vertebral motion segment model by Cunningham et al.[23] allows for in vitro comparison of different spinal systems with regard to fatigue testing and mechanism of failure. *A,* An oblique view of the Cotrel-Dubousset standard system demonstrating a screw fatigue fracture. In all cases, this system exhibited fracture within the screw shank. *B,* A posterior view of the VSP plate system fatigue fracture located at the machine thread portion of the pedicle screw. The use of a universal testing mechanism allows for the implant to fail at its "weak link," thereby permitting an unconstrained testing environment. This is best seen by rotation of the UHMWP cylinders, which exposes the cylindrical steel testing fixtures. *C,* Oblique view of the Compact Cotrel-Dubousset system exhibiting the characteristic fatigue failure: fracture of the spinal rod adjacent to the pedicle screw. In all cases, the rods were weak links in the construct.

Table 33–5. RADIOGRAPHIC EVALUATION

	Intact	Injured	After Posterior Reduction	Reduction Rate
Harrington Instrumentation				
Angle (degrees)	1, lordosis	13, kyphosis	5, lordosis	18
ID (%)	100	109.5	106.6	3
ABH (%)	100	60.8	100.9	40.1
PBH (%)	100	78.8	98.6	19.8
Canal clearance (%)	100	44.2	56.5	12.3*
Midsagittal anterior-posterior diameter (%)	100	51.9	61.4	9.5*
AO Fixateur Interne				
Angle (degrees)	2, kyphosis	16, kyphosis	3, kyphosis	13
ID (%)	100	107.7	104.3	3.4
ABH (%)	100	52	95.8	43.8
PBH (%)	100	74.6	94.2	19.6
Canal clearance (%)	100	40.4	58.9	18.5*
Midsagittal anterior-posterior diameter (%)	100	49.1	66.6	17.5†
Total				
Angle (degrees)	1, kyphosis	14, kyphosis	1, lordosis	15
ID (%)	100	108.6	105.4	3.2
ABH (%)	100	56.2	98.2	42
PBH (%)	100	76.6	96.3	19.7
Canal clearance (%)	100	42.3	57.7	15.4
Midsagittal anterior-posterior diameter (%)	100	50.5	64	13.5

ABH, anterior vertebral body height of L1; Angle, sagittal angle between the inferior endplate of T12 and superior endplate of L2; ID, interpedicular distance of L1; PBH, posterior vertebral body of L1.
*$p < .05$; significant difference between the two posterior instrumentation systems.
†$p < .02$; significant difference between the two posterior instrumentation systems.
Except for the angle measurement, all data represent percentage values that have been normalized to the values of the intact specimen (100%).

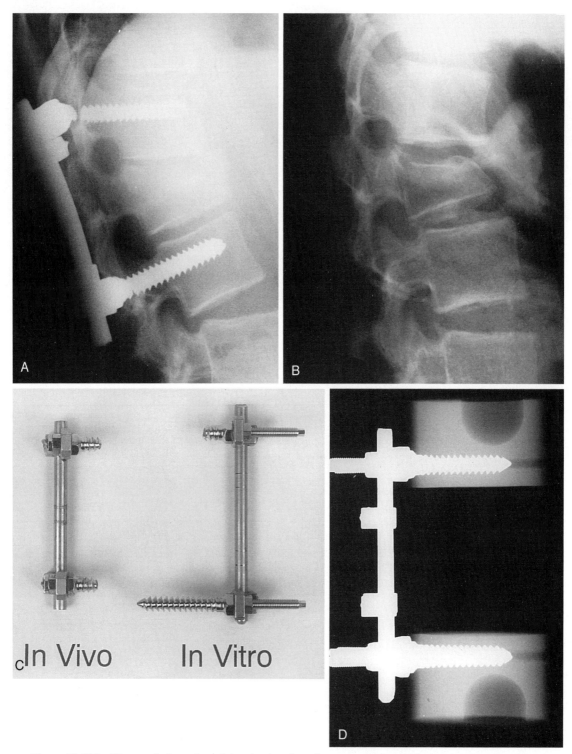

Figure 33–108. The predictive value of the simulated motion segment model is demonstrated by this clinical correlation. *A,* This 16-year-old patient presented with an L2 compression fracture (Denis type B) resulting from a two-story fall off a rope swing. Posterior reconstruction was performed with the ISOLA spinal system. Minimal ventral augmentation used local bone graft. *B,* The patient returned six months postoperatively with two superior screw fractures. *C* and *D,* The identical fracture patterns were observed in the ISOLA system under in vitro fatigue testing conditions.

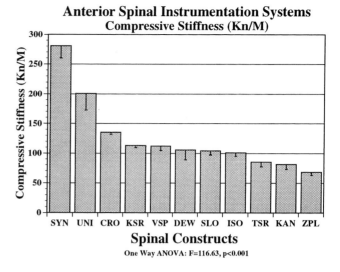

Figure 33–109. Compressive stiffness levels of 11 thoracolumbar spinal implant systems. A one-way analysis of variance and post hoc student-Newman-Keuls multicomparison test highlighted, among other comparisons, the Synthes and University Plate systems as exhibiting statistically higher stiffness properties compared with the remaining implants.

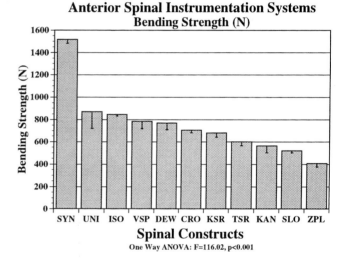

Figure 33–110. Bending strength values demonstrated the Synthes Plate system as statistically different from the 10 other devices. The plate thickness combined with a low profile was thought to account for the increased stiffness and bending strength properties.

Nomenclature for Anterior Spinal Constructs:

Plate Systems	Rod Systems
SYN = Synthes Plate	ISO = ISOLA
UNI = University Plate	CRO = Synergy System
VSP = Variable Screw	KSR = Kaneda Smooth Rod
Placement	Device
DEW = DeWald Plate	TSR = TSRH
ZPL = Z-Plate	KAN = Kaneda Standard Device
	SLO = Slot-Zielke Device

Figure 33–111. Fatigue failure mechanism of the anterior Z-plate device. The Z-plate fractured within the plate at the screw nest. In contrast to the bulky Synthes and University Plate systems, the Z-plate allows for a lower profile system and easily permits compression of the selected graft material spanning the defect site. Most of the plate systems fractured at the screw-plate junction.

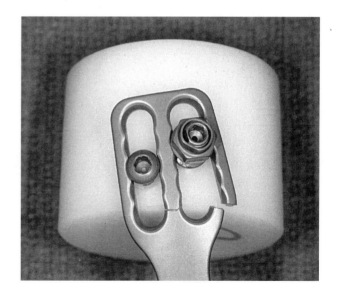

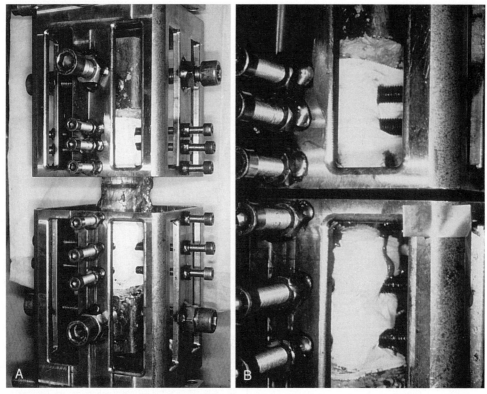

Figure 33–112. *A,* Impact loading apparatus used to create the L1 burst fracture. The L1 vertebra and adjacent discs are isolated by the upper and lower box-shaped fixtures. *B,* The resulting L1 burst fracture created by high-speed vertical compression.

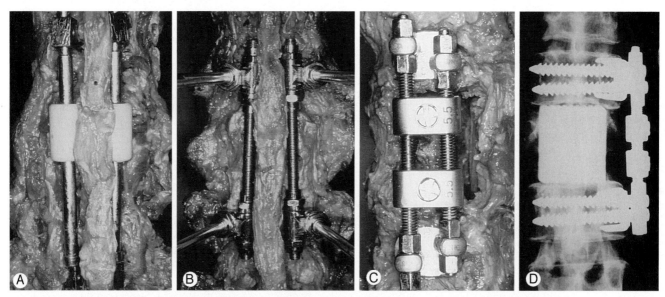

Figure 33–113. Burst fractures at L1 were created and reconstructed using three spinal implant systems. *A,* Posterior view of a specimen stabilized with Harrington dual distraction rods with sleeves (fixation range, T11–L3). *B,* Posterior view of a specimen stabilized with the AO Fixateur Interne (fixation range, T12–L2). *C,* Lateral view of a specimen reconstructed with iliac crest strut graft and the threaded rod Kaneda device (fixation range, T12–L2). *D,* Anteroposterior radiograph of a specimen stabilized with a ceramic vertebral prosthesis and the threaded rod Kaneda device (fixation range, T12–L2).

rior fixateur interne systems. The findings of this study indicate that a one-stage anterior decompression and reconstruction procedure with instrumentation effectively decompresses intracanal bone fragments and offers superior mechanical stability compared with indirect reduction and stabilization of posterior instrumentation.

Reconstruction of the fractured specimens was performed using three systems: (1) Harrington dual distraction rods with sleeves, (2) AO Fixateur Interne, and (3) anterior reconstruction with the Kaneda device and strut graft (Fig. 33–113). The posterior reconstruction methods relied on indirect decompression of the retropulsed bone fragments and restoration of spinal alignment by posterior distraction of the anterior and middle columns. Anterior decompression allowed for direct visualization and complete resection of the retropulsed bone fragments. Testing of the intact and reconstructed specimens quantified segmental stiffness under axial compression, rotation, and flexion-extension modes (Fig. 33–114).

There were no statistical differences between the two posterior reconstruction methods with respect to reduction of the interpedicular distance, kyphotic angular deformity, or correction of the vertebral body heights (see Table 33–5; Fig. 33–115). Potential canal clearance depends mainly on the extent of canal encroachment before posterior reduction (Fig. 33–116). CT scans from two cases are presented (Figs. 33–117 and 33–118).

Biomechanical testing indicated that anterior reconstruction with the Kaneda device provided more stability under all testing modalities, particularly axial compression and axial rotation (Fig. 33–119). Although the Harrington and AO constructs were typically more stable than the injured spine in these testing modes, the multisegmental stiffness afforded by these constructs was significantly less than with the anterior Kaneda device. Reconstruction with the Kaneda device was more stable than with the posterior instrumentation systems in all loading conditions and was significantly more rigid in axial compression and rotation.

Although the Harrington instrumentation had a fixation range that extended two vertebral levels cephalad and two levels caudal to the injured vertebra, it was less rigid compared with the AO internal fixator, which required incorporation of only two motion segments. Despite sleeve application, the conventional hook-based system merely provides fixation to the posterior column and lacks anterior and middle column fixation mechanisms. Therefore, it appears incapable of providing stability to the severely destructed spinal segment with anterior and middle column instabilities.

One-stage anterior decompression and reconstruction with anterior instrumentation effectively decompresses the intracanal bone fragments and offers superior mechanical stability compared with the indirect reduction and stabilization of posterior instrumentation.

In Vivo Models of Thoracolumbar Spinal Instrumentation

Maturation Process of the Posterolateral Spinal Fusion

Although several studies have examined sequential stages of bone graft healing, the healing mechanism of the posterolateral spinal fusion remains controversial and unclear.[9, 48, 52, 113] Furthermore, it remains poorly understood how the histologic properties of the posterolateral fusion mass correlate with its mechanical strength during the healing process.

Kanayama et al.[57] have studied the temporal relationship between the biomechanical, radiographic, and histologic properties of posterolateral spinal fusions with respect to the load-sharing changes, if any, between spinal instrumentation and the fusion mass throughout the healing process. Sheep underwent destabilization of the posterior spinal column and transpedicular screw fixation at the L3–L4 and L5–L6 segments (Fig. 33–120). A posterolateral spinal arthrodesis was performed at one segment with autologous corticocancellous bone. The other segment (without bone graft) served as the unfused instrumented control. The posterolateral fusion has increased stiffness after the fourth postoperative week, with no differences between the eight-, 12-, and 16-week time periods (Fig. 33–121A). Hardware strain, measured using rods af-

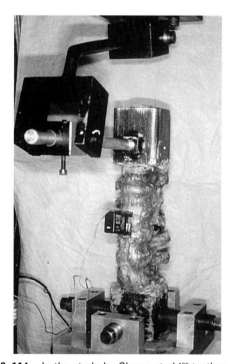

Figure 33–114. In the study by Shono et al.[106] testing of the intact and reconstructed specimens quantified segmental stiffness under axial compression, rotation, and flexion-extension modes. The configuration for a flexion-extension test is demonstrated. An extensometric displacement gauge bridges the anterior aspects of the T12 and L2 vertebrae and continuously measures longitudinal strain across the L1 vertebrae and adjacent intervertebral levels.

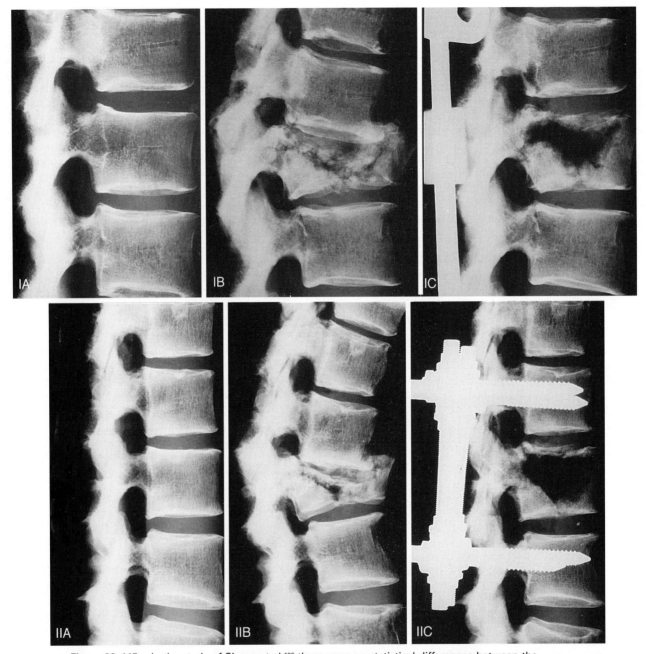

Figure 33–115. In the study of Shono et al.[106] there were no statistical differences between the Harrington dual distraction rods with sleeves and the AO Fixateur Interne with respect to reduction of the interpedicular distance, kyphotic angular deformity, or correction of the vertebral body heights. Lateral radiographs of the intact spine (IA), injured spine (IB), and after reduction and stabilization with Harrington instrumentation (IC) are shown. A kyphotic deformity of 14 degrees was corrected to 5 degrees of lordosis. Posterior vertebral body height was restored from 86 per cent to 93 per cent. Residual bony defect in the anterior and middle spinal columns is observed following posterior reduction. Lateral radiographs of the intact spine (IIA), injured spine (IIB), and after reduction and stabilization with AO Fixateur Interne (IIC) are shown. A kyphotic deformity of 19 degrees was corrected to 3 degrees of lordosis, and posterior vertebral body height was restored from 71 per cent to 100 per cent. Note the bony defect despite posterior reduction.

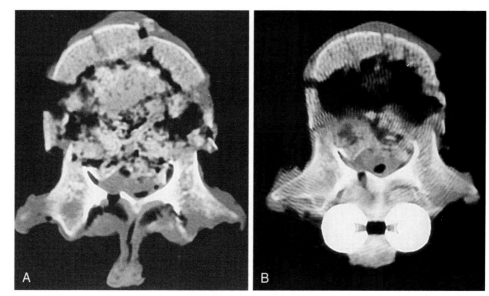

CANAL CLEARANCE
Injured Versus After Posterior Reduction

$R^2 = 0.803$

After Posterior Reduction (%)

Injured (%)

Figure 33–116. Shono et al.[106] demonstrated that potential canal clearance depends mainly on the extent of canal encroachment before posterior reduction. Comparison of canal clearance of the injured spine and after indirect posterior reduction. Linear regression analysis yielded a significant correlation.

Figure 33–117. Shono et al.[106] created burst fractures at L1 and quantified the degree of canal clearance using indirect reduction and posterior stabilization using Harrington instrumentation. Computed tomography scans of injured spine (A) and after reduction and stabilization with Harrington instrumentation (B). Preoperative canal clearance is 34 per cent. After reduction it is 45 per cent. Note the residual bone fragments following indirect reduction.

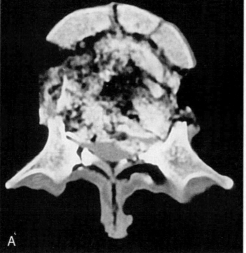
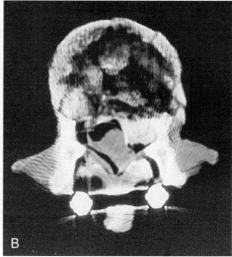

Figure 33–118. Shono et al.[106] created burst fractures at L1 and quantified the degree of canal clearance using indirect reduction and posterior stabilization using the Fixateur Interne. Computed tomography scans of injured spine (A) and after reduction and stabilization with the AO Fixateur Interne (B). Preoperative canal clearance is 27 per cent, and 57 per cent after reduction. Note the rotational migration of a large bone fragment into the spinal canal after indirect reduction.

AXIAL COMPRESSION STIFFNESS (KN/M)

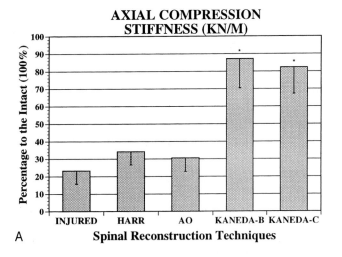

A

Spinal Reconstruction Techniques

The load-sharing properties of spinal instrumentation decreased concurrently with the developing spinal fusion mass. In the early period after posterolateral spinal arthrodesis with instrumentation, the load across the fused segment is mainly shared by the hardware, since the fusion mass had no contribution to the initial strength or stability of the operative segment. As the fusion mass develops and achieves increasing strength with time, the load across the fused segment is primarily distributed to the solid fusion mass, resulting in unloading of the instrumentation. Importantly, these load-sharing changes occurred at the time when the fusion mass achieved mechanical maturation—before solid fusion was confirmed radiologically and histologically. This study revealed discrepancy between biomechanical stability and histologic maturation of the pos-

AXIAL ROTATION STIFFNESS (NM/DEG)

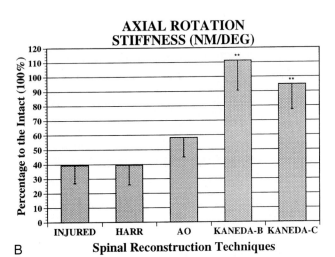

B

Spinal Reconstruction Techniques

Figure 33–119. Shono et al.[106] compared the peak axial compressive *(A)* and rotational *(B)* stiffness of the injured spine and four reconstruction techniques. All values are normalized to the value of the intact specimen (intact = 100%). HARR, Harrington instrumentation; AO, AO Fixateur Interne; Kaneda-B, iliac strut bone graft augmented with the Kaneda device; Kaneda-C, Kaneda device with a ceramic vertebral prosthesis. Error bar signifies one standard deviation and asterisk (*) indicates no statistical difference. Although the Harrington and AO constructs were typically more stable than the injured spine in these testing modes, the multisegmental stiffness afforded by these constructs was significantly less than the anterior Kaneda device. Reconstruction with the Kaneda device was more stable than the posterior instrumentation systems in all loading conditions and was significantly more rigid in axial compression and rotation.

fixed with strain gauges (Fig. 33–122), decreases significantly starting at eight weeks (Fig. 33–121*B*). Radiographically, although all of the four-month fusions were solid (Fig. 33–121*A*; Fig. 33–123). Mineralization in the fusion mass increased in a linear fashion even after eight weeks, despite having achieved sufficient mechanical strength (Figs. 33–124 and 33–125). Woven bone formation was observed within the fusion mass at eight weeks; thereafter, the fusion mass was gradually trabeculated (Fig. 33–126).

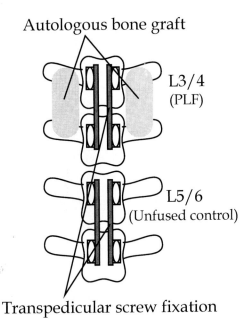

Autologous bone graft

L3/4 (PLF)

L5/6 (Unfused control)

Transpedicular screw fixation

Figure 33–120. Kanayama et al.[57] undertook a study designed to investigate the temporal relationship between the biomechanical, radiographic, and histologic properties of posterolateral spinal fusions, and to elucidate the load-sharing changes, if any, between spinal instrumentation and the fusion mass throughout the healing process. The current study revealed a great discrepancy between biomechanical stability, histologic maturation, and radiographic appearance of the posterolateral fusion mass. The biomechanical properties of a stable spinal fusion preceded the radiographic appearance of a solid fusion by at least eight weeks, suggesting that immature woven bone provided substantial stiffness to the fusion mass. These findings suggest that maturation of the posterolateral fusion mass occurs around eight weeks postoperatively and precedes the solid bony union as confirmed radiographically. Specifically, mineralization in the fusion mass continues despite having achieved sufficient mechanical strength. Transpedicular screw fixation was performed at the L3–L4 and L5–L6 segments in the sheep model after destabilization of the posterior spinal columns. Posterolateral spinal arthrodesis was then carried out with autologous corticocancellous bone randomly at either the L3–L4 or L5–L6 segment. No bone was grafted at the other segment, which served as the unfused control level. In this case, the posterolateral arthrodesis level was the L3–L4 segment.

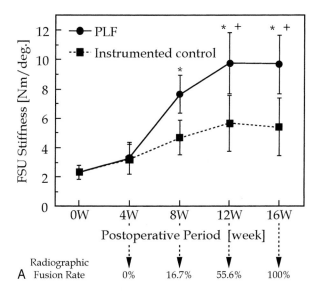

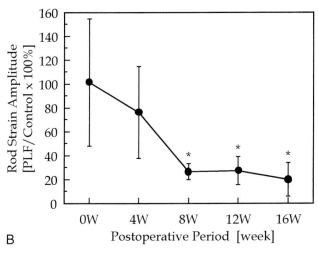

Figure 33–121. *A,* Time-related change in torsional stiffness of the posterolateral fusion (PLF) and unfused control segments. Kanayama et al.[57] demonstrated that posterolateral fusion levels became significantly stiffer at eight weeks after surgery (p < 0.01, one-way ANOVA and Scheffe's F-test). *, p < .01 versus zero and four weeks; +, p < .05 versus respective unfused control levels. FSU, functional spinal unit. *B,* Time-related change in medial surface rod strain under lateral bending. Strain is represented as the strain amplitude of the posterolateral fusion (PLF) level normalized to the respective unfused control level. Strain within instrumentation significantly decreased at eight weeks after surgery (p < .01, one-way ANOVA and Scheffe's F-test). *, p < .01 versus zero weeks. Radiographic fusion rate (%) is based on readings from three independent observers.

terolateral fusion mass. The biomechanical properties of a stable spinal fusion preceded the radiographic appearance of a solid fusion by at least eight weeks, suggesting that immature woven bone provides substantial stiffness to the fusion mass. These findings suggest that maturation of the posterolateral fusion

mass occurs around eight weeks postoperatively and precedes the solid bony union as confirmed radiographically. Specifically, mineralization in the fusion mass continues after mechanical integrity is achieved.

Influence of Rigid Spinal Instrumentation on the Healing Process

Numerous studies have documented that rigid spinal instrumentation leads to a higher rate of fusion, as compared with uninstrumented fusions[10, 81, 122] and, in fact, serves to augment the functional spinal unit stability even after fusion has occurred.[64] It remains unclear, however, whether spinal instrumentation influences the healing process itself. Kanayama et al.[57] investigated the effect of spinal instrumentation on the healing process of a posterolateral spinal fusion by comparing instrumented and uninstrumented fusions.

Adult sheep underwent posterior spinal column destabilization and posterolateral spinal arthrodeses with autologous bone at the L2–L3 and L4–L5 segments. Randomly, one of those segments was augmented bilaterally with TSRH transpedicular screw fixation. Animals were sacrificed at eight or 16 weeks. Biomechanical testing was performed for each fusion segment following instrumentation removal. Fusion status was assessed by manual palpation and plain radiographs. Mineralized volume of the fusion mass was quantified using CT scan images. Histologic evaluation was performed using undecalcified sagittal sections of the fusion masses.

At eight weeks after surgery, the instrumented fusion demonstrated significantly higher flexural stiffness

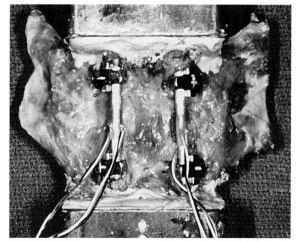

Figure 33–122. Kanayama et al.[57] evaluated the healing mechanism of the posterolateral spinal fusion using the sheep model. Uniaxial strain gauges measured hardware strain. Gauges were affixed using a waterproof coating on two opposing surfaces of 4.76-mm stainless steel rods. Rods were replaced with the strain-gauged rods before mechanical testing. The gauges were positioned equidistant from the screw-rod junctions and aligned sagittally on either rod and coronally on the other. Hardware strain decreases significantly starting at eight weeks.

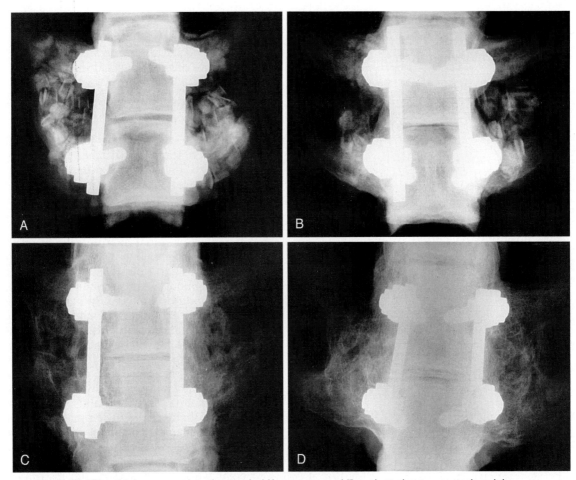

Figure 33–123. At the appropriate time period Kanayama et al.[57] evaluated anteroposterior plain radiographs of the posterolateral arthrodesis segments taken after sacrifice. *A*, Four weeks after surgery. All three observers graded this fusion as "D" (definitely not solid). *B*, Eight weeks after surgery. One observer graded this fusion as "B" (possibly solid), but the other two graded it as "C" (probably not solid) or "D". *C*, Twelve weeks after surgery. All observers graded this fusion as "A" (definitely solid). *D*, Sixteen weeks after surgery. All observers graded this fusion as "A".

than the uninstrumented fusion. At 16 weeks postoperatively, although instrumented fusions had a tendency to be stiffer than uninstrumented fusions, no statistical difference was observed between the two fusions. Using manual palpation, 85.7 per cent of instrumented fusions and 57.1 per cent of instrumented fusions were solid at eight weeks after surgery (Fig. 33–127A). All of the 16-week fusions were solid. Radiographically, fusion rates in the instrumented and uninstrumented segments were 47.2 ± 8.5 per cent versus 38.1 ± 29.8 per cent at eight weeks and 95.8 ± 7.2 per cent versus 91.7 ± 7.2 percent at 16 weeks postoperatively. Quantitative CT analysis showed that instrumented fusions had a greater mineralized fusion mass volume than the uninstrumented segments at eight and 16 weeks postoperatively (Fig. 33–127B). Histologically, the eight-week fusion mass at the instrumented level had more woven bone formation and less fibrous stroma than the uninstrumented fusion segment (Fig. 33–128). At 16 weeks, both instrumented and uninstrumented levels were demonstrated as trabeculated bony bridges.

Internal fixation has not been shown to accelerate the healing process in long-bone fractures[96]; however, recent clinical studies suggest that rigid spinal instrumentation not only increases the fusion rate but also shortens the time to union of a posterolateral spinal fusion.[62, 121] To our knowledge, there is a paucity of biomechanical and histologic data regarding whether instrumentation speeds up the spinal fusion process. Our study demonstrated that instrumented fusions had higher stiffness, higher union rate, and better histologic properties than uninstrumented fusions in the early postoperative period (eight weeks after surgery). Moreover, this suggests that transpedicular screw fixation expedites the healing process of the posterolateral spinal fusion.

Effects of Spinal Fixation and Destabilization on the Biomechanical and Histologic Properties of Lumbar Spinal Ligaments

The combination of these studies highlighting maturation of the instrumented and uninstrumented postero-

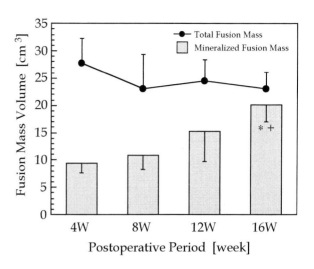

Figure 33–124. Kanayama et al.[57] demonstrated that mineralization of the fusion mass increased in a linear fashion even after eight weeks despite having achieved sufficient mechanical strength. Quantitative CT analysis of the posterolateral spinal fusion mass (p < .01, one-way ANOVA and Scheffe's F-test). There were no significant changes in the total fusion mass volume (p = .257, one-way ANOVA). +, p < .01 versus eight weeks; *, p < .01 versus four weeks.

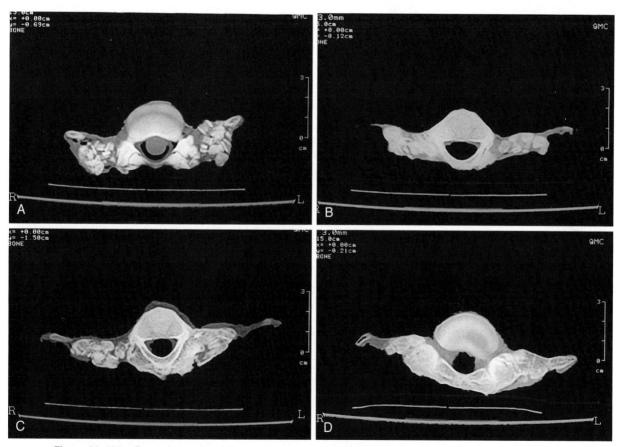

Figure 33–125. From the study of Kanayama et al.,[57] CT scans of the posterolateral arthrodesis segments at the four-, eight-, 12-, and 16-week postoperative periods were obtained. CT sections were taken at the intervertebral disc level. Although the four-week fusion mass was only morselized bone chips surrounded by soft tissue (A), bone graft was gradually incorporated at eight (B) and 12 weeks (C) after surgery. Solid bony fusion mass was confirmed at 16 weeks after surgery (D).

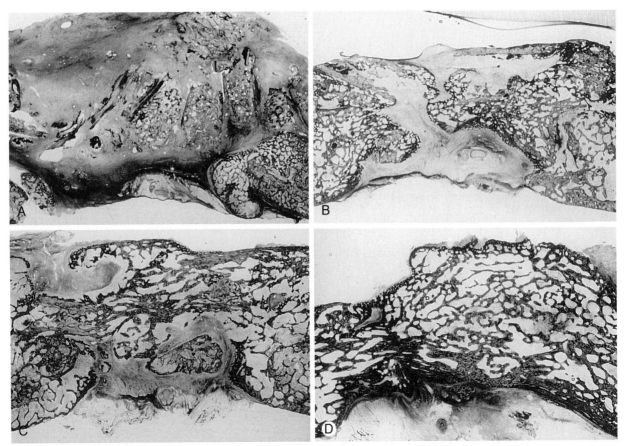

Figure 33–126. Kanayama et al.[57] obtained histologic parasagittal section of the posterolateral fusion mass (Osteochrome Villanueva Bone Stain, × 1). *A,* At four weeks, the fusion mass was primarily composed of bone graft chips and fibrous stroma. *B,* At eight weeks, woven bone formation was predominantly observed within the fusion mass. *C,* At 12 weeks, partly trabeculated bony fusion mass bridged between the transverse processes but was still immature. *D,* At 16 weeks, the entire fusion mass area was composed of trabeculated bone.

lateral arthrodesis and others[18, 57, 58, 80, 81, 111] provides an extensive survey of the functional spinal unit stability following arthrodesis of the two-vertebrae motion segment. No studies have investigated the effects of spinal destabilization and instrumentation on the biomechanical and histologic properties of spinal ligaments. Recent studies have documented neuronal innervations of several spinal ligaments, suggesting the importance of their neurosensory role for determining and controlling vertebral motions.[95, 120] Spinal ligaments serve a vital role in the structural stability of the spine, and these passive structures, abundantly supplied with pain-sensitive nerve endings (nociceptors),[47, 98] may possibly be a source of pain if overstretched or ruptured. Although several authors have reported on the biomechanical properties of spinal ligaments,[98, 121] there have been no studies investigating changes in spinal ligament properties secondary to conditions of spinal destabilization and instrumentation.

To analyze the effects of spinal fixation and destabilization as well as surgical intervention itself on the biomechanical and histologic properties of spinal ligaments, Kotani et al.[66] developed an in vivo animal model of spinal destabilization and instrumentation. In this study, mature sheep were divided into four groups: Group I, nonsurgical control; Group II, sham operation consisting of bilateral posterolateral exposure at L4–L5; Group III, spinal fixation using transpedicular screws and plates and bilateral posterolateral bone graft at L4–L5; and Group IV, spinal destabilization consisting of bilateral facetectomies and anterior discectomy at L4–L5. Four months postoperatively, biomechanical analysis of specimens included destructive tensile testing of four different bone-ligament-bone complexes (Fig. 33–129): anterior longitudinal ligament (ALL), posterior longitudinal ligament (PLL), ligamentum flavum (LF), and supraspinous and interspinous ligaments combined (SSL & ISL) at the operative and proximal adjacent levels, with calculation of ultimate tensile load and elastic modulus. Quantitative histomorphometric analyses of the vertebral body and spinal ligaments were also performed.

Biomechanical analysis demonstrated remarkable changes in the structural and mechanical properties of the operative level ligament. The fixation group ligaments demonstrated significant decreases in the ul-

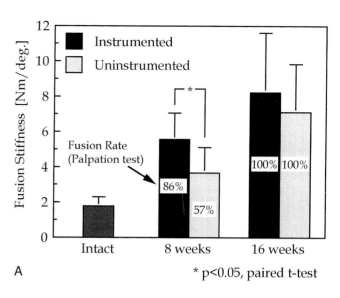

Figure 33–127. Kanayama et al.[58] investigated the effect of spinal instrumentation on the healing process of posterolateral spinal fusion, through the biomechanical, radiographic, and histologic comparison of instrumented versus uninstrumented fusions. A total of 15 adult sheep underwent posterior spinal column destabilization and posterolateral spinal arthrodesis with autologous bone at the L2–L3 and L4–L5 segments. Randomly, one of those segments was augmented bilaterally with TSRH transpedicular screw fixation. The current study demonstrated that instrumented fusions had higher stiffness, higher union rate, and better histologic properties than uninstrumented fusions in the early postoperative period (eight weeks after surgery). Moreover, this suggests that transpedicular screw fixation expedites the healing process of the posterolateral spinal fusion. *A,* This chart compares the functional spinal unit stiffness of instrumented and uninstrumented posterolateral spinal fusions under flexion-extension loading. At the eight-week postoperative time period, differences are observed between the two fusion techniques ($p < .05$, paired t-test). However, no differences are discernible at the 16-week postoperative time interval. The manual palpation fusion rates (%) are based on assessment from three independent observers. *B,* Quantitative CT analysis by Kanayama et al.[58] showed the instrumented fusions as having greater mineralized fusion mass volume than the uninstrumented fusions at both eight and 16 weeks postoperatively ($p < .05$).

Quantitative CT Evaluation of the Posterolateral Spinal Fusion Mass:

Mineralized Fusion Mass Volume (% to Total Volume)			
	Instrumented		Uninstrumented
8 Weeks	61 +- 8.6%	---*---	52.6 +- 9.7%
16 Weeks	83.0 +- 5.9%	---*---	76.0 +- 6.5%

* $p < 0.05$ Paired T-Test

B

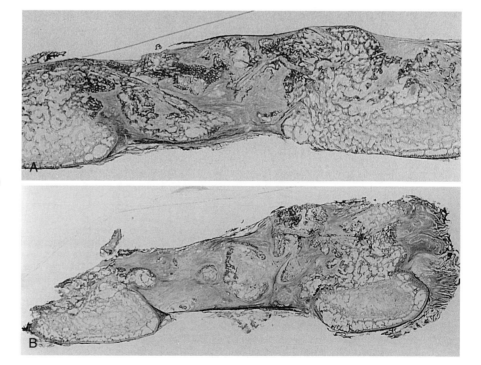

Figure 33–128. Undecalcified histologic sagittal sections of the eight-week instrumented fusion mass *(A)* from Kanayama et al.[58] demonstrated more woven bone formation and less fibrous stroma than the uninstrumented fusion sites *(B)* at the same time interval. At 16 weeks postoperatively, both the instrumented and uninstrumented fusions were observed as trabeculated bony bridges.

Figure 33–129. The biomechanical testing set-up used by Kotani et al.[66] for destructive tensile testing of four different spinal bone-ligament-bone complexes.

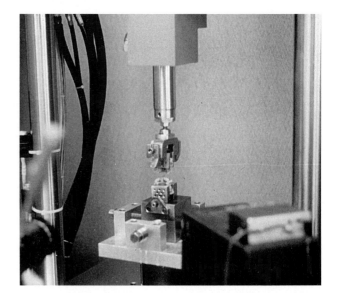

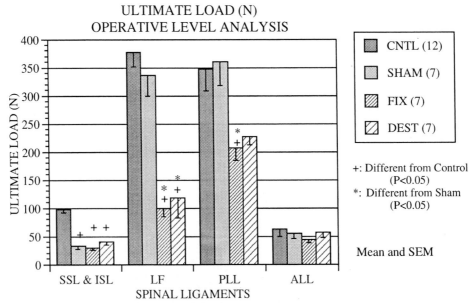

Figure 33–130. Kotani et al.[66] developed an in vivo animal model of spinal destabilization and instrumentation to analyze the effects of spinal fixation and destabilization as well as surgical intervention itself (SHAM) on the biomechanical and histologic properties of spinal ligaments. This serves as the first study to demonstrate changes in the biomechanical and histologic properties of spinal ligaments secondary to the surgical procedures of spinal fixation, destabilization, and surgical intervention itself. The "stress shielding" effects of spinal instrumentation occur not only in the vertebral bone, but also within spinal ligaments. This investigation demonstrated that posterior spinal instrumentation and fusion lead to decreases in cross-sectional area, tensile strength, elastic stiffness, and elastic modulus of the operative level ligamentum flavum, posterior longitudinal ligament, and interspinous and supraspinous ligaments. Comparison of the ultimate or peak tensile failure load of four different operative level bone-ligament-bone complexes. Importantly, changes in the tensile strength properties of the fixation group ligaments are demonstrated (p < .05). The fixation group ligaments demonstrated significant decreases in the ultimate failure load, compared with the control. The failure load of the fixation group operative level ligaments exhibited stress-shielded values of 26 per cent for LF, 30% for SSL and ISL, and 59% for the PLL when compared with the control. ALL, anterior longitudinal ligament; PLL, posterior longitudinal ligament; LF, ligamentum flavum; SSL & ISL, supraspinous and interspinous ligaments combined. Four groups included a nonsurgical control (CNTL) (n = 12). SHAM, sham operation consisting of bilateral posterolateral exposure at L4–L5 (n = 8); FIX, spinal fixation using transpedicular screws and plates and bilateral posterolateral bone graft at L4–L5 (n = 8); DEST, spinal destabilization consisting of bilateral facetectomies and anterior diskectomy at L4–L5 (n = 8).

Table 33–6. CORRECTION OF KYPHOSIS

Author (Year)	Surgical Technique	Mean Follow-up (in Months)	Number of Patients	Mean Kyphosis in Degrees		
				Preop	Postop	Follow-up
Convery (1978)	Harrington rods	16	24	17	5	15
McEvoy (1985)	Harrington rods	12	53	16		16
Edwards (1986)	Rod-sleeve	12	135	14	0	0.5
Roman (1986)	Harrington rod	36	36	28	10	14
Kinnard (1986)	Plates	24	21	Loss of correction greater than 10° in 5 patients		
Aebi (1987)	Fixateur	12	30	15.8	3.5	7.1
Karlström (1990)	Olerud	24	37	11.0	−2.0	7.0
Crutcher (1991)	Jacobs		44	13.3	−1.0	?
Daniaux (1991)	VSP plate	38	172	Mean loss of correction of 9.3°		
Ebelke (1991)	VSP plate	17	21	12.7	0.0	7.4
Esses (1991)	Fixateur	17	89	18.8	2.7	?
Lindsey (1991)	Fixateur	35	80	17	6.0	14.5
Sasso (1991)	Plates	20	23	10.8	6.2	13.0
Chang (1992)	RF system	24	33	21	0.0	0.0
Hardaker (1992)	Harrington	43	58	15	5	8
Sim (1992)	Fixateur	25	27	8.6	−2.7	6.4
Willen (1992)	Harrington	12	26	18	7	?
McLain (1993)	CD screws	15	19	Mean loss of correction of 7.4°		

From McAfee, P.C., Levine, A.M., and Anderson, P.A.: Surgical management of thoracolumbar fractures. AAOS Instructional Course Lectures *44*:49, 1995.

timate failure load compared to the control. The failure load of the fixation group operative level ligaments exhibited stress-shielded values of 26 per cent for LF, 30 per cent for SSL & ISL, and 59 per cent for the PLL when compared to the control (Fig. 33–130). Histologically, the fixation group ligamentum flavum revealed a marked vacuolation in the ligament substance, while the ISL demonstrated remarkable insertion changes compared with small substance changes.

The adaptation and regulating mechanisms of musculoskeletal soft tissues other than the spine have been extensively investigated.[68, 94, 120] Kotani et al.[66] showed a maximum decrease of 74 per cent in the ultimate failure load and 91 per cent decrease in the elastic modulus for the fixation group ligamentum flavum in lieu of only a 36 per cent decrease in volumetric density of bone for the spanned vertebral body. These findings may indicate that spinal ligaments are more responsive to mechanical changes when compared with vertebral bone. This serves as the first study to demonstrate changes in the biomechanical and histologic properties of spinal ligaments secondary to the surgical procedures of spinal fixation, destabilization, and surgical intervention itself. The stress-shielding effects of spinal instrumentation occur not only in the vertebral bone[80] but also within spinal ligaments. In this investigation, Kotani et al.[66] found that posterior spinal instrumentation and fusion led to decreases in cross-sectional area, tensile strength, elastic stiffness, and elastic modulus of the operative level ligamentum flavum, posterior longitudinal ligament, and interspinous and supraspinous ligaments. The altered biomechanical environment produced by spinal fixation, surgical intervention itself, or, conversely, unphysiologic immobilization can effect the ligamentous properties in vivo, possibly serving as the impetus for low back pain.

CONCLUSION

The goals of surgical treatment are to protect the neural structures from further injury, reduce fractures and dislocations, stabilize the spine, and, in the long term, achieve a stable, painless spine. The surgeon must accurately identify the fracture pattern and plan a technique that best reverses the abnormal biomechanics. The specific procedure should reduce the malalignment in all three planes and provide sufficient stability to allow fracture and bone graft healing without redisplacement. This should be accomplished with a minimal number of levels fused. Postoperative braces are used in most cases, although patients are rapidly mobilized. Second-stage decompressive or stabilization procedures are indicated to maximize neurologic recovery or maintain alignment. Complications are avoided by meticulous technique, selection of appropriate procedures, and careful postoperative care.

References

1. Aebi, M., Etter, C., Kehl, T., Thalgott, J.: Stabilization of the lower thoracic and lumbar spine with internal spinal skeletal fixation system: Indications, techniques and first results of treatment. Spine *12*:544–551, 1987.
2. Akbarnia, B. A., Mardjetko, S. M., Kostial, P. N.: Results of anterior spinal fusion and Kaneda instrumentation using tricorticate iliac allograft, a two year follow up. Ortho. Trans. *17*:123, 1993.
3. An, H., Simpson, J., Ebraheim, N., Jackson, W., et al.: Low lumbar burst fractures: Comparison between conservative and surgical treatments. Orthopedics *15*:367–373, 1992.
4. Ashman, R. B., Johnston, C. E., Corin, J. D.: Pedicle screw plate junction: Susceptibility to fatigue fracture. Transactions of the Scoliosis Research Society 145, 1987.
5. Bell, G. H., Dunbar, O., Beck, J. S., Gibb, A.: Variation in strength of vertebrae with age and their relation to osteoporosis. Calcif. Tiss. Res. *1*:75, 1967.
6. Benson, D. R., Burkus, J. K., Montesano, P. X., et al.: Unstable

thoracolumbar and lumbar burst fractures treated with the AO fixateur interne. J. Spinal Disord. 5:335–343, 1992.

7. Berlanda, P., Bassi, G.: Surgical treatment of traumatic spinal injuries with cord damage: Clinical review of 12 years of experience with Roy-Camille technique. Ital. J. Orthopaed. Trauma 17:491–498, 1991.

8. Blumenthal, S., Gill, K.: Complications of the Wiltse pedicle screw fixation system. Spine 18:1867–1871, 1993.

9. Boden, S. D., Schimandle, J. H., and Hutton, W. C.: An experimental lumbar intertransverse process spinal fusion model. Radiographic, histologic, and biomechanical healing characteristics. Spine 20:412–420, 1995.

10. Bridwell, K. W., et al.: Role of fusion and instrumentation in the treatment of degenerative spondylolisthesis. J. Spinal Disord. 6:461–472, 1993.

11. Broom, M., Jacobs, R. R.: Current status of internal fixation of thoracolumbar fractures. J. Orthop. Trauma 3:148–155, 1989.

12. Camissa, F. P., Eismont, F. J., Green, A. B.: Dural laceration occurring with burst fractures and associated laminar fractures. J. Bone Joint Surg. 71A:1044–1052, 1989.

13. Carl, A., Thromanhauser, S., Roger, D.: Pedicle screw instrumentation for thoracolumbar burst fractures and fracture-dislocations. Spine 17:S317–S324, 1992.

14. Chang, K.: A reduction-fixation system for unstable thoracolumbar burst fractures. Spine 17:879–886, 1992.

15. Cigliano, A., de Falco, R., Scarano, E., et al.: A new instrumentation system for the reduction and posterior stabilization of unstable thoracolumbar fractures. Neurosurgery 30:208–216; discussion, 216–217, 1992.

16. Convery, F., Minteer, M., Smith, R., Emerson, S.: Fracture-dislocation of the dorsal-lumbar spine, acute operative stabilization by Harrington instrumentation. Spine 3:160–166, 1978.

17. Cotterill, P. C., Kostuik, J. P., Wilson, J. A., et al.: Production of a reproducible spinal burst fracture for use in biomechanical testing. J. Orthop. Res. 5:462–465, 1987.

18. Craven, T. G., Carson, W. L., Asher, M. A., Robinson, R. G.: The effects of implant stiffness on the bypassed bone mineral density and facet fusion stiffness of the canine spine. Spine 19(15):1664–1673, 1994.

19. Crutcher, J. P. Jr., Anderson, P. A., King, H. A., Montesano, P. X.: Indirect spinal canal decompression in patients with thoracolumbar burst fractures treated by posterior distraction rods. J. Spinal Disord. 4:39–48, 1991.

20. Cunningham, B. W., Kanayama, M., Parker, L. M., et al.: Osteogenic protein versus autologous fusion in the sheep thoracic spine. A comparative endoscopic study using the BAK interbody fusion device. Trans. Orthopaed. Res. Soc. 21:117–120, 1996.

21. Cunningham, B. W., Sefter, J. C., Shono, Y., McAfee, P. C.: Static and cyclical biomechanical analysis of pedicle screw spinal constructs. Spine 18(12):1677–1688, 1993.

22. Daniaux, H., Seykora, P., Genelin, A., et al.: Application of posterior plating and modifications in thoracolumbar spine injuries: Indication, techniques and results. Spine 16:S125–S133, 1991.

23. Dekutoski, M. B., Conlan, E. S., Salciccioli, G. G.: Spinal mobility and deformity after Harrington rod stabilization and limited arthrodesis of thoracolumbar fractures. J. Bone Joint Surg. 75A:168–176, 1993.

24. Denis, F.: The three column spine and its significance in the classification of acute thoracolumbar spinal injuries. Spine 8:817–831, 1983.

25. Denis, F.: Spinal instability as defined by the three-column spine concept in acute spinal trauma. Clin. Orthop. 189:65–76, 1984.

26. Dickson, J. H., Harrington, P. R., Erwin, W. D.: Results of reduction and stabilization of the severely fractured thoracic and lumbar spine. J. Bone Joint Surg. 60A:799–805, 1978.

27. Doer, T., Montesano, P. X., Burkus, J., Benson, D. R.: Spinal canal decompression in traumatic thoracolumbar burst fractures: Posterior distraction rods versus transpedicular screw fixation. J. Orthopaed. Trauma 6:403–411, 1991.

28. Ebelke, D. K., Asher, M. A., Neff, J. R., Kraker, D. P.: Survivorship analysis of VSP spine instrumentation in the treatment of thoracolumbar and lumbar burst fractures. Spine 16:S428–S432, 1991.

29. Edwards, C. C.: Thoracolumbar trauma: Posterior reduction and fixation with a modular spinal system. Semin. Spine Surg. 2:8–18, 1990.

30. Edwards, C. C., Levine, A. M.: Early rod-sleeve stabilization of the injured thoracic and lumbar spine. Orthop. Clin. North Am. 17:121–145, 1986.

31. Eismont, F. J., Garfin, S. R., Abitbol, J. J.: Thoracic and upper lumbar spine injuries. In Browner, B. D., Levine, A. M., Jupiter, J. B., and Trafton, P. G. (eds.): Skeletal Trauma. Philadelphia, W. B. Saunders, 1992, pp. 729–804.

32. Esses, S. I., Botsford, D. J., Wright, T., et al.: Operative treatment of spinal fractures with the AO internal fixator. Spine 16:S146–S150, 1991.

33. Floman, Y., Fast, A., Pollack, D., et al.: The simultaneous application of an interspinous compressive wire and Harrington distraction rods in the treatment of fracture-dislocation of the thoracic and lumbar spine. Clin. Orthop. 205:207–215, 1986.

34. Frederickson, B. E., Edwards, W. T., Rauschning, W., et al.: Vertebral burst fractures: An experimental, morphologic and radiographic study. Spine 17:1012–1021, 1992.

35. Frederickson, B. E., Mann, K. A., Yuan, H. A., Lubicky, J. P.: Reduction of the intracanal fragment in experimental burst fractures. Spine 13:267–271, 1988.

36. Garfin, S. R., Mowery, C. A., Guerra, J., Jr., Marshall, L. F.: Confirmation of the posterolateral technique to decompress and fuse thoracolumbar spine burst fractures. Spine 10:218–223, 1985.

37. Gellad, F. E., Levine, A., Joslyn, J. N., et al.: Pure thoracolumbar facet dislocation: Clinical features and CT appearance. Radiology 161:505–508, 1986.

38. Goldstein, J. A., McAfee, P. C.: Video-assisted thoracic surgery of the spine. Curr. Opin. Orthopaed. 7:54–60, 1996.

39. Goldstein, J. A., McAfee, P. C.: Minimally invasive endoscopic surgery of the lumbar spine. Operative Techniques in Orthopaedics 7(1):27–35, 1997.

40. Greenfield, R., III, Grant, R., Bryant, D.: Pedicle screw fixation in the management of unstable thoracolumbar spine injuries. Orthopaedic Review 21:701–706, 1992.

41. Gurr, K. R., McAfee, P. C., Shih, C. M.: Biomechanical analysis of anterior and posterior instrumentation systems following corpectomy. A calf spine model. J. Bone Joint Surg. 70A:1182–1191, 1988.

42. Gurwitz, G. S., Dawson, J. M., McNamara, M. J., et al.: Biomechanical analysis of three surgical approaches for lumbar burst fractures using short-segment instrumentation. Spine 18:977–982, 1993.

43. Guyer, D. W., Yuan, H. A., Werner, F., et al.: Biomechanical comparison of seven internal fixation devices for the lumbosacral junction. Spine 12:569, 1987.

44. Hardaker, W. T., Jr., Cook, W. A., Jr., Friedman, A. H., Fitch, R. D.: Bilateral transpedicular decompression and Harrington rod stabilization in the management of severe thoracolumbar burst fractures. Spine 17:162–171, 1992.

45. Harrington, P. R.: Surgical instrumentation for management of scoliosis. J. Bone Joint Surg. 42A:1448, 1960.

46. Harrington, R. M., Budorick, T., Hoyt, J., et al.: Biomechanics of indirect reduction of bone retropulsed into the spinal canal in vertebral fracture. Spine 18:1–8, 1993.

47. Hirsh, L., Ingelmark, B. E., Miller, M.: The anatomical basis for low back pain. Studies on the presence of sensory nerve endings in ligamentous, capsular and intervertebral disc structures in the human lumbar spine. Acta Orthop. Scand. 33:1–17, 1963.

48. Hurley, L. A., Stinchfield, F. E., Bassett, C. A. L., and Lyon, W. H.: The role of soft tissues in osteogenesis: An experimental study of canine spine fusions. J. Bone Joint Surg. 41A:1243–1254, 1959.

49. Jacobs, R. R., Casey, M. P.: Surgical management of thoracolumbar spinal injuries: General principles and controversial considerations. Clin. Orthop. 189:22–35, 1984.

50. Jacobs, R. R., Montesano, P. X.: Development of the locking hook spinal rod system. Orthopaedics 11:1415–1421, 1988.

51. Jinnah, R. H., Amstutz, H. C., Tooke, S. M., et al.: The UCLA Charnley Experience: A long term followup study using survival analysis. Clin. Orthop. 211:164–172, 1986.

52. Kahanovitz, N., Arnoczky, S. P., Hulse, D., and Shires, P. K.: The effect of postoperative electromagnetic pulsing on canine posterior spinal fusions. Spine *9:*273–279, 1984.

53. Kahonovitz, N., Bullough, P., Jacobs, R. R.: The effect of internal fixation without arthrodesis on human facet joint cartilage. Clin. Orthop. *189:*204, 1984.

54. Kaneda, K.: Anterior approach and Kaneda instrumentation for lesions of the thoracic and lumbar spine. *In* Bridwell, K. H., and DeWald, R. L (eds.): The Textbook of Spinal Surgery, Vol. 2. Philadelphia, J. B. Lippincott Co., 1991, pp. 959–990.

55. Kaneda, K., Abumi, K., Fujiya, K.: Burst fractures with neurologic deficits of the thoracolumbar spine, results of anterior decompression and stabilization with anterior instrumentation. Spine *9:*78–95, 1984.

56. Kanayama, M., Cunningham, B. W., Ng, J. T. W., et al.: Biomechanical analysis of anterior versus circumferential spinal reconstruction for various anatomical stages of tumor lesions. Unpublished Data.

57. Kanayama, M., Cunningham, B. W., Weis, J. C., et al.: Maturation of the posterolateral spinal fusion and its effect on strain within spinal instrumentation: An in vivo study. Trans. Orthopaed. Res. Soc. *21:*673, 1996.

58. Kanayama, M., Cunningham, B. W., Weis, J. C., et al.: Does rigid spinal instrumentation influence the healing process of posterolateral spinal fusion? An in vivo sheep model. Unpublished Data.

59. Karjalainen, M., Aho, A., Katevuo, K.: Operative treatment of unstable thoracolumbar fractures by the posterior approach with the use of Williams plates or Harrington rods. Int. Orthopaed. *16:*219–222, 1992.

60. Karlstrom, G., Olerud, S., Sjostrom, L.: Transpedicular fixation of thoracolumbar fractures. Contemp. Orthopaed. *20:*285–300, 1990.

61. Kinnard, P., Ghibely, A., Gordon, D., et al.: Roy-Camille plates in unstable spinal conditions: A preliminary report. Spine *11:*131–135, 1986.

62. Kornblatt, M. D., Casey, M. P., Jacobs, R. R.: Internal fixation in lumbosacral spine fusion. Clin. Orthop. Rel. Res. *203:*141–150, 1986.

63. Kotani, Y., Cunningham, B. W., Abumi, K., McAfee, P. C.: Biomechanical analysis of cervical stabilization systems: An assessment of transpedicular screw fixation in the cervical spine. Spine *19(22):*2529–2539, 1994.

64. Kotani, Y., Cunningham, B. W., Cappuccino, A., McAfee, P. C.: The role of spinal instrumentation in augmenting posterolateral fusion. Spine *21(3):*278–287, 1996.

65. Kotani, Y., Cunningham, B. W., Parker, L. M., et al.: Intrinsic biomechanical strength of anterior thoracolumbar spinal implant systems. Transactions of the Scoliosis Research Society, Asheville, North Carolina, 1995.

66. Kotani, Y., Cunningham, B. W., Cappuccino, A., McAfee, P. C.: The effect of spinal fixation and destabilization on the biomechanical and histological properties of spinal ligaments. An in vivo study. Trans. Orthopaed. Res. Soc. *20:*48, 1995.

67. Krag, M. H.: Biomechanics of thoracolumbar spinal fixation: A review. Spine *16:*S84–S99, 1991.

68. Laros, G. S., Tipton, C. M., and Cooper, R. R.: Influence of physical activity on ligament insertions in the knees of dogs. J. Bone Joint Surg. *53-A:*275–286, 1971.

69. Lemons, V., Wagner, J., Jr., Montesano, P. X.: Management of thoracolumbar fractures with accompanying neurologic injury. Neurosurgery *30:*667–671, 1992.

70. Levine, A. M.: Chap 30: Lumbar and sacral spine trauma. *In* Browner, B. D., Levine, A. M., Jupiter, J. B., and Trafton, P. G. (eds.): Skeletal Trauma. Philadelphia, W. B. Saunders, 1992, pp. 805–848.

71. Levine, A. M.: Dural lacerations associated with low lumbar burst fractures. American Academy of Orthopaedic Surgeons Meeting, Washington, DC, February 1992.

72. Levine, A. M., Bosse, M., and Edwards, C. C.: Bilateral facet dislocations in the thoracolumbar spine. Spine *13:*630–640, 1988.

73. Lindsey, R. W., Dick, W.: The Fixateur Interne in the reduction and stabilization of thoracolumbar spine fractures in patients with neurologic deficit. Spine *16:*S140–S145, 1991.

74. Liu, Y. K., Goel, V. K., DeJong, A., et al.: Torsional fatigue of the lumbar intervertebral joints. Spine *10:*894–900, 1985.

75. Lucas J. T., Ducker, T. B.: Motor classification of spinal cord injuries with mobility, morbidity and recovery indices. Am. Surg. *45:*151–158, 1979.

76. Mack, M. J., Regan, J. J., McAfee, P. C., et al.: Video-assisted thoracic surgery for the anterior approach to the thoracic spine. Ann. Thorac. Surg. *59:*1100–1106, 1995.

77. McAfee, P. C.: Complications following anterior approaches to the thoracolumbar spine: Emphasis on Kaneda instrumentation. Clin. Orthop. Rel. Res. *306:*110–119, 1996.

78. McAfee, P. C., and Bohlman, H. H.: Complications of Harrington instrumentation for fractures of the thoracolumbar spine. J. Bone Joint Surg. (Am) *67A(5):*672–686, 1985.

79. McAfee, P. C., Bohlman, H. B., and Yuan, H. A.: Anterior decompression of traumatic thoracolumbar fractures with incomplete neural deficit using a retroperitoneal approach. J. Bone Joint Surg. (Am) *67A(1):*89–104, 1985.

80. McAfee, P. C., Farey, I. D., Sutterlin, C. E., et al.: 1989 VOLVO Award for basic science research in low back pain. Device-related osteoporosis with spinal instrumentation. A canine model. Spine *14(9):*919–926, 1989.

81. McAfee, P. C., Farey, I. D., Sutterlin, C. E., et al.: The effect of spinal implant rigidity on vertebral bone density: A canine model. Spine *16(6S):*S190–S197, 1991.

82. McAfee, P. C., Regan, J. R., Fedder, I. L., et al.: Anterior thoracic corpectomy for spinal cord decompression performed endoscopically. Surg. Laparoscop. Endoscop. *5:*339–348, 1995.

83. McAfee, P. C., Regan, J. R., Zdeblick, T., et al.: The incidence of complications in endoscopic anterior thoracolumbar spinal reconstructive surgery. A prospective multicenter study comprising the first 100 consecutive cases. Spine *20:*1624–1632, 1995.

84. McAfee P. C., Weiland, D. J., Carlow, J. J.: Survivorship analysis of pedicle spinal instrumentation. Spine *16S:*S422–427, 1991.

85. McAfee, P. C., Yuan, H. A., Fredrickson, B. E., Lubicky, J. P.: The value of computed tomography in thoracolumbar fractures: An analysis of one hundred consecutive cases and a new classification. J. Bone Joint Surg. *65A:*461–473, 1983.

86. McBride, G. G.: Cotrel-Dubousset rods in surgical stabilization of spinal fractures. Spine *18:*466–473, 1993.

87. McCord, D. H., Cunningham, B. W., Shono, Y., et al.: Biomechanical analysis of lumbosacral fixation. Spine *17(8S):*S235–S243, 1992.

88. McEvoy, R. D., Bradford, D. S.: The management of burst fractures of the thoracic and lumbar spine: Experience in 53 patients. Spine *10:*631–637, 1985.

89. McLain, R. F., Sparling, E., Benson, D. R.: Early failure of short-segment pedicle instrumentation for thoracolumbar fractures: A preliminary report. J. Bone Joint Surg. *75:*162–167, 1993.

90. Mumford, J., Weinstein, J. N., Spratt, K. F., Goel, V. K.: Thoracolumbar burst fractures: The clinical efficacy and outcome of nonoperative management. Spine *18:*955–970, 1993.

91. Nachemson, A. L.: The influence of spinal movement on the lumbar intradiscal pressure and on the tensile stresses in the annulus fibrosis. Acta Orthop. Scand. *33:*183, 1963.

92. Nachemson, A. L.: Lumbar intradiscal pressure. Acta Orthop. Scand. Suppl. *43:*76–78, 1960.

93. Nachemson, A. L., and Evans, J. H.: Some mechanical properties of the third human lumbar interlaminar ligament. J. Biomechanics *1:*211–220, 1968.

94. Noyes, F. R.: Functional properties of knee ligaments and alterations induced by immobilization. A correlative biomechanical and histological study in primates. Clin. Orthop. *123:*210–242, 1977.

95. Panjabi, M. M.: The stabilizing system of the spine. Part I. Function, dysfunction, adaptation, and enhancement. J. Spinal Disord. *5:*383–389, 1992.

96. Perren, S. M.: Physical and biological aspects of fracture healing with special reference to internal fixation. Clin. Orthop. Rel. Res. *138:*175–196, 1979.

97. Perry, O.: Resistance and compression of the lumbar vertebrae. Encyclopedia of Medical Radiology. New York, Springer-Verlag, 1974.

98. Rhalmi, S., Yahia, L., Neuman, N., Isler, M.: Immunohistochemi-

cal study of nerves in lumbar spine ligaments. Spine 18:264–267, 1993.

99. Riebel, G. D., Yoo, J. U., Frederickson, B. E., Yuan, H. A.: Review of Harrington rod treatment of spinal trauma. Spine 18:479–491, 1993.

100. Rosenthal, R., Lowery, E.: Unstable fracture-dislocations of the thoracolumbar spine: Results of surgical treatment. J. Trauma 20:485–490, 1980.

101. Roy-Camille, R.: Posterior screw plate fixation in thoracolumbar injuries. A.A.O.S. Instructional Course Lectures 41:157–163, 1992.

102. Roy-Camille, R., Saillant, G., Mazel, C.: Plating of thoracic, thoracolumbar and lumbar injuries with pedicle screw plates. Orthop. Clin. North Am. 17:147–159, 1986.

103. Sasso, R. C., Cotler, H. B., Reuben, J. D.: Posterior fixation of thoracic and lumbar spine fractures using DC plates and pedicle screws. Spine 16:S134–S139, 1991.

104. Shirado, O., Zdeblick, T. A., McAfee, P. C., Cunningham, B. W., DeGroot, H., Warden, K. E.: Quantitative histologic study of the influence of anterior spinal instrumentation and biodegradable polymer on lumbar interbody fusion after corpectomy: A canine model. Spine 17(7):795–803, 1992.

105. Shono, Y., Cunningham, B. W., McAfee, P. C.: 1991 CSRS Resident Award Paper: A biomechanical analysis of decompression and reconstruction methods in the cervical spine—Emphasis on a carbon fiber composite. J. Bone Joint Surg. 75A(11):1674–1684, 1993.

106. Shono, Y., McAfee, P. C., Cunningham, B. W.: Experimental study of thoracolumbar burst fractures: A radiographic and biomechanical analysis of anterior and posterior instrumentation systems. Spine 19(15):1711–1722, 1994.

107. Sim, E.: Location of transpedicular screws for fixation of the lower thoracic and lumbar spine: Computed tomography of 45 fracture cases. Acta Orthop. Scand. 64:28–32, 1993.

108. Sim, E., Stergar, P.: The Fixateur Interne for stabilizing fractures of the thoracolumbar and lumbar spine. Intern. Orthop. 16:322–329, 1992.

109. Simpson, J., Ebraheim, N., Jackson, W., Chung, S.: Internal fixa-tion of the thoracic and lumbar spine using Roy-Camille plates. Orthopaedics 16:663–672, 1993.

110. Sjostrom, L., Jacobsson, O., Karlstrom, G., et al.: CT analysis of pedicles and screw tracts after implant removal in thoracolumbar fractures. J. Spinal Disorders 6:225–231, 1993.

111. Smith, K. R., Hunt, T. R., Asher, M. A., et al.: The effect of a stiff spinal implant on the bone-mineral content of the lumbar spine in dogs. J. Bone Joint Surg. 73A(1):115–123, 1991.

112. Steffee, A. D., Brantigan, J.: The VSP spinal fixation system: Report of a prospective study of 250 patients enrolled in FDA clinical trials. Ortho. Trans. 18:250, 1994.

113. Thomas, I., Kirkaldy-Willis, W. H., Singh, S., and Paine, K. W.: Experimental spinal fusion in guinea pigs and dogs: The effect of immobilization. Clin. Orthop. 112:363–375, 1975.

114. Viale, G., Silvestro, C., Francaviglia, N., et al.: Transpedicular decompression and stabilization of burst fractures of the lumbar spine. Surg. Neurol. 40:104–111, 1993.

115. Tkaczuk, H.: Tensile properties of human lumbar longitudinal ligaments. Acta Orthop. Scand. Suppl. 115:1–69, 1968.

116. West, J. L., Bradford, D. S., Ogilvie, J. W.: Steffee instrumentation: Two year results. Transactions of the Scoliosis Research Society, Baltimore, Maryland, 1988.

117. West, J. L., Ogilvie, J. W., Bradford, D. S.: Complications of the variable screw plate pedicle screw fixation. Spine 16:576–579, 1991.

118. Willen, J.: Unstable thoracolumbar injuries. Orthopaedics 15:329–335, 1992.

119. Willen, J., Lindahl, S., Irstam, L., Nordwall, A.: Unstable thoracolumbar fractures: A study by CT and conventional roentgenography of the reduction effect by Harrington instrumentation. Spine 9:214–219, 1984.

120. Woo, S. L. Y., Gomez, M. A., Sites, T. J., et al.: The biomechanical and morphological changes in the medial collateral ligament of the rabbit after immobilization and remobilization. J. Bone Joint Surg. 69-A:1200–1211, 1987.

121. Yuan, H. A., Garfin, S. R., Dickman, C. A., Mardjetko, S. M.: A historical cohort study of pedicle screw fixation in thoracic, lumbar, and sacral spinal fusions. Spine 20S:2279S–2296S, 1994.

122. Zdeblick, T. A.: A prospective, randomized study of lumbar fusion: Preliminary results. Spine 18:983–991, 1993.

34

Biomechanical Considerations of Spinal Stability

Mark Bernhardt, M.D.

Augustus A. White III, M.D., D. Med. Sci.

Manohar M. Panjabi, Ph.D., D. Tech.

The spine is a mechanical structure. The vertebrae articulate with one another in a controlled manner through a complex system of levers (vertebrae), pivots (facets and discs), passive restraints (ligaments), and activators (muscles). A comprehensive knowledge of spinal biomechanics is of paramount importance for the understanding of all aspects of the clinical analysis and management of spinal problems. A basic understanding of the terms and engineering concepts applicable to orthopedic biomechanics is a prerequisite. A short glossary of these terms and concepts is presented at the end of the chapter as a foundation for the discussion to follow.

PHYSICAL PROPERTIES AND FUNCTIONAL BIOMECHANICS OF THE INTERVERTEBRAL DISC

The three basic functions of the spine are to transmit load, allow motion, and protect the vital spinal cord. The anatomy of the spine appears to optimally provide for these functions. The spine consists of seven cervical vertebrae, twelve thoracic vertebrae, five lumbar vertebrae, five fused sacral vertebrae, and three to four fused coccygeal segments. When viewed in the frontal plane, the spine generally appears straight and symmetric. The sagittal plane reveals four normal curves. These curves are anteriorly convex in the cervical and lumbar regions and posteriorly convex in the thoracic and sacrococcygeal regions. There is a mechanical basis for these normal anatomic curves; they give the spinal

column increased flexibility and augmented shock-absorbing capacity while maintaining adequate stiffness and stability at the intervertebral joint level.

The intervertebral disc is subjected to a variety of forces and moments. Along with the facet joints, it is responsible for carrying all the compressive loading to which the trunk is subjected.[29, 52] Certain portions of the disc are subjected to tensile stresses during the physiologic motions of flexion, extension, and lateral bending. Axial rotation of the torso with respect to the pelvis causes torsional loads that result in shear stresses in the disc. Because rotation and bending are known to be coupled, the stresses in the disc are a combination of tensile, compressive, and shear stresses with these motions.

Compression Characteristics of the Disc

The compressive load is transferred from one vertebral body end plate to the other by way of the nucleus pulposus and the annulus fibrosus. In the early years of life (up to age 30), the nucleus has sufficient moisture to act like a gelatinous mass.[4, 44, 53] As the load is applied, a certain pressure is developed within the nucleus. This fluid pressure pushes the surrounding structures in all directions away from the nucleus center (Fig. 34-1A). The compression produces complex stresses within the annular ring, as shown in Figure 34-1B. The situation is different when the nucleus is dry (Fig. 34-2). The load-transferring mechanism is significantly altered, because the nucleus is not capable of building sufficient fluid pressure. As a result, the end plates are subjected to less pressure at the center, and the loads are distributed more around the periphery. The stresses in the annular ring are also changed (see Fig. 34–2*B*.) In the outer layers of the annulus of a degenerated disc, there is less peripheral tension, more axial stress, and much more fiber stress.

Virgin observed that although discs showed permanent deformation when subjected to high compressive loads, there was no herniation of the nucleus pulposus.[63] Even when a longitudinal incision was made in the posterolateral part of the annulus fibrosus all the way to the center and the specimen was loaded in compression, there was little change in the elastic properties and definitely no disc herniation. This work, as

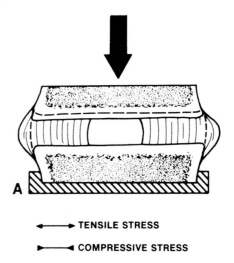

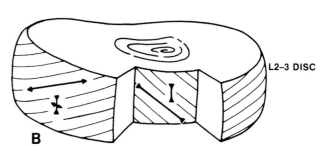

TENSILE STRESS

COMPRESSIVE STRESS

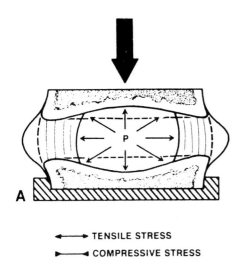

TENSILE STRESS

COMPRESSIVE STRESS

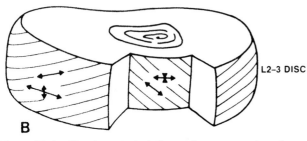

L2–3 DISC

Figure 34–1. Nondegenerated disc under compression. *A,* Pressure within the nucleus is produced by compression. This pressure pushes the disc annulus and the two end plates outward. The disc bulges out in the horizontal plane, and the end plates deflect in the axial direction. *B,* The annulus is subjected to varying amounts of stresses in different directions and at different depths. In the outer layers there is a large tensile stress along the annulus fibers and a relatively small tensile stress in the axial direction. In the inner layers of the annulus the stresses are generally smaller in magnitude but are of the same type, except for the axial stress, which is now compressive. (Based on mathematical simulations by Kulak, R. F., Belytschko, T. B., Schultz, A. B., and Galante, G. O.: Nonlinear behavior of the human intervertebral disc under axial load. J. Biomech. *9:*377, 1976. From White, A. A., III, and Panjabi, M. M.: Clinical Biomechanics of the Spine. 2nd ed. Philadelphia, J. B. Lippincott Co., 1990.)

Figure 34–2. Degenerated disc under compression. *A,* The compressive load is carried through a different mechanism. The load is transferred from one end plate to the other by way of the annulus only, thus loading the end plates at the periphery. *B,* The stresses in the degenerated disc annulus are significantly different from those in the nondegenerated disc (see Fig. 34–1). In the outer layers of the disc, tangential (peripheral) stress is much smaller, but the annulus fibers are subjected to nearly twice as much stress. Further, the axial stress is smaller but compressive. In the inner layers the fiber stress remains very high, but now it is compressive. (Based on mathematical simulations by Kulak, R. F., Belytschko, T. B., Schultz, A. B., and Galante, G. O.: Non-linear behavior of the human intervertebral disc under axial load. J. Biomech. *9:*377, 1976. From White, A. A., III, and Panjabi, M. M.: Clinical Biomechanics of the Spine. 2nd ed. Philadelphia, J. B. Lippincott Co., 1990.)

well as additional experiments by Hirsch,[29] Markolf and Morris,[40] and Farfan and associates,[19] suggests that disc herniation is not caused by excessive compressive loading, although Schmorl's nodes may be the result of such loading. This implies that the tendency for the disc to herniate posterolaterally, as seen in the clinical situation, is *not* inherent in the structure of the disc but must depend on certain loading situations other than compression.

Tensile Properties of the Disc

Although clinically the disc is never loaded purely in tension, tensile forces are applied to parts of the disc during physiologic motions. Markolf studied the tensile properties of the disc as a structure and found that the disc was less stiff in tension than under compression.[39] This was attributed to the buildup of fluid pressure within the nucleus under compression loading. Also, because of both the fluid nature of the nucleus and Poisson's effect, the disc bulges during compression and contracts in tension.

Bending Characteristics of the Disc

The spine is subjected to tension on its convex side and compression on its concave side when bending loads are applied during flexion, extension, and lateral bending. Thus, bending loads can be thought of as a combination of tensile and compressive loads, each applied to about half of the disc.

Bending and torsional loads are of particular interest, because experimental findings suggest that these and not the compression loads are the most damaging to the disc.[19] Bending 6 to 8 degrees in the sagittal, frontal, and other vertical planes did not result in failure of the lumbar disc; however, after removal of the posterior elements and with 15 degrees of bending (flexion), failure did occur.[6]

Torsional Behavior of the Disc

When the disc is subjected to torsion, there are shear stresses in the horizontal as well as the axial plane. The magnitude of these stresses varies in direct proportion to the distance from the axis of rotation (Fig. 34–3). In the planes between the horizontal and axial, there are other combinations of stresses.

The hypothesis that torsion may be the major injury-causing load was put forward by Farfan in 1973.[18] A vertebra-disc-vertebra construct (including posterior elements) was subjected to torsional loading around a fixed axis passing through the posterior aspect of the

disc. Torque was applied, and a continuous record was made of the applied torque and the angle of deformation until failure occurred. The torque angle curves were found to be sigmoidal, with three distinct phases. In the initial phase, 0 to 3 degrees of deformation could be produced by little torque. In the intermediate phase, consisting of 3 to 12 degrees of rotation, there was a linear relationship between the torque and the angular deformation. In the final phase, about 20 degrees of rotation was generally required to produce failure. The angle of failure was somewhat less for degenerated discs. Sharp cracking sounds emanating from the specimen were always noted before failure occurred. Farfan and associates found that the average failure torque for the normal discs was 25 per cent higher than that for the abnormal discs.[19]

Shear Characteristics of the Disc

Shear is the force that acts in the horizontal plane, perpendicular to the long axis of the spine. It produces shear stresses that are about equal in magnitude over the entire annulus and are parallel to the applied shear force.

The shear stiffness in the horizontal plane (anteroposterior and lateral directions) was found to be about 260 N/mm.[39] This is a high value and is clinically significant, showing that a large force is required to cause an abnormal horizontal displacement of a normal vertebral disc unit. This means that it is relatively rare for the annulus to fail clinically because of pure shear loading. Clinical evidence of annular disruption implies that the disc has most likely failed because of some combination of bending, torsion, and tension.

Creep and Relaxation Properties of the Disc

The intervertebral disc exhibits creep and relaxation.[30] Kazarian performed creep tests on functional spinal

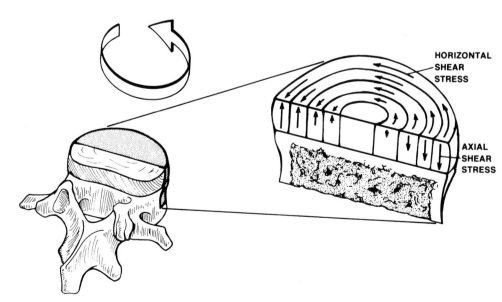

Figure 34–3. Disc stresses with torsion. Application of a torsional load to the disc produces shear stresses in the disc. These are in the horizontal plane as well as in the axial direction, and both are always of equal magnitude. However, they vary at different points in the disc in proportion to the distance from the instantaneous axis of rotation. (From White, A. A., III, and Panjabi, M. M.: Clinical Biomechanics of the Spine. 2nd ed. Philadelphia, J. B. Lippincott Co., 1990.)

HORIZONTAL SHEAR STRESS

AXIAL SHEAR STRESS

units (FSUs) and classified the discs of the specimens into four grades, from 0 to 3 according to their degree of degeneration.[33] He observed that the creep characteristics and the disc grades are related, as shown in Figure 34–4. The nondegenerated discs (Grade 0) creep slowly and reach their final deformation value after considerable time, compared with the degenerated discs (Grades 2 and 3). The Grade 0 curve is characteristic of a more viscoelastic structure, compared with the curves of Grades 2 and 3. Thus, the process of degeneration makes the disc less viscoelastic. This implies that as the disc degenerates, it loses the capability to attenuate shocks and to distribute the load over the entire end plate.

Hysteresis Properties of the Disc

All viscoelastic structures, including the disc and functional spinal unit, exhibit hysteresis. This is a phenomenon in which there is loss of energy when a structure is subjected to repetitive load and unload cycles. Hysteresis seems to vary with the load applied and the age of the disc, as well as its level: the larger the load, the greater the hysteresis. It is largest in very young people and least in the middle-aged. Virgin observed that the lower thoracic and upper lumbar discs showed less hysteresis than lower lumbar discs and that hysteresis decreased when the same disc was loaded a second time.[63]

Fatigue Tolerance of the Disc

Short-duration loading causes irreparable structural damage of the intervertebral disc when a stress of higher value than the ultimate failure stress is generated at a given point. The mechanism of failure during long-duration loading of relatively low magnitude is entirely different and is caused by fatigue failure. A tear develops at a point where the nominal stress is relatively high (but much less than the ultimate or even yield stress), and it eventually enlarges and results in complete disc failure.

Intradiscal Pressure

Nachemson and Morris first determined the actual loads to which a disc is subjected in vivo.[43] They measured the loads on the disc when a person is resting in different body postures or performing certain tasks. Some of their data are presented in Figure 34–5. Observe that the load carried by the disc is rather large. Although the portion of the body around the L3–L4 disc constitutes 60 per cent of the total body weight, the load in the L3–L4 disc, in sitting and standing positions with 20 degrees of flexion, is about 200 per cent. It becomes nearly 300 per cent with the addition of 20 kg of weight in the hands (Fig. 34–6).

KINEMATICS OF THE SPINE

The right-handed orthogonal (90-degree angle) coordinate system has been recommended for precise orientation about the body. Its orientation in space and its conventions are shown in Figure 34–7. Understanding the text is not dependent on following the conventions used here; however, they are helpful for more precise communication and understanding of the biomechanics literature.

Occipital–Atlantoaxial Complex (C0–C1–C2)

The occipital–atlantoaxial complex contains the most complex structures; they are unique and highly specialized. It is the transitional zone between the more standard vertebral design and the radically different skull. The three units maintain structural stability and at the same time combine to allow sizable quantities of motion in flexion-extension, lateral bending, and especially axial rotation. More free space for the spinal cord

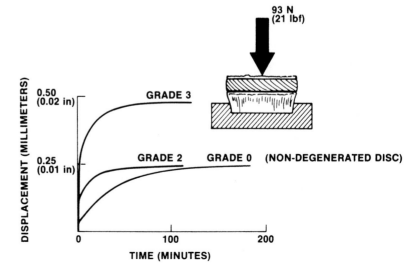

Figure 34–4. Creep behavior of the disc. The creep behavior of a structure is documented by applying a sudden load and maintaining it. The deformation of the structure as a function of time is recorded. This behavior seems to correlate with the degree of degeneration of the intervertebral disc. Sample creep curves for discs with different grades of degeneration are shown. The nondegenerated disc (Grade 0) has smaller overall deformation, and this deformation is reached over a relatively longer period, compared with the degenerated disc (Grade 3). (Based on data of Kazarian, L. E.: Creep characteristics of the human spinal column. Orthop. Clin. North Am. *6*:3, 1975. From White, A. A., III, and Panjabi, M. M.: Clinical Biomechanics of the Spine. 2nd ed. Philadelphia, J. B. Lippincott Co., 1990.)

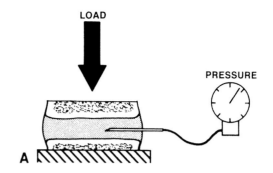

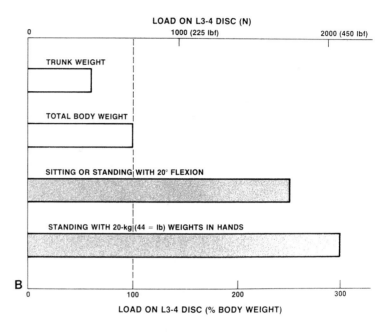

Figure 34–5. Intradiscal pressure and loads on the disc. *A,* The needle pressure transducer is calibrated by introducing it into the nucleus pulposus of cadaveric functional spinal units. A correlation is obtained between the compressive load applied and the pressure within the nucleus. *B,* Using the same needle transducers, in vivo measurements were made at the L3–L4 disc in volunteers performing physiologic tasks. The bar graphs record the compressive load on the disc. Note that the disc load during standing with a 20-kg weight in the hands is about three times the weight of the whole body. (Results based on those of Nachemson, A.: Electromyographic studies on the vertebral portion of the psoas muscle. Acta Orthop. Scand. *37:*177, 1966. From White, A. A., III, and Panjabi, M. M.: Clinical Biomechanics of the Spine. 2nd ed. Philadelphia, J. B. Lippincott Co., 1990.)

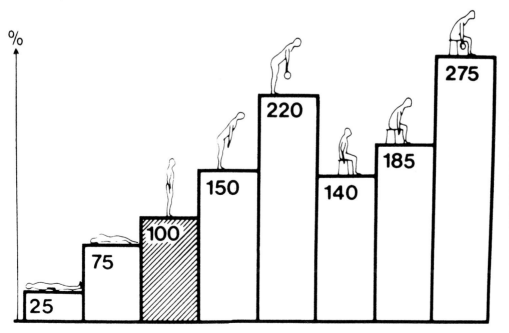

Figure 34–6. Diagrammatic comparison of in vivo loads (disc pressures) in the third lumbar disc during various activities. Note that sitting pressures are greater than standing pressures. (From Nachemson, A. L.: The lumbar spine, an orthopaedic challenge. Spine *1:*59, 1976.)

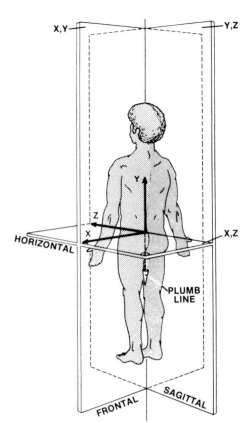

Figure 34–7. The suggested central coordinate system with its origin between the cornua of the sacrum is shown. Its orientation is as follows. The −Y axis is described by the plumb line dropped from the origin, and the +X axis points to the left at a 90-degree angle to the Y axis. The +Z axis points forward to a 90-degree angle to both the Y axis and the X axis. The human body is shown in the anatomic position. Some basic conventions are observed that make this a useful system. The planes are as shown: the sagittal plane is the Y, Z plane; the frontal plane is the Y, X plane; and the horizontal plane is the X, Z plane. Movements are described in relation to the origin of the coordinate system. The arrows indicate the positive direction of each axis. The origin is the zero point, and the direction opposite to the arrows is negative. Thus, direct forward translation is +Z; up is +Y; to the left is +X and to the right is −X; down is −Y; and backward is −Z. The convention for rotations is determined by imagining oneself at the origin of the coordinate system looking in the positive direction of the axis. Clockwise rotations are +θ and counterclockwise rotations are −θ. Thus, +θX is roughly analogous to flexion; +θZ is analogous to right lateral bending; and +θY is axial rotation toward the left. A coordinate system may be set up at any defined point parallel to the master system described. The location of the coordinate system should be clearly indicated for precise, accurate communications. In spinal kinematics, the motion is usually described in relation to the subjacent vertebra. The secondary coordinate system may be established in the body of the subjacent vertebra. For in vivo measurements, the tip of its spinous process may be used. (Reprinted from Journal of Biomechanics, Volume 7, M. M. Panjabi, A. A. White, and R. A. Brand, A note on defining body parts configurations, page 385, Copyright 1974, with kind permission from Elsevier Science Ltd, The Boulevard, Langford Lane, Kidlington OX5 IGB, UK.

is present here than anywhere else in the spine, thereby decreasing the risk of injury to the vital medullary structures in the area. Additionally, an anatomic mechanism for axial rotation has evolved in which the instantaneous axis of rotation is placed as close as possible to the spinal cord, permitting a large magnitude of rotation without any bony impingement on the spinal cord.

The representative figures for the ranges of motion for the units of the occipital–atlantoaxial complex are shown in Table 34–1. Both joints of the complex participate about equally during flexion-extension in total motion in the sagittal plane. The major axial rotation in the region is between C1 and C2, which contributes 40 to 50 per cent of the axial rotation of the entire cervical spine and occiput.

It is generally accepted that there is a strong coupling pattern at the atlantoaxial joint (Fig. 34–8). The axial (± θ Y axis) rotation of C1 is associated with vertical (± Y axis) translation. In 1858 Henke described it as a "double-threaded screw" joint.[28] This coupling is probably the result of the biconvex design of the C1–C2 articulation.

The instantaneous axes of rotation (IARs) for the CO–C1 articulation pass through the centers of the mastoid processes for flexion-extension and through a point 2 to 3 cm above the apex of the dens for lateral bending. Although until recently there was thought to be no horizontal plane (± θ Y) rotation at CO–C1, we now appreciate that there is a slight amount (5 degrees) of axial rotation, but no IAR has been determined to our knowledge. The IARs for the C1–C2 articulation

Table 34–1. REPRESENTATIVE VALUES OF THE RANGES OF ROTATION OF THE OCCIPITAL–ATLANTOAXIAL COMPLEX

Unit of Complex	Type of Motion	Degrees of Motion
Occipital–atlantal joint (C0–C1)	Combined flexion-extension (± ΘX)	25
	One-side lateral bending (ΘZ)	5
	One-side axial rotation (ΘY)	5
Atlantoaxial joint (C1–C2)	Combined flexion-extension (± ΘX)	20
	One-side lateral bending (ΘZ)	5
	One-side axial rotation (ΘY)	40

From White, A. A., III, and Panjabi, M. M.: Clinical Biomechanics of the Spine. 2nd ed. Philadelphia, J. B. Lippincott Co., 1990.

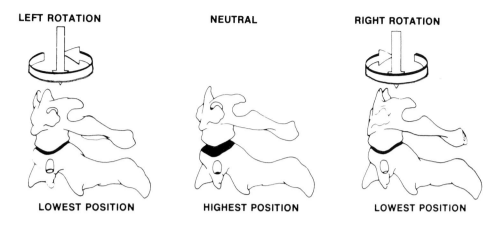

Figure 34–8. Atlantoaxial coupling pattern. Because of the anatomic design of the lateral articulations, C1 is highest in the middle position and lowest with the extremes of axial rotation to the right or the left. (From White, A. A., III, and Panjabi, M. M.: Clinical Biomechanics of the Spine 2nd ed. Philadelphia, J. B. Lippincott Co., 1990.)

are somewhere in the region of the middle third of the dens for flexion-extension and in the center of the dens for axial rotation. Lateral bending is negligible at C1–C2, making IAR determination moot.

Middle and Lower Cervical Spine (C2–T1)

The second cervical vertebra is also part of the middle cervical spine. In the middle and lower cervical re-

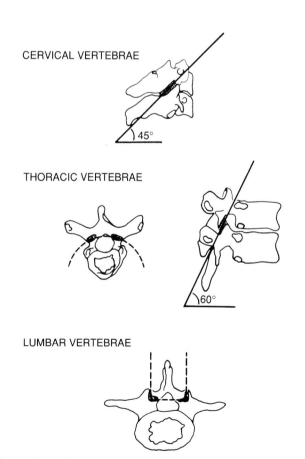

Figure 34–9. Characteristic facet orientation in the cervical, thoracic, and lumbar regions. The spatial alignment of the facet joints determines to a large extent, but not completely, the characteristic kinematics of different regions of the spine. (From White, A. A., III, and Panjabi, M. M.: Clinical Biomechanics of the Spine. 2nd ed. Philadelphia, J. B. Lippincott Co., 1990.)

gions, stability and mobility must be provided; at the same time, the vital spinal cord and, in most of this region, the vertebral arteries must be protected. There is a good deal of flexion-extension and lateral bending in this area.

The sagittal orientation of the facet joints (Fig. 34–9) is probably the cause of the distinct coupling pattern seen in this region (lateral bending and axial rotation). Because these joints are oriented at about a 45-degree angle to the vertical in the sagittal plane, the lateral bending results in axial rotation. During lateral bending to the left ($-\theta Z$), as the left inferior articular process of the upper vertebra moves down the 45-degree incline to the left, it is also displaced somewhat posteriorly. As the corresponding articular process on the right moves up the 45-degree incline on the right, it is displaced somewhat anteriorly. The total effect is an axial rotation such that the spinous process points to the right ($+\theta Y$).

Ranges of motion for the middle and lower cervical spine are shown in Table 34–2. Most of the flexion-extension motion is in the central region, with the C5–C6 FSU generally considered to have the greatest range. The maximal sagittal plane translation (Z axis) occurring in the lower cervical spine under physiologic loads is 2 to 2.7 mm.[66]

The coupling patterns in the middle and lower cervical spine are dramatic. The coupling is such that with lateral bending the spinous processes go to the convexity of the curve (Fig. 34–10).[38] At C2, there are 2 degrees of coupled axial rotation for every 3 degrees of lateral bending. Between C2 and C7, there is a gradual cephalocaudal decrease in the amount of axial rotation associated with lateral bending. This may be the result of a gradual cephalocaudal increase in the angle of incline of the facets in the sagittal plane in this area.

For sagittal and horizontal plane motion of the middle and lower cervical spine, the IARs are believed to lie in the anterior portion of the subjacent vertebrae. For lateral bending, they are probably in the middle of the subjacent vertebrae.

Thoracic Spine

The thoracic spine is a transitional region between the relatively more mobile cervical and lumbar regions. It

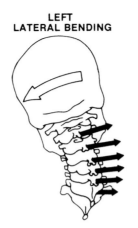
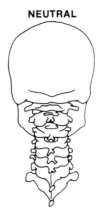
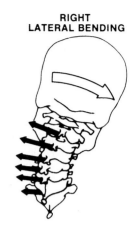

LEFT LATERAL BENDING   **NEUTRAL**   **RIGHT LATERAL BENDING**

Figure 34–10. An important, major cervical spine coupling pattern. When the head and neck are bent to the right, the spinous processes go to the left. The converse is also shown. Expressed in the coordinate system, +Z axis rotation is coupled with −Y axis rotation, and −Z axis rotation is coupled with +Y axis rotation. (From White, A. A., III, and Panjabi, M. M.: Clinical Biomechanics of the Spine. 1st ed. Philadelphia, J. B. Lippincott Co., 1978.)

appears to have been designed for rigidity, which is vital for general, erect bipedal support and for protection of the cord and the other organs in the thoracic cavity, and to facilitate the mechanical activities of the lungs and rib cage.

The upper thoracic spine is similar to the cervical region, and the lower thoracic spine is similar to the lumbar region. The upper thoracic vertebrae are relatively small, similar to those in the cervical spine. The spatial orientation of the facet joints is similar to that of the cervical spine, but the angulation in the sagittal plane is greater (see Fig. 34–9). The spatial orientation of the facet in the thoracic spine changes from the upper to the lower region. In a given individual, the spatial orientation of the facet joints may change abruptly to that seen in the lumbar region anywhere between T9 and T12.[26, 55] Because of these differences in facet orientation, the upper thoracic spine exhibits more axial rotation than the lower thoracic spine. In the lower thoracic spine, the vertebral bodies and the discs are larger.

The ranges of normal flexion-extension, lateral bend-

ing, and axial rotation for the thoracic spine are given in Table 34–3. There are approximately 4 degrees of flexion-extension at each level in the upper portion, 6 degrees in the middle segments, and 12 degrees in the lower portion (T11–T12 and T12–L1). With lateral bending, there are approximately 6 degrees of motion in the upper thoracic spine and 8 to 9 degrees in the middle and lower segments. In the horizontal plane (axial rotation), there are 8 to 9 degrees of motion in the upper half and 2 degrees for the three lower segments. This decreased range of axial rotation of the lower segments is undoubtedly because of the transition of the facet joints into a more constricting orientation, as seen in the lumbar spine.

The pattern of coupling in the thoracic spine is similar to that observed in the cervical spine. Lateral bending is coupled with axial rotation, such that the spinous processes move toward the convexity of the lateral curvature. In the upper portion of the thoracic spine, the two motions are strongly coupled, although not as strongly as in the cervical spine. In the middle and lower portions, the coupling patterns are by no means

Table 34–2. LIMITS AND REPRESENTATIVE VALUES OF RANGES OF ROTATION OF THE MIDDLE AND LOWER CERVICAL SPINE

Interspace	Combined Flexion-Extension (± X Axis Rotation)		One-Side Lateral Bending (Z Axis Rotation)		One-Side Axial Rotation (Y Axis Rotation)	
	Limits of Ranges (degrees)	Representative Angle (degrees)	Limits of Ranges (degrees)	Representative Angle (degrees)	Limits of Ranges (degrees)	Representative Angle (degrees)
Middle						
C2–C3	5–16	10	11–20	10	0–10	3
C3–C4	7–26	15	9–15	11	3–10	7
C4–C5	13–29	20	0–16	11	1–12	7
Lower						
C5–C6	13–29	20	0–16	8	2–12	7
C6–C7	6–26	17	0–17	7	2–10	6
C7–T1	4–7	9	0–17	4	0–7	2

From White, A. A., III, and Panjabi, M. M.: Clinical Biomechanics of the Spine. 2nd ed. Philadelphia, J. B. Lippincott Co., 1990.

Table 34–3. LIMITS AND REPRESENTATIVE VALUES OF RANGES OF ROTATION OF THE THORACIC SPINE

Interspace	Combined Flexion-Extension (± X Axis Rotation)		One-Side Lateral Bending (Z Axis Rotation)		One-Side Axial Rotation (Y Axis Rotation)	
	Limits of Ranges (degrees)	Representative Angle (degrees)	Limits of Ranges (degrees)	Representative Angle (degrees)	Limits of Ranges (degrees)	Representative Angle (degrees)
T1–T2	3–5	4	5	5	14	9
T2–T3	3–5	4	5–7	6	4–12	8
T3–T4	2–5	4	3–7	5	5–11	8
T4–T5	2–5	4	5–6	6	5–11	8
T5–T6	3–5	4	5–6	6	5–11 ·	8
T6–T7	2–7	5	6	6	4–11	7
T7–T8	3–8	6	3–8	6	4–11	7
T8–T9	3–8	6	4–7	6	6–7	6
T9–T10	3–8	6	4–7	6	3–5	4
T10–T11	4–14	9	3–10	7	2–3	2
T11–T12	6–20	12	4–13	9	2–3	2
T12–L1	6–20	12	5–10	8	2–3	2

From White, A. A., III, and Panjabi, M. M.: Clinical Biomechanics of the Spine. 2nd ed. Philadelphia, J. B. Lippincott Co., 1990.

distinct. Note that the physiologic coupling motion is in the direction opposite to that of the coupling seen in the deformity of idiopathic scoliosis.

Lumbar Spine

The unique characteristic of the lumbar spine is that it must bear tremendous loads. This is because of the large, superimposed body weight that interacts with additional forces generated by lifting and other activities that involve powerful forces. The lumbar spine and the hips are responsible for the mobility of the trunk. These impose formidable mechanical demands on this region. Kinematically, because of the spatial orientation of the facets (see Fig. 34–9), there is relatively little axial rotation in this region.

The representative rotations in flexion-extension, lateral bending, and axial rotation are shown in Table 34–4. In flexion-extension, there is usually a cephalo-caudal increase in the range of motion in the lumbar spine. The L5–S1 joint offers more sagittal plane motion than the other joints. For lateral bending, each level is about the same except for L5–S1, which shows a relatively small amount of motion.[37] It is not unreasonable to speculate that the high incidence of clinically evident disc disease at L4–L5 and L5–S1 is related to mechanics. These two areas bear the highest loads and tend to undergo the most motion.

Several coupling patterns have been observed in the lumbar spine. In stereoradiographic studies of the lumbar spine, Pearcy observed coupling of 2 degrees of axial rotation and 3 degrees of lateral bending with flexion-extension (i.e., X axis rotation coupled with Y axis rotation as well as Z axis rotation).[49] One of the strongest coupling patterns is that of lateral bending (Z axis rotation) with flexion-extension. Moreover, there is also a coupling pattern described by Miles and Sullivan in which axial rotation is combined with lateral bend-

Table 34–4. LIMITS AND REPRESENTATIVE VALUES OF RANGES OF ROTATION OF THE LUMBAR SPINE

Interspace	Combined Flexion-Extension (± X Axis Rotation		One-Side Lateral Bending (Z Axis Rotation)		One-Side Axial Rotation (Y Axis Rotation)	
	Limits of Ranges (degrees)	Representative Angle (degrees)	Limits of Ranges (degrees)	Representative Angle (degrees)	Limits of Ranges (degrees)	Representative Angle (degrees)
L1–L2	5–16	12	3–8	6	1–3	2
L2–L3	8–18	14	3–10	6	1–3	2
L3–L4	6–17	15	4–12	8	1–3	2
L4–L5	9–21	16	3–9	6	1–3	2
L5–S1	10–24	17	2–6	3	0–2	1

From White, A. A., and Panjabi, M. M.: Clinical Biomechanics of the Spine. 2nd ed. Philadelphia, J. B. Lippincott Co., 1990.

ing, such that the spinous processes point in the same direction as the lateral bending.[41] This pattern is the opposite of that in the cervical and upper thoracic spines.

In 1930, Calve and Galland suggested that the center of the intervertebral disc is the site of the axes for flexion-extension;[8] however, Rolander showed that when flexion is simulated from a neutral position, the axes are in the region of the anterior portion of the disc.[56] In lateral bending (frontal plane rotation), the axes fall in the region of the right side of the disc with left lateral bending and in the region of the left side of the disc with right lateral bending. For axial (Y axis) rotation, the IARs are in the region of the posterior nucleus and annulus.[10]

A SYSTEMATIC APPROACH TO CLINICAL INSTABILITY OF THE SPINE

Clinical instability is defined as the loss of the ability of the spine under physiologic loads to maintain relationships between vertebrae in such a way that there is neither initial nor subsequent damage to the spinal cord or nerve roots and there is no development of incapacitating deformity or severe pain.

Physiologic loads are those incurred during normal activity of the particular patient being evaluated. *Incapacitating deformity* is defined as gross deformity that the patient finds intolerable. *Incapacitating pain* is defined as pain that cannot be controlled by nonnarcotic analgesic medications. Clinical instability can occur as a result of trauma, disease, surgery, or some combination of the three.

In the diagnosis of clinical instability or clinical stability in any region of the spine, several crucial anatomic, biomechanical, and clinical factors come into play. The evaluative approach that follows takes all these factors into account and provides the clinician with a rational, systematic, and objective basis for the treatment of spinal problems, given the current clinical and biomechanical knowledge. We do not purport to provide physicians with ideal judgment and wisdom. Our goal with the system presented here is to have patients realize the maximal benefit of treatment with an absolute minimum of risks and inconvenience. We are aware that the problem of clinical instability of the spine is unsolved. There are several alternative and significantly different approaches to the problem (Denis,[11, 12] Dunsker and associates,[3] Gertzbein and associates,[23, 24] Kirkaldy-Willis and Farfan,[35] and Louis[36]). A symposium by the International Society for the Study of the Lumbar Spine presented several of these approaches.[34] We present this method as our best opinion based on currently available clinical and biomechanical information.

It is prudent to clarify our focus in this chapter with respect to the concept of clinical instability. *Clinical instability is not a diagnosis per se.* It has been estimated that 85 to 90 per cent of patients seeking medical care for complaints of low back pain suffer from "idiopathic" low back pain.[22] That is, for the vast ma-

jority of low back pain sufferers, a definite, diagnosable cause of their symptoms is not known. The term *instability* has sometimes been used as a "diagnosis" in efforts to explain the cause of idiopathic low back pain. Instability in this vein has been hypothesized to include certain quantitative or qualitative abnormalities of the FSU, such as abnormal kinetics (abnormal stiffness of an FSU[16, 17, 50]) or abnormal kinematics (abnormal coupling patterns[45, 60] or scattering of the IARs[23, 24]). However, we suggest that we be purists and limit *instability* to the concept of component ablation instability. It is therefore fitting and not by chance that this chapter is located in the Trauma section of this textbook (although component ablation instability analyses can be used in other clinical settings, such as surgical trauma, tumors, or developmental conditions such as spondylolisthesis).

Specific injuries are not discussed in this chapter. General characteristics and components of stability are discussed for each region of the spine. Because of the unique characteristics of the occipital–atlantoaxial complex and specific patterns of instability in this region, a checklist is not presented for this area. The specific injuries and instabilities of the C0–C1–C2 region are discussed in Chapter 28.

The Checklist Approach

The checklist approach is intended to assure the patient that all pertinent factors are considered and reasonably balanced. An attempt has been made to set the sensitivity of the system at the proper level (Fig. 34–11). The goal of the setting is to avoid overtreatment and undertreatment and to provide reasonable insurance against the development of any sequelae from the basic clinical problem. A total of five or more points in the checklist for each region of the spine is necessary to confirm the diagnosis of clinical instability.

Injuries to the spinal column involve a wide spectrum, from minimal structural injury without neurologic deficit to complete loss of structural integrity, large displacements, and complete neurologic deficit. The checklist approach is an attempt to grade injuries along this spectrum. It is implied that the greater the number of points assigned to a particular patient's spinal injury, the more unstable the injury. Treatment recommendations should take into consideration this spectrum of instability (see the clinical stability scale in Fig. 34–11). A total of five or more points in the checklist does not indicate the need for surgery. By the same token, a total of less than five points does not imply that treatment is unnecessary for that particular patient. Thorough serial clinical and radiographic follow-up evaluations of patients with suspected or diagnosed spinal injuries are required to optimize their treatment. At the bottom of Figure 34–11, two broad areas of treatment are proposed for various point totals along the clinical stability scale on a theoretic basis. The Cervical Spine Research Society has an ongoing prospective multicenter study to test the validity of the

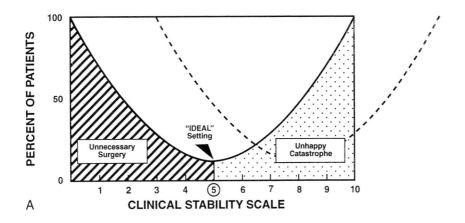

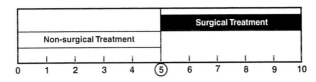

Figure 34–11. *A,* Theoretic sensitivity setting of checklist for the evaluation of clinical instability. One of the goals with regard to clinical instability is to determine the less obvious needs for protection and provide it through appropriate management of the patient in need of treatment. This is a theoretic graph depicting conceptually the choice of 5 as an "ideal" sensitivity setting. The ordinate shows percentages of improperly treated patients. The improper treatment could result in unnecessary surgery or catastrophe. The ideal setting should be the point at which the lowest percentage of patients is treated improperly. In our best judgment, that point is 5 on the clinical stability scale. We believe that this theoretical curve is correct; however, the real curve may be shifted to the right or to the left. For example, if it is shifted to the right, as shown by the dotted curve, a cutoff of 5 on the stability scale would result in a significantly large percentage of improperly treated patients. Assuming that the curve is as indicated on the graph, a setting of 1 would involve a large percentage of unnecessary surgery and no catastrophe. A setting of 9 would avoid any unnecessary surgery but permit a large percentage of catastrophes. *B,* Theoretic initial treatment recommendations for various point totals along the clinical stability scale. The patient's point total is derived after evaluating multiple critical anatomic, biomechanical, and clinical factors from the checklist of the specific region of the spine. The clinical stability scale is an attempt to grade spinal injuries along a spectrum of decreasing stability; the more points assigned to a particular patient's spinal injury, the less stable the injury. Thorough serial clinical and radiographic follow-up evaluations of patients with suspected or diagnosed spinal injuries are often required to optimize their treatment. Patients with low point totals (0, 1, or 2) are probably best treated with relative rest, sometimes protection with an orthosis, and close observation. A high percentage of patients with high point totals (7, 8, 9, or 10) are best treated by surgical decompression, reduction, and/or fusion. Patients with 3 or 4 points on the clinical stability scale are probably best treated initially with an orthosis or cast; if these patients' injuries prove to be unstable with close follow-up (failure to maintain satisfactory reduction or alignment), surgical management is indicated. Patients with 5 or 6 points on the clinical stability scale have unstable injuries; some of these patients may be best treated with bed rest, traction, and/or an orthosis or cast, while others are best managed initially by surgical means. (Adapted from White, A. A., III, and Panjabi, M. M.: Clinical Biomechanics of the Spine. 2nd ed. Philadelphia, J. B. Lippincott Co., 1990.)

checklist criteria and approaches to cervical spine–injured patients.

Anatomic Considerations

For each region of the spine, the checklist includes anatomic considerations for the evaluation of clinical instability. Schematic representations of the cogent anatomy of each region are also given.

Holdsworth[31] conceptualized the spine into two columns: anterior—disc and vertebra and both longitudi-

nal ligaments; and posterior—all elements posterior to the posterior longitudinal ligament. The checklists use the two-column model of the spine because of its validation in component ablation experimental studies on functional spinal units.[27, 48, 51, 66] A three-column model of the spine has been proposed by Denis;[11, 12] the anterior and middle columns are created by dividing Holdsworth's anterior column into two halves, and the posterior column is the same as Holdsworth described. Denis suggested that the middle column of the three-column spine is the primary determinant of mechanical stability. Since the three-column model's introduction, one biomechanical study by Panjabi and colleagues has supported the hypothesis that the middle column is the primary determinant of stability.[47] Another study by James and colleagues concluded that the posterior column was a more influential determinant of stability.[32] Until further experimental and clinical research better defines the critical determinants of mechanical stability, we suggest using the two-column model because of its ease of application, simplicity, and experimental validation.

Radiographic Considerations

The evaluation of radiographs is a critical step in the assessment of clinical stability and instability. Criteria based on the current knowledge of vertebral alignment, kinematics, and normal and pathologic anatomy are given in the checklists for each region of the spine. Because flexion-extension radiographs are helpful and commonly used in evaluating clinical stability in the cervical and lumbar regions, criteria for the evaluation of both dynamic (flexion-extension) and static (resting) radiographs are given for these regions. Translation and rotation refer to measurements on dynamic radiographs, whereas displacement and angulation refer to measurements on static radiographs.

Clinical Considerations

For each region of the spine, the checklist accounts for the critically important clinical element. This is, above all, the neurologic picture. Point values are given to various levels of neurologic dysfunction (i.e., spinal cord, nerve root, or cauda equina damage), and these play an important role in the evaluation of clinical instability.

Occipital–Atlantoaxial Complex (C0–C1–C2)

Although no checklist for the evaluation of clinical instability of this region is presented, some of the pertinent clinical biomechanics related to the C0–C1–C2 complex are given here to help clinicians in the evaluation of specific injuries and instability patterns discussed in Chapter 28.

One of the key variables in the problem of clinical instability is that of allowable displacement without neurologic deficit. This is partially dependent on the normal sagittal diameter of the spinal canal, which was studied in 200 healthy adults by Wolf and colleagues.[69] These results are presented in Figure 34–12. Note that there is more space available for the cord at C1 and C2 than in the middle and lower cervical spine.

A schematic illustration of the major ligaments involved in the clinical stability of the upper cervical spine is presented in Figure 34–13.

Because of the level of the anatomic lesion, dislocations at C0–C1 are usually fatal. Unless resuscitation is begun immediately at the scene of the accident, the

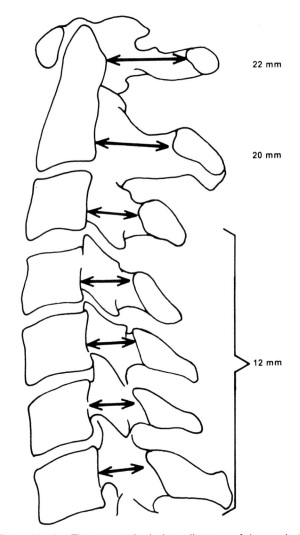

Figure 34–12. The true sagittal plane diameter of the cervical spine canal. The upper portion has relatively more space for the spinal cord, even though the cord is larger there. (From White, A. A., III, and Panjabi, M. M.: Clinical Biomechanics of the Spine. 1st ed. Philadelphia, J. B. Lippincott Co., 1978.)

victim dies of respiratory paralysis. Any patient who survives should be considered clinically unstable and should be fused, occiput to C2.

With transection of the tectorial membrane and the alar ligaments, there is an increased flexion of the units of the C0–C1–C2 complex and a subluxation of the occiput.[64] Dvorak and Panjabi demonstrated that transection of the alar ligament on one side causes increased axial rotation to the opposite side by approximately 30 per cent.[15] On the basis of measurements of in vivo functional computed tomography (CT) scans of the C0–C1–C2 region in 43 spine-injured patients and 9 healthy individuals, guidelines were suggested for measuring and identifying normal and abnormal rotations.[14] The suggestion is that axial rotation between C0 and C1 greater than 8 degrees or rotation between C1 and C2 greater than 56 degrees is abnormal. Also, a right-left difference in rotation at C0–C1 greater than

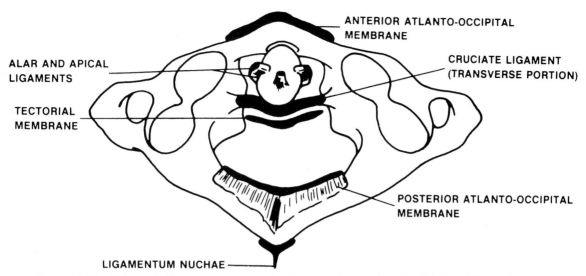

Figure 34–13. Schematic illustration of the major ligaments involved in the clinical stability of the upper cervical spine. (From White, A. A., III, and Panjabi, M. M.: Clinical Biomechanics of the Spine. 1st ed. Philadelphia, J. B. Lippincott Co., 1978.)

5 degrees or at C1–C2 greater than 8 degrees represents excessive motion. These findings may constitute a clinically significant rotatory instability, but a complete clinical entity has not yet been fully defined.

The major stability at the C1–C2 articulation is provided by the dens and the intact transverse ligament.[21] The articular capsules between C1 and C2 are designed loosely, to allow a large amount of rotation and provide a small amount of stability. Although the C1–C2 segment is clinically unstable after failure of the transverse ligament, the tectorial membrane, the alar, and the apical ligaments probably provide some resistance against gross dislocation. Additionally, with a Jefferson fracture, the transverse ligament should be presumed to be ruptured if the total overhang of the lateral masses of C1 in relation to the lateral borders of the body of C2, as viewed on an open-mouth anteroposterior radiograph (with the head in the neutral rotatory position), is as great as 7 mm.[57] The clinical problem of subluxation and dislocation at C1–C2 is complicated, controversial, and often difficult to diagnose. The possible types of displacement have not been completely described and documented. When clinical instability owing to ligamentous injury at C1–C2 is diagnosed, because of the potential risks of displacement in this area (resulting in quadriplegia and death), C1–C2 fusion is probably the treatment of choice.

Middle and Lower Cervical Spine (C2–T1)

The middle and lower cervical spine has received the most attention with regard to clinical instability. In the cervical spine, major neurologic deficit is most frequently associated with trauma,[54] but the instability checklist has been designed for use in any clinical setting (Table 34–5).

Anatomic Considerations

A schematic representation of the anatomy of the middle and lower cervical spine is presented in Figure 34–14. At the level of the intervertebral disc, the annulus fibrosus appears to be the crucial stabilizing structure.[68] Bailey emphasized the importance of this structure in several studies.[2, 3] Munro carried out experimental studies on cadaver spines and concluded that

Table 34–5. CHECKLIST FOR THE DIAGNOSIS OF CLINICAL INSTABILITY IN THE MIDDLE AND LOWER CERVICAL SPINE

Element	Point Value
Anterior elements destroyed or unable to function	2
Posterior elements destroyed or unable to function	2
Positive stretch test	2
Radiographic criteria	4
A. Flexion-extension radiographs	
1. Sagittal plane translation >3.5 mm or 20% (2 pts)	
2. Sagittal plane rotation >20° (2 pts)	
or	
B. Resting radiographs	
1. Sagittal plane displacement >3.5 mm or 20% (2 pts)	
2. Relative sagittal plane angulation >11° (2 pts)	
Developmentally narrow spinal canal	1
1. Sagittal diameter <13 mm	
2. Pavlov's ratio <0.8	
Abnormal disc narrowing	1
Spinal cord damage	2
Nerve root damage	1
Dangerous loading anticipated	1

Total of 5 or more = unstable.

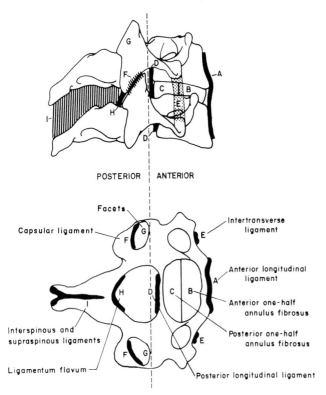

POSTERIOR | ANTERIOR

Facets

Capsular ligament

Intertransverse ligament

Anterior longitudinal ligament

Anterior one-half annulus fibrosus

Posterior one-half annulus fibrosus

Interspinous and supraspinous ligaments

Ligamentum flavum

Posterior longitudinal ligament

Figure 34–14. A schematic illustration of the ligamentous structures that participate in the stabilization of the middle and lower cervical spine. The components are divided into anterior and posterior elements. In experiments on clinical stability, ligaments were cut in the alphabetic order indicated in the diagram from anterior to posterior and in reverse alphabetic order from posterior to anterior. (From White, A. A., III, and Panjabi, M. M.: Clinical Biomechanics of the Spine. 2nd ed. Philadelphia, J. B. Lippincott Co., 1990.)

cervical spine stability comes mainly from the intervertebral discs and the anterior and posterior longitudinal ligaments.[42]

White and Panjabi and colleagues performed experiments on cervical spine FSUs in high-humidity chambers using physiologic loads to simulate flexion and extension.[48, 66] They defined the *anterior elements* as the posterior longitudinal ligament and all structures anterior to it. The *posterior elements* were defined as all structures behind the posterior longitudinal ligament. On the basis of these studies, it was suggested that if an FSU has all its anterior elements plus one additional structure or all its posterior elements plus one additional structure, it will probably remain stable under physiologic loads. Therefore, to provide for some clinical margin of safety, we suggest that any FSU in which all the anterior elements or all the posterior elements are either destroyed or unable to function should be considered potentially unstable. Two points in the checklist are given for the loss of each of these anatomic elements.

Controlled, monitored axial traction (the "stretch test") may be helpful to evaluate the integrity of the ligamentous structures of the middle and lower cervi-

cal spine. Figure 34–15 and Table 34–6 provide a diagrammatic synopsis of this test and details of the procedure. An abnormal test is indicated by either a greater than 1.7-mm difference in interspace separation or a greater than 7.5-degree change in angle between vertebrae, comparing the prestretch condition with the situation after application of axial traction equivalent to one third of body weight.[67] Two points in the checklist are given for a positive stretch test.

One final anatomic consideration should be noted. If all other considerations are the same, patients with the anterior elements destroyed or unable to function are more clinically unstable in extension, whereas patients with the posterior elements destroyed or unable to function are more unstable in flexion. These factors should be considered during patient transfers and when a patient's neck is immobilized after injury.

Radiographic Considerations

The measurement of translation and displacement is shown in Figure 34–16. This method takes into account variations in magnification and should be useful when there is a tube-to-film distance of 72 inches. Sagittal plane displacement or translation greater than 3.5 mm on either static (resting) or dynamic (flexion-extension) lateral radiographs should be considered potentially unstable. This value was determined from an experimentally obtained value of 2.7 mm and an assumed radiographic magnification of 30 per cent.[66] Two points in the checklist are given for abnormal sagittal plane displacement or translation.

Angular measurements are shown in Figure 34–17. There is no magnification problem in measuring rotation or angulation. More than 20 degrees of sagittal plane rotation on dynamic (flexion-extension) radiographs should be considered abnormal and potentially unstable. This value was based on a review of the literature on in vitro and in vivo cervical spine ranges of motion.[68] When dynamic radiographs are unable to be obtained (e.g., in an acute traumatic setting), a static (resting) lateral radiograph that shows more than 11 degrees of relative sagittal plane angulation should be considered potentially unstable. Note that 11 degrees of relative angulation means 11 degrees more than the amount of angulation at the FSU above or below the FSU in question. This standard of comparison takes into account the normal angulation between FSUs (i.e., normal posture). Two points in the checklist are given for abnormal sagittal plane rotation or abnormal relative sagittal plane angulation.

Note that a total of four points in the cervical checklist is given for these radiographic measurements: either dynamic (flexion-extension) or static (resting) radiographs are used in the checklist, not both. When both dynamic and static radiographs have been obtained, the measurements should be made on the dynamic films. Static radiographs should be used in the cervical checklist only when flexion-extension films cannot be obtained.

The radiographic interpretation in general, espe-

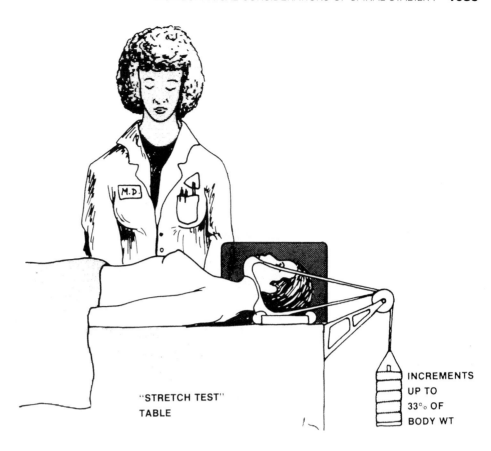

Figure 34–15. Diagrammatic synopsis of the stretch test. A physician who is knowledgeable about the test is in attendance. The neurologic status is monitored by following signs and symptoms. Incremental loads up to 33 per cent of body weight or 65 pounds are applied. Each lateral radiograph is checked before augmentation of the axial load. Note the neurologic hammer to symbolize neurologic examination and the roller platform under the head to reduce friction. Despite the cartoon-like presentation, this is a serious test. (From White, A. A., III, and Panjabi, M. M.: Clinical Biomechanics of the Spine. 2nd ed. Philadelphia, J. B. Lippincott Co., 1990.)

"STRETCH TEST" TABLE

INCREMENTS UP TO 33% OF BODY WT

cially for sagittal plane translation and displacement, is decidedly different in children up to 7 years old.[9] It is risky to interpret radiographs of patients in this age group without a knowledge of some of the normal findings that may appear to be pathologic to the inexperienced physician.

Two final radiographic considerations should be noted. First, Bailey remarked and we have observed that in the traumatized spine there is frequently narrowing of the disc at the damaged FSU.[2] In patients younger than 35 years of age, we submit that posttraumatic disc narrowing is modestly suggestive of disruption of the annulus fibrosus and of possible instability. Second, if all other considerations are the same, patients with a developmentally narrow spinal canal are more apt to develop neurologic deficit, because less

---

Table 34–6. PROCEDURE FOR STRETCH TEST TO EVALUATE CLINICAL STABILITY IN THE MIDDLE AND LOWER CERVICAL SPINE

1. It is recommended that the test be done under the supervision of a physician.
2. Traction is applied through secure skeletal fixation or a head halter. If the latter is used, a small portion of gauze sponge between the molars improves comfort.
3. A roller is placed under the patient's head to reduce frictional forces.
4. The radiographic film is placed 0.36 m (14 in) from the patient's spine. The tube distance is 1.82 m (72 in) from the film.
5. An initial lateral radiograph is taken, carefully evaluating for C0–C1–C2 subluxation. Abnormal displacement in this region should be looked for on each film, as it can often be difficult to identify.
6. A 10-lb weight is added (if the initial weight is 10 lb, this is omitted).
7. Traction is increased by 10-lb increments. A lateral radiograph is taken and measured.
8. Step 7 is repeated until one third of body weight or 65 lb is reached.
9. After each additional weight application, the patient is checked for any change in neurologic status. The test is stopped and considered positive should this occur. The radiographs are developed and read after each weight increment. Any abnormal separation of the anterior or posterior elements of the vertebrae is the most typical indication of a positive test. There should be at least 5 minutes between incremental weight applications; this will allow for the developing of the film, necessary neurologic checks, and creep of the viscoelastic structures involved.
10. The test is contraindicated in a spine with obvious clinical instability.

From White, A. A., III, and Panjabi, M. M.: Clinical Biomechanics of the Spine. 2nd ed. Philadelphia, J. B. Lippincott Co., 1990.

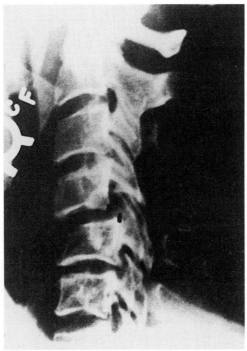
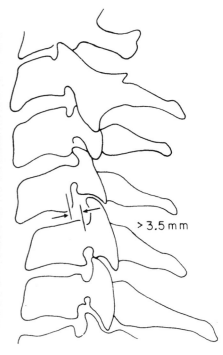

Figure 34–16. The method of measuring translatory displacement. A point at the posteroinferior angle of the lateral projection of the vertebral body above the interspace in question is marked. A point at the posterosuperior angle of the projection of the vertebral body below is also marked. The distance between the two in the sagittal plane is measured. A distance of 3.5 mm or greater is suggestive of clinical instability. This distance is to be measured on a lateral radiograph. It is computed from an experimentally obtained value of 2.7 mm and an assumed radiographic magnification of 30 per cent. (From White, A. A., Johnson, R. M., Panjabi, M. M., and Southwick, W. O.: Biomechanical analysis of clinical stability in the cervical spine. Clin. Orthop. *109:* 85, 1975.)

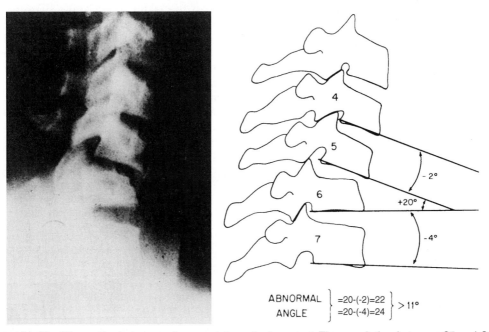

Figure 34–17. The method of measuring angulatory displacement. The angulation between C5 and C6 is 20 degrees, which is more than 11 degrees greater than that at either adjacent interspace. The angle at C4 and C5 measures −2 degrees, and the one at C6 and C7 measures −4 degrees. This finding of abnormal angulation is based on a comparison of the interspace in question with either adjacent interspace. This is to allow for the angulation that is present as a result of the normal lordosis of the cervical spine. We interpret a difference of 11 degrees or greater from either adjacent interspace as evidence of clinical instability. (From White, A. A., Johnson, R. M., Panjabi, M. M., and Southwick, W. O.: Biochemical analysis of clinical stability in the cervical spine. Clin. Orthop. *109:*85, 1975.)

space is available for the spinal cord. A developmentally narrow canal is defined as one measuring less than 13 mm in its anteroposterior (AP) dimension on a lateral radiograph[7, 20] or one with a Pavlov's ratio of less than 0.8.[2, 62] The 13-mm absolute value accounts for some radiographic magnification, whereas the Pavlov's ratio need not consider magnification, because it is the ratio of the AP diameter of the canal to the AP diameter of the vertebral body. One point is given for abnormal disc narrowing and one for a developmentally narrow canal.

Clinical Considerations

Is the presence of distinct medullary or root damage associated with spinal trauma or disease evidence of clinical instability? This question deserves some discussion with regard to our definition of clinical instability. We stated that clinical instability concerns the prediction of subsequent neurologic damage. Therefore, is the presence of initial neurologic damage a significant indicator of the probability of subsequent neurologic damage? We believe that if the trauma is severe enough to cause initial neurologic damage, the support structures probably have been altered sufficiently to allow subsequent neurologic damage, and thus the situation is clinically unstable. It should be noted, however, that Gosch and colleagues showed that in animals it is possible to produce medullary damage with intact supporting structures.[25] In general, despite a few exceptions, we believe that neurologic deficit is an important consideration in the evaluation of clinical instability. Evidence of root involvement is a weaker indicator of clinical instability. For example, a unilateral facet dislocation may cause enough foraminal encroachment to result in root symptoms or signs, but not enough ligamentous damage to render the FSU unstable. Two points in the checklist are given for spinal cord damage and one point for nerve root damage.

The final consideration involves the important individual variation in physiologic load requirements, especially with regard to differences in habitual activities. The clinician uses judgment to anticipate the magnitude of loads that the particular patient's spine will be expected to maintain after injury. Anticipating dangerous loads can be especially helpful when other available criteria are inconclusive. One point in the checklist is given if dangerous loading is anticipated.

Thoracic and Thoracolumbar Spine

There are several unique considerations in the evaluation of clinical instability in the thoracic and thoracolumbar spine. This region of the spine is mechanically stiffer and less mobile than the cervical and lumbar regions. There is less free space and a more precarious blood supply for the spinal cord in this region of the spine. It is well stabilized by the costovertebral articulations and the rib cage structure. Therefore, greater forces are required to disrupt it. The instability checklist (Table 34–7) is an attempt to summarize and inter-

Table 34–7. CHECKLIST FOR THE DIAGNOSIS OF CLINICAL INSTABILITY IN THE THORACIC AND THORACOLUMBAR SPINE

Element	Point Value
Anterior elements destroyed or unable to function	2
Posterior elements destroyed or unable to function	2
Disruptions of costovertebral articulations	1
Radiographic criteria	4
1. Sagittal plane displacement >2.5 mm (2 pts)	
2. Relative sagittal plane angulation >5° (2 pts)	
Spinal cord or cauda equina damage	2
Dangerous loading anticipated	2

Total of 5 or more = unstable.

pret the basic evidence regarding the important question of thoracic and thoracolumbar clinical instability.

Anatomic Considerations

There are several anatomic characteristics that relate to the biomechanics of this region and affect its clinical stability. There is a normal thoracic kyphosis owing to the slight wedged configuration of both the vertebral bodies and the intervertebral discs. Because of this physiologic kyphosis, the thoracic spine is more prone to be unstable in flexion.

A schematic representation of the major ligaments of the thoracic spine is presented in Figure 34–18. The anterior and posterior longitudinal ligaments, as well as the yellow ligaments, are well-developed structures in the thoracic spine. Laboratory studies suggest that with all the anterior elements cut, the loaded thoracic and thoracolumbar spine in extension is either unstable or on the brink of instability.[27, 67] These studies also suggest that with all the posterior elements cut, there is likely to be enough abnormal displacement to cause additional neural damage. Kinematic studies have shown that there can be abnormal movements in flexion, extension, lateral bending, and axial rotation when the posterior elements are removed.[27, 65, 67] All these motions are potentially injurious to the spinal cord.

The capsular ligaments in the thoracic region, in contrast to those in the cervical region, are thin and loose, which means that the support provided by these structures against flexion is minimal and is much less than might be expected in the cervical spine, where there are well-developed capsules on the articular facets. In addition to the effects of the capsular structure of the facet articulations, their spatial orientation has some significance (see Fig. 34–9). In the middle and upper portions of the thoracic spine, the facets provide stability primarily against anterior translation. When the orientation changes, which may happen anywhere between T9 and T12, the facets provide less stability against anterior and posterior displacement. The joints become oriented more in the sagittal plane and provide

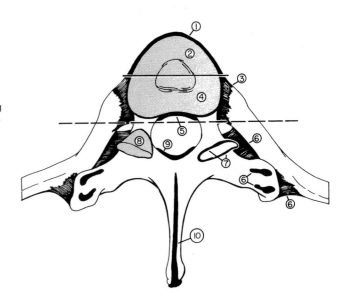

Figure 34–18. Schematic representation of the major ligaments involved in the thoracic spine. Ligaments are numbered according to the order in which they were cut in biomechanical experiments used to evaluate instability. Anterior elements: 1, anterior longitudinal ligament; 2, anterior half of annulus fibrosus; 3, radiate and costovertebral ligaments; 4, posterior half of annulus fibrosus; 5, posterior longitudinal ligament. Posterior elements: 6, costotransverse and intertransverse ligaments; 7, capsular ligaments; 8, facet articulation; 9, ligamentum flavum; 10, supraspinous and interspinous ligaments. (From White, A. A., III, and Panjabi, M. M.: Clinical Biomechanics of the Spine. 2nd ed. Philadelphia, J. B. Lippincott Co., 1990.)

stability against axial rotation. Therefore, in the presence of rotatory displacement in the lower thoracic or thoracolumbar region, facet dislocations or fracture-dislocations must be present.

There are two mechanisms through which the ribs tend to increase the stability of the thoracic spine. The first involves the articulation of the head of the rib to the articular facets of the adjacent vertebral bodies (Fig. 34–19). The second is related to the presence of the entire thoracic cage (Fig. 34–20). The thoracic cage effectively increases the moment of inertia, resulting in added resistance to bending in the sagittal and frontal planes, as well as to axial rotation. Andriacchi and colleagues, in computer simulation studies of the human thoracic spine, found that the greatest increase in stiffness was 132 per cent during extension, 45 per cent in lateral bending, and 31 per cent for flexion and axial rotation.[1]

Two points in the checklist are given for the loss of the anterior elements' ability to contribute to stability. Two points are also given for the loss of the posterior elements' contribution. In addition, one point is given if there is evidence of disruption of the costovertebral articulation.

Radiographic Considerations

The measurements of displacement and angulation are made in the same manner as in the cervical region. Because there is less free space for the cord and a more precarious blood supply to the spinal cord in this region, there is less tolerance for displacement before neurologic injury occurs. Sagittal plane displacement greater than 2.5 mm in the thoracic spine on a lateral radiograph should be considered potentially unstable. This criterion is based on experimental biomechanical studies completely analogous to those on which the criteria for the cervical spine were based.[27] Relative sagittal plane angulation greater than 5 degrees is in-

dicative of clinical instability in the thoracic spine.[27] Note that 5 degrees of relative angulation means 5 degrees more than the amount of angulation at the FSU above or below the FSU in question. This standard of comparison takes into account the normal angulation between FSUs. Two points in the checklist are given for abnormal sagittal plane displacement or abnormal relative sagittal plane angulation.

Clinical Considerations

One might consider giving spinal cord or cauda equina damage a full five points on the checklist. There are situations, however, in which there is no recognizable structural damage yet there is neurologic deficit. Some of these may be overlooked structural lesions, but it is also possible to have cord damage with a truly intact column. This is not a clinically unstable situation. This entity is given a high value but requires other evidence of instability to make the diagnosis of clinical instability. Two points in the checklist are given for spinal cord or cauda equina damage.

Anticipating dangerous loads is evaluated in the same way as recommended in the cervical spine. It is even more crucial in this region, however. The forces applied to this region are likely to be greater because of the superincumbent weight, and the operative moment arms are greater. Two points in the checklist are given if dangerous loading is anticipated.

Lumbar Spine

In the lumbar spine, there are some unique considerations related to the definition of clinical instability. The associated neurologic deficits in the lumbar spine are less frequent, less disabling, and more likely to recover than in the cervical and thoracic regions. The second consideration is related to the phenomena of subse-

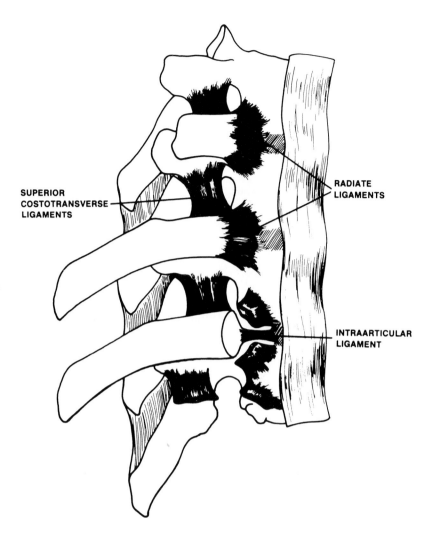

Figure 34–19. Costovertebral articulation. This diagram highlights ligamentous structures in the costovertebral articulation that contribute to the clinical stability of the thoracic spine. Note the radiate ligaments attaching to the head of the rib and to both adjacent vertebral bodies. There are also costotransverse ligaments, which may offer some secondary stability. (From White, A. A., III, and Panjabi, M. M.: Clinical Biomechanics of the Spine. 2nd ed. Philadelphia, J. B. Lippincott Co., 1990.)

SUPERIOR COSTOTRANSVERSE LIGAMENTS

RADIATE LIGAMENTS

INTRAARTICULAR LIGAMENT

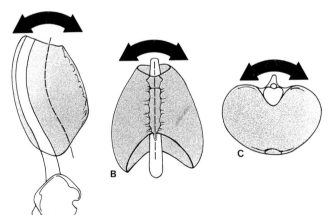

Figure 34–20. The thoracic cage effectively increases the transverse dimensions of the spine structure. This, in turn, increases its moment of inertia and therefore its stiffness and strength in all modes of rotation: *A,* bending in sagittal plane (flexion-extension); *B,* bending in frontal plane (lateral bending); and *C,* axial rotation. (From White A. A., III, and Panjabi, M. M.: Clinical Biomechanics of the Spine. 2nd ed. Philadelphia, J. B. Lippincott Co., 1990.)

Table 34–8. CHECKLIST FOR THE DIAGNOSIS OF CLINICAL INSTABILITY IN THE LUMBAR SPINE

Element	Point Value
Anterior elements destroyed or unable to function	2
Posterior elements destroyed or unable to function	2
Radiographic criteria	4
A. Flexion-extension radiographs:	
1. Sagittal plane translation >4.5 mm or 15% (2 pts)	
2. Sagittal plane rotation >15° at L1–L2, L2–L3, and L3–L4 (2 pts)	
>20° at L4–L5 (2 pts)	
>25° at L5–S1 (2 pts)	
or	
B. Resting radiographs	
1. Sagittal plane displacement >4.5 mm or 15% (2 pts)	
2. Relative sagittal plane angulation >22° (2 pts)	
Cauda equina damage	3
Dangerous loading anticipated	1

Total of 5 or more = unstable.

quent pain, deformity, and disability and to the high loads that must be borne by this region of the spine.

The physician's goal is to take full advantage of the recuperative power of the cauda equina and minimize the possibility of prolonged disability associated with low back pain. With use of the checklist, fusion in the lumbar spine purely as a treatment for pain is not indicated.

To provide some perspective, the rationale and experimental basis of the checklist (Table 34–8) are re-

viewed briefly. The goal was to establish reproducible guidelines based on anatomy, biomechanics, and clinical observations. It was considered desirable to establish criteria that would be applicable to all types of instability analyses. The list is designed with some internal checks and balances, some partially overlapping criteria, and some latitude for "gray zone" weighting of a given criterion (e.g., if a criterion is weighted two points and it is not possible to arrive at a definitive yes or no, it is assigned one point). Finally,

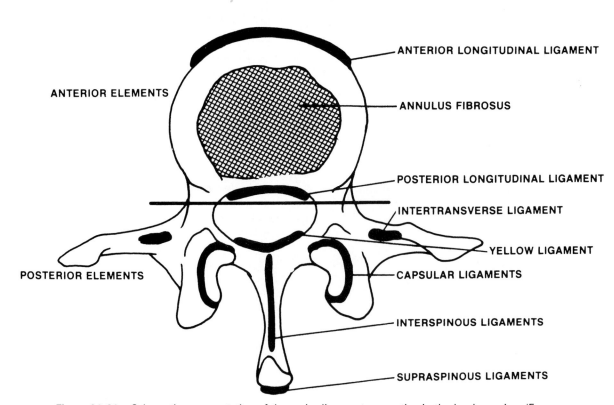

Figure 34–21. Schematic representation of the major ligaments operative in the lumbar spine. (From White, A. A., III, and Panjabi, M. M.: Clinical Biomechanics of the Spine. 2nd ed. Philadelphia, J. B. Lippincott Co., 1990.)

the checklist was based largely on an experiment designed explicitly to address the issue of lumbar spine instability.[51] Eighteen FSUs from three levels of the lumbar spine (L1–L2, L3–L4, and L5–S1) were preloaded to stimulate the load calculated to be present for a person lying supine and standing, each with maximal physiologic flexion and extension. The sagittal plane translations were then measured using linear variable differential transformers and a minicomputer. Sequential transection of components in the posterior to anterior direction was performed until failure occurred. From this it was possible to determine the upper limits of physiologic motion of the intact FSU and the effect of component ablation on normal motion. In addition, it was possible to determine the point in the sequence of component ablation at which the FSU either was on the brink of failure or failed.

Anatomic Considerations

A schematic representation of the major ligaments and the facet orientation in the lumbar spine is presented in Figure 34–21. The anterior longitudinal ligament is a well-developed structure in this region. The annulus fibrosus, which has received an enormous amount of attention in the literature, constitutes 50 to 70 per cent of the total area of the intervertebral disc. As in other regions of the spine, it contributes in a major way to the clinical stability of the FSU. The posterior longitudinal ligament is less developed than its anterior counterpart. The facets play a crucial role in the stability of the lumbar spine. The well-developed capsule of these joints play a major part in stabilizing the FSU against axial rotation and lateral bending. When these displacements are observed, fracture or fracture-dislocation of the facet articulations must be suspected. Sullivan and Farfan showed that axial rotation of the lumbar spine of 30 degrees or more caused failure of the neural arch, progressing from facet joint dislocation to fracture of the articular process.[59]

The annulus fibrosus or vertebral body may be compromised or rendered unable to function by surgery, trauma, tumor, or infection. The annulus can also be compromised by chemonucleolysis. Extensive plastic deformation of the annulus may occur in long-standing spondylolisthesis and contribute to instability. Excessive vertebral body wedging can contribute to instability, particularly if the posterior ligaments are not intact. Surgery, trauma, tumor, and infection may also destroy the posterior elements or render them unable to function. Two points in the checklist are given for the loss of the contribution of the anterior or posterior elements to stability.

Radiographic Considerations

The method of measuring translation and displacement in the lumbar spine is the same as in the cervical spine. Figure 34–22 also depicts the measurement of translation and displacement as a percentage of the width of the vertebral body.

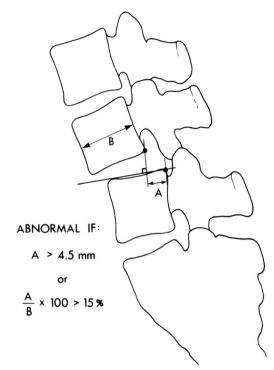

ABNORMAL IF:

A > 4.5 mm

or

$\dfrac{A}{B} \times 100 > 15\%$

Figure 34–22. A method of measuring sagittal plane translation or displacement. If the translation or displacement is as much as 4.5 mm or 15 per cent of the sagittal diameter of the adjacent vertebra, it is considered abnormal. These criteria are included in Table 34–8. (From White, A. A., III, and Panjabi, M. M.: Clinical Biomechanics of the Spine. 2nd ed. Philadelphia, J. B. Lippincott Co., 1990.)

When readily apparent residual displacement remains after the recoil and rebound of injury, the structural damage is obvious. Where there is little or no residual displacement of the position of the vertebrae after injury to the cauda equina, however, clinical instability must be suspected. The physician should look for other evidence of clinical instability to make a diagnosis when there is no residual displacement.

Measurements can be made directly from resting or flexion-extension radiographs. In the acute traumatic setting, resting radiographs are usually taken. Sagittal plane displacement greater than 4.5 mm or 15 per cent of the anteroposterior diameter of the vertebral body on a static (resting) lateral radiograph should be considered potentially unstable. These values were obtained from the aforementioned biomechanical experiment.[53] Relative sagittal plane angulation on a static lateral radiograph greater than 22 degrees is abnormal and potentially unstable at any level in the lumbar spine. Note that 22 degrees of relative angulation means 22 degrees more than the amount of angulation at the FSU above or below the FSU in question (Fig. 34–23). This value was obtained from a review of the literature on the normal resting sagittal posture of the lumbar spine.[5, 58] This value was tested on the data of 102 normal subjects,[5] and this standard of comparison takes into account the normal angulation between FSUs.

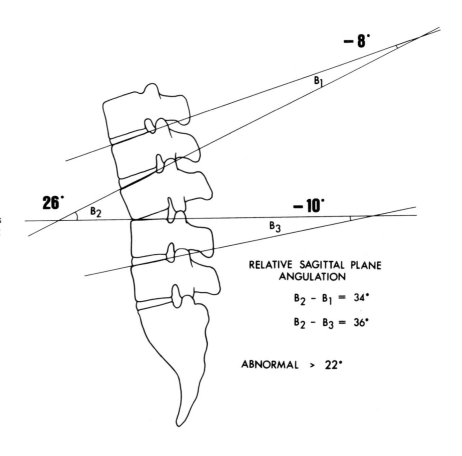

Figure 34–23. A method of measuring relative sagittal plane angulation of the L3–L4 functional spinal unit (FSU) on a static (resting) lateral radiograph. Relative sagittal plane angulation greater than 22 degrees is abnormal and potentially unstable in the lumbar spine. Note that this means 22 degrees greater than the amount of angulation at the FSU above or below the FSU in question. By convention, negative values denote lordosis and positive values kyphosis. (From White, A. A., III, and Panjabi, M. M.: Clinical Biomechanics of the Spine. 2nd ed. Philadelphia, J. B. Lippincott Co., 1990.)

After evaluating the resting radiographs, additional information may be gained by obtaining flexion-extension radiographs. Sagittal plane translation greater than 4.5 mm or 15 per cent of the anteroposterior diameter of the vertebral body on dynamic (flexion-extension) radiographs should be considered potentially unstable. These values were obtained from the aforementioned experimental study.[51] Sagittal plane rotation on dynamic radiographs greater than 15 degrees at L1–L2, L2–L3, and L3–L4; greater than 20 degrees at L4–L5; or greater than 25 degrees at L5–S1 is abnormal and potentially unstable (Fig. 34–24). These values were based on a review of the literature on in vitro and in vivo lumbar spine ranges of motion.[68]

Two points in the checklist are given for abnormal sagittal plane translation or displacement. Two points

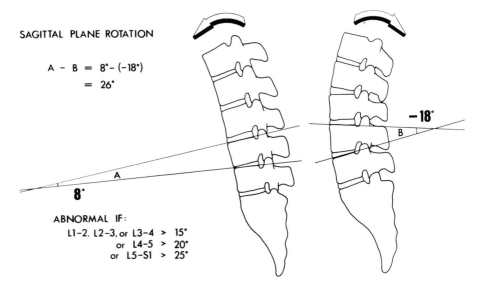

Figure 34–24. A method of measuring sagittal plane rotation of the L4–L5 functional spinal unit on dynamic (flexion-extension) lateral radiographs. The sagittal plane rotation is the difference between the Cobb measurements taken in flexion (A) and in extension (B). Sagittal plane rotation greater than 15 degrees at L1–L2, L2–L3, and L3–L4; greater than 20 degrees at L4–L5; or greater than 25 degrees at L5–S1 is abnormal and potentially unstable. Note that negative values denote lordosis and positive values kyphosis. (From White, A. A., III, and Panjabi, M. M.: Clinical Biomechanics of the Spine. 2nd ed. Philadelphia, J. B. Lippincott Co., 1990.)

in the checklist are also given for abnormal sagittal plane rotation or abnormal relative sagittal plane angulation. Note that a total of four points in the lumbar checklist are given for radiographic measurements; either dynamic (flexion-extension) or static (resting) radiographs are used in the checklist, not both. When both dynamic and static radiographs have been obtained, the measurements should be made on the dynamic films. Static radiographs should be used in the lumbar checklist only in the acute traumatic setting when flexion-extension films cannot be obtained.

Clinical Considerations

There is a relatively large margin of safety in the lumbar spine, because the space available for the neural elements usually amply exceeds the space occupied by them. Therefore, the presence of neurologic deficit is likely to be the harbinger of clinical instability. In other words, if there is enough displacement to cause neural damage, it is generally the case that enough displacement has occurred to cause significant ligamentous or bony failure. Three points in the checklist are given for cauda equina damage.

Anticipating dangerous loads was discussed previously. Because of the normally heavy loading in this region and the socioeconomic considerations (workers' compensation, disability, and medicolegal issues), this criterion is important in the evaluation of the clinical stability of the lumbar spine. One point in the checklist is given if dangerous loading is anticipated.

CONCLUSION

Our approach has been to take what is known of anatomy, biomechanics, and documented clinical experience and to analyze it in a manner that is clinically useful. A major anatomic consideration is the significance of regional variations of several structural characteristics. The relative size of the neural elements and the space in which they are enclosed is a valid consideration. Regional variations also exist in mechanical properties such as kinematics, stiffness, and physiologic loads. We have emphasized the importance of a proper interpretation of the significance of neurologic deficit in the determination of clinical stability. Generally, when a deficit is associated with significant structural damage, clinical instability should be suspected.

Our goal in managing these patients is to gain maximal recovery as rapidly as possible, to avoid unnecessary treatment (surgical or nonsurgical), and to prevent initial or subsequent neurologic damage. There is no convincing evidence that a diagnosis of clinical instability demands that the treatment should be surgical reduction, fusion, or fixation. However, the management of a patient with such a diagnosis should definitely differ from that of a clinically stable patient. Surgical treatment is reasonable and is indicated for many clinically unstable patients.

Checklists have been presented to organize and summarize the information conveniently; to stimulate others to criticize and improve on them; and to provide clinical protocols for systematic evaluation, management, and study. More research in the area of spinal instability is necessary. We believe that with well-designed and well-executed clinical protocols, we can improve our knowledge and base our decisions on solid scientific evidence.

GLOSSARY*

Allowable Stress. A stress value that is higher than that from normal loads but is lower than the yield stress of the material.

Bending. The deformation that occurs when a load is applied to a long structure that is not directly supported at the point of application of the load.

Bending Moment. A quantity at a point in a structure equal to the product of the force applied and the shortest distance from the point to the force direction.

Biomechanical Adaptation. Biologically mediated changes in the mechanical properties of tissues (material properties or structural changes) in association with the application of mechanical variables to those tissues.

Biomechanical Stability. The ability of the ex vivo spine or spine construct, when subjected to biomechanical testing under physiologic loads, to limit patterns of displacement within physiologic ranges of motion.

Clinical Stability. The ability of the spine under physiologic loads to limit patterns of displacement so as not to damage or irritate the spinal cord, cauda equina, or nerve roots and, in addition, to prevent incapacitating deformity or pain owing to structural changes.

Compression. The normal force that tends to push together material fibers.

Coordinate System. A reference system that makes it possible to define position and motion of rigid bodies in space or with respect to each other.

Coupling. A phenomenon of consistent association of one motion (translation or rotation) about an axis with another motion about a second axis. One motion cannot be produced without the other.

Creep. The phenomenon of a viscoelastic material deforming with time when it is subjected to a constant, suddenly applied load. The deformation-time curve approaches a steady state asymptomatically.

Deformation. Change in length or shape; generally represented in the form of strain.

Degrees of Freedom. The number of independent coordinates in a coordinate system required to completely specify the position of an object in space. The term is loosely applied to specify the independent motion components involved in the characteristic movements of a given rigid body. The motion of a

---

*Adapted from White, A. A., III, and Panjabi, M. M.: Clinical Biomechanics of the Spine. 2nd ed. Philadelphia, J. B. Lippincott Co., 1990, pp. 635–696.

rigid body in space has six degrees of freedom, three translations (expressed by linear coordinates), and three rotations (expressed by angular coordinates).

Dynamic Load. A load applied to a specimen is called dynamic if it varies with time. A dynamic load with a repetitive pattern of variation is called a cyclic load.

Dynamics. A branch of mechanics that consists of the study of the loads and the motions of interacting bodies.

Elastic Range. A range of loading within which a specimen or a structure remains elastic.

Elastic Stability. The ability of a loaded structure, given an arbitrary small elastic deformation, to return to its original position.

Elasticity. The property of a material or a structure to return to its original form after the removal of the deforming load.

Energy. The amount of work done by a load on a body. If the load deforms or displaces the body, the energy is called the strain or potential energy, respectively. If the load imparts motion to the body, it is called kinetic energy.

Equilibrium. A body is said to be in a state of equilibrium if it is at rest or in uniform motion under a given set of forces and moments.

Fatigue. A process of birth and growth of cracks in structures subjected to repetitive load cycles. The load is generally below the failure load of the structure.

Flexibility Coefficient. The ratio of the amount of displacement produced to the load applied. It is a quantity that characterizes the responsiveness of a structure to the applied load.

Force. Any action that tends to change the state of rest or motion of a body to which it is applied.

Functional Spinal Unit (FSU). The smallest unit of the spine, representing the inherent biomechanical characteristics of the entire bony-ligamentous spine. Physically, it consists of two adjacent vertebrae and the interconnecting soft tissue, devoid of musculature. In the thoracic region, two articulating heads of ribs with their connecting ligaments are also included.

Hysteresis. A phenomenon associated with energy loss exhibited by viscoelastic materials when they are subjected to loading and unloading cycles.

Inertia. The property of all material bodies to resist change in the state of rest or motion under the action of applied loads.

Instantaneous Axis of Rotation (IAR). When a rigid body moves in a plane, at every instant there is a point in the body or some hypothetical extension of it that does not move. An axis perpendicular to the plane of motion and passing through that point is the instantaneous axis (center) of rotation for that motion at that instant.

Kinematics. The division of mechanics (dynamics) that deals with the geometry of the motion of bodies (displacement, velocity, and deceleration) without taking into account the forces that produce the motion.

Kinetics. A branch of mechanics (dynamics) that studies the relations between the force system acting on a body and the changes it produces in the body motion.

Load. A general term describing the application of a force or moment (torque) to a structure.

Mass. The quantitative measure of inertia for linear motion.

Mass Moment of Inertia. The quantitative measure of inertia for change in angular velocity.

Modulus of Elasticity. The ratio of normal stress to normal strain in a material.

Motion. The relative displacement with time of a body in space, with respect to other bodies or some reference system.

Neutral Axis. A longitudinal line in a long structure where normal axial stresses are zero when the structure is subjected to bending.

Neutral Zone.[46] There is no single neutral position for a given functional spinal unit, but there exists a zone in the load-displacement curve of an FSU within which movement occurs with a minimal application of external load. This is called the neutral zone. Increasingly higher loads are required to produce motion outside the neutral zone.

Normal Stress. The intensity of force perpendicular to the surface on which it acts.

Plastic Range. If a specimen is loaded beyond its elastic range, it enters the plastic range. The larger the plastic range failure, the higher the ductility and energy absorption capacity of the material.

Plasticity. The property of a material to permanently deform when it is loaded beyond its elastic range.

Polar Moment of Inertia. A property of the cross section of a long structure that gives a measure of the distribution of the material about its axis so as to maximize its torsional strength.

Range of Motion. Quantities that indicate two points at extremes of physiologic ranges of translation and rotation of a joint for each of its six degrees of freedom.

Relative Motion. Between two moving objects, the motion of one object observed from the perspective of the second object.

Relaxation. The decrease in stress in a deformed structure over time when the deformation is held constant.

Rotation. Motion of a rigid body in which a certain straight line of the body or its rigid extension remains motionless. This line is the axis of rotation.

Shear Stress. The intensity of force parallel to the surface on which it acts.

Static Load. A load applied to a specimen is called static if it remains constant with respect to time. Its antonym is dynamic.

Statics. The branch of mechanics that deals with the equilibrium of bodies at rest or in motion with zero acceleration.

Stiffness. A measure of resistance offered to external

loads by a specimen or structure as it deforms. This phenomenon is characterized by the stiffness coefficient. Stiffness and elasticity are two similar but different concepts. The former represents mechanical behavior of a structure, including the material, shape, and size, whereas the latter is a pure material property.

Stiffness Coefficient. The property of a structure defined by the ratio of force applied to the deformation produced. It quantifies the resistance that a structure offers to deformation.

Strain. The change in unit length or angle in a material subjected to load.

Stress. The force per unit area of a structure and a measurement of the intensity of the force.

Stress-Strain Diagram. The plot of stress, usually on the ordinate or Y axis, versus strain, usually on the abscissa or X axis. The relationship represents mechanical behavior of a material.

Tension. A normal force that tends to elongate the fibers of a material.

Torsion. A type of load that is applied by two forces (parallel and directed opposite to each other) about the long axis of a structure. The load is called torque. It produces relative rotation of different axial sections of the structure with respect to each other.

Torsional Rigidity. The torque per unit of angular deformation. Torsional rigidity means rotatory stiffness.

Translation. Motion of a rigid body in which a straight line in the body always remains parallel to itself.

Ultimate Load. The final load reached by a structure subjected to failure.

Viscoelastic Stability. The type of stability in which the critical load is a function of time as well as the geometric and material properties of the structure.

Viscoelasticity. The property of a material to show sensitivity to the rate of loading or deformation.

Work. The amount of energy required to move a body from one position to another. Mechanical work is defined as the product of force applied and the distance moved in the direction of the force.

Yield Stress. That point of stress on the load-deformation curve at which appreciable deformation takes place without any appreciable increase in load.

ACKNOWLEDGMENT. This work is supported in part by the Daniel E. Hogan Spine Fellowship Program, Beth Israel Deaconess Medical Center, Augustus A. White III, M.D., D.Med.Sci., Director; and the St. Luke's Hospital of Kansas City Division of Research Support.

References

1. Andriacchi, T. P., Schultz, A. B., Belytschko, T. B., and Galante, G. O.: A model for studies of mechanical interactions between the human spine and rib cage. J. Biomech. *7:*497, 1974.
2. Bailey, R. W.: Fractures and dislocations of the cervical spine: Orthopedic and neurosurgical aspects. Postgrad. Med. *35:*588, 1964.
3. Bailey, R. W.: Observations of cervical intervertebral disc lesions in fractures and dislocations. J. Bone Joint Surg. [Am:] *45:*461, 1963.
4. Beadle, O. A.: The intervertebral disc: Observations on their normal and morbid anatomy in relation to certain spinal deformities. Med. Res. Counc. Spec. Rep. Serv. (London) no. 161, 1931.
5. Bernhardt, M., and Bridwell, K. H.: Segmental analysis of the sagittal plane alignment of the normal thoracic and lumbar spines and thoracolumbar junction. Spine *14:*717, 1989.
6. Brown, T., Hanson, R., and Yorra, A.: Some mechanical tests on the lumbo-sacral spine with particular reference to the intervertebral discs. J. Bone Joint Surg. [Am.] *39:*1135, 1957.
7. Calliet, R.: Neck and Arm Pain. 2nd ed. Philadelphia, F. A. Davis Co., 1981.
8. Calve, J., and Galland, M.: Physiologie pathologique du mal de Pott. Rev. Orthop. *17:*5, 1930.
9. Catteil, H. S., and Filtzer, D. L.: Pseudo-subluxation and other normal variations of the cervical spine in children. J. Bone Joint Surg. [Am.] *47:*1295, 1965.
10. Cossette, J. W., Farfan, H. F., Robertson, G. H., and Wells, R. V.: The instantaneous center of rotation of the third intervertebral joint. J. Biomech. *4:*149, 1971.
11. Dennis, F.: Spinal instability as defined by the three-column spine concept in acute spinal trauma. Clin. Orthop. *189:*65, 1984.
12. Denis, F.: The three-column spine and its significance in the classification of acute thoracolumbar spine injuries. Spine *8:*817, 1985.
13. Dunsker, S. B., Schmidek, H. H., Frymoyer, J. W., and Kahn, A.: The Unstable Spine. Orlando, Grune & Stratton, 1986.
14. Dvorak, J., Hayek, J., and Zehnder, R.: CT-functional diagnostics of the rotatory instability of the upper cervical spine. Spine *12:*726, 1987.
15. Dvorak, J., and Panjabi, M. M.: Functional anatomy of the alar ligaments. Spine *12:*83, 1987.
16. Dvorak, J., Panjabi, M. M., Novotny, J. E., et al.: Clinical validation of functional flexion-extension roentgenograms of the lumbar spine. Spine *16:*943, 1991.
17. Esses, S. I., Botsford, D. J., and Kostuik, J. P.: The role of external spinal skeletal fixation in the assessment of low back disorders. Spine *14:*594, 1989.
18. Farfan, H. F.: Mechanical Disorders of the Low Back. Philadelphia, Lea & Febiger, 1973.
19. Farfan, H. F., Cossette, J. W., Robertson, G. H., et al.: The effects of torsion on the lumbar intervertebral joints: The role of torsion in the production of disc degeneration. J. Bone Joint Surg. [Am.] *52:*468, 1970.
20. Ferguson, R. J. L., and Caplan, L. R.: Cervical spondylitic myelopathy. Neurol. Clin. *3:*373, 1985.
21. Fielding, J. W., Cochran, G. V. B., Lansing, J. F., and Hohl, M.: Tears of the transverse ligament of the atlas: A clinical biomechanical study. J. Bone Joint Surg. [Am.] *56:*1683, 1974.
22. Frymoyer, J. W., and Gordon, S. L.: New Perspectives on Low Back Pain. American Academy of Orthopaedic Surgeons, 1988.
23. Gertzbein, S. D., Seligman, J. H., Holtby, R., et al.: Centrode characteristics of the lumbar spine as a function of segmental instability. Clin. Orthop. *208:*48, 1986.
24. Gertzbein, S. D., Seligman, J., Holtby, R., et al.: Centrode patterns and segmental instability in degenerative disc disease. Spine *10:*267, 1985.
25. Gosch, H. H., Gooding, E., and Schneider, R. C.: An experimental study of cervical spine and cord injuries. J. Trauma *12:*570, 1972.
26. Gray, H.: Descriptive and Applied Anatomy. 34th ed. Davies, D. V. (ed.). London, Longmans, Green & Co., 1967.
27. Hausfeld, J. N.: A biomechanical analysis of clinical stability in the thoracic and thoracolumbar spine [thesis]. Yale University School of Medicine, New Haven, CT, 1977.
28. Henke, W.: Hanbuch der Anatomie and Mechanik der Gelanke. Leipzig and Heidelberg, 1863.
29. Hirsch, C.: The reaction of intervertebral discs to compression forces. J. Bone Joint Surg. [Am.] *37:*1188, 1955.
30. Hirsch, C., and Nachemson, A.: A new observation on the mechanical behavior of lumbar discs. Acta Orthop. Scand. *23:*254, 1954.
31. Holdsworth, F. W.: Fractures, dislocations, and fracture dislocations of the spine. J. Bone Joint Surg.[Br.] *45:*6, 1963.
32. James, K. S., Wenger, K. H., Schlegel, J. D., and Dunn, H. K.: Biomechanical evaluation of the stability of thoracolumbar burst fractures. Spine *19:*1731, 1994.

33. Kazarian, L. E.: Creep characteristics of the human spinal column. Orthop. Clin. North Am. 6:3, 1975.

34. Kirkaldy-Willis, W. H.: Symposium: Instability of the lumbar spine. Spine 10:253, 1985.

35. Kirkaldy-Willis, W. H., and Farfan, H. F.: Instability of the lumbar spine. Clin. Orthop. 165:110, 1982.

36. Louis, R.: Spinal stability as defined by the three-column spine concept. Anat. Clin. 7:33, 1985.

37. Lumsden, R. M., and Morris, J. M.: An in vivo study of axial rotation and immobilization at the lumbosacral joint. J. Bone Joint Surg. [Am.] 50:1591, 1968.

38. Lysell, E.: Motion in the cervical spine. Acta Orthop. Scand. Suppl. 123, 1969.

39. Markolf, K. L.: Stiffness and damping characteristics of the thoracic-lumbar spine. In Proceedings of Workshop on Bioengineering Approaches to the Problems of the Spine. NIH, September 1970.

40. Markolf, K. L., and Morris, J. M.: The structural components of the intervertebral disc. J. Bone Joint Surg. [Am.] 56:675, 1974.

41. Miles, M., and Sullivan, W. E.: Lateral bending at the lumbar and lumbosacral joints. Anat. Rec. 139:387, 1961.

42. Munro, D.: Treatment of fractures and dislocations of the cervical spine complicated by cervical cord and root injuries: A comparative study of fusion vs. nonfusion therapy. N. Engl. J. Med. 264:573, 1961.

43. Nachemson, A., and Morris, J. M.: In vivo measurements of intradiscal pressure. J. Bone Joint Surg. 46:1077, 1964.

44. Naylor, A., Happey, F., and MacRae, T.: Changes in the lumbar intervertebral disc with age: A biophysical study. J. Am. Geriatr. Soc. 3:964, 1955.

45. Olsson, T. H., Selvik, G., and Willner, S.: Vertebral motion in spondylolisthesis. Acta Radiol.: Diagnosis 17:861, 1976.

46. Panjabi, M. M., Goel, V. K., and Takata, K.: Physiologic strains in the lumbar spinal ligaments: An in vitro biomechanical study. Spine 7:19, 1982.

47. Panjabi, M. M., Oxland, T. R., Kifune, M., et al.: Validity of the three-column theory of thoracolumbar fractures. Spine 20:1122, 1995.

48. Panjabi, M. M., White, A. A., and Johnson, R. M.: Cervical spine mechanics as a function of transection of components. J. Biomech. 8:327, 1975.

49. Pearcy, M. J.: Stereoradiography of lumbar spine motion. Acta Orthop. Scand. Suppl. 56:212, 1985.

50. Pearcy, M., Portek, I., and Sheperd, J.: The effect of low-back pain on lumbar spinal movements measured by three-dimensional x-ray analysis. Spine 10:150, 1985.

51. Posner, I., White, A. A., Edwards, W. T., and Hayes, W. C.: A biomechanical analysis of clinical stability of the lumbar lumbosacral spine. Spine 7:374, 1982.

52. Prosad, P., King, A. I., and Ewing, C. L.: The role of articular facets during +Gz acceleration. J. Appl. Mech. 41:321, 1974.

53. Puschel, J.: Der Wassergehalt normaler und degenerierter zwischen Wirbelscheiben. Beitr. Path. Anat. 84:123, 1930.

54. Riggans, R. S., and Kraus, J. F.: The risk of neurological damage with fractures of the vertebra. J. Trauma 17:126, 1977.

55. Rockwell, H., Evans, F. G., and Pheasant, H. C.: The comparative morphology of the vertebral spinal column: Its form as related to function. J. Morphol. 63:87, 1938.

56. Rolander, S. D.: Motion of the lumbar spine with special reference to the stabilizing effect of posterior fusion. Acta Orthop. Scand. Suppl. 99, 1966.

57. Spence, K. F., Decker, S., and Sell, K. W.: Bursting atlantal fracture associated with rupture of the transverse ligament. J. Bone Joint Surg. [Am.] 52:543, 1970.

58. Stagnara, P., DeMauroy, J. C., Dran, G., et al.: Reciprocal angulation of vertebral bodies in a sagittal plane: Approach to references for the evaluation of kyphosis and lordosis. Spine 7:335, 1982.

59. Sullivan, J. D., and Farfan, H. F.: The crumpled neural arch. Orthop. Clin. North Am. 6:199, 1975.

60. Tibrewal, S. B., Pearcy, M. J., Portek, I., and Spivey, J.: A prospective study of lumbar spinal movements before and after discectomy using biplanar radiography. Spine 10:455, 1985.

61. Torg, J. S.: Pavlov's ratio: Determining cervical spinal stenosis on routine lateral roentgenograms. Contemp. Orthop. 18:153, 1989.

62. Torg, J. S., Pavlov, H., Genuario, S. E., et al.: Neuropraxia of the cervical spinal cord with transient quadriplegia. J. Bone Joint Surg. [Am.] 68:1354, 1986.

63. Virgin, W.: Experimental investigations into physical properties of intervertebral disc. J. Bone Joint Surg. [Br.] 33:607, 1951.

64. Werne, S.: Studies in spontaneous atlas dislocation. Acta Orthop. Scand. Suppl. 23, 1957.

65. White, A. A., III: Analysis of the mechanics of the thoracic spine in man. Acta Orthop. Scand. Suppl. 127, 1969.

66. White, A. A., Johnson, R. M., Panjabi, M. M., and Southwick, W. O.: Biomechanical analysis of clinical stability in the cervical spine. Clin. Orthop. 109:85, 1975.

67. White, A. A., III, and Panjabi, M. M.: Clinical Biomechanics of the Spine. 1st ed. Philadelphia, J. B. Lippincott Co., 1977.

68. White, A. A., III, and Panjabi, M. M.: Clinical Biomechanics of the Spine. 2nd ed. Philadelphia, J. B. Lippincott Co., 1990.

69. Wolf, B. S., Khilnami, M., and Malis, L.: The sagittal diameter of the bony cervical spinal canal and its significance in cervical spondylosis. J. Mt. Sinai Hosp. N.Y. 23:283, 1956.

Spinal Orthoses for Traumatic and Degenerative Disease

Michael J. Botte, M.D.

Steven R. Garfin, M.D.

Kel Bergmann, C.P.O.

Thomas P. Byrne, O.T.C.

Alexander R. Vaccaro, M.D.

Orthosis is defined as an external device that is applied to the body in order to restrict motion in a body segment.[3] Although numerous terms have been used throughout the years to describe the different braces used, the terminology was not standardized until 1973.[3] Spinal orthoses have been divided into five categories: sacroiliac (SIO), lumbosacral (LSO), thoracolumbosacral (TLSO), cervicothoracic (CTO), and cervical (CO) (Fig. 35–1).[3]

Spinal orthoses are classified by the Food and Drug Administration (FDA) as Class I devices. They are not subject to the strict regulations and scrutiny that apply to implantable devices.[76] Because of this, there are a plethora of orthotic devices, multiple claims about their degrees of immobilization, and numerous terms that describe the braces. Unfortunately, limited scientific research has been done to document the actual motion allowed by the different devices, and strict criteria for their uses have not been developed.[6, 15–17, 23, 24, 36, 39–41, 47, 51, 53, 54, 57, 58, 66, 72, 73, 78, 79]

This chapter focuses on the accepted terminology and biomechanics of generally used, commercially available orthoses for immobilizing the spine. The discussion is restricted to those employed in the treatment of traumatic and degenerative disease. Bracing for scoliosis is not covered. Those scientific studies that are available can help the reader generate his or her own ideas regarding the utility of the various devices. Because the halo device has the most scientific background, as well as the most concerns about its use, it is discussed in more detail than the others. We ac-

knowledge that there may be a lack of scientific basis for some of our recommendations and that there are a number of braces currently available that we have not evaluated. The guidelines given should be used with that in mind.

HISTORIC BACKGROUND

The first recorded use of orthotic devices can be found in the chronicles of the Fifth Egyptian Dynasty.[70] Most early spinal bracing efforts were directed at the correction of spinal deformities. Gale was the first physician to advocate braces for the correction of spinal deformity.[21] He described the use of chest strappings and exercises in the treatment of scoliosis. In the early 1700s, Nicholas Andry designed the "iron cross" for immobilization of the cervical spine.[21] This was a flat, straight, metal upright with a cross and a metal ring attached to the top for support of the head. In the early 1800s, the first spinal supports of American origin were developed.[3] A popular orthosis, the Knight brace, is still in use today.[3]

The materials used in spinal braces in the eighteenth century consisted mostly of wood, iron, and leather. During the nineteenth and early twentieth centuries, a proliferation of spinal braces were developed in Germany. Most of these were made of iron, wood, paper cellulose, and glue. With the advent of new composites, polymer resins, and, recently, thermoplastics, the number of orthoses available has markedly increased. The most common rigid, high-temperature plastic used to-

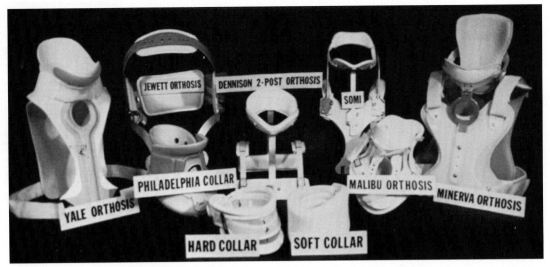

Figure 35–1. Samples of orthotic devices discussed in the text.

day is polypropylene, with various copolymers.[9] Thermoplastics have allowed the development of inexpensive and rapidly fabricated custom orthoses.[9] For an excellent historic review of the development of braces, the reader is referred to the *Orthopedic Appliances Atlas.*[21]

BIOMECHANICS OF SPINAL BRACING

Spinal bracing involves the use of external forces to control the position of the spine for purposes of protection, immobilization, support, and correction and prevention of deformity, as well as for diagnostic trials.[79] In order to achieve this, a bony ligamentous structure that is relatively stiff must be supported or immobilized by applying external forces through an envelope of soft, compliant tissue.

The elastic and viscoelastic characteristics of the different anatomic structures differ widely from the cervical spine to the sacrum. These components, however, are all linked and behave as a unit. The classic example of the effects of the surrounding tissues on the stiffness of the spine is the ribs. These have been reported to stiffen the spine up to 200 percent.[6]

The successful application of forces to the spine is highly dependent on the soft tissue anatomy of the individual patient. Although not specifically addressed in many studies, most authors agree that obese patients have significantly increased bony motion when compared with slender patients immobilized with the same device.[79]

Pressure measurements on the soft tissues with orthotic application have been evaluated and remain a significant area of controversy in the bracing of deformities. Some studies have shown a correlation between the magnitude of the applied forces and the correction achieved,[14] whereas others have reported no correlation between the magnitude of the applied external pressure and the ultimate correction in bracing

for scoliosis.[82] Pressure measurements, however, appear to be an objective way to assess the fit, as well as control the amount of force in the restrained spine.

Applying rigid forces to immobilize the spine is not without side effects.[72] The most common and troublesome include skin breakdown, local pain, skin rash, weakening and atrophy of the axial musculature, contracture of soft tissues, decrease in vital capacity, increase in the lower extremity venous pressure (which may aggravate hemorrhoids and varicose veins), and psychologic dependence on the device.[72] In order to minimize these and other side effects of immobilization when a spinal orthosis is prescribed, an activity or exercise regimen should be recommended, if appropriate.

In the strict engineering sense, there are six degrees of freedom of each segment of the spine (translation and rotation around the X, Y, and Z axes). However, the clinically significant degrees of freedom in describing motion of the spine can be classified in three broader terms: flexion-extension, lateral bending, and rotation.[79] Because these latter terms are used in the clinical setting, we limit the discussion to these more clinically relevant degrees of freedom.

CERVICAL ORTHOSES

The soft tissue structures around the neck, particularly those located anteriorly (e.g., esophagus, trachea, carotid arteries, jugular veins), seriously compromise the safe application of significant external forces to the cervical spine. Complicating the problem further is the fact that the neck has multiple, extremely mobile motion segments that are difficult to control.[24, 36, 39, 43, 54, 66, 79] This is particularly important when an unstable injury to the neck occurs, and excess motion can lead to catastrophic consequences. Although the cervical spine has been the most carefully investigated area of the spine in terms of immobilization by orthoses, the pro-

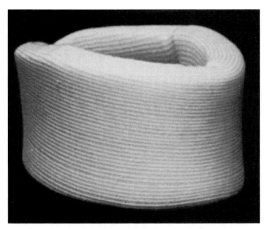

Figure 35–2. Example of a soft collar. Typically, the Velcro strap goes posteriorly; this, however, keeps the neck somewhat extended. Reversing the collar and wearing the strap in front allows some degree of flexion.

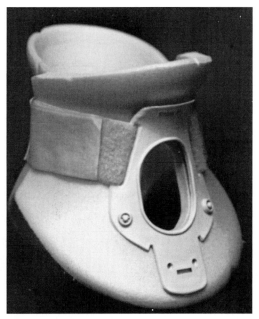

Figure 35–4. Philadelphia collar. The anterior hole is for a tracheotomy tube.

liferation of available devices and the lack of consensus in the analyses make it extremely difficult for a physician to select an orthosis.

Cervical orthoses can be divided into two basic types: cervical (CO) and cervicothoracic (CTO) (Fig. 35–1). The former are cylinders that fit around the neck and can be anchored to the mandible and/or the occiput to increase their stiffness. Many of these devices, in addition to restricting motion to a variable degree, serve as a proprioceptive reminder to the patient to limit neck activity. Typical examples of these include the soft collar (Fig. 35–2), the hard collar (Fig. 35–3), the Philadelphia collar (Fig. 35–4), the Thomas brace, the Camp orthosis, the Mayo collar, and, more recently, the Malibu (Fig. 35–5), the Miami J (Fig. 35–6), the Aspen (Fig. 35–7), and the Canadian braces.[35, 43, 58] The differences among these devices include the material used to fabricate them, as well as the design. The materials used include polyethylene, which is perhaps the most comfortable (Table 35–1).[9]

The effectiveness of these collars in immobilizing the

spine has been studied by the use of roentgenography, goniometry, and cineradiography.[24, 36, 39] Roentgenographic methods are accurate, reproducible, and perhaps the most clinically significant.[15, 39, 54, 66, 79] All these devices somewhat restrict flexion-extension motion of the neck but provide limited control of lateral bending and rotational components of motion.[39] No single study has compared all the available collars, and some have not been tested in any rigorous scientific manner.

CTOs use chin and occiput fixations affixed to the

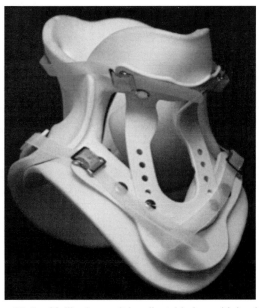

Figure 35–5. Malibu brace. It is adjustable in multiple planes.

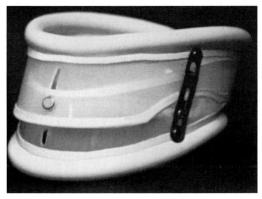

Figure 35–3. Hard collar. It is shaped similar to a soft collar but is more rigid. Its height is adjustable.

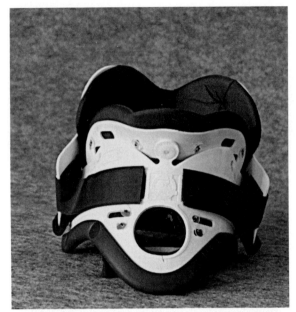

Figure 35–6. Miami "J" cervical orthosis. It has a two-piece design and is made out of polyethylene with a soft lining. The orthosis has an anterior opening for a tracheotomy tube.

Table 35–1. COMMONLY USED MATERIALS IN THE FABRICATION OF ORTHOSES

Material	Product Name
Oliphin	Polypropylene
Ionomer	Thermovac Surlyn
Polyethylene	Vitrathene
Polycarbonate	Lexan
PVC	Kydex
Resins	Epoxy, polyester
Polyethylene foam	Plastazote, Aliplast

brace (Fig. 35–10), the Minerva brace (Fig. 35–11), the L-200 (Fig. 35–12), and the halo-brace. These devices, compared with collars, improve control in all planes. However, they are often less comfortable for the patient.

The mechanics of these devices were first report by Jones in 1960.[41] He used cineradiography to analyze the effect of various collars on the restriction of motion. Hartman and colleagues[36] published the first biomechanical comparison of cervical orthoses in the orthopedic literature. In this study, the cervical spines of five volunteers were evaluated with cineradiography before and after the application of five different cervical orthoses. They concluded that the soft cervical collar restricted less than 10 per cent of the total motion in flexion-extension (FE) and lateral bending (LB), and it provided no rotational restriction (RR).[36] They also observed that the Thomas collar, which restricted motion about 75 per cent in FE and LB, was not as effective as the four- and two-poster CTOs. A long, two-poster brace was found to restrict up to 95 per cent of

trunk by means of straps or circumferential supports. CTOs can have from two (Fig. 35–8) to four rigid uprights to increase their stiffness. Typical of these orthoses are the sterno-occipito-mandibular immobilizer (SOMI) (Fig. 35–9), the Guilford brace, the Yale

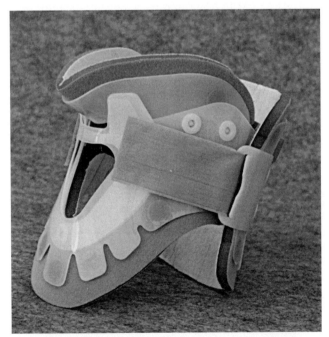

Figure 35–7. Aspen cervical orthosis, designed to provide circumferential control of the spine. The Aspen is a two-piece orthosis manufactured out of polyethylene with a soft foam liner.

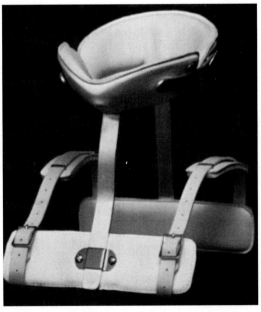

Figure 35–8. Dennison brace. This is an example of a "two-poster" brace.

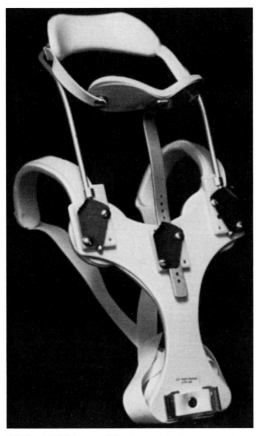

Figure 35–9. SOMI brace. The long anterior support can be seen, and the lack of significant posterior extension support should also be noted. The three uprights attach anteriorly on this orthosis.

Camp collar does not have any attachment to the thoracic wall. They pointed out that comfort would probably be an important determinant of compliance; because it was the most restrictive, the Camp collar was poorly tolerated by patients and perhaps would not be worn regularly. Additionally, they studied the pressure on the chin and the occiput after application, as well as with forced motion. They concluded that this pressure was an extremely important determinant of the limitation of motion. Fisher and coauthors[24] also noted poor correlation between goniometric measurements and total bony motion on radiographs.

Johnson and associates, in what is probably the most rigorous study to date, evaluated immobilization techniques in the cervical spine (Fig. 35–13).[39, 40] They compared a soft collar, a Philadelphia collar, a four-poster CO, a four-poster CTO, a Yale brace, and a halo-brace affixed to a vest in 44 volunteers. Each subject served as his or her own control. Cervical radiographs were used to assess motion (except for rotation, for which goniometry was used). A statistical analysis was provided, as well as a level-by-level assessment. Unfortunately, the halo-brace studies were done with only seven subjects, all of whom had cervical fusions. The investigators reported detailed recommendations for the use of these devices for each level of the cervical spine. Of interest is the finding that the motion between the occiput and C1 increased from the normal motion of the unrestricted spine for all the braces. This paradoxic or "snake" motion has been noted by

cervical motion and to provide the best immobilization. Unfortunately, the authors provided no specific quantitative information and no statistical analysis, and the number of subjects was small. In addition, cineradiography has been demonstrated to lack the reproducibility and resolution of other techniques.[15, 24] This study, however, made a useful contribution and prompted further investigations. Their conclusion on the soft cervical collar has been corroborated by other studies.[39]

Colachis and associates[17] used flexion-extension radiographs to study four types of collars and verified some of Hartman's results. Additionally, they noted that by adding chin and occiput supports, significant FE control could be achieved. This report did not provide any statistical analysis.

Fisher and coauthors[24] studied two COs (Philadelphia collar and Camp brace) and two CTOs (SOMI and a four-poster orthosis) using FE radiographs and goniometry techniques. This study provided detailed information on a level-by-level basis with some statistical validation. They observed that of the orthoses tested, the SOMI brace provided the best immobilization in the prevention of FE motion in four of seven cervical levels. They also noted that the Camp brace provided the best restriction at the C1–C2 level; the

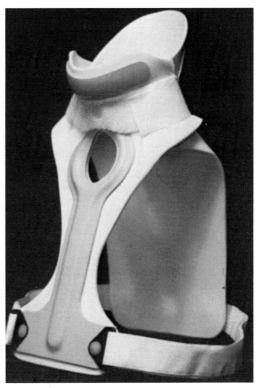

Figure 35–10. Yale brace. This is classified as a cervicothoracic orthosis.

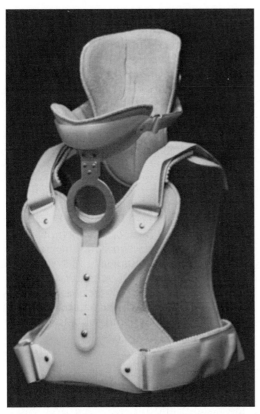

Figure 35–11. Minerva brace. The jacket component is similar to that of a halo-vest. The occipital and mandibular supports have thick pads and encompass the head more than most other available braces.

numerous authors in the cervical as well as the lumbosacral spine.[16, 36, 50, 79] Johnson and associates also noted that, in general, increasing the length of the orthosis and the rigidity of the connection improved the rotational and flexion control, but LB and total FE motions were not affected by these factors. They concluded that the halo-brace provided the best overall control of the cervical spine and should be used for truly unstable injuries. They also reported very little difference (less than 2 degrees) in the immobilization of the C2–C3 interspace with a halo-brace, a four-poster, and a Yale brace.

The halo-vest was described by Perry and Nickel in the late 1950s.[64] Since then, numerous investigations have been done on various aspects of the vest.[7, 26, 32, 37, 44, 50, 52, 59, 60, 64, 65] Unfortunately, but understandably, all the investigations of the immobilization characteristics of this device have been done in patients with cervical spine pathology. The range of allowed total motion with the halo-vest has been reported to be from 4 to 30 per cent of normal.[44, 50] Although conflicting in some conclusions, most reports agree that the halo device provides the least restriction above the C2 level and is best below C4–C5. A careful review of the literature failed to identify the thoracic level at which it becomes ineffective. Our recommendation for the lowest effec-

tive level for a halo with a prefabricated vest is T1. Below this point, we attach the halo-ring and superstructure to a custom-fabricated TLSO. The complications associated with the use of a halo-vest have been described in the literature and exceed the severity of the complications associated with other devices.[7] Despite these complications, general agreement exists that only the halo device should be used in truly unstable fractures of the cervical spine. A detailed description of the halo-brace is included later in this chapter.

Table 35–2 lists our modifications of recommendations made by Johnson and associates.[39, 40, 54] It must be pointed out that all devices lose effectiveness at the ends of the immobilized segments.

Devices to immobilize the cervical spine in the field have also been studied.[15, 19, 66] Cline and coworkers[15] studied 92 volunteers using the Hare extrication collar, the Philadelphia collar, and their own system for immobilization, which consists of a short board with forehead and chin straps. They concluded that a board with straps (Kerlix rolls) provided the best acute immobilization. They did not provide a level-by-level statistical analysis of motion. Podolsky and colleagues[66] used goniometry to assess the immobilization provided by a Hare device, a Philadelphia collar, a soft collar, and their technique of using a board, two sandbags, and forehead tape. They concluded that the Philadelphia collar provided the best immobilization against FE motion, but provided almost no restriction of rotation or

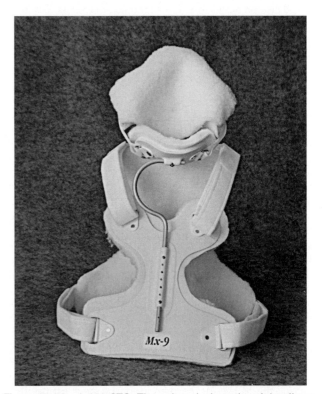

Figure 35–12. L-200 CTO. The unique L-shaped upright allows a patient with a tracheotomy tube to be fitted without disconnecting the tube. Auto-aligning chin and occipital pieces help prevent skin breakdown in nonambulatory patients.

Table 35–2. RECOMMENDED ORTHOSES FOR IMMOBILIZATION OF THE CERVICAL SPINE

	Total Flexion-Extension	Flexion	Extension
0CC–C1	Halo	Halo	Halo
C1–C2	Halo	Halo	Halo
	CTO	SOMI	CTO
C2–C3	Halo	Halo	Halo
		CTO	CTO
C3–C7	Halo	Halo	Halo
	CTO	CTO	CTO
	CO	CO	CO
C7–T2	Halo	CTO	CTO
	CTO		

CO, cervical orthosis; CTO, cervicothoracic orthosis; halo, halo-brace.

lateral bending. They thought that their extrication-immobilization system was the best way to immobilize the cervical spine in the acute setting. These recommendations have also been made by others.[19]

THORACOLUMBAR AND SACRAL ORTHOSES

SIOs, LSOs, and TLSOs can be classified into flexible or rigid devices. The flexible orthoses are made similar to the rigid ones in terms of the overall architecture. Flexible sacral orthoses usually encircle the pelvis, between the iliac crests and the trochanters. Additionally, they have perineal straps that prevent upward displacement. LSOs are similar in coverage but extend to the xiphoid process anteriorly and to the inferior angle of the scapula. The flexible TLSO extends higher, with the posterosuperior border at the midscapular level and the anterosuperior border remaining at the xiphoid process. These garments are circumferentially adjustable by means of side, front, and back laces or hooks, or more recently by Velcro straps.

A proposed use of the flexible SIO is to provide support for postpartum traumatic separation of the sacroiliac joint. The flexible LSO and TLSO are often used for low back pain. They reportedly decrease the myoelectric activity of the paraspinal muscle groups and increase intra-abdominal pressures, thus diminishing the loads on the discs and the low back.[47, 54, 57, 61, 78] These claims, however, are controversial; some authors report that these corsets lead to increased myoelectric activity in certain muscle groups when specific activities are performed.[47] Although corsets (flexible LSOs and TLSOs) do provide some degree of immobilization, the support is minimal, and they should not be used when rigid external fixation is necessary.[47, 51, 78] Newer versions of these corsets are made out of elastic, with Velcro closures and a heat-moldable plastic back panel. The low-temperature thermoplastic panel is heated and custom molded to fit the affected area as closely as possible. After molding, the plastic panel is fitted into a pocket in the elastic corset, which wraps around the torso and is fastened with Velcro. Although this type of garment cannot provide as much abdominal compression as the traditional corset, it is well received by patients. It is light, less bulky, easy to fit, and affordable.

Rigid Thoracolumbosacral and Lumbosacral Orthoses

Rigid TLSOs and LSOs have not received nearly as much attention in the scientific literature as cervical orthoses. Conventional TLSOs exert most of their control in the FE axis and are less rigid in preventing rotational and lateral bending motions. A typical, non-custom-molded TLSO is the Jewett hyperextension brace (Fig. 35–14). It applies a three-point truncal force with two anterior pads, one on the symphysis pubis and another at the sternomanubrial junction. The third point of control is a posterior pad held in place with rigid straps. Positioning of this pad is usually midway between the levels of the anterior sternal and pubic pads. The posterior pad provides the counterforce that enables this orthosis to place the spine in a hyperextended position. The Knight-Taylor brace (Fig. 35–15) is another example of a commonly prescribed TLSO. This style of orthosis can be prefabricated out of Kydex (polyvinyl chloride [PVC]) or can be custom fabricated out of aluminum with a leather covering. The device uses a corset-type front and has lateral and posterior uprights with over-the-shoulder straps to limit LB and FE. Adding crossed uprights makes these devices more rigid. However, the rotational control, even with uprights, is poor.

A relatively new entry into this class of orthosis is the prefabricated TLSO such as the Atlantic International (Fig. 35–16). These devices are usually fabricated out of 1/8- to 3/16-inch low-density polyethylene with a full 1/4-inch foam liner. Using a bivalve or clamshell design, they are fastened in place with three Velcro closures per side. The orthoses can be ordered to measurements or in a series of prefabricated sizes. Some manufacturers include pneumatic bladders in the abdominal and/or lumbar areas to aid in fit and for use in volume changes. Although these bladders do help increase the tightness of the orthosis, patients often find them confusing and difficult to use.

A prefabricated TLSO provides better control for lateral side bending than does the Knight-Taylor orthosis, as well as better rotational control. Most of the motion restriction in this class of orthosis is in the FE axis.

To obtain optimal control of motion in all planes, a TLSO should be fully custom molded. An example of this is a high-temperature thermoplastic TLSO that is custom fitted from a plaster shell taken from the patient. These devices should not be used to immobilize the thoracic spine above T5.[79] To gain control of this area, a cervical extension should be added to the thermoplastic jacket.[79] The distal extent of immobilization of these orthoses is at L4.[61, 73, 79]

LSOs are frequently prescribed. Their main use is in

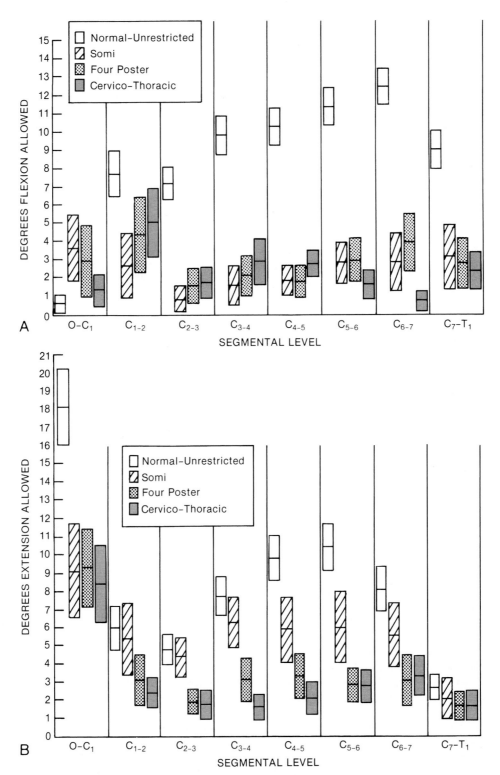

Figure 35–13. Graphs of motion allowed in the normal cervical spine compared with related cervical orthotics. *A,* Degrees of flexion allowed in SOMI, four-poster, and cervicothoracic braces compared with the normal unrestricted cervical spine. *B,* Degrees of extension allowed in SOMI, four-poster, and cervicothoracic braces compared with the normal unrestricted cervical spine.

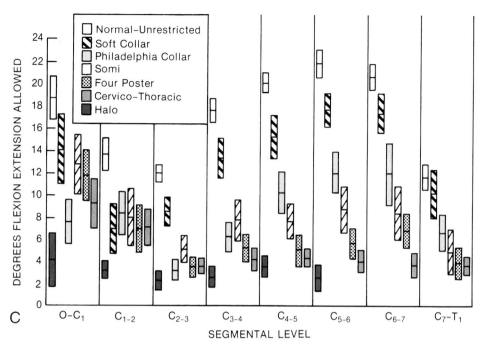

Figure 35-13 *Continued C,* Degrees of flexion-extension allowed at each cervical segmental level in a normal spine compared with a variety of orthotics. (From Johnson, R. M., Hart, D. L., Simmons, E. F., et al.: Cervical orthoses: A study comparing their effectiveness in restricting cervical motion in normal subjects. J. Bone Joint Surg. Am. *59*:332, 1977.)

the treatment of low back pain, as well as following lumbosacral surgical instrumentation and fusion. The typical rigid LSO is similar in shape to a corset, with the addition of anterior, posterior, and lateral uprights to achieve control in FE, rotation, and LB. Again, these devices exert the poorest control against rotation.[61, 73, 79] The effect of an LSO on the abdominal and paraspinal musculature has been debated.[47, 78] Waters and Morris[78] analyzed 10 subjects using a chairback brace as well as a corset. They implanted wire electrodes in the erector spinae and external abdominal musculature and monitored myoelectric activity. They reported that with subjects at rest, neither a corset nor a chairback brace had any effect on the activity of the erector spinae muscles. They noted that at high levels of activity, the paraspinal muscles actually had increased activity. They also noted that abdominal muscles had decreased activity with both braces when subjects were at rest as well as during limited activity. In this report, however, the electrical activity was only qualitatively assessed, and no statistical analysis was done.

Lantz and Schultz looked at the same braces (chairback and corset) plus a thermoplastic molded TLSO.[47] They studied five volunteers who performed various tasks. Muscle activity was monitored through surface electrodes. They concluded that, depending on the task performed, the myoelectric activity of the "restricted" subjects was higher than in controls, and that no consistent pattern could be observed. Unfortunately, only five subjects were used, and part of the variability reported could be attributed to the sample size. Despite the effort expended, the effects of these orthoses on the myoelectric activity of the erector spinae muscles have not been conclusively demonstrated. Most authors, however, agree that the myoelectric activity in the ab-

dominal musculature appears to be decreased with all braces.[54, 55, 78]

Motion in the lumbar spine has been studied extensively.[2, 23, 33, 47, 51, 73, 83] The effect of bracing on this motion has received some attention.[47, 51, 61] Norton and Brown[61] published the earliest scientific study on the use of braces to restrict motion in the lumbar spine. They studied four types of LSO (three rigid and one flexible), as well as a TLSO. The specific types of orthoses studied were the Jewett (see Fig. 35-14), Goldthwait, Taylor, Arnold-Abbott, and Williams braces, as well as their own design and a custom-fitted plaster brace. To measure motion, they placed Kirschner wires in the spinous processes of subjects and measured the angles between the wires. Additionally, radiographic measurements were made. They reported that motion across the lumbosacral junction actually increased with the use of each of the braces. They also observed increased motion at the L4–L5 level while the subjects were sitting in these braces. All the braces studied also caused some degree of flexion at the L4–L5 and L5–S1 levels when standing, as compared with the unbraced state. Additionally, the investigators attempted to measure the forces exerted between the body and the braces. They modified the pressure points in their experimental brace and succeeded in eliminating some of the flexion observed in volunteers wearing the standard braces in the lower spine. Although some of the observations made by this group remain useful, they did not analyze motion above the L3 level and limited the study to flexion and extension.

Lumsden and Morris[51] studied the rotational motion at the lumbosacral joint. In their study, subjects had instrumented Steinmann pins inserted in the posterior superior iliac spine. Measurements were done as a

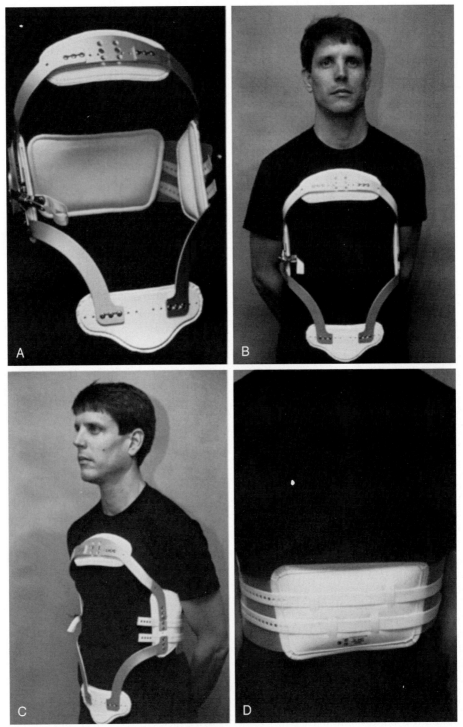

Figure 35–14. *A,* Jewett brace. This is an example of a thoracolumbosacral orthosis. Anteriorly, there are pads that cross the sternum and the pubic symphysis. The posterior pad crosses the upper lumbar spine. This is designed to provide three-point fixation and some degree of extension. *B,* Frontal, *C,* oblique, and *D,* posterior projections of a model in a Jewett brace.

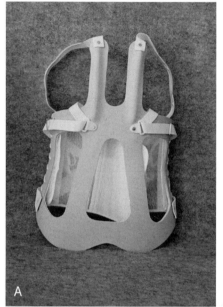

Figure 35–15. *A,* Knight-Taylor orthosis. It is available in prefabricated sizes, or it can be custom made to measurements. The corset front provides abdominal compression, and the axilla straps provide thoracic control. *B,* Frontal, *C,* oblique, and *D,* posterior projections of a model in a Knight-Taylor orthosis.

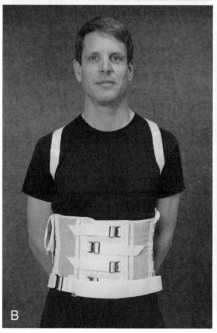

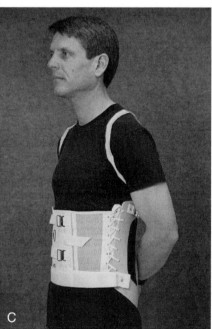

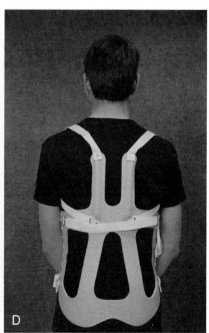

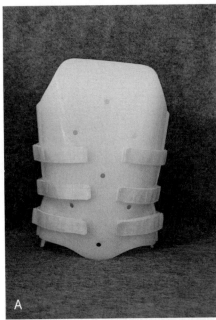

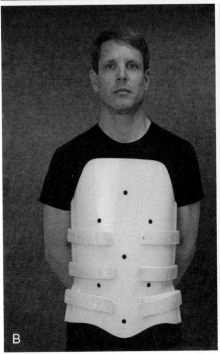

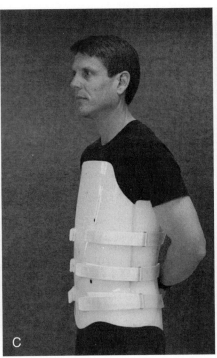

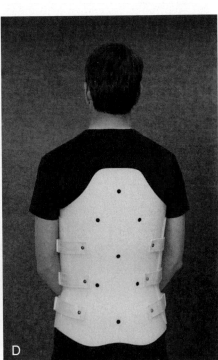

Figure 35–16. *A,* Atlanta International Pre-Fab TLSO. This is a bivalve design prefabricated TLSO made from polyethylene with a full foam liner. *B,* Frontal, *C,* oblique, and *D,* posterior projections of a model in an Atlanta International Pre-Fab TLSO.

Table 35–3. RECOMMENDED ORTHOSES FOR RIGID IMMOBILIZATION OF THE THORACOLUMBOSACRAL SPINE

T2–T5	Plastic TLSO with attached chin and occiput support
T6–L3	Plastic TLSO
L4–S1	Plastic TLSO with a thigh cuff

TLSO, thoracolumbosacral orthosis.

combination of pin rotations and radiographic studies. A chairback brace as well as an LSO corset were used to restrict motion. They concluded that these conventionally used braces increased the motion at the lumbosacral level.

Fidler and Plasmans[23] reported their observations on the limitation of lumbosacral motion obtained with a corset, a brace, and a plaster jacket with and without a thigh cuff. Radiographs were used to assess motion. They concluded that a custom-molded plaster jacket was the most effective way of restricting motion at L1–L3, but to immobilize the L4–S1 levels, a thigh cuff must be included. In this study, however, only five volunteers were used, and a very limited statistical analysis was provided.

Lantz and Schultz[47] investigated the effects of a corset, a chairback brace LSO, and a TLSO on the motion of the lumbosacral spine. They concluded that the per cent of restriction of motion was greatest with the plastic-molded TLSO. These authors, unfortunately, did not provide segmental information and had no statistical analysis.

As can be inferred from this review, no brace provided ideal immobilization. Table 35–3 lists our recommendations for immobilization at the various levels in the thoracic and lumbosacral spine.

Thoracic Spine

For the thoracic spine there are few available devices. The most commonly used is the Jewett brace (see Fig. 35–14). It has a proximal sternal and distal pubic symphysis support, as well as posterior and lateral components that provide three-point fixation. This orthosis attempts to extend the thoracic and upper lumbar spine and requires some degree of bony contact. It is best used for symptomatic relief of compression fractures, when there is not significant fear or risk of further collapse. It does not provide strong rigidity against flexion and is poorly tolerated by elderly patients.

For rigid immobilization, a custom-molded body jacket of Kydex (PVC) or a custom-fitted plaster jacket (or synthetic plaster) is required. A TLSO provides restriction of motion up to approximately the T5 level and distally to approximately L4. If the injury is in the upper thoracic spine, a cervical extension should be included; if the injury is below, one hip or thigh should be included in the orthosis to prevent pelvic rotation and motion.

Corsets (thoracolumbar or lumbosacral) should be considered for the symptomatic treatment of back pain, or perhaps osteoporotic compression fractures. Although abdominal muscle electromyographic (EMG) changes do occur in a patient wearing a corset for six weeks, the corset does not structurally stabilize the bony column of the spine.

CERVICAL SPINE

Soft (Fig. 35–17) and hard (Fig. 35–18) cervical collars are available. For the most part, these serve as reminders to the patient not to flex and extend, but they do not provide significant rigid support. Soft collars are used primarily in whiplash-type injuries, where some mild degree of cervical support is necessary but it is

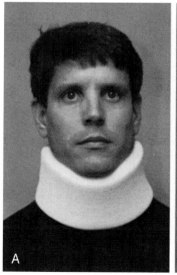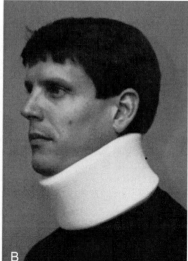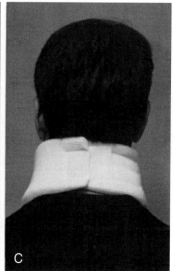

Figure 35–17. *A,* Frontal, *B,* oblique, and *C,* posterior projections of a model in a soft cervical collar.

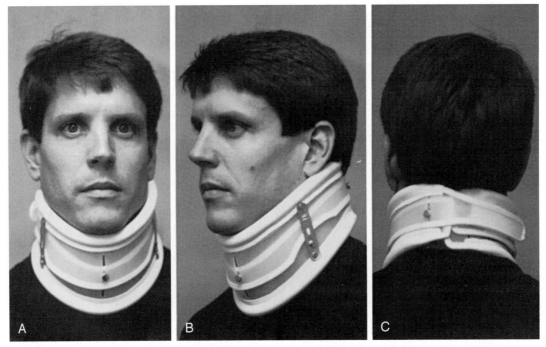

Figure 35–18. *A*, Frontal, *B*, oblique, and *C*, posterior projections of a model in a hard cervical collar.

not necessary to provide rigid restriction against flexion, extension, or rotation. Hard collars are similar to soft collars but have slightly more rigid support mechanisms. They do not, however, provide the occipital, mandibular, or shoulder contouring and motion restriction that other cervical orthoses do. Soft collars have very little role in cervical spine injuries.

One of the most commonly used cervical orthoses is the Philadelphia collar (Fig. 35–19). This is made of polyethylene and PVC. It is a circumferential device, with anterior and posterior shells united with Velcro straps. The collar fits on the shoulders. There is no significant extension anterior or posterior onto the thorax. There are multiple sizes for the anterior and posterior pieces. When fitted well, most of these collars keep the neck in some degree of flexion. Therefore, if a flexion force needs to be resisted, a Philadelphia collar is not the ideal orthotic device.

An infrequently used orthosis is a four-poster, which has an upper thoracic support and two anterior and two posterior metal struts, affixing to the chin and occipital rests, respectively. These are relatively heavy devices and, for the most part, have been replaced by the Philadelphia collar and other orthoses. Two-posters (Fig. 35–20) with one midline anterior support and one midline posterior support are not effective in rotation and have, for the most part, been replaced. The Guildford brace is essentially a modification of the two-poster brace. In this case, the head (chin and occiput) support includes a circumferentially fitting metal support that decreases the likelihood of a patient rotating out of the device and prevents flexion and extension. Johnson and coworkers[39, 40] showed that this orthotic

device provided one of the highest degrees of immobilization in the midcervical spine.

A newer cervical orthosis is the Malibu brace (Fig. 35–21), which is made of polyethylene and PVC. It extends further onto the thorax anteriorly and posteriorly, and the construction is more rigid than that of the Philadelphia collar; it appears to control flexion and extension more rigidly than does the Philadelphia collar. It fits the chin and the occiput tightly. In our opinion, when a cervicothoracic brace is not needed but it is important to rigidly protect a midcervical injury, the Malibu brace provides more support and restriction than the Philadelphia collar.

Other cervical orthoses that need to be considered are the Miami J orthosis (Fig. 35–22) and the Aspen orthosis (Fig. 35–23). Both are two-piece braces, fabricated out of polyethylene with soft interface materials. The Aspen comes in six sizes, and the Miami J is available in five; both brands are radiolucent.

A frequent problem associated with all cervical orthoses is the occurrence of skin breakdown over bony prominences, particularly in nonambulatory patients requiring long-term immobilization. In an effort to study this concern, Plaisier and associates[65a] compared the pressure exerted by four cervical collars on the chin, occiput, and mandible in the upright and supine positions. Both the Miami J and the Aspen were under the capillary closing pressure in the supine and upright positions. The Philadelphia collar exposed the wearer to high pressure while supine, and the stiff neck exceeded the capillary closing pressure on most contact points in both positions. Their conclusions were that the Aspen and Miami J were more "skin-friendly" and

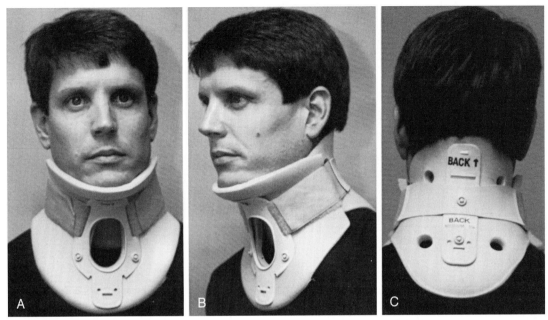

Figure 35–19. *A,* Frontal, *B,* oblique, and *C,* posterior projections of a model in a Philadelphia collar. Multiple sizes (caudad to cephalad height) and lengths (anterior/posterior dimensions of the chin occipital prominences) are available, as is a hole for a tracheotomy tube.

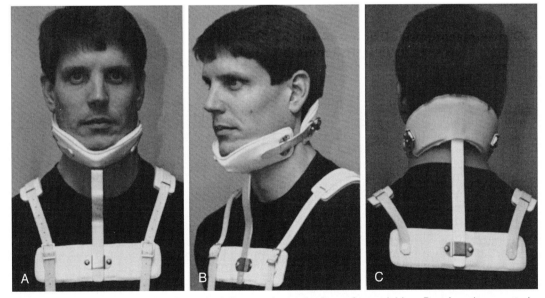

Figure 35–20. *A,* Frontal, *B,* oblique, and *C,* posterior projections of a model in a Dennison (two-poster) brace.

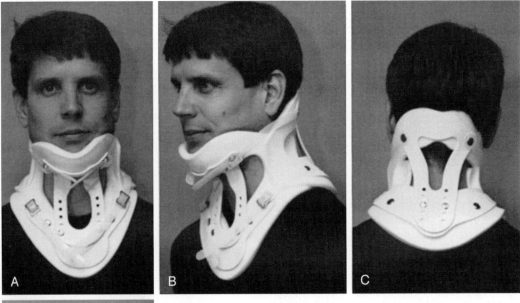

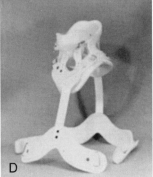

Figure 35–21. *A,* Frontal, *B,* oblique, and *C,* posterior projections of a model in a Malibu brace. *D,* Extensions can be added to the caudal aspect of this cervical orthosis to extend the fixation to the thorax and to provide more rigid fixation across the cervicothoracic junction and perhaps also cephalically.

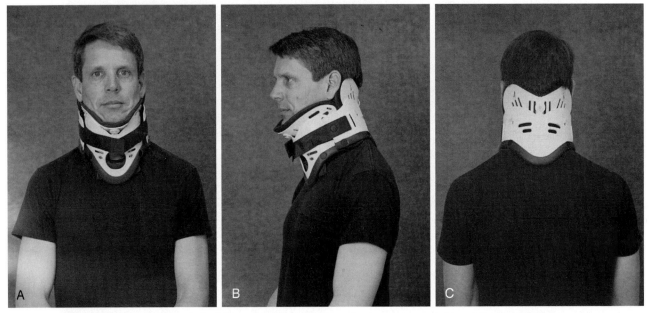

Figure 35–22. *A,* Frontal, *B,* oblique, and *C,* posterior projections of a model in a Miami J cervical orthosis.

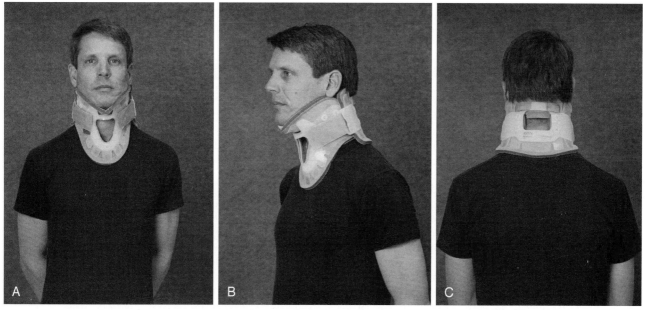

Figure 35–23. *A,* Frontal, *B,* oblique, and *C,* posterior projections of a model in an Aspen cervical orthosis.

more comfortable to wear; these orthoses are now their primary choices in nonambulatory patients requiring long-term immobilization.

The SOMI brace (Fig. 35–24) structurally qualifies as a cervicothoracic orthosis, because there is an anterior thoracic extension. However, the posterior support extends only slightly distal to the shoulders. Straps connect the posterior to the anterior piece. There is one anterior upright for chin-mandibular support, and two posterior uprights for occipital support. The anterior and posterior connection is relatively weak. This device does not extend posteriorly over the back, making it relatively easy for a patient to rotate his or her neck out of this device. Extensions can be added to the standard SOMI brace to help control the cervicothoracic region and provide more rigidity across the thorax.

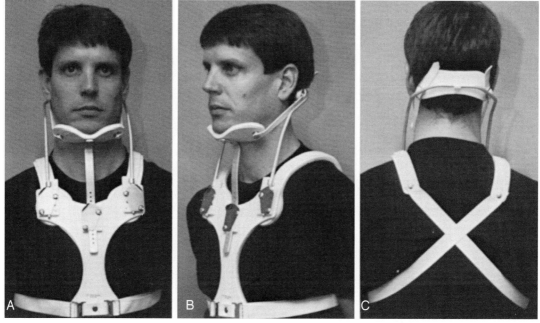

Figure 35–24. *A,* Frontal, *B,* oblique, and *C,* posterior projections of a model in a SOMI.

Additionally, the occipital piece can be extended proximally, and a band can be attached around the forehead to control rotation and further restrict flexion.

The next most-rigid devices for cervical immobilization are cervicothoracic orthoses. The Yale brace (Fig. 35–25) is made of Kydex and Aliplast. It is similar to a Philadelphia collar, with an extension anteriorly down the sternum and posteriorly over the scapula and thoracic spine. Velcro bands connect the anterior to the posterior struts. This provides fairly rigid fixation, particularly at the upper and lower levels of the cervical spine. Although encompassing the thoracic spine, it should not be used to provide rigid immobilization below C7–T1. The Minerva brace (Fig. 35–26) is thicker, broader, and more restrictive than the Yale brace. The posterior cervical portion extends over the occiput. Anteriorly, a rigid plastic piece, which supports the mandible, is fixed to a metal rod and secured to the thoracic vest portion. The occipital and chin supports are united with straps. The thoracic component fits broadly over the chest, as well as the thoracic spine and scapula posteriorly. It is shaped similar to a halo-vest. A strap applied to the occipital extension fits around the forehead and provides rotational and further flexion-extension control.

A new orthosis for the cervicothoracic region is the L-200 CTO (Fig. 35–27). The thoracic portion is similar in contact area and strap configuration to the Minerva orthosis, but the L-200 utilizes replaceable sheepskin liners where it contacts the body. The anterior upright has a unique configuration, which allows fitting of the orthosis on an intubated patient without requiring the disconnection and reconnection of the ventilator tube. Nonambulatory patients who require long-term immo-

bilization in CTOs are frequently at risk for skin breakdown in the chin and occipital regions. This is usually caused by a tendency of the orthosis to "ride up" on the supine patient, resulting in increased pressures over these bony prominences. The L-200 CTO has been designed with "auto-aligning" chin and occipital pieces that pivot slightly and may lessen the risk of decubitus ulcers in this patient population.

The halo-brace provides the most rigid cervical immobilization. It is frequently used for fractures that are not surgically stabilized. It is most successfully used when the injury is primarily bony, because pure ligamentous injuries (dislocations, transverse ligament disruptions, occipitoatlantal dislocations, and so forth) do not heal as well as bone, are difficult to maintain aligned even with halo-ambulatory traction, and frequently require surgery to create short- and long-term stability. Unstable surgical fusions may also have to be maintained in a halo device while healing progresses. Additionally, if there is any question regarding the patient's ability to cooperate, the halo-brace is the most difficult orthosis for a patient to remove and is the safest if there is any risk of spinal cord injury. Finally, early application of a halo-brace allows the patient to become ambulatory and aids rehabilitation if surgery is not indicated and rigid external stabilization is required. This allows the maintenance of cervical traction and immobilization in most patients while they are upright and mobile.

FINANCIAL ASPECTS

Currently, with insurance cutbacks and restrictions on the availability and type of medical care based on

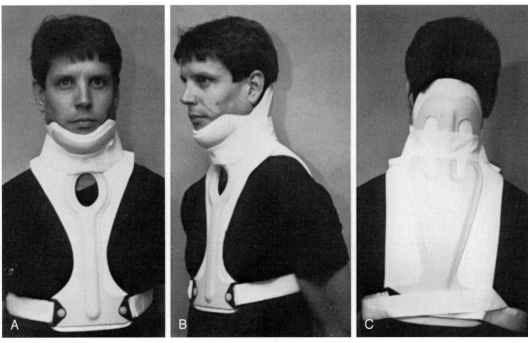

Figure 35–25. *A,* Frontal, *B,* oblique, and *C,* posterior projections of a model in a Yale brace.

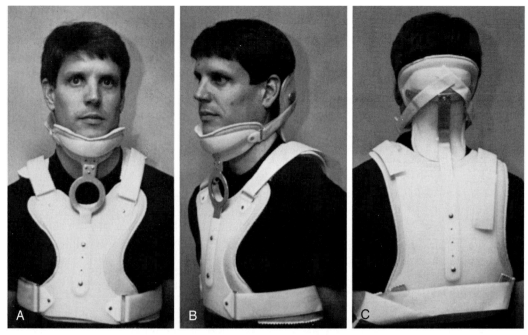

Figure 35–26. *A,* Frontal, *B,* oblique, and *C,* posterior projections of a model in a Minerva brace. Additionally, a strap can be placed around the most proximal aspect of the occipital support to encircle the forehead.

economic factors, physicians have to be aware of the financial impact of a brace prescription. Table 35–4 lists the approximate costs for fitting a patient with some of the most common spinal orthoses in the San Diego area in 1996. When using some of the newer, untested orthoses, physicians should be aware of the advantages in terms of restriction of motion and comfort, as well as their relative cost.

RECOMMENDATIONS FOR FUTURE RESEARCH

Spinal orthotic studies have significant limitations in scientific validity. Based on a review of this literature, we conclude that there is a growing need for better, more rigorous studies. Future work should use modern radiographic techniques that minimize radiation to

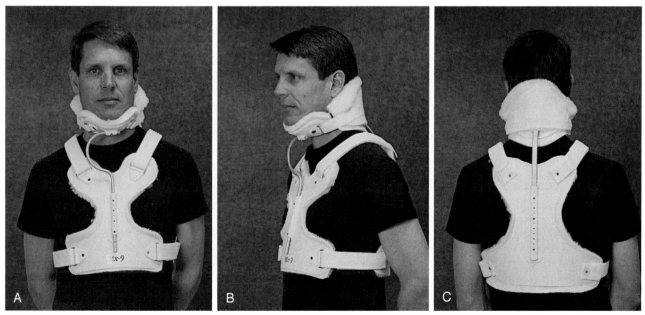

Figure 35–27. *A,* Frontal, *B,* oblique, and *C,* posterior projections of a model in an L-200 CTO.

Table 35–4. RELATIVE PRICES OF SELECTED ORTHOSES

Brace	Average Cost*
Soft collar	$50
Philadelphia collar	$125
Malibu collar	$235
SOMI	$480
Polyform TLSO	$1250
Halo with standard vest	$2800

*1996 prices, San Diego, CA.
SOMI, sterno-occipito-mandibular immobilizer; TLSO, thoracolumbosacral orthoses.

study various braces. A large number of individuals should be studied, and an adequate statistical analysis should be provided. The fit and maximal effort of the braces should be normalized with pressure measurements. Additionally, further studies on the halo-brace should be done on the normal spine and used as a baseline to compare with other orthoses. Lastly, the effect of body fat on fit should be correlated with limitation of motion. This can be done by the use of objective fat-quantifying techniques, such as triceps skin fold thickness.

THE HALO SKELETAL FIXATOR

The halo skeletal fixator provides the most rigid type of immobilization of all the orthoses that stabilize the cervical spine. Since its introduction by Perry and Nickel in 1959,[64] its effectiveness in immobilization has been well established.[1, 8, 18, 32, 42, 44–46, 56, 59, 63, 65, 67, 71, 74, 80] For many years following its introduction, few changes were made in the design or recommended method of application.[8, 37, 59, 60, 64] Despite the halo-braces's demonstrated effectiveness, problem areas, especially with pin loosening and infection, became apparent.[7, 11, 27, 28, 63, 71, 81] More recent studies on these and other potential problems, as well as studies on skull anatomy, biomechanical aspects, and pin insertion techniques, have resulted in more scientifically derived guidelines for application and maintenance.[8, 10–25, 26, 29–31, 68, 75, 85]

Development of the Halo

A device similar to the current halo-brace, but consisting of an incomplete ring that was open posteriorly, was conceived by orthopedic surgeon Frank Bloom during World War II. This device was used to treat pilots who had sustained inwardly displaced facial fractures with overlying skin burns. The device stabilized and applied traction to these fractures by the use of pins placed into the facial bones, with outward traction applied through the incomplete ring. The pin design was similar to those used today.

Bloom's device subsequently led to the development of the well-known halo skeletal fixator by Vernon Nickel, which was first reported by Perry and Nickel

in 1959.[64] The halo-brace originally consisted of a complete ring attached to a body cast. It used skeletal pins placed through holes in the ring to anchor the skull to the ring. The device was initially used for cervical spine immobilization following arthrodesis in patients with paralytic cervical muscles from poliomyelitis.[59, 60, 64] The halo-brace was subsequently adapted to stabilize the cervical spine in both adults and children following trauma, infection, tumors, inflammatory and degenerative diseases, congenital malformation, and surgical fusion.[1, 8, 18, 22, 32, 38, 42, 44–46, 55, 56, 59, 63, 65, 67, 68, 71, 74, 80]

The Halo-Ring. The original halo-ring was manufactured out of metal and was available in different sizes. It had multiple holes for pin insertion. The ring curved upward in the rear to afford greater surgical exposure to the upper cervical spine with the ring in place. The halo-ring was connected to a plaster body jacket by two upright anterior posts.[64]

Subsequent improvements in materials and design have resulted in several different halo fixators, which are now available from a variety of manufacturers. Lightweight metals and composite materials have led to radiolucent rings, adjustable rings, convertible tong-to-ring devices, and open rings or crown-type devices that encircle only part of the head. These later designs are open posteriorly and avoid the need to pass the head through the ring, thus easing application and improving safety. In some of the incomplete rings, the posterior ends are prudently angled inferiorly to ensure posterior pin placement below the equator of the skull (see later).

The Halo-Vest. Advancement in plastics technology has allowed the development of lightweight, durable, quickly applied, adjustable vests that have replaced plaster body casts.[37, 64] Cross-straps and supports stabilize and decease shear stress between the anterior and posterior portions. A low-profile design for the metal uprights and connecting rods provides a more manageable and patient-livable frame. Anodizing or special coating of the metal upright rods helps prevent metal seizing during tightening. Additionally, connecting bolts on the vest can be tightened with torque wrenches that ratchet or "give way" at a set amount of torque (i.e., 28 ft/lb). These wrenches can potentially save time and minimize overtightening and bolt stripping. Current plastic vests and connecting-rod systems allow cervical spine adjustment in virtually any plane. Safety-knurled adjustment knobs, two-point flexion-extension supports with ratchets, and lightweight metals have allowed fine adjustments for fracture alignment.

Despite their easy application, the prefabricated vests do not always fit adequately, especially if limited sizes are available. If a vest fits poorly (especially in an extremely thin or obese patient), use of a form-fitting plaster body cast or custom-molded plastic halo-vest should be considered. This is particularly true if there are skin problems or multiple injuries that require custom fitting to the trunk.

The Halo-Pin. Few changes have been made in the pin design since its original description. It has been shown, however, that altering this design can significantly improve the mechanical qualities of the pin-bone interface.[30] A pointed, bullet-type pin with a broad shoulder may provide more rigidity at the pin-bone interface than currently available pins. This design and others, including a peg-type tip with a broad shoulder, are still under investigation and are not commercially available.

Recently, "breakaway" torque wrench handles designed for one-time use to insert halo-pins have been introduced. These wrenches break off at set amount of torque (e.g., 8 inch/lb, 0.90 N/m) and can save time. They are smaller than standard wrenches and allow pin tightening despite limited access to the posterior aspect of the skill (e.g., when the patient is on a Rotobed). Although preliminary results show these wrenches to be accurate, rechecking the pin torque with a calibrated torque screwdriver is prudent. Some desirable features of a halo apparatus are listed in Table 35–5.[13]

Pin Insertion Techniques

Pin Site Selection. The preferred sites for halo-pin insertion have been evaluated in cadaver skull studies, radiographic studies, and clinical reviews of pin-related complications.[8, 11, 12, 25, 26, 28, 31, 84] The optimal position for anterior halo-pin placement, based on anatomic structures at risk and skull thickness, is in the anterolateral aspect of the skull, approximately 1 cm superior to the orbital rim (eyebrow), cephalad to the lateral two thirds of the orbit, and below the greatest circumference (equator) of the skull. This area can be considered a "safe zone" (Figs. 35–28 through 35–30). Placement of the pin above the supraorbital rim prevents displacement or penetration into the orbit. Placement of the pin below the level of the greatest skull diameter helps prevent cephalad migration of the pin.[8, 13, 25, 26, 28, 31, 84]

On the lateral aspect of the safe zone lies the temporalis muscle and fossa. Avoidance of the temporalis muscle and fossa is desirable for two reasons: (1) penetration of the temporalis muscle by the halo-pin can be painful and may impede mandibular motion during mastication, and (2) the bone in this area is very thin, often consisting of a single thin cortical shell without a cancellous component, making skull penetration or pin loosening more likely (Fig. 35–31). Although placement of pins in the temporalis region has the advantage of hiding the pin scar behind the hairline, the anatomic and mechanical disadvantages of this site do not seem to warrant choosing this location if other areas are available.[13, 25, 26, 28, 31]

Along the medial aspect of the safe zone lie the supraorbital and supratrochlear nerves and underlying frontal sinus. Placement of the pin lateral to the medial one third of the orbit avoids injury to these nerves and decreases the risk of penetration into the frontal sinus (see Figs. 35–28 through 35–30).[13, 25, 26, 28, 31]

Posterior pin placement seems to be less critical, because vulnerable neuromuscular structures are lacking, the skull is thick, and the bony contours are more uniform. The posterolateral aspects of the skull appear optimal at approximately the four o'clock and eight o'clock positions (directly anterior = twelve o'clock) (see Figs. 35–28 through 35–30).[8, 13, 25, 26, 28, 31, 84]

Angle of Pin Insertion. The angle of pin insertion influences pin fixation.[71] Cyclic loading of pins inserted at different angles demonstrated that perpendicularly inserted pins have superior fixation compared with those placed at 15 or 30 degrees to the skull surface. This is probably because of the broader pin-bone interface, with increased contact area achieved with the perpendicularly placed pins. With any angulation, the shoulder of the pin may intercept the skull's outer cortex before the tip is fully seated.[8, 75] Because the pin angle is fixed or predetermined by the ring in many current halo devices, placement of the ring over a relatively flat portion of the skull (i.e., below the equator) is desirable in order to help obtain a perpendicular insertion at the pin-bone interface.

Use of Skin Incisions. Clinical studies comparing the use of skin incisions prior to pin placement with direct insertion of the pin into the skin indicate that there are no advantages to skin incision.[11] Loosening, infection, comfort, and resultant scars were not altered by creating a small skin incision before inserting the pins. A

Table 35–5. DESIRABLE FEATURES OF THE HALO SKELETAL FIXATOR

Ring and pins
  Maximum number of threaded holes structurally possible
    (to ease pin site selection)
  Occipital area open (to ease ring placement)
  Radiolucent
  MRI compatible (nonferrous, nonmagnetic)
  Pins placed with breakaway wrenches set at 8 in/lb
  Easy connections to upright posts
  Holes allow pin placement at 90 degrees to skull
  Pins have shoulder
Upright posts
  Low profile with length above ring kept to minimum
  Do not interfere with lateral roentgenograms
    (radiolucent or strategically placed)
  Multiplane adjustment of head and neck
  Fine-tuning not essential
Vest
  Lightweight, conforming, yet rigid enough to provide support
  Compatible sizes with additional pediatric and extra-large
    sizes available
  Bridges or cross-straps connecting anterior and posterior
    components to prevent shear motion
  Radiolucent buckles and attachments
  Easy to apply, particularly in an unstable or anesthetized
    patient
  Provision for emergency access to the anterior chest

From Botte, M. J., Garfin, S. R., Byrne, T. P., et al.: The halo skeletal fixator: Principles of application and maintenance. Clin. Orthop. *239*:12–18, 1989.

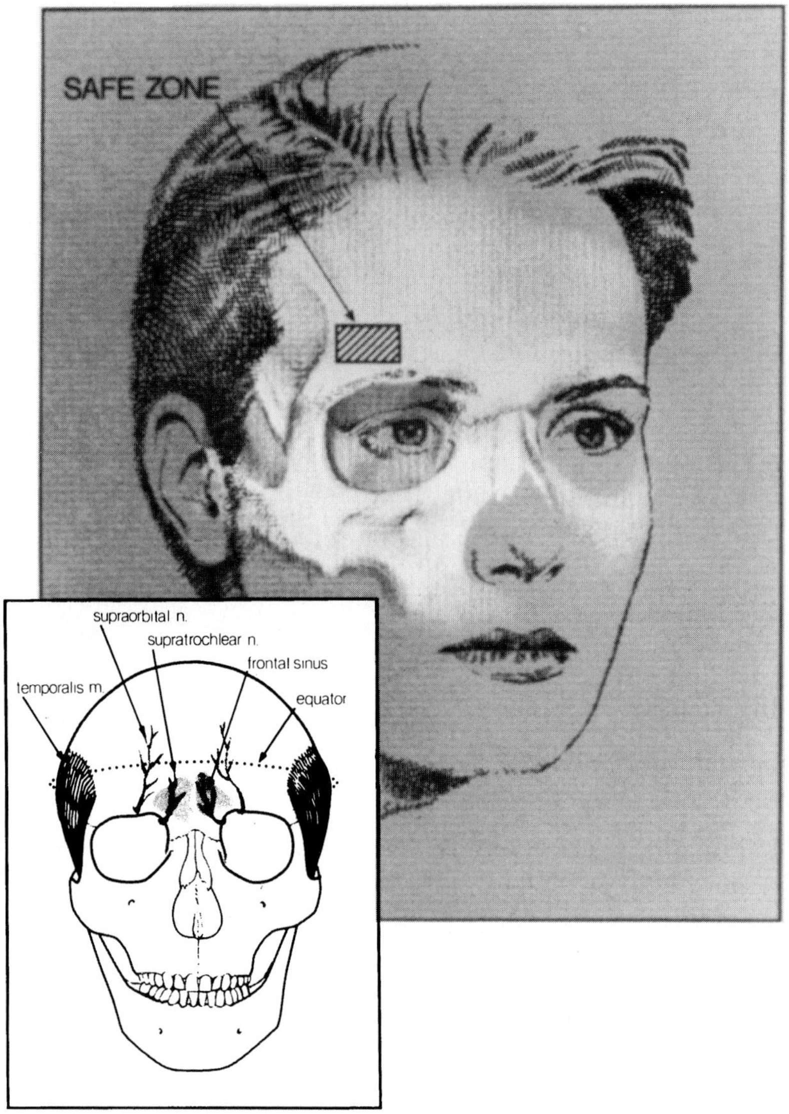

Figure 35–28. The "safe zone" for placement of halo fixator pins. The anterior pins are placed anterolaterally, approximately 1 cm above the orbital rim, below the equator of the skull, and cephalad to the lateral two thirds of the orbit. The safe zone avoids the temporalis muscle and fossa laterally and the supraorbital and supratrochlear nerves and the frontal sinus medially. (From Garfin, S. R., Botte, M. J., Nickel, V. L., and Waters, R. L.: Complications in the use of the halo fixation device. J. Bone Joint Surg. Am. *68*:320, 1986.)

skin incision does, however, cause occasional problems with bleeding, which momentarily delays the halo-application procedure. Therefore, routine placement of skin incisions for halo-pin placement does not seem warranted.[11]

Pin Insertion Torque. The pin insertion torque originally recommended was 5 to 6 inch/lb (0.57 to 0.68 N/m).[60, 63, 64] These recommendations were based primarily on empiric observations. Because of problems with pin loosening, anatomic studies on cadaver human skulls have been performed and demonstrate that halo-pins inserted at up to 10 inch/lb (1.13 N/m) barely penetrate the outer table of the skull.[10] Mechanical testing of the pin-bone interface (cyclic loading and load-to-failure) revealed that a torque of 8 inch/lb (0.90 N/m) significantly improved the mechanical qualities over those achieved with 6 inch/lb (0.68 N/m).[30] Clinically, the use of 8 inch/lb (0.90 N/m) was shown to be safe

and effective in lowering the incidence of pin loosening and infection when compared with application at 6 inch/lb (0.68 N/m).[10] From these studies, 8 inch/lb (0.90 N/m) appears to be preferable to the 5 or 6 inch/lb originally recommended.

Method of Application

Preparation and Selection of Equipment. At least three persons are desirable for halo application.[13, 25] Positioning pins and mechanical head holders are also helpful. The person holding the patient's head should be aware of the nature of the fracture and be comfortably situated while maintaining the unstable cervical spine and halo in position. This task should not be left to an inexperienced member of the team.

Ring and vest sizes are checked, and all materials and equipment inspected.[13, 85] Suggested materials are listed in Table 35–6. Ring size is determined by selec-

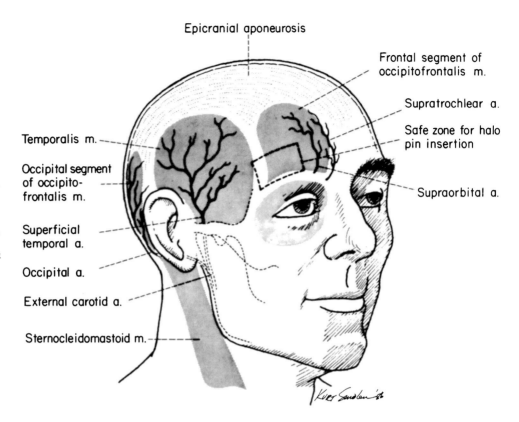

Epicranial aponeurosis

Frontal segment of occipitofrontalis m.

Supratrochlear a.

Safe zone for halo pin insertion

Supraorbital a.

Temporalis m.

Occipital segment of occipito-frontalis m.

Superficial temporal a.

Occipital a.

External carotid a.

Sternocleidomastoid m.

Figure 35–29. Oblique diagram of the safe zone for placement of halo fixator pins. (From Ballock, R. T., Botte, M. J., and Garfin, S. R.: Complications of halo immobilization. *In* Garfin, S. R. [ed.]: Complications of Spine Surgery. Baltimore, Williams & Wilkins, 1989, p. 376. © 1989 Williams & Wilkins Co.)

tion of a ring that provides 1 to 2 cm of clearance around every aspect of the head perimeter. Vest size is determined by measurement of chest circumference using a tape measure. A crash cart with resuscitation equipment must be available throughout the procedure.

Preparation of the Patient. If the medical and neurologic status permit, the patient is lightly sedated but kept awake to report any changes in neurologic status during head and neck manipulation. General anesthesia is not recommended, unless required for concomitant surgical procedures.

The patient is placed supine on the bed or gurney, with the head held beyond the edge. If a crown-type halo is employed (with the posterior portion of the ring removed), the patient's head can remain on the bed. A head-ring support aids application.[13, 25]

The anterior pin sites are selected in the anterolateral aspect of the skull (approximately 1 cm superior to the supraorbital rim, medial to the temporalis muscle and fossa, and cephalad to the lateral two thirds of the orbit) (see Figs. 35–28 through 35–30). The skin sites for pin insertion are prepped with a povidone-iodine solution.

The posterior pins sites are then selected. These sites are located in the posterolateral aspects of the skull at the approximate clock positions of four and eight o'clock (occiput = six o'clock). Although these specific site locations are less critical, it is desirable to place the posterior pins approximately diagonal to the corres-

ponding contralateral anterior pins (i.e., right posterolateral to left anterolateral). The posterior sites should be inferior to the equator of the skull, yet superior enough to prevent ring impingement on the upper helix of the ear. Optimally, the ring passes approximately 1 cm cephalad to the top of the ear. The hair is shaved at the posterior pin sites, and the skin is prepped with povidone-iodine solution.[13, 25, 85]

Application of the Halo-Ring. The ring or crown (incomplete ring) is slipped over the head and held in position. Optimal ring position is below the equator of the skull, but above the top of the ear, as described earlier. The center hole (if presented) is in the anterior portion of the ring. The skin is prepped, then infiltrated with 1 per cent lidocaine hydrochloride solution. Pins are advanced directly through the skin using a torque screwdriver, inserting the pins perpendicular to the skull surface, if possible. During anterior pin advancement, the patient is asked to close the eyes and relax the forehead. This helps prevent skin or eyebrow tenting, which can hinder eyelid closing after pin insertion. Alternating in a diagonal fashion, the pins are tightened in 2-inch/lb intervals until an 8 inch/lb (0.90 N/m) torque is reached. If one-time, break-off handles are used, the torque should be verified with a calibrated torque screwdriver. Once the halo is secured, manual traction on the ring can be used to control the cervical spine. Areas of tented skin surrounding the pins are released with a scalpel.

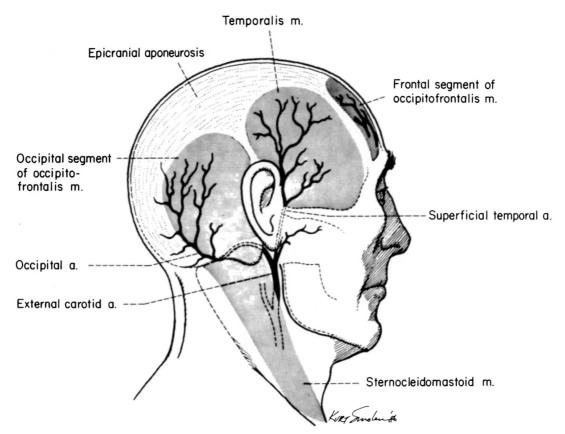

Figure 35–30. Posterior diagram of the safe zone for placement of halo fixator pins. (From Ballock, R. T., Botte, M. J., and Garfin, S. R.: Complications of halo immobilization. *In* Garfin, S. R. [ed.]: Complications of Spine Surgery. Baltimore, Williams & Wilkins, 1989, p. 376. © 1989 Williams & Wilkins Co.)

CHILD   ADULT

Figure 35–31. Transverse sections through the skull (as shown by computed tomography at the level of halo-pin site insertion) in children and adults. A, anterior; AL, anterolateral; T, temporal fossa; PL, posterolateral; P, posterior. (From Garfin, S. R., Roux, R., Botte, M. J., et al.: Skull osteology as it affects halo pin placement in children. J. Pediatr. Orthop. *6*:434, 1986.)

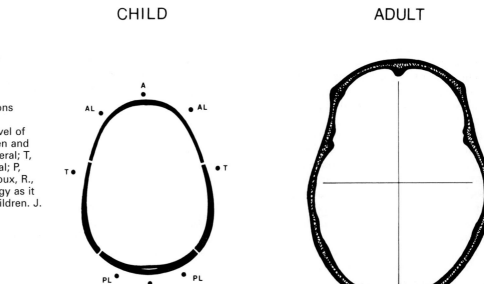

Table 35–6. MATERIALS FOR HALO APPLICATION

Three-person minimum recommended
Halo-ring or crown (in preselected size)
Sterile halo-pins (5, including 1 spare)
Halo torque screwdrivers (2) or "breakaway" wrenches (4)
Halo-vest (in preselected size)
Halo upright post and connecting rods
Head board
Spanners or ratchet wrenches (3)
Preparation razors (2)
Povidone-iodine solution
Sterile gloves (2 pairs)
Sterile gauze (4 packs of 2, 4″ × 4″ size)
Syringes (2, 10 ml)
Needles (4, 25 gauge)
Lidocaine hydrochloride (10 ml of 1% solution)
Crash cart (including manual resuscitator, endotracheal tube)

From Botte, M. J., Garfin, S. R., Byrne, T. P., et al.: The halo skeletal fixator: Principles of application and maintenance. Clin. Orthop. *239*:12–18, 1989.

Application of the Vest. With continued manual cervical traction, the patient's trunk is elevated to allow placement of the posterior part of the vest. The anterior half of the vest is placed, and the head and neck are positioned and the bolts secured. Ratchet-type wrenches that give way at a set torque (i.e., 28 ft/lb) can speed application of the bolts and prevent stripping. The application tools should be kept at the bedside in case emergency removal of the vest is required. A roentgenogram of the cervical spine is repeated.

Following initial application, the pins are retightened once to 8 inch/lb (0.90 N/m) 24 to 28 hours after application. Dressings are not used routinely around the pin sites. The sites are kept clean with hydrogen peroxide, cleansing every other day or as needed. Table 35–7 summarizes the steps in halo fixator application.

Biomechanical Aspects

Although the halo is the treatment of choice for many types of cervical spine instabilities, the device has been shown to allow motion and variation of forces across the cervical spine. Motion and force variations are dependent on patient position and activity with the halo-brace in place.

Initial studies on motion of the cervical spine with the halo-brace in place demonstrated only 4 per cent of normal motion during flexion and extension movements of the head and neck. Further studies, however, revealed that more significant motion occurs, especially when the patient moved from an upright to a supine position.[5, 44] The greatest absolute amount of motion occurred at the C4–C5 level (7.2 degrees). However, the greatest per cent of normal motion is at the C2–C3 level (42 per cent of normal), and the least amount was shown at the C7–T1 level (20 per cent of normal). The mean overall amount was 31 per cent of normal.

Although the halo-brace was designed to provide distraction across the cervical spine, individual varia-

tion of force occurs, with both distraction and compression forces demonstrated across the neck. The average distraction forces vary with different body positions and different activities.[77] The average distraction force was shown to vary in different positions by nearly 20 lb when the vest was employed and by over 30 lb when a cast was employed. The forces across the cervical spine change owing to changes in gravity forces when the head changes attitude (e.g., during bending over) or with vest distortion from changes in body shape, from direct pushing from the lower abdomen, arms, or shoulders, or from supporting surfaces. Bending forward from a seated position and reaching over sideways while lying significantly change forces across the cervical spine when the halo-brace is in place. Medial-lateral forces have been found to be small in comparison with vertical and anterior-posterior forces.

Treatment of Complications

Despite its effectiveness, substantial complications can occur following application of the halo skeletal fixator (Table 35–8).[7, 11, 12, 20, 27, 28, 63, 71, 81] Pin loosening and pin site infection are the two most common complications.

Loosening. If a pin becomes loose during the course of treatment, the loose pin and remaining pins are retightened to 8 inch/lb once, as long as resistance is met within the first two complete rotations of the pin. If no resistance is met, the pin should be removed following placement of a new pin in an adjacent or nearby location.[12, 13, 25, 27] Placement of a new pin prior

Table 35–7. PROCEDURE SUMMARY FOR APPLICATION OF THE HALO SKELETAL FIXATOR

1. Determine ring or crown size (hold ring or crown over head, visualize proper fit)
2. Determine vest size (from chest circumference measurement)
3. Identify pin site locations (while holding ring in place)
4. Shave hair at posterior pin sites
5. Prepare pin sites with povidone-iodine solution
6. Anesthetize skin at pin sites with 1% lidocaine hydrochloride
7. Advance sterile pins to level of skin
8. Have patient close eyes
9. Tighten pins at 2 in/lb increments in diagonal fashion
10. Seat and tighten pins to 8 in/lb torque
11. Apply lock nuts to pins
12. Maintain cervical traction and raise patient trunk to 30 degrees
13. Apply posterior portion of vest
14. Apply anterior portion of vest
15. Connect anterior and posterior portions of vest
16. Apply upright posts and attach ring to vest
17. Recheck fittings, screws, and nuts
18. Tape vest-removing tools to vest or keep at bedside
19. Obtain cervical spine roentgenograms

From Botte, M. J., Garfin, S. R., Byrne, T. P., et al.: The halo skeletal fixator: Principles of application and maintenance. Clin. Orthop. *239*:12–18, 1989.

Table 35–8. COMPLICATIONS ASSOCIATED WITH THE HALO IMMOBILIZATION DEVICE

Complication	Percentage of Patients
Pin loosening	36
Pin site infection	20
Severe pin discomfort	18
Pressure sores	11
Severe scars	9
Nerve injury	2
Dysphagia	2
Bleeding at pin sites	1
Dural puncture	1

From Garfin, S. R., Botte, M. J., Nickel, V. L., and Waters, R. L.: Complications in the use of the halo fixation device. J. Bone Joint Surg. Am. *68*:320, 1986.

to removal of the loose pin helps maintain ring fixation of the skull during pin site change.

Infection. If drainage around a pin develops, bacterial cultures should be obtained, appropriate oral antibiotic therapy started, and local pin care initiated. If the drainage does not respond to treatment, or if cellulitis or an abscess develops, the pin should be removed following insertion of a new pin at a different site. Parenteral antibiotic therapy should be instituted, and incision, drainage, and irrigation performed as needed.[12, 13, 25, 26, 28]

Pin Site Bleeding. Slow, continuous bleeding at pin sites has been shown to occur in patients taking anticoagulants. Tapering the anticoagulant may be required. Pin site packing has not been shown to be effective in these cases, as long as anticoagulant medication is continued.[12, 13, 26]

Difficulty in Swallowing. Difficulty in swallowing may occur if the head and neck are placed in exaggerated extension. Readjustment of the halo to provide less cervical extension usually relieves this problem.[12, 26]

Dural Puncture. Dural puncture may occur if the patient falls on the halo.[12, 13, 25, 26, 28] The patient may complain of headache, malaise, visual disturbances, or other local or systemic symptoms. Clear cerebrospinal fluid leakage around loose or deeply seated pins should alert one to this possibility. Roentgenograms may disclose previously unnoticed skull fractures. Treatment includes hospitalization, prophylactic parenteral antibiotics, and pin removal following placement of a new pin at a different site (assuming no skull fractures are present). Elevation of the head of the bed decreases cranial cerebrospinal fluid pressure and helps alleviate leakage. The dural tear should heal in four to five days. If the leak does not respond, surgical exploration and dural repair may be required. If a subdural abscess develops, this requires surgical incision, drainage, and irrigation.[12, 28]

Pressure Sores. Pressure sores under the halo-vest or cast may develop if it is not appropriately padded or if the patient is not appropriately turned or positioned.[12, 26] Patients with neurologic compromise or sensory deprivation are particularly at risk. Surgical stabilization of the cervical spine may be considered to avoid use of the halo in selected patients with spinal cord injury or in patients with sensory dysfunction. This minimizes skin problems and aids in rapid rehabilitation.

Loss of Reduction. Loss of reduction of fractures or dislocations has been shown to occur with the halo in place.[12, 44, 59, 81] Injuries of the posterior ligaments appear to be more likely than other cervical spine instabilities to lose reduction. Fracture of the superior aspect of the inferior facet has also been associated with loss of reduction with the halo-brace in place. An additional predisposing factor may be poor vest fit, especially in large or stout patients, because the vest may not be long enough to exert sufficient control on the unstable cervical motion segments. Inability to maintain reduction can be treated with open reduction, internal fixation, or arthrodesis of the unstable segments.

Halo-Brace Application in Children

Successful use of the halo-brace in children and infants has been demonstrated.[20, 45, 55, 69] Recommended pin application torques are between 2 and 5 inch/lb.[45, 55] In children younger than 3 years old, a multiple-pin, low-torque technique has been recommended to allow a greater range of pin placement sites in areas where the infant skull might be considered too thin or too weak to accept limited, high-torque forces.[20, 55] With the exception of component size and pin torque, halo-brace application for children in this age group requires similar hardware and techniques as those used for older patients. However, because of the patient's small size and the infrequent use of the halo-brace in this age group, manufacturers may not carry an inventory of parts. Therefore, custom-made components may be required.[55] Custom fabrication of the halo can be accomplished by the following steps, as outlined by Mubarak and associates:[55] (1) size and configuration of the head are obtained with the use of flexible lead wire placed around the head; (2) the halo-ring is fabricated by constructing it 2 cm larger in diameter than the wire impression; (3) a plaster mold of the trunk is obtained for manufacture of the bivalved polypropylene vest; and (4) linear measurements are made to ensure appropriate length of the superstructure, which is made of lightweight anodized material. Ten to 12 standard skull pins can be used. The custom-constructed halo-ring is applied under general anesthesia, placing the halo below the skull equator. Ten pins can be inserted to finger or torque tightness of 2 inch/lb circumferentially, avoiding the thinner temporal regions as well as the frontal sinus areas, where thinner cortical bone may be present.[31, 84] The vest and superstructure are then applied. A computed tomography (CT) scan helps visualize bone structure to plan pin scan sites, avoiding suture lines or bone "fragments" (found in congenital malformations).[55, 84] Postoperatively, the halo-pin sites should be cleaned daily, as needed, by the patient's parents. If the pin sites become infected, oral or parenteral antibiotics should be started. If drainage persists in spite of antibiotics, removal of the infected pin is necessary.

The chronology of skull development is pertinent in the consideration of potential complications related to halo-brace application in patients younger than 2 years old.[55] In this group, cranial suture interdigitation may be incomplete, and fontanelles may be open anteriorly (in those younger than 18 months) or posteriorly (in those younger than 6 months). Cranium distortion and cranial bone shifting can be minimized by short halo-brace application periods, custom-fitted halo-rings, and evenly distributed, low cranial pressure accomplished through numerous pins.[55]

Conclusion

The halo skeletal fixator is a proven, effective device for stabilization of many types of cervical instabilities in both adults and children. Proper application and maintenance are necessary to minimize problems or complications.

ACKNOWLEDGMENT. The photographs of the orthoses in this chapter were supplied by Southern California Orthotics and Prosthetics Inc., San Diego, CA. The model wearing the braces in the photographs is Kel Bergmann, C.P.O., of Southern California Orthotics and Prosthetics. We appreciate their contribution to this chapter. The costs shown in Table 35-4 were also obtained from that company. A sampling of orthotic and prosthetic companies in San Diego was not performed.

References

1. Abitbol, J. J., Botte, M. J., Garfin, S. R., and Akeson, W. H.: The treatment of multiple myeloma of the cervical spine with a halo vest. J. Spinal Disord. 2:263, 1989.
2. Allbrook, D.: Movement of the lumbar spinal column. J. Bone Joint Surg. Br. 39:339, 1957.
3. American Academy of Orthopedic Surgeons: Atlas of Orthotics. St. Louis, C. V. Mosby Co., 1975.
4. American Academy of Orthopedic Surgeons: Atlas of Orthotics. St. Louis, C. V. Mosby Co., 1985.
5. Anderson, P. A., Budorick, T. E., Easton, K. B., et al.: Failure of halo vest to prevent in vivo motion in patients with injured cervical spines. Spine 16:S501, 1991.
6. Andriacchi, T., Schults, A., Belytschoco, T., and Galante, J.: A model for students of the mechanical interaction between the human spine and the ribcage. J. Biomech. 7:497, 1974.
7. Ballock, R. T., Botte, M. J., and Garfin, S. R.: Complications of halo immobilization. In Garfin, S. R. (ed.): Complications of Spine Surgery. Baltimore, Williams & Wilkins, 1989, p. 376.
8. Ballock, R. T., Thay, Q. L., Triggs, K. J., et al.: The effect of pin location on the rigidity of the halo pin-bone interface. Neurosurgery 26:238, 1990.
9. Barnes, J. W., and Harwell, A. D.: Technical note: The use of low heat thermoplastics in vacuum forming. Orthotics and Prosthetics 40:58, 1986.
10. Botte, M. J., Byrne, T. P., and Garfin, S. R.: Application of the halo fixation device using an increased torque pressure. J. Bone Joint Surg. Am. 69:750, 1987.
11. Botte, M. J., Byrne, T. P., and Garfin, S. R.: Use of skin incisions in the application of halo skeletal fixator pins. Clin. Orthop. 246:100, 1989.
12. Botte, M. J., Byrne, T. P., Reid, A. A., and Garfin, S. R.: The halo skeletal fixator: Current concepts of application and maintenance. Orthopedics 18:463, 1995.
13. Botte, M. J., Garfin, S. R., Byrne, T. P., et al.: The halo skeletal fixator: Principles of application and maintenance. Clin. Orthop. 239:12, 1989.
14. Chase, A. P., Bader, D. L., and Houghton, G. R.: The biochemical effectiveness of the Boston brace in the management of adolescent idiopathic scoliosis. Spine 14:646, 1989.
15. Cline, J. R., Scheidel, E., and Bigsby, E. F.: A comparison of methods of cervical immobilization used in patient extrication and transport. J. Trauma 25:7, 1985.
16. Colachis, S. C., and Strohm, B. R.: Radiographic studies of cervical spine motion in normal subjects. Arch. Phys. Med. Rehabil. 46:253, 1965.
17. Colachis, S. C., Strohm, B. R., and Ganter, E. L.: Cervical spine motion in normal women: A radiographic study of effect of cervical collars. Arch. Phys. Med. Rehabil. 54:161, 1973.
18. Cooper, P. R., Maravilla, K. R., Sklar, F. H., et al.: Halo immobilization of the cervical spine fractures: Indications and results. J. Neurosurg. 50:603, 1979.
19. Dick, T., and Land, R.: Spinal immobilization devices. J. Emerg. Serv. 14:26, 1982.
20. Dormans, J. P., Criscitiello, A. A., Drummond, D. S., and Davidson, R. S.: Complications in children managed with immobilization in a halo vest. J. Bone Joint Surg. Am. 77:1370, 1995.
21. Edwards, J. W.: Orthopedic Appliances Atlas. St. Louis, American Academy of Orthopedic Surgeons, 1952.
22. Ewald, F. C.: Fracture of the odontoid process in a seventeen-month-old infant treated with a halo. J. Bone Joint Surg. Am. 53:1636, 1971.
23. Fidler, M. W., and Plasmans, C. M. T.: The effect of four types of support on the segmental mobility of the lumbosacral spine. J. Bone Joint Surg. Am. 65:943, 1983.
24. Fisher, S. V., Bower, J. F., Awad, E. A., and Gullickson, G.: Cervical orthoses' effect on cervical spine motion: Roentgenographic and goniometric method of study. Arch. Phys. Med. Rehabil. 58:109, 1977.
25. Garfin, S. R., Botte, M. J., Byrne, T. P., and Woo, S. L. Y.: Application and maintenance of the halo skeletal fixator. Update on Spinal Disorders 2:1, 1987.
26. Garfin, S. R., Botte, M. J., Centeno, R. S., and Nickel, V. L.: Osteology of the skull as it affects halo pin placement. Spine 10:697, 1985.
27. Garfin, S. R., Botte, M. J., Nickel, V. L., and Waters, R. L.: Complications in the use of the halo fixation device. J. Bone Joint Surg. Am. 68:320, 1986.
28. Garfin, S. R., Botte, M. J., Triggs, K. J., and Nickel, V. L.: Subdural abscess associated with halo-pin traction. J. Bone Joint Surg. Am. 70:1338, 1988.
29. Garfin, S. R., Botte, M. J., Woo, S. L. Y., and Nickel, V. L.: Reliability after repeated use of a torque screwdriver employed for halo pin fixation. J. Orthop. Res. 3:121, 1985.
30. Garfin, S. R., Lee, T. O., Roux, R. D., et al.: Structural behavior of the halo orthosis pin-bone interface: Biomechanical evaluation of standard and newly designed stainless steel halo fixation pins. Spine 11:97, 1986.
31. Garfin, S. R., Roux, R., Botte, M. J., et al.: Skull osteology as it affects halo pin placement in children. J. Pediatr. Orthop. 6:434, 1986.
32. Garret, A., Perry, J., and Nickel, V. L.: Stabilization of the collapsing spine. J. Bone Joint Surg. Am. 43:474, 1961.
33. Gianturco, C.: A roentgen analysis, of the motion of the lower lumbar vertebrae in normal individuals and in patients with low back pain. AJR Am. J. Roentgenol. 52:261, 1944.
34. Glaser, J. A., Whitehall, R., Stamp, W. G., and Jane, J. A.: Complications associated with the halo-vest. J. Neurosurg. 65:762, 1986.
35. Hannah, R. E., and Cottrill, S. D.: The Canadian collar: A new cervical orthosis. Am. J. Occup. Ther. 39:171, 1985.
36. Hartman, J. T., Palumbo, F., and Hill, J. B.: Cineradiography of the braced normal cervical spine. Clin. Orthop. 109:97, 1975.

37. Houtkin, S., and Levine, D. B.: The halo yoke: A simplified device for attachment of the halo to a body cast. J. Bone Joint Surg. Am. 54:881, 1972.

38. James, J. I. P.: Fracture dislocation of the cervical spine. J. R. Coll. Surg. Edinb. 5:232, 1960.

39. Johnson, R. M., Hart, D. L., Simmons, E. F., et al.: Cervical orthoses: A study comparing their effectiveness in restricting cervical motion in normal subjects. J. Bone Joint Surg. Am. 59:332, 1977.

40. Johnson, R. M., Owen, J. R., Hart, D. L., and Callahan, R. A.: Cervical orthoses. Clin. Orthop. 154:34, 1981.

41. Jones, M. D.: Cineradiographic studies of the collar-immobilized cervical spine. J. Neurosurg. 17:633, 1960.

42. Kalamachi, A., Yau, A. C. M. C., O'Brien, J. P., and Hodgson, A. R.: Halo-pelvic distraction apparatus: An analysis of one hundred and fifty consecutive patients. J. Bone Joint Surg. Am. 58:1119, 1976.

43. Kaufman, W. A., Lunsford, T. R., Lundsford, B. R., and Lance, L. L.: Comparison of three prefabricated cervical collars. Orthotics and Prosthetics 39:4, 1986.

44. Koch, R. A., and Nickel, V. L.: The halo vest: An evaluation of motion and forces across the neck. Spine 3:103, 1978.

45. Kopits, S. E., and Steignass, M. H.: Experience with the "halo-cast" in small children. Surg. Clin. North Am. 50:935, 1970.

46. Kostuik, J. P.: Indications for the use of the halo immobilization. Clin. Orthop. 154:46, 1981.

47. Lantz, S. A., and Schultz, A. B.: Lumbar spine orthosis wearing. Spine 11:838, 1986.

48. Levine, A. M.: Spinal orthoses. Am. Fam. Physician 29:3, 1984.

49. Lind, B., Nordwall, A., and Sihlbom, H.: Odontoid fractures treated with halo-vest. Spine 12:173, 1987.

50. Lind, B., Sihlbom, H., and Nordwall, A.: Forces and motions across the neck in patients treated with the halo vest. Spine 13:162, 1988.

51. Lumsden, R. M., and Morris, J.: An in vivo study of axial rotation and immobilization at the lumbosacral joint. J. Bone Joint Surg. Am. 50:1591, 1968.

52. Lyddon, D. W.: Experience with the halo and body cast in the ambulatory treatment of cervical spine fractures. Ill. J. Med. 146:458, 1974.

53. Morris, J. M., Benner, G., and Lucas, D. B.: An electromyographic study of the intrinsic muscles of the back in man. J. Anat. 96:509, 1962.

54. Morris, J. M., and Lucas, D. B.: Biomechanics of spinal bracing. Ariz. Med. 2:170, 1964.

55. Mubarak, S. J., Camp, J. F., Vuletich, W., et al.: Halo application in the infant. J. Pediatr. Orthop. 9:612, 1989.

56. Muller, I., Varmuzkova, O., Vlach, O., and Messner, P.: Halo: Another method of treatment and care for cervical spine injuries. Acta Chir. Orhtop. Traumatol. Cech. 46:161, 1979.

57. Nachemson, A., Schultz, A., and Anderson, G. B.: Mechanical effectiveness of the lumbar spine orthoses. Scand. J. Rehab. Med. Suppl. 9:139, 1983.

58. Nakamura, T., Oh-Hama, M., and Shingu, H.: A new orthosis for fixation of the cervical spine: Fronto-occipito-zygomatic orthosis. Orthotics and Prosthetics 38:41, 1984.

59. Nickel, V. L., Perry, J., Garrett, A., and Heppenstall, M.: The halo: A spinal skeletal traction fixation device. J. Bone Joint Surg. Am. 50:1400, 1968.

60. Nickel, V. L., Perry, J., Garrett, A. L., and Snelson, R.: Application of the halo. Orthop. Pros. App. J. 14:31, 1960.

61. Norton, P. L., and Brown, T.: The immobilizing efficiency of back braces. J. Bone Joint Surg. Am. 39:111, 1957.

62. Olson, B., Ustanko, L.: Self-care needs of patients in the halo brace. Orthop. Nursing 9:28, 1990.

63. Perry, J.: The halo in spinal abnormalities: Practical factors and avoidance of complications. Orthop. Clin. North Am. 3:69, 1972.

64. Perry, J., and Nickel, V. L.: Total cervical spine fusion for neck paralysis. J. Bone Joint Surg. Am. 41:37, 1959.

65. Pieron, A. P., and Welpy, W. R.: Halo traction. J. Bone Joint Surg. Br. 52:119, 1970.

65a. Plaisier, B., Gabram, S. G., Schwartz, R. J., and Jacobs, L. M.: Prospective evaluation of craniofacial pressure in four different cervical orthoses. J. Trauma 37:714, 1994.

66. Podolsky, S., Baraf, L. J., Simon, R. R., et al.: Efficacy of cervical spine immobilization methods. J. Trauma 23:6, 1983.

67. Prolo, D. J., Rennels, J. B., and Jameson, R. M.: The injured cervical spine: Immediate and long-term immobilization with the halo. JAMA 224:591, 1973.

68. Sears, W., and Fazi, M.: Prediction of stability of cervical spine fracture managed in the halo vest and indications for surgical intervention. J. Neurosurg. 72:426, 1990.

69. Sherk, H. H., Nicholson, J. T., and Chung, S. M. K.: Fractures of the odontoid process in young children. J. Bone Joint Surg. Am. 60:921, 1978.

70. Smith, G. E.: The most ancient splint. Br. Med. J. 1:732, 1908.

71. Sneddon, M. H., and Giammatei, F.: Pitfalls in halo application and management. Scientific exhibit at the annual meeting of the American Academy of Orthopedic Surgeons, Anaheim, CA, March 10–15, 1983.

72. Sypert, G. W.: External spinal orthotics. Neurosurgery 20:4, 1987.

73. Tanz, S. S.: Motion of the lumbar spine: A roentgenologic study. AJR Am. J. Roentgenol. 69:399, 1953.

74. Thompson, H.: Halo traction apparatus: A method of external splinting of the cervical spine after surgery. J. Bone Joint Surg. Br. 44:655, 1962.

75. Triggs, K. J., Ballock, R. T., Lee, T. Q., et al.: The effect of angel insertion on halo pin fixation. Spine 14:781, 1989.

76. U.S. Food and Drug Administration: Medical Device Amendments. 2nd ed. 1986.

77. Walker, P. S., Lamser, D., Hussey, R. W., et al.: Forces in the halo-vest apparatus. Spine 9:773, 1984.

78. Waters, R. L., and Morris, J. M.: Effect of spinal supports on the electrical activity of muscles of the trunk. J. Bone Joint Surg. Am. 52:51, 1970.

79. White, A. A., and Panjabi, M. M.: Clinical Biomechanics of the Spine. Toronto, J. B. Lippincott, 1978.

80. White, R.: Halo traction apparatus. J. Bone Joint Surg. Br. 48:592, 1966.

81. Whitehall, R., Richman, J. A., and Glaser, J. A.: Failure of immobilization of the cervical spine by the halo vest. J. Bone Joint Surg. Am. 68:326, 1986.

82. Wilner, F.: The effect of the Boston brace on the frontal sagittal curves of the spine. Acta Orthop. Scand. 55:457, 1984.

83. Wiltse, L. L., Kirkaldy-Willis, W. H., and McIvor, G. W.: The treatment of spinal stenosis. Clin. Orthop. 115:83–91, 1976.

84. Wong, W. B., and Haynes, R. J.: Osteology of the pediatric skull: Considerations of halo pin placement. Spine 19:1451, 1994.

85. Young, R., and Thomassen, E. H.: Step-by-step procedure for applying the halo ring. Orthop. Rev. 3:62, 1974.

86. Zwerling, M. T., and Riggins, R. S.: Use of the halo apparatus in acute injuries of the cervical spine. Surg. Gynecol. Obstet. 138:189, 1974.

CHAPTER 36

Spinal Cord Injury Rehabilitation

David F. Apple, Jr., M.D.

Spinal cord injury (SCI) is defined as an insult to the spinal cord that partially or completely interrupts the three main functions of the cord—motor, sensory, and reflex activities. The insult is most commonly traumatic but may be produced by infection, tumor, or vascular compromise. Paralysis of the upper and lower extremities—quadriplegia—accounts for 54 per cent of patients, and paraplegia accounts for the remaining 46 per cent. The problem occurs predominantly in men, only 18 per cent of patients being women.

The incidence of traumatic spinal cord injury varies according to the source.[7, 12] Most data analyzers believe that there is underreporting and that many individuals with spinal cord injury die at the accident scene or shortly thereafter. The most accurate reports place the annual rate at 30 to 35 per million people, or about 10,000 new injuries per year. The incidence of nontraumatic spinal cord paralysis is even more difficult to determine, and in this group cancer is a leading cause of paralysis.

Traumatic injury is more than twice as common as nontraumatic disease in patients under 40, but in those over 40, cancer is four times as common as traumatic injury.[7, 22] Fifty-eight per cent of traumatic SCI occurs between the ages of 16 and 30 (Table 36–1). SCI occurs most frequently in July, followed closely by August. Twenty per cent of injuries occur on Saturday, with 19 per cent and 15 per cent happening on Sunday and Friday, respectively (Table 36–2).

HISTORICAL PERSPECTIVE

Egyptian physicians, because of their fear of being put to death by the Pharaoh for allowing a patient to die, labeled spinal cord injury as "an ailment not to be treated." This approach continued during World War I, with only minor improvements in care because of better recognition and institution of urinary drainage. In spite of the recognition by orthopedic centers of the necessity for preventing contractures and bedsores, there was no carryover into the treatment of spinal cord injury. During this period, the mortality rate declined from 95 to 80 per cent, with predominantly only those with partial lesions surviving.

During the early part of World War II there was little improvement, but gradually it was recognized that the situation could be improved. Breslau in Germany, Munro in Boston, and Botterell in Canada, along with Guttmann in England, were developing ideas of care that would drastically change the prognosis for

Table 36–1. AGE AT SPINAL CORD INJURY

Age Group (years)	Percentage of Patients
0–15	5
16–30	58
31–45	21
46–60	10
61–75	5
76–90	1

From Go, B. K., DeVivo, M. J., and Richards, J. S.: The epidemiology of spinal cord injury. *In* Stover, S. L., DeLisa, J. A., and Whiteneck, G. G. (eds.): Spinal Cord Injury: Clinical Outcomes from the Model Systems. Gaithersburg, MD, Aspen Publications, 1995, pp. 21–55. © 1995, Aspen Publishers, Inc.

Table 36–2. SPINAL CORD INJURY OCCURRENCE

Day of Week		Month of Injury	
Monday	13%	January	6%
Tuesday	11%	February	6%
Wednesday	11%	March	7%
Thursday	12%	April	8%
Friday	15%	May	9%
Saturday	20%	June	10%
Sunday	19%	July	12%
		August	11%
		September	9%
		October	8%
		November	8%
		December	7%

From Go, B. K., DeVivo, M. J., and Richards, J. S.: The epidemiology of spinal cord injury. In Stover, S. L., DeLisa, J. A., and Whiteneck, G. G. (eds.): Spinal Cord Injury: Clinical Outcomes from the Model Systems. Gaithersburg, MD, Aspen Publications, 1995, pp. 21–55. © 1995, Aspen Publishers, Inc.

spinal cord injuries. Guttmann[10] believed that the first step to improve the management of spinal cord injuries was taken by the Peripheral Nerve Committee of the Medical Research Council when it decided to set up special units. In February 1944, the spinal unit at the Ministry of Pensions Hospital at Stoke Mandeville, Aylesbury, England, opened and became the model for all subsequent centers. Later in the same year a similar unit opened at Lyndhurst Lodge in Toronto, and in 1945 the United States Veterans Administration opened eight units. The first civilian center in the United States opened in 1964 at Rancho Los Amigos Hospital in California.

The special spinal cord units were set up using the guidelines developed by Sir Ludwig Guttmann. They are:

1. Transfer to a specialized unit as soon after injury as possible.
2. Unit management by a physician who is knowledgeable and dedicated to spinal care.
3. A team of allied health professionals who are trained in the intricacies of spinal cord problems.
4. A commitment to vocational pursuits.
5. An emphasis on psychosocial and recreational needs.
6. Provision for follow-up care for the life-time of the individual.

Experience has shown that omitting any of these elements dooms the unit to failure.

Spinal cord care received a significant boost in the United States when the Rehabilitation Services Administration began supporting research and demonstration projects for the development of model systems of care. The first federally sponsored system was established at Good Samaritan Hospital in Phoenix in 1970. In addition to providing care, another objective was to develop a database that would document cost effectiveness and rehabilitation outcome. The model system grew over the years as federal funding became avail-

able and at its peak numbered 17 centers. The national database continues but is now at the University of Alabama, where over 10,000 patients are monitored.

The model system centers make a commitment to coordinate a patient's care from the moment of injury to the acute-care setting, through the rehabilitation process and continuing into follow-up care for both acute and chronic problems. Included in this commitment are attention to quality-of-life issues, an education and participation effort toward prevention, and an emerging involvement in solving some of the issues surrounding aging.

CLINICAL HIGHLIGHTS

Urinary Drainage

Before the early 1900s the inability of the bladder to empty after a spinal cord injury often caused the patient's death within five to ten days. Some survived if overflow incontinence occurred and was not complicated by infection. Another small group lived if an early reflex bladder developed. When the technique of urinary drainage was developed, mortality rates improved, and those who died did so at a longer time after injury.

Antibiotic Usage

The introduction of antibiotics around 1940 further reduced the mortality and morbidity. The most common cause of death in the early postinjury period was respiratory infection. In the later postinjury periods, urinary tract infections led to destruction of the kidneys and renal death. The development of pressure sores provided a focus of infection and often produced a septic death. Antibiotics positively affected the outcome of these three infectious complications.

Team Care

Development of team care in the middle and late 1940s created the biggest advance in treatment of SCI. This remains true today. Physicians and paramedical personnel developed expertise in the vagaries of spinal care that prevented contractures, stopped muscle wasting, reduced the incidence of pressure sores, and taught techniques that allowed the patient to be as functional as possible according to the level of paralysis. By introducing quality-of-life issues into the rehabilitation process, the patient could see that life was worth living.

Halo-Brace

Before the 1950s, stabilization of the bony spine after a spine injury was accomplished by keeping the patient in bed in a postural reduction position or by applying a traction device to immobilize the spine. The immobilization had to be maintained at least six weeks but was usually necessary for 12 weeks. Attaching a halo-ring to the skull and connecting the ring to a body jacket enabled the cervical spine to be immobilized sufficiently to hold the fractured spine in alignment while healing occurred and get the patient out of bed. This allowed the patient to start rehabilitation earlier and lessened the likelihood of many of the common complications.

Internal Fixation

In the 1960s methods to fix the spine internally were introduced. These methods are still undergoing refinements and modifications. Wiring the cervical spine and placing rods in the thoracic and lumbar spine not only immobilized the spine, allowing the patient to get out of bed earlier, but also freed patients from restrictive external devices. This allowed earlier and more vigorous rehabilitation.

Emergency Medical Services

During the 1970s, an intensive effort developed to better train the personnel who were manning ambulances. They were taught correct techniques for extraction of patients at the scene of accidents. Instruction was given in proper immobilization of the spine for transport to the hospital. This improved care increased the number of incomplete spinal cord injuries.

Space-Age Electronics

Computerization and miniaturization have many applications for the SCI patient. The patient with high quadriplegia who requires a ventilator can have a wheelchair with a portable ventilator and a drive control that can be operated by the mouth, the eyebrows, or a blink. An environmental control device can also be fitted with similar controls so the patient can manipulate light switches, TVs, and other electronic devices. Muscle stimulators have been developed that are programmed to stimulate walking and can be attached to trained and properly motivated individuals, allowing them to "walk." A nerve stimulator can be attached to the phrenic nerve and programmed to pace the diaphragm, allowing the patient to be freed from the ventilator, often for as long as 24 hours.

Managed Care

As the 1990s progressed and shorter hospital stays resulted from managed care, the program for SCI patients began undergoing re-engineering. Those with paraplegia were in rehabilitation less than 30 days, and those with quadriplegia less than 56 days. In response, subacute care, day hospital, and expanded outpatient services were developed.

PRESENT STATUS OF PATIENT MANAGEMENT

Systems of care have developed in all federally designated SCI centers, and it is hoped that the system

model will be duplicated wherever there is a commitment to manage spinal cord injury.[11] When a system is used, the patient can expect a certain quality of care that produces a good result.

At the time the injury occurs, the emergency medical services (EMS) team that arrives at the accident scene will know how to extract the injured person from the vehicle safely and immobilize the spine for safe transport to the emergency room. After arrival in the emergency room, the physician and other personnel conduct an examination directed toward preserving life while at the same time protecting the spinal cord from further damage. To assess spinal cord function, the recorded examination should include an accurate sensory examination that includes the rectal area, a precise motor examination that includes toe function, and a reflex evaluation that includes the bulbocavernosus reflex. Roentgenographic examination must include routine views of the areas of the spine shown to be injured by the results of the physical examination. More specialized roentgenographic evaluation should be determined by the spinal cord treatment team, usually an orthopedist or neurosurgeon. Computed tomography (CT) with or without myelographic dye or magnetic resonance imaging (MRI) may be indicated.

The SCI treatment team physician should be capable of managing the initial care to enhance spinal cord function and determine the most appropriate method of spinal stabilization. That same physician should be able to provide the correct rehabilitation program or should consult a rehabilitation physician to start providing rehabilitation input within the first 48 to 72 hours of injury. While the decisions are being made regarding spinal cord and spinal column management, the therapy part of the team can keep the joints mobile and preserve the strength of those muscles that are still functioning. The nursing staff can begin bowel and bladder training and work to prevent the development of pressure sores.

After the implementation of the spinal column treatment plan, the rehabilitation team can develop individualized patient goals. These goals are reviewed and updated at a team conference, which is held at least weekly and is directed by the patient's program manager, usually the physician. The team functions best by solving the problems and achieving the patient's goals using an interdisciplinary or transdisciplinary approach.

At discharge from the inpatient facility, with family training having been accomplished, the patient's rehabilitation program is often incomplete. In those instances, the patient's program is completed in a day hospital setting. An outpatient program can be used if only one discipline is required or if a daily program is not necessary. Final delivery of equipment occurs after discharge. Recreational therapy and most of the vocational program is finalized in an outpatient setting. Even though the program is not totally accomplished during the inpatient stay, the individual program goal is still to achieve the highest level of functioning consistent with the neurologic damage and to reintegrate the patient back into the community.

ANATOMY AND PHYSIOLOGY OF SPINAL CORD INJURY

The spinal cord is a continuation of neural tissue from the brain occupying the upper two thirds of the spinal canal and ending behind the first lumbar vertebra. At that level the cord broadens to form the conus medullaris. Neural tissue identified as nerve roots constitutes the cauda equina, which occupies the remainder of the lumbar canal. The average length of the spinal cord is 43 to 45 cm. The average dimensions of the oval-shaped cord are 8 by 10 mm, but there are two enlarged areas. Between the second and seventh cervical vertebrae, the cord measures 8 by 14 mm, and between the tenth and twelfth thoracic vertebrae the measurement is 8 by 12 mm. The cross-sectional area of the cord at C1 is 80 mm^2; it widens to 100 mm^2 at C6–C7. At T6 the cord is 60 mm^2; at L3, 70 mm^2; and at S2, 50 mm^2.

The cord, conus medullaris, and cauda equina are surrounded by the meninges, which consist of the dura, arachnoid, and pia. The epidural contents include fat, arteries, and the venous plexus of Batson. Surrounding all these structures is the vertebral canal, which is lined by the ligamentum flavum and the anterior and posterior longitudinal ligaments, which connect the vertebral bodies.

The spinal cord is the continuation of the medulla oblongata and extends from the occiput to the lower border of the first lumbar vertebra or the upper border of the second vertebra. Thirty-one pairs of spinal nerves leave the cord as anterior and posterior roots. The eight cervical roots leave the cord in an almost horizontal plane to enter the foramina, but below this level the course of the roots becomes increasingly horizontal, entering the foramina one or two vertebrae lower. At the lumbar level, the roots are coursing in almost a true vertical plane. The anterior roots contain the efferent fibers for control of the skeletal muscles, and the posterior roots contain the afferent fibers.

The vertebral column is composed of 33 vertebrae, seven cervical, 12 thoracic, five lumbar, five sacral, which are fused, and three to five coccygeal vertebrae. The bodies of the vertebrae are separated by discs, which contribute about one fourth of the length of the vertebral column. The typical vertebra consists of a body and an arch, with the spinal cord lying within the arch. The arch has three parts The pedicles form the sides connecting to the body. The roof, or lamina, unites the pedicles. The third part is the transverse processes, which protrude from the junction of the lamina with the pedicle. The superior articular process projects forward and upward from the pedicles to articulate with downward and posteriorly directed inferior articular facets of the vertebrae above. The palpable spinous process is a continuation of the lamina. All these bony structures serve as muscular attachments.

The blood supply of the spinal cord is derived mainly from the anterior spinal artery, which originates from the coalescing of two branches of the vertebral artery. The anterior spinal artery runs along the cord in the anterior median fissure. There are two posterior spinal arteries, derived from the posterior inferior cerebellar arteries or the vertebral arteries. All three of these arteries receive branches of radicular arteries at various intervals. The anterior spinal artery supplies the anterior two thirds of the spinal cord, and the posterior spinal arteries supply the remainder. The communicating branches that enter the vertebral canal with the anterior spinal roots contribute to the circulation of the spinal cord. The artery of Adamkiewicz, which is usually on the left side in the thoracic region, contributes to cord dysfunction when injured.

Pathophysiology

There are two basic types of physiologic injuries that can occur to the spinal cord. One is concussion, which is uncommon and is believed to be totally reversible. In this instance, cord functions can be either totally or partially shut down. Recovery is usually quick, occurring within two to four weeks. In the other type of injury, laceration or transection, which is caused by contusion, cord function is totally absent. Contusion[26] is the most common type of injury, and the cord damage is caused by the impact of the inflicting violence. Three stages of pathologic changes ensue. In the acute stage the cord is swollen and bluish with dural petechial hemorrhages. Microscopically there are hemorrhages that are more prominent in the gray matter but extend into the white matter. In the intermediate stage there are absorption and attempts at reorganization. The late stage demonstrates the formation of fibrous and glial scarring. During this stage the cord is more pale and shrunken. A final stage that may develop is the formation of cysts, which may occur months or years after the injury, causing late myelopathy.

When an anatomic or physiologic transection of the cord occurs, there is immediate cessation of all ascending and descending function. In addition to paralysis and loss of deep tendon reflexes, sensation and autonomic function are eliminated below the level of injury. This is the state of "spinal shock" that continues until the reflex function of the cord starts to recover, usually within 24 to 48 hours. The bladder and bowel are paralyzed, leading to urinary retention and ileus. Without vasomotor control, the blood pressure falls temporarily, sweat is absent below the level of injury, and temperature control is affected because of loss of vasoconstriction. With the resolution of spinal shock during the four to six weeks after the injury, reflex activity returns. The motor and sensory function does not recover unless the insult to the cord has produced an incomplete injury. Complete recovery is rare.

Cause

The National Spinal Cord Injury Statistical Center at the University of Alabama has the records of 14,791 patients in its database. The most common cause of spinal cord injury is motor vehicle accidents (44.5 per cent). Following in descending order are falls (18.1 per cent), acts of violence (16.6 per cent), sports (12.7 per cent), and other (8 per cent) (Table 36–3). In those under 15 years of age, vehicular accidents accounted for 38 per cent, increasing to 49 per cent in the 16–30 age group. In those over 60, the most common etiology is falls at 48 per cent.

MANAGEMENT OF SPINAL CORD INJURY

The management of spinal cord injury is a continuum of care and should not be separated into acute and rehabilitation segments, because rehabilitation should start shortly after the time of the injury and continue for a lifetime. This continuum of care is more easily accomplished if a system has been developed, which starts at the time of injury with an effective EMS delivery, continues into the hospital phase for both early management and the restorative phase, and culminates with follow-up coordination. If the system is effectively developed, the time it takes for the individual to return to productivity is shortened because of strict attention to details in early management, which decreases the number and severity of complications as the patient progresses through the various phases of care. Society benefits from this by decreased cost of care, and the injured person benefits because of an improved perspective on an altered life style.

At the time of the injury, the EMS personnel should be summoned for the safest management of the patient. After the efforts in the late 1970s, EMS personnel training was intensively upgraded. The management at the time of the accident has greatly improved so that the spine is carefully protected whether the patient is conscious or unconscious, resulting in a higher percentage of incomplete injuries. The goal of early management is first preservation of life, which means establishing

an airway, monitoring cardiac activity, and establishing an effective means of administering appropriate medications with the establishment of an adequate intravenous line.

The second priority is to further reduce injury and to preserve whatever function is still present. In the spine this means providing sufficient external support to both the cervical and thoracic spine by the use of a cervical collar, a spine board, or appropriately applied traction. This must be accomplished while extracting the individual from the injury circumstances. If these two priorities are obtained, reversing the severity of the spinal cord injury may be possible in some cases, although this is infrequent.

Once effective spinal immobilization has been instituted in the unconscious or conscious patient, safe transport can be carried out to the closest hospital capable of managing spinal cord injury. In some states it has been legislatively mandated that an EMS vehicle may bypass the closest hospital and proceed without fear to the appropriately designated trauma center that can handle spinal cord injuries. Unfortunately, this situation does not prevail in most areas of the country.

Because of the complexity of managing a patient with a spinal cord injury; which affects virtually all systems of the body, it is imperative that the patient reach a team of medical and paramedical personnel trained in the care of spinal cord injury. The team concept of care mandates that the team be led by a single physician whose responsibility it is to be involved in the patient's care by directing the other members of the team with their various areas of expertise so that the patient receives a coordinated, balanced program. The team takes on a varied composition, depending on the needs of the patient, but in general, it includes the following members: a physician skilled in providing spinal cord care, nursing staff trained in the management of the spinal cord injured patient, occupational therapist, physical therapist, social worker, psychologist, recreational therapist, and vocational rehabilitation specialist. Additional medical disciplines often needed are orthopedic surgery; neurosurgery; urology; internal medicine, especially respiratory medicine; plastic surgery; psychiatry, and neurology.

After the patient's arrival in the emergency department, the attending physician should complete a thorough physical examination, as would be expected for any patient. When a spinal cord injury is suspected or identified by either loss of motor function or a sensory deficit, a more detailed neurologic examination should be performed. Emergency department physicians should be cognizant of the various sensory dermatomes and major motor levels of the cervical, thoracic, and lumbar spine. In this examination, two areas are often overlooked and are critical in the assessment of spinal cord function. One is rectal sensation and tone and the presence or absence of a bulbocavernosus reflex. The other area often ignored is toe flexion.

Once the normal life-support measures have been taken and the general physical and more detailed neurologic examinations completed, radiologic examina-

Table 36–3. ETIOLOGY OF SPINAL CORD INJURY

Motor vehicular	44.5%
Falls	18.1%
Acts of violence	16.6%
Sports	12.7%
Diving	8.5%
Football	0.7%
Snow skiing	0.5%
Trampoline	0.3%
Other sports	2.0%
Wrestling	0.3%
Gymnastics	0.3%
Horseback	0.4%
Other	1.4%
Other	8.0%
Total patients	14791

From Go, B. K., DeVivo, M. J., and Richards, J. S.: The epidemiology of spinal cord injury. *In* Stover, S. L., DeLisa, J. A., and Whiteneck, G. G. (eds.): Spinal Cord Injury: Clinical Outcomes from the Model Systems. Gaithersburg, MD, Aspen Publications, 1995, pp. 21–55. © 1995, Aspen Publishers, Inc.

Table 36–4. ASIA MOTOR INDEX SCORE

Right	Key Muscle Segment	Left
5	C5	5
5	C6	5
5	C7	5
5	C8	5
5	T1	5
5	L2	5
5	L3	5
5	L4	5
5	L5	5
5	S1	5
50	Total score	50

Each key muscle is graded 0, absent; 1, trace; 2, poor; 3, fair; 4, good; 5, normal. The grade is put in the table and totaled, producing the score used to compare admission, discharge, and follow-up status.

tion should take place if it can be performed safely. The initial films obtained should be anteroposterior (AP) and lateral views of the suspected injured area of the spine. Gross assessment of these films will normally indicate the bony level of injury, which should roughly correlate with the physical findings.

After identification of a spinal cord injury the appropriate treating physician is requested, who, whether orthopedist or neurosurgeon, should be thoroughly familiar with both operative and nonoperative management of spinal column injuries associated with spinal cord injury.

The treating physician should document the spinal cord injury accurately from both motor and sensory standpoints, as well as the status of reflex activity. Knowing these levels accurately often aids judgments regarding management of the bony spine in the first two weeks after injury.

Chart documentation of the neurologic function should include at least an accurate sensory map; an accurate muscle grading using the 0 to 5 scale, 0 being absent and 5 being normal; and the rectal examination. For data purposes, the patient should be assigned a motor index score as developed by the American Spinal Injury Association (Table 36–4) and graded according to the ASIA Scale:

ASIA A. Sensory incomplete.
ASIA B. Sensory incomplete.
ASIA C. Useless distal motor function.
ASIA D. Useful distal motor function.
ASIA E. Normal.

During this initial phase, an indwelling catheter should be inserted pending more definitive bladder management. At this time, associated injuries, such as head, chest, and abdominal injuries and long bone fractures, should be evaluated.

The patient should be ready for transfer from the emergency department to the hospital bed, whether in the intensive care unit or on the orthopedics/neurology

floor. At this time, if the patient has a thoracic or lumbar injury, anatomic postural positioning is all that is necessary. However, if the patient has a cervical injury, tong traction, the most popular being Gardner-Wells, with the attachment of the appropriate amount of weight, is appropriate. Generally this is calculated as 10 pounds for the head and 5 pounds for each cervical level. An injury at C5, for instance, would require 35 pounds.

The attending physician's next task is to determine the appropriate care for the bony spine. Much information can be obtained by a thorough analysis of the plain films of the spine. These help in identifying the mechanism of injury. Knowing the mechanism of the injury allows the most appropriate management.

Classification of the Spinal Cord Injury Neurologically

From a neurologic standpoint, there are two types of spinal cord injury: complete and incomplete. If the patient has a complete injury, little neurologic return can be expected. To determine the completeness of injury, the spinal cord must be recovering from spinal shock. At the time of spinal cord injury, all functions of the spinal cord cease (i.e., motor, sensory, and reflex function). As spinal shock begins to resolve, reflex function, a function of the cord itself, returns. The return of reflex function is heralded by the appearance of the bulbocavernosus reflex (BCR), which is elicited by genital stimulation that triggers the reflex arc, producing an anal contraction or puckering. If this reflex is present or if the patient is exhibiting priapism, the spinal cord is out of shock and thus, if there is no motor or sensory function below the injury level, by definition the injury is complete. Occasionally, there is undetected but present deep rectal sensation that may make the initial impression of complete injury incorrect. Thus, it is incumbent on the examining physician to be sure to ascertain the presence of deep rectal sensation rather than just superficial sensation. The determination of a complete injury can usually be made within the first 72, if not the first 24, hours after injury (Table 36–5).

Table 36–5. NEUROLOGIC CLASSIFICATION OF SPINAL CORD INJURY

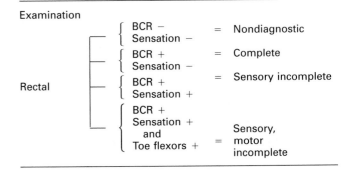

Incomplete Syndromes

There are four incomplete spinal cord injury syndromes. These are all characterized by the presence of some spinal cord function below the level of injury but have varying prognoses.

Anterior Cord Syndrome. Anterior cord syndrome is characterized by injury to the anterior horn cells in the gray matter opposite the area of spinal injury. There is alteration in the function in the long tracts in the white matter in the anterolateral aspect of the spinal cord. The posterior columns and the posterior horn area of the gray matter are variously spared. Clinically, this type of injury is more common in the cervical region, characterized by paralysis of portions of the upper limbs with an upper motor neuron paralysis of the lower extremities. In the lower extremities, the only preserved function is deep pressure and position sense, with no motor function below the area of injury. Lost below the injury level are light touch, sharp/dull, and temperature sensation as well as motor function. The mechanism of injury is usually a compression or flexion injury, commonly seen in diving injuries. The prognosis in this type of incomplete injury is the worst of all the incomplete syndromes. Return of any muscle function below the anatomic site of injury is rare.

Posterior Cord Syndrome. Posterior cord syndrome is rare. In this injury, most damage is in the posterior columns, which results in the preservation of motor function with loss of sensory function below the injury level. This injury is so rare that it is impossible to predict the outcome.

Central Cord Syndrome. Central cord syndrome is common and occurs when the central gray matter containing the motor horn cells of the upper extremities with extension into the adjacent white matter, involving the central long tracts, is injured. The mechanism of injury is usually an extension injury that occurred in an older patient with a more rigid spine, producing a central hematomyelia. Because the motor and sensory impulses in the sacral segments of the spinal cord are in the peripheral white matter, the perianal sensation is preserved. Return of motor and sensory function in the lower extremities usually occurs early. Control of the bowel and bladder also may return. Occasionally the patient ends up with good function in the lower extremities, although there may be spasticity. Because of the damage to the central matter of the cord at the anatomic site of injury, upper extremity function usually does not improve significantly.

Brown-Séquard Syndrome. Brown-Séquard syndrome is produced by a penetrating object in which half of the cord is injured and the other half remains intact. Because of the crossing over of the spinal tracts, the clinical picture below the level of injury is different on each side. On the ipsilateral side of the injury site, there will be paresis or paralysis with hypalgesia on the contralateral side. Prognosis for recovery is the most promising of the incomplete syndromes. The weak side should become stronger and usually has normal sensation, whereas the contralateral limb regains some sensibility and has good motor power.

Conus Medullaris Syndrome

The conus medullaris is usually posterior to the bodies from T12 to L1 but may be at T11 or L2. Isolated injury to this portion of the cord produces loss of bowel and bladder control. The physical findings are loss of perirectal sensation and poor rectal muscle tone. The prognosis is poor for significant return of bowel and bladder control (Table 36–6).

Cauda Equina Syndrome

The cauda equina is in the spinal canal from L1 to L5 and is composed entirely of the lumbar and sacral nerve roots. Thus, an injury in this region does not produce a spinal cord injury but one more similar to a peripheral nerve injury. The physical findings are variable sensory and motor loss. Because of the peripheral nerve similarity, the prognosis for motor nerve recovery is good. This is an area of the spine where more aggressive surgical management may produce the best results.

Radiologic Evaluation

Cervical Region

When evaluating the cervical spine region for injury, there are seven checkpoints the physician should observe. First, the roentgenogram should be an adequate one of the cervical spine, meaning that all seven cervical vertebrae plus the superior portion of T1 should be visualized. Second, the soft tissue should be examined. The most important area in this examination is the evidence of any swelling at the anteroinferior border of C3. If the soft tissue shadow at that area measures more than 5 mm, it is indicative of swelling in the cervical region, which is presumptive evidence of injury. The third checkpoint is evaluation of the configuration of the cervical bodies. Fourth is assessment of the overall alignment of the spine. This can be determined by observing the congruity of the posterior aspect of the cervical bodies and checking the alignment of the spinolaminar line. Fifth is assessment of the alignment and configuration of the facet joints at each level. The sixth is checking the spinous processes for fracture or widening between the processes. The final observation should be checking the atlantoaxial articulation for bony integrity and alignment (Table 36–7).

Where there is a loss of alignment, the amount of alignment should be measured. If there is offset of one body on the other in the range of 25 to 50 per cent, this indicates a unilateral facet dislocation. If there is more than 50 per cent malalignment, bilateral facet dislocation is suspected. Assessment of bony abnor-

Table 36–6. INCOMPLETE SPINAL CORD INJURIES

Syndrome	Physical Findings	Prognosis
Anterior cord syndrome Diving Compression flexion	Motor loss Pain/temperature loss Partial pain	Poor for any functional return
Central cord syndrome Older patient Flexion	Distal motor function better than proximal Sensory function altered Usually cervical	Variable return of upper extremity function Spasticity
Brown-Séquard syndrome Penetrating object	Paresis or paralysis ipsilateral side Pain and temperature loss contralateral	Significant return usually occurs
Posterior cord syndrome Rare Extension	Variable motor loss Pain intact	Unknown
Conus medullaris	Injury at T11–L2 Loss of bowel and bladder control	Usually not much improvement
Cauda equina	Injury at L1–L5 Variable motor loss	Usually some return of motor function

malities should give an indication of the mechanism of injury, i.e., flexion, extension, and/or rotation. The ability to determine this is helpful in making the decisions that lead to restoration of spinal stability.

Thoracolumbar Region

Roentgenograms in the upper thoracic spine from T1 to T8 are often difficult to see because of the overlying hard and soft tissues. Therefore, special adjunctive radiologic techniques may be needed to delineate the injury further. In the lower thoracic and upper lumbar spine, routine roentgenograms usually demonstrate the pathology. Areas that should be noted are the configuration of the bodies; the extension of fracture lines into the pars interarticularis, lamina, and spinous process; and the angulation of the spine. On AP films, the observation should include any translation to either side, any widening of the pedicles, or any spreading of the spinous processes.

Tomography

Before the development of CT, tomographs of the spine were an important part of a more definitive examination of all areas of the spine. Tomography has been supplanted by CT and MRI; however, there are still

Table 36–7. CERVICAL SPINE ROENTGENOGRAM REVIEW

1. Adequate film of C1–T1
2. Soft tissue swelling at anteroinferior C3 body—5 mm or less
3. Body configuration
4. Alignment of posterior bodies
5. Facet joints
6. Spinous process (fracture—spread)
7. Atlantoaxial relationship

times when tomography is helpful. This is particularly true for attempts to evaluate the lower cervical spine and the upper thoracic spine, where either a complete tomographic series or a midline tomograph may help determine fracture and facet joint abnormalities.

CT has proved valuable in evaluating the bony spine. With the developing computer programs, CT is capable of reconstructing the spine at any level in both the AP and lateral views as well as three-dimensional views, producing a good visual image of the damaged spinal column. Also, the size of the spinal canal can be ascertained, as well as the presence of any foreign material within the spinal column and canal.

CT with Metrizamide

If CT is combined with metrizamide myelography, better delineation of soft tissues, especially the cord and disc, can be achieved, as well as a determination of the degree of obstruction to the spinal canal.

MRI

With MRI it is possible to assess the damage to the spinal cord as well as the disc space. Each advance in computer programs brings the opportunity to obtain more information on the soft tissues in the injury area.

Spinal Column Management

Management of the bony injury of the spine is discussed in depth in Chapter 28. There are some general comments that need to be made about how the management of spinal column injury relates to the rehabilitation process. The general goals in approaching a fractured spine should be to re-establish spinal stability, to cause no further neurologic damage, and if possible to enhance neurologic return. These goals can be met either operatively or nonoperatively, depending on an analysis of the mechanism of injury, the extent of altered bony anatomy, and the safety of reconstructing the altered anatomy to a better state.

Spinal Stability

Spinal stability may be re-established by either operative or nonoperative means. The clinical judgement is whether there is instability. This may be difficult to determine, and for this judgment to be made, abnormal motion must be demonstrated. Often this can be done using motion films that compare flexion and extension views. This is most easily accomplished in the cervical spine, is difficult in the thoracic spine, and may be demonstrated in the thoracolumbar spine. In any type of motion demonstration, testing should be directly supervised by the responsible physician and not delegated.

If the spinal column is judged to be stable, it must be protected to maintain good alignment until bony healing has occurred. In previous years in countries other than the United States, traction in bed accomplished that goal. There are many positive effects of getting the patient immobilized as quickly as possible. Use of something as simple as a cervicothoracic orthosis may be all that is required; however, usually the injury is of such magnitude that a halo-jacket provides more effective immobilization and maintains alignment with more certainty. A well-applied and professionally maintained halo is a safe and effective means to allow bony healing.

Operative treatment should be used when it is a more effective way of immobilizing the spine than nonoperative means. The chosen method of internal fixation should be easy to accomplish, should be expertly performed, and should minimize any risks of further neurologic damage. The method chosen for internal fixation should provide the internal stability needed until healing has occurred. For instance, if an operative procedure for stability with internal fixation is done in the cervical spine and a halo is still needed, little has been gained by proceeding with an operative method. In the thoracolumbar spine, if the internal fixation devices do not provide enough stability so that external support can be discontinued within four to six weeks, little has been gained in terms of mobilization and rehabilitation. In many instances the fracture could have been treated just as effectively nonoperatively with the same activity restrictions.

The second goal of the spine surgeon should be to cause no further neurologic damage. If there is an operative approach that provides spinal stability, that procedure should be used in the management of the spine rather than an operative method that works but may entail additional general and neurologic risks to the patient. It is a good rule to avoid introducing any type of instrument or metal part of a stabilization device within the confines of the spinal canal.[17] Wires under the lamina, screws that have the opportunity to violate the cortex of the pedicle and thus the canal, and hooks that take up space within the canal have

been known to create the potential for neurologic compromise, either to the cord or to the nerve roots. In patients who have lost considerable neurologic function because of their injury, additional neurologic loss secondary to an operative procedure is a considerable price to pay for a gain that may only allow them to get up a few weeks earlier. The more proximal the neurologic damage, the greater is the loss, even if it is only part of the function of a nerve root.

The third goal of the spine surgeon should be to enhance neurologic return. The surgeon has two opportunities to fulfill this goal. If the patient has a complete neurologic lesion as determined by the physical examination but does not have function of the appropriate nerve roots for the level of injury, the surgeon should try to obtain return of that nerve root function. For instance, if the patient has a C5–C6 fracture-dislocation and the neurologic level of function is at C5, the surgeon should strive to achieve return of the sixth nerve root function. This may be accomplished by realigning the spine, decreasing tension on the nerve root, and with the passage of time allowing the nerve root function to return. It may require the removal of bony fragments or disc fragments causing pressure on the nerve root.[2] These statements are particularly true for cervical injuries in which one additional nerve root is critical in eventual physical functioning. In the thoracic spine, there is virtually no benefit to additional motor function attributed to one nerve root. In the lumbar spine, however, an additional functioning nerve root can be significant in relation to the patient's ability to ambulate.

The second area in which the surgeon has the potential for enhancing the neurologic outcome has not been completely evaluated: re-establishing the size of the bony canal. At the present time an adequate size for the bony canal has not been completely ascertained. In a complete injury, with the expected nerve roots already functioning, an operative procedure to remove bone from the canal and re-establish more normal canal size has not demonstrated consistent enough improvement to be recommended. In the case of an incomplete spinal cord injury, researchers suggest that re-establishing an adequate spinal canal improves the chances of neurologic return, but again the definition of "adequate" has not been determined. There is also gathering evidence based on CT studies that canal size may be enlarged as healing progresses because of remodeling of bony fragments as the spinal bone responds to stress in the healing process.

Finally, the spine surgeon should be reminded that in spinal column injuries that have no neurologic deficit, the patient cannot be neurologically better than normal. Thus, when planning any surgery the main requirement should be re-establishment of spinal stability. Any canal compromise should be noted, but surgical attempts to improve it should take into account that neurologic compromise may result from trying to improve a roentgenographic finding.

In summary, the spine surgeon's first goal should be attempting to provide spine stability. Attempts to do more than that should be tempered by the knowledge of the patient's neurologic function, weighing the risks against potential benefits.

Restorative Management

This section discusses the management of those entities produced by loss of spinal cord integrity. In some texts these have been listed as "complications" and in others as "problems." Alteration of innervation owing to the spinal cord injury causes alteration of certain physiologic areas, and thus the management of these functions must be addressed.

Urinary Function

The injury change in the urinary system is the loss of active control of the patient's ability to urinate. In the early injury, bladder drainage is most effectively accomplished by insertion of an indwelling catheter, used for 24 hours to 10 days, until the period of diuresis has passed and the blood pressure, cardiac function, urinary output, and fluid intake have been stabilized. At that time urinary tract management is best accomplished by intermittent catheterization every four hours around the clock until the volumes obtained indicate that a less frequent schedule can be instituted.

As spinal cord shock clears and reflex function returns, and if the patient has an upper motor neuron lesion, a reflex bladder program can be developed. As reflex activity increases, the bladder reflex can be stimulated by tapping the abdomen or stroking the inner thigh; the bladder sphincter relaxes and the bladder contracts, emptying the bladder of its contents. During the early phases, the intermittent catheterization program is continued until the bladder contains less than 50 ml after it has been reflexively emptied.[13] From that time on, bladder function can be managed with an external collecting device until the reflex voiding pattern has become established enough to be trusted.

If the cord is injured in the region of the conus and a lower motor neuron bladder develops, the bladder will continue to accept fluid until it becomes so distended that overflow incontinence develops. This is not a good situation, and the patient needs to either continue to use intermittent catheterization or else void by the Credé maneuver or pressure on the abdomen, causing the bladder to empty.

Under either of these types of bladder programs, the bladder should never be allowed to accumulate more than 450 to 500 ml of urine. All patients should be taught to catheterize themselves whether they are using a reflex program or the Credé maneuver, because occasionally they will need to check residual urine to be sure they are maintaining an effective emptying program. The external collecting devices for men are satisfactory and function well. This is not the case for women, who often opt for an indwelling Foley or suprapubic catheter rather than use a moisture-collecting pad or pant. Some individuals with a reflex bladder develop significant spasticity that cannot be controlled by appropriate medications. In these patients an indwelling Foley or suprapubic tube may be indicated.

In summary, the goal of an effective bladder program should be to perform a complete urologic evaluation, including urodynamic studies and possibly bladder muscle electromyographic studies, to determine the best functioning method of urinary control, to achieve and maintain a controlled pattern of urine elimination, to prevent complications, to educate the family and the patient in the bladder program, and to develop patient independence regarding the bladder system.

Maintaining a noninfected state for the upper and lower genitourinary tract should be the goal of the urologic team. Placing a foreign body into the bladder on an intermittent or chronic basis commonly causes bladder infections in the rehabilitation setting as well as after discharge. During the early hospital phase, sterile technique should be used for inserting catheters. If the ultimate bladder program is to be intermittent catheterization, the patient or family must be taught the technique. Using a sterile technique at home is impractical, but a clean technique should be taught as part of the rehabilitation process. During this time, frequent infections may occur. Suppressive antibiotic therapy has been recommended in the past but is currently losing favor. Focus for prevention is on improving technique.

Infection is manifested by cloudy, thick urine. Fever is often present. If the patient has spasticity, the first sign of infection may be worsening of the spasticity. A culture should be obtained, with antimicrobial sensitivity requested. Antibiotic treatment is generally withheld until the reports are received. If the culture count is not greater than 100,000 per ml, treatment is usually not indicated. Treatment should last long enough to produce a negative culture.

Bowel Function

Bowel function is affected in a way similar to urinary function, in that sphincter control is lost with the spinal cord injury. The distal bowel can be trained in a reflex bowel elimination program. Stimulating the anal reflex causes sphincter relaxation and bowel contraction, causing the bowel contents to be emptied. Stimulating the bowel reflex is done by stretching the external anal sphincter, which relaxes the reflexively controlled internal anal sphincter, allowing the bowel to empty. The patient is taught to take the proper amount of fluids, eat the correct foods, and engage in sufficient exercise to develop a regular bowel elimination program. Because of time restraints and to avoid interference with other critical functions, it is best to develop the bowel program on an every-other-night schedule, preferably an hour or two after ingestion of the evening meal. The use of laxatives or enemas is discouraged, because eventually these bowel irritants lose their effectiveness on the intestinal wall and chronic constipation may develop, with increasing need for more effective stimulants.

It should be the goal of a bowel program to develop a regulated program, to educate the family and the patient in how the bowel functions to prevent complications, and finally to promote as much patient independence as possible.

Skin

Those areas below the anatomic level of injury to the spinal cord will lose sensation, and thus the skin is at risk. Without sufficient pressure relief on a periodic basis, the skin will break down, causing a skin sore, bedsore, or decubitus ulcer. To prevent this, the nursing staff needs to be encouraged to turn the patient every two hours during the early postinjury period and to pad the appropriate bony prominences, depending on the bed position. As the patient improves and starts sitting in a wheelchair, a weight-shift program must be developed. Initially, when in the sitting position, the patient should shift weight every 15 minutes, relieving the pressure on the ischium for at least 1 minute. The weight shifts are gradually increased at 15-minute increments so that ultimately the patient can sit for one hour between weight shifts. Similarly, when the patient is in bed, the time between turns can be gradually increased so that eventually the patient can lie in one position from six to seven hours, making it possible to sleep through the night without needing a position change. These general guidelines may need to be altered for each patient, depending on the skin texture and blood supply of individual areas.

It should be the goal of any skin program to increase the tolerance to pressure, to maintain skin integrity, to educate the family and the patient regarding the risk factors, to develop an effective discharge plan for skin maintenance, and to promote the patient's independence in performing good skin care.

Challenges in Restorative Management

The skin, bowel, and bladder are areas involved in all spinal cord injuries. The following sections discuss challenges that are potentially present for all patients with spinal cord injury but may not become problems.

Deep Venous Thrombosis—Pulmonary Embolus

Deep venous thrombosis occurs in 25 to 95 per cent of patients, depending on the study reviewed and, more specifically, on the tests used for diagnosis of thrombophlebitis. Clinically, it is a problem in about 25 to 30 per cent of patients, causing a delay in rehabilitation programs. The initial presentation is a swollen leg. This can be detected early if the nursing staff performs routine thigh and calf measurements. When these indicate an enlarging thigh, the therapy program should be stopped, and the patient kept at bed rest until a more definitive diagnostic test can be made. Tests that

can be considered are Doppler test, impedance plethysmography, radionuclide scanning, or ultrasound venography. The last is the most diagnostic test, but it may produce phlebitis. If the selected test is positive for thigh clot, the patient should be kept at bed rest for seven days and heparin should be administered. After seven days the medication should be switched to warfarin (Coumadin) and maintained for three months. If the clot is in the calf, some protocols call for heparinization followed quickly by warfarin. When the appropriate clotting level is obtained, the patient's rehabilitation can be continued. Because of the high incidence of clotting, prophylaxis has been attempted.[9, 16] Low-dose aspirin, low-dose heparin (Lovenox), sequential compression hose, and early exercise have been advocated as methods of preventing or reducing the incidence of thrombophlebitis. There is no good evidence that any of these alter the incidence, however.

An even more devastating problem is pulmonary embolus. Spinal cord injured patients are at significant risk for this potentially lethal complication for several months after their injury. Depending on the person's neurologic level, there may be no presenting symptoms. In higher quadriplegic patients, the physiologic alteration may be an increase in oxygen requirements. Diagnosis should be confirmed by the appropriate test, which may be a lung scan or a ventilation-perfusion study. Once the diagnosis is made, anticoagulants should be given and therapy programs stopped until the patient's general condition warrants resumption.

The use of preventive measures for thrombophlebitis, such as anticoagulation, aspirin, minidose heparin, and sequential compression hose, appears to have been more effective in reducing the incidence of pulmonary embolism than in reducing phlebitis. With either of these diagnoses, if there is any contraindication to the use of anticoagulation, consideration should be given to the placement of a vena cava filter.

Autonomic Dysreflexia

Autonomic dysreflexia can develop into the most significant emergency in spinal cord injury.[8] Primary symptoms of dysreflexia are headache and hypertension up to 300/180. The symptom complex may develop in a patient with a neurologic lesion above T6 because of increased stimulation into the afferent centers of spinal reflex activity, stimulating an overreaction at the sympathetic nervous system. Other symptoms that can develop are increased sweating, pupil dilation, and bradycardia down to a rate of 50. This clinical symptom complex usually does not occur before six weeks, until the reflex activity of the cord is returning, and in many patients, it runs its course within three years.

The most common cause of dysreflexia is distention of the bowel or bladder. Thus, the initial treatment is aimed at relief of any obstruction. In the case of the bladder, the catheter should be checked, and if a catheter is not in place, intermittent catheterization should be performed to completely empty the bladder. If the symptoms continue, the bowel should be checked for an impaction. If these measures do not relieve the hypertension and headache, drug therapy should be considered. Short-acting agents such as amyl nitrate and nitroglycerin or longer-acting agents such as mecamylamine and guanethidine can be administered. In very severe cases spinal anesthesia has been necessary.

Special consideration should be given to pregnant women, because development of a headache during a normal vaginal delivery may be misinterpreted. The obstetrician must keep in mind that a headache during labor may mark the onset of dysreflexia, and failure to recognize this problem and treat it may be lethal to the mother.

Pulmonary

Respiratory complications are a potential challenge in any spinal cord injured patient whose injury is at T10 or above, but they are more significant the more proximal the cord injury.[4] The act of respiration involves four muscle groups, the most significant being the diaphragm. The abdominal muscles, the muscles of the chest wall, and the accessory neck muscles also support respiratory effort. If the injury occurs at C3 or above, phrenic nerve and thus diaphragmatic function are lost. In this case, a ventilator is necessary. Patients injured at C4 frequently require a ventilator initially, but after development of accessory muscle function, unless there is pre-existing lung or chest wall disease, the ventilator can be discontinued. Most C5 injury patients do not require ventilation support even in the early period unless there is pre-existing chronic lung disease.

Because of the decreased respiratory capabilities in all spine-injured patients and in the period of recumbency immediately after the injury, development of secretion problems, including mucous plugs, makes it mandatory that the respiratory system be examined daily until the patient is up and active in rehabilitation programs. A mucous plug is potentially life-threatening, causing respiratory arrest. Cord-injured patients, especially quadriplegic patients, with their inability to cough and clear secretions, may need bronchoscopy. To minimize the necessity for bronchoscopy, the respiratory and nursing staff should routinely perform assisted coughing. This technique should be taught to the family so it can be used at home.

Initially, the quadriplegic patient can use diaphragmatic contraction only, producing a vital capacity of 1000 to 1500 ml, which is approximately 25 per cent of normal. As the accessory muscles of respiration and those intercostals that remain strengthen, vital capacity may increase to 3000 ml, approximately 50 per cent of normal.

A phrenic nerve stimulator can be used in high quadriplegic patients on a ventilator.[18] The phrenic nerves should be tested to determine their capability of conducting electrical impulse, and if this is present, phrenic nerve pacing is feasible, although expensive. With successful pacing and an appropriate training program, the patient can develop enough respiratory effort to be off the ventilator for eight hours. Some achieve 24 hours off the ventilator, which allows them to be completely free.

Cardiovascular

After spinal cord injury, especially if it is above the thoracic sympathetic outflow between T6 and T12, a physiologic situation similar to a sympathectomy below the level of the injury develops.[25] There is dilation of the blood vessels, resulting in hypotension because of blood pooling in the extremities. The blood remains in this pool because there is no effective muscle pump working to help free the limbs of blood. Hypotension in the 90/60 range and tachycardia around 100 develop and may remain for several days. The patient is in no danger if the hypotension and tachycardia have been differentiated from blood loss and if an adequate urinary output is maintained by administration of appropriate fluids. Four days after injury, sympathetic tone begins to return, causing potential overload of the cardiovascular system and producing significant diuresis. During this time, diuretic and cardiotrophic agents may be necessary to support the cardiovascular system.

As the patient begins to be mobilized, orthostatic hypotension may develop. The patient may experience lightheadedness, dizziness, or even sudden loss of consciousness. Short-term treatment consists of lowering of the head and elevation of the extremities. Long-term treatment includes gradual positioning of the patient in the upright position, encouraging fluid intake before sitting, and use of abdominal and leg binders. In refractory cases, mild hypertensive and mineralocorticoid agents can be used to increase peripheral fluid volume.

Succinylcholine should not be used in patients with spinal cord injury who are under anesthesia. In a matter of minutes in the susceptible patient, succinylcholine can increase the serum potassium to a level over 12 or 13 mEq/liter, which is potentially lethal.

Spasticity

As the spinal cord recovers from shock and reflex arcs begin to function again, spasticity may develop in patients with injuries at the middle and upper thoracic and cervical levels.[3] Spasticity is divided into three classes. Mild spasticity is manifested by hyperactive reflexes and unsustained clonus. Moderately spastic patients demonstrate involuntary contractions they cannot control and a sustained clonus that does not interfere with activities. Patients with marked spasticity have unpredictable and uncontrolled paroxysms of spasm and involuntary clonus, both of which may cause them to be thrown out of the wheelchair or make them unable to lie quietly in bed. Such spasticity significantly interferes with functional activity such as sitting, balance, ability to use the wheelchair, and transfers.

With prolonged marked spasticity, contractures may develop so that neither lying nor sitting can be accomplished without undue pressure on bony prominences. This leads to skin breakdown and chronic pressure sores. In the management of some pressure sores, spasticity relief may be the first step in treatment.

Treatment of spasticity is frustrating for both patient and physician. Four medications are commonly used. Baclofen is the most popular and works at the spinal reflex arc level. Dosage levels start at 5 mg twice a day and are progressively increased to a maximum of 30 mg four times a day. The second medication used is sodium dantrolene, which acts at the neuromuscular junction. It is prescribed in dosages beginning with 25 mg four times a day and progressing to a maximum of 100 mg four times a day. This medication tends to produce drowsiness, is not as effective a muscle relaxant, and risks liver toxicity. The third medication, diazepam (Valium), works centrally and is an effective muscle relaxant but is addictive and subject to abuse. It can be used in dosages starting with 2 mg twice a day and progressing to 10 mg four times a day. The fourth medication is clonidine, which can be used in dosages of 1 mg twice a day, progressing to 2 mg three times a day.[5]

In the future, the use of baclofen intrathecally via an implantable pump may have significant application in patients with severe spasticity. An operative procedure that has proved effective in many patients is thermal rhizotomy, used in patients with marked lower extremity spasticity who have no sensation. The amount and duration of spasticity relief are not predictable, however.

The negative aspects of spasticity are its unexpectedness, its uncontrollability, its role in developing contractures, and its interference with functional activity such as transfers. There are positive aspects to spasticity, however. A low level of spasticity maintains some muscle bulk in the spastic muscles, which provides further protection over bony prominences. In some patients who become ambulatory, spasticity may assist function, and with ablation of the spasticity, the ability to ambulate or perform certain other activities is lost.

Contractures

Contractures can develop in any joint that is paralyzed and not being used. Early in the injury phase, nurses and therapists should participate in daily range of motion and stretching exercises for the joints subject to paralysis to prevent tightness, and thus contractures, from developing. In the early treatment phase, particular attention should be focused on shoulder range of motion.[20] Positioning in bed while the patient is in traction or when a halo-jacket is used for stabilization of the bony spine often leads to significant tightness of the shoulders, which becomes painful and is difficult to relieve. This situation can be lessened or prevented from developing by early attention to proper positioning and range of motion to the shoulder joints three times daily.

In the lower extremities, the foot and ankle are most

prone to developing contractures early because positioning in the supine or prone position favors dorsiflexion. The foot and ankle are the most common joints affected in the early rehabilitation phase. All joints should have range of motion performed daily from the time of injury. In the restorative phase of rehabilitation, prevention of contractures is of paramount importance. In function of the hand, however, development of myostatic tightness is beneficial for developing the tenodesis effect for gross grasp and release in C6 and C7 quadriplegic patients.

It is important to teach the patient a range of motion program, because it will need to be continued at home on a regular basis. Most range of motion is done by the patient in a functional manner. For instance, when the patient transfers from the bed to the wheelchair, the elbows need to go into full extension, the wrists need to be dorsiflexed, and after the sitting position is assumed, the hips and knees go from full extension to flexion. Thus, one or two transfers a day keep these joints mobile.

Heterotopic Ossification

Heterotopic ossification (HO) occurs in 20 to 30 per cent of spinal cord injured patients. There is development of ossification around a major joint, most commonly the hip, followed in order by the knee, shoulder, and other joints. Ossification usually appears one to four months after injury but has been reported earlier and later. The process may be heralded by leg swelling and thus be part of the differential diagnosis of thrombophlebitis. Another early symptom is a subtle loss of motion in the affected joint. The physical therapist may be first to note the symptoms. Roentgenograms of the affected joint should be obtained but are often negative until seven to 21 days after onset of swelling or loss of range of motion. Alkaline phosphatase level should be obtained, because it is usually elevated in the early stages of the process.

Because of the significance of the development of HO, especially if it occurs in the hip with a significant loss of range of motion, treatment should begin on suspicion. The only treatment currently available is the administration of disodium etidronate, which may prevent deposition of calcium around the affected joint. It is recommended that this medication be continued for three months.

In patients in whom the diagnosis is not made or the medication is ineffective who proceed to significant joint range of motion restrictions, surgery may become necessary. Surgery should not be done while the patient is in the acute phase, however. The end of the acute phase is determined by the alkaline phosphatase level returning to normal, the bony mass looking mature on roentgenogram (i.e., with smooth edges rather than a fuzzy outline), and a negative radionuclide uptake scan. When these conditions have been met, the ossification can be excised either in a wedge manner or by circumferentially excising the mass coupled with continued administration of disodium etidronate for at least a year. When the patient recovers from the surgical process, gentle range of motion can be reinstituted with the goal of establishing enough range of motion so that the patient can sit safely in a wheelchair.

Fractures

Because many spinal cord injured patients have suffered significant trauma, fractures may also occur to the long bones. Treatment of long bone fractures in the acute spinal injury phase varies from that in the later chronic stages. In general, long bone fractures in the acute phase are best managed by rapid internal fixation so that the patient can be mobilized as quickly as possible. Treating a fracture in traction with the added problem of skin insensitivity makes the likelihood of developing skin problems significant. Similarly, if the patient is treated in a cast, unless the padding is appropriate, development of skin sores is likely.

Conversely, when a fracture of a long bone occurs later than six to nine months after injury, the bone is osteoporotic, and obtaining adequate internal fixation is often difficult. The long bones of the longer-term spinal cord injured patients tend to form callus more quickly and heal at a rapid rate. Therefore, if adequate positioning can be obtained, external immobilization either with a well-padded cast or splint or using a pillow splint is often all that is required. For instance, with a fractured femur that has been sustained as a spinal cord injured person does a transfer, a callus may be seen as early as three or four weeks and becomes reasonably mature by six or eight weeks. The patient or family can be taught how to remove either the anterior or posterior half of a bivalved cast to inspect the skin during the course of fracture immobilization. If a skin problem develops, the physician must assist in devising alternative ways of immobilization.

Fever

Spinal cord injured patients are subject to body temperature elevations from two primary sources. In the immediate postinjury period, respiratory problems are the most common cause of an elevation of body temperature. As the patient progresses from the second week to the fourth to sixth month, urinary tract infections become the most common cause of temperature elevation. Thus, these two areas should be investigated as the primary source of temperature elevation before more sophisticated testing is attempted. Another not so obvious possibility is the development of a subcutaneous abscess over a pressure point. If these possibilities have been ruled out and temperature elevation persists, even to 106°F, a complete work-up for fever of unknown origin should be done. This includes culture of all orifices, appropriate scanning techniques, and appropriate viral antigen studies. Occasionally, all of these are normal and the fever persists. In some patients with spinal cord injury, the temperature-regulating mechanisms of the body are also altered and a fever may persist on this basis alone.

If a thorough work-up for a fever of unknown origin has been conducted and no cause found, the patient should be encouraged to continue in the rehabilitation program in spite of a significantly elevated temperature. If the temperature persists for four to six weeks, the fever of unknown origin work-up should be repeated. If it is normal at that time, the patient should continue with the rehabilitation program. Usually, fevers attributed to the spinal cord injury decrease over time. In the course of such a problem, it is necessary that the physician maintain good communication with the patient and the family.

Spinal Cyst (Syringomyelia)

Spinal cysts can occur at the level of injury as early as three months after injury but may occur at any time.[6] The incidence has been reported to be as high as 3 per cent, but with the advent of MRI, the incidence may prove to be greater than that. The cyst may vary in size from a few millimeters to the entire length of the cord. Presence of a cyst is not significant unless it is causing symptoms. However, the cyst can be responsible for significant functional losses.

The initial presenting symptom is often increasing pain. The patient may notice increased spasticity or there may be an ascending level of numbness and loss of motor strength in previously functioning muscles. There may be no symptoms unless an activity that causes increased pressure, such as coughing or sneezing, produces the symptoms. Deep tendon reflexes may be altered. There may be excessive sweating even below the level of the spinal cord injury. An additional physical finding may be Horner's syndrome, produced by having the patient lie on either side and observing the pupils for unequal size.

The diagnosis is becoming increasingly easy. The physician must have a high index of suspicion if a previously stable patient starts to complain of changes. Because many patients with spinal cord injury have pain, and increasing pain is often the presenting complaint, it may be difficult to determine a cyst as the cause. If one is suspicious after a complaint of pain, checking for other alterations such as increased spasticity, reflex loss, sensory aberrations, or Horner's syndrome may pinpoint the diagnosis.

Previously the diagnosis was made by doing a metrizamide myelogram and taking a delayed roentgenogram 12 to 24 hours later. Often the dye would be concentrated within the cyst, but now, with MRI, even very small cysts can be readily outlined. If the symptoms are severe enough and there is documentation of progressive loss of neurologic function, particularly sensation and strength, surgical relief may be necessary. The approach is to drain the cyst and install a shunt, which is usually drained into the peritoneum. A surgical complication was inadequate drainage, but with the use of intraoperative ultrasonography, the limits of the cyst can be ascertained and the complete drainage procedure performed. If the surgery is timed appropriately, there is a good chance of return of the lost function.

Pain

Pain is a frequent complication of spinal cord injury.[19] It is seen more commonly in patients who have been injured by a gunshot wound. The pain may be localized in the area of the injured portion of the spinal column. The pain may be radicular in nature, with a sharp quality, radiating in the distribution of the intercostal nerves. There may be radiation of pain into the dermatomal distribution. The pain may be distal from the level of injury, commonly occurring in the rectal region. There may be phantom pain going into the extremities, often described as burning pain.

Treatment of pain is difficult and encompasses all the usual treatments for chronic pain. Reassurance, relaxation techniques, transcutaneous nerve stimulation, tricyclic antidepressants, and biofeedback can be used. Analgesics, specifically narcotics, should not be used in the management of the pain syndrome. From the surgical standpoint, the dorsal root entry zone (DREZ) surgical approach has been advocated by some but is largely unpredictable and therefore unreliable. Cordotomy has been tried in many patients with marginal success.

Sexual Functioning

Spinal cord injury occurs most frequently in patients under 30, and sexual functioning is an important area in overall patient management. Spinal cord injured patients, both male and female, can be assured that some sexual functioning is generally possible. In men, if the injury level is above L1, normal erection potential is lost but reflex erections are possible. With proper external stimulus an erection is possible, much as the normal male gets when his bladder becomes distended. A normal ejaculation is not possible but can be stimulated by electroejaculation procedures,[14] which in many individuals produces sufficient quantity and quality of sperm to allow artificial impregnation. A high percentage of men with spinal cord injury are sterile. It is believed that this occurs because of the loss of temperature-regulating mechanisms. Without proper scrotal control, the narrow range of safe temperature for the testes is not maintained.

For women, the ability to achieve orgasm is limited, but fertility is not altered. There may be lubrication problems requiring use of artificial lubrication techniques.

With proper counseling, good instruction in alternative sexual techniques, and assistance in developing a strong feeling of sexuality, a sexual pattern can be developed that is gratifying to both the spinal cord injured patient and the significant other.

Rehabilitation Considerations

Functional Expectations

The rehabilitation team develops functional goals for each patient based on the preserved neurologic function. The experienced team is cognizant of the expected degree of root return and how the goals will be changed when and if that occurs. Wheelchair use and activities of daily living (ADL) can be achieved on four basic levels: dependent, partially dependent, stand with assistance, and independent. Gross functional goals corresponding to the neurologic level are listed in Table 36–8. Tables 36–9 and 36–10 list the motor and sensory levels of the general rehabilitation goals for frequent neurologic levels.

Orthotic Use. The use of orthoses in both the upper and lower extremities is a consideration that the rehabilitation team must address. Orthoses are available for use by quadriplegics in the upper extremities, especially patients who are functional at C6 or C7. This type of splint can be used for assisting in feeding, writing, typing, and many other areas of ADL. It is best to fit the strongest hand if they are unequal. If they are equal, the brace should be fitted for the domi-

Table 36–8. FUNCTIONAL CHART

	C1–C4	C5	C6	C7	C8	T1	T2–T7	T8–T12	L1–T3	L4–S1
Wheelchair manual		±	+	+	+	+	+	+	+	NA
Wheelchair power	+	+	±							
Transfers	a	a	+	+	+	+	+	+	+	+
Ambulation household							+	+	+	+
Ambulation community								±	+	+
ADLs										
Eating	a	a	±	+	+	+	+	+	+	+
Dressing	a	a	±	+	+	+	+	+	+	+
Driving			±	+	+	+	+	+	+	+
Grooming	a	a	±	+	+	+	+	+	+	+
Bath/toilet	a	a	±	+	+	+	+	+	+	+
Communication	±	+	+	+	+	+	+	+	+	+
Sexual	±	±	±	±	±	±	±	±	±	+

+, Yes; ±, Maybe; a, assistance; NA, not applicable.

Table 36–9. CERVICAL REGION

	Sensory	Motor	Test	Goals
C1—C3	To the neck	Cervical flexors and extensors	Trapezius Shoulder shrug	Respiratory dependent Blink or head control wheelchair Environmental control unit Computer Mouth stick
C4	Shoulder mantle	Deltoid Diaphragm	Shoulder abduction Breathing	Dependent Electric wheelchair with chin control
C5	Lateral arm Thumb	Biceps	Elbow flexion	Partial independence with adaptive equipment Electric wheelchair with arm control
C6	Index, long fingers	Wrist extensors	Wrist extension	Independent with equipment Driving hand controls Manual wheelchair with pegs
C7	Long, index fingers	Triceps Wrist flexor Finger extensors	Elbow extension Finger extension	Independent transfers and ADLs Standard manual chair
C8	5th finger	Finger flexors Interosseous	Flex fingers Spread fingers	Independent ADLs without splints Independent transfers

nant hand. There is little indication for bilateral bracing. Most patients find the braces useful early in the rehabilitation course, but as time passes and myostatic contractures develop in the fingers, producing a more effective tenodesis, patients gradually discontinue brace use.

In some patients who continue to be effective brace users, who have undergone a thorough physical and psychologic evaluation, and who have the appropriate motivation, surgical reconstruction of the upper extremity is a consideration. It should not be performed earlier than 12 months after injury. In the case of the functional C5 patient, the brachioradialis tendon can be transferred into the extensor carpi radialis longus to provide a functional wrist extensor. In the case of pa-

tients functional at the C6 level, the key grip procedure can be considered. In the case of the C7 functional patient, tendon transfers can be done to provide finger flexion and extension. A surgeon considering these types of procedures must be aware of the ways in which proposed tendon transfers may interfere in functional ADLs such as dressing.

Bracing the lower extremities is a consideration in the paraplegic patient. Some patients with a T3–T4 injury level are capable of using long leg braces. These patients usually attempt to use the braces, use them for a short time, and discard them, using them only occasionally for standing. Even patients with lower level injuries, such as at T12 and L1, who have enough truncal stability to effectively use long leg braces usu-

Table 36–10. THORACOLUMBAR REGION

	Sensory	Motor	Test	Goals
T1–T10	Chest to umbilicus	Intercostals Spine extensors	Normal upper extremity	Independent in all skills for living
T11–T12	Inguinal ligament	Rectus abdominis	Elevate trunk	Independent stand in long leg braces
L1–L2	Anterior and medial thigh	Iliopsoas adductors	Hip flexion	Ambulation with long leg braces in household
L3–L4	Medial calf	Quadriceps Hamstrings	Knee extension	Community ambulation with long leg (possibly short leg) braces
L4–L5	Dorsum foot	Anterior tibial	Dorsiflexion of foot	Community ambulation with short leg braces
L5–S1	Lateral foot	Gastrocnemius Toe flexors	Plantar flexion of foot	Community ambulation with short leg braces
S2–S5	Perianal region	Gluteus Sphincters	Hip extension Anal tone	Community ambulation, possibly without braces

ally discard the braces because the energy requirements for their continued use outside the home are too great.

If the injury level is below L1 and there is some hip stabilization, long leg bracing is likely to be more acceptable. To effectively use short leg bracing, the patient needs to have good quadriceps control. At this level, orthoses are usually well accepted and used by patients.

Reconstructive surgery in the lower extremities that attempts to decrease the amount of bracing necessary and improve the patient's function has not been successful. Surgical stabilizations of joints to provide better platforms for gaiting or ambulation usually create problems with skin breakdown because of the loss of flexibility. The only reconstructive surgery occasionally required is lengthening the Achilles tendon when it has become contracted secondary to spasticity or improper positioning of the foot and ankle in the wheelchair or bed. Achilles tendon lengthening should be undertaken for improvement of foot and ankle relationships so that the foot will fit comfortably in a wheelchair.

Orthoses are available for both the upper and lower extremities and can improve function. It is the experience of most spinal cord centers, however, that use of the brace beyond the rehabilitation hospital setting diminishes as the years from the time of injury pass. Thus the rehabilitation team should be selective and precise in its evaluation of the patient and the proposed orthoses or surgical reconstruction.

Psychosocial Considerations

The patient who has sustained a spinal cord injury goes through a process that one hopes will lead to a positive readaptation to the injury and its alterations. Immediately after the injury the patient experiences a time of denial of its severity. During this time, cooperation is common, because the patient believes that the situation is not permanent.

As the patient gets further into the rehabilitation process and starts to deal with the daily use of a wheelchair, reality sets in and attention focuses on the skills that are lost.

After this period of grief, which occurs after the realization that the injury and consequences may be permanent, almost all patients go into a period of depression. Attitudes toward family and the rehabilitation program may become negative. The depression phase may start as early as two to three months after injury and may last up to a year. During this time, outside support is necessary. Most patients with spinal cord injury are not mentally ill and do not require psychiatric help, but they do need the help of a well-trained social worker or clinical psychologist.

The final stage is one of coping. It is probably true that no spinal cord injured patient ever accepts the injury, but he or she does learn to cope with it. The job of the rehabilitation team is to try to make this positive rather than negative coping in which the patient turns to drugs, alcohol, or even suicide. In the coping phase the patient has learned to capitalize on remaining abili-

ties and develops an interest in the things that he or she is still capable of performing. In this phase the patient again becomes cooperative with those who are trying to help and sees life as a series of challenges that must be met and conquered.

It is appropriate to say that spinal cord injury does not change the patient's basic personality. Therefore, by examining the patient's history to determine how problems have been managed, information can be gained about how the patient will learn to cope with this anatomic problem. If the patient has successfully dealt with problems previously, he or she will successfully handle the problems of spinal cord injury. Additionally, patients who have a good support system and good family involvement will do well, not only in the rehabilitation program but in managing life effectively.

Home Modifications

As soon as the discharge location is determined, a home evaluation should be obtained. Using this evaluation, the team should determine the necessary modifications. Many modifications may be identified, but a few are essential. The home should have two accessible entrances, one for routine use and the second in case of emergency. The most frequently used doorways should be appropriately wide. At least one bathroom should be adapted for daily use. It is nice, but not as necessary, if the kitchen can be totally accessible, but often this can be managed by the use of extension aids, grippers, and other equipment. The necessary modifications should be completed by the time of discharge.

Leisure and Recreation

Fourteen per cent of spinal cord injuries occur as a result of recreation and leisure pursuits. Most other patients had preinjury recreation and leisure interests that should be evaluated as part of the rehabilitation process. An assessment of leisure skills should be performed. Armed with this assessment, and a knowledge of recreational interests, the therapeutic recreationist can develop a program, which should provide the patient with the necessary adaptations for pursuing the same recreation, or with a suitable alternative. Most spinal cord injured patients have unoccupied time after the injury that can be constructively and enjoyably used for adapted pursuits. Showing a patient that participation is possible and that competence can be developed is often the first and most important step in returning the patient to work and re-establishing a meaning to life.

Follow-up Care

The spinal cord rehabilitation team should commit itself to lifetime follow-up care. The initial rehabilitation team does not need to provide this care but should make appropriate community referrals to see that care is continuous. It is incumbent on the rehabilitation team to make the patient aware of those potential long-term problems that are common and to provide the patient with enough knowledge either to prevent these problems or to know when and where to seek the appropriate help should they arise.

Generally the patient should be re-evaluated eight to 12 weeks after discharge from the rehabilitation center and yearly thereafter. However, most patients, once they return to the community, develop more of their coping mechanisms, and return to a useful life, will probably not be any more successful in continuing annual follow-up care than is the general population.

References

1. Apple, D. F., and Hudson, L. M.: Spinal cord injury: The model Proceedings of the National Consensus Conference on Catastrophic Illness and Injury, Atlanta, Georgia: The Georgia Regional Spinal Cord Injury Care System. Shepherd Spinal Center. December 1989.
2. Apple, D. F., McDonald, A. P., and Smith, R. A.: Identification of herniated nucleus pulposus in spinal cord injury. Paraplegia 25:78–85, 1987.
3. Barolat, G., and Maiman, D.: Spasms in spinal cord injury. A study of 72 patients. Paraplegia 10:35–38, 1987.
4. Carter, R. E.: Respiratory aspects of spinal cord injury management. Paraplegia 23:262–266, 1987.
5. Donovan, W. H., Carter, R. E., Rossi, D., and Wilkerson, M. A.: Effect of clonidine on spasticity: A clinical trial. Arch. Phys. Med. Rehabil. 69:188–192, 1988.
6. Dworkin, G. E., and Staas, W. E.: Post traumatic syringomyelia. Arch. Phys. Med. Rehabil. 66:329–331, 1985.
7. Fine, P. R., Kuhlemeier, K. V., De Vivo, M. J., and Stover, S. L.: Spinal cord injury: An epidemiologic perspective. Paraplegia 17:237–250, 1979.
8. Gellman, H., Eckert, R., Bothe, M. J., et al.: Reflex sympathetic dystrophy in cervical spinal cord injury patients. Clin. Orthop. 233:126–131, 1988.
9. Green, D., Lee, M. Y., Ito, V., et al.: Fixed vs adjusted dose heparin in the prophylaxis of thromboembolism in spinal cord injury. JAMA 260:1255–1258, 1988.
10. Guttmann, L.: History of the National Spinal Injuries Centre, Stoke Mandeville Hospital, Aylesbury. Paraplegia 5:115–126, 1967.
11. Heinemann, A. W., Yarkony, G. M., Roth, E. J., et al.: Functional outcome following spinal cord injury: A comparison of specialized spinal cord injury center versus general hospital care. Arch. Neurol. 46:1098–1102, 1989.
12. Kraus, J. F., Fronti, C. E., Riggins, R. S., et al: Incidence of traumatic spinal cord lesions. J. Chronic Dis. 28:471–492, 1975.
13. Kuhlemeier, K. V., Lloyd, L. K., Stover, S. L., et al.: Frequency and volume of urination in patients with spinal cord injuries. Int. J. Rehabil. Res. 4:536–538, 1981.
14. Linsenmeyer, T., Wilmot, C. B., and Anderson, R. U.: The effects of electroejaculation procedure on sperm motility. Paraplegia 27:465–469, 1989.
15. Matsuura, P., Waters, R. L., Adkins, R. H., et al.: Comparison of CT parameters of the cervical spine in normals and spinal cord injured patients. J. Bone Joint Surg. [Am.] 71:183–188, 1989.
16. Merli, G. J., Herbison, G. J., Ditunno, J. F., et al.: Deep venous thrombosis prophylaxis in acute spinal cord injured patients. Arch. Phys. Med. Rehabil. 69:661–664, 1988.
17. Meyer, P. R., Cotter, H. B., and Giresan, G. T.: Operative neurological complications resulting from thoracic and lumbar spine internal fixation. Clin. Orthop. 237:125–131, 1988.
18. Miller, J. I., Farmer, J., Stewart, W., and Apple, D. F.: Phrenic nerve pacing in the quadriplegic patient. J. Thorac. Cardiovasc. Surg. 99:35–40, 1990.
19. Nepomuceno, C. S., Fine, P. R., Richards, J. S., et al.: Pain in patients with spinal cord injury. Arch. Phys. Med. Rehabil. 60:605–609, 1979.
20. Scott, J. A., and Donovan, W. H.: The prevention of shoulder pain and contracture in the acute tetraplegic patient. Paraplegia 19:313–319, 1981.
21. Seibert, C. E., Dreisback, J. N., Hahn, H. R., and Brown, C.: The contribution of computerized tomography in diagnostic skeletal imaging in acute spinal cord injury. Paraplegia 23:197, 1985.
22. Stover, S. L., and Fine, P. R.: Spinal Cord Injury, The Facts and Figures. University of Alabama Press, University of Alabama at Birmingham, 1986, pp. 20, 32.
23. Stover, S. L., Lloyd, L. K., Waites, K. B., and Jackson, A. B.: Urinary tract infections in spinal cord injury. Arch. Phys. Med. Rehabil. 70:47–54, 1989.
24. Waters, R. L., Adkins, R. H., Nelson, R., and Garland, D.: Cervical spinal cord trauma: Evaluation and nonoperative treatment with halo-rest immobilization. Contemp. Orthop. 12:35–45, 1987.
25. Winston, C. B., Lelsch, M., Talano, J. R., and Meyer, P. R.: Spinal cord injuries associated with cardiopulmonary complications. Spine 11:809–812, 1986.
26. Young, W.: The post-injury responses in trauma and ischemia: Secondary injury or protective mechanisms. Centr. Nerv. Syst. Trauma 4:27–51, 1987.
27. Young, J. S., Burns, P. E., Bowen, A. M., and McCutchen, R.: Spinal Cord Injury Statistics. Good Samaritan Medical Center, 1982.

37

Experimental Spinal Cord Injury: Pathophysiology and Treatment

Alberto Martinez-Arizala, M.D.

Barth A. Green, M.D.

Richard P. Bunge, M.D.

Interest in exploring the basis of spinal cord function by utilizing experimental models of spinal cord injury (SCI) dates back to the time of Galen (A.D. 130–201). He noted that following longitudinal cord incisions, animals retained respiration and limb movement; following cord transection, however, animals exhibited paralysis distal to the level of the lesion.[296] Only through skillfully planned laboratory research have we been able to accumulate the knowledge and expertise that have dramatically improved our understanding of the pathophysiology of SCI. The combination of this knowledge with the advancement in surgical techniques for spinal stabilization, the specialized care of patients in dedicated SCI units, and the availability of neuroprotective drugs has effectively reduced the morbidity and mortality associated with spinal injuries. In spite of these advances, SCI remains a complex and challenging problem, because our capability to prevent the loss or promote the restoration of neural function following spinal trauma remains limited.

The development of effective therapies for SCI will depend on our ability to further refine our understanding of the associated pathophysiologic changes. The size of the human cord, its complexity, and its encasement in a protective bony structure have made documenting the changes associated with its acute injury a difficult task, particularly in the areas of blood flow and metabolic changes. The current neurophysiologic and neuroimaging methods used for assessing the pathophysiology of acute human SCI have significant limitations. Therefore, our progress in understanding the pathophysiology of SCI and the development of novel treatments will continue to rely on experimental animal models. Strategic studies in animal models of experimental SCI have already stimulated the development of one effective therapeutic intervention for certain types of human spinal cord injuries.[48] Specifically, it was the beneficial effect of methylprednisolone noted in animal models of SCI that resulted in its use in the Second National Acute Spinal Cord Injury Study. Results from this study revealed that methylprednisolone was also efficacious in the treatment of selected cases of acute SCI in humans.[48] This landmark study was the first documented successful pharmacologic treatment of human SCI. We can expect that recent advances in our understanding of factors influencing successful nerve regeneration and central nervous system transplantation will offer therapeutic alternatives for the acute, subacute, and chronic spinal cord–injured patient.

In order to obtain useful data from the study of the pathophysiology of SCI in animals, the lesions produced must resemble the human lesion as closely as possible. Unfortunately, there are many kinds of human injury inflicted at various cord levels. These injuries may be open (rarely) or closed; they may rarely involve direct severance of cord tissue or, commonly, derive from contusive forces that do not interrupt the continuity of the cord but lead to internal tissue loss.[195] This latter instance, in which hemorrhage and tissue damage lead to a central necrotic area that evolves into a fluid-filled cyst, is, in its gross aspects, mimicked in most animal models of contusive injury, as illustrated in the rat (Fig. 37–1). This type of pathologic change, however, is not uniformly representative of the human injury (for a review, see reference 60a). There are, however, essentially no studies of the pathology of human SCI using the best modern fixation, embedding, and cytologic techniques. Our own efforts in studying recently obtained autopsy specimens from spinal cord–injured patients suggest that the spectrum of cord in-

jury in the human includes more subtle injuries to cord tissues than are now represented in the animal models commonly used. Thus, only certain types of human injury are reasonably modeled in animals.

EXPERIMENTAL SPINAL CORD INJURY MODELS

The task of designing a clinically relevant animal model of SCI is extremely difficult, because human

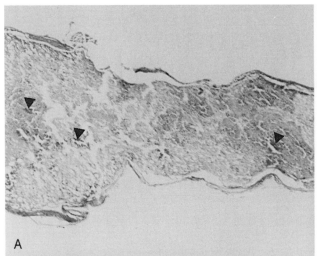

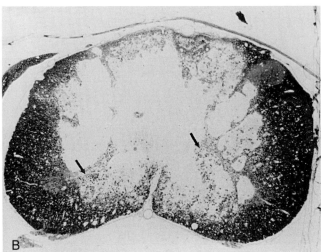

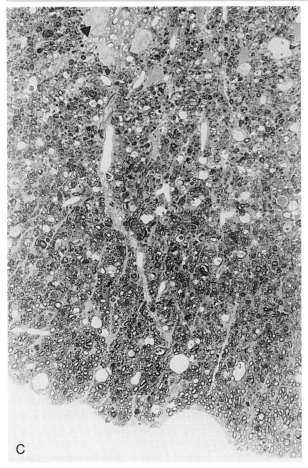

Figure 37–1. Morphologic characteristics of weight-drop contusions in the rat spinal cord produced by the weight-drop apparatus. *A,* A severe thoracic spinal cord lesion three days after injury. The spinal cord tissue was totally obliterated at the epicenter. This section, taken one segment away from the epicenter, shows extensive necrosis and edema. Scattered small hemorrhages still remain *(arrowheads).* (H&E stain.) *B,* A moderate contusive cervical lesion one month after injury. The typical cystic cavity has formed in the center of the lesion. There is a moderate amount of tissue preservation in the ventral and lateral aspects of the spinal cord. In this stage, the cyst still contains numerous macrophages *(arrows).* (Toluidine blue–stained thin plastic section.) *C,* High-power view of the ventral white matter in a moderate cervical contusive lesion one month after injury. Several motor neurons have survived *(arrowhead),* and the surviving white matter contains scattered microcysts and injured axon-myelin units.

injuries are multifactorial (Table 37–1). Some variables involved in human injury, such as age and sex, can be easily controlled in an animal model, but other variables are difficult to mimic.

First, it must be realized that all animal models of SCI require anesthesia, which itself changes the physiologic characteristics of the nervous system and may interact with any therapeutic agent under evaluation. In fact, halothane anesthesia has been reported to have a neuroprotective effect in experimental SCI.[325] Second, although most human injuries occur from the anterior and lateral displacement of the vertebral elements, most animal models use a posterior approach via a laminectomy to create the injury. This obviates the need to invade a major body cavity (such as the thorax or the abdomen), which would be required to produce an anterior injury. Third, a number of complex forces are active at the time of human injury (flexion, extension, compression, rotation).[75, 365] The velocity of the deformation of the tissue produced by these forces varies according to the nature of the force that caused the lesion. Forces involved in an injury sustained during a diving accident are markedly different from those sustained in a high-speed motor vehicle accident. Fourth, a significant interval usually occurs between the time of the injury and the time the patient is evaluated and treated medically and surgically. The degree and duration of the compressive forces applied to the spinal cord during this interval are variables that no animal model could be expected to reproduce. Last, human injuries occur in a closed vertebral system, whereas most animal models use an open laminectomy to produce the lesion. Although some closed-injury

systems have been attempted, the results have not been consistent.[196, 308]

Considering these variables, it is not surprising that a variety of experimental models of SCI have been developed (Table 37–2).[94, 132] All experimental models can be classified into those that allow some quantification of the forces involved in producing the injury and those that do not.

Although early models of experimental SCI provided information about the neurologic and histopathologic changes associated with experimental spinal cord lesions, they were primitive, and the quality of the data obtained was limited. Histopathologic changes, consisting of areas of degeneration and cavitation in the spinal cord of rabbits subjected to SCI, were initially described by Schmaus in 1890.[333] In 1907, Stcherback[352] also described necrosis of the spinal cord gray matter in rabbits following SCI. The hemorrhagic nature of the lesion was noted by Marinesco[248] in 1918 and by McVeigh[258] in 1923. Although some early models of SCI attempted to simulate the biomechanics of human SCI (see Table 37–2), most of these methods were crude and did not produce graded injuries or results that could be easily duplicated.

The modern era of experimental SCI was heralded by A. R. Allen in 1911, when he introduced a model that was reproducible and whose force could be grossly measured.[2] Allen's method created spinal injuries in dogs by dropping a known weight through a tube that was placed on the exposed thoracic cord.[2] Henceforth, the Allen technique also became known as the weight-drop model of SCI. In this model, the severity of the spinal injury is graded by varying either the weight or the height of its drop. By recording the height in centimeters and the weight in grams, the magnitude of the injury is expressed as its product in gram-centimeters (g-cm). For example, a 20-g weight dropped 20 cm would produce a 400 g-cm injury. In dogs, Allen noted that an impact of approximately 340 g-cm produced transient (7 to 10 days) paraplegia, whereas a 420 g-cm injury produced permanent deficits. He described the pathologic changes in these lesions as consisting of intramedullary hemorrhages and edema.[3] The weight-drop technique has since been modified by numerous investigators and successfully used to create contusive spinal cord lesions in a variety of animals, including cats,[42, 43, 142, 373] primates,[56, 104] and rats.[160, 389] In spite of its popularity, the weight-drop technique has potential disadvantages. The g-cm product is not a true representation of the energy imparted to the cord; for example, a 50-g mass dropped 8 cm transfers much more energy to the cord when compared with a 5-g mass dropped 80 cm, even though both are 400 g-cm injuries.[95] In addition, the cord is compressed from the posterior aspect, which differs from the more common anterior or circumferential compression seen in human injuries. The weight-drop method has also been reported to produce variable results.[199, 222] In spite of these drawbacks, however, the weight-drop closely simulates some of the biomechanics of the human SCI, and it has been used effectively by investigators who carefully

Table 37–1. VARIABLES INVOLVED IN HUMAN SPINAL CORD INJURY

Age
Sex
Level of injury
Open vs. closed injury
Completeness of the injury
Point of impact (anterior, posterior)
Force of impact
Type of force
    Flexion
    Extension
    Compression
    Distraction
    Rotation
Velocity of deformation of the spinal cord tissue
Associated bony and ligamentous damage producing vertebral column disruption and instability
Vertebral canal compromise by the presence of bony and foreign fragments
Duration of compression
Other associated injuries
Pre-existing conditions
    Vascular disease
    Hypertension
    Diabetes
    Spinal stenosis
    Rheumatoid arthritis

Table 37–2. SPINAL CORD INJURY MODELS: NONQUANTIFIABLE AND QUANTIFIABLE

		Nonquantifiable	
Study	*Year*	*Animal*	*Method*
Galen	Second century	Various	Incised the cord
Schmaus[333]	1890	Rabbit	Suspended them vertically attached to boards and struck the boards
Watson[378]	1891	Dog	Dropped them from various heights in a specially constructed apparatus
Spiller[351]	1899	Kitten	Squeezed them in a swinging door
Stcherbak[352]	1907	Rabbit	Applied a vibrating device to the cord
D'Abundo[78]	1916	Small animals	Centrifuged the animals
Marinesco[248]	1918	Dog	Used explosive forces
Ayer[16]	1919	Cat	Injected paraffin into the epidural space
Roussy et al.[320]	1920	Rabbit, guinea pig	Struck the thoracic vertebral column
McVeigh[258]	1923	Dog	Pressed the cord with a finger
Ferraro[135]	1927	Rabbit	Delivered blows to the back with an iron rod
Groat et al.[159]	1945	Cat	Suspended them vertically and struck them with a board
Fontaine et al.[141]	1954	Dog	Crushed the spinal cord with a Kocher clamp
Kajiwara[203]	1961	Rabbit	Dropped them secured in a wooden cylinder
Allen[2]	1911	Dog	Dropped a weight onto the exposed cord
Tarlov et al.[363]	1953	Dog	Inflated a hydraulic balloon in the epidural space
Croft et al.[76]	1972	Cat	Placed a static load on the exposed cord
Rivlin and Tator[310, 311]	1978	Rat	Applied an aneurysm clip to the spinal cord
Watson et al.[380]	1986	Rat	Produced a photochemical lesion with a laser
Bresnahan et al.[55]	1987	Rat	Used a weight-drop device, OSU impactor
Gruner[160]	1992	Rat	Used a weight-drop device, NYU impactor

controlled experimental variables.[55, 136, 149, 160, 276, 278, 287, 389] The latest generation of weight-drop devices produces highly reproducible injuries by incorporating computer software for monitoring the degree of cord compression and vertebral movement and provides an immediate feedback of the mechanical properties of the impact.[55, 160, 281] The most widely utilized instrument is the New York University (NYU) device, which is depicted in Figure 37–2. This model is presently being used in a multicenter trial for the development of new pharmacologic treatments in experimental SCI.[32, 33] Although a variety of other models to impact the cord have been developed, they have not been used as extensively as the weight-drop.

Balloon or cuff compression techniques have also been employed to create spinal cord lesions. This was first described in detail by Tarlov and colleagues,[363] who inserted an inflatable balloon into the spinal extradural space of dogs to produce paralysis. This technique has been applied to create spinal cord injuries in monkeys[364] and in rats.[199, 250] The disadvantages of this technique are that (1) it is difficult to verify proper balloon position in some animals, (2) the pressure on the cord itself cannot be measured, (3) the techniques are more difficult to perform in small animals (e.g., rodents), and (4) they do not closely mimic the biomechanics of the human injury. Similar effects have been obtained in static load compression models in which large weights are placed for varying times on the exposed cords of cats,[76] ferrets,[108] or rats.[41]

In 1978, Rivlin and Tator[310] introduced a rat model in which a spinal lesion was created by compressing the spinal cord with a modified Kerr-Lougheed aneurysm clip. This model offered the precise delivery of a known force, and graded injuries were produced by varying either the force or the duration of the compression.[100, 310] Unlike the weight-drop, it causes a circumferential compression of the cord, but it has been reported to produce greater hemorrhagic changes than the weight-drop injury.[200] The disadvantages of this method are that (1) it requires more manipulation of the cord, because the clip must be placed under its ventral aspect; (2) the biomechanics of the initial component of the injury do not mimic the human condition; and (3) the histopathologic and functional correlates of this injury have not been defined as extensively as in the weight-drop method.

Our laboratories have adapted laser technology to produce experimental nontraumatic spinal cord injuries.[60] In this model, spinal lesions are created by means of a photochemical reaction induced by a rose bengal–laser beam interaction. The reaction causes an acute vascular thrombosis associated with extensive tissue injury, which eventually results in cavity formation. Although this model yields reproducible lesions that can be created without performing a laminectomy, it does not share the biomechanics of the human injury and relies more on ischemic mechanisms.

The preceding observations pertain to acute traumatic spinal injury; therefore, they should not be generalized to models of other types of spinal injury, such as slow-graded cord compressions that are used to mimic tumor masses, or to models of spinal ischemia.[406] Furthermore, it must be noted that certain aspects of

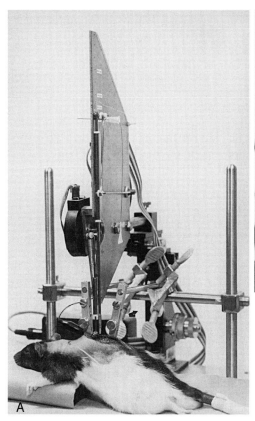

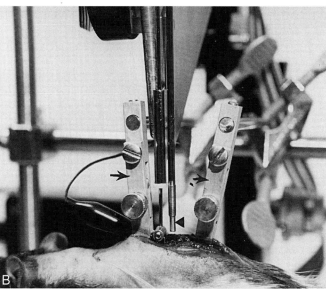

Figure 37–2. *A,* The NYU impounder (weight-drop apparatus) used to produce spinal trauma in rats. *B,* The clamps *(arrows)* are used for spinal fixation. The impounder unit *(arrowhead)* is lowered onto the dorsal surface of the cord in preparation for injury.

cord function and plasticity are often better addressed in transection or in vitro models.

PATHOPHYSIOLOGY OF THE ACUTE EXPERIMENTAL SPINAL CORD INJURY

Our basic understanding of the pathophysiology of SCI is based on studies of the evolution of the lesion in experimental models of SCI. These studies have produced evidence to support the division of the injury into primary and secondary components. The primary injury, which is clinically manifested by acute paralysis, is accompanied by shifts in electrolytes, decreases in the membrane-bound sodium-potassium adenosine triphosphatase (Na^+-K^+ ATPase), loss of energy stores, and early morphologic alterations.[23, 101, 156, 397] The secondary components of SCI consist of a series of autodestructive processes (which are activated following trauma) that promote neural dysfunction and tissue damage for hours or days following SCI.[23, 397]

Primary Mediators of Spinal Cord Injury

Electrolytes. Significant injuries of the spinal cord are accompanied by conduction block, which is a loss of neurophysiologic conduction across the lesion site.[76, 79, 111, 251, 346] This has been hypothesized to be associated with the intracellular leakage of sodium.[215] However,

Eidelberg and colleagues[111] reported large increases in the potassium concentration in superfusants obtained from spinal cords subjected to prolonged compression. Because extracellular potassium levels above 10 mM can block axonal conduction,[371] their findings suggested that axonal conduction block was caused by the rise in extracellular potassium. These findings were corroborated by two other laboratories.[358, 401] Using ion-sensitive microelectrodes, Young and colleagues recorded acute rises in extracellular potassium from a preinjury level of less than 4 mM to a postinjury mean level of 54 mM in the white matter of the lateral columns.[401] Furthermore, they found that evoked potentials, which disappeared immediately after injury, returned as the extracellular potassium levels fell below 15 mM. Following the return of extracellular potassium levels toward normal, there were no further potassium increases, even though white matter blood flow decreased to significant levels. A decrease in total tissue potassium occurs at the lesion site within one hour of injury.[400]

The failure of calcium homeostasis is also associated with acute SCI. Calcium has an integral role in the regulation of sodium and potassium conductance during neuronal excitation, in the regulation of critical enzymes such as protein kinase C, in the modulation of the neuronal cytoskeleton, and in the storage and release of neurotransmitters at synaptic junctions.[1, 144, 191, 210, 245] Normal intracellular calcium concentrations are a thousand-fold less than extracellular concentrations (<1 μM compared with > 1 mM), and normal neuronal function depends on the maintenance of this gradient.[19] The extracellular calcium concentration in injured spinal cords falls within a few minutes from levels of 1.2 mM to levels of about 0.01 mM, which implies a brisk and significant movement of calcium into the intracellular compartment.[358, 398, 403] Therefore, the intracellular accumulation of calcium has been implicated in the mediation of secondary injury.

Metabolites. Numerous studies have documented marked metabolic alterations following experimental spinal trauma. Rawe and colleagues[300] described increases in both gray and white matter glucose utilization for up to one hour after moderate traumatic spinal injuries in dogs. Following this initial increase, gray matter glucose utilization progressively decreased and remained low from three to eight hours after injury, whereas white matter glucose utilization returned toward baseline. Severe traumatic injuries caused similar transient increases in white matter glucose utilization and a subsequent progressive deterioration to levels below baseline from four to eight hours after injury. Gray matter glucose utilization also progressively decreased after the initial trauma in severe injuries. The transient increase in glucose utilization was hypothesized to be secondary to the continued delivery of substrate in the face of ischemia and an enhancement in anaerobic glycolysis.

A rapid decline in tissue pO_2 has also been documented to occur in both the gray and white matter of the spinal cord as early as 15 minutes following trauma.[358, 359] Decreases in tissue oxygen tension are not unexpected in view of the reduction in spinal cord blood flow (SCBF) that occurs in spinal trauma. The decrease in tissue oxygen tension has been reported to last for several hours following injury, indicating that tissue hypoxia is a major factor in SCI.[106, 175, 207, 208] Studies of energy metabolism in SCI have shown that a rapid and marked depletion of high-energy phosphates (adenosine triphosphate and phosphocreatinine) occurs following injury.[9, 201, 375, 376] This is associated with spinal cord tissue lactic acidosis and oxidative shifts of NAD:NADH ratios.[9, 201, 238, 313, 375, 376, 394] Marked reductions in the specific activity of Na^+-K^+ ATPase, a critical membrane-bound enzyme, have been reported to occur as early as five minutes after injury.[71]

Morphology. Within minutes of spinal injury, a variety of morphologic changes become evident. These consist of petechial hemorrhages in the gray matter, small ruptures in the walls of the muscular venules, increases in the size of the extracellular spaces in the gray and white matter, attenuation of the myelin sheaths, enlarged periaxonal spaces, tubulovesicular invaginations into the axoplasm, and disruption of the axoplasm.[3, 20, 21, 96, 97, 104] By one hour after SCI, changes characteristic of central chromatolysis and ischemia begin to appear in the anterior ventral horn cells.[372] By four hours after injury, the hemorrhagic changes progress centrifugally and coalesce to form an area of hemorrhagic necrosis that extends along the longitudinal axis of the cord in a spindle-shaped form.[20, 101, 104, 258] The acute damage is located more centrally, and depending on the severity of the injury, it may progress to involve the adjacent white matter.[104, 156] Although minor white matter changes have been identified at the ultrastructural level as early as 15 minutes after injury,[97] progressive edema is eventually manifested at the level of light microscopy as spongiform changes. These are secondary to axonal fragmentation and axonal and periaxonal swelling.[21] The axonal enlargements contain multiple organelles (mitochondria, neurofilaments, lysosomes, and smooth endoplasmic reticulum), which Bresnahan and colleagues attributed to the occurrence of axoplasmic stasis.[21, 54, 56] Increases in beta-amyloid precursor protein can be detected in damaged axons at four hours after injury and appear to be related to the degree of injury.[234] Changes in the white matter begin in the areas adjacent to the gray matter and spread outward in a centrifugal fashion.[54, 56] Frank demyelination in the dorsal columns has been observed as early as 21 hours after injury.[152] Initially, an acute cellular infiltration by polymorphonuclear leukocytes occurs, and it is replaced by an invasion of macrophages within days of the injury.[44, 259] By the end of first week after injury, cystic degeneration of the necrotic areas begins to become evident, particularly in animals that receive more severe injuries.[104] At four weeks, the cyst is better defined, and the surviving white matter displays demyelination and microcysts.[276, 373] At four months, the cyst is surrounded by astrocytic gliosis, and the region of injury shows thickening of the dura matter. An increased cellularity of the leptomeninges is apparent, especially in the more severe injuries.[373] An example of the histologic evolution of the lesions is shown in Figure 37–1.

Secondary Mediators of Spinal Cord Injury

The progressive nature of the morphologic changes that occur following spinal trauma suggests that damage to the spinal cord evolves over time.[20, 104, 156] This evidence, by itself, is insufficient to prove the existence of secondary injury processes, because cells within the lesion may lose vitality in spite of their initial normal appearance. A period of time may be required before the tissue displays the histologic manifestations of cell death. Additional data from SCI studies, however, support the existence of secondary injury processes that promote further tissue destruction. The onset of significant decreases in white matter blood flow is delayed until one to four hours following severe SCI,[169, 175, 176, 239, 338, 399] and evoked potentials, which transiently recover after acute SCI in some animals, disappear again hours or days later.[105, 138, 402] Treatment of the acute phase of SCI (e.g., with steroids, naloxone, excitatory amino acid antagonists) directed against these secondary processes has been successful, which suggests that the deleterious effects of these processes can be ameliorated.[35, 40, 118–121, 127, 138, 154, 166, 167, 260, 387, 399] The existence of secondary processes in human SCI has been speculative, because the progressive deterioration of neurologic deficits following SCI in humans is uncommon.[249, 290] Until recently, the application of these findings to the human condition remained a significant question. However, the beneficial effects of steroids in certain types of human spinal cord injuries reported in the second cooperative study demonstrate that these treatments can be effective in the human condition.[48]

Ischemia. Because alterations in the spinal cord vasculature have been evident in the histopathology of SCI,[13, 20, 99] numerous investigations have focused on the role of spinal ischemia in the pathogenesis of traumatic SCI.[326] Several lines of evidence support a role for ischemia in experimental SCI. First, the deprivation of oxygen causes a shift to anaerobic metabolism, and significant elevations in the level of lactate have been documented following SCI.[238] Second, spinal cord ischemia models produce pathologic changes comparable to those produced by spinal trauma.[145, 406] Third, the degree of posttraumatic hypoperfusion correlates with changes in evoked potentials recorded from the spinal cord.[133] Last, tissue oxygen content decreases significantly after trauma.[106, 175, 207, 208]

Unfortunately, results from studies of posttraumatic spinal ischemia are not all in agreement. Their differences are probably due to the various experimental conditions used by each laboratory, such as the animal species and the injury model used, the severity of injury produced, the method chosen to measure SCBF, the anesthetic utilized, and changes in systemic blood pressure. The normal spinal cord autoregulates blood flow within the same arterial pressure range (approximately 50 to 130 mm Hg) as the brain.[181, 217, 247] Systemic blood pressure is important, because the autoregulation of SCBF is impaired following SCI.[339, 348]

Earlier techniques for measuring SCBF relied on qualitative methods. Examples of these are the description of changes in the vessels of the cord recorded under direct visualization,[102] or the outlining of spinal blood vessels via fluorescent tracers or microangiographic techniques.[98, 129, 146] The first quantitative techniques relied on the clearance of inert gases such as xenon or argon.[105, 106] These methods were invasive and offered poor resolution between the white and gray

matter. The current methods used, which are shown in Table 37–3, are adaptations of techniques that were initially utilized to measure cerebral blood flow. They offer a better degree of resolution and accuracy. The relative value of each technique varies according to the questions each particular study is attempting to answer and according to the model employed. For example, although C^{14} iodoantipyrine offers the best resolution, it allows only one measurement from each animal and requires that the animal be sacrificed. The technique of H^2 clearance allows multiple measurements over time and offers an adequate degree of resolution in large animals (monkeys, cats), but it is more invasive and offers a lesser degree of resolution in small animals (rats) because of the smaller size of their spinal cords. Laser Doppler flowmetry is a more recent innovation that allows continuous on-line measurement of SCBF, but it is limited to reporting relative changes in SCBF instead of absolute values.

Although not all studies of posttraumatic SCBF agree in their results (Table 37–4), the occurrence of posttraumatic hypoperfusion of the gray matter has been a consistent finding. Many investigators have concentrated on studying the changes in white matter SCBF following SCI, because this area contains the critical fibers for controlling function below the level of the lesion and is the last to undergo histologic changes. In addition, the detrimental effect of ischemia on the white matter is suggested in models of spinal cord contusion in which evoked potentials transiently recover but are subsequently lost concomitantly with the onset of white matter hypoperfusion.[169, 239, 338, 399] However, reports of posttraumatic white matter blood flow have conflicted, with both hyperemia and ischemia being reported by different investigators (see Table 37–4). Even in studies disclosing posttraumatic white matter hypoperfusion, it must be emphasized that ischemic levels for the spinal cord white matter have not been defined. In fact, several experiments suggest that the spinal cord white matter is rather resistant to the effects of ischemia or hypoxia.[150, 219, 220]

The origin of the delayed white matter hypoperfusion is unclear. Osterholm and Mathews[284, 285] proposed that an alteration in catecholamines (norepinephrine in particular) occurred with SCI and caused vasoconstriction. Unfortunately, their findings could not be sub-

Table 37–3. METHODS USED TO MEASURE SPINAL CORD BLOOD FLOW

Method	Invasive	Multiple Measurements	Resolution
Radiolabeled microspheres*	No	Yes	Poor
H^2 clearance†	Yes	Yes	Fair
C^{14} iodoantipyrine‡	No	No	Good
Laser Doppler flowmetry§	No	Yes	Fair

*References 180, 348.
†References 14, 175, 216.
‡References 38, 303.
§References 236, 356.

Table 37–4. POSTTRAUMATIC ALTERATIONS IN SPINAL CORD BLOOD FLOW

Study	Year	Animal	Model	Technique	Severity	Spinal Cord Blood Flow		
						Time	*Gray*	*White*
Bingham et al.[39]	1975	Monkey	Weight drop	C¹⁴ iodo.	Moderate	5′	↓	—
						15′	—	↑↑
						1°	↓↓	—
						2–4°	↓↓	↑
Kobrine et al.[218]*	1975	Monkey	Weight drop	H² w.o.	Severe	1°	↓	↑↑
						4°	↓↓	↑
						8–24°		—
Sandler and Tator[326]	1976	Monkey	Cuff compression	C¹⁴ iodo.	Moderate	15′	↓↓	↓↓
						1–6°	↓	↓
						24°	↓	↑
					Severe	2°	↓↓↓	↓↓↓
						24°	↓↓↓	↓↓↓
Ducker et al.[106]†	1978	Dog	Weight drop	Xe w.o.	Severe	1°		
						1–3°	↓↓	
Rivlin and Tator[311]	1978	Rat	Clip compression	C¹⁴ iodo.	Severe	15′	↓↓↓	↓↓
						2°	↓↓↓	↓↓
						24		
Senter and Venes[338]‡	1978	Cat	Weight drop	H² w.o.	Severe	<1°		—
						1–6°		↓
Lohse et al.[239]	1980	Cat	Weight drop	H² w.o.	Mild	1–6°		—
					Moderate	1–6°		↑
Cawthon et al.[66]§	1980	Cat	Weight drop	C¹⁴ iodo.	Severe	1°		—
				H² w.o.		2–6°		↓
Young et al.[401]	1982	Cat	Weight drop	H² w.o.	Severe	30′–1°		—
						2–3°		↓
Hall and Wolf[169]	1987	Cat	Weight drop	H² w.o.	Moderate	<30′		↑
						30′–4°		
					Severe	30′		↓
						2–4°		↓↓

C¹⁴ iodo., C¹⁴ iodoantipyrine; H² w.o., H² washout (clearance); Xe w.o., xenon washout.
—, no significant change from baseline; ↓, mild decrease; ↓ ↓, moderate decrease; ↓ ↓ ↓, marked decrease; ↑, mild increase; ↑ ↑, moderate increase; ↑ ↑ ↑, marked increase.
*the reported gray matter blood flows were low, which suggests they also reflect white matter flow.
†flow was measured at the center of the cord, but the low values suggest it also reflects white matter flow.
‡some animals had hyperemic values at <1°.
§some animals had hyperemic values at 1°.

stantiated by other investigators.[4, 39, 59, 82, 134, 178, 301, 302] Changes in the levels of other transmitters, including dopamine and serotonin, have been investigated, but the results are inconsistent.[39, 57, 82, 178, 271, 284, 302, 407] Thus, the etiology of the hypoperfusion in SCI remains unclear, but the actions of other vasoactive transmitters or peptides can not be excluded. It is clear that the bulk of the data supports the theory that posttraumatic spinal ischemia is more than just an epiphenomenon; however, its precise contribution to the neurologic deficits and to the resultant pathologic changes remains to be elucidated.

Edema. Traumatic injuries of the brain and spinal cord produce a disruption of the blood-brain barrier or, in the case of the spinal cord, the blood–spinal cord barrier, thereby impairing the selective permeability of the normal endothelium of the central nervous system. Damage to the endothelium promotes the formation of vasogenic edema, which is the accumulation of plasma-like fluid rich in protein in the extravascular space.[211] Although cytotoxic edema (cellular edema) has not been emphasized in SCI, it is commonly seen in central nervous system ischemia, and it is reasonable to suspect that it also occurs in SCI in view of the associated reductions in SCBF. It has been theorized that the formation of edema in SCI is detrimental because it leads to compression of neural tissues and maintains an abnormal electrolyte environment.[23] The temporal association of the onset of white matter edema with the onset of white matter hypoperfusion has implicated edema in the promotion of secondary tissue injury. Although the presence of edema in SCI had been identified histologically,[3, 13, 157] the details of its formation were delineated later with the use of fluorescent tracers such as albumin conjugated to Evans blue or fluorescein. These conjugated complexes are excluded by the normal blood-brain barrier and can be detected in the extravascular space following alterations in blood-brain barrier function. In addition, more detailed analysis can now be performed using quantitative autoradiography with vascular tracers such as C¹⁴-aminobutyric acid.[294]

Immediately following SCI, edema is confined to the central portions of the cord, after which it progressively spreads into the white matter in a centrifugal fashion.[156, 158, 274] The severity of spinal injury has correlated with the longitudinal extension of the edema.[374] In acute studies, edema is maximized at six to eight hours after injury, but significant increases in spinal cord tissue water occurring at three to five days after injury have been reported.[294, 395] In support of this finding, Nemecek and colleagues[274] described the existence of a secondary type of edema in SCI, which had the characteristics of a plasma ultrafiltrate, appeared more gradually, and outlasted vasogenic edema.

Several processes have been proposed to explain the pathogenesis of posttraumatic edema, including capillary leakage secondary to loosening of the endothelial cell tight junctions[360] and an increase in vesicular transport across the endothelium.[34, 182] However, the occurrence of these specific derangements has not been fully studied in experimental traumatic SCI.

Calcium. Besides its critical role in the regulation of normal neuronal function, calcium has an equally important role in the mediation of cell injury and cell death.[70, 131, 329] Calcium overload was first suggested as a mechanism of cellular injury in liver cells.[257] This finding was corroborated by Schanne and colleagues,[329] who described the viability of hepatocytes after exposure to several membrane toxins in the absence of extracellular calcium. An even more interesting phenomenon, the calcium paradox, was noted in studies of heart tissue by Zimmerman and colleagues.[404, 405] In a series of experiments, it was demonstrated that perfusion of isolated rat hearts with a calcium-free medium produced electromechanical dissociation without significant morphologic changes. However, the introduction of calcium into the medium produced substantial intracellular calcium influx, cellular contracture, and death.

The initial observation of calcium's potential involvement in SCI was made by Balentine in 1977, who described the occurrence of selective intra-axonal calcification in SCI in rats.[21, 26] He noted that the accumulation of calcium occurred as early as 30 minutes after trauma and became more profuse in the late necrotic phases of the injury. Similar findings have been reported in injured spinal cords of monkeys, cats, and humans.[22] Several observations support the role of calcium in spinal cord injury: (1) the extracellular calcium concentration in the injured cord rapidly decreases;[358, 398, 403] (2) total calcium concentration in the injured spinal cord segment becomes significantly elevated at 45 minutes, maximizes at eight hours, and remains elevated for at least one week after injury;[173] (3) morphologic alterations and behavioral deficits similar to those seen following spinal cord trauma have been produced by dripping calcium chloride onto the exposed spinal cord;[24, 25] and (4) increased concentrations of calcium have been shown to produce alterations in the peripheral nervous system that are similar to those seen in experimental SCI.[330–332] Since calcium has also been implicated as a mediator of cellular death in central nervous system hypoxic-ischemic injury, posttraumatic spinal cord ischemia is likely to potentiate the role of calcium in SCI.[88, 342]

Potential mechanisms for calcium accumulation in the injured spinal cord tissue are (1) leakage through the damaged membrane, the voltage-dependent calcium channels, or the excitatory amino acid N-methyl-D-aspartate (NMDA) receptor channels; (2) failure of Ca^{2+}-ATPase mediated calcium extrusion; and (3) release of calcium from intracellular organelles, i.e., endoplasmic reticulum and mitochondria, which normally bind cytosolic calcium.[70]

Excess intracellular calcium produces deleterious effects on cellular function and may culminate in cellular death. An increase in free cytosolic calcium disrupts the normal regulation of the function of calcium-dependent protease and nucleases. The activation of calcium-dependent protease can lead to the degradation of neurofilament and myelin proteins.[28, 29] Increases in both the activity and the immunoreactivity of calpain (calcium-activated neural proteinase) have been documented in the rat spinal cord following trauma.[27, 235] In addition, elevations in the levels of calcium adversely affect mitochondrial performance, which results in a decrease in energy production.[231] Activation of the calcium-dependent phospholipase enzymes, phospholipase C and phospholipase A_2, also occurs with elevations of intracellular calcium. The activation of these phospholipases results in the breakdown of cellular membranes and the production of arachidonate by phospholipase A_2.[299] The metabolism of arachidonate yields thromboxanes, leukotrienes, and free radicals, which promote tissue injury via their effects on the vasculature and the inflammatory response (see later).

Free Radicals. Free radicals are molecules with an unusual reactivity secondary to the presence of unpaired electrons in their outer orbitals. A peculiar aspect of this reactivity is their ability to propagate via chain reactions.[83] The involvement of fatty acids in oxygen free radical chain reactions is known as lipid peroxidation. The phospholipid and cholesterol components of biologic membranes are very susceptible to damage by free radical reactions.[85] The normal cellular metabolic pathways for oxygen reduction generate oxygen free radicals: superoxide anion (O^-_2), hydroxyl radical OH, and hydrogen peroxide (H_2O_2). In the normal state, cells control the harmful effects of free radical production with a number of naturally occurring antioxidant compounds (Table 37–5). For example, superoxide dismutases scavenge the superoxide anion by catalyzing its conversion into hydrogen peroxide and

Table 37–5. NATURALLY OCCURRING ANTIOXIDANTS

Superoxide dismutases
Catalases
Glutathione peroxidase
Ascorbic acid
Alpha-tocopherol
Steroids
Cysteine
Selenium

oxygen, and catalases reduce hydrogen peroxide to water. Pathologic states that cause the generation of excess free radicals can lead to lipid peroxidation and result in the fragmentation of cellular membranes.

The generation of free radicals and their deleterious actions have been implicated in the pathophysiology of central nervous system ischemia,[85, 379, 396] as well as of brain and spinal cord trauma.[30, 85] Findings in acute SCI that support the role of free radical lipid peroxidation are (1) increases in peroxidized polyunsaturated fatty acid breakdown products,[229, 264] (2) decreases in cholesterol in conjunction with the appearance of cholesterol oxidation products,[10, 86] (3) the activation of guanylate cyclase and the corresponding increase in cyclic guanosine monophosphate (cGMP),[168, 229] (4) decreases in tissue antioxidants such as alpha-tocopherol and ascorbic acid,[292, 328] (5) inhibition of the phospholipid-dependent membrane-bound $Na^+ - K^+$ ATPase,[71] (6) increases in lipid peroxidation products,[30] and (7) the efficacy of antioxidants in the treatment of experimental SCI.[6, 10, 167]

There are a number of potential sources for the formation of oxygen radicals following SCI. As in models of cerebral ischemia, spinal trauma and posttraumatic ischemia deplete ATP and produce an accumulation of adenosine monophosphate (AMP), which is degraded to hypoxanthine.[212] During ischemia, xanthine dehydrogenase converts to its oxidase form and, in the presence of hypoxanthine, catalyzes the formation of O_2^-.[256] Coenzyme Q, an important component of the electron transport chain, also produces oxygen free radicals in the setting of ischemia.[85] In addition, both trauma and ischemia cause increases in arachidonic acid, and arachidonate's metabolism in the cyclooxygenase pathway generates superoxide radicals.[269] This effect is probably enhanced by the calcium-mediated activation of phospholipase A_2 that occurs following injury. Other possible sources of oxygen free radicals are the respiratory burst of invading neutrophils[255] and the auto-oxidation of catecholamines.[266] The hemorrhagic nature of acute SCI contributes hemoglobin, which itself can stimulate lipid peroxidation or provide a source of iron to catalyze oxygen radical and lipid peroxidation reactions.[7, 15, 323] Besides injury to cellular membranes by lipid peroxidation, free radicals have also been documented to disrupt lysosomal membranes,[140] promote tissue edema,[67, 68] and inhibit mitochondrial function.[85]

Endogenous Opiates. Based on the observation that the opioid antagonist naloxone reversed the hypotension produced by cervical spinal cord transection,[185] it was hypothesized that naloxone could ameliorate SCI by raising arterial pressure and thereby improving SCBF. Indeed naloxone was found to be beneficial in the treatment of experimental SCI.[118, 399] It also improved posttraumatic SCBF, but this was independent of its effect on systemic blood pressure.[399] These data and the findings of large elevations in plasma β-endorphin (an endogenous opiate) after SCI suggested the possibility of endogenous opiate involvement in SCI.[121]

Three principal types of opioid receptors have been identified: the mu, the delta, and the kappa receptors.[289] Although naloxone is more selective for the mu receptor, the high doses used to treat SCI make it active at all three receptors.[241] The work of Faden and colleagues suggests that the endogenous opioid dynorphin A (1–17), the ligand for the kappa opioid receptor, is the opioid most likely to be involved in SCI.[113] Dynorphin immunoreactivity selectively increases following SCI, and the increase correlates with the severity of injury.[125] Preprodynorphin messenger RNA is elevated after SCI,[393] and significant time-dependent increases in kappa opioid receptor binding have also been documented following spinal trauma.[226] Furthermore, opiate antagonists that are more selective for the kappa receptor have been increasingly effective in the treatment of experimental SCI and ischemia.[116, 126, 128] Dynorphin is unique among the endogenous opioids, because it is the only one that produces hindlimb paralysis in the rat following intrathecal injection in the lumbar subarachnoid space.[115, 242, 298] However, dynorphin-induced hindlimb paralysis appears to be in part a nonopiate effect, as it is not reversible by either naloxone or other more specific kappa antagonists.[243, 357] Dynorphin-induced paralysis is associated with marked reductions in SCBF, and this may in part explain its paralytic actions.[240, 244] Unlike the paralysis produced by traumatic injury, dynorphin-induced paralysis is not affected by pretreatment with thyrotropin-releasing hormone.[253] Although the evidence collected to date suggests that dynorphin A may participate in the secondary mechanisms of SCI, the precise role of endogenous opioids and their receptors need further elucidation.

Excitatory Amino Acids. In 1969, Olney[282] introduced the term "excitotoxicity" to describe the neurotoxic effects of systemically administered glutamate on the endocrine hypothalamus. Excitotoxic effects consist of the mediation of neuronal injury via the actions of the excitatory amino acid transmitters glutamate and aspartate at their receptors. Extensive evidence has now accumulated to implicate excitotoxicity in the pathophysiology of central nervous system hypoxic-ischemia[319] and of brain and spinal trauma.[114, 127, 387, 390, 391]

There are three well-characterized excitatory amino acid receptors: the NMDA receptors and the non-NMDA receptors kainate and quisqualate. Although glutamate is an agonist at all three receptors, most experimental evidence implicates glutamate's actions at the NMDA receptor complex as the major component of excitotoxicity in central nervous system trauma and ischemia.[318, 343] Several observations support the role of excitatory amino acid toxicity in SCI: (1) significant spinal ischemia occurs following spinal trauma, and excitotoxicity has been shown to occur in other models of central nervous system ischemia; (2) the concentrations of excitatory amino acids are elevated after spinal trauma;[288] and (3) treatment of experimental spinal cord injury and ischemia with excitatory amino acid receptor antagonists has been effective in improving outcome.[126, 221, 244, 254]

Eicosanoids.   Several investigators have invoked a role for the eicosanoids (thromboxane, leukotrienes) in SCI. In accordance with this, elevated levels of thromboxane, which stimulates platelet aggregation and vasoconstriction, have been reported in SCI.[84, 190, 269] The interaction of calcium, phospholipases, arachidonic acid production, and lipid peroxidation contributes significantly to the increases in thromboxane. Leukotrienes, which are potent mediators of inflammation, have been reported to either increase or remain unchanged after SCI.[84, 268]

Inflammation.   SCI is associated with an inflammatory component that involves the ingress of inflammatory cells and the release of their products. An early infiltration by polymorphonuclear leukocytes, which appear to be involved in neuronophagia acutely after spinal injury, has been documented in SCI.[107, 259] In addition to this effect, polymorphonuclear leukocytes can contribute to the injury, because their respiratory burst can serve as a source of free radicals.[255] In 1985, Blight[44] documented the infiltration of the cat spinal lesion by macrophages, and he raised a possible role for the macrophage in the demyelination that occurs following SCI. Blight[44a] also showed that decreasing the macrophage component of the inflammatory response increases the number of myelinated axons and retards the onset of secondary loss of function in a guinea pig model of SCI. Activated macrophages can serve as a potential source of quinolinic acid, an excitotoxin.[45, 295] Recent evidence has also implicated tumor necrosis factor (TNF), a cytokine that can mediate inflammatory responses, in the pathophysiology of secondary injury processes. Increases in the levels of both TNF and its messenger RNA have been observed following SCI.[377, 393] This cytokine stimulates the proliferation and hypertrophy of astrocytes, which can lead to the formation of glial scarring,[336] enhances endothelial cell permeability, which contributes to blood-brain barrier breakdown,[367] and has cytotoxic activity against oligodendrocytes.[337] Its precise role is equivocal, because it

may also enhance repair and regeneration by promoting angiogenesis and inducing growth factors.[130, 148]

THERAPEUTIC APPROACHES TO ACUTE EXPERIMENTAL SPINAL CORD INJURY

In order to develop novel therapies for the treatment of SCI, it is useful to relate the different possible approaches to the timing of the different events in SCI. An example of such a scheme is illustrated in Figure 37–3. Although advances in preventive measures and clinical management have had a significant impact in SCI, it is in the areas of pharmacotherapy and regeneration that most future gains lie. The majority of these advances will rely on data obtained from well-designed laboratory studies in SCI. In order to interpret therapeutic studies of SCI, however, one must critically evaluate the injury model, the animal species, the anesthetic, the drug regimen, and the methods used to measure the outcome. Although the weight-drop technique remains the most popular model in experimental SCI, it is often performed under different conditions by each laboratory. This must be taken into account when comparing results from different investigators. A major effort was recently undertaken to develop and utilize a standardized model of the weight apparatus to create spinal injuries in rats.[32, 160] Different laboratories also employ various parameters to evaluate outcome in SCI studies, such as motor and sensory function, evoked potentials, SCBF, degree of edema, and histopathologic changes. To measure neurologic or behavioral outcome, the two most commonly used tests are the modified Tarlov scale and the inclined plane. The Tarlov scale consists of the subjective assignment of scores to the performance of a motor task, usually walking.[362] Although a number of variations of the Tarlov score have been used, a fairly reliable and reproducible scoring system has been developed and is being extensively utilized in a rat SCI multicenter therapeutic trial.[31, 33] The inclined plane is another widely used method that grades motor function by assessing a rat's ability to hold its position on a surface whose slope is progressively increased.[309]

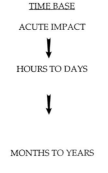

Figure 37–3.   Approaches to the treatment of spinal cord injury.

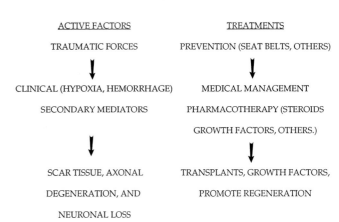

An equally important consideration in the recovery of function following SCI is the anatomic and physiologic basis for recovery. A therapeutic modality may improve the return of function after SCI by limiting tissue death, enhancing neurophysiologic function, or enhancing the regenerative capacities of the cord. Unfortunately, most studies on the therapy of experimental SCI do not include detailed morphologic analyses, because these are time consuming and labor intensive. Therefore, our present understanding of the anatomic requirements for the preservation of locomotive capacity in animals is sparse. Experimental data from studies done in cats suggest that as little as 10 per cent of the white matter will permit locomotion.[42, 109, 110, 382] Blight[42] found that after SCI in the cat, there was a preferential loss of the large-diameter axons that were located toward the center of the lesion. He also showed that for the surviving axons, conduction across the spinal lesion was absent or abnormal.[43] His findings support the role of demyelination in the pathophysiology of SCI. A good understanding of the basis for recovery of function in SCI requires a more precise elucidation of the pathways responsible for different spinal cord functions and of the time course and extent of demyelination produced by these injuries.

The first therapeutic interventions employed in experimental SCI were not pharmacologic. When describing the weight-drop technique in dogs, Allen[2, 3] also reported the beneficial effects of myelotomies. The second major intervention developed was the application of hypothermia. This evolved from the observation that hypothermia decreased cerebral metabolic demand and reduced brain volume.[261, 314] The beneficial effects of hypothermia include (1) reducing central nervous system metabolic activity and the cerebral metabolic rate for oxygen,[162, 163, 315] (2) markedly decreasing the rate of ATP loss,[224, 263] and (3) protecting against the loss of phosphocreatinine and the accumulation of lactate and NADH following hypoxia.[163, 262] Other beneficial actions of spinal cord cooling include the attenuation of edema and hemorrhage formation that occurs in SCI[155] and the possible dialyzation of toxins by opening the dura and perfusing with solutions. Furthermore, in models of central nervous system ischemia, hypothermia reduces the release of neurotransmitters, such as glutamate, which can mediate secondary injury processes.[61] Although initial results of the application of hypothermia to SCI were positive,[5] subsequent studies were unfavorable, and this technique has been technically difficult to implement in humans.[40, 155, 189, 252] Interest in hypothermia has been rekindled by the findings of Busto and colleagues,[61–63] who showed the protective effects of mild hypothermia in certain models of rodent brain ischemia. Studies in which brain temperature was monitored showed that a drastic lowering of central nervous system temperature was unnecessary to lessen the degree of tissue damage occurring after brain ischemic injury. Modest temperature changes (1 to 3°C) in models of brain ischemia critically alter the extent of neuronal injury and blood-brain barrier alterations.[62, 91–93]

Because brain temperature can be easily manipulated with local cooling, mild hypothermia has been successfully applied in animal models of traumatic brain injury.[73, 90] Pilot studies using mild systemic hypothermia in human traumatic brain injuries have produced encouraging results.[72, 340] Based on this, prospective clinical trials continue to be organized. Similar applications for the treatment of SCI are still under consideration.

Monoamines Antagonists. Although the monoamine theory of SCI proposed by Osterholm and Mathews[284, 285] could not be confirmed, it kindled interest in the biochemical changes associated with SCI and in identifying therapies that intervened against the actions of these processes. Attempts at treating experimental SCI with catecholamine blockade using substances such as α-methyltyrosine, phenoxybenzamine, clonidine, and mianserin have produced mixed results or results that were difficult to interpret secondary to methodologic difficulties.[179, 189, 272, 285, 324, 327]

Steroids. The treatment of both experimental and human SCI with steroids was initially based on their anti-inflammatory actions and their effectiveness in treating cerebral edema.[137, 177] Results from studies of the treatment of experimental SCI with steroids are presented in Table 37–6. This table includes only studies that assessed some form of functional outcome, such as the neurologic status of the animal, and the majority show a beneficial effect. It is difficult to draw detailed conclusions, however, because of the many differences in methodology and treatment protocols. For example, some investigators combined other drugs with steroids; others used steroids in conjunction with different surgical modalities.[103, 321] Moreover, the steroid preparation and the doses used by the different laboratories were dissimilar. The use of either dexamethasone or methylprednisolone is an important variable, because methylprednisolone is a stronger inhibitor of lipid peroxidation.[49] Recent studies showing that high doses of methylprednisolone (30 mg/kg) were necessary to improve neurologic recovery following SCI led to its incorporation in the second human SCI cooperative study.[48]

Several mechanisms have been proposed to explain the beneficial effects of steroids in SCI.[167] Although steroids may not necessarily affect posttraumatic edema, they have been documented to prevent the loss of potassium from the injured cord tissue and facilitate extracellular calcium ionic recovery[233, 398]; ameliorate posttraumatic spinal cord hypoperfusion[8, 170, 398]; enhance the postinjury activity of neuronal Na^+-K^+ ATPase;[51] enhance the excitability of the central nervous system, including the motor neuron;[51, 165, 385] inhibit lipid peroxidation;[51, 166] and reduce the release of excitatory amino acids.[237] The effect on lipid peroxidation is perhaps the most significant beneficial action of steroids in SCI. To capitalize on this finding, the 21-aminosteroids, a new class of steroidal compounds, have been developed.[50, 194] These compounds, such as

Table 37–6. EFFECTS OF STEROIDS IN EXPERIMENTAL SPINAL CORD INJURY

Study	Year	Animal	Model	End Point	Drug	Results
Ducker and Hamit[103]	1969	Dog	WD	BEH	DEX and MP	+ *
Black and Markowitz[40]	1971	Monkey	WD	BEH	DEX	+ †
Campbell et al.[65]	1973	Cat	WD	BEH	MP	+ ‡
Hedeman and Sil[179]	1974	Dog	WD	BEH	MP	−
Hansebout et al.[172]	1975	Dog	BAL	BEH	DEX	+
de la Torre et al.[81]	1975	Dog	WD	BEH	DEX	+
Eidelberg et al.[108]	1976	Ferret	SL	BEH	DEX	−
				HISTO		+
Green et al.[154]	1980	Monkey	WD	BEH	MP and DEX	+
Means et al.[260]	1981	Cat	SL	BEH, HISTO	MP	+
Rucker et al.[321]	1981	Dog	WD	BEH	DEX	− §
Young and Flamm[398]	1982	Cat	WD	SCBF, SEP	MP	+
Faden et al.[122]	1984	Cat	WD	BEH, HISTO	MP and DEX	−
Braughler et al.[51a]	1987	Cat	SL	BEH	MP	+
				HISTO		?

WD, weight drop; SL, static load compression; BAL, balloon compression; BEH, behavioral (neurologic) scores of function; HISTO, histopathologic analysis; SCBF, spinal cord blood flow; SEP, somatosensory evoked potentials; MP, methylprednisolone; DEX, dexamethasone.
* Some animals were treated with intrathecal steroids.
† Some animals were subjected to different surgical therapeutic modalities.
‡ Used a myelotomy or dural decompression in addition to steroids.
§ Animals subjected to multiple drugs and surgical treatments.

tirilazad, are potent inhibitors of lipid peroxidation, lack glucocorticoid activity, and have already shown efficacy in the treatment of experimental brain and spinal trauma.[6, 171] In fact, tirilazad has been incorporated into the third national human SCI multicenter trial.

Opiate Antagonists. Based on the initial observation that naloxone reversed spinal shock, it was also used successfully in the treatment of experimental SCI. Following these early reports, a series of studies confirming the beneficial action of naloxone in SCI ensued (Table 37–7). Although earlier investigations reported positive results, more recent ones have been negative. As with steroids, the methodology, the therapeutic regime, and the models varied with each study, and this must be taken into consideration when interpreting differences in results.

Besides its actions at opiate receptors, naloxone has also been demonstrated to (1) reverse posttraumatic calcium and ascorbic acid derangements,[291, 358] (2) inhibit neutrophil superoxide release and iron-catalyzed lysosomal lipid peroxidation,[223, 344] and (3) inhibit proteolysis and stabilize lysosomal membranes.[77] The evidence gathered to date has implicated the endogenous opioid dynorphin A in the pathophysiology of SCI, and more selective kappa opiate receptor (the receptor for dynorphin A) antagonists have been developed and used successfully in the treatment of experimental SCI.[126, 128] The recent cooperative study of the use of naloxone or steroid for the treatment of human SCI did not show naloxone to be beneficial,[48] but antagonists more selective for the kappa receptor may be efficacious.

Thyrotropin-releasing hormone (TRH), like naloxone, was shown to be beneficial in models of circulatory shock and spinal injury.[119, 184] In fact, subsequent experiments by the same investigators showed that TRH was more effective than naloxone.[124] Since the major limitation of this peptide is its short half-life,

Table 37–7. EFFECTS OF NALOXONE IN EXPERIMENTAL SPINAL CORD INJURY

Study	Year	Animal	Model	End Point	Results
Faden et al.[118]	1981	Cat	WD	BEH	+
Young et al.[399]	1981	Cat	WD	SCBF, SEP	+
Faden et al.[121]	1981	Cat	WD	SCBF, SEP	+
Faden et al.[120]	1982	Cat	WD	BEH	+
Flamm et al.[138]	1982	Cat	WD	BEH, SEP	+ *
Wallace and Tator[376a]	1986	Rat	CLIP	BEH	−
Black et al.[41]	1986	Rat	SL	BEH, HISTO	−
Haghighi et al.[163a]	1987	Cat	WD	SEP	−

WD, weight drop; SL, static load compression; CLIP, clip compression; BEH, behavioral (neurologic) scores of function; HISTO, histopathologic analysis; SEP, somatosensory evoked potentials.
* Low doses (1 mg/kg) showed no effect; high doses (10 mg/kg) were effective.

more stable analogues have been synthesized and used with positive results in experimental SCI.[35, 36, 112, 117] The positive effects of TRH have not been universal, as some investigators have reported TRH to be of no benefit in SCI.[186] It was initially hypothesized that TRH acted as a physiologic opiate antagonist that spared the analgesic system.[184] However, as with naloxone, the mechanisms by which TRH improves neurologic function in SCI are unknown. TRH has been documented to potentiate spinal reflexes and to have trophic effects on cholinergic spinal neurons.[147, 334] Thus, after spinal injury, TRH may be active in the recovery phase rather than in the prevention of the acute evolution of the injury.

Excitatory Amino Acid Antagonists. The actions of the excitatory amino acids glutamate and aspartate have also been implicated in the pathophysiology of SCI. Antagonists at both the NMDA and non-NMDA receptors have been shown to improve outcome in experimental SCI. Besides the binding site for glutamate, the NMDA receptor contains a noncompetitive binding site in its ion channel.[209] Therapeutically, antagonists at this noncompetitive site are important, because they function in an agonist-dependent fashion (i.e., the receptor must be activated in order for the antagonist to bind). This type of situation is favorable for the treatment of pathologic conditions, such as central nervous system ischemia, in which excessive receptor activation is thought to occur.[384] Both competitive and noncompetitive NMDA receptor antagonists have been shown to be protective in models of spinal cord trauma and ischemia.[127, 221, 254, 391] The prototype noncompetitive NMDA receptor antagonist drugs are phencyclidine and ketamine, and they both share significant anesthetic effects. It has also been shown that dextrorotatory opioid compounds such as dextrorphan or dextromethorphan inhibit NMDA receptor channel function and may be beneficial in models of central nervous system ischemia.[230, 355] These compounds are attractive because they lack the psychotomimetic effects of phencyclidine-like compounds. In addition, various non-NMDA receptor antagonists have been shown to be beneficial in the treatment of experimental SCI.[387, 388]

Calcium Channel Antagonists. Based on the observation that the intracellular accumulation of calcium is a critical event in the mediation of neural injury, calcium channel blockers were used successfully in certain models of brain ischemia.[353, 354] The beneficial effects of these compounds cannot be ascribed specifically to the prevention of calcium movement into the neuron. First, the presence of calcium channels in the vascular smooth muscle imparts a significant degree of vascular reactivity to most calcium channel blockers,[261a] and the protective effects could be mediated through a vasodilatory improvement in perfusion. The pronounced effect of calcium channel blockers on the circulation, however, may produce a hypotension that can be detrimental to the injured cord because of the loss

of autoregulation. This is more of a concern in cervical and high thoracic cord lesions, where neurogenic hypotension frequently occurs and can be worsened by these compounds. Second, after injury, calcium may enter cells via other receptor channels (such as the NMDA receptor) or by nonspecific leakage through the damaged cell membrane. And third, the calcium that is normally bound to intracellular organelles may be released into the cytosol after injury. Although nimodipine has been reported to increase blood flow in the traumatized spinal cord and improve neurologic recovery,[133, 316, 317] it has not improved neurologic function in most studies of spinal cord trauma or ischemia.[123, 143, 164, 187]

Gangliosides. The glycolipid GM-1 ganglioside is a normal component of mammalian cells and is found in high concentrations in the axons, myelin sheaths, and glial cells of the central nervous system.[11] This glycolypid maybe beneficial in central nervous system injury, because it has been reported to (1) increase neurite outgrowth in vitro,[87, 197, 232, 312] (2) reduce retrograde and anterograde fiber degeneration,[47, 322, 349] (3) induce regeneration and sprouting in neurons,[321a] and (4) reduce amino acid–induced neurotoxicity.[275] GM-1 ganglioside has been found to be effective in models of central nervous system ischemia,[204, 361] in clinical stroke trials,[12] and, on a more limited basis, in models of SCI.[47, 153, 192] Although its mechanisms of action are unclear, it has been shown that exogenously administered GM-1 ganglioside is incorporated into myelin sheaths and axons.[192] These limited positive observations led to a clinical trial in a small number of human spinal injuries in which a positive result was noted.[149a] An interesting aspect was that it appeared to be of benefit when administered up to 72 hours after injury. This study had several limitations, and its results have been questioned. Negative results were noted by investigators who assessed GM-1 ganglioside's effect on lesion volume in rodent SCI model[74] and in a clinical stroke trial in a limited number of patients.[183] Nevertheless, a major study of the effects of GM-1 ganglioside in human SCI has been undertaken in the hope of resolving this issue.

Neurotrophic Factors. Neurotrophic factors were originally found to be target secreted molecules that provided support for their respective innervating neurons. Nerve growth factor (NGF) was the first one discovered and represents the classic factor that regulates neuronal survival, neurite outgrowth, and differentiation.[46] Recently, major advances in the discovery of new factors have occurred. The NGF neurotrophin (NT) family now includes brain-derived neurotrophic factor (BDNF), NT-3, NT-4/5, and NT-6. These and other factors such as ciliary neurotrophic factor (CNTF), leukemia inhibitory factor (LIF), insulin-like growth factor (IGF), and the acidic or basic fibroblast growth factors (aFGF and bFGF) are being extensively studied for use in the acute phase of SCI and in the chronic phase for stimulating central nervous system regeneration.[37]

Some evidence suggests a possible role for these factors in SCI. Messenger RNA expression and protein levels of bFGF have been noted to increase following spinal trauma.[139, 267] In addition, the exogenous application of these factors in experimental SCI has been observed to have beneficial effects. Methylprednisolone combined with bFGF has been reported to enhance neurologic recovery following SCI in the rat,[17] and BDNF, NT-3, and NFG have been observed to prevent retrograde cell death in the red nucleus following spinal cord hemisection in the newborn rat.[89] Schnell and colleagues[335] also noted an increase in the regenerative sprouting of the transected rat corticospinal tract when treated with NT-3.

Other Therapies. Although other pharmacologic therapies have been used in the treatment of acute experimental SCI, they have provided either limited data or conflicting results (Table 37–8). It can be expected that as we gain further insight into the pathophysiologic changes that occur in SCI, newer drugs with more specific actions will be developed. As the therapeutic time window for the application of these compounds is better identified, we will be able to create the proper combination for the treatment of specific injuries.

INTERVENTIONS DESIGNED TO INFLUENCE RECOVERY IN CHRONIC LESIONS

Chronic spinal injuries constitute a major challenge in the treatment of SCI. Whereas 10,000 acute spinal injuries occur every year, the prevalence of chronic injuries has been estimated at approximately 250,000. The effective repair of these chronic lesions relies on transplantation methods and techniques that stimulate regeneration of the damaged spinal pathways. Recent advances in the fields of neural transplantation and regeneration have shed a positive outlook on what once appeared to be an impossible task. The following observations support this positive view: (1) animal experiments using selective spinal lesions have demonstrated that functional locomotion is possible with as little as 10 per cent of the white matter,[42, 43, 109, 110, 382] (2) the recovery of one or two segments in cervical or lumbar lesions would convey great functional gains, (3) central nervous system neurons can regenerate under appropriate conditions, (4) the availability and the number of nerve growth factors continue to increase, and (5) advances in genetic engineering can now successfully provide cells tailored to fit specific needs.

Subsequent to the tissue injury and loss occurring during the acute and subacute phases of cord injury, the region of the lesion stabilizes. Our own experience suggests that certain aspects of the lesion site reflect the nature of the initial injury. Penetrating injuries, such as those caused by tissue aspiration, develop border regions dominated by multiple layers of astrocytes.[227, 228] Contusion lesions leading to central cystic spaces within the cord parenchyma have borders along the cyst wall, with less conspicuous astrocyte content. At this point, several problems mitigate against effective repair. First, essential neuronal machinery may be lost. For example, several segments of spinal cord gray matter may be destroyed so that both interneurons and motor neurons essential for muscle control are no longer present at the level of injury. Second, ascending and descending fiber tracts are interrupted (or suffer loss of myelin); thus, even though the motor apparatus below a level of injury may be retained, it may fail to receive signals that are useful in programming motor activity. Third, neurons whose axons are interrupted by the injury may not survive the major loss of connection to their target areas. For certain neuronal groups, this last problem is known to be more acute when cord injury occurs in the neonatal period.[53]

Repair of Spinal Cord Injuries in Lower Vertebrates. Space allows only a brief review of the remarkable ability of fish, tailed amphibians, and reptiles to regenerate injured central nervous system axons and, in some cases, neuronal populations in the adult animal.[381] Regeneration has been described in the spinal cord of each of these three vertebrate orders. Regeneration of the amputated tail in reptiles and amphibians includes restoration of spinal cord tissue deriving from

Table 37–8. OTHER PHARMACOLOGIC THERAPIES FOR EXPERIMENTAL SPINAL CORD INJURY

Drug	Study	Year	Rationale
Urea	Joyner and Freeman[198]	1963	Osmotic agent
L-thyroxine	Harvey and Srebnik[174]	1967	Enhance regeneration
	Tator and van der Jagt[365a]	1980	
Dimethyl sulfoxide	Kajihara et al.[202]	1973	Multiple effects
	de la Torre et al.[81]	1975	
Enzymes*	Guth et al.[161]	1980	Enhance regeneration
Phenytoin	Gerber et al.[151]	1980	Multiple effects
Leupeptin	Iwasaki et al.[193]	1985	Protease inhibitor
Electrical fields	Politis and Zanakis[293]	1989	Enhance regeneration

* Multiple enzymes were used (lidase, trypsin, elastase).

retained ependymal cells. In reptiles, these ependymal cells do not form new neurons but guide and support new axons originating above the lesion site. Sensory fibers also invade from above.[345] In urodele amphibians, the ependymal cells that bud into the regenerating tail differentiate into both glia and neurons, with formation of new motor and sensory neurons.[279]

Common themes in this regenerative activity are the ability of the ependymal region to generate new cellular stock, which acts as a guide to the growth of regenerating axons; the retention of neurons whose axons are damaged; and the rapidity and vigor of axonal regrowth. The retention of damaged neurons is essential but has not been studied in detail in the spinal cord. Differences in the degree of neuronal loss are particularly striking in studies of the reaction of retinal ganglion cells to section of the optic nerve. Transection of retinal ganglion cell axons close to the eye does not induce retrograde cell death in fish,[270] whereas approximately 90 per cent of these cells die after optic nerve transection in the rat.[265]

Thus, neuronal loss after injury appears to be less of a factor in lower vertebrate forms, and the neuron is able to mount a prompt and effective regenerative response. The glial and connective tissue cells encountered by the regrowing axons appear to provide little impediment to axonal regrowth, and restoration of substantial function has been demonstrated. Functional return has been extensively studied in the regenerated visual system of fish.[350]

Regeneration in Mammals.   It has been recognized since the days of Cajal[64] that after axonal injury in the adult mammal, an initial axonal sprouting and regenerative effort is initiated, but this regeneration aborts after several days, even though the neuron and proximal part of the axon are retained. For several decades, there has been a general assumption that this failure of regeneration represented an inability of the neuronal soma to mount an effective regenerative effort for its amputated axon. It has been demonstrated over the last decade, however, that if the environment of the tip of this severed axon is altered so that it is exposed to the cellular content normally present in the peripheral nerve trunk, substantial regeneration of surviving axons is possible.[80, 370] This has been most convincingly demonstrated in the optic system of the rat, where it has been possible to elicit substantial regeneration of retinal ganglion cell axons into transplants of sciatic nerve placed in the back of the eye and led through the skull and subcutaneous tissue to be implanted into the region of the superior colliculus. Although many retinal ganglion cells die under these conditions, those that survive have been shown to grow over distances of more than 4 cm to reach the region of the superior colliculus. In similar experiments undertaken in the hamster, these axons have been shown to make effective synapses in that target tissue.[206] These experiments have clearly demonstrated that those neurons of the adult mammalian central nervous system that survive the shock of axotomy have the capability of expressing a substantial regenerative effort if provided with an altered environment in the region of the severed axonal tip. In addition, modification of the substrate can substantially enhance cell survival and axonal regeneration, as has been shown in retinal ganglion cells.[18]

Thus it seems clear that central nervous system neurons have the capacity to regenerate but do not normally express this capacity within the parenchyma of the central nervous system. This clearly suggests that there are inhibitory factors that normally prevent regeneration within the mature mammalian central nervous system. The older concept that this inhibition resulted from astrocyte scarring has been questioned,[304] as astrocytic scar tissue displays both inhibitory (such as keratin and chondroitin sulfate) and permissive (such as heparin sulfate) influences.[205, 246, 341] Inhibitory factors have also been ascribed to the presence of oligodendrocytes, which are the dominant cellular constituents in white matter, where it is known that central regeneration is particularly poor.[304] Schwab and colleagues[304] demonstrated that central nervous system myelin and oligodendrocyte membranes contain two minor proteins with strong inhibiting effects on growing neurites. These workers suggested that with the development of the oligodendrocyte population (which occurs in many mammals shortly after birth), a definitive inhibitory influence is deposited within the central nervous system parenchyma, which mitigates against the regeneration of axons in the mature mammal. These investigators prepared antibodies to these inhibitory molecules and found evidence that in the presence of these antibodies, oligodendrocytes' inhibition of growth cone motility is neutralized.[328a] They further demonstrated that adult rats carrying tumors of myeloma cells secreting these antibodies show a degree of axonal regeneration after cord lesions that is substantially greater than that in controls.[335]

Efforts to Improve Recovery After Chronic Cord Injury.   The majority of neural transplantation techniques in the past used fetal tissue and produced limited results. However, the field has rapidly advanced due to the availability of innovative methodologies such as using specific nerve bridges combined with substances to promote growth,[286, 392] transplanting genetically modified cells,[283] or transplanting cells that have been genetically engineered to deliver growth factors.[368] The development of antibodies to inhibitory molecules that may be present within the mammalian central nervous system is an important step in efforts to influence regenerative activity after SCI. This tool alone is hardly adequate, however, to overcome the spectrum of problems present. For example, in severe SCI, there are substantial regions of the cord tissue that are lost, and the central part of the cord is often occupied by a fluid-filled cyst. Here the problem is to provide terrain that allows regeneration of nerve fibers through the region of damage; it is well known that nerve fiber growth can occur only on solid substratum. There have been a number of efforts to provide transplants into the region of injury that may beneficially influence the regenerative processes. Pioneering work with adult cord was undertaken utilizing transplants of segments of peripheral nerve into regions of spinal cord transections. Wrathall and associates[386] demonstrated ingrowth of nerve fibers in peripheral nerve segments placed in damaged regions of cat spinal cord but did not establish the origin of these fibers. Richardson and coworkers[307] clearly showed that axons from central nervous system neurons entered similar grafts placed in adult rat spinal cord.

Some of the most successful of these transplantation experiments have been undertaken after SCI in the newborn rat. The work of Bregman and Reier[53] illustrated that the implantation of embryonic spinal cord tissue into regions of injury in the neonatal spinal cord provides trophic support, which prevents the loss of neurons in the red nucleus of the brain stem. Normally, following axotomy of the rubrospinal tract in the neonatal rat, most of the neurons of this nucleus undergo cell death. The presence of embryonic implants is effective in preventing essentially all this cell death. The same degree of cell death is not observed when the rubrospinal tract is severed in adult rats. It has also been shown that the presence of these embryonic implants in neonatal rat spinal cord lesions allows serotonergic fibers to traverse the region of the lesion to reach the cord distal to the injury.[52]

Reier and colleagues[305] undertook a series of experiments to influence regions of SCI in adult rats with the implantation of embryonic spinal cord. Their work has shown that in adult rats, these implants have the capacity to survive and grow and to effectively fill defects caused by lesions. Furthermore, these implants have the ability to suppress the astrocytic scarring that normally forms at the lesion border; this reaction is suppressed in areas where the implant and the host tissue are in close proximity after the transplantation procedure.[188] These workers have also shown that axonal connections develop between the host tissue and the implanted embryonic cord, as well as connections that go between the implant and the host.[366] The degree of this connectivity is sparse, however, and these implants have not been shown to affect functional recovery after lesions in the adult cord. Kuhlengel and colleagues[227, 228] attempted to influence axonal growth after injury in the neonatal cord by implanting combinations of dorsal ganglion neurons and Schwann cells that had been prepared and modeled into cellular prosthetic constructs in tissue culture dishes. Their hope was that these implants would extend sensory axons into the dorsal columns of the injured cord, carrying with them Schwann cells that would provide beneficial terrain for axonal growth through the region of the lesion. After extensive experimentation, however, they observed that intrinsic axons of the spinal cord did not enter these implants, which remained separated from the cord parenchyma by a substantial astrocytic interface. These implants did influence the nature of this adjacent astrocytic tissue, and axons growing into the region of injury seemed to prefer growth on the paraexplant astrocytic substratum where it was in contact with the implanted material. No functional benefits of the implants were noted. Several laboratories are also studying the effects of placing pure populations of Schwann cells into spinal cord lesions in adult rats.[250, 286] This technique has proved effective in encouraging regeneration of severed septohippocampal axons in the adult rat brain.[225] Initial observations after cord lesions indicate that the presence of this cellular population engenders a considerable axonal ingrowth into the region of injury and decreases posttraumatic gliosis, but it remains to be shown whether this kind of cellular construct acts as an effective bridge for the intrinsic neurons of the spinal cord.

An alternative approach has been to introduce implants of embryonic neurons below the level of the spinal lesion. The aim is to provide new sources of transmitters to replace those no longer available because the injury has severed axons normally delivering these transmitters from brain stem sources. Nornes and colleagues[280] showed that reinnervation of the adult rat spinal cord below a lesion can be observed after implantation of catecholamine neurons obtained from the embryonic brain stem. These implants enhanced hindlimb flexion reflexes in the recipient animals.[58] Using a similar approach, Privat and colleagues[297] transplanted serotonergic brain stem neurons to the isolated distal cord of the rat and demonstrated a significant change in penile reflex activity in these injured animals.

The most recent area in the field of regeneration and transplantation involves the use of growth factors. Fibroblasts are now being genetically modified to secrete factors such as NGF, BDNF, NT-3, or bFGF,[273, 368] and these in turn can be grafted into the spinal cord. Grafting of NGF-producing fibroblasts into lesioned spinal cords has been reported to elicit a robust growth of sensory and noradrenergic neurites.[368] More recently, investigators using a model of spinal cord transection in the rat grafted multiple intercostal nerves placed in a manner that redirected specific pathways.[69] These grafts were stabilized with a fibrin glue containing aFGF and were observed to promote corticospinal tract regeneration and improve hindlimb motor function. Whereas these pioneering efforts at tissue transplantation after SCI have not yet resulted in effective restoration of major axon pathways in the adult mammalian spinal cord, they show considerable promise and point the way toward future experimentation.

References

1. Abood, L. G., and Hoss, W.: Excitation and conduction in the neuron. In Siegel, G. J., Albers, R. W., Katzman, R., and Agranoff, B. W. (eds.): Basic Neurochemistry. Boston, Little, Brown, 1976, pp. 103–124.
2. Allen, A. R.: Surgery of experimental lesion of spinal cord equivalent to crush injury of fracture dislocation of spinal column. JAMA 57:878–880, 1911.
3. Allen, A. R.: Remarks on the histopathological changes in the spinal cord due to impact: An experimental study. J. Nerv. Ment. Dis. 41:141–147, 1914.
4. Alvin, M. S., and Bunegin, L.: Catecholamine synthesis rates in traumatized spinal cord. Anat. Rec. 178:296–297, 1974.
5. Alvin, M. S., White, R. J., Acosta-Rua, G., and Yashon, D.: Study

of functional recovery produced by delayed localized cooling after spinal cord injury in primates. J. Neurosurg. *29*:113–120, 1968.

6. Anderson, D. K., Braughler, J. M., Hall, E. D., et al.: Effects of treatment with U-74006F on neurological outcome following experimental spinal cord injury. J. Neurosurg. *69*:562–567, 1988.

7. Anderson, D. K., and Means, E. D.: Lipid peroxidation in the spinal cord: FeCl$_2$ induction and protection with antioxidants. Neurochem. Pathol. *1*:249–264, 1983.

8. Anderson, D. K., Means, E. D., Waters, T. R., and Green, E. S.: Microvascular perfusion and metabolism in injured spinal cord after methylprednisolone treatment. J. Neurosurg. *56*:106–113, 1982.

9. Anderson, D. K., Means, E. D., Waters, T. R., and Spears, C. J.: Spinal cord energy metabolism following compression trauma to the feline spinal cord. J. Neurosurg. *53*:375–380, 1980.

10. Anderson, D. K., Saunders, R. D., Demediuk, P., et al.: Lipid hydrolysis and peroxidation in injured spinal cord: Partial protection with methylprednisolone or vitamin E and selenium. CNS Trauma *2*:257–267, 1985.

11. Ando, S.: Gangliosides in the nervous system. Neurochem. Int. *5*:507–537, 1983.

12. Argentino, C., Sachetti, M. L., Toni, D., et al.: GM1 ganglioside therapy in acute ischemic stroke. Italian acute stroke study—hemodilution + drug. Stroke *20*:1143–1149, 1989.

13. Assenmacher, D. R., and Ducker, T. B.: Experimental traumatic paraplegia: The vascular and pathological changes seen in reversible and irreversible spinal-cord lesions. J. Bone Joint Surg. *53*:671–680, 1971.

14. Auckland, K., Bower, B. F., and Berliner, R. W.: Measurement of local blood flow with hydrogen gas. Circ. Res. *14*:164–187, 1964.

15. Aust, S. D., Morehouse, L. A., and Thomas, C. E.: Role of metals in oxygen radical reactions. J. Free Radic. Biol. Med. *1*:3–25, 1985.

16. Ayer, J. B.: Cerebrospinal fluid in experimental compression of the spinal cord. Arch. Neurol. Psychiat. *2*:158–164, 1919.

17. Baffour, R., Achanta, K., Kaufman, J., et al.: Synergistic effect of basic fibroblast growth factor and methylprednisolone on neurological function after experimental spinal cord injury. J. Neurosurg. *83*:105–110, 1995.

18. Bahr, M., Hopkins, J. M. and Bunge, R. P.: In vitro myelination of regenerating adult rat retinal ganglion cell axons by Schwann cells. Glia *4*:529–533, 1991.

19. Baker, P. F.: The regulation of intracellular calcium. Symp. Soc. Exp. Biol. *30*:67–88, 1976.

20. Balentine, J. D.: Pathology of experimental spinal cord trauma. I. The necrotic lesion as a function of vascular injury. Lab. Invest. *39*:236–253, 1978.

21. Balentine, J. D.: Pathology of experimental spinal cord trauma. II. Ultrastructure of axons and myelin. Lab. Invest. *39*:254–266, 1978.

22. Balentine, J. D.: Axonal calcification in spinal cord injury of humans, monkeys and cats. Lab. Invest. *42*:99, 1980.

23. Balentine, J. D.: Hypotheses in spinal cord trauma research. *In* Becker, D. P., and Povlishock, J. T. (eds.): Central Nervous System Trauma Status Report. Bethesda, National Institute of Neurological and Communicative Disorders and Stroke, National Institutes of Health, 1985, pp. 455–461.

24. Balentine, J. D., and Dean, D. L., Jr.: Calcium induced spongiform and necrotizing myelopathy. Lab. Invest. *47*:286–295, 1982.

25. Balentine, J. D., and Hilton, C. W.: Ultrastructural pathology of axons and myelin in calcium-induced myelopathy. J. Neuropathol. Exp. Neurol. *39*:339–345, 1980.

26. Balentine, J. D., and Spector, M.: Calcifications of axons in experimental spinal cord trauma. Ann. Neurol. *2*:520–523, 1977.

27. Banik, N. L., Hogan, E. L., Fischer, I., et al.: Calpain activity in spinal cord injury. J. Neurochem. *61*:S112B, 1993.

28. Banik, N. L., Hogan, E. L., Powers, J. M., and Whetstine, L. J.: Degradation of cytoskeletal proteins in experimental spinal cord injury. Neurochem. Res. *7*:1465–1475, 1982.

29. Banik, N. L., Hogan, E. L., Whetstine, L. J., and Balentine, J. D.: Changes in myelin and axonal proteins in CaCL$_2$-induced myelopathy in rat spinal cord. CNS Trauma *1*:131–137, 1984.

30. Barut, S., Canbolat, A., Bilge, T., et al.: Lipid peroxidation in experimental spinal cord injury: Time-level relationship. Neurosurg. Rev. *16*:53–59, 1993.

31. Basso, D. M., Beattie, M. S., and Bresnahan, J. C.: A sensitive and reliable locomotor rating scale for open field testing in rats. J. Neurotrauma *12*:1–21, 1995.

32. Basso, D. M., Beattie, M. S., and Bresnahan, J. C.: Graded histological and locomotor outcomes after spinal cord contusion using the NYU weight-drop device versus transection. Exp. Neurol. *139*:244–256, 1996.

33. Basso, D. M., Beattie, M. S., Bresnahan, J. C., et al.: MASCIS evaluation of open field locomotor scores: Effects of experience and teamwork on reliability. Multicenter Animal Spinal Cord Injury Study. J. Neurotrauma *13*:343–359, 1996.

34. Beggs, J. L., and Waggener, J. D.: Transendothelial vesicular transport of protein following compression injury to the spinal cord. Lab. Invest. *34*:428–439, 1976.

35. Behrmann, D. L., Bresnahan, J. C., and Beattie, M. S.: A comparison of YM-14673, U-50488H, and nalmefene after spinal cord injury in the rat. Exp. Neurol. *119*:258–267, 1993.

36. Behrmann, D. L., Bresnahan, J. C., and Beattie, M. S.: Modeling of acute spinal cord injury in the rat: Neuroprotection and enhanced recovery with methylprednisolone, U-74006F and YM-14673. Exp. Neurol. *126*:61–75, 1994.

37. Bhatt, D. H., and Green, B. A.: The molecular biology of regeneration in the CNS. *In* Rassel, C., and Harsh, G. R., IV (eds.): The Molecular Basis of Neurosurgical Diseases. New York, Williams & Wilkins, 1996, pp. 304–338.

38. Bingham, W. G., Goldmans, H. G., Friedman, S., et al.: Blood flow in normal and injured monkey spinal cord. J. Neurosurg. *43*:162–171, 1975.

39. Bingham, W. G., Rufflo, R., and Friedman, S. J.: Catecholamine levels in the injured spinal cord of monkeys. J. Neurosurg. *42*:174–178, 1975.

40. Black, P., and Markowitz, R. S.: Experimental spinal cord injury in monkeys: Comparison of steroids and local hypothermia. Surg. Forum *22*:409–411, 1971.

41. Black, P., Markowitz, R. S., Cooper, V., et al.: Models of spinal cord injury: Part 1. Static load technique. Neurosurgery *19*:752–762, 1986.

42. Blight, A. R.: Cellular morphology of chronic spinal cord injury in the cat: Analysis of myelinated axons by line-sampling. Neuroscience *10*:521–543, 1983.

43. Blight, A. R.: Axonal physiology of chronic spinal cord injury in the cat: Intracellular recording in vitro. Neuroscience *10*:1471–1486, 1983.

44. Blight, A. R.: Delayed demyelination and macrophage invasion: A candidate for secondary cell damage in spinal cord injury. CNS Trauma *2*:299–315, 1985.

44a. Blight, A. R.: Effects of silica on the outcome from experimental spinal cord injury: Implication of macrophages in secondary tissue damage. Neuroscience *60*:263–273, 1994.

45. Blight, A. R., Saito, K., and Heyes, M. P.: Increased levels of the excitotoxin quinolinic acid in spinal cord following contusion injury. Brain Res. *632*:314–316, 1993.

46. Blottner, D., and Baumgarten, H. G.: Neurotrophy and regeneration in vivo. Acta Anat. *150*:235–245, 1994.

47. Bose, B., Osterholm, J. L., and Kalia, M.: Ganglioside-induced regeneration and reestablishment of axonal continuity in spinal cord-transected rats. Neurosci. Lett. *63*:165–169, 1986.

48. Bracken, M. B., Shepard, M. J., Collins, W. F., et al.: A randomized, controlled trial of methylprednisolone or naloxone in the treatment of acute spinal-cord injury. N. Engl. J. Med. *322*:1405–1411, 1990.

49. Braughler, J. M.: Lipid peroxidation-induced inhibition of τ-aminobutyric acid uptake in rat brain synaptosomes: Protection by glucocorticoids. J. Neurochem. *44*:1282–1288, 1985.

50. Braughler, J. M., Chase, R. L., Neff, G. L., et al.: A new 21-aminosteroid antioxidant lacking glucocorticoid activity stimulates adrenocorticotropin secretion and blocks arachidonic acid release from mouse pituitary tumor (AtT-20) cells. J. Pharmacol. Exp. Ther. *244*:423–427, 1988.

51. Braughler, J. M., and Hall, E. D.: Correlation of methylprednisolone levels in cat spinal cord with its effects on (Na$^+$ + K$^+$)-ATPase, lipid peroxidation, and alpha motor neuron function. J. Neurosurg. *56*:838–844, 1982.

51a. Braughler, J. M., Hall, E. D., Means, E. D., et al.: Evaluation of an intensive methylprednisolone sodium succinate dosing regimen in experimental spinal cord injury. J. Neurosurg. 67(1):102–105, 1987.

52. Bregman, B. S.: Spinal cord transplants permit the growth of serotonergic axons across the site of neonatal spinal cord transection. Dev. Brain Res. 34:265–279, 1987.

53. Bregman, B. S., and Reier, P. J.: Neural tissue transplants rescue axotomized rubrospinal cells from retrograde death. J. Comp. Neurol. 244:86–95, 1986.

54. Bresnahan, J. C.: An electron-microscopic analysis of axonal alterations following blunt contusion of the spinal cord of the rhesus monkey (Macaca mulatta). J. Neurol. Sci. 37:59–82, 1978.

55. Bresnahan, J. C., Beattie, M. S., Todd, F. D., and Noyes, D. H.: A behavioral and anatomical analysis of spinal cord injury produced by a feedback-controlled impaction device. Exp. Neurol. 95:548–570, 1987.

56. Bresnahan, J. C., King, J. S., Martin, G. F., and Yashon, D.: A neuroanatomical analysis of spinal cord injury in the rhesus monkey. J. Neurol. Sci. 28:521–542, 1976.

57. Brodner, R. A., Dohrmann, G. J., and Roth, R. H.: Intramedullary serotonin patterns following experimental spinal cord trauma. Mt. Sinai J. Med. 44:213–217, 1977.

58. Buchanan, J. T., and Nornes, H. O.: Transplants of embryonic brain stem containing the locus coeruleus into the spinal cord enhance the hindlimb flexion reflex in adult rats. Brain Res. 381:225–236, 1986.

59. Bunegin, L., Albin, M. S., and Jannetta, P. J.: Catecholamine responses to experimental spinal cord impact injury. I. Intrinsic spinal cord synthesis rates. Exp. Neurol. 53:279–280, 1976.

60. Bunge, M. B., Holets, V. R., Bates, M. L., et al.: Characterization of photochemically induced spinal cord injury in the rat by light and electron microscopy. Exp. Neurol. 127:76–93, 1994.

60a. Bunge, R. P., Puckett, W. R., Becerra, J. L., et al.: Observations on the pathology of human spinal cord injury. A review and classification of 22 new cases with details from a case of chronic cord compression with extensive focal demyelination. Adv. Neurol. 59:75–89, 1993.

61. Busto, R., Dietrich, W. D., Globus, M. Y. T., and Ginsberg, M. D.: Postischemic moderate hypothermia inhibits CA1 hippocampal ischemic neuronal damage. Neurosci. Lett. 101:299–304, 1989.

62. Busto, R., Dietrich, W. D., Globus, M. Y. T., et al.: Small differences in intraischemic brain temperature critically determine the extent of ischemic neuronal injury. J. Cereb. Blood Flow Metab. 7:729–738, 1987.

63. Busto, R., Globus, M. Y. T., Dietrich, W. D., et al.: Effect of mild hypothermia on ischemia-induced release of neurotransmitters and free fatty acids in rat brain. Stroke 20:904–910, 1989.

64. Cajal, R. S.: Degeneration and Regeneration of the Nervous System. New York, Hafner, 1928, pp. 329–353 (reprinted in 1968).

65. Campbell, J. B., DeCrescito, V., Tomasula, J. J., et al.: Experimental treatment of spinal contusion in the cat. Surg. Neurol. 1:102–106, 1973.

66. Cawthon, D. F., Senter, H. J., and Stewart, W. B.: Comparison of hydrogen clearance and C^{14}-antipyrine autoradiography in the measurement of spinal cord blood flow after severe impact injury. J. Neurosurg. 52:801–807, 1980.

67. Chan, P. K., and Fishman, R. A.: Brain edema: Induction in cortical slices by polyunsaturated fatty acids. Science 201:358–360, 1978.

68. Chan, P. K., and Fishman, R. A.: Transient formation of superoxide radicals in polyunsaturated fatty acid-induces brain swelling. J. Neurochem. 35:1004–1007, 1980.

69. Cheng, H., Cao, Y., and Olson, L.: Spinal cord repair in adult paraplegic rats: Partial restoration of hind limb function. Science 273:510–513, 1996.

70. Cheung, J. Y., Bonventre, J. V., Malis, C. D., and Leaf, A.: Calcium and ischemic injury. N. Engl. J. Med. 314:1670–1676, 1986.

71. Clendenon, N. R., Allen, N., Gordon, W. A., and Bingham, G. W., Jr.: Inhibition of Na$^+$ − K$^+$-activated ATPase activity following experimental spinal cord trauma. J. Neurosurg. 49:563–568, 1978.

72. Clifton, G. L., Allen, S., Barrodale, P., et al.: A phase II study of moderate hypothermia in severe brain injury. J. Neurotrauma 10:263–271, 1993.

73. Clifton, G. L., Jiang, J. Y., Lyeth, B. G., et al.: Marked protection by moderate hypothermia after experimental traumatic brain injury. J. Cereb. Blood Flow Metab. 11:114–121, 1991.

74. Constantini, S., and Young, W.: The effects of methylprednisolone and the ganglioside GM1 on acute spinal cord injury in rats. J. Neurosurg. 80:97–111, 1994.

75. Cook, P. L.: Radiology of spine and spinal cord injury. In Illis, L. S. (ed.): Spinal Cord Dysfunction: Assessment. New York, Oxford University Press, 1988, pp. 41–103.

76. Croft, T. J., Brodkey, J. S., and Nulsen, F. E.: Reversible spinal cord trauma: A model for electrical monitoring of spinal cord function. J. Neurosurg. 36:402–406, 1972.

77. Curtis, M. T., and Lefer, A. M.: Protective actions of naloxone in hemorrhagic shock. Am. J. Physiol. 239:H416–H421, 1980.

78. D'Abundo, G.: Alterazioni nel sistema nervoso centrale consecutive a particolari commozioni traumatiche. Riv. Ital. Neuropat. 9:145–171, 1916.

79. D'Angelo, C. M., Vangilder, J. C., and Taub, A.: Evoked clinical potentials in experimental spinal cord trauma. J. Neurosurg. 38:332–336, 1973.

80. David, S., and Aguayo, A. J.: Axonal elongation into peripheral nervous system bridges after central nervous system injury in adult rats. Science 214:931–933, 1981.

81. de la Torre, J. C., Johnson, C. M., Goode, D. J., and Mullan, S.: Pharmacologic treatment and evaluation of permanent experimental spinal cord trauma. Neurology 25:508–514, 1975.

82. de la Torre, J. C., Johnson, C. M., Harris, L. H., et al.: Monoamine changes in experimental head and spinal cord trauma: Failure to confirm previous observations. Surg. Neurol. 2:5–11, 1974.

83. del Maestro, R.: An approach to free radicals in medicine and biology. Acta Physiol. Scand. Suppl. 492:153–168, 1980.

84. Demediuk, P., and Faden, A. I.: Traumatic spinal cord injury in rats causes increases in tissue thromboxane but not peptidoleukotrienes. J. Neurosci. Res. 20:115–121, 1988.

85. Demopoulos, H. B., Flamm, E. S., Pietronegro, D. D., and Seligman, M. L.: The free radical pathology and the microcirculation in the major central nervous system disorders. Acta Physiol. Scand. Suppl. 492:91–119, 1980.

86. Demopoulus, H. B., Flamm, E. S., Seligman, M. C., et al.: Further studies on free radical pathology in the major central nervous system disorders: Effects of very high doses of methylprednisolone on the functional outcome, morphology and chemistry of experimental spinal cord impact injury. Can. J. Physiol. Pharmacol. 60:1415–1424, 1985.

87. Di Gregorio, F., Ferrari, G., Marini, P., et al.: The influence of gangliosides on neurite outgrowth and regeneration. Neuropediatrics 15:93–96, 1984.

88. Diener, G. A.: Regional accumulation of calcium in post-ischemic rat brain. J. Neurochem. 43:913–925, 1984.

89. Diener, P. S., and Bregman, B. S.: Neurotrophic factors prevent the death of CNS neurons after spinal cord lesions in newborn rats. Neuroreport 5:1913–1917, 1994.

90. Dietrich, W. D., Alonso, O., Busto, R., et al.: Post-traumatic brain hypothermia reduces histopathological damage following concussive brain injury in the rat. Acta Neuropathol. 87:250–258, 1994.

91. Dietrich, W. D., Busto, R., Halley, M., and Valdes, I.: The importance of brain temperature in alterations of the barrier following cerebral ischemia. J. Neuropathol. Exp. Neurol. 49:486–497, 1990.

92. Dietrich, W. D., Busto, R., Valdes, I., and Loor, Y.: Effects of normothermic versus mild hyperthermic forebrain rats. Stroke 21:1318–1325, 1990.

93. Dietrich, W. D., Halley, M., Valdes, I., and Busto, R.: Interrelationships between increased vascular permeability and neuronal damage following temperature-controlled brain ischemia. Acta Neuropathol. 81:615–625, 1991.

94. Dohrmann, G. J.: Experimental spinal cord trauma. Arch. Neurol. 27:468–473, 1972.

95. Dohrmann, G. J., Panjabi, M. M., and Banks, D.: Biomechanics of experimental spinal cord trauma. J. Neurosurg. 48:993–1001, 1978.

96. Dohrmann, G. J., Wagner, F. C., Jr., and Bucy, P. C.: The microvasculature in transitory traumatic paraplegia: An electron microscopic study in the monkey. J. Neurosurg. 35:263–271, 1971.

97. Dohrmann, G. J., Wagner, F. C., Jr., and Bucy, P. C.: Transitory traumatic paraplegia: Electron microscopy of early alterations in myelinated nerve fibers. J. Neurosurg. 36:407–415, 1972.

98. Dohrmann, G. J., and Wick, K. M.: Intramedullary blood flow patterns in transitory traumatic paraplegia. Surg. Neurol. 1:209–215, 1973.

99. Dohrmann, G. J., Wick, K. M., and Bucy, P. C.: Spinal cord blood flow patterns in experimental traumatic paraplegia. J. Neurosurg. 38:52–58, 1972.

100. Dolan, E. J., and Tator, C. H.: A new method for testing the force of clips for aneurysms of experimental spinal cord compression. J. Neurosurg. 51:229–233, 1979.

101. Ducker, T. B.: Experimental injury of the spinal cord. In Vinken, P. J., and Bruyn, G. W. (eds.): Handbook of Clinical Neurology. New York, American Elsevier Publishing Co., 1976, pp. 9–26.

102. Ducker, T. B., and Assenmacher, D. R.: Microvascular response to experimental spinal cord trauma. Surg. Forum 20:429–430, 1969.

103. Ducker, T. B., and Hamit, H. F.: Experimental treatments of acute spinal cord injury. J. Neurosurg. 30:693–697, 1969.

104. Ducker, T. B., Kindt, G. W., and Kempe, L. G.: Pathological findings in acute experimental spinal cord trauma. J. Neurosurg. 35:700–708, 1971.

105. Ducker, T. B., Saleman, M., Lucas, J. T., et al.: Experimental spinal cord trauma. II. Blood flow, tissue oxygen, evoked potentials in both paretic and plegic monkeys. Surg. Neurol. 10:64–70, 1978.

106. Ducker, T. B., Saleman, M., Perot, P. L., and Balentine, D.: Experimental spinal cord trauma. I. Correlation of blood flow, tissue oxygen and neurologic status in the dog. Surg. Neurol. 10:60–63, 1978.

107. Dusart, I., and Schwab, M. E.: Secondary cell death and the inflammatory reaction after dorsal hemisection of the rat spinal cord. Eur. J. Neurosci. 6:712–724, 1994.

108. Eidelberg, E., Staten, E., Watkins, C. J., and Smith, J. S.: Treatment of experimental spinal cord injury in ferrets. Surg. Neurol. 6:243–246, 1976.

109. Eidelberg, E., Story, J. L., Walden, J. G., and Meyer, B. L.: Anatomical correlates of return of function after partial spinal cord lesions in cats. Exp. Brain Res. 42:81–88, 1981.

110. Eidelberg, E., Straehley, D., and Ersparmer, R.: Relationship between residual hindlimb assisted locomotion and surviving axons after incomplete spinal cord injuries. Exp. Neurol. 56:213–322, 1977.

111. Eidelberg, E., Sullivan, J., and Brigham, A.: Immediate consequences of spinal cord injury: Possible role of potassium in axonal conduction block. Surg. Neurol. 3:317–321, 1975.

112. Faden, A. I.: TRH analog YM-14673 improves outcome following traumatic brain and spinal cord injury in rats: Dose-response studies. Brain Res. 486:228–235, 1989.

113. Faden, A. I.: Opioid and nonopioid actions mechanisms may contribute to dynorphin's pathophysiological actions in spinal cord injury. Ann. Neurol. 27:67–74, 1990.

114. Faden, A. I., Demediuk, P., Panter, S. S., and Vink, P.: The role of excitatory amino acids and NMDA receptors in traumatic brain injury. Science 244:798–800, 1989.

115. Faden, A. I., and Jacobs, T. P.: Dynorphin-related peptides cause motor dysfunction in the rat through a non-opiate action. Br. J. Pharmacol. 81:271–276, 1983.

116. Faden, A. I., and Jacobs, T. P.: Opiate antagonist WIN44,441–3 stereospecifically improved neurological recovery after ischemic spinal injury. Neurology 35:1311–1315, 1985.

117. Faden, A. I., and Jacobs, T. P.: Effect of TRH analogs on neurologic recovery after experimental spinal trauma. Neurology 35:1331–1334, 1985.

118. Faden, A. I., Jacobs, P. T., and Holaday, J. W.: Opiate antagonist improves neurologic recovery after spinal injury. Science 211:493–494, 1981.

119. Faden, A. I., Jacobs, T. P., and Holaday, J. W.: Thyrotropin-releasing hormone improves neurologic recovery after spinal trauma in cats. N. Engl. J. Med. 305:1063–1067, 1981.

120. Faden, A. I., Jacobs, T. P., and Holaday, J. W.: Comparison of early and late naloxone treatment in experimental spinal injury. Neurology 32:677–681, 1982.

121. Faden, A. I., Jacobs, T. P., Mougey, E., and Holaday, J. W.: Endorphins in experimental spinal injury. Ann. Neurol. 10:326–332, 1981.

122. Faden, A. I., Jacobs, T. P., Patrick, D. H., and Smith, M. T.: Megadose corticosteroid therapy following experimental spinal injury. J. Neurosurg. 60:712–717, 1984.

123. Faden, A. I., Jacobs, T. P., and Smith, M. T.: Evaluation of the calcium channel antagonist nimodipine in experimental spinal cord ischemia. J. Neurosurg. 60:796–799, 1984.

124. Faden, A. I., Jacobs, T. P., Smith, M. T., and Holaday, J. W.: Comparison of thyrotropin-releasing hormone (TRH), naloxone and dexamethasone treatments on experimental spinal cord injury. Neurology 33:673–678, 1983.

125. Faden, A. I., Molineaux, C. J., Rosenberger, J. C., et al.: Endogenous opioid immunoreactivity in rat spinal cord following traumatic injury. Ann. Neurol. 17:386–390, 1985.

126. Faden, A. I., Sacksen, I., and Noble, L. J.: Opiate receptor antagonist nalmefene improves neurological recovery after traumatic spinal cord injury in rats through a central mechanism. J. Pharmacol. Exp. Ther. 245:742–748, 1988.

127. Faden, A. I., and Simon, R. P.: A potential role for excitotoxins in the pathophysiology of spinal cord injury. Ann. Neurol. 23:623–626, 1988.

128. Faden, A. I., Takemori, A. E., and Portoghese, T. S.: k-Selective opiate antagonist nor-binaltorphimine improves outcome after traumatic spinal cord injury in rats. CNS Trauma 4:227–237, 1987.

129. Fairholm, D. J., and Turnbull, I. M.: Microangiographic study of experimental spinal cord injuries. J. Neurosurg. 35:277–286, 1971.

130. Fajardo, L. F., Kwan, H. H., Kowalski, J., et al.: Dual role of tumor necrosis factor alpha in angiogenesis. Am. J. Pathol. 140:539–544, 1992.

131. Farber, J. L.: Biology of disease: Membrane injury and calcium homeostasis in the pathogenesis of coagulative necrosis. Lab. Invest. 47:114–123, 1982.

132. Fehlings, M. G., and Tator, C. H.: A review of models of acute experimental spinal cord injury. In Illis, L. S. (ed.): Spinal Cord Dysfunction: Assessment. New York, Oxford University Press, 1988, pp. 3–33.

133. Fehlings, M. G., Tator, C. H., and Linden, R. D.: The relationship among the severity of spinal cord injury, motor and somatosensory evoked potentials and spinal cord blood flow. Electroencephalogr. Clin. Neurophysiol. 74:241–259, 1989.

134. Felten, D. L., Hall, P. V., Campbell, R. L., and Kalsbeck, J. E.: A histochemical investigation of catecholamines in spinal cord injury. J. Neural Transm. 39:209–221, 1976.

135. Ferraro, A.: Experimental medullary concussion of the spinal cord in rabbits: Histologic study of the early stages. Arch. Neurol. Psychiatry 18:357–373, 1927.

136. Finkelstein, S. D., Gillespie, J. A., Markowitz, R. S., et al.: Experimental spinal cord injury: Qualitative and quantitative histopathologic evaluation. J. Neurotrauma 7:29–40, 1990.

137. Fishman, R. A.: Cerebrospinal Fluid in Diseases of the Nervous System. Philadelphia, W. B. Saunders Co., 1980, pp. 107–128.

138. Flamm, E. S., Young, W., Demopoulus, H. B., et al.: Experimental spinal cord injury: Treatment with naloxone. Neurosurgery 10:227–231, 1982.

139. Follesa, P., Wrathall, J. R., and Mocchetti, I.: Increased basic fibroblast growth factor mRNA following contusive spinal cord injury. Brain Res. Mol. Brain Res. 22:1–8, 1994.

140. Fong, K. L., McCay, P. B., Poyer, J. L., et al.: Evidence that peroxidation of lysosomal membranes is initiated by hydroxyl free radicals produced during flavin enzyme activity. J. Biol. Chem. 248:7792–7797, 1973.

141. Fontaine, R., Mandel, P., Dany, A., et al.: Etude du déséquilibre biochimique provoqué, par les traumatisme médullaires, chez l'homme et chez le chein. Lyon Chir. 49:395–408, 1954.

142. Ford, R. W.: A reproducible spinal cord injury model in the cat. J. Neurosurg. 59:268–275, 1983.

143. Ford, R. W., and Malm, D. N.: Failure of nimodipine to reverse acute experimental spinal cord injury. CNS Trauma 2:9–17, 1985.

144. Forscher, P.: Calcium and phosphoinositide control of cytoskeletal dynamics. Trends Neurol. Sci. *12*:468–474, 1989.

145. Fried, L. C., and Aparicio, O.: Experimental ischemia of the spinal cord—histological studies after anterior spinal artery occlusion. Neurology *23*:289–314, 1973.

146. Fried, L. C., and Goodkin, R.: Microangiographic observations of the experimentally traumatized spinal cord. J. Neurosurg. *35*:709–714, 1971.

147. Fukuda, H., and Ono, H.: Ventral root depolarization and spinal reflex augmentation by a TRH analog in spinal cord. Neuropharmacology *21*:739–744, 1982.

148. Gadient, R. A., Cron, K. C., and Otten, U.: Interleukin-1 and tumor necrosis factor synergistically stimulate nerve growth factor (NGF) release from cultured rat astrocytes. Neurosci. Lett. *117*:335–340, 1990.

149. Gale, K., Kerasidis, H., and Wrathall, J. R.: Spinal cord contusion in the rat: Behavioral analysis of functional neurologic impairment. Exp. Neurol. *88*:123–134, 1985.

149a. Geisler, F. H., Dorsey, F. C., and Coleman, W. P.: Recovery of motor function after spinal-cord injury—a randomized, placebo-controlled trial with GM-1 ganglioside. N. Engl. J. Med. *324*:1829–1838, 1991.

150. Gelfan, S., and Tarlov, I. M.: Differential vulnerability of spinal cord structures to anoxia. J. Neurophysiol. *18*:170–188, 1955.

151. Gerber, A. M., Olson, W. L., and Harris, J. H.: Effect of phenytoin on functional recovery after experimental spinal cord injury in dogs. Neurosurgery *7*:472–476, 1980.

152. Gledhill, R. F., Harrison, B. M., and McDonald, W. I.: Demyelination and remyelination after acute spinal cord compression. Exp. Neurol. *38*:472–487, 1973.

153. Gorio, A., Guillo, A. M., Young, W., et al.: GM$_1$ effects on chemical, traumatic and peripheral nerve induce lesions to the spinal cord. *In* Goldberger, M. E., Gorio, A., and Murray, M. (eds.): Development and Plasticity of the Mammalian Spinal Cord. Padua, Liviana Press, 1986, pp. 227–242.

154. Green, B. A., Kahn, T., and Klose, K. J.: A comparative study of steroid therapy in acute experimental spinal injury. Surg. Neurol. *13*:91–97, 1980.

155. Green, B. A., Khan, T., and Raimondi, A. J.: Local hypothermia as a treatment of experimentally induced spinal cord contusion: Quantitative analysis of beneficent effect. Surg. Forum *24*:436–438, 1973.

156. Green, B. A., and Wagner, F. C., Jr.: Evolution of edema in the acutely injured spinal cord: A fluorescence microscopic study. Surg. Neurol. *1*:98–101, 1973.

157. Green, B. A., Wagner, F. C., Jr., and Bucy, P. C.: Oedema formation within the spinal cord. Trans. Am. Neurol. Assoc. *96*:244–245, 1971.

158. Griffith, I. R., and Miller, R.: Vascular permeability to protein and vasogenic oedema in experimental concussive injuries to the canine spinal cord. J. Neurol. Sci. *22*:291–304, 1974.

159. Groat, R. A., Wambach, W. A., Jr., and Windle, W. F.: Concussion of the spinal cord. Surg. Gynecol. Obstet. *81*:63–74, 1945.

160. Gruner, J. A.: A monitored contusion model of spinal cord injury in the rat. (Review.) J. Neurotrauma *9*:123–126, 1992.

161. Guth, L., Albuquerque, E. X., Deshpande, S. S., et al.: Ineffectiveness of enzyme therapy on regeneration in the transected spinal cord of the rat. J. Neurosurg. *52*:73–86, 1980.

162. Hägerdal, M., Harp, J., Nilsson, L., and Siesjö, B. K.: The effect of induced hypothermia upon oxygen consumption in the rat brain. J. Neurosci. *24*:311–316, 1975.

163. Hägerdal, M., Welsh, F. A., Keykhah, M. M., et al.: Protective effects of combinations of hypothermia and barbiturates in cerebral hypoxia in the rat. Anesthesiology *49*:165–169, 1978.

163a. Haghighi, S. S., and Chehrazi, B.: Effect of naloxone in experimental acute spinal cord injury. Neurosurgery *20*:385–388, 1987.

164. Haghighi, S. S., Stiens, T., Oro, J. J., and Madsen, R.: Evaluation of the calcium channel antagonist nimodipine after experimental spinal cord injury. Surg. Neurol. *39*:403–408, 1993.

165. Hall, E. D.: Glucocorticoid effects on the electrical properties of spinal motor neurons. Brain Res. *240*:109–116, 1982.

166. Hall, E. D., and Braughler, J. M.: Acute effects of intravenous glucocorticoid pre-treatment on the in vitro peroxidation of spinal cord tissue. Exp. Neurol. *72*:321–324, 1981.

167. Hall, E. D., and Braughler, J. M.: Glucocorticoid mechanisms in acute spinal injury: A review and therapeutic rationale. Surg. Neurol. *18*:320–327, 1982.

168. Hall, E. D., and Braughler, J. M.: Effects of intravenous methylprednisolone on spinal cord lipid peroxidation and Na$^+$-K$^+$-ATPase activity: Dose-response analysis during 1st hour after contusion injury in the cat. J. Neurosurg. *57*:247–253, 1982.

169. Hall, E. D., and Wolf, D. L.: Post-traumatic spinal cord ischemia: Relationship to injury severity and physiological parameters. CNS Trauma *4*:15–25, 1987.

170. Hall, E. D., Wolf, D. L., and Braughler, J. M.: Effects of a single large dose of methylprednisolone sodium succinate on experimental posttraumatic spinal cord ischemia. J. Neurosurg. *61*:124–130, 1984.

171. Hall, E. D., Yonkers, P. A., McCall, J. M., and Braughler, J. M.: Effect of the 21-aminosteroid U74006F on experimental head injury in mice. J. Neurosurg. *68*:456–461, 1988.

172. Hansebout, R. R., Kuchner, E. F., and Romero-Sierra, C.: Effects of local hypothermia and of steroids upon recovery from experimental spinal cord compression injury. Surg. Neurol. *4*:531–535, 1975.

173. Hapel, R. D., Smith, K. P., Banik, N. L., et al.: Ca^{2+}-accumulation in experimental spinal cord trauma. Brain Res. *211*:476–479, 1981.

174. Harvey, J. E., and Srebnik, H. H.: Locomotor activity and axon regeneration following spinal cord compression in rats treated with L-thyroxine. J. Neuropathol. Exp. Neurol. *26*:661–668, 1967.

175. Hayashi, N., de la Torre, J. C., and Green, B. A.: Regional spinal cord blood flow and tissue oxygen content after spinal cord trauma. Surg. Forum *31*:461–463, 1980.

176. Hayashi, N., de la Torre, J. C., Green, B. A., and Mora, J.: Rat spinal cord laminar blood flows of gray and white matter using multiple micro-electrode hydrogen clearance. Neurology *30*:406, 1980.

177. Haynes, R. C., and Murad, F.: Adrenocortical steroids and their synthetic analogs: Inhibitors of adrenocortical steroid biosynthesis. *In* Goodman, A. G., Goodman, L. S., Rall, T. W., and Murad, F. (eds.): *The Pharmacological Basis of Therapeutics.* New York, Macmillan, 1985, pp. 1459–1489.

178. Hedeman, L. S., Shellenberger, M. K., and Gordon, J. H.: Studies in experimental spinal cord trauma. Part 1. Alterations in catecholamine levels. J. Neurosurg. *40*:37–43, 1974.

179. Hedeman, L. S., and Sil, R.: Studies in experimental spinal cord trauma. Part 2. Comparison of treatment with steroids, low molecular weight dextran, and catecholamine blockade. J. Neurosurg. *40*:44–51, 1974.

180. Heymann, J. I., Payne, B. B., Hoffman, J. I., and Rudolph, A. M.: Blood flow measurements with radionuclide-labeled particles. Prog. Cardiovasc. Dis. *20*:55–79, 1977.

181. Hickey, R., Allen, M. S., Bunegin, L., and Gelineau, J.: Autoregulation of spinal cord blood flow: Is the cord a microcosm of the brain? Stroke *17*:1183–1189, 1986.

182. Hirano, A., Becker, N. H., and Zimmerman, H. M.: Pathological alterations in the cerebral endothelial cell barrier to peroxidase. Arch. Neurol. *20*:300–308, 1969.

183. Hoffbrand, B. I., Bingley, P. J., Oppenheimer, S. M., and Sheldon, C. D.: Trial of ganglioside GM1 in acute stroke. J. Neurol. Neurosurg. Psychiatry *51*:1213–1214, 1988.

184. Holaday, J. W., D'Amato, R. J., and Faden, A. I.: Thyrotropin-releasing-hormone improves cardiovascular function in experimental endotoxic and hemorrhagic shock. Science *213*:216–218, 1981.

185. Holaday, J. W., and Faden, A. I.: Naloxone acts at central opiate receptors to reverse hypotension, hypothermia and hypoventilation in spinal shock. Brain Res. *189*:295–299, 1980.

186. Holtz, A., Nystrom, B., and Gerdin, B.: Blocking weight-induced spinal cord injury in rats: Effects of TRH or naloxone on motor function recovery and spinal cord blood flow. Acta Neurol. Scand. *80*:215–220, 1989.

187. Holtz, A., Nystrom, B., and Gerdin, B.: Spinal cord injury in rats: Inability of nimodipine or anti-neutrophil serum to improve spinal cord blood flow or neurologic status. Acta Neurol. Scand. *79*:460–467, 1989.

188. Houlé, J. D., and Reier, P. J.: Transplantation of fetal spinal cord

tissue into the chronically injured adult rat spinal cord. J. Comp. Neurol. 269:535–547, 1988.

189. Howitt, W. M., and Turnbull, I. M.: Effects of hypothermia and methysergide on recovery from experimental paraplegia. Can. J. Surg. 15:179–186, 1972.

190. Hsu, C. Y., Halushka, P. V., Hogan, E. L., et al.: Alteration of thromboxane and prostacyclin levels in experimental spinal cord injury. Neurology 35:1003–1009, 1985.

191. Huang, K. P.: The mechanism of protein kinase C activation. Trends Neurol. Sci. 12:425–432, 1989.

192. Imanaka, T., Hukuda, S., and Maeda, T.: The role of GM1-ganglioside in the injured spinal cord of rats: An immunohisto-chemical study using GM1-antisera. J. Neurotrauma 13:163–170, 1996.

193. Iwasaki, Y., Iizuka, H., Yamamoto, T., et al.: Alleviation of axonal damage in acute spinal cord injury by a protease inhibitor: Automated morphometric analysis of drug effects. Brain Res. 347:124–126, 1985.

194. Jacobson, E. J., McCall, J. M., Ayer, D. E., et al.: Novel 21-aminosteroids that inhibit iron-dependent lipid peroxidation and protect against central nervous system trauma. J. Med. Chem. 33:1145–1151, 1990.

195. Jellinger, K.: Neuropathology of spinal cord injuries. In Vinken, P. J., and Bruyn, G. W. (eds.): Handbook of Clinical Neurology. Vol. 25. New York, American Elsevier Publishing Co., 1976, pp. 43–121.

196. Jones, M., and Keenan, R. W.: A biochemical investigation of spinal cord after contusive injury. Exp. Neurol. 78:67–82, 1982.

197. Jonsson, G., Gorio, A., Hallman, H., et al.: GM1 ganglioside treatment enhances regrowth of central and peripheral nor-adrenaline neurons after selective 6-hydroxydopamine-induced lesions. In Gilad, G. M., Gorio, A., and Kreutzberg, G. W. (eds.): Processes of Recovery From Neural Trauma. Berlin, Springer-Verlag, 1986, pp. 275–293.

198. Joyner, J. J., and Freeman, L. W.: Urea and spinal cord trauma. Neurology 13:69–72, 1963.

199. Kahn, M., and Gabriel, R.: Acute spinal cord injury in the rat: Comparison of three experimental techniques. Can. J. Neurosci. 10:161–165, 1983.

200. Kahn, M., Griebel, R., Rozdilsky, and Politis, M.: Hemorrhagic changes in experimental spinal cord injury models. Can. J. Neurol. Sci. 12:259–262, 1985.

201. Kahn, T., Green, B., and Raimondi, A. J.: Energy metabolism of acutely injured spinal cord of cat. J. Neuropathol. Exp. Neurol. 34:84–85, 1975.

202. Kajihara, K., Kawanaga, H., de la Torre, J. C., and Mullan, S.: Dimethyl sulfoxide in the treatment of experimental acute spinal cord injury. Surg. Neurol. 1:16–22, 1973.

203. Kajiwara, K.: An experimental study on the spinal cord injury. Juntendo Med. J 7:612–618, 1961.

204. Karpiak, S. E., Li, Y. S., and Mahadik, S. P.: Gangliosides (GM1 and AGF2) reduce mortality due to ischemia: Protection of membrane function. Stroke 18:184–187, 1987.

205. Kawaguchi, S.: Axonal regeneration in the spinal cord with functional restoration in young rats. In Axonal Regrowth in the Mammalian Spinal Cord and Peripheral Nerve. Normandy, France, IRME, 1995.

206. Keirstead, S. A., Rasminsky, M., Fukuda, I., et al.: Electrophysiologic responses in hamster superior colliculus evoked by regenerating retinal axons. Science 246:255–257, 1989.

207. Kelly, D. L., Lassiter, R. R. L., Calogero, J. A., and Alexander, E., Jr.: Effects of local hypothermia and tissue oxygen studies in experimental paraplegia. J. Neurosurg. 33:554–563, 1970.

208. Kelly, D. L., Lassiter, R. R. L., Vongsvivut, A., and Smith, J. M.: Effects of hyperbaric oxygenation and tissue oxygen studies in experimental paraplegia. J. Neurosurg. 36:425–429, 1972.

209. Kemp, J. A., Foster, A. C., and Wong, E. H.: Non-competitive antagonists of excitatory amino acid receptors. Trends Neurosci. 10:294–298, 1987.

210. Kennedy, M. B.: Regulation of neuronal function by calcium. Trends Neurosci. 12:417–420, 1989.

211. Klatzo, I.: Presidential address: Neuropathological aspects of brain edema. J. Neuropathol. Exp. Neurol. 26:1–14, 1967.

212. Kleihus, P., Kobayashi, K., and Hossman, K. A.: Purine nucleo-tide metabolism in the cat brain after one hour of complete ischemia. J. Neurochem. 23:417–425, 1974.

213. Kleitman, N., Simon, D. K., Schachner, M., and Bunge, R. P.: Growth of embryonic retinal neurites elicited by contact with Schwann cell surfaces is blocked by antibodies to L1. Exp. Neurol. 102:298–306, 1988.

214. Kleitman, N., Wood, P., Johnson, M. I., and Bunge, R. P.: Schwann cell surfaces but not extracellular matrix support neurite outgrowth from cultured embryonic rat retina. J. Neurosci. 8:653–663, 1988.

215. Kobrine, A. I.: The neuronal theory of experimental spinal cord dysfunction. Surg. Neurol. 3:317–321, 1975.

216. Kobrine, A. I., Doyle, T. F., and Martins, A. N.: Spinal cord blood flow in the rhesus monkey by the hydrogen clearance method. Surg. Neurol. 2:197–200, 1974.

217. Kobrine, A. I., Doyle, T. F., and Martins, A. N.: Autoregulation of spinal cord blood flow. Clin. Neurosurg. 22:573–581, 1975.

218. Kobrine, A. I., Doyle, T. F., and Martins, A. N.: Local spinal cord blood flow in experimental traumatic myelopathy. J. Neurosurg. 42:144–149, 1975.

219. Kobrine, A. I., Evans, D. E., and Rizzoli, V.: The effects of ischemia on long-tract neural conduction in the spinal cord. J. Neurosurg. 50:639–644, 1979.

220. Kobrine, A. I., Evans, D. E., and Rizzoli, V.: Effects of progressive hypoxia on long tract neural conduction in the spinal cord. Neurosurgery 7:369–375, 1980.

221. Kochlar, A., Zivin, J. A., Lyde, P. D., and Mazarella, V.: Glutamate antagonist therapy reduces neurologic deficits produced by focal central nervous system ischemia. Arch. Neurol. 45:148–153, 1988.

222. Koozekanani, S. H., Vise, M., Hashemi, R., and McGhee, R.: Possible mechanisms for observed pathophysiological variability in experimental spinal cord injury by the method of Allen. J. Neurosurg. 44:429–434, 1976.

223. Koreh, K., Seligman, M. L., Flamm, E. S., and Demopoulus, H. B.: Lipid antioxidant properties of naloxone in vitro. Biochem. Biophys. Res. Commun. 102:1317–1322, 1984.

224. Kramer, R. S., Sanders, A. P., Lesage, A. M., et al.: The effect of profound hypothermia on preservation of cerebral ATP content during circulatory arrest. J. Thorac. Cardiovasc. Surg. 56:699–709, 1968.

225. Kromer, L. F., and Cornbrooks, C. J.: Transplants of Schwann cell cultures promote axonal regeneration in the adult mammalian brain. Proc. Natl. Acad. Sci. USA 82:6330–6334, 1985.

226. Krumins, S. A., and Faden, A. I.: Traumatic injury alters opiate receptor binding in rat spinal cord. Ann. Neurol. 19:498–501, 1986.

227. Kuhlengel, K. R., Bunge, M. B., and Bunge, R. P.: Implantation of cultured sensory neurons and Schwann cells into lesioned neonatal rat spinal cord. I. Methods for preparing implants from dissociated cells. J. Comp. Neurol. 293:63–73, 1990.

228. Kuhlengel, K. R., Bunge, M. B., Bunge, R. P., and Burton, H.: Implantation of cultured sensory neurons and Schwann cells into lesioned neonatal rat spinal cord. II. Implant characteristics and examination of corticospinal tract growth. J. Comp. Neurol. 293:74–91, 1990.

229. Kurihara, M.: Role of monoamines in experimental spinal cord injury. Relationship between Na$^+$-K$^+$-ATPase and lipid peroxidation. J. Neurosurg. 62:743–749, 1985.

230. Lehmann, J., Sills, M. A., Tsai, C., et al.: Dextromethorphan modulates the NMDA-type receptor-associated ion channel by binding to its closed state. In Cavalheiro, E. A., et al. (eds.): Frontiers in Excitatory Amino Acid Research. New York, A. R. Liss, 1988, pp. 571–578.

231. Lehninger, A. L.: Mitochondria and calcium ion transport. Biochem. J. 119:129–138, 1970.

232. Leon, A., Facci, L., Benvegnu, D., and Toffano, G.: Morphological and biochemical effects of gangliosides in neuroblastoma cells. Dev. Neurosci. 5:108, 1982.

233. Lewin, M. G., Hansebout, R. R., and Pappius, H. M.: Chemical characteristics of traumatic spinal cord edema in cats: Effects of steroids on potassium depletion. J. Neurosurg. 40:65–75, 1974.

234. Li, G. L., Farooque, M., Holtz, A., and Olsson, Y.: Changes of beta-amyloid precursor protein after compression trauma to the

spinal cord: An experimental study in the rat using immunohistochemistry. J. Neurotrauma 12:269–277, 1995.

235. Li, Z., Hogan, E. L., and Banik, N. L.: Role of calpain in spinal cord injury: Increased calpain immunoreactivity in rat spinal cord after impact trauma. Neurochem. Res. 21:441–448, 1996.

236. Lindsberg, P. J., O'Neill, J. T., Paakkari, I. A., et al.: Validation of laser-Doppler flowmetry in measurement of spinal cord blood flow. Am. J. Physiol. 257:H674–H680, 1989.

237. Liu, D., and McAdoo, D. J.: Methylprednisolone reduces excitatory amino acid release following experimental spinal cord injury. Brain Res. 609:293–297, 1993.

238. Locke, G. E., Yashon, D., and Feldman, R. A.: Ischemia in primate spinal cord injury. J. Neurosurg. 34:614–617, 1971.

239. Lohse, D. C., Senter, H. J., Kauer, J. S., et al.: Spinal cord blood flow in experimental transient paraplegia. J. Neurosurg. 52:335–345, 1980.

240. Long, J. B., Kinney, R. C., Malcolm, D. S., et al.: Intrathecal dynorphin A 8(1–13) and dynorphin A (3–13) reduce rat spinal cord blood flow by non-opioid mechanisms. Brain Res. 436:374–379, 1987.

241. Long, J. B., Martinez-Arizala, A., Petras, J. M., and Holaday, J. W.: Endogenous opioids in spinal cord injury: A critical evaluation. CNS Trauma 4:295–315, 1986.

242. Long, J. B., Petras, J. M., Mobley, W. C., and Holaday, J. W.: Neurological dysfunction following intrathecal injection of Dyn A-(1–13) in the rat. II. Non-opioid mechanisms mediate loss of motor function, sensory and autonomic function. J. Pharmacol. Exp. Ther. 246:1167–1174, 1988.

243. Long, J. B., Rigamonti, D. D., deCosta, B., et al.: Dynorphin A–induced rat hindlimb paralysis and spinal cord injury are not altered by the k opioid antagonist nor-binaltorphimine. Brain Res. 497:155–162, 1989.

244. Long, J. B., Rigamonti, D. D., Oleshansky, M. A., et al.: Dynorphin A–induced rat spinal cord injury: Evidence for excitatory amino acid involvement in a pharmacological model of ischemic spinal cord injury. J. Pharmacol. Exp. Ther. 269:358–366, 1994.

245. Malenka, R. C., Kauer, J. A., Perkel, D. J., and Nicoll, R. A.: The impact of post-synaptic calcium on synaptic transmission—its role in long-term potentiation. Trends Neurol. Sci. 12:444–450, 1989.

246. Malhotra, S. K., Svensson, M., and Aldskogious, H.: Diversity among reactive astrocytes: Proximal reactive astrocytes in lacerated spinal cord preferentially react with monoclonal Ab J1-31. Brain Res. Bull. 30:395–404, 1993.

247. Marcus, M. L., Heistad, D. D., Ehrhardt, J., and Abboud, F. M.: Regulation of total and regional spinal cord blood flow. Circ. Res. 41:128–134, 1977.

248. Marinesco, G.: Lésions commotionnelles expérimentales. Rev. Neurol. 34:329–331, 1918.

249. Marshall, L. F., Knowlton, S., Garfin, S. R., et al.: Deterioration following spinal cord injury. J. Neurosurg. 66:400–404, 1987.

250. Martin, D., Schoenen, J., Delree, P., et al.: Experimental acute traumatic injury of the adult rat spinal cord by a subdural inflatable balloon: Methodology, behavioral analysis, and histopathology. J. Neurosci. Res. 32:539–550, 1992.

251. Martin, S. H., and Bloedel, J. R.: Evaluation of experimental spinal cord injury using cortical evoked potentials. J. Neurosurg. 39:75–81, 1973.

252. Martinez-Arizala, A., and Green, B. A.: Hypothermia in spinal cord injury. (Review.) J. Neurotrauma 9(Suppl. 2):S497–505, 1992.

253. Martinez-Arizala, A., Long, J. B., and Holaday, J. W.: TRH fails to antagonize the paralytic effects of intrathecal dynorphin A and substance P antagonists. Brain Res. 473:385–388, 1988.

254. Martinez-Arizala, A., Rigamonti, D. D., Long, J. B., et al.: Effects of NMDA receptor antagonists following spinal ischemia in the rabbit. Exp. Neurol. 108:232–240, 1990.

255. McCord, J. M.: Oxygen-derived radicals: A link between reperfusion injury and inflammation. Fed. Proc. 46:2402–2406, 1987.

256. McCord, J. M., and Fridovich, I.: The reduction of cytochrome C by milk xanthine oxidase. J. Biol. Chem. 243:5753–5760, 1968.

257. McLean, A. E. M., McLean, E., and Judah, J. D.: Cellular necrosis in the liver induced and modified by drugs. Int. Rev. Exp. Pathol. 4:127–157, 1965.

258. McVeigh, J. F.: Experimental cord crushes with special references to the mechanical factors involved and subsequent changes in the areas affected. Arch. Surg. 7:573–600, 1923.

259. Means, E. D., and Anderson, D. K.: Neuronophagia by leukocytes in experimental spinal cord injury. J. Neuropathol. Exp. Neurol. 42:707–719, 1983.

260. Means, E. D., Anderson, D. K., Waters, T. R., and Kalaf, L.: Effect of methylprednisolone in compression trauma to the feline spinal cord. J. Neurosurg. 55:200–208, 1981.

261. Meyer, J. S., and Hunter, J.: Effects of hypothermia on local blood flow and metabolism during cerebral ischemia and hypoxia. J. Neurosurg. 14:210–227, 1957.

261a. Michalewicz, L., and Messerli, F. H.: Cardiac effects of calcium antagonists in systemic hypertension. Am. J. Cardiol. 79(10A):39–46, 1997.

262. Michenfelder, J., Milde, J., and Sundt, T.: Cerebral protection by barbiturate anesthesia: Use after middle cerebral artery occlusion in Java monkeys. Arch. Neurol. 33:345–350, 1976.

263. Michenfelder, J. D., and Theye, R. A.: The effects of anesthesia and hypothermia on canine cerebral ATP and lactate during anoxia produced by decapitation. Anesthesiology 33:430–439, 1970.

264. Milvy, P., Kakari, S., Campbell, J. B., and Demopoulos, H. B.: Paramagnetic species and radical products in cat spinal cord. Ann. N. Y. Acad. Sci. 222:1102–1111, 1973.

265. Misantone, L. J., Gershenbaum, M., and Murray, M.: Viability of retinal ganglion cells after optic nerve crush in adult rats. J. Neurocytol. 13:449–465, 1984.

266. Misra, H. P., and Fridovich, I.: The role of superoxide anion in the autooxidation of epinephrine and a simple assay for superoxide dismutase. J. Biol. Chem. 247:3170–3175, 1972.

267. Mocchetti, I., Rabin, S. J., Colangelo, A. M., et al.: Increased basic fibroblast growth factor expression following contusive spinal cord injury. Exp. Neurol. 141:154–164, 1996.

268. Moreland, D. B., Soloniuk, D. S., and Feldman, M. J.: Leukotrienes in experimental spinal cord injury. Surg. Neurol. 31:277–280, 1989.

269. Murphy, E. J., Behrmann, D., Bates, C. M., and Horrocks, L. A.: Lipid alterations following impact spinal cord injury in the rat. Mol. Chem. Neuropathol. 23:13–26, 1994.

270. Murray, M.: A quantitative study of regenerative sprouting by optic axons in the goldfish. J. Comp. Neurol. 209:352–362, 1982.

271. Naftchi, N. E., Demeny, M., DeCrescito, V., et al.: Biogenic amine concentrations in traumatized spinal cord of cats: Effects of drug therapy. J. Neurosurg. 40:52–57, 1974.

272. Naftchi, N. F.: Functional restoration of the traumatically injured spinal cord in cats by clonidine. Science 217:1042–1047, 1982.

273. Nakahara, Y., Gage, F. H., and Tuszynski, M. H.: Grafts of fibroblasts genetically modified to secrete NGF, BDNF, NT-3, or basic FGF elicit differential responses in the adult spinal cord. Cell Transplant. 5:191–204, 1996.

274. Nemecek, S., Petr, R., Suba, P., et al.: Longitudinal extension of oedema in experimental spinal cord injury: Evidence for two types of post-traumatic oedema. Acta Neurochir. 37:7–16, 1977.

275. Nicoletti, F., Cavallaro, S., Bruno, V., et al.: Gangliosides attenuate NMDA receptor-mediated excitatory amino acid release in cultured cerebellar neurons. Neuropharmacology 28:1283–1286, 1989.

276. Noble, L. J., and Wrathall, J. R.: Spinal cord contusion in the rat: Morphometric analyses of alterations in the cord. Exp. Neurol. 88:135–149, 1985.

277. Noble, L. J., and Wrathall, J. R.: An inexpensive apparatus for producing graded spinal cord contusive injuries in the rat. Exp. Neurol. 95:530–533, 1987.

278. Noble, L. J., and Wrathall, J. R.: Correlative analyses of the lesion development and functional status after graded spinal cord injuries in the rat. Exp. Neurol. 103:34–40, 1989.

279. Nordlander, R., and Singer, M.: The role of ependyma in regeneration of the spinal cord in the urodele amphibian tail. J. Comp. Neurol. 180:349–373, 1978.

280. Nornes, H. O., Bjorklund, A., and Stenevi, U.: Reinnervation of the denervated spinal cord of rats by intraspinal transplants of embryonic brain stem neurons. Cell Tissue Res. 230:15–35, 1983.

281. Noyes, D. H.: Electromechanical impactor for producing experi-

mental spinal cord injury in animals. Med. Biol. Eng. Comput. 25:335–340, 1987.

282. Olney, J. W.: Brain lesions, obesity and other disturbances in mice treated with monosodium glutamate. Science 164:719–721, 1969.

283. Onifer, S. M., Whittemore, S. R., and Holets, V. R.: Variable morphological differentiation of a raphe-derived neuronal cell line following transplantation into the adult rat CNS. Exp. Neurol. 122:130–142, 1993.

284. Osterholm, J. L., and Mathews, G. J.: Altered norepinephrine metabolism following experimental spinal cord injury. Part 1. Relationship to hemorrhagic necrosis and post-wounding neurological deficits. J. Neurosurg. 36:386–394, 1972.

285. Osterholm, J. L., and Mathews, G. J.: Altered norepinephrine metabolism following experimental spinal cord injury. Part 2. Protection against traumatic spinal cord hemorrhagic necrosis by norepinephrine synthesis blockade with alpha methyl tyrosine. J. Neurosurg. 36:395–401, 1972.

286. Paino, C. L., Fernandez-Valle, C., Bates, M. L., and Bunge, M. B.: Regrowth of axons in lesioned adult rat spinal cord: Promotion by implants of cultured Schwann cells. J. Neurocytol. 23:433–452, 1994.

287. Panjabi, M. M., and Wrathall, J. R.: Biomechanical analysis of experimental spinal cord injury and functional loss. Spine 13:1365–1370, 1988.

288. Panter, S. S., Yum, S. W., and Faden, A. I.: Alteration in extracellular amino acids after traumatic spinal cord injury. Ann. Neurol. 27:96–99, 1990.

289. Patterson, S. J., Robson, L. E., and Kosterlitz, H. W.: Classification of opioid receptors. Br. Med. Bull. 39:31–36, 1983.

290. Philipi, R., Kuhn, W., Zach, G. A., et al.: Survey of the neurological evaluation of 300 spinal cord injuries seen within 24 hours after injury. Paraplegia 18:337–346, 1980.

291. Pietronigro, D. D., DeCrescito, V., Tomasula, J. J., et al.: Ascorbic acid: A putative biochemical marker or irreversible neurologic functional loss following spinal cord injury. CNS Trauma 2:85–90, 1985.

292. Pietronigro, R. D., Hovsepian, M., Demopoulus, H. B., and Flamm, E. S.: Loss of ascorbic acid from injured feline spinal cord. J. Neurochem. 41:1072–1076, 1983.

293. Politis, M. J., and Zanakis, M. F.: The short-term effects of delayed application of electric fields in the damaged rodent spinal cord. Neurosurgery 25:71–75, 1989.

294. Popovich, P. G., Horner, P. J., Mullin, B. B., and Stokes, B. T.: A quantitative spatial analysis of the blood-spinal cord barrier. I. Permeability changes after experimental spinal contusion injury. Exp. Neurol. 142:258–275, 1996.

295. Popovich, P. G., Reinhard, J. F., Jr., Flanagan, E. M., and Stokes, B. T.: Elevation of the neurotoxin quinolinic acid occurs following spinal cord trauma. Brain Res. 633:348–352, 1994.

296. Prindergast, J. S.: The background of Galen's life and activities, and influences on his achievements. Proc. R. Soc. Med. 23:1131–1148, 1930.

297. Privat, A., Mansour, H., and Geffard, M.: Transplantation of fetal serotonin neurons into the transected spinal cord of adult rats: Morphological development and functional influence. Prog. Brain Res. 78:155–166, 1988.

298. Przewlocki, R., Shearman, G. T., and Herz, A.: Mixed opioid/non-opioid effects of dynorphin and dynorphin related peptides after their intrathecal injection in rats. Neuropeptides 3:233–240, 1983.

299. Rasmussen, H.: The calcium messenger system (first of two parts). N. Engl. J. Med. 314:1094–1101, 1986.

300. Rawe, S. E., Lee, W. A., and Perot, P. L.: Spinal cord glucose utilization after experimental spinal cord injury. Neurosurgery 9:40–47, 1981.

301. Rawe, S. E., Roth, R. H., Boadle-Biber, M., and Collins, W. F.: Norepinephrine levels in spinal cord trauma. Part 1. Biochemical study of hemorrhagic necrosis. J. Neurosurg. 46:350–357, 1977.

302. Rawe, S. E., Roth, R. H., and Collins, W. F.: Norepinephrine levels in experimental spinal cord trauma. Part 2. Histopathological study of hemorrhagic necrosis. J. Neurosurg. 46:350–357, 1977.

303. Reicvich, M., Jehle, J., Sokoloff, L., et al.: Measurement of regional cerebral blood flow with antipyrine-^{14}C in awake cats. J. Appl. Physiol. 27:296–300, 1969.

304. Reier, P. J., Stensaas, L. J., and Guth, L.: The astrocytic scar as an impediment to regeneration in the central nervous system. In Kao, C. C., Bunge, R. P., and Reier, P. J. (eds.): Spinal Cord Reconstruction. New York, Raven Press, 1983, pp. 163–195.

305. Reir, P. J., Bregman, B. S., and Wujek, J. R.: Intraspinal transplantation of embryonic spinal cord tissue in neuronal and adult rats. J. Comp. Neurol. 247:275–296, 1986.

306. Richardson, P. M., Issa, V. M. K., and Aguayo, A. J.: Regeneration of long spinal axons in the rat. J. Neurocytol. 13:165–182, 1984.

307. Richardson, P. M., McGuinness, U. M., and Aguayo, A. J.: Axons from CNS neurons regenerate into PNS grafts. Nature 284:264–265, 1980.

308. Rigamonti, D. D., Mena, H., Long, J. B., et al.: Percussive injury to the rat spinal cord: A model of axonal damage. Soc. Neurosci. Abs. 14:620, 1988.

309. Rivlin, A. S., and Tator, C. H.: Objective clinical assessment of motor function after experimental spinal cord injury in the rat. J. Neurosurg. 47:577–581, 1977.

310. Rivlin, A. S., and Tator, C. H.: Effect of duration of acute spinal cord compression in a new acute cord injury model in the rat. Surg. Neurol. 9:39–43, 1978.

311. Rivlin, A. S., and Tator, C. H.: Regional spinal cord blood flow in rats after severe cord trauma. J. Neurosurg. 49:844–853, 1978.

312. Roisen, F. J., Bartfeld, H., Nagele, R., and Yorke, G.: Ganglioside stimulation of axonal sprouting in vitro. Science 214:577–578, 1981.

313. Rosenthal, M., Lamanna, J., Yamada, S., et al.: Oxidative metabolism, extracellular potassium, and sustained potential shifts in cat spinal cord in situ. Brain Res. 162:113–127, 1979.

314. Rosomoff, H. L., and Gilbert, R.: Brain volume and cerebrospinal fluid pressure during hypothermia. Am. J. Physiol. 183:19–22, 1955.

315. Rosomoff, H. L., and Holaday, D. A.: Cerebral blood flow and cerebral oxygen consumption during hypothermia. Am. J. Physiol. 179:85–88, 1954.

316. Ross, I. B., and Tator, C. H.: Spinal cord blood flow and evoked potential responses after treatment with nimodipine or methylprednisolone in spinal cord–injured rats. Neurosurgery 33:470–476, 1993.

317. Ross, I. B., Tator, C. H., and Theriault, E.: Effect of nimodipine or methylprednisolone on recovery from acute experimental spinal cord injury in rats. Surg. Neurol. 40:461–470, 1993.

318. Rothman, S. M., and Olney, J. W.: Excitotoxicity and the NMDA receptor. Trends Neurol. Sci. 10:299–302, 1987.

319. Rothman, S. M., and Olney, J. W.: Glutamate and the pathophysiology of hypoxic-ischemic brain damage. Ann. Neurol. 19:105–111, 1988.

320. Roussy, G., Lhermitte, J., and Cornil, L.: Etude expérimentale des lésions commotionnelles de la moella épinière. Ann. Méd. 8:335–353, 1920.

321. Rucker, N. C., Lumb, W. V., and Scott, R. J.: Combined pharmacologic and surgical treatments for acute spinal cord trauma. Am. J. Vet. Res. 42:1138–1142, 1981.

321a. Sabel, B. A., and Schneider, G. E.: Enhanced sprouting of retinotectal fibers after early superior colliculus lesions in hamsters treated with gangliosides. Exp. Br. Res. 71:365–376, 1988.

322. Sabel, B. A., Del Mastro, R., Dunbar, G. L., and Stein, D. G.: Reduction of anterograde degeneration in brain damaged rats by GM1-gangliosides. Neurosci. Lett. 77:360–366, 1987.

323. Sadrzadeh, S. M., Graf, E., Panter, S. S., et al.: Hemoglobin, a biological Fenton reagent. J. Biol. Chem. 259:14354–14356, 1984.

324. Salzman, S. K., Kelly, G., Chavin, J., et al.: Characterization of mianserin neuroprotection in experimental spinal trauma: Dose/route response and late treatment. J. Pharmacol. Exp. Ther. 269:322–328, 1994.

325. Salzman, S. K., Lee, W. A., Sabato, S., et al.: Halothane anesthesia is neuroprotective in experimental spinal cord injury: Early hemodynamic mechanisms of action. Res. Commun. Chem. Pathol. Pharmacol. 80:59–81, 1993.

326. Sandler, A. N., and Tator, C. H.: Review of the effect of spinal

cord trauma on the vessels and blood flow in the spinal cord. J. Neurosurg. *45*:638–646, 1976.

327. Saruhashi, Y., and Young, W.: Effect of mianserin on locomotory function after thoracic spinal cord hemisection in rats. Exp. Neurol. *129*:207–216, 1994.

328. Saunders, R. D., Dugan, L. L., Demediuk, P., et al.: Effects of methylprednisolone and the combination of alpha tocopherol and selenium on arachidonic acid metabolism and lipid peroxidation in traumatized spinal cord tissue. J. Neurochem. *49*:24–31, 1987.

328a. Schnell, L., and Schwab, M. E.: Axonal regeneration in the rat spinal cord produced by an antibody against myelin-associated neurite growth inhibitors. Nature *343*:269–272, 1990.

329. Schanne, F. A. X., Kane, A. B., Young, E. E., and Farber, J. L.: Calcium dependence of toxic cell death: A final common pathway. Science *206*:700–702, 1979.

330. Schlaepfer, W. W.: Vesicular disruption of myelin simulated by exposure of nerve to calcium ionophore. Nature *265*:734–736, 1977.

331. Schlapfer, W. W.: Nature of mammalian neurofilaments and their breakdown by calcium. *In* Zimmerman, H. M. (ed.): *Progress in Neuropathology*. Vol. 4. New York, Raven Press, 1979, pp.101–123.

332. Schlaepfer, W. W., and Bunge, R. P.: Effects of calcium ion concentration on the degeneration of amputated axons in tissue culture. J. Cell Biol. *59*:456–470, 1973.

333. Schmaus, H.: Beiträge zur pathologischen anatomie der rückenmarkserschütterung. Virchows Arch. *122*:470–495, 1890.

334. Schmidt-Achert, K. M., Askansas, V., and Engel, W. K.: Thyrotropin-releasing hormone enhances choline acetyl transferase and creatine kinase in cultured spinal ventral horn neurons. J. Neurochem. *43*:586–589, 1984.

335. Schnell, L., Schneider, R., Kolbeck, R., et al.: Neurotrophin-3 enhances sprouting of corticospinal tract during development and after adult spinal cord lesion. Nature *367*:170–173, 1994.

336. Selmaj, K. W., Faroog, M., Norton, W. T., et al.: Proliferation of astrocytes in vitro in response to cytokines: A primary role for tumor necrosis factor. J. Immunol. *144*:129–135, 1990.

337. Selmaj, K. W., and Raine, C. S.: Tumor necrosis factor mediates myelin and oligodendrocyte damage in vitro. Ann. Neurol. *23*:339–346, 1988.

338. Senter, H. J., and Venes, J. L.: Altered blood flow and secondary injury in experimental spinal cord trauma. J. Neurosurg. *49*:569–578, 1978.

339. Senter, H. J., and Venes, J. L.: Loss of autoregulation and posttraumatic ischemia following experimental spinal cord trauma. J. Neurosurg. *50*:198–206, 1979.

340. Shiozaki, T., Sugimoto, H., Taneda, M., et al.: Effect of mild hypothermia on uncontrollable intracranial hypertension after severe head injury. J. Neurosurg. *79*:363–368, 1993.

341. Silver, J.: Inhibitory molecules in development and regeneration. J. Neurol. *241*:S22–S24, 1994.

342. Simon, R. P., Griffiths, T., Evans, M. C., et al.: Calcium overload in selectively vulnerable neurons of the hippocampus during and after ischemia: An electron microscopy study in the rat. J. Cereb. Blood Flow Metab. *4*:350–361, 1984.

343. Simon, R. P., Swan, J. H., Griffith, T., and Meldrum, B. S.: Blockade of N-methyl-D-aspartate receptors may protect against ischemic damage in the brain. Science *226*:850–852, 1984.

344. Simpkins, C. O., Alailima, S. T., and Tate, E. A.: Inhibition by naloxone of neutrophil superoxide release: A potentially useful anti-inflammatory effect. Circ. Shock *20*:181–191, 1986.

345. Simpson, S.: Fasciculation and guidance of regenerating central axons by the ependyma. *In* Kao, E., Bunge, R., and Reier, P. (eds.): *Spinal Cord Reconstruction*. New York, Raven Press, 1983, p. 151.

346. Singer, J. M., Russel, G. V., and Coe, J. E.: Changes in evoked potentials after experimental cervical spinal cord injury in the monkey. Exp. Neurol. *29*:449–461, 1970.

347. Smith, A. J. K., McCreery, D. B., Bloedel, J. R., and Chou, S. N.: Hyperemia, CO_2 responsiveness, and autoregulation in the white matter following experimental spinal cord injury. J. Neurosurg. *48*:239–251, 1978.

348. Smith, D. R., Smith, H. J., and Rajjoub, R. K.: Measurement of spinal cord blood flow by the microsphere technique. Neurosurgery *2*:27–30, 1978.

349. Sofroniew, M. V., Pearson, R. C. A., Cuello, A. C., et al.: Parenterally administered GM1 ganglioside prevents retrograde degeneration of the rat basal forebrain. Brain Res. *398*:393–396, 1986.

350. Sperry, R. W.: Optic nerve regeneration with return of vision in anurans. J. Neurophysiol. *7*:57–69, 1944.

351. Spiller, W. G.: A critical summary of recent literature on concussion of the spinal cord with some original observations. Am. J. Med. Sci. *118*:190–198, 1899.

352. Stcherbak, A.: Des altérations de la moella épinière chez le lapin sous l'influence de la vibration intensive: Valeur diagnostique du clonus vibratoire: Contribution a l'étude de la moella épinière. Encephale *2*:521–535, 1907.

353. Steen, P. A., Gisvold, S. E., Milde, J. H., et al.: Nimodipine improves outcome when given after complete cerebral ischemia in primates. Anesthesiology *62*:406–414, 1985.

354. Steen, P. A., Newberg, L. A., Milde, J. H., and Michefelder, J. D.: Nimodipine cerebral blood flow and neurologic recovery after complete global ischemia in the dog. J. Cereb. Blood Flow Metab. *3*:38–43, 1982.

355. Steinberg, G. K., Saleh, J., and Kunis, D.: Delayed treatment with dextromethorphan and dextrorphan reduces cerebral damage after transient focal ischemia. Neurosci. Lett. *89*:193–197, 1988.

356. Stern, M. D.: In vivo evaluation of microcirculation by coherent light scattering. Nature *254*:56–58, 1975.

357. Stevens, C. W., and Yaksh, T. L.: Dynorphin A and related peptides administered intrathecally in the rat: A search for putative kappa opiate receptor activity. J. Pharmacol. Exp. Ther. *238*:833–838, 1986.

358. Stokes, B. T., Fox, P., and Hollinden, G.: Extracellular metabolites: Their measurement and role in the acute phase of spinal cord injury. *In* Dacey, R. G., Jr., Winn, H. R., Rimmel, R. W., and Jane, J. A. (eds.): *Trauma of the Central Nervous System*. New York, Raven Press, 1985, pp. 309–323.

359. Stokes, B. T., and Garwood, M.: Traumatically induced alterations in the oxygen fields in the canine spinal cord. Exp. Neurol. *75*:665–677, 1982.

360. Studer, R. K., Welch, D. M., and Siegel, B. A.: Transient alteration of the blood-brain barrier: Effect of hypertonic solutions administered via carotid artery injection. Exp. Neurol. *44*:266–273, 1974.

361. Tanaka, K., Dora, E., Urbanics, R., et al.: Effect of the ganglioside GM1, on cerebral metabolism, microcirculation, recovery kinetics of EcoG and histology, during the recovery period following focal ischemia in cats. Stroke *17*:1170–1178, 1986.

362. Tarlov, I. M.: *Spinal Cord Compression: Mechanism of Paralysis and Treatment*. Springfield, IL, Thomas, 1957.

363. Tarlov, I. M., Klinger, H., and Vitale, S.: Spinal cord compression studies. I. Experimental techniques to produce acute and gradual compression in dogs. Arch. Neurol. Psychiatry *70*:813–819, 1953.

364. Tator, C. H.: Acute spinal cord injury in primates produced by an inflatable extradural cuff. Can. J. Surg. *16*:222–231, 1972.

365. Tator, C. H.: Spine–spinal cord relationships in spinal cord trauma. *In Clinical Neurosurgery*. Baltimore, Williams & Wilkins, 1982, pp. 479–494.

365a. Tator, C. H., and van der Jagt, R. H.: The effect of exogenous thyroid hormones on functional recovery of the rat after acute spinal cord compression injury. J. Neurosurg. *53*:381–384, 1980.

366. Tessler, A., Hiones, B., Houle, J., and Reier, P.: Regeneration of adult dorsal root axons into transplants of embryonic spinal cord. J. Comp. Neurol. *270*:537–548, 1988.

367. Tracey, K. J.: Tumor necrosis factor. *In* Thomson, A. W. (ed.): *The Cytokine Handbook*. 2nd ed. New York, Academic Press, 1994, pp. 289–304.

368. Tuszynski, M. H., Gabriel, K., Gage, F. H., et al.: Nerve growth factor delivery by gene transfer induces differential outgrowth of sensory, motor, and noradrenergic neurites after adult spinal cord injury. Exp. Neurol. *137*:157–173, 1996.

369. Van Neuten, J. M., Wauquier, A., De Clerk, F., and Van Reempts, J.: Vascular reactivity of selective calcium-entry blockers. *In* Lenzi, S., and Descovich, G. C. (eds.): *Atherosclerosis and Cardiovascular Disease*. Boston, MTP Press Ltd., 1984, pp. 93–105.

370. Vidal-Sanz, M., Bray, G. M., Villegas-Perez, M. P., et al.: Axonal regeneration and synapse formation in the superior colliculus by retinal ganglion cells in the adult rat. J. Neurosci. 7:2894–2909, 1987.

371. Vyklicky, L., and Sykova, E.: The effects of increased extracellular potassium in the isolated spinal cord on the flexor reflex of the frog. Neurosci. Lett. 19:203–207, 1975.

372. Wagner, F. C., Dohrmann, G. J., and Bucy, P. C.: Histopathology of transitory traumatic paraplegia in the monkey. J. Neurosurg. 35:272–276, 1971.

373. Wagner, F. C., Jr., VanGilder, J. C., and Dohrmann, G. J.: Pathological changes from acute to chronic in experimental spinal cord trauma. J. Neurosurg. 48:92–98, 1978.

374. Wagner, F. C., Jr., and Stewart, W. B.: Effect of trauma dose on spinal cord edema. J. Neurosurg. 54:802–806, 1981.

375. Walker, J. G., Yates, R. R., O'Neill, J. J., and Yashon, D.: Canine spinal cord energy state after experimental trauma. J. Neurochem. 29:929–932, 1977.

376. Walker, J. G., Yates, R. R., and Yashon, D.: Regional canine spinal cord energy state after experimental trauma. J. Neurochem. 33:397–401, 1979.

376a. Wallace, M. C., and Tator, C. H.: Failure of blood transfusion or naloxone to improve clinical recovery after experimental spinal cord injury. Neurosurgery 19:489–494, 1986.

377. Wang, C. X., Nuttin, B., Heremans, H., et al.: Production of tumor necrosis factor in spinal cord following traumatic injury in rats. J. Neuroimmunol. 69:151–156, 1996.

378. Watson, B. A.: An experimental study of lesions arising from severe concussions. Zentralbl. Allgem. Pathol. 2:74, 1891.

379. Watson, B. D., Busto, R., Goldberg, W., et al.: Lipid peroxidation in vivo induced by reversible global ischemia in rat brain. J. Neurochem. 42:268–274, 1984.

380. Watson, B. D., Prado, R., Dietrich, W. D., et al.: Photochemically induced spinal cord injury in the rat. Brain Res. 367:296–300, 1986.

381. Windle, W.: Regeneration in the Central Nervous System. Springfield, Il, Thomas, 1955.

382. Windle, W. F., Smart, J. O., and Beers, J. J.: Residual function after subtotal spinal cord transection in adult cats. Neurology 8:518–521, 1958.

383. Wolman, L.: The disturbance of circulation in traumatic paraplegia in acute and late stages: A pathological study. Paraplegia 2:213–226, 1965.

384. Wong, E. H., Knight, A. R., and Woodruff, G. N.: [³H]MK-801 labels a site on the N-methyl-D-aspartate receptor channel complex in rat membrane. J. Neurochem. 50:274–281, 1988.

385. Woodbury, D. M., and Vernadakis, A.: Effects of steroids on the central nervous system. Methods Horm. Res. 5:1–56, 1966.

386. Wrathall, J. D., Rigamonti, D. D., Braford, M. R., and Kao, C. C.: Reconstruction of the contused cat spinal cord by the delayed nerve graft technique and cultured peripheral non-neuronal cells. Acta Neuropathol. (Berl.) 57:59–69, 1982.

387. Wrathall, J. R., Bouzoukis, J., and Choiniere, D.: Effect of kynurenate on functional deficits resulting from traumatic spinal cord injury. Eur. J. Pharmacol. 218:273–281, 1992.

388. Wrathall, J. R., Choiniere, D., and Teng, Y. D.: Dose-dependent reduction of tissue loss and functional impairment after spinal cord trauma with the AMPA/kainate antagonist NBQX. J. Neurosci. 14:6598–6607, 1994.

389. Wrathall, J. R., Pettegrew, R. K., and Harvey, F.: Spinal cord contusion in the rat: Production of graded, reproducible, injury groups. Exp. Neurol. 88:108–122, 1985.

390. Wrathall, J. R., Teng, Y. D., and Choiniere, D.: Amelioration of functional deficits from spinal cord trauma with systemically administered NBQX, an antagonist of non-N-methyl-D-aspartate receptors. Exp. Neurol. 137:119–126, 1996.

391. Wrathall, J. R., Teng, Y. D., Choiniere, D., and Mundt, D. J.: Evidence that local non-NMDA receptors contribute to functional deficits in contusive spinal cord injury. Brain Res. 586:140–143, 1992.

392. Xu, X. M., Guenard, V., and Kleitman, N.: Methylprednisolone and neurotrophin treated rat/rat syngeneic transplants. J. Comp. Neurol. 351:145–160, 1995.

393. Yakovlev, A. G., and Faden, A. I.: Sequential expression of c-fos protooncogene, TNF-alpha, and dynorphin genes in spinal cord following experimental traumatic injury. Mol. Chem. Neuropathol. 23:179–190, 1994.

394. Yamada, S., Sanders, D., and Maeda, G.: Oxidative metabolism during and following spinal cord ischemia. Neurol. Res. 3:1–16, 1981.

395. Yashon, D., Bingham, G., Jr., Faddoul, E., and Hint, W. E.: Edema of the spinal cord following experimental impact trauma. J. Neurosurg. 38:693–697, 1973.

396. Yoshida, S., Abe, K., Busto, R., et al.: Influence of transient ischemia on lipid soluble antioxidants, free fatty acids and energy metabolites in the rat brain. Brain Res. 245:307–316, 1982.

397. Young, W.: Blood flow, metabolic and neurophysiological mechanisms in spinal cord injury. In Becker, P. B., and Povlishock, J. T. (eds.): Central Nervous System Trauma Report. Bethesda, National Institute of Neurological and Communicative Disorders and Stroke, National Institutes of Health, 1985, pp. 463–473.

398. Young, W., and Flamm, E. S.: Effect of high dose corticosteroid therapy on blood flow, evoked potentials, and extracellular calcium in experimental spinal injury. J. Neurosurg. 57:667–673, 1982.

399. Young, W., Flamm, E. S., Demopoulos, H. B., et al.: Effect of naloxone on posttraumatic ischemia in experimental spinal contusion. J. Neurosurg. 55:209–219, 1981.

400. Young, W., and Koreh, I.: Potassium and calcium changes in injured spinal cords. Brain Res. 365:42–53, 1986.

401. Young, W., Koreh, I., Yen, V., and Lindsay, A.: Effect of sympathectomy on extracellular potassium activity and blood flow in experimental spinal cord contusion. Brain Res. 253:115–125, 1982.

402. Young, W., Tomasula, J. J., Decrescito, V., et al.: Vestibulospinal monitoring in experimental spinal trauma. J. Neurosurg. 52:64–72, 1980.

403. Young, W., Yen, V., and Blight, A. R.: Extracellular calcium activity in experimental spinal cord contusion. Brain Res. 253:115–125, 1982.

404. Zimmerman, A. N. E.: Paradoxical influence of calcium ions on the permeability of the cell membranes of the isolated rat heart. Nature 211:646–647, 1966.

405. Zimmerman, A. N. E., Daems, W., Hülsmann, W. C., et al.: Morphological changes of heart muscle caused by successive perfusion with calcium-free and calcium-containing solutions (calcium paradox). Cardiovasc. Res. 1:201–209, 1967.

406. Zivin, J. A., and Degirolami, V.: Spinal cord infarction: A highly reproducible stroke model. Stroke 11:200–204, 1980.

407. Zivin, J. A., Doppman, J. L., Reid, J. L., et al.: Biochemical and histochemical studies of biogenic amines in spinal cord trauma. Neurology 26:99–107, 1976.

Afflictions of the Vertebra

38

Tumors of the Spine

Robert F. McLain, M.D.

James N. Weinstein, D.O., M.S.

The treatment of spinal column tumors has changed dramatically over the past three decades and continues to evolve rapidly. Improved systemic therapy, more sophisticated preoperative evaluation and staging, the availability of new surgical implants and biomaterials, and a more aggressive surgical approach have led to improvements in both the short- and long-term outcomes for patients with spinal tumors. Unfortunately, there is currently no uniform approach to treatment in these patients and little uniformity in reporting outcome measures. This makes direct comparison of treatment protocols difficult and conclusions regarding definitive management somewhat tenuous. In appropriately selected patients, however, surgical treatment now offers a reasonable likelihood of functional improvement, pain relief, and, in some cases, cure of the disease.

Because of the opportunity to provide patients with such significant improvement, it is imperative that treating physicians appreciate the symptoms and characteristics of spinal neoplasia and that the principles of tumor staging and management be followed closely whenever such a lesion is suspected. As in extremity surgery, biopsy should be planned with definitive surgery in mind and carried out by the surgeon who will ultimately deliver that treatment. The goals of treatment are to obtain a definitive diagnosis through biopsy or primary excision, to institute appropriate surgical or medical treatment according to tumor type and the patient's condition at presentation, to preserve neurologic function, and to maintain spinal column stability. Although patients with spinal tumors must be treated as individuals, we can outline general principles for managing specific tumor types in order to meet these goals.

GENERAL INFORMATION

Neoplastic disease of the spine may arise from local lesions developing within or adjacent to the spinal column or from distant malignancies spreading to the spine or paraspinous tissues by hematogenous or lymphatic routes. Local involvement of the spine may result from primary tumors of bone, primary lesions arising in the spinal cord or its coverings, or contiguous spread of tumors of the paraspinous soft tissues and lymphatics. Regional or distant spread of metastatic disease to the spine may occur with almost any of the solid tumors of the body, with osseous malignancies of the appendicular skeleton, and with systemic lymphoreticular malignancies such as multiple myeloma and lymphoma. The likelihood that any one of these tumors will account for any given lesion depends on intrinsic patient-related and tumor-related characteristics. Understanding these relationships allows the surgeon faced with an unknown spinal lesion to formulate a useful differential diagnosis and appropriately direct subsequent examinations. Such a directed approach allows the physician to quickly establish a definitive diagnosis and treatment plan.

Incidence

Although both metastatic and primary tumors can be found in all age groups and at all levels of the spinal column, metastatic tumors are far more common than primary lesions. Metastatic carcinoma accounts for skeletal lesions in 40 times as many patients as are affected by all other forms of bone cancer combined.[66] It has been estimated that between 50 and 70 percent of patients with carcinoma will develop skeletal metastases prior to death, and this number may be as high as 85 percent for women with breast carcinoma.[75] Primary tumors of the spine are very rare, and for the most part, their relative incidence reflects that of the skeleton in general. Certain tumors (chordoma, osteoblastoma) show a predilection for the spinal column, but these still make up a very small proportion of all spinal tumors.

Presentation

The interval between the onset of symptoms and presentation to the physician has both diagnostic and prognostic significance. Although tumors of the spinal column may remain asymptomatic for some time, when symptoms do develop, they are usually a consequence of one or more of the following: (1) expansion of the cortex of the vertebral body by tumor mass, with fracture and invasion of paravertebral soft tissues; (2) compression or invasion of adjacent nerve roots; (3) pathologic fracture owing to vertebral destruction; (4) development of spinal instability; and (5) compression of the spinal cord.[64] Obviously, rapidly progressive symptoms of pain or neurologic compromise are associated with the more malignant, rapidly destructive tumors. Patients who present with symptoms that have gradually progressed over the years typically have slow-growing tumors with a better long-term prognosis. The caveat to this point is that slowly growing, locally aggressive tumors that might be easily managed in the extremities may prove inexorable and lethal when extensively established in the spine.

Age

The age of the patient at diagnosis is an important prognosticator, in that age is highly correlated with malignancy in both primary and metastatic disease. The relationship between age and metastatic disease is well known, as most carcinomas demonstrate a peak incidence in the fourth, fifth, and sixth decades. Systemic diseases such as myeloma and lymphoma are also predominant in the fifth, and sixth decades. Primary spinal neoplasms also show a strong correlation between age and malignancy, though the break point is somewhat lower. In patients older than 21 years of age, over 70 percent of primary tumors prove to be malignant, whereas benign lesions produce the majority of lesions in patients under 21.[169] Clearly, in a patient presenting in middle age with an undiagnosed lesion of the spine, the suspicion of malignancy must be very high.

Location

Location of the lesion within the vertebra is another important prognosticator for benign or malignant disease. The majority of malignant tumors, both primary and metastatic, originate anteriorly, involving the vertebral body and possibly one or both pedicles. Strictly posterior localization, even when more than one level is involved, is far more typical of benign lesions.

DIAGNOSIS

The clinical presentation usually provides clues that alert the physician to the presence of a spinal neoplasm. In a review of 82 primary neoplasms of the spine, pain and weakness were the most common presenting complaints (Table 38–1); pain was present in nearly 85 percent of these patients, including 10 percent who reported radicular symptoms.[169] At the time of initial evaluation, over 40 percent of patients had subjective complaints of weakness, and objective neurologic deficits could be identified in 35 percent of patients with benign tumors and 55 percent of those with malignancies. A palpable mass was detectable in only 16 percent of patients.

Symptoms

The most consistent complaint of patients presenting with spinal column neoplasia is pain. Although back pain is an exceedingly common and nonspecific complaint, pain associated with neoplasia tends to be progressive and unrelenting and does not have such a close association with activity as does mechanical back pain. Pain at night is particularly worrisome. Pain symptoms may localize to a specific spinal segment and may be reproduced by pressure or percussion over the involved segment. Radicular symptoms are less common but are frequently seen in patients with cervical or lumbar involvement. Radicular pain in the tho-

Table 38–1. SYMPTOMS AND SYMPTOM COMPLEXES IN PATIENTS PRESENTING WITH NEOPLASTIC SPINAL DISEASE

Presenting Symptom	Number of Patients	Percentage
Pain (localized or radicular)	69	84.0
Back pain	25	30.5
Radicular pain	8	10.0
Pain and weakness	28	28.0
Pain and mass	9	11.0
Pain and autonomic dysfunction	4	5.0
Weakness	34	41.5
Weakness	7	8.5
Weakness and pain	23	28.0
Mass	13	16.0
Mass	4	5.0
Mass and pain	9	11.0
Asymptomatic	2	2.5

racic region may result in "girdle" pain forming a belt of dysesthesias and paresthesias circumferentially from the level of vertebral involvement.

Pain usually arises from one of several causes. Local tumor growth may expand the cortex of the vertebral body, resulting first in thinning and remodeling of the cortex and later in pathologic fracture and invasion of paravertebral soft tissues. As the cortex expands, the overlying periosteum is distorted and stretched, stimulating pain receptors in that tissue. Local tumor extension from a paravertebral mass or following fracture may compress or invade adjacent nerve roots, resulting in radicular symptoms of pain or paresthesias. Pathologic fracture resulting from extensive vertebral body destruction may produce acute pain symptoms similar to those seen in traumatic compression fractures. Fractures may also produce mechanical instability and subsequent pain. Finally, any of these causes of back pain may be associated with acute or chronic compression of the spinal cord, resulting in focal and radicular symptoms of pain, paraparesis, or paraplegia.[64]

Radicular symptoms similar to those seen in herniated nucleus pulposus may be caused by either benign or malignant spinal tumors, leading to confusion in diagnosis and treatment. In reviewing 38 cases of bone tumors simulating lumbar disc herniation, Sim and colleagues identified 23 patients with lumbar or sacral neoplasm and noted that the pain associated with these lesions was usually unremitting and progressive and was not relieved by rest or recumbency.[147]

Spinal deformity may be associated with the onset of pain and usually results from paraspinous muscular spasm. Scoliosis is sometimes associated with osteoid osteoma or osteoblastoma and typically presents with localized paravertebral pain, paravertebral muscle spasm, and limitation of motion. The onset of such a scoliosis may be rapid. The tumor is found on the concave side of the deformity and usually at the apex of the curve.[80] Although these deformities are usually correctable early in the process, curves neglected for prolonged periods will become structural. The bone scan is highly sensitive to osteoid osteoma and can significantly improve the efficiency of treatment by providing an earlier diagnosis and accurate localization of the tumor.[121]

Neurologic deficits are fairly common in patients presenting with spinal tumors; they are most common in rapidly expanding malignant lesions, but any slowly progressive, expansile neoplasm may produce a deficit if left alone long enough. Weakness, usually in the lower extremities, may become apparent months or years after the onset of pain and is rarely the first symptom seen. Nonetheless, as many as 70 percent of patients manifest clinical weakness by the time the correct diagnosis is made. To avoid this complication, the clinician should maintain a high index of suspicion in patients with persistent back or radicular pain, particularly in those with a history of known systemic malignancies.[9, 51, 142]

Bowel and bladder dysfunction may develop prior to diagnosis in as many as half of patients with cord compression.[51] Patients with compression at the level of the conus medullaris may present with isolated sphincter dysfunction, but it is far more common to see associated lower extremity impairments. The neurologic assessment in these patients must be thorough and should include an evaluation of bladder function if any deficits are suspected.

Imaging Techniques

Plain Films

Plain roentgenograms should be the first test whenever a neoplasm is suspected. Anteroposterior (AP) and lateral views of the involved vertebra can provide considerable information about the nature and behavior of the lesion and may be sufficient to identify some characteristic tumor types. Even when the specific tumor type is not implicated, the benign or malignant nature of the lesion may be deduced from the pattern of bony destruction. Geographic patterns of bone destruction suggest a slowly expanding lesion, typically benign; more rapidly growing tumors produce a moth-eaten appearance; and highly malignant, aggressive lesions produce a permeative pattern of destruction.[90] However, as radiographic evidence of bone destruction is not apparent until between 30 and 50 percent of the trabecular bone has been destroyed, early lesions may be hard to detect.[40] Twenty-six percent of patients with spinal metastases have occult lesions undetectable on plain radiographs.[177]

The most classic early sign of vertebral involvement is the "winking owl" sign seen on the AP view. The loss of the pedicle ring unilaterally results from the destruction of the cortex of the pedicle, usually by tumor invading from the vertebral body proper. Vertebral collapse secondary to erosion of bone by tumor is another common radiographic finding. A pathologic compression fracture may be difficult to differentiate from a traumatic injury, particularly in patients with osteoporosis; but a periosteal reaction that seems too old the acute trauma, or the presence of a soft tissue mass or soft tissue calcifications, should alert the physician to obtain more definitive diagnostic tests. Distinguishing neoplastic vertebral destruction from that of pyogenic osteomyelitis may also prove tricky; the differential diagnosis is based on the preservation of the intervertebral disc in patients with neoplasms. The disc is highly resistant to tumor invasion and usually maintains its height even after extensive collapse of the vertebral body. In the presence of infection, the disc is frequently destroyed along with the adjacent vertebral body.[9]

Bone Scan

The most sensitive test for neoplastic disease of the musculoskeletal system is the technetium 99m bone scan. Technetium scans are sensitive to any area of increased osteoid formation and can detect lesions as small as 2 mm, whether in trabecular bone or cortical, provided there is some osteoblastic response in the surrounding bone. When an isolated lesion is detected by scintigraphy, the differential diagnosis must include fracture, infection, neoplasm, or local soft tissue inflammation, and further evaluation with plain films or tomography is necessary to make a diagnosis. Although scans have a high incidence of false-positive findings, their sensitivity makes them a valuable tool in assessing symptomatic patients with negative or equivocal radiographs or as a method of determining the extent of dissemination in those patients with systemic disease.[19, 167] Although bone scans lack specificity, patterns of uptake showing multiple areas of skeletal involvement are virtually diagnostic for metastatic disease in a patient with a known primary malignancy. In patients in whom a primary malignancy has not been identified, such a pattern is still very suggestive and enables the surgeon to choose the most accessible lesion for biopsy. It should be remembered, however, that even in patients with known malignancies, a solitary abnormality on bone scan may prove falsely positive in a third of all cases. The most common source of false-positive scans is osteoarthritis, which is frequently present in the older population most commonly seen with metastatic disease.[26]

Computed Tomography

Computed tomography (CT) offers improved sensitivity in the detection of spinal neoplasms. CT has proved highly sensitive to alterations in bone mineralization and is able to demonstrate neoplastic involvement far more reliably than plain radiographs. Lesions may be visualized at an earlier time in their development, before extensive bony destruction or intramedullary extension has occurred, and before cortical erosion has progressed to the point of impending fracture. However, CT is effective only when the right area is studied; a preliminary bone scan may help identify the correct level for CT scanning, improving the yield in diagnostically difficult cases.

Myelography

Once the only reliable way to assess spinal cord and nerve root compression, myelography has now given way to magnetic resonance imaging (MRI) in most instances. In combination with CT, however, it remains a valuable tool for detecting cord compression owing to fracture and bony impingement. Myelography provides some dynamic information, in that a complete block on myelography conclusively demonstrates pressure on the neural structures, evidence that can only be inferred from MRI. Myelography also may be easier to interpret in patients with complex spinal deformities, multiple operations, or spinal instrumentation. Cerebrospinal fluid removed at the time of examination should be submitted for cytologic examination and determination of protein and glucose levels.

There are drawbacks to myelography. The procedure is invasive and uncomfortable, and it can lead to un-

pleasant and, rarely, life-threatening complications. In cases of complete myelographic block, a second injection of contrast is usually necessary to demonstrate the proximal extent of the tumor. Finally, myelography can only detect lesions that are displacing contents of the spinal canal; tumor contained within the vertebral body is not apparent on myelography.

Magnetic Resonance Imaging

Although myelography was the gold standard for the evaluation of epidural metastases and cord compression in the past, MRI has proved both sensitive and accurate and has largely replaced the older test in spinal diagnosis. MRI has proved useful in evaluating a variety of spinal diseases, and it is well tolerated, noninvasive, and safe. The superior soft tissue contrast provided by MRI and the ability to obtain multiplanar images enhance the surgeon's diagnostic and treatment planning capabilities considerably. MRI provides better delineation of soft tissue tumor extension and adherence or invasion of paravertebral structures than does CT.[105] Direct sagittal and coronal images are far superior to reconstructions available through CT, and MRI can directly depict the spinal cord without the aid of intrathecal contrast material.[52]

Spinal MRI is also more sensitive than bone scanning for some tumor types. Kattapuram and associates recently reported three cases of biopsy-proved spinal metastasis identified on spinal MRI in patients with negative radionuclide bone scans.[79] Because the entire spine is imaged at one sitting, MRI is a practical screening study for spinal disease and should be considered the most sensitive study for neoplasm of the spinal column. Newer techniques such as short T1 inversion recovery (STIR) and fat-suppressed fast spin echo (FSE) may provide valuable information on the character of tumor tissue and help identify the specific tumor type prior to biopsy.

Tumor foci may be sclerotic (low in signal intensity on T1- and T2-weighted images) or lytic (low in signal intensity on T1- and high in intensity on T2-weighted images). In routine spin-echo studies, the low-signal-intensity neoplasm is easily delineated from the normal, high signal intensity of adjacent fatty marrow. Gadolinium-enhanced T1 images generally do not show tumor as well, because the enhanced tumor tissue may be rendered inconspicuous against the background fat signal. STIR and fat-suppressed FSE are approximately equal in their ability to detect marrow lesions, but STIR imaging is more time consuming. When used in concert, fat-suppressed and contrast-enhanced imaging can detect the vast majority of lesions displacing normal marrow, whether focal or diffuse, and can distinguish between pathologic and osteoporotic compression fractures.[4, 53, 126]

Biopsy Techniques

Once the biopsy incision has been made, there are few choices left in planning the definitive tumor removal.

Once an approach for biopsy is selected, the surgeon is committed to that approach. For instance, if a posterolateral incision has been made for the biopsy, tumor excision must be completed through that incision, and the incision must be excised with the tumor; it would not be possible to switch to a posterior approach for the definitive excision without violating several principles of good surgical technique. The importance of a carefully planned biopsy cannot be overemphasized.

The hazards of biopsy in musculoskeletal tumors of the extremities are doubly apparent in the axial skeleton. The incidence of inadequate or inappropriate biopsy that significantly alters a patient's care is greater than one in three overall and is probably higher in lesions of the spine.[97] This risk is reduced significantly when the biopsy is performed by the *treating*, rather than the *referring*, physician.

Three forms of biopsy are available to the surgeon: excisional, incisional, and needle biopsy or aspiration. On occasion, a posterior lesion may prove suitable for an excisional biopsy, but most lesions of the spinal column require either an incisional or a needle biopsy. Needle biopsies are subject to sampling errors and provide a small specimen for evaluation (Fig. 38–1). The primary role of needle biopsy is confirmation—confirmation of metastatic disease, of recurrence of a known lesion, or of sarcomatous histology in an otherwise classic clinicoradiologic presentation of osteosarcoma.[109] Culture results may also be obtained when infection must be ruled out. When the differential diagnosis is narrow and limited to lesions that are easily distinguished histologically, a needle biopsy may be ideal. In more complex lesions and those with a more subtle differential diagnosis, the specimen obtained most often proves inadequate.[150]

The incisional biopsy should be the last step in the staging of the patient, performed just before the definitive surgical resection. Both procedures may be performed under the same anesthetic if proper preoperative staging has been completed and the frozen section provides a clear diagnosis. The surgical technique used during biopsy influences both the yield of the procedure and the risk of postoperative complications. A number of basic principles should be observed when performing the biopsy. The biopsy incision is placed so that it may be excised with the tumor during the definitive procedure. *Transverse incisions must be avoided,* and the tumor is approached in the most direct manner possible. Tissues are handled carefully, and hemostasis is meticulous. Bone is not removed or windowed unless absolutely necessary. Bleeding from exposed bone or from uncauterized vessels and injured muscle will form a postoperative hematoma that may carry tumor cells beyond the margins of the intended excision and contaminate tissues far proximal or distal to the primary lesion. All tissue contaminated during biopsy or by hematoma must be excised if surgical control is expected. Even a moderate-sized hematoma may make this impractical.[150] Once the tumor is exposed, an adequate sample of tissue must be obtained. The specimen obtained should be large enough to allow histologic and ultrastructural analysis, as well as immunologic stains. The margin of the soft tissue mass is most helpful, as central portions are often necrotic. The surgeon should take care not to crush or distort the specimen, so as to maintain its architecture. If a soft tissue component exists, a frozen section should be obtained.

Finally, if the definitive excision is to follow the biopsy under the same anesthetic, it is essential that all instruments used during the biopsy be discarded. The field is redraped, and the surgeons change gowns and

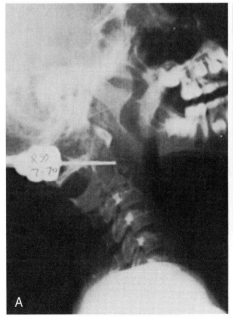
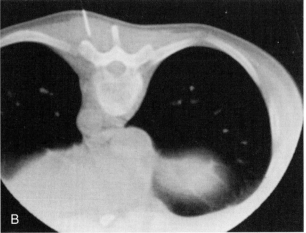

Figure 38–1. *A,* Percutaneous needle biopsy of C2 osteoblastoma. *B,* CT scan–directed needle biopsy of T6 metastatic breast cancer.

gloves before the excision is begun. This same precaution should be followed in obtaining the bone graft for spinal reconstruction.

TUMORS

Primary Tumors of Bone

Primary bone or soft tissue tumors arising in the spine are uncommon. In a review of 82 primary neoplasms of the spine seen over a 50-year period at one center, 31 benign and 51 malignant lesions were identified, representing eight benign and nine malignant tumor types (Fig. 38–2). Seventy-five percent of tumors found in the vertebral body were malignant, compared with only 35 percent of those in the posterior elements. In patients older than 18 years, 80 percent of primary tumors proved to be malignant; in children and adolescents only 32 percent of lesions were malignant. The five-year survival in this series was 86 percent in patients with benign tumors and 24 percent in patients with malignancies.[169] Bohlman's review of 23 patients with primary neoplasms of the cervical spine also showed a marked difference in tumor type with patient age. In that series, all patients younger than 21 years old had benign tumors, whereas 10 of 14 patients (71 percent) over 21 had malignancies.[10]

Benign

Osteochondroma. Multiple osteochondromatosis is the most common of the skeletal dysplasias, and osteochondromas, either single or multiple, are among the most common lesions of bone encountered.[95, 118] Vertebral involvement occurs in approximately 7 percent of these patients, but neurologic compromise is rarely seen.[92] When symptoms of cord compression do occur, routine imaging studies may not be adequate. Tomography outlines the bony lesion and establishes its point of origin, but the radiolucent cartilage cap that causes the compressive symptoms may not be visualized without myelography or MRI. In 16 cases of osteochondroma with symptomatic cord compression, over 60 percent of lesions arose in the cervical spine, and another 19 percent arose in the thoracic spine at or above the T6 level.[18, 78, 95, 149] Although 14 patients (88 percent) experienced good neurologic recovery following decompression, the other two died because of cervical cord compression and respiratory failure. One experienced sudden death from an odontoid lesion, and the other had symptoms of compression months before expiring from C1 compression by a lesion of the foramen magnum. Because of the very slow progression of the compressive cord lesion, excision of the tumor, en bloc or piecemeal, provides excellent recovery of neurologic function, with little likelihood of recurrence (Fig. 38–3).

Osteoblastoma and Osteoid Osteoma. Osteoblastoma and osteoid osteoma are osteoblastic lesions differentiated primarily by size. These benign lesions show a propensity for spinal involvement, usually involving the posterior elements. In one review of 36 patients with osteoid osteoma, nine lesions (25 percent) occurred in the spine, all located in the posterior elements.[80] Osteoblastoma shows an even greater propensity for the spine. In a review of 197 osteoblastomas, Marsh and coworkers noted that 41 percent were located within the spine and that these lesions always originated in the posterior elements.[99] Patients usually

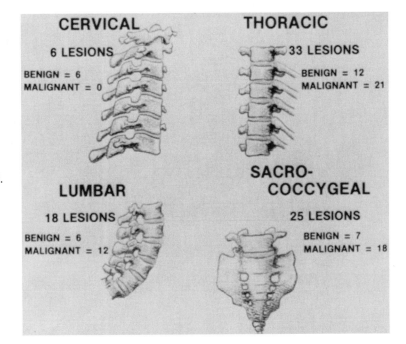

Figure 38–2. Primary spine tumors by vertebral level.

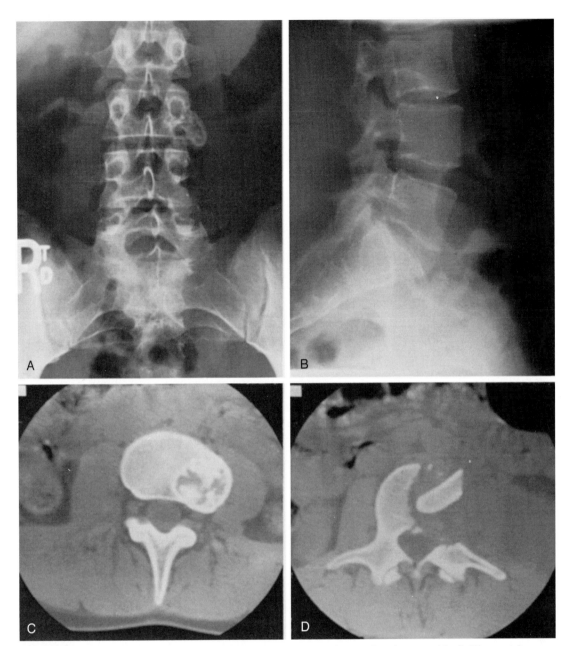

Figure 38–3. *A, B,* Anteroposterior and lateral radiographs of osteochondroma at L3. *C,* CT scan of osteochondroma at L3. *D,* CT scan after en bloc anterior resection and strut-craft reconstruction.

present in the second or third decade of life, and the most common complaint is back pain. The pain is typically persistent and unrelated to activity and is often most noticeable at night. Although aspirin classically provides dramatic relief of symptoms, this is not universal. Lack of a response to aspirin does not rule out the diagnosis.

Radiographic demonstration of osteoid osteoma is difficult (Fig. 38–4). The lesion, by definition less than 2 cm in diameter, is easily obscured among the overlapping shadows of the vertebral column. CT demonstrates the lesion very well, but if the cuts are at the wrong level or too wide, the tumor may be missed

completely. The most sensitive method of locating an osteoid osteoma is by bone scan. The technetium bone scan provides accurate localization of the lesion, decreasing the average duration of symptoms by providing an early diagnosis and allowing prompt treatment.[121] Osteoblastomas become considerably larger than osteoid osteomas and may be quite apparent on plain radiographs (Fig. 38–5). The lesion is characterized radiographically by the expansion of the cortical bone, maintaining a thin rim of reactive bone between the lesion and the surrounding soft tissue. There is often a rim of reactive bone separating the tumor from the rest of the medullary bone. Although the tumor

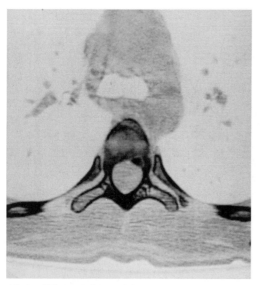

Figure 38–4. CT scan of osteoid osteoma at T4. Plain radiographs were interpreted as negative.

may show stippling in some cases, there is rarely if ever a lobulated or soap-bubble appearance to these lesions.[99] When there is involvement of the vertebral body, it is limited and results from extension of tumor into the body from the pedicle.

Although benign, either of these lesions can produce significant spinal deformity. In Marsh's review, scoliosis was present in approximately 50 percent of the

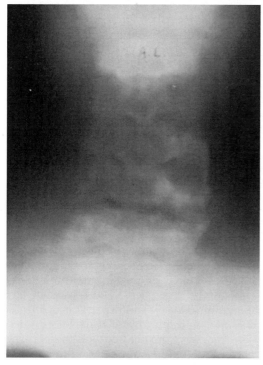

Figure 38–5. Tomogram of osteoblastoma at C5.

patients whose tumors arose from the thoracolumbar spine or from the ribs.[99] Pettine and Klassen reported that of 41 patients with osteoid osteoma or osteoblastoma of the spine, 63 percent had a significant scoliosis. Nearly all patients in that series had improvement or resolution of their scoliosis when the tumor was removed within 15 months of the onset of symptoms, but only one of 11 had any improvement when symptoms had been present for more than 15 months.[121] Ransford and colleagues saw similar results in 15 patients with scoliosis but noted that skeletally mature patients did not develop a structural scoliosis even when the duration of symptoms was more than two years.[127]

The treatment for either of these lesions is excision (Fig. 38–6). Excision provides reliable pain relief, and the spinal deformity is improved or disappears in the majority of patients.[80] Although a complete excision is desirable, it is not always feasible in the spine. Curettage and bone grafting of vertebral osteoblastomas have provided satisfactory long-term results in the vast majority of cases.[58, 99] Some authors advocate instrumentation and posterior spine fusion for large scoliotic curves present for two years or more, but this need not be done at the time of excision.[1]

Aneurysmal Bone Cyst. Aneurysmal bone cysts (ABCs) involving the spine are very rare lesions. They are most common in the lumbar spine and involve the posterior elements approximately 60 percent of the time (Fig. 38–7). These lesions have a tendency to involve adjacent vertebrae and may involve three or more vertebrae in sequence. Radiographs typically demonstrate an expansile, osteolytic cavity with strands of bone forming a bubbly appearance. The cortex is often eggshell thin and blown out. When total excision is not feasible, curettage provides a high rate

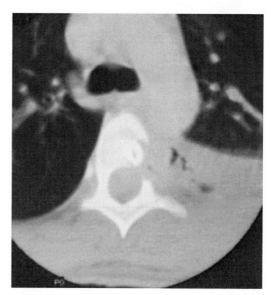

Figure 38–6. CT scan of the T4 osteoid osteoma in Figure 38–4, after resection and rib grafting.

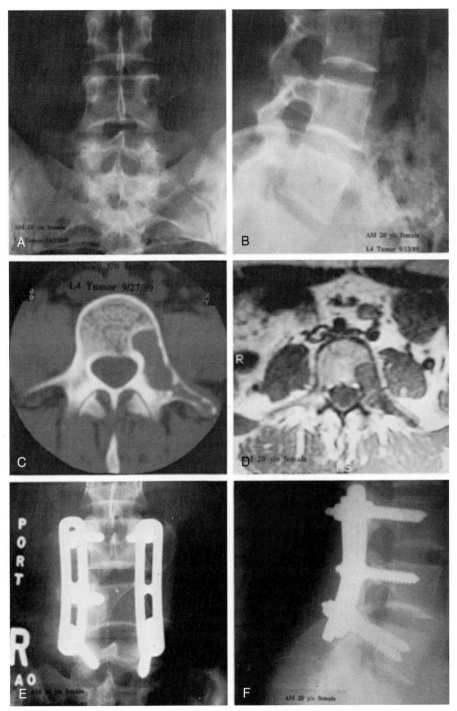

Figure 38–7. *A, B,* Plain anteroposterior and lateral radiographs of L4 tumor involving the left L4 transverse process and pedicle. Diagnosis was osteoblastoma/aneurysmal bone cyst (solid). *C, D,* Preoperative CT and MRI scans of lesion. *E, F,* Anteroposterior and lateral radiographs after resection of tumor involving Zones II, III, and IVA (see Fig. 38–13).

of cure. Recurrence developed in 13 percent of cases in Hay's review, but these were all successfully treated by a second curettage or excision.[68]

Hemangioma.   Vertebral hemangiomas are common lesions, occurring in approximately 10 percent of all patients, but they are rarely symptomatic or of clinical importance. Reports of deformity or pain associated with vertebral hemangiomas are uncommon, but cases of nerve root and cord compression have been documented (Fig. 38–8). The diagnosis of vertebral body hemangioma can usually be made on plain radiographs, although CT imaging provides more information about cord impingement or fracture. Plain films classically show prominent vertical striations produced by the abnormally thickened trabeculae of the involved vertebral body. These lesions are radiosensitive and frequently respond to radiotherapy alone. When cord compression develops and surgical treatment is considered, angiography is indicated to establish the vascular source for the tumor, to identify the primary vascular supply to the cord (the artery of Adamkiewicz), and for consideration of preoperative embolization or operative ligation.[15] Surgical excision may be difficult because of the vascularity of the tumor itself and may be further complicated by a consumptive coagulopathy, occasionally encountered in cavernous hemangiomas.[93]

Giant Cell Tumor.   Although rare reports of malignant giant cell tumors exist, the vast majority of these lesions are slow-growing, locally aggressive tumors that do not metastasize. Spinal involvement is usually seen in patients in their third and fourth decades, and symptoms may exist for many months before the patient sees a physician. Plain radiographs usually demonstrate an area of focal rarefaction, although some have a more geographic lytic appearance and show marginal sclerosis. Giant cell tumors are most commonly found in the vertebral body and may expand the surrounding cortical bone extensively as the tumor enlarges (Fig. 38–9). CT is especially important in the evaluation of these tumors preoperatively, as complete resection is very important to the eradication of local disease. CT is also crucial in the early identification of recurrences and should be used in postoperative follow-up on a routine basis. Complete excision is the treatment of choice and should be attempted whenever feasible. This requires an anterior approach and vertebrectomy, and if an adequate resection can be obtained, radiotherapy is not necessary.

Our experience has been that giant cell tumors involving the spine have a particularly bad prognosis because of their locally invasive nature. Two of five patients in our series died as a result of recurrent and invasive local disease. In our experience, curettage or intralesional resection appears to be contraindicated.[169] Other authors have reported better results in treating these tumors and have even suggested that lesions of the spine are less aggressive than those in the extremities.[30, 134] Prolonged disease-free survivals have

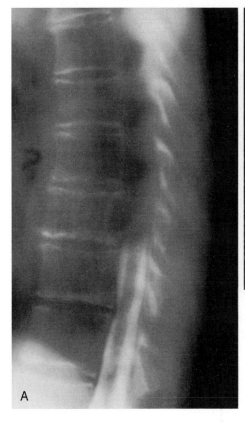
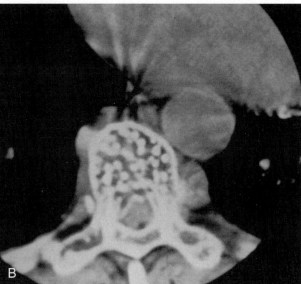

Figure 38–8.   *A,* Lateral thoracic myelogram demonstrating obstruction of contrast flow. The diagnosis was hemangioma of T8 with soft tissue extension. *B,* CT scan T8 hemangioma with extradural extension.

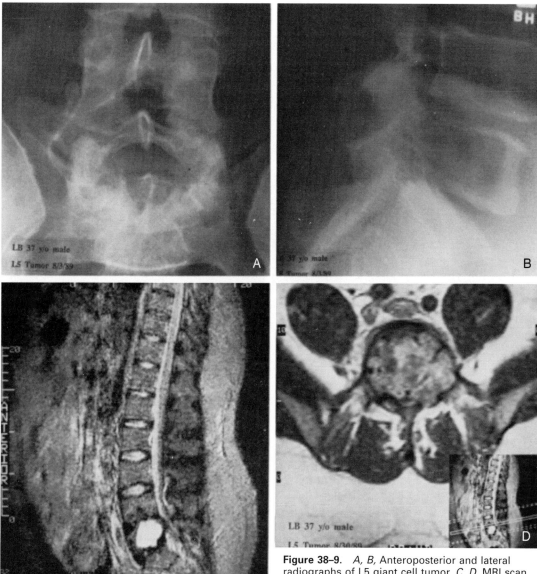

Figure 38–9. *A, B,* Anteroposterior and lateral radiographs of L5 giant cell tumor. *C, D,* MRI scan of the tumor (T2-weighted sagittal and axial images).

been reported following resection or curettage and radiotherapy, although some patients require two or three additional procedures because of local recurrence.[36] With more aggressive surgical resection, radiotherapy is unnecessary, and good disease-free survivals have been obtained without the risks of irradiation[134] (Fig. 38–10).

Stener and Johnsen describe a resection of three adjacent vertebrae in a young woman with a giant cell tumor of the twelfth thoracic vertebra.[154] Resection of such a lesion requires great care to avoid leaving any tissue behind, as recurrence is very common. Lubicky and associates describe a two-stage vertebrectomy for an L4 giant cell tumor, with the anterior vertebrectomy performed one week following laminectomy, biopsy, and posterior stabilization with Harrington rods and

methyl methacrylate. Although the rods did not supply adequate stability, and the anterior iliac crest grafts collapsed into kyphosis, the graft united and the patient had no evidence of recurrence at one year.[94] These reports emphasize the technical demands of vertebrectomy and stabilization required to obtain a disease-free margin in this locally aggressive tumor.

Eosinophilic Granuloma. Eosinophilic granuloma is a benign, self-limited condition that produces focal destruction of bone. A process of unproved etiology, eosinophilic granuloma is most commonly seen in children before the age of 10 years. Lesions of the skull are most common, but any bone may be affected; vertebral involvement occurs in approximately 10 to 15 percent of cases. Spinal involvement can be seen in any of the

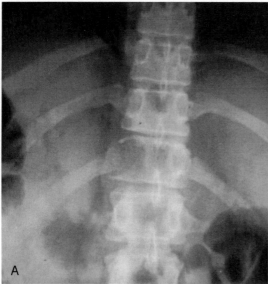

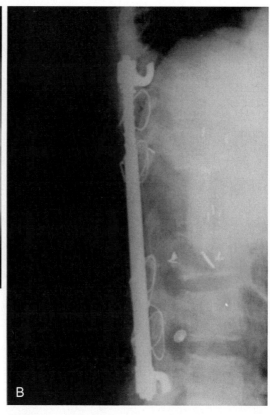

Figure 38–10. *A,* Giant cell tumor T12. *B,* Lateral radiograph five years after total vertebrectomy with no recurrence.

triad of syndromes in which the disease manifests itself: isolated eosinophilic granuloma; the multifocal, chronic, and disseminated form, Hand-Schüller-Christian disease; or the acute disseminated or infantile form, Letterer-Siwe disease.[46, 112] The vertebral body is typically involved, usually in the thoracic or lumbar spine, and the ensuing bony destruction may produce cavitation, partial vertebral collapse, or a classic vertebra plana following complete collapse of the vertebral body (Fig. 38–11). Vertebral collapse produces pain, focal spasm (torticollis is common in cervical lesions), and mild to moderate kyphosis. Neurologic compromise develops in a significant number of patients and may be severe. Neurologic symptoms may develop with or without associated vertebral collapse. If treatment is instituted without delay, recovery of neurologic function is usually excellent.

Early in the disease process, radiographs show a central lytic lesion with poorly defined margins and permeative bone destruction. At this point, the lesion may produce a marked periosteal reaction, and distinguishing it from osteomyelitis or a high-grade sarcoma may be impossible. As the vertebral body collapses and settles, radiographs demonstrate the flattened disc of dense cortical bone retained between the two intact intervertebral discs.[23, 140] This "coin on end" appearance of vertebra plana is a classic finding in eosinophilic granuloma but is not pathognomonic; a similar appearance can be produced by either infection or Ewing's sarcoma. With such a broad differential diagnosis, the

importance of obtaining an adequate biopsy specimen before beginning treatment cannot be overstated. Open biopsy is preferable, to ensure an adequate specimen and to allow definitive treatment at the same procedure.[46, 56, 140]

The treatment of eosinophilic granuloma is somewhat controversial, but it is clear that in many patients the lesions heal without any treatment other than biopsy. Low-dose radiotherapy (500 to 1000 rads) has been advocated in the past, but this may be avoided in most patients. In those who present with a neurologic deficit, the established course of biopsy followed by irradiation and immobilization remains the most widely accepted.[56]

Malignant

Multiple Myeloma and Solitary Plasmacytoma. Most authors today consider multiple myeloma and solitary plasmacytoma to be two manifestations in a continuum of B-cell lymphoproliferative diseases. Because the natural history of these two lesions differs so significantly, the clinical distinction between solitary plasmacytoma and multiple myeloma remains pertinent.

Multiple myeloma is an uncommon neoplastic process, with an incidence of 2 to 3 per 100,000 among the general population. True solitary plasmacytoma is a rare entity, constituting only 3 percent of all plasma cell neoplasms.[27] Patients with solitary and multiple myeloma differ in terms of age and sex distributions

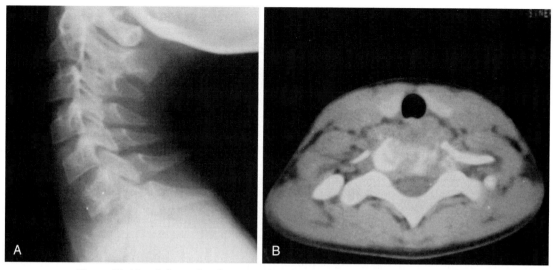

Figure 38–11. *A,* Lateral radiograph of eosinophilic granuloma at C7. *B,* CT scan.

and in terms of survival.[7] Although the course of multiple myeloma is usually rapidly progressive and lethal, patients with solitary plasmacytoma may have prolonged survival, despite eventual progression. The treatment of solitary plasmacytoma must therefore be somewhat different from the treatment of a spinal focus of multiple myeloma.[176] Solitary plasmacytoma is an isolated lesion, the treatment of which may provide long-term disease-free survival or cure. The spinal lesion in multiple myeloma represents a metastasis in a progressive, systemic disease that commonly results in death within two to three years, despite local or systemic treatment. Both the overall survival and the five-year survival in solitary plasmacytoma of the spine are significantly increased when compared with multiple myeloma.[103]

The prognosis for survival of patients with disseminated myeloma is poor, with a five-year survival of 18 percent and a median survival of 24 months. In cases involving the spinal column, the outcome is even worse. Valderrama and Bullough reported that 76 percent of such patients were dead within a year of their diagnosis, and all were dead within four years.[165] The prognosis is significantly improved for patients with solitary plasmacytoma of the spine. Bergsagel and Rider reported a 35 percent disease-free five-year survival for patients with solitary plasmacytoma of bone, with a median survival of 86 months.[8] The five-year disease-free survival in 84 cases of spinal solitary plasmacytoma was roughly 60 percent, with a median survival of 92 months (Table 38–2). Survivals of 20 years and more were seen both in our group and in previous case reports.[81, 136, 169]

The treatment of choice in solitary plasmacytoma and in multiple myeloma is radiation. Because of the radiosensitivity of this tumor, surgical treatment has less influence in determining outcome than it does in other tumor types. Hoping to prevent vertebral body collapse and cord compression, some reviewers have recommended prophylactic laminectomy and stabilization prior to radiotherapy.[91] We have not seen any case of onset or progression of neurologic deficit during radiotherapy and do not recommend surgical intervention unless cord compromise or spinal instability is present. Dissemination of myeloma may occur after many years of disease-free survival, and routine follow-up is indicated for an indefinite period. Serum protein immunoelectrophoresis has proved to be the

Table 38–2. SURVIVAL AND CHARACTERISTICS OF PATIENTS WITH MULTIPLE MYELOMA, SOLITARY PLASMACYTOMA OF BONE, AND SOLITARY PLASMACYTOMA OF THE SPINE

Disease	Percent Male	Age At Pres'n	Disease-Free Interval (Months)	Median Survival (Months)	Five-Year Survival (%)
Multiple myeloma	51	M = 60 F = 61	—	24	18
Solitary plasmacytoma of bone	68	M = 50 F = 55	78	86	35
Solitary plasmacytoma of the spine	74	M = 51 F = 57	76	92	60

most accurate indicator of dissemination and should be followed closely after therapy is introduced. If dissemination does occur, systemic chemotherapy should be instituted.

Osteosarcoma. Approximately 2 percent of all primary osteogenic sarcomas arise in the spine. Treatment of lesions in the spinal column is usually difficult, and the outcome in these tumors has traditionally been very poor. In a review of 27 cases of osteosarcoma of the spine, median survival was 10 months from the time of diagnosis; only seven patients survived more than one year, and one patient survived over five years.[142] Similar results were seen by Barwick and coworkers, who reported a median survival of 6 months for 10 patients.[5]

Vertebral osteosarcoma arises from the anterior elements in more than 95 percent of cases. The radiographic findings include both lytic and sclerotic lesions, with cortical destruction, soft tissue calcification, and collapse in advanced cases. CT demonstrates intraspinal and paraspinal soft tissue masses more clearly, allowing more accurate preoperative planning. Traditionally, therapy has consisted of limited tumor excision and radiotherapy. As noted earlier, the outcomes associated with this approach have been poor. In hopes of improving survival in this and other spinal malignancies, a more aggressive surgical approach has been advocated by some authors.[159, 169] In reviewing treatment results in a larger group of patients, Sundaresan and colleagues reported seven cases undergoing wide resection or vertebral body resection combined with radiotherapy.[159] Three of these patients had died of their disease at a mean follow-up of 11 months after operation, but four others were still alive, and three had no evidence of disease at a mean of 52 months. Although the early indication is that more aggressive management may result in longer survival, longer follow-up is needed before assumptions can be made about our ability to cure these tumors.

Secondary Osteosarcoma. This subgroup of the osteosarcoma tumor type arises secondarily in pagetoid or previously irradiated bone. Patients presenting with secondary osteosarcoma are significantly older than those with primary osteosarcoma; in patients over the age of 60, over 60 percent of cases of osteosarcoma of bone were secondary lesions.[73] The majority of patients with postirradiation sarcoma present in the fourth or fifth decade of life, whereas those with Paget's sarcoma are usually in their sixth. Although secondary lesions account for between 3.6 and 5.5 percent of all intramedullary osteosarcomas,[31, 74] these patients represent approximately 30 percent of all osteosarcomas of the spine.[5, 142]

Most patients with Paget's disease who develop an osteosarcoma have polyostotic disease. Tumors typically arise in diseased, pagetoid bone and progress rapidly. They are aggressive lesions, producing extensive bony destruction and metastasizing early. These lesions are typically very anaplastic. The prognosis for

long-term survival in patients with sarcomatous transformation of Paget's disease is dismal, with less than 5 percent long-term survival.[125]

The association between irradiation and osteosarcoma has been appreciated for many years.[16, 110] Although it has been reported in patients with low levels of radiation exposure, most patients who develop postirradiation sarcoma have received in excess of 5000 rads. Many demonstrate radiographic evidence of radiation osteitis. The majority of these patients were originally irradiated for nonosseous disease—Hodgkin's lymphoma, breast carcinoma, and cervical carcinoma. Of those receiving irradiation for skeletal disease, the most common underlying neoplasms are giant cell tumor and Ewing's sarcoma. The survival in these patients is only slightly better than for those with Paget's; the five-year disease-free survival is approximately 17 percent.

Even though most victims are older, postradiation osteosarcoma has been reported in childhood, occurring in a 14-year-old who had undergone radiation for a cervical astrocytoma and later posterior fusion to correct a progressive scoliosis. This case was typical in the long latency (11 years) between irradiation and presentation of the tumor and in the rapid progression of the lesion, resulting in paraplegia and death three weeks after the onset of symptoms.[38] Sundaresan and associates reported a case of postradiation osteosarcoma occurring in a woman 31 years after treatment for Hodgkin's disease. Progression was rapid, and there was limited response to chemotherapy.[158] Considering the prolonged latency between exposure and the development of disease, patients with a history of irradiation or of Paget's disease warrant added vigilance in the evaluation of acute back pain or spinal pathology.

Ewing's Sarcoma. Approximately 3.5 percent of all Ewing's tumors arise in the spinal column, with the majority originating in the sacrum.[172] Although the prognosis is generally poorer than for those with extremity lesions, long-term survivals have been reported.[131] Neurologic compromise is common in the presentation of either primary or metastatic Ewing's. Pilepich and coworkers reported 22 cases of primary vertebral Ewing's and noted that 14 of these patients had neurologic deficits at the time of diagnosis.[122] The permeative appearance of Ewing's tumors on radiographs can make diagnosis difficult, even in advanced disease, and collapse of the vertebral body may produce a vertebra plana indistinguishable from that seen in eosinophilic granuloma.[123] Metastatic Ewing's sarcoma arising in the spinal epidural space, without bony involvement, is a rare but documented phenomenon.[135, 138] Surgical treatment is indicated for decompression of neural elements and stabilization of the vertebral column, but the treatment of choice for Ewing's sarcoma involves multiagent chemotherapy and high-dose radiotherapy. Although surgical treatment in combination with systemic therapy has improved survival in some extremity lesions, this improvement has not been seen in spinal Ewing's.[156] With current regimens of therapy, excellent local control and encouraging disease-free survivals are obtainable in the spine, although the long-term outlook for most patients remains grim.[82]

Chordoma. Chordoma is a relatively rare malignancy occurring in all age groups but predominantly found in patients in the fifth or sixth decade of life. The tumor arises from remnants of the primitive notochord found in the sacrococcygeal and suboccipital regions of the spine, and occasionally from notochordal rests within the vertebral body in the thoracic or lumbar region.[77, 108] Although this tumor is characterized by its slow but relentless local spread, it is a fully malignant lesion capable of distant metastases. Initial symptoms are usually mild and progress slowly as the tumor expands. Chordomas may reach a considerable size before metastasizing, and symptoms of constipation, urinary frequency, or nerve root compression may appear before patients present to their physician. A firm, fixed presacral mass can usually be palpated on rectal examination.

Patient survival depends on local control of the tumor. Surgical extirpation of the tumor is the only curative procedure, and a wide margin must be obtained (Fig. 38–12). Biopsy should be performed only after all appropriate staging studies have been completed, after which an open biopsy through a direct posterior approach is preferred. The biopsy incision must be excised en bloc with the tumor at the time of the definitive resection. Local recurrence of a chordoma is a grim prognostic sign, dramatically reducing the likelihood of cure. Kaiser and associates found that simply exposing the tumor during resection increased the recurrence rate of this tenacious lesion from 28 to 64

percent.[77] The indicated surgical procedure for sacrococcygeal chordoma is a high sacral amputation, maintaining a cuff of normal tissue over the tumor. Sacral nerve roots are sacrificed as necessary.[153] This radical surgical approach results in surprisingly little morbidity or functional loss if the S2 roots can be spared bilaterally and has provided a significant improvement in survival.[49, 128] Samson and coworkers reported 15 of 21 patients free of disease at a mean of 4.5 years.[133]

Chondrosarcoma. Approximately 10 percent of chondrosarcomas arise in the spinal column.[31] These tumors are slow growing and relatively resistant to radiotherapy and chemotherapy, and because of their tendency to recur locally, lesions of the vertebral column have a relatively poor prognosis. Long-term survivals have been reported in low-grade chondrosarcomas when patients have been treated with repeated local excisions of recurrent disease, but few lesions can be managed this way with any success.[72]

Radiographically, chondrosarcoma has a fairly characteristic appearance. In advanced disease, there is a large area of bone destruction, an associated soft tissue mass, and flocculent calcifications of the soft tissue mass. If there is no soft tissue mass, the vertebral lesion may be primarily lytic, with sclerotic margins and with no mottled calcification.[70] CT scanning is invaluable in demonstrating the extent of the lesion and evaluating cord compromise.

Complete surgical excision is required to cure a patient with chondrosarcoma, and this may be impossible to obtain in a vertebral lesion. Stener described a thoracic vertebrectomy for chondrosarcoma with en bloc excision of the T6–T8 vertebral bodies and a large T7 tumor. This combined anterior and posterior procedure

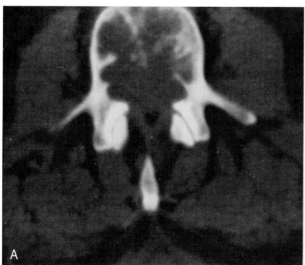
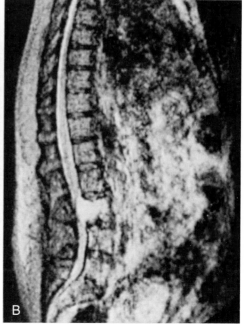

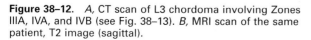
Figure 38–12. *A,* CT scan of L3 chordoma involving Zones IIIA, IVA, and IVB (see Fig. 38–13). *B,* MRI scan of the same patient, T2 image (sagittal).

produced good postoperative stability without evidence of recurrent disease at 15 months.[152]

Lymphoma. Lymphoma may present as a systemic disease with skeletal manifestations or as an isolated bony tumor referred to in the past as a reticulum cell sarcoma. Because the lesion has been considered a metastatic lesion by some authors, it is not consistently included in reviews of primary bone tumors. Whether considered primary or metastatic, lymphomas account for a fair number of spinal neoplasms requiring treatment. Ostrowsky and colleagues reviewed 422 cases of malignant lymphoma involving bone and identified 49 cases of spinal involvement (12 percent). Twenty-one (5 percent) of these appeared to be primary lesions arising in the spine.[115] The thoracic spine was involved in over 60 percent of cases. Patients with lymphoma arising primarily from bone have a distinctly better prognosis than those with disseminated disease that affects bone secondarily.

Treatment of the rare well-localized lesion consists of radiotherapy alone, with 40 Gy delivered to the tumor and 10 Gy to the surrounding nodes.[3] As most lesions include a soft tissue mass, and many are multifocal at the time of diagnosis, adjuvant chemotherapy is often indicated.[34] Surgical treatment is limited primarily to biopsy, cord decompression, or stabilization of pathologic fractures, although some recurrences after radiation treatment may need to be surgically resected.

Metastatic Tumors

Metastases are by far the most common skeletal tumors seen by orthopedists, and the spine is the most common site of skeletal involvement.[31, 66] Skeletal metastases are produced by almost all forms of malignant disease but are most often secondary to carcinomas of the breast, lung, or prostate and less frequently from renal, thyroid, or gastrointestinal carcinomas (Table 38–3).[9, 20, 55, 59, 64, 104, 106, 107] Breast cancer is the most common source of bony metastasis; between 65 and 85 percent of women with breast cancer develop skeletal disease prior to death.[75, 166] Among men, bronchogenic and prostatic carcinomas are the most common causes of bony metastases. Multiple myeloma and lymphoma

Table 38–3. LOCATION OF PRIMARY NEOPLASMS PRODUCING METASTATIC LESIONS OF BONE: A REVIEW OF 5006 CASES

Primary Site	Number	Percentage
Breast	2020	40
Lung	646	13
Prostate	296	6
Kidney	284	6
Gastrointestinal tract	255	5
Thyroid	110	2
Bladder	160	3

Table 38–4. LOCATION OF PRIMARY TUMORS PRODUCING METASTATIC DISEASE OF THE SPINAL COLUMN: A REVIEW OF 2748 CASES

Primary Neoplasm	Number	Percentage
Breast	576	21
Lung	377	14
Prostate	211	7.5
Thyroid	73	2.5
Kidney	154	5.5
Lymphoma	180	6.5
Myeloma	245	9
Gastrointestinal	113	5

are common sources of disseminated skeletal lesions, although whether they are considered metastatic or primary lesions varies from author to author.

In the spinal column, metastatic disease usually arises from one of three primary tumor types: carcinoma of bronchogenic or breast origin, or the lymphoreticular malignancies lymphoma and myeloma. Metastases from these tumor types account for approximately half of the spinal lesions seen in most clinical studies, but the relative prevalence of specific primary tumors varies significantly among series (Table 38–4).[9, 35, 39, 66, 111, 120, 179] When only the solid tumor primaries are considered, breast, lung, and prostate carcinomas are cited as the most common sources of spinal metastases, followed by renal, gastrointestinal, and thyroid carcinomas. Although rarely mentioned in reviews of metastatic disease, tumors of the gastrointestinal system result in significantly more spinal metastases (and skeletal metastases in general) than do thyroid carcinomas, which are more often included in the "textbook" differential diagnosis.

Estimating the true incidence of metastasis for each tumor type is difficult. Depending on whether one looks at the absolute incidence of metastasis (as recorded in most autopsy studies) or the incidence of clinically significant metastasis (the data available from clinical reviews), the disease profile that emerges differs significantly.[164] The clinical behavior of the primary tumor dictates the perceived prevalence of metastasis and ultimately determines the clinical importance of that lesion for each patient. Hence, patients with breast, renal, and prostate carcinoma frequently survive long enough to require treatment of their spinal disease, whereas patients with pulmonary malignancies frequently succumb so rapidly that little more than supportive care can be offered. Because gastrointestinal carcinoma tends to involve the liver and lungs long before it involves the spine, these patients often die before their spinal lesions become clinically apparent.

Pathophysiology

Tumor emboli entering the bloodstream tend to arrest in the natural filters of the vascular tree—the capillary beds of the liver, lungs, and bone marrow.[155] To become established in the medullary canal, tumor emboli must either bypass the capillary beds of the liver and lungs, usually by establishing a metastasis there first, or circumvent these filters and reach the medullary sinusoids by an entirely different route. Tumors of the lung may seed the vertebral column directly through the segmental arteries, and carcinomas of the breast, gastrointestinal tract, and prostate are thought to reach the vertebral system through communications with the paravertebral venous plexus originally described by Batson.[6] Venous drainage from the breast by the azygous veins communicates with the paravertebral venous plexus in the thoracic region, and the prostate drains through the pelvic plexus in the lumbar region. Retrograde flow through Batson's plexus has been shown to occur during Valsalva's maneuver and may allow direct implantation of tumor cells in the vascular sinusoids of the vertebral body without passing through the usual capillary networks.

A second factor thought to be important in tumor distribution involves the nature of the tissue bed in which the embolus comes to rest. Certain tissues probably provide a more favorable environment for the survival of the tumor embolus. This "seed and soil" theory postulates that the red marrow of bone provides a biochemically and hemodynamically suitable environment for the implantation and proliferation of tumor cells.[175] Because the capillary network of the vertebral red marrow is particularly susceptible to tumor implantation and invasion, tumor cells find it easier to escape from the circulation and multiply within the fine network of cancellous bone.[64] Finally, there are intrinsic factors inherent to the tumor cells themselves that may give one cell line a particular advantage in surviving and growing in the medullary space. Specifically, the elaboration of prostaglandins and the stimulation of osteoclast activating factors by breast cancer cells have been associated with the establishment of lytic metastases in bone.[48, 124] These cells may also produce a protective fibrin sheath, which further isolates them within the marrow.

Diagnosis

The first symptom, and the most universal symptom of osseous metastasis, is pain. Pain usually begins insidiously, progresses relentlessly, and persists despite the patient's attempts to limit activity. It is usually localized, at least initially, and often seems worse at night. Patients may associate the onset of pain with some minor trauma, but the temporal relationship is usually loose and inconsistent. Because of the ubiquitous nature of back pain in the elderly population, patients are frequently treated empirically for arthritis or may see a number of physicians before a correct diagnosis is made.

In many patients the primary cancer will have been diagnosed months or years before symptoms of spinal involvement become apparent. In Gilbert and colleagues' review of 130 patients with spinal cord compression, only 10 patients (8 percent) presented with neurologic involvement as the first symptom of cancer.[51] Siegal and coworkers reported that 16 of 113 patients (14 percent) with cord compression presented similarly.[146] Patients may present with back symptoms many years after the treatment of their primary disease, particularly in cases of breast carcinoma or slowly growing tumors such as chondrosarcoma.[51] Regardless of how remote the history of malignancy may be, metastatic disease must be ruled out whenever unexplained and persistent pain develops in a patient with a previous primary cancer.

The medical evaluation of patients with spinal metastases may be more complicated than for patients with isolated malignancies. Patients with metastatic disease are by definition systemically ill. The extent of this illness is variable and may not become apparent until a detailed clinical examination is completed. Patients with advanced disease may be cachectic and anemic and have little respiratory reserve or gastrointestinal function. Those receiving chemotherapy may be immunosuppressed and thrombocytopenic, and those who have been radiated may have regions of skin unsuitable for surgical incision. Preoperative renal function should be assessed and serum calcium and phosphorus followed serially to avoid the development of malignant hypercalcemia.[66] When possible, such abnormalities should be corrected and the patient's medical fitness maximized before any surgical procedure. In patients who remain severely compromised, the risk of surgical mortality must be weighed carefully against the risks of incapacitating pain, paralysis, and a shortened life expectancy if surgical treatment is withheld.

Prognosis

Outcome and survival in metastatic disease depend on several interrelated factors, the most important of which is the primary tumor type. Although sex, age, location of metastases, and interval between diagnosis of disease and appearance of metastases have all been correlated with differences in outcome, each of these variables is influenced in turn by tumor type. For instance, women may have a better overall survival and greater percentage of satisfactory treatment results than men because of the relative predominance of breast carcinoma in women and pulmonary carcinoma in men. Similarly, because thoracic metastases frequently arise from pulmonary tumors in men and breast tumors in women, men with thoracic spine metastases have a significantly worse outcome than women with thoracic disease.[141]

Treatment

Radiotherapy. Radiotherapy has historically been the treatment of choice for osseous metastases involving the spine and remains the most reasonable treatment option for many patients. Patients with spinal pain or neurologic compromise without vertebral collapse may receive significant benefit from radiotherapy without any surgical intervention. The preoperative neurologic status of the patient dictates the likely outcome following radiotherapy. Although 70 percent of ambulatory patients retain that functional ability following radiotherapy, rarely do patients who have lost the ability to walk regain it following radiation alone.[163] The nature of the metastasis is also important to the outcome following radiotherapy. There is a significant difference in radiosensitivity among tumor types and among different clones of the same tumor type. Prostatic and lymphoreticular tumors are usually quite radiosensitive, and excellent clinical results can be obtained in most patients.[14, 107, 163] Metastases from breast carcinoma are usually responsive to irradiation, but as many as 30 percent of patients may not demonstrate a clinical response with radiation alone.[57, 163] Gastrointestinal and renal tumors may prove relatively recalcitrant when radiotherapy is used alone.

Surgery. In patients with bony instability or those who have failed radiation therapy, surgical treatment offers the only hope of pain relief and neurologic recovery. In a review of 33 patients with metastatic lesions of the thoracic and lumbar spine treated variably with anterior, posterior, or combined resections, O'Neil and associates found that 94 percent had good to excellent pain relief. Of 24 patients unable to walk preoperatively, 75 percent regained the ability to walk independently.[114] In a report of 100 consecutive tumor cases, Kostuik and colleagues reviewed 71 metastatic lesions of the cervical, thoracic, and lumbar spine. Both anterior and posterior surgical approaches were used, and stabilization was augmented with methyl methacrylate. Good to excellent pain relief was obtained in 81 percent. Significant improvement of neurologic deficits was obtained in 40 percent of patients undergoing posterior decompression and in 71 percent of patients decompressed anteriorly. Survival in metastatic disease was 11.3 months.[84] In a series reported by Harrington, 72 of 77 patients (94 percent) treated by anterior decompression and stabilization experienced good to excellent pain relief. Sixty-two patients had major neurologic impairment preoperatively, of which 68 percent experienced significant improvement after surgery; 26 had complete recoveries, and 16 others had significant improvement after decompression.[65]

Bracing. The halo vest is an important option for neurologically intact patients with cervical metastasis, instability, and pain. Used in conjunction with appropriate radiotherapy, symptomatic relief is reasonably good, and bony healing of the lesion occurs in many cases. Most importantly, neurologic injury can be prevented while medical therapy is instituted. In patients with metastatic prostate carcinoma, Danzig and associates reported good maintenance of neurologic function and no morbidity using the halo vest. In the end, however, these patients wore the halo for roughly a third of their remaining lives.[32] Thoracolumbar sacral orthosis and lumbosacral orthosis are also viable and important tools in the management of thoracolumbar metastases.

Extradural Tumors

Extradular, extraosseous tumors are very uncommon. The majority are benign soft tissue lesions that expand slowly and have little invasive potential.

Epidural Hemangioma. Epidural hemangiomas represent approximately 4 percent of all epidural tumors and 12 percent of all intraspinal hemangiomas.[117] They are almost always located in the upper thoracic spine and are characterized by slowly progressive spinal cord compression, usually present for some months before presentation. Acute progression and increase in symptoms may be precipitated if hemorrhage occurs and an epidural hematoma forms.

Epidural Lipoma. Epidural lipomas are an unusual cause of spinal cord compression, but their occurrence is well documented, and the increased risk in patients with Cushing's syndrome should be appreciated. Failure to appreciate the extensive nature of these benign tumors can lead to inadequate excision, which can be disastrous.[54]

Steroid-induced lipomatosis usually involves the thoracic spine. Signs of cord compression can appear quite acutely, even though the process has usually been ongoing for many months. Patients may present with rapidly progressive weakness and a myelographic block that involves the entire thoracic canal. Lesions have been misdiagnosed as epidural abscesses or as vertebral metastases, and some patients have even undergone irradiation, with a dismal outcome.[54] MRI has proved useful in demonstrating the full extent and character of these lesions, the severity of cord compression, and the relative location anteriorly or posteriorly in the canal.[69, 173] Although regression of lipomatosis may occur after decreasing or discontinuing steroid medications, laminectomy and surgical decompression are the treatment of choice in progressive lesions, providing neurologic improvement in 90 percent of cases.[60]

External Meningioma. External meningiomas represent approximately 7 percent of meningiomas treated. These are rare tumors that are almost always associated with an intradural component, although a communication between the two cannot always be demonstrated.[88] The extradural lesions tend to be vascular and may erode bone, giving an appearance of an extradural metastasis. When excised, these tumors have a tendency to recur, but neurologic recovery is usually satisfactory following decompression. Whenever an extradural meningioma is encountered, an intradural lesion must be ruled out, possibly through intradural exploration.

Neurofibroma. Neurofibromas are a relatively common spinal cord tumor, accounting for approximately a quarter of all spinal tumors. Although 80 percent are intradural lesions, approximately 10 percent are entirely extradural, and another 10 percent have both intradural and extradural components.[89] The tumors are usually solitary but may be multiple, and they usually arise from the spinal nerve root. They are the most common cause of an hourglass or dumbbell lesion (a tumor with a mass both internal and external to the canal, connected by a narrow isthmus through the neural foramen), although other neoplasms can produce this appearance. As 20 per cent of these lesions may undergo malignant degeneration, and as they may produce significant cord compression, excision is indicated. Whenever an extradural neurofibroma is encountered, intradural exploration to rule out an intradural tumor should be strongly considered.

Lymphoma. The most common malignancy found in the epidural space is lymphoma. Although extension from paraspinous nodes or from the vertebral body is thought to account for most lymphomas of the spinal canal, there are a number of cases of primary lymphoma reported to arise within the epidural space.[17] Plain radiographs may show some bony erosion in these cases or may be completely normal. Myelography has traditionally been most reliable for demonstrating the presence and extent of the lesion. Surgical decompression usually involves laminectomy, and neurologic improvement depends to a great extent on the preoperative grade of neurologic deficit.

TUMORS IN CHILDREN

Spinal tumors are uncommon in children, but when they occur, they present both short-term and long-term challenges. Aside from the usual complexities of treating the neoplasm itself, the added dimension in the care of children's tumors is the prevention or management of spinal deformities that often develop as a result of treatment.

Tumors of the immature spine differ in type from those seen in adults, particularly in terms of the malignant lesions. Nearly 70 per cent of primary bone tumors in children are benign. Osteoid osteomas and osteoblastomas, osteochondromas, and aneurysmal bone cysts account for over 40 per cent of all primary spinal lesions seen in pediatric patients. Ewing's sarcoma is the most common primary malignancy (Table 38–5).[169] Although the metastatic lesions of adulthood are generally absent, metastasis or contiguous invasion from neuroblastoma, embryonal carcinoma, and sarcoma predominates. These highly aggressive lesions have a poor prognosis regardless of treatment. Ewing's sarcoma may arise primarily in the spine but is more commonly a metastatic lesion. If intramedullary spinal cord tumors are excluded, 37 per cent of spinal lesions in Tachdjian and Matson's series were malignant,[161] with neuroblastoma accounting for 20 per cent of the lesions seen. In Fraser and coworkers' review of 40 pediatric spine tumors, neuroblastoma accounted for nearly 30 per cent of all tumors, and in Leeson and colleagues' review of metastatic tumors, neuroblastoma accounted for 41 per cent of lesions seen.[47, 85] Diagnosis in these patients may be challenging; nearly 70 per cent of the patients in Tachdjian and Matson's series

Table 38–5. PRIMARY BONE TUMORS FOUND IN THE SPINAL COLUMN IN 31 PATIENTS YOUNGER THAN 18 YEARS OF AGE

Tumor	Number
Benign	
Osteoblastoma	4
Osteochondroma	4
Aneurysmal bone cyst	4
Giant cell tumor	3
Eosinophilic granuloma	2
Osteoid osteoma	2
Hemangioma	1
Angiolipoma	1
Malignant	
Ewing's sarcoma	3
Chordoma	1
Osteosarcoma	1
Malignant giant cell tumor	1
Chondrosarcoma	1
Other	3

had been misdiagnosed originally, and treatment delay played a major role in determining their survival and the deformities associated with treatment.

Leukemia

Another disease presenting in pediatric patients is leukemia. In 6 per cent of children with leukemia, back pain and vertebral collapse are the initial findings at the time of presentation. During the course of the disease, 10 per cent will sustain a pathologic vertebral fracture, sometimes involving multiple levels.[129] When first seen, these children manifest a variety of nonspecific constitutional symptoms, and the correct diagnosis is often hard to make. Lethargy, anemia, and fever occur commonly and often in combination. The peripheral leukocyte count is elevated in 60 per cent of patients, and the erythrocyte sedimentation rate is also elevated. Radiographs may not demonstrate any focal abnormality, or they may show focal lytic lesions, occasional sclerotic lesions, or isolated periosteal reactions. It is important to keep in mind that radionucleotide scans are unreliable in patients with leukemia, in some cases showing no uptake in areas of obvious bony destruction.[22] These symptoms and signs mimic those seen in patients with osteomyelitis or joint sepsis, and this misdiagnosis is common. Key to making the correct diagnosis in these confusing presentations are the identification of anemia, the recognition of those 40 per cent of patients who are leukopenic at presentation, the presence of inconsistent bone scan results, and a high index of suspicion on the part of the examining physician.

Spinal Deformity

Progressive deformity may occur for any number of reasons after treatment of pediatric spinal tumors. As in adults, deformity may result from structural deficiencies caused by the erosion of bone by tumor or by aggressive surgical resection. These deformities may be more severe or progressive in children, however, particularly in the case of postlaminectomy kyphosis, and particularly in the thoracic spine. The younger the child at the time of laminectomy, the more severe the eventual deformity is likely to be.[47] Irradiation and rib resection are well-known factors in the development of iatrogenic scoliosis. Deformity following congenital or acquired paraplegia is also common and tends to be more severe in children with earlier onset of paralysis and higher levels of cord injury. Fully two thirds of patients with spinal cord compromise will develop spinal deformity, irrespective of treatment and neurologic recovery.[24] Surgical management of pediatric tumor patients must anticipate the later development of deformity and seek to minimize it. Deformities that are certain to progress must be identified early on, and treatment instituted to halt this progression.

SPINAL CORD COMPRESSION

Spinal cord compression is reported to occur in 5 to 20 per cent of patients with widespread cancer.[25, 145] Spinal cord compression results from one of four types of processes: direct compression from an enlarging soft tissue mass, pressure owing to fracture and retropulsion of bony fragments into the canal, severe kyphosis following vertebral collapse, and pressure from intradural metastases.[11] The most common cause of cord compression is mechanical pressure from tumor tissue or bone extruded from the collapsing vertebral body.[64] Experimental studies have shown that tumor cells invade the spinal canal from the marrow cavity by migrating through the foramina of the vertebral veins. Once in the canal, cell lines that manifest infiltrative growth tend to migrate dorsally, producing cord compression from a posterior direction. Tumor cell lines that form compact tumors tend to implant at the point where they emerge from the vertebral body, compressing the cord from an anterior direction.[2] Because of the flexion moment acting on the vertebrae of the thoracic spine, erosion of the vertebral body tends to produce collapse into kyphosis, extruding tumor and the posterior cortex of the vertebral body dorsally into the spinal canal. Direct compression of the cord may occur without vertebral erosion if the tumor expands directly into the canal. The spinal cord is well protected from tumor invasion by the dura, which is quite resistant to tumor infiltration. In the presence of an epidural metastasis, the dura is often found to be considerably thickened.[64] Compression of the spinal cord or a nerve root may occasionally result from extension of a paraspinal tumor through the intervertebral foramen. Intradural metastases are very rare, although they have been reported.[71]

Although the pathologic cause of spinal cord compression may vary, the symptoms of compression remain constant.[61] Early recognition of these symptoms is crucial to early intervention, preventing progressive and permanent neurologic injury. The first symptoms to appear are back pain, radicular or "girdle" pain, followed by weakness in the lower limbs, sensory loss, and loss of sphincter control. Although nearly all patients experience some localized back pain, patients with cervical and lumbosacral lesions are also likely to experience radicular pain. Patients with thoracic lesions occasionally experience radicular pain bilaterally, producing a segmental band or "girdle" of pain.[51] Persistent, progressive back pain and radicular pain are the most useful warning symptoms of impending spinal cord compression but may precede actual cord compromise by days or years.[9] Although bowel and bladder dysfunction may be seen at initial presentation, they are almost never isolated findings. When autonomic dysfunction occurs in the absence of motor or sensory loss, it is usually associated with a lesion of the T10–T12 vertebral body.

Important factors in determining the prognosis for neurologic outcome include tumor biology, pretreatment neurologic status, and tumor location within the spinal canal.[145]

Tumor Biology

The intrinsic nature of each specific primary or metastatic neoplasm determines which will have slow or rapid growth, which will be invasive, and which will produce metastases. Although metastatic lesions usually demonstrate behavior similar to their parent lesions, this is not always true; some metastases are more invasive or grow more rapidly than the primary lesions they come from. Rapid tumor expansion or vertebral erosion and fracture produce acute cord compression and a poorer prognosis for improvement. Slower expansion produces gradual cord impingement, from which the patient has a much better chance of recovering. Understanding the tumor type and its biology allows the surgeon to reasonably predict when and if a specific lesion will endanger neurologic structures.

Neurologic Status

The neurologic status before treatment correlates strongly with posttreatment outcome, whether in terms of likelihood of recovery, extent of recovery, or ability to maintain or regain ambulation or bowel and bladder function. Between 60 and 95 per cent of the patients who can walk at the time of diagnosis will retain that ability following treatment. By comparison, only 35 to 65 per cent of paraparetic patients will regain the ability to walk, and less than 30 per cent of paraplegic patients will regain ambulation.[9, 42, 61, 65, 84, 96, 111] The rate of progression of the neurologic deficit also has clear prognostic significance. A patient who progresses from the earliest onset of symptoms to a major deficit in less than 24 hours has a poor prognosis for recovery, irrespective of treatment. Conversely, if compression has evolved over a course of months, the patient has a far more favorable prognosis for recovery following treatment.[64]

Cord decompression can provide dramatic improvement in neurologic function, even in advanced states, depending on the rate of progression, the interval from paralysis to treatment, and the appropriate approach to cord decompression. Radiation therapy has been the traditional treatment for cord impingement, particularly in metastatic disease. Surgical decompression in the past consisted of laminectomy, with removal of whatever tumor could be reached laterally in the gutters or through the pedicle. Unfortunately, the results of laminectomy are often no better than those of radiotherapy alone, and posterior decompression has often resulted in iatrogenic instability postoperatively.[51, 64, 141] Constans and coworkers reported that 46 per cent of their patients treated with decompressive laminectomy and radiotherapy experienced significant neurologic improvement, compared with 39 per cent of patients treated with radiotherapy alone.[25] Gilbert and associates reported that satisfactory results were obtained in 46 per cent of patients treated with laminectomy and radiotherapy, as compared with 49 per cent of patients treated with radiotherapy alone.[51] They concluded that surgical decompression provided no benefit to these patients. Still, less than half the patients treated by either method were obtaining satisfactory results.[139]

The results of surgical decompression through the anterior approach have been far more favorable and now offer a genuine improvement over treatment with radiotherapy alone (Table 38–6).

Tumor Location

Location of the neoplasm within the vertebral body or spinal canal determines what symptoms and signs may be produced and dictates the surgical approach required for treatment. Metastatic tumors and primary malignancies commonly arise in the vertebral body. When tumor from an anterior lesion encroaches on the spinal cord, the anterior columns of the cord are compressed first. This leads to loss of motor function early on, and progressive loss of sensory function as the cord is pressed back against the lamina. As the mechanical loading of the vertebral elements differs from anterior to posterior, location also has value in predicting which lesions will cause vertebral collapse and segmental instability. For both of these reasons, tumors of the anterior and middle columns are associated with more frequent and more profound neurologic injury.

Location within the spinal column is also a factor in the development of cord compression. Neural compression occurs most commonly in the thoracic region of the spine, where the cord is relatively large with respect to the vertebral canal; it is less common in the thoracolumbar region. It occurs late in lower lumbar lesions, usually long after pain symptoms have become prominent.

SURGICAL APPROACHES AND TREATMENT

General

Indications for surgical treatment have been outlined by a number of different authors. Gilbert suggested that decompressive laminectomy was indicated in metastatic disease when (1) the nature of the primary tumor was not known or the diagnosis was in doubt; (2) relapse of tumor occurred following maximal radiotherapy to that segment; and (3) symptoms progressed inexorably during radiotherapy treatments.[35, 51] With the acceptance of more aggressive surgical methods, these indications have been expanded; recent authors have recommended surgical intervention in instances of (1) an isolated primary or metastatic lesion or a solitary site of relapse, (2) pathologic fracture or deformity producing neurologic symptoms or pain, (3) radioresistant tumors—metastatic or primary, and (4) segmental instability following radiotherapy.[45, 64, 67, 84, 96, 145, 157, 169] All of these presume a patient who is healthy enough to survive surgery but are not incumbent on a

Table 38–6. NEUROLOGIC RECOVERY IN CORD DECOMPRESSION

Author	Number of Patients	% with Improvement	% with Satisfactory Outcome
Anterior decompression			
Manabe et al.[96]	28	82	89
Fidler[42]	17	73	78
Harrington[65]	77	84	73
Kostuik et al.[84]	70	73	84
Siegal and Siegal[144]	75	80	80
Sundaresan et al.[157]	160	80	78
Posterior decompression			
Hall and Mackay[61]	123	30	29
Kostuik et al.[84]	30	36	37
Nather and Bose[111]	42	13	29
Siegal and Siegal[144]	25	39	39
Gilbert et al.[51]	65	45	46
White et al.[171]	226	38	37
Wright et al.[178]	86	35	33
Sherman and Waddell[141]	149	27	48

long expected survival. Any patient with expectations of surviving six weeks or longer who is not hopelessly bedridden should be given consideration.

There are a number of different surgical approaches available to the spine surgeon, and variations to each have been described (Table 38–7). Choosing the correct approach for the given situation is perhaps the most important step in treating these conditions.

Tumor Care

Although some authors have advised that attempts at surgical extirpation are fruitless and should not be attempted,[10] it is clear from others that the ability to completely resect the primary tumor plays a role in overall patient survival and in recovery of neurologic function.[142, 152, 154, 169] Although true anatomic compartments (as defined by Enneking) do not exist in the spinal column, anatomic structures do provide natural planes for dissection and wide excision. The vertebral body, anterior and posterior longitudinal ligaments, intervertebral discs, and dura may all be resected to avoid leaving residual tumor behind. Neural, muscular, and vascular structures may all be sacrificed to obtain an adequate surgical margin in primary malignancies. Such an aggressive approach is justified: as in extremity surgery, a complete resection provides the best prognosis for both local control and cure of the disease.

To treat spinal neoplasms appropriately, an organized, calculated approach must be applied in preoperative planning. In planning the surgical approach, the anatomic extent of the lesion must be understood in three dimensions, and the stabilization and reconstruction needed must be anticipated in planning the surgical approach.

The vertebral body may be divided into four zones, I–IV. Tumor extension is designated as A–C for intraosseous, extraosseous, and distant tumor spread (Fig. 38–13).[168] Zone IA includes the spinous process to the pars interarticularis and the inferior facets. Zone IIA includes the superior articular facet, the transverse process, and the pedicle from the level of the pars to its junction with the vertebral body. Zone IIIA includes the anterior three fourths of the vertebral body, and Zone IVA designates involvement of the posterior one fourth of the body, that segment immediately anterior to the cord. Zones IB–IVB are the extraosseous extensions of tumor beyond the boundaries of the cortical bone, and Zones IC–IVC designate associated regional or distant metastatic involvement. Surgical outcome is determined by the zones involved, the extent of the local or distant tumor spread, and the type and grade of tumor.

Complete radiographic evaluation, including CT and MRI, allows accurate determination of the tumor location and extension and a more informed prediction of the tumor grade, if not its actual tissue type. Additional laboratory and screening studies focus the differential diagnosis further, allowing the surgeon to plan an operation that will adequately treat the tumor without exposing the patient to needless risks. Accurately determining the most likely tumor type before surgery is important; overtreatment of benign disease can be nearly as disastrous as undertreatment of malignancy. An algorithm has been developed for the evaluation of patients presenting for the first time with a spinal lesion (Fig. 38–14).

Obtaining the widest margin possible is essential in many locally aggressive or malignant tumors, particularly those that do not respond well to irradiation. A wide margin can be obtained in most isolated lesions in Zones IA–IIIA, as the tumor can usually be completely resected. Lesions in Zone IVA can be resected cleanly, but only by removing the surrounding compartments as well. An adequate margin can be extremely difficult to obtain in Type B lesions. Zone IB–IVB lesions may not be completely resectable without producing serious neurologic deficits. In these cases, surgery is marginal at best and usually intralesional. The decision to attempt a wide or radical resection in these cases must be weighed against the risk of neurologic deficit.

The surgical approach selected must provide sufficient access for both tumor excision and stabilization of the spine thereafter. If both operations cannot be performed through the same incision, the surgeon must plan for a combined approach. An ill-planned approach may leave the surgeon unable to complete the excision of the tumor, a situation to be avoided if at all possible. Zone I lesions are best approached posteriorly, and the extent of excision must be based on any soft tissue extension seen on preoperative studies. Zone

Table 38–7. SURGICAL APPROACHES TO SPINAL NEOPLASM

Level	Anterior	Posterior
Cervical (C1–C2)	Transoral	Midline posterior
(C1–T2)	Anterolateral	Posterolateral
	Trans-sternal	
Thoracic	Thoracotomy	Midline posterior
		Costotransversectomy
Thoracolumbar (T11–L2)	Thoracoabdominal tenth to twelfth rib resection, detachment of diaphragm	Midline posterior Posterolateral
Lumbar	Retroperitoneal	Midline posterior
	Transabdominal	

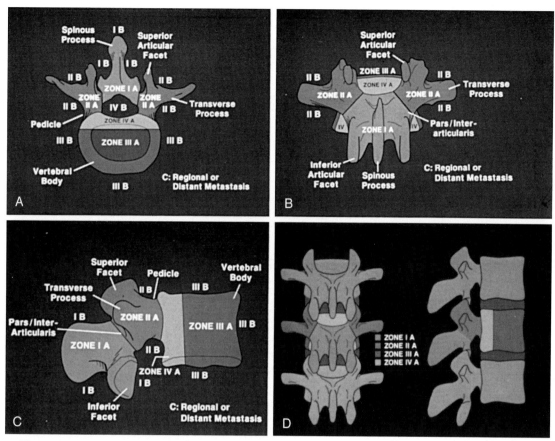

Figure 38–13. Anatomic extent of spine tumors by zone. *A,* Axial cut through L1 Zones I–IVA: intraosseous lesions confined within the boundaries of the cortical spine. *B,* Posterior view of L1 Zones I–IVB: extraosseous extension beyond the boundaries of the cortical spine. *C,* Lateral views of L1. *D,* Posterior views of L1 through L3.

II lesions are also more easily excised through a posterior or posterolateral approach[86] and should be similarly stabilized. The need for stabilization following Zone I and II resections depends to a great extent on the spinal segment involved. Extensive or multilevel laminectomies in the cervical or thoracic spine routinely lead to progressive and severe kyphosis, and posterior instrumentation prevents this by restoring a posterior column tension band to combat the normal tensile loads seen in these segments. In the lumbar segments, kyphosis is less of a concern than translational deformities and back pain. Iatrogenic spondylolisthesis may occur any time an entire facet is removed or more than 50 per cent of both facets are removed at any one level.

Lesions in Zone III should be approached anteriorly. Adequate resection of Zone IIIA lesions can usually be obtained throughout the spinal column, but Zone IIIB lesions should be carefully analyzed preoperatively to anticipate possible invasion of or adherence to the great vessels of the thoracic cavity, retroperitoneal structures of the abdomen, or critical neurovascular elements, esophagus, or trachea in the cervical region. Reconstruction may be performed with or without internal

fixation, depending on the extent of the resection and the inherent stability of the residual elements.

Zone IV lesions that require a complete or en bloc excision must be managed through a combined anterior and posterior surgical approach. These lesions involve the most inaccessible region of the vertebral body and are the most difficult lesions to reconstruct; they provide major technical challenges to the surgeon before, during, and after the actual tumor resection. Zones I, II, and/or III must be crossed at some point to provide access to Zone IV lesions, and frequently more than one zone may be involved with tumor. Complete excision can be obtained, although tumor margins must often be crossed. Excision requires vertebrectomy, essentially separating Zone II from Zones III and IV through combined approaches (Figs. 38–15 and 38–16). In such cases, both anterior and posterior stabilization is usually necessary. Failure to provide sure fixation and an adequate bone graft may result in loss of fixation, with catastrophic neurologic complications if hardware migrates into the canal or if excessive kyphosis develops.[102, 152]

In planning tumor treatment, the zones involved must be clearly identified. The surgeon can then estab-

Approach to Spine Tumors

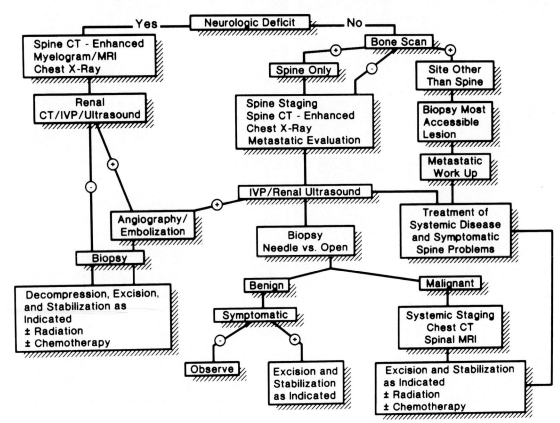

Figure 38–14. Algorithm for the evaluation of patients presenting with spinal lesions.

lish a coherent treatment plan that addresses the three elements of importance: decompression, resection, and reconstruction.

Decompression

Metastatic

In situations in which conservative therapy is not feasible or has proved ineffective in treating neural impingement, surgical decompression is indicated. Below the level of T2, anterior stabilization should be used to restore stability; above T2, posterior instrumentation is indicated. Laminectomy should be restricted to those rare cases in which the site of compression has been shown to be primarily posterior.[42] In lesions of the cervical spine above the level of C3, a posterior approach is advocated. In a series of 11 patients with pathologic fracture resulting from high cervical metastases, posterior decompression and stabilization provided good to excellent pain relief in all patients but was not adequate to prevent collapse in one patient with severe anterior vertebral destruction.[41] An anterior approach with decompression and methyl methacrylate stabilization has been recommended for metastatic lesions involving one or two levels, but Kostuik prefers a posterolateral approach to lesions involving multiple adjacent levels. A single nerve root may need to be sacrificed to allow adequate anterior decompression by this approach. Stabilization following a posterolateral decompression is with segmental fixation and sublaminar wiring, augmented with methyl methacrylate as needed.[83, 84] In contrast, Harrington reported good results with anterior stabilization using longitudinal rods and methyl methacrylate in lesions involving up to seven vertebral levels.[63]

Metastatic tumors of the upper thoracic spine are particularly difficult to approach anteriorly. Either a high, right-sided thoracotomy or a sternotomy may be used, but the approach is challenging, and potential complications are severe. The posterolateral approach circumvents the problem of thoracotomy, but access to the tumor is limited. Video-assisted vertebrectomy promises improvement in tumor resection and reconstruction in this difficult region.

Renal tumors present special challenges to the surgical oncologist; patients frequently present with osseous metastases at the time of initial diagnosis and demonstrate a highly variable course in terms of survival.[132, 148] Sundaresan and associates reported on 43 patients with renal cell carcinoma—32 undergoing anterior resection for cord compression, and 11 having radiation only.

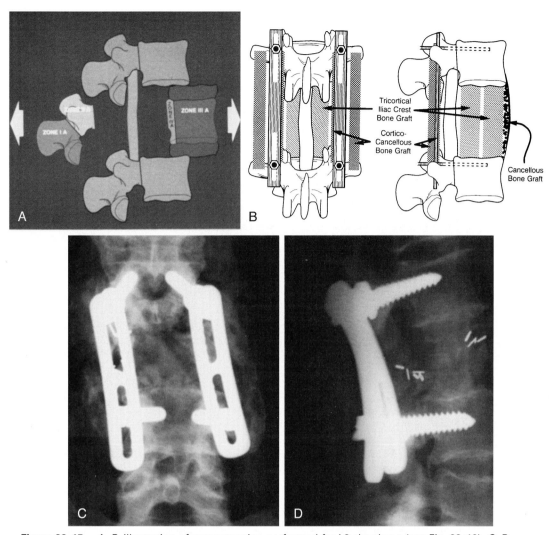

Figure 38–15. *A, B,* Illustration of reconstruction performed for L3 chordoma (see Fig. 38–12). *C, D,* Anteroposterior and lateral radiographs taken three years postoperatively. No signs of recurrence to date.

The median survival of the surgical group was 13 months, compared with three months for those treated with radiation alone. Patients undergoing complete resection of tumor anteriorly had a 37 per cent survival at two years, whereas none of those treated with radiotherapy alone survived two years. Significant neurologic improvement was seen in 70 per cent of surgical patients, compared with 45 per cent of radiated patients.[160] Other authors have reported survival rates of 30 per cent or more at five years following aggressive resection of solitary renal metastases.[162] In the surgical management of these patients, preoperative angiography and embolization may prove lifesaving, as the extensive neovasculature of renal cell tumors produces dramatic hemorrhage during resection. Two courses of embolization are sometimes necessary to identify all the major vessels feeding the lesion.

Renal cell metastases can recur aggressively, leading to cord or cauda equina compression, construct failure, and intractable pain. Whenever possible, a complete resection of tumor is indicated. Combined anterior and posterior reconstruction allows rapid mobilization.

Posterior Approach

Whether laminectomy provides any greater benefit to patients with cord compression than radiotherapy is debatable. In one uncontrolled, retrospective review of 38 patients treated by laminectomy, only 24 per cent demonstrated any improvement in neurologic function.[113] Results were no better in a review of 27 cases of osteosarcoma of the spine; biopsy combined with laminectomy or root decompression provided only transient relief in patients with neurologic deficits, and the survival of these patients was dismal.[142] Although Constans and colleagues showed some improvement in results using laminectomy with radiotherapy, Gilbert and associates found very little difference between patients treated with radiotherapy alone and those treated with both laminectomy and radiation.[25, 51] The

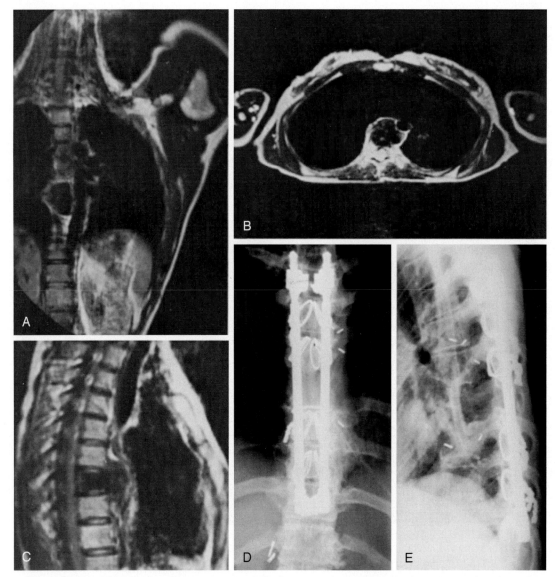

Figure 38–16. MRI scan: anteroposterior (*A*), axial (*B*), and sagittal (*C*) views of T7 metastatic clear cell sarcoma adherent to the descending aorta. *D, E,* Anteroposterior and lateral radiographs three years after tumor resection. A vascularized rib graft was used anteriorly off the internal mammary artery.

proportion of satisfactory outcomes was less than 50 per cent in either case.

The classification of Brice and McKissock,[13] based on mild, moderate, and severe neurologic deficits, defined satisfactory outcome as restoration of ambulation and bowel and bladder function. It is not directly comparable to the Frankel classification widely used today, and this lack of continuity makes comparison of data for anterior and posterior approaches more difficult. The trend seen in comparison is still quite clear, however (see Table 38–6): of 746 reported cases, only 38 per cent of patients undergoing posterior decompression had a satisfactory neurologic outcome, and fewer of those with a severe deficit showed significant improvement.[51, 61, 84, 111, 141, 171, 178] Although stabilization significantly improved the pain relief and maintenance of

neurologic function compared with laminectomy alone, the overall results were still disappointing.[141]

Laminectomy may be distinctly detrimental to neurologic outcome in patients with anterior cord compression. If the cord is manipulated in an effort to reach anterior tumor tissue, the risk of neurologic injury is high, particularly in the thoracic region.[100] Findlay reviewed the results of laminectomy in patients with and without vertebral collapse and noted a poorer rate of recovery and twice the rate of postoperative paraplegia in patients with collapse.[44] Laminectomy fails in these patients because adequate decompression of the cord is impossible if retropulsed vertebral fragments cannot be removed from the canal. Furthermore, even if adequate decompression is obtained, the resulting instability puts these patients at high risk of postoperative kyphosis, cord compression, and paraplegia. Combining a destabilizing posterior decompression with an already unstable anterior column is clearly unwise.

Costotransversectomy combined with posterior segmental instrumentation has been used to debulk and stabilize metastatic tumors, but the results have not been as good as with the anterior approach. Only one of five patients reported by DeWald and colleagues regained the ability to walk, and survival was only five months.[35] Somewhat better results have been reported after a modified costotransversectomy approach with anterolateral decompression, but access to the tumor is always limited anteriorly, and results are still inferior to those obtained by a formal anterior approach.[116] An endoscope may be used to directly visualize the spinal cord and posterior longitudinal ligament during posterolateral resection.[103a] This allows the surgeon to carefully resect all pathologic tissue from the vertebra and to directly decompress the spinal cord without having to manipulate it. After completing the vertebrectomy and removing the adjacent discs, a strut graft or prefabricated cage may be introduced posterolaterally to provide anterior stability. The endoscope allows optimal positioning of the cage without cord impingement (Fig. 38–17).

Anterior Approach

Anterior decompression has been successfully used to treat cord compression caused by fracture, neoplasm, infection, and congenital deformity. Of 25 patients reviewed by Johnson and coworkers, 17 had a partial recovery and five a complete recovery from their neurologic deficits. Patients with early intervention had the best outcomes.[76] Similarly, Fidler and Harrington observed significant neurologic improvement in 93 and 75 per cent of patients, respectively, decompressed anteriorly for metastatic disease.[42, 63]

In one of the few prospective studies of surgical decompression of epidural tumors, Siegal and Siegal chose an anterior approach and decompression for lesions located ventral to the cord and a posterior laminectomy for lesions located dorsally. Patients who did not satisfy the indications for surgical decompression were treated with radiotherapy. Only 30 per cent of patients treated with radiotherapy retained or regained the ability to walk, as opposed to 40 per cent of the laminectomy patients and 80 per cent of the vertebrectomy patients. Of 13 paraplegic patients treated by anterior decompression, all but one improved at least one grade in neurologic function, whereas five of 25 patients treated with laminectomy actually deteriorated as a result of treatment. The operative mortality was similar for both approaches, but postoperative complications were far more frequent in the laminectomy group, commonly owing to poor wound healing after operations performed through irradiated tissue.[144] In 427 cases of anterior decompression in which objective grading of neurologic recovery was reported, 79 per cent had a significant improvement in functional grade, and 77 per cent obtained a satisfactory outcome—independent ambulation and intact autonomic function (see Table 38–6).

Resection

When patients present with a solitary primary malignancy, a benign but locally aggressive tumor, or a solitary metastasis, decompression is only part of the problem. Resection of the tumor may determine both local control and eventual cure. Although some radiosensitive tumors (solitary plasmacytoma) are relatively forgiving of intralesional resection,[103] others (notably chordoma and chondrosarcoma) distinctly are not. In these cases, resection of the tumor determines the patient's outcome.

Zone I and II lesions may be resected through a posterior or posterolateral approach. A cuff of normal tissue is retained with the tumor mass, and the previous biopsy incision is resected as well. To reach the base of the pedicle, the transverse process may be removed through a posterolateral approach. The pedicle can then be amputated at the level of the vertebral body.

If the posterior soft tissue mass is large, a curvilinear incision may be needed to allow dissection around the lateral tumor margins. Both bony and soft tissue margins should be checked for tumor.

Zone III lesions may be amenable to a purely anterior approach, but reconstruction may require combining this with a posterior stabilization. Small Zone IIIA lesions may be resectable through a hemivertebrectomy approach. Zone IIIB lesions may require a more formal vertebrectomy, removing one pedicle and both discs to allow mobilization of the vertebral body.

Zone IV lesions require a combined approach if the tumor is to be removed en bloc. Posterior laminectomy provides access to the vertebral pedicles at the involved level. The pedicles can then be drilled out to release the anterior vertebral body from the posterior restraints and transverse processes. Bleeding from the pedicles should be controlled with bone wax or, if persistent, may be stopped by packing the pedicle with a small amount of PMMA. The spine can then be stabilized prior to repositioning the patient for the anterior approach.

With locally aggressive Zone III or IVB malignancies, the surgeon must balance the risks of radical resection against the likelihood of a lethal recurrence. Preoperative staging sometimes alerts the physician to problems of vascular or dural adhesion, but these may be encountered in any case. The dura may be excised and patched with a fascial graft, if necessary, and individual nerve roots may be sacrificed to permit en bloc excision. Invasion of the great vessels has a dire prognosis; segmental resection of the aorta with synthetic replacement is possible, but morbidity and mortality are significant. Tumor invasion and irradiation may leave the aorta friable, and dissection may result in rents or tears that cannot be repaired as in normal tissues. Catastrophic bleeding can occur.

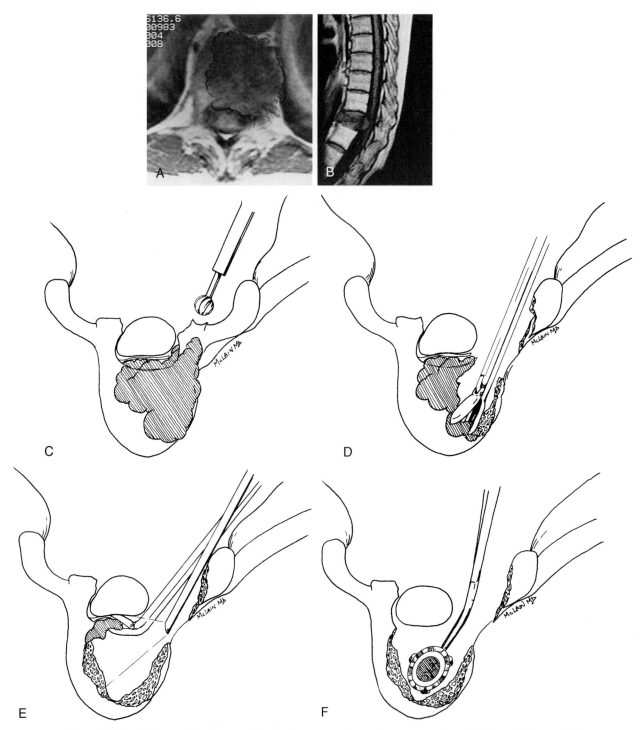

Figure 38–17. Video-assisted transpedicular decompression and reconstruction of T11 metastases. *A, B,* Axial and sagittal MRI scans of T11 metastasis producing pain and spinal cord compression. Posterolateral surgical approach allows combined anterior-posterior decompression and reconstruction through a single incision. *C,* After posterior laminectomy, a left-sided transpedicular resection is carried out to expose the anterior lateral tumor mass and vertebral body. *D,* Transpedicular tumor resection is carried out with rongeurs and curets. *E,* Under endoscopic control, tumor adjacent to the anterior spinal cord is resected with rongeurs and Epstein curets. *F,* After wide decompression and vertebrectomy, a Moss cage with autograft bone is introduced posterolaterally.

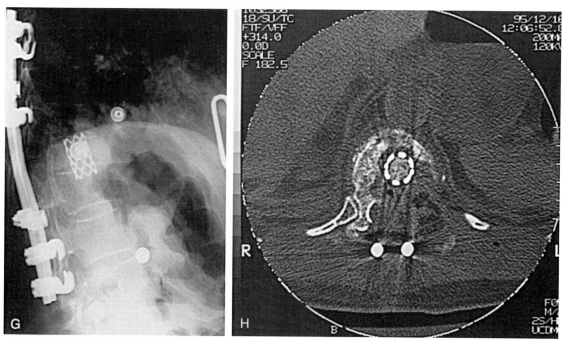

Figure 38–17 *Continued. G,* Lateral radiograph demonstrating anterior cage placement with posterior stabilization. *H,* Postoperative CT scan shows wide decompression with central placement of titanium strut.

Reconstruction Biomechanics

Whether a tumor is resected posteriorly or anteriorly, posterior stabilization is frequently indicated to prevent early, progressive deformity and to allow incorporation of bone graft. A wide variety of instrumentation systems have been used successfully, and the surgeon must choose the hardware that will meet the challenges of each individual case.

Harrington distraction and compression rods have been used for many years to stabilize lesions of the thoracic and lumbar spine. Distraction rods are sufficient to stabilize the vertebral column following laminectomy or in cases of compression fracture. When both the anterior and the middle columns are involved, as is seen in extensive vertebral fracture or erosion,[33] the three-point fixation of the Harrington system cannot counter the excessive bending and tension loads and is at risk for failure.[50, 170] Although the Harrington system can restore proper alignment and in some cases restore appropriate vertebral height to the spinal elements, retropulsed vertebral fragments responsible for cord impingement are not reduced. Even with an intact posterior longitudinal ligament, reduction of the fracture is associated with a 25 per cent residual stenosis.[174]

Stabilization with Luque instrumentation and sublaminar wiring has been successful in cervical, thoracic, and lumbar segments. Although there are risks involved in passing sublaminar wires, this technique may provide better fixation in soft bone than the Harrington system.[29, 35]

Newer instrumentation systems for posterior stabilization have been applied with good short-term results.

Although the indications for the use of the Cotrel-Dubousset instrumentation system[28] and the variety of pedicle fixation systems[130, 151] have been established for scoliosis, segmental instability, and trauma, experience with these systems in tumor care is limited (Fig. 38–18).

Even when fusion and stabilization are obtained posteriorly, excessive motion of the anterior elements may still occur if there is no attempt to reconstruct the anterior and middle columns. It has been shown that even when the posterior elements are rigidly fixed, there can be significant motion anteriorly in response to physiologic compression and bending loads.[170] Because of the increased incidence of infection and wound breakdown associated with posterior instrumentation, Harrington has recommended posterior stabilization only when (1) combined anterior and posterior decompression is necessary, (2) lengthy anterior fixation is inadequate to restore stability, (3) posterior instability is produced by tumor lysis of posterior elements, and/or (4) lesions are either anteriorly or posteriorly distal to the L3 vertebral body.[65]

To deal with this dilemma, a number of techniques of anterior stabilization have been developed, some depending on methyl methacrylate or other synthetic spacers and others using bone graft in anticipation of a solid arthrodesis. Some authors have advocated the use of autogenous or allograft bone, with or without internal fixation, to fill even very large postoperative defects.[152, 154] Such an approach is clearly favored in the treatment of benign or slowly growing tumors, when patient survival is expected to be measured in years. Even when radiotherapy is required postoperatively, incorporation of the graft can be expected.

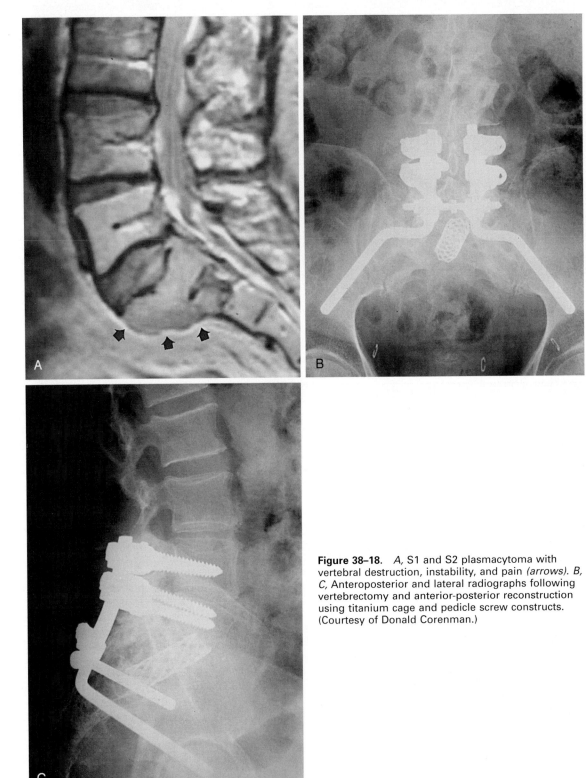

Figure 38–18. *A*, S1 and S2 plasmacytoma with vertebral destruction, instability, and pain *(arrows)*. *B, C*, Anteroposterior and lateral radiographs following vertebrectomy and anterior-posterior reconstruction using titanium cage and pedicle screw constructs. (Courtesy of Donald Corenman.)

Spinal reconstruction using methyl methacrylate remains somewhat controversial. Although its use in traumatic spinal instability has led to significant complications and failure, most authors agree that there is a role for cement in stabilizing metastatic spinal lesions. This role has become more limited, however, as better alternatives have become available.

Methyl methacrylate functions as an adjunct to stabilization, providing a temporary internal splint in anticipation of eventual bony arthrodesis. If arthrodesis is not obtained, it is only a matter of time before the methacrylate construct fails; only patients with a very limited life expectancy should undergo methacrylate fixation without bone grafting.[21] The way in which methyl methacrylate is used also determines the likelihood of failure. Methyl methacrylate has proved quite resilient and dependable for anterior vertebral reconstructions, where it is exposed to primarily compressive loads.[119, 170] Reinforcing methyl methacrylate with wire or wire mesh increases its tensile strength and improves its ability to withstand bending loads. Longitudinal Steinmann pins may be used anteriorly to enhance both the bending resistance of the construct and its fixation to the adjacent vertebral bodies. Two or more Steinmann pins, 1 to 5 mm in diameter, may be inserted into the adjacent vertebral bodies prior to instilling liquid cement into the defect.[157] Siegal and colleagues had advocated the use of Harrington distraction rods and, more recently, Moe sacral hooks and threaded rods to obtain anterior purchase,[146] and Harrington has used Knodt rods for several years to the same purpose.[63, 64]

Reconstruction of the vertebral body with methyl methacrylate requires care to avoid contact of the cement with the dural sac. Although thermal injury to the cord is unlikely, reports of postoperative dural compression suggest that space must be maintained between the cement mass and the posterior longitudinal ligament. Cement is applied in the dough phase to allow better control of placement, and a sheet of Gelfoam is interposed anterior to the dural elements to further shield them.[37] A steady flow of saline irrigation minimizes the heat transmitted to surrounding tissues.

Several prosthetic spacers have become available over the past five years that can provide both the mechanical support necessary for axial stability and the potential for bone ingrowth or arthrodesis, without the morbidity of harvesting large tricortical autografts. Matsui and coworkers described encouraging results using a modular ceramic spacer system for vertebral replacement, although migration of the spacer was noted in 20 per cent of patients.[101] Carbon fiber and titanium cages are also available, and biomechanical and animal studies have shown that these are capable of providing superior sagittal stability and more rapid graft incorporation than allograft bone struts.[12, 143] Anterior plate fixation may be combined with anterior column reconstruction to restore sagittal, coronal, and torsional rigidity following vertebrectomy, eliminating the need for posterior instrumentation in some patients.[62] Plate fixation also minimizes the likelihood that the strut graft or cage will displace. There is less need to key the graft into the adjacent vertebral bodies, and the graft can be impacted directly into the hard vertebral end plates. Because the graft or cage rests on the end plates, there is less chance of subsidence over time.

Cervical Spine Tumors

In a review of 20 cases of cervical spine tumors treated by anterior vertebrectomy and bone grafting, there were no cases of graft failure through either collapse or extrusion.[43] Iliac crest, fibular, and tibial grafts were all used, and posterior fusions were used in 13 cases to augment stability. In patients with primary benign tumors, anterior resection and grafting eliminated symptoms in each case, and there were no recurrences. In primary malignancies and in metastatic lesions, there was excellent stability, with resolution of neurologic symptoms and pain. Quality of life and longevity were improved in these patients. Because a recurring tumor is likely to involve the vertebrae above and below the site of previous resection, it is recommended that the posterior fusion span two levels above and below the site of fusion. In a review of 13 benign and 10 malignant primary neoplasms of the cervical spine, anterior excision with iliac crest autograft, supplemented with posterior grafting in some cases, proved to be reliable in relieving pain and neurologic symptoms, providing stability, and improving quality of life. Large tumors involving anterior, lateral, and posterior elements of the vertebral body were excised through staged anterior and posterior approaches. An intralesional margin was obtained in all malignant tumors. Only two patients with malignancy survived more than three years.[10]

Involvement of local structures can severely limit the potential for radical resection of extradural cervical tumors. Involvement of the vertebral arteries on one or both sides may render a tumor essentially unresectable. In a case in which local control would provide a significant likelihood of cure or improved quality of life, preservation or reconstruction of the vertebral artery can be achieved through an anterolateral approach.[137]

Palliative treatment, involving neural decompression, segmental stabilization, but incomplete tumor resection, is indicated for patients with unremitting neck pain, vertebral destruction with loss of spinal stability, and/or cord or root compression caused by tumor. Anterior surgery, combining vertebrectomy with strut grafting and plate fixation, is appropriate for tumors involving one level between C3 and T1 (Fig. 38–19). A combined approach, adding posterior instrumentation and fusion, should be selected for multilevel resections or combined anterior and posterior decompressions.[98] Some benign lesions may respond to intralesional curettage, but the diagnosis must be confirmed before committing to this course.[87]

Complications

A number of series have shown that iatrogenic instability and deformity impede neurologic improvement and

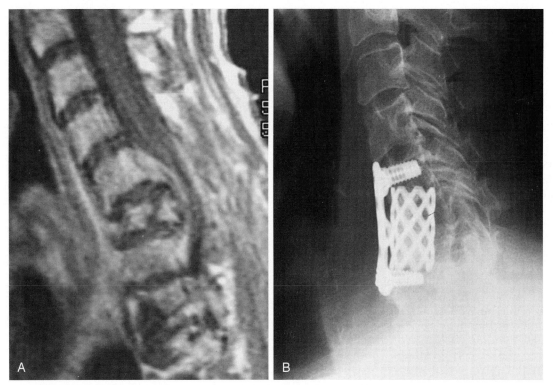

Figure 38–19. *A,* Lateral MRI of 69-year-old with metastatic lung carcinoma of the cervical spine. *B,* Lateral radiograph showing reconstruction with Moss titanium cage and methyl methacrylate. Anterior plate fixation allowed this patient to be mobilized in a brace immediately after surgery. Pain relief was immediate, and function was excellent for the remainder of the patient's life.

may result in progressive neurologic dysfunction.[102, 141] Prevention of postoperative kyphosis and instability is crucial to maintaining neurologic integrity. Instability may result from inadequate reconstruction or stabilization at the time of initial surgery or from late fixation failure owing to progression of disease or hardware failure. In Harrington's series of 77 patients treated with posterior stabilization and methyl methacrylate, five patients suffered loss of fixation requiring restabilization. In addition, six patients subsequently developed spinal instability owing to metastatic disease at other levels of the spine.[65]

There is a higher complication rate when methyl methacrylate is used with posterior rather than anterior stabilization.[102] Of 24 complications reported by McAfee and colleagues, only five occurred after anterior stabilization using methyl methacrylate. Of the 19 patients with posterior stabilization, 15 suffered loss of fixation, and a number of these subsequently developed a significant kyphosis. Six patients developed deep infections, three of whom suffered significant neurologic deterioration.[102]

SUMMARY

The prognosis for survival has improved dramatically for cancer patients over the past three decades. New approaches to treating systemic disease have pro-

longed survival and improved quality of life, even in those who cannot be cured. As survival has increased, the importance of managing spinal column disease and protecting the spinal cord has also increased. Any patient presenting with some residual neurologic function and enough physical reserve to withstand an operation will benefit from a stable spine, relief of pain, and spinal cord decompression; there are very few exceptions.

Advances in surgical technique and biomaterials have not only improved survival and functional outcome but also limited many of the postoperative complications that plagued earlier treatment techniques. Methods of correcting acquired deformity and of reliably preventing iatrogenic deformity have improved outcome. Newer fixation techniques promise to eliminate many of the causes of hardware failure and loss of fixation previously seen.

Surgeons have long known that neurologic function has a much better chance of improving when treatment is begun early. Improved medical management, antibiotics, and preoperative planning, along with techniques of preoperative embolization and early postoperative mobilization, have made surgical management much less risky. Vertebrectomy, a last-ditch effort used in very selected cases in the past, is now coming to be seen as the "conservative" approach to management in many situations. The results of numerous clinical series bear this out.

References

1. Akbarnia, B. A., and Rooholamini, S. A.: Scoliosis caused by benign osteoblastoma of the thoracic or lumbar spine. J. Bone Joint Surg. [Am.] *63*:1146–1155, 1981.
2. Arguello, F., Baggs, R. B., Duerst, R. E., et al.: Pathogenesis of vertebral metastasis and epidural spinal cord compression. Cancer *65*:98–106, 1990.
3. Bacci, G., Jaffe, N., Emiliani, E., et al.: Therapy for primary non-Hodgkin's lymphoma of bone in comparison to results of Ewing's sarcoma. Cancer *57*:1468–1472, 1986.
4. Baker, L. L., Goodman, S. B., and Peckash, I.: Benign versus pathological compression fractures of vertebral bodies: Assessment with conventional spin-echo, chemical shift, and STIR MR imaging. Radiology *174*:495–502, 1990.
5. Barwick, K. W., Huvos, A. G., and Smith, J.: Primary osteogenic sarcoma of the vertebral column. Cancer *46*:595–604, 1980.
6. Batson, O. V.: The role of the vertebral veins in metastatic processes. Ann. Intern. Med. *16*:38–45, 1942.
7. Bergsagel, D. E., Bailey, A. J., Langley, G. R., et al.: The chemotherapy of plasma-cell myeloma and the incidence of acute leukemia. N. Engl. J. Med. *301*:743–748, 1979.
8. Bergsagel, D. E., and Rider, W. D.: Plasma cell neoplasms in cancer. In De Vita, V. T., Hellman, S., and Rosenberg, S. A. (eds.): Principles and Practice of Oncology. 2nd ed. Philadelphia, J. B. Lippincott, 1985, pp. 1753–1795.
9. Black, P.: Spinal metastasis: Current status and recommended guidelines for management. Neurosurgery *5*(6):726–746, 1979.
10. Bohlman, H. H., Sachs, B. L., Carter, J. R., et al.: Primary neoplasms of the cervical spine. J. Bone Joint Surg. [Am.] *68*:483–494, 1986.
11. Boland, P. J., Lane, J. M., and Sundaresan, N.: Metastatic disease of the spine. Clin. Orthop. *169*:95–102, 1982.
12. Brantigan, J. W., McAfee, P. C., Cunningham, B. W., et al.: Interbody lumbar fusion using a carbon fiber cage implant versus allograft bone. Spine *19*:1436–1444, 1994.
13. Brice, J., and McKissock, W.: Surgical treatment of malignant extradural spinal tumors. Br. Med. J. *1*:1341–1344, 1965.
14. Bruckman, J. E., and Bloomer, W. D.: Management of spinal cord compression. Semin. Oncol. *5*:135–140, 1978.
15. Bucknill, T., Jackson, J. W., and Kendall, B. E.: Hemangioma of a vertebral body treated by ligation of the segmental arteries. J. Bone Joint Surg. [Br.] *55*:534–539, 1973.
16. Cahan, W. G., Woodward, H. Q., Higinbotham, N. L., et al.: Sarcoma arising in irradiated bone. Cancer *1*:3–29, 1948.
17. Cappellani, G., Giuffre, F., Tropea, R., et al.: Primary spinal epidural lymphoma. J. Neurosurg. Sci. *30*:147–151, 1986.
18. Chiurco, A. A.: Multiple exostoses of bone with fatal spinal cord compression. Neurology *20*:275–278, 1970.
19. Citrin, D. L., Bessent, R. G., and Greig, W. R.: A comparison of sensitivity and accuracy of the 99mTc phosphate bone scan and skeletal radiograph in the diagnosis of bone metastases. Clin. Radiol. *28*:107–111, 1977.
20. Clain, A.: Secondary malignant disease of bone. Br. J. Cancer *19*:15–29, 1965.
21. Clark, C. R., Keggi, K. J., and Panjabi, M. M.: Methylmethacrylate stabilization of the cervical spine. J. Bone Joint Surg. [Am.] *66*:40–46, 1984.
22. Clausen, N., Gotze, H., Pedersen, A., et al.: Skeletal scintigraphy and radiography at onset of acute lymphocytic leukemia in children. Med. Pediatr. Oncol. *11*:291–296, 1983.
23. Compere, E. L., Johnson, W. E., and Coventry, M. B.: Vertebra plana (Calve's disease) due to eosinophilic granuloma. J. Bone Joint Surg. [Am.] *36*:969–980, 1954.
24. Conrad, E. U., III, Olszewski, A. D., Berger, M., et al.: Pediatric spine tumors with spinal cord compromise. J Pediatr. Orthop. *12*:454–460, 1992.
25. Constans, J. P., Divitiis, E., Donzelli, R., et al.: Spinal metastases with neurological manifestations: Review of 600 cases. J. Neurosurg. *59*:111–118, 1983.
26. Corcoran, R. J., Thrall, J. H., Kyle, R. W., et al.: Solitary abnormalities in bone scans of patients with extraosseous malignancies. Radiology *121*:663–667, 1976.
27. Corwin, J., and Lindberg, R. D.: Solitary plasmacytoma of bone vs. extramedullary plasmacytoma and their relationship to multiple myeloma. Cancer *43*:1007–1013, 1979.
28. Cotrel, Y., Dubousset, J., and Guillaumat, M.: New universal instrumentation in spinal surgery. Clin. Orthop. *227*:10–23, 1988.
29. Cybulski, G. R., Von Roenn, K. A., D'Angelo, C. M., and DeWald, R. L.: Luque rod stabilization for metastatic disease of the spine. Surg. Neurol. *28*:277–283, 1987.
30. Dahlin, D. C.: Giant-cell tumor of vertebrae above the sacrum. Cancer *39*:1350–1356, 1977.
31. Dahlin, D. C.: Bone Tumors: General Aspects and Data on 6221 Cases. 3rd ed. Springfield, IL, Charles C. Thomas, 1978.
32. Danzig, L. A., Resnick, D., and Akeson, W. H.: The treatment of cervical spine metastasis from the prostate with a halo cast. Spine *5*(5):395–398, 1980.
33. Denis, F.: The three column spine and its significance in the classification of acute thoracolumbar spine injuries. Spine *8*(8):817–831, 1983.
34. Devita, V. T., Canellos, G. P., Chabner, B., et al.: Advanced diffuse histiocytic lymphoma, a potentially curable disease: Results with combined chemotherapy. Lancet *1*:248–250, 1975.
35. DeWald, R. L., Bridwell, K. H., Prodromas, C., and Rodts, M. F.: Reconstructive spinal surgery as palliation for metastatic malignancies of the spine. Spine *10*(1):21–26, 1985.
36. Di Lorenzo, N., Spallone, A., Nolletti, A., and Nardi, P.: Giant-cell tumors of the spine: A clinical study of six cases, with emphasis on the radiological features, treatment, and follow-up. Neurosurgery *6*(1):29–34, 1980.
37. Dolin, M. G.: Acute massive dural compression secondary to methylmethacrylate replacement of a tumorous lumbar vertebral body. Spine *14*(1):108–110, 1989.
38. Dowdle, J. A., Winter, R. B., and Dehner, L. P.: Postradiation osteosarcoma of the cervical spine in childhood. J. Bone Joint Surg. [Am.] *59*:969–971, 1977.
39. Drury, A. B., Palmer, P. H., and Highman, W. J.: Carcinomatous metastases to the vertebral bodies. J. Clin. Pathol. *17*:448–460, 1964.
40. Edelstyn, G. A., Gillespie, P. J., and Grebell, E. S.: The radiologic demonstration of osseous metastases: Experimental observations. Clin. Radiol. *18*:158–164, 1967.
41. Fidler, M. W.: Pathologic fractures of the cervical spine. J. Bone Joint Surg. [Br.] *67*:352–357, 1985.
42. Fidler, M. W.: Anterior decompression and stabilization of metastatic spinal fractures. J. Bone Joint Surg. [Br.] *68*:83–90, 1986.
43. Fielding, J. W., Pyle, R. N., and Fietti, V. G.: Anterior cervical vertebral body resection and bone grafting for benign and malignant tumors. J. Bone Joint Surg. [Am.] *61*:251–253, 1979.
44. Findlay, G. F. G.: The role of vertebral body collapse in the management of malignant spinal cord compression. J. Neurol. Neurosurg. Psychiatry *50*:151–154, 1987.
45. Flatley, T. J., Anderson, M. H., and Anast, G. T.: Spinal instability due to malignant disease. J. Bone Joint Surg. [Am.] *66*:47–52, 1984.
46. Fowles, J. V., and Bobechko, W. P.: Solitary eosinophilic granuloma of bone. J. Bone Joint Surg. [Br.] *52*:238–243, 1970.
47. Fraser, R. D., Paterson, D. C., and Simpson, D. A.: Orthopaedic aspects of spinal tumours in children. J. Bone Joint Surg. [Br.] *59*:143–151, 1977.
48. Galasko, C. S. B.: The development of skeletal metastases. In Weiss, L., and Gilbert, H. A. (eds.): Bone Metastases. Boston, G. K. Hall Medical Publishers, 1981, pp. 157–168.
49. Gennari, L., Azzarelli, A., and Quagliuolo, V.: A posterior approach for the excision of sacral chordoma. J. Bone Joint Surg. [Br.] *69*:565–568, 1987.
50. Gertzbein, S. D., MacMichael, D., and Tile, M.: Harrington instrumentation as a method of fixation in fractures of the spine. J. Bone Joint Surg. [Br.] *64*:526–529, 1982.
51. Gilbert, R. W., Kim, J. H., and Posner, J. B.: Epidural spinal cord compression from metastatic tumor: Diagnosis and treatment. Ann. Neurol. *3*(1):40–51, 1978.
52. Godersky, J. C., Smoker, W. R. K., and Knutzon, R.: Use of magnetic resonance imaging in the evaluation of metastatic spinal disease. Neurosurgery *21*(5):676–680, 1987.
53. Golfieri, R., Baddeley, H., and Pringle, J. S.: The role of STIR sequence in magnetic resonance imaging examination of bone tumors. Br. J. Radiol. *63*:251–256, 1990.

54. Goyal, R. N.: Epidural lipoma causing compression of the spinal cord. Surg. Neurol. *14*:77–79, 1980.
55. Graham, W. D.: Metastatic cancer to bone. *In* Graham, W. D. (ed.): Bone Tumours. London, Butterworths, 1966, pp. 94–100.
56. Green, N. E., Robertson, W. W., and Kilroy, A. W.: Eosinophilic granuloma of the spine with associated neural deficit. J. Bone Joint Surg. [Am.] *62*:1198–1202, 1980.
57. Greenberg, H. S., Kim, J. H., and Posner, J. B.: Epidural spinal cord compression from metastatic tumor. Ann. Neurol. *8*:361–366, 1980.
58. Griffin, J. B.: Benign osteoblastoma of the thoracic spine. J. Bone Joint Surg. [Am.] *60*:833–835, 1978.
59. Habermann, E. T., Sachs, R., Stern, R. E., et al.: The pathology and treatment of metastatic disease of the femur. Clin. Orthop. *169*:70–82, 1982.
60. Haid, R. W., Kaufmann, H. H., Schochet, S. S., and Marano, G. D.: Epidural lipomatosis simulating an epidural abscess. Neurosurgery *21*(5):744–747, 1987.
61. Hall, A. J., and MacKay, N. N. S.: The results of laminectomy for compression of the cord or cauda equina by extradural malignant tumor. J. Bone Joint Surg. [Br.] *55*:497–505, 1973.
62. Hall, D. J., and Webb, J. K.: Anterior plate fixation in spine tumor surgery: Indications, technique, and results. Spine *16*:580–583, 1991.
63. Harrington, K. D.: The use of methylmethacrylate for vertebral-body replacement and anterior stabilization of pathologic fracture-dislocations of the spine due to metastatic malignant disease. J. Bone Joint Surg. [Am.] *63*:36–46, 1981.
64. Harrington, K. D.: Current concepts review: Metastatic disease of the spine. J. Bone Joint Surg. [Am.] *68*:1110–1115, 1986.
65. Harrington, K. D.: Anterior decompression and stabilization of the spine as a treatment for vertebral collapse and spinal cord compression from metastatic malignancy. Clin. Orthop. *233*:177–197, 1988.
66. Harrington, K. D.: Metastatic disease of the spine. *In* Harrington, K. D. (ed.): Orthopaedic Management of Metastatic Bone Disease. St. Louis, C. V. Mosby, 1988, pp. 309–383.
67. Harrington, K. D., Sim, F. H., Enis, J. E., et al.: Methylmethacrylate as an adjunct in internal fixation of pathological fractures. J. Bone Joint Surg. [Am.] *58*:1047–1055, 1976.
68. Hay, M. C., Paterson, D., and Taylor, T. K. F.: Aneurysmal bone cysts of the spine. J. Bone Joint Surg. [Br.] *60*:406–411, 1978.
69. Healy, M. E., Hesselink, J. R., Ostrup, R. C., and Alksne, J. F.: Demonstration by magnetic resonance of symptomatic spinal epidural lipomatosis. Neurosurgery *21*(3):414–415, 1987.
70. Hermann, G., Sacher, M., Lanzieri, C. F., et al.: Chondrosarcoma of the spine: An unusual radiographic presentation. Skeletal Radiol. *14*:178–183, 1985.
71. Hirsh, L. F., Thanki, A., and Spector, H. B.: Spinal subdural metastatic adenocarcinoma. Neurosurgery *10*(5):621–625, 1982.
72. Hirsh, L. F., Thanki, A., and Spector, H. B.: Primary spinal chondrosarcoma with eighteen-year follow-up. Neurosurgery *14*(6):747–749, 1984.
73. Huvos, A.: Osteogenic sarcoma of bones and soft tissues in older persons: A clinico-pathologic analysis of 117 patients older than 60 years. Cancer *57*:1442–1449, 1986.
74. Huvos, A. G., Woodward, H. Q., Cahan, W. G., and Higinbotham, N. L.: Postirradiation osteogenic sarcoma of bone and soft tissue: A clinico-pathologic study of 66 patients. Cancer *55*:1244–1255, 1985.
75. Jaffe, H. L.: Tumors and Tumorous Conditions of the Bones and Joints. Philadelphia, Lea & Febiger, 1958.
76. Johnson, J. R., Leatherman, K. D., and Holt, R. T.: Anterior decompression of the spinal cord for neurologic deficit. Spine *8*(4):396–405, 1983.
77. Kaiser, T. E., Pritchard, D. J., and Unni, K. K.: Clinicopathologic study of sacrococcygeal chordoma. Cancer *54*:2574–2578, 1984.
78. Kak, V. J., Prabhakar, S., Khosla, V. K., and Banerjee, A. K.: Solitary osteochondroma of spine causing spinal cord compression. Clin. Neurol. Neurosurg. *87*(2):135–138, 1985.
79. Kattapuram, S. V., Khurana, J. S., Scott, J. A., and El-Khoury, G. A.: Negative scintigraphy with positive magnetic resonance imaging in bone metastases. Skeletal Radiol. *19*:113–116, 1990.
80. Keim, H. A., and Reina, E. G.: Osteoid-osteoma as a cause of scoliosis. J. Bone Joint Surg. [Am.] *57*:159–163, 1975.
81. Knowling, M., Harwood, A., and Bergsagel, D. E.: A comparison of extramedullary plasmacytoma with multiple and solitary plasma cell tumors of bone. J. Clin. Oncol. *1*:255–262, 1983.
82. Kornberg, M.: Primary Ewing's sarcoma of the spine. Spine *11*(1):54–57, 1986.
83. Kostuik, J. P.: Anterior spinal cord decompression for lesions of the thoracic and lumbar spine: Techniques, new methods of internal fixation, results. Spine *8*(5):512–531, 1983.
84. Kostuik, J. P., Errico, T. J., Gleason, T. F., and Errico, C. C.: Spinal stabilization of vertebral column tumors. Spine *13*(3):250–256, 1988.
85. Leeson, M. C., Makley, J. T., and Carter, J. R.: Metastatic skeletal disease in the pediatric population. J. Pediatr. Orthop. *5*:261–267, 1985.
86. Lesoin, F., Rousseaux, M., Lozes, G., et al.: Posterolateral approach to tumours of the dorsolumbar spine. Acta Neurochir. (Wien) *81*:40–44, 1986.
87. Levine, A. M. Boriani, S., Donati, D., and Companacci, M.: Benign tumors of the cervical spine. Spine *17*(5):399–406, 1992.
88. Levy, W. J., Bay, J., and Dohn, D.: Spinal cord meningioma. J. Neurosurg. *57*:804–812, 1982.
89. Levy, W. J., Latchaw, J., Hahn, J. F., et al.: Spinal neurofibromas: A report of 66 cases and a comparison with meningiomas. Neurosurgery *18*(3):331–334, 1986.
90. Lodewick, G. S.: Determining growth rates of focal lesions of bone from radiographs. Radiology *134*:577–583, 1980.
91. Loftus, C. M., Michelsen, C. B., Rapoport, F., and Antunes, J. L.: Management of plasmacytomas of the spine. Neurosurgery *13*:30–36, 1983.
92. Loftus, C. M., Rozario, R. A., Prager, R., and Scott, R. M.: Solitary osteochondroma of T4 with thoracic cord compression. Surg. Neurol. *13*:355–357, 1980.
93. Lozman, J., and Holmblad, J.: Cavernous hemangiomas associated with scoliosis and a localized consumptive coagulopathy. J. Bone Joint Surg. [Am.] *58*:1021–1024, 1976.
94. Lubicky, J. P., Patel, N. S., and DeWald, R. L.: Two-stage spondylectomy for giant cell tumor of L4. Spine *8*(1):112–115, 1983.
95. Malat, J., Virapongse, C., and Levine, A.: Solitary osteochondroma of the spine. Spine *11*(6):625–628, 1986.
96. Manabe, S., Tateishi, A., Abe, M., and Ohno, T.: Surgical treatment of metastatic tumors of the spine. Spine *14*(1):41–47, 1989.
97. Mankin, H. J., Lange, T. A., and Spanier, S. S.: The hazards of biopsy in patients with malignant primary bone or soft tissue tumors. J. Bone Joint Surg. [Am.] *64*:1121–1127, 1982.
98. Marchesi, D. G., Boos, N., and Aebi, M.: Surgical treatment of tumors of the cervical spine and first two thoracic vertebrae. J. Spinal Disord. *6*:489–496, 1993.
99. Marsh, B. W., Bonfiglio, M., Brady, L. P., and Enneking, W. F.: Benign osteoblastoma: Range of manifestations. J. Bone Joint Surg. [Am.] *57*:1–9, 1975.
100. Martin, N. S., and Williamson, J.: The role of surgery in the treatment of malignant tumours of the spine. J. Bone Joint Surg. [Br.] *52*:227–237, 1970.
101. Matsui, H., Tatezaki, S., and Tsuji, H.: Ceramic vertebral body replacement for metastatic spine tumors. J. Spinal Disord. *7*:248–254, 1994.
102. McAfee, P. C., Bohlman, H. H., Ducker, T., and Eismont, F. J.: Failure of stabilization of the spine with methylmethacrylate. J. Bone Joint Surg. [Am.] *68*:1145–1157, 1986.
103. McLain, R. F., and Weinstein, J. N.: Solitary plasmacytomas of the spine: A review of 84 cases. J. Spinal Disord. *2*(2):69–74, 1989.
103a. McLain, R.F.: Endoscopically assisted decompression for metastatic thoracic neoplasms. Spine *23*:1130–1135, 1998.
104. Meissner, W. A., and Warren, S.: Neoplasms. *In* Anderson, W. A. D. (ed.): Pathology. 5th ed. Vol. 1. St. Louis, C. V. Mosby, 1966, pp. 534–540.
105. Meyers, S. P., Yaw, K., and Devaney, K.: Giant cell tumor of the thoracic spine: MR appearance. Am. J. Neuroradiol. *15*(5):962–964, 1994.
106. Milch, A., and Changus, G. W.: Response of bone to tumor invasion. Cancer *9*(2):340–351, 1956.
107. Millburn, L., Hibbs, G. C., and Hendrickson, F. R.: Treatment of spinal cord compression from metastatic carcinoma. Cancer *21*:447–452, 1968.

108. Mindell, E. R.: Current concepts review: Chordoma. J. Bone Joint Surg. [Am.] *63*:501–505, 1981.

109. Mirra, J. M., Gold, R. H., and Picci, P.: General considerations. *In* Mirra, J. M. (ed.): Bone Tumors. Philadelphia, Lea & Febiger, 1989, pp. 31–33.

110. Mirra, J. M., Gold, R. H., and Picci, P.: Osseous tumors of intramedullary origins. *In* Mirra, J. M. (ed.): Bone Tumors. Philadelphia, Lea & Febiger, 1989, pp. 350–358.

111. Nather, A., and Bose, K.: The results of decompression of cord or cauda equina compression from metastatic extradural tumors. Clin. Orthop. *169*:103–108, 1982.

112. Nesbit, M. E., Kieffer, S., and D'Angelo, G. J.: Reconstitution of vertebral height in histiocytosis X: A long-term follow-up. J. Bone Joint Surg. [Am.] *51*:1360–1368, 1969.

113. Nicholls, P. J., and Jarecky, T. W.: The value of posterior decompression by laminectomy for malignant tumors of the spine. Clin. Orthop. *201*:210–213, 1985.

114. O'Neil, J., Gardner, V., and Armstrong, G.: Treatment of tumors of the thoracic and lumbar spinal column. Clin. Orthop. *227*:103–112, 1988.

115. Ostrowsky, M. L., Krishnan, K. U., Banks, P. M., et al.: Malignant lymphoma of bone. Cancer *58*:2646–2655, 1986.

116. Overby, M. C., and Rothman, A. S.: Anterolateral decompression for metastatic epidural spinal cord tumors. J. Neurosurg. *62*:344–348, 1985.

117. Padovani, R., Poppi, M., Pozzati, E., et al.: Spinal epidural hemangiomas. Spine *6*(4):336–340, 1981.

118. Palmer, F. J., and Blum, P. W.: Osteochondroma with spinal cord compression: A report of three cases. J. Neurosurg. *52*:842–845, 1980.

119. Panjabi, M. M., Goel, V. K., Clark, C. R., et al.: Biomechanical study of cervical spine stabilization with methylmethacrylate. Spine *10*(3):198–203, 1985.

120. Perrin, R. G., and McBroom, R. J.: Anterior vs. posterior decompression for symptomatic spinal metastasis. Can. J. Neurol. Sci. *14*(1):75–80, 1987.

121. Pettine, K. A., and Klassen, R. A.: Osteoid-osteoma and osteoblastoma of the spine. J. Bone Joint Surg. [Am.] *68*:354–361, 1986.

122. Pilepich, M. V., Vietti, T. J., Nesbit, M. E., et al.: Ewing's sarcoma of the vertebral column. Int. J. Radiat. Oncol. Biol. Phys. *7*:27–31, 1981.

123. Poulsen, J. O., Jensen, J. T., and Tommesen, P.: Ewing's sarcoma simulating vertebra plana. Acta Orthop. Scand. *46*:211–215, 1975.

124. Powles, T. J.: Breast cancer osteolysis, bone metastasis, and the antiosteolytic effect of aspirin. Lancet *1*:608–610, 1976.

125. Price, C. H. G., and Goldie, W.: Paget's sarcoma of bone: A study of 80 cases. J. Bone Joint Surg. [Br.] *51*:205–224, 1969.

126. Rahmonni, A., Divintz, M., and Mathieu, D.: Detection of multiple myeloma involving the spine: Efficacy of fat-suppression and contrast-enhanced MR imaging. Am. J. Radiol. *160*:1049–1052, 1993.

127. Ransford, A. O., Pozo, J. L., Hutton, P. A. N., and Kirwan, E. O.: The behavior pattern of the scoliosis associated with osteoid osteoma or osteoblastoma of the spine. J. Bone Joint Surg. [Br.] *66*:16–20, 1984.

128. Rich, T. A., Schiller, A., Suit, H. D., and Mankin, H. J.: Clinical and pathological review of 48 cases of chordoma. Cancer *56*:182–187, 1985.

129. Rogalsky, R. J., Black, G. B., and Reed, M. H.: Orthopaedic manifestations of leukemia in children. J. Bone Joint Surg. [Am.] *68*:494–501, 1986.

130. Roy-Camille, R., Saillant, G., and Mazel, C.: Internal fixation of the lumbar spine with pedicle screw plating. Clin. Orthop. *203*:7–17, 1986.

131. Russin, L. A., Robinson, M. J., Engle, H. A., and Sonni, A.: Ewing's sarcoma of the lumbar spine. Clin. Orthop. *164*:126–129, 1982.

132. Saitoh, H., and Hida, M.: Metastatic processes and a potential indication of treatment for metastatic lesions of renal adenocarcinoma. J. Urol. *128*:916–918, 1982.

133. Samson, I. R., Springfield, D. S., Suit, H. D., and Mankin, H. J.: Operative treatment of sacrococcygeal chordoma: A review of twenty-one cases. J. Bone Joint Surg. [Am.] *75*:1476–1484, 1993.

134. Savini, R., Gherlinzoni, F., Morandi, M., et al.: Surgical treatment of giant-cell tumor of the spine. J. Bone Joint Surg. [Am.] *65*:1283–1289, 1983.

135. Savitz, M. H., Goldstein, H. B., Jaffrey, I. S., et al.: Ewing's sarcoma arising in the sacral epidural space. Mt. Sinai J. Med. *55*(4):339–342, 1988.

136. Schajowicz, F.: Tumors and Tumorlike Lesions of Bones and Joints. New York, Springer-Verlag, 1981, pp. 281–302.

137. Sen, C., Eisenberg, M., Casden, A. M., et al.: Management of the vertebral artery in excision of extradural tumors of the cervical spine. Neurosurgery *36*:106–115, 1995.

138. Sharma, B. S., Khosla, V. K., and Banerjee, A. K.: Primary spinal epidural Ewing's sarcoma. Clin. Neurol. Neurosurg. *88*(4):299–302, 1986.

139. Shaw, M. D. M., Rose, J. E., and Paterson, A.: Metastatic extradural malignancy of the spine. Acta Neurochir. (Wien) *52*:113–120, 1980.

140. Sherk, H. H., Nicholson, J. T., and Nixon, J. E.: Vertebra plana and eosinophilic granuloma of the cervical spine in children. Spine *3*(2):116–121, 1978.

141. Sherman, R. M. P., and Waddell, J. P.: Laminectomy for metastatic epidural spinal cord tumors. Clin. Orthop. *207*:55–63, 1986.

142. Shives, T. C., Dahlin, D. C., Sim, F. H., et al.: Osteosarcoma of the spine. J. Bone Joint Surg. [Am.] *68*:660–668, 1986.

143. Shono, Y., McAfee, P. C., Cunningham, B. W., and Brantigan, J. W.: A biomechanical analysis of decompression and reconstruction methods in the cervical spine: Emphasis on a carbon-fiber-composite cage. J. Bone Joint Surg. [Am.] *75*:1674–1684, 1993.

144. Siegal, T., and Siegal, T.: Surgical decompression of anterior and posterior malignant epidural tumors compressing the spinal cord: A prospective study. Neurosurgery *17*(3):424–432, 1985.

145. Siegal, T., and Siegal, T.: Current considerations in the management of neoplastic spinal cord compression. Spine *14*(2):223–228, 1988.

146. Siegal, T., Tiqva, P., and Siegal, T.: Vertebral body resection for epidural compression by malignant tumors. J. Bone Joint Surg. [Am.] *67*:375–382, 1985.

147. Sim, F. H., Dahlin, D. C., Stauffer, R. N., and Laws, E. R.: Primary bone tumors simulating lumbar disc syndrome. Spine *2*(1):65–74, 1977.

148. Skinner, D. G., and Colvin, R. B: Diagnosis and management of renal cell carcinoma. Cancer *28*:1165–1177, 1971.

149. Slepian, A., and Hamby, W. B.: Neurologic complications associated with hereditary deforming chondrodysplasia. J. Neurosurg. *8*:529–535, 1951.

150. Springfield, D. S., Enneking, W. F., Neff, J. R., and Makley, J. T.: Principles of tumor management. Instr. Course Lect. *33*:1–25, 1984.

151. Steffee, A. D., Biscup, R. S., and Sitkowski, D. J.: Segmental spinal plates with pedicle screw fixation: A new internal fixation device for disorders of the lumbar and thoracolumbar spine. Clin. Orthop. *203*:45–53, 1986.

152. Stener, B.: Total spondylectomy in chondrosarcoma arising from the seventh thoracic vertebra. J. Bone Joint Surg. [Br.] *53*:288–295, 1971.

153. Stener, B., and Gunterberg, B.: High amputation of the sacrum for extirpation of tumors. Spine *3*:351–366, 1978.

154. Stener, B., and Johnsen, O. E.: Complete removal of three vertebrae for giant cell tumour. J. Bone Joint Surg. [Br.] *53*:278–287, 1971.

155. Stoll, B. A.: Natural history, prognosis, and staging of bone metastases. In Stoll, B. A., and Parbhoo, S. (eds.): Bone Metastases: Monitoring and Treatment. New York, Raven Press, 1983, pp. 1–20.

156. Sudanese, A., Toni, A., Ciaroni, D., et al.: The role of surgery in treatment of localized Ewing's sarcoma. Chir. Organi Mov. *75*(3):217–230, 1990.

157. Sundaresan, N., Galicich, J. H., Lane, J. M., et al.: Treatment of neoplastic epidural cord compression by vertebral body resection and stabilization. J. Neurosurg. *63*:676–684, 1985.

158. Sundaresan, N., Huvos, A. G., Rosen, G., and Lane, J. M.: Postradiation osteosarcoma of the spine following treatment of Hodgkin's disease. Spine *11*(1):90–92, 1986.

159. Sundaresan, N., Rosen, G., Huvos, A. G., and Krol, G.: Combined treatment of osteosarcoma of the spine. Neurosurgery 23(6):714–719, 1988.

160. Sundaresan, N., Scher, H., DiGiacinto, G. V., et al.: Surgical treatment of spinal cord compression in kidney cancer. J. Clin. Oncol. 4:1851–1856, 1986.

161. Tachdjian, M. O., and Matson, D. D.: Orthopaedic aspects of intraspinal tumors in infants and children. J. Bone Joint Surg. [Am.] 47:223–248, 1965.

162. Tolia, M. B., and Whitmore, W. R.: Solitary metastasis from renal carcinoma. J. Urol. 224:836–838, 1975.

163. Tomita, T., Galicich, J. H., and Sundaresan, N.: Radiation therapy for spinal epidural metastases with complete block. Acta Radiol. Oncol. 22:135–143, 1983.

164. Torma, T.: Malignant tumors of the spine and the spinal epidural space: A study based on 250 histologically verified cases. Acta Chir. Scand. Suppl. 225:1–138, 1957.

165. Valderrama, J. A. F., and Bullough, P. G.: Solitary myeloma of the spine. J. Bone Joint Surg. [Br.] 50:82–90, 1988.

166. Viadana, E.: Autopsy study of metastatic sites of breast cancer. Cancer Res. 33:179–181, 1973.

167. Waxman, A. D.: Bone scans are of sufficient accuracy and sensitivity to be part of the routine work up prior to definitive surgical treatment of cancer. In Van Scoy-Mosher, M. B. (ed.): Medical Oncology—Current Controversies in Cancer Treatment. Boston, G. K. Hall Medical Publishers, 1981, pp. 69–76.

168. Weinstein J. N.: Surgical approach to spine tumors. Orthopaedics 12(6):897–905, 1989.

169. Weinstein, J. N., and McLain, R. F.: Primary tumors of the spine. Spine 12(9):843–851, 1987.

170. White, A. A., III, and Panjabi, M. M.: Surgical constructs employing methylmethacrylate. In White, A. A., Panjabi, M. M. (eds.): Clinical Biomechanics of the Spine. Philadelphia, J. B. Lippincott, 1978, pp. 423–431.

171. White, W. A., Patterson, R. H., and Bergland, R. M.: Role of surgery in the treatment of spinal cord compression by metastatic neoplasm. Cancer 27(3):558–561, 1971.

172. Whitehouse, G. H., and Griffiths, G. J.: Roentgenologic aspects of spinal involvement by primary and metastatic Ewing's tumor. J. Can. Assoc. Radiol. 27:290–297, 1976.

173. Wiedemayer, H., Nau, H. E., Reinhardt, V., and Hebestreit, H. P.: Spinal cord compression by extensive epidural lipoma. Eur. Neurol. 27:46–50, 1987.

174. Willen, J., Lindahl, S., Irstam, L., and Nordwall, A.: Unstable thoracolumbar fractures: A study by CT and conventional roentgenology of the reduction effect of Harrington instrumentation. Spine 9(2):214–219, 1984.

175. Willis, R. A.: The Spread of Tumours in the Human Body. 3rd ed. London, Butterworths, 1973.

176. Wiltshaw, E.: The natural history of extramedullary plasmacytoma and its relation to solitary myeloma of bone and myelomatosis. Medicine 55:217–238, 1976.

177. Wong, D. A., Fornasier, V. L., and MacNab, I.: Spinal metastases: The obvious, the occult, and the imposters. Spine 15:1–4, 1990.

178. Wright, R. L.: Malignant tumors in the spinal extradural space: Results of surgical treatment. Ann. Surg. 157(2):227–231, 1963.

179. Young, R. F., Post, E. M., and King, G. A.: Treatment of spinal epidural metastases. J. Neurosurg. 53:741–748 1980.

39

Infections of the Spine

Bradford L. Currier, M.D.

Frank J. Eismont, M.D.

Historically, spine infections were devastating diseases with exceedingly high morbidity and mortality rates. With the advent of antimicrobial chemotherapy and powerful new diagnostic techniques, the prognosis has improved dramatically in recent years. There still are many pitfalls in the management of spine infections, however, and they still deserve great respect. Close cooperation between the orthopedist and the infectious disease specialist is essential because of the changing patterns of pathogenic organisms and the emergence of resistant strains. Successful management of spine infections includes maintaining a high level of diagnostic acuity to avoid delays in diagnosis, using antibiotic therapy as directed by biopsy results, and instituting appropriate surgical intervention, when indicated.

There are numerous ways to classify spine infections. The most basic is by the histologic response of the host to the specific organism. Most bacteria cause a pyogenic response, whereas *Mycobacteria*, fungi, *Brucella*, and syphilis induce a granulomatous reaction. Infections may be classified by their primary anatomic location—vertebral osteomyelitis, discitis, or epidural abscess. Another way to categorize spine infections is by cause; the main routes of infection are hematogenous, direct inoculation (postoperative and traumatic), and spread from a contiguous source. Finally, age may be the determinant, and infections may be classified as occurring in pediatric or adult populations. Each of these classifications has implications with regard to evaluation, treatment, and prognosis.

HISTORIC PERSPECTIVE

The first recorded descriptions of spine infections were those in the Hippocratic texts on tuberculous spondylitis written between the fourth century B.C. and the first century A.D. Sir Percival Pott's description of paralysis in association with tuberculosis of the spine in the 18th century led to the eponym *Pott's paraplegia*. His frustration with the inadequate treatment options available to him was shared by physicians for another 150 years: "To attend to a distemper from its beginning through a long and painful course, to its last fatal period, without even the hope of being able to do anything which shall be really serviceable, is of all tasks the most unpleasant."[261]

Prior to the advent of antimicrobial therapy, the treatment of tuberculosis of the spine was based on bed rest, often in a plaster cast, with attention to diet and exposure to fresh air and sunlight. Laminectomy was the mainstay of surgical treatment in the late 1800s and the early part of this century, but was later condemned by Seddon and others because it did not address the anterior disease and led to further instability.[237] In 1911, Hibbs[146] and Albee[7] independently described the use of posterior fusion to hasten recovery. The idea evolved from the demonstration that ankylosis of peripheral joints led to remission of local disease. Unfortunately, posterior fusion did not prevent progressive kyphosis or address the lesion that was causing paralysis, and the technique was later abandoned. The mortality rate for children treated by these various techniques was 40 per cent.[2] In 1894, Menard[226] described a series of patients with Pott's paraplegia who were successfully treated with decompression by costotransversectomy. The technique fell into disfavor because of a high rate of secondary infection, and it did not gain acceptance until Girdlestone reintroduced it in 1931 with aseptic technique.[123]

Ito and associates[163] described the anterior approach to the lumbar spine in 1934 and demonstrated that it provided wider exposure and allowed more radical débridement and fusion. Hodgson and colleagues[150–155] popularized the anterior approach for the management of tuberculosis of the spine and stressed radical excision and strut-graft fusion to prevent kyphosis and late-onset paraplegia.

Antituberculous chemotherapy became available in 1945 and was found to be capable of curing the disease even without surgery.[80, 109, 183, 184, 312] Faced with a number of wildly divergent regimens for the treatment of the disease, a group of investigators formed the British Medical Research Council Working Party on Tuberculosis of the Spine. This group set out to perform a number of large-scale, controlled prospective trials of treatment methods. These studies, and others to be described later, helped to determine the current treatment recommendations for this disease.

The first recorded description of a pyogenic spine infection was by Lannelongue in 1897.[191] Although pyogenic spine infections differ in many ways from tuberculous spondylitis, the surgical treatment of the former has been influenced a great deal by the developments in the management of tuberculosis. The introduction of penicillin and streptomycin revolutionized the treatment of all spine infections. As more powerful antimicrobial agents were developed and combinations and dosages were refined, the relative effectiveness of surgical treatment decreased.

The introduction of needle biopsy of the spine obviated the need for open biopsy in many cases. Greater awareness of spine infections and greater availability of better diagnostic modalities have shortened the delay in diagnosis and have diminished the role of surgery in the prevention or treatment of deformity. Patients with a neurologic deficit still are best managed with prompt surgical decompression, however, and, although the indications for surgery in other patients now are more limited, surgery still plays an important role in the management of spine infections.

PYOGENIC INFECTIONS

Postoperative Wound Infections and Disc Space Infections

These disorders are dealt with in Chapter 54.

Pediatric Discitis

Please refer to Chapter 14.

Vertebral Osteomyelitis

Epidemiology

Although the incidence of tuberculous spondylitis has decreased dramatically in recent years, the incidence of pyogenic vertebral osteomyelitis appears to have increased.[58, 305] Various reports have stated that vertebral osteomyelitis represents 2 to 7 per cent of all cases of osteomyelitis.[188, 276, 317, 326] The disease may occur from infancy to old age but has a predilection for the elderly.[32, 51, 58, 81, 106, 129, 174, 188, 277, 282, 317, 318] Approximately one half of patients with spine infections are more than 50 years old and two thirds are male.[282] The incidence may be higher in younger patients who are intravenous drug abusers.[237]

Etiology

Any condition that causes a bacteremia may lead to hematogenous vertebral osteomyelitis. The most frequent sources are urinary tract infections and the transient bacteremia caused by genitourinary procedures.[51, 106, 113, 117, 277, 305, 319] Of 198 cases in the literature in which the probable source of infection was noted, it was the genitourinary tract in 29 per cent, soft tissue infections in 13 per cent, and respiratory tract infections in 11 per cent; 1.5 per cent of the infections occurred in intravenous drug abusers,[282] but this association is being reported with increasing frequency.[158, 185, 190, 228, 282, 283, 294] Vertebral osteomyelitis also may be caused by direct inoculation of bacteria into the spine by penetrating wounds, spine surgery, chemonucleolysis, or discography (Fig. 39–1).[25, 84, 91, 200, 256, 264, 270, 282, 285, 306, 310] The source of infection could not be identified in 37 per cent of cases.[282]

Immunocompromised hosts appear to be particularly susceptible to spine infections.[51, 113, 282, 319] In particular, diabetic persons have a high incidence of vertebral osteomyelitis.[32, 61, 113, 305]

Kulowski[188] thought that trauma was a predisposing factor in pyogenic vertebral osteomyelitis. More recent studies have not supported that association.[113, 237, 277] In Sapico and Montgomerie's review of 207 cases in the literature in which the presence or absence of blunt trauma was discussed, in only 5 per cent was there a history of trauma.[282]

Bacteriology

In 1931, Hatch[142] reviewed the literature and reported that the causative organism was almost exclusively *Staphylococcus aureus*. There has been an increase in the number of gram-negative bacillary infections.[106] From data reported in the postantibiotic era, Sapico and Montgomerie[282] found that 67 per cent of 222 patients were infected with gram-positive aerobic cocci; *S. aureus* constituted 55 per cent of the total. The emergence of tolerant *S. aureus* is a concern, and such strains may become more prevalent with the widespread use of antibiotics.[236] The most frequently isolated gram-negative organisms are *Escherichia coli*, *Pseudomonas* species, and *Proteus* species. These frequently are found in association with genitourinary tract infection[106, 113, 117, 143, 144, 272] *Pseudomonas aeruginosa* is frequently isolated from heroin abusers.[158, 164, 190, 196, 283, 325] In a review of 67 reported cases, gram-negative aerobic bacilli were

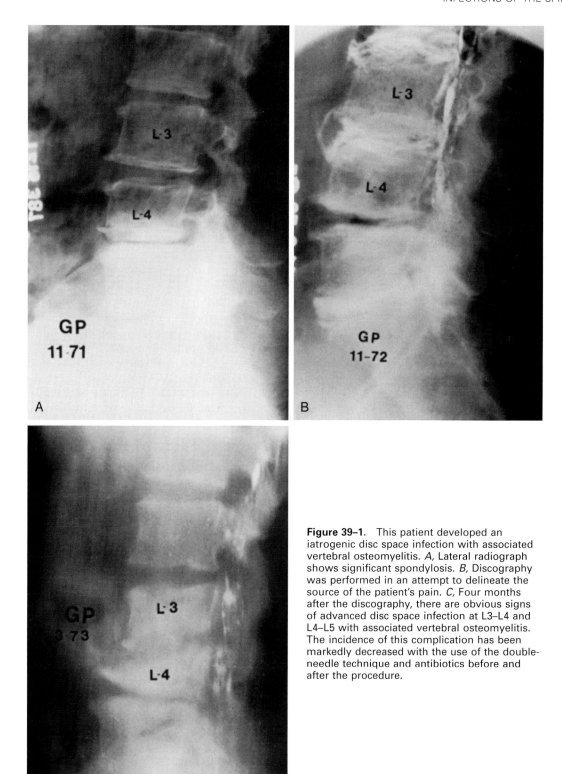

Figure 39–1. This patient developed an iatrogenic disc space infection with associated vertebral osteomyelitis. *A,* Lateral radiograph shows significant spondylosis. *B,* Discography was performed in an attempt to delineate the source of the patient's pain. *C,* Four months after the discography, there are obvious signs of advanced disc space infection at L3–L4 and L4–L5 with associated vertebral osteomyelitis. The incidence of this complication has been markedly decreased with the use of the double-needle technique and antibiotics before and after the procedure.

isolated in 82 per cent of the cases and *Pseudomonas* was the pathogen in 66 per cent.[283] However, one series included 15 intravenous drug abusers with pyogenic vertebral osteomyelitis, and all 11 with positive cultures were infected with *Staphylococcus aureus.*[51]

Salmonella osteomyelitis is uncommon. It generally occurs after an acute intestinal infection, but the interval between the gastroenteritis and the onset of osteomyelitis may be quite long[52]; in some cases, no previous infection can be identified.[229] *Salmonella* has a strong tendency to localize in tissues where there is pre-existing disease.[52, 281]

Infection with anaerobic bacteria is unusual and is generally associated with foreign bodies, open fractures, infected wounds, diabetes, or human bites.[162, 282]

Infection caused by multiple organisms is rarely encountered.[55, 282] Infection with *Haemophilus* species has been reported but is extremely rare in adults.[246, 253] Low-virulence organisms such as diphtheroids and coagulase-negative staphylococci may cause indolent infections with delayed diagnosis.[287] These organisms may grow slowly, and cultures should be held for 10 days before they are considered to be negative. Low-virulence organisms should not be dismissed as contaminants in patients suspected clinically to have vertebral osteomyelitis.[287] In one series of 111 cases of pyogenic vertebral osteomyelitis, low-virulence organisms caused 48 per cent of the infections in the 61 patients who were 60 years of age or older and 55 per cent of the 44 patients who had an impaired immune system.[51]

Pathogenesis and Pathology

Although the nucleus pulposus is an avascular tissue, it is relatively active metabolically.[43] It receives its nutrition via diffusion across the end plates and from blood vessels at the periphery of the annulus fibrosus.[43, 141] In the developing spine, very orderly arranged cartilage canals within the end plate contain vascular organs resembling glomeruli.[67, 322] Earlier studies suggested that blood vessels penetrate the nucleus pulposus in human fetuses and neonates.[141] However, elegant studies by Whalen and coauthors demonstrated that the nucleus pulposus is always avascular.[322] Coventry and colleagues[65] demonstrated that, after birth, the cartilage end plates become progressively thinner and the vessels within the cartilage canals become obliterated. Some persist up to the age of 30 years, but by adulthood most of the vessels within the end plate itself have disappeared.

Wiley and Trueta[327] demonstrated the rich arterial anastomosis within the vertebral body, with end arterioles in the metaphyseal region. Spinal arteries enter the canal through the intervertebral foramen at the level of the disc. Branches ascend and descend, supplying the vertebral bodies above and below. Through their injection studies, Wiley and Trueta[327] demonstrated how bacteria could easily spread hematogenously to the metaphyseal region of adjacent vertebrae. The infection also could start in the metaphyseal region of one vertebra and spread either across the avascular disc by lysosomal destruction of the nucleus pulposus or through vessels anastomosing on the periphery of the annulus fibrosus.

It has been suggested that Batson's plexus may be the route of hematogenous spread of infection. Batson[23] demonstrated, in injection studies, that dye flows into the valveless vertebral venous plexus when pressure is applied to the lower abdominal wall. The distribution of veins within the vertebral body is an arborization of

vessels. Minute tributaries draining the metaphyseal region empty into large, valveless, venous channels that drain into the loose plexus lining the canal. Wiley and Trueta[327] demonstrated that it takes considerable force to fill the very small metaphyseal vessels in a retrograde fashion, compared with the ease of injection of the metaphyseal arterioles; this suggests that the former is an unlikely route of hematogenous seeding.

Once microorganisms lodge in the low-flow vascular arcades in the metaphysis, infection spreads. The disc is destroyed by bacterial enzymes in a manner similar to the destruction of cartilage in septic arthritis. This is in contrast to tuberculous infections (to be described later), in which the end plates and bone are destroyed but the disc frequently is preserved.[60] In children, the cartilage canals allow microorganisms nearly direct access to the disc, which probably explains the clinical differences between spine infections in children and those in adults. In adults, disc space infection may occur by direct inoculation of the disc as a result of surgery, chemonucleolysis, or discography, but is unlikely to occur spontaneously.[124, 303]

Some authors have suggested that discitis in adults is a separate entity from vertebral osteomyelitis.[119, 174] Ghormley and associates[119] stressed the benign nature of this variation, but in Kemp and coworkers' series,[174] the disease was quite severe with a high rate of irreversible paralysis. It is conceivable that adult discs could receive blood directly through persistent vascular channels in the end plate, degenerative defects in the end plate, or vessels anastomosing on the peripheral annulus fibrosus and perhaps gaining access through rents in the annulus. If adult discitis occurs at all, it appears that hematogenous involvement of the metaphysis is far and away the most common mechanism and, whether the infection begins in the metaphysis and spreads across the disc or vice versa, the clinical manifestations and treatment are the same.

The upper cervical spine has a peculiar blood supply. Parke and associates[252] demonstrated a venous plexus around the odontoid, called the *pharyngeal vertebral vein*, which frequently has lymphovenous anastomoses. This venous plexus may be responsible for hematogenous spread to the upper cervical spine.[252, 337]

Abscesses may drain into the soft tissues surrounding the spine or into the spinal canal itself. In the cervical spine, a retropharyngeal abscess may invade the mediastinum.[188, 243] In the thoracic spine, an abscess may be paraspinous or retromediastinal.[188] Infection in the lumbar spine may cause a psoas abscess or, less commonly, an abscess pointing through Petit's triangle.[188] Occasionally, an abscess may create a tract through the greater sciatic foramen and appear in the buttock beneath the piriform fascia, in the perirectal region, or even in the popliteal fossa.[188] The more virulent organisms may not follow fascial planes and may extend into visceral structures. They also are more likely to produce spinal deformity. An abscess that enters the spinal canal is considered to be an epidural abscess and will be discussed later. Infection may cross the dura, causing a subdural or intradural abscess or meningitis.[104, 188]

The pathogenesis of neural compromise may be related to direct compression by epidural pus, by granulation tissue, or by bone and disc from the development of spinal deformity and instability. In addition, the cord or nerve roots may suffer ischemic damage from septic thrombosis or may be damaged by inflammatory infiltration of the dura (Figs. 39–2 and 39–3).[174, 188, 282]

An unusual association between vertebral osteomyelitis and compression fractures secondary to osteoporosis has been described. It is theorized that the osteomyelitis may develop as a complication of the fracture because the fracture creates a favorable environment for the hematogenous infection. Alternatively, the osteomyelitis may develop within the central portion of an osteoporotic vertebral body, perhaps because the bone is more hyperemic or because of vascular stasis. Infection may then lead to a pathologic fracture of the vertebra without the usual involvement of the disc space.[213]

Clinical Presentation

The clinical manifestations of spine infection are determined by the virulence of the organism and the resistance of the host. The presentation may be acute, subacute, or chronic.[174, 188] Before the antibiotic era, most patients had acute osteomyelitis, and in 68 per cent of the cases the disease was fulminant with severe toxemia.[142] The mortality rate ranged from 25 to 71 per cent.[142, 188] A literature review in 1979 found that only 20 per cent of the patients had symptoms for less than three weeks before presentation, 30 per cent had them for three weeks to three months, and 50 per cent had them for longer than three months.[282] Greater awareness of the disease and improved diagnostic modalities (especially magnetic resonance imaging [MRI]) have shortened the delay in diagnosis. In one series reported in 1997, 68 of 111 patients were diagnosed within 28 days of the onset of their symptoms and only eight patients were diagnosed more than three months after their symptoms began.[51]

Fever is present in only 52 per cent of the patients overall; pain in the back or neck is a much more common finding, occurring in approximately 90 per cent of patients.[282] Patients with acute infection present with fever, local spine pain, severe muscle spasm, and limitation of motion of the spine. With lumbar spine involvement, there may be a positive straight leg raising test, reluctance to bear weight, and hip flexion contracture due to psoas irritation. Hamstring tightness and loss of lumbar lordosis may be noted. Torticollis and fever may be the only presenting signs with cervical osteomyelitis.[316, 337]

Subacute and chronic infections may be much more insidious, and patients with such infections have a vague history. Pain may be the only symptom, especially with an occult infection by a low-virulence organism.[287] Approximately 15 per cent of the patients

have atypical symptoms, such as chest pain, abdominal pain, hip pain, radicular symptoms, or meningeal irritation.[133, 282, 305] These unusual and often vague complaints have led to unnecessary exploratory laparotomies before the diagnosis was made.[133, 282] A significant delay in diagnosis is common with chronic infections.[29, 32, 81, 106, 129, 176, 282, 305]

Vertebral osteomyelitis is more common in the lumbar region. In Sapico and Montgomerie's literature review,[282] in 48 per cent of 294 cases the involvement was lumbar, in 35 per cent thoracic, in 6.5 per cent cervical, and in approximately 5 per cent thoracolumbar and lumbosacral. Vertebral osteomyelitis at noncontiguous levels is uncommon (Fig. 39–4).

Abscesses are not encountered as frequently now as they were before the antibiotic era but should still be sought, both in the paraspinous region and in remote areas.[188] Abscess formation is more likely in the cervical and thoracic regions than in the lumbar spine.[113] A tender or pulsatile abdominal mass may be caused by a mycotic aneurysm, a dilatation of the wall of an artery resulting from an infection.[278]

Approximately 17 per cent of the patients present with a neurologic deficit secondary to nerve root or spinal cord involvement.[282] Eismont and others identified several factors that predisposed patients to paralysis, including diabetes,[61, 87, 188, 305] rheumatoid arthritis,[87] increased age,[87, 88] and a more cephalad level of infection.[87, 228] Patients on systemic steroid therapy are more likely to be paralyzed, and those infected with *S. aureus* seem to have the most severe degree of paralysis.[87] Some authors have noted that neurologic involvement is uncommon in patients infected with *Pseudomonas*.[164, 325]

With the advent of antibiotics, significant spine deformity is not as common as it was in the past, but significant kyphosis still may occur.[106, 188]

Infants and intravenous drug abusers are two subsets of patients who have slightly different presentations. Infants generally present acutely with high temperature, septicemia, and generalized signs of systemic illness (Fig. 39–5).[88, 262] Heroin abusers also present earlier than most patients. In a review of the literature, 81 per cent of heroin abusers presented within three months after the onset of their symptoms, compared with 50 per cent in the general population with vertebral osteomyelitis.[88, 262, 282, 283] The authors postulated that the earlier presentation may be related to infection with more virulent organisms, or perhaps to the fact that their patients have less tolerance to pain or may be using their back pain as an excuse to receive more narcotics.[283]

Diagnostic Evaluation

The erythrocyte sedimentation rate, Gram stain, and culture are the laboratory studies that are most useful in the diagnosis of pyogenic spine infections.[81, 113, 124, 282] The leukocyte count is increased on presentation in only 42 per cent of cases and usually is normal in patients with chronic disease.[113, 124, 282] Conversely, the

Text continued on page 1217

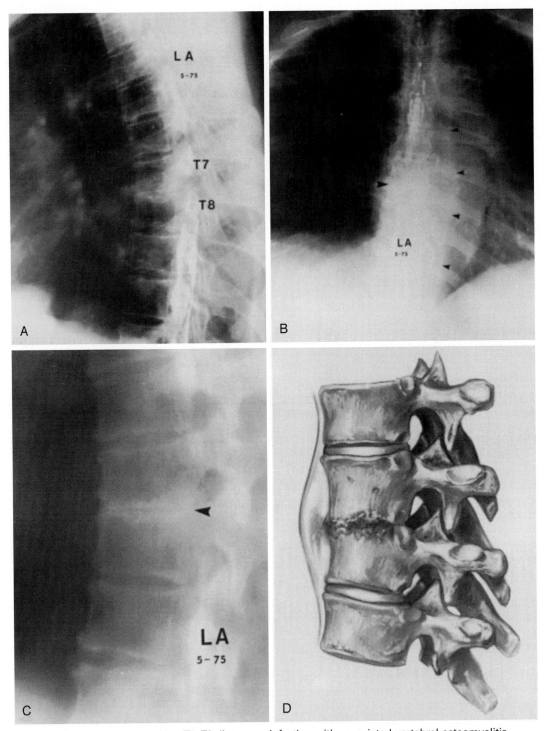

Figure 39–2. This patient with a T7–T8 disc space infection with associated vertebral osteomyelitis developed progressive paraplegia as a result of overwhelming sepsis associated with antibiotic-induced neutropenia. *A,* An early myelogram reveals a decreased disc space with associated sclerosis at the T7–T8 level. *B,* This anteroposterior radiograph reveals a significant associated paraspinal abscess *(arrowheads)* associated with this disc space infection and associated vertebral osteomyelitis. The T7–T8 interspace *(large arrowhead)* is at the center of the paraspinal abscess. *C,* This lateral tomogram best demonstrated the marked narrowing and sclerosis at the T7–T8 interspace. *D,* Artist's rendition of the pathology shows the collapse centered at the T7–T8 interspace and the associated paraspinal abscess.

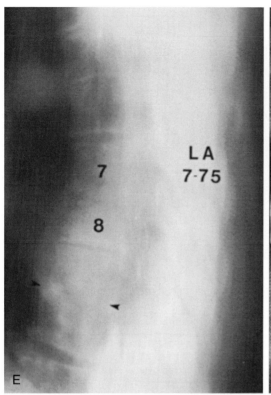

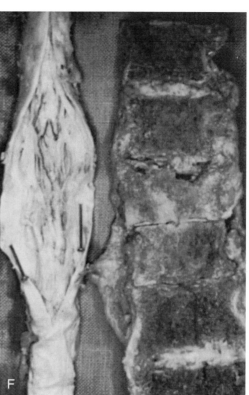

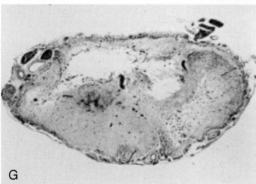

Figure 39–2 *Continued* *E,* Two months later, it is apparent that there has been spread of infection down to the T9–T10 interspace, with marked narrowing at that level. *F,* Gross destruction of the disc can be seen on this gross pathology specimen at the T7–T8, T8–T9, and T9–T10 levels. *G,* This microscopic section of the spinal cord has been taken at 11.5 times normal magnification. The dorsal aspect of the spinal cord is at the top of this figure. The patient was completely paraplegic. This is consistent with the changes seen within the spinal cord. (Courtesy of Dr. H. H. Bohlman, Cleveland, Ohio.)

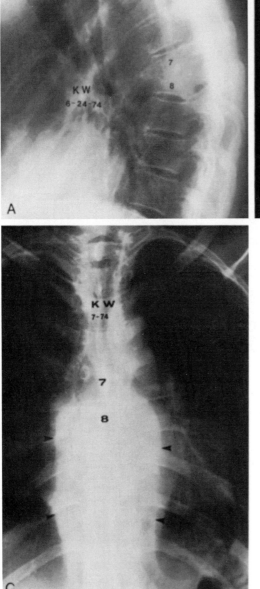
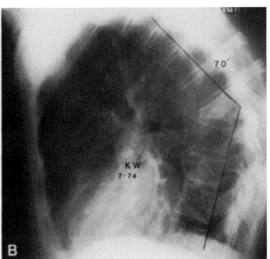

Figure 39–3.   This patient died with thoracic vertebral osteomyelitis secondary to overwhelming meningitis associated with the spine infection. *A,* The patient developed a T7–T8 disc space infection with associated vertebral osteomyelitis following a urologic operation with associated postoperative sepsis. He was treated initially with oral antibiotics. *B,* One month later, there is an obvious increasing kyphosis secondary to the spine infection. The patient is still being mobilized despite this deformity. *C,* This anteroposterior radiograph taken at the time of transfer to our institution reveals a large paraspinous abscess *(arrowheads).* At this time the patient had an incomplete paraplegia.

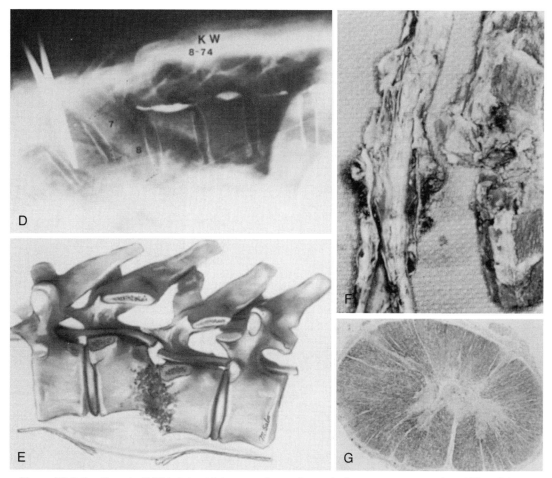

Figure 39–3 *Continued* *D,* This lateral intraoperative radiograph demonstrates gross instability of the thoracic spine with the T7 vertebra 50 per cent retrolisthesed on the T8 vertebra. At this time the patient still had an incomplete paraplegia. Surgery was undertaken to drain the paraspinal abscess. *E,* This drawing shows the extent of destruction at the T7–T8 interspace. The retrolisthesis of T7 on T8 is well demonstrated. The paraspinous abscess is also shown. *F,* The gross destruction of the anterior vertebral column is well demonstrated in this pathology specimen. *G,* This transverse section of the spinal cord has been magnified 11.5 times. Although there are significant changes within the neural tissue, this patient had an incomplete paraplegia at the time of death. (Courtesy of Dr. H. H. Bohlman, Cleveland, Ohio.)

Figure 39–4. Although this is uncommon, some patients present with vertebral osteomyelitis at noncontiguous levels. This diabetic patient had an infection of the cervical spine as well as the lumbar spine secondary to *Staphylococcus aureus. A,* The patient has an obvious disc space infection at L2–L3, with an associated vertebral osteomyelitis. *B,* This lateral radiograph of the cervical spine demonstrates a disc space infection at C5–C6 with destruction of the adjacent bone. The patient had a quadriparesis as a result of this infection.

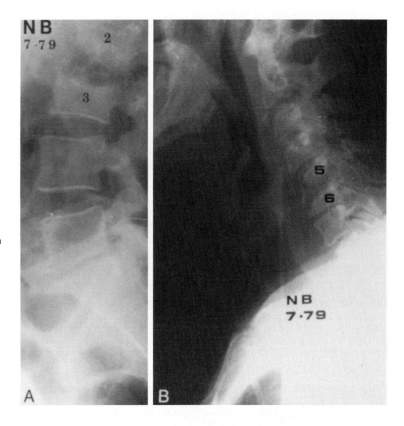

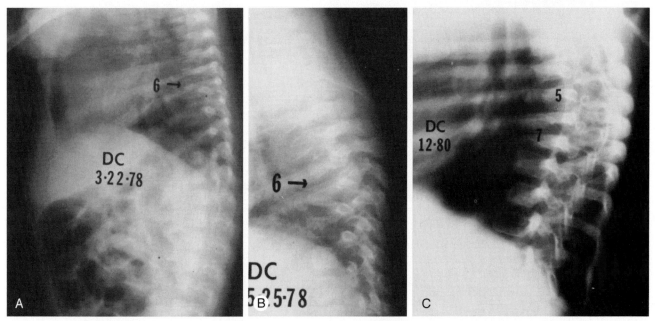

Figure 39–5. This infant developed vertebral osteomyelitis and life-threatening sepsis. Unlike the relatively benign disc space infection of childhood, this infection of infancy follows a much more destructive course. *A,* At the time the infant became septic, the T6 vertebral body could be visualized *(arrow). B,* Two months later, despite aggressive antibiotic treatment, there is gross destruction of the T6 vertebral body *(arrow). C,* This lateral roentgenogram taken 2.5 years after the spine infection reveals that the patient has a kyphotic deformity from T5 to T7. This deformity behaves very much like an anterior failure of formation of the T6 vertebral body. (From Eismont, F.J., Bohman, H.H., Soni, P.L., et al.: Vertebral osteomyelitis in infants. J Bone Joint Surg *64B*:32–35, 1982.)

sedimentation rate was increased in 92 per cent of 184 patients reported in the literature.[282] It is a very nonspecific test, however, and the rate may be increased in pregnancy, malignancy, other infections, dysproteinemias, and connective tissue diseases. In addition, it is influenced by serum levels of fibrinogen and globulin.[282] The sedimentation rate may be normal in occult infections with low-virulence organisms.[287]

The sedimentation rate is useful in follow-up to assess the response to treatment.[58, 81, 106, 174, 177, 209, 282] In one small series, the sedimentation rate decreased to at least two thirds of the original value at the completion of successful antibiotic therapy in all patients, and decreased to half of the original value in the majority.[282] In another series of 30 cases, the sedimentation rate returned to normal after resolution of the infection.[81] The C-reactive protein value is helpful in the diagnosis of postoperative discitis[288] and may prove to be beneficial in the diagnosis of hematogenous vertebral osteomyelitis.

The findings on plain radiographs are characteristic but do not appear for at least two to four weeks.[60, 81, 113, 144, 277, 318] The earliest and most constant radiographic finding, narrowing of the disc space, is present in 74 per cent of patients at presentation.[282] Tomograms frequently show abnormalities earlier than plain radiographs (Fig. 39–6) and may show local osteopenia of the end plates at 10 to 14 days.[113] Widening of the retropharyngeal space in the cervical spine, enlargement of the paravertebral shadow in the thoracic spine, or changes in the psoas shadow in the lumbar spine may indicate either abscess or granulation tissue surrounding the infection. After three to six weeks, destructive changes in the body can be noted, usually beginning as a lytic area in the anterior aspect of the body adjacent to the disc and diffusely in the end plate.

Reactive bone formation and sclerosis are present in 11 per cent of patients on presentation, and most patients will have sclerosis when the disease resolves.[282] Depending on the virulence of the organism and the response to treatment, progressive bony destruction, collapse, and kyphosis may develop. The radiographic findings generally lag behind the clinical response by one to two months. With healing, new bone formation and hypertrophic changes at the vertebral margins eventually may produce spontaneous fusion. Fusion occurs in just over 50 per cent of cases[179, 282] but may take up to five years.[10] If a solid fusion does not occur, a fibrous ankylosis may be achieved.[106, 179]

Although the radiographic findings are characteristic, they are not specific, and a definite diagnosis is possible only by biopsy.[179] An unusual radiographic finding that may help with the diagnosis is gas in the disc space; this may represent infection with a gas-forming organism (Fig. 39–7).[55]

An atypical presentation of vertebral osteomyelitis was reported by McHenry and colleagues.[213] They described a series of six patients with osteomyelitis in an osteoporotic vertebral compression fracture. The vertebral end plates were intact on the initial plain radiographs. This presentation occurred in 13 per cent of all hospitalized patients with vertebral osteomyelitis and 2.4 per cent of in-patients with osteoporotic compression fractures at one institution over a five-year pe-

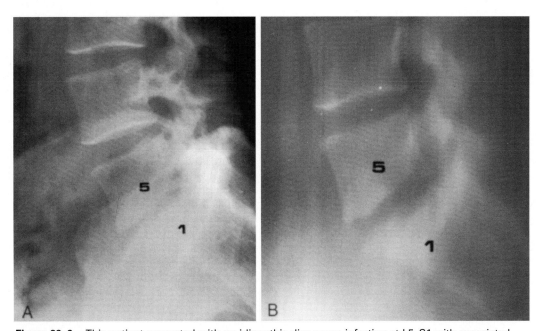

Figure 39–6. This patient presented with an idiopathic disc space infection at L5–S1 with associated vertebral osteomyelitis. His main complaint was low back pain. *A,* This lateral radiograph demonstrates marked narrowing of the disc space at L5–S1; however, nothing is seen that would demonstrate this to be a spine infection. *B,* This lateral tomogram better demonstrates the destruction of the end plates at L5–S1 and the rarefaction of the adjacent bone. The only diagnosis consistent with these findings is a disc space infection with associated vertebral osteomyelitis.

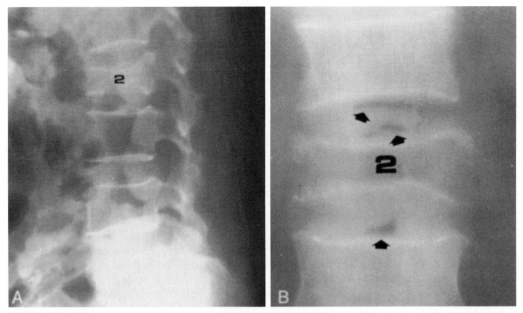

Figure 39–7. This patient presented with a significant paraparesis and associated sepsis. *A,* This lateral radiograph demonstrates marked diminution in the height of the L2 vertebral body. It is surprising that the disc heights at L1–L2 and L2–L3 appear to be relatively normal. *B,* Tomogram of the lumbar spine reveals gas shadows *(arrows)* within the disc spaces at L1–L2 and L2–L3. At the time of surgical debridement, *Escherichia coli* was cultured.

riod.[71] Chest radiographs may reveal atelectasis, pleural effusion, and soft tissue masses that may be confused with a tumor.[29]

The radiographic findings of vertebral osteomyelitis in infants is very striking, with almost complete dissolution of the involved vertebral bodies and nearly normal adjacent end plates. The late radiographic appearance may be identical to that of congenital kyphosis.[88, 262]

Radionuclide studies are useful for early detection and localization of infection, before plain films become positive.[45, 106, 174, 176, 209, 231, 302, 318] Clinical studies have suggested that gallium scans become positive before technetium scans do,[45] and this has been confirmed in experimental studies.[241] Technetium scans show increased uptake diffusely in the region of the infection, whereas gallium scans may show increased uptake in a butterfly area around the infected spine.[136] Gallium scanning has been found to have a sensitivity of 89 per cent, a specificity of 85 per cent, and an accuracy of 86 per cent in the diagnosis of disc space infections.[45] In a separate study,[231] technetium scans were found to have a sensitivity of 90 per cent, a specificity of 78 per cent, and an accuracy of 86 per cent. The accuracy of combined technetium and gallium scans was 94 per cent.[231] These two scans combined are currently the authors' preferred nuclear medicine studies.

In experimental disc space infection, bone scans were positive in 23 per cent of patients at three to five days, in 29 per cent at six to eight days, and in 71 per cent at 13 to 15 days.[308] The probability of technetium bone scans becoming abnormal increases with the duration of symptoms, to almost 100 per cent, but false-negative scans have been reported in young children and also in the elderly. This has been postulated to be the result of regional ischemia.[287]

The major mechanism of gallium localization is thought to be neutrophil labeling followed by migration to the inflammatory focus. False-negative gallium scans have been reported in leukopenic patients.[302] Both technetium and gallium scans may be negative with occult infection by low-virulence organisms.[287] Two cases have been reported in which the technetium scan was negative but the gallium scan was positive, and the authors postulated that this represented pyogenic discitis without vertebral osteomyelitis.[85] Technetium scans remain positive for a long time after resolution of the disease, whereas gallium scans become normal during healing and, therefore, may be useful in following the response to treatment.[247]

Indium-111–labeled leukocyte imaging has been found to be helpful in the evaluation of sepsis in the appendicular skeleton.[227] Unfortunately, it is not sensitive in the spine.[97, 321, 331] This may be related to the fact that most cases of vertebral osteomyelitis are chronic by the time the patients are studied, and the inflammatory response may have fewer leukocytes. The overall sensitivity of indium scanning for infections of the spine is 17 per cent, the specificity is 100 per cent, and the accuracy is only 31 per cent.[321] A correlation was found between prior antibiotic therapy and false-negative indium scans and photon-deficient indium uptake.[321] Photon-deficient lesions may be detected by indium-111–labeled leukocyte imaging in many other conditions, including previous surgery, radiation therapy, or metastatic disease.[42] Palestro and colleagues[250] reported that the specificity was 52 per cent and the sensitivity was 54 per cent when decreased activity was the criterion for osteomyelitis with indium-111 scanning.

Single-photon emission computed tomography is a sensitive bone scintigraphic modality for early detection of spondylitis. It is more sensitive than planar scintigraphy and has the advantage of increased contrast resolution and the capability of three-dimensional localization.[307] The role of this modality has not yet been defined.

Computed tomography (CT) may show cystic changes in the bone as well as soft tissue masses, gas in the soft tissues or within the bone and disc, and, later, lytic destruction of the body.[125, 170, 192] The prevertebral soft tissue involvement seen on CT usually completely surrounds the spine anteriorly, and the destruction of the vertebra is generally an osteolytic process around the disc space. This is in contrast to neoplasms, which are characterized by no or only partial paravertebral soft tissue swelling and by changes that may be osteoblastic and are more likely to involve the posterior elements than in infection.[314]

Computed tomography is valuable in differentiating pyogenic spondylitis from a tuberculous or fungal infection; in the latter, the soft tissue components tend to be more prominent.[38] The finding of disc hypodensity on CT is relatively specific for infection in the lumbar spine but is less useful in the thoracic and cervical region.[192] CT with contrast medium is helpful to delineate the boundary between abscesses and swollen paravertebral muscles.[125, 170, 192] CT after intrathecal administration of metrizamide provides exquisite detail for the spinal canal.[38] CT-guided biopsies of the spine have been shown to be very safe and can be done at all levels of the spine (Fig. 39–8).[3, 118, 125, 156]

Myelography and postmyelography CT are indicated in cases of neurologic deficit and radicular pain to rule out epidural and subdural abscesses. Cerebrospinal fluid should also be examined to rule out meningitis.[104] (The evaluation of epidural abscesses is described in a later section.)

The imaging modality of choice for the evaluation of spine infections is magnetic resonance imaging (MRI). MRI permits early diagnosis of infection and recognition of paravertebral or intraspinal abscesses without the risk associated with myelography.[44, 258] In a prospective study of 37 patients suspected clinically of having vertebral osteomyelitis, MRI was found to be at least as accurate and as sensitive as gallium and bone scanning combined: MRI had a sensitivity of 96 per cent, a specificity of 93 per cent, and an accuracy of 94 per cent.[231] MRI has the advantage of providing more anatomic information than radionuclide studies and is capable of differentiating degenerative and neoplastic disease from vertebral osteomyelitis.[1] The changes on MRI occur at about the same time as the changes on gallium scans.[231]

Disadvantages of MRI are that it is more sensitive to motion degradation, and there are problems with patient positioning and claustrophobia. MRI has a lim-

ited field of view, whereas radionuclide scans can image the entire skeleton. MRI findings may be falsely negative in cases of epidural abscess without involvement of the adjacent bone because the signal intensity of the inflammatory exudate is similar to that of cerebrospinal fluid.[114, 231]

The MRI changes in vertebral osteomyelitis are characteristic (Fig. 39–9). On T1-weighted sequences, there is a confluent decreased signal intensity of the vertebral bodies and adjacent disc, making the margin between the two structures indistinct. On T2-weighted sequences, the signal intensity of the vertebral bodies in the involved disc is higher than normal, and there generally is an absence of the intranu cleft normally seen within the adult disc.[44, 231] The disc and the involved portions of the vertebral bodies generally enhance after administration of gadolinium.[259] The typical T1 changes in the vertebral body and end plates and the T2 changes in the disc space were seen in 95 per cent of the 37 cases of vertebral osteomyelitis described by Dagirmanjian and associates.[70] Only 56 per cent of their cases had typical T2 vertebral body changes. Isointense or decreased signal in the vertebral body on T2-weighted images is consistent with infection if the other typical findings are present. The cause of the signal intensity changes seen in vertebral osteomyelitis is uncertain but is thought to parallel the pathogenesis of the disease. The earliest changes are thought to be related to ischemia and the increased water content of the inflammatory process. As the infection crosses the end plate, a confluent signal intensity occurs on MRI. The normal finding of an intranu cleft within adult discs is thought to be related to fibrous tissue within the nucleus pulposus. This cleft is lost at the time of inflammatory involvement of the disc.[231]

In a comparison of MRI, bone scans, and plain radiographic evaluations in an animal model of disc space infection, MRI was found to have a sensitivity of 93 per cent, a specificity of 97 per cent, and an accuracy of 95 per cent, corresponding very well to results of clinical studies in humans.[231, 308]

The findings are time related. In one study, scans of rabbits made three to five days after injection of bacteria all showed a decreased signal from the nucleus pulposus on both T1-weighted and short T1-inversion recovery (STIR) sequences. Scans at six to eight days also showed increased signal from the adjacent end plates on the STIR sequence and blurring of the disc margins on the T1 image. Scans at 13 to 18 days showed more florid end plate changes, and in several scans at 21 days there was increased signal from the vertebral end plates and the disc on STIR sequences.[308] The MRI findings slowly return to normal after successful treatment of vertebral osteomyelitis.[231] Gallium scans revert to normal much more rapidly and are better indications of appropriate therapy. Post and associates[259] noted that abnormal gadolinium enhancement of the disc, vertebral bodies, and paraspinal soft tissues progressively decreases with successful treatment of the infection. Gillams and others described some patients who were improving clinically and had

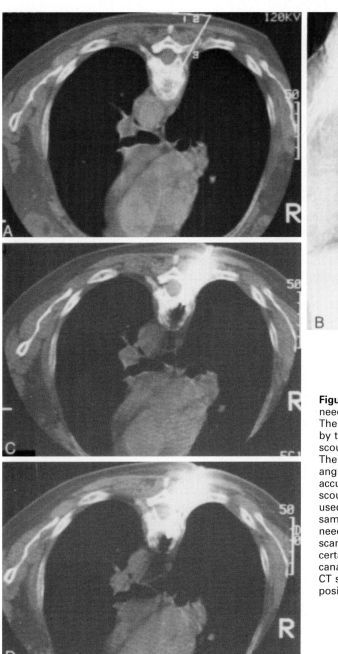
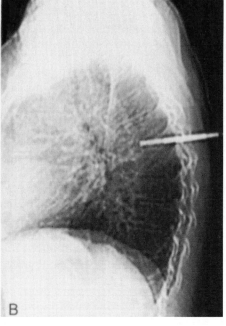

Figure 39–8. The technique of Craig needle biopsy in the thoracic spine. *A,* The course of the needle is determined by the measurements obtained on the scout computed tomographic (CT) scan. The distance from midline as well as the angle from the vertical position can be accurately determined. *B,* The lateral scout film from the CT scan should be used to determine the exact level to be sampled. *C,* As the trocar and the biopsy needles are advanced, transverse CT scans are routinely obtained to make certain that the thoracic cavity and spinal canal are not being compromised. *D,* A CT scan is taken to confirm the final position of the biopsy needle.

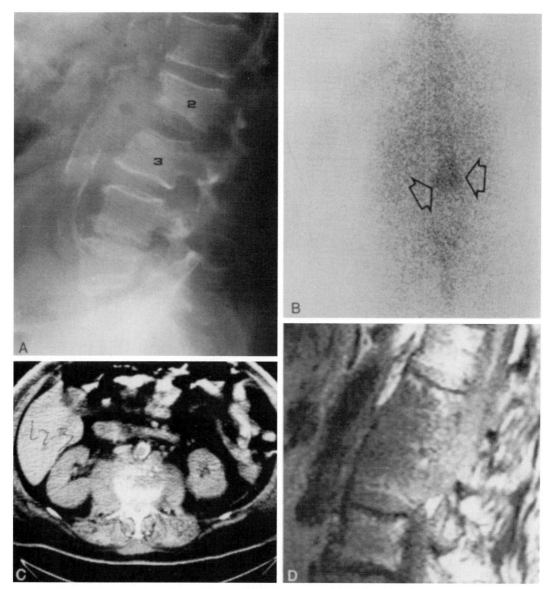

Figure 39–9. This diabetic patient with severe arteriosclerotic vascular disease developed a disc space infection with associated vertebral osteomyelitis at the L2–L3 interspace. *A,* This lateral radiograph demonstrates the destruction of the end plates at L2–L3. At this point, the patient was severely osteoporotic. *B,* A gallium scan demonstrates increased uptake in the region of the midlumbar spine, which is consistent with a disc space infection and vertebral osteomyelitis *(arrows). C,* A computed tomographic (CT) scan at the L2–L3 interspace reveals significant destruction of the vertebral body of L3. This irregular erosion is most consistent with vertebral osteomyelitis. *D,* This sagittal magnetic resonance (MR) image shows a decrease in signal intensity in the L2 and L3 vertebral bodies. This is a T1-weighted image. It is extremely difficult to determine the room available for the neural tissue.

Illustration continued on following page

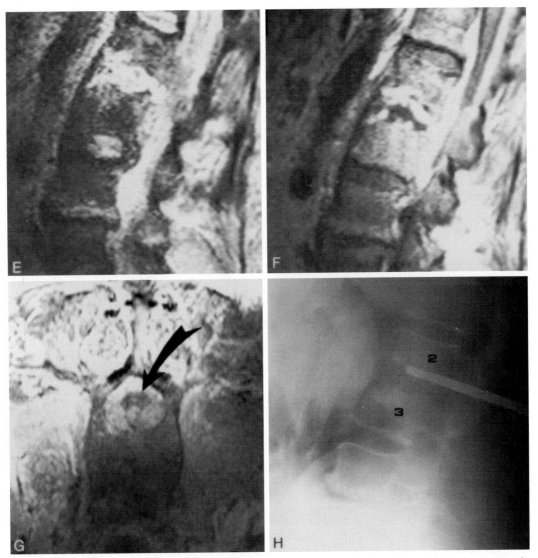

Figure 39–9 *Continued* *E,* This sagittal MR image shows an increase in signal intensity in the region of the L2–L3 disc space and also reveals a lack of the normal disc cleft that can be seen at the other disc levels. This is consistent with disc space infection and adjacent vertebral osteomyelitis. This T2-weighted image still fails to visualize the room available for the neural elements. *F,* This sagittal MR scan has been done after an injection of gadolinium. This allows visualization of the neural elements and shows that there is extensive epidural constriction secondary to the spine infection. This is a T1-weighted image. *G,* This transverse section at the level of the superior L3 vertebral body demonstrates the space available for the neural elements *(arrow).* This was not apparent on MR imaging studies performed without gadolinium enhancement. This is a T1-weighted image. *H,* The patient underwent a Craig needle biopsy under fluoroscopic control, which would be routinely performed for any infection at the L1 level or below. Above the L1 level, CT control would normally be used. The Craig needle biopsy cultured positive for *Staphylococcus aureus.*

stable or increasing enhancement patterns and concluded that such findings should not be interpreted as treatment failure.[50, 122]

Unfortunately, even MRI findings may be negative in surgically documented occult infections by low-virulence organisms.[287] Despite the accuracy of MRI, an absolute diagnosis must be based on bacteriologic or microscopic examination of the tissue.[90, 188, 238] The only situation in which the diagnosis can be made without a tissue biopsy is when a positive blood culture is obtained from a patient with signs and symptoms of spondylitis. Blood cultures are positive in 24 to 59 per cent of patients with pyogenic spine infections.[51, 282] Urine cultures are less reliable, because patients with vertebral osteomyelitis may have a coexistent urinary tract infection with a different organism.[51, 106]

Needle biopsy of the spine was first reported by Ball in 1934. In 1956, Craig[66] described a set of instruments designed to increase the percentage of successful closed-needle biopsies, especially in sclerotic or softened bone, in discs, or in fibrous tissue. Needle biopsies have been shown to be safe in the cervical and thoracic spine as well as in the lumbar spine.[248, 249] A definite diagnosis is possible by closed-needle biopsy in 68 to 86 per cent of cases.[14, 113, 118, 249, 282] CT-guided closed biopsy of the spine should provide a margin of safety and allow biopsy of the area most likely to yield the diagnosis. In a series of 22 patients with a mass or destructive lesion who underwent this procedure, 17 biopsies provided a definite diagnosis; only one was false negative and in four cases the specimens were insufficient. All areas of the spine were sampled, including one lesion at C2. The patient with the C2 lesion had a transient increase in quadriparesis but returned to baseline, and no other complications were reported.[3]

Closed biopsies of the spine often have false-negative results in patients who are being treated with antibiotics at the time of the biopsy. If a biopsy is nondiagnostic, it would be reasonable to observe the patient off the antibiotic regimen and repeat the biopsy if the clinical situation allows such a delay. If the second closed biopsy also is nondiagnostic, an open biopsy should be considered. This will provide larger tissue samples and selection of grossly pathologic tissue, and should have a lower false-negative rate. In their review of the literature, Sapico and Montgomerie[282] found that 30 per cent of needle biopsy specimens and aspirates were sterile, compared with only 14 per cent of surgical specimens.

The differential diagnosis of pyogenic vertebral osteomyelitis includes tuberculosis, fungal infections, metastatic carcinoma, multiple myeloma, localized Scheuermann's disease, trauma, degenerative disease, epidural abscess, and fractures associated with osteoporosis.[57, 58, 213, 282] Less common disorders in the differential diagnosis are leukemia, perinephric abscess, neuropathic spinal arthropathy, and sarcoidosis, as well as erosive arthritides in rare cases of facet joint involvement.[124, 167, 251, 255, 262, 277] With such a wide variety of diseases that can present with signs and symptoms similar to those of vertebral osteomyelitis, diagnostic acuity is important. As Kulowski said in 1936, "Knowledge of the disease is the primary factor in the diagnosis."[188]

Management

Before the advent of antibiotic therapy, treatment of pyogenic vertebral osteomyelitis involved drainage of abscesses, rest on a frame or plaster bed, and attention to nutrition and general hygiene. The mortality rate with this approach was between 25 and 70 per cent.[142, 188] The use of antibiotics has drastically changed the prognosis with this disease, but attention to good general medical care still is a vital part of the treatment. Associated conditions that compromise wound healing or immune response should be managed aggressively. Attention to proper nutrition and the reversal of metabolic deficits and hypoxia are essential. Diabetes and other systemic illnesses should be brought under control.[87] Any underlying focus of infection in the urinary tract, lungs, skin, or elsewhere must be treated concurrently with the spine infection.[286]

The goals of treatment are to establish tissue and bacteriologic diagnoses, to prevent or reverse neurologic deficits, to relieve pain, to establish spinal stability, to eradicate the infection, and to prevent relapses. Biopsy, by either a closed or an open method, is mandatory in any case of spine infection before the institution of antibiotic therapy. The only exceptions to this rule are straightforward cases of pediatric discitis (see Chapter 14) and cases with positive blood cultures in association with strong clinical evidence of spine infection.

Changes in patterns of pathogenic organisms and antimicrobial agents necessitate an accurate bacteriologic diagnosis. If possible, treatment should be withheld until an organism is identified, in case a second biopsy is necessary. However, patients who are systemically toxic should be treated with maximal doses of broad-spectrum antibiotics as soon as the biopsy has been completed. Most patients with vertebral osteomyelitis are not septic and will not be harmed by a delay in treatment for several days. Conversely, if the biopsy is nondiagnostic and antibiotic therapy has been started, a second biopsy is unlikely to yield the organism. Patients with clinical evidence of vertebral osteomyelitis but negative cultures from open biopsy should be treated with a full course of broad-spectrum antibiotics. When possible, the choice of antibiotics should be based on the culture and sensitivity test results, so that more specific and less toxic agents can be used.

Daly and others have demonstrated that antibiotic penetration of osteomyelitic bone parallels serum concentrations for all classes of antibiotics.[73, 99] The penetration of antibiotics into inflammatory exudates and the intervertebral disc is less certain.[69, 89, 105, 121, 130, 138] Vancomycin, gentamycin, tobramycin, clindamycin, and teicoplanin all penetrate the nucleus pulposus reasonably well.[69, 89, 274, 291] The data regarding cephalosporins are inconclusive, but if penetration does occur, it appears to be at a relatively low level.[89, 105, 121] The penetration of cephalosporins into inflammatory exudates appears to be inversely proportional to the degree of serum protein binding.[130] Riley and colleagues[274] have shown that the penetration and distribution of antibiotics into the nucleus pulposus is significantly influenced by the charge of the antibiotic.

The route of administration of the antibiotics and the duration of therapy are somewhat empiric because little research has been done to clarify these topics. At the present time, it is recommended that parenteral antibiotic therapy be used in maximal dosage for six weeks and followed with an oral course of antibiotics until resolution of the disease. It may be reasonable to switch from parenteral to oral therapy at four weeks.[106] Parenteral therapy for less than four weeks results in a higher rate of failure.[282] Oral ciprofloxacin therapy has been used successfully in the management of patients with chronic osteomyelitis of the tibia or femur.[203] It is possible that ciprofloxacin and other new agents for oral use may supplant parenteral treatment of vertebral osteomyelitis in the future, but general use of these agents should await evidence of their effectiveness.

The erythrocyte sedimentation rate has been found to be a reasonable guide to the response to therapy[58, 81, 106, 174, 177, 209, 282] and can be expected to decrease to one half to two thirds of pretherapy levels by the completion of successful treatment.[282] If the sedimentation rate does not decrease with treatment, consideration should be given to a repeat biopsy. C-reactive protein may prove to be a useful laboratory test to follow resolution of the infection. Antibiotic administration must be carefully monitored to avoid toxicity, especially in diabetic patients and others who might have impaired renal function.[61]

Patients should be immobilized for pain control and prevention of deformity or neurologic deterioration. The length of time a patient should remain at bed rest, the type of orthosis, and the duration of its use all depend on the location of the infection in the spine, the degree of bone destruction and deformity, and the response to treatment. Thoracic and thoracolumbar lesions are best treated initially with bed rest on a Rotorest or similar device, at least until a good response to treatment is obtained, as judged by the sedimentation rate and pain control. Thoracic and thoracolumbar lesions are more likely to cause deformity, and, if neurologic deficits occur, the prognosis is worse with these lesions than with lumbar spine involvement.[87, 106]

Cervical and cervicothoracic lesions should be immobilized with a halo device. Upper thoracic lesions are best immobilized in a thoracolumbosacral orthosis device with a chin piece, and lower thoracic and lumbar lesions should be immobilized in a thoracolumbosacral orthosis device without a chin piece. Frederickson and coworkers[106] found that immobilization was most important in those patients with destruction of greater than 50 per cent of a vertebra and recommended immobilization for the first three months. In five of their 17 cases, significant deformity developed in the first six to eight weeks, all at the thoracolumbar junction or above; those patients with the greatest deformity had 50 per cent or more vertebral body destruction at presentation. Most authors recommend bracing for at least three to four months. Garcia and Grantham[113] recommend that the duration of immobilization should be individualized and based on the response to treatment.

Surgery is indicated in the following circumstances: (1) to obtain a bacteriologic diagnosis when closed biopsy is negative or deemed unsafe; (2) when a clinically significant abscess is present (spiking temperatures and septic course); (3) in cases refractory to prolonged nonoperative treatment, where the sedimentation rate remains high or pain persists; (4) in cases with spinal cord compression causing a neurologic deficit; and (5) in cases with significant deformity or with significant vertebral body destruction, especially in the cervical spine.[87, 92, 101] Upper cervical osteomyelitis is rare but generally requires fusion because of the associated instability.[337] In cases of lumbar lesions with root deficits, the final outcome is satisfactory with or without surgical treatment, but patients with spinal cord compression have a better prognosis with surgery.[87] Surgery should be carried out as soon as possible in these cases, but when doubt exists regarding the chances of a reversible spinal cord lesion, decompression should be carried out because recovery has been noted in patients with paralysis who underwent decompression as late as five months after the onset of weakness.[87]

In nearly all cases, the spine should be approached anteriorly (Fig. 39–10), because this allows direct access to the infected tissues and adequate débridement. Anterior exposure allows stabilization of the spine by bone grafting, which promotes rapid healing without collapse and facilitates rehabilitation.[87, 152, 173, 175, 186, 301] Laminectomy is contraindicated in most cases because it may lead to neurologic deterioration and increased instability.[87, 175, 293] The situation is similar to that in acute trauma.[31] Laminectomy may be performed in the lumbar spine below the level of the conus, provided there is no psoas abscess or extensive anterior destruction of the bodies that would require extensive débridement. If laminectomy is carried out, the facets should be preserved and discectomy should be performed.

Anterior approaches to the spine have been described elsewhere[30, 301] and are reviewed in Chapter 49. For lesions in the thoracic or thoracolumbar spine, the transthoracic approach has the advantage of better exposure, allowing more extensive débridement and better decompression of the cord and more effective bone grafting.[102, 154, 173, 186] The disadvantage is the potential increased morbidity after a thoracotomy in the presence of a purulent infection. Costotransversectomy or the slightly more extensive lateral rachiotomy described by Capener[48] is recommended when a spine biopsy or minimal decompression with limited grafting is necessary or when gross purulence is expected.

After débridement of the infected focus, autogenous iliac crest grafting can be performed during the same procedure. The graft should extend from healthy bone above to healthy bone below.[102, 154, 173, 186] Autogenous bone grafting after vertebral body resection in the presence of active infection was first reported by Wiltberger in 1952, and has since been demonstrated to be safe and effective regardless of the causative organism.[212, 328] Grafting with iliac crest generally is better than grafting with rib.[152, 173, 266] If a good quality rib is excised in the process of a transthoracic approach, however, it is often adequate as long as a large segment does not need to be spanned and there is no significant kyphotic deformity.[266] Revascularization of a cortical graft may not be complete even after one year.[93] Vascularized rib grafts have been used with good success for the stabilization of kyphosis.[37] Louw[201] reports successful fusions in 95 per cent of cases at 6 months and 100 per cent at one year when vascularized rib grafts were used for tuberculous kyphosis. Fibular grafts have been shown to be effective for reconstruction of multiple-level anterior decompressions of the cervical spine[324]; however, the large amount of cortical bone in fibular

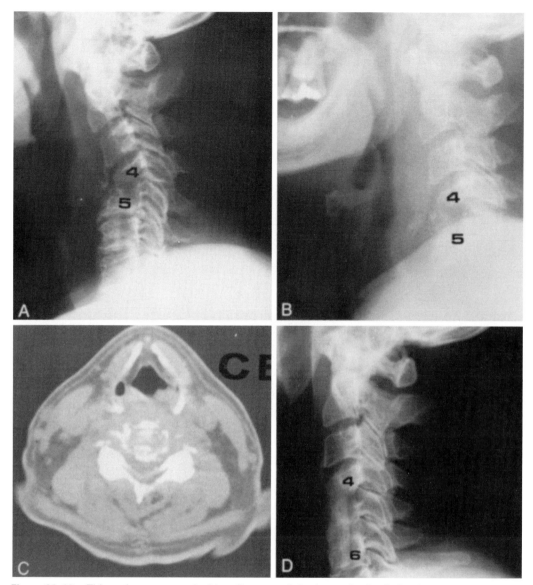

Figure 39-10. This patient presented with a disc space infection at the C4–C5 level with quadriparesis and sepsis. *A,* This lateral radiograph demonstrates an increase in the retropharyngeal space and also demonstrates destruction of the end plates at the C4–C5 interspace. This should have been diagnosed as a spine infection. *B,* Without any treatment, the infection can be seen to have progressed, with an increase in the retropharyngeal space and further destruction of the C4 and C5 vertebral bodies. The interspace is grossly widened compared with that seen in part *A,* because the patient has now been placed in Tong traction. *C,* This transverse computed tomographic scan demonstrates anterior bone destruction. *D,* The patient was taken to surgery for an anterior decompression with resection of the inferior portion of the C4 vertebral body, the entire C5 vertebral body, and the superior portion of the C6 vertebral body with insertion of an autogenous iliac bone graft to provide support anteriorly. Excellent incorporation of the graft can be seen.

grafts makes them less ideal in the presence of infection.

In the past, cervical spine vertebral osteomyelitis was managed effectively without bone grafting by drainage, antibiotics, and skull traction for 6 to 12 weeks.[228] Prolonged hospitalization can be avoided by débridement, bone grafting, halo immobilization, and outpatient antibiotics. Posterior stabilization performed as a second stage may be reasonable to avoid a halo.

In cases with significant kyphotic deformity, anterior reconstruction with autogenous bone grafts after débridement should be carried out as a first stage.[173, 186, 266] Posterior stabilization and fusion can be performed in a second-stage procedure if necessary (Fig. 39–11).[19, 102, 173, 175, 266] Posterior instrumentation has been shown to be safe and effective after anterior débridement and fusion.[51, 128, 315] The long-term fate of the hardware is not known and those patients should be followed long-term or consideration given to removing the hardware after the fusion is solid.

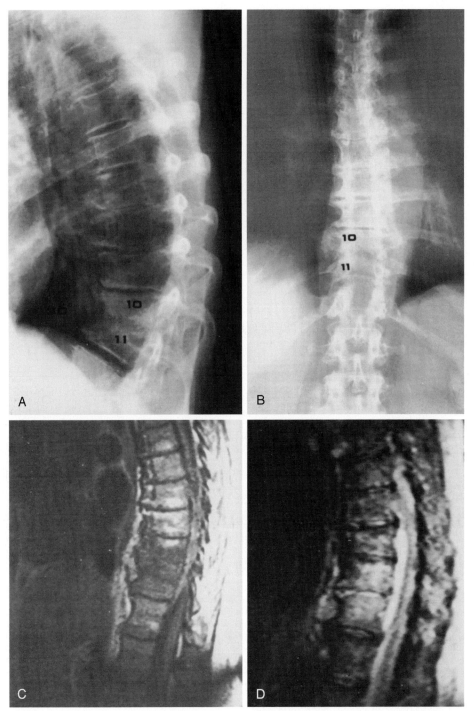

Figure 39–11. This patient with significant paraparesis was referred for evaluation and treatment. The patient had already undergone a wide posterior multilevel laminectomy; it was noted at the time of previous surgery that there was significant granulation tissue causing spinal cord compression. *A,* This lateral radiograph reveals 30-degree kyphosis at the T10–T11 interspace with complete destruction of the end plates. This is consistent with the diagnosis of disc space infection with adjacent vertebral osteomyelitis. *B,* This anteroposterior radiograph reveals that a wide laminectomy has been performed from T6 down through T11. *C,* A review of the original T1-weighted preoperative sagittal magnetic resonance (MR) image shows that there is a decrease in signal intensity at the T10–T11 interspace, which is consistent with a disc space infection and adjacent vertebral osteomyelitis. *D,* This original preoperative T2-weighted sagittal MR image was reviewed and revealed that there was an anterior epidural abscess present from approximately T9 through T11, causing severe compromise of the spinal canal. The original diagnosis should have been that the patient had a disc space infection with vertebral osteomyelitis and an associated epidural abscess.

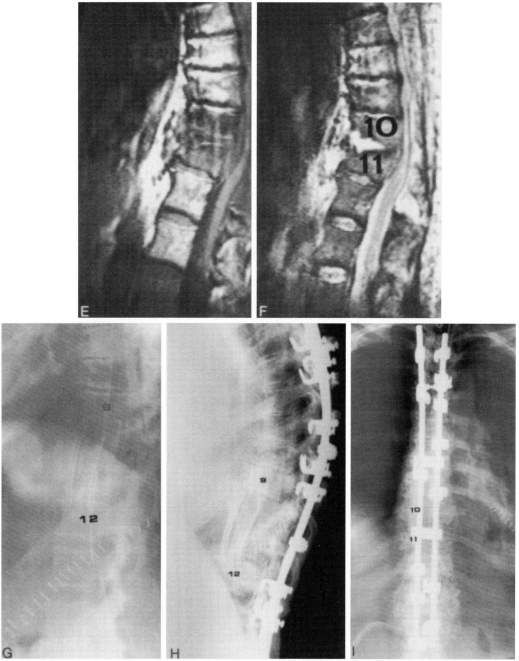

Figure 39–11 *Continued   E,* At the time of transfer, a new sagittal magnetic resonance image was obtained. This T1-weighted image again shows a marked decrease in the signal intensity in the T10 and T11 vertebral bodies and still shows significant anterior neural compression. *F,* At the time of transfer, this sagittal MR T2-weighted image was obtained. This also shows that there is significant compromise of the spinal canal at the T10–T11 interspace. It can also be appreciated that there is a marked increase in the signal intensity at the level of the T10–T11 interspace. This is consistent with either purulent material or granulation tissue. *G,* After full evaluation, it was determined that this condition would best be treated with an anterior decompression and fusion and posterior stabilization. The anterior decompression was performed first, and a resection of the T10 and T11 vertebral bodies was performed along with a fusion from the level of T9 to T12. A combination of iliac crest bone graft and rib graft was used. *H,* The patient was later taken back to surgery for the insertion of posterior segmental instrumentation. The posterior instrumentation and fusion extended above and below the level of the previous decompression so as to allow the patient to be mobilized. The patient has had significant improvement of her paraparesis to the near-normal level. The infection was adequately treated with a 6-week course of parenteral antibiotics. *I,* This anteroposterior radiograph demonstrates the extent of posterior segmental spinal instrumentation that was necessary to adequately immobilize and stabilize the spine. Because of the patient's age and osteopenia due to prolonged bed rest, the application of fixation at nearly every level of the spine was necessary to achieve adequate stabilization.

When vertebral osteomyelitis occurs in a patient who has undergone a surgical procedure on the spine or sustained a penetrating trauma of the spine, a fistula should be suspected (Fig. 39–12). Depending on the level of the spine infection, the appropriate imaging study (barium swallow or gastrointestinal series) or endoscopic examination should be ordered to rule out a fistula. If a fistula is identified, it must be repaired along with treatment of the spine infection.

Prognosis

Relapse of infection occurs in up to 25 per cent of cases but is much less common if antibiotics are adminis-

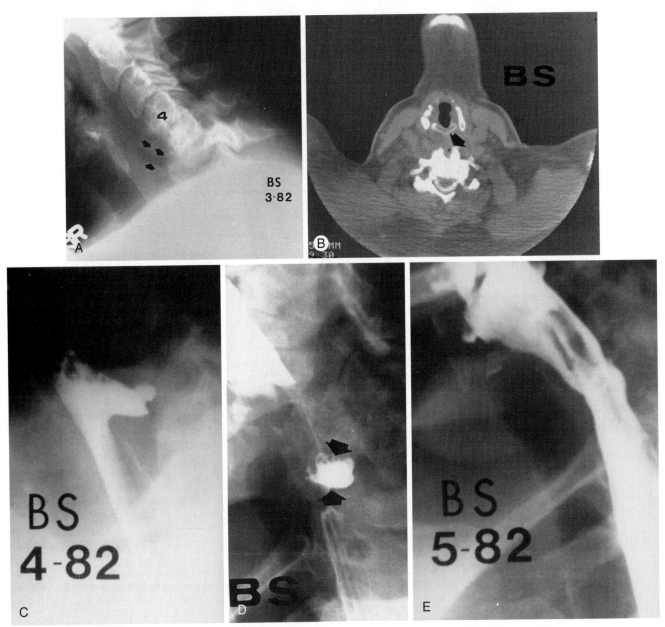

Figure 39–12. This patient had undergone a multilevel anterior discectomy and fusion 2 months previously and was referred for evaluation of a persistent low-grade fever and increasing neck pain. *A,* This lateral radiograph shows destruction of the C6 vertebral body and a fistula (between the *arrows*) going into the vertebra. *B,* This postmyelogram computed tomographic scan shows free air leading into the anterior aspect of the C6 vertebral body. *C,* This barium swallow scan shows that there is a defect in the back of the esophagus with barium extravasating and leading directly to the vertebral body. *D,* The pocket of barium is well seen (between the *arrows*) just anterior to the spine. *E,* The patient was treated with an anterior cervical debridement and bone grafting and by excision of the fistula tract and primary repair of the esophagus. She was treated with 6 weeks of parenteral antibiotics. This follow-up barium swallow scan shows that the esophagus is now competent. Her vertebral osteomyelitis successfully resolved.

tered for more than 28 days.[87, 282] Nonoperative treatment has a higher failure rate in patients with an impaired immune system.[51] The mortality rate is less than 5 to 16 per cent, depending on the average age and comorbidities of the patients in the series. Death is much more likely in the elderly and in those with an underlying disease.[51, 87, 113, 282] In one series, *Staphylococcus aureus* infection was associated with a higher mortality rate than infection with other pathogens.[51]

Factors that have been found to predispose a patient to paralysis include increased age, a more cephalic level of infection, and a history of diabetes mellitus or rheumatoid arthritis.[87] In one series, a neurologic deficit occurred in 45 per cent of the 44 patients who had an impaired immune system, whereas only 19 per cent of the remaining 67 patients developed a deficit.[51] Less than 7 to 15 per cent of patients overall have residual neurologic deficits.[51, 282] Diabetic patients are more likely to have permanent neurologic deficits, and patients with thoracic involvement are the least likely to recover.[87, 282] Eismont and associates[87] described the results of operation in 14 patients with spinal cord paralysis. Three of the seven patients who underwent a laminectomy deteriorated and four remained unchanged. In contrast, half of the patients treated by an anterior procedure recovered normal or nearly normal function, and no patient was made worse by the procedure. The patients with root lesions alone had an excellent outcome with or without operation.[87]

In selected patients who require surgical treatment for pyogenic osteomyelitis, the prognosis is very good after the anterior débridement and primary bone grafting in conjunction with a full course of antibiotics. In a recent series of 21 patients, of whom six had neurologic deficits, there were no deaths and no relapses, and all of the patients with neurologic deficit recovered. All but one of the patients who underwent fusion had a solid fusion, and one of the two patients who did not have a graft had spontaneous fusion. The mean increase in kyphosis was three degrees.[92]

Garcia and Grantham[113] found that spontaneous interbody fusion was the rule and occurred in less than one year in most patients and in two years in almost all other cases. Some studies have found that the chance of spontaneous fusion in patients treated nonoperatively is 50 per cent or less.[106, 179, 282] Fortunately, those who do not develop a bony union achieve a fibrous ankylosis, which generally is painless.[10, 106, 113, 179] Occasionally, a patient complains of persistent back pain from localized degenerative changes at the site of previous infection.[106, 113, 179]

The more cephalad the level of infection, the higher the rate of spontaneous fusion; almost all cases of cervical infection will fuse spontaneously.[58, 228] In one series, six of six cervical lesions went on to solid interbody fusion, compared with 22 of 29 thoracic lesions and five of 21 lumbar lesions.[58] One of the patients with cervical infection and one with thoracic involvement had undergone posterior fusion. Fifteen of the patients with thoracic disease underwent costotrans-

versectomy, and five patients with lumbar involvement had anterior débridement without fusion.[58]

Although deformities are much less common with pyogenic infection than with tuberculous infection, they still may occur.[106, 204] Deformities have been reported to occur in the cervical spine[204] but are more common in the thoracic and thoracolumbar areas and in those cases with involvement of more than 50 per cent of one or more vertebral bodies.[106]

Infants with vertebral osteomyelitis have a poor prognosis and a very high recurrence rate.[88, 262] The late radiographic appearance in these cases may be identical to that of congenital kyphosis and should be treated in a similar fashion.[88]

Interestingly, intravenous drug abusers have an excellent prognosis. Ninety-two per cent responded to parenteral antibiotic therapy for four weeks or more, and those who relapsed responded to a second course. In 67 cases reported in the literature, there were no deaths or permanent neurologic sequelae.[283]

EPIDURAL ABSCESS

Epidemiology

Most cases of epidural abscess occur in adults (mean age, 57 years; range, two to 81 years).[76] Occurrence in children under 12 years of age is rare.[21] The male-to-female ratio is approximately 1:1.[76] The incidence of the disease is 0.2 to 1.2 per 10,000 hospital admissions per year.[20] At the University of Miami/Jackson Memorial Hospital Medical Center, 137 spine infections were treated by the orthopedic service over an eight-year period and, of these, epidural abscess occurred in 10 (7.3 per cent).[114]

Danner and Hartman[76] noted an increased frequency of epidural abscess at their hospital between 1971 and 1982. This increase was disproportionate to the small increase in admissions and laminectomies performed at that hospital. The authors' proposed explanations were an increased use of medical instrumentation, an increase in frequency of intravenous drug abuse, and an aging population. Other investigators have also documented an increasing incidence in the condition in the last decade.[147, 242]

Etiology

The primary source of infection can be identified in approximately 60 per cent of the cases.[76] Infection may occur by hematogenous spread from a remote focus of infection,[20, 76, 131, 140, 145, 171] by spread from a contiguous focus of vertebral osteomyelitis or a disc space infection,[20, 40, 76, 114, 145] or from direct inoculation at the time of operation, epidural steroid injection, lumbar puncture, or epidural catheterization.[20, 25, 53, 76, 98, 145, 268] In 136 cases compiled from five series in the literature, skin and soft tissue infections were thought to be the source in 21 per cent, bone or joint infections in 13 per cent (up to 28 per cent if vertebral osteomyelitis is included), spine surgery or other procedures in 10 per cent, upper respiratory tract infection in 6 per cent, abdominal sources in 4 per cent, urinary tract infection in 2 per cent, and intravenous drug abuse in 4 per cent.[20, 76, 140, 146, 171]

Factors that may be associated with a higher incidence of infection include diabetes mellitus, intravenous drug abuse, prior back trauma, and pregnancy.[20, 40, 76, 114] Between 12 and 30 per cent of patients reported an episode of trauma preceding the infection.[20, 40, 76]

Bacteriology

In 1948, Heusner reported on 20 patients with an epidural abscess; *S. aureus* was the pathogen in all of the cases in which the organism was known.[145] In more recent series, *S. aureus* accounts for approximately 60 per cent of cases in which the organism is known.[20, 76, 171] From the results in 166 patients from five series, *S. aureus* accounted for 62 per cent, aerobic streptococci for 8 per cent, *Staphylococcus epidermidis* for 2 per cent, aerobic gram-negative rods for 18 per cent, anaerobes for 2 per cent, and other bacteria for 1 per cent; 6 per cent of the organisms were unidentified.[20, 76, 140, 145, 171] Gram-negative organisms have been reported with increasing frequency.[20, 131, 171] One study found that intravenous drug abusers were frequently infected with gram-negative organisms[171]; in another series, 12 of 18 intravenous drug abusers were infected with *S. aureus* and only one with *Pseudomonas*.[185]

Pathogenesis and Pathology

In an effort to elucidate the pathophysiology of epidural abscesses, Dandy[74] performed cadaver dissections and provided much of the present knowledge on the anatomy of the epidural space. The epidural space is filled with fat and loose areolar tissue containing numerous veins. The size and shape of this space is determined by the variations in size of the spinal cord. In the cervical region, the space is potential with almost no fat between bone and dura. The epidural space is present only dorsal to the origin of the spinal nerves. Ventrally, the dura is closely applied to the canal from C1 to S2. Posteriorly, the space begins to appear at C7 and gradually deepens along the thoracic vertebrae to a depth of 0.5 to 0.75 cm between T4 and T8. The space tapers again and becomes shallow between T11 and L2 and attains its greatest depths below L2. Below S2, the epidural space surrounds the dura on all sides.[74] The epidural space communicates with the retroperitoneal and posterior mediastinal spaces through the intervertebral foramina.[77] As would be expected by this description of the anatomy, most epidural abscesses are in the thoracic and lumbar spine and generally are posterior.[20, 76, 137, 140, 145, 171, 254, 279] In six series in the literature, the thoracic spine was involved in 51 per cent of cases, the lumbar spine in 35 per cent, and the cervical spine in 14 per cent.[20, 76, 137, 145, 171, 254] The abscess was anterior in 21 per cent and posterior in 79 per cent of the 133 patients from four series in which the location was recorded.[20, 76, 140, 145] An abscess is more likely to be located anteriorly if the infection is in the lumbar spine and if it is secondary to vertebral osteomyelitis.[76, 140] Because there is no anatomic boundary within the space, the infection may extend the entire length of the canal but generally covers only three or four segments (Fig. 39–13).[21, 76, 114, 145, 171, 254]

The pathogenesis of the neurologic manifestations is related either to direct compression from epidural pus or granulation tissue or to embarrassment of the intrinsic circulation of the cord.[20, 40, 41, 145] A microangiographic study in a rabbit model demonstrated that the initial neurologic deficit is related to compression rather than to ischemia. The spinal arteries and epidural venous plexus remained patent in cases of mild to moderate spinal cord compression. The vessels became occluded only with extreme spinal cord compression.[95] On the basis of postmortem examinations, Russell and others identified thrombosis and thrombophlebitis of the veins of the cord and epidural space without involvement of the arteriolar supply[40, 279]; however, others have found thrombosis of the arteriolar supply as well as of the veins.[20]

Several authors have identified a correlation between the duration of infection and the gross appearance at operation or postmortem examination. Corradini and associates described a very early presuppurative phase in which the inflammatory lesion was characterized by an epidural mass of swollen, red, friable fat without any gross pus.[64] In patients who have had symptoms for less than two weeks, gross pus with varying amounts of red granulation tissue has been identified.[20, 40, 64, 76, 279] Above and below the level of the pus, the epidural fat may undergo reactive changes and appear swollen and necrotic.[40] In patients with symptoms of longer duration, granulation tissue is often identified on the dura. There frequently are small beads of pus imbedded in the granulation tissue.[20, 64, 76, 279] In delayed cases with symptoms for 150 days or longer, grayish white granulation tissue or maturing fibrous tissue has been found.[279] Some authors have thought that it is not always possible to predict whether pus or granulation tissue is likely to be found at operation.[140, 145, 171] Hancock[140] described patients in whom granulation tissue was found one day after the onset of symptoms, and other patients who had had symptoms for up to four weeks and had no granulation tissue at operation.

Subdural extension of infection is possible but uncommon.[20, 104] With spinal cord involvement, there may be evidence of vessel thrombosis, inflammatory response of glial cells, and myelomalacia with liquefaction and vacuolization of the white matter.[40, 41]

Clinical Presentation

Patients with an epidural abscess have a highly variable presentation, which causes initial misdiagnosis in approximately 50 per cent of cases.[76] The difficulty in making the correct diagnosis frequently leads to long delays between presentation and definitive treatment.[20, 41, 76, 137, 140, 145, 161, 171, 254, 269] Patients who present acutely

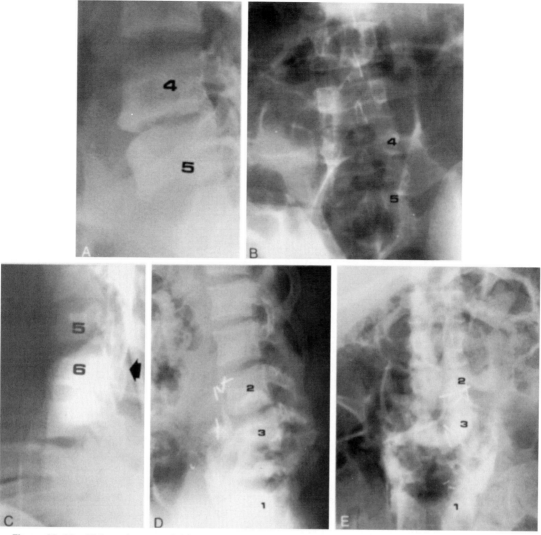

Figure 39–13. This patient was initially treated for a herniated disc at the L4–L5 level. He subsequently developed an epidural abscess and paraplegia that was progressing to quadriplegia. At this time he was transferred to our institution. *A,* This lateral radiograph demonstrates narrowing at the L4–L5 interspace that was present at the time of transfer. This narrowing is consistent with a previous discectomy. *B,* This anteroposterior radiograph of the lumbar spine does not show any abnormality other than the presence of an ileus, which was associated with the new-onset quadriplegia. *C,* At the time of transfer, a C1–C2 puncture was performed, and a myelogram was performed at that level. It can be seen that there is a block to the dye at the level of the C6 vertebral body; it also can be seen that there is marked compression from posterior *(arrow).* This is consistent with a posterior epidural abscess extending from L4 up to C6. This corresponded to the patient's level of quadriplegia. He was taken to surgery for an emergency laminectomy from C5 through L5. The patient had resolution of the paralysis of the arms and upper trunk; however, he had a persistent paraparesis at the level of the thoracolumbar junction. *D,* At final follow-up, this lateral roentgenogram reveals marked destruction of the lower lumbar spine. The patient was found to have multiorganism vertebral osteomyelitis associated with the initial spine infection and an epidural abscess, which caused this destruction. After several operative procedures, the infection was resolved and the lumbosacral spine was stable. *E,* This anteroposterior radiograph taken at final follow-up similarly demonstrates the fusion from L2 to the sacrum. At this time, the patient was a functional paraplegic and limited to a wheelchair for most activities.

and who have had symptoms for less than two to three weeks generally have a better-defined syndrome than do patients with chronic disease. The differentiation between acute and chronic disease is somewhat arbitrary and probably relates to the virulence of the organism, the resistance of the host, and the type of treatment received prior to definitive diagnosis. Most patients with an acute epidural abscess present with fever, back pain, and spine tenderness. These signs and symptoms may be lacking in patients with chronic disease.[20, 40, 114, 127, 137, 140, 145, 254, 279]

Without treatment, the disease frequently progresses

through four stages. The patients complain of local spine pain initially, followed by radicular pain and weakness and, finally, by paralysis. Heusner frequently is given credit for defining these stages of progression; however, Browder described the same syndrome in 1937, and a number of other authors reiterated the pattern before Heusner's report in 1948.[40, 64, 127, 145, 269] The transition from one stage to another is highly variable, and weakness or paralysis may not develop for many months or may occur suddenly and unpredictably in a matter of hours.[76, 114, 254]

The location of the pain depends on the site of disease and, therefore, pain is more common in the thoracic than in the lumbar or cervical spine.

If the abscess penetrates the dura, a subdural abscess or meningitis may result.[20, 104] Many patients with an epidural abscess have nuchal rigidity, and this sign is not helpful in differentiating an epidural abscess from meningitis.[20] Fraser and colleagues[104] suggested that a patient with a subdural abscess presents exactly like one with an epidural abscess, except that often there is no spinal percussion tenderness. Butler and coauthors[46] reviewed 16 patients with subdural abscesses described in the literature and found that only four had spinal tenderness. Unfortunately, this feature is not pathognomonic because not all patients with an epidural abscess have spine tenderness.[137, 140]

Heusner thought that it was possible to differentiate patients with acute hematogenous epidural abscess from those whose abscess developed secondary to vertebral osteomyelitis: the latter patients had a predictable delay between the phases of spine pain and radicular pain followed by rapid progression of the illness.[145]

Diagnostic Evaluation

Patients with an acute epidural abscess generally have more systemic illness than those with vertebral osteomyelitis. The leukocyte count and the erythrocyte sedimentation rate generally are increased. In one study by Gardner and associates,[114] the mean sedimentation rate was 86.3 mm in one hour, and the mean leukocyte count was 22,000 cells/mm^3 (range, 11,700 to 41,400 cells/mm^3). Patients with chronic disease usually have less systemic illness, and their leukocyte count often is normal.[20] The definitive diagnosis is based on identification of the organism. Pus from the abscess tests positive in approximately 90 per cent of the cases, blood cultures are positive in 60 per cent, and cultures of spinal fluid yield the organism in approximately 17 per cent.[20, 76, 140, 145, 171]

Plain radiographic findings frequently are normal unless vertebral osteomyelitis or disc space infection is

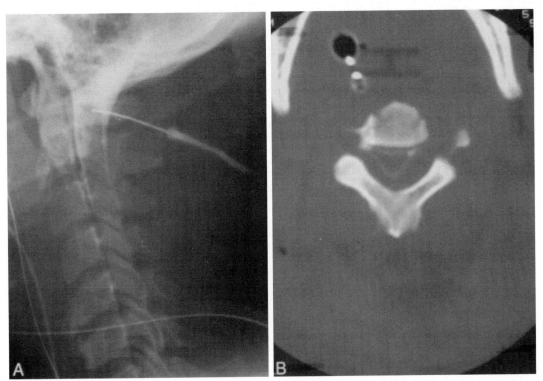

Figure 39–14. This patient presented with a fever and quadriparesis. It was suspected from his history that this was a spine infection. *A*, A C1–C2 puncture was performed, and a myelogram revealed a block at the level of the midcervical spine. From this view, it is suspected that there is a collection of purulent material posteriorly shifting the dye column more anteriorly than normal. *B*, This computed tomographic scan at the level of the upper cervical spine reveals that the dural sac is closely approximated to the vertebral bodies anteriorly but is shifted away from the posterior elements. This is consistent with an epidural abscess.

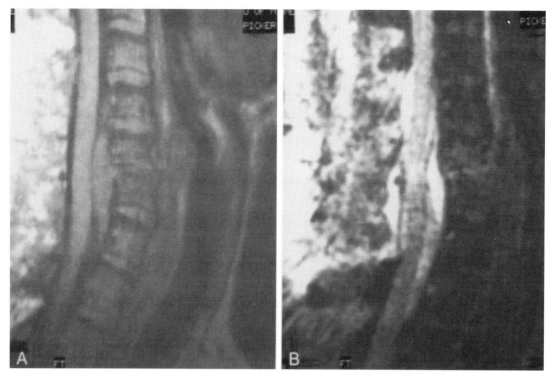

Figure 39–15. This patient presented with quadriparesis; an epidural abscess was suspected. A magnetic resonance (MR) imaging scan was performed. *A,* This T1-weighted midsagittal MR image shows that there is an anterior epidural mass, which is consistent with an epidural abscess. There is also a decrease in the signal intensity at the disc space at C5–C6 in the central region of the abscess. *B,* This T2-weighted sagittal MR image again shows an anterior epidural mass, and the intensity is consistent with an epidural abscess. Also note that there is an increased intensity in the signal from the disc space at the C5–C6 level, consistent with an associated disc space infection.

present and enough time has elapsed for the radiographic finding to become positive.[185, 279]

Radionuclide studies often are helpful but are nonspecific and may be falsely negative.[185] The gallium scan may be slightly more sensitive than the technetium scan.[185]

Until recently, myelography was the standard imaging tool for the diagnosis of an epidural abscess. The puncture site should be placed at a level remote from the expected area of infection. It may be necessary to perform injections at two sites to demonstrate both the cranial and caudal extents of compression. The findings are those of an extradural mass, and generally there is a high-grade or complete block. The lateral myelogram will demonstrate whether the abscess is anterior or posterior.[20, 171, 279] In one series, myelography was accurate to within one vertebral level in both the cephalic and caudal extents of the abscess in 10 of 12 cases, as compared with findings at operation.[114]

The needle should be inserted slowly, and, if pus is encountered, a specimen should be taken for culture without entering the thecal sac; myelography can then be performed at a different level. At the time of myelography, cerebrospinal fluid should be studied for cell total and differential counts, glucose, protein, and culture and sensitivities. The cerebrospinal fluid findings generally reflect a parameningeal infection with mark-

edly increased protein content and no bacteria unless there is an associated subdural abscess or meningitis.[20, 171, 279] If a CT scan can be done expeditiously after the myelogram is obtained, the degree of neural compression will be defined more accurately (Fig. 39–14).

Plain CT scans may be helpful if they demonstrate an extradural mass.[185] Plain CT has a high false-negative rate, and in one study was diagnostic in only four of nine cases.[76] The CT scan may demonstrate hypodense tissue in the epidural space.[53] If gas-forming organisms are present, gas may be seen within the epidural space.[180] When positive, CT could be useful to guide epidural puncture for isolation of the organism.[197]

Contrast-enhanced CT has been found to be helpful by some authors.[11, 15, 36, 197] Positive findings include the loss of physiologic epidural fat and fixation of contrast at the level of the dura surrounded by an area of higher density between the bone and the dura.[197] One major limitation of CT without a preceding myelogram is that the area of interest may be missed unless a large number of cuts are taken.

Magnetic resonance imaging has proved extremely useful and is now the imaging study of choice (Fig. 39–15).[11, 27, 94, 114] It is noninvasive and safe and is able to visualize the degree of cord compression and extent of abscess in all directions. In addition, it has the capability of diagnosing disc space infection or vertebral osteomyelitis. Areas of infection have a characteristic high signal intensity on T2-weighted images. One potential disadvantage of MRI is that the cerebrospinal fluid also has a high signal intensity on T2-weighted images; therefore, there is very little contrast between the cerebrospinal fluid and the epidural abscess. This has led to false-negative MRI results, especially with very long abscesses that do not have a discrete abnormality.[114] MRI findings may also be falsely negative in patients with concomitant epidural abscess and meningitis because the signal changes in the abscess may not be distinct from those in the infected cerebrospinal fluid.[258]

The sensitivity of MRI in detecting an epidural abscess is increased by administration of gadolinium.[187, 259] The pus in the epidural space will enhance with gadolinium, whereas the cerebrospinal fluid will have a low signal intensity on the T1-weighted sequence. Patients who have abundant epidural lipomatous tissue may have false-negative scan results because fat has a bright signal on T1-weighted images before administration of gadolinium and the contrast enhancement of the epidural pus may be obscured.[187] The epidural venous plexus normally enhances with gadolinium administration and may be mistaken for an epidural abscess.[187] The plexus is characteristically more prominent in the cervical spine and it should be symmetric and extend into the neural foramens.

Myelography followed by CT should be performed in patients with negative MRI findings if they are suspected clinically to have an epidural abscess.[258] Repeat MRI with gadolinium enhancement may also detect an infection missed on the first study, since there is a short time delay between the onset of clinical symptoms and the MRI appearance of an abnormality.[50, 187]

Two other conditions to consider in the differential diagnosis of an epidural abscess are epidural metastasis and subdural abscess. It is much more critical to make the appropriate diagnosis in the case of epidural metastasis because the treatment of the two disorders is distinctly different. Subdural abscesses are uncommon. A review of the literature in 1988 revealed only 16 reported cases.[46] Myelography will reveal an intradural extramedullary filling defect, usually with a complete spinal block, and may demonstrate defects at several levels.[46, 104, 202, 309] CT with intrathecal contrast provides better definition of the process than does myelography alone.[185, 309]

Management

An epidural abscess is a medical and surgical emergency. The goals of treatment are eradication of infection, preservation or improvement of the neurologic status, relief of pain, and preservation of spinal stability. The standard approach to an epidural abscess in the early part of this century was immediate laminectomy for spinal decompression. In 1941, Browder and Meyers[41] suggested that chemotherapy might be a

helpful adjunct to surgery. Heusner[145] found survival rates of 63 per cent in patients managed surgically without antibiotics and 90 per cent in those who received antibiotics in addition.

A review of the literature from 1970 to 1990 revealed 37 cases of epidural abscess that had been treated conservatively.[323] Sixty-three per cent of the cases had a successful result; however, some of the patients had disastrous outcomes.[20, 76, 127, 145, 147, 161] Even the most ardent proponents of nonsurgical management of epidural abscesses recommend this approach only in selected cases: (1) poor surgical candidates, (2) abscess involves a considerable length of the vertebral canal, (3) no significant neurologic deficit, and (4) complete paralysis for more than three days. These authors think that the patients who are deteriorating neurologically should undergo surgery.[197, 205]

The surgical approach depends on the location of the abscess. Because the abscess is posterior in most cases, laminectomy generally is the treatment of choice.[20, 145] The facet joints should be left intact for spinal stability. Intraoperative ultrasonography after laminectomy allows localization of epidural masses and differentiation of them from the adjacent spinal cord.[258] When the abscess is secondary to vertebral osteomyelitis, it may be necessary to perform both anterior and posterior decompression. Instrumentation and fusion may be necessary in those cases in which spinal stability has been compromised by the decompression. In these cases, long-term follow-up is mandatory because of the risk of pseudoarthrosis and persistent infection.

The wound may be closed over drains or packed open.[20, 76, 145] Garrido and Rosenwasser[115] recommended closure of the wound and continuous suction-irrigation for five days after decompressive laminectomy. Baker and associates[20] recommended open wound treatment in cases with gross purulence followed by closure of the wound only when granulation tissue is identified. If the wound is left open, delayed closure may be carried out when the leukocyte count, sedimentation rate, and temperature return to normal and the wound shows good granulation tissue.[145]

In children, an extensive laminectomy is undesirable because of the risk of postoperative spinal deformity.[99, 161] Hulme and Dott[161] suggest two limited procedures for children. They recommend first a laminoplasty type of en bloc removal of the lamina and ligaments with replacement after drainage. Alternatively, they advise exploration of the canal through a small fenestration made by removing ligamentum flavum and portions of adjacent lamina and insertion of thin rubber catheters. They believe that this technique is appropriate when gross purulence is encountered, but recommend laminectomy if granulation tissue is found to be compressing the dura.[161] de Villiers reported on four children successfully managed by a modification of Hulme's second technique. A single-level laminectomy was performed, catheters were passed cranially and caudally, and the epidural space was irrigated with antibiotic solution. None of the children required reoperation, and no sinus tract developed with this technique.[77]

A variation of Hulme's technique was reported by Cardan and Nanulescu[49] in 1987. A 2½-year-old boy with an extensive epidural abscess was treated by epidural lavage using Mancao needles. Three hundred milliliters of isotonic saline was flushed through the epidural space over a 30-minute period while the patient was under general anesthesia. A multiple-hole catheter was then inserted from the sacral hiatus to the midthoracic spine, and a solution of 2.5 mg of gentamicin in 5 ml of isotonic saline was administered every 12 hours for five days. The patient improved clinically and, at 18 months postoperatively, was neurologically intact without any sequelae.

As soon as the diagnosis is made, specimens should be obtained and antibiotic therapy started immediately based on the Gram stain results and the known bacteriologic basis of the disease. Initial therapy should include a first-line antistaphylococcal agent. Gram-negative organisms should be suspected if there is a history of a spinal procedure or in intravenous drug abusers. *S. epidermidis* also should be considered after spinal procedures.[76] The definitive antibiotic therapy should be based on the culture and sensitivity results. Antibiotics should be given in maximal dosages for at least two weeks, and most authors recommend three to four weeks of parenteral therapy.[20, 76] Antibiotics must be administered parenterally for at least six to eight weeks for coexistent vertebral osteomyelitis.[20, 76]

Prognosis

The natural history of an untreated epidural abscess is relentless progression of symptoms and eventual paralysis and possibly death. Before the advent of antibiotics, the overall mortality rate was between 55 and 70 per cent.[40, 41, 127, 230] Mixter and Smithwick reported on 10 cases; all three patients treated nonoperatively died.[230] With surgery, the mortality rate decreased to between 30 and 57 per cent[41, 230]; 50 per cent of the survivors were left with residual neurologic deficit.[41] From the data on 168 patients reported in six early series since the introduction of antibiotics, 38 per cent made a complete recovery, 29 per cent had residual weakness, 21 per cent were paralyzed, and 12 per cent died.[20, 41, 76, 137, 140, 171, 254] The data from six series published since 1990[62, 68, 147, 211, 242, 271] indicated that 78 per cent of patients undergoing surgery recover fully or with minimal weakness. The prognosis is similar for patients with acute or with chronic disease as long as they are managed appropriately.[20]

The prognosis for neurologic recovery depends on the duration and severity of the neurologic deficit.[76, 114, 137, 145, 171, 254] Heusner found that most patients with paresis of less than 36 hours' duration had a complete recovery. No patient with complete paralysis for more than 36 to 48 hours recovers significant neurologic function.[137, 145, 332] Complete sensory loss also is a poor prognostic factor.[137] Patients who have an acute progressive syndrome with complete paraplegia occurring within the first 12 hours have a poor prognosis; it is postulated that these patients have spinal cord infarction rather than mechanical compression as the pathogenesis of the neurologic deficit.[185]

Other associated conditions thought to be poor prognostic factors are diabetes,[114] advanced age,[114] female gender,[114] human immunodeficiency virus infection,[185] and associated vertebral osteomyelitis.[145]

The prognosis with subdural abscess is relatively similar—two thirds of the patients in reported cases made a complete or good recovery after surgical treatment in association with antibiotic therapy.[195, 202]

GRANULOMATOUS INFECTIONS

Granulomatous infections may be caused by fungi, certain bacteria, and spirochetes. They are grouped together because they are uncommon lesions with similarities in clinical presentation and in histologic features. If a granuloma is identified on the frozen section, appropriate studies should be initiated to facilitate an accurate diagnosis.[263]

The most common granulomatous spine infection in the world by far is tuberculosis. Tuberculous spondylitis will be described in detail; the fungal and other granulomatous infections will be briefly reviewed by outlining the differences between them and tuberculous infection.

Bacteria in the order Actinomycetales cause chronic infections. This order includes the following families of pathogens: Mycobacteriaceae (genus: *Mycobacterium*), Actinomycetaceae (genera: *Actinomyces, Arachnia*), and Nocardiaceae (genus: *Nocardia*).[194]

Tuberculosis

Epidemiology

The incidence of tuberculous spondylitis varies considerably throughout the world and is usually proportional to the quality of public health services available. It is extremely common in underdeveloped countries where malnutrition and overcrowding are major problems. In affluent countries, the incidence has decreased dramatically in the last 30 years, and it now is uncommon.[58] Bone and joint involvement develops in approximately 10 per cent of patients with tuberculosis,[126] and half of these affected patients have tuberculosis of the spine.[56, 313] A neurologic deficit will develop in 10 to 47 per cent of those with tuberculous spondylitis.[2, 4, 19, 34, 56, 82, 96, 108, 154, 169, 206, 207] In developing countries, the disease is still a significant source of morbidity and mortality and remains the most common cause of nontraumatic paraplegia.[290]

In North America, Europe, and Saudi Arabia, the disease primarily affects adults; in Asia and Africa, a large percentage of the patients are children.[5, 108, 149, 199, 206, 207, 218, 220, 225, 232] These patterns are changing, and a decrease in the incidence of infection in infants and young children has been noted in Hong Kong.[232]

The age incidence of paraplegia corresponds with

the general age incidence of tuberculosis of the spine, except for the first decade in which the incidence of paraplegia is significantly less.[34]

Etiology

Spinal tuberculosis may occur from hematogenous spread from well-established foci outside the spine. The pulmonary and genitourinary systems are the most frequent sources, but spinal tuberculosis also may arise from other skeletal lesions.[60, 108] At presentation, the primary focus of infection may be quiescent. Spinal involvement may develop from visceral lesions by direct extension.[60]

Bacteriology

Infection most commonly is caused by *Mycobacterium tuberculosis*, but any species of *Mycobacterium* may be responsible.[257]

Pathogenesis and Pathology

The pathogenesis of the early stages of spinal tuberculosis is similar to that of pyogenic infections of the spine and may result from hematogenous spread or from direct extension of disease.[60] One study has suggested that the venous or lymphatic routes may be more important than the arterial system for dissemination of this disease. Blacklock[28] was unable to produce spinal disease by injection of mycobacteria into a vertebra or into the left ventricle of experimental animals.

There are three major types of spinal involvement: peridiscal, central, and anterior.[83] In one series of 914 cases, the disease was peridiscal in 33 per cent, central in 11.6 per cent, and anterior in 2.1 per cent; in 52.8 per cent, the disease was too widespread at presentation for identification of the primary focus.[82] Atypical forms of spinal tuberculosis include those with neural arch involvement only and rare cases in which granulomas occur in the spinal canal without bony involvement.[18, 82, 239]

The actual incidence of tuberculosis primarily involving the posterior elements is unknown but probably is between 2 and 10 per cent.[18, 189, 239]

With peridiscal disease, the infection begins in the metaphyseal area and spreads under the anterior longitudinal ligament to involve the adjacent bodies. In contrast to pyogenic infections, the disc is relatively resistant to infection and may be preserved, even with extensive bone loss.[60, 273] Disc space narrowing has been postulated to occur either as a result of extension of disease or from dehydration of the disc secondary to the altered functional capacities of the end plate.

In cases with primarily anterior involvement, the infection spreads beneath the anterior longitudinal ligament and may extend over several segments. The radiographic features include scalloped anterior erosion of several vertebral bodies. This pattern is said to result from aortic pulsations transmitted via a prevertebral abscess beneath the anterior longitudinal liga-

ment.[120] Similar changes have been seen in the cervical spine, however, and another hypothesis is that the scalloping may be due to changes in local vertebral body blood supply.[19]

In cases classified as central involvement, the disease begins within the middle of the vertebral body and remains isolated to one vertebra. These lesions are frequently mistaken for a tumor. They tend to lead to vertebral collapse and therefore are the most likely type to produce significant spinal deformity.[83]

The pathologic findings in tuberculous spondylitis differ in several ways from those in pyogenic infections. The disc is relatively resistant to tuberculous infection. The pathologic changes generally take longer to develop and frequently are associated with greater deformity. Large paraspinal abscesses are more common with tuberculous infections.[60, 81, 154, 273, 277]

There are numerous mechanisms by which a neurologic deficit may develop in a patient with tuberculous spondylitis. The focus of disease may be within the bone or, occasionally, within the spinal canal without osseous involvement.[18, 107, 112, 199, 208, 239, 260] Seddon[293] recognized that neurologic deficits may occur either acutely or chronically (i.e., after healing of the disease). He classified acute disease as "paraplegia of active disease" and recognized that this was due either to external pressure or to invasion of the dura. Pressure on the spinal cord may arise from an epidural granuloma or abscess, from sequestered bone and disc, or from pathologic subluxation or dislocation of the vertebra. The paraplegia in chronic cases is related to pressure on the cord from epidural granulomas or fibrosis or from a ridge of bone anteriorly caused by a progressive kyphotic deformity. Several other authors have confirmed these pathogenetic mechanisms at operation or postmortem examination.[19, 112, 126, 150, 159, 183, 292]

An epidural granuloma is analogous to a pyogenic epidural abscess. Most frequently, the granuloma arises by spread from the adjacent bone. Because the primary bony lesion is anterior in the majority of cases, spinal cord compression occurs anteriorly. With posterior arch involvement, however, the cord may be compressed from behind.[17, 189, 239] Although isolated involvement of the neural arch is uncommon, posterior compression from arch involvement occurs in approximately 10 per cent of cases associated with paralysis.[312]

Rarely, an epidural granuloma may occur directly by hematogenous seeding without any bony involvement.[18, 107, 112, 197, 199, 239, 256] Other lesions that may cause a neurologic deficit without bony involvement are intradural tuberculomas and tuberculous arachnoiditis.[107, 199, 208] Paraplegia from extraosseous disease occurs in no more than 5 per cent of cases.[199]

Transdural extension of tuberculous inflammation was first described by Michod in 1871.[150] Since then, it has been described by other authors.[19, 107, 112, 150, 154] Presumably, transdural extension can occur regardless of whether the process originates within the bone.

The pathologic features of tuberculous spondylitis may be altered by secondary pyogenic infection, which may occur through sinus tracts or after débridement procedures.[60] Secondary infections were the dreaded sequelae of many attempted débridement procedures before antibiotics were available.

Clinical Presentation

The clinical presentation of tuberculous spondylitis is variable and depends on many factors. In the classic presentation, the patient complains of spine pain and exhibits manifestations of chronic illness, such as weight loss, malaise, and intermittent fever. The physical findings include local tenderness, muscle spasm, and restricted motion. The patient also may have a spinal deformity and neurologic deficit. The duration of symptoms before a definitive diagnosis is made varies from months to years; most cases are diagnosed in less than two years.[19] In affluent countries, presentation generally is early, whereas in underdeveloped countries the complications of neglected disease, such as paraplegia, kyphosis, and draining sinuses, may be the presenting complaints.[154, 220, 221, 223]

The location of the pain corresponds to the site of the disease, which is most frequent in the thoracic region, less common in the lumbar region, and rare in the cervical spine and sacrum.[19, 82, 154, 169]

Patients may present with an abscess in any one of many locations, including the groin and buttocks.[83]

In 10 to 47 per cent of patients, neurologic deficits develop during the course of their disease.[2, 4, 19, 34, 56, 82, 96, 108, 154, 169, 206] The incidence of paraplegia is higher with spondylitis in the thoracic and the cervical spine.[82, 160]

The manifestations of cervical spine involvement vary with the age of the patient. Children under 10 years of age usually have extensive disease, with large abscesses and a relatively low (17 per cent) incidence of paralysis. In patients older than this, the disease is more localized with less pus, but the incidence of paraplegia is 81 per cent.[160]

A distinct syndrome has been reported in heroin addicts with tuberculous spondylitis. All five patients in one series had an acute toxic reaction with fever, back pain, weight loss, night sweats, and rapidly evolving neurologic deficits. All patients had disseminated tuberculosis with involvement of extravertebral sites.[100]

Diagnostic Evaluation

The sedimentation rate generally is increased with tuberculous spondylitis, but this is nonspecific. The tuberculin purified protein derivative skin test usually is positive and indicates either past or present exposure to *Mycobacterium*.[199] Cultures of early morning urine samples may be helpful in cases of renal involvement, and sputum specimens and gastric washings may be positive with active pulmonary disease. These laboratory findings are helpful in the diagnosis, but an absolute diagnosis can be made only by biopsy of the spine lesion.[186] Aspiration of a subcutaneous abscess on occasion may reveal the organism and obviate the need for spine biopsy.

Isolation of mycobacterium from clinical specimens takes several weeks, and the sensitivity of culture may be as low as 50 per cent.[75] Polymerase chain reaction has been used to amplify specific DNA sequences and rapidly identify the presence of mycobacterium in formaldehyde solution–fixed, paraffin-embedded tissue specimens.[26] This promising technique may achieve widespread use in the detection of mycobacterium and other spinal infections.

The findings on plain radiographs of the spine (Fig. 39–16) will vary depending on the pathologic type and chronicity of the infection. The earliest finding may be bone rarefaction, regardless of type. With peridiscal involvement, disc space narrowing is followed by bone destruction, similar to pyogenic infections. With anterior multilevel spine involvement, the anterior aspect of several adjacent vertebrae may be eroded in a scalloped fashion. Central body involvement resembles a tumor, with central rarefaction and bone destruction followed by collapse. The initial radiographs often show far advanced bony changes, in contrast to pyogenic infections in which radiographs may be normal on first presentation. The central type is more common in the thoracic area and the peridiscal variant is more common in the lumbar region. The central type causes greater and earlier bone collapse than the peridiscal type.[83] Although these radiographic changes are characteristic, a diagnosis based on radiologic changes alone is inadequate in 10 per cent of cases.[275]

Chest radiographs are helpful in demonstrating pulmonary involvement and may show a paraspinal abscess. It is not possible to differentiate fibrosis and paravertebral edema from abscess formation on the basis of plain radiographs.[19] Occasionally, lumbar spine radiographs will demonstrate calcification in the psoas muscle in cases with a long-standing abscess.[19]

Sclerotic reactive bone formation occurs with healing of tuberculous infection, but is seen much later and is less marked than with pyogenic infection.[133]

Heroin addicts with Pott's disease may have atypical radiographs. In one study, four of five patients had atypical radiographs, including two with an ivory vertebra.[100]

Radionuclide scanning with technetium or gallium may help to define the extent of disease.[284] Gallium scanning has been recommended for diagnosing extrapulmonary tuberculosis and also to monitor the response to treatment.[284] Unfortunately, radionuclide scans are not sensitive for tuberculous infection; technetium bone scan results are negative in 35 per cent of cases and gallium scans are negative in 70 per cent.[199]

Computed tomography is useful to delineate soft tissue changes around the spine and in the canal but is not capable of differentiating an abscess from granulation tissue.

Magnetic resonance imaging is the imaging modality of choice because it demonstrates both bony and soft tissue involvement. The MRI findings in tuberculous spondylitis may be indistinguishable from pyogenic infections, but there are some differences that are characteristic of tuberculosis and reflect the different pathologic types described earlier.[299] The intervertebral

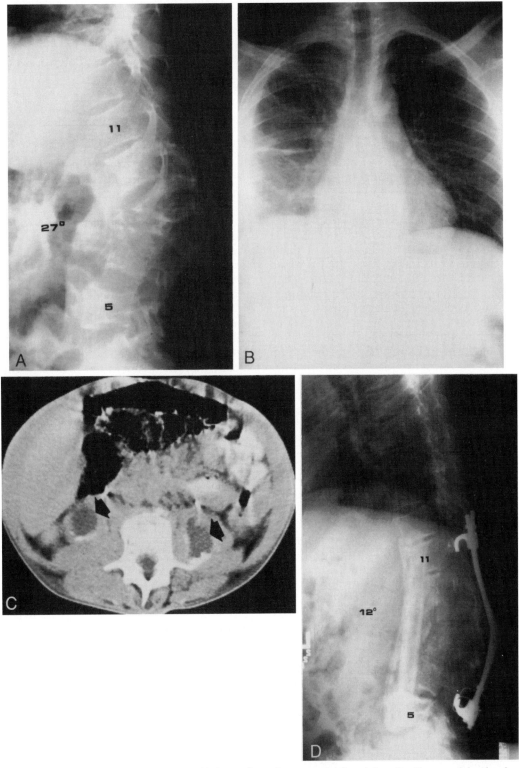

Figure 39–16. This patient presented with intermittent fevers and spine deformity. He complained only of relatively minor spine pain. He was neurologically intact. Tuberculosis was suspected and confirmed by culture. *A,* This lateral radiograph shows a 27-degree kyphosis from the inferior portion of T12 to the superior end plate of L5. The intervening vertebrae are grossly destroyed. *B,* An anteroposterior chest radiograph reveals chronic changes in the right lung and an effusion, which are also consistent with tuberculosis. *C,* This computed tomographic (CT) scan of the lumbar spine reveals bilateral psoas abscesses *(arrows).* There is also a significant paraspinal mass, which is most likely granulation tissue. This was later verified at surgery. *D,* This postoperative lateral radiograph reveals that the kyphosis at the thoracolumbar spine has been reduced to 12 degrees. The intervening neural elements have been decompressed with complete corpectomies from T12 through L4. The patient's fibula was used for an autogenous bone graft and supplemented with autogenous cancellous iliac bone graft. The patient remained neurologically intact. At the time of surgery, gross purulence was found, which corresponded with the psoas abscesses identified on the CT scan.

disc may have normal height and a normal signal on MRI, reflecting the resistance of the disc to tuberculous infection. Involvement of the anterior aspect of several contiguous vertebral bodies (see Fig. 39–16) or involvement of posterior elements suggests a diagnosis of tuberculous spondylitis. Paraspinal masses tend to be longer in tuberculous spondylitis than in pyogenic infections and can be imaged well with plain or gadolinium-enhanced MRI. Enhanced scans can distinguish abscesses from granulation tissue. A mass with near-total enhancement is generally granulation tissue, whereas a mass with enhancement only at the periphery is generally an abscess (Fig. 39–17).[178] As the infection resolves, the T1-weighted images of the vertebral body characteristically have progressively greater signal intensity.[71] Even the MRI findings are not completely characteristic, and a biopsy is necessary in all cases. Central body tuberculosis very closely resembles a neoplasm[298, 299]; an epidural tuberculous granuloma without osseous involvement cannot be differentiated from an epidural neoplastic metastatic lesion. The distinction between these conditions can be made only at operation.[18]

The differential diagnosis should include other bacterial and fungal infections as well as sarcoidosis and neuropathic spine disease. Sarcoidosis rarely involves the spine but may produce paraspinal masses and circumscribed lytic spine lesions with or without a sclerotic rim. Purely sclerotic lesions occur less frequently.[124] Neuropathic disease of the spine usually is limited to one to three contiguous vertebrae and is characterized by marked reactive sclerosis or destruction. Sclerosis associated with neuropathic disease of the spine parallels the base of the vertebral body and commonly involves the posterior arch. It is associated with paraspinal debris but not masses.[124]

Management

The goals of management are to eradicate the infection and to prevent or to treat neurologic deficits and spinal deformity. The modern era in the treatment of spinal tuberculosis began in 1943 with the discovery of streptomycin by Waxmin. The first major paper on the use of streptomycin in tuberculous bone and joint lesions was published by Bosworth and colleagues in 1950.[33] The drug had a tremendous influence on the mortality rate from tuberculosis. Between the five years before streptomycin was used and the five years after its introduction, the mortality rate at Sea View Hospital in New York decreased by 72.5 per cent.[15] Kondo and Yamada[182] reported a decrease in the mortality rate from 42.9 to 9.3 per cent with the addition of streptomycin to the regimen for patients treated nonoperatively. In patients undergoing Albee's fusion, the mortality rate was 32 per cent without streptomycin and none with streptomycin. In patients undergoing focal débridement, the mortality rate decreased from 71.4 per cent without streptomycin to 2.1 per cent with streptomycin.[182]

In 1952, Bosworth and associates[35] published a preliminary report showing encouraging results with the use of isoniazid. These drugs and others eliminated the risk of dissemination of disease and the development of chronic sinuses after surgical débridement and allowed radical procedures to be performed in relative safety.[151, 166] Both drugs were found to be effective without surgery when the patients were kept immobilized in the hospital for long periods.[168]

In Nigeria, a shortage of medical beds and poor medical facilities forced Konstam and Konstam to use chemotherapy on an ambulatory basis.[183, 184] Although many patients in their study were lost to follow-up, 96

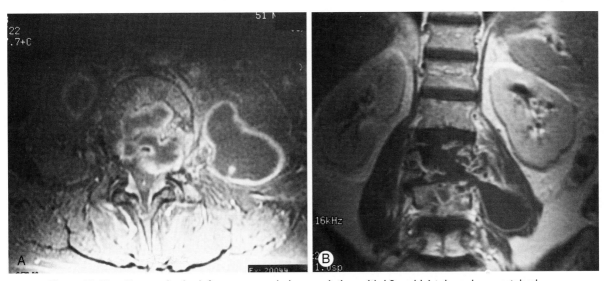

Figure 39–17. Abscess in the left psoas muscle in association with L3 and L4 tuberculous vertebral osteomyelitis. The periphery of the abscess enhances after administration of gadolinium, suggesting that the mass is an abscess rather than granulation tissue. The psoas abscess was found to be a sterile loculation of pus. *A,* axial image; *B,* coronal image.

per cent of those returning were thought to be healed and free of disease. Spinal deformity was found to be a problem with this form of treatment; only 75 per cent developed a bony fusion, 49 per cent had between 0 and 10 degrees of increased kyphosis, and 18 per cent had 30 degrees or more of kyphosis.[183] Other authors found reasonably good results with chemotherapy alone.[80, 108, 233]

Hodgson and Stock had excellent results with their procedure of radical débridement and anterior strut graft fusion in association with chemotherapy (the Hong Kong operation).[151, 153]

In 1963, the Medical Research Council Committee for Research on Tuberculosis in the Tropics began to investigate these widely divergent forms of treatment. A subcommittee was established that later became known as the Working Party on Tuberculosis of the Spine. This group initiated a number of large-scale controlled prospective trials of treatment methods. The design of each study was based on the available resources in areas where tuberculosis was endemic. The first studies, carried out in Korea and Rhodesia, established that chemotherapy is highly effective in ambulatory patients.[218, 221, 222] These investigations showed that there was no advantage to an initial period of bed rest in the hospital,[218] application of a plaster of Paris jacket,[222] or addition of streptomycin to the chemotherapy regimen.[218, 221, 222] These results were maintained after five years[224] and 10 years[216] of follow-up. Other studies comparing the effectiveness of débridement with that of more radical resection and bone grafting were carried out at three different centers. In Hong Kong, where the radical procedure was popularized, resection and fusion were found to have advantages in terms of less deformity and earlier bony fusion.[219] Patients with extensive disease and neurologic deficit were excluded from that study. In two concurrent studies in Africa in which patients with more severe disease were included, there was no significant difference between the two surgical approaches.[220] Most of the patients in the three centers were doing well by the three-year follow-up, and these results were maintained with up to five years of follow-up.[225] No changes were found at 10 years in the Hong Kong series.[215]

The Medical Research Council then set out to determine whether short courses of chemotherapy would be as effective as the standard 18-month regimen (used in all previous studies). In Hong Kong, patients underwent the radical operation and either a six-month or nine-month chemotherapy regimen of isoniazid and rifampin supplemented with streptomycin for six months. The six-month and nine-month courses were equally effective and at least as successful as the standard 18-month regimen when assessed at three years.[223] In South India, ambulatory chemotherapy alone with six- or nine-month regimens was compared with radical surgery plus six months of chemotherapy.[217] Ninety-seven per cent of the patients treated by the nine-month regimen achieved a favorable status at three years compared with 93 per cent for the patients in the six-month ambulatory group. Surprisingly only 85 per cent of the patients in the surgical series achieved a favorable status.[217]

The conclusion of the Research Council was that the treatment of choice for spinal tuberculosis in developing countries is ambulatory chemotherapy with six- or nine-month regimens of isoniazid and rifampicin. Surgery should be considered only for biopsy or the management of myelopathy, abscesses, and sinuses. Even in technically advanced countries they advised against surgery in all cases.[217]

When surgery is felt to be necessary, the Hong Kong operation was recommended.[215, 223] Although the results of the studies in Hong Kong and Africa on radical débridement and fusion versus débridement alone were at variance, the overall conclusion was that the Hong Kong operation allows anterior bony fusion to occur earlier and in a higher percentage of patients. Kyphotic deformity was less common and not progressive in those patients undergoing the more radical procedure.[215]

Other independent studies have demonstrated the effectiveness of débridement and fusion, and they support the philosophy of the Medical Research Council.[12, 132, 173, 186, 296, 328] The group in Hong Kong has written extensively on this approach and are responsible for its popularity.[149, 151–155, 160, 335] Another advantage of anterior decompression and fusion compared with nonoperative treatment that has been demonstrated by a number of authors is the higher recovery rate in patients with neurologic deficit.[19, 96, 199, 206]

Refinements in antituberculosis chemotherapy have permitted a more selective approach to the surgical management of spinal tuberculosis. Rather than operate in every case, Tuli described a "middle-path" regimen of operating only when medical management failed.[312, 313] The first line of treatment was drug therapy. Surgery was considered for the following: decompression in patients with neurologic deficit who failed to respond to conservative therapy, posterior spinal lesions, failure of response after three to six months of nonoperative treatment, doubtful diagnosis, instability after healing, or recurrence of disease or of neurologic complications. In cases without neurologic involvement, healing occurred in 94 per cent with antibiotics alone. In 200 cases with neurologic involvement, 38 per cent of the patients recovered with drugs alone; of those patients requiring operation, 69 per cent recovered completely. The overall success rate in patients with neurologic complications treated by this regimen was 78.5 per cent.[312]

The indications for surgery outlined by Tuli are similar to our current recommendations, except that patients with a neurologic deficit would be operated on urgently rather than after a delay to see whether drug therapy alone would be effective. In general, the indications for operation are the same as with pyogenic infection.

Lifeso and associates[199] think that patients with mild neurologic deficits should not undergo operation because medical therapy alone with close observation is safe. Two of their 23 patients became worse with conservative treatment; both recovered completely after anterior decompression and fusion. They also thought that patients with slight kyphosis could be treated with medical therapy alone because the increase in kyphosis and in the number of affected vertebral bodies reported in children was not found in adults treated medically.

When an operation is indicated, it is easier to do it early because abscesses tend to dissect along tissue planes. If operation is delayed, fibrosis makes the procedure technically much more difficult. Hodgson and Stock[152] found a direct correlation between the duration of neurologic symptoms before the operation and the time for recovery from paraplegia. Others have confirmed this finding.[96] Operation also is advised in late-onset paralysis associated with cord compression by a hard bony ridge in association with kyphosis. Hsu and coworkers[159] think that, in patients with mild or moderate paraplegia, stabilization alone may be indicated, with decompression reserved for those patients with severe paralysis.

Regardless of whether an operation is performed or not, chemotherapy is an integral part of the management of spinal tuberculosis. The only cases in which chemotherapy is not indicated are those in which late-onset paraplegia from progressive deformity has occurred in a patient with healed inactive disease. Drug therapy usually is started preoperatively but may be started after operation if a biopsy is necessary. The first line of drugs currently in use includes isoniazid, rifampin, pyrazinamide, streptomycin, and ethambutol. A number of second-line agents that occasionally are used in special circumstances include ethionamide, cycloserine, kanamycin, capreomycin, prothionamide, and para-aminosalicylic acid.[135] The choice of agents, dosages, and duration of therapy should be directed by an infectious disease expert.

Multiple drugs are used because of the potential for resistance to a single agent. Selection of rational combinations of drugs is based on the mechanism of action and toxicity of the agents.[135] The organisms may be in several different environments and therefore not accessible to all agents. They may reside in the extracellular space, either in the hyperoxic neutral environment of the pulmonary cavity or in the hypoxic acidic environment of caseous material in the spine. They also may exist in the highly suppressive acidic environment inside the activated macrophage. Isoniazid and rifampin are bactericidal against both intracellular and extracellular organisms.[22, 135] Rifampin may have an advantage against bacilli with very low metabolic activity, as are present in caseous material. Pyrazinamide is bactericidal only in an acidic environment and therefore is effective against intracellular organisms or within caseous lesions. Conversely, streptomycin is active only in the extracellular space and therefore is often used to complement pyrazinamide. Ethambutol is bacteriostatic against both intracellular and extracellular organisms and often is used in multiple-drug regimens in place of the once-popular para-aminosalicylic acid.

All these agents have the potential for significant toxicity.[135] Hepatitis can be caused by both isoniazid and rifampin, and is four times more common in patients receiving both agents than in those receiving isoniazid alone. Isoniazid can also cause dose-dependent peripheral neuritis. The major toxicity of streptomycin is nerve VIII damage; that of ethambutol is optic neuritis.

Antimicrobial resistance may occur from the multiplication of resistant mutants under the selective pressure of single-drug therapy.[135] Resistance developing during the course of treatment in a patient with an initially drug-sensitive infection is termed *secondary resistance. Primary resistance*, defined as infection with drug-resistant organisms in a previously untreated patient, may be transmitted to other patients. The prevalence of primary resistance rose from less than 3 per cent in the United States during the 1970s to approximately 9 per cent by 1986.[300] Resistance is much more common in certain urban areas and in patients who are homeless, drug abusers, or infected with human immunodeficiency virus.[135] The patterns of drug resistance are variable throughout the world, re-emphasizing the need for close follow-up during treatment.[183, 199, 223, 232] Resistance generally is not a problem with multiple-drug regimens as long as the patient is in compliance.

A six-month, three-drug regimen including isoniazid, rifampin, and pyrazinamide is used for most cases of drug-sensitive infection in Western nations.[135] Atypical mycobacterial species are often resistant to standard drug regimes.[257] Because spinal tuberculosis carries a significant risk, maximal chemotherapy should be used.

Surgery

An operation may be performed to drain abscesses, to débride sequestered bone and disc, to decompress the spinal cord, or to stabilize the spine for the prevention or correction of deformity.

In 1779, Pott described the drainage of a tuberculous abscess: "The remedy for this most dreadful disease consists merely in procuring a large discharge of matter, by suppuration from underneath the membrana adiposa on each side of the curvature, and in maintaining such discharge until the patient shall have perfectly recovered the use of his legs."[261] His statement was rather optimistic—many patients did not recover neurologic function after this procedure and many others died of secondary pyogenic infection. In general, abscess drainage is indicated only if the patient is septic from the abscess or has a neurologic deficit from an epidural abscess or when the abscess is extremely extensive. After drainage of an abscess, the tissues may be closed in layers or the wound may be packed open. Paravertebral abscesses in the thoracic spine can be drained effectively by a costotransversectomy.[48] Large psoas abscesses may be drained by a retroperitoneal approach.[320]

Simple débridement of the spine without fusion is advocated by some surgeons[182, 220]; however, most authors agree with the conclusions of the Medical Research Council that the Hong Kong procedure of anterior radical débridement and strut graft fusion is superior.[19, 103, 132, 152–154, 173, 186, 296, 328] Surgery performed when the disease is active is safer and the response is faster and better than that performed in patients with resolved disease.[159]

In the Hong Kong procedure, the spine is approached anteriorly so that the affected area may be dealt with most directly. The sequestered bone and caseous material must be débrided back to bleeding bone above and below and back to the posterior longitudinal ligament. The decompression should go back to the dura in cases of neurologic deficit when spinal cord decompression is necessary.[225] The angular deformity is corrected by insertion of a strut graft. Autogenous bone grafting at the time of the primary débridement is reliable in both adults and children.[8, 9, 19, 96, 132, 154, 163, 173, 186, 215, 296] The incidence of fusion with a bone graft is 97 per cent at 10 years, compared with 90 per cent with débridement alone.[215] Medical management with chemotherapy alone may yield a solid fusion in 65 to 79 per cent of cases.[80, 179, 183]

The choice of graft material is based on considerations of graft incorporation and structural support. The grafts used most frequently are iliac crest and ribs. Fibular grafts provide good structural support, but the large amount of cortical bone is undesirable in cases of infection. In addition, long segments of fibula are likely to fracture. In a study of 4 cm long canine fibular grafts, the grafts were markedly weakened between six weeks and six months after implantation. The total incorporation may take several years; at 48 weeks, approximately 60 per cent of the necrotic matrix had been remodeled. Despite that, the strength of the graft is nearly normal at one year.[93] Bradford and Daher[37] described the use of vascularized rib grafts for stabilization of kyphosis. Incorporation of the grafts occurred between four and 16 weeks (mean, 8.5 weeks). They described three patients in whom the graft was placed 4 cm or more anterior to the apical vertebra for mechanical advantage, and none of these grafts fractured. High fusion rates have been reported when vascularized rib grafts are used in the treatment of tuberculous kyphosis.[201]

Kemp and associates found that rib grafting was inadequate in adults. They reported a 32 per cent incidence of graft fracture and a mean increase in kyphosis of 20 degrees. Partial collapse occurred in some cases because the ribs penetrated the end plate. The overall fusion rate was 62 per cent with rib grafts and 94.5 per cent when autogenous, full-thickness iliac crest grafts were inserted, as long as they crossed the coronal diameter of the vertebra.[173] Iliac crest may be preferable to rib, especially in patients with large defects.[152, 173, 266]

McCuen described the first case of tuberculous spondylitis treated by laminectomy in 1882. In the early part of this century it had become a common procedure for patients with Pott's paraplegia. In 1935, Seddon condemned the procedure, claiming that "laminectomy is futile" because it removes the integrity of the poste-

rior arch and may lead to instability and further neurologic damage.[293]

The opinion that laminectomy is contraindicated is shared by many authors.[34, 96, 112, 132, 154, 166, 175, 267] Patients actually may improve considerably immediately after laminectomy but, as Bosworth and colleagues[33] noted, paraplegia inevitably recurs unless fusion is performed both anteriorly and posteriorly. They described 14 patients who had had laminectomies: all died except four who had "circumduction" fusions. Currently, the only indication for laminectomy in the treatment of Pott's paraplegia is atypical disease involving the neural arch and causing posterior spinal cord compression.[112, 175, 238, 239, 293] It also is reasonable in rare circumstances with posterior epidural tuberculoma without bony involvement.[18]

Débridement, decompression, and fusion in the thoracic spine may be performed through a transthoracic approach, through a costotransversectomy, or by an extrapleural anterolateral approach. The last has the theoretic benefit of avoiding the tuberculous empyema.[132] However, no studies have demonstrated any actual advantage of an extrapleural approach over a standard thoracotomy. Kirkaldy-Willis and Thomas[186] demonstrated that the transthoracic approach is more successful than lateral rachiotomy (modified costotransversectomy). The fusion rate was 95 per cent in the former and 78 per cent in the latter; the mortality rate was 3 per cent and 8 per cent, respectively. They recommended thoracotomy in cases of early tuberculosis, with lateral rachiotomy reserved for late-onset paraplegia associated with a large kyphotic deformity requiring lateral exposure of the dura. Kemp and coworkers support this concept.[173]

This technique of decompression through a transthoracic approach is described in Chapter 49. With tuberculosis, the periosteum generally is thicker and frequently adherent to the pleura. Therefore, it often is necessary to dissect in a subperiosteal plane for exposure. If a lung abscess is found at the time of thoracotomy, the abscess may be débrided by scooping out the necrotic material. Yau and Hodgson[334] rarely found an air leak in this situation and had good success by insufflating the cavity with streptomycin and suturing the visceral pleura. Because of the potential for wound dehiscence in these patients, who are frequently immunocompromised and have poor wound-healing potential, the wounds should be closed in layers with interrupted nonabsorbable sutures. In patients with lesions involving more than two vertebral bodies, a period of bed rest followed by external support in a thoracolumbosacral orthosis device is recommended until the fusion becomes consolidated.[266]

Posterior fusion alone, without instrumentation, does not control progressive kyphosis,[139] but it may be performed in addition to anterior strut grafting for added stability (Fig. 39–18).[19, 266] If a laminectomy is performed for posterior neural compression, a fusion also should be performed if any of the facets are removed.[175]

Progressive kyphosis may occur in the immature

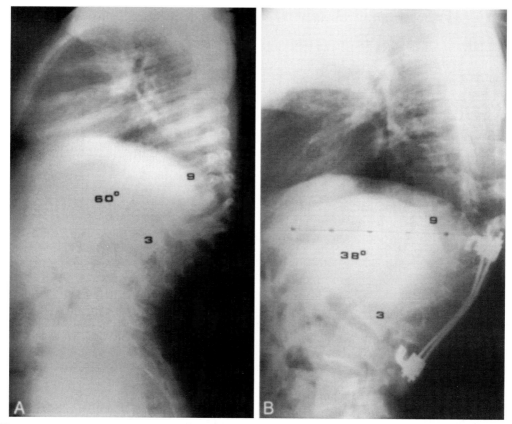

Figure 39–18. This 10-year-old boy complained of intermittent thoracolumbar spine pain. He had a history of an unknown infection in early childhood that was treated with a prolonged course of antibiotics for several years. *A,* At this time, the patient has the complaint of intermittent pain at the thoracolumbar spine, and the lateral radiograph reveals 60-degree kyphosis from T9 to L2. It was suspected that, with further growth, this deformity would increase significantly. *B,* The patient was taken to surgery for an anterior multibody corpectomy from T10 through L2 and a fusion from T9 to L3. The patient's final kyphosis measures 38 degrees several years after the fusion. At this time the patient has no particular complaints and is able to participate in all normal activities of childhood.

spine in spite of a solid anterior fusion. Some authors recommend that a posterior fusion be performed in addition to an anterior fusion to eliminate the risk of increasing deformity.[175, 233] Fountain and associates[103] found that progressive kyphosis developed in only three of 31 children with solid anterior fusions. They recommended performing a supplementary posterior fusion only if progressive deformity is noted.

Anterior grafts may not provide stable fixation, especially in cases in which the graft spans more than two disc spaces.[266] To prevent loss of correction, some authors recommend a two-stage procedure with an instrumented posterior fusion followed by anterior débridement and fusion.[178, 193, 234] Moon and others[234] reported on 39 adults undergoing the two-stage procedure in the same operative setting or in a delayed fashion. The infection was cured in all cases and they achieved excellent deformity correction without a prior anterior release. The loss of correction did not exceed 3 degrees.

Güven and others[134] recommend a single-stage posterior approach without any anterior procedure in cases without paralysis, multisegmental involvement,

or large abscesses. They reported on 10 patients who underwent the procedure. All patients had resolution of the infection and the mean loss of correction was only 3.4 degrees.

Oga and others[245] studied the risk of using spinal instrumentation despite active tuberculous infection. All 11 of their patients had resolution of the infection and none developed a kyphotic deformity after operation. They also evaluated the adherence properties of *Mycobacterium tuberculosis* and *S. epidermidis* to stainless steel. The *Staphylococcus* heavily colonized the rods and was covered with a thick biofilm, whereas only a few biofilm-covered colonies of *Mycobacterium tuberculosis* were seen.

The incidence of cord compression with cervical tuberculous spondylitis is more than 40 per cent overall and much higher in adults[160]; therefore, an infection in this region requires aggressive treatment. Hsu and Leong[160] reported excellent results from using the Hong Kong procedure via a Southwick-Robinson approach in conjunction with medical management. With C1–C2 involvement, drainage may be performed by the transoral route with or without a supplementary posterior occiput-to-C2 fusion.[94] Isolated involvement of the arch of the atlas has been treated successfully in one case by chemotherapy, needle aspiration of an abscess, and halo-brace immobilization.[63] Lesions between C3 and C7 may be approached through either the anterior triangle[301] or the posterior triangle. The latter may be preferable in some cases because pus often tracks and points in the posterior triangle, making dissection easier.[148]

When cervical disease is complicated by kyphosis, staged procedures may be necessary. Strut grafting may be performed at the time of débridement if the deformity can be reduced. If the deformity is too great, traction may be necessary before final anterior grafting. Anterior reconstruction should be followed by posterior stabilization and fusion.[335] Laminectomies are contraindicated in the cervical spine because subluxation and further neurologic deficits may occur.[60]

Complications of surgical treatment are frequent. The operative risk is greatest in elderly patients with extensive disease. In one series, the operative mortality was 2.9 per cent and an additional 1 per cent of the patients died of the disease later.[153] Early complications include wound sepsis, pleural effusion, pulmonary embolism, cerebrospinal fluid fistula into the pleural cavity, ileus, progressive neurologic deficit, damage to the ureter, loss of graft fixation or graft fracture, atelectasis, pneumonia, air leak, Horner's syndrome, and injury to one of the great vessels.[155] When streptomycin is placed directly on exposed dura, convulsions may occur.[155] Late complications include graft resorption, graft fracture, nonunion, and progressive kyphosis.[173, 265, 266] Adrenal insufficiency may occur secondary to tuberculous involvement of the adrenal glands. Adrenal suppression should be suspected, especially if calcification is noted on radiographic studies.[96]

Prognosis

With tuberculous spondylitis, the prognosis depends on the age and general health of the patient, the severity and duration of the neurologic deficit, and the treatment selected.

Mortality

Before the advent of chemotherapy, the mortality rate in patients treated nonoperatively was 12 to 43 per cent.[2, 82, 169, 182] The rate in patients with a neurologic deficit was close to 60 per cent.[34] In one study, the mortality rate was found to be linked directly to associated pulmonary involvement: 9.4 per cent of the patients with spine infections and inactive pulmonary tuberculosis died, in contrast to 51.3 per cent of those who had active pulmonary disease or metastatic spread to other organs.[56] Attempted débridement of the spine without antibiotic coverage was associated with a mortality rate as high as 71 per cent.[182] With the chemotherapeutic regimens now available, the mortality rate should be less than 5 per cent if the disease is diagnosed early, the patients comply with the regimen, and follow-up is close.[5, 199] The mortality rate in pa-

tients treated with the Hong Kong procedure in addition to antibiotics is directly proportional to the severity of the neurologic deficit. In one study, among patients undergoing surgery, the mortality rate was 2 per cent in those with mild neurologic deficit, 6 per cent in those with moderate neurologic deficit, and 11 per cent in those with a severe deficit.[5]

Relapse

The relapse rate in patients treated with the antibiotics available between 1952 and 1962 was 21 per cent.[108] With current medical regimens and close follow-up, the rate should approach zero.[199]

Kyphosis

Progressive kyphosis is a significant cosmetic deformity, but more important is the fact that it may cause a neurologic deficit or respiratory and cardiac failure due to restriction of pulmonary function (Fig. 39–19). Rajasekaran and Soundarapandian[266] reported the results of a prospective controlled study performed in collaboration with the Medical Research Council. The treatment groups included chemotherapy alone for either six or nine months or radical surgery in combination with six months of chemotherapy. Ninety patients (98 per cent of the study group) were followed for a minimum of six years. Those who underwent nonsurgical treatment had a statistically significantly higher rate of kyphotic deformity than those treated surgically. There was a direct correlation between the final angle of the deformity and the amount of initial loss of vertebral body. The angle increased severely in 10 per cent of the surgical group and in 32 per cent of the nonsurgical group. Severe deformity in the surgical group was related to graft failure.

To predict the angle of deformity expected, the researchers devised a formula[265]; $Y = a + bX$, in which Y is the final angle of the deformity, X is the amount of initial loss of vertebral body, and a and b are constants (5.5 and 30.5, respectively). With their formula, the final angle of the gibbus was predictable, with 90 per cent accuracy in the patients treated nonsurgically.[265] If the predicted angle is excessive, early operation should be considered.

Rajasekaran and Soundarapandian[266] provided additional information on 81 patients treated by the Hong Kong operation and followed for a minimum of eight years; 19 per cent of these patients had an increase in the gibbous angle of up to 20 degrees, and in 22 per cent it was more than 20 degrees. The major risk factor for increasing deformity was extensive involvement of the vertebral bodies, which resulted in a large defect after débridement and necessitated a graft spanning more than two disc spaces. Patients with lesions of the thoracic vertebrae and those with marked kyphosis preoperatively were also more likely to have progression. These authors concluded that when the length of the graft exceeds two disc spaces, surgical treatment should be augmented by prolonged bed rest, bracing, or posterior arthrodesis. Rib strut grafts were used in many of the patients with progressive deformities, and

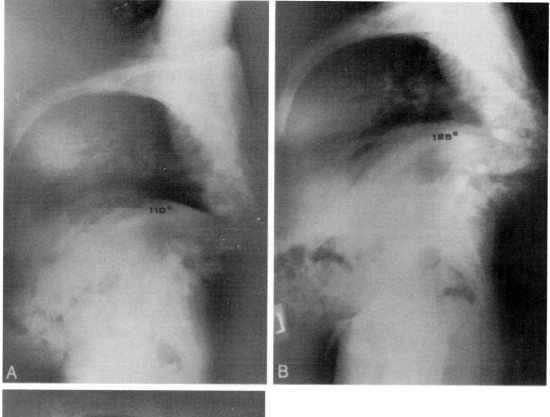

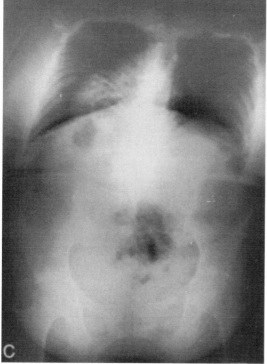

Figure 39–19. This young adult patient was known to have had tuberculosis of the spine as a child. At this time, she presented with a history of spine pain that was relieved with bed rest and aggravated by increasing activities. *A,* At the time of first presentation, the patient was seen to have kyphosis of 110 degrees. It is apparent that she has had extreme shortening of the trunk caused by the combination of kyphosis and vertebral body destruction. *B,* Over a period of 5 years, it can be seen that the patient has had an increase in the kyphosis from 110 degrees to 125 degrees. At this point, she remained neurologically normal. *C,* This anteroposterior radiograph of the thoracic and lumbar spine is consistent with the gross deformity seen on the lateral radiographs and obvious on clinical inspection. This is the type of deformity that is best prevented with surgical intervention.

it was proposed that iliac crest graft may be preferable in patients with large defects.[266] Iliac crest grafts were used exclusively by Hodgson and Stock[152] and may explain the very low incidence of progressive kyphosis in their series. Others also have recommended the use of iliac crest grafts rather than rib struts.[173] In patients

with small defects, however, the availability of rib graft and avoidance of additional donor site problems make rib grafts a more attractive alternative.

In addition to graft failure, children are at risk of progressive deformity after anterior débridement and fusion because of persistent growth posteriorly and growth retardation anteriorly. Close follow-up is necessary, and a supplementary posterior fusion should be performed if progressive kyphosis occurs.[19, 103] A study comparing the radiographs of 117 children operated on for spinal tuberculosis at the age of two to six years showed that anterior fusion alone leads to greater kyphotic angulation than a posterior fusion, a combined anterior and posterior fusion, or anterior débridement alone.[289]

Neurologic Deficit

Patients with neurologic deficit may improve spontaneously without surgery or chemotherapy[112, 169] or with chemotherapy alone,[108, 183, 312] but, in general, the prognosis is improved with early surgery.[19, 199, 206] In one study, 94 per cent of neurologically impaired patients recovered normal function after anterior decompression; only 79 per cent totally recovered after nonsurgical management.[199] When patients with a neurologic deficit were operated on only if they failed to respond to an initial course of antibiotics, the overall success rate was 78.5 per cent.[312] As expected, patients with less severe neurologic deficit and those who were treated early after the development of neurologic signs had a better outcome.[4, 5, 126, 154, 181, 312] In one study of 64 patients, only 48 per cent of those with severe neurologic deficits recovered, whereas 83 per cent of patients with moderate deficits recovered; only four of ten patients with late-onset paraplegia had a satisfactory recovery.[5]

Patients with paraplegia of long duration should be treated aggressively. Hodgson and coworkers[154] found that the chances of complete recovery are good after surgical treatment, although it may take longer for these patients to recover. They documented recovery in a patient who had had a neurologic deficit for five years. In patients with late-onset paraplegia, the response to the operation is faster, better, and safer in patients who have active disease than in those with resolved disease and a hard, bony ridge compressing the cord.[159] Overall, most patients with a neurologic deficit recover within six months, but those who have direct involvement of the meninges (pachymeningitis) may recover more slowly.[154]

Govender and colleagues[126] found that patients who have an atrophic cord as seen on CT myelography preoperatively usually do poorly after decompression.

Patients with cervical spine involvement are at high risk of neurologic deficit but do very well after anterior débridement and fusion.[160]

The only indication for laminectomy is posterior cord involvement. In 19 patients with posterior element disease undergoing laminectomy, 16 had good results and three had fair results in one series. Six of ten patients undergoing laminectomy for epidural tuberculomas without bony involvement had good results, three patients had fair results, and one had a poor result.[18] The overall prognosis with posterior spinal tuberculosis is better in those patients who have less severe neurologic deformity of shorter duration and slower progression, and are younger and in good general health.[189]

Age

In general, children have a better prognosis than adults.[19, 154, 173, 206]

Fusion

Bosworth and associates[34] thought that solid fusion was essential for permanent recovery from tuberculous spondylitis. They described five patients who initially recovered but became paralyzed again with the development of pseudarthrosis. These patients recovered once again after repair of the pseudarthrosis.

Spontaneous bony fusion occurred in 27 per cent of patients treated with bed rest in a plaster shell, without surgery or chemotherapy.[82] With chemotherapy alone, spontaneous fusion occurred in 24 per cent at 18 months and in 36 per cent at 36 months.[233] In the prospective study by the Medical Research Council, the fusion rate in patients treated by the Hong Kong procedure was 28 per cent by six months, 70 per cent by 12 months, 85 per cent by 18 months, and 92 per cent at five years. The corresponding values for the patients undergoing débridement without fusion were 3, 23, 52, and 84 per cent, and the fusion rates in patients treated by ambulatory chemotherapy alone were 9, 26, 50, and 85 per cent, respectively.

Actinomycosis

Actinomyces israelii is a slowly growing, facultative or anaerobic, filamentous, gram-positive bacterium. The diseases it causes mimic those produced by true fungi. It is noted for causing chronic suppurative infections with external sinuses that discharge distinctive aggregates of organisms ("sulfur granules").[263, 280] The organism, an endogenous, oral saprophyte, requires trauma, surgery, or other infection to penetrate the mucosa. Infections involving *Actinomyces* frequently are polymicrobic.[280]

The lesions are characterized by hard, fibrotic walls with granulation tissue surrounding loculations of pus. Sinus tracts extending to the skin or into other organs are commonly seen in more chronic infections.[280]

Bone is involved in approximately 15 per cent of cases, most commonly in the mandible and spine.[124] Before 1950, vertebral actinomycosis was the most common form of osseous involvement. With the advent of antibiotics, vertebral infection is becoming less common. Vertebral infection occurs by extension from retropharyngeal, mediastinal, or retroperitoneal soft tissue abscesses or by hematogenous dissemination. Unlike *M. tuberculosis,* the organism has a predilection for the cervical spine from retropharyngeal spread.

As in tuberculosis, the radiographs may demonstrate prominent paraspinal abscesses and involvement of several vertebral bodies. Distinctive features include simultaneous vertebral body and posterior element involvement, spread to adjacent ribs, periosteal new bone formation outlining the vertebra, and a mixture of lytic and sclerotic changes that may produce a honeycomb appearance of the bone.[124] The vertebral body collapse and disc space narrowing that are common in tuberculosis are uncommon in actinomycosis.[124]

Epidural abscesses may occur by extension from a vertebral source or through an intervertebral foramen from a cervical, pulmonary, or abdominal focus.[280] The dura generally resists penetration, but neurologic deficit may occur by epidural compression.[280]

Before the introduction of penicillin, most cases of actinomycosis were fatal. The current treatment is still penicillin in large doses given over extended periods in association with abscess drainage and excision of sinus tracts when necessary.[280] Other first-line antibiotics that are effective are tetracycline, erythromycin, clindamycin, and the cephalosporins. When response to penicillin is poor, the possible reasons include an undrained abscess, polymicrobial infection, and perhaps bacterial resistance.

Nocardiosis

Nocardia asteroides is the most common human pathogen in this family of aerobic, weakly gram-positive bacteria. It is a natural soil saprophyte often found in decaying organic matter.[194] Infection most commonly occurs through the respiratory tract, although other modes of infection may occur. This infection now is seen most frequently in immunocompromised hosts.

Nocardiosis may initiate a chronic granulomatous response, but more frequently the histologic features are suppurative necrosis and abscess formation, typical of pyogenic infections.[280]

The most frequent primary site is the pulmonary system, but dissemination to almost any organ occurs in 45 per cent of cases. Dissemination to the brain, meninges, and spinal cord occurs in 23 per cent, but hematogenous involvement of the vertebrae is uncommon.[333] Epidural spinal cord compression from vertebral osteomyelitis has been reported.[16, 297] Rapidly growing bacteria in mixed cultures may obscure the growth of *Nocardia* spp., and the laboratory should be alerted if *Nocardia* infection is suspected.

Sulfonamides, in conjunction with appropriate surgery, have been the mainstay of treatment since 1944. Many other antibiotics—including minocycline, trimethoprim sulfate, methoxazole, amikacin, imipenem, ceftriaxone, cefuroxime, and cefotaxime—have been used either alone or in combination. The optimal duration of therapy is uncertain but, because of the possibility of relapse, treatment is often continued for many months after apparent cure. A poor response to treatment may be related to the presence of a second pathogen.[280]

Brucellosis

Brucellosis is caused by an aerobic, gram-negative coccobacillus commonly found in domestic animals and transmitted to humans by direct contact, by ingestion of contaminated products, and, possibly, by inhalation

of aerosols.[172, 198, 263, 336] The disease affects approximately 500,000 persons per year worldwide.[336] Its incidence is decreasing throughout the United States, primarily because of pasteurization of milk. In 1976, 75.6 million dollars were spent to maintain the brucellosis control program and the incidence in the United States is now less than 0.5 cases per 100,000 population.[330, 336] The causative organisms include *Brucella abortus* (cattle), *B. melitensis* (goats), *B. suis* (swine), and *B. canis* (dogs). The infection spreads via lymphatics and blood vessels and produces acute systemic infection as well as chronic relapsing disease (undulant fever).

The clinical presentation of patients with brucellosis varies widely. After an incubation period of days to several weeks, low-grade fever, weakness, headaches, lymphadenopathy, hepatosplenomegaly, and generalized musculoskeletal complaints may develop insidiously.[235, 263] Approximately one third of the patients have a more fulminant illness with acute onset of systemic toxicity.[336] Some infections are asymptomatic initially. After the initial illness, which may last for several days to weeks, relapses occur in about 5 per cent of patients. Relapses seldom occur in patients who receive appropriate treatment, and often are the result of focal suppurative complications such as spondylitis.[336] The classic feature of an undulating fever is not present in most cases.[172, 336] Late complications may affect almost any organ system and include septic arthritis, central nervous system involvement, osteomyelitis, and spine infection. The statistics on brucellosis vary widely depending on the source of the information. Between 11 and 80 per cent of patients with brucellosis have bone and joint involvement and, of these, 6 to 54 per cent have spinal column involvement,[59, 111, 198, 235, 336] most commonly in the lumbar spine.[172, 263] Localized spine pain is the earliest sign of spondylitis.[172] Of those with spondylitis, between 10 and 43 per cent have some degree of neurologic compromise,[198, 235] and in 10 to 20 per cent a paraspinal abscess develops.

In one series of 593 patients with brucellosis, neurologic deficits occurred in five (71 per cent) of the patients with cervical spondylitis, two (11 per cent) of the patients with thoracic involvement, and nine (21 per cent) of the patients with lumbar disease. The patients with cervical and thoracic disease had significantly more paraspinal and epidural abscesses than the patients with lumbar infection. Patients with cervical spine involvement had a much worse prognosis than those with disease in other areas.[59]

Blood cultures are positive in less than half the cases overall,[172, 198] but are positive in 70 per cent of patients with acute *B. melitensis* infection.[336] An agglutination reaction with a brucella antibody titer of 1:160 or greater is presumptive evidence of infection, but an increasing titer is a more helpful sign of active infection.[172, 198, 336] If *B. canis* infection is suspected, a specific agglutination test must be used because the standard test does not react with antibodies against *B. canis*.[336]

The characteristic radiologic features of brucellar spondylitis include predilection for the lower lumbar spine, intact vertebral architecture despite evidence of diffuse vertebral osteomyelitis, disc space involvement, minimal associated paraspinal soft tissue involvement, and absence of gibbous deformity.[6, 198, 295] Bone scintigraphy is not helpful in differentiating brucellar from tubercular spondylitis. The MRI findings are similar in the two, except that tuberculosis often produces more severe changes with more deformity and abscess formation.[295]

The current World Health Organization treatment of choice for brucellosis is doxycycline at 200 mg/day and rifampin at 600 to 900 mg/day for at least six weeks.[336] A randomized, double-blind study comparing doxycycline plus rifampin with doxycycline plus streptomycin for 45 days showed that the latter was more effective in the treatment of spondylitis.[13] Some authors recommend that treatment should be continued for at least three months in cases of spondylitis because high relapse rates have been reported with shorter courses.[198] After single-agent therapy with tetracycline, streptomycin, rifampin, or trimethoprim-sulfamethoxazole, the relapse rates are between 5 and 40 per cent.[336] Response to treatment is monitored with repeated agglutination tests. Lifeso and associates[198] recommend continuing antibiotic therapy until the titer is 1:160 or less and there is clinical and radiographic evidence of resolution. Surgery usually is unnecessary.[198]

Fungal Infections

Fungal infections of the spine are uncommon, although they frequently occur in immunosuppressed hosts with multiple medical problems. There often is a long delay in diagnosis, mainly because other medical conditions may mask the diagnosis and because fungal spondylitis characteristically runs an indolent course.[47]

In one series of 11 cases, the source of infection was hematogenous seeding from septic episodes in five, postoperative osteomyelitis in three, local extension from an adjacent fungal infection in two, and direct traumatic implantation in one.[47]

Although certain radiographic features are characteristic of each type of infection, the diagnosis rests on the evaluation of a tissue specimen. Biopsies must be evaluated with fungal stains as well as cultures, because the latter may be negative or take several weeks or months before identification is possible. Closed biopsy was reported to be positive in only 50 per cent of cases, whereas open biopsy was positive in all cases in the series of Campbell and coworkers.[47]

The treatment of fungal infection involves correcting host factors that may compromise wound healing or immune defense capabilities. Antifungal agents are the mainstay of treatment, but surgery frequently is necessary. The approach should be based on the pathologic features encountered, but in general anterior débridement and stabilization is preferred.[47]

The prognosis for patients with fungal vertebral osteomyelitis depends on the organism as well as on the host. As with bacterial infections, it appears that pa-

tients with diabetes mellitus or neurologic deficits have a poorer prognosis.[47]

The unique characteristics of the fungi causing vertebral osteomyelitis are discussed in the sections following.

Coccidioidomycosis

Coccidioides immitis is endemic in parts of the southwestern United States (especially the San Joaquin Valley in central California), Central America, and parts of South America.[263, 329]

The fungus exists in its mycelial phase in the soil of desert areas. The saprophytic cycle includes the formation of spores that become airborne. Humans become infected most commonly by inhalation of the spores or, less commonly, through abrasions of the skin. The spores swell and become spherules, which reproduce by the formation of internal spores known as "endospores." When the spherule ruptures, endospores are released and each may develop into a new spherule, completing the parasitic cycle. The saprophytic cycle can begin again only when the spores are returned to the soil. The disease is not contagious, because person-to-person transmission can occur only in rare circumstances when the fungus reverts from its tissue phase to its airborne form in contaminated secretions.[304]

The primary focus of disease is the lung, but infection may become disseminated in 0.5 per cent of the cases; osseous manifestations occur in 10 to 50 per cent of those with disseminated disease.[210] Histologically, coccidioidomycosis causes a granulomatous tissue reaction resembling tuberculosis.[304] Extrapulmonary disease is uncommon if the infection has been quiescent in the year after the initial pulmonary infection, unless the host is immunocompromised.[304] Bone lesions are multifocal in 40 per cent of cases overall and in most cases of vertebral involvement.[304] The bones most commonly involved are the skull, metacarpals, metatarsals, spine, and tibia. Spine infection occurs in 10 to 60 per cent of patients with osseous involvement.[124]

Serum IgM precipitins can be detected by a variety of methods. These antibodies occur in 75 per cent of cases, one to three weeks after onset of symptoms of primary infection, and they disappear within four months.[304]

Skin tests with coccidioidal antigens are positive within three weeks after the onset of symptoms. Anergy is common in disseminated coccidioidomycosis, and therefore skin testing is unreliable in systemic disease. A negative skin test in a patient with a primary infection suggests that dissemination will occur.[304]

An increased complement-fixing antibody titer indicates disseminated disease. Sixty-one per cent of patients with disseminated disease have titers of at least 1:32, and 41 per cent have titers of at least 1:64. In contrast, 95 per cent of patients without disseminated disease have titers below 1:32, and 99 per cent have titers below 1:64.[304]

Spine lesions frequently are multiple (Fig. 39–20) and generally are lytic.[72, 124, 263, 304] The entire vertebra,

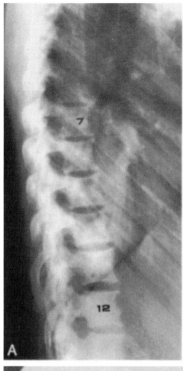

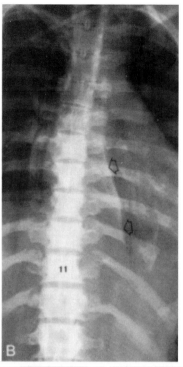

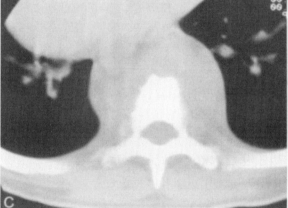

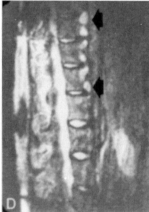

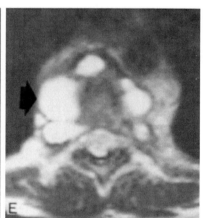

Figure 39–20. This patient had a long-standing history of spine pain and spontaneous draining fistulas through the skin in the paraspinous region. At the time of presentation to our institution, she had symptoms of a low-grade meningitis. *A,* This lateral radiograph of the thoracic spine reveals marked scalloping of the anterior aspect of the vertebral bodies; this is especially apparent at the T12 level. *B,* This anteroposterior radiograph reveals marked sclerosis of the thoracic vertebrae from T7 down through T12. It can also be appreciated that there is a very large left-sided paraspinous mass *(arrows),* which is consistent with paraspinal abscess. *C,* This transverse computed tomographic image reveals gross paraspinous swelling, which is consistent with infection. *D,* This T2-weighted sagittal magnetic resonance (MR) image reveals increased signal intensity *(arrows)* anterior to the vertebral bodies. This is consistent with pockets of purulent material. It is interesting that all the discs appear normal. *E,* This T2-weighted transverse MR image reveals multiple loculations in the paraspinous region *(arrow).* At surgery this proved to be a chronic coccidioidomycosis infection of the spine with an associated meningitis. This was adequately treated with surgical débridement and appropriate antibiotic therapy.

including the arch, often is involved, but the disc usually is spared. Paraspinal masses are frequent, and contiguous rib involvement may be seen.[72, 304] Vertebral collapse occurs late.[72]

Although most patients with symptomatic primary infection recover without therapy, chemotherapy is indicated in patients with severe primary infection and in all patients with dissemination. The standard treatment of coccidioidomycosis has been a total dose of 1 to 2.5 g of amphotericin B intravenously given over a period of many weeks. Alternative agents include miconazole, an azole available for intravenous therapy, or the oral azole ketoconazole. The oral triazole drugs, itraconazole and fluconazole, are under evaluation in clinical trials.[304] Relapse rates are high and azole therapy should probably be continued for six months after the disease is inactive.[304]

The response to treatment may be followed by measuring complement-fixing antibody titers. The treatment program should be reassessed if the titers are increasing.[304] The indications for surgery are the same as in other spine infections.[329] The local use of antifungal agents may add to the success of treatment.[304]

Blastomycosis

Blastomyces dermatitidis is a dimorphic fungus endemic in areas bordering the Mississippi and Ohio rivers, the Great Lakes, and the St. Lawrence River. Cases have also been reported in Central and South America, Africa, and the Middle East.[54, 124, 263] The organism exists in warm, moist soil rich in organic debris.[54]

Primary infection in humans occurs by inhalation of conidia, which then covert to the yeast phase in the lung. The inflammatory response resembles coccidioidomycosis, with clusters of neutrophils and noncaseating granulomas. The incubation period for acute pulmonary infection is 30 to 45 days. The symptoms are nonspecific, and acute infection may go unrecognized. Dissemination by hematogenous spread occurs frequently. The skin is the most common extrapulmonary site, being affected in 40 to 80 per cent of the patients. Skeletal blastomycosis is seen in 10 to 50 per cent of cases, and the long bones, vertebrae, and ribs are the most common sites of osseous involvement.[54, 124]

The radiographic findings in vertebral blastomycosis resemble those in tuberculosis: disc space narrowing, anterior involvement of the vertebral body, and development of large abscesses. Collapse and gibbous deformity are more common with blastomycosis than with the other fungal diseases.[54, 116, 124] The thoracic and lumbar regions are more commonly involved than the cervical spine. Unlike the situation in tuberculosis, lesions frequently invade adjacent ribs, cause draining sinuses, and involve the posterior elements.[116, 124, 263]

Unfortunately, serum complement-fixation tests are not sensitive or specific. An immunodiffusion test is more sensitive and more specific and is more likely to be positive in patients with disseminated disease. A radioimmunoassay and an enzyme immunoassay are available and are quite sensitive but lack specificity. An enzyme-linked immunosorbent assay is commercially available and is often used for initial screening.[54]

Before the availability of effective antimicrobial therapy, the mortality rate exceeded 60 per cent.[54] The present recommended treatment is ketoconazole in a single daily dose of 400 mg. The dose should be increased in 200 mg increments to a maximum of 800 mg/day if the response to treatment is not satisfactory. Itraconazole has less toxicity and is at least as effective as ketoconazole, and some authors consider itraconazole to be the oral azole of choice.[54] The role of fluconazole is under investigation. Chemotherapy should be continued for six months, although the optimal duration of treatment has not been determined. Amphotericin B is reserved for patients with life-threatening disease or involvement of the central nervous system or when ketoconazole treatment fails. A total dose of 1.5 to 2.5 g of amphotericin B is recommended. Ketoconazole cannot be used in patients with central nervous system blastomycosis because it does not cross the blood-brain barrier.[54] The roles of miconazole and itraconazole are under investigation. The role of surgery in blastomycosis is the same as in other spine infections.

Cryptococcosis

Cryptococcus neoformans, a yeastlike fungus, is surrounded by a thick, gelatinous capsule. It is found throughout the world, most commonly in pigeon feces and soil.[79] The disease is more common in males, whites, and immunocompromised hosts. Cryptococcosis is the fourth most common life-threatening infection in patients with acquired immunodeficiency syndrome (AIDS).[79]

Infection is acquired by inhalation after the organism is aerosolized. There are no known instances of direct human-to-human or animal-to-human transmission.[79, 263] The inflammatory response is variable and generally is made up of chronic inflammatory cells, but neutrophils may predominate. The cellular reaction usually is minimal, and there is very little suppuration and necrosis.[263] The exudate in cryptococcal lesions is quite mucoid, giving the granuloma a gelatinous appearance so that it may be mistaken for a myxomatous tumor.[263] Well-formed granulomas are uncommon.[79]

Cryptococcosis may be localized to the lung or generalized. Central nervous system involvement is common in the disseminated form. Osseous involvement occurs in approximately 5 to 10 per cent of patients and resembles cold abscesses, similar to tuberculosis.[79] Unlike the findings in other fungal infections, sinus tracts and abscess formation are rare.[124]

Radiographically, the lesions resemble those of coccidioidomycosis. Lucent lesions of the vertebral bodies and posterior elements are sharply defined, but lack reactive sclerosis or periosteal new bone formation.[124] The disc spaces frequently are spared, but involvement of the posterior elements is common.[124]

A latex agglutination procedure for the detection of cryptococcal polysaccharide capsular antigen is available. Both serum and cerebrospinal fluid should be tested. The tests detect antigen in 90 per cent of patients with cryptococcal meningitis, but is much less sensitive in patients without central nervous system involvement.[79] Rheumatoid factor also causes agglutination in this procedure, necessitating a test for rheumatoid factor as a control on all samples.[79] Definitive diagnosis is made by culture of the organism.

The current recommended medical treatment of cryptococcosis is a combination of amphotericin B (0.3 mg/kg/day, intravenously) and flucytosine (37.5 mg/kg every six hours by mouth) for six weeks. The dose of flucytosine can be adjusted based on serum levels to reduce the risk of drug accumulation. Alternatively, amphotericin B alone in doses of 0.5 to 0.7 mg/kg/day for at least 10 weeks can be given. Flucytosine is limited by the development of drug resistance when used alone. Ketoconazole and itraconazole both penetrate cerebrospinal fluid poorly and therefore cannot be used in cases of central nervous system involvement. Twenty to 25 per cent of the patients initially cured of the disease have a relapse. Patients who also have AIDS rarely are cured of the cryptococcal infection, and the goal of treatment in these patients is suppression of disease.[79]

Candidiasis

There are 10 species of *Candida* that are regarded as pathogens for humans. *Candida* organisms are small, thin-walled yeast cells that reproduce by budding. The organisms are normal commensals of humans and are found throughout the gastrointestinal tract, in sputum, in the female genital tract, on diseased skin, and in the urine of patients with indwelling catheters. Human-to-human transmission is possible, but most infections are endogenous.[86]

For *Candida* organisms to become pathogenic, the host must be immunocompromised. *Candida* may gain access to the vascular system of susceptible patients via intravenous lines or monitoring devices and the implantation of prosthetic materials. Intravenous drug abusers also are at risk.[86, 110, 244]

The initial cellular reaction is by polymorphonuclear leukocytes. Chronic inflammatory cells appear early, causing a granulomatous response. In severely immunocompromised patients, the reaction may be minimal.[86]

Spinal involvement (Fig. 39–21) is rare, with only 14 cases reported in the literature as of 1987. Most of these patients had complex multisystem medical problems, and the disease occurred after prolonged hospitalization.[110]

The treatment of choice is amphotericin B; a total dose of 1 to 1.2 g may be adequate, given over a period of weeks. Flucytosine and ketoconazole are alternative agents in selected patients but comparative studies with amphotericin B have not been done.[110] Patients

who have persistent back pain should undergo another biopsy to confirm resolution of the disease.

Aspergillosis

Aspergillus is a mold found throughout the world. The organism is pathogenic only in immunocompromised hosts.[24, 39, 98] The one report of aspergillosis occurring in a previously healthy young man without immunocompromise is an enigma.[214] Infection occurs by inhalation of small spores (conidia). Vascular invasion is common in immunosuppressed patients, and leads to necrosis of tissues with abundant hyphae from proliferation of the organism. In patients with chronic granulomatous disease, vascular invasion is uncommon and hyphae are sparse.[24]

Osseous involvement may occur by direct extension from the lung or by hematogenous spread.[24, 98] It also has been reported as a complication after lumbar discectomy.[24] Spine involvement is uncommon, with only 12 cases in the literature by 1988.[157]

The radiographic findings are similar to those in tuberculosis of the spine. Disc space narrowing,

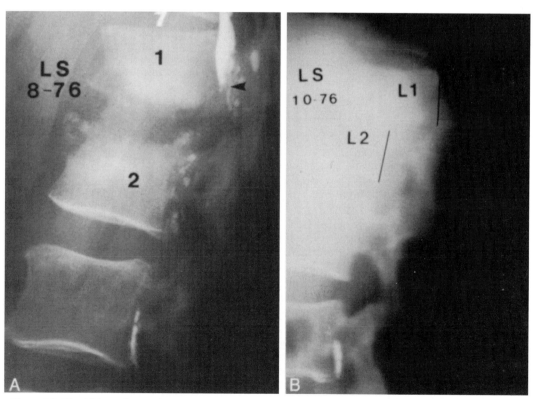

Figure 39–21. This patient, who had been chronically ill, developed a *Candida* disc space infection at the L1–L2 interspace. *A,* This lateral radiograph reveals erosion of the end plates at the inferior portion of L1 and superior portion of 12 vertebral bodies, which is consistent with a standard disc space infection and adjacent vertebral osteomyelitis. This cannot be differentiated from a standard pyogenic disc space infection. *B,* The patient was inappropriately treated with a wide laminectomy posteriorly and subsequently developed retrolisthesis of L1 on L2. The paraparesis never improved, and he subsequently died of a gastrointestinal hemorrhage while still under treatment for this spinal condition. (From Eismont, F.J., Bohlman, H.H., Soni, P.L., et al.: Pyogenic and fungal vertebral osteomyelitis with paralysis. J Bone Joint Surg *65A:*19–29, 1983.)

involvement of adjacent vertebrae, and the presence of paraspinal abscesses are characteristic.[124] Dense new bone formation with small lytic lesions without sequestration may be seen.[98]

Clinically, sinus tract formation is characteristic. The incidence of epidural abscess formation in association with neurologic deficits is quite high.[98]

The diagnosis is made by microscopic examination of tissue and by culture. *Aspergillus* may be isolated in culture due to contamination or colonization, so the culture results must be correlated with the clinical situation.

The drug of choice for the treatment of aspergillosis is amphotericin B, although the response may be poor in markedly immunosuppressed patients.[24] Itraconazole has been effective in some of the more indolent cases of aspergillosis.[24, 78]

The prognosis of patients with *Aspergillus* spondylitis is guarded. Surgery has been used in the past in almost all cases. In 10 cases in adults reported in the literature, all were treated by posterior decompression and antifungal therapy; four recovered and two died. The four patients with epidural abscess and paraplegia did not improve, and one died. Of five children with aspergillosis but without paraplegia, four died.[98] There have been several reports of successful treatment with antifungal agents alone, without surgery.[98, 157] If surgery is thought to be indicated, the principles of treatment outlined for tuberculosis should be followed.[39, 240] Posterior segmental instrumentation and fusion may be necessary in some cases of spinal instability.[39]

SYPHILITIC DISORDERS OF THE SPINE

The spirochete *Treponema pallidum*, the organism responsible for syphilis, causes two types of spine lesions. Charcot's spine is the most common lesion and tends to occur in the thoracolumbar or lumbar spine.[124, 165] It may be detected coincidentally or may produce low back pain or root involvement if destruction and hypertrophic changes are severe. The pathophysiology of the lesion is a manifestation of posterior column involvement of the spinal cord, and not a primary lesion of the bone itself. It is related to defective protective sensation. The treatment should be bracing to limit excessive movement and to prevent further injury. The role of fusion is undetermined.

Infection of the spine causes gummatous lesions, syphilitic granulomas representing the local reaction of the tissues to the organism and its products. Gummata are rare, destructive, and usually symptomatic, causing collapse and neurologic deficits. Syphilis is the "great imitator" and must be differentiated from a host of other disorders, including tuberculosis of the spine. It is difficult to distinguish the clinical features of spinal gumma from coincident neuropathy that is frequently present, and biopsy is necessary for the diagnosis.[165]

The treatment of choice for syphilis is penicillin. Effective alternative agents are tetracycline, chloramphenicol, ceftriaxone, and other cephalosporins.[311]

References

1. Abram, S.R., Tedeschi, A.A., Partain, C.L., et al.: Differential diagnosis of severe back pain using MRI. South Med J 81:1487–1492, 1988.
2. Adams, Z.B.: Tuberculosis of the spine in children: A review of sixty-three cases from the Lakeville State Sanatorium. J Bone Joint Surg 22:860–861, 1940.
3. Adapon, B.D., Legada, B.D., Lim, E.V.A., et al.: CT guided closed biopsy of the spine. J Comput Assist Tomogr 5:73–78, 1981.
4. Adendorff, J.J., Boeke, E.J., and Lazarus, C.: Pott's paraplegia. S Afr Med J 71:427–428, 1987.
5. Adendorff, J.J., Boeke, E.J., and Lazarus, C.: Tuberculosis of the spine: Results of management of 300 patients. J R Coll Surg Edinb 32:152–155, 1987.
6. Al-Shahed, M.S., Sharif, H.S., Haddad, M.C., et al.: Imaging features of musculoskeletal brucellosis. Radiographics 14:333–348, 1994.
7. Albee, F.H.: Transplantation of a portion of the tibia into the spine for Pott's disease: A preliminary report. JAMA 57:885–886, 1911.
8. Allen, A.R., and Stevenson, A.W.: Follow-up notes on articles previously published in the Journal: A ten-year follow-up of combined drug therapy and early fusion in bone tuberculosis. J Bone Joint Surg 49A:1001–1003, 1967.
9. Allen, A.R., and Stevenson, A.W.: The results of combined drug therapy and early fusion in bone tuberculosis. J Bone Joint Surg 39A:32–42, 1957.
10. Ambrose, G.B., Alpert, M., and Neer, C.S.: Vertebral osteomyelitis. A diagnostic problem. JAMA 197:101–104, 1966.
11. Angtuaco, E.J., McConnell, J.R., Chadduck, W.M., et al.: MR imaging of spinal epidural sepsis. Am J Radiol 149:1249–1253, 1987.
12. Arct, W.: Operative treatment of tuberculosis of the spine in old people. J Bone Joint Surg 50A:255–267, 1968.
13. Ariza, J., Gudiol, F., Pallares, R., et al.: Treatment of human brucellosis with Doxycycline plus rifampin or Doxycycline plus Streptomycin. Ann Intern Med 117:25–30, 1992.
14. Armstrong, P., Green, G., and Irving, J.D.: Needle-aspiration/biopsy of the spine in suspected disc space infection. Br J Radiol 51:333–337, 1978.
15. Arnott, G., and Delfosse, J.M.: Acute spinal epidural abscess. J Neurol 213:343–344, 1985.
16. Awad, I., Bax, J.W., and Petersen, J.M.: Nocardial osteomyelitis of the spine with epidural spine cord compression: A case report. Neurosurgery 15:254–256, 1984.
17. Azzam, N.I., and Tammawy, M.: Tuberculosis spondylitis in adults: Diagnosis and treatment. Br J Neurosurg 2:85–91, 1988.
18. Babhulkar, S.S., Tayade, W.B., and Babhulkar, S.K.: Atypical spinal tuberculosis. J Bone Joint Surg 66B:239–242, 1984.
19. Bailey, H.L., Gabriel, S.M., Hodgson, A.R., et al.: Tuberculosis of the spine in children: Operative findings and results in one hundred consecutive patients treated by removal of the lesion and anterior grafting. J Bone Joint Surg 54A:1633–1657, 1972.
20. Baker, A.S., Ojemann, R.G., Swartz, M.N., et al.: Spinal epidural abscess. N Engl J Med 293:463–468, 1975.
21. Baker, C.J.: Primary spinal epidural abscess. Am J Dis Child 121:337–339, 1971.
22. Barclay, W.R., Ebert, R.H., LeRoy, G.V., et al.: Distribution and excretion of radioactive isoniazid in tuberculosis patients. JAMA 151:1384–1388, 1953.
23. Batson, O.V.: The function of the vertebral veins and their role in the spread of metastasis. Ann Surg 112:138–149, 1940.
24. Bennett, J.E.: Aspergillus species. In Mandell, G.L., Bennett, J.E., and Dolin, R. (eds.): Principles and Practice of Infectious Diseases. New York, Churchill Livingstone, 1995, pp 2306–2311.
25. Bergman, I., Wald, E.R., Meyer, J.D., et al.: Epidural abscess and vertebral osteomyelitis following serial lumbar punctures. Pediatrics 72:476–480, 1983.
26. Berk, R.H., Yazici, M., Atabey, N., et al.: Detection of mycobacterium tuberculosis in formaldehyde solution-fixed, paraffin-embedded tissue by polymerase chain reaction in Pott's disease. Spine 21:1991–1995, 1996.
27. Bertino, R.E., Porter, B.A., Stimac, G.K., et al.: Imaging spinal

osteomyelitis and epidural abscess with short T1 inversion recovery (STIR). AJNR *9*:563–564, 1988.

28. Blacklock, J.W.S.: Injury as an aetiological factor in tuberculosis: President's address. Proc R Soc Med *50*:61–68, 1957.

29. Bloom, R., Yeager, H., and Garagusi, V.F.: Pleuropulmonary complications of thoracic vertebral osteomyelitis. Thorax *35*:156–157, 1980.

30. Bohlman, H.H., and Eismont, F.J.: Surgical techniques of anterior decompression and fusion for spinal cord disorders. Clin Orthop *154*:57–67, 1981.

31. Bohlman, H.H., Freehafer, A., and Dejak, J.: The results of treatment of acute injuries of the upper thoracic spine with paralysis. J Bone Joint Surg *67A*:360–369, 1985.

32. Bonfiglio, M., Lange, T.A., and Kim, Y.M.: Pyogenic vertebral osteomyelitis: Disc space infections. Clin Orthop *96*:234–247, 1973.

33. Bosworth, D.M., Pietra, A.D., and Farrell, R.F.: Streptomycin in tuberculous bone and joint lesions with mixed infection and sinuses. J Bone Joint Surg *32A*:103–108, 1950.

34. Bosworth, D.M., Pietra, A.D., and Rahilly, G.: Paraplegia resulting from tuberculosis of the spine. J Bone Joint Surg *35A*:735–740, 1953.

35. Bosworth, D.M., Wright, H.A., and Fielding, J.W.: The treatment of bone and joint tuberculosis: Effect of 1-isonicotinyl-2-isopropylhydrazine. J Bone Joint Surg *34A*:761–771, 1952.

36. Bouchez, B., Arnott, G., and Delfosse, J.M.: Acute spinal epidural abscess. J Neurol *231*:343–344, 1985.

37. Bradford, D.S., and Daher, Y.H.: Vascularized rib grafts and stabilization of kyphosis. J Bone Joint Surg *68B*:357–361, 1986.

38. Brant-Zawadrzki, M., Burke, V.D., and Jeffery, R.B.: CT in the evaluation of spine infection. Spine *8*:358–364, 1983.

39. Bridwell, K.H., Campbell, J.W., and Barenkamp, S.J.: Surgical treatment of hematogenous vertebral Aspergillus osteomyelitis. Spine *15*:281–285, 1990.

40. Browder, J., and Meyers, R.: Infection of the spinal epidural space. An aspect of vertebral osteomyelitis. Am J Surg *37*:4–26, 1937.

41. Browder, J., and Meyers, R.: Pyogenic infections of the spinal epidural space: A consideration of the anatomic and physiologic pathology. Surgery *10*:296–308, 1941.

42. Brown, M.D., Hauser, M.F., Aznarez, A., et al.: Indium-111 leukocyte imaging: The skeletal photopenic lesions. Clin Nucl Med *11*:611–613, 1986.

43. Brown, M.D., and Tsaltas, T.T.: Studies on the permeability of the intervertebral disc during skeletal maturation. Spine *1*:240–244, 1976.

44. Bruns, J., and Maas, R.: Advantages of diagnosing bacterial spondylitis with magnetic resonance imaging. Arch Orthop Trauma Surg *108*:30–35, 1989.

45. Bruschwein, D.A., Brown, M.L., and McLeod, R.A.: Gallium scintigraphy in the evaluation of the disc space infections: Concise communication. J Nucl Med *21*:925–927, 1980.

46. Butler, E.G., Dohrmann, P.J., and Stark, R.J.: Spinal subdural abscess. Clin Exp Neurol *25*:67–70, 1988.

47. Campbell, D.R., Eismont, F.J., Garvey, T., et al.: Diagnosis and treatment of fungal infections of the spine: Report of eleven patients. Submitted for publication, 1998.

48. Capener, N.: The evolution of lateral rhachiotomy. J Bone Joint Surg *36B*:173–179, 1954.

49. Cardan, E., and Nanulescu, M.: Epidural lavage for extensive epidural suppuration. Anaesthesia *42*:1023, 1987.

50. Carragee, E.J.: The clinical use of magnetic resonance imaging in pyogenic vertebral osteomyelitis. Spine *22*:780–785, 1997.

51. Carragee, E.J.: Pyogenic vertebral osteomyelitis. J Bone Joint Surg *79A*:874–880, 1997.

52. Carvell, J.E., and Maclarnon, J.C.: Chronic osteomyelitis of the thoracic spine due to *Salmonella typhi*: A case report. Spine *6*:527–530, 1981.

53. Chan, S.-T., and Leung, S.: Spinal epidural abscess following steroid injection for sciatica: Case report. Spine *14*:106–108, 1989.

54. Chapman, S.W.: Blastomyces dermatitidis. *In* Mandell, G.L., Bennett, J.E., and Dolin, R. (eds.): Principles and Practice of Infectious Diseases. New York, Churchill Livingstone, 1995, pp. 2353–2365.

55. Charles, R.W., Mody, G.M., and Govender, S.: Pyogenic infection of the lumbar vertebral spine due to gas-forming organisms: A case report. Spine *14*:541–543, 1989.

56. Cleveland, M.: Tuberculosis of the spine. A clinical study of 203 patients from Sea View and St. Luke's Hospital. Am Rev Tuberculosis *41*:215–321, 1940.

57. Cohn, S.L., Akbarnia, B.A., Luisiri, A., et al.: Disk space infection versus lumbar Scheuermann's disease. Orthopedics *11*:330–335, 1988.

58. Collert, S.: Osteomyelitis of the spine. Acta Orthop Scand *48*:283–290, 1977.

59. Colmenero, J.D., Cisneros, J.M., Orjuela, D.L., et al.: Clinical course and prognosis of brucella spondylitis. Infection *20*:42–46, 1992.

60. Compere, E.L., and Garrison, M.: Correlation of pathologic and roentgenologic findings in tuberculosis and pyogenic infections of the vertebra: The fate of the intervertebral disk. Ann Surg *104*:1038–1067, 1936.

61. Cooppan, R., Schoenbaum, S., Younger, M.D., et al.: Vertebral osteomyelitis in insulin-dependent diabetics. S Afr Med J *50*:1993–1996, 1976.

62. Corboy, J.R., and Price, R.W.: Myelitis and toxic, inflammatory, and infectious disorders. Curr Opin Neurol Neurosurg *6*:56, 1993.

63. Corea, J.R., and Tamimi, T.M.: Tuberculosis of the arch of the atlas: A case report. Spine *12*:608–611, 1987.

64. Corradini, E.W., Turney, M.F., and Browder, E.J.: Spinal epidural infection. NY State J Med *48*:2367–2370, 1948.

65. Coventry, M.B., Ghormley, R.K., and Kernohan, J.W.: The intervertebral disc: Its microscopic anatomy and pathology. Part I: Anatomy, development, and physiology. J Bone Joint Surg *27*:105–112, 1945.

66. Craig, F.: Vertebral body biopsy. J Bone Joint Surg *38A*:93–102, 1956.

67. Crock, H.V., and Goldwasser, M.: Anatomic studies of the circulation in the region of the vertebral end-plate in adult greyhound dogs. Spine *9*:702–706, 1984.

68. Curling, O.D., Gower, D.J., and McWhorter, J.M.: Changing concepts in spinal epidural abscess: A report of 29 cases. Neurosurgery *27*:185, 1990.

69. Currier, B.L., Banovak, K., and Eismont, F.J.: Gentamicin penetration into normal rabbit nucleus pulposus. Spine *19*:2614–2618, 1994.

70. Dagirmanjian, A., Schils, J., McHenry, M., et al.: Vertebral osteomyelitis revisited. Am J Roentgenol *167*:1539–1543, 1996.

71. Dagirmanjian, A., Schils, J., McHenry, M., et al.: Spinal osteomyelitis. Sem Spine Surg *9*:38–50, 1997.

72. Dalinka, M.K., Dinnenberg, S., Greendyke, W.H., et al.: Roentgenographic features of osseous coccidioidomycosis and differential diagnosis. J Bone Joint Surg *53A*:1157–1164, 1971.

73. Daly, R.C., Fitzgerald, R.H., and Washington, J.A.: Penetration of cefazolin into normal and osteomyelitic canine cortical bone. Antimicrob Agents Chemother *22*:461–469, 1982.

74. Dandy, W.E.: Abscesses and inflammatory tumors in the spinal epidural space (so-called pachymeningitis externa). Arch Surg *13*:477–494, 1926.

75. Daniel, T.M.: The rapid diagnosis of tuberculosis: A selective review. J Lab Clin Med *116*:277–282, 1990.

76. Danner, R.L., and Hartman, B.J.: Update of spinal epidural abscess: 35 cases and review of the literature. Rev Infect Dis *9*:265–274, 1987.

77. de Villiers, J.C., and de Clüver, P.F.: Spinal epidural abscess in children. S Afr J Surg *16*:149–155, 1978.

78. Denning, D.W., and Stevens, D.A.: Antifungal and surgical treatment of invasive Aspergillosis in review of 2,121 published cases. Rev Infect Dis *12*:1147–1201, 1990.

79. Diamond, R.D.: Cryptococcus neoformans. *In* Mandell, G.L., Bennett, J.E., and Dolin, R., eds. Principles and Practice of Infectious Diseases. New York: Churchill Livingstone, 1995, pp. 2331–2340.

80. Dickson, J.A.S.: Spinal tuberculosis in Nigerian children: A review of ambulant treatment. J Bone Joint Surg *49B*:682–694, 1967.

81. Digby, J.M., and Kersley, J.B.: Pyogenic nontuberculous spinal

infection: An analysis of thirty cases. J Bone Joint Surg 61B:47–55, 1979.

82. Dobson, J.: Tuberculosis of the spine. An analysis of the results of conservative treatment and of the factors influencing the prognosis. J Bone Joint Surg 33B:517–531, 1951.

83. Doub, H.P., and Badgley, C.E.: The roentgen signs of tuberculosis of the vertebral body. Am J Radiol 27:827–837, 1932.

84. Dripps, R.D., and Vandam, L.D.: Hazards of lumbar puncture. J Am Med Assoc 147:1118–1121, 1951.

85. Dux, S., Halevi, J., Pitlik, S., et al.: Early diagnosis of infective spondylitis with gallium-67. Isr J Med Sci 17:451–452, 1981.

86. Edwards, J.E.: Candida species. In Mandell, G.L., Bennett, J.E., and Dolin, R. (eds.): Principles and Practice of Infectious Diseases. New York, Churchill Livingstone, 1995, pp. 2289–2306.

87. Eismont, F.J., Bohlman, H.H., Soni, P.L., et al.: Pyogenic and fungal vertebral osteomyelitis with paralysis. J Bone Joint Surg 65A:19–29, 1983.

88. Eismont, F.J., Bohlman, H.H., Soni, P.L., et al.: Vertebral osteomyelitis in infants. J Bone Joint Surg 64B:32–35, 1982.

89. Eismont, F.J., Wiesel, S.W., Brighton, C.T., et al.: Antibiotic penetration into rabbit nucleus pulposus. Spine 12:254–256, 1987.

90. Eismont, R.J., Green, B.A., Brown, M.D., et al.: Coexistent infection and tumor of the spine: A report of three cases. J Bone Joint Surg 69A:452–458, 1987.

91. El-Gindi, S., Aref, S., Salama, M., et al.: Infection of intervertebral discs after operation. J Bone Joint Surg 58B:114–116, 1976.

92. Emery, S.E., Chan, D.P.K., and Woodward, H.R.: Treatment of hematogenous pyogenic vertebral osteomyelitis with anterior debridement and primary bone grafting. Spine 14:284–291, 1989.

93. Enneking, W.F., Burchardt, H., Puhl, J.J., et al.: Physical and biological aspects of repair in dog cortical-bone transplants. J Bone Joint Surg 57A:237–252, 1975.

94. Erntell, M., Holtas, S., Norlin, K., et al.: Magnetic resonance imaging in the diagnosis of spinal epidural abscess. Scand J Infect Dis 20:323–327, 1988.

95. Feldenzer, J.A., McKeever, P.E., Schaberg, D.R., et al.: The pathogenesis of spinal epidural abscess: Microangiographic studies in an experimental model. J Neurosurg 69:110–114, 1988.

96. Felländer, M.: Paraplegia in spondylitis: Results of operative treatment. Paraplegia 13:75–88, 1975.

97. Fernandez-Ulloa, M., Vasavada, P.J., Hanslits, M.L., et al.: Diagnosis of vertebral osteomyelitis: Clinical, radiological and scintigraphic features. Orthopedics 8:1144–1150, 1985.

98. Ferris, B., and Jones, C.: Paraplegia due to aspergillosis: Successful conservative treatment of two cases. J Bone Joint Surg 67B:800–803, 1985.

99. Fischer, E.G., Greene, C.S., and Winston, K.R.: Spinal epidural abscess in children. Neurosurgery 9:257–260, 1981.

100. Forlenza, S.W., Axelrod, J.L., and Grieco, M.H.: Pott's disease in heroin addicts. J Am Med Assoc 241:379–380, 1979.

101. Forsythe, M., and Rothman, R.H.: New concepts in the diagnosis and treatment of infections of the cervical spine. Orthop Clin N Am 9:1039–1051, 1978.

102. Fountain, S.S.: A single stage combined surgical approach for vertebral resections. J Bone Joint Surg 61A:1011–1017, 1979.

103. Fountain, S.S., Hsu, L.C.S., Yau, A.C.M.C., et al.: Progressive kyphosis following solid anterior spine fusion in children with tuberculosis of the spine: A long term study. J Bone Joint Surg 57A:1104–1107, 1975.

104. Fraser, R.A.R., Ratzan, K., Wolpert, S.M., et al.: Spinal subdural empyema. Arch Neurol 28:235–238, 1973.

105. Fraser, R.D., Osti, O.L., and Vernon Roberts, B.: Iatrogenic discitis: The role of intravenous antibiotics in prevention and treatment. An experimental model. Spine 14:1025–1032, 1989.

106. Frederickson, B., Yuan, H., and Orlans, R.: Management and outcome of pyogenic vertebral osteomyelitis. Clin Orthop 131:160–167, 1978.

107. Freilich, D., and Swash, M.: Diagnosis and management of tuberculous paraplegia with special reference to tuberculous radiculomyelitis. J Neurol Neurosurg Psychiatry 42:12–18, 1979.

108. Friedman, B.: Chemotherapy of tuberculosis of the spine. J Bone Joint Surg 48A:451–474, 1966.

109. Friedman, B., and Kapur, V.N.: Newer knowledge of chemotherapy in the treatment of tuberculosis of bones and joints. Clin Orthop 97:5–15, 1973.

110. Friedman, B.C., and Simon, G.L.: Candida vertebral osteomyelitis: Report of three cases and a review of the literature. Diagn Microbiol Infect Dis 8:31–36, 1987.

111. Ganado, W., and Craig, A.J.: Brucellosis myelopathy. J Bone Joint Surg 40A:1380–1388, 1958.

112. Garceau, G.J., and Brady, T.A.: Pott's paraplegia. J Bone Joint Surg 32A:87–95, 1950.

113. Garcia, A., and Grantham, S.A.: Hematogenous pyogenic vertebral osteomyelitis. J Bone Joint Surg 42A:429–436, 1960.

114. Gardner, R.D., Cammisa, F.P., Eismont, F.J., et al.: Nongranulomatous spinal epidural abscesses. Orthop Trans 13:562–563, 1989.

115. Garrido, E., and Rosenwasser, R.H.: Experience with the suction-irrigation technique in the management of spinal epidural infection. Neurosurgery 12:678–679, 1983.

116. Gehweiler, J.A., Capp, M.P., and Chick, E.W.: Observations on the roentgen patterns in blastomycosis of bone: A review of cases from the blastomycosis cooperative study of the Veterans Administration and Duke University Medical Center. Am J Radiol 108:497–510, 1970.

117. Genster, H.G., and Andersen, M.J.F.: Spinal osteomyelitis complicating urinary tract infection. J Urol 107:109–111, 1972.

118. Ghelman, B., Lospinuso, M.F., Levine, D.B., et al.: Percutaneous CT guided biopsy of the thoracic and lumbar spine. Orthop Trans 14:635, 1990.

119. Ghormley, R.K., Bickel, W.H., and Dickson, D.D.: A study of acute infectious lesions of the intervertebral discs. South Med J 33:347–352, 1940.

120. Ghormley, R.K., and Bradley, J.I.: Prognostic signs in the x-rays of tuberculous spines in children. J Bone Joint Surg 10:796–804, 1928.

121. Gibson, M.J., Karpinski, M.R.K., Slack, R.C.B., et al.: The penetration of antibiotics into the normal intervertebral disc. J Bone Joint Surg 69B:784–786, 1987.

122. Gillams, A.R., Chaddha, B., and Carter, A.P.: MR appearances of the temporal evolution and resolution of infectious spondylitis. Am J Roentgenol 166:903–907, 1996.

123. Girdlestone, G.R.: The operative treatment of Pott's paraplegia. Br J Surg 9:121–141, 1931.

124. Goldman, A.B., and Freiberger, R.H.: Localized infectious and neuropathic diseases. Semin Roentgenol 14:19–32, 1979.

125. Golimbu, C., Firooznia, H., and Rafii, M.: CT of osteomyelitis of the spine. Am J Radiol 142:159–163, 1984.

126. Govender, S., Charles, R.W., Naidoo, K.S., et al.: Results of surgical decompression in chronic tuberculous paraplegia. S Afr Med J 74:58–59, 1988.

127. Grant, F.C.: Epidural spinal abscess. J Am Med Asoc 128:509–511, 1945.

128. Graziano, G.P., and Sidhu, K.S.: Salvage reconstruction in acute and late sequelae from pyogenic thoracolumbar infection. J Spinal Disorders 6:199–207, 1993.

129. Griffiths, H.E.D., and Jones, D.M.: Pyogenic infection of the spine: A review of twenty-eight cases. J Bone Joint Surg 53B:383–391, 1971.

130. Guerrero, I.C., and MacGregor, R.R.: Comparative penetration of various cephalosporins into inflammatory exudate. Antimicrob Agents Chemother 15:712–715, 1979.

131. Guerrero, I.C., Slap, G.B., MacGregor, R.R., et al.: Anaerobic spinal epidural abscess: Case report. J Neurosurg 48:465–469, 1978.

132. Guirguis, A.R.: Pott's paraplegia. J Bone Joint Surg 49B:658–667, 1967.

133. Guri, J.P.: Pyogenic osteomyelitis of the spine: Differential diagnosis through clinical and roentgenographic observations. J Bone Joint Surg 28:29–39, 1946.

134. Güven, O., Kumano, K., Yalcin, S., et al.: A single stage posterior approach and rigid fixation for preventing kyphosis in the treatment of spinal tuberculosis. Spine 19:1039–1043, 1994.

135. Haas, D.W., and Des Prez, R.M.: Mycobacterium tuberculosis. In Mandell, G.L., Bennett, J.E., and Dolin, R., eds. Principles and Practice of Infectious Diseases. New York: Churchill Livingstone, 1995, pp. 2213–2243.

136. Haase, D., Martin, R., and Marrie, T.: Radionuclide imaging in pyogenic vertebral osteomyelitis. Clin Nucl Med 5:533–537, 1980.

137. Hakin, R.N., Burt, A.A., and Cook, J.B.: Acute spinal epidural abscess. Paraplegia *17*:330–336, 1979.
138. Hall, W.H., Gerding, D.N., and Schierl, E.A.: Penetration of tobramycin into infected extravascular fluids and its therapeutic effectiveness. J Infect Dis *135*:957–961, 1977.
139. Halpern, A.A., Rinsky, L.A., Fountain, S., et al.: Coccidioidomycosis of the spine: Unusual roentgenographic presentations. Clin Orthop *140*:78–79, 1979.
140. Hancock, D.O.: A study of 49 patients with acute spinal extradural abscess. Paraplegia *10*:285–288, 1973.
141. Hassler, O.: The human intervertebral disc: A microangiographical study on its vascular supply at various ages. Acta Orthop Scand *40*:765–772, 1970.
142. Hatch, E.S.: Acute osteomyelitis of the spine: Report of case with recovery. Review of the literature. N Orleans Med Surg J *83*:861–873, 1931.
143. Henriques, C.Q.: Osteomyelitis as a complication in urology: With special reference to the paravertebral venous plexus. Br J Surg *46*:19–28, 1958.
144. Henson, S.W., and Coventry, M.B.: Osteomyelitis of the vertebrae as a result of infection of the urinary tract. Surg Gynecol Obstet *102*:207–214, 1956.
145. Heusner, A.P.: Nontuberculosis spinal epidural infections. N Engl J Med *239*:845–854, 1948.
146. Hibbs, R.A.: An operation for progressive spinal deformities. N Y State Med J *93*:1013–1016, 1911.
147. Hlavin, M.L., Kaminski, H.J., Ross, J.S., et al.: Spinal epidural abscess: A 10 year prospective. Neurosurgery *27*:177, 1990.
148. Hodgson, A.R.: An approach to the cervical spine (C3–C7). Clin Orthop *39*:129–134, 1965.
149. Hodgson, A.R.: Report of the findings and results in 300 cases of Pott's disease treated by anterior fusion of the spine. J West Pacific Orthop Assoc *1*:3, 1964.
150. Hodgson, A.R., Skinsnes, O.K., and Leong, C.Y.: The pathogenesis of Pott's paraplegia. J Bone Joint Surg *49A*:1147–1156, 1967.
151. Hodgson, A.R., and Stock, F.E.: Anterior spinal fusion: A preliminary communication on the radical treatment of Pott's disease and Pott's paraplegia. Br J Surg *44*:266–275, 1956.
152. Hodgson, A.R., and Stock, F.E.: Anterior spine fusion for the treatment of tuberculosis of the spine: The operative findings and results of treatment in the first one hundred cases. J Bone Joint Surg *42A*:295–310, 1960.
153. Hodgson, A.R., Stock, F.E., Fang, H.S.Y., et al.: Anterior spinal fusion: The operative approach and pathological findings in 412 patients with Pott's disease of the spine. Br J Surg *48*:172–178, 1960.
154. Hodgson, A.R., Yau, A., Kwon, J.S., et al.: A clinical study of one hundred consecutive cases of Pott's paraplegia. Clin Orthop *36*:128–150, 1964.
155. Hodgson, A.R., and Yau, A.C.M.C.: Anterior surgical approaches to the spinal column. Recent Adv Orthop *1*:289–323, 1969.
156. Hoffer, F.A., Strand, R.D., and Gebhardt, M.C.: Percutaneous biopsy of pyogenic infection of the spine in children. J Pediatr Orthop *8*:442–444, 1988.
157. Holmes, P.F., Osterman, D.W., and Tullos, H.S.: *Aspergillus* discitis. Report of two cases and review of the literature. Clin Orthop *226*:240–246, 1988.
158. Holzman, R.S., and Bishko, F.: Osteomyelitis in heroin addicts. Ann Intern Med *75*:693–696, 1971.
159. Hsu, L.C.S., Cheng, C.L., and Leong, J.C.Y.: Pott's paraplegia of late onset: The cause of compression and results after anterior decompression. J Bone Joint Surg *70B*:534–538, 1988.
160. Hsu, L.C.S., and Leong, J.C.Y.: Tuberculosis of the lower cervical spine (C2 to C7): A report on 40 cases. J Bone Joint Surg *66B*:1–5, 1984.
161. Hulme, A., and Dott, N.M.: Spinal epidural abscess. Br Med J *1*:164–168, 1954.
162. Incavo, S.J., Muller, D.L., Krag, M.H., et al.: Vertebral osteomyelitis caused by *Clostridium difficile*: A case report and review of the literature. Spine *13*:111–113, 1988.
163. Ito, H., Tsuchiya, J., and Asami, G.: A new radical operation for Pott's disease: A report of ten cases. J Bone Joint Surg *16*:499–515, 1934.
164. Jabbari, B., and Pierce, J.F.: Spinal cord compression due to pseudomonas in heroin addict. Case report. Neurology *27*:1034–1037, 1977.
165. Johns, D.: Syphylitic disorders of the spine: Report of two cases. J Bone Joint Surg *52B*:724–731, 1970.
166. Johnson, R.W., Hillman, J.W., and Southwick, W.O.: The importance of direct surgical attack upon lesions of the vertebral bodies, particularly in Pott's disease. J Bone Joint Surg *35A*:17–25, 1953.
167. Kalen, V., Isono, S.S., Cho, C.S., et al.: Charcot arthroplasty of the spine in long-standing paraplegia. Spine *12*:42–47, 1987.
168. Kaplan, C.J.: Conservative therapy in skeletal tuberculosis: An appraisal based on experience in South Africa. Tubercle *40*:355–368, 1959.
169. Kaplan, C.J.: Pott's disease in South African Bantu children. An analysis of results and comparison with Lancashire figures. Br J Tuberculosis *46*:209–213, 1952.
170. Kattapuram, S.V., Phillips, W.C., and Boyd, R.: CT in pyogenic osteomyelitis of the spine. Am J Radiol *140*:1199–1201, 1983.
171. Kaufman, D.M., Kaplan, J.G., and Litman, N.: Infectious agents in spinal epidural abscesses. Neurology *30*:844–850, 1980.
172. Keenan, J.D., and Metz, C.W.: Brucella spondylitis: A brief review and case report. Clin Orthop *82*:87–91, 1972.
173. Kemp, H.B.S., Jackson, J.W., Jeremiah, J.D., et al.: Anterior fusion of the spine for infective lesions in adults. J Bone Joint Surg *55B*:715–734, 1973.
174. Kemp, H.B.S., Jackson, J.W., Jeremiah, J.D., et al.: Pyogenic infections occurring primarily in intervertebral discs. J Bone Joint Surg *55B*:698–714, 1973.
175. Kemp, H.B.S., Jackson, J.W., and Shaw, N.C.: Laminectomy in paraplegia due to infective spondylosis. Br J Surg *61*:66–72, 1974.
176. Kern, R.Z., and Houpt, J.B.: Pyogenic vertebral osteomyelitis: Diagnosis and management. Can Med Assoc J *130*:1025–1028, 1984.
177. Kersley, J.B.: Nontuberculous infection of the spine. Proc R Soc Med *70*:176–181, 1977.
178. Kim, N.H., Lee, H.M., and Suh, J.S.: Magnetic resonance imaging for the diagnosis of tuberculous spondylitis. Spine *19*:2451–2455, 1994.
179. King, D.M., and Mayo, K.M.: Infective lesions of the vertebral column. Clin Orthop *96*:248–253, 1973.
180. Kirzner, H., Oh, Y.K., and Lee, S.H.: Intraspinal air: A CT finding of epidural abscess. Am J Radiol *151*:1217–1218, 1988.
181. Kohli, S.B.: Radical surgical approach to spinal tuberculosis. J Bone Joint Surg *49B*:668–673, 1967.
182. Kondo, E., and Yamada, K.: End results of focal debridement in bone and joint tuberculosis and its indications. J Bone Joint Surg *39A*:27–31, 1957.
183. Konstam, P.G., and Blesovsky, A.: The ambulant treatment of spinal tuberculosis. Br J Surg *50*:26–38, 1962.
184. Konstam, P.G., and Konstam, S.T.: Spinal tuberculosis in southern Nigeria: With special reference to ambulant treatment of thoraco-lumbar disease. J Bone Joint Surg *40B*:26–32, 1958.
185. Koppel, B.S., Tuchman, A.J., Mangiardi, J.R., et al.: Epidural spinal infection in intravenous drug abusers. Arch Neurol *45*:1331–1337, 1988.
186. Kirkaldy-Willis, W.H., and Thomas, T.G.: Anterior approaches in the diagnosis and treatment of infections of the vertebral bodies. J Bone Joint Surg *47A*:87–110, 1965.
187. Küker, W., Mull, M., Mayfrank, L., et al.: Epidural spinal infection. Variability of clinical and magnetic resonance imaging findings. Spine *22*:544–551, 1997.
188. Kulowski, J.: Pyogenic osteomyelitis of the spine. An analysis and discussion of 102 cases. J Bone Joint Surg *18*:343–364, 1936.
189. Kumar, K.: A clinical study and classification of posterior spinal tuberculosis. Int Orthop *9*:147–152, 1985.
190. Kurtzman, R.S.: Complications of narcotic addiction. Radiology *96*:23–30, 1970.
191. Lannelongue, O.: On Acute Osteomyelitis, Miscellaneous, Pathological, and Practice Medicine Tracts. Paris, 1897.
192. Lardé, D., Mathieu, D., Frija, J., et al.: Vertebral osteomyelitis: Disk hypodensity on CT. Am J Radiol *139*:963–967, 1982.
193. Lee, E.Y., and Hahn, M.S.: A study of influences of the anterior

intervertebral fusion upon the correct ability of kyphosis in tuberculous spondylitis. J Korena Orthop Assoc 3:31–40, 1968.

194. Lerner, P.I.: Nocardia species. *In* Mandell, G.L., Bennett, J.E., and Dolin, R. (eds.): Principles and Practice of Infectious Diseases. New York: Churchill Livingstone, 1995, pp. 2273–2280.

195. Levy, M.L., Wieder, B.H., Schneider, J., et al.: Subdural empyema of the cervical spine: Clinical pathologic correlates and magnetic resonance imaging. J Neurosurg 79:929, 1993.

196. Lewis, R., Gorbach, S., and Altner, P.: Spinal pseudomonas chondro-osteomyelitis in heroin users. N Engl J Med 286:1303, 1972.

197. Leys, D., Lesoin, F., Viaud, C., et al.: Decreased morbidity from acute bacterial spinal epidural abscesses using computed tomography and nonsurgical treatment in selected patients. Ann Neurol 17:350–355, 1985.

198. Lifeso, R.M., Harder, E., and McCorkell, S.J.: Spinal brucellosis. J Bone Joint Surg 67B:345–351, 1985.

199. Lifeso, R.M., Weaver, P., and Harder, E.H.: Tuberculous spondylitis in adults. J Bone Joint Surg 67A:1405–1413, 1985.

200. Lindholm, T.S., and Pylkkänen, P.: Discitis following removal of intervertebral disc. Spine 7:618–622, 1982.

201. Louw, J.A.: Spinal tuberculosis with neurologic deficit. Treatment with vascularized rib grafts, posterior osteotomies and fusion. J Bone Joint Surg 72B:686–693, 1990.

202. Lownie, S.P., and Ferguson, G.G.: Spinal epidural empyema complicating cervical discography. Spine 14:1415–1417, 1989.

203. Mader, J.T., Cantrell, J.S., and Calhoun, J.: Oral ciprofloxacin compared with standard parenteral antibiotic therapy for chronic osteomyelitis in adults. J Bone Joint Surg 72A:104–110, 1990.

204. Malik, G.M., Crawford, A.H., and Halter, R.: Swan-neck deformity secondary to osteomyelitis of the posterior elements of the cervical spine: Case report. Neurosurgery 50:388–390, 1979.

205. Mampalam, T.J., Rosegay, H., Andrews, B.T., et al.: Nonoperative treatment of spinal epidural infections. J Neurosurg 71:208–210, 1989.

206. Martin, N.S.: Pott's paraplegia: A report of 120 cases. J Bone Joint Surg 53B:596–608, 1971.

207. Martin, N.S.: Tuberculosis of the spine: A study of the results of treatment during the last twenty-five years. J Bone Joint Surg 52B:613–628, 1970.

208. Mathuriya, S.N., Khosla, V.K., and Banerjee, A.K.: Intradural extramedullary tuberculous spinal granulomas. Clin Neurol Neurosurg 90:155–158, 1988.

209. McCain, G.A., Harth, M., Bell, D.A., et al.: Septic discitis. J Rheumatol 8:100–109, 1981.

210. McGahan, J.P., Graves, D.S., and Palmer, P.E.S.: Coccidioidal spondylitis: Usual and unusual radiographic manifestations. Radiology 136:5–9, 1980.

211. McGee-Collett, M., and Johnston, I.H.: Spinal epidural abscess: Presentation and treatment. Med J Australia 155:14, 1991.

212. McGuire, R.A., and Eismont, F.J.: The fate of autogenous bone graft in surgically treated pyogenic vertebral osteomyelitis. J Spinal Disorders 7:206–215, 1994.

213. McHenry, M.C., Duchesneau, P.M., Keys, T.F., et al.: Vertebral osteomyelitis presenting as spinal compression fracture: Six patients with underlying osteoporosis. Arch Intern Med 148:417–423, 1988.

214. McKee, D.F., Barr, W.M., Bryan, C.S., et al.: Primary aspergillosis of the spine mimicking Pott's paraplegia. J Bone Joint Surg 66A:1481–1483, 1984.

215. Medical Research Council Working Party on Tuberculosis of the Spine: A 10 year assessment of a controlled trial comparing debridement and anterior spinal fusion in the management of tuberculosis of the spine in patients on standard chemotherapy in Hong Kong. J Bone Joint Surg 64B:393–398, 1982.

216. Medical Research Council Working Party on Tuberculosis of the Spine: A 10 year assessment of controlled trials of inpatient and outpatient treatment and of plaster of Paris jackets for tuberculosis of the spine in children on standard chemotherapy: Studies in Masan and Pusan, Korea. J Bone Joint Surg 67B:103–110, 1985.

217. Medical Research Council Working Party on Tuberculosis of the Spine: A comparison of 6 or 9 month course regime of chemotherapy in patients receiving ambulatory treatment or undergoing radical surgery for tuberculosis of the spine. Indian J Tuberculosis (Suppl) 36:1–21, 1989.

218. Medical Research Council Working Party on Tuberculosis of the Spine: A controlled trial of ambulant out-patient treatment and in-patient rest in bed in the management of tuberculosis of the spine in young Korean patients on standard chemotherapy. A study in Masan, Korea. J Bone Joint Surg 55B:678–697, 1973.

219. Medical Research Council Working Party on Tuberculosis of the Spine: A controlled trial of anterior spinal fusion and debridement in the surgical management of tuberculosis of the spine in patients on standard chemotherapy: A study in Hong Kong. Br J Surg 61:853–866, 1974.

220. Medical Research Council Working Party on Tuberculosis of the Spine: A controlled trial of anterior spinal fusion and debridement in the surgical management of tuberculosis of the spine in patients on standard chemotherapy: A study in two centers in South Africa. Tubercle 59:79–105, 1978.

221. Medical Research Council Working Party on Tuberculosis of the Spine: A controlled trial of debridement and ambulatory treatment in the management of tuberculosis of the spine in patients on standard chemotherapy. A study in Bulawayo, Rhodesia. J Trop Med Hyg 77:72–92, 1974.

222. Medical Research Council Working Party on Tuberculosis of the Spine: A controlled trial of plaster of Paris jackets in the management of ambulant outpatient treatment of tuberculosis of the spine in children on standard chemotherapy: A study in Pusan, Korea. Tubercle 54:261–282, 1973.

223. Medical Research Council Working Party on Tuberculosis of the Spine: A controlled trial of six month and nine month regimens of chemotherapy in patients undergoing radical surgery for tuberculosis of the spine in Hong Kong. Tubercle 67:243–259, 1986.

224. Medical Research Council Working Party on Tuberculosis of the Spine: A five year assessment of controlled trials in in-patient and out-patient treatment and of plaster of Paris jackets for tuberculosis of the spine in children on standard chemotherapy: Studies in Masan and Pusan, Korea. J Bone Joint Surg 58B:399–411, 1976.

225. Medical Research Council Working Party on Tuberculosis of the Spine: Five year assessments of controlled trials of ambulatory treatment, debridement and anterior spinal fusion in the management of tuberculosis of the spine: Studies in Vulawayo (Rhodesia) and in Hong Kong. J Bone Joint Surg 60B:163–177, 1978.

226. Menard, V.: Causes de paraplégie dans le mal de Pott. Son traitement chirurgical par l'ouverture directe du foyer tuberculeux des vertébres. Rev Orthoped 5:47–64, 1984.

227. Merkel, K.D., Fitzgerald, R.H., and Brown, M.L.: Scintigraphic evaluation in musculoskeletal sepsis. Orthop Clin N Am 15:401–416, 1984.

228. Messer, H.D., and Litvinoff, J.: Pyogenic cervical osteomyelitis. Chondro-osteomyelitis of the cervical spine frequently associated with parenteral drug use. Arch Neurol 33:571–576, 1976.

229. Miller, M.E., Fogel, G.R., and Dunham, W.K.: Salmonella spondylitis: A review and report of two immunologically normal patients. J Bone Joint Surg 70A:463–466, 1988.

230. Mixter, W.J., and Smithwick, R.H.: Acute intraspinal epidural abscess. N Engl J Med 207:126–131, 1932.

231. Modic, M.T., Feiglin, D.H., Piraino, D.W., et al.: Vertebral osteomyelitis: Assessment using MR. Radiology 157:157–166, 1985.

232. Moodie, A.S.: Tuberculosis in Hong Kong. Tubercle 4:334–345, 1963.

233. Moon, M.-S., Kim, I., Woo, Y.-K., et al.: Conservative treatment of tuberculosis of the thoracic and lumbar spine in adults and children. Int Orthop 11:315–322, 1987.

234. Moon, M.S., Woo, Y.K., Lee, K.S., et al.: Posterior instrumentation and anterior interbody fusion for tuberculous kyphosis of dorsal and lumbar spines. Spine 20:1910–1916, 1995.

235. Mousa, A.R.M., Muhtaseb, S.A., Almudallal, D.S., et al.: Osteoarticular complications of brucellosis: A study of 169 cases. Rev Infect Dis 9:531–543, 1987.

236. Musher, D.M., and Fletcher, T.: Tolerant Staphylococcus aureus causing vertebral osteomyelitis. Arch Intern Med 142:632–634, 1982.

237. Musher, D.M., Thorsteinsson, S.B., Minuth, J.N., et al.: Vertebral osteomyelitis still a diagnostic pitfall. Arch Intern Med 136:105–110, 1976.

238. Nagel, D.A., Albright, J.A., Keggi, J.K., et al.: Closer look at spinal lesions: Open biopsy of vertebral lesions. J Am Med Assoc 191:103–106, 1965.

239. Naim-ur-Rahman, Al Arabi, K.M., and Khan, F.A.: A typical form of spinal tuberculosis. Acta Neurochir 88:26–33, 1987.

240. Nasca, R.J., and McElvein, R.B.: Aspergillus fumigatus osteomyelitis of the thoracic spine treated by excision and interbody fusion. Spine 10:848–850, 1985.

241. Norris, S., Ehrlich, M.G., and McKusick, K.: Early diagnosis of disk space infection with 67 Ga in an experimental model. Clin Orthop 144:293–298, 1979.

242. Nussbaum, E.S., Rigamonti, D., Standiford, H., et al.: Spinal epidural abscess: A report of 40 cases and review. Surg Neurol 38:225, 1992.

243. Nyberg, D.A., Jeffrey, R.B., Brant Sawakzki, M., et al.: Computed tomography of cervical infections. J Comp Assist Tomogr 9:288–296, 1985.

244. O'Connell, C.J., Cherry, A.V., and Zoll, J.G.: Osteomyelitis of cervical spine: Candida guilliermondii [letter to the editor]. Ann Intern Med 79:748, 1973.

245. Oga, M., Arizono, T., Takasita, M., et al.: Evaluation of the risk of instrumentation as a foreign body in spinal tuberculosis. Spine 18:1890–1894, 1993.

246. Oill, P.A., Chow, A.W., Flood, T.P., et al.: Adult Haemophilus influenzae Type B vertebral osteomyelitis: A case report and review of the literature. Clin Orthop 136:253–256, 1978.

247. Onofrio, B.M.: Intervertebral discitis: Incidence, diagnosis and management. Clin Neurosurg 27:481–516, 1980.

248. Ottolenghi, C.E.: Aspiration biopsy of the spine: Technique for the thoracic region and results of twenty-eight biopsies in this region and overall results of 1050 biopsies of other spinal segments. J Bone Joint Surg 51A:1531–1544, 1969.

249. Ottolenghi, C.E., Schajowicz, F., and DeSchant, F.A.: Aspiration biopsy of the cervical spine: Technique and results in thirty-four cases. J Bone Joint Surg 46A:715–733, 1964.

250. Palestro, C.J., Kim, C.K., Swyer, A.J., et al.: Radionuclide diagnosis of vertebral osteomyelitis: Indium-111-leukocyte and technetium-99m-methylene diphosphonate bone scintigraphy. J Nucl Med 32:1861–1865, 1991.

251. Park, Y., Taylor, J.A.M., Szoller, S.M., et al.: Imaging findings in spinal neuroarthropathy. Spine 19:1499–1504, 1994.

252. Parke, W.W., Rothman, R.H., and Brown, M.D.: The pharyngovertebral veins: An anatomical rationale for Grisel's syndrome. J Bone Joint Surg 66A:568–574, 1984.

253. Petty, B.G., Burrow, C.R., Robinson, R.A., et al.: Hemophilus aphrophilus meningitis followed by vertebral osteomyelitis and suppurative psoas abscess. Am J Med 78:159–162, 1985.

254. Phillips, G.E., and Jefferson, A.: Acute spinal epidural abscess. Observations from fourteen cases. Postgrad Med J 55:712–715, 1979.

255. Piazza, M.R., Bassett, G.S., and Bunnell, W.P.: Neuropathic spinal arthropathy in congenital insensitivity to pain. Clin Orthop 236:175–179, 1988.

256. Pilgaard, S.: Discitis closed space infection following removal of lumbar intervertebral disc. J Bone Joint Surg 51A:713–716, 1969.

257. Pirofsky, J.G., Huang, C.T., and Waites, K.B.: Spinal osteomyelitis due to mycobacterium avium-intracellulare in an elderly man with steroid-induced osteoporosis. Spine 18:1926–1932, 1993.

258. Post, M.J.D., Quencer, R.M., Montalvo, B.M., et al.: Spinal infection: Evaluation with MR imaging and intraoperative US. Radiology 169:765–771, 1988.

259. Post, M.J.D., Sze, G., Quencer, R.M., et al.: Gadolinium enhancing MR in spinal infection. J Comput Assist Tomogr 14:721–729, 1990.

260. Postacchini, F., and Montanaro, A.: Tuberculous epidural granuloma simulating a herniated lumbar disc: A report of a case. Clin Orthop 148:182–185, 1980.

261. Pott, P.: Remarks on That Kind of Palsy of the Lower Limbs Which Is Frequently Found to Accompany a Curvature of the Spine and Is Supposed to Be Caused by It. Together with Its Method of Cure. London: J Johnson, 1779, pp. 1–84.

262. Pritchard, A.E., and Thompson, W.A.L.: Acute pyogenic infections of the spine in children. J Bone Joint Surg 42B:86–89, 1960.

263. Pritchard, D.J.: Granulomatous infections of bones and joints. Orthop Clin N Am 6:1029–1047, 1975.

264. Puranen, J., Mäkela, J., and Lähde, S.: Postoperative intervertebral discitis. Acta Orthop Scand 55:461–465, 1984.

265. Rajasekaran, S., and Shanmugasundaram, T.K.: Prediction of the angle of gibbus deformity in tuberculosis of the spine. J Bone Joint Surg 69A:503–509, 1987.

266. Rajasekaran, S., and Soundarapandian, S.: Progression of kyphosis in tuberculosis of the spine treated by anterior arthrodesis. J Bone Joint Surg 71A:1314–1323, 1989.

267. Rand, C., and Smith, M.A.: Anterior spinal tuberculosis: Paraplegia following laminectomy. Ann R Coll Surg Engl 71:105–109, 1989.

268. Rangell, L., and Glassman, F.: Acute spinal epidural abscess as a complication of lumbar puncture. J Nerv Ment Dis 102:8–18, 1945.

269. Rankin, R.M., and Flothow, P.G.: Pyogenic infection of the spinal epidural space. West J Surg Obstet Gynecol 54:320–323, 1946.

270. Rawlings, C.E., Wilkins, R.H., Gallis, H.A., et al.: Postoperative intervertebral disc space infection. Neurosurgery 13:371–376, 1983.

271. Redekop, G.J., and DelMaestro, R.: Diagnosis and management of spinal epidural abscess. Can J Neurol Sci 19:180, 1992.

272. Redfern, R.M., Cottam, S.N., and Phillipson, A.P.: Proteus infection of the spine. Spine 13:439–441, 1988.

273. Resnick, D., and Niwayama, G.: Osteomyelitis septic arthritis and soft tissue infection: The axial skeleton. In Resnick, D., and Niwayama, G. (eds.): Diagnosis of Bone and Joint Disorders with Emphasis on Articular Abnormalities. Philadelphia: WB Saunders Co, 1981, pp. 2130–2153.

274. Riley, L.H., Banovac, K., Martinez, O.V., et al.: Tissue distribution of antibiotics in the intervertebral disc. Spine 19:2619–2625, 1994.

275. Roaf, R., Kirkaldy Willis, W.H., and Cathro, A.J.M.: Surgical Treatment of Bone and Joint Tuberculosis. Edinburgh: Churchill Livingstone, 1959.

276. Robinson, B.H.B., and Lessof, M.H.: Osteomyelitis of the spine. Guy Hosp Rep 110:303–318, 1961.

277. Ross, P.M., and Fleming, J.L.: Vertebral body osteomyelitis: Spectrum and natural history: A retrospective analysis of 37 cases. Clin Orthop 118:190–198, 1976.

278. Rubery, P.T., Smith, M.O., Cammisa, F.P., et al.: Mycotic aortic aneurysm in patients who have lumbar vertebral osteomyelitis. A report of two cases. J Bone Joint Surg 77A:1729–1732, 1995.

279. Russell, N.A., Vaughan, R., and Morley, T.P.: Spinal epidural infection. Can J Neurol Sci 6:325–328, 1979.

280. Russo, T.A.: Agents of Actinomycosis. In Mandell, G.L., Bennett, J.E., and Dolin, R., eds. Principles and Practice of Infectious Diseases. New York: Churchill Livingstone, 1995, pp. 2280–2288.

281. Sandiford, J.A., Higgins, G.A., and Blair, W.: Remote salmonellosis: Surgical masquerader. Am Surg 48:54–58, 1982.

282. Sapico, F.L., and Montgomerie, J.Z.: Pyogenic vertebral osteomyelitis: Report of nine cases and review of the literature. Rev Infect Dis 1:754–776, 1979.

283. Sapico, F.L., and Montgomerie, J.Z.: Vertebral osteomyelitis in intravenous drug abusers: Report of three cases and review of the literature. Rev Infect Dis 2:196–206, 1980.

284. Sarkar, S.D., Ravikrishnan, K.P., Woodbury, D.H., et al.: Gallium 67-citrate scanning: A new adjunct in the detection and follow-up of extrapulmonary tuberculosis: Concise communication. J Nucl Med 20:833–836, 1979.

285. Schaefer, S.D., Bucholz, R.W., Jones, R.E., et al.: The management of transpharyngeal gunshot wounds to the cervical spine. Surg Gynecol Obstet 152:27–29, 1981.

286. Scherbel, A.L., and Gardner, W.J.: Infections involving the intervertebral discs: Diagnosis and management. J Am Med Assoc 174:370–374, 1960.

287. Schofferman, L., Schofferman, J., Zucherman, J., et al.: Occult infections causing persistent low-back pain. Spine 14:417–419, 1989.

288. Schulitz, K.P., and Assheuer, J.: Discitis after procedures on the intervertebral disc. Spine 19:1172–1177, 1994.

289. Schulitz, K.P., Kothe, R., Leong, J.C.Y., et al.: Growth changes of solidly fused kyphotic bloc after surgery for tuberculosis. Spine 22:1150–1155, 1997.

290. Scrimgeour, E.M., Kaven, J., and Gajdusek, D.C.: Spinal tuberculosis: The commonest cause of nontraumatic paraplegia in Papua New Guinea. Trop Georg Med 39:218–221, 1987.

291. Scuderi, G.J., Greenberg, S.S., Banovac, K., et al.: Penetration of glycopeptide antibiotics in nucleus pulposus. Spine 18:2039–2042, 1993.

292. Scully, R.E., Mark, E.J., and McNeely, B.U.: Case records of the Massachusetts General Hospital. N Engl J Med 306:729–737, 1982.

293. Seddon, H.J.: Pott's paraplegia: Prognosis and treatment. Br J Surg 22:769–799, 1934–1935.

294. Selby, R.C., and Pillay, K.V.: Osteomyelitis and disc infection secondary to Pseudomonas aeruginosa in heroin addiction. J Neurosurg 37:463–466, 1972.

295. Sharif, H.S., Aideyan, O.A., Clark, D.C., et al.: Brucellar and tuberculous spondylitis: Comparative imaging features. Radiology 171:419–425, 1989.

296. Shaw, N.E., and Thomas, T.G.: Surgical treatment of chronic infective lesions of the spine. Br Med J 1:162–164, 1963.

297. Siao, P., McCabe, P., and Yagnik, P.: Nocardial spinal epidural abscess. Neurology 39:996, 1989.

298. Singer, J., and Sundaram, M.: Tuberculosis of the vertebra. Orthopedics 2:1222–1224, 1988.

299. Smith, A.S., Weinstein, M.A., Mizushima, A., et al.: MR imaging characteristics of tuberculous spondylitis vs vertebral osteomyelitis. Am J Radiol 153:399–405, 1989.

300. Snider, D.E., Cauther, G.M., and Farer, L.S.: Drug-resistant tuberculosis. Am Rev Respir Dis 144:732, 1991.

301. Southwick, W.O., and Robinson, R.A.: Surgical approaches to the vertebral bodies in the cervical and lumbar regions. J Bone Joint Surg 39A:631–644, 1957.

302. Staab, E.V., and McCartney, W.H.: Role of gallium 67 in inflammatory disease. Semin Nucl Med 8:219–234, 1978.

303. Stauffer, R.N.: Pyogenic vertebral osteomyelitis. Orthop Clin N Am 6:1015–1027, 1975.

304. Stevens, D.A.: Coccidioides immitis. In Mandell, G.L., Bennett, J.E., and Dolin, R., eds. Principles and Practice of Infectious Diseases. New York: Churchill Livingstone, 1995, pp. 2365–2375.

305. Stone, D.B., and Bonfiglio, M.: Pyogenic vertebral osteomyelitis: A diagnostic pitfall for the internist. Arch Intern Med 112:491–500, 1963.

306. Sullivan, C.R., Bickel, W.H., and Svien, H.J.: Infections of vertebral interspaces after operations on intervertebral discs. J Am Med Assoc 166:1973–1977, 1958.

307. Swayne, L.C., Dorsky, S., Caruana, V., et al.: Septic arthritis of a lumbar facet joint: Detection with bone SPECT imaging. J Nucl Med 30:1408–1411, 1989.

308. Szypryt, E.P., Hardy, J.G., Hinton, C.E., et al.: A comparison between magnetic resonance imaging and scintigraphic bone imaging in the diagnosis of disc space infection in an animal model. Spine 13:1042–1048, 1988.

309. Theodotou, B., Woosley, R.E., and Whaley, R.A.: Spinal subdural empyema: Diagnosis by spinal computed tomography. Surg Neurol 21:610–612, 1984.

310. Thibodeau, A.A.: Closed space infection following removal of lumbar intervertebral disc. J Bone Joint Surg 50A:400–410, 1968.

311. Tramont, E.C.: Treponema pallidum (syphilis). In Mandell, G.L., Bennett, J.E., and Dolin, R., eds. Principles and Practice of Infectious Diseases. New York, Churchill Livingstone, 1995, pp. 2117–2133.

312. Tuli, S.M.: Results of treatment of spinal tuberculosis by "middle-path" regime. J Bone Joint Surg 57B:13–23, 1975.

313. Tuli, S.M., Srivastava, T.P., Varma, B.P., et al.: Tuberculosis of spine. Acta Orthop Scand 38:445–458, 1967.

314. VanLom, K.J., Kellerhouse, L.E., Pathria, M.N., et al.: Infection versus tumor in the spine: Criteria for distinction with CT. Radiology 166:851–855, 1988.

315. Versca, J.M., Leung, K.Y., Wagner, T.A., et al.: Primary infections of the spine treated surgically: Instrumented versus noninstrumented. 10th Annual Meeting of the North American Spine Society. Washington, DC, 1995.

316. Visudhiphan, P., Chiemchanya, S., Somburanasin, R., et al.: Torticollis as the presenting sign in cervical spine infection and tumor. Clin Pediatr 21:71–76, 1982.

317. Waldvogel, F.A., Medoff, G., and Swartz, M.N.: Osteomyelitis: A review of clinical features, therapeutic considerations and unusual aspects. N Engl J Med 282:198–206, 260–266, 316–322, 1970.

318. Waldvogel, F.A., and Vasey, H.: Osteomyelitis: The past decade. N Engl J Med 303:360–370, 1980.

319. Wedge, J.H., Oryschak, A.F., Robertson, D.E., et al.: Atypical manifestations of spinal infections. Clin Orthop 123:155–163, 1977.

320. Weinberg, J.A.: The surgical excision of psoas abscesses resulting from spinal tuberculosis. J Bone Joint Surg 39A:17–27, 1957.

321. Whalen, J.L., Brown, M.L., McLeod, R., et al.: Limitations of indium leukocyte imaging for diagnosis of spine infections. Spine 16:193–197, 1991.

322. Whalen, J.L., Parke, W.W., Mazur, J.M., et al.: The intrinsic vasculature of developing vertebral and plates and its nutritive significance to the intervertebral discs. J Pediatr Orthop 5:403–410, 1985.

323. Wheeler, D., Keisser, P., and Rigamonte, D.: Medical management of spinal epidural abscesses: Case report and review. Clin Infect Dis 15:22–27, 1992.

324. Whitecloud, T.S., and LaRocca, H.: Fibular strut graft in reconstructive surgery of the cervical spine. Spine 1:33–43, 1976.

325. Wiesseman, G.J., Wood, V.E., and Kroll, L.L.: Pseudomonas vertebral osteomyelitis in heroin addicts. Report of five cases. J Bone Joint Surg 55A:1416–1424, 1973.

326. Wilensky, A.O.: Osteomyelitis of the vertebrae. Ann Surg 89:561–570, 1929.

327. Wiley, A.M., and Trueta, J.: The vascular anatomy of the spine and its relationship to pyogenic vertebral osteomyelitis. J Bone Joint Surg 41B:796–809, 1959.

328. Wiltberger, B.R.: Resection of vertebral bodies and bone grafting for chronic osteomyelitis of the spine. J Bone Joint Surg 34A:215–218, 1952.

329. Winter, W.G., Larson, R.K., Zettas, J.P., et al.: Coccidioidal spondylitis. J Bone Joint Surg 60A:240–244, 1978.

330. Wise, R.I.: Brucellosis in the United States. Past, present and future. J Am Med Assoc 224:2318–2322, 1980.

331. Wukich, D.K., Van Dam, B.E., and Abreu, S.H.: Preoperative indium-labeled white cell scintigraphy in suspected osteomyelitis of the axial skeleton. Spine 13:1168–1170, 1988.

332. Yang, S.Y.: Spinal epidural abscess. N Z Med J 95:302–304, 1982.

333. Yanoff, D.B., and Church, M.L.: Nocardial vertebral osteomyelitis. Clin Orthop 175:223–226, 1983.

334. Yau, A.C.M.C., and Hodgson, A.R.: Penetration of the lung by the paravertebral abscess in tuberculosis of the spine. J Bone Joint Surg 50A:243–254, 1968.

335. Yau, A.C.M.C., Hsu, L.C.S., O'Brien, J.P., et al.: Tuberculous kyphosis: Correction with spinal osteotomy, halo-pelvic distraction, and anterior posterior fusion. J Bone Joint Surg 56A:1419–1434, 1974.

336. Young, E.J.: Brucella specia. In Mandell, G.L., Bennett, J.E., and Dolin, R., eds. Principles and Practice of Infectious Diseases. New York, Churchill Livingstone, 1995, pp. 2053–2060.

337. Zigler, J.E., Bohlman, H.H., Robinson, R.A., et al.: Pyogenic osteomyelitis of the occiput, the atlas, and the axis: A report of five cases. J Bone Joint Surg 69A:1069–1073, 1987.

40

Metabolic Bone Disorders of the Spine

Joseph M. Lane, M.D.

Joseph Bernstein, M.D.

No metabolic bone diseases affect the spine exclusively: as systemic processes, these diseases can appear in all bones. However, because the spine represents a major portion of the body's bone mass, contains the largest quantity of metabolically active (cancellous) bone, and specifically loads this trabecular bone in compression during upright posture, metabolic bone diseases, although affecting the entire skeleton, are often encountered as diseases primarily of the spine.

The spinal skeleton is more than mere inert, mechanical tissue. Rather, as in all bones, its component cells are physiologically active and responsive to an assortment of metabolic and mechanical stimuli. These activities serve the biochemical role of mineral balance (through the storage and release of Ca^{2+}, Mg^{2+}, HPO_4^{2-}, and H^+), as well as the bones' obvious structural role of remodeling and repair according to skeletal demands. Bone is thus a homeostatic organ and, perforce, a metabolically active one.

Metabolic bone disease, then, results when the bone constituents (cells and matrices) behave abnormally, when the stimuli to which bone responds are inappropriately interpreted, or when systemic processes derange the bones' environment, leading to impairment of either the biomechanical or the structural tasks.

Accordingly, this section on metabolic bone disease begins with an understanding of the norm: the characteristic interplay of cells, ions, and proteins; the effects of the various bone stimuli; and the organ's role in skeletal and mineral homeostasis. Next, we consider the abnormal—metabolic bone pathology and patho-physiology. For each major metabolic bone disease as it appears in the spine, we discuss epidemiology, its causes and clinical appearance, and its possible prevention and treatment. Within that, we present an overview of current radiologic, serologic, and histologic diagnostic tests in metabolic bone disease, discussing their indications, benefits, and limitations. Finally, we describe some less commonly encountered metabolic or parametabolic bone diseases of the spine.

NORMAL BONE

Unlike other organ systems, bone is primarily extracellular. Nevertheless, healthy bones, just like healthy livers and spleens, demand proper cellular function: the cells of the skeletal system, although proportionally few in number, synthesize, modify, and maintain the extracellular matrix. All metabolic bone events take place on the surface of the osseous matrix: either on its exterior side, or within the matrix, in lacunae that connect to the outer surface.

Bone Cells

There are four families of cells that combine to create biomechanically functional and mechanically sound bone tissue. These include the osteoprogenitor cell; its derivative, the osteoblast; the incorporated mature form, the osteocyte; and, finally, the osteoclast. Together, these cells fabricate new osseous tissue, maintain it, and resorb and remodel it; in short, they determine mechanical stability and mineral homeostasis. Healthy bone metabolism results from equilibrating these competing forces. Some forms of metabolic bone disease, therefore, can be viewed as the pathologic imbalance—in either number, power, or degree of differentiation—of bone-forming cells and bone-resorbing ones.[12, 68]

The osteoprogenitor cells[89]—either inducible or differentiated—are components of the bone marrow stromal system, approximating the surfaces of bone (periosteum and endosteum). These potentially mitotic cells, under appropriate stimulation and conditions, can give rise to either the bone-forming osteoblast or the cartilage-producing chondroblast. Its natural history, and the precise signals for its differentiation and modulation, are not yet fully elucidated.

Osteoblasts[13, 14, 86, 115] sit on the forming surface of bone in an adherent row, where they synthesize and release osteoid—the yet unmineralized bone matrix. They further participate in the mineralization of the osteoid by releasing packets of ions, as well as by synthesizing regulatory and crystal-nucleating noncollagenous proteins. These cells are characterized by high levels of alkaline phosphatase, the ability to manufacture Type I collagen and osteocalcin, and the presence of numerous receptor sites for parathyroid hormone (PTH) and estrogen, to name two. Furthermore, they seem to govern the actions of osteoclasts (described later), thus regulating and coupling both bone formation and bone resorption. The osteoblast is also found in a quiescent state—the so-called resting cell. Flatter than an active osteoblast and possessing fewer organelles, the resting cell does not make osteoid. In spite of its shape, however, it is not totally metabolically inactive either: along with osteocytes, these cells regulate the local ionic environment. Furthermore, they can be stimulated to become osteoblasts.

The osteocyte,[13, 14] the terminal cell of the osteogenic cell line, is derived immediately from osteoblasts. As this latter cell synthesizes matrix, it ensconces itself within its product. The cell is now termed an *osteocyte*, and the space in which it sits is termed a *lacuna*. There is one osteocyte per lacuna. Nevertheless, the osteocyte is not completely isolated from other cells, because its cell processes extend out to the surface by means of the osteocytic canaliculi and connect to others through gap junctions. These cells are believed to maintain the micro matrix that envelops them, regulate local ionic concentrations, and govern the degree of mineralization.

Osteoclasts[4, 19] resorb bone. Unlike the other mesenchymally derived cells so far described, osteoclasts arise from the monocyte line. These large multinucleated cells are found on the rough, resorbing surfaces of bone, where they bind to a bone-specific integrin[118] and form an isolated macrocavity. At this attachment cavity site, release of carbonic anhydrase creates an acidic microenvironment, which causes the dissolution of the hydroxyapatite mineral. Subsequent release of acid hydrolases degrades the organic collagen matrix as well. The resultant resorption cavity is called a

Howship lacuna. Osteoclasts, accordingly, participate in both the mechanical and biochemical tasks of bone tissue: remodeling formed bone, as well as dispensing calcium into the circulation. Surprisingly, the osteoclast is devoid of PTH receptors, even though it functionally responds to that hormone. Indeed, the hormonal response is found only in those osteoclasts approximated to functional osteoblasts (which do possess PTH receptors), demonstrating that the osteoclast actually responds to a coupling effector mediated by the osteoblast.

Bone Matrices

Beyond the cellular component, two matrices (organic and inorganic) constitute the remainder of the tissue (Fig. 40–1). The inorganic matrix, representing two thirds of the bone's dry weight, is primarily calcium phosphate,[91] found in three forms: (1) the predominant, crystalline hydroxyapatite $[Ca_{10}(PO_4)_6(OH)_2]$; (2) the rarer octacalcium phosphate $[Ca_8H_2(PO_4)_6 \cdot 3H_2O)]$; and (3) brushite $[CaHPO_4 \cdot 2H_2O]$. The hydroxyapatite forms platelike crystals 40 nm long and 3 nm thick. The crystals are not pure, with carbonate at times interposed for a phosphate or with fluoride for a hydroxy group. (Other potential inclusions comprise lead and arsenic.) These contaminants alter the physical properties of the matrix and may affect the biologic characteristics as well. The mineral crystal closely associates with the organic matrix, initially deposited in the hole zones of the collagen fibril. Later, it surrounds itself with ground substance (proteoglycan), as well as with water and other ions.

The initial formation of hydroxyapatite is under osteoblast control, which is replete with alkaline phosphatase. This enzyme catalyzes, among others, reactions that release phosphate from pyrophosphate. The conversion of pyrophosphate has two effects: it creates higher local concentrations of phosphate—levels that

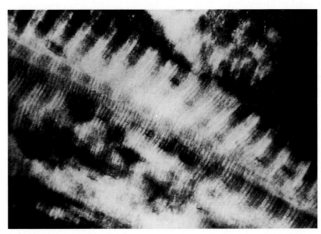

Figure 40–1. Collagen-mineral relationship: the hydroxyapatite forms in the hole zone between collagen molecules (Anatomy II. Orthop. Science. Park Ridge, IL, AAOS, 1986.)

permit the calcium and phosphate to precipitate—and it destroys pyrophosphate, an inhibitor of calcification. Thus, through the action of this enzyme, bone can calcify at serum concentrations of calcium and phosphate at which dystrophic (extraskeletal) calcification does not occur.

Nonetheless, concentration alone does not dictate mineral deposition. To assist with mineralization, as well as to regulate it, the body uses an organic matrix.[96] The organic matrix of bone is primarily composed of proteins, of which over 90 per cent is collagen. Collagen, a rigid macromolecule, employs tropocollagen as its basic structural unit. Tropocollagen, in turn, is composed of three polypeptide chains, each of approximately 1000 amino acids.[95] In bone collagen (Type I), two of these chains are of identical amino acid sequence; the α_2 is of similar but not identical sequence. All three chains contain unusually high concentrations of glycine, proline, alanine, hydroxyproline, and hydroxylysine. These chains are wound into right-handed helices. The presence of the small, neutral glycine in every third spot in the chain permits dense winding of the helix. Numerous hydrogen bonds between the chains hold the helix in place. Within the chains, hydroxylysine residues are oxidized to form aldehydes, which bond covalently in the form of complex cross links to further stabilize the helix. These polypeptide chains are then wound into a left-handed superhelix 300 nm in length—the tropocollagen molecule.

Tropocollagen contributes to collagen fibers by linking both horizontally (to the sides of other tropocollagen molecules) as well as vertically (i.e., carboxy end to amino terminus), thus creating a longer, wider macromolecule. The tropocollagen molecules standing side to side are staggered such that the end of one tropocollagen cable begins at approximately the 200th amino acid of the molecule next to it, yielding a stairlike configuration. In addition, the ends of the molecules are not tightly opposed; rather, a 40-nm gap remains. This space plays a central role in the mineralization of the fiber, serving as a nidus for mineral nucleation: closely aligned with these hole zones are proteins with the potential to nucleate the original hydroxyapatite crystal.

Type I collagen synthesis occurs in the osteoblast. The cytoplasmic product is procollagen, which, on cleavage of signal sequences at its ends, is then extruded. After secretion, many modifications are made to the procollagen molecule. Notably, this precursor molecule loses extensive nonhelical regions from both its amino and carboxy termini, and key proline and lysine residues are hydroxylated by an iron-containing enzyme. (The iron in this hydroxylase functions only in the ferrous state; therefore, ascorbic acid, functioning as a reducing agent, is needed.) This hydroxylation occurs after the proline and lysine enter the chain; consequently, free hydroxyproline in the serum represents lysis of collagen or its precursors. Accordingly, measurements of urinary hydroxyapatite excretion give the clinician a qualitative indication of bone breakdown or turnover. The hydroxylation of these two

amino acids facilitates cross linking, and the cross linking, accordingly, lowers the collagen's solubility and increases its tensile strength. Indeed, collagen is one of its strongest—in bone, its tensile strength exceeds the compressive strength of the bone mineral by 2000 N/cm^2. Pyrodinoline, deoxypyrodinoline, and N-telopeptides are cross-link breakdown products and are better markers of bone resorption than hydroxyproline.[94, 105] They are elevated in high-turnover osteoporosis and decline rapidly with successful antiresorptive therapy (see later).

Type I collagen is found not only in the bones of the spine but also in the intervertebral discs. There it is accompanied by Type II collagen. These homologous molecules differ only in the chains that compose the triple helix. Each type of collagen within the disc has its own anatomic domain: Type I collagen outnumbers the Type II in the annulus fibrosus, whereas Type II represents more of the nucleus pulposus.[16]

Proteoglycans form the ground substance of bone. In it, the glycosaminoglycans keratin sulfate and chondroitin sulfate attach to a core protein. Keratin and chondroitin sulfate form through the polymerization of disaccharide units, one sugar of which is always a hexosamine possessing an anionic group. This negatively charged group imbibes water, expanding the tissue volume in which it is found. When the bone mineralizes, the water content is reduced, leading to denser, more compact tissue. In addition, the relative concentration of water in the organic matrix (due to a proteoglycan effect) dictates the relative flux of ions through the substance, diffusion being proportional to water content. Thus, in bone, proteoglycans exert regulatory as well as structural forces. The spinal discs contain proteoglycans, too, with 30 to 60 per cent of the dry weight of the nucleus pulposus due to that class of molecules. Proteoglycan concentration drops with age, and with it water concentration drops as well; as noted, the anionic groups in the proteoglycan bind water. At all times, though, osmotic forces retain at least some water.[63]

Osteocalcin[93] is a bone-specific protein that, like Type I collagen, is synthesized by osteoblasts. Unlike collagen, it is a small protein (5800 daltons); although its molar concentration is that of collagen, it makes up only 2 per cent of the organic matrix by weight. This protein is widespread throughout the bone. Vitamin D enhances the synthesis of this protein, but it is not an absolute requirement. Osteocalcin contains three γ-carboxyglutamic amino acid residues, post-translationally produced by a vitamin K–dependent carboxylase. These negatively charged residues (termed "Gla") allow the osteocalcin (also known as bone Gla protein [BGP]) to bind the cationic calcium. Osteocalcin prefers to bind to calcium within hydroxyapatite. The spacing of the Gla residues in the BGP molecule aligns with the Ca^{2+} ions on the hydroxyapatite surface, promoting attachment of the protein to the bone. The precise function of this widely found osseous protein is not known, although its levels are correlated with bone mineral content. Possible roles include the attraction of osteoclasts to sites of bone resorption, regulation of the rate of mineral turnover, and determination of the morphology of the mineral crystal. Osteocalcin, derived from new bone synthesis, circulates in plasma in concentrations proportional to osteoblast activity. One study demonstrated a correlation between abnormal osteocalcin levels and radiographic evidence of metabolic bone disease.

Osteonectin, a 32-kd phosphoprotein secreted by osteoblasts, is the second most prevalent protein in bone. It binds to both collagen and hydroxyapatite,[123] as well as to carbohydrate moieties. Putative roles for osteonectin include calcium phosphate nucleation and stabilization of the newly formed crystal.

Bone morphogenetic protein (BMP), as the name implies, induces osteoprogenitor cells to form bone.[39] A small structure, it accounts for only 0.1 per cent of the total bone protein mass in cortical bone, and even less in the spine. It is now known that there are several BMPs, some of which are related to the transforming growth factors. Experimentally, BMP implanted in ectopic sites (in the absence of bone collagen) induces perivascular mesenchymal cells to become osteoprogenitor cells and form bone. The absence of this protein—or the blocking of its activity—might play a part in diseases of decreased bone mass, failures of bone remodeling, or impaired bone repair. Likewise, now that the genes for the expression of the BMPs have been cloned,[39, 126] the protein may have a potential pharmacologic role as well in repairing bone.

There are still other proteins found in bone that are synthesized not by osteoblasts but rather by the liver, such as α_2 HS-glycoprotein and albumin, among others. These proteins circulate in the bloodstream and incorporate themselves into the bone on mineralization. Although few in number, the protein growth factors occupy significant places in metabolic bone pathways. Specifically, they may couple cycles of bone lysis to bone synthesis: the dissolution of bone tissue concomitantly releases these stored proteins, which in turn influence bone regeneration.

Bone Tissue

Bone tissue[15] may be categorized either grossly or microscopically (Fig. 40–2). Grossly, we recognize bone as either cortical or cancellous (trabecular). The assignment of a given bone to either category relates to its density, which, in turn, reflects the presence of intraosseous cavities—only trabecular bone has them. Bone of both types can be demonstrated in the spine: the vertebrae are predominantly trabecular, whereas the spinous and transverse processes and articulating facets are cortical.

Cortical bones are dense bones; over 90 per cent of their volume is hard tissue. There are no intraosseous cavities, and the surface linings are smooth. Although the labeling of a bone as cortical can be made with the naked eye, there are microscopic correlates. For example, cortical bones organize around haversian systems, or osteons. In these, concentric, parallel lamellae

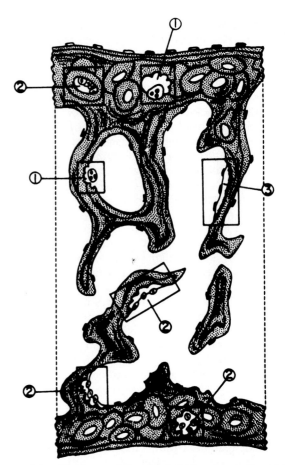

Figure 40–2. Bone remodeling in cortical and cancellous bone. 1, Osteoclast; 2, active osteoblast; 3, flattened inactive lining cell. (Disorders of Bone 3. Orthop. Science. Park Ridge, IL, AAOS, 1986.)

of collagen fibers gather about a central cavity. This central cavity was made by the burrowing of osteoclasts, and within it lies a blood vessel. Along the walls of the osteon, new bone is made by osteoblasts. The osteon communicates with its neighbors via Volkmann's canals—transverse tunnels that connect the haversian systems. Cortical bones resist torque forces and thus usually function as lever arms; the diaphyses of the femur, tibia, and fibula are all predominantly cortical bone.

Trabecular bone, the other gross category, has only rare concentric lamellae but rather shows a spicular pattern, lattices organized along lines of compressive force. By dint of these platelike spicules, ordered in parallel sheets, trabecular bone is adapted to a unique physical task: the resistance to crushing and shearing. Unlike cortical bone, trabecular bone has a high surface-to-volume ratio; because metabolism characteristically occurs on the bone surface, it is especially metabolically active.

"Trabecular" and "cortical" are gross descriptions. The microscopic appearance divides bone into two other categories: woven (immature) and lamellar (mature) bone. Compared with lamellar bone, woven bone is rich: it has increased metabolic activity, greater cellularity, high mineral concentration, and thicker collagen fibrils. Still, it is the weaker of the two because it lacks organization and orientation—the collagen whorls in all directions. Woven bone is found in growing organisms, in fracture calluses, and in the involucrum of osteomyelitis, as well as in certain metabolic diseases, to be discussed later; it is the bone of high turnover. It is functionally imperfect, one might suggest, because it was made to be only a temporary constituent of (adult) bone: the normal sequence of events has woven bone replaced by the longer-lasting lamellar variety.

Lamellar bone, the mature form, is a study of mechanical efficiency. Although lacking thick collagen fibrils (here they are one fourth the size of woven bone's fibrils) and the high cell and mineral content characteristic of woven bone, it is stronger and functionally superior. It achieves this supremacy by orienting its collagen along lines of greatest load. Its mineral is distributed uniformly and its cells are spaced out evenly. In between the lamellae sits a thin seam of interlamellar cement—an extracellular material with a high mineral-to-collagen content. These cement lines provide a histologic record of the bone's growth and development. When these lines are irregular, they indicate bone deposition atop regions of resorbed bone—the irregularity represents the remains of osteoclastic lacunae. Smooth cement lines imply bone growth applied to areas where bone has previously grown but then stopped. These are accordingly termed *arrest lines*, whereas the former types are *reversal lines*. The structural strength of bone is related not only to its mass but also to the distribution of the mass and to the degree of trabecular interconnectedness within bone.[24, 29, 67] As a consequence, the ultimate strength of a specific bone is a function of its type (cortical venous trabecular); the architectural distribution of the mass within the bone; and the structural integrity and connectivity of the bone.[24, 29, 67]

OSTEOGENESIS AND MINERALIZATION

Spinal bones form by endochondral ossification; that is, the mineralized tissue replaces a cartilaginous model.[48, 67, 83] (The classic textbook description of this process is applied to the long bones. In the spine, which has proportionally greater horizontal growth than, say, the femur, the process is similar but not identical.) The mineralization of the spine begins at three months in utero, and although essentially complete at birth, the process continues in newly formed bone throughout life. The epiphyseal plates of the vertebral bodies provide longitudinal axial growth and do not fuse until the end of the second decade.[54] Osteoblasts control the mineralization process both indirectly (by synthesizing the organic matrix that anchors the mineral) and directly (through the release of mineral-rich matrix vesicles). Furthermore, osteoblasts promote

the deposition of hydroxyapatite by creating and maintaining the requisite alkaline environment.

The scheme can be viewed as follows: On the smooth, forming surface of bone, osteoblasts synthesize collagen-rich osteoid. Through chemical and physical changes, such as the loss of water, the formation of cross links, and the creation of osteocytic lacunae, the osteoid "matures." This maturation provides a nucleation surface for mineral deposition—an absolute requirement at physiologic concentrations of the mineral ions. Mature osteoid, with its correctly aligned collagen fibrils, proper hydration, and active calcium-binding proteins located in collagen hole zones, functions well as a nucleation surface for the initial crystal formation and promotes its further mineralization. Nearly all the mineralization occurs within days of osteoid formation by the process of osteoblast deposition. This is termed *primary ossification*. The small remainder of growth, the *secondary ossification*, occurs over months by way of crystal growth and expansion. Because this demands motion of ions through dense substance, it is an understandably slow process.

The strength of bone depends on both osteoid synthesis and mineral deposition; the osteoid offers tensile strength, and compressive strength comes from the mineral. Furthermore, as we have seen, mineralization requires more osteoid. Thus, skeletal health demands not only the presence of both processes but also their correct synchronization. Even if the mechanisms for both are found, if they are not temporally coupled correctly, inferior tissue results.

Bone, therefore, is made by the tight coupling of two processes: osteoid synthesis and mineralization. Still, they do not occur simultaneously: mineralization, promoted by and dependent on matrix synthesis, must lag behind. That gap in time creates a visible artifact: a seam of yet unmineralized osteoid between the osteoblasts and the front of already mineralized tissue. By using fluorescent markers that are deposited at that line (tetracycline is the prototype), one can locate and measure regions of new bone formation.

SKELETAL HOMEOSTASIS

Bone growth occurs at all phases of the organism's life.[13, 14] Functionally, this growth can be divided into two types. The first kind, the deposition of new bone in regions not first cleared by resorption or, conversely, the resorption of old bone without the concomitant deposition of new tissue, is termed *modeling*. Modeling results in change in either the shape, volume, or mass of existing bone. The second form of bone growth creates little, if any, change in the microbone dimensions. This balanced synthesis and lysis is called *remodeling*, the process by which bone replaces itself. This turnover releases ions into the circulation and prevents accumulation of aged or fatigued bone.

The predominance of scalloped cement lines in lamellar bone (indicating osteoclastic activity before osteoblastic) implies that remodeling is the more common practice. Indeed, modeling creates only a scant minority of the adult bone tissue mass. As with de novo synthesis, remodeling follows a characteristic sequence of steps. First osteoclasts, responding to a yet precisely undefined signal, arrange themselves into a multicellular "drill" and burr their way into existing bone. When the cavity attains a depth of 5 to 10 μm, the osteoclasts rest. Then, at some distance behind and some time later, osteoblasts enter onto the surface of this defect and begin the synthesis of replacement bone, following the normal pattern of matrix synthesis and subsequent mineralization. This continues until the defect has been fully reconstituted. This remodeling process can be viewed as two heads on the same zipper: as one moves along opening, the second one follows and closes. The key aspect of remodeling is that the new structure is only similar but not identical to the original—and there are reversal lines to prove it.

In the remodeling cycle, osteoclasts work as much as four times faster than osteoblasts. Thus the clastic phase usually requires 20 days in the typical remodeling unit, whereas the blastic phase carries over 80 days. After this period elapses, the tissue is almost exactly restored, notably with younger, aptly mineralized bone. The preferential remodeling of older tissue leads to an overall younger skeleton, one better suited to current mechanical demands. Conversely, if the body were to either stochastically choose its remodeling sequence or opt to remodel young, healthy tissue, these improper processes would lead to a structurally poorer skeleton. Thus, remodeling affects the quality of bone in a given individual. Furthermore, it can alter the quantity of bone if total bone formation lags but slightly behind resorption, as is commonly the case. High-frequency remodeling, in that case, leads to a net loss of skeletal tissue.

In sum, remodeling, a process that ordinarily prevents structural demise by repairing old or damaged regions in bone, can be responsible for eroding the bones' mechanical integrity. First, the remodeling can occur too frequently, magnifying what would ordinarily be an inconsequential net loss. Second, the remodeling can be poorly focused, inefficiently replacing that bone which requires no replacement and letting stand the weaker, older tissue. Finally, even within the confines of a normal remodeling cycle frequency and proper focus of that action, the process can contribute to overall skeletal debilitation if the formation cycle does not fully replace the bone lost during resorption.

MINERAL HOMEOSTASIS

Calcium

Bone exchanges calcium, magnesium, and phosphate and participates in acid-base balance. Of all of these, calcium[9, 67, 82, 83] is the most important in bone. This importance derives from calcium's vertex position in both homeostatic tasks of bone; skeletal and metabolic function depend on proper storage and release of this ion more than any other. The skeletal role of calcium is played in the hydroxyapatite mineral crystal, where it provides mechanical strength. Its metabolic functions occur as a free divalent cation. These include transducing hormonal signals within the cytoplasm ("second messenger" function), coupling neural excitation with muscular contraction, and effecting homeostasis by interacting with both vascular smooth muscle and platelets.

Body stores of calcium in the typical, 70-kg man total approximately 1300 g. More than 98 per cent of this resides in the teeth and bones. The remainder divides itself between the cytoplasmic and extracellular fluids. The serum concentration centers around 9 mg per dl. It is found in three states: (1) free (ionized and diffusible), (2) complexed to citrate and other anions (and thus nonionic but still diffusible), and (3) bound to proteins (neither ionic nor diffusible). Only the free and diffusible ion (normally about 45 per cent of the total) possesses physiologic activity. At normal body pH, albumin and other anionic proteins bind 50 per cent of the total. The proportion of bound calcium increases with increasing alkalinity. Accordingly, as the pH rises, the individual becomes effectively hypocalcemic, even though the total amount—and, importantly, the amount typically reported by standard laboratory tests—remains normal. Conversely, in states of liver and kidney failure, when albumin is either not synthesized or lost in the urine, even though the absolute levels of total serum calcium may be depressed, the effective physiologic calcium concentration may be near normal. Finally, calcium-anion complexes account for the remaining 5 per cent of serum calcium. Abnormal levels of these anions, likewise, may cause a physiologic calcium disturbance, one not necessarily obvious from the serum calcium concentration. Thus, unless ionic calcium is directly measured, attention should be directed at albumin levels and pH state before inferring functional calcium levels from the total serum measurement.

The body poorly tolerates variance in its serum calcium concentration. When the levels are low, cell membrane permeability for sodium increases and we see increased neural activity, beginning with twitching and progressing to seizures. High levels, conversely, lead to neural depression, found first peripherally (decreased reflexes) and then centrally (coma, at the extreme). Furthermore, the cardiac cycle, dependent on calcium channels for proper rhythm and contraction, is in turn disturbed by derangements of the serum calcium levels. Accordingly, calcium is among the most stringently regulated of all serum substances.

Maintenance of calcium concentration is the task of three organ systems: the gut, to absorb it; the kidney, to excrete it; and the bone, to store it. Each of these systems can alter the magnitude of the calcium contribution in response to a number of regulatory substances.

The gut—duodenum and jejunum specifically—absorbs calcium from the diet, taken in primarily as dairy products. Despite the critical need for calcium absorption, the gut does so with marked inefficiency: of the recommended daily allowance of 800 mg, only half will ever cross the luminal border, and of that fraction, more than half will be returned to the lumen with the secretion of intestinal fluids. Thus, less than one fourth of the daily intake (about 150 mg) finds its way into the system.

Absorption in the duodenum[121] takes place by means of a protein-dependent transport system. In the jejunum, passive diffusion brings in the rest. Clearly, the jejunal phase depends more on concentration gradients and intestinal transit times. In addition, dietary composition affects absorption: diets high in fiber and oxalate (both found in green vegetables) allow for less calcium absorption. In times of increased calcium demand, such as the growth years, or during pregnancy, the duodenal fractional absorption can be augmented by increased carrier protein synthesis (in turn stimulated by the active vitamin D metabolite [see later]). The efficiency of calcium absorption decreases with aging.[56, 67]

The bone stores calcium. Like the fat-storing adipocyte, which constantly synthesizes and hydrolyzes triglycerides even when the body is in energy balance, the bone tissue exchanges calcium into the plasma at all times, even when intake matches excretion. This daily, 400-mg exchange results from the nearly balanced activity of osteoclasts and osteoblasts (remodeling), as well as the movement of ions between intracellular and extracellular compartments at the osteocyte plasma membrane.

The bone functions as a metabolic calcium bank. Like a bank, it takes deposits and uses them—here to make skeletal tissue. And like a bank, it keeps a small fraction of the deposits on hand for rapid withdrawals. Thus, bone maintains its calcium in two distinct functional states. One is in mature matrix as hydroxyapatite. This is most structurally useful, at the cost of decreased liquidity; this calcium is not available for immediate dispensation into the circulation. At the surface of bone and along the canaliculi sits another, less mature mineral pool that is readily exchangeable with the plasma calcium. The significance of the two calcium pools is that only long-term disturbance of calcium concentration, not the minute-to-minute flux, affects skeletal stability. The bone tries to meet demands of both mineral and mechanical homeostasis, but under chronic imbalance it will uniformly sacrifice the latter for the former. When the long-term (structural) deposits of calcium are mobilized, those regions under least mechanical stress primarily are affected. This further protects the body against skeletal instability, even as the calcium providing mechanical strength is mobilized.

The kidneys are the prime excreters of systemic calcium. The glomerular load of calcium is almost 10,000 mg. Most of it is resorbed proximally, following sodium-driven bulk flow. Some calcium remains in the lumen until the distal nephron, where it can be selectively resorbed by calcium-specific transport processes: it follows not only the dictates of calcium-regulating agents but also the demands of salt and water balance and acid-base control. For example, when volume depletion demands increased sodium resorption, proportionally more calcium will be retained proximally, regardless of the serum levels. Diet can also affect renal calcium handling, with both high-protein and high-carbohydrate loads augmenting spillage into the urine. Under normal conditions, the kidneys resorb 98 per cent of the filtered load, excreting increasing amounts commensurate with increased intake or resorption from bone. One deleterious consequence of this renal response to high calcium is the formation of stones. Although there is no precise threshold at which stones will form—because other factors, such as urinary flow rate, influence the process—the risk of stone formation climbs with increasing hypercalciuria.

Phosphate

The second important ion in bone metabolism is phosphate.[72] Like calcium, phosphate has disparate functions throughout the body. As a component of adenosine triphosphate, phosphate participates in the interconversion of the energy of metabolism; as a constituent of nucleotides, phosphate partakes in the transmission and expression of genetic information; and in 2,3-diphosphoglycerate, it regulates the oxygen affinity of hemoglobin.

Phosphate is found in two forms: $H_2PO_4^-$ and PO_4^{2-}. The ratio of this dissociation, like that of any acid, depends on the pK_a of the system (a constant) and at local pH, which, obviously, can vary. Thus, in the extracellular fluid, whose pH is 7.4, the ratio of $H_2PO_4^-$ to PO_4^{2-} is about 4:1; whereas in the slightly less alkaline cytosol, the ratio is closer to 2.5:1. But unlike calcium, which is physiologically sensed only as the free ion, phosphate is internally measured as a sum of both forms. Again, unlike that of calcium, phosphate's role outside of bone is less dependent on concentration; and thus alterations in its level cause few immediate effects. Nevertheless, the quantity of phosphate, normally about 4 mg/dl, is regulated.

The body stores of phosphate sum to 700 g, about half that of calcium. As with calcium, most of it (perhaps 85 per cent of the total) resides in bone. The typical intake is about 1000 mg per day, with about two thirds of this absorbed. The presence of substances in the gut that can bind phosphate, such as aluminum salts, determines in a major way the amount of phosphate absorbed. Under normal circumstances, the amount absorbed rises linearly with increasing intake.

As with calcium, the kidney is responsible for maintaining phosphate balance,[61] and it does so by a similar mechanism: proximal sodium bulk-driven flow, with distal control. When phosphate intake is high, it excretes increasing amounts by spilling the excess phosphate into the urine. When concentrations in the serum are low, the kidney can avidly conserve it by changes effected in calcium concentration by vitamin D. In addition to calcium balance, dietary load, volume status, and acid-base balance also all affect renal phosphate handling.

REGULATORS OF BONE AND MINERAL METABOLISM

Parathyroid Hormone

Parathyroid hormone is an 84 amino acid polypeptide secreted by the parathyroid gland's chief cells in response to low serum calcium.[125] Its physiologic objective is to restore that low level to normal by stimulating all three organs of calcium homeostasis. The kidney and the bone are affected directly,[67, 87] whereas the intestine is affected only indirectly, by means of the synthesis of the active vitamin D metabolite $1,25(OH)_2$–vitamin D.

PTH promotes calcium conservation in the kidney.[92] There, increased serum calcium is achieved through a twofold mechanism; both steps depend on stimulation of adenylate cyclase, the enzyme that forms cyclic adenosine monophosphate (AMP). First, PTH increases calcium resorption in the distal nephron. In addition, it promotes the loss of phosphate. This phosphaturic effect prevents the recently resorbed calcium from being deposited into the bone hydroxyapatite or into ectopic calcium-phosphate deposits. Moreover, the excretion of phosphate lowers the levels of circulating calcium-anion complexes, causing more of the serum calcium to stand in the physiologically useful, ionic and diffusible form.

PTH also blocks the resorption of bicarbonate in the proximal nephron, thus causing a slight renal tubular acidosis. Although of slight magnitude, this hyperchloremic acidosis helps to raise the effective calcium concentration, because acidosis causes albumin binding of calcium to decrease. Also, the bone buffers acidosis directly by exchanging calcium in the matrix for protons from the circulation, leading to net increase in total serum calcium as well.

In the kidney, PTH further promotes elevation of calcium level by stimulating additional synthesis of 1α-hydroxylase, a key enzyme in the formation of active vitamin D, which in turn enhances calcium absorption in the digestive system. In this manner, PTH indirectly affects gut handling of calcium as well.

In the bone, PTH affects calcium metabolism by increasing the surface resorption of the mineral by osteoclasts, by promoting ion flux by osteocytes, and through the inhibition of calcium "consumption" by osteoblasts, by decreasing their bone synthetic activity. PTH increases the number of resorptive surfaces in bone and, within them, the density of osteoclasts. The precise mechanism of this osteoclastic action is unknown, because no receptors to the hormone have been detected on those cells. The osteoblast, conversely, does possess such receptors. It is postulated that PTH induces the osteoblast to produce a coupling agent, which stimulates osteoclastic bone resorption. Surprisingly, these catabolic effects are reversed at low, intermittent doses of PTH, after long-term administration. This delayed anabolic effect is consistent with the concept of the bone as calcium bank: responding to PTH, the bone first "lends" calcium to the plasma by augmenting resorption and then "collects" it back (presumably after dietary ingestion) by stimulating osteoblastic synthesis.

Vitamin D

Unlike the polypeptide hormone PTH, vitamin D is a steroid.[87] As such, it defies rapid proteolytic inactivation and thus functions best as a longer-acting regulator of calcium homeostasis. The principal effect of this hormone is to increase intestinal absorption of calcium from the diet, a process that is usually only 25 per cent efficient. Secondarily, it complements PTH in the promotion of calcium resorption from the bone, again by promoting transport across cell membranes (in this case, bone cells, not intestinal cells).

Cholecalciferol (inactive vitamin D_3) forms in the skin from the ultraviolet light activation of 7-dehydrocholesterol, an intermediate of cholesterol synthesis.[6a] 7-Dehydrocholesterol can degrade and re-form cholecalciferol; therefore, once formed, cholecalciferol is removed from the local environment by a transport protein to generate equilibrium pressure favoring its formation. As little as 15 minutes of sunlight exposure allows the synthesis of a fair-skinned individual's vitamin D_3 requirement; the total need for sunlight increases with melanin concentration. Cod liver oil and enriched milk can provide usable precursors of the hormone in the absence of sun exposure.

In the liver, vitamin D_3 undergoes 25-hydroxylation,[23] forming $25(OH)_2D_3$. 1-Hydroxylation of this prehormone to the active form, $1,25(OH)_2D_3$, takes place in the kidney, a reaction promoted by PTH. In the presence of low PTH, an alternative hydroxylation occurs at the 24 position, which yields $24,25(OH)_2D_3$, an inactive form of the hormone. Unlike PTH, which is functionally regulated at the level of secretion (calcium levels do not cause minute-to-minute changes in messenger RNA activity but rather control the release of PTH), vitamin D is regulated at the level of biosynthesis. The 1-hydroxylation reaction is the rate-limiting step; and it is regulated by feedback inhibition as well as by PTH levels.

Vitamin D, also known as calcitriol, promotes increased transport across cell borders. A steroid maturation hormone, such as vitamin D, works as follows: First it crosses the cell membrane; then it enters the nucleus. There it binds to DNA to promote its translation, thus increasing the synthesis of the target proteins. In this case specifically, vitamin D mediates increased expression of calcium-transport proteins, although the nucleic receptor has not yet been identified. In the gut, $1,25(OH)_2D_3$ causes increased calcium transport; additionally, phosphate absorption increases as well. In the bone, $1,25(OH)_2D_3$ complements the action of PTH by increasing calcium transport across bone cell membranes, thus assisting with the resorption of calcium from the bone and into the circulation. As such, it functions as an agent of bone resorption. But it can indirectly assist with bone formation as well, because the tasks of mineral homeostasis and skeletal homeostasis are not always at odds with each other. That is, calcium needs usually can be met through the diet, not by bone resorption. Vitamin D also functions as a maturation hormone by increasing the villous membrane of the gut and augments PTH recruitment of osteoclast for bone resorption by acting as a maturation hormone for the macrophage stem cells. Accordingly, vitamin D, which promotes the uptake of dietary calcium, typically also serves as an agent of bone maintenance.

Calcitonin

Calcitonin is a 32 amino acid polypeptide secreted by the parafollicular cells in the thyroid in response to rises in serum calcium concentrations. It works to lower serum calcium levels by actions in the bone and the kidney. Still, its precise physiologic role awaits determination.[52, 119]

In the bone, at pharmacologic doses, calcitonin rapidly inhibits osteoclastic action. Direct calcitonin-binding sites are present on osteoclasts. Calcitonin affects individual osteoclasts by decreasing their adherence to the resorptive surfaces and their activity once they adhere. Furthermore, calcitonin decreases not only the activity of osteoclasts but also their absolute numbers. The hormone affects osteocytes, causing decreased calcium ion flux across their cell membranes. In the kidney, calcitonin blocks the reuptake from the glomerular fluid of calcium and phosphate, as well as that of other ions, notably sodium (which influences calcium uptake by the passive mechanisms described earlier). In the gut,[1] calcitonin may influence calcium handling; in addition, other processes there (such as water balance) can be altered by pharmacologic doses.

In patients with medullary carcinoma of the thyroid (a malignancy of the parafollicular cells), calcitonin levels are many orders of magnitude higher than in healthy cohorts. Nevertheless, such patients demonstrate neither long-term derangements of calcium metabolism nor loss of skeletal integrity. This suggests a minor role, if one at all, for calcitonin in overall mineral homeostasis. (High levels of calcitonin may cause transient hypocalcemia, but the bone seemingly escapes that effect in a short time.) Furthermore, patients who have had a complete thyroidectomy, and are thus completely calcitonin-deficient, show no persistent hypercalcemia. Such evidence further bolsters the hypothesis of a small physiologic role for calcitonin.

Despite a perhaps minor physiologic role, calcitonin is very important medically. First, in patients with medullary carcinoma of the thyroid, measurement of serum calcitonin levels provides an assessment of tumor burden, much in the way that CEA-125 informs physicians about neoplasms of the colon. For example, changes in CEA-125 levels postoperatively may herald a recurrence long before it is clinically apparent. Similarly, calcitonin levels can be measured as a screening test in those patients at risk for medullary carcinoma, namely, relatives of patients with multiple endocrine neoplasia Type II. Finally, calcitonin (most often as a salmon-derived analogue) is also used as a drug to inhibit osteoclasts, as in Paget's disease and osteoporosis, or to quell the hypercalcemia accompanying a variety of malignancies. In addition, it has analgesic properties that enhance its therapeutic use.

Estrogen

The bone-regulating effects of estrogen[72] have been known clinically for many years: pathologic fractures were long associated with menopause.[100] We now know that estrogen-deficient patients have a decreased bone mass due to increased resorption of bone. We further know that the skeletal effects of menopause or castration can be mitigated by pharmacologic administration of estrogen.[59] Nevertheless, the precise mechanism for these phenomena still has not been elucidated.

Several investigators have demonstrated that a limited number of estrogen-binding sites are on osteoblasts as well as osteoclasts.[32] Other evidence suggests that the effect of estrogen may be, in part, indirect. Putative intermediates include PTH, vitamin D, and calcitonin. Because laboratory animals that are deficient in estrogen show increased bone resorption on PTH stimulation, it is thought that this hormone may underlie the sex steroid effect.[66] Similarly, because menopausal women absorb calcium from the diet less efficiently than those still menstruating, vitamin D might play a major role in bringing about the metabolic consequences of estrogen deficiency. Confounding the investigation into the role of estrogen is the interplay of the suspected participants: PTH levels are affected by vitamin D activity, and vice versa. Adding still further to the confusion is the finding that calcitonin levels are lowered by estrogen deficiency. Despite this complex interplay of potential participants, the net effect of estrogen is to inhibit bone resorption. Its decline at menopause ushers in a rapid bone loss. Owing to the increased metabolic rate of cancellous bone, this loss is greater in trabecular bones. Thus, the spine is particularly vulnerable in the estrogen-deficient state.

Corticosteroids

Glucocorticoids, used over prolonged periods, decrease the individual's bone mass.[42, 46] They achieve this undesirable effect by blocking bone formation and promoting its dissolution. Glucocorticoids disrupt the normal reactive bone synthesis occurring during remodeling and inhibit the intestinal effects of vitamin D. Indeed, patients on chronic steroid therapy excrete fractionally more calcium in their feces than untreated individuals.[96] Because the mechanism of steroid action is by nuclear modifications, a possible explanation of the vitamin D–blocking effect is that it works through inhibition of calcium-transport protein synthesis or the blockade of intestinal villus maturation. Steroids also increase urinary excretion of calcium.

Osteoblasts have receptors to glucocorticoids; the steroid binds to the osteoblast, enters the nucleus, and alters its normal, bone-forming apparatus. It thus has a direct effect on these bone-making cells by inhibiting collagen synthesis. By blocking calcium uptake, it causes a reactive hyperparathyroidism, which further undermines skeletal integrity. Still, because there is less organic matrix formed, this reactive hyperparathyroidism does not lead to noticeable defective mineralization (osteomalacia); the proportion of mineral to matrix is relatively normal, because both are depressed.

The steroid-induced bone loss is not reserved for only patients taking it pharmacologically. High levels of endogenously produced glucocorticoids, as in Cushing's syndrome, impede bone formation, especially in trabecular regions. Thus, cushingoid patients have, among all else, a propensity for vertebral compression fractures. Internal spine (as well as in the ribs and pelvis) crush fractures due to steroid-caused bone loss form a pseudocallus, a hyperdense but failed attempt at normal healing. These lead to well-known radiographic changes and are deemed specific to this condition.

Thyroid Hormones

Excess thyroxine leads to hypermetabolic states. In the bone, this is seen as an increase in both bone formation and resorption. On the whole, however, hyperthyroidism causes decreased bone mass,[2] because there is an additional stimulatory effect on resorption alone. In direct contrast to calcitonin, iatrogenic hyperthyroidism is common with thyroid supplementation and can lead to osteopenia,[84] which decreases both the absolute number of osteoclasts and their activity, thyroxine stimulates both the activity and proliferation of osteoclasts. The mechanism of action of thyroxine rests on an increase in cytosolic cyclic AMP. This augmentation permits an especially potent response to circulating PTH; but because hyperthyroidism can lead to hypercalcemia, and thus low circulating PTH, this action must be independent of the hormone. Unlike corticosteroids, thyroxine does not cause a permanent loss of bone mass; once the primary disorder is contained, its skeletal manifestations abate. This is true for the hypercalcemia that may ensue from high levels of thyroid function as well.

Prostaglandins and Other Local Factors

Prostaglandins, the cyclooxygenase products of arachidonic acid metabolism, are implicated in an ever-growing list of biologic processes. One of the earliest entries on that list was bone metabolism. The prostaglandin E line is made by osteoblasts and has an effect on bone similar to that of PTH: it elevates intracellular cyclic AMP and thus stimulates the resorption of bone. Chambers and colleagues[19] found that isolated osteoclasts do not resorb bone in response to prostaglandins. This finding implies that the observed osteolytic response to prostaglandins involves either other cells or additional signals.

Unlike PTH and some other regulators of bone resorption, prostaglandins are produced locally, in proximity to the cells on which they act. This is balanced, in part, by their short half-life. One case in which their effect might be at a greater distance is malignancy. Some neoplasms, such as hypernephroma, are known to destroy bone by a mechanism different from direct invasion into the tissue. In these cases, the osteolysis might ensue from a prostaglandin effect: the tumor produces a prostaglandin-like substance, which then dissolves the bone.

Growth factors,[17, 31] like prostaglandins, also work across short distances. These polypeptides, stored in the organic matrix, profoundly influence cell replication and differentiation. These factors originate in both the bone cells themselves and from adjacent tissues. Transforming growth factor-β is one that is made within bone cells,[113] and it is both mitogenic and stimulatory on osteoblasts; that is, it instructs the osteoblast to proliferate and thereafter to increase its synthetic activity. Bone-derived growth factor (BDGF) and platelet-derived growth factor (PDGF) are others synthesized by bone cells. BDGF stimulates DNA and collagen synthesis, too, and might modulate the effects of other factors by receptor interaction. PDGF is synthesized primarily by platelets but also by bone cells. Like the others, it stimulates DNA and matrix synthesis within the osteoblast. Its particular significance might be in the healing of fractures, when many platelets aggregate and release it. BMP is now considered the primary bone differentiation factor.[29, 31]

Another important class of local regulators is that made not by bone cells but rather by cells nearby. In this category are interleukins[71] and cachectins. These macrophage-derived factors have a wide spectrum of effects. Interleukin-1 stimulates bone resorption as well as bone formation. Cachectin, like interleukin-1, stimulates bone resorption. Additionally, it promotes osteoblast replication, but it can also inhibit collagen synthesis. These factors might work not only by a direct effect but also by stimulating the synthesis and release of still other factors.

Electrical and Mechanical Forces

Wolff's law that bone will grow by appositional growth in areas of increased stress implies the existence of some factor or process that can translate a mechanical signal into an osteoinductive one. That coupling factor might be locally generated electrical potentials.

When bone is compressed, the surfaces directly receiving the forces develop an electronegative potential with respect to the remaining bone.[5] This voltage arises from a strain on the organic matrix (most likely the highly organized collagen fibrils). This electronegativity, in turn, stimulates osteogenesis.[11] Furthermore, in all bones undergoing modeling the regions actively synthesizing bone become electronegative by dint of that metabolic activity alone. Thus, the original signal from a stress force is amplified: the primary signal (electronegativity) becomes translated into a process (osteogenesis), which yields as a byproduct more of the signal and perpetuates the process.

At the osteoblast level, electronegativity stimulates proteoglycan synthesis (which, as described, has a regulatory effect itself) and may also promote collagen biosynthesis and alkaline phosphatase activity. Accordingly, electrical phenomena might underlie the skeletal benefits of impact exercise[31]: impact loading and other movements like it create stresses in the bone, which in turn create potential differences and thus stimulate osteogenesis. Persons who exercise retard the normal tendency to lose bone by inducing their osteoblasts to make more bone.

OSTEOPOROSIS

Osteoporosis is a condition of reduced bone mass and impaired skeletal function.[67, 83] Affecting as many as 15 to 20 million people in the United States, osteoporosis is the most prevalent metabolic bone disease.[85] Its toll on health care spending was measured at billions of dollars in 1992, a figure sure to rise with the expanding elderly population. In postmenopausal women and in the elderly, osteoporosis is a major underlying cause of pathologic fractures. At least 1.2 million fractures each year are attributable to the disease, and almost half of these occur in the spine. Moreover, one third of all American women older than 65 years of age suffer vertebral fractures.[100]

Like all metabolic bone diseases, osteoporosis is not limited to the spine. In addition to the annual 538,000 vertebral fractures caused by osteoporosis, the disease claims 200,000 hip fractures and 172,000 Colles' fractures.[59] In the elderly, hip fractures, most due to osteoporosis, result in death, disability, and dependency: the mortality rate of older patients with hip fractures can be as much as 20 per cent higher than in persons of similar age[37]; up to 50 per cent require long-term nursing home care, and fewer than 30 per cent return to a life style comparable to their prefracture state.[81]

The National Institutes of Health (NIH) Consensus Conference defined primary osteoporosis as an age-related disorder characterized by decreased bone mass and increased susceptibility to fractures in the absence of other recognizable causes of bone loss.[85] (Similar bone loss in the presence of a precipitating cause is termed *secondary osteoporosis*.) Several risk factors for osteoporosis have been identified. A typical patient is a slim, white, postmenopausal woman of northwestern European descent.[21] She may have a history of premature menopause, cigarette or heavy alcohol use,[83] a sedentary life style, use of anticonvulsants,[51] or poor calcium intake. Seventy-five per cent of women with scoliosis older than 65 years of age have at least one osteopenic wedge fracture.[47]

Clinically, one sees fractures of the vertebral bodies and of the extremities. Radiographically, osteopenia is evident; there is a "washed-out" skeletal appearance, with attenuation of the horizontal trabecular pattern. Although primary osteoporosis is a common cause of osteopenia in the elderly, it is only one in a spectrum of causes. The clinician must consider endocrinopathies, neoplastic and hematologic diseases, disturbances of the bone's organic matrix, mechanical disuse or immobilization, nutritional deficiencies, and perturbations of vitamin D metabolism. These conditions must be ruled out before a diagnosis of primary osteoporosis can be made.

Pathology

Osteoporosis is a disease of decreased bone mass in the absence of mineralization defect. It is a disease of lost bone mass; the bone that remains contains a normal matrix and a normal degree of calcification. Declining bone mass is now thought to be a universal phenomenon of aging.[25] Peak bone mass is attained in the mid 30s for both sexes. Gender, nutrition, race, exercise habits, and overall health all influence bone mass. It is 30 per cent higher in men than in women and 10 per cent higher in blacks than in whites.[85] After the fourth decade, all people lose bone mass from the skeleton (Fig. 40–3). Two phases of this loss have been identified: slow and accelerated. The slow phase, related to the inexact balance between resorption and formation leading to negative calcium balance, is equal in both men and women. It results in an annual loss of 0.3 per cent bone volume.[75] The accelerated phase, a phenomenon found in women exclusively, is responsible for a bone mass loss of 2 to 3 per cent per year. This loss is on top of the slow phase losses, which continue during the accelerated phase. The accelerated phase begins after surgical or natural menopause and lasts for 6 to 10 years.[108] Thereafter, bone loss continues at the basal slow phase rate of 0.3 to 0.5 per cent. Multiple studies have shown the importance of estrogen deficiency in the causation of the accelerated phase.[62, 98]

The spine is composed of primarily trabecular bone. Compared with cortical bone, it has a high surface-to-volume ratio. Because metabolic activity (remodeling) occurs on bone surfaces, trabecular bones in general

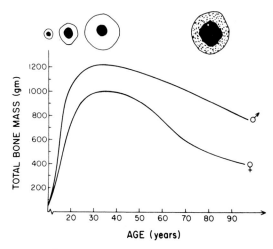

Figure 40–3. Bone mass as a function of age in men and women. (Disorders of Bone 9. Orthop. Science. Park Ridge, IL, AAOS, 1986.)

and the vertebral bodies in particular are resorbed preferentially in times of skeletal loss.[102] Osteoporosis is thus characterized by trabeculae of decreased size and number. Work by Dempster and others has demonstrated in osteoporosis that there is a thinning of the cortex as well as a change in the shape of the trabecular bone from plates to narrow bars.[29] Within the trabecular bone these are areas where osteoclasts have created a loss of connectivity of the trabecular bone, leading to a significant weakening of the bone in that local area.[24, 29] In the phases of bone loss, vertebral body density declines before a similar loss is detected in cortical areas. The body accommodates bone loss by redistribution. As people grow older the diameter of the long bones gradually increases both in women and in men. Concurrently, the medullary diameter also increases, leading to a net thinning of the cortical bone. A 10 per cent shift of bone mass outward from the epicenter through an enlargement of the bone diameter will compensate for a 30 per cent decrease in the bone mass against applied bending and torque stresses but not against axial loading. This differential resorption explains the timing and patterns of the fracture syndromes seen in osteoporosis.[100] The incidence of vertebral crush fractures rises immediately after menopause, whereas the hip (with its higher proportion of cortical bone) fractures later in life, when cortical bone loss accumulates over one or two additional decades. The distal forearm, like the spine, has a high trabecular content, so Colles' fractures are also seen closer to menopause.

Riggs and Melton[101] have subclassified primary osteoporosis based on these patterns of bone loss and fracture (Table 40–1). Type I or postmenopausal osteoporosis occurs in women aged 51 to 65 years, involves areas of predominantly trabecular bone, and is characterized by vertebral and Colles' fractures. Estrogen plays a primary role in the causation of Type I osteoporosis. In contrast, Type II osteoporosis, known also as senile osteoporosis, occurs in both men and women aged 75 years and older and involves areas of predominantly cortical bone. Clinically, fractures of the hip, pelvis, proximal humerus, and proximal tibia are seen. The causes of senile osteoporosis are the aging process itself and chronic calcium deficiency. Senile osteoporosis may also involve decreased vitamin D and increased PTH activity or impaired bone formation. Osteoporosis in patients between the ages of 66 and 74 years may represent a combination of these two syndromes.

Table 40–1. TYPE I VERSUS TYPE II OSTEOPOROSIS

	Type I	Type II
Female-male ratio	6 : 1	2 : 1
Calcium deficiency	No	Yes
Estrogen deficiency	Yes	No
Fractures	Spine	Spine Appendicular

Because bone loss is considered to be a universal phenomenon of aging, peak bone density might determine which patients develop clinically significant osteoporosis. The rationale is that individuals with more bone mass before the bone-losing phases can endure much greater negative bone balance before fractures occur. The peak bone mass an individual attains depends on many facts. Studies of twins showed greater concordance of radial bone density between identical as compared with dizygotic twins, thus implying a genetic influence.[112] Additionally, deficiencies in dietary calcium have been demonstrated to cause decreased peak bone mass.[73] White women on average have less bone than either white men or blacks of either sex.[69] Thus, the risk of clinically significant osteoporosis depends on hereditary factors, gender, race, and nutrition, which are responsible for peak bone mass as well as aging, which causes progressive bone loss. Although the formation of good bone in sufficient quantity in young adulthood is no doubt important, it is the aging process that remains the most important cause of involutional osteoporosis.

Aging leads to bone loss independent of menopause, but the rapid subtraction of skeletal mass after estrogen deficiency implies that this hormone prevents the dissolution of the skeleton.[80] Nonetheless, its precise mechanism is unclear. Some investigators believe that the action is mediated by estrogen receptors on osteoblasts.[32] Others contend that estrogen antagonizes PTH activity[66] or that it stimulates endogenous calcitonin release. Decreased calcitonin levels have been found in oophorectomized and postmenopausal patients, and increased calcitonin levels are noted after estrogen administration. Regardless of the mechanism, estrogen deficiency leads to bone loss and plays a major role in the pathogenesis of Type I osteoporosis: in a state of estrogen deficiency, the body loses 2 to 3 per cent of its total bone mass per year for up to 10 years after menopause.

The age-related ("slow phase") bone loss is not dependent on estrogen. Rather, it probably represents impaired vitamin D metabolism. As an individual ages, the kidney slowly loses its ability to hydroxylate vitamin D into its active form, $1,25(OH)_2$–vitamin D.[120] This active vitamin D is needed to transport calcium in the gut; therefore, decreased hydroxylation, often coupled with poor dietary intake, leads to lowered serum calcium levels and, in turn, to elevated parathyroid secretion of PTH. Beyond secondary hyperparathyroidism, older people are usually more likely to take drugs (such as diuretics) that cause calcium losses. Also, there is some evidence that the mechanism in remodeling that couples the action of osteoclasts to that of osteoblasts functions suboptimally in old age: after the fourth decade, at a given site of remodeling, less bone is laid down than is resorbed.[69] Accordingly, normal bone turnover in the elderly leads to calcium depletion as well.

Life style, too, can influence the risk of becoming osteoporotic. Cigarette smokers have greater bone loss and more frequently fracture their hips and vertebral bodies than do nonsmokers.[27] This effect might be due to increased estrogen degradation in smokers.[32] Similarly, heavy alcohol consumers have decreased bone density in the iliac crest,[51] femoral neck, and vertebral bodies relative to nondrinkers of the same demographics.[108] Alcohol is believed to directly suppress osteoblasts,[8] blocking the body's ability to compensate for normal turnover losses. The presence of other illnesses, such as renal failure or hepatic disease, or the use of many medications, especially steroids, likewise adds to the risk. Impact exercise protects against bone loss[64]; this protection is often lost in old age, when people become even more sedentary. Young women who develop amenorrhea due to chronic high levels of exercise suffer bone loss far beyond that of individuals who do not exercise yet maintain normal menstrual cycles.[36] Excess body fat, perhaps surprisingly, reduces the relative risk of osteoporosis. This benefit results from either a stimulatory effect on the bones produced by weight loading or perhaps by peripheral production of estrogens in the adipose tissue.

Clinical Course

End-stage osteoporosis culminates in fracture.[58, 67, 83] Still, for most of its course osteoporosis is a silently progressive disease. It typically comes to the attention of a physician, usually late in its course, in one of a limited number of ways. First, the patient may present with an acute painful fracture, usually of the spine (Fig. 40–4) but also of the rib, wrist, or hip. In the spine, normal activity (or barely any at all) may exceed the depleted bones' stress tolerance and lead to fracture. The acute fracture can be severely painful, with the pain remaining over the affected area or radiating across the thorax. The pain from a vertebral fracture does not radiate down the legs. Symptoms such as leg pain that suggest involvement of the spinal cord obligate the physician to search for another or concomitant process to explain the complaint. Osteoporosis, even if established in that case, is probably not the only disease present. The acute pain usually abates when the fracture heals. Nonetheless, the patient rarely returns to the pre-event status. At a minimum, there may be point tenderness over the fracture site. The patient may note constant abdominal pain, often brought about by the constraining forces on the viscera in the now smaller abdominal cavity. Other patients complain of generalized backache. The backache may be due to changing muscular demands brought on by altered spinal curvature. Furthermore, some patients, out of fear of reinjury, strictly limit their activities. Others develop chronic pain syndromes, dysthymic states, or even overt clinical depression. Osteoporosis, therefore, often has a profound effect on the patient's life beyond the acute fracture episode.

Not every patient has an acute episode. Alternatively, an asymptomatic thoracic wedge or lumbar compression fracture of the spine may be noted on a radiographic examination performed for an unrelated purpose. These compression fractures may present subacutely, with twinge pain noted on minimal strain or exercise over a period of time, or the patient may even have no complaints at all. The macroscopic fracture observed on radiography, then, represents integration over time of a series of small, individually insignificant microfractures.

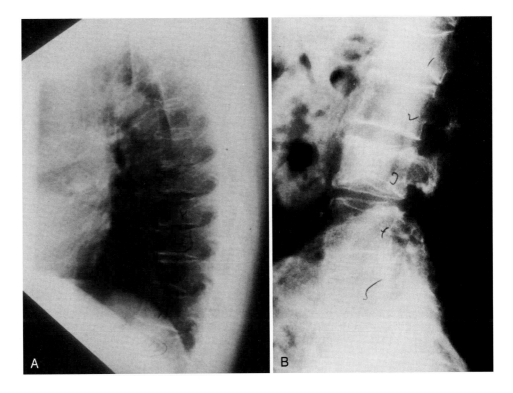

Figure 40–4. Spinal fractures associated with osteoporosis. *A,* Thoracic wedge fracture. *B,* Lumbar crush fracture.

In the thoracic spine, both asymptomatic and painful fractures have a predilection for the anterior aspect of the bone. Progressive fracture thus leads to progressive shortening of the anterior height of the vertebral body relative to the posterior. The resultant shape of the body suggests the name of this process: wedge fracture. The wedge shape of the body, when summed over two or more vertebrae, causes dorsal kyphosis. In the lumbar region, the fractures are distributed equally throughout the vertebral body; no wedge is formed, and the process is thus termed *compression* or *collapse fracture*. The combined effects of compression and wedge fractures lead to an unfortunate but frequent skeletal deformity: lost height coupled with excessive dorsal kyphosis. A vertebral body deformation due to an osteoporotic fracture can be difficult to determine. The technique of Genant requires a 25 per cent change in one dimension or a 40 per cent change in total cross section.[117]

Finally, generalized osteopenia without fracture may be noted on plain radiographs. This is not a different disease but an earlier phase of the same process that leads to fracture and deformity. These patients are merely those who suffer from bone loss but who have not yet crossed the critical point of stress tolerance.

By the time any one of these three scenarios comes to pass, the patient has lost a significant amount of bone. The physician must discover two things: (1) what caused this bone loss and (2) how much bone remains. Because primary osteoporosis is a diagnosis of exclusion, the other causes of osteopenia must be ruled out. The differential diagnosis includes endocrine disease, neoplasms, disturbances of either the bone's two matrices or the marrow, osteomalacia, and drug or mechanical effects. The medical history is used explicitly to discover risk factors for these disorders or for primary osteoporosis itself. Beyond the medical interview, two diagnostic modalities may be employed. Invasive tests, including blood tests but possibly bone biopsy as well, best answer the question of the cause of the osteopenia. The noninvasive tests, once the diagnosis is secured, establish the extent of the disease.

Diagnosis

The sine qua non for the diagnosis of osteoporosis is osteopenia (see later for determination). Accordingly, the diagnostic work-up of osteoporosis follows recognition of osteopenia, often on plain radiographs or by densitometry. Diagnostic studies then move on to laboratory tests. The common blood tests comprise a complete blood cell count; sedimentation rate; serum protein electrophoresis; measurements of serum glucose, alkaline phosphatase, calcium, phosphate, and blood urea nitrogen; thyroid function tests; and quantitation of 25(OH)–vitamin D and PTH. Twenty-four-hour urine specimens can be assayed for collagen breakdown products (pyrodinoline and N-telopeptides) and calcium, phosphate, and creatinine levels. They also may be tested for the presence of Bence Jones

proteins, which are the immunoglobins excreted in multiple myeloma.[67, 83]

Currently, the best markers for bone formation are bone-specific alkaline phosphatase and osteocalcin; for bone resorption, the markers are pyrodinoline, deoxypyrodinoline, and N-telopeptides.[105] Normal results from the complete blood cell count, sedimentation rate, and serum electrophoresis effectively rule out a myelophthisic cause of the osteopenia. If these test results are abnormal, a hematologic disorder is suggested and a bone marrow biopsy is indicated. In the documented absence of a malignancy, the clinician should then measure PTH, glucose, and cortisol levels and assess thyroid function (thyroid-stimulating hormone) to rule out an endocrinopathy. Bone biopsies are indicated in individuals younger than 60 years of age who are 2.5 to 3.0 standard deviations (SDs) below their peers in bone density, individuals younger than the age of 65 who sustain low-energy fractures without apparent metabolic abnormalities, and patients with complex medical problems and osteoporosis. For patients without an endocrinologic or hematologic abnormality, the differential diagnosis of osteopenia is essentially limited to osteomalacia (defective mineralization) versus osteoporosis (lost bone mass). Low serum phosphate or high serum alkaline phosphatase levels suggest osteomalacia; but after fracture in osteoporosis, the repair process might cause an elevation of the alkaline phosphatase levels in patients with no mineralization defect. Measurements of 25(OH)–vitamin D_3 also can assist in the differentiation, but older people may have low levels of active hormone (without defective mineralization) merely as a function of age. Often in osteoporosis the laboratory values are all within normal limits. Still, there is sufficient overlap between those values seen in osteomalacia that serum tests can at best only suggest the pathophysiology underlying the osteopenia. Should the physician demand a definitive diagnosis, a transilial biopsy may be needed. Only undecalcified iliac bone specimens subjected to histomorphometry can qualify and quantitate bone formation, resorption, and mineralization.

The transilial bone biopsy[67] allows the histopathologist to examine a core of bone (often taken from a region near the anterior superior iliac crest), from which he or she can observe and measure bone volume, the extent of mineralization, and the approximate rate of bone turnover. The histopathologist is not looking for tissue markers of osteoporosis—there are none—but rather wishes to document the absence of mineralization pathology, namely, osteomalacia. Even under the microscope, primary osteoporosis is a diagnosis of exclusion: the patient with osteopenia and normal laboratory studies who has been proved free of osteomalacia has osteoporosis.

Although there are no pathognomonic findings of osteoporosis on bone biopsy, these specimens are not entirely normal either. For example, trabecular bone volume is lower in this population. Other osteoporotic patients have altered rates of bone resorption or formation. Many show regions of decreased trabecular density; within these or normal regions, the trabeculae are of decreased size. Most important, these patients do not have pathologic osteoid measurements suggestive of osteomalacia, or any findings characteristic of other metabolic bone disease, such as the tunneling resorption seen in hyperparathyroidism. Quantitative histomorphometry should place the patient into the class of high-turnover osteoporosis with increased osteoclastic resorption or low-turnover osteoporosis with decreased osteoblastic bone formation.

The bone biopsy coupled with laboratory tests (the combined invasive approach) serves well to identify the cause of osteopenia. To measure it accurately, non-invasive measures work best. Quantitative analysis helps physicians determine response to therapy, as well as offering prognostic indicators in those cases in which the quantitative loss has not yet been translated into a qualitative, that is, clinically apparent, one.

Noninvasive, quantitative bone density determinations are of greatest value in conditions in which there is a quantitative decrease in bone mass without a qualitative defect, as in osteoporosis. Several radiologic methods are available today for the noninvasive evaluation of bone mineral content.[106] Each of these modalities is useful for measuring specific skeletal sites and specific types of bone. This is important to keep in mind for two reasons. First, trabecular bone, with its higher metabolic activity and turnover, may be a more sensitive site for measuring changes in bone mineral content. In addition, there is a poor correlation between measurements of bone mineral density of the appendicular and axial skeleton.[107] Thus, the assessment of fracture risk at a particular site is best achieved by direct measurements of that site, rather than from extrapolation from a different site.[76] Thus, spinal fracture risk is best predicted from noninvasive studies of the spine.

Techniques are available to quantify bone mass using simple radiographs. Radiogrammetry measures the thickness of the cortex of metacarpal or other tubular bones on standard anteroposterior radiographs of the hand. This study is widely available and easy to perform but does not reflect absolute bone mineral content or intracortical porosity. Radiogrammetry has mainly been applied to the appendicular skeleton and provides information only on relative changes in bone volume. Radiographic photodensitometry attempts to estimate bone mass by measuring the optical density of the bone image on a standard radiograph, thereby indirectly measuring bone mineral content. This technique is limited by the inability to correct for soft tissue thickness. Finally, although decreased radiodensity with attenuation of the horizontal trabecular pattern on plain radiographs may suggest osteopenia, up to 40 per cent of skeletal bone mass may be lost before this finding becomes evident.[57]

Single-energy photon absorptiometry (SPA) makes use of the difference in photon absorption between bone and soft tissue to determine bone mineral content. It is usually performed on the radius or calcaneus and measures the mineral content of the appendicular

skeleton. The radiation dose is small (2 to 5 mrad), and precision (3 to 5 per cent) and reliability (1 to 4 per cent) are good.[60] Limitations of this technique include reliance on exact positioning of the examination site during sequential studies; the fact that cortical bone is measured, which may be less sensitive to metabolic changes than trabecular bone; and the fact that mineral content of the radius or calcaneus may not accurately reflect mineral content in the spine and proximal femur, as noted earlier. Specific juxtawrist sites are richer in trabecular bone but have lower precision and are still under investigation.

Dual-photon absorptiometry (DPA) is a modification of SPA that uses a radioisotope that emits photons at two energy levels. This modification eliminates the need for constant soft tissue density (which SPA requires), thereby allowing use in the spine and proximal femur. It incorporates the total of both cortical and trabecular bone into a single measurement. Radiation dosage is low (5 to 15 mrad), and precision (1 to 3 per cent) and reliability (4 to 6 per cent) are good. Because this technique directly measures the femoral neck and spine, it is a more reliable predictor of risk of fracture at these sites than SPA. Limitations of this method include the possibility of falsely elevated values in patients with scoliosis, compression fractures, and extraosseous calcifications such as from osteophytes, degenerative changes, and vascular calcifications. In addition, DPA cannot independently evaluate high-turnover cancellous bone; both cortical and trabecular bone density values are included in the measurement. Finally, the gallium energy source decays appreciably with time, leading to potential problems in long-term studies. Dual-beam x-ray (DXA), using a new energy source vehicle, obviates this problem while at the same time improving precision (1 per cent) and decreasing radiation dose (5 to 10 mrad). DXA has become the method of choice for determining and observing bone mass not only for the spine but also for the hip (3 to 4 per cent precision).

Computed tomography may also be used to measure bone mineral density. The midportion of the vertebral bodies is scanned, and total, cortical, or trabecular bone mineral density can be calculated.[109] Radiation doses (200 to 250 mrad) are ten times higher, and reliability (4 to 10 per cent) and precision (3 to 15 per cent) are inferior to those with DXA. The advantage of this technique is that it allows evaluation of isolated trabecular bone, which may be a more sensitive indicator of change in bone mineral content. Limitations of this technique include higher cost and radiation dose, poorer reliability and precision, and underestimation of trabecular bone in elderly patients with fat replacement of the bone marrow; its use at present is limited to larger centers.

A new method centered on ultrasound is now becoming available. It offers a measurement of bone mass and connectivity. Currently its limitations rest with its wider precision and measurement of a bone (calcaneus) far from the hip and spine.

The rationale for the use of quantitative bone density determinations centers on the ability of these studies to predict which patients are at high risk for sustaining fractures. However, there are many factors that determine whether a fracture will occur. These include, but are not limited to, the structural geometry as well as the density of the bone, the force (magnitude and direction) of the insult, and the ability of the soft tissues to absorb the trauma. Quantitative bone density measurements evaluate only one of these factors. In spite of this limitation, studies have demonstrated a significant correlation between bone mineral density and fracture risk,[53] and a fracture threshold of 1.0 gm/cm^2 has been described, with 90 per cent of nontraumatic vertebral fractures occurring in patients with a bone mineral density below this level. However, a significant overlap between diseased and healthy populations has been noted at the Hospital for Special Surgery Metabolic Bone Disease Unit, rendering bone mineral density measurements of limited value in predicting which specific individuals will sustain fractures. Having mentioned these limitations, it is important to point out that we have found quantitative bone mineral density values very useful in determining those patients at increased risk of fracture and for longitudinally following the efficacy of therapeutic intervention. Fifty-year-old women with bone density measurements 1 SD below those of their peers have a 30% fracture rate, and women with measurements 2.5 SD below those of their peers have a 60% lifetime fracture rate.[58] The World Health Organization has defined bone status based on peak bone mass. Individuals within 1 SD of peak bone mass are normal; between 1.5 SD and 2.4 SD, below the mean, osteopenic; lower than −2.5 SD, osteoporotic; and severely osteoporotic if they also have a low-energy fracture.

Treatment and Prevention

Therapy in osteoporosis defies easy categorization. For one thing, the disease is heterogeneous, with multiple causes. Moreover, many patients—even those with significant osteopenia—are symptom-free. And those symptoms that do present, such as fracture pain, might abate even in the absence of intervention. This obviously limits the measurement of a given regimen's efficacy: if both valid and invalid therapies relieve symptoms, then they cannot be distinguished on that basis. Therefore, the treatment of osteoporosis is both complex and controversial. However, one aspect of therapy that is clear is that all patients likely to develop the disease as well as those currently afflicted would do well to remove all risk factors from their lives. Notably, those patients who smoke cigarettes or have heavy alcohol intake should be strongly encouraged to stop. As discussed earlier, these two habits are clearly detrimental to bone mass, as well as health in general. Concurrent illness that erodes skeletal integrity must be recognized and treated. Medicines that induce bone loss must be used carefully and judiciously. And clearly, nutritional influence should not be ignored either.

Prevention and therapy of osteoporosis go hand in hand (Table 40–2). The end point of both is to endow or replete the patient with sufficient bone mass to avoid fracture. The amount of bone mass in an individual is a function of the starting bone mass, as well as the rate and duration of its loss. Therapy and prevention of osteoporosis, therefore, point at increasing bone mass and delaying the onset of bone loss and, finally, curtailing its rate. Therapy can be viewed in this context as a reversal of prior loss tied to prevention of further loss. The result of that approach will give the treated individual a greater bone mass and a lower risk of fracture at any given time relative to an untreated one.

Exercise

A comprehensive general rehabilitation program that stresses spine extension and abdominal strengthening exercises without flexion, as well as impact-loading activities such as walking, should be part of all treatment plans for osteoporotic patients. Prospective studies have demonstrated that one hour of exercise two or three times per week can increase both bone mineral content in the lumbar spine and total body calcium in postmenopausal women. Conversely, sedentary control subjects in both studies continued to lose bone and have an increased risk for hip fracture.[26] Other studies have found a significant correlation between muscle mass and bone mass,[67] suggesting that increased skeletal loading leads to increased bone mass. Furthermore,

Table 40–2. PROTOCOL TO TREAT OSTEOPOROSIS

Patient Category	Treatment
Premenopausal, age 13–25	Elemental calcium, 1200–1500 mg/day Vitamin D (400–800 IU/day)
Premenopausal, age 25 or older	Elemental calcium, 1000 mg/day Vitamin D (400–800 IU/day)
Pregnant and nursing	Elemental calcium, 1200–1500 mg/day Vitamin D (400–800 IU/day)

Postmenopausal	Elemental calcium
	    1000 mg/day (on estrogen)
	    1500 mg/day (off estrogen)
	Vitamin D (400–800 IU/day)
	
	Estrogen (conjugated)
	                        + Progestin
	    (nonconjugated)
	        or
	Raloxifene, 60 mg/day
	    (wait 5 years after menopause)
	        or
	Alendronate
	    5 mg/day—DXA 0–2.0 SD below peak
	    10 mg/day—DXA > 2.0 SD below peak
	        or
	Nasal calcitonin, 1 spray (200 units) per day

it is known that immobilization leads to increased bone resorption[30, 32] and that astronauts in space with decreased mechanical loading lose bone.

These data suggest that exercise is beneficial in maintaining bone mass. Therefore, conservative management of osteoporotic patients should include an exercise program to minimize the effects of the more sedentary life style that the elderly are more likely to lead. Of course, the prescribing physician should tailor the exercise regimen to the patient's overall fitness, most specifically the cardiac tolerance. Accordingly, exercises that deliver high impact for a given aerobic effort, such as walking, are preferable to those, such as swimming, that have little effect. Young women, however, who become amenorrheic due to chronic high levels of exercise suffer bone loss far beyond that of individuals who do not exercise yet maintain a normal menstrual cycle.[36]

Falls increase the risk for osteoporotic fractures. Consequently, fall prevention programs are beneficial. Of all the interventions, tai chi appears to be most effective in decreasing falls (47 per cent).

Calcium

The role of calcium supplementation in the treatment of osteoporosis remains controversial. Evidence as to its benefit has been controversial, while the amount of money spent on calcium preparations in the United States has risen dramatically. One study suggested that the average woman does not ingest enough calcium in her diet to achieve a net neutral calcium balance.[83] This study concluded that 1.2 g per day of elemental calcium was necessary to prevent net calcium decline in this premenopausal population. In addition, a specific transmenopausal deterioration in calcium balance performance has been described, resulting in an average requirement of 1.5 g of elemental calcium daily after menopause.

Despite this body of data suggesting that most women have a calcium-deficient diet, the protective effects of calcium on bone loss remain unproved. Data that suggested that 1.5 g of calcium daily decreased bone loss have been contradicted by two prospective studies that failed to demonstrate that calcium (1.5 g daily in one study, 2.0 g in the other) prevented significant bone loss in the early postmenopausal period.[33, 103]

Data collected at the Osteoporosis Center at the Hospital for Special Surgery demonstrate not only the protective effects of calcium on overall skeletal bone loss but also its ability to increase femoral bone mass. The patients in this study group were placed on 1500 mg of calcium and 800 U of vitamin D daily, as well as an exercise program. The patients were divided into three groups: premenopausal, early postmenopausal (0 to 15 years status postmenopause), and late postmenopausal (more than 15 years). Bone mass was evaluated using dual-photon absorptiometry in the spine and proximal femur.

Calcium therapy was clearly shown to have beneficial effects in the proximal femur at all ages studied, increasing bone mass by 3 to 5 per cent in the first year of treatment. In the spine, where a 0.3 to 0.5 per cent loss is expected in the premenopausal population, calcium was shown to prevent that bone loss and to increase bone mass slightly in the late postmenopausal population. The 2.2 per cent annual bone loss observed in the early postmenopausal patients is consistent with that expected in an untreated group; that is, in this group calcium was no help. This suggests that in the early postmenopausal period of rapid bone loss, the effects of estrogen deficiency far outweigh those of calcium supplementation. Although these results may not be the definitive word on the subject, they provide strong evidence for the use of calcium in all patients with osteoporosis or at risk for it, in the absence of any contraindication. Therefore, all premenopausal women at risk for osteoporosis should receive 1200 mg of elemental calcium daily in diet and supplement, and postmenopausal women similarly at risk should ingest 1500 mg of calcium daily. Addition of 400 to 800 units of vitamin D daily in the form of a multivitamin is likewise advised; vitamin D is especially important in the elderly population because of their impaired metabolism of this vitamin to its active metabolite. A study in France demonstrated that low replacement calcium and vitamin D reduced the rate of hip fractures significantly in the elderly.[20] Combined studies suggest an overall decrease of 25 per cent. The form of the ingested calcium is a matter of individual preference. High-calcium food is clearly the most natural source, but with it comes perhaps unwanted calories and fat. Calcium carbonate requires the least number of pills to achieve the needed dose, but there may be absorption difficulty in some patients. In that case, calcium citrate may be preferable. Calcium citrate does not require acidity for absorption, and the citrate decreases the risk for kidney stones.

Estrogen

Estrogen is the cornerstone of support for the skeletal system, and its deficiency plays a prominent role in the pathogenesis of osteoporosis.[122] It can correct calcium balance primarily through a direct mechanism of the estrogen receptors on bone.

Every postmenopausal white woman (up to age 65 years) should be considered for estrogen replacement therapy aimed at preventing osteoporosis. To avoid excess bone mineral loss, estrogens should be started as soon as possible after the onset of menopause. As noted, bone loss is markedly accelerated during the 6 to 10 years after menopause, and it has been estimated that 50 per cent of the total postmenopausal bone loss occurs during the first 7 years of estrogen deficiency.[28] Numerous studies have demonstrated that low-dose estrogen therapy, if begun shortly after menopause, can arrest or retard spinal bone loss and significantly reduce the incidence of radial, vertebral, and proximal femur fractures by approximately 50 per cent.[33, 34, 50, 53,

[59, 122] Bone mass augmentation is 2 to 3 per cent per year in the spine and 1 to 2 per cent per year in the hip.

The use of estrogen replacement therapy, however, is not without risks. A 1989 study in over 23,000 Swedish women who used estradiol alone showed a nearly doubled relative risk of breast cancer over a five-year period.[7] More recent studies provide breast cancer risk rates from 30 per cent to none.[6, 22] Other studies have shown that estrogen use alone results in a significant increased in the risk of endometrial cancer.[111] Still, the combination therapy with estrogen and progesterone seems to eradicate this increased risk and may even result in a decreased incidence of endometrial cancer compared with that in controls who receive no replacement therapy.[18, 38]

Estrogen increases the risk for breast cancer up to 40 per cent after 10 years of use. Other problems related to estrogen include venous thrombosis and pulmonary embolism, hypertension, and cholelithiasis. These side effects are potentially secondary to the high portal levels of estrogen associated with oral dosing, causing excessive liver production of coagulation factors and bile acids. The effect of estrogens on atherosclerotic heart disease is yet another variable that must be added to the cost-benefit equation. Although there have been studies offering conflicting views on this issue,[3, 114, 124] the latest evidence is that replacement therapy is beneficial by improving the cardiac lipid profile (R42,43)[49, 74] and that survival is superior to controls, even considering the increased breast cancer risk. Other benefits to estrogen are better cognitive skills, limitation of Alzheimer's disease, better dentition, and improved urinary function.

Absolute contraindications to estrogen therapy include breast cancer, regardless of estrogen-receptor status, as well as any other estrogen-sensitive tumor, a history of pulmonary embolism, acute liver disease, and severe uncontrolled hypertension. Gallbladder and thromboembolic disease represent relative contraindications. Indications for hormonal replacement therapy include premature menopause (surgical or natural) and recently postmenopausal women (within six years) who are victims of severe bone loss. The 1984 NIH Consensus Conference on Osteoporosis report recommended combination therapy for all women younger than the age of 60 years if none of the above contraindications are present. The indications to consider for estrogen therapy are a family history of marked osteoporosis, a bone mass 2 SD or more below normal, and evidence of accelerated bone loss (defined as greater than 5 per cent per year) in the presence of adequate calcium and exercise. If estrogen therapy is chosen, we recommend a combined therapy with a progestin. Transdermal estrogen patches are available, possibly with fewer side effects because the portal circulation is bypassed. Clearly, perimenopausal intervention with hormonal replacement is significantly more cost effective than treatment of clinically overt osteoporosis.

Although hormonal replacement therapy may be a boon to the patient's skeletal system, it may exact a price in other areas. Accordingly, the prescription of hormonal replacement must never be used as a blanket panacea, but rather as a treatment tailored to the individual and carefully monitored once initiated. For each patient, all the risks of the therapy must be noted and weighed against the potential benefits, both for the bones and for other organ systems. Stepping into this dilemma are the selective estrogen receptor modulators (SERMs). Raloxifene (Evista),[28a] the first SERM approved by the Food and Drug Administration (FDA), increases bone mass 60 per cent as effectively as estrogen, has some cardiolipid benefits, but does not increase the risk of breast or uterine cancer. There are no fracture prevention data at this time. Raloxifene appears to be a second-line alternative to estrogen and biphosphonates.

Calcitonin

Calcitonin has been approved by the FDA for treatment of osteoporosis. Salmon calcitonin is the typical pharmacologic preparation, but amino acid differences with the human form render it immunogenic.[78] Calcitonin is a polypeptide hormone that has been shown to inhibit bone resorption. Acutely, calcitonin therapy inhibits osteoclast function, whereas in the long term, it may actually decrease the number of osteoclasts.[77] The rationale for calcitonin therapy also stems from the fact that decreased calcitonin levels have been observed postmenopausally.[109] Calcitonin already has an established role in the treatment of Paget's disease, a disease characterized by increased bone turnover. Calcitonin is available in injectable and nasal spray form.[97]

Studies using 100 Medical Research Council (MRC) units of calcitonin given in daily or alternate-day injections have demonstrated that postmenopausal osteoporotic women can increase total body calcium, iliac crest bone volumes, and the bone mineral content of the lumbar vertebrae and femoral diaphysis.[41, 43] One of these studies showed that most of the beneficial effects of calcitonin on bone mass were observed in the first six months of treatment.[77] Nasal calcitonin increases spinal bone mass and decreases spine fractures by 37 per cent (as compared with 50 per cent for estrogen and alendronate). There are no data proving that calcitonin prevents hip fractures.

Problems with subcutaneous calcitonin therapy[78] center on the injectable route and side effects. Many patients are unable to tolerate this route of administration. Side effects include nausea, flushing, anorexia, and, especially if the injection is given too deep, bruising and rash at the injection site. In light of these symptoms, nasal calcitonin is the agent of choice because its only complication is nasal irritation in 2 per cent of patients, yet it is effective for osteoporosis. Indications for calcitonin use include evidence of a high bone turnover state on bone biopsy in postmenopausal women who are unable to take estrogen. It has a significant analgesic property either working through elevated endorphins or through an inhibition of neuropeptide release. It is the agent of choice for the acute painful compression fracture. We recommend giving calcitonin to postmenopausal women who have evidence of significant bone loss on serial bone density while on estrogen studies and again in patients unable to take estrogen. Estrogen and alendronate are preferred to nasal calcitonin for the usual postmenopausal nonfracture care. If nasal calcitonin is employed, a typical course would be 200 MRC units given daily for six months, when indicated. Calcium and vitamin D (physiologic doses) are included in this regimen.

Bisphosphonates

Bisphosphonates are stable active analogues of pyrophosphate that inhibit osteoclastic resorption and depress bone turnover.[67] Etidronate, long employed to treat Paget's disease, and newer bisphosphonates including alendronate, pamidronate, residronate, taludrinate, and clinodrate are currently the most investigated agents in osteoporosis.[79, 88] Intermittent cyclic etidronate may eliminate the untoward histologic abnormalities that can accompany long-term etidronate therapy. Etidronate is most effective when given during the first two years of therapy.[45, 116] This agent has not gained FDA approval. There are more promising second-generation agents that are more potent and yet cause less inhibition of mineralization than etidronate. Alendronate, released by the FDA (10 mg for treatment, 5 mg for prevention), appears to increase vertebral bone

mass in osteoporotic spine (2 to 3 per cent per year; hip, 1 to 2 per cent per year), decreases fractures by 50 per cent in spine and hip, and does not alter the mechanical properties of bone. It continues to work even after the agent has been stopped.[104] Alendronate appears to have few or no side effects except for esophagitis and is an excellent alternative to estrogen. Women with low bone loss, postmenopausal symptoms, poor cardiolipid profile, and no family history of breast cancer should consider estrogen. Women with normal cardiolipid profile, a family history of breast cancer, a history of thrombophlebitis, and manageable postmenopausal symptoms would prefer alendronate. Because there is some concern about bone turnover (bone formation) with bisphosphonates, alendronate may not be ideal for fresh fractures. Esophagitis can be limited by gradual dosing. Half-dosing gives 85 per cent of the drug benefit.

Fluoride

Sodium fluoride has been shown to increase bone mass in many patients with osteoporosis (Fig. 40–5).[44, 99] Although fluoride-treated bone is denser than untreated bone, whether it has the same strength as normal bone remains to be established.[79] However, several studies have demonstrated a significant decrease in fracture rates in patients on a fluoride and calcium regimen

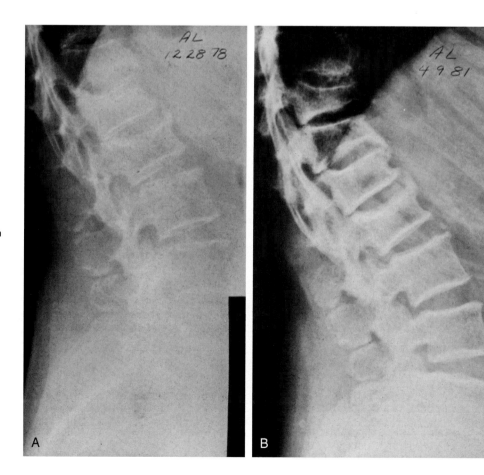

Figure 40–5. Fluoride effect on the spine before *(A)* and after *(B)* treatment.

alone, as well as in combination with estrogen or vitamin D.[10, 35] A study by Riggs and associates[99] in 165 osteoporotic women demonstrated a vertebral fracture rate of 834 per 1000 person-years in untreated patients, 419 in patients on calcium therapy, 304 in patients treated with calcium and fluoride, 181 with estrogen and calcium therapy, and 53 in patients on a regimen of fluoride, calcium, and estrogen. In a study by Lane and colleagues,[65] osteoporotic patients on calcium, fluoride, and vitamin D suffered no vertebral fractures after 18 months of treatment.

A study comparing two Finnish communities, one with fluoridated water of 1.0 ppm and the other with only trace amounts of fluoride in the drinking water, demonstrated that the community with fluoridated water had a significantly lower hip fracture rate.[110] Further study of the same group implied that bone formation due to fluoride therapy decreased the vertebral fracture rate as long as the bone deposition is slow enough to allow proper mineralization and fluoride levels do not exceed a toxic threshold. Studies by Pak indicated that cyclical low-dose slow-release fluoride markedly decreased fracture rate.[90] Riggs,[102] in 1990, reported a random study of very high fluoride doses in which the spine fracture rate was no better than with calcium alone, and there was an increased hip fracture rate. But within that group those patients given adequate calcium fared the best. Although the mechanism of fluoride action is not clear, it is thought to act predominantly through stimulation of osteoblastic function and possibly in part by stabilization of the hydroxyapatite crystal.

Sodium fluoride therapy is not without risks. Fluoride therapy without calcium supplementation can result in secondary hyperparathyroidism and poorly mineralized bone. In patients with underlying hyperosteoidosis or hyperosteoclastosis, fluoride treatment leads to the development of brittle bone[65]; accordingly, patients should begin this therapy regimen only after bone biopsy has ruled out the presence of these conditions. Side effects of fluoride are dose-related and include nausea, indigestion, and transient arthralgias of the lower extremities. The gastrointestinal problems can often be avoided by taking the drug with meals and by starting patients on a low dose initially and increasing to therapeutic doses over the course of several weeks. The lower-extremity arthralgias respond well to nonsteroidal anti-inflammatory drugs, temporary discontinuance of the fluoride, and concurrent calcitonin therapy. The keys to fluoride therapy are to convert the patient to low turnover osteoporosis, use a low dose of fluoride, and give 1500 to 2000 mg elemental calcium. Slow-release sodium fluoride developed by Pak will be approved by the FDA.

References

1. Austin, L. A., and Heath, H.: Calcitonin: Physiology and pathophysiology. N. Engl. J. Med. 304:269, 1981.
2. Auwerx, J., and Bouillon, R.: Mineral and bone metabolism in thyroid disease: A review. Q. J. Med. 232:737, 1986.
3. Bailor, J. C.: When research results are in conflict. N. Engl. J. Med. 313:1080, 1985.
4. Bartriewicz, M., Hernando, N., Reddy, S. V., et al.: Characterization of the osteoclast vacuolar, H(+)-ATPase B-subunit. Gene 160:157–164, 1995.
5. Basset, H. C.: Orthopedic aspects of Paget's disease of bone. Arthritis Rheum. 23:1128, 1980.
6. Belchetz, P. E.: Hormonal treatment of postmenopausal women. N. Engl. J. Med. 330:1062–1071, 1994.
6a. Bell, N. H.: Vitamin D endocrine system. J. Clin. Invest. 76:1, 1985.
7. Bergkvist, L, Adami, H., Persson, I., et al.: The risk of breast cancer after estrogen and estrogen-progestin replacement. N. Engl. J. Med. 321:293, 1989.
8. Bikle, D. D., Genant, H. K., Cann, C., et al.: Bone disease in alcohol abuse. Ann. Intern. Med. 103:42, 1985.
9. Boden, S. D., and Kaplan, F. S.: Calcium homeostasis. Orthop. Clin. North Am. 21:31, 1990.
10. Briancon, D., and Meunier, P. J.: Treatment of osteoporosis with fluoride, calcium, and vitamin D. Orthop. Clin. North Am. 12:629, 1981.
11. Brighton, C. T., and McClusky, W. P.: Cellular response and mechanisms of action of electrically induced osteogenesis. In Peck, W. A. (ed.): Bone and Mineral Research. Vol. 4. Amsterdam, Elsevier, 1986, p. 213.
12. Bruder, S. P., Fink, D. J., and Caplan, A. I.: Mesenchymal stem cells in bone development, bone repair, and skeletal regeneration therapy. J. Cell. Biochem. 56:283–294, 1994.
13. Buckwalter, J. A., Glimcher, M. J., Cooper, R. R., Recker, R.: Bone biology: I. Structure, blood supply, cells, matrix, and in mineralization. Instructional Course Lectures 45:371–386, 1996.
14. Buckwalter, J. A., Glimcher, M. J., Cooper, R. R., Recker, R.: Bone biology: II. Formation, form, modeling, remodeling and regulation of cell function. Instructional Course Lectures 45:387–399, 1996.
15. Bullough, P. G., and Vigorita, V. J.: Atlas of Orthopedic Pathology. New York, Gower Medical Publishing, 1984.
16. Bullough, P. G., and Boachie-Adjei, O.: Atlas of Spinal Diseases. New York, Gower Medical Publishing, 1988.
17. Canalis, E., McCarthy, T., and Centrella, M.: Growth factors and the regulation of bone remodeling. J. Clin. Invest. 81:277, 1988.
18. The Cancer and Steroid Hormone Study of the Centers for Disease Control and the National Institute of Child Health and Human Development: Combination oral contraceptive use and the risk of endometrial cancer. JAMA 257:796, 1987.
19. Chambers., T. J.: The origin of the osteoclast. In Peck, W. A. (ed.): Bone and Mineral Research. Vol. 6. Amsterdam, Elsevier, 1989, p. 1.
20. Chapun, M. C., Arlot, M. E., Duboeuf, F., et al.: Vitamin D₃ and calcium to prevent hip fractures in elderly women. N. Engl. J. Med. 327:1637–1642, 1992.
21. Cohn, S. H., Abesamis, C., Yasumura, S., et al.: Comparative skeletal mass and radial bone mineral content in black and white women. Metabolism 26:171, 1977.
22. Colditz, G. A., Egan, R. M., Stampfer, M. J.: Hormone replacement therapy and risk of breast cancer: Results of epidemiologic studies. Am J. Obstet. Gynecol. 168:473–1480, 1993.
23. Compston, J. E.: Hepatic osteodystrophy: Vitamin D metabolism in patients with liver disease. Gut 27:1073, 1986.
24. Compston, J. E.: Connectivity of cancellous bone: Assessment and mechanical implications. Bone 15:463–466, 1994.
25. Cummings, S. R., Kelsey, J. L., Nevitt, M. C., and O'Dowd, K. J.: Epidemiology of osteoporosis and osteoporotic fractures. Epidemiol. Rev. 7:178, 1985.
26. Cummings, S. R., Nevett, M. C., Browner, W. S., et al.: Risk factors for hip fracture in white women: Study of osteoporotic fracture research group. N. Engl. J. Med. 332:767–773, 1995.
27. Daniell, H. W.: Osteoporosis of the slender smoker: Vertebral compression fracture and loss of metacarpal cortex in relation to postmenopausal cigarette smoking and lack of obesity. Arch. Intern. Med. 136:298, 1976.
28. DeFazio, J., and Speroff, L.: Estrogen replacement therapy: Current thinking and practice. Geriatrics 40:32, 1985.
28a. Delmas, P. D., Bjar Nason, N. H., Mitlak, B. H., et al.: Effects of

raloxifene on bone mineral density, serum cholesterol concentrations and uterine endometrium in postmenopausal women. N. Engl. J. Med. *337*:164–47, 1997.

29. Dempster, D. W., Ferguson-Pell, M. W., Cochran, G. V. B., and Lindsay, R.: A new manual method for assessing two-dimensional cancellous bone structure comparison between iliac crest and lumbar vertebra. J. Bone Miner. Res. *6*:689–696, 1991.

30. Doty, S. B., and DiCarlo, E. F.: Pathophysiology of immobilization osteoporosis. Curr. Opin. Orthop. *6*:45–49, 1995.

31. Einhorn, T. A.: Current concepts review: Enhancement of fracture healing. J. Bone Joint Surg. Am. *77*:940–956, 1995.

32. Eriksen, E. F., Berg, N. J., Graham, M. L., et al.: Evidence of estrogen receptors in human bone cells. J. Bone Miner. Res. *2*(I):238, 1987.

33. Ettinger, B., Genant, H. K., and Cann, C. E.: Long-term estrogen replacement therapy prevents bone loss and fractures. Ann. Intern. Med. *102*:319, 1985.

34. Ettinger, B., Genant, H. K., and Cann, C. E.: Postmenopausal bone loss is prevented by treatment with low-dosage estrogen with calcium. Ann. Intern. Med. *106*:40, 1987.

35. Farley, S. M., Libanati, C. R., Smith, L., et al.: Long-term fluoride therapy corrects the spinal bone density defect in osteoporosis. Presented at the 67th annual meeting of the Endocrine Society, Baltimore, June 19–21, 1985.

36. Flawn, L. B.: Amenorrhea, anorexia, and osteoporosis—the female triad. Curr. Opin. Orthop. *5*:16–20, 1994.

37. Gallagher, J. C., Melton, L. J., III, Riggs, B. L., et al.: Epidemiology of fractures of the proximal femur in Rochester, Minnesota. Clin. Orthop. *150*:163, 1980.

38. Gambrell, R. D., Jr.: Breast disease in the postmenopausal years. Semin. Reprod. Endocrinol. 1:27, 1983.

39. Gazdag, A. R., Lane, J. M., Glaser, D., Forster, R. A.: Alternatives to autogenous bone graft: Efficacy and indications. J. Am. Acad. Orthop. Surg. *3*:1–8, 1995.

40. Genant, H. K., and Boyd, D. P.: Quantitative bone mineral analysis using dual energy computed tomography. Invest. Radiol. *12*:545, 1977.

41. Gennari, C., and Agnusdei, D.: Calcitonin, estrogen, and the bone. J. Steroid Biochem. Mol. Biol. *37*:451, 1990.

42. Gennari, C.: Glucocorticoids and bone. *In* Peck, W. A. (ed.): Bone and Mineral Research. Vol. 3. Amsterdam, Elsevier, 1985, p. 213.

43. Gruber, H. E., Ivey, J. L., and Baylink, D. J.: Long-term calcitonin therapy in postmenopausal osteoporosis. Metabolism *33*:295, 1984.

44. Hansson, T., and Roos, B.: The effect of fluoride and calcium on spinal bone mineral content: A controlled prospective (3 years) study. Calcif. Tissue Int. *40*:315, 1987.

45. Harrer, S. T., Watts, N. B., Jackson, R. D., et al.: Four year study of intermittent cyclic etidronate treatment of postmenopausal osteoporosis: Three years of blinded therapy followed by one year of open therapy. Am. J. Med. *95*:557–597, 1993.

46. Healey, J. H.: Glucocorticoid induced osteoporosis. Curr. Opin. Orthop. *5*:33–38, 1994.

47. Healey, J. H., and Lane, J. M.: Structural scoliosis in osteoporotic women. Clin. Orthop. *195*:216–223, 1985.

48. Heersche, J. N. M.: Bone cells and bone turnover: The basis of pathogenesis. *In* Tam, C. S., Heersche, J. N. M., and Murray, T. M. (eds.): Metabolic Bone Disease: Cellular and Tissue Mechanisms. Boca Raton, CRC Press, 1989, p. 2.

49. Hemminki, E., Topo, P., Molin, M., and Kongas, I.: Physicians' views on hormone therapy around and after menopause. Maturitas *16*:163–173, 1993.

50. Horsman, A., Gallagher, J. C., Simpson, M., and Nordin, B. E. C.: Prospective trial of estrogen and calcium in postmenopausal women. BMJ *2*:789, 1977.

51. Hunt, P. A., Wu-Chen, M. L., Handal, N. J., et al.: Bone disease induced by anticonvulsant therapy and treatment with calcitriol. Am. J. Dis. Child. *140*:715, 1986.

52. Hurley, D. L., Tiegs, R. D., Wahner, H. W., and Heath, H. III: Axial and appendicular bone mineral density in patients with long-term deficiency or excess of calcitonin. N. Engl. J. Med. *317*:537, 1987.

53. Hutchinson, T. A., Polansky, S. M., and Feinstein, A. R.: Post-

menopausal estrogens protect against fractures of hip and distal radius: A case control study. Lancet *2*:705, 1979.

54. Iannotti, J. P.: Growth plate physiology and pathology. Orthop. Clin. North Am. *21*:1, 1990.

55. Johnston, C. C. Jr., and Epstein, S.: Clinical, biochemical, epidemiologic, and economic features of osteoporosis. Orthop. Clin. North Am. *12*:559, 1981.

56. Johnston, C. C., and Slemenda, C. W.: Peak bone mass, bone loss and risk of factor. Osteoporos. Int. *4*:43–45, 1994.

57. Johnston, C. C. Jr., Smith, D. M., Yu, P. L., and Deiss, W. P. Jr.: In vivo measurement of bone mass in the radius. Metabolism *17*:1140, 1968.

58. Kanis, J. A., Melton, L. J. III, Christiansen, C., et al.: Perspective: The diagnosis of osteoporosis. J. Bone Miner. Res. *9*:1137–1141, 1994.

59. Kiel, D. P., Felson, D. T., Anderson, J. J., et al.: Hip fracture and the use of estrogens in postmenopausal women. N. Engl. J. Med. *317*:1169, 1987.

60. Kimmel, P. L.: Radiologic methods to evaluate bone mineral content. Ann. Intern. Med. *100*:908, 1984.

61. Klahr, S., and Hruska, K.: Effects of parathyroid hormone on the renal reabsorption of phosphorus and divalent cations. *In* Peck, W. A. (ed.): Bone and Mineral Research. Vol. 2. Amsterdam, Elsevier, 1983, p. 65.

62. Klibanski, A., Neer, R. M., Beitins, I. Z., et al.: Decreased bone density in hyperprolactinemic women. N. Engl. J. Med. *303*:1511, 1980.

63. Kraemer, J., Kolditz, D., and Gowin, R.: Water and electrolyte content of human intervertebral discs under variable load. Spine *10*:69, 1985.

64. Krolner, B., Toft, B., Pors Nielsen, S., and Tondevold, E.: Physical exercise as prophylaxis against involutional vertebral bone loss: A controlled trial. Clin. Sci. *64*:541, 1983.

65. Lane, J. M., Healey, J. H., Schwartz, E., et al.: The treatment of osteoporosis with sodium fluoride and calcium: Effects on vertebral fracture incidence and bone histomorphometry. Orthop. Clin. North Am. *15*:729, 1984.

66. Lane, J. M., Healey, J. H., Vigorita, V. J., and Werntz, J. R.: Orthopaedic management of osteoporosis: Effects of nutrition and exercise on the skeleton. *In* Uhthoff, H. K. (ed.): Current Concepts of Bone Fragility. Berlin, Springer-Verlag, 1986, pp. 429–447.

67. Lane, J. M., Riley, E. H., and Wirganowicz, P. Z.: Osteoporosis: Diagnosis and treatment. J. Bone Joint Surg. *78A*(4):618–632, 1996.

68. Lazarus, H. M., Haynesworth, S. E., Gerson, S. L., et al.: Ex vivo expansion and subsequent infusion of human bone marrow–derived stromal progenitor cells (mesenchymal progenitor cells), implications for therapeutic use. Bone Marrow Transplant. *16*:557–564, 1995.

69. Lips, P., Courpron, P., and Meunier, P. J.: Mean wall thickness of trabecular bone packets in human iliac crest: Changes with age. Calcif. Tissue Res. *26*:13, 1978.

70. Lontbardi, A., and Sontora, A. C. Clinical trials with bisphosphonate. J. Bone Miner. Res. *22*:559–570, 1993.

71. Lorenzo, J. A., Sousa, S. L., and Centrella, M.: Interleukin-1 in combination with transforming growth factor alpha produces enhanced bone resorption in vitro. Endocrinology *123*:2194, 1988.

72. Marcus, R.: Endocrine control of bone and mineral metabolism. *In* Manolagas, S. C., Olefsky, J. M. (eds.): Metabolic Bone and Mineral Disorders. New York, Churchill Livingstone, 1988, p. 13.

73. Matkovic, V., Kostial, K., Simonovic, I., et al.: Bone status and fracture rates in two regions of Yugoslavia. Am. J. Clin. Nutr. *32*:540, 1979.

74. Matthews, K. A., Meilahn, F., Kuller, L. H., et al.: Menopause and risk factors for coronary heart disease. N. Engl. J. Med. *321*:641, 1989.

75. Mazess, R. B.: On aging bone loss. Clin. Orthop. *165*:239, 1982.

76. Mazess, R. B.: The non-invasive measurement of skeletal mass. *In* Peck, W. A. (ed.): Bone and Mineral Research Annual I. Amsterdam, Excerpta Medica, 1983, p. 223.

77. Mazzuoli, G. F., Passeri, M., Gennari, C., et al.: Effects of salmon

calcitonin in postmenopausal osteoporosis: A controlled double-blind clinical study. Calcif. Tissue Int. *38*:3, 1986.

78. Anonymous: Human calcitonin for Paget's disease. Med. Lett. *29*:47, 1987.

79. Anonymous: Prevention and treatment of postmenopausal osteoporosis. Med. Lett. *29*:75, 1987.

80. Meema, S., Bunker, M. L., and Meema, H. E.: Preventive effect of estrogen on postmenopausal bone loss: A follow-up study. Arch. Intern. Med. *135*:1436, 1975.

81. Melton, L. J. III, and Riggs, B. L.: Epidemiology of age-related fractures. *In* Avioli, L. V. (ed.): The Osteoporotic Syndrome. New York, Grune & Stratton, 1987, pp. 1–30.

82. Minaire, P., Meunier, P., Edouard, C., et al.: Quantitative histological data on disuse osteoporosis: Comparison with biological data. Calcif. Tissue Res. *17*:57, 1974.

83. Mohler, D. G., Lane, J. M., Cole, B. J., and Weinerman, S. A.: Skeletal failure in osteoporosis. *In* Lane, J. M., and Healey, J. H. (eds.): Diagnosis and Management of Pathological Fractures. New York, Raven, 1993.

84. Mosekilde, L., Eriksen, E. F., and Charles, P.: Effects of thyroid hormone on bone and mineral metabolism. Endocrinol. Metab. Clin. North Am. *19*:35–63, 1990.

85. National Institutes of Health Consensus Development Conference: Statement on osteoporosis. JAMA 252:799, 1984.

86. Nijweide, P. J., Burger, E. H., and Feyen, J. H.: Cells of bone proliferation, differentiation and hormonal regulation. Physiol. Rev. *66*:855, 1986.

87. Norman, A. W., Roth, J., and Orci, L.: The vitamin D endocrine system: Steroid metabolism, hormone receptors and biological response. Endocr. Rev. *3*:331, 1982.

88. Ott, S. M.: Clinical effects of bisphosphonates in involutional osteoporosis. J. Bone Miner. Res. *8*(Suppl. 2):S597–606, 1993.

89. Owen, M.: Lineage of osteogenic cells and their relationship to the stromal system. *In* Peck, W. A. (ed.): Bone and Mineral Research. Vol. 3. Amsterdam, Elsevier, 1985, p. 1.

90. Pak, C. Y. C., Sakhall, K., Adams-Huet, B., et al.: Treatment of postmenopausal osteoporosis with slow release sodium fluoride: Final report of a randomized controlled trial. Ann. Intern. Med. *123*:401–408, 1995.

91. Posner, A. S.: Bone mineral and the mineralization process. *In* Peck, W. A. (ed.): Bone and Mineral Research. Vol. 5. Amsterdam, Elsevier, 1987, p. 65.

92. Potts, J. T., Kronenberg, H. M., and Rosenblatt, M.: Parathyroid hormone: Chemistry, biosynthesis, and mode of action. Adv. Protein Chem. *35*:323, 1982.

93. Price, P.: Osteocalcin. *In* Peck, W. A. (ed.): Bone and Mineral Research Annual I. Amsterdam, Excerpta Medica, 1983, p. 157.

94. Price, C. P., Thompson, P. W.: The role of biochemical tests in the screening and monitoring of osteoporosis. Ann. Clin. Biochem. *32*:244–260, 1995.

95. Prockop, D. J., Kivirikko, I., Tuderman, L., and Guzman, N. A.: The biosynthesis of collagen and its disorders: N. Engl. J. Med. *301*:13, 1979.

96. Raisz, L. G., and Kream, B. E.: Regulation of bone formation. N. Engl. J. Med. *309*:29, 1983.

97. Reginster, J. Y., Denis, D., Deroisy, R., et al.: Long term (three years) prevention of trabecular postmenopausal bone loss with low dose intermittent nasal salmon calcitonin. J. Bone Miner. Res. *9*:69–73, 1994.

98. Richelson, L. S., Wahner, H. W., Melton, L. J. III, and Riggs, B. L.: Relative contributions of aging and estrogen deficiency to postmenopausal bone loss. N. Engl. J. Med. *311*:1273, 1984.

99. Riggs, B. L., Seeman, E., Hodgson, S. F., et al.: Effect of the fluoride/calcium regimen on vertebral fracture occurrence in post-menopausal osteoporosis: Comparison with conventional therapy. N. Engl. J. Med. *306*:446, 1982.

100. Riggs, B. L., and Melton, L. J. III: Evidence for two distinct syndromes of involutional osteoporosis. Am. J. Med. 75:899, 1983.

101. Riggs, B. L., and Melton, L. J. III: Involutional osteoporosis. N. Engl. J. Med. 314:1676, 1986.

102. Riggs, B. L., Hodgson, S., O'Fallon, W., et al.: Effect of fluoride

treatment on the fracture rate in postmenopausal women with osteoporosis. N. Engl. J. Med. 322:802, 1990.

103. Riis, B., Thomsen, K., and Christiansen, C.: Does calcium supplementation prevent postmenopausal bone loss? A double-blind, controlled clinical study. N. Engl. J. Med. 316:173, 1987.

104. Rossini, M., Gatti, D., Zomberlan, N., et al.: Long term effects of a treatment course with oral alendronate of post menopausal osteoporosis. J. Bone Miner. Res. 9:1833–1837, 1994.

105. Sanchez, C. P., Salusky, I. B: Biochemical marker in metabolic bone disease. Curr. Opin. Orthop. 5:43–49, 1994

106. Schneider, R., and Math, K.: Bone density analysis, an update. Curr. Opin. Orthop. 5:66–72, 1994.

107. Seeman, E., Wahner, H. W., Offord, K. P., et al.: Differential effects of endocrine dysfunction on the axial and the appendicular skeleton. J. Clin. Invest. 69:1302, 1982.

108. Seeman, E., Melton, L. J. III, O'Fallon, W. M., and Riggs, B. L.: Risk factors for spinal osteoporosis in men. Am. J. Med. 75:977, 1983.

109. Shamonki, I. M., Frumar, A. M., Tataryn, I. V., et al.: Age-related changes of calcitonin secretion in females. J. Clin. Endocrinol. Metab. 50:437, 1980.

110. Simonen, O., and Laitinen, O.: Does fluoridation of drinking water prevent bone fragility and osteoporosis? Lancet 2:432, 1985.

111. Smith, D. C., Prentice, R., Donovan, J. T., et al.: Association of exogenous estrogen and endometrial carcinoma. N. Engl. J. Med. 293:1164, 1975.

112. Smith, D. M., Nance, W. E., Kang, K. W., et al: Genetic factors in determining bone mass. J. Clin. Invest. 52:2800, 1973.

113. Sporn, M. B., and Roberts, A. B.: Transforming growth factor beta: Multiple actions and potential clinical applications. JAMA 262:938, 1989.

114. Stampfer, M. J., Willett, W. C., Colditz, G. A., et al: A prospective study of postmenopausal estrogen therapy and coronary heart disease. N. Engl. J. Med. *313*:1044, 1985.

115. Stein, G. S., and Lian, J. B.: Molecular mechanisms mediating proliferation/differentiation interrelationships during progressive development of the osteoblast phenotype. Endocr. Rev. *14*:424–442, 1993.

116. Storm, T., Steiniche, T., Thamsborg, G., and Melsen, F.: Changes in bone histomorphometry after long term treatment with intermittent cyclic etidronate for postmenopausal osteoporosis. J. Bone Miner. Res. *8*:199–208, 1993.

117. Storm, T., Thamsborg, G., Steiniche, T., et al.: Effects of intermittent cyclical etidronate therapy on bone mass and fracture rate in women with postmenopausal osteoporosis. N. Engl. J. Med. *322*:1265–1271, 1990.

118. Teitelbaum, S. L., Abu-Amer, Y., Ross, F. P.: Molecular mechanisms of bone resorption. J. Cell. Biochem. *59*:1–10, 1995.

119. Tiegs, R. D., Body, J. J., and Wahner, H. W.: Calcitonin secretion in postmenopausal osteoporosis. N. Engl. J. Med. *312*:1097, 1985.

120. Tsai, K. S., Heath, H. III, Kumar, R., and Riggs, B. L.: Impaired vitamin D metabolism with aging in women: Possible role in the pathogenesis of senile osteoporosis. J. Clin. Invest. *73*:1668, 1984.

121. Wasserman, R. H., and Chandler, J. S.: Molecular mechanisms of intestinal calcium absorption. *In* Peck, W. A. (ed.): Bone and Mineral Research. Vol. 3. Amsterdam, Elsevier, 1985, p. 181.

122. Weiss, N. S., Ure, C. L., Ballard, J. H., et al.: Decreased risk of fractures of hip and lower forearm with postmenopausal use of estrogen. N. Engl. J. Med. *303*:1195, 1980.

123. Whyte, M. P.: Alkaline phosphatase: Physiological role explored in hypophosphatasia. *In* Peck, W. A. (ed.): Bone and Mineral Research. Vol. 6. Amsterdam, Elsevier, 1989, p. 175.

124. Wilson, P. W. F., Garrison, R. J., and Castelli, W. P.: Postmenopausal estrogen use, cigarette smoking, and cardiovascular morbidity in women over 50: The Framingham study. N. Engl. J. Med. *313*:1038, 1985.

125. Wong, G. L.: Skeletal effects of parathyroid hormone. *In* Peck, W. A. (ed.): Bone and Mineral Research. Vol. 4. Amsterdam, Elsevier, 1986, p. 103.

126. Wozney, J. M., Rosen, V., Celeste, A. J., et al.: Novel regulators of bone formation: Molecular clones and activities. Science *242*:1528, 1988.

CHAPTER

41

Rheumatoid Arthritis: Surgical Considerations

Charles R. Clark, M.D.

Arnold H. Menezes, M.D.

The majority of patients afflicted with rheumatoid arthritis have cervical spine involvement. In the past, such involvement was thought to be relatively innocuous. The lack of correlation between the severity of rheumatoid subluxations of the upper cervical spine and the supposed absence of neurologic damage has led to the erroneous supposition that this finding was clinically benign.[59] Progressive instability of the upper cervical spine may lead to cord, medullary, and vertebral artery compression, with resultant severe neurologic deficit or even death.[3, 52, 77] The ultimate consequence, "sudden death in rheumatoid patients," may occur as a result of this recurrent traumatization of the spinal cord.[25, 61, 90]

The most common sites of involvement in rheumatoid arthritis are the metatarsophalangeal joints, followed by the metacarpophalangeal joints and the cervical spine.[3] In 1969, Matthews reported that 25 to 30 per cent of rheumatoid patients admitted to the hospital had radiographic evidence of cervical spine involvement.[51] Conlon and associates retrospectively reviewed a large series of patients with rheumatoid arthritis and found that 60 per cent had neck involvement varying from mild to severe.[18] The frequency of radiographic and clinical cervical spine involvement has been reported to be greater than 80 per cent.[4, 19] Despite this, the cervical spine may be easily overlooked in a patient with severe rheumatoid arthritis. Indeed, rheumatoid arthritis may involve the cervical spine with little or no clinical or radiographic manifestations.[4, 45, 70] The activity of rheumatoid arthritis in the cervical spine appears to begin early in the disease and progresses in relation to the peripheral involvement.[41] The physician must be cognizant of the possibility of cervical spine involvement in rheumatoid arthritis. Prompt recognition of such involvement and the initiation of appropriate treatment may avoid the grave consequences of significant cervical spine instability with resultant neurologic deficit and even death.[3]

This chapter describes the current understanding of the natural history of this condition, which is still quite limited. The diagnostic evaluation of a patient with rheumatoid involvement of the cervical spine is presented, followed by a lengthy discussion of various operative interventions, including indications and operative techniques.

PATHOPHYSIOLOGY AND NATURAL HISTORY

The cervical spine has multiple synovial-lined articulations that are susceptible to rheumatoid involvement. Consequently, the cervical spine is frequently affected.[2, 3, 6, 18, 39] The pathology of rheumatoid arthritis in the cervical spine resembles that in the peripheral joints. Synovitis in the small apophyseal joints and bursae, as well as involvement of the ligamentous apparatus, may lead to instability via a loss of articular cartilage, bone erosion, and laxity of the ligaments. The T lymphocyte is the predominant cell found in focal infiltrates in the cervical spine ligamentous tissue. Mononuclear cell infiltrates lead to the production of interleukin-1, which in turn may cause ligamentous damage, laxity, and subluxation.[40] Synovitis in the apophyseal joints erodes the articular cartilage and subchondral bone, leading to anterior, posterior, and lateral instability. Further instability can occur in rotation. In addition, rheumatoid discitis may occur at the discovertebral junction.[33] The primary joints involved include the atlanto-occipital, atlantoaxial, atlantodental, and neurocentral joints or joints of Luschka,[12] with a predilection for involvement of the craniocervical junction.[84, 87] Lesions from the joints of Luschka extend into the disc spaces and into the vertebral bodies, but without osteophytosis; this is pathognomonic of the rheumatoid process, in contradistinction to osteoarthrosis.[56]

The three most common lesions resulting from rheumatoid involvement of the cervical spine are atlantoaxial subluxation (C1–C2), subaxial subluxation (subluxation below the level of C2), and cranial settling (destruction of the occipitoatlantal and atlantoaxial joints, with resultant settling of the cranium on the dens). Synonymous terms for cranial settling include upward migration of the dens,[64] translocation of the dens,[68, 69] atlantoaxial impaction,[85] vertical settling,[38] vertical subluxation of the dens,[91] upward migration of the odontoid,[62] and basilar invagination.[77] The term cranial settling[23] most accurately represents the pathology and is our preferred terminology.[12] The terms basilar invagination and basilar impression are often used erroneously. Basilar invagination refers to the primary form of basilar impression, which consists of a distinct developmental defect of the chondral cranium, often associated with other anomalies of the notochord in the region of the craniovertebral junction, such as occipitalization of the atlas and Klippel-Feil syndrome. Basilar invagination is also associated with anomalies of development of the epicaudal neural axis, such as the Chiari malformation, syringobulbia, and syringomyelia.[59] Basilar impression refers to the secondary, acquired form of basilar invagination that is caused by softening of the bone,[61] which occurs in such conditions as hyperparathyroidism and osteomalacia.[56] Consequently, neither of these two terms (basilar invagination and basilar impression) are appropriate when referring specifically to rheumatoid involvement of the cervical spine.

It is important to differentiate between cranial settling and atlantoaxial subluxation.[77] Atlantoaxial subluxation with resultant instability may have a more benign natural history, with less than 20 per cent of patients showing progressive instability in one series.[52] Cranial settling, however, has been shown to progress in 35 to 50 per cent of patients in another series.[61]

In addition to the problems posed by the destruction of cartilage, bone, and ligamentous apparatus, problems may result from severe osteopenia. All these factors must be considered when contemplating operative intervention. Not only is the spinal cord and/or brain stem at risk from direct compression secondary to subluxation of the vertebrae, but there can also be compression of the cord by the rheumatoid granulation tissue. A mass of rheumatoid pannus within the confines of the spinal canal may cause significant compression. This may occur despite relatively minimal evidence of radiographic instability. This process is most evident at the level of C2, where there frequently is substantial periodontal pannus.

The presence of rheumatoid granulation tissue or pannus may be partially related to the presence of instability. Larsson and colleagues[44] performed pre- and postoperative magnetic resonance imaging (MRI) of the craniovertebral junction in patients with rheumatoid arthritis and found a substantial decrease in the periodontoid pannus after stabilizing surgery. Similarly, Grob and coworkers documented a series of 21 rheumatoid patients with retrodental tissue present on preoperative MRIs. All patients underwent fusion of the atlantoaxial segment, and no patient underwent anterior decompression. All patients had a minimum follow-up of 36 months and a successful fusion of the atlantoaxial segment. These authors noted resolution of the pannus after operative immobilization.[25] The results of this investigation indicate that transoral decompression is not required in cases of neural compression caused by retrodental pannus alone, without bony obstruction.[25] This is consistent with the finding of Larsson and colleagues that the reduction in pannus seems to result from immobilization of the instability by posterior fusion.[44]

Although rheumatoid involvement of the cervical spine may appear early in the course of the disease and cervical spine subluxation may develop within two years, in most cases, subluxation occurs later.[74] Patients with arthritis mutilans deformities of the hands and fingers often have accompanying changes in the cervical spine.[37] Any synovial joint in the cervical spine may be involved, but the earliest changes are usually seen in the occipitoatlantoaxial complex.[8] Atlantoaxial subluxation is the most common instability, followed by cranial settling and then subaxial subluxation. However, in many cases there is combined involvement, particularly atlantoaxial subluxation and cranial settling.

Atlantoaxial subluxation results primarily from involvement of the transverse atlantal ligament as well as the paired alar ligaments. Secondary involvement of the atlantoaxial apophyseal joints also occurs. The most common plane of instability is sagittal, with anterior subluxation of the atlas on the axis being the most common form of involvement. Early in the disease, synovitis and effusion in the atlantodental joint permit an abnormally large excursion of the atlas on the axis. Later, progressive erosion of the dens often accompanies attenuation or destruction of the transverse and alar ligaments. Instability of the atlas becomes greater, and the effective canal diameter decreases as these changes progress.[12, 77] The width of the cervical canal and the degree of synovial proliferation are among the most important determinants of neural deterioration.[10] As the predental interval increases, the space available for the cord is diminished, assuming the ring of the atlas is intact. As the predental interval (normally 3 mm or less in adults) approaches 10 mm, the extra space available for the cord is taken up, and cord compression may be imminent. However, the critical dimension for the spinal cord is the space available for the cord, which represents the posterior atlantodental interval. When this space measures 13 mm on a plain, magnified film or 10 mm in absolute dimension, cord compression is likely. The presence of rheumatoid granulation tissue may cause additional compression of the cord.

Although most subluxation occurs in the anteroposterior (AP) plane, lateral and rotatory subluxation may be noted. This is often best seen on a computed tomography (CT) scan. Weissman and coauthors[85] showed that cord compression is most likely to result when lateral subluxation is present, when atlantoaxial subluxation is combined with cranial settling, in males, and when the predental interval is greater than 8 mm.

Substantial involvement of the atlanto-occipital as well as atlantoaxial joints may lead to destruction of the occipitoatlantoaxial complex, allowing the cranium to settle on the cervical spine and the dens to project above the level of the foramen magnum.[12, 50, 52, 68, 77] Neurologic compromise results from impingement of the brain stem and the upper cervical cord by the dens. The vertebral arteries may also be occluded as they converge to enter the skull between the dens and the margins of the foramen magnum.[23] Cranial settling results primarily from bone and cartilage destruction, as opposed to ligamentous laxity.[80]

Involvement of the neurocentral as well as apophyseal joints by the rheumatoid inflammatory process may lead to instability and subluxation and is the primary pathologic process leading to subaxial subluxation. In addition, the pachymeningitis that may occur secondary to rheumatoid inflammatory tissue may cause further compromise of the cord within the confines of the spinal canal.

Our knowledge of the natural history of cervical involvement with rheumatoid arthritis is quite limited. Indeed, it is difficult to determine the natural history of any condition when attempts are made to treat patients, because such treatment necessarily alters the natural history. Therefore, one might argue that it is virtually impossible to obtain such information, because practically all rheumatoid patients are treated in some manner.[16] Therefore, one must be skeptical when viewing reports that are labeled "natural histories." Further, one must keep in mind that many reports of treatment of this condition may suffer from selection bias, because many of these series represent "selected" series of patients undergoing operative or nonoperative management rather than representing a truly randomized series.[17]

Rana and coworkers reported a series of 41 patients with atlantoaxial subluxation followed over a 12-year period. Sixty-one per cent of the patients had no change in the radiographic degree of involvement, 27 per cent had progression, and 12 per cent apparently had decreased involvement.[68] With further follow-up of this same group of patients, Rana reported that 12 patients died, two with evidence of neurologic damage. Further, he found that four patients who had had a

decrease in the extent of atlantoaxial subluxation by 2 to 9 mm had developed cranial settling.[67]

Pellicci and colleagues reviewed a series of 106 rheumatoid patients followed over a five-year period.[65] At the onset, 43 per cent had cervical spine involvement, after five years, 70 per cent of these patients had such involvement. Thirty-six per cent of patients had neurologic progression, and 80 per cent had radiographic progression. Mortality was 17 per cent, compared with 9 per cent for the same age group without rheumatoid disease. In a postmortem study of 104 patients with rheumatoid arthritis, Mikulowski found atlantoaxial dislocation with cervical medullary compression in 11.[61] Seven of these 11 patients died suddenly, indicating an estimated 10 per cent rate of fatal medullary compression.

Zoma and coworkers reviewed a series of patients with rheumatoid cervical involvement and neurologic deficit. When the neurologic deficit was severe, death or failure occurred in 97 per cent of patients.[91] When there was a lesser degree of involvement, 80 per cent of patients had good results from operative intervention. Santavirta and associates[74] reported on 34 patients with cervical involvement; 16 were treated nonoperatively, and only one of eight had a decrease in pain. Neurologic function slowly worsened in the nonoperatively treated group. The authors concluded that nonoperative treatment does not always decrease pain and does not prevent progression of existing disease.

Untreated atlantoaxial subluxation may have severe consequences. Upper cord and medullary compression may occur. In addition, there may be occasional vertebral artery insufficiency, and there have been several reports of sudden death because of this lesion.[20, 78, 83] Once myelopathy is established secondary to rheumatoid involvement of the cervical spine, death is common.[49] Indeed, the best results of operative management of the rheumatoid spine have occurred in patients who were treated before profound myelopathy was present.[17, 32, 75, 91]

Because the natural history of rheumatoid involvement of the cervical spine is unknown, outcome studies of operative management are needed.[15] Despite this lack of knowledge, there are several basic aspects of rheumatoid involvement that are known. First of all, the cervical spine is frequently involved, and neurologic compromise may progress without treatment. The presence of myelopathy is a bad prognostic sign, and the results of operative management appear to be better with early neurologic involvement rather than after the development of profound myelopathy.[16]

CLINICAL FEATURES

The clinical evaluation of a patient with severe rheumatoid arthritis may be difficult because of multifocal involvement. This is further confounded by the "silent" nature of involvement of the cervical spine. Involvement of the hands, peripheral nerve root entrapment, root involvement by foraminal encroachment, and cord or brain stem compression by bony displacement may all lead to weakness and neurologic deficit.[12] A review of a series of 45 rheumatoid patients with cranial settling by Menezes and associates[59] revealed the following clinical findings in order of prevalence: occipital pain (45 patients), myelopathy (36), blackout spells (24), brain stem signs (17), and lower cranial nerve palsies (10); four patients had previous tracheostomies, and four previously asymptomatic patients presented acutely quadriparetic.

Rana and coworkers[68] pointed out the very subtle and often overlooked signs of impairment of the fifth cranial nerve, which may be seen in patients with involvement of the craniovertebral junction. Depression of pain sensation and light touch, especially in the first division of the trigeminal nerve, and absence of the corneal reflex are the most common findings. These signs may indicate involvement of the descending tract of the nerve, which reaches as low as C2.

Despite the problems associated with the neurologic examination, a careful examination of the patient should be performed. Pyramidal tract signs, including hyperactive reflexes, a positive Babinski's sign, and loss of proprioception, are early manifestations of myelopathy and are indications of impending compression of the spinal cord.[75] Other nonspecific findings may indicate the presence of cervical involvement. An abrupt increase in neck pain may be a clue to such involvement. Compression of the greater occipital nerve (posterior ramus of C2) may result in suboccipital pain.[91] Irritation of the lesser occipital nerve (C1 root) may also produce pain in this region. Other nonspecific findings include the onset of bowel or bladder incontinence; the development of spasticity, particularly in the lower extremities; and a change in walking ability. A patient who has been walking for many years with crutches or a walker and then progresses to a wheelchair should arouse the suspicion of cervical spine involvement.

Because the neurologic examination may be difficult in a patient with polyarticular involvement, objective assessment of the cervical spine by somatosensory evoked potentials has gained interest and is discussed in the section on diagnostic evaluation. Somatosensory evoked potentials may be particularly valuable in confirming a diagnosis of cervical myelopathy.[43, 81]

Rheumatoid arthritis may involve other levels of the spine. Subcervical rheumatoid spondylitis is more common than generally believed, although much less common than involvement of the cervical spine. Heywood and Meyers[33] reported seven patients with rheumatoid arthritis of the thoracic and lumbar spine and demonstrated histologic corroboration in four patients.

In summary, clinical signs and symptoms of cervical involvement range from none to quadriplegia. The early symptoms include suboccipital pain, and the earliest findings are nonspecific. Certain findings, however, should arouse the suspicion of the physician: an abrupt increase in the severity of neck pain, the development of bowel or bladder incontinence, increase in weakness, spasticity of the lower extremities, or change in ambulatory status. One must always consider the possibility of cervical involvement when one of these entities appears.[12]

The most frequent symptom of occipitoatlantoaxial involvement is occipital pain with radiation toward the vertex. This was present in 90 per cent of patients with cranial settling and in 60 per cent of patients with atlantoaxial subluxation in Menezes's series.[56] Myelopathy was found in 75 per cent of individuals with cranial settling and in 60 per cent of patients with atlantoaxial subluxation. Brain stem dysfunction was present in 50 per cent of patients with cranial settling. The cranial nerves most affected were the hypoglossal, glossopharyngeal, and trigeminal nerves.

In patients with rheumatoid arthritis, an erroneous diagnosis of entrapment neuropathy, rheumatoid peripheral neuropathy, vasculitis, or progression of rheumatoid disease is not uncommon. Because of the severe deformity effects of rheumatoid arthritis, hyperreflexia and Babinski's sign are of major importance in identifying those patients who have myelopathy.[59]

DIAGNOSTIC EVALUATION

Initial radiographic evaluation consists of plain radiographs: AP, transoral odontoid, and lateral flexion and extension dynamic views. Diffuse osteopenia and overlap of bony structures at the craniovertebral junction often make interpretation of radiographs difficult. In many cases, advanced diagnostic studies are indicated; polytomography in the AP and lateral planes is particularly advantageous. Lateral midline flexion and extension polytomograms are helpful in defining the pathologic anatomy. CT may provide additional data, particularly when evaluating for the presence of lateral or rotatory subluxation.

Instability of the cervical spine is determined radiographically. The criteria described by White and associates[86] are useful for defining AP instability of the subaxial spine (more than 3.5 mm of mobile AP displacement is considered unstable). Bear in mind, however, that these authors determined this parameter in the laboratory setting and that they were evaluating acute trauma to the spine, not rheumatoid arthritis. Therefore, extrapolation to the rheumatoid patient has its limitations. Atlantoaxial subluxation is defined as a predental interval of greater than 3 mm that is not fixed on lateral flexion and extension views. The predental interval is the distance between the posterior edge of the anterior ring of C1 and the anterior surface of the dens measured along the transverse axis of the ring of C1.[17] The posterior atlantodental interval, which represents the space available for the cord at this level, is perhaps the most important parameter to consider.[5] This interval is the distance between the posterior edge of the dens and the anterior aspect of the posterior arch of C1 measured along the transverse axis of the ring of C1. The posterior atlantodental interval as well as the AP diameter of the subaxial sagittal canal measured on cervical radiographs demonstrated statistically significant correlations with the presence and severity of paralysis in a report by Boden and colleagues.[5] All patients who had Ranawat Class 3 neurologic deficit had a posterior atlantodental interval or subaxial canal diameter that was less than 14 mm. In contrast, the anterior atlantodental interval, which traditionally has been reported as the predictor of potential paralysis, did not correlate with paralysis.

Intrusion of the tip of the dens above the transverse diameter of the foramen magnum (McRae's line) defines cranial settling. Polytomography, however, is often required to view McRae's line accurately and to determine where the tip of the dens is. Several other radiographic parameters are often used to define cranial settling. These include Chamberlain's line and Wackenheim's line (Fig. 41–1), the measurement described by Ranawat and associates (Fig. 41–2),[70] and the measurement described by Redlund-Johnell and Pettersson (Fig. 41–3).[72]

Clark and colleagues[17] defined a term known as "station of the atlas," which notes the relationship of the anterior ring of C1 to the axis (Fig. 41–4). The station of C1 is determined by dividing the second cervical vertebra into thirds in the sagittal plane, noting the relationship of the anterior ring of C1 to C2. Normally, the anterior ring of C1 should be adjacent to the upper third of C2. This is defined as Station 1. If the ring of C1 is adjacent to the middle third of C2, this is considered Station 2 and is indicative of mild cranial settling. If the anterior arch of C1 is adjacent to the base of C2, this is called Station 3 and is considered

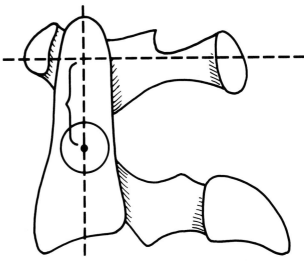

Figure 41–2. The distance described by Ranawat and colleagues is between the sclerotic ring, which represents the pedicle of the axis, and the transverse axis of the atlas, as measured along the longitudinal axis of the dens. As this interval becomes shorter, the severity of cranial settling increases. (From Clark, C. R., Goetz, D. D., and Menezes, A. H.: Arthrodesis of the cervical spine in rheumatoid arthritis. J. Bone Joint Surg. [Am.] 71:381–392, 1989.)

evidence of severe cranial settling. The methods described by both Clark and Ranawat are particularly useful, because plain radiographs can be used. Abnormal Ranawat and Clark values are often associated with problems in the C1–C2 segment, whereas an abnormal Redlund-Johnell value reflects problems associated with the entire occipitoatlantoaxial complex.[62]

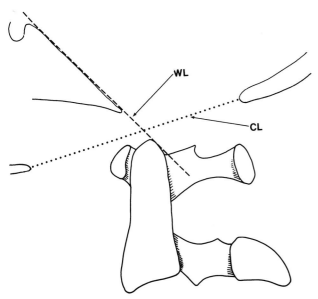

Figure 41–1. The Chamberlain line (CL) is drawn from the posterior edge of the hard palate to the posterior rim of the foramen magnum. Normally, the tip of the dens should not protrude more than 3 mm above this line. The Wackenheim line (WL) is drawn along the cranial surface of the clivus. It should normally be tangent to, or intersect the tips of, the dens. Protrusion of the dens posterior to this line is indicative of cranial settling. (From Clark, C. R., Goetz, D. D., and Menezes, A. H.: Arthrodesis of the cervical spine in rheumatoid arthritis. J. Bone Joint Surg. [Am.] 71:381–392, 1989.)

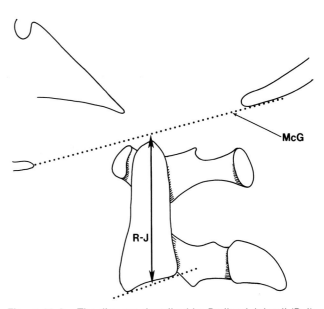

Figure 41–3. The distance described by Redlund-Johnell (R-J) is the minimal distance between the sagittal midpoint of the base of the axis and the McGregor (McG) line.

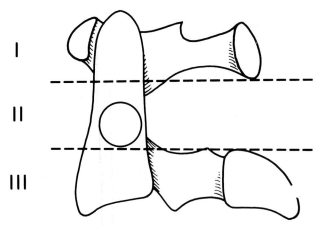

Figure 41–4. The station of the atlas is determined by noting the relationship of the anterior arch of the atlas to the area by dividing the axis into thirds in the sagittal plane (see text). (From Clark, C. R., Goetz, D. D., and Menezes, A. H.: Arthrodesis of the cervical spine in rheumatoid arthritis. J. Bone Joint Surg. [Am.] 71:381–392, 1989.)

These values are not substantially changed in flexion, extension, or neutral views.

Ranawat determined the normal range of his distance (the distance from the sclerotic ring representing the pedicle of C2 to the transverse axis of the first cervical vertebra measured along the longitudinal axis of C2) to be 17 ± 2 mm for men and 15 ± 2 mm for women. As this interval becomes shorter, the severity of cranial settling increases. Normal values for the Redlund-Johnell method are greater than or equal to 34 mm in men and greater than or equal to 29 mm in women.[72] Advanced radiographic studies are required to determine the presence of cord compression. In addition, these studies are useful in determining whether there is multilevel involvement. Cervical myelography, CT with intrathecal contrast, and polytomomyelography have all been used to evaluate the craniovertebral junction and cervical cord. However, these studies often necessitate placing the patient head down and allowing the dye to pass through the foramen magnum into the cranium. This may lead to complications secondary to irritation of the meninges by the contrast agent. Profound headaches as well as seizures may result. In addition, myelography may be painful in patients with advanced rheumatoid arthritis. It may even be impossible to perform in some cases.[66] MRI provides detailed information about soft tissue lesions, vertebral displacement, and narrowing of the spinal canal. It is also useful when multilevel involvement is present, to determine the most important level. MRI has already been established as the best method for evaluation of the craniocervical region.[66] Indeed, this advanced diagnostic procedure appears to be the procedure of choice to evaluate the neural structures in the rheumatoid cervical spine. Periodontoid soft tissue pannus is particularly well visualized on MRI. The moderately increased signal intensity of the mass seen on the T2-weighted image is consistent with an increased amount of water as in edema. Pettersson and associates believe that the soft tissue mass may represent not only rheumatoid inflammatory tissue but also fibrous tissue resulting from chronic mechanical irritation and edema.[66]

Electrophysiologic modalities appear to have limited usefulness in the rheumatoid patient. The electromyogram may be useful in differentiating radicular or myelopathic involvement from peripheral nerve or brachial plexus involvement. Somatosensory evoked potentials (SSEPs) are gaining popularity not only during the intraoperative management of patients undergoing spinal surgery but also for clinical evaluation. The presence or absence of appropriate evoked potentials and their latencies is the major feature of SSEPs used in clinical interpretations. Lachiewicz and colleagues[43] evaluated medial nerve SSEPs in 24 consecutive patients with unstable rheumatoid cervical spines. Fifty-eight per cent of patients with irreducible atlantoaxial subluxation or cranial settling demonstrated abnormal cervical cord conduction latencies. These investigators believed that patients with these radiographic findings may be at high risk for the development of overt myelopathy. All patients with reducible atlantoaxial subluxation or subaxial subluxation had normal SSEPs. Toolanen and coworkers[81] reported on the use of SSEPs in 34 rheumatoid patients. They had 18 patients with abnormal subluxation and 16 patients without subluxation. They found pathologic SSEPs in the subluxation group and believed that it was secondary to the subluxation. These authors concluded that SSEPs may be particularly valuable in confirming a diagnosis of cervical myelopathy, because neurologic signs and symptoms are difficult to evaluate in these often severely disabled patients.

Motor evoked potentials by means of fractionated magnetic stimulation of motor pathways to the upper limbs have also been used to assess cervical spine disorders.[22] Dvorak and associates found that 67 per cent of the 55 patients with rheumatoid arthritis in their series showed a pathologic delay of central motor latency. These authors recommended this method in the diagnosis of cervical spine disorders in patients with suspected compression of neural structures. The technique is nonevasive and has sensitivity.

Because the neurologic examination is often difficult in patients with polyarticular involvement, an objective test such as evoked potentials is desirable. Evoked potentials may be of great value in the management of patients with rheumatoid subluxation and early myelopathy, for both diagnostic and follow-up evaluation.

In summary, the initial approach to the diagnostic evaluation of a patient with rheumatoid arthritis consists of plain radiographs with emphasis on the lateral flexion and extension dynamic views. Particular attention is paid to the craniocervical junction, noting the station of the atlas as well as the predental interval. If significant abnormalities are noted, AP and lateral polytomograms are useful in defining bony anatomy, and MRI defines the neurologic structures. A dynamic lateral flexion and extension MRI of the craniovertebral junction and upper cervical spine is particularly helpful in evaluating the status of the cord and brain stem (Fig. 41–5).

INDICATIONS FOR OPERATIVE INTERVENTION

Despite frequent cervical involvement, an operation on the cervical spine is indicated only in a small percentage of rheumatoid patients. Treatment is based on the presence of signs and symptoms in addition to the radiographic findings. The presence of subluxation on dynamic radiographs does not by itself warrant fusion.

Symptoms must be sufficiently important to warrant the hazards of surgery.[1] Patients with mild instability of the cervical spine who complain of intermittent suboccipital headaches are often treated symptomatically. A cervical orthosis may be prescribed when such patients ride in a car. Such patients, however, must be followed carefully with periodic examinations, including lateral and flexion-extension radiographs.

The goals of operation are to stabilize the spine, relieve neurologic compression, and relieve pain.[14] The indications for arthrodesis are pain; instability; neurologic deficit, either actual or impending; or a combination of these. Instability is the most frequent indication for operation. In addition, an impending neurologic deficit may be a valid indication for operation. An impending deficit is defined as severe instability combined with cord or thecal sac compression on neural radiographic studies.[17]

Dynamic lateral flexion and extension radiographs are the primary studies used to quantitate the degree of instability. Greater than 3 mm of mobile atlantoaxial subluxation is considered unstable. When the anterior atlantodental interval is greater than 8 or 9 mm, the cord is at potential risk. Many authors agree that more than 9 mm of mobile atlantoaxial subluxation, despite the presence of objective neurologic signs, is an indica-

tion for surgery.[17, 72] As previously mentioned, Boden and colleagues described the importance of the posterior atlantodental interval and recommended operative stabilization of the rheumatoid cervical spine, in the presence or absence of a neurologic deficit, for patients who had atlantoaxial subluxation and a posterior atlantodental interval of 14 mm or less. In addition, they recommended stabilization in patients who had atlantoaxial subluxation and at least 5 mm of cranial settling and in patients who had subaxial subluxation and an AP sagittal diameter of the spinal canal of 14 mm or less.[5]

Therefore, when the following are present, one should consider operative intervention: atlantoaxial subluxation greater than 8 mm with neuroradiographic evidence of cord compression on dynamic flexion-extension views or a posterior atlantodental interval less than or equal to 14 mm; cranial settling of 5 mm or greater plus neuroradiographic evidence of cord compression; or more than 3.5 mm of mobile subaxial subluxation with evidence of cord compression on neuroradiographic studies or a sagittal diameter of the spinal canal of 14 mm or less.[5] A progressive neurologic deficit is a strong indication for possible operative intervention. An overriding factor when considering a patient for operation, however, is the overall status of the patient. Many severely involved rheumatoid patients suffer from chronic anemia and may be malnourished. It is advisable to attempt to correct as many of these problems as possible preoperatively. A patient with profound involvement with severe osteopenia of the cervical vertebrae may not be a candidate for operation because of insufficiency of the bone. One requires solid bone to provide the foundation for a cervical arthrodesis. Wire, cement, screws, and plates will not provide stability if there is not firm fixation to the bone. A realistic operative construct must be carefully planned preoperatively.

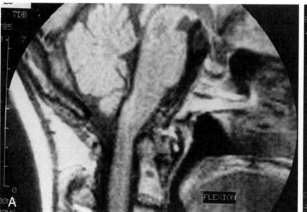
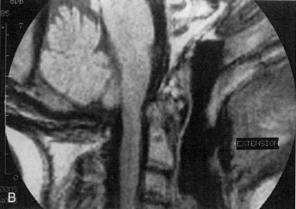

Figure 41–5. Dynamic sagittal MRI scans of a rheumatoid patient with atlantoaxial subluxation. *A,* Flexion image demonstrating an increase in the predental interval. *B,* Extension image demonstrating a decrease in the predental interval. (From Clark, C. R.: The cervical spine. *In* Pos, R. [ed.]: Pediatric and reconstructive aspects. Orthopaedic Knowledge Update. Vol. 3. Park Ridge, IL, American Academy of Orthopaedic Surgeons, 1990, pp. 379–393.)

OPERATIVE PROCEDURES

Preoperative planning is the first step in successful operative management. Preoperative radiographic studies should be carefully evaluated to assess not only the presence of multilevel involvement but also the quality of the bone stock. Operative constructs should be carefully planned.

Patients with severe subluxation that does not completely reduce are considered for preoperative skeletal traction. We prefer to use a halo ring for traction, because traction can best be controlled with this device. Traction may be indicated for three to seven days, and halo wheelchair traction is advisable to avoid prolonged immobilization in bed. Traction should be applied gently; 7 to 12 pounds is generally sufficient. Typically, traction is applied along the midline longitudinal axis of the patient, and hyperflexion or hyperextension of the craniovertebral junction is avoided. The patient is monitored neurologically and radiographically during the process. Overdistraction must be avoided in these very unstable patients.

Most patients with subluxations and instability can be managed with stabilization procedures alone. Indeed, the report by Grob and coworkers[25] clearly demonstrates that rheumatoid pannus may resorb when a satisfactory fusion is obtained. However, patients with irreducible subluxation, profound compression, and/or profound myelopathy may require decompression in addition to the stabilization procedure. Patients who have substantial improvement of their neurologic status in skeletal traction are considered for stabilization procedures. Patients with a profound or progressive deficit that is unimproved by traction may be candidates for a major decompressive procedure.

Patients undergo an awake nasal or endotracheal intubation. If used, spinal cord monitoring electrodes are applied next, and a baseline SSEP tracing is obtained. Obtaining the baseline SSEP preoperatively, before entering the operating room, is more efficient. Patients are carefully logrolled into position while awake, and a lateral radiograph is obtained before the induction of anesthesia to verify satisfactory alignment of the spine. Awake intubation, interoperative skeletal traction, and interoperative spinal cord monitoring are employed to maximize the protection of neurologic structures. A neurologic examination is then performed, and anesthesia is induced.

Atlantoaxial Arthrodesis: Wire Technique

The patient is positioned in the prone position in skeletal traction (Fig. 41–6). The torso is supported on a Wilson-type frame, and the shoulders are pulled and taped distally for countertraction. Approximately 5 to 10 pounds of skeletal traction are applied in the longitudinal axis. The posterior head and neck are shaved from the inion distally. The neck and iliac crest region are then sterilely prepped and draped. The proposed skin incision and underlying subcutaneous tissues are infiltrated with approximately 10 ml of 1:500,000 epinephrine in saline solution. A skin incision is made from just below the level of the inion to the midcervical level. The approach is made in the midline, with the inion and the posterior spinous process of C2 as landmarks. The dissection is carried down in the midline plane to the level of the posterior spinous process of C2. Soft tissues are carefully dissected off the posterior elements of C2 from the midline laterally. Dissection is then carefully performed in a cephalad direction, starting at the midline and dissecting out laterally. The posterior tubercle of the atlas is identified, and a careful dissection of the soft tissues off the posterior arch is performed. Care is taken to protect the vertebral arteries; the dissection should not extend more than 1 to 1.5 cm lateral to the posterior tubercle. A towel clip is useful to stabilize the posterior spinous of C2 during the soft tissue dissection of the posterior arch of the axis. Soft tissues may need to be reflected from the midline laterally off the basiocciput to allow adequate exposure of the posterior ring of C1. A dental elevator is used to dissect subposteriorly underneath the anterior aspect of the posterior arch of C1, as well as underneath the lamina of C2. A curved Mayo needle, placed in a reverse manner with the blunt end of the needle forward, is used to pass the suture underneath the arch of C1 and under the lamina of C2. Two sutures are placed on either side of the midline at each level, for a total of eight sutures. The two sets of sutures on either side are then secured underneath C1 and C2 so that there are two continuous sutures underneath C1 and C2 on either side. Then wires are passed with each of the sutures from cephalad to caudad. Twenty-four-gauge, double-twisted wire with approximately two to three twists per centimeter is durable yet flexible. The posterior aspects of C1 and C2 are then lightly decorticated with a diamond burr. A cortical cancellous graft is obtained from the posterior iliac crest. One large piece of graft approximately 2 by 4 cm in size is preferable; a small notch is prepared to receive the posterior spinous process of C2. The graft is then secured in a method similar to that described by Brooks and Jenkins[9] by securing the graft on either of the midline with the wires. It is important to obtain secure fixation of the graft to the posterior arches of C1 and C2. The large graft may be supplemented with small chips of cancellous iliac crest graft. If necessary, a small drain is left for approximately 24 hours, and the wound is closed. If a dural leak occurs during the procedure, the drain should be placed in the subcutaneous tissues above the level of the fascia. Patients are typically maintained postoperatively in a halo-vest, which is left in place approximately six to 12 weeks, followed by a cervical orthosis if necessary.

Atlantoaxial Arthrodesis: Transarticular Screw Fixation

Posterior transarticular screw fixation is an excellent way to facilitate fusion and can be used in conjunction with interspinous wiring and bone grafting to provide three-point atlantoaxial fixation.[26, 30] The transarticular

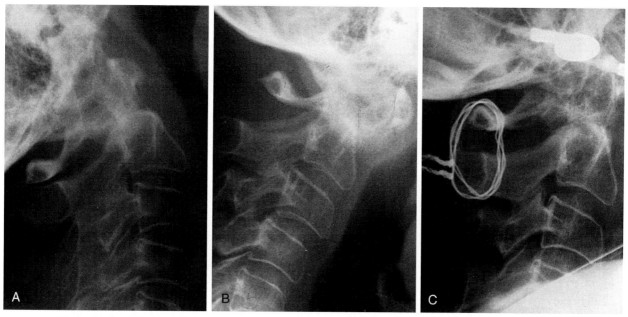

Figure 41–6. A rheumatoid patient with significant atlantoaxial subluxation. *A,* Extension lateral radiograph demonstrating reduction of the atlantoaxial complex. *B,* Flexion lateral radiograph showing a significant increase of the predental interval. *C,* Postoperative lateral radiograph demonstrating an atlantoaxial arthrodesis.

screw fixation rigidly couples the facets of the axis and atlas vertebrae, providing immediate internal fixation. Thus, a postoperative halo-brace is unnecessary.[27, 48] Before posterior atlantoaxial transarticular screw fixation is attempted, the atlantoaxial subluxation must be reduced satisfactorily. The superior facet of C2 and the lateral masses of C1 must be aligned properly to obtain adequate purchase of the screw.[47] The morphology and pathologic anatomy of the atlas and axis, as well as the third cervical vertebra, must be carefully defined by CT. Collapse of the lateral atlantal masses, as with rheumatoid cranial settling, comminuted fractures of the atlas and axis vertebrae, anomalous course of the vertebral artery, and marked osteoporosis and osteopenia, are contraindications to posterior atlantoaxial screw fixation.[48, 57]

Menezes prefers application of crown halo traction before the operative procedure to achieve reduction of the atlantoaxial subluxation. At operation, an awake fiberoptic oral endotracheal intubation is performed, after which continuous traction is maintained with the patient awake. The patient is then transferred onto the operating table. The chest is elevated on laminectomy rolls, and the crown of the halo ring rests on a padded Mayfield horseshoe headrest, with traction being maintained over a pulley bar at 6 pounds.[54] There is mild controlled flexion of the patient's neck to obtain the proper trajectory for insertion of the drills and screws. Lateral fluoroscopic C-arm visualization is used and positioning is done before draping. Once satisfactory alignment and position are achieved, general endotracheal and intravenous anesthesia ensues.[55]

The operative field is prepared from just above the external occipital protuberance to about the third thoracic spinous process. The cervical incision extends from the external occipital protuberance to the spinous process of T1. Subperiosteal exposure gains access to the squamous-occipital bone, foramen magnum, and upper three cervical vertebrae. This is carried fairly far laterally to the facet joints. The spinous process of C2 is transfixed with a towel clip during dissection to provide manual control of the vertebra and to stabilize the craniocervical articulation. Rotational abnormalities of C1 and C2 must be manually corrected at this point, and if need be, a wire can be placed around the posterior ring of C1 for traction and subsequently fixation.

The ligamentum flavum between the atlas and the axis, as well as between the axis and the third cervical vertebra, must be removed to identify the laminae, the pedicles, and the facet joints. The anatomic landmarks of the C2 pedicle, the atlantoaxial facet joint, and the C2 nerve root and venous plexus must be identified, and the nerve root is elevated with a retractor. It is advantageous to lower the head of the operative field to be able to gain proper trajectory. A K-wire is used for the initial drilling. The drill enters the posterior C2 cortex 3 mm above the C2–C3 facet joint and 2 to 3 mm lateral to the medial border of the C2 facet. The drill trajectory is aimed toward the dorsal cortex of the anterior arch of C1 with a 0- to 10-degree medial alignment (Fig. 41–7). The posterior bone cortex of C2 is penetrated with a high-speed drill or bone awl to direct the K-wire drill insertion. The guidewire skims just beneath the C1–C2 articular facet to enter into the lateral atlantal mass, pointing toward the anterior cortex of the anterior arch of C1 on lateral fluoroscopy.

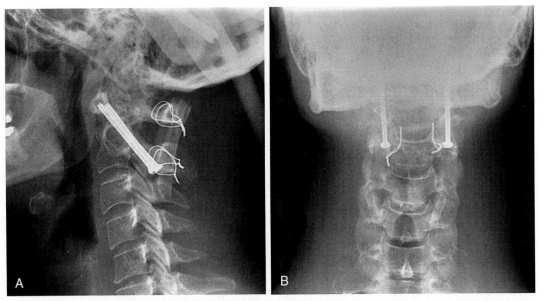

Figure 41–7. *A,* Lateral cervical radiograph made two weeks after posterior atlantoaxial facet–transarticular screw fixation for rheumatoid C1–C2 dislocation. Note the apex of the screws in the lateral atlantal masses. A dorsal interlaminar rib graft fusion completes the fusion construct. *B,* Frontal cervical radiograph of the same patient. Note the screw trajectory from C2 into C1.

This guidewire should stop short of the anterior cortex of C1 by 3 mm. A cannulated drill guide then follows the K-wire, which is still in position and is visualized on continuous fluoroscopy. Menezes prefers a partially threaded, cannulated, self-tapping lag screw. As the screw crosses the joint space into C1, the atlas and the axis become rigidly coupled. Satisfactory fixation can be achieved using a minimum number of operative steps by inserting the screw directly into the hole without tapping the hole. Ideally, the screw is placed bilaterally; thus, prior to placement of the first screw, the second guidewire should be passed to make sure that the wires are parallel to each other on lateral fluoroscopy. Only then should the self-tapping screws be placed over each guidewire. In most instances, a screw can be placed on either side. However, this may become difficult owing to incongruous bone density as well as position. In any case, the C1–C2 facet screw fixation must be supplemented with an interlaminar bone fusion including the posterior arches of C1 and C2. This three-point fixation of C1–C2 provides mechanical stability that is superior to either procedure alone. Thus, the screw and wire technique are complementary. An advantage of posterior atlantoaxial facet screw fixation is that it can be used even when the posterior ring of the atlas is fractured or incompetent.

Preoperative CT studies are essential, and the precise screw trajectory is mandatory to avoid vertebral artery injury and injury to the nerve roots. Should injury occur to the vertebral artery, the K-wire is removed and the bony opening filled with microfibrillar collagen. No further attempt should be made at screw fixation. An alternative arthrodesis is performed. It is prudent to obtain a vertebral angiogram postopera-

tively to document vessel status and possibly identify pseudoaneurysm or a subintimal flap. These require analysis of the posterior fossa circulation, with the aim of balloon occlusion of the damaged vessel.

Postoperative immobilization is provided with a modified custom-contoured occipitocervical brace that is an extension of the "Philadelphia collar."[59] We believe that this is an important addition to the armamentarium of atlantoaxial arthrodesis given the proper indications.[24, 27, 47, 48, 55]

Occipitocervical Arthrodesis: Wire and Graft Technique

The procedure is performed in a similar manner to that of atlantoaxial arthrodesis (Fig. 41–8).[13] The skin incision extends from just above the level of the inion proximally to approximately the C5 level distally. In addition to the dissection of the soft tissues from the posterior elements of C1 and C2, the soft tissues are elevated from the base of the occiput up to the level of the inion. Soft tissues should be dissected with sharp dissection and gentle blunt dissection. A towel clip placed through the posterior spinous process of C2 is useful in stabilizing the axis while soft tissues are dissected. Occasionally patients may have associated atlantoaxial subluxation with anterior displacement of C1 on C2. If the preoperative neuroradiographic studies demonstrate posterior impingement of the thecal sac by the posterior arch of the atlas, the central portion of the posterior arch of C1 is removed at this time. Note that it is dangerous to pass sublaminar wires underneath the posterior arch of C1 if there is irreducible anterior atlantoaxial subluxation. In addition, re-

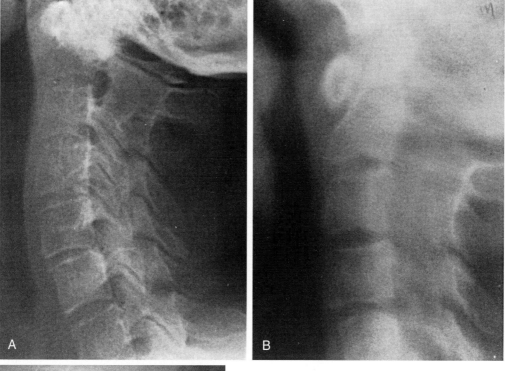

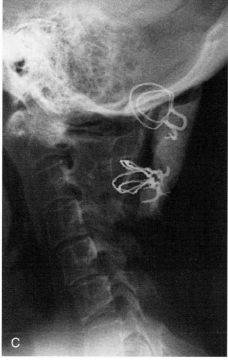

Figure 41–8. A rheumatoid patient with significant cranial settling. *A,* Lateral radiograph demonstrating moderate settling. The atlas is between Stations 2 and 3. *B,* Lateral midline tomogram depicting protrusion of the dens through the foramen magnum. *C,* Postoperative lateral radiograph demonstrating solid posterior occipitocervical fusion. (From Clark, C. R., Goetz, D. D., and Menezes, A. H.: Arthrodesis of the cervical spine in rheumatoid arthritis. J. Bone Joint Surg. [Am.] *71:*381–392, 1989.)

moval of the central portion of the posterior arch of C1 facilitates exposure of the base of the foramen magnum. The posterior 2 cm of the arch is generally removed, leaving a small portion laterally on either side just medial to the vertebral arteries to allow fixation for wire (Fig. 41–9).[13]

A small portion of the posterior aspect of the foramen magnum is removed. This portion typically has a small ventral lip, which interferes with the passage of wires. A semicircle of bone is removed from the posterior aspect of the foramen magnum until the posterior lip is removed and a dural elevator can easily be passed. Generally, the semicircle is approximately 2 cm across, and approximately 7 mm of the rim of the foramen magnum is removed in the midline. The dura is then separated off the inner aspect of the occiput

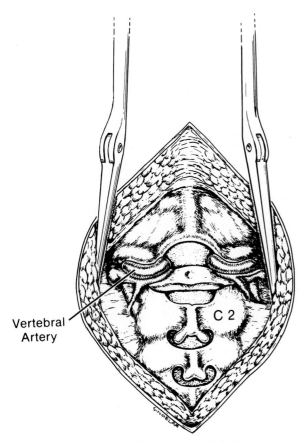

Figure 41–9. Posterior surgical exposure of the base of the occiput, atlas, and axis. (From Clark, C. R.: Occipitocervical fusion for the unstable rheumatoid neck. Orthopedics *12:*469–473, 1989.)

Vertebral Artery

C 2

strips of corticocancellous graft, approximately 1.5 by 5 cm, are harvested from the iliac crest. Three small drill holes are placed in the grafts to accept the wires at the three levels (occiput, C1, C2). The posterior aspect of the base of the occiput and the remnants of C1 and C2 are then lightly decorticated with a diamond burr. The grafts are secured from occiput to C2 on either side of the midline, and the cancellous graft is packed underneath the cortical struts (Fig. 41–11). It is important to have good contact between the struts and the underlying host bone. If necessary, small drains are left in place, but if a dural leak is present, the drain should be placed in the subcutaneous region above the fascial closure. Typically, patients are maintained in a halo orthosis postoperatively for approximately 12 weeks.

Occipital Cervical Arthrodesis: Contoured Loop/Rod Technique

When immediate fixation of the occiput to the upper cervical spine is required for severe instability, a contoured threaded loop of stainless steel is custom fitted to the occiput and upper cervical spine and anchored with cables or wires.[35, 53, 55] The contoured loop was first proposed by Ransford and colleagues in 1986.[71]

The exposure is as previously described for the occipitocervical arthrodesis. A horseshoe loop of 5/32 threaded stainless steel (Steinmann) rod is used. It is custom contoured as a loop to fit the occiput and

with a dural elevator. Two burr holes are then placed approximately 1 cm from the midline and 7 mm from the posterior opening in the foramen magnum. Each hole is approximately 7 mm in diameter. A carbide bit is used to remove the outer cortex, and then a diamond-tipped burr is used to remove the inner table of the occipital bone. A small, angled curet is used to carefully enlarge the opening, and then a dural separator is used to separate the dura from the inner table of the occiput. An extradural tunnel is made from this hole down to the foramen magnum. A reverse curved suture needle is used to pass sutures from these two holes in the occiput out through the foramen magnum. A small drill hole is placed in the remnant of the posterior arch of C1 if a posterior decompression of the arch has been performed. If the arch is intact, sublaminar wires are placed at this level, as in the atlantoaxial arthrodesis. Sublaminar wires are placed at C2 using a reverse curved needle. Double-twisted, 24-gauge wire is then attached to each level of the sutures, one at each level. If the posterior arch of C1 has been decompressed, the small drill hole in the remnant of C1 may be too small to receive a double-twisted wire; consequently, a single strand of 24- or 22-gauge wire is applied to this level (Fig. 41–10). Two

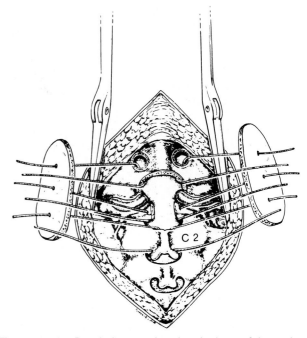

Figure 41–10. Burr holes are placed at the base of the occiput, and a small drill hole is placed on either side of the remnant of the decompressed atlas to accept fixation wires. Additional sublaminar wires are placed at C2. (From Clark, C. R.: Occipitocervical fusion for the unstable rheumatoid neck. Orthopedics *12:*469–473, 1989.)

C 2

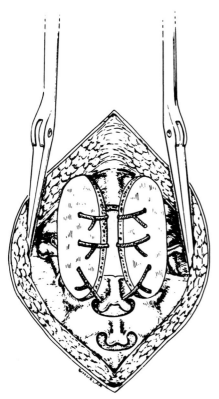

Figure 41–11. Corticocancellous grafts are secured with 24-gauge wire at each level. (From Clark, C. R.: Occipitocervical fusion for the unstable rheumatoid neck. Orthopedics *12*:469–473, 1989.)

the occipitocervical articulation so that the descending limbs flow down the upper cervical spine along the laminae to the C3 level. It is imperative that the horizontal limb of the contoured loop be approximately 3.5 to 4 cm. The height of the occipital portion of the loop is between 2.5 and 3 cm. A craniectomy is made to remove the posterior rim of the foramen magnum for approximately 1 cm to either side of the midline and ascending by 1 cm. This removes the inner occipital ridge.[29, 63] The bone can be saved for use in the subsequent bone construct. Trephines are then made 2 cm to either side of the midline and 1 cm above the foramen magnum. Two other trephines are made, one on either side of the midline, 3 cm above the foramen magnum. These trephines allow for passage of epidural cable or wire between the trephine and the craniectomized midline at the foramen magnum, to gain purchase of the occipital bone. In Menezes's experience, stainless steel cable or braided stainless steel wire can be used. Sublaminar cable is passed beneath C1, C2, and C3 bilaterally. The contoured loop is fixated to the skull and upper cervical spine, and the braided wire or stainless steel cables are tightened starting at the C2 or C3 level and then at the occiput to maintain proper fixation and position. This may be combined with posterior decompression of C1. A transverse crossbar fixation between the descending loops may be used to

augment the biomechanical strength of the construct. It is imperative that the horizontal limb of the contoured loop instrumentation be fixated and supported by cables superiorly and laterally to the occiput. This construct is then supplemented with bone. One hundred six such constructs have been made with success.

Since 1991, a custom-contoured threaded titanium loop has been used for dorsal occipitocervical instrumentation and titanium threaded cables for fixation. The bone has been harvested from the diploic occipital bone or rib for the osseous construct (Fig. 41–12A). Postoperative immobilization is accomplished in a custom-contoured occipitocervical orthosis, as with transarticular screw fixation patients. The quality of postoperative MRIs is excellent, with little image distortion and minimal scatter. Menezes has found this technique ideal for assessing alignment, regression of pannus, or neural decompression (Fig. 41–12B). Integration of bone with an osseous construct has occurred within three months (Fig. 41–13).[53, 55, 57]

Subaxial Arthrodesis

Patients with subaxial subluxation are best managed with a posterior stabilization procedure. Despite evidence of anterior compression from the subluxation, removal of the intervertebral disc and anterior longitudinal ligament with application of bone graft may make the spine more unstable. Therefore, a posterior procedure is usually preferred. Some patients, however, have profound subluxation and may require anterior decompression as well as posterior stabilization. Posterior stabilization is typically performed with a modification of Roger's interspinous wiring technique and posterior iliac crest graft. However, in patients with gross deficiency of the posterior elements, modification of the facet arthrodesis described by Callahan and associates[11] may be required to provide stability. Autogenous bone graft and postoperative immobilization in a halo device are preferred.

Transoral Resection of the Dens

The primary indication for an anterior midline transoral approach to the craniovertebral junction in rheumatoid arthritis patients is irreducible ventral extradural compression of the cervicomedullary junction.[59, 60] This is common with irreducible cranial settling and secondary odontoid invagination into the posterior fossa, odontoid fracture with complex compression, and fracture fragments with a large fibrous pannus (Fig. 41–14A). Pathology located within the subarachnoid space is best approached from a lateral or posterolateral route, unless this has proved ineffective on a previous attempt.

Preoperative Assessment

It is extremely important to obtain a working distance of 2.5 to 3 cm between the upper and lower incisor teeth. When there is immobilization of the temporo-

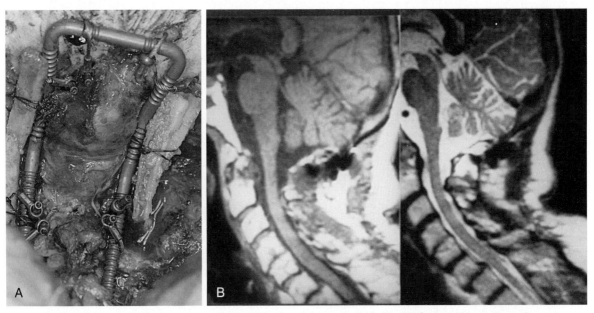

Figure 41–12. *A,* Operative photograph of dorsal occipitocervical (O–C2–C3) fusion with contoured threaded titanium loop and cables. This patient had previously undergone foramen magnum and posterior atlantal decompression for rheumatoid cranial settling with worsening. The invagination was reduced prior to fusion. Note the rib grafts. *B,* Composite of midsagittal T1- (L) and T2- (R) weighted MRI of craniocervical region made three months after dorsal O–C3 titanium loop instrumentation with rib graft fusion. Note the satisfactory alignment, posterior decompression, and lack of artifact.

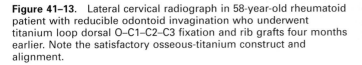

Figure 41–13. Lateral cervical radiograph in 58-year-old rheumatoid patient with reducible odontoid invagination who underwent titanium loop dorsal O–C1–C2–C3 fixation and rib grafts four months earlier. Note the satisfactory osseous-titanium construct and alignment.

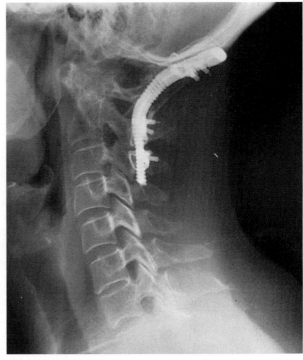

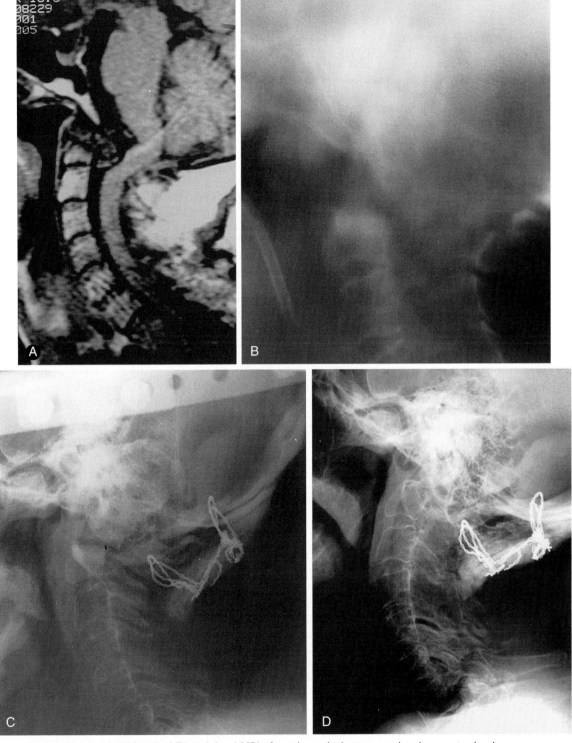

Figure 41–14. *A,* Midsagittal T1-weighted MRI of craniocervical area reveals a large extradural mass ventral to the cervicomedullary junction and dorsal occipitocervical dislocation. *B,* Midline lateral tomogram of the craniovertebral junction (CVJ) made four days after transoral resection of the odontoid fracture and pannus mass. A nasogastric feeding tube is in place. Note the resection of the anterior atlantal arch and dens, with restoration of alignment. *C,* Lateral radiograph of CVJ made two months after dorsal O–C2 fusion with rib grafts and braided wires, supplemented with methyl methacrylate. The bone fusion has not matured. *D,* Lateral cervical roentgenogram made one year after fusion. Note the more than adequate osseous fusion beneath the methyl methacrylate and into the occiput and dorsal atlantoaxial bone.

mandibular joint, a straightforward transoral approach may be limited and may require median mandibular splitting with midline glossotomy or an alternative route.[28, 34, 36, 82] It is imperative that a complete general medical and nutritional evaluation be made prior to the operative procedure. Nasopharyngeal and oropharyngeal cultures are obtained three days before the ventral operation, and a complete dental assessment is mandatory.[53] Antibiotics are contraindicated unless pathologic flora are present. It is imperative that a preoperative assessment of swallowing and respiratory function be made. Rheumatoid involvement of the larynx is not uncommon, nor is rheumatoid involvement of the upper respiratory tree. Compromise of lower cranial nerves mandates prolonged postoperative intubation or even the consideration of tracheostomy at the time of the ventral operative procedure.

It is important to remember that 78 per cent of rheumatoid patients with cranial settling have a reducible lesion that requires only primary dorsal occipitocervical fixation.[53, 55, 59, 60] Thus, only one in five patients with rheumatoid cranial settling in Menezes's series required a ventral decompression.

Operative Technique

The patient is transported supine to the operating suite with the head in neutral position. An awake fiberoptic oral endotracheal intubation is performed. The patient is then positioned supine with very mild extension. The head rests on a padded Mayfield horseshoe headrest. Traction is maintained using a pulley bar with mild extension of the neck. Skull clamps are avoided because of the potential instability that may arise during the operative procedure and also because fixation of only the head still allows the distal segment to move. Once it has been established that no neurologic deficit has occurred as a result of intubation and positioning maneuvers, general endotracheal and intravenous and anesthesia ensues.

A modified Dingman self-retaining mouth retractor secures the oral endotracheal tube and allows for exposure of the entire oral cavity as well as the oropharynx and the nasopharynx. Operative procedures that involve the foramen magnum and clivus make it essential to split the soft palate to obtain necessary exposure. Otherwise, the soft palate may be retracted upward with a palatal retractor or with a rubber catheter sutured to the soft palate and brought out through the nostrils, lifting up the soft palate.

A throat pack is placed to occlude the laryngopharynx and the esophagus. Ten per cent PVP-iodine is used to cleanse the pharynx and oral cavity. This is then rinsed with hydrogen peroxide and saline.

The median raphe of the soft palate is infiltrated with 0.5 per cent lidocaine (Xylocaine) solution with 1:200,000 epinephrine. The palatal incision starts to the right of the uvula and immediately comes to the midline, hence ascending along the median raphe toward the hard palate. The leaves of the soft palate are held apart with stay sutures to expose the nasopharynx

and the oropharynx. The posterior pharyngeal wall is topically anesthetized with 2.5 per cent cocaine, and the median raphe is infiltrated with 0.5 per cent Xylocaine solution with 1:200,000 epinephrine. The midline posterior pharyngeal incision extends from the clivus to the upper border of the third cervical vertebra, and the pharyngeal flaps are swept to either side. Self-retaining stay sutures hold apart the pharynx. The longus capitis and longus colli muscles are dissected free of the osseous and ligamentous attachments to expose the upper cervical vertebrae and the clivus as necessary. The lateral exposure is limited to approximately 1.5 cm to either side of the midline to prevent injury to the eustachian tubes, the vertebral artery, and the hypoglossal nerves superiorly.

The microscope is used for magnification and a concentrated light source throughout the operative procedure. The position of the operating surgeon is at the head of the table. The anterior arch of the atlas is removed with a high-speed drill, as is the caudal clivus. Soft tissue ventral to the odontoid process is now removed, and the odontoid process is then resected. This resection starts from rostral to caudal, using a high-speed carbide burr under constant saline irrigation. Once the offending odontoid mass is reduced to a shell, this is resected with a diamond burr. Sharp dissection is done in a subperiosteal manner to free the frayed alar and apical ligaments. The odontoid resection needs to be carried down to at least 1 cm below the slopes of the superior facets of the axis vertebra. Fine angled curets and Kerrison rongeurs facilitate the removal of the bony mass and the tough pannus.

The extent of the bone resection is governed by the preoperative diagnostic studies (see Fig. 41–14B). It may be prudent to transect a bony spicule that might have a subarachnoid location or be adherent to the brain stem or the vertebrobasilar vascular system. In such a situation, detachment of this prevents neurologic or vascular injury, as well as cerebrospinal fluid (CSF) leakage. Resection of tough pannus should be done after cauterization. The tectorial membrane is decompressed to allow for dural pulsations, which herald completion of the extradural decompression.

Opening of the dura on the ventral aspect of the upper cervical spine and along the clivus may be accompanied by bleeding from the circular sinus. This is controlled with titanium dural clips. Closure of the dura should be attempted in a primary fashion, backed with fascial graft and subsequently fat. The fat pad is reinforced with plasma glue and a subsequent careful closure of the wound. When intra-arachnoid pathology is suspected preoperatively, a lumbar subarachnoid drain should be installed prior to the operative procedure and drainage maintained for 10 days after the operation. If the dura has been violated, metronidazole, nafcillin, and cefotaxime are continued for five days after the operative procedure. Should there be no CSF leak, the cefotaxime is discontinued, and nafcillin and metronidazole are continued for another five days.

When the subarachnoid space has not been violated, the closure of the posterior wound is started with the approximation of the longus colli and longus capitis muscles in the midline, followed by a layered closure of the posterior pharyngeal musculature. This is accomplished with 3-0 polyglycolic suture in interrupted fashion. The mucosa of the posterior pharynx is then brought together with interrupted sutures of a similar strength. The throat pack is removed, and under direct vision, a nasal oropharyngeal-gastric feeding tube is passed. This is anchored to the alar of the nostril. The soft palate is approximated in two layers, first bringing together the nasal mucosa with interrupted sutures and then bringing the muscularis together with the oral mucosa with interrupted vertical mattress sutures.

Menezes used brain stem evoked potentials and direct bipolar recordings in his first 100 transoral procedures[79, 88] but has not found them useful. Hence, the subsequent 230 transoral craniovertebral resections were made without such recordings.

Postoperative Care for Transoral Procedures

No oral intake is permitted postoperatively. The head of the bed is elevated, and the endotracheal tube is left in place for at least 48 to 72 hours until the lingual and pharyngeal soft tissue swelling has receded. A cervical collar is placed around the neck, and the patient is gradually elevated before the commencement of feedings by the nasogastric tube. Oral intake is permitted at the end of the first week, beginning with a clear liquid diet and followed by a gradual increase in feedings to a regular diet by the end of 21 days. Postoperative intravenous antibiotics are maintained only for the first 24 hours and consist of penicillin.

Rheumatoid cranial settling implies occipitoatlantoaxial instability. Thus, these patients require a dorsal fixation (see Fig. 41–14C and D). Depending on the surgeon and the patient's general medical condition, this may be carried out immediately after the ventral transoral procedure, which has been the recent trend in our management. However, it is not uncommon to delay the fusion procedure to a later date.

Complications

The most dreaded complication is CSF leakage and meningitis. The technique of closure of the pharyngeal wall and prevention of dural leak has been described.[7, 31, 54, 89] Bleeding during the transoral operation at the level of the circular sinus can be stopped only by clipping the two leaves of the dura, which houses the venous sinuses. Careful packing with microfibrillar collagen or oxidized cellulose may bring the situation under control. If the vertebral artery branches bleed, hemostasis has to be obtained with bipolar cauterization and occlusion with an aneurysm clip. This does not always spell disaster, because the opposite vertebral artery can accomplish adequate posterior circulation.

In rheumatoid patients, severe postoperative tongue swelling may occur. Intermittent release of the tongue retractor during the operation and maintenance of endotracheal intubation postoperatively are essential until the swelling recedes. Palatal dehiscence requires immediate reclosure. However, pharyngeal wound dehiscence that occurs after the first week implies retropharyngeal infection, as with abscess. This requires an extrapharyngeal approach and drainage.

The most unrecognized complication is postoperative craniovertebral instability, and this is always present in patients with rheumatoid cranial settling.

Neurologic worsening after the transoropharyngeal operation signifies loss of alignment, retained bone or tumor, the possibility of abscess formation, and possible meningitis. In rare circumstances, the vertebrobasilar system may occlude as a complication of the operation or coincidentally.

GENERAL COMMENTS

For most patients, there should be an attempt to realign the osseous anatomy to relieve the neural compression. This is done by cervical traction and position. All individuals undergoing cervical traction should be monitored in a care facility for neurologic status, respiratory status, and radiographic alignment.[56] In individuals with gross instability or complex forms of craniovertebral involvement, instrumentation of the craniovertebral junction may be necessary. Contoured loop instrumentation is used to fixate the skull to the upper cervical vertebrae.[46, 58, 71, 74] As in all fusions, it is essential to obtain stability with the osseous construct, and the instrumentation is only a temporary feature until bony integration takes place.[70] It is important to include all unstable segments in the fusion construct.

Methyl methacrylate or a contoured loop or rod may be a valuable adjunct in selected cases. Long-term success of cervical arthrodesis requires solid bony union. Therefore, autogenous bone graft, either locally from the cranium or distally from the iliac crest or rib, is the preferred means of stabilization. Patients with substantial osteopenia and those requiring multilevel constructs may benefit from the addition of methacrylate or an internal fixation device. Bear in mind that the methacrylate or device should be considered a temporary internal splint, used to provide stability during incorporation of the graft. The surgeon must not rely on methacrylate as the primary stabilizer, because it will fatigue and fail. Young patients with relatively normal bone can be managed successfully without the use of methacrylate. When used, methacrylate must be applied with great caution. A minimal amount of material should be used to provide stability and avoid the problems associated with wound closure.

Because of problems associated with nonunion, particularly at the C1–C2 level, patients are typically managed with a halo device postoperatively. Fixation with contoured rods and loops may be a reasonable alternative, because the results appear promising.

The decision to remove a cervical orthosis postoperatively is based on dynamic lateral flexion and extension radiographs.

CLINICAL EXPERIENCE

As previously noted, definitive long-term studies on the natural history of cervical spine involvement are not available. Therefore, the indications for operative management of this condition are controversial.[14] There are several reports in the literature, however, detailing the results of operative management. Zoma and associates[91] described the results of 40 operative procedures in 32 patients with rheumatoid arthritis. They had a 57 per cent success rate, with 35 per cent failures and 8 per cent early operative deaths. Overall, these results were discouraging; however, the authors found that the most important factor for success was the severity of neurologic involvement. Eighty-seven per cent of patients with severe deficit had failure or early death, whereas 80 per cent of patients with lesser grades of neural involvement had good clinical results.[91] The authors used as their indication for operation progressive neurologic impairment and progressive instability. An occasional indication for operation in their series was intractable pain. Complications included four infections and nine graft fractures or rib resorption. On the basis of these findings, the authors questioned the wisdom of operating on such patients and concluded that early recognition of potentially serious instability was the most important factor.[91]

Santavirta and colleagues[75] reported 32 patients with rheumatoid involvement; 18 were treated operatively and 14 nonoperatively. Of their operative patients, 13 underwent atlantoaxial arthrodesis and five had occipitocervical arthrodesis. Pain relief was obtained in 12 of 15 patients treated operatively, compared with only one of eight treated nonoperatively. Neurologic status was either unchanged or improved in the operated group, compared with an overall slight decrease in patients treated nonoperatively. The authors believed that despite the lack of clear indications for operative intervention, arthrodesis of the unstable rheumatoid spine relieved pain and prevented progression of existing neurologic lesions without undue risk.[14, 75] Heywood and coworkers[32] described a similar positive clinical experience. They reported on 26 patients who underwent 30 operative procedures. Twelve of 15 patients who underwent atlantoaxial arthrodesis were reviewed for follow-up. Patients with occipitocervical fusions and subaxial posterior cervical fusions did well. There was an 8 per cent mortality rate in this series. The authors concluded that early intervention was the key to success. They advised against the use of anterior cervical fusion in these patients. They found that most of their patients could be managed by stabilization alone and recommended early intervention in the presence of significant instability.[33]

Clark and coauthors[17] reported a series of 41 consecutive patients who underwent cervical arthrodesis with a minimum follow-up of 23 months. Twenty patients underwent atlantoaxial arthrodesis, 16 occipitocervical arthrodesis, and five posterior arthrodesis of the subaxial spine. In addition, two patients had transoral odontoidectomies, and one had an anterior cervical verte-brectomy. Overall the authors reported an 88 per cent rate of osseous union. There were two fibrous unions that were clinically stable and three nonunions. All problems with union occurred in patients who underwent isolated atlantoaxial arthrodesis. Clinically, 66 per cent of patients were improved, 34 per cent were unchanged, and none were worse. Complications included a transient hemiparesis in one patient that occurred before the institution of intraoperative skeletal traction and spinal cord monitoring. Other complications included superficial wound infection in two patients, displacement of the anterior graft in one, broken wires in three, and erosion of the methacrylate into the outer part of the occipital cortex in one. Four patients died of causes unrelated to the operation. The authors cautioned about the development of instability at additional levels following arthrodesis and recommended that patients be monitored carefully for the development of further instability. The authors concluded that rheumatoid patients who are operatively managed by posterior cervical arthrodesis are at risk for early operative morbidity and mortality; however, with early recognition and appropriate management, this risk may be very low.[14, 17]

Krieg and associates[42] provided a long-term follow-up of the same series of patients described by Clark and coworkers.[17] At a minimum follow-up of seven years, 13 patients were known to be dead, and one patient could not be located. Of the remaining patients, 18 underwent full examination, including physical examination and radiographs. All patients considered the operation a success. Only one patient at follow-up had a nonunion, and this was stable over time. No patient had deteriorated neurologic function. There was no significant degeneration or instability seen at levels adjacent to the fused segments as compared with the rest of the cervical spine. The authors concluded that posterior cervical spine arthrodesis for rheumatoid involvement of the neck is a safe, efficacious procedure with no significant deterioration of effects over time.[42]

Menezes's series of more than 600 fusions at the craniovertebral junction included 335 patients who underwent occipitocervical fixation. The majority of rheumatoid patients had methyl methacrylate for supplemental internal stabilization and were immobilized with an occipital cervical brace.[53, 56, 59] Fusion was achieved in 98 per cent. A fibrous union occurred in 2 per cent. An additional 106 patients had occipital cervical bony fusion and halo immobilization.

Boden and colleagues, in their long-term analysis of the predictors of paralysis and recovery in patients with rheumatoid arthritis of the cervical spine, found that the prognosis for neurologic recovery following operation was not affected by the duration of the paralysis but was influenced by the severity of paralysis at the time of operation.[5] The most important predictor of the potential for neurologic recovery after the operation was the preoperative posterior atlantodental interval. In patients who had paralysis caused by atlantoaxial subluxation, no recovery occurred if the posterior atlantodental interval was less than 10 mm, whereas recovery of at least one neurologic class always occurred when the posterior atlantodental interval was at least 10 mm. When cranial settling was superimposed, clinically important neurologic recovery occurred only when the posterior atlantodental interval was at least 13 mm. All patients who had paralysis and a posterior atlantodental interval or an AP diameter of the subaxial canal of 14 mm had complete motor recovery after operation.

SUMMARY

The physician must be aware that rheumatoid arthritis frequently involves the cervical spine. In many cases, such involvement may be silent and the clinical findings fairly nonspecific. Certain signals should alert the physician to the possibility of cervical involvement, including an abrupt increase in neck pain, development of spasticity or hyperreflexia, bowel or bladder incontinence, and change in ambulatory status.[12] Such patients should be carefully studied with dynamic radiographs to rule out instability. Advanced radiographic studies, including polytomography and MRI, may be required to fully delineate the problem.

Most patients with rheumatoid involvement of the cervical spine can be managed nonoperatively. Such patients, however, should be followed on a periodic basis with dynamic flexion and extension radiographs. In addition, all rheumatoid patients who are undergoing general anesthesia should have preoperative lateral flexion and extension cervical radiographs to rule out occult instability. In patients with significant instability, severe pain, progressive neurologic deficit, or impending neurologic deficit, operative management may be indicated. Most patients can be managed effectively with a posterior arthrodesis. Early recognition and prompt appropriate management are paramount to the successful management of these patients.

References

1. Bailey, R. W.: Dislocation from conditions other than trauma—postlaminectomy and in rheumatoid arthritis. *In* Bailey, R. W. (ed.): The Cervical Spine. Philadelphia, Lea & Febiger, 1974, pp. 197–210.
2. Ball, J.: The articular pathology of rheumatoid arthritis. *In* Carter, M. E. (ed.): Radiological Aspects of Rheumatoid Arthritis. Amsterdam, Exerpta Medica, 1964, pp. 25–39.
3. Bland, J. H.: Rheumatoid arthritis of the cervical spine. J. Rheumatol. 1:319–342, 1974.
4. Bland, J. H., Davis, P. H., London, M. G., et al.: Rheumatoid arthritis of the cervical spine. Arch. Intern. Med. *112:*892–898, 1963.
5. Boden, S. D., Dodge, L. D., Bohlman, H. H., and Rechtine, G. R.: Rheumatoid arthritis of the cervical spine: A long term analysis with predictors of paralysis and recovery. J. Bone Joint Surg. [Am.] *75:*1282–1297, 1993.
6. Bohlman, H. H.: Atlantoaxial dislocations in the arthritic patient: Report of 45 cases. Orthop. Trans. *2:*197, 1978.
7. Bonkowski, J. A., Gibson, R. D., and Snape, L.: Foramen magnum meningioma. Transoral resection with a bone baffle to prevent CSF leakage. Case report. J. Neurosurg. *72:*493–496, 1990.
8. Boyle, A. C.: The rheumatoid neck. Proc. R. Soc. Med. *64:*1161, 1971.
9. Brooks, A. L., and Jenkins, E. B.: Atlanto-axial arthrodesis by the wedge compression method. J. Bone Joint Surg. [Am.] *60:*279–284, 1978.
10. Cabot, A., and Becker, A.: The cervical spine in rheumatoid arthritis. Clin. Orthop. *131:*130–140, 1978.
11. Callahan, R. A., Johnson, R. M., Margolis, R. N., et al.: Cervical facet fusion for control of instability following laminectomy. J. Bone Joint Surg. [Am.] *59:*991–1002, 1977.
12. Clark, C. R.: Cervical spine involvement in rheumatoid arthritis: A primer for the practitioner. Iowa Med. *74:*57–62, 1984.
13. Clark, C. R.: Occipitocervical fusion for the unstable rheumatoid neck. Orthopedics *12:*469–473, 1989.
14. Clark, C. R.: The cervical spine: Pediatric and reconstructive aspects. *In* Poss, R. (ed.): Orthopaedic Knowledge Update. Vol. 3. Park Ridge, IL, American Academy of Orthopaedic Surgeons, 1990, pp. 379–393.
15. Clark, C. R.: Rheumatoid involvement of othe cervical spine: An overview. Spine *19:*2257–2258, 1994.
16. Clark, C. R.: Cervical spine and rheumatoid arthritis: Natural history and diagnostic criteria for operation. *In* Baumgartner H., et al. (eds.): Rheumatoid Arthritis: Current Trends and Diagnostics, Conservative Treatment, and Surgical Reconstruction. Stuttgart, George Thieme Verlag, 1995, pp. 132–138.
17. Clark, C. R., Goetz, D. D., and Menezes, A. H.: Arthrodesis of the cervical spine in rheumatoid arthritis. J. Bone Joint Surg. [Am.] *71:*381–392, 1989.
18. Conlon, P. W., Isdale, I. C., and Rose, B. S.: Rheumatoid arthritis of the cervical spine: An analysis of 33 cases. Ann. Rheum. Dis. *25:*120–126, 1966.
19. Cregan, J. C. F.: Internal fixation of the unstable rheumatoid cervical spine. Ann. Rheum. Dis. *25:*242–252, 1966.
20. Davis, F. W., Jr., and Markley, H. E.: Rheumatoid arthritis with death from medullary compression. Ann. Intern. Med. *35:*451–454, 1951.
21. Dvorak, J.: The retrodental pannus after posterior atlanto-axial fusion in rheumatoid arthritis [abstract]. Twenty-second annual meeting, CSRS, Baltimore, 1994.
22. Dvorak, J., Herdmann, J., Janssen, B., et al.: Motor evoked potentials in patients with cervical spine disorders. Spine *15:*1013–1016, 1990.
23. El Khoury, G. Y., Wener, M. H., Menezes, A. H., et al.: Cranial settling in rheumatoid arthritis. Radiology *137:*637–642, 1980.
24. Goel, V. K., Clark, C. R., Galles, K., et al.: Movement-rotation relationship of the ligamentous occipito-atlanto-axial complex. J. Biomech. *17:*363–376, 1984.
25. Grob, D.: Surgical interventions in the cervical spine: Where and how? *In* Baumgartner, H., et al. (eds.): Rheumatoid Arthritis: Current Trends and Diagnostics, Conservative Treatment, and Surgical Reconstruction. Stuttgart, George Thieme Verlag, 1995, pp. 150–157.
26. Grob, D., Crisco, J. J., III, Panjabi, M. M., et al.: Biomechanical evaluation of four different posterior atlantoaxial fixation techniques. Spine *17:*480–490, 1992.
27. Grob, D., Jeanneret, B., Aebi, M., et al.: Atlantoaxial fusion with transarticular screw fixation. J. Bone Joint Surg. [Br.] *73:*972–976, 1991.
28. Hall, J. E., Denis, F., and Murray, J.: Exposure of the upper cervical spine for spinal decompression by a mandible and tongue splitting approach. J. Bone Joint Surg. [Am.] *59:*121–123, 1977.
29. Hamblen, D. L.: Occipitocervical fusion: Indications, technique and results. J. Bone Joint Surg. [Br.] *49:*33–45, 1967.
30. Hanson, P. B., Montesano, P. X., Sharkey, N. A., et al.: Anatomic and biomechanical assessment of transarticular screw fixation for atlantoaxial instability. Spine *16:*1141–1145, 1991.
31. Hayakawa, T., Kamakawa, K., Osnishi, T., et al.: Prevention of postoperative complications after a transoral transclival approach to basilar aneurysms. J. Neurosurg. *54:*699–703, 1981.
32. Heywood, A. W. B., Learmonth, I. D., and Thomas, M.: Cervical spine instability in rheumatoid arthritis. J. Bone Joint Surg. [Br.] *70:*702–707, 1988.
33. Heywood, A. W. B., and Meyers, O. L.: Rheumatoid arthritis of the thoracic and lumbar spine. J. Bone Joint Surg. [Br.] *68:*362–368, 1966.
34. Honma, A., Murota, K., Shiba, R., et al.: Mandible and tongue

splitting approach for giant cell tumor of axis. Spine *14*:1204–1210, 1989.

35. Itoh, T., Tsuji, H., Katoh, Y., et al.: Occipito-cervical fusion reinforced by Luque's segmental spinal instrumentation for rheumatoid disease. Spine *13*:1234–1238, 1988.

36. James, D., and Crockard, H. A.: Surgical access to the base of the skull and upper cervical spine by extended maxillotomy. Neurosurgery *29*:411–416, 1991.

37. Kankaanpaa, U., and Santavirta, S.: Cervical spine involvement in rheumatoid arthritis. Ann. Chir. Gynaecol. *198*:117, 1985.

38. Kawaida, H., Sakov, T., and Morizono, Y.: Cervical settling in rheumatoid arthritis. Clin. Orthop. *239*:128–135, 1989.

39. Konttinnen, Y., Santavirta, S., Bergroth, V., et al.: Inflammatory involvement of the cervical spine ligaments in rheumatoid arthritis. Acta Orthop. Scand. *57*:587, 1986.

40. Konittinen, Y. T., Bergroth, V., Santavirta, S., and Sandelin, J.: Inflammatory involvement of cervical spine ligaments in patients with rheumatoid arthritis and atlanto-axial subluxation. J. Rheumatol. *14*:531–534, 1987.

41. Krane, S. M., and Simon, L. S.: Rheumatoid arthritis: Clinical features and pathogenetic mechanisms. Med. Clin. North Am. *70*:263–284, 1986.

42. Krieg, J. C., Clark, C. R., and Goetz, D. D.: Cervical spine arthrodesis and rheumatoid arthritis: A long term follow-up. Yale J. Biol. Med. *6*:257–262, 1993.

43. Lachiewicz, P. F., Schoenfeldt, R., and Inglis, A.: Somatosensory evoked potentials in the evaluation of the unstable rheumatoid cervical spine: A preliminary report. Spine *11*:813–817, 1986.

44. Larsson, E. M., Holtas, S., and Zygmont, S.: Pre- and postoperative MR imaging of the craniocervical junction in rheumatoid arthritis. Am. J. Radiol. *152*:561–566, 1989.

45. Lawrence, J. S., Laine, U. A. F., and DeGraft, R.: The epidemiology of rheumatoid arthritis in northern Europe. Proc. R. Soc. Med. *54*:454–462, 1961.

46. MacKenzie, A. L., Uttley, D., Marsh, H. T., et al.: Craniocervical stabilization using Luque/Hartshill rectangles. Neurosurgery *26*:32–36, 1990.

47. Magerl, F., and Seemann, P. S.: Stable posterior fusion of the atlas and axis by transarticular screw fixation. *In* Kehr, P., and Weidner, A. (eds.): Cervical Spine. Vol. 1. New York, Springer Verlag, 1987, pp. 322–327.

48. Marcotte, P., Dickman, C. A., Sonntag, V. K. H., et al.: Posterior atlantoaxial facet screw fixation. J. Neurosurg. *79*:234–237, 1993.

49. Marks, J. S., and Sharp, J.: Rheumatoid cervical myelopathy. O. J. Med. *50*:307, 1981.

50. Martel, W., and Page, J. W.: Cervical vertebral erosions and subluxation in rheumatoid arthritis and ankylosing spondylitis. Arthritis Rheum. *3*:546–556, 1960.

51. Mathews, J. A.: Atlanto-axial subluxation in rheumatoid arthritis. Ann. Rheum. Dis. *28*:260–266, 1969.

52. Mathews, J. A.: Atlanto-axial subluxation in rheumatoid arthritis. Ann. Rheum. Dis. *33*:526–531, 1974.

53. Menezes, A. H.: Surgical approaches to the craniocervical junction. *In* Frymoyer, J. (ed.): The Adult Spine: Principles and Practice. Vol. 2. New York, Raven Press, 1991, pp. 967–986.

54. Menezes, A. H.: Complications of surgery at the craniovertebral junction: Avoidance and management. Pediatr. Neurosurg. *17*:254–266, 1992.

55. Menezes, A. H.: Occipitocervical fusions: Indications, technique and avoidance of complications. *In* Hitchon, P. W. (ed.): Techniques of Spinal Fusion and Stabilization. New York, Thieme Medical Publishers, 1994, pp. 82–91.

56. Menezes, A. H.: Congenital and acquired abnormalities of the craniovertebral junction. *In* Youmans, J. R. (ed.): Neurological Surgery: A Comprehensive Reference Guide to the Diagnosis and Management of Neurosurgical Problems. 4th ed. Philadelphia, W. B. Saunders Co., 1996, pp. 1035–1089.

57. Menezes, A. H.: Posterior occipital C1–C2 fusion. *In* Menezes, A. H., and Sonntag, V. K. H. (eds.): Principles of Spinal Surgery. New York, McGraw-Hill, 1996, pp. 1051–1066.

58. Menezes, A. H., and Ryken, T. C.: Instrumentation of the craniocervical region. *In* Benzel, E. (ed.): Spinal Instrumentation. Park Ridge, IL, American Association of Neurological Surgeons, 1994, pp. 47–62.

59. Menezes, A. H., VanGilder, J. C., Clark, C. R., and El Khoury, G. Y.: Odontoid upward migration in rheumatoid arthritis. J. Neurosurg. *63*:500–509, 1985.

60. Menezes, A. H., VanGilder, J. C., Graf, C. J., et al.: Craniocervical abnormalities: A comprehensive surgical approach. J. Neurosurg. *53*:444–455, 1980.

61. Mikulowski P.: Sudden death in rheumatoid arthritis with atlanto-axial dislocations. Acta Med. Scand. *198*:445–451, 1975.

62. Morizono, Y., Sakou, T., and Kawaida, H.: Upper cervical involvement in rheumatoid arthritis. Spine *12*:721–725, 1987.

63. Newman, P., and Sweetman, R.: Occipitocervical fusion: An operative technique and its indications. J. Bone Joint Surg. [Br.] *51*:423–431, 1969.

64. Park, W. M., O'Neil, M., and McCall, I. W.: The radiology of rheumatoid involvement of the cervical spine. Skeletal Radiol. *4*:107, 1979.

65. Pellicci, P. M., Ranawat, C. S., and Tsairis, P.: A prospective study of the progression of rheumatoid arthritis of the cervical spine. J. Bone Joint Surg. *63*:342–346, 1981.

66. Pettersson, H., Larrson, E. M., Holtas, S., et al.: MR imaging of the cervical spine in rheumatoid arthritis. Am. J. Neuroradiol. *9*:573–577, 1988.

67. Rana, N. A.: Natural history of atlanto-axial subluxation in rheumatoid arthritis. Spine *14*:1054–1056, 1989.

68. Rana, N. A., Hancock, D. O., Taylor, A. R., et al.: Upward translocation of the dens in rheumatoid arthritis. J. Bone Joint Surg. [Br.] *55*:471–477, 1973.

69. Rana, N. A., and Taylor, A. R.: Upward migration of the odontoid peg in rheumatoid arthritis. Proc. R. Soc. Med. *64*:717–718, 1971.

70. Ranawat, C. S., O'Leary, P., Pellicci, P., et al.: Cervical spine fusion in rheumatoid arthritis. J. Bone Joint Surg. [Am.] *61*:1003–1010, 1979.

71. Ransford, A. O., Crockard, H. A., Pozo, J. L., et al.: Craniocervical instability treated by contoured loop fixation. J. Bone Joint Surg. [Am.] *68*:173–177, 1986.

72. Redlund-Johnell, I., and Pettersson, H.: Radiographic measurements of the cranio-vertebral region. Acta Radiol. *25*:23–28, 1984.

73. Sakou, T., Kawaida, H., Morizono, Y., et al.: Occipitoatlantoaxial fusion utilizing a rectangular rod. Clin. Orthop. *239*:136–144, 1989.

74. Santavirta, S., Kankaanpaa, U., Sandelin, J., et al.: Evaluation of patients with rheumatoid cervical spine: Review article. Scand. J. Rheumatol. *16*:9–16, 1987.

75. Santavirta, S., Slatis, P., Kankaanpaa, U., et al.: Treatment of the cervical spine in rheumatoid arthritis. J. Bone Joint Surg. [Am.] *70*:658–667, 1988.

76. Sharp, J., Purser, D. W., and Lawrence, J. S.: Rheumatoid arthritis of the cervical spine in the adult. Ann. Rheum. Dis. *17*:303–313, 1958.

77. Sherk, H. H.: Atlantoaxial instability and acquired basilar invagination in rheumatoid arthritis. Orthop. Clin. North Am. *9*:1053–1063, 1978.

78. Smith, H. P., Chalia, V. R., and Alexander, E., Jr.: Odontoid compression of the brain in a patient with rheumatoid arthritis: Case report. J. Neurosurg. *53*:841–845, 1980.

79. Solazzo, D., and Bruni, P.: Brainstem auditory evoked potentials (BAEP) abnormalities in subjects with craniovertebral malformation. Int. J. Neurol. Sci. *6*:185–189, 1985.

80. Swinson, D. R., Hamilton, E. B., Mathews, J. A., et al.: Vertical subluxation of the axis in rheumatoid arthritis. Ann. Rheum. Dis. *31*:359–363, 1972.

81. Toolanen, G., Knibestol, M., Larsson, S. E., and Landman, K.: Somatosensory evoked potentials (SSEPs) in rheumatoid cervical subluxation. Scand. J. Rheumatol. *16*:18–25, 1987.

82. Uttley, D., Moore, A., and Arch, D. J.: Surgical management of midline skull base tumors: A new approach. J. Neurosurg. *71*:705–710, 1989.

83. Voigelsand, H. Z., Zeidler, H., Wittenberg, A., and Weidner, A.: Rheumatoid cervical luxations with fatal neurological complications. Neuroradiology *6*:87–92, 1973.

84. Weisel, S. W., and Rothman, R. H.: Occipitoatlantal hypermobility. Spine *4*:187, 1979.

85. Weissman, B. N. W., Alibad, P., Weinfeld, M. S., et al.: Prognostic features of atlantoaxial subluxation in rheumatoid arthritis patients. Radiology *144*:745–751, 1982.

86. White, A. A., III, Johnson, R. M., Panjabi, M. M., and Southwick, W. O.: Biomechanical analysis of clinical stability of the cervical spine. Clin. Orthop. *109:*85–96, 1975.

87. Winfield, J., Cooke, D., Brook, A. S., et al.: A prospective study of the radiological changes in the cervical spine in early rheumatoid arthritis. Ann. Rheum. Dis. *42:*613–618, 1983.

88. Yamada, T., Ishida, T., Kudo, Y., et al.: Clinical correlates of abnormal P14 in median SEP's. Neurology *36:*765–771, 1986.

89. Yamarura, A., Makino, H., Isobe, K., et al.: Repair of cerebrospinal fluid fistula following transoral transclival approach to a basilar aneurysm: Technical note. J. Neurosurg. *50:*834–836, 1979.

90. Yaszemski, M. J., and Shepler, T. R.: Sudden death from cord compression associated with atlanto-axial instability in rheumatoid arthritis: A case report. Spine *15:*338–341, 1990.

91. Zoma, A., Sturroch, R. D., Fisher, W. D., et al.: Surgical stabilization of the rheumatoid cervical spine. J. Bone Joint Surg. [Br.] *69:*8–12, 1987.

CHAPTER

42

Ankylosing Spondylitis: Surgical Considerations

Edward H. Simmons, M.D., B.Sc.(Med), F.R.C.S.(C), M.S.(Tor), F.A.C.S.

Although orthopedic surgeons may commonly consider the problems of ankylosing spondylitis and rheumatoid arthritis together, it should be emphasized that they are different diseases. Ankylosing spondylitis has often been described as "rheumatoid spondylitis," but it is a different disease with a different serology. It is more common in males, with a predilection for the spine and major joints, whereas rheumatoid arthritis is more common in females, with a predilection for the joints of the appendicular skeleton. Clinical manifestations of ankylosing spondylitis occur with an incidence of two to three per thousand, representing a significant patient population in a country the size of the United States.

Surgeons should be aware that ankylosing spondylitis, as a seronegative spondylitis, is a systemic disease and may have extra-articular manifestations. These include iridocyclitis,[8] aortitis,[6, 8, 68] cardiac conduction abnormalities,[25, 68] arachnoiditis,[25, 68] and cauda equina syndrome.[5, 48] There is a recognized association with ulcerative colitis,[37] regional enteritis,[37] psoriasis,[37] multiple sclerosis,[20] Reiter's disease,[37] and Behçet's disease.[37]

Typically, in its early stages, ankylosing spondylitis is a disease of young men presenting with an insidious onset of low back pain that is worse in the morning and better with activity. It is not unusual for the low back symptoms to be interpreted as being caused by "disc disease," and on occasion, inappropriate surgery may be performed for what was thought to be discogenic back pain.

The author's careful review of the histories of North Americans referred for correction of fixed deformities indicates that the average time from onset of symptoms to diagnosis is 5.5 years.

Clinicians should be alert to young men presenting with an insidious onset of low back pain that is worse in the morning and better as the day progresses. Such patients should be assessed for decreased lengthening of the spine on forward bending, as indicated by tape measure; decreased lateral bending; decreased chest expansion, and sacroiliac or costochondral tenderness. Early radiographic changes with "squaring" of lumbar vertebrae; changes in the sacroiliac joints, with a positive bone scan related to the sacroiliac joints; and a positive HLA-B27 antigen test will allow a correct diagnosis for a knowledgeable observer.

The main presenting clinical problems related to the spine in ankylosing spondylitis are gross fixed deformities. The main problems of the spine in rheumatoid arthritis are those of local destruction and instability.

ATLANTOAXIAL INSTABILITY

Atlantoaxial subluxation and dislocation may occur in both rheumatoid arthritis and ankylosing spondylitis, and its possible presence justifies a constant awareness by clinicians in managing patients with these diseases. It is essential to rule out its presence when planning any operative procedure under general anesthesia on patients with these conditions, in which manipulation

1303

of the neck might be required during intubation or positioning of the patient.

In ankylosing spondylitis, a solid column of bone below the atlas (C1) may place increased stress at the craniocervical junction. This, along with attritional effects of inflammation of the transverse ligament or the associated effects of hyperemia on its bony attachments, may result in atlantoaxial subluxation and dislocation. Subluxation may occur, and the joint may then become stabilized in the subluxed position without significant subsequent symptoms. It is a wise precaution to have routine radiographs of the cervical spine, including flexion and extension lateral films, done preoperatively on these patients to determine whether any subluxation exists and whether it is stable or unstable.

First described in 1890 by Garod,[16] rheumatoid involvement of the cervical spine has a reported incidence of 25 to 95 per cent in rheumatoid patients, depending on the particular study and diagnostic criteria.[4, 9, 33, 35, 46] The types of involvement in order of decreasing frequency are atlantoaxial subluxation, atlantoaxial subluxation combined with subaxial subluxation, and subaxial subluxation alone. Combinations of superior migration of the odontoid process with the preceding constitute the remainder. The pathologic changes usually cause neck pain that, with atlantoaxial involvement, radiates to the occiput. The soreness tends to be aggravated by flexion or extension of the neck, and there is usually tenderness in the suboccipital area. In the more advanced phases of subluxation, vague paresthesias in the upper and lower extremities and a feeling of weakness and instability in an otherwise grossly disabled patient may not always give rise to any particular suspicion. The neurologic symptoms and signs are more ominous. Radiating paresthesias, hyperreflexia, and posterior column dysfunction indicate cord involvement that may progress to serious disability.

The natural history of rheumatoid arthritis of the cervical spine is one of progression.[4, 45, 46] Radiographic disease progresses to a greater degree than does neurologic involvement.

The majority of patients with radiographic involvement have atlantoaxial subluxation. The recognition of atlantoaxial instability or dislocation requires a clinical index of suspicion, and flexion and extension lateral radiographs of the cervical spine are frequently required to diagnose it. When gross instability is present, particularly in an individual who is still reasonably active and disposed to injury, stabilization is warranted.

Pellicci and colleagues have graded neurologic defi-

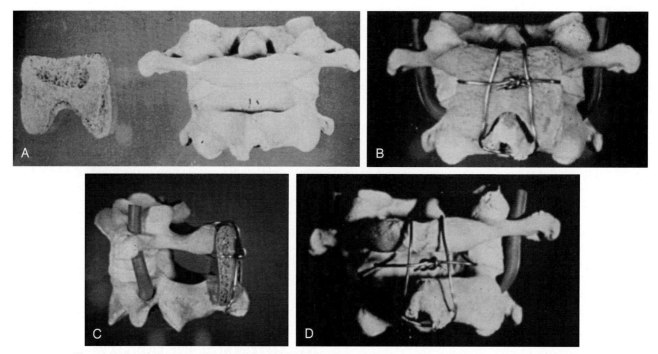

Figure 42–1. *A,* Bone model showing cancellous surface of Gallie modified H graft, contoured from the posterior iliac crest to fit over the arches of C1 and C2, sitting astride the spinous process of C2. *B,* Posterior view with the graft in position, the cortical surface being superficial. The Gallie wire is passed through the interspinous ligament of C2–C3 inferior to the spinous process of C2, and carried upward over the graft on each side. It is brought out below the arch of C1 laterally and tied firmly posteriorly. *C,* Lateral view showing the modified H graft in position, with the wire pulling back C1 into normal relationship with the odontoid. The inferior portion of the wire is passed below the spinous process of C2 through the interspinous ligament of C2–C3. It is important to preserve the interspinous ligament during exposure and wiring, because it assists in maintaining the wire in position until it is tightened. *D,* Posterior view of bone model showing the wire configuration without the graft in position.

cit as Grade 0, no neurologic involvement; Grade I, hyperreflexia and dysesthesias; Grade II, mild weakness and posterior column deficit; and Grade III, severe weakness resulting in significant functional disability. The results of their study suggested that approximately 10 per cent of patients with radiographic evidence of disease deteriorate to a level requiring surgery.[45]

The indications for surgery include uncontrolled pain associated with neurologic deterioration, progression to Grade II neurologic dysfunction when caused by superimposition of subaxial subluxation or superior migration on a pre-existing atlantoaxial subluxation, and progression to Grade III neurologic dysfunction.[4, 45, 46]

Surgical Stabilization

When gross atlantoaxial instability is present, particularly if symptomatic and associated with long tract signs, surgical stabilization is required. Although different techniques are available to achieve this, the inflammatory and often osteoporotic nature of the bone makes the author's surgical preference the Gallie posterior atlantoaxial arthrodesis.[38, 55, 66] Gallie employed a modified H graft from the iliac crest, contoured to fit over the posterior aspect of the arches of C1 and C2 and sitting astride the spinous process of C2. A single piece of 22-gauge stainless steel wire is passed inferior to the spinous process of C2 through the interspinous ligament between C2 and C3. The two ends of the wire are carried upward, posterior to the graft around a notch cut in its upper border, and under the arch of C1 on each side of the graft. The two ends of the wire are tied over the posterior aspect of the graft, locking it into position and pulling back the arch of C1 into normal relationship with the arch of C2 (Fig. 42–1). An essential instrument is a wire-tightening apparatus such as that developed by the late R. I. Harris.[21] The wire tightener grasps the wire and allows one to put forceful tension on it, tying the knot quite firmly in the narrow confines of the wound with gentle pressure exerted by the hand (Fig. 42–2).

The deep cancellous surface of the graft should be contoured to fit over the curved posterior surfaces of the arch of C1 and C2, so that the graft is in intimate contact with the underlying vertebrae (Fig. 42–3). In addition to the main graft, it is important to place cancellous bone chips over the laminae on both sides as far laterally as possible. The technique immobilizes the involved C1–C2 segment and avoids fusing to the occiput, thereby preserving motion at the atlanto-occipital joints. It should be emphasized that despite the presence of internal fixation, the fusion should be protected for an adequate interval (10 to 12 weeks) by an efficient form of external immobilization. The halo-cast is most effective for this, and if it is used with a well-performed fusion, success is almost certain.[13, 51, 55, 63] If a halo-jacket is used, it should fit the patient well and give immobilization similar to that of a halo-cast.

A clear knowledge of the anatomy of the upper cervical spine is essential. The vulnerability of the vertebral arteries and the neural elements must be recog-

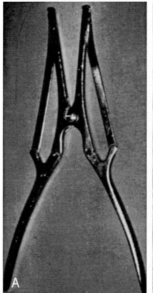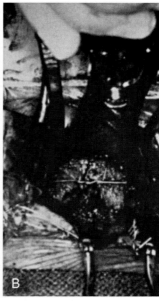

Figure 42–2. *A,* The Harris wire tier allows the surgeon to grasp the wire and tighten it firmly in the depths of the wound. *B,* Posterior view showing the wire tier tightening the first knot with the graft in position. The first knot is tightened firmly, compressing the graft against the two vertebrae, and restoring normal alignment. The first knot is held with a needle driver when tight, and the second loop of a square knot is added, the knot being tightened by the tier.

nized. The vertebral arteries are carefully avoided while dissecting the ligamentum flavum from the anterior surface of the posterior arch of C1. A flat curve guide may be inserted between the arch and the underlying ligamentum flavum as a safeguard when the wire is being passed. The end of the wire may be bent back on itself to prepare a blunt end, and then directed around the arch with a needle driver.

When C1–C2 subluxation is combined with superior migration of the odontoid process, the occiput may have to be incorporated into the fusion with an occipitocervical fusion. The subluxation at C1–C2 may be reduced by preoperative halo traction, and fusion may then be performed to the occiput. These procedures are usually adequate for most cases of C1–C2 subluxation combined with superior migration of the odontoid process. However, in certain instances in which the odontoid is producing significant spinal cord or brain stem compression that cannot be reduced, transoral resection of the odontoid may have to be considered. This is more hazardous than posterior decompression and stabilization procedures and is indicated less frequently.[15] Transoral surgery is reserved for patients with significant anterior cord or brain stem compression associated with myelopathy. Two types of abnormalities can be differentiated. In the first, basilar invagination alone is present without gross atlantoaxial instability. In the second, there is concomitant atlantoaxial instability and luxation. Posterior column involvement may occur in the second type, caused by posterior compression of

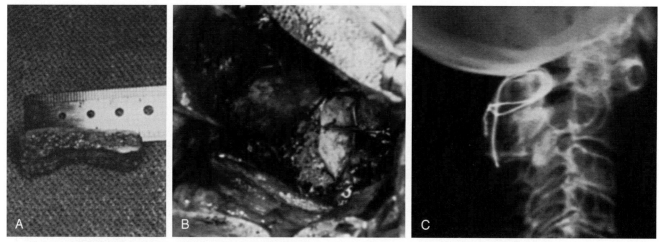

Figure 42–3. *A,* Superior view of modified H graft. The contoured deep cancellous surface allows intimate contact with the underlying vertebrae. *B,* Operative view with the main graft in position. Adequate cancellous bone is placed over the laminae on both sides. *C,* Lateral radiograph three years postoperatively of a rheumatoid patient who had presented with cord compression associated with gross subluxation that was not completely reducible. The Gallie graft is well incorporated with solid fusion. The neurologic deficit recovered completely.

the spinal cord by the posterior arch of C1 as it slides anteriorly. Isolated basilar invagination with narrowing of the anterior cerebellomedullary system is the primary indication for transoral decompression. Anterior decompression may involve the removal of not only the odontoid process but also the body of C2 and a portion of the clivus. In patients with isolated atlantoaxial instability, a stable posterior atlantoaxial arthrodesis is preferred. Results of primary anterior decompression combined with simultaneous anterior fusion are suboptimal, and it is preferable to perform a posterior occipitocervical fusion as a secondary procedure after the primary anterior decompression.

Preoperative examination should identify and treat oral infection or dental sepsis. Nasal, oral, and pharyngeal swabs should be taken for bacterial culture and sensitivity, and the most appropriate parenteral antibiotic combination should be administered preoperatively, intraoperatively, and in the immediate postoperative period.

Surgery is performed with the patient in the supine position and the neck extended. Lateral radiographic visualization is necessary. Routine tracheostomy with endotracheal anesthesia has been recommended by some.[15] However, the presence of an endotracheal tube without concomitant tracheostomy does not constitute an obstacle at surgery and in some ways is preferable. Patients not having a tracheostomy should have a nasogastric tube inserted postoperatively, with normal oral nutrition commenced seven to eight days postoperatively. If tracheostomy is employed, it is performed at the beginning of the procedure with ventilation through a cuffed tracheal tube. After preparation of the oral cavity, a Whitehead retractor is introduced, and the tongue is depressed. The nasopharynx and hypopharynx are packed off. The procedure can usually be

done without division of the soft palate. The soft palate is folded back on itself and sutured to the junction of the hard and soft palates to expose the lower portion of the nasopharynx. The sutures are released at the end of the procedure (Fig. 42–4*A*). If division of the soft palate is considered necessary, it is incised on one side of the midline to avoid the uvula, and the flaps are retracted laterally (Fig. 42–4*B*). Palpation of the posterior pharyngeal wall localizes the prominence of the anterior tubercle of the atlas. In atlantoaxial dislocation, this is quite evident.

A 5-cm midline incision is made from the lower portion of the clivus to the lower portion of C2. The incision is centered a finger breadth below the anterior tubercle of the atlas. The incision is carried down to bone. The soft tissues are stripped laterally to the outer margin of the lateral masses of the atlas and axis. The soft tissues may be anchored with retraction stay sutures. The anterior arch of the atlas and the body of the axis are exposed. If fusion of the atlantoaxial joints is to be done, these are completely exposed. The anterior arch of the atlas is removed with sharp rongeurs, and the odontoid is exposed (Fig. 42–5). The odontoid process is removed. A high-speed drill is necessary, and a diamond burr is recommended. Removal of the displaced upward and backward projecting odontoid process is the most complicated part of the procedure. It should be carefully and gently freed of its soft tissue attachments, using sharp dissection as necessary.

Difficulty in resection of the odontoid may be encountered owing to its elevation and the angle of approach required to visualize it. It may therefore be necessary to initiate the odontoid resection in the central part of the body of the axis. The lower portion of the clivus (anterior margin of the foramen magnum) is removed only when necessary, and a diamond burr

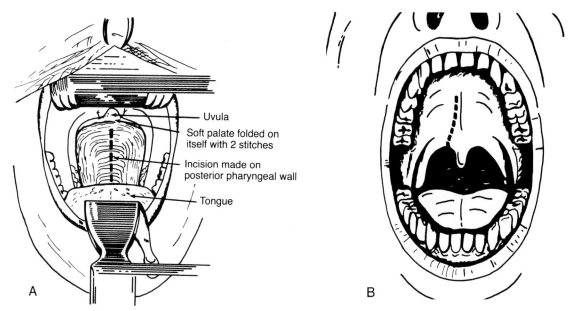

Figure 42–4. *A,* Artist's view of transoral exposure. Two stay sutures pulled the soft palate on itself, keeping it in position. A vertical incision is made in the midline of the posterior pharyngeal wall. *B,* Diagram of exposure showing soft palate incision on one side, avoiding the uvula.

and upward cutting bone forceps are recommended to facilitate this portion of the procedure. If fusion of the lateral C1–C2 joints is performed, the articular cartilage is cleared away from the joints and an iliac graft is wedged between the lateral masses. Anterior C1–C2 anthrodesis is ordinarily not recommended, because of increased morbidity. A subsequent posterior fusion is preferable. The posterior pharyngeal wall is then closed. Some authors recommend a multilayer closure involving the anterior ligament, the buccal pharyngeal fascia and constrictor muscles, and the pharyngeal mu-

cosa. However, many recommend a loose, single-layer closure that allows wound secretions to drain more easily.[15, 17] The latter has technical advantages, and the results appear satisfactory. Some have recommended a double incision of the posterior pharyngeal wall and deeper structures to promote better healing and safe closure.[44] Although this has some theoretic advantages, it has technical disadvantages and has been shown to produce clinically superior results. Oral feedings should be delayed six to seven days to allow adequate healing and should start with liquids.

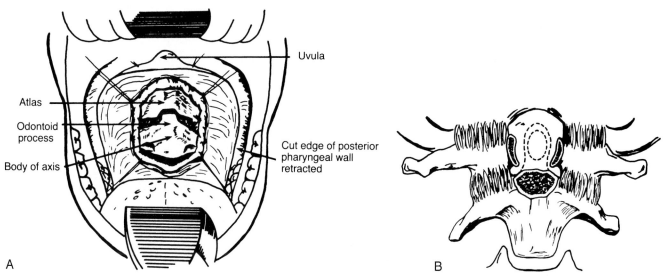

Figure 42–5. *A,* The atlas and axis are shown exposed anteriorly, with the soft tissues stripped laterally. *B,* Diagram showing excision of the anterior arch of the atlas, allowing exposure of the odontoid.

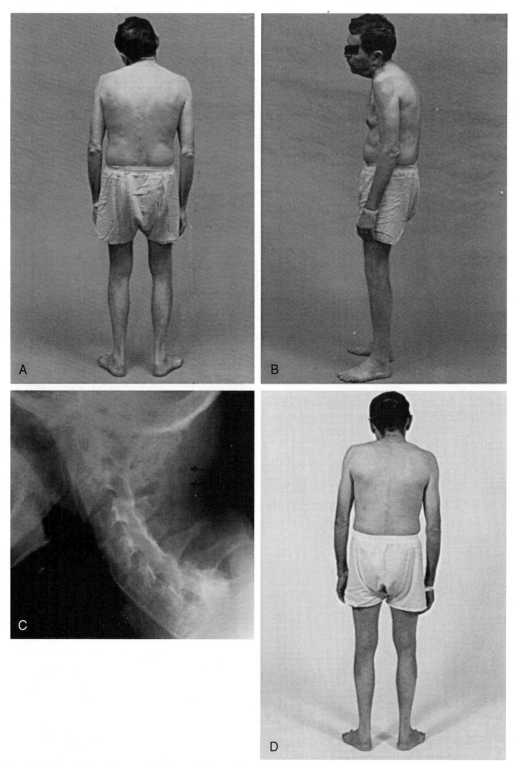

Figure 42–6. *A,* Posterior and *B,* lateral views of a patient with severe painful torticollis associated with occipitoatlantal joint destruction. Scars in the lumbar area mark the site of three operations for "low back pain" during the early stages of the disease. *C,* Postoperative lateral radiograph of the cervical spine after reduction of the deformity with halo-dependent traction, immobilization in a halo-cast, and successful occipitocervical fusion using onlay technique. *D,* Postoperative view showing correction of the deformity, the painful symptoms having been completely relieved.

Atlanto-Occipital Disability

Occasionally, protracted pain and disability in ankylosing spondylitis may arise from destructive changes at the atlanto-occipital joint. In many patients, this is the last joint in the spine to be significantly involved; therefore, some mobility is often preserved. Destructive changes may exist, with intractable pain and minimal motion occurring. When this is not responsive to medication and bracing, stabilization by occipitocervical fusion is indicated.

Occasionally, destructive changes at the atlanto-occipital joints may contribute to deformity as well as pain. Most commonly, flexion deformity occurs, but on occasion rotatory or lateral angulatory deformity occurs as well. When this problem is not responsive to conservative management, gradual reduction of the deformity should be attempted by halo-dependent traction along the line of the neck, and then stabilization with occipitocervical fusion with the head and neck in normal alignment (Fig. 42–6).

The author has used simple onlay grafting (see Fig. 42–6) but prefers a modified Dewar technique,[11, 12, 56] fixing the double-onlay grafts to the base of the skull and the upper cervical spine, reinforced by multiple cancellous bone grafts (Fig. 42–7A). After stripping the base of the skull, a wire is passed through small burr holes in the skull to be used to fix the grafts against the skull. Double iliac cortical and cancellous onlay grafts are contoured to fit over the posterior arches of the upper cervical vertebrae (usually down to C4), the cancellous surfaces of the graft being contoured to fit over the posterior arches. The grafts are also contoured to fit accurately against the skull and are held firmly

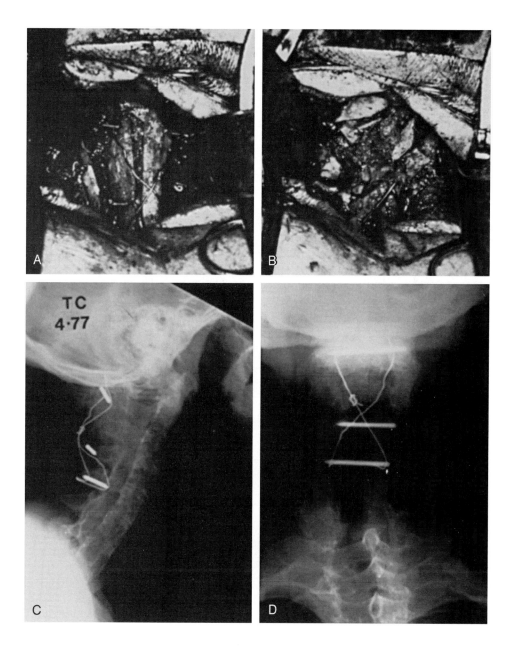

Figure 42–7. *A,* Posterior operative view with double-onlay cortical and cancellous iliac grafts in position. The grafts are fixed to the upper cervical posterior arches using transfixing Compere threaded pins reinforced with an overtying loop of stainless wire that has been passed through the skull, keeping the grafts in contact with the skull and compressing them against the posterior aspect of the spine. *B,* Posterior operative view showing additional onlay cancellous bone grafts reinforcing the main grafts, extending from the cervical spine to the skull. *C,* Lateral postoperative radiograph showing solid fusion from the occiput to the cervical spine. The wire passes through the skull. The threaded Compere pins fix the onlay grafts to the posterior arches of the cervical spine. *D,* Anteroposterior postoperative radiograph showing configuration of the wire loop, Compere threaded pins, and grafts. The threaded pins are inserted percutaneously from the lateral aspect of the neck on one side, through the graft on that side, the base of the spinous process, and the graft on the opposite side. The pins are divided laterally on the side from which they were inserted, and the excess portion is removed. It is important when preparing the patient to drape the neck well laterally to allow easy lateral percutaneous insertion.

in this position, being fixed to the posterior arches of the cervical vertebrae by passing threaded Compere wires percutaneously from one side of the spine, through the base of the spinous process, and then through the graft on the opposite side. The Compere wire is then cut free on the side of its entrance, lateral to the graft. The wire that has been passed through the skull is then used to fix the grafts against the skull, as well as to tie the grafts against the posterior arches, passing the wire around the ends of the threaded Compere wires. The main grafts are reinforced by cancellous grafts placed between the skull and the cervical spine about the main grafts (Fig. 42–7B).

Dewar used a full-thickness graft from the posterior portion of the superior margin of the iliac crest. This was divided in a straight line from the superior aspect into equal portions, allowing the cancellous surfaces of the grafts to be contoured to fit astride the posterior arches of the upper cervical spine, and the broad cancellous posterior margins of the grafts to be contoured to fit in firm apposition with the skull (see Fig. 42–7A).

Although plate fixation to the skull may be considered, patients with this disease often have exceedingly thin bone in the occiput, which could make screw fixation tenuous and difficult. Postoperative immobilization by a well-fitting halo-cast for three months is essential to protect the area of fusion from abnormal stress owing to the rigidity of the remainder of the spine.

SUBAXIAL SUBLUXATION

For rheumatoid arthritis with painful destructive subaxial subluxation without neurologic involvement, the author prefers an attempt at reduction with halo traction, followed by posterior stabilization using onlay cortical and cancellous iliac grafts contoured to fit the posterior arch structures as recommended by Dewar[11, 12, 56] (similar to the technique shown in Fig. 42–7).

Again, the grafts are prepared by removing the full-thickness superior portion of the posterior iliac crest and then splitting the graft from its superior aspect into equal portions in a straight fashion so that the cancellous surfaces can be contoured and fitted to the posterior arches in the same manner, with an overtying figure-of-eight stainless steel wire passed around the ends of the Compere wires, fixing the grafts to the spine (Fig. 42–8). Further cortical and cancellous grafts are placed laterally on the laminae and around the posterior facet joints, lateral to the main grafts.

When subaxial subluxation is not completely reducible and is associated with spinal cord compression, anterior decompression and stabilization are required. This is performed by excision of the involved disc space and the vertebral body below the displacement, since it is the inferior vertebral body that projects into the spinal cord and compresses the spinal cord between the posterosuperior border of the inferior vertebral body and the posterior arch of the vertebra above.

Gentle halo traction is attempted for reduction, and the reduction is confirmed by lateral radiography. Spinal cord monitoring is used to identify any change that may occur during the positioning of the patient on the operating table. If any significant change in the tracing is noted, the traction is altered and the position of the neck adjusted. An anterior approach is made to the cervical spine, with excision of the involved disc space followed by careful removal of the inferior vertebral body. Using a small oscillating saw and power burrs, the surgeon removes the inferior end plate of the vertebra above the subluxation and the superior end plate of the vertebra below the subluxation, as well as the upper part of that vertebral body, and creates a keystone defect.[60] This is done by beveling upward into the inferior portion of the vertebra above and downward into the superior portion of the vertebra below, leaving a step of the posterior vertebral cortex of the superior and inferior vertebrae on which the keystone

Figure 42–8. *A,* Axial view demonstrating insertion of threaded pins percutaneously from the lateral aspect of the cervical spine. The threaded pin passes through the graft, which has been closely applied to the spine, through the base of the spinous process, and the graft on the opposite side. It is important to contour the grafts carefully so that their cancellous surfaces lie close to the posterior arches of the spine. An overtying wire loop adds to the fixation. Additional cortical and cancellous onlay grafts are placed laterally on both sides. *B,* Posterior view showing onlay grafts applied to the spine with an overtying loop of wire further holding the wires closely applied to the spine.

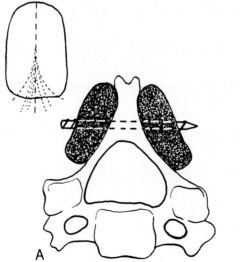

A

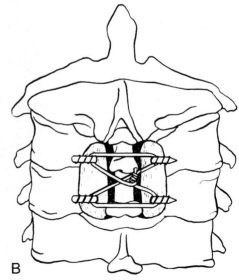

B

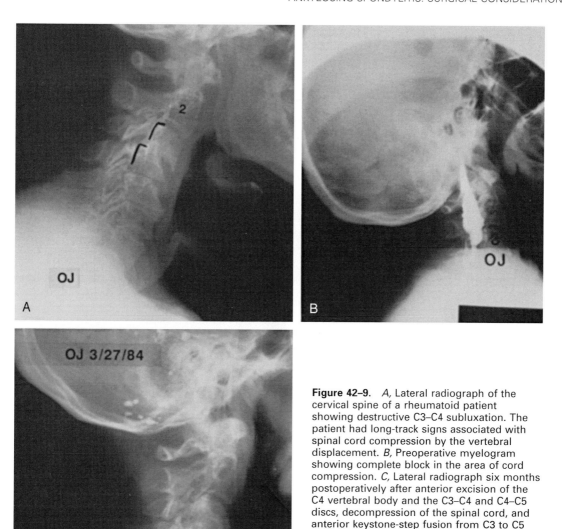

Figure 42–9. *A,* Lateral radiograph of the cervical spine of a rheumatoid patient showing destructive C3–C4 subluxation. The patient had long-track signs associated with spinal cord compression by the vertebral displacement. *B,* Preoperative myelogram showing complete block in the area of cord compression. *C,* Lateral radiograph six months postoperatively after anterior excision of the C4 vertebral body and the C3–C4 and C4–C5 discs, decompression of the spinal cord, and anterior keystone-step fusion from C3 to C5 using autogenous iliac graft. The spinal canal has been decompressed. Normal vertebral alignment has been established with a solid bony fusion. The patient was relieved of the neurologic deficit and continued to do well seven-and-a-half years postoperatively.

graft will rest. The spinal cord is completely decompressed in the area of its impingement. The neck is distracted by the anesthetist by traction on the halo, and an iliac crest keystone graft is placed into the defect, maintaining fixed distraction and immobilization.[60] The distraction is accomplished by the patient's being fixed to the table with restraints around the ankles, which are applied during positioning. The anesthetist is thus able to apply manual traction on the halo when desired, opening up the defect to its maximum and allowing initial measurements for preparation of the graft, with the traction applied again at the time of insertion of the graft. Additional cancellous bone is placed in the remaining empty area of the disc space on each side about the main graft. When two segmental levels are involved, the graft can be extended further distally, removing the upper portion of the most inferior vertebra. This technique provides stabilization and a high rate of fusion. Postoperative immobilization with a halo-jacket for three months is recommended (Fig. 42–9).

SPONDYLODISCITIS

A characteristic radiographic feature of ankylosing spondylitis is erosion and sclerosis of bone adjacent to the sacroiliac joints. Occasionally, this erosive sclerotic process extends into the intervertebral disc and adja-

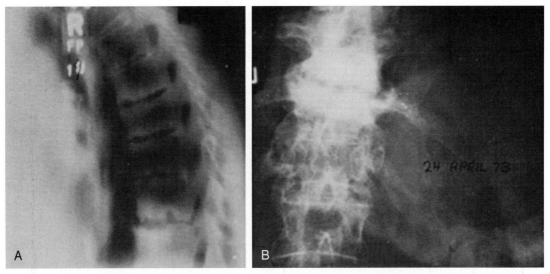

Figure 42–10. *A,* Lateral radiograph of a patient with ankylosing spondylitis showing areas of spondylodiscitis. The main typical lesion is in the lower thoracic spine, the most frequent location. Erosive sclerotic changes involve the vertebral end plates adjacent to the disc space. *B,* Anteroposterior radiograph of the area of spondylodiscitis in the lower thoracic spine, again showing erosive sclerotic changes at the level of the disc space.

cent bone; it is then called spondylodiscitis. These erosive lesions of vertebral bodies were first reported by Andersson in 1937.[3] Initially, the lesions were considered to be infective. Wholey and colleagues in 1960 reported on biopsies of the lesions showing chronic inflammatory changes without bacteriologic evidence of infection. They reported that although the lesions showed striking destructive changes resembling infection, they failed to show the progression that would be expected of infectious processes; in addition, spontaneous healing could occur without specific treatment. They stated that the lesion was merely another manifestation of rheumatoid spondylitis.[71] Coste and associates in 1963 further described this lesion as an inflammatory process.[10] Kanefield and coworkers in 1969, on the basis of three patients studied, acknowledged that the cause of the lesions was unknown but suggested that they represent a response to delayed union or nonunion of fractures occurring in rheumatoid spondylitis.[27]

Speculation on the nature of the lesions, confusion related to the process itself, and the possible effect of trauma have given rise to two opposing views. The first is that spondylodiscitis is an expression of an inflammatory process that affects the intervertebral disc and the surrounding bone; detailed assessment and biopsy specimens support this view. The second, less commonly held view is that spondylodiscitis is caused by trauma, with excessive forces localized to one intervertebral segment, resulting in mechanical destruction of that motion segment and a functional pseudarthrosis. This lesion has been described by Little and others as an asymptomatic abnormality on routine radiographic examination.[33, 47]

The ossified spine in ankylosing spondylitis is susceptible to fracture, and the findings are usually fairly typical. It is routinely noted at surgery that the ossified interspinous ligaments, ligamentum flavum, and disc are much harder and stronger than the bone itself. Fractures are, therefore, more prone to occur through the vertebral body than through the disc space. They are usually associated with a significant traumatic incident with acute onset of pain.

Spondylodiscitis as a manifestation of ankylosing spondylitis arises as a destructive lesion of the disc space that is frequently asymptomatic and noted on routine radiographic studies, but it may become symptomatic with minor injury or stress. Significant bone destruction anteriorly makes the posterior elements vulnerable to injury and even stress fracture. These factors should be considered in attempting to decide the true nature of a fracture, pseudarthrosis, or spondylodiscitis with or without superimposed injury in a patient.

The radiographic appearance of spondylodiscitis is fairly typical (Fig. 42–10). The erosive process widens the disc space, breaking down the subchondral bony end plates. The surrounding bone becomes sclerotic and radiodense. Either erosion or sclerosis may appear more prominent. Spondylodiscitis has had a reported incidence of 5 to 6 per cent.[33, 47, 49] Most lesions develop in the lower thoracic spine. About half the cases present with back pain, and a little over half are asymptomatic and are discovered incidentally on routine radiographs.[33] It appears that the lesion generally follows a benign course and usually responds to conservative management. However, surgical stabilization occasionally may be required for intractable pain, particularly when there is an associated fracture or disruption of the posterior fused spine at the same level. Figure 42–11 shows the radiographs of a man with a longstanding history of ankylosing spondylitis. He had gone onto bilateral involvement of the hip joints. He was admitted to the hospital, and total right hip replacement arthroplasty was performed. Immediately postoperatively, he had severe back pain aggravated by

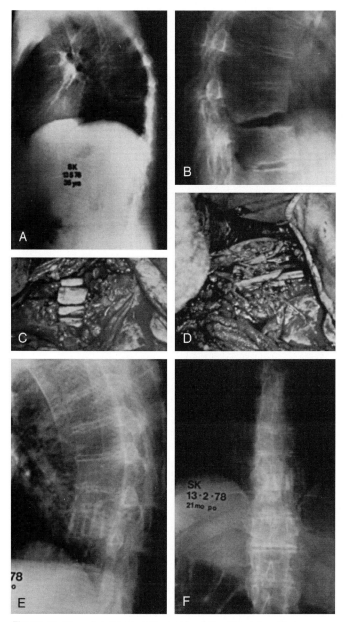

Figure 42–11. *A,* Lateral radiograph of the thoracic spine showing absence of deformity but extensive destructive change of spondylodiscitis at T9–T10. The patient suffered a stress crack fracture of the posterior fusion area due to lack of bony support anteriorly, causing severe pain with movement. *B,* Lateral view showing the extent of end plate destruction and absorption at the disc space. *C,* Anterior exposure of the spine showing excision of the area of spondylodiscitis with multiple fibular strut grafting. *D,* Final operative view showing addition of further onlay cortical and cancellous bone grafts. *E,* Lateral radiograph 21 months postoperatively showing successful grafting and normal spinal alignment. *F,* Anteroposterior postoperative radiograph showing fusion 21 months postoperatively. The pain was relieved by stabilization of the spine with anterior strut grafts.

any movement, and ambulation was therefore difficult. Radiographs showed extensive destructive spondylodiscitis anteriorly at T9–T10, with an area of breakdown of the posterior fusion related to the disease. The disability was of such magnitude as to require surgical treatment. Anterior transthoracic resection of the area of spondylodiscitis was performed, with insertion of fibular strut grafts. This provided almost immediate relief of pain because of the stability obtained. He went on to a satisfactory fusion, with relief of his pain. He was able to undergo replacement arthroplasty of the opposite hip joint and return to full-time work on an assembly line (Fig. 42–11*E* and *F*). The spinal lesion was typical of spondylodiscitis, with pain induced by the minor trauma of the operative management for total hip replacement arthroplasty.

Figure 42–12 shows a 58-year-old physician with a 22-year history of symptoms related to ankylosing spondylitis. For three to four years, he had noted increasing flexion deformity of his thoracolumbar spine but was able to function adequately. Nine months earlier he had stepped down some steps forcefully, suffering pain in the lower thoracic spine. This was relatively mild at first, but it persisted and increased, and he noted progression of the flexion deformity. Radiographs showed a typical area of spondylodiscitis at the T12–L1 level (Fig. 42–12*B* and *C*). The destructive changes were through the disc space, consistent with pre-existing spondylodiscitis. His chief complaint was pain interfering with daily activity and his medical practice and, to a lesser degree, his deformity. The lesion was under a flexion-shear strain, owing to the kyphotic deformity and the weight-bearing line being situated far anteriorly to the T12–L1 spondylodiscitis (Fig. 42–12*D*). He was treated by extension-resection osteotomy of the midlumbar spine under local anesthesia, thereby correcting the deformity and shifting the weight-bearing line posterior to the osteotomy site. This transformed the shear forces acting on the area of spondylodiscitis to a compression force. The lesion went on to uneventful healing (Fig. 42–12*E* and *F*). The deformity was fully corrected, with relief of pain, allowing the patient to return to work with a normal posture (Fig. 42–12*G*).

In contrast to spondylodiscitis as described earlier, Figure 42–13*A* demonstrates the typical findings of a fracture pseudarthrosis. The patient was a 56-year-old man who had long-standing ankylosing spondylitis, but without major complaint. Two and a half years earlier, he had suffered a major injury when the jack of his car slipped and the car fell on him while he was changing a tire. He had severe back pain and went on to increasingly painful deformity aggravated by any motion. The radiographic appearances showed a typical area of pseudarthrosis through the upper body of L1, rather than through the disc space (Fig. 42–13*B* and *C*). The lesion was under shear stress owing to the kyphotic deformity. He was treated with extension osteotomy of the lumbar spine under local anesthesia, thereby correcting the deformity and transferring the shear stress to a compression force and allowing heal-

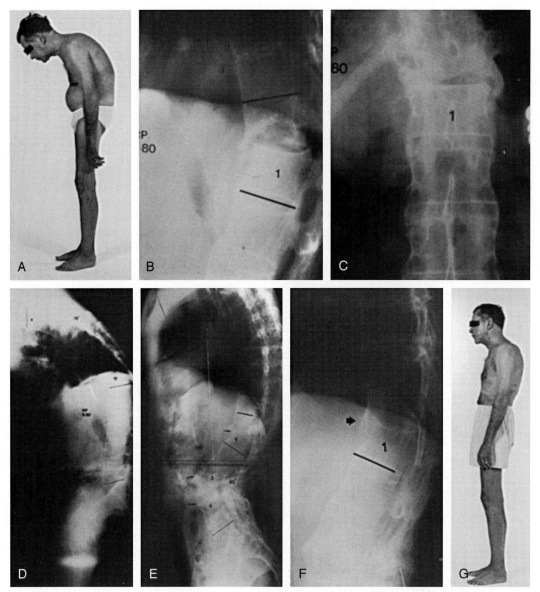

Figure 42–12. *A,* Lateral view of a physician with painful increasing flexion deformity of the thoracolumbar spine associated with spondylodiscitis. Note the thoracolumbar apex. *B,* Lateral radiograph showing gross destructive spondylodiscitis at T12–L1 with end plate destruction and bone absorption. *C,* Anteroposterior radiograph showing changes at the T12–L1 disc space. *D,* Standing lateral 3-foot radiograph of the spine showing the weight-bearing line well anterior to the area of destructive spondylodiscitis. *E,* Postoperative standing lateral 3-foot radiograph showing resection-extension osteotomy of the midlumbar spine shifting the weight-bearing line posteriorly, converting shear force at the site of the spondylodiscitis to compression force. *F,* Lateral radiograph at T12–L1 four months postoperatively, showing spontaneous healing of the area of spondylodiscitis as a result of conversion of shear stress to compression by lumbar osteotomy. *G,* Lateral view of the patient after union of the osteotomy and area of spondylodiscitis, showing correction of the deformity.

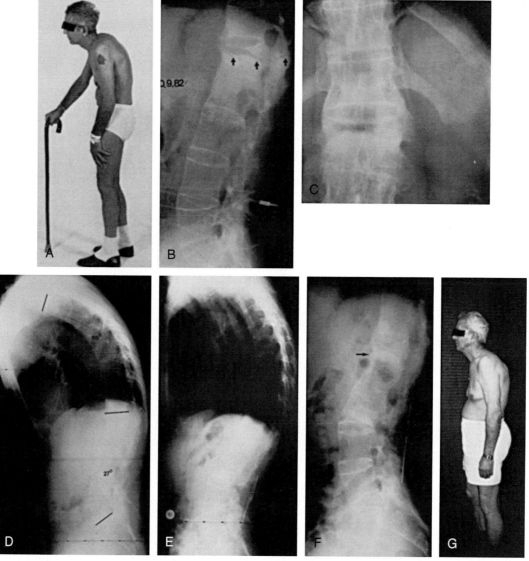

Figure 42–13. *A,* Lateral view of a 56-year-old man with painful fracture pseudarthrosis at L1. Note the need to support the weight of the upper trunk with a cane and hand on the thigh owing to weight-bearing distress. He suffered increasing painful deformity with the apex at the fracture site. Note the weight-bearing line anterior to the area of the fracture. *B,* Lateral radiograph of the thoracic spine showing fracture through the upper body of L1 and the posterior elements. The lesion is away from the disc space. It extended on recumbency and collapsed in flexion on weight bearing. *C,* Anterior view showing the fracture involving the vertebral body. *D,* Standing lateral 3-foot radiograph of the spine showing loss of lumbar lordosis with the weight-bearing line well anterior to the fracture site. *E,* Postoperative standing lateral 3-foot film of the spine showing correction of deformity with the weight-bearing line shifted well posterior to the fracture site. Both the osteotomy and the fracture have healed. *F,* Postoperative lateral radiograph of the lumbar spine showing healed osteotomy as well as spontaneous healing of the fracture pseudarthrosis. *G,* Lateral view eight years postoperatively showing erect posture with normal chin-brow to vertical angle. The patient works full time as a barber.

ing of the nonunion (Fig. 42–13D–G). The radiographic appearances of spondylodiscitis and fracture pseudarthrosis, although superfically similar, are different when carefully assessed, with the primary lesion being in different locations. There is less erosive change with pseudarthrosis and a greater tendency to heal than with spondylodiscitis.

The incidence of spondylodiscitis may be greater than the literature suggests, and undoubtedly its recognition requires a high index of suspicion. Of 141 cases of ankylosing spondylitis referred for evaluation and surgical correction of spinal deformity, 124 had radiographs of the entire spine suitable for study. Of these, 26, or 21 per cent, were found to have spondylodiscitis.[64] This high incidence may be partly attributable to the severity of the cases analyzed. The chief complaint was progressive kyphotic deformity in 23 of the 26 cases. Nine of the 26 patients recalled a traumatic episode that resulted in increasing pain and deformity in the area of spondylodiscitis. There were no neurologic deficits secondary to the lesions. The site of the spondylodiscitis ranged from T7 to L5, most commonly occurring at T11–L1. There were seven cases of multiple-level involvement. Twenty-four of the 26 patients had surgical correction of the primary deformity. The goal of surgery was to shift the weight-bearing line of the upper body posteriorly to the site of spondylodiscitis to produce a balanced spine. When the spondylodiscitis was at the site of the deformity and contributed to it, correction of the deformity resulted in fusion of the spondylodiscitis. This occurred when the plane of the disc space was shifted from a vertical to a more transverse position, converting shear forces to compression forces. There were two cases that required multiple-level thoracic anterior strut grafting with posterior Harrington compression instrumentation for severe angular thoracic kyphotic deformities associated with destructive spondylodiscitis. Another patient in the study required anterior fibular strut grafting at the site of gross destructive spondylodiscitis, not associated with deformity (see Fig. 42–11).

Most patients with spondylodiscitis are asymptomatic, with the lesion being noted on routine radiologic examination. However, when the area of involvement is under shear stress, it may become painful and can contribute significantly to kyphotic deformity. The treatment in severe cases of deformity is surgical correction to produce a balanced spine and to result in fusion at the site of the spondylodiscitis. Rarely, anterior grafting is indicated for grossly painful destructive lesions without deformity.

FLEXION (KYPHOTIC) DEFORMITIES OF THE SPINE

It is well known that severe flexion deformities of the spine may occur in patients suffering from Marie-Strümpell spondylitis and ankylosing spondylitis associated with psoriasis. Prevention of these deformities by early recognition of the disease process and adequate medical treatment should be the main goal of treatment. However, despite these conservative treatment measures, we too often see patients with advanced kyphotic deformities of the trunk who are grossly disabled and who present a major surgical dilemma for correction of the deformity.

Indications for Surgical Correction

The indications for surgical correction of spinal deformity are variable and depend on the extent of the deformity, the degree of functional disability, the age and general condition of the patient, the feasibility of correction, and, perhaps above all else, the willingness of the patient to accept the risks and rehabilitative measures required for correction.

Assessment of the Deformity

In assessing patients for possible surgical correction, it is important to recognize and identify the primary site of the deformity. In some instances, the surgeon may attempt to improve spinal alignment and improve patient function by operating at a site somewhat removed from the area of primary deformity. In most cases, however, particularly if any major correction is to be attempted, the correction must be done at the site of the main deformity. If this is not done, disturbance of balance and of the ability to walk and stand upright could occur. Patients who present with apparent spinal deformity may have the main deformity in the hip joints rather than in the spine. The spinal deformity, even when the primary cause of the patient's symptoms, may be in the lumbar spine, the thoracic spine, or even the cervical spine.

Figure 42–14A shows a 57-year-old woman who was referred for correction of her "spinal" deformity. Once a woman of normal height, she was flexed so much that the distance from her nose to the floor was only 32 inches. She had been held rigidly in this position for 16 years. Her knees were held rigidly together in adduction, and as a result of impingement of one knee against the other, she wore a protective pad on her right knee. The spine and hip joints were both solidly ankylosed so that she could be moved up and down in a teeter-totter fashion by either lifting up on her extremities or pushing down on her head (Fig. 42–14B–D). Although she did have a forward curvature of the lumbar spine, the thoracic spine, and, to a degree, the neck, it was evident that her main flexion deformity was at the fused hip joints. If her lower limbs could be positioned below her, in line with her trunk, her main deformity would be corrected. She was therefore treated by bilateral total hip replacement arthroplasties rather than spinal osteotomy. The hip flexion deformities were corrected, and the lower limbs were placed in more normal alignment below the trunk. After this, she was able to stand and look straight ahead (Fig. 42–14E). As far as she is concerned, her main problem had been relieved. She continued to progress well, walking with canes, and was able to look after her own home.

Accurate assessment and measurement of any trunk

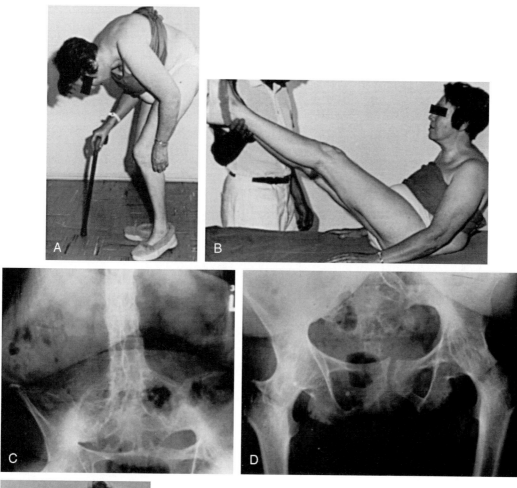

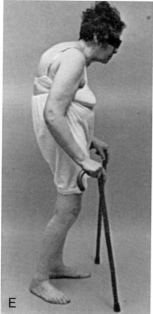

Figure 42–14.   *A,* Lateral view of a 57-year-old woman referred for correction of "spinal" deformity. She had been deformed in this position for 16 years. The distance between the floor and her nose was 32 inches. *B,* Lateral view showing the effect of the fused hip joint, creating trunk deformity and "teeter-totter" movement. *C,* Anteroposterior radiograph showing ankylosis of the spine and sacroiliac joints. *D,* Radiograph demonstrating complete ankylosis of both hip joints. *E,* Early postoperative standing view after bilateral total replacement arthroplasties, with correction of the main clinical deformity.

deformity are required in planning treatment and to assess its results. The most effective and consistent measure of trunk flexion deformity is the chin-brow to vertical angle. This is a measure of the angle formed by a line from the brow to the chin through the vertical, when the patient stands with the hips and knees fully extended and the neck in its neutral or fixed position (Fig. 42–15).

Kyphotic Deformity of the Lumbar Spine

This was the first type of deformity corrected surgically in arthritic disease and was reported by Smith-Petersen and colleagues in 1945.[67] The initial procedure was done under general anesthesia with the patient prone. This has been further reported by LaChappelle,[28] Herbert,[22, 23] Nunziata,[43] Wilson,[73] Law,[29–31] and others.[2, 14, 19, 26, 40–42, 50] To avoid difficulties with the prone position, Adams recommended that the operation be performed with the patient on his or her side, and he used a three-point rack to manipulate the spine and allow correction.[2]

Some have recommended a two-stage procedure or a double-exposure procedure with division of the longitudinal ligament anteriorly. In the author's experience, this is not required, and correction can be done from the posterior approach alone. The double-exposure technique has the drawback of extending the operative procedure and anesthesia time.

A major complication of lumbar osteotomy is gastric dilatation and abdominal ileus. As the spine is extended, the superior mesenteric artery is stretched over the third part of the duodenum, predisposing to gastric dilatation. If this hazard is not anticipated, patients may vomit a large amount in the postoperative interval, and with a stiff, rigid neck and lying supine, there is a significant risk of aspiration. As a result, it is necessary to insert a nasogastric tube with suction drainage until intestinal motility is established postoperatively. The irritation of a nasogastric tube and the

accumulation of secretions caused by it may contribute to pulmonary complications, particularly under general anesthesia.

Kallio[26] stated that "anesthetization is no easy task," in patients with kyphotic deformity. Emneus[14] stated that general anesthesia is contraindicated owing to the prone position at operation, the completely rigid thoracic cage, and the difficulty with intubation. He performed the operation on three patients under local analgesia and subsequently on two other patients using extradural analgesia.

A review of all the reported cases of lumbar osteotomy performed with the patients under general anesthesia prior to 1969 revealed a mortality rate of 8 to 10 per cent and some degree of neurologic deficit, including paraplegia, in 30 per cent. An analysis of the causes of death in these cases revealed that two thirds appeared to be related to the use of general anesthesia. As a result of this background knowledge and the author's experience correcting kyphotic deformity of the cervical spine under local anesthesia, the possibility of carrying out correction on the lumbar spine under local anesthesia was investigated extensively in 106 patients beginning in 1969. This investigation revealed local anesthesia to be a relatively safe, reliable, and practical procedure.[54–56, 72]

With improvements in anesthesia, particularly with the ability to carry out fiberoptic intubation with the patient awake and the development of spinal cord and electromyographic (EMG) monitoring, the risks of surgery under general anesthesia have markedly decreased. As a result, the author's current technique is for the patient to be intubated while awake. With the endotracheal tube in place, the patient positions himself or herself on an adjusted Tower table with the hips and knees flexed and with supports for the pelvis, chest, and head. The supports are adjusted until the patient is comfortable, avoiding any strain on the neck or elsewhere. When the patient indicates that he or she is comfortable, general anesthesia is introduced. Spinal

Figure 42–15. Technique for measuring the degree of kyphotic or flexion deformity of the spine in ankylosing spondylitis. The angle formed by a line from the brow to the chin to the vertical is measured with the patient standing with the hips and knees extended and the neck in either its fixed or neutral position. *A,* Chin-brow to vertical angle measuring thoracolumbar deformity. *B,* Chin-brow to vertical angle measuring cervical deformity.

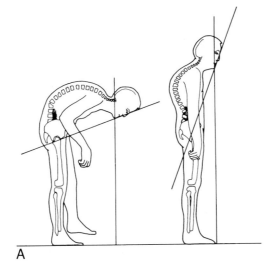

A

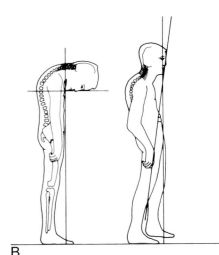

B

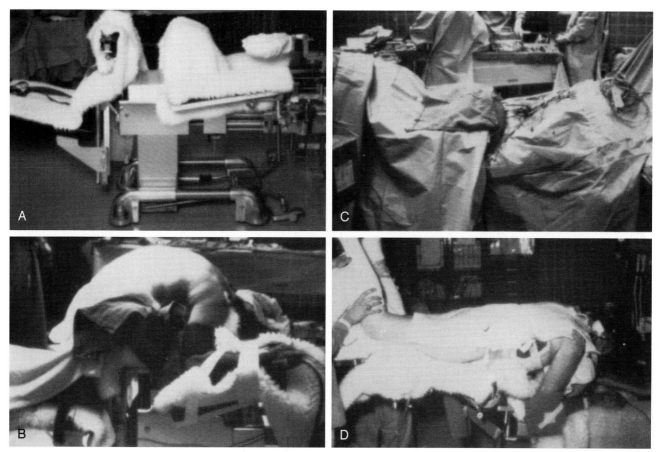

Figure 42–16. *A,* Side view of a Tower table prepared for lumbar osteotomy under general anesthesia. The patient is intubated while awake and positioned on the table awake. Adjustments are made so that the head is supported in a comfortable position with the eyeballs free of pressure. The chest and pelvis are supported with the abdomen free. The knees bear part of the patient's weight, with the hips and knees flexed. When the patient is comfortable, general anesthesia is begun. *B,* Lateral view of a patient with lumbar flexion deformity in position on a Tower table with the knees flexed at 90 degrees. C, Operative view showing correction of the flexion deformity after lumbar resection-extension osteotomy. The hips are extended with the spine fracturing anteriorly and the resected defect closing posteriorly. The knees are kept flexed to avoid stretching of the sciatic nerves and interference with spinal cord monitoring. The resected defect closes, allowing Luque instrumentation with Wisconsin buttons, and grafting. *D,* Postoperative view with application of posterior shell to support the patient when turned supine.

cord and EMG monitoring are performed throughout the procedure. It is important to have valid preoperative tracings for comparison with the findings during surgery. The use of general anesthesia makes the resection easier for the surgeon and allows easier undercutting of the pedicles above and below, with a more thorough decompression of the L3 nerve roots. The amount of decompression is determined preoperatively, and the laminar margins are undercut above and below the osteotomy site to avoid neural impingement. When the decompression has been completed in a symmetric fashion, the hips are extended to produce extension correction. While this is done, the knees are kept flexed to avoid any changes in the evoked spinal response recordings if posterior tibial nerve stimulation is used at the ankles (Fig. 42–16).

The initial recommendation of Smith-Petersen and colleagues[67] was to carry out a posterior wedge resec-

tion osteotomy of the midlumbar spine in a V fashion, with manipulative fracturing of the anterior longitudinal ligament. The osteotomy was performed under general anesthesia with the patient in the prone position. The osteotomy resection was carried through the superior articular facet of the vertebra below and the inferior articular facet of the vertebra above in an oblique fashion, its angle being approximately 45 degrees to the horizontal plane. The obliquity of the osteotomy was to allow locking of the vertebrae following correction in an effort to prevent displacement. The technique of osteotomy as recommended by Smith-Petersen is still sound and requires little alteration. It is the basis for the author's current procedure.

Technique of Lumbar Osteotomy

Patients are selected whose primary flexion deformities are in the lumbar spine, with a loss of lumbar lordosis.

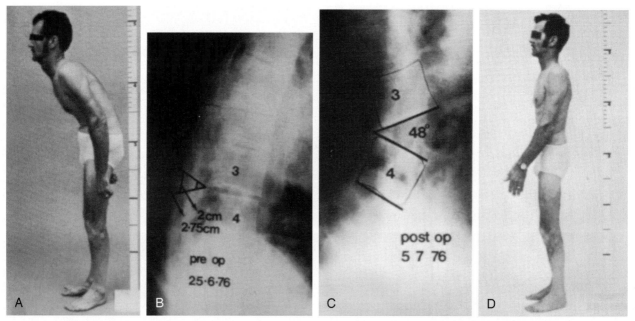

Figure 42–17. *A,* Preoperative lateral view of a patient standing with hips and knees extended showing flexion deformity of the lumbar spine. When the patient closed his eyes and placed his neck in a comfortable position, the chin-brow to vertical angle measured 42 degrees. *B,* Lateral preoperative radiograph of the kyphotic lumbar spine showing the planned angle of resection at the L3–L4 level with the amount of bone required for resection. *C,* Postoperative radiograph showing extension correction of 48 degrees after closure of the posterior resection defect with anterior osteoclasis at L3–L4. *D,* Postoperative lateral view showing complete correction of preoperative deformity. (From Simmons, E. H.: Kyphotic deformity of the spine in ankylosing spondylitis. Clin. Orthop. *128*:65–77, 1977.)

This is determined by clinical and radiologic assessment. The angle of correction that will be required to straighten the deformity is determined by having the patient stand with the hips and knees extended and then measuring the angle of flexion of the spine from the vertical when viewed from the lateral aspect (Fig. 42–17). If the patient's neck is placed in a neutral position or if it is in a fixed position, the chin-brow to vertical angle can be determined, and this is the amount of correction that should be obtained. This angle is transposed to a lateral radiograph of the lumbar spine, the apex of the angle being at the level of the posterior longitudinal ligament at the L3–L4 disc space (on rare occasions, L4–L5). The L3–L4 level is ordinarily selected for extension osteotomy of the lumbar spine because it represents the apex of the normal lumbar lordosis and is below the termination of the spinal cord. It is located at or below the bifurcation of the aorta.

One of the concerns with extension osteotomy of the lumbar spine is the possibility of injury to the major vessels, particularly the abdominal aorta.[2, 32, 70] The author has reviewed all the reported cases of major vascular injury associated with resection-extension osteotomy of the lumbar spine for ankylosing spondylitis. The level at which the osteotomy was performed in each case was documented. It was noted that in all the cases with injury to the abdominal aorta, the osteotomy was done at T12–L1, L1–L2, or L2–L3. No case of aortic injury was reported with osteotomy performed at L3–L4 or L4–L5. One hundred sixteen consecutive lumbar osteotomies performed by the author were also reviewed. Of these, 113 were done at L3–L4, two at L4–L5, and only one at L2–L3. There was no incidence of major arterial injury. Previous radiation or atheromatous change did not result in major injury. Extent of correction was also not a factor. Correction ranged from 40 to 104 degrees, with an overall average of 58 degrees (Fig. 42–18). The anatomic basis for greater vascular safety of osteotomies done at L3–L4 or L4–L5 is the increased mobility of the aortic bifurcation and iliac arteries necessitated by lower limb motion required for ambulation. Segmental vessels of L5 arise from the internal iliac arteries, and the segmental vessels of L5 and L4 are smaller than higher segmental arteries. The greater vascular risk of osteotomies at higher levels is related to the decreased mobility of the aorta proximally. The renal arteries arise at L2–L3, adding to fixation of the aorta, and the segmental vessels increase in size proximally.

To date, the only vascular injury encountered by the author was an inferior vena cava thrombosis extending above the renal veins. This occurred in a markedly obese man who had undergone previous extension osteotomy to L2–L3 but still had major deformity. Thrombosis was likely induced by the weight of the patient's corpulent abdomen resting on his stretched vena cava after extension correction. The patient did well in the early postoperative period, but four to five days postoperatively, gradually increasing edema developed, which later became massive and extended to the midchest and produced a "football sized" scrotum. There was no change in arterial pulses or evidence of arterial insufficiency. Routine Doppler studies of the lower extremities did not reveal the diagnosis initially, and the diagnosis of inferior vena cava thrombosis was ultimately made by venography. With the associated increased interspinal venous pressure, neurologic deficit developed on the basis of venous stasis of the conus, as described by Aboulker and coworkers.[1] The degree of neurologic deficit was maximal when the edema was greatest. Fortunately, most patients with this condition are relatively thin, which would likely decrease the incidence of this complication.

EVOLUTION OF THE AUTHOR'S CURRENT TECHNIQUE FOR LUMBAR RESECTION-EXTENSION OSTEOTOMY IN ANKYLOSING SPONDYLITIS

Initial Technique

Initially the operation was done under local anesthesia. This avoided pulmonary complications and pulmonary-associated mortality. It provided the best intraoperative monitoring of neurologic, vascular, and other vital functions.[52, 53, 56, 57] The results of the first 64 cases done under local anesthesia were reported by D. G. Wills in 1945.[72] When performed under local anesthesia, stabilization was initially based on a V-shaped locking osteotomy, plaster shells, and a turning frame for six to eight weeks. Wire loop fixation was later added to the osteotomy site to increase postoperative stability (Fig. 42–19). Later a Luque rectangle was used with Drummond buttons and wires for fixation (Fig. 42–20). This was followed by Cotrel-Dubousset instrumentation (Fig. 42–21). All this was possible with the procedure performed under local anesthesia. Regardless of whether internal fixation is used and what type of fixation is used, it should be clearly understood that the most important factor in the successful maintenance of correction is to correct the deformity completely, which shifts the weight-bearing line posteriorly to the osteotomy site, where gravity maintains correction. This stimulates bone formation through the weight-bearing lines of the fusion masses posterolaterally. Postoperative management included the use of well-molded posterior and anterior body shells extending from head to knee. The patient was firmly strapped in and turned with the use of a Circ-O-Lectric bed, later a Stryker turning frame, and finally a Roto-Rest bed (Fig. 42–22).[36, 39, 41]

Current Technique

The author's current technique uses fiberoptic intubation with the patient awake, as described previously. The awake patient is assisted and placed on an ad-justed Tower table. When the patient is comfortable, anesthesia is commenced. Spinal cord monitoring is utilized throughout the procedure. Titanium screws are placed into the pedicles at the appropriate levels above and below the planned osteotomy site. Electrical stimulation of the screws and EMG monitoring are used to confirm satisfactory screw placement.[7, 18, 34] The posterior resection is done with the laminae and pedicles undercut to avoid nerve root compression and dural sac impingement following extension correction. The hips are extended, producing anterior osteoclasis and closure of the posterior osteotomy. The screw-rod instrumentation is completed.

Posterolateral and posterior bone grafting is performed using the removed morselized bone, which is quite adequate. A well-molded posterior plaster shell is applied from head to knee. The patient is strapped into the shell to allow transfer to a Roto-Rest bed. The importance of a well-molded posterior supporting shell should be emphasized. Following extension osteotomy, the rigid thoracic kyphosis will be more prominent than the pelvis. If the patient lies on a flat surface, gravity will push the thorax forward and allow the pelvis and lower lumbar spine to move posteriorly. If the trap door of the bed is removed for a bowel movement, the spine will be unsupported. The well-contoured, rigid posterior plaster shell provides a well-fitted surface on which the rigid trunk can lie, protecting the osteotomy site (Fig. 42–23).

It is essential that a nasogastric suction tube be in position before the patient leaves the operating room. It should be recognized that following extension correction, tension on the mesentery and superior mesenteric artery may produce a functional block of the duodenum, with associated gastric distention. If this is allowed to occur, the patient may vomit, and with a rigid cervical spine, the risks of aspiration are significant. Nasogastric suction should be maintained until the patient is passing gas and has normal gastric function.

The current technique provides the advantages of allowing easier and more liberal decompression. It allows the use of more rigid pedicle screw-rod internal fixation with less risk of loss of correction postoperatively. It provides easier and more rapid mobilization of the patient with greater comfort. The disadvantages of such internal fixation are increased operative time; the presence of altered anatomy, which makes screw insertion into the pedicles more difficult; and the potential risks of bone screws. Correct screw positioning is determined both radiographically and with electrical pedicle screw stimulation with EMG monitoring.[7, 18, 34] Experience to date indicates that the advantages of pedicle fixation outweigh the disadvantages, and the technique seems to provide excellent results (Fig. 42–24).

Kyphotic Deformity of the Thoracic Spine

A certain amount of thoracic kyphosis is fairly common in ankylosing spondylitis, but rarely does it present to

Text continued on page 1328

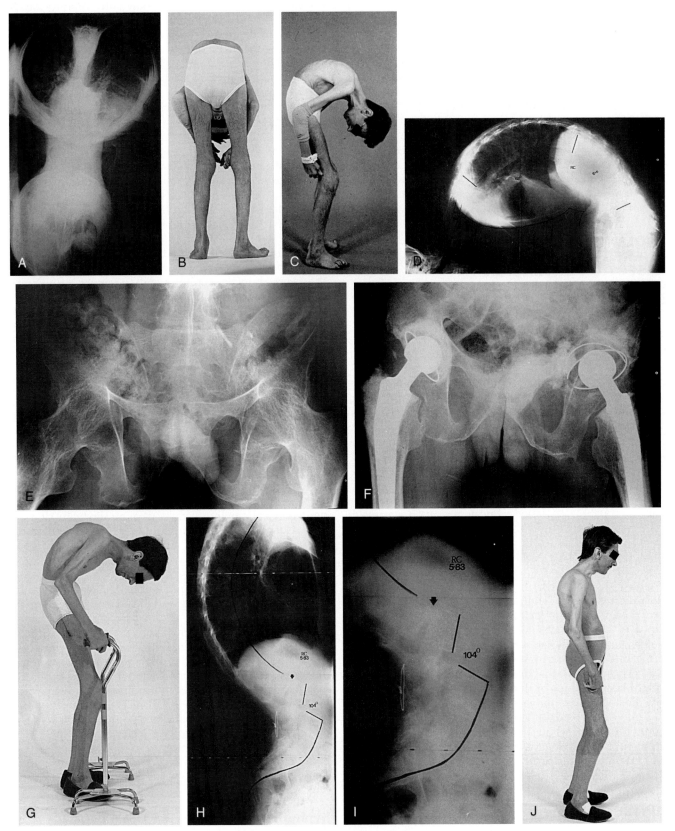

Figure 42–18. See legend on opposite page

Figure 42–18. Illustrations of a 36-year-old man with an 18-year history of ankylosing spondylitis demonstrating the complexity of spinal deformity and its assessment. *A,* Anteroposterior standing radiograph of the patient's spine. The thorax resembles a CT axial view. *B, C,* Posterior and lateral standing views. He could look only backward and therefore had to walk backward. The lateral view shows a chin-brow to vertical angle of 134 degrees. He has combined deformities of thoracic kyphosis, lumbar kyphosis, cervical kyphosis, and hip flexion deformities. *D,* Lateral standing radiograph showing neck flexion deformity, thoracic kyphosis of 68 degrees, complete loss of lumbar lordosis with superimposed 47 degrees of lumbar kyphosis, and hip flexion deformities. *E,* Anteroposterior radiograph of the pelvis showing fused hip joints. The patient was treated with bilateral total hip replacement arthroplasties at one sitting, under regional anesthesia. *F,* Anteroposterior view of hip joints following total replacement arthroplasties. *G,* Lateral standing view of the patient following bilateral hip arthroplasties. His deformity was improved, but he could not look either backward or forward while walking. *H,* Postoperative standing lateral radiograph of the spine following resection-extension osteotomy of 104 degrees at L3–L4 done under local anesthesia. The weight-bearing line is shifted well posterior to the osteotomy site. *I,* Close-up lateral radiograph of the lumbar spine showing the extent of lumbar osteotomy. The patient had associated spondylodiscitis *(arrow)* above the area of osteotomy, which went on to spontaneous healing. *J,* Standing lateral postoperative view of the patient showing correction of his major deformities. He still has some flexion of the knees and neck and is able to stand and look ahead. He walks in a normal fashion and is able to enjoy the activities of normal daily living with his family.

Figure 42–19. *A,* Operative view showing posterior resection in the midline extending upward and laterally on both sides in symmetric fashion. A 20-gauge stainless steel wire loop has been passed through drill holes in the bases of the spinous process and the ossified interspinous ligaments above and below. *B,* After extension of the spine, the posterior defect is closed, the lateral masses coming together. The encircling wire has been tied with wire tier. *C,* Posterior view showing completion of the operative fusion using the resected bone, which is placed posterolaterally on both sides, creating an effective autogenous fusion mass. *D,* Postoperative anteroposterior radiograph showing locking of the posterior V-shaped resection osteotomy.

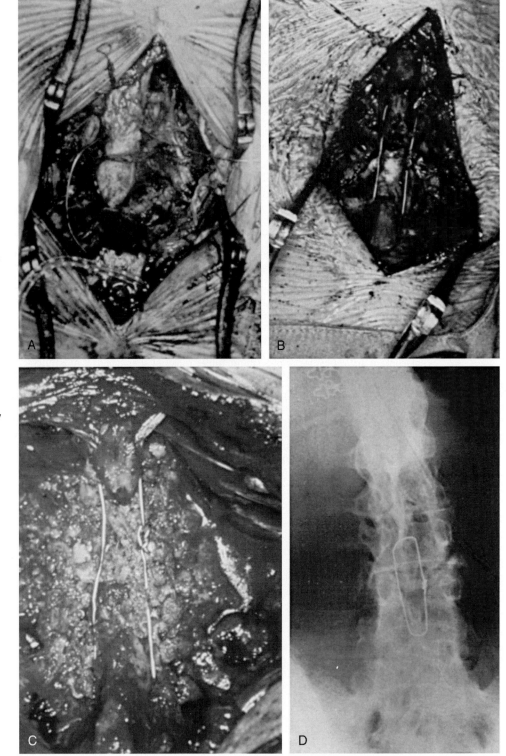

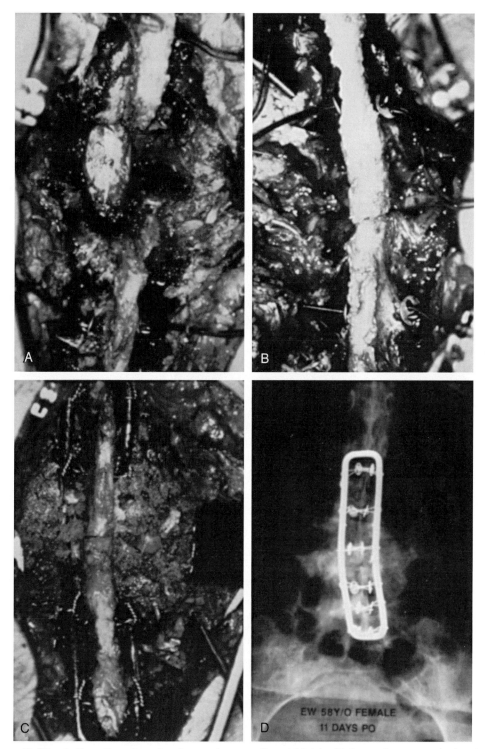

Figure 42–20. *A,* Operative view showing wedge resection at L3–L4 with Luque buttons and wires in position above and below the osteotomy site. *B,* Operative view after extension correction. Symmetrically resected bone margins have come together. *C,* The Luque rectangle is in position and wired to the spine. The osteotomy defect is closed. The resected bone is used for an autograft and may be supplemented by crushed cancellous allograft bone to give an adequate fusion mass. *D,* Postoperative anteroposterior view showing Luque rectangle with Drummond buttons and wires.

Illustration continued on following page

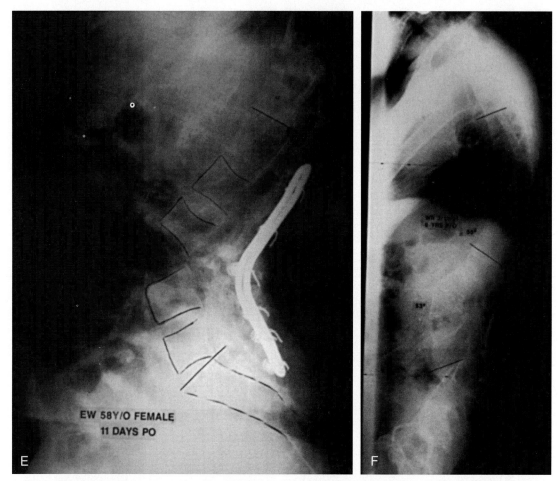

Figure 42–20. *Continued.* *E,* Early postoperative lateral radiograph showing extension correction with the weight-bearing line well posterior to the osteotomy site. The Luque instrumentation is fixed to the posterior elements without invasion of the spinal canal. *F,* Standing lateral 3-foot radiograph of a spine six years after resection-extension osteotomy of the lumbar spine with Luque instrumentation. There is a solid bony mass posterior to the weight-bearing line as well as fusion anteriorly.

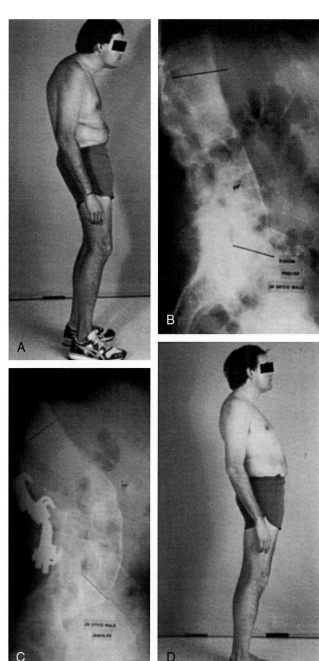

Figure 42–21.   *A,* Preoperative lateral view of a 37-year-old physician with thoracolumbar flexion deformity. With his knees extended the chin-brow to vertical angle was 40 degrees. He had pain and fatigue on attempting to hyperextend the neck and flex the knees to look ahead. He had increase in the thoracic kyphosis and loss of lumbar lordosis. *B,* Preoperative lateral radiograph of the lumbar spine showing loss of normal lordosis. *C,* Postoperative lateral radiograph of the lumbar spine showing healed extension osteotomy at L3–L4 with Cotrel-Dubousset instrumentation. The correction was adequate to balance the spine. *D,* Postoperative standing lateral view showing normal chin-brow to vertical angle. The extension correction of the lumbar spine has balanced the increased kyphosis and corrected the loss of lumbar lordosis. The patient is normally active with relief of preoperative discomfort.

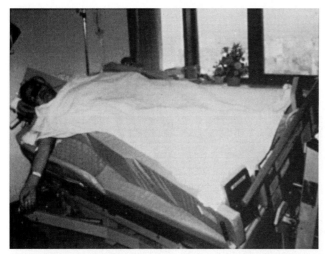

Figure 42–22. Postoperative management of a patient in a Roto-Rest bed. The bed provides secure fixation with slow constant rotation, avoiding the necessity of turning the patient from prone to supine positions. The patient's spine is supported with a well-molded posterior shell, applying even contact to the spine and protecting it on removal of the trap door for bedpan use.

such a major degree that definitive correction is required. It is in an area of the spine that has generally been avoided because of serious potential risks.

Patients with thoracic kyphosis can be classified into two groups, according to the characteristics of their spinal deformity. The first group has a primary deformity in the thoracic spine, but also has loss of lumbar lordosis and spinal rigidity. If the thoracic kyphosis is

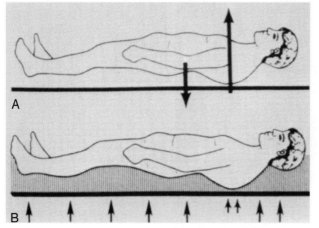

Figure 42–23. *A,* Diagrammatic view showing the lateral outline of a patient's contour after extension correction of the lumbar spine. The spine is rigid. The diagram illustrates the areas of relative pressure contact difference. Most of the pressure is against the thoracic hump, pushing it forward, with the lumbar spine tending to translate posteriorly. *B,* Inferior diagram shows the effect of a well-molded rigid shell providing equal support throughout the spine, avoiding uneven contact forces that would favor displacement.

mild or moderate in degree and the lumbar spine is rigid and flattened, correction of the overall spinal deformity in this group may be accomplished by a compensating osteotomy in the lumbar spine. By extending the lumbar spine sufficiently, compensation for thoracic kyphosis can be achieved. To achieve spinal balance, the lumbar spine is overcorrected to compensate for the thoracic kyphosis, thereby providing the individual with a horizontal gaze and erect posture.

Figure 42–25 shows a 43-year-old man who has had ankylosing spondylitis for 17 years. He had a severe flexion deformity, primarily in the thoracic spine. He had associated flattening of the lumbar spine and a height loss of 4 inches. He had a thoracic kyphosis of 108 degrees from T3 to T12. Under local anesthesia, a posterior wedge resection osteotomy of the lumbar spine was done at the L3–L4 level, creating an anterior spinal opening wedge of 58 degrees. Postoperatively, the torso is well balanced over the pelvis. He is now able to stand erect with a horizontal gaze. The correction was well maintained five years after surgery.

The second group of patients with thoracic kyphosis is distinguished by maintenance of cervical and lumbar lordoses. The surgical treatment of these patients poses several problems. Further extending the lumbar spine by lumbar extension osteotomy would produce an unphysiologic hyperlordosis. The cardiopulmonary function of these individuals may be severely compromised, thereby constituting an indication for correction of the thoracic deformity. The primary deformity is in the thoracic spine, and correction must be obtained in this region. However, a single major angular correction of the spine in this area could cause significant spinal cord injury. There are several reasons for this. The spinal canal is relatively small in the thoracic region. The amount of available free canal space not occupied by the neural elements is relatively small. In addition, the cord and nerve roots in the thoracic spine have relatively little mobility. Finally, the blood supply to the thoracic spinal cord is very precarious. To circumvent these problems, alternative surgical approaches are required. It has been established in the treatment of rigid deformities of the spine secondary to Scheuermann's disease and congenital thoracic kyphosis that combinations of preoperative traction and staged anterior and posterior osteotomies of the spine with interval traction provide satisfactory results. Employing these surgical principles with certain modifications, we have found it feasible to correct severe flexion deformities of the thoracic spine secondary to ankylosing spondylitis.

Patients with thoracic kyphosis who maintain their lumbar and cervical lordoses can be further divided into two subgroups, according to the amount of residual spinal flexibility that exists. The first subgroup is distinguished by incomplete ossification of the spine or extensive areas of destructive spondylodiscitis, resulting in areas of relative mobility. The second subgroup has a rigid thoracic kyphosis with relatively complete ossification.

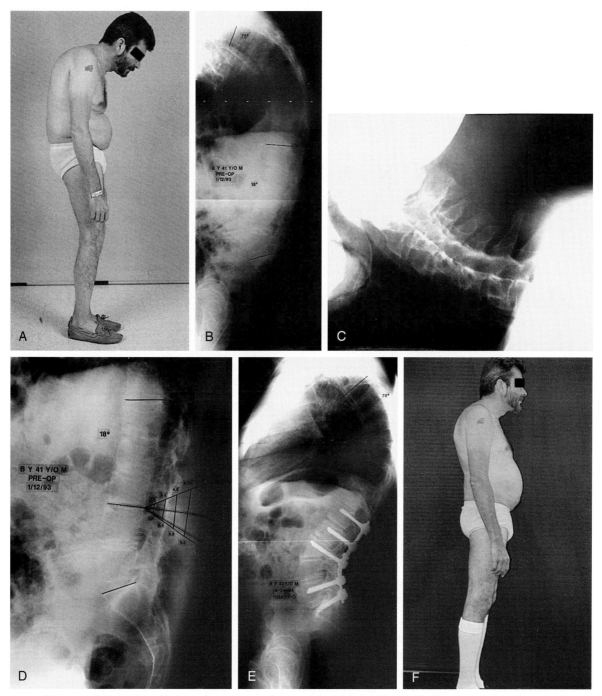

Figure 42–24. *A*, Lateral view of a 41-year-old man with a 21-year history of ankylosing spondylitis. He had suffered with a major kyphotic deformity for 10 years, which prevented him from working for five to six years. His chin-brow to vertical angle measured 55 degrees. *B*, Lateral standing 3-foot film of the spine showing increased thoracic kyphosis measuring 75 degrees but decreased lumbar lordosis measuring 18 degrees. His weight-bearing line is well anterior to the midlumbar spine. *C*, Lateral standing radiograph of the cervical spine showing a compensatory increase in cervical lordosis with ossification from C2 distally. *D*, Preoperative lateral radiograph of the lumbar spine showing planned resection-osteotomy at L3–L4 of 50 to 55 degrees. *E*, Lateral standing 3-foot radiograph 16 months postoperatively showing healed osteotomy with lumbar lordosis measuring 74 degrees. Thoracic kyphosis was corrected slightly to 70 degrees. The spine is in balance. The main weight-bearing line is posterior to the osteotomy site. *F*, Standing lateral view of the patient 16 months postoperatively. He has returned to a normal lifestyle. His correction prompted an uninformed observer to state that his wife was living with "different man."

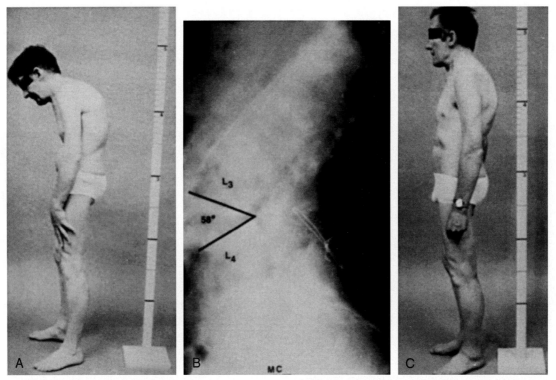

Figure 42–25. *A,* Lateral view of a patient with thoracic kyphosis of 108 degrees from T3 to T12. There is some loss of lumbar lordosis. *B,* Postoperative lateral radiograph of the lumbar spine after resection-extension osteotomy of 58 degrees, producing lordosis to balance the thoracic kyphotic deformity. *C,* Postoperative lateral standing view showing a well-balanced trunk and normal chin-brow to vertical angle.

Incomplete Anterior Ossification

Figure 42–26 shows a 32-year-old woman with ankylosing spondylitis associated with psoriasis for 14 years. She developed iritis, for which she was placed on steroid therapy. During the previous 12 years, she noted a progressive loss in height of 6 inches. She developed a severe thoracic kyphosis of 120 degrees, extending from T2 to T12. She had gross rib impingement against the pelvis and an obvious area of destructive spondylodiscitis at the T8–T9 region anteriorly. She had a sharp angular kyphosis with pressure changes and impending skin breakdown over the area of the kyphos. Pulmonary function was 34 per cent of the predicted normal. With further increase in the kyphos, there was a significant risk of increased pulmonary insufficiency, as well as spinal cord compression. There was also a mild degree of C1–C2 subluxation.

The areas of destructive spondylodiscitis indicated the potential for correction of the deformity with preliminary traction. Accordingly, a period of careful halo-femoral traction was instituted, and the kyphosis decreased to 68 degrees. Multiple posterior resection osteotomies were then performed from T4 to T12. Stabilization and further correction were obtained using bilateral Harrington compression rods with posterior fusion. This resulted in reduction of the kyphosis to 50 degrees. Two weeks later, a right transthoracic approach to the spine was performed, with resection of the areas of spondylodiscitis. A trough was cut in the spine anteriorly throughout the area of the kyphosis, extending from T6 to T11. A 6-inch section of the right fibula was beveled to lock into place in the prepared trough, producing a solid strut to support the spine anteriorly. The fibular strut was reinforced with multiple strips of rib grafting. The pleura was closed, and the patient was left with a solid strut supporting her spine anteriorly (Fig. 42–26*F*). She gained 5 inches in height. The grafts incorporated anteriorly, and she had maintained her correction at her last follow-up eight years postoperatively (Fig. 42–26*I*).

Rigid Spine

Figure 42–27 shows a 34-year-old woman who had a 14-year history of increasing kyphosis and lateral curvature of the thoracic spine associated with ankylosing spondylitis. Her height had diminished 5 inches over the preceding five years. She complained of constant back and neck pain. Pulmonary function was 54 per cent of the predicted normal. Radiographs revealed a primary thoracic kyphosis, with a compensatory increase in lumbar lordosis and cervical lordosis. The thoracic kyphosis measured 110 degrees (Fig. 42–27*D*). Halo-dependent traction was carried out with the pa-

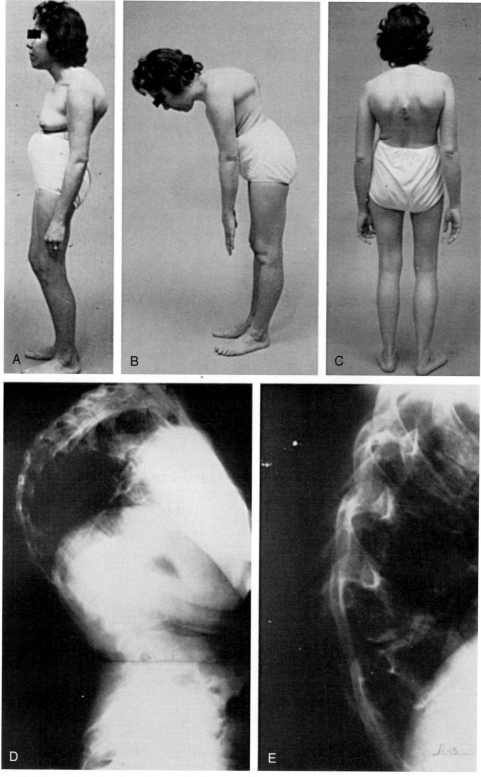

Figure 42–26. *A,* Standing lateral view of a 32-year-old woman with severe thoracic kyphosis associated with ankylosing spondylitis and steroid treatment. Her height had decreased by 6 inches with rib impingement against the pelvis. *B,* Lateral bending view demonstrating angular thoracic kyphosis. *C,* Posterior view showing skin changes over the apex of the deformity. *D,* Lateral standing radiograph showing thoracic kyphosis of 120 degrees with exaggerated lumbar lordosis. *E,* Lateral radiograph of the thoracic spine showing destructive spondylodiscitis at the apex of the deformity.

Illustration continued on following page

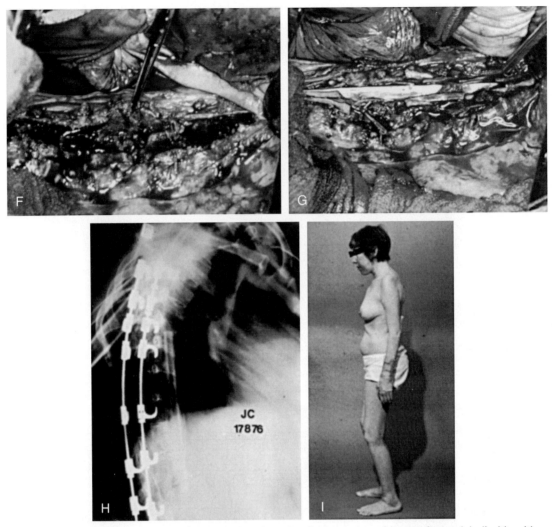

Figure 42–26. *Continued.* *F,* Anterior operative view showing resection of areas of spondylodiscitis with a trough prepared from T6 to T11 for the fibular strut graft. *G,* Operative view with the fibular strut graft locked into position from T6 to T11 with onlay rib grafts. *H,* Postoperative lateral radiograph showing the strut graft and posterior Harrington compression instrumentation. The areas of spondylodiscitis have healed. *I,* Postoperative lateral standing view showing correction of deformity with an increase in height of 5 inches.

tient in a Circ-O-Lectric bed for 10 days, with only 15 degrees of improvement in the thoracic kyphosis owing to the rigidity of the deformity. Attempts to intubate the patient were unsuccessful because of the deformity. A tracheostomy was therefore performed preoperatively, and multiple anterior transthoracic osteotomies were performed from T11 to L1. Division of the ossified spine was carried out with an oscillating saw, and careful curettement of the residual disc material to the level of the posterior longitudinal ligament was performed. Rib grafts were cut into small pieces and packed into the osteotomy sites. She was returned to the Circ-O-Lectric bed with halo-dependent traction for two weeks, during which time the kyphosis reduced another 10 degrees—to 85 degrees. Multiple posterior resection thoracic osteotomies were then performed from T3 to L1. The spine was further

straightened and stabilized using bilateral Harrington compression rods with posterior fusion augmented by autogenous iliac bone. The kyphosis was corrected to 50 degrees, with some correction of the scoliosis. She was recumbent for six weeks postoperatively, then ambulatory in a plaster body jacket for six months. She wore a Jewett hyperextension brace for nine months postoperatively. Her height increased by 4 inches, and her ribs moved from below and inside the iliac crest to four finger breadths above the pelvis. She returned to work and maintained the correction (Fig. 42–27*F, G,* and *H*).

Correction of a primary thoracic kyphosis is undoubtedly more hazardous than correction of a lumbar kyphosis. It requires a general anesthetic, with all its potential hazards and complications. Forty per cent of patients require a tracheostomy. In general, the patients are younger than those with incomplete ossification, thereby decreasing the anesthetic risk. It should be remembered that these patients breathe almost entirely with the diaphragm, and care should be taken to avoid injury to it during surgery. They are at greater risk of pulmonary compromise, and correction of the deformity should be approached with caution. The principles of surgical treatment of this condition are as follows:

1. Multiple osteotomies are performed in the thoracic region of the spine so that correction at any one level is minimal, although the cumulative effect of the osteotomies provides a substantial correction.
2. Two-stage surgical correction of the deformity with osteotomies of both the posterior and the anterior aspects of the spine, combined with interval traction, is essential in achieving maximal correction. The distractive forces are applied progressively and

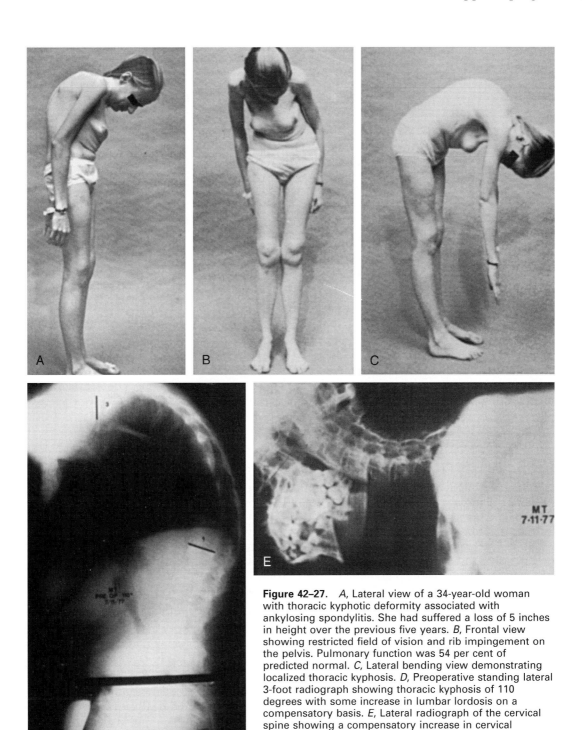

Figure 42–27.   *A,* Lateral view of a 34-year-old woman with thoracic kyphotic deformity associated with ankylosing spondylitis. She had suffered a loss of 5 inches in height over the previous five years. *B,* Frontal view showing restricted field of vision and rib impingement on the pelvis. Pulmonary function was 54 per cent of predicted normal. *C,* Lateral bending view demonstrating localized thoracic kyphosis. *D,* Preoperative standing lateral 3-foot radiograph showing thoracic kyphosis of 110 degrees with some increase in lumbar lordosis on a compensatory basis. *E,* Lateral radiograph of the cervical spine showing a compensatory increase in cervical lordosis.

Illustration continued on following page

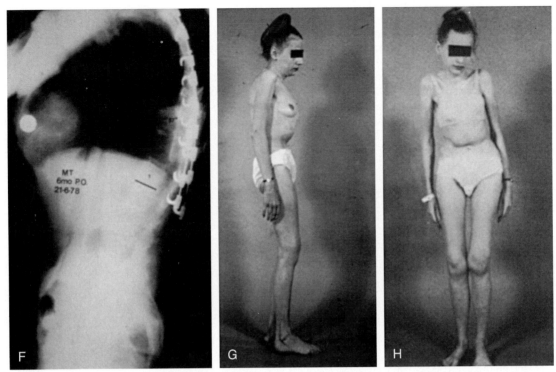

Figure 42–27. *Continued.* *F,* Postoperative lateral 3-foot radiograph showing correction of the major deformity, with cervical kyphosis and lumbar lordosis producing a balanced spine. *G,* Postoperative lateral view showing correction of deformity. *H,* Postoperative frontal view showing elevation of the ribs from the pelvis and restoration of more normal field of vision.

gradually with the patient awake and in traction to minimize neurologic risk. If the spine does not appear to be entirely ossified, or if there are areas of destructive spondylodiscitis, preliminary halo-dependent traction may be attempted and is followed by posterior resection osteotomies with bilateral compression instrumentation and fusion. This may then be followed by anterior resection of the areas of spondylodiscitis, with fibular strut grafting to support the spine anteriorly. With a rigid thoracic kyphosis, initial halo-dependent traction will not produce significant initial correction, and anterior transthoracic osteotomies will be necessary, with rib grafting of the osteotomy sites. This should be followed by halo-dependent traction, followed by multiple posterior resection osteotomies with compression instrumentation and fusion (Fig. 42–28). The staging of the surgeries probably decreases the risk of producing vascular insufficiency of the spinal cord by allowing collateral circulation, from postoperative hyperemia, to develop in the interval between the procedures. Harrington instrumentation was used in most of the author's patients admitted for correction of thoracic deformities. The compression rod worked effectively in permitting graduated correction to be applied at surgery. More recently, Cotrel-Dubousset instrumentation has been used, and Texas Scottish Rite Hospital (TSRH) instrumentation has also been effective. These systems are

currently more popular and more readily available than Harrington instrumentation, but they can be more prominent beneath the skin and muscle of thin patients. To date, there has not been enough experience to indicate whether such fixation methods are really more effective for the treatment of this condition.

Kyphotic Deformity of the Cervical Spine

There are few patients with ankylosing spondylitis in whom kyphotic deformity of the spine occurs primarily in the cervical region. This deformity can be severely disabling, with restricted field of vision and interference with skin care under the chin and shaving difficulties in men; it may even progress to the point of interfering with opening of the mouth. There may be major difficulty in swallowing, including episodes of choking; this may be the chief symptom that leads some patients to request correction of the deformity. The indications for and technique of correcting flexion deformity of the neck are less well understood than for lumbar or thoracic kyphoses. The procedure is also fraught with significantly greater hazards than is surgical correction of other kyphotic deformities. A thorough review of the results of cervical osteotomy under general anesthesia is not available. However, the author's conversations with other surgeons and centers indicate that isolated attempts at correction of cervical kyphoses made at such centers have resulted in a high rate of serious complications, some of which resulted in death. For the few severely afflicted patients with this particular problem, the indications for and principles related to surgical correction should be clearly established.

Selection of Patients for Cervical Osteotomy

It is important to recognize that not all patients with a chin-on-chest deformity in ankylosing spondylitis re-

quire a cervical osteotomy. Those who present with painful flexion deformity are unlikely to require osteotomy. A patient with ankylosing spondylitis whose trunk alignment was stable and relatively unchanged over time and who was previously relatively pain-free but who subsequently sustains minimal trauma with development of a painful and progressive flexion deformity of the neck must be considered to have a fracture of the cervical spine until it is proved otherwise. The site of fracture is usually at the base of the neck, at the cervicothoracic junction. Fractures of the

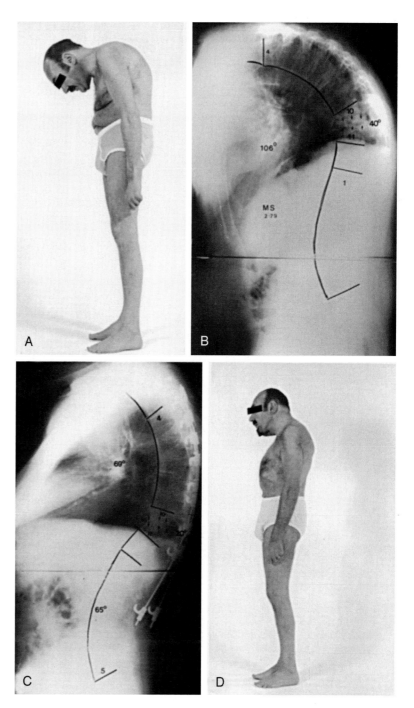

Figure 42–28. *A*, Lateral preoperative view of a 48-year-old surgeon with major thoracic deformity. Cervical and lumbar lordosis are near normal. *B*, Preoperative standing lateral 3-foot radiograph showing fixed kyphosis of 106 degrees with normal lordosis. Despite an area of localized spondylodiscitis, the deformity was rigid, with no correction obtained on halo-dependent traction. This required initial anterior disc space resection and grafting. *C*, Postoperative standing 3-foot radiograph after staged anterior and posterior osteotomies with posterior compression instrumentation. The thoracic kyphosis of 106 degrees has been reduced to 69 degrees, balanced by lordosis of 65 degrees. The area of spondylodiscitis has healed. *D*, Postoperative lateral view showing correction of the major deformity. The patient was able to return to the practice of surgery and a normal lifestyle.

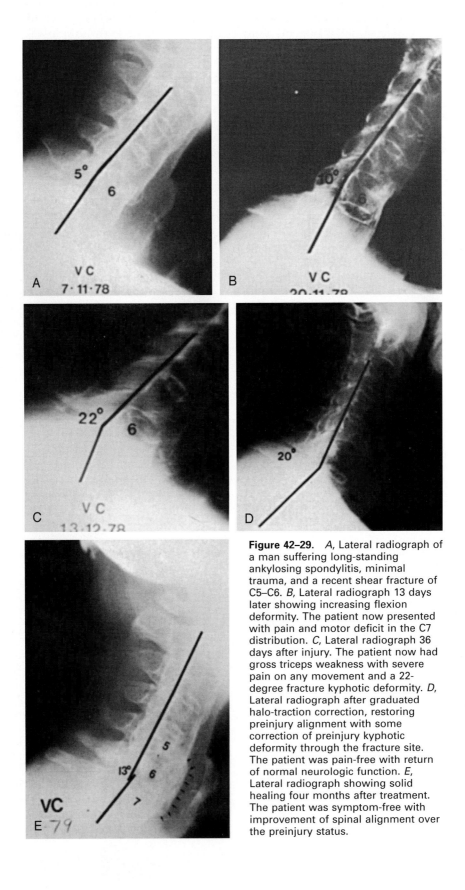

Figure 42–29.   *A,* Lateral radiograph of a man suffering long-standing ankylosing spondylitis, minimal trauma, and a recent shear fracture of C5–C6. *B,* Lateral radiograph 13 days later showing increasing flexion deformity. The patient now presented with pain and motor deficit in the C7 distribution. *C,* Lateral radiograph 36 days after injury. The patient now had gross triceps weakness with severe pain on any movement and a 22-degree fracture kyphotic deformity. *D,* Lateral radiograph after graduated halo-traction correction, restoring preinjury alignment with some correction of preinjury kyphotic deformity through the fracture site. The patient was pain-free with return of normal neurologic function. *E,* Lateral radiograph showing solid healing four months after treatment. The patient was symptom-free with improvement of spinal alignment over the preinjury status.

spine in ankylosing spondylitis are similar to fractures of an osteoporotic tubular bone, with a transverse shear pattern being predominant. It is often difficult to recognize the fracture with routine radiographs, because the fracture, which usually occurs between C6 and T2 and is most common at C7–T1, may be obscured by the shoulders. The fracture undergoes gradual erosion with collapse anteriorly, thereby allowing the chin to approach the chest. The patient typically notices that the position of the head varies during the day, being more upright in the morning and approaching the chest as the day progresses. On presentation, the patient may hold his or her head with the hands to ease the pain. It is sometimes necessary to use lateral tomography at the cervicothoracic junction to diagnose this fracture.

These patients do not require cervical osteotomy. A cranial halo-ring should be applied with traction along the patient's typical alignment of the neck, slowly restoring normal alignment by altering the vector of traction with careful neurologic assessment, until the head is restored to its normal functional position. This is most efficiently accomplished with the patient supported on a Circ-O-Lectric bed. A fairly normal chinbrow to vertical angle can usually be obtained, and the alignment can at least be restored to the preinjury state. When satisfactory alignment has been achieved, the patient should be immobilized in a well-molded halocast for four months or until the fracture has healed. Rigid immobilization in a halo-cast, rather than in a less rigid halo-vest, is essential, because a routine halovest does not permit adequate immobilization. In the author's experience, if rigid immobilization is provided in this manner, union occurs consistently (Fig. 42–29). Under unusual circumstances, fracture healing may not occur, and anterior cervical fusion using a keystone graft[60] or posterior fusion will be required.

Although shear fractures are most common at the base of the neck, they may occur at any level. If the displacement is significant, patients may initially present with evidence of spinal cord injury, or this may occur relatively rapidly during the course of their early management as a result of fracture displacement. It should be recognized that patients with this problem are at major risk for neurologic deterioration and are prone to disastrous results when conventional treatment methods used for fracture-dislocations in patients without ankylosing spondylitis are employed. The spine in these patients is rigid both above and below the fracture site. Any movement of the trunk translates all the force of motion to the fracture site. A common observation from relatives of such patients when they first see them after admission to the emergency department with a fracture of the cervical spine is that "the neck is straight," whereas before the injury the patient had a well-known forward flexion alignment. This indicates that the patient had an extension displacement at the fracture site when lying flat in bed. Information should be obtained from the patient or family members about the preinjury alignment of the neck, and attempts should be made to simulate this position with

the application of a halo and gentle traction along what was believed to be the patient's normal alignment. The patient should be protected with a halo-vest before obtaining any radiographic studies that might cause fracture displacement. Lateral tomography is a valuable diagnostic aid to visualize alignment at the fracture site.

When an incomplete spinal cord injury occurs and incomplete reduction has been obtained, open reduction and internal fixation may be required to decompress the cord and stabilize the spine to protect the cord from further injury caused by motion. It is important to recognize the dangers of attempting operative reduction under general anesthesia. The movement of the neck required for intubation of a patient with a rigid upper cervical spine can cause further spinal cord injury. Transferring patients to the operating table and positioning them present significant risks if they are asleep. They are most safely operated on while awake and in the sitting position. After the neck has been stabilized with a firmly applied halojacket, surgery can be performed with the patient in the sitting position, with traction applied along the line of the neck. The posterior cervical spine can be exposed under local anesthesia and the fracture accurately reduced and fixed internally with methyl methacrylate if needed. This may be accomplished by passing threaded Compere wires percutaneously through the bases of the spinous processes above and below the fracture site. Methyl methacrylate can then be applied, incorporating the threaded pins (Fig. 42–30). This provides instantaneous fixation, thereby relieving the patient's pain and maintaining accurate alignment of the spinal canal until healing occurs anteriorly. Following the surgery, the halo-vest should be changed to a well-molded halo-cast that will supply more rigid and accurate immobilization. The cast must be molded below the costal cage and over the iliac crests to prevent any upward or downward motion. This is worn for four months.

The restoration of accurate alignment of the spinal canal is the main factor in providing neural decompression. In more long-standing cases with residual displacement, or in the presence of a small spinal canal, additional decompression can be accomplished by removing the adjacent neural arches at the fracture site. Immobilization is then accomplished by placing the methyl methacrylate laterally on each side, thereby acting as a bridge from the segments above and below.

The other area where lesions of the cervical spine may occur, causing patients to present with painful flexion deformity, is the craniocervical junction. Patients with erosive fractures through the posterior arch of C1 and subluxation at C1–C2 may present with painful neck flexion with or without neurologic symptoms. Destructive arthritis at the atlanto-occipital joints may result in the patient flexing the neck at these joints with the chin held downward. The lateral radiograph of the cervical spine is a clue to these diagnoses. It shows a relatively normal lordosis, with flexion deformity at the craniocervical junction. These conditions

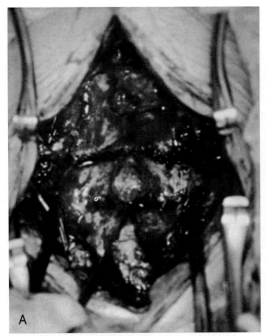

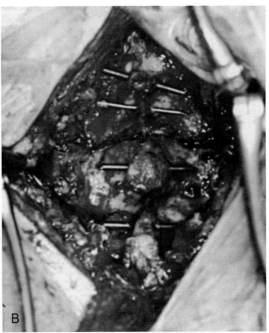

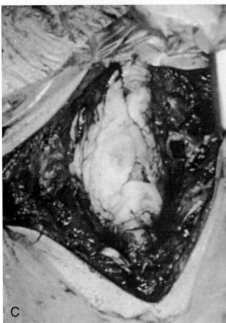

Figure 42–30. *A*, Operative view of the posterior aspect of the cervical spine of a 32-year-old male spondylitic suffering fracture-dislocation at C6–C7 with partial quadriplegia after a motor vehicle injury. The patient was immobilized in a halo-vest with some residual displacement. The effect of the displacement and instability in this type of patient is magnified by the solid column of bone above and below. Surgery was performed under local anesthesia with the patient in the sitting position. The halo was suspended along the line of the neck, adding to the immobilization. The fracture has been reduced. The C5 and C6 spinous processes are exposed above, and the spinous processes of C7 and T1 below. *B*, Operative view showing reduction of shear fracture-dislocation and the threaded Compere pins in position through the posterior arches of C5, C6, C7, and T1 below. The pins were inserted percutaneously through the left lateral side of the neck, transfixing the bases of the spinous processes. The pins were then cut lateral to the spine. *C*, Posterior surgical view after methyl methacrylate application, incorporating the Compere pins and spinous processes. This maintains reduction and provides "instant" fixation of the unstable shear fracture. The accurate reduction provides normal alignment of the spinal canal. The rigid fixation prevents the deleterious effect of any motion on the neural elements until bony healing occurs. If midline decompression is required, bridges of methyl methacrylate can be placed laterally on each side, leaving the midline free.

should be recognized and the deformity corrected by graduated halo traction, initially applied along the line of the neck, restoring a normal chin-brow to vertical angle, followed by posterior stabilization. If reduction of a C1–C2 dislocation is obtained, posterior atlantoaxial arthrodesis, such as by the Gallie technique, may be all that is required. For occipitocervical destructive changes and erosive fractures through the arch of C1, occipitocervical fusion is required and, if necessary, excision of the posterior fragmented arch of C1 (Fig. 42–31).

Unrecognized fractures at the base of the cervical spine may proceed to gradual erosion and collapse anteriorly until the chin reaches the chest. They ultimately heal, at which time the pain disappears, but the patient is left with a painless, fixed flexion deformity of the cervical spine. At this stage, cervical osteotomy is required for correction (Fig. 42–32).

In a review of patients referred for cervical osteotomy, 36 per cent showed evidence of previous cervical fracture. In 31 per cent, the fracture contributed significantly to the final deformity. In only 14 per cent of those who presented with evidence of fracture had the fracture been diagnosed previously. This highlights the fact that early recognition of the fracture and adequate immobilization are essential if the risk of increased deformity is to be avoided. If the fracture is still mobile, some correction of the deformity may be obtained through the fracture site if caution is exercised. If, however, it is solidly united and the spine is fused, osteotomy is required for correction.

An unrecognized factor in the development of spinal deformity in ankylosing spondylitis may be involvement of the muscle itself. Ankylosing spondylitis is a systemic disease involving connective tissue, and muscle tissue is likely to be involved. It is a frequent

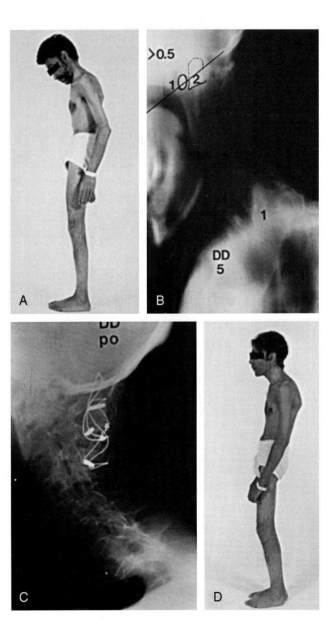

Figure 42–31. *A,* Preoperative lateral view of a male physicist with painful chin-on-chest deformity. The patient used his hands to hold his head when sitting, to control the pain. *B,* Lateral tomogram showing normal cervical lordosis and normal alignment at the cervicothoracic junction. The C1–C2 relationships are normal. The mandible approximates the cervical spine, indicating flexion at the occipitoatlantal junction. The dense posterior arch of C1 was found to be eroded and loose at surgery, probably causing dural irritation with any attempt at extension. There also were destructive changes at the occipitoatlantal joints. *C,* Postoperative lateral radiograph after graduated reduction of the deformity with halo traction, operative excision of the loose posterior arch of C1, and solid posterior occipitocervical fusion. Double-onlay cortical and cancellous iliac grafts were used, fixed to the skull and upper cervical spine, and augmented with cancellous grafts. *D,* Postoperative lateral view showing correction of chin-on-chest deformity with restoration of normal chin-brow to vertical angle. The pain was relieved.

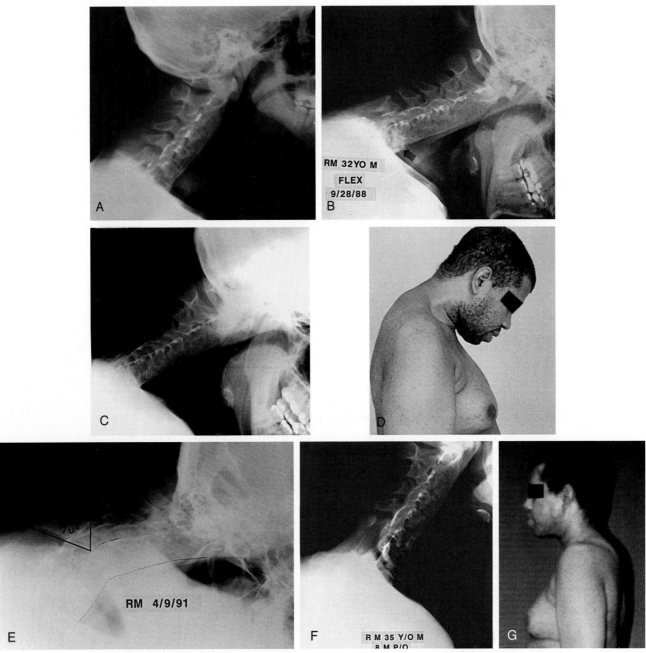

Figure 42–32. *A,* Lateral emergency department radiograph of the cervical spine of a 32-year-old man with a known history of ankylosing spondylitis who presented with pain in the neck after a minor injury. The radiograph was interpreted as "normal," and the patient was told that he had a "sprain" but no major bony injury. The undetected area of fracture is indicated by the arrow. *B,* Lateral radiograph of the same patient four months later showing development of kyphotic deformity of the cervical spine. The area of fracture erosion is indicated by the arrow. The patient was treated with a collar support. *C,* Lateral radiograph of the cervical spine one year after injury. By this time, the patient had gone on to healing and relief of pain, but with a fixed kyphotic deformity and a chin-on-chest deformity. *D,* Lateral view of the patient presenting with a painless fixed kyphotic deformity of the cervical spine following the missed fracture at the base of the neck and healing with the chin approaching the chest. *E,* Preoperative lateral tomogram outlining the 70-degree wedge resection that was required for extension osteotomy. *F,* Lateral radiograph of the cervical spine showing the healed osteotomy eight months postoperatively. *G,* Postoperative lateral standing view of the patient showing correction of the deformity with normal chin-brow to vertical angle. Early recognition of the fracture would have prevented progression of deformity and the need for osteotomy correction.

observation at operation that the paraspinal muscles appear pale and atrophied. The author has described flexion deformity of the cervical spine developing on the basis of occult myopathy in patients without ankylosing spondylitis.[61] In patients with flexion deformity and ankylosing spondylitis, we have identified neurogenic atrophy of the extensor muscles of the spine based on histologic examination and EMG studies.[65] This is now being studied prospectively in all patients. If this is recognized in the earlier stages of the disease before the spine is ossified, intensive medical management and bracing may decrease the risk of deformity. The presence or absence of neurogenic atrophy of the extensor muscles of the spine may have important prognostic value (Fig. 42–33).

Technique of Cervical Osteotomy

It should be recognized that cervical osteotomy is not required for mobile kyphotic deformity when the cervical spine is not solidly fused. It is required for fixed major deformity with a completely ossified cervical spine that will not respond to traction. Surgical correction of fixed major kyphotic deformity of the cervical spine in ankylosing spondylitis by resection-extension osteotomy poses a significant potential risk in patients who have a major systemic disease with its associated medical risks. When making the decision to perform a corrective osteotomy, the surgeon and patient must fully understand the risks involved, and the surgeon must follow established basic principles to allow major correction of deformity with the least risk to the patient.

Since 1966, the author has carried out osteotomy correction using a consistent and reliable technique that has allowed gratifying correction of deformity with an acceptable level of risk. Following the recommendation of Urist,[69] the operation is performed under local anesthesia with the patient in the sitting position. This minimizes major anesthetic hazards, allows accurate spinal cord monitoring and assessment of vital functions with the patient awake, minimizes the likelihood

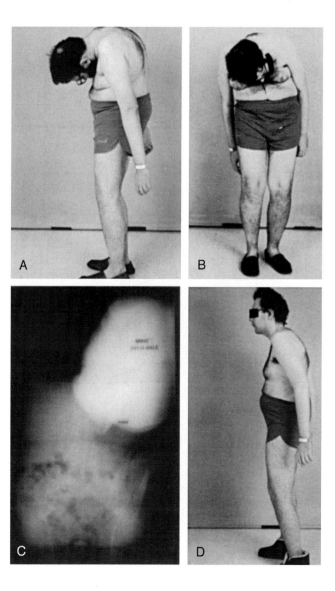

Figure 42–33. *A*, Lateral view of a 34-year-old man with severe chin-on-chest deformity developing over five years. There was an established diagnosis of ankylosing spondylitis and a positive HLA-B27 antigen test. *B*, Frontal view showing rotation of the head and neck to the left, to relieve the chin-on-chest impingement. *C*, Standing anteroposterior 3-foot radiograph showing obliteration of the sacroiliac joints, with the nose just above the level of the iliac crest. There is gross osteopenia. EMG studies of the spinal extensor muscles showed changes of myopathy. At biopsy the extensor muscles were pale and atrophic; histologic studies indicated neurogenic atrophy. *D*, Lateral view six months later. The patient was treated with halo-dependent traction, which allowed correction of the deformity, restoring the chin-brow to vertical angle to normal. He was immobilized in a halo-cast in the corrected position for four months. Calcium, vitamin D, and calcitonin were administered to decrease the osteopenia. He then wore a protective brace for two months and performed isometric extension exercises of the neck. The chin-brow to vertical angle was normal. Histologic studies of the hip extensor muscles also showed neurogenic atrophy. Extensor muscle involvement of the spine has been a consistent finding in patients presenting for correction of major deformity.

of any major neurologic complications, and allows the patient to assist with anatomic localization during the decompression, which is of significant value to the surgeon. The level between the C7 and T1 vertebrae is selected for correction of the deformity (Fig. 42–34). As Mason and coworkers[36] and Urist[69] indicated, this interspace is more amenable to surgical treatment than other levels in the cervical region. The spinal canal is relatively wide, and the cervical cord and eighth cervi-

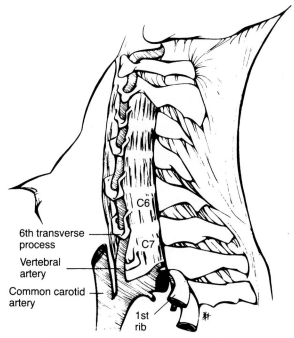

Figure 42–35. Lateral anatomic diagram showing passage of the vertebral arteries and veins in front of the transverse process of the seventh vertebra, entering the transverse foramen at the sixth vertebra. (From Simmons, E. H.: Kyphotic deformity of the spine in ankylosing spondylitis. Clin. Orthop. *128*:65, 1977.)

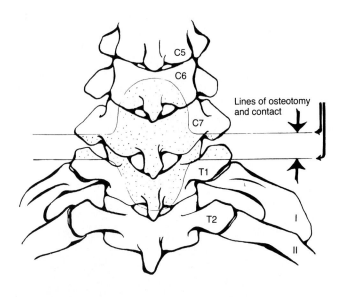

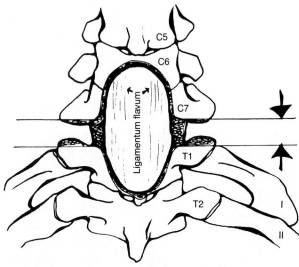

Figure 42–34. *A*, Diagrammatic outline of the posterior aspect of the spine in the area of resection. The lines of resection of the fused posterior joints are beveled away from each other posteriorly, so that after correction the two surfaces will be parallel and in apposition. *B*, Posterior view showing the extent of the midline and lateral resections. It is important that the pedicles be undercut to avoid impingement of the C8 nerve roots. The midline resection is beveled on its deep surface above and below to avoid impingement against the dura after extension correction. (From Simmons, E. H.: Kyphotic deformity of the spine in ankylosing spondylitis. Clin. Orthop. *128*:65, 1977.)

cal nerve roots are relatively mobile in this area. Furthermore, any inadvertent injury to the eighth cervical nerve root would likely cause less disability than would injury to other roots. Fortunately, the vertebral artery and veins usually pass anterior to the transverse process of the seventh vertebra and enter the transverse foramen at the level of the sixth vertebra. The position of these vessels above the level of the first thoracic vertebra protects them from serious injury during osteotomy at the C7–T1 level (Fig. 42–35). Adequate laminectomy and facetectomy are performed, with subsequent fracturing of the longitudinal ligament and extension of the spine at the cervicothoracic junction (Fig. 42–36).

One or two days before the operation, the patient is fitted with a plaster body jacket incorporating the supports for a halo unit. The plaster jacket must be well molded below the costal margins and over the iliac crests, so that it will not move freely upward or downward. A halo-ring is fitted to the skull. The patient is allowed to adjust to the cast and the sensation of the halo on the head. The halo-ring is used to control the head during the procedure and to serve as a basis for stability immediately after the operation. It is suspended with 9 pounds of balanced traction along the axis of the neck. A dental-type chair is used to allow the patient to be placed in a recumbent position if necessary (Fig. 42–37).

Exposure is carried out posteriorly under local infiltration (1 per cent lidocaine and epinephrine 1:200,000).

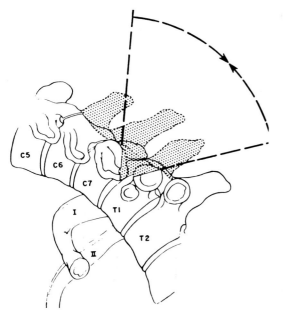

Figure 42–36. Lateral diagram of the area of resection. (From Urist, M. R.: Osteotomy of the cervical spine. Report of a case of ankylosing rheumatoid spondylitis. J. Bone Joint Surg. Am. *40*:833, 1958.)

The last bifid spinous process of C6 is usually easily identified (Fig. 42–38). If difficulty is encountered, radiographic confirmation of the level is obtained. The C7 spinous process and laminae are completely removed, along with the inferior portion of the spine of C6 and the upper portion of T1 with their associated laminae. The bone is preserved for grafting. The entire posterior arch of C7 is resected, along with the inferior half of the arch of C6 and the superior half of the arch of T1. The spinal canal is opened, and the dura and spinal cord are protected with cottonoid patties. The eighth nerve root canal is identified. The patient may be able to assist by indicating the distribution of any paresthesias associated with traction or displacement of the root. Bone is then removed laterally through the

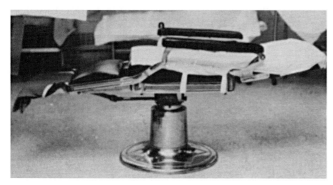

Figure 42–37. Dental chair as used during the cervical osteotomy, showing capacity to extend to the horizontal position if required.

fused area of the posterior joints, thereby decompressing the eighth nerve root thoroughly.

The amount of bone to be resected is indicated by the angle of correction that is desired. This is assessed by the degree the neck is flexed from the vertical (chin-brow to vertical angle) when the patient stands with the hips and knees extended. If the patient still has some mobility in the upper cervical spine, the amount that the neck is flexed from the vertical is measured when the neck is in a neutral or comfortable position (see Fig. 42–15). This angle is then transposed to a lateral radiograph with the apex at the posterior longitudinal ligament at C7–T1. The angle is centered over the posterior arch of C7. The amount of bone to be resected in the area of the fused posterior joints is estimated and varies from 1.5 to 2.5 cm, depending on the extent of correction required.

The lines of resection are slightly beveled upward and downward, so that after correction the two surfaces will be parallel to each other and in apposition (Fig. 42–38B). The inferior surfaces of the bases of the pedicles of C7 and the superior surfaces of the bases of the pedicles of T1 are rongeured away sufficiently and undercut, to avoid impingement or a pincher effect on the eighth nerve roots after extension correction of the cervical spine. Ideally, a recess should be cut into the base of the pedicles of C7 and T1, to avoid any pressure on the nerve roots and to protect them when the neck is extended. The amount of bone resected should be carefully assessed and planned to avoid any compression of the nerve roots. The lateral masses must be completely and symmetrically resected posteriorly.

Supplemental oxygen is usually administered by the anesthetist during the procedure, either by nasal catheter or by face mask. The patient is allowed to enjoy the music of a radio or tape recorder. This, together with an ongoing, reassuring conversation between the anesthetist or attendant and the patient, is an important part of anesthetic management. When this is done well, the amount of discomfort or concern expressed by the patient is minimal. Fentanyl and midazolam (Versed) are used by the anesthetist as indicated to supplement the local anesthesia. Pulse oximetry, a carbon dioxide analyzer, and systematic blood gases are used by the anesthetist to monitor the patient. A Doppler apparatus is fixed to the patient's chest to detect any possible air embolism.

When the decompression has been completed, the patient is given a small dose of a short-acting barbiturate. Either methohexital sodium (Brevital Sodium) or sodium pentothal (thiopental sodium) may be used. Brevital Sodium is preferred for cervical osteotomy because of its shorter duration. The anesthetist administers the barbiturate very slowly while conversing with the patient. When the patient is no longer able to converse effectively, the neck is extended by the surgeon, who grasps the halo through the drapes and tilts the neck backward. The surgeon keeps the head and upper cervical spine in the same relationship to each other, so that stresses are at the base of the neck rather

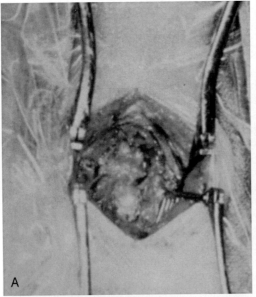

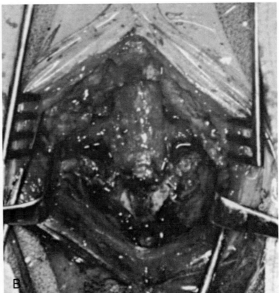

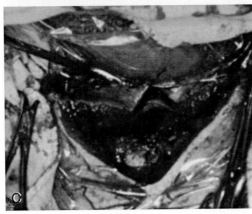

Figure 42–38. *A*, Operative exposure showing the last bifid spinous process of C6 at the upper end of the wound. *B*, Operative view demonstrating posterior midline decompression and decompression of C8 nerve roots. *C*, View of the wound after osteoclasis and extension correction, showing the vertical wound becoming transverse. The lateral masses come together on each side.

than at the upper cervical spine. An audible snap may be heard, and a sense of fracture will be appreciated by the surgeon. The neck is extended until resistance occurs. The lateral masses can be palpated coming together posteriorly on each side (Fig. 42–38C). The patient is given supplemental 100 per cent oxygen until he or she is fully awake, which should be almost instantly, and the patient should be able to confirm normal neurologic function of the extremities with the ability to move the upper and lower limbs without sensory complaint. With the surgeon holding the patient's head firmly in the corrected position, an assistant stabilizes the head by connecting the anterior supports for the halo to the cast. Portions of the bone that have been removed during the course of the decompression are then placed posterolaterally on both sides over the approximated resected remains of the lateral bony masses. An attempt is made not to place any bone in the midline area, where it could impinge on the dura. Deep closing sutures are loosely applied, and a suction drain is inserted before the osteoclasis is carried out in order to facilitate rapid wound closure (Fig. 42–38C).

After correction, the deep muscle sutures are tied, and the wound is closed in layers. The skin is usually closed with interrupted nylon sutures. The surgeon can then supervise any adjustment or alteration in the position of the head while assistants make the final connections of the halo to the halo supports in the plaster cast. When this is completed, the patient is able to stand and walk toward the Circ-O-Lectric bed, which is turned to the vertical position to allow the patient to back into it easily. The bed is then tilted to the horizontal position with the patient supine. It may be partly flexed if desired for increased comfort. The surgeon must be certain not to overcorrect the neck deformity, particularly in individuals with a rigid cervical spine and no significant compensatory motion at the occipitocervical junction. These patients must accept a compromise between looking ahead for walking and being able to work at a desk (Figs. 42–39 and 42–40).

Excessive force is not required to straighten the neck, provided there has been complete decompression posteriorly. If the spine does not fracture readily, the surgeon must be certain that there is not a bridge of bone

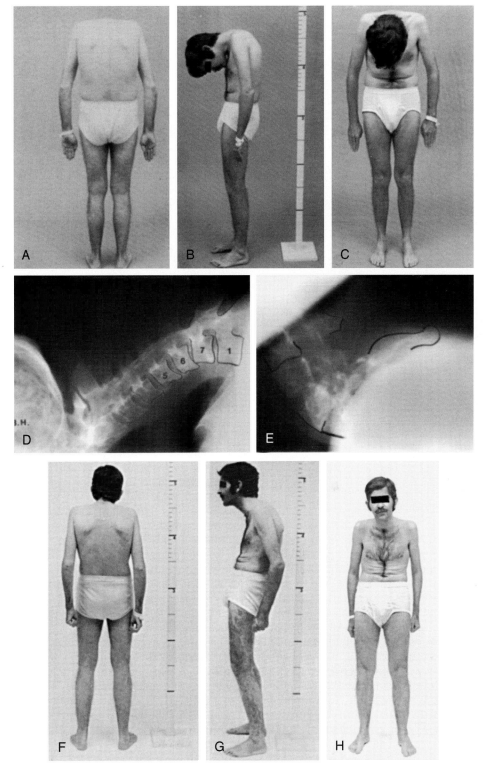

Figure 42–39.   *A,* Posterior aspect of a man with severe fixed kyphotic deformity of the cervical spine of sufficient degree that the head is not visible on the posterior view. *B,* Side view showing the chin rigidly fixed against the chest, with severe restriction of the field of vision and interference with ability to open the mouth. *C,* Frontal view showing complete loss of forward field of vision. *D,* Lateral radiograph of the cervical spine showing ossification of posterior joints and previous subluxation of C6–C7. *E,* Postoperative lateral radiograph after extension osteotomy correction. *F,* Postoperative rear view showing restoration of the head to a normal trunk configuration. *G,* Postoperative lateral view showing normal chin-brow to vertical angle. *H,* Postoperative frontal view showing normal forward field of vision.

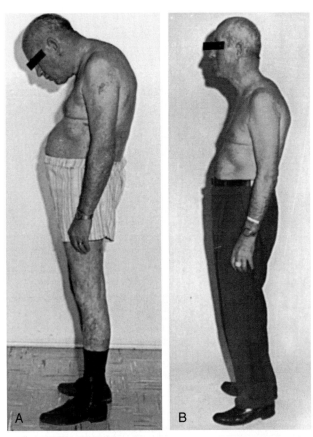

Figure 42–40.   *A*, Lateral view of a man with flexion deformity of the cervical spine associated with ankylosing spondylitis and psoriasis. *B*, Postoperative lateral view after correction of deformity with restoration of normal chin-brow to vertical angle.

remaining laterally and that the correct level of C7–T1 has been operated on, rather than a level below. Although an attempt is made to obtain full or nearly full correction at the time of the procedure, this is sometimes limited by tightness of the musculature anteriorly or by apprehension on the part of the patient. If necessary, further correction can be carried out about seven days later, when the soft tissues have had an opportunity to stretch. At that time, with the patient supine and under midazolam and fentanyl sedation, the head may be supported by the surgeon while the attachments for the halo-ring are released by assistants. The neck is allowed to carefully extend, and full correction is obtained. The head is then stabilized in its new position.

Patients are nursed in the immediate postoperative period on a Circ-O-Lectric frame. This allows them to be brought to the vertical position easily and safely, to stand and walk about, and to return to the recumbent position without difficulty. When sufficiently mobile to get in and out of a regular bed, patients are transferred to a hospital bed with or without a trapeze attachment. The importance of a well-molded halo-cast with shoulder straps should again be emphasized. If the patient

loses weight, the straps tend to keep the cast from migrating distally, thereby preventing the weight of the cast from being transferred to the osteotomy site. Also, the halo-cast can be adjusted to allow some graduated lengthening of the distance between the halo-ring and the cast if symptoms occur as a result of the weight of the cast. This usually relieves any C8 nerve root discomfort or paresthesias until union of the osteotomy occurs. The patient is immobilized in a halo-cast for four months, after which time it is removed and careful radiographic studies are performed, including lateral tomography centered at C7–T1. Clinical evidence of union, such as lack of pain on attempted motion, is assessed. Further bracing is then carried out, using a Somi orthosis for an additional two months or until evidence of solid clinical and radiographic union is confirmed.

The technique just described has been followed in a consistent fashion without any major deviation from protocol since it was first initiated in 1966.[24, 52–56, 58, 59, 64] The long-term results were recently reviewed and reported.[62] The results have been very satisfactory, with relatively few complications related to the surgery, considering the nature of the deformity and the associated disease process. The average desired angle of correction was 60 degrees. The average amount of local anesthetic used was 54 ml of 1 per cent lidocaine with 1:200,000 epinephrine. Union after osteotomy appears to have occurred fairly readily in most instances. However, in four patients nonunion occurred, for an incidence of 4 per cent. Three of these patients responded to anterior cervical fusion at the C7–T1 level with a keystone iliac strut graft,[60] and one of these procedures was performed under local anesthesia. This patient was a 50-year-old physician who had been unable to drive a car for 10 years and whose private practice had been curtailed for seven years. He progressed well from the initial surgery and was discharged home. Shortly before he returned for his four-month postoperative checkup, he suffered a fall and felt a "crack" in his neck. He developed definite evidence of nonunion at the osteotomy site. During his subsequent anterior surgery, there was difficulty with intubation, and under local anesthesia an anterior cervical fusion using the keystone technique was performed at the C7–T1 level. He went on to solid union without any postoperative complications and returned to his medical practice (Fig. 42–41). The fourth patient with a nonunion required both an anterior cervical fusion and a posterior segmental instrumentation and fusion to obtain solid union.

Patients on steroids or high doses of nonsteroidal anti-inflammatory drugs have a greater risk of developing a nonunion, and these medications should be stopped preoperatively, if possible. The most frequent postoperative neurologic symptoms were paresthesias or muscle weakness in the C8 dermatomal distribution, which occurred in 10 per cent of cases. This usually subsided following gentle distraction between the halo-ring and the cast. The symptoms gradually resolved following bony union, even when there was some tran-

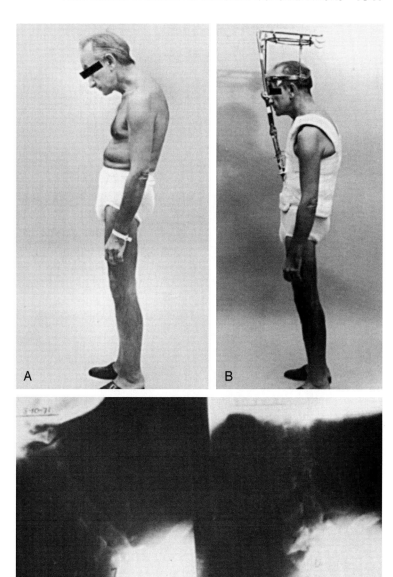

Figure 42–41. *A*, Lateral view of a 50-year-old physician with rigid kyphotic deformity of the cervical spine. *B*, Postoperative lateral view showing correction of deformity with the patient immobilized in a halo-cast. *C*, Lateral radiographs in flexion and extension showing gross motion with nonunion at the osteotomy site.

Illustration continued on following page

sient weakness. Only one patient required further decompression of the C8 nerve roots. That patient now plays golf without difficulty.

There has been no major permanent injury to the spinal cord following cervical osteotomy. One patient, however, exhibited a dramatic intraoperative event that demonstrated the importance of performing surgery under local anesthesia. This was a 70-year-old man with severe flexion deformity of the cervical spine accentuated by an unrecognized fracture that had healed in severe flexion, resulting in a chin-on-chest deformity. Preoperatively, his chief complaint was a fear of choking, because he had experienced several episodes of difficulty in swallowing owing to the deformity. Correction was planned under local anesthesia with the

patient in the sitting position. There was dense scarring about the dura related to his previous fracture. As his spinal canal was decompressed, the patient experienced increasing weakness of his right lower limb followed by his left, and he finally developed difficulty with his speech. Because the dura was exceedingly tense with dense scarring about it, it was split longitudinally down to the arachnoid. As this was done, there was an immediate and dramatic return of the patient's neurologic function in the lower extremities, and his speech returned to normal. The operation was continued, and as the decompression was being completed on the left side, he again began to develop weakness of his right lower limb. The remaining exposed dura was split further distally, with immediate recovery of

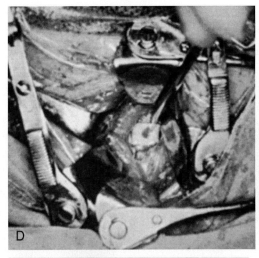

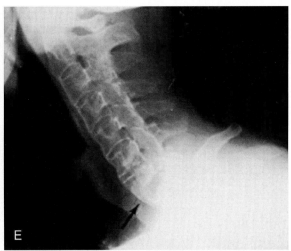

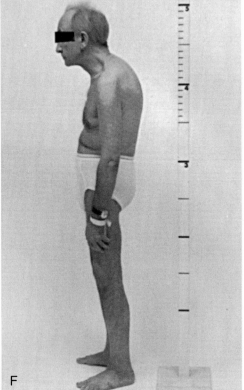

Figure 42–41. *Continued. D,* Surgical view of anterior keystone fusion at the C7–T1 level, performed under local anesthesia. *E,* Postoperative lateral radiograph showing solid bony fusion with incorporation of the keystone graft. *F,* Postoperative lateral view showing complete correction of deformity with restoration of normal chin-brow to vertical angle. (From Simmons, E. H.: The surgical correction of flexion deformity of the cervical spine in ankylosing spondylitis. Clin. Orthop. *86*:132, 1972.)

neurologic function being noted. The operation was then completed without difficulty, and the patient had a satisfactory result without neurologic deficit (Fig. 42–42). This observation is in keeping with the report of McKenzie and Dewar,[39] which described the results of laminectomy for cord compression associated with kyphoscoliosis. They reviewed the reported literature and their own cases, and the only patients who did not become worse after laminectomy, or in whom any benefit was noted following surgery, were those in whom there was extensive splitting of the dura. The authors felt that this was related to the compression effect of the dura in kyphosis. They recommended that

the dura be split both longitudinally and transversely. Surgeons undertaking this type of surgery should be cognizant of this fact. If intraoperative symptoms or signs develop, adequate splitting of the dura should be performed, longitudinally and possibly transversely as well.

During the operative procedure, no significant difficulties occurred during or after the osteoclasis. Toward the end of the decompression in one patient, however, a sudden cardiac arrest occurred. The operating chair was leveled out, and the patient responded well to resuscitation. The possibility of air embolism was considered, but there was no gross venous bleeding, and aspiration of the heart revealed no air. The cause of the cardiac arrest in this case was unknown. To detect the presence of air embolism, we routinely monitor the patient with a Doppler apparatus fixed to the patient's chest.

Despite the procedure being performed under local anesthesia, the possibility of pulmonary embolism must be considered. Interestingly, one patient suffered a fatal pulmonary embolism before the osteotomy was done. Autopsy revealed multiple thrombi in the leg veins, with evidence of previous pulmonary infarctions. One 79-year-old woman died suddenly 21 days

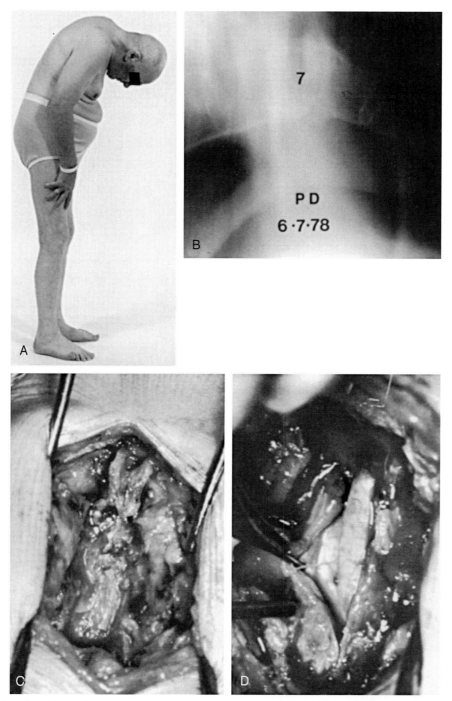

Figure 42–42. *A,* Lateral presentation of a 70-year-old man with severe kyphotic deformity accentuated by an unrecognized fracture three years previously. The fracture had healed with chin-on-chest deformity. *B,* Lateral tomogram of C7–T1 showing previous compression fracture. *C,* Surgical view showing decompression of the cervical spinal cord with extensive scarring of the dura. *D,* Operative view after incision of the scar in the dura down to the arachnoid. The scar in the dura was later split further at the lower end of the operative site for a recurrent neurologic complaint, with relief of symptoms and signs.

postoperatively of pulmonary embolism. Her lungs showed multiple areas of embolism that had not been recognized clinically. In retrospect, she had had some pulmonary symptoms that were thought to be caused by a mild pneumonitis, and anticoagulant therapy had therefore not been instituted.

Other complications can occur and are related to the age of the patient and associated disease processes. These include one nonfatal pulmonary embolism, a perforated peptic ulcer, a perforated abdominal viscus, and a myocardial infarction. Considering the age of and medical risk factors associated with these patients,

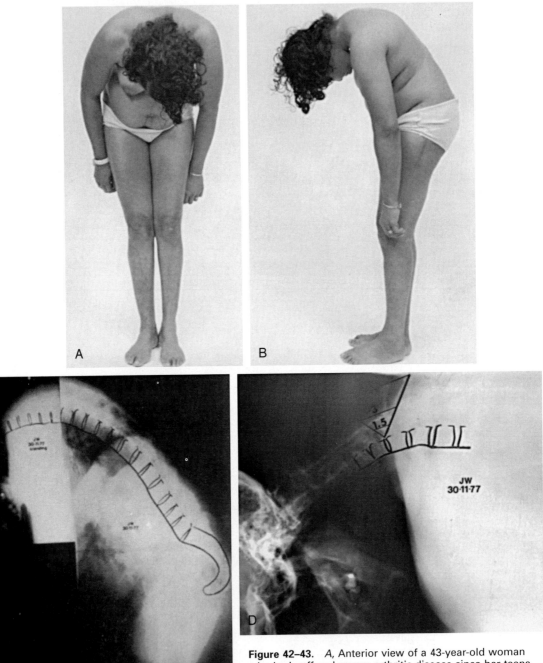

Figure 42–43. *A*, Anterior view of a 43-year-old woman who had suffered severe arthritic disease since her teens. She had gross restriction of field of vision. *B*, Standing lateral view demonstrating combined severe kyphotic deformity of the cervical spine and lumbar spine. *C*, Lateral radiographic study showing combined kyphotic deformity. *D*, Lateral cervical radiograph demonstrating the extent and site of cervical osteotomy required.

the results and complication rate of surgery compare favorably with those of other types of major reconstructive procedures in a similar group of patients with a similar disease process. These patients have an increased tendency to develop peptic ulcers. In view of the potentially fatal nature of any intra-abdominal catastrophe in these patients and the increased tendency for peptic ulcers in these individuals, all patients are now routinely placed on ranitidine (Zantac).

In 21 patients, cervical osteotomy was combined with lumbar osteotomy for major deformity in both areas.[58] In one third of these patients, the secondary procedure was done during a separate admission owing to development of an unanticipated deformity in the other area. In two thirds of these cases, correction of both areas was planned, since the patients initially presented with severe combined deformity in both areas, and was therefore performed during the same admission.

When correction of both kyphotic deformities is required, the cervical osteotomy is done first, followed by the lumbar osteotomy approximately 10 days later. Both procedures were performed under local anesthesia in 17 patients. Following the cervical osteotomy, the patient is placed on his or her side, and the posterior lumbar portion of the plaster cast is removed to allow the lumbar osteotomy to be performed. The remaining plaster serves to immobilize the cervical spine. After the lumbar osteotomy, the lower portion of the cast is reapplied in the new position (Fig. 42–43). With the development of the author's technique for lumbar osteotomy under general anesthesia with awake fiberoptic intubation, the same technique has been applied to the lumbar spine after the cervical osteotomy has been done under local anesthesia (Fig. 42–44).

Resection-extension osteotomy of the cervical spine for severe flexion deformity, when carefully planned and executed, is a valid technique with acceptable

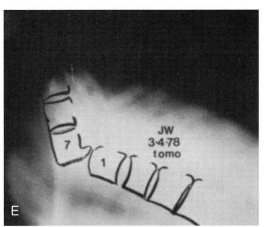

Figure 42–43. *Continued.* E, Lateral tomograph showing postoperative osteotomy correction. F, Postoperative lateral standing 3-foot radiograph showing combined resection-extension osteotomy of the cervical and lumbar spine. The weight-bearing line of the upper trunk is posterior to the lumbar osteotomy site. G, Postoperative lateral view showing correction of combined deformities with a normal chin-brow to vertical angle. H, Postoperative frontal view showing normal field of vision with ability to look straight ahead.

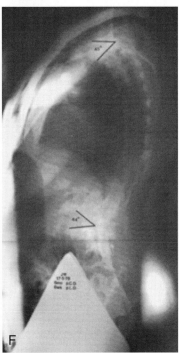

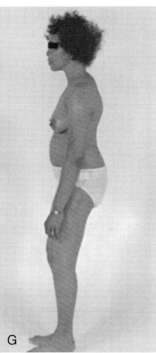

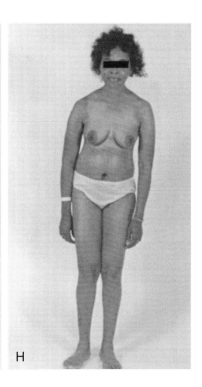

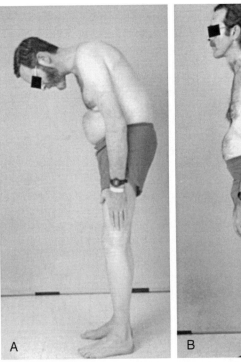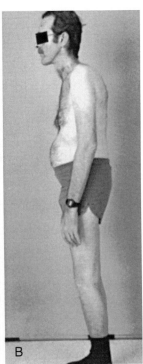

Figure 42–44. *A,* Lateral view of a 47-year-old man standing with hips and knees extended. The spine is rigid, with a fixed chin-brow to vertical angle of 80 degrees. He was unable to get about by himself owing to severe restriction of field of vision. *B,* Postoperative lateral view after resection-extension osteotomies of the cervical and lumbar spine. The cervical osteotomy was done under local anesthesia. In this instance a Lev-Tec halo-brace was firmly applied to the patient. Twelve days after the cervical osteotomy the patient was intubated awake. He placed himself on a Tower table, and when comfortable was anesthetized. Extension osteotomy of the lumbar spine was performed with the patient under general anesthesia with spinal cord monitoring. A plaster cast was applied incorporating the brace. There was complete correction of both deformities, with restoration of a normal chin-brow to vertical angle and a normal lifestyle. Histologic studies of the extensor muscles of the cervical and lumbar spine showed neurogenic atrophy in both areas.

risks. It is emphasized that it is essential that the surgery be performed under local anesthesia with the patient awake. This provides the surgeon with accurate and continual monitoring of the patient's neurologic functions, allowing instantaneous corrective action if any major dysfunction should occur. It should also be emphasized that an essential part of the technique is the preoperative application of a halo-ring and a well-fitted plaster cast that is molded to the patient so that it does not move and that incorporates the supports for the halo-ring. This allows instantaneous immobilization of the osteotomy site following extension-correc-tion. Internal fixation is provided by the tension-band effect of the contracted soft tissue anteriorly and firm opposition of the carefully resected lateral masses posteriorly.

MUSCLE DISEASE RELATED TO THE PATHOGENESIS OF KYPHOTIC DEFORMITY IN ANKYLOSING SPONDYLITIS

As stated previously, ankylosing spondylitis has well-recognized extra-articular manifestations, including

Figure 42–45. *A,* Lateral view of a 34-year-old man referred for surgical correction for cervical kyphotic deformity. He had a four-year history of ankylosing spondylitis followed by rapid progression of kyphotic deformity. His chin-brow to vertical angle was 97 degrees. *B,* Standing lateral radiograph of the patient demonstrating severe osteopenia, multiple compression fractures, chin-on-chest deformity, and a thoracic kyphosis of 100 degrees. The lack of fusion suggested the possibility of correction with traction alone and raised a question about the pathogenesis of the deformity. *C,* Muscle biopsy from the paracervical extensor muscles showing an abnormality of small scattered angular fibers, the majority of which reacted as Type II fibers in ATPase stain. The findings were consistent with neuropathic atrophy. Biopsy of the gluteal musculature revealed similar findings. EMG studies were interpreted as being consistent with a nonspecific neuropathic abnormality. *D,* Lateral view of the patient five months after correction with halo-dependent traction, including four months in a halo-cast. The patient was treated concurrently with calcium, vitamin D, and calcitonin. *E,* Lateral 3-foot radiograph five months following initiation of treatment showing correction of deformity and increase in bone density. *F,* Lateral view of the patient one year after initiation of treatment. Recurrence of deformity is noted in the thoracic spine, associated with weakness of the extensor musculature. Fortunately, correction was maintained in the cervical spine, which showed progressing ossification. *G,* Lateral radiograph of the thoracic spine showing increased kyphotic deformity. *H,* Postoperative lateral radiograph following Cotrel-Dubousset instrumentation with correction of thoracic kyphosis. *I,* Final lateral postoperative view of the patient showing correction of thoracic kyphotic deformity and maintenance of correction of his severe cervical kyphosis.

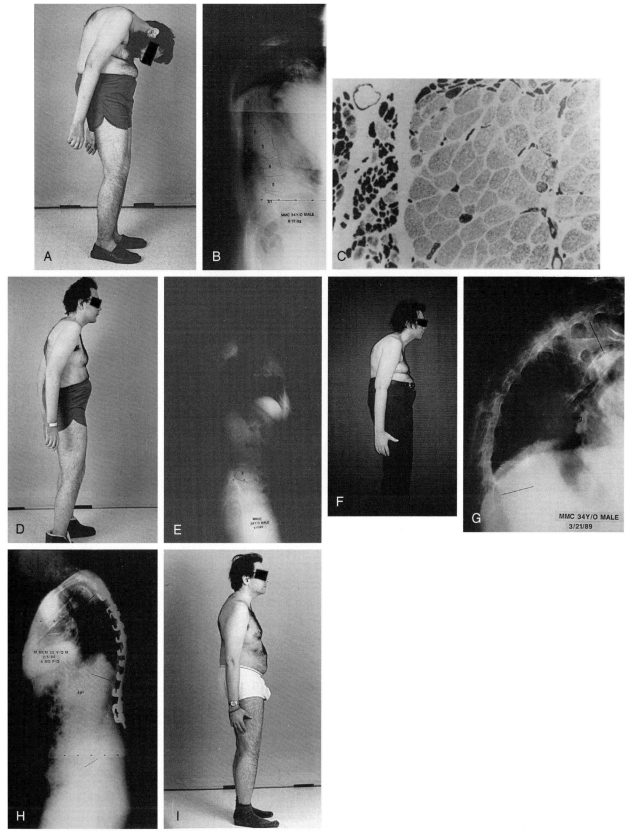

Figure 42–45. *See legend on opposite page*

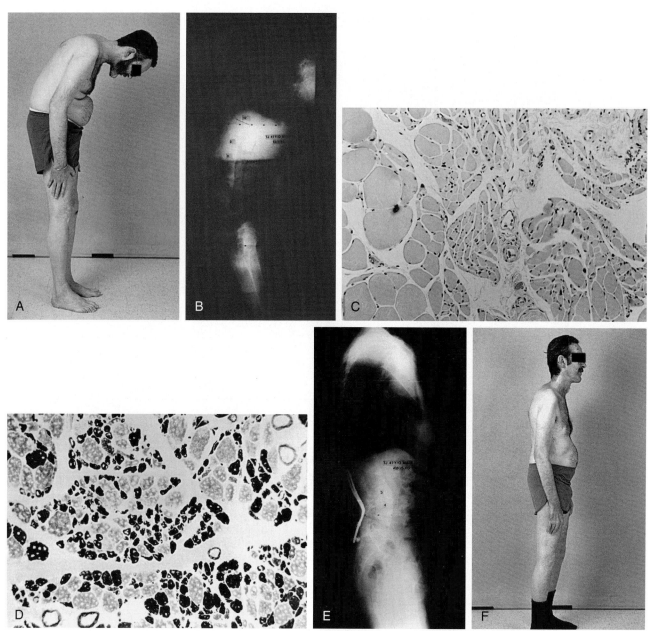

Figure 42–46. *A,* Lateral view of a 47-year-old man with severe spinal kyphosis restricting his field of vision and causing difficulty swallowing. His chin-brow to vertical angle was 82 degrees. He had obvious combined kyphotic deformity of the cervical spine and lumbar spine. *B,* Lateral standing 3-foot radiograph showing lumbar lordosis reduced to 3 degrees with thoracic kyphosis of 57 degrees. Cervical extension-resection osteotomy was performed, followed by lumbar extension osteotomy. *C,* Biopsy of the cervical extensor musculature. The muscle was pale and atrophic in appearance. It was poorly contractile to tactile stimulation. The musculature showed grouped atrophy of small angular fibers, indicating chronic denervation. *D,* Histologic studies showing target fibers with central pale area surrounded by rim of increased enzyme activity. Numerous target fibers were visualized. The changes were consistent with a severe atrophic process, suggesting chronic denervation. EMG studies were consistent with neuropathic change. *E,* Lateral standing 3-foot radiograph of the spine four months postoperatively showing extension osteotomy correction of the lumbar spine. Note that the weight-bearing line has shifted posterior to the osteotomy site. Cervical osteotomy had been done under local anesthesia with the patient in the sitting position, followed by extension osteotomy of the lumbar spine under local anesthesia. Luque segmental instrumentation and Drummond buttons were used for fixation. *F,* Postoperative lateral standing view of the patient indicating normal chin-brow to vertical angle. The patient has been able to return to a normal lifestyle.

neurologic abnormalities, cardiac conduction defects, arachnoiditis, cauda equina syndrome, and an association with multiple sclerosis.

When patients present with fixed deformity, the main treatment concern is to correct the gross fixed deformity. It is generally assumed that the patient's deformity is a manifestation of inflammatory disease of the spine, associated with osteopenia, painful kyphotic deformity, and later ossification. Other possible etiologies for the deformity, such as involvement of the extensor muscles of the spine, are generally not considered. However, patients have been referred to the author for correction of kyphotic deformities of the neck that were not caused by ankylosing spondylitis but were proved instead to be caused by myopathic flexion deformities of the cervical spine. Such patients exhibited an electrodiagnostic abnormality of the extensor muscles, suggesting a myopathy, and had findings on muscle biopsy and laboratory tests consistent with extensor muscle disease.[61]

It was consistently noted at surgery in patients with fixed deformities associated with ankylosing spondylitis that the extensor muscles were pale and atrophic compared with muscles in normal patients. The occurrence of myopathic kyphotic deformities of the neck in patients without ankylosing spondylitis suggested the possibility of such muscle disease contributing to kyphotic deformities in patients with ankylosing spondylitis. Some patients were identified with ankylosing spondylitis associated with major kyphotic deformity of the cervical spine that was not fixed and that responded to halo-dependent traction. Electrodiagnostic studies, creatine kinase studies, and isometric muscle biopsies illustrated consistent extensor muscle disease with atrophy of Type I and Type II muscle fibers (Fig. 42–45).

A prospective study was carried out on all patients presenting for correction of kyphotic deformity in ankylosing spondylitis.[65] Consistent abnormality of the extensor muscles of the spine as described earlier was noted. The findings were consistent with a denervating process of the paraspinal extensor muscles, suggesting a neuropathic abnormality.[65]

The same findings have been consistent in an ongoing study of all patients since that time (Fig. 42–46). It seems evident that chronic denervation of the spinal extensor musculature is related to the development of kyphotic deformity in ankylosing spondylitis. The presence of extensor muscle involvement may have prognostic significance in patients with this disease, since patients at risk for spinal deformity could possibly be identified earlier. More aggressive medical management might also be indicated in order to slow the progression of the disease and to decrease the likelihood of the deformity. Early aggressive strengthening exercises for the extensor musculature and bracing might be indicated in patients who were noted early on to have evidence of extensor muscle involvement. Prospective studies of patients with and without such deformity will be required to establish this. Physicians should therefore be aware of potential paraspinal muscle involvement as part of the systemic disease process in ankylosing spondylitis.

ACKNOWLEDGMENT.   The author would like to acknowledge the significant contribution of, and express his gratitude to, Mary E. Smith for her assistance in preparation of the manuscript.

References

1. Aboulker, J., Aubin, M. L., Leriche, H., et al.: L'Hypertension Veineuse Intra-Rachidienne par Anomalies Multiples du Systeme Cave. Acta Radiol. Suppl. 347:395–401, 1975.
2. Adams, J. C.: Technique, dangers, and safeguards in osteotomy of the spine. J. Bone Joint Surg. Br. 34:226–232, 1952.
3. Andersson, O.: Rontgenbilden vid spondylarthrosis ankylopoetica. Nord. Med. 14:2000, 1937.
4. Bland, J. H.: Rheumatoid arthritis of the cervical spine. J. Rheumatol. 3:319, 1974.
5. Bove, E. A., and Glasgow, G. L.: Cauda equina lesions associated with ankylosing spondylitis: Report of 3 cases. Br. Med. J. 2:24–27, 1961.
6. Buckley, B. H., and Robert, W. C.: Ankylosing spondylitis and aortic regurgitation: Description of the characteristic cardio-vascular lesion from study of 8 necropsy patients. Circulation 18:1014–1027, 1978.
7. Calancie, B., Lebwohl, N., Madsen, P., et al.: Intraoperative evoked EMG monitoring in an animal model: A new technique for evaluating pedicle screw placement. Spine 17:1229–1235, 1992.
8. Calin, A.: Ankylosing spondylitis. In Kelly, W. N., Harris, E. D., Ruddy, S., and Sledge, C. B. (eds): Textbook of Rheumatology. Philadelphia, W. B. Saunders Co., 1981, pp. 1017–1032.
9. Conlon, P. W., Isdale, I. C., and Rose, B. S.: Rheumatoid arthritis in the cervical spine: An analysis of 333 cases. Ann. Rheumatol. Dis. 25:120, 1966.
10. Coste, F., Delbarre, F., Cayla, J., et al.: Spondylites destructives dans la spondylarthrite ankylosante. Presse Med. 71:1013–1016, 1963.
11. Davey, J. R., Rorabeck, C. H., Bailey, S. I., et al.: A technique of posterior cervical fusion for instability of the cervical spine. Spine 10:722, 1985.
12. Dewar, F. P.: Personal communication, 1955.
13. Donovan, M. M.: Efficacy of rigid fixation of fractures of the odontoid process—historical review of treatment and retrospective analysis of 54 cases. Thesis, University of Texas, Houston. Submitted to American Orthopaedic Association.
14. Emneus, H.: Wedge osteotomy of spine in ankylosing spondylitis. Acta Orthop. Scand. 39:321–336, 1968.
15. Fang, H. S. Y., and Ong, G. B.: Direct approach to the upper cervical spine. J. Bone Joint Surg. Am. 44:1588, 1962.
16. Garod, A. W.: A Treatise on Rheumatism and Rheumatoid Arthritis. London, Griffin, 1890.
17. Gilsbach, J.: Transoral operations for cranio-spinal malformations. Neurosurg. Rev. 6:199, 1983.
18. Glassman, S. D., Dimar, J. R., Puno, R. M., et al.: A prospective analysis of intraoperative electromyographic monitoring of pedicle screw placement with computed tomographic scan confirmation. Spine 20:1375–1379, 1995.
19. Goel, M. K.: Vertebral osteotomy for correction of fixed flexion deformity of the spine. J. Bone Joint Surg. Am. 50:287, 1968.
20. Hanrachan, P., Russell, A., and McLean, P.: Ankylosing spondylitis and multiple sclerosis: An apparent association. J. Rheum. 15:1512–1514, 1988.
21. Harris, R. I.: New investigations: Instrument for tightening knots in steel wire. Lancet 1:504, 1944.
22. Herbert, J. J.: Vertebral osteotomy for kyphosis, especially in Marie-Strumpell arthritis: A report on 50 cases. J. Bone Joint Surg. Am. 41:291, 1959.
23. Herbert, J. J.: Vertebral osteotomy, technique, indications and results. J. Bone Joint Surg. Am. 30:680, 1948.
24. Hruska, J. S., and Simmons, E. H.: Review of cervical extension osteotomy in ankylosing spondylitis. Orthopedic residents an-

nual graduation presentation, State University of New York at Buffalo, May 27, 1994.

25. Isenbery, D. A., and Smith, M. L.: Muscle disease in systemic lupus erythematosus: A study of its nature, frequency, and cause. J. Rheumatol. 18:917–924, 1981.
26. Kallio, K. E.: Osteotomy of the spine in ankylosing spondylitis. Ann. Chir. Gynaecol. 52:615, 1963.
27. Kanefield, D. G., Mullins, B. P., Freehafer, A. A., et al.: Destructive lesions of the spine in rheumatoid ankylosing spondylitis. J. Bone Joint Surg. Am. 51:1369–1375, 1969.
28. LaChapelle, E. H.: Osteotomy of the lumbar spine for correction of kyphosis in a case of ankylosing spondylarthritis. J. Bone Joint Surg. Am. 28:270, 1959.
29. Law, W. A.: Lumbar spinal osteotomy. J. Bone Joint Surg. Br. 41:270, 1959.
30. Law, W. A.: Osteotomy of the spine. J. Bone Joint Surg. Am. 44:1199, 1962.
31. Law, W. A.: Osteotomy of the spine. Clin. Orthop. 66:70, 1969.
32. Lichtblau, P. O., and Wilson, P. D.: Possible mechanism of aortic rupture in orthopaedic correction of rheumatoid spondylitis. J. Bone Joint Surg. Am. 38:123–127, 1956.
33. Little, H., Urowitz, M. B., Smythe, H. A., et al.: Asymptomatic spondylodiscitis: An unusual feature of ankylosing spondylitis. Arthritis Rheum. 17:487–493, 1974.
34. Maguire, J., Wallace, S., Madiga, R., et al.: Evaluation of intrapedicular screw position using intraoperative evoked electromyography. Spine 20:1068–1074, 1995.
35. Martel, W., Duff, I. F., Preston, R. E., et al.: The cervical spine and rheumatoid arthritis: Correlation of radiographic clinical manifestations (Abstract.) Arthritis Rheum. 7:326, 1964.
36. Mason, C., Cozen, L., and Adelstein, L.: Surgical correction of flexion deformity of the cervical spine. Calif. Med. 79:244, 1953.
37. McEwen, C. D., Tata, D., Ling, C., et al.: Ankylosing spondylitis and spondylitis accompanying ulcerative colitis, regional enteritis, psoriasis, and Reiter's disease. Arthritis Rheum. 14:291–318, 1971.
38. McGraw, R. W., and Rusch, R. M.: Atlanto-axial arthrodesis. J. Bone Joint Surg. Br. 55:482–489, 1973.
39. McKenzie, K. G., and Dewar, F. P.: Scoliosis with paraplegia. J. Bone Joint Surg. Br. 31:162–174, 1949.
40. McMaster, P. E.: Osteotomy of the spine for fixed flexion deformity. J. Bone Joint Surg. Am. 44:1207, 1962.
41. McMaster, P. E.: Osteotomy of the spine for fixed flexion deformity. Pacific Med. Surg. 73:314, 1965.
42. McMaster, M. J., and Coventry, M. B.: Spinal osteotomy in ankylosing spondylitis. Mayo Clin. Proc. 48:476, 1973.
43. Nunziata, A.: Osteotomia de la columna, Operacio de Smith-Petersen. Prensa Med. Argent. 35:1536, 1948.
44. Pasztor, E.: Transoral approach for epidural craniocervical pathological processes. Adv. Tech. Stand. Neurosurg. 12:125, 1985.
45. Pellicci, P. M., Ranawat, C. S., Tsarairis, P., et al.: Progression of rheumatoid arthritis of the cervical spine. J. Bone Joint Surg. Am. 63:342, 1981.
46. Ranawat, C. S., O'Leary, P., Pellicci, P. M., et al.: Cervical spine fusion in rheumatoid arthritis. J. Bone Joint Surg. Am. 61:1003, 1979.
47. Rosen, P. S., and Graham, D. C.: Ankylosing spondylitis (a clinical review of 128 cases). Arch. Int. Am. Rheumatol. 5:158–233, 1962.
48. Russell, M. L., Gorder, D. A., Orgryzlo, M. A., et al.: The cauda equina syndrome of ankylosing spondylitis. Ann. Intern. Med. 78:551–554, 1973.
49. Schulitz, K. P.: Destruktive Veranderungen an Wirbelkorpern bei der Spondyliarthritis Ankylopoetica. Arch. Orthop. Unfall. Chir. 64:116–134, 1968.
50. Scudese, V. A., and Calabro, J. J.: Vertebral wedge osteotomy. JAMA 186:104, 1963.
51. Simmons, E. H.: Alternatives in the surgical stabilization of the upper cervical spine. In Tator, C. H. (ed.): Early Management of Acute Spinal Cord Injury. New York, Raven Press, 1982, pp. 393–434.
52. Simmons, E. H.: Ankylosing spondylitis: Surgical considerations. In The Spine. 3rd ed. Philadelphia, W. B. Saunders Co., 1992, pp. 1447–1511.
53. Simmons, E. H.: Kyphotic deformity of the spine in ankylosing spondylitis. Clin. Orthop. 128:65, 1977.
54. Simmons, E. H.: Surgery of Rheumatoid Arthritis. Philadelphia, J. B. Lippincott Co., 1971, pp. 100–104.
55. Simmons, E. H.: Surgery of rheumatoid arthritis. In Cruess, R. L., and Mitchell, N. (eds.): Surgery of the Spine in Rheumatoid Arthritis and Ankylosing Spondylitis. Philadelphia, J. B. Lippincott Co., 1971, pp. 93–110.
56. Simmons, E. H.: Surgery of the spine in ankylosing spondylitis and rheumatoid arthritis. In Chapman, M. (ed.): Operative Orthopaedics. Vol. 3. Philadelphia, J. B. Lippincott Co., 1988, pp. 2077–2114.
57. Simmons, E. H.: Surgery of the spine in rheumatoid arthritis and ankylosing spondylitis. In Evarts, C. M. (ed.): Surgery of the Musculoskeletal System. Vol. 2. New York, Churchill Livingstone, 1983, p. 85.
58. Simmons, E. H.: The surgical correction of flexion deformity of the cervical spine. In Cervical Spine Research Society (ed.): Ankylosing Spondylitis in the Cervical Spine. 2nd ed. Philadelphia, J. B. Lippincott Co., 1989, pp. 573–598.
59. Simmons, E. H.: The surgical correction of flexion deformity of the cervical spine in ankylosing spondylitis. Clin. Orthop. 86:132, 1972.
60. Simmons, E. H., and Bhalla, S. K.: Anterior cervical discectomy and fusion (keystone technique). J. Bone Joint Surg. Br. 51:225, 1969.
61. Simmons, E. H., and Bradley, D. D.: Neuro-myopathic flexion deformity of the cervical spine. Spine 13:756–762, 1988.
62. Simmons, E. H., and DiStefano, R. J.: Long-term review of cervical spinal extension osteotomy for kyphotic deformity in ankylosing spondylitis. Presented to the Association of Bone and Joint Surgeons, Cape Cod, MA; the Canadian Orthopaedic Association, Quebec City, Quebec, Canada; the American Orthopaedic Association, Colorado Springs, CO; and the North American Spine Society, Vancouver, British Columbia, Canada, 1996.
63. Simmons, E. H., and Fielding, J. W.: Atlanto-axial arthrodesis. J. Bone Joint Surg. Am. 49:1022, 1967.
64. Simmons, E. H., and Goodwin, C. B.: Spondylodiscitis: A manifestation of ankylosing spondylitis. Orthop. Trans. 8:165, 1984.
65. Simmons, E. H., Graziano, G. P., and Heffner, R., Jr.: Muscle disease as a cause of kyphotic deformity in ankylosing spondylitis. Spine 16(Suppl.):351–360, 1991.
66. Simmons, E. H., and Mouradian, W. H.: Unusual malunion of the odontoid process. J. Bone Joint Surg. Am. 59:552–553, 1977.
67. Smith-Petersen, M. N., Larson, C. B., and Aufranc, O. E.: Osteotomy of the spine for correction of flexion deformity in rheumatoid arthritis. J. Bone Joint Surg. 27:1, 1945.
68. Tucker, C. R., Fowles, R. E., Calin, A., et al.: Aortitis in ankylosing spondylitis: Early detection of aortic root abnormalities with 2-dimensional echocardiography. Am. J. Cardiol. 9:680–686, 1982.
69. Urist, M. R.: Osteotomy of the cervical spine: Report of a case of ankylosing rheumatoid spondylitis. J. Bone Joint Surg. Am. 41:833, 1958.
70. Weatherley, C., Jaffray, D., and Terry, A.: Vascular complications associated with osteotomy in ankylosing spondylitis: A report of two cases. Spine 13:43–46, 1988.
71. Wholey, M. H., Pugh, D. G., and Bickel, W. H.: Localized destructive lesions in rheumatoid spondylitis. Radiology 74:54–56, 1960.
72. Wills, D. G.: Anesthetic management of posterior lumbar osteotomy. Can. Anesth. Soc. J. 32:248–257, 1985.
73. Wilson, M. J., and Turkell, J. H.: Multiple spinal wedge osteotomy: Its use in the case of Marie-Strumpell spondylitis. Am. J. Surg. 77:777, 1949.

Spinal Cord

43

Intradural Tumors

Frederick A. Simeone, M.D.

The surgical treatment of intradural tumors, historically, began in 1887, when Sir Victor Horsley removed a tumor compressing the spinal cord and the patient improved substantially.[22] This was at the urging of neurologist William Gowers, who encouraged the surgeon to attempt this pioneering operation.

Since then, the removal of intradural tumors has become routine. In 1925 Charles Elsberg reported the first large series of intradural tumors treated surgically. Despite the high mortality rate, difficulty with clinical localization, and poor instrumentation, surgical results gradually improved. Eventually, successful removal of intramedullary tumors became possible, and large series were reported as early as 1963. Improved results in the treatment of intraspinal tumors has followed greater sophistication in diagnostic modalities and surgical technical devices. Whereas originally the tumor could be diagnosed radiographically only by bone erosion seen on plain x-ray films, myelography, computed tomography (CT), and magnetic resonance imaging (MRI) now provide precise localization. Indeed, MRI is the stand-alone diagnostic preoperative study for virtually all intradural tumors.

With the advent of the operating microscope, microsurgical instruments, bipolar cautery, intraoperative ultrasonography, ultrasonic cavitation, and other technical modalities, surgeons can approach these tumors safely. Although it is of some value in certain intradural tumors, laser dissection has not kept its promise of safety or precision.

Finally, intraoperative care is enhanced by evoked response monitoring, both sensory and motor, which can warn the surgeon during the operation should his or her manipulations alter the function of normal ascending and descending spinal pathways.

Despite these technologic improvements, the skill and experience of the surgeon remain critical factors in determining the result. The size, location, and histologic type of the tumor are predetermined factors that affect outcome. Although obvious to experienced surgeons, the following anatomic predictors apply to intradural tumors: dorsally placed tumors do better than ventrally placed tumors; extramedullary tumors do better than intramedullary tumors; small tumors do better than large tumors. These obvious generalizations have their exceptions, but with the precision of modern MRI scanning, an experienced surgeon should be able to assess the surgical risks after a history and examination.

INCIDENCE, TYPE, AND LOCATION

The reported incidence of intradural spinal cord tumors ranges from 3 to 10 per 100,000 population. Intramedullary tumors are substantially more common in children, where they represent about half of intradural tumors; in adults, they represent less than one third of intradural tumors. Sex distribution is roughly equal, although meningiomas at all locations in the central nervous system (spinal and cranial) are more common in women.

Complete resection with cure is possible with all

extramedullary intradural tumors. Similarly, ependymomas, although histologically malignant, can be cured by complete resection. Aggregately, at least 90 per cent of all intradural spinal cord tumors can be cured by modern surgical techniques. Intradural tumors have classically been divided anatomically as to their location within or without the spinal cord substance:

1. Extramedullary/intradural (84 per cent of all intradural tumors)
   a. Neurofibroma (29 per cent)
   b. Meningioma (25 per cent)
   c. Exophytic ependymoma (13 per cent)
   d. Sarcoma (12 per cent)
   e. Exophytic astrocytoma (6 per cent)
   f. Other (e.g., vascular tumors, epidermoid tumors, lipomas—15 per cent)
2. Intramedullary (16 per cent of all intradural tumors)
   a. Ependymoma (56 per cent)
   b. Astrocytoma (29 per cent)
   c. All others (less than 4 per cent each, including lipoma, epidermoid, teratoma, dermoid, meningioblastoma, oligodendroglioma)

Extradural tumors are beyond the scope of this discussion. Most are metastatic and spread into the spinal canal from contiguous structures. Their surgical treatment is entirely different from that of intradural tumors and is discussed elsewhere.

NEUROLOGIC EVALUATION IN PATIENTS WITH INTRADURAL TUMORS

Because intradural tumors are generally slow growing, patients may be symptomatic for years prior to discovery of the tumor. A common symptom of all types of intradural tumor is pain. The pain can be related to compression of a spinal nerve, in which case it is radicular. Back pain may result from compression of surrounding structures. Symptoms from spinal cord compression include upper motor neuron deficits, weakness, lack of coordination, loss of sphincter control (and sensory abnormalities), decrease in pain and temperature perception, loss of position sense with gait difficulties, and disturbed sexual sensation. Surprisingly, large tumors that grow slowly over a long period of time can produce few symptoms, although early neurologic signs can be discovered. Neurologic signs relate specifically to the site of compression.

Intramedullary tumors can be associated with syringomyelia either above or below the bulk of the tumor mass. The syringomyelia itself can cause symptoms that may be more prominent than those of the tumor. Tumors at all levels can produce bladder and bowel involvement, which as an isolated symptom is not usually attributed to spinal cord tumor.

Intradural extramedullary tumors may present with some specific signs and symptoms. For reasons that are not fully understood, the patient may suffer pain at night but be totally pain-free during the day. Radicular night pain should alert the examiner, particularly when it is associated with gait difficulty, urinary retention, or evidence of myelopathy. Extramedullary intradural lesions near the foramen magnum may present with suboccipital or neck pain, upper extremity dysesthesias, and loss of dexterity. These tumors are particularly difficult to diagnose and frequently have reached appreciable size at the time of initial discovery, despite the patient's long history of vague complaints.

The combination of night pain in a radicular distribution and gait and bladder problems in the presence of myelopathy can progress over such a long interval that the patient's complaints may be masked by his or her ability to cope. Occasionally the compressed nerve root sends pain radiating to the chest, in which case angina pectoris may be diagnosed. Pain in a right T7–T10 distribution can lead to surgical excision of a gallbladder, whereas pain from T10–T12 may trigger abdominal exploration for appendicitis.

A slow and painless progression is typical of intramedullary tumors. Because they destroy structures near the center of the spinal cord, crossing pain and temperature fibers are damaged, and segmental sensory deficits may be discovered. This is noticed earlier in the upper extremities, when the patient may have sensory abnormalities best appreciated in the fingertips. Long tract signs, weakness, and incontinence subsequently develop. Patients initially complain of burning dysesthesias in the upper extremities, particularly the hands. Because the lumbosacral pain and temperature conducting fibers are located on the outer surface of the spinothalamic tract, so-called sacral sparing has been described on occasion as characteristic of intramedullary tumors.

In general, extramedullary tumors are eccentric and may be associated with a Brown-Séquard syndrome. This consists of corticospinal tract signs ipsilateral to the tumor and contralateral spinothalamic tract signs. Upper cervical spine tumors can produce a loss of position and vibration sense in the upper extremities, as well as a loss of similar sensations in the lower extremities. Tumors near the cervicomedullary junction may produce nystagmus and rarely papilledema. In the thoracic region, a bandlike sensory loss, Horner's syndrome, or symptoms of visceral disease may result.

Lumbosacral tumors can affect bowel, bladder, and sexual function and frequently mimic genitourinary or gastrointestinal disorders. When painful, they are frequently confused with degenerative disorders of the lumbar spine and its intervertebral discs.

In children, spinal cord tumors may present as kyphoscoliosis, gait abnormalities, foot deformities, bedwetting, and a variety of other abnormalities observed by the concerned parent but frequently ignored by the patient.

PATHOLOGIC FEATURES OF INTRADURAL TUMORS

Over three quarters of intraspinal meningiomas occur in women, predominantly in the thoracic region, proba-

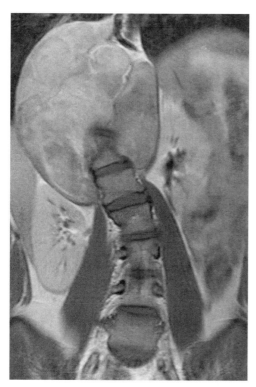

Figure 43–1. Large neurofibroma enveloping the spine anteriorly and laterally.

When a clear-cut cystic margin is visible, they can be completely excised. However, some intramedullary astrocytomas have a malignant histology, and their borders cannot be clearly distinguished from normal neural tissue. Under these circumstances, complete excision is not possible, and one has to be satisfied with an internal debulking procedure followed by some form of adjuvant oncologic therapy.[18] Most of the other less common intradural tumors are completely excisable and are benign histologically.

Hemangioblastomas of the spinal cord, occurring as an independent tumor or as part of von Hippel-Lindau disease, are benign, and complete excision should be attempted.

Specific clinical features for each histologic type of tumor may be vague. A slow-growing tumor in a middle-aged woman raises suspicion of a meningioma. Any tumor with a dumbbell configuration radiographically associated with enlargement of the bony exit foramen of the spinal nerve suggests a neurofibroma (Figs. 43–1 to 43–4).[2] This tumor can be associated with marked elevated cerebrospinal fluid protein whether or not a myelographic block is present. Tumors at the level of the cauda equina, particularly in adults (60 per cent occur in males), are often intraspinal ependymomas.

MRI has illuminated many of the preoperative diagnostic concerns in the treatment of these tumors, and rarely does one rely on these clinical features to make

bly because there are more thoracic vertebrae than at any other level. They are more common after the fifth decade of life. Because they grow from cellular remnants in the arachnoid, they are almost invariably attached to the dura by a base from which they get their blood supply.

Tumors of spinal nerve sheaths (neurofibroma, neurilemoma, schwannoma) usually arise from dorsal sensory roots near the exit of the root from the spinal canal. Of all intraspinal tumors, they are the most likely to be multiple, particularly when associated with von Recklinghausen's disease. Sometimes the tumor follows the nerve root sleeve out of the spinal canal and produces a so-called dumbbell tumor, with the narrowest portion being at the level of the root exit in the bony spine. In extremely rare instances, these tumors can be entirely intramedullary, in which case total removal should be attempted.

Ependymomas within the spinal canal usually arise inside the substance of the spinal cord, although they may arise from the tip of the conus medullaris at its juncture with the filum terminale, particularly in adults. In this location they may be partially intramedullary and predominantly extramedullary. These tumors may run a benign or a malignant course; in the latter case, they may be associated with "seeding" anywhere in the craniospinal axis. Complete excision should be attempted whenever possible.

Spinal cord astrocytomas are intramedullary and may or may not be associated with syringomyelic cysts.

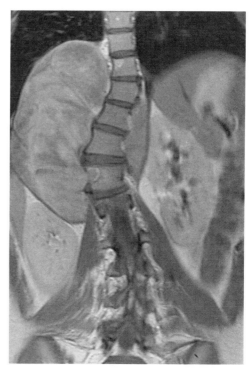

Figure 43–2. The same neurofibroma as in Figure 43–1 in a more posterior section. Despite the large extraspinal component of this tumor, there was little intraspinal and minimal spinal cord compression.

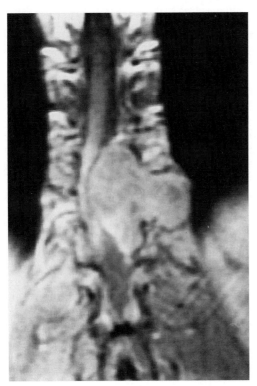

Figure 43–3. A neurofibroma compressing the thoracolumbar spinal cord. In this case, the intraspinal portion is greater than the extraspinal portion, which is exiting the intervertebral foramen and not entering the paraspinal tissue. This is in contrast to the neurofibroma depicted in Figures 43–1 and 43–2.

a specific diagnosis. It is the MRI that reveals the most definitive preoperative information.

SPECIFIC POINTS ABOUT RARE TUMORS

Epidermoid tumors most frequently occur in the lumbar region. They arise from epidermal rests that may

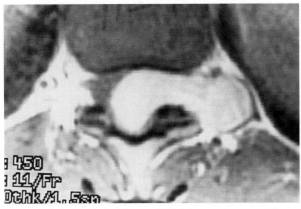

Figure 43–4. The classic "dumbbell" shape of a neurofibroma that has interspinal and extraspinal components of approximately equal dimensions.

be present congenitally but that can be induced, according to some investigators, by a lumbar puncture carrying a plug of viable epidermis. In the lumbar region, these extramedullary tumors are cheesy and easily excised.

Pure intramedullary lipomas are extremely rare in adults, but lipomas of the cauda equina may be present well into the later years. They consist of a large, fatty, fibrous mass that ultimately fills most of the lumbar theca. They are usually associated with a cutaneous angiolipoma or a dimple that communicates with the fibrofatty tissue through a spina bifida. Surgical excision in adulthood may be associated with worsening of any preoperative sphincter or sexual disturbances. Tethering of the spinal cord is part of the pathophysiologic mechanism and may not be helped by simple excision of the lipoma. These tumors should be treated surgically only by those experienced with their peculiarities and in a framework of great conservatism.

Hemangioblastomas are usually intramedullary, relatively small, and well encapsulated. Intramedullary cysts are frequently associated. Their benign nature favors complete surgical excision. They are rarely subject to spontaneous internal hemorrhage and should be excised only when there is clear evidence of progressive neurologic deficit.

Recently, central neurocytomas of the cervical spinal cord have been identified. The central neurocytoma is a benign primary tumor that can be seen in the lateral or third ventricles of the brain. Tetter and colleagues described central neurocytomas arising in two men, aged 65 and 49, who had progressive neurologic deficits secondary to intramedullary tumors in the cervical spinal canal.[45] In those instances the tumors revealed cells that were positive for synatpophysin and neuron-specific neolace and negative for glial fibrillary acidic protein, all characteristics of a neuronal tumor. These tumors apparently have an excellent prognosis if totally excised.

Sonneland and associates reviewed reports of paragangliomas of the spinal cord, which occur predominantly in the cauda equina.[42] They usually become symptomatic in midlife and are about twice as frequent in men as in women. They may be opposite the L2–L3 interspace in a stereotypic fashion, and they commonly present with back pain. Although they are embryologically and histologically related to catecholamine-secreting tumors, flushing, tachycardia, and hypertension have not been reported with spinal paragangliomas.

Rarely, leukemias, sarcomas, lymphomas, and metastatic cancers can occur within the spinal cord. In view of the tendency for aggressive cancers to spread to the brain, it is surprising that intramedullary metastases are extremely unusual. Although primary brain neoplasms occur five times more commonly than primary spinal cord tumors, intramedullary metastases are rarely suspected, even in patients with known cancer. Metastases to the spinal cord constitute a tiny fraction of all central nervous system secondary tumors.

Occasionally, malignant tumors "seed" from other sites in the central nervous system. The most common

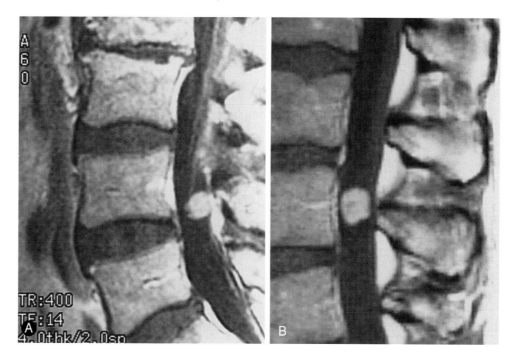

Figure 43–5. *A, B,* These two enhanced MRI scans show paragangliomas in two different patients. The size, enhancement characteristics, and location (midlumbar) demonstrate the stereotypic morphology of this rare tumor.

are medulloblastomas in children and malignant astrocytomas and ependymomas in adults. Meningeal carcinomatosis is not rare, despite the unusual incidence of metastases to the parenchyma of the spinal cord.

Acute demyelinating diseases may be associated with transverse myelitis and myelographic widening of the spinal cord. Their abrupt history and MRI appearance differentiate them from intramedullary tumors.

Not unlike the usual disparity between intracranial and intramedullary metastases, the extreme rarity of spinal cord infarction compared with the ubiquitous occurrence of stroke is remarkable. Occasionally, ante-

rior spinal artery syndromes can mimic intramedullary or extramedullary spinal cord lesions, and afflicted patients usually undergo a full set of radiographic studies in search of a compressive etiology. Severe diabetes, myeloproliferative disorders, diseases of the aorta, and other associated afflictions may be discovered.

RADIOLOGIC DIAGNOSIS OF INTRADURAL TUMORS

With the advent of MRI, the diagnosis of intradural tumors has been markedly altered (Figs. 43–5 to 43–

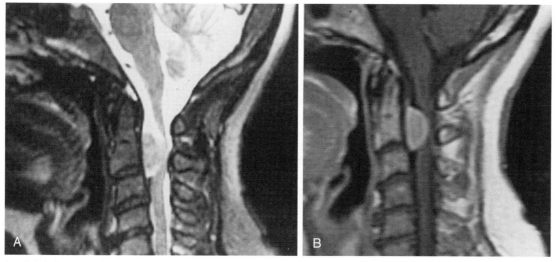

Figure 43–6. An anteriorly placed meningioma opposite the second cervical vertebra. *A,* The tumor on the T2-weighted image without enhancement. *B,* The gadolinium-enhanced tumor on a T1-weighted imaging sequence.

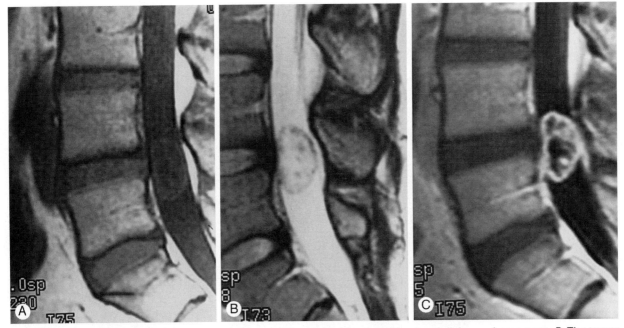

Figure 43–7. *A,* A lumbar neurofibroma barely visible on a T1-weighted image without gadolinium enhancement. *B,* The tumor shows up better on the T2-weighted image without gadolinium enhancement. *C,* Gadolinium enhancement clearly outlines the tumor and demonstrates its necrotic nature yet thick capsule, all of which strongly suggest a schwannoma.

13). In virtually all instances, MRI is a stand-alone diagnostic test. The principal role of CT in the diagnosis of intradural tumors is in patients in whom MRI procedures cannot be performed or are contraindicated (such as in the presence of implanted ferromagnetic devices). These scans must be directed specifically toward the presumed site of the intraspinal tumor. With the administration of intravenous iodinated contrast material, tumors may be better demonstrated on CT, and cystic lesions may be defined from their solid components.[3, 25]

Previously, intramedullary cavities associated with spinal cord tumors could be diagnosed only by "delayed" myelograms or CT scans that could visualize only portions of the spinal cord in axial sections.[47] The MRI scan is capable of readily defining intraspinal cysts and demonstrating the extent in a composite sagittal view.

Because many intraspinal tumors enhance with gadolinium, they are readily distinguishable from surrounding spinal cord structures. Even enhancement characteristics may be histologically specific. Detailed MRI can discern the relationship between certain intradural tumors and specific nerve roots. In some instances, MRI may define the surgical approach, the potential for complete resection, the degree of vascularity, and so forth. Furthermore, the MRI scan is an excellent way to follow patients after surgery, particularly if residual tumor is suspected.

Not only is myelography less effective in diagnosing spinal cord tumors, but in some instances, it may be dangerous, particularly in the presence of a complete myelographic block secondary to a tumor associated with neurologic deficit. In some instances, drainage of the spinal fluid during myelography below the level of the block has enhanced the neurologic deficit and necessitated emergency surgery. Although the CT scan, particularly with enhancement by iodinated contrast medium, can clearly delineate a spinal cord tumor, the image quality simply does not compare with that of MRI. Finally, a patient being "scanned" for a suspected tumor in the thoracic region can best be evaluated with a long sagittal image of the spine.

For this reason, this chapter focuses on MRI of spinal cord tumors, because all other diagnostic modalities, whether clinical or radiographic, ultimately rely on MRI as the final word before making treatment decisions.

As mentioned earlier, MRI has become the study of choice for virtually all spinal tumors.[29] Longitudinal information demonstrated particularly in the sagittal plane, with gadolinium enhancement, provides the most diagnostic information in virtually all instances.[5] Both T1- and T2-weighted images are used in the sagittal plane. On T2-weighted images, the spinal fluid has more signal intensity than the spinal cord, and intramedullary abnormalities can be well demonstrated. On T1-weighted images, vertebral structures are best delineated. T2-weighted images, a combination of long TR and long TE sequences, show soft tissue better and also specifically detect intramedullary lesions. On T2-weighted images, the spinal fluid has a high signal intensity and clearly outlines extramedullary intradural lesions.[5, 19, 20]

Intravenously administered paramagnetic ions (gadolinium) reduce T1 relaxation times. These compounds

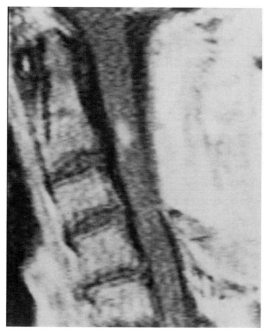

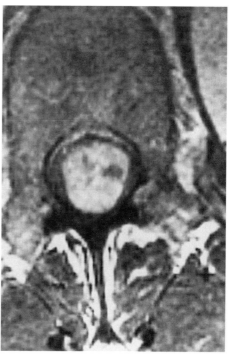

Figure 43–8. With gadolinium enhancement, intramedullary tumors generally stand out within the substance of the spinal cord. This small astrocytoma, shown after gadolinium enhancement, is about the smallest sized tumor that would be accessible surgically. In this case, serial scans were recommended to follow the progress of the mass lesion. Surgery at this stage could be of more harm than good, although early excision is generally more favorable.

Figure 43–10. Despite enhancement, spinal cord tumors are difficult to visualize, even on T2-weighted images in the axial plane. The margins of this tumor in the lumbar spinal canal can barely be differentiated from the normal contents of the lumbar theca.

Figure 43–9. *A,* An ependymoma of the conus medullaris without enhancement. *B,* Following gadolinium injection, the tumor enhances uniformly. This well-encapsulated, uniformly enhanced appearance, particularly in association with the tumor at the conus medullaris, strongly suggests an ependymoma.

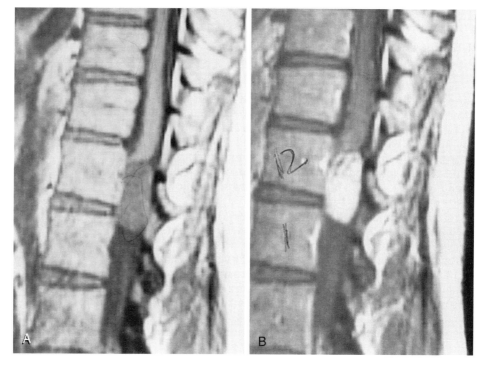

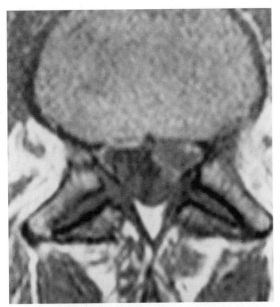

Figure 43–11. Following gadolinium enhancement, a small extradural meningioma is clearly visible in the lateral aspect of the spinal canal. Without enhancement, this lesion could have easily been mistaken for a lumbar disc herniation.

remain intravascular in intact tissue but provide enhancement of tumors or other lesions when the blood–spinal cord barrier is disturbed. Increased signal intensity is therefore seen on T1-weighted images obtained soon after contrast administration. Lesions that cannot be detected on conventional and echo sequences are better defined after enhancement by paramagnetic ions.[36, 39]

MRI Characteristics of Specific Tumor Types

A detailed analysis of specific MRI characteristics of tumor types is beyond the scope of this discussion. Some basic observations, however, may be of value.

Astrocytomas and ependymomas are intramedullary (except when present at the conus medullaris). Both have low to intermediate signal intensity on T1-weighted images and generally produce a diffuse swelling of the spinal cord over several segments. Both the tumor and the adjacent edema have prolonged T2 relaxation times on T2-weighted images. Following gadolinium enhancement, ependymomas tend to enhance noticeably more homogeneously, with clearer margins than astrocytomas. Intramedullary cysts can be present in both lesions. Hemangioblastomas have similar radiographic characteristics and are difficult to differentiate because they can be highly enhancing and are present with or without cystic cavities. When there are small nodular tumors in the posterior fossa, the index of suspicion for hemangioblastoma is increased.[36]

The MRI characteristics of schwannomas are not consistent. Although they do enhance intensely, they may or may not be associated with a low signal intensity within the mass. Heterogeneous enhancement is sometimes seen, but a peripheral enhancement is not uncommon. Meningiomas also appear as rounded, sharply marginated masses, most often isointense to the spinal cord on T1-weighted images but hyperintense on T2-weighted images. They usually enhance intensely. Calcification may be present, and this may help distinguish them from nerve sheath tumors. Unless there is a dumbbell configuration or clear-cut evidence of attachment to a nerve root, the differentiation between nerve sheath tumors and meningiomas may be difficult on MRI scans.

TREATMENT OF INTRASPINAL TUMORS

This volume will be published 110 years after Horsley performed the first successful intraspinal tumor resection. Despite certain technical advancements, his basic concept that there was only one form of treatment for intraspinal tumors has not changed. That treatment was and is, in his words, "removal of the source of pressure by operation."

There is no doubt that the results have improved since Horsley's time, and even since the landmark reports of Elsberg in 1924[11] and Greenwood in 1963.[16] In the many years since Greenwood's report of the

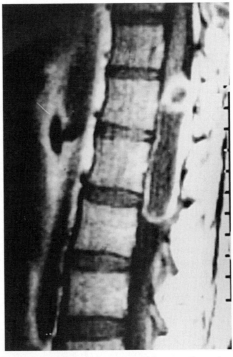

Figure 43–12. Tumors can present with a cystic and a solid component, as seen in this thoracolumbar tumor following gadolinium enhancement. The superior portion of the tumor enhances and appears somewhat "solid," as is typical of an ependymoma. However, the inferior portion has become necrotic and is now somewhat cystic in appearance, with a brightly enhancing capsule.

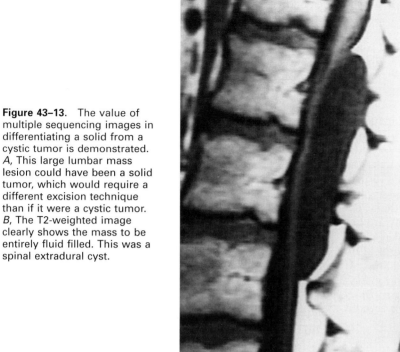

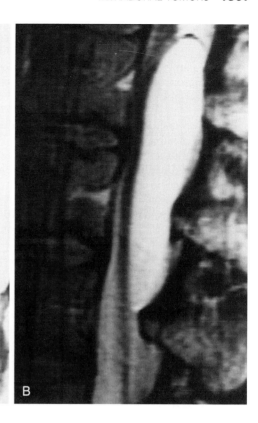

Figure 43–13. The value of multiple sequencing images in differentiating a solid from a cystic tumor is demonstrated. *A,* This large lumbar mass lesion could have been a solid tumor, which would require a different excision technique than if it were a cystic tumor. *B,* The T2-weighted image clearly shows the mass to be entirely fluid filled. This was a spinal extradural cyst.

first successful complete removal of an intramedullary tumor, no viable alternatives to surgery have been found. All developments have been technical, and to some extent they have been effective in lesions such as meningiomas and neurofibromas, for which complete, safe removal of the intraspinal portion is the rule. These technical developments have come on the heels of the more remarkable and extremely innovative neuroradiologic techniques that make the precise localization of intraspinal tumors routine.

TECHNICAL ADVANCES IN THE TREATMENT OF SPINAL CORD TUMORS

Several technical advances have significantly improved the results of surgical treatment of intraspinal tumors. They are discussed briefly here, but the reader is referred to the reference list, which contains publications that highlight each of the described techniques.

The addition of the *operating microscope* in the treatment of intraspinal tumors probably marked the dawn of modern therapy for those lesions. Its application to excision of small lesions in or near the neural tissue has significantly reduced the complication rate while fostering more aggressive surgery.

The *microsurgical instrumentation* that accompanied the surgical microscope evolved from other specialties. An experienced microsurgeon may have a complete set of otolaryngologic surgical instruments on the table. Precise instrumentation complemented the better view and illumination afforded by the surgical microscope.

The pioneering role of Greenwood's application of *bipolar coagulation* was mentioned earlier.[17] There are various types of *surgical lasers,* but those used commonly are the CO_2 laser, whereas Nd:YAG may be effective in gently debulking the mass of the tumor.[4, 10, 13, 48] In a preliminary report on the use of the argon laser in neurosurgery, Powers and associates described 10 patients treated with a 150-micron spot diameter and between 3 and 5 watts of laser power.[30] There was gross total removal in all four ependymoma patients, and also gross total removal in each patient with thoracic hemangioblastoma, cervical intramedullary schwannoma, and thoracic astrocytoma. These authors also advise using lasers to perform an accurate midline myelotomy. In recent years, finer surgical instruments have replaced the laser in the hands of many neurosurgeons.[46]

Ultrasonic surgical aspiration has a limited but significant role in the debulking of intraspinal tumors.[12] This device consists of a hollow tube that vibrates at high frequencies and physically cavitates tumor tissue to an emulsion that is irrigated and aspirated through the tube. Gentle removal of abnormal tissue, even near the tumor–spinal cord interface, is possible.

Localization with *intraoperative ultrasonography* has now become a routine surgical technique whereby an ultrasonic transducer is placed over the exposed spinal cord.[8, 15, 32, 37] Intramedullary cysts or solid masses, which leave no visible clues on the exposed surface of the spinal cord, can be localized with this technique.[23, 31] Recently, Kawakami and colleagues developed an ultrasonic microprobe that overcomes some of the limitations of normal spinal sonography.[24] These tiny transducers can assess intramedullary spinal cord lesions, and they can monitor the surgical procedure. The tip of the microprobe is 5 mm wide and 13 mm long. These hand-held devices can be placed directly on the spinal cord for accurate intraoperative recording.

Continuous *evoked response monitoring* during spinal surgery is a subject of some controversy. During surgery for a thoracic intramedullary tumor, for instance, continuous stimuli are given to the posterior tibial nerve and recorded from the brain. Within 15 seconds, changes in evoked potential can be observed, and the operation can be halted until normal potentials return. Cooper and Epstein use this technique routinely, but they suggest that the operative results are the same with or without monitoring.[7] Furthermore, they are not certain that motor pathways are protected even when the operation is stopped in response to deterioration of the somatosensory evoked response. Stimulation of descending pathways, as described by Levy and associates, may be a better way to monitor spinal cord function during surgery.[26] With this technique, motor pathways are stimulated centrally, and responses are recorded directly from extremity muscles. This method measures conduction in the descending motor pathways, whereas somatosensory evoked responses are transmitted primarily up the dorsal columns.

RESULTS OF TREATMENT OF INTRAMEDULLARY TUMORS

Despite the historic importance of those investigators who pioneered in the treatment of spinal cord tumors, only recent series are discussed here with reference to results and complications.

In 1985, Cooper and Epstein reported 29 patients: 14 had ependymomas, 11 had astrocytomas, two had lipomas, and there was one case each of intramedullary "fibrosis" and "astrogliosis." Complete tumor removal was achieved in 14 patients, and "99 per cent removal" was accomplished in seven others. In 21 of the 29 patients, the neurologic condition stabilized or improved after surgery. Postoperative deterioration was seen only in patients who had advanced motor deficits before surgery.[7]

Stein's series of 31 intramedullary tumors was characterized by postoperative deterioration in only seven patients. If incomplete tumor removal was achieved, the subsequent course depended on the rate of growth of the tumor. In highly malignant tumors, rapid growth and seeding of the tumor were devastating. In up to 10 years of follow-up, Stein has had no incidence of recurrence in cases of total removal.[43]

RESULTS OF TREATMENT OF EXTRAMEDULLARY INTRADURAL TUMORS

Regardless of cell type and location, the results of surgery for intradural extramedullary spinal cord tumors are usually gratifying. When the previously men-

tioned neurosurgical techniques are employed, neurologic complications as a result of surgery are uncommon, and if they do occur, ultimate improvement can be expected.

Progressive improvement of preoperative deficits can proceed for months, not reaching a plateau until over one year after the operation. If gross total removal is observed under the operating microscope, recurrence is rare.[38]

With the advent of fine radiologic techniques, it is possible to follow patients radiologically, as well as clinically. Previously, accurate radiologic evaluation could be performed only with periodic myelography. Even if subsequent MRI shows evidence of recurrent or residual tumor, reoperation may not be indicated immediately. Such a decision should consider the patient's neurologic status, age, health, response to previous surgery, and tumor growth rate on serial MRI scans. When treatment of a recurrent tumor is indicated, it is generally managed operatively.

THE VALUE OF RADIOSURGERY IN INTRASPINAL TUMORS

Radiotherapy appears to have no role in the treatment of benign tumors. Radiation therapy has occasionally been advised in patients with nonresectable neurofibromas, but there is sparse evidence that this treatment is effective.

Initially there were reports of a salutary response to radiation on intramedullary tumors. Since the reports of Wood and associates in 1954[49] and Schwade and associates in 1978,[40] there has been a gradual but significant change in philosophy. Some patients improved, but this could have been attributable to the decompressive laminectomy that inevitably preceded radiation. In other instances, radiation necrosis of the spinal cord complicated therapy. Every effort should be made to excise ependymomas completely.[35] Low-grade astrocytomas, although they may be partially resected, are probably better treated by repeat surgery than solely by radiation treatment. Malignant astrocytomas of the spinal cord have a poor prognosis. Their spread through the intraspinal axis is relatively rapid and usually fatal. Complete cure does not seem to be possible, even with aggressive resection.[28, 35] Radiation of the spinal cord may be palliative and is frequently recommended in this relatively small group of patients.

Radiation therapy may be valuable in patients with metastatic intraspinal lesions such as lymphomas and carcinomatous meningitis, and in those with seeding from malignant primary central nervous system tumors. In some of these patients, chemotherapy is of additional value.

COMPLICATIONS OF SURGERY

History

Early in the twentieth century, mortality figures of almost 20 per cent were reported in association with surgical excision of spinal cord tumors. In 1925 Elsberg said that a responsible investigator could determine the role of surgery, if any, in the treatment of intraspinal tumors.[11] At that time, the mortality rate was high, and incomplete removal and postoperative paraplegia were frequent. Elsberg's 100 patients were the subject of his 422-page textbook. The mortality rate in those 100 cases was 10 per cent. This covered both intra- and extradural tumors. In his last 52 operative procedures, however, there was only one operative fatality.

Elsberg states, "a critical study of the histories of the fatalities in my series shows that most of the deaths occurred either in patients with inoperable and irremovable tumors, or from complications that were only indirectly connected with the operative procedure." Since these 100 patients were all operated on before January 1924, it is likely that the "indirect" complications were indeed a significant factor.[1]

Mortality figures improved dramatically as neurosurgery developed. In 1922 Frazier and Spiller reported 14 cases of surgery for spinal cord tumor with one death,[14] and in 1922 Adson and Ott reported 85 laminectomies for spinal cord tumor with a 14 per cent mortality.[1] In their text *Intraspinal Tumors of Childhood*, Rand and Rand mention that among nine patients with astrocytomas of the spinal cord who were subjected to surgery, only one showed no postoperative deficit.[34] The neurologic condition invariably worsened when astrocytomas were treated, compared with the seven children with ependymomas, some of whom were apparently cured, with one survival up to 25 years. They concluded that only 20 per cent of the 64 verified tumors in their series could be totally removed.

Failure to Find the Tumor

Despite the accuracy of modern neuroimaging techniques, some surgeons subject their patients to an unnecessarily prolonged or extensive operative procedure because the tumor is not directly under the initially planned operative site. The technical beauty of MRI of a spinal cord tumor is both aesthetic and practical, but it is of little help to a surgeon who is searching in the midthoracic region for a vertebra whose landmarks are now obscured by surgical drapes. This problem could have been avoided by a much simpler device—a paper clip or ordinary hypodermic needle. When such a radiopaque device is placed over the site of the tumor, subsequent films and the marked skin will guide the surgeon to the proper place. In the lumbar and cervical regions, there are sufficient landmarks so that the surgeon can usually plan the operative procedure without preoperative localization films.

Postoperative Spinal Fluid Leak

Postoperative spinal fluid fistulas, paradoxically, are more likely to occur when there are small openings in the dura than when the dura is left wide open. In general, a patient who has had previous radiation therapy is more likely to develop a spinal fluid leak, re-gardless of the nature of the tumor. Spinal fluid leakage seems to occur more commonly in the upper thoracic region, where wound dehiscence caused by stretching of the skin and muscle is also most common. Leakage of spinal fluid should be treated promptly. If there is any doubt, the incision should be reopened and the dura closed properly.

An alternative form of treatment, developed empirically by some surgeons, is the insertion of a local epidural drain. By continuous drainage of cerebrospinal fluid, the fistulous tract is kept dry, and natural healing may ultimately result. Continuous spinal fluid drainage, however, is an uncomfortable procedure associated with bed confinement, headaches, and the potential for infection. It is not invariably successful, and its ultimate effectiveness may take several days to ascertain. Re-exploration and proper closure of the dura should not be delayed.

Postoperative Instability After Extensive Laminectomy For Spinal Cord Tumor

Postoperative subluxation and instability are most common in young patients, usually younger than 18 years of age; extensive, wide laminectomies, perhaps involving some facet joints; and laminectomies in the cervical region. Even in adults, wide laminectomies, particularly in patients without chronic disc degeneration, may be associated with mechanical instability or alterations of vertebral alignment. The earlier this developing problem is identified, the easier it can be arrested with a stabilization procedure. Raimondi and associates recommend avoiding this problem in children who have continued expected growth potential by suturing the posterior elements back in place.[33]

The late development of swan-neck deformity in children and in adults requires early recognition. For children who have had extensive cervical laminectomy, x-ray films taken every three months for the first year are advisable.

The procedure of choice is stabilization of the affected segments before bony molding has taken place. Because the weight of the head favors the anterior surface of the spine, wedge-shaped deformities with narrowing of the anterior portion of the vertebral bodies may evolve in association with a permanent kyphotic deformity. This problem can be prevented by earlier anterior fusion, particularly if one segment is involved predominantly. Anterior fusion procedures inherently destabilize the spine in the immediate postoperative period because, in addition to the previously resected laminae and interspinous ligaments, the anterior operation may destroy the anterior longitudinal ligament.[21] The use of firm bracing procedures, such as a halo apparatus, is advisable in such cases.

Attempts to fuse the spine primarily at the time of initial decompressive laminectomy have been recommended. I have been pleased with the results in multilevel laminectomies of lateral mass screws and plates with bone graft. The bone does not impinge on the spinal canal, and the fusion incorporates quickly with adequate postoperative immobilization.

Postoperative Pain

Pain after surgery for removal of spinal cord tumors can be conveniently categorized as acute postoperative pain (somatic) and chronic pain (central). Little has to be said about acute postoperative pain after such surgery. Persistent radicular pain, particularly after removal of a thoracic neurofibroma, may be related to ligation of the proximal portion of the dorsal sensory root. This root should be cut sharply, and if the radicular artery bleeds inordinately, it should be cauterized directly. Under magnification it is easy to avoid the radicular artery.

Other forms of postoperative pain are treated similarly to that experienced after any other spinal operation. Prolonged narcotics are avoided. Steroids such as dexamethasone are excellent pain relievers and should be used liberally in the first two to three days after surgery. When used for short intervals, they are free of complications and provide the patient relief of inflammation, ease of pain, and a feeling of well-being, which is important after a serious operation.

Chronic pain after spinal cord tumor surgery, particularly after removal of intramedullary tumors, is a different and more difficult problem. As Stein reiterates, the physiologic mechanisms for this phenomenon are poorly understood, and treatment generally fails.[43] The pain may involve extensive portions of the body, and it is difficult to control. The pain has more of a "central quality." It can be a burning, gnawing discomfort that spreads beyond the area of stimulus and is a uniform response to various stimuli, including light touch. Often it is strongly affected by mood. There appear to be no consistent results from the use of drugs or stimulators. Interestingly, "incessant" pain followed Sir Victor Horsley's first successful removal of a spinal cord tumor. Such patients should not be given narcotics but rather should be enrolled in an effective pain treatment program that includes psychologic as well as physical therapeutic techniques.

Postoperative Hematoma

Postoperative hematomas are recognized by progressive deterioration of spinal cord function in the minutes to hours after the operation. This requires immediate attention, with emergency MRI or CT. If these studies are not immediately available and the patient is deteriorating rapidly, the surgeon should not hesitate to open the incision, even though a hematoma has not been demonstrated radiologically. An overnight stay in the intensive care unit is recommended, with periodic checks of neurologic function to ensure early recognition of this problem.

Spinal Cord Ischemia or Infarction Secondary to Spinal Tumor Surgery

Great controversy exists over the relative importance of individual blood vessels that supply the spinal cord.

In 1939, Suh and Alexander noted that "much of what has been written in the past forty years about the circulation of spinal cord is either inaccurate or incomplete."[44] In the same year, Bolton determined that the vessels that supply the spinal cord are end-arteries, and there are no anastomoses between the capillary beds.[6] Individual vessels that travel with the spinal nerves into the spinal canal do not seem important. Scoliosis surgeons have ligated 13 to 16 segmental arteries in one patient without neurologic loss. Great attention was given in the past to the artery of Adamkiewicz (arteria radicularis anterior magna), which is the largest of the feeders of the lumbar spinal cord.[41] It occurs on the left side in 80 per cent of patients between T7 and L4, with the greatest incidence at T9 to T11. It usually enters the spinal canal as at least one feeder.

Dommisse and Enslin noted four cases of paraplegia in a series of 68 spinal procedures, most for scoliosis, three of which occurred between T5 and T9; only one occurred with surgery below T10.[9] The authors emphasized a "critical zone of the spinal cord" extending from T5 to T9. In this study, they demonstrated that the spinal canal was also narrower in this region, which could predispose to surgical complications, particularly in the face of a chronic low reserve state of spinal fluid circulation.

Laminectomy Trauma

The term "laminectomy trauma" describes the neurologic deficit caused by removing the lamina over the tumor and the spinal cord. The existence of significant spinal cord trauma secondary to laminectomy alone, without opening of the dura, is well known. Love and Schorn presented the distressing statistics of neurologic deterioration in patients who underwent simple laminectomy for thoracic disc disease.[27] Simply removing the lamina in a tight spinal canal with ordinary rongeurs was associated with a high incidence of neurologic worsening, and often postoperative paraplegia, even when there was no attempt to retract the intradural contents after the laminectomy was done. This is avoided today by lateral approaches to the thoracic spine. Similarly, the potential for patients to become neurologically worse after a cervical laminectomy for conditions such as cervical spondylosis is well known. Our routine when spinal cord compression is present is to drill bilateral gutters over the borders of the spinal canal and then gently lift off the lamina.

CONCLUSION

This has been an overview of some of the peculiarities and advancements in the diagnosis and treatment of intraspinal tumors. No attempt has been made to detail the specifics of diagnosis or treatment, but these are covered in the references given. Readers should understand that intradural tumors are rarely diagnosed at the first presentation to a medical generalist. The diagnosis is becoming more common, however, because of the availability of better imaging techniques, notably MRI.

The overall prognosis of benign tumors is excellent if they are not too far advanced at the time of treatment. An array of technical devices has made safe surgical cure of these tumors routine, although malignant tumors remain a challenge.

References

1. Adson, A. W., and Ott, W. O.: Results of removal of tumors of the spinal cord. Arch. Neurol. Psych. 8:520, 1922.
2. Akwari, O. E., Payne, W. S., Onofrio, B. M., et al.: Dumbbell neurogenic tumors in the mediastinum. Mayo Clin. Proc. 53:353, 1978.
3. Aubi, M. L., Jardin, C., Bar, D., and Vignaud, J.: Computerized tomography in 32 cases of intraspinal tumor. J. Neuroradiol. 6:81–92, 1979.
4. Beck, O. J.: Use of the Nd-Yag laser in neurosurgery. Neurosurg. Rev. 7:151–157, 1984.
5. Bluemm, R. G., Baleriaus, D., Lausberg, G., and Brotchi, J.: Initial experience with MR imaging of intracranial midline lesions and lesions of the cervical spine at half tesla. Neurosurg. Rev. 7:287–302, 1984.
6. Bolton, B.: The blood supply of the human spinal cord. J. Neurol. Psych. 2:137, 1939.
7. Cooper, P. R., and Epstein, F.: Radical resection of intramedullary spinal cord tumors in adults. J. Neurosurg. 63:492–499, 1985.
8. Dohrmann, G. J.: Intraoperative ultrasound imaging of the spinal cord: Syringomyelia, cysts, and tumors—a preliminary report. Surg. Neurol. 18:395–399, 1982.
9. Dommisse, G. F., and Eslin, T. B.: Hodgson's circumferential osteotomy in the correction of spinal deformity. J. Bone Joint Surg. 52B:778, 1970.
10. Edwards, M. S.: Argon laser surgery of pediatric neural neoplasms. Childs Brain 11:171–175, 1984.
11. Elsberg, C. A.: Tumors of the spinal cord and symptoms of irritation and compression of the spinal cord and nerve roots. In Pathology, Symptomatology, Diagnosis and Treatment. New York, Paul B. Hoeverg, 1925, pp. 206–239.
12. Epstein, F.: The cavitron ultrasonic aspirator in tumor surgery. Clin. Neurosurg. 31:497–505, 1983.
13. Fasano, V. A., Benc, F., and Ponzio, R. M.: Observations on the simultaneous use of CO_2 Nd:Yag lasers in neurosurgery. Lasers Surg. Med. 2:155–161, 1982.
14. Frazier, C. H., and Spiller, W. G.: Analysis of 14 consecutive cases of spinal cord tumors. Arch. Neurol. Psych. 8:455, 1922.
15. Gooding, G. A. W., Edward, M. S. B., Rabkin, A. E., and Powers, S. K.: Intraoperative real-time ultrasound in the localization of intracranial neoplasms. Radiology 146:459–462, 1983.
16. Greenwood, J., Jr.: Intramedullary tumors of spinal cord: A follow-up study after total surgical removal. J. Neurosurg. 20:665–668, 1963.
17. Greenwood, J.: Surgical removal of intramedullary tumors. J. Neurosurg. 26:276–282, 1967.
18. Guidetti, B., Mercuri, S., and Vagnozzi, R.: Long-term results of the surgical treatment of 129 intramedullary spinal gliomas. J. Neurosurg. 54:323, 1981.
19. Han, J. S., Benson, J. E., and Yoon, Y. S.: Magnetic resonance imaging in the spinal column and craniovertebral junction. Radiol. Clin. North Am. 22:805, 1984.
20. Han, J. S., Kaufman, B., and Yousef, S. J.: NMR imaging of the spine. AJR Am. J. Roentgenol. 141:1137–1145, 1151–1159, 1983.
21. Hodgson, A. R., and Stock, F. E.: Anterior spine fusion for the treatment of tuberculosis of the spine: The operative findings and results of treatment in the first one hundred cases. J. Bone Joint Surg. Am. 42:295–310, 1960.
22. Horsley, V., and Gowers, W. R.: A case of tumors of the spinal cord: Removal-recovery. Med. Chit. Tr. London 71:3277, 1888.
23. Hutchins, F.: Differentiation of tumor from syringohydromyelia:

Intraoperative neurosonography of the spinal cord. Radiology 151:171–174, 1984.
24. Kawakami, R., et al.: New transducers for intraoperative spinal sonography: Technical note. J. Neurosurg. 79:787–790, 1993.
25. LaPoint, J. S., Grabe, D. A., and Neugent, R. A.: Value of intravenous contrast enhancement in the CT evaluation of intraspinal tumors. AJNR Am. J. Neuroradiol. 6:939–943, 1985.
26. Levy, W. J., York, D. H., McCaffrey, M., et al.: Motor evoked potentials from transcranial stimulation of the motor cortex in humans. Neurosurgery 15:287–302, 1984.
27. Love, J. G., and Schorn, V. G.: Thoracic disc protrusions. JAMA 191:267, 1965.
28. Marsa, G. W., Goffinet, D. R., Rubenstein, L. J., et al.: Megavoltage irradiation in the treatment of gliomas of the brain and spinal cord. Cancer 36:1681–1689, 1975.
29. Norman, D., Mills, C. M., Brant-Zawadzki, M., et al.: Magnetic resonance imaging of the spinal cord and canal: Potentials and limitations AJR Am. J. Roentgenol. 141:1147–1152, 1983.
30. Powers, S. K., Edwards, M. S. B., Boggan, J. E., et al.: Use of argon surgical laser in neurosurgery. J. Neurosurg. 62:523–530, 1984.
31. Quencer, R. M.: Intraoperative spinal sonography of soft tissue masses of the spinal cord and spinal canal. Am. J. Radiol. 143:1307–1315, 1984.
32. Raghavendra, B. N., Epstein, F. J., and McCleary, L.: Intramedullary spinal cord tumors in children: Localization by intraoperative sonography. AJNR Am. J. Neuroradiol. 5:395–397, 1984.
33. Raimondi, J., Gutierez, F. A., and DiRocco, C.: Laminotomy and total reconstruction of the posterior spinal arch with spinal canal in childhood. J. Neurosurg. 45:555–560, 1976.
34. Rand, R. W., and Rand, C. W.: Intraspinal Tumors of Childhood. Springfield IL, Charles C. Thomas, 1960.
35. Read, G.: The treatment of ependymoma of the brain or spinal canal by radiotherapy: A report of 79 cases. Clin. Radiol. 35:163–166, 1984.
36. Rothwell, C. I., Jaspin, T., Worthington, B. S., et al.: Gadolinium enhanced magnetic resonance imaging of spinal tumors. Br. J. Radiol. 62:1067–1074, 1989.
37. Rubin, J. M., and Dohrmann, G. W.: Work in progress: Intraoperative ultrasonography of the spine. Radiology 146:173–175, 1983.
38. Rutichelli, P., Scoditti, U., Moretti, G., et al.: Retrospective study of 50 cases of spinal meningioma. Acta Biomed. Ateneo Parmense 55:255–260, 1984.
39. Schroth, G., Thron, A., and Guhl, L.: Magnetic resonance imaging of spinal meningiomas and neurinomas. J. Neurosurg. 66:695–700, 1987.
40. Schwade, J., Wara, W. W., and Scheiline, G. E.: Management of primary spinal cord tumors. Rad. Oncol. Biol. Phys. 4:389–391, 1978.
41. Seddon, H. H.: Antero-lateral decompression for Pott's paraplegia. J. Bone Joint Surg. Br. 33:461, 1951.
42. Sonneland, S., Scheithauer, B. W., LeChago, J., et al.: Paragangliomas of the cauda equina region: Clincopathologic study of 31 cases with special reference to immunocytology and ultrastructure. Cancer 58:1720–1735, 1986.
43. Stein, B. M.: Intramedullary spinal cord tumors. Clin. Neurosurg. 30:717–741, 1983.
44. Suh, T. H., and Alexander, L.: Vascular system of the human spinal cord. Arch. Neurol. Psych. 41:659–677, 1939.
45. Tetter, S. B., Borges, L. F., and Lewis, D. N.: Central neurocytomas of the cervical spinal cord. J. Neurosurg. 81:288–293, 1994.
46. Twe, J. M., Jr., and Tobler, W. D.: The laser: History, biophysics and neurosurgical applications. Clin. Neurosurg. 31:506–549, 1983.
47. Van Der Tas, C.: Importance of computer assisted myelography in diseases affecting the vertebral column. Diagn. Imaging 48:71–79, 1979.
48. Walter, G. F.: The effect of carbon dioxide and neodynium YAG lasers on the central and peripheral nervous systems and cerebral blood vessels. J. Neurosurg. Psych. 47:745–749, 1984.
49. Wood, E. H., Berne, A. S., and Traveras, J. M.: The value of radiation therapy in the management of intrinsic tumors of the spinal cord. Radiology 63:11–24, 1954.

44

Intraspinal Infections

Ann Marie Flannery, M.D.

Marshall B. Allen, M.D.

The spinal epidural abscess is an uncommon but potentially severe infection that occurs at a frequency of about one per 13,000 admissions,[20] or about one per year at large referral hospitals.[88] Because of the close proximity of the infection to the spinal cord, conus medullaris, and nerve roots, patients with epidural abscesses are at significant risk for permanent neurologic dysfunction. For the diagnosis to be made, intraspinal infection must be considered in the differential diagnosis of patients who have fever, back pain, and localized spinal tenderness.[5] The diagnosis is established by magnetic resonance imaging (MRI).[33] Myelograms, computed tomography (CT), plain spine radiographs, and bone scanning may also be useful.[20] Once the diagnosis of epidural abscess has been made, the appropriate therapy often results in a good outcome for patients who are treated before paralysis occurs.

Although osteomyelitis has long been known because of its chronicity and tendency to result in long-term survivors with spinal deformities,[61] the nature of epidural infections was not well understood until 1926, when Dandy described the epidural abscess in its acute and chronic form.[19] He identified the propensity of this disorder to be a dorsal spine disease, based on his two cases and a review of the literature. Additionally, he described the extradural space that is present dorsally, except for below the second bony sacral segment. Dandy noted that in the cervical region, the epidural space is only a potential space.[19] The actual epidural space extends from the seventh cervical vertebra caudally, becoming prominent between the fourth and dally, becoming prominent between the fourth and

eighth thoracic vertebrae, and again widening and becoming more prominent below the second lumbar vertebra.

The acute and chronic forms of epidural abscess were recognized and differentiated in 1931 and 1932.[69, 92] In 1948, Heusner contributed greatly to the understanding of the clinical presentation of this disorder.[45] He divided the clinical presentation into four phases. Phase 1 includes localized spinal ache; Phase 2, root pain; Phase 3, loss of sensation, loss of sphincter control, or muscle weakness; and Phase 4, paralysis. Other names for spinal epidural abscess include spinal pachymeningitis or peripachymeningitis.[25]

CLINICAL PRESENTATION

Epidural abscess must be considered as part of the differential diagnosis of a febrile patient who has limb weakness and of a patient with point tenderness over the spine, fever, and back pain or radiculopathy.[93] Ataxia has also been reported as a presenting symptom of cord compression.[42] Variations in the acuity of presentation are based on the underlying pathophysiology of the infection. In cases of hematogenous spread, the systemic signs of infection are more pronounced and the overall clinical course of the patient is more acute. In these patients, frank pus is likely to be present. Other patients have a more chronic or indolent course.[93] Progression between the first two phases is usually prolonged in this chronic group.[88]

The differential diagnosis of patients with spinal

epidural abscess may include musculoskeletal strain, transverse myelitis, neoplasia, spontaneous extradural hematoma, and epidural lipomatosis, as well as poliomyelitis, meningitis, and arthritis.[5, 41, 45, 59, 65, 88]

The erythrocyte sedimentation rate is usually elevated in cases of spinal epidural abscess,[73] and patients may be disoriented.[5] Fever is present 57 per cent of the time and back pain 89 per cent of the time.[20] Even in recent series, however, patients are only occasionally admitted with epidural abscess as their diagnosis or even as part of the differential diagnosis.[88] This serious infectious disorder must be considered early, especially in patients with impaired immunocompetence, such as renal transplant patients; drug addicts, especially those who are HIV positive; alcoholics; and the very elderly. The clinical picture has been noted to be subtle in alcoholics and patients on hemodialysis.[74, 85] Sources of infection have included osteomyelitis, urinary tract infections, pneumonia and other pulmonary infections, dental abscesses, psoas abscesses, sacral decubitus,[5] paravertebral injections for back pain,[86] lumbar punctures,[47] epidural catheters,[28, 29] and from sites as distant as the foot.[81] An epidural abscess has even presented as a rectal fistula[52] and has arisen from a J-pouch ileal-anal anastomosis[71] and a cervical esophagogastric anastomosis.[49]

PATHOPHYSIOLOGY

Dandy's original work in defining the dural space was significant in noting that the anterior epidural space is a potential space at most vertebral levels.[19] This observation predicted that anterior epidural infections are relatively uncommon, and when they do occur, they are usually spread from osteomyelitis.

Between 1930 and 1982, seven large series reported a total of 28 anterior epidural abscesses and 105 posterior (dorsal) abscesses. Of these, 20 were cervical, 71 were thoracic, and 48 were lumbar.[20] A more recent review of 43 cases found an equal distribution of anterior and posterior abscesses.[21] Hematogenous spread is implicated 25 to 50 per cent of the time, the usual source being the skin. Many patients report an incidence of minor trauma before the onset of the initial discomfort.[48, 53] The most common causative organism is *Staphylococcus aureus*. In a series of 35 patients and a review of the literature, Danner and Hartman found *S. aureus* in 54 per cent of the cases.[20] Other etiologic organisms found have included *Staphylococcus epidermidis, Streptococcus pneumoniae,* alpha- and beta-hemolytic streptococci, *Streptococcus milleri, Escherichia coli, Pseudomonas aeruginosa, Listeria monocytogenes, Salmonella typhi,[77] Brucella,[75] Blastomyces,[43, 60] Aspergillus,[44] Actinomyces, Echinococcus,* guinea worm,[13, 36, 59] *Fusobacterium necrophorum,[40]* mucormycosis,[14, 90] and *Haemophilus parainfluenzae.[43, 60, 84]*

The mechanisms cited to explain the damage to the spinal cord have included simple compression, compression with thrombosis and thrombophlebitis, and venous infarction.[5, 12, 45, 48] In 1932, Allen and Kahn reported an autopsy that showed necrosis of the cord with swelling.[2] Feldenzer and associates, who used an experimental rabbit model, found white matter vascularization, loss of myelin, and external swelling with relative preservation of gray matter.[27] In this model of an *S. aureus* epidural infection, no evidence of thrombosis or vasculitis was found. Pathologic changes were related primarily to compression. This observation may explain why early treatment can reverse neurologic deficits.

DIAGNOSTIC MODALITIES

Patients with a suspected epidural abscess are generally diagnosed by one or more of the following tests: MRI, CT, and myelography. Lumbar punctures and plain spine radiographs are often performed as part of the initial work-up of a patient with spine pain and fever and may provide diagnostic clues.

Magnetic Resonance Imaging

Its increasing availability, its high resolution of soft tissue entities, and its noninvasive nature have made MRI the most effective method of diagnosing epidural abscesses. Whenever available, MRI should be the primary diagnostic test. Epidural abscesses may be clearly outlined on both T1- and T2-weighted images. Intravenous administration of the paramagnetic agent gadolinium helps delineate areas of inflammation. The MRI often includes abnormal signal in the bone marrow of adjacent vertebral bodies and adjacent epidural enhancement. The epidural abscess often demonstrates peripheral enhancement (Fig. 44–1A–C). Spinal cord compression can be seen on T2 fast-spin-echo sequences.[33] Homogeneous and heterogeneous enhancement of the solid portion of the spinal epidural abscess have also been reported.[72] The abscess has been isointense or hypointense on T1-weighted spin-echo images and hyperintense on T2-weighted images.[58] Gas within the epidural abscess has been reported by Kokes and colleagues.[56]

The advantages of MRI include its superior ability to visualize the degree of cord compression and the extent of the epidural mass. MRI can be performed on those with only vague symptoms before the infectious process has progressed to a potentially irreversible neurologic deficit. When linked with a high index of suspicion, the potential ability to achieve an early diagnosis with MRI should allow for improved outcomes in infected patients.

Myelography

Myelography has long been the standard test for imaging of epidural abscesses. As expected by its pathophysiology, the abscess presents as an extradural defect, often a complete or near-complete block. A cervical myelogram may facilitate preoperative planning by showing the upper limits of the abscess. Myelography with or without CT is the most effective

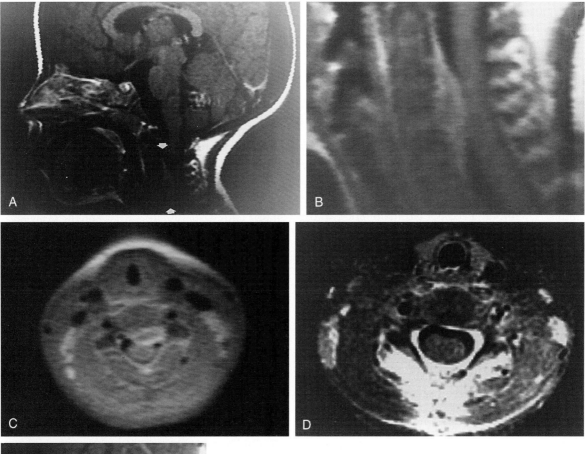

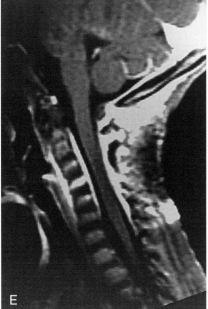

Figure 44–1. A 2-year-old girl was admitted with a history of fever, irritability, sore throat, and stiff neck. Physical examination showed nuchal rigidity. Lumbar puncture showed an elevated white cell count, no organisms on Gram's stain, and normal glucose and protein. *A,* Sagittal section MRI (T1) with contrast shows a ventral mass with an enhancing rim extending from C3 to C5. *B,* Enlargement of the area noted in *A* by the arrows. *C,* A transaxial view demonstrates the relationship of the mass to the spinal cord. After a cervical laminectomy that revealed granulation tissue, antibiotics were continued. *D, E,* Follow-up MRI with gadolinium shows a resolution of the mass and enhancement of the ventral and dorsal dura, C3–C4 disc space, and prevertebral space. Infection may have originated from the pharynx.

means of diagnosing an epidural abscess in patients undergoing hemodialysis.[74]

Computed Tomography

CT is useful after myelography. When myelography is not safe or is unavailable, CT is used after the injection of intravenous contrast material to outline the epidural space. Characteristic findings include loss of epidural fat and fixation of contrast at the level of dural sheath, surrounded by an area of higher-density granulation tissue of higher attenuation situated between the bone and the dural sheath.[62] Gas has also been noted at the level of an epidural abscess on CT.[55]

Lumbar Puncture

Frank pus is occasionally encountered, especially in a lumbar abscess during placement of the lumbar puncture needle. Therefore, needle placement should be slow, with frequent removal of the stylet to check for pus.[5] A lumbar puncture performed below the level of the epidural abscess is often associated with a protein level greater than 350 mg/dl.[20] The cerebrospinal fluid (CSF) cell count is often elevated, with lymphocytes making up most of the total cells. Polymorphonuclear cells may predominate. Glucose content is usually normal. The CSF culture may or may not be positive.[53]

Plain Radiographs of the Spine

Plain radiographs of the spine are often unrevealing. When osteomyelitis or disc space infection is present, however, characteristic findings may include erosion of bone surrounding the disc space. Posterior elements may also be involved but may not be visualized on plain films.[1]

TREATMENT

Once the diagnosis of epidural abscess is suspected, definitive treatment is initiated without delay to minimize the risk of neurologic complications. Intravenous antibiotics are started early. The choice of drugs is tailored by clinical factors. For a person with an unknown source in an uncomplicated setting, drugs that treat *S. aureus* are most appropriate. If the patient has a known potential source, such as a skin lesion, urinary tract infection, pneumonia, or endocarditis, or positive blood cultures, antibiotics effective for the known infection are given. Immunocompromised hosts should probably be treated not only for the most common suspected organisms but also with antituberculous agents if there is a clinical suspicion warranting the toxicity of the appropriate medications.[57] Kaufman and colleagues call attention to the relative predominance of gram-negative infections among intravenous drug abusers and suggest that a history of drug abuse may warrant the use of drugs to cover gram-negative organisms as well as *Staphylococcus*.[53] Duration of drug therapy is generally four to six weeks, often with additional

prolonged oral therapy. Shorter courses of antibiotics were found by Del Curling and colleagues to be effective after surgery.[22]

Surgical decompression is the standard therapy for both acute and chronic epidural abscesses.[5, 19, 45, 46, 53] Chronic epidural abscesses require a laminectomy over the extent of the granulation tissue, with removal of as much of the granulation tissue as possible. Extensive laminectomies are reported to be well tolerated and effective.[78] The wound may be closed primarily. To treat acute epidural abscess, enough lamina should be removed to afford adequate decompression of pus. Drains may be left in the epidural space, or the wound may be packed open and allowed to granulate in.[5] Use of a closed suction-irrigation system has been reported as an alternative to open healing by secondary intention for acute epidural abscesses.[34] Suction must be maintained to be certain that all fluid is removed. Patients with associated anterior infection, and especially those with osteomyelitis, may benefit from an anterior débridement and decompression alone or combined with posterior decompression.[1, 39] Although extensive operations are known to be effective, in selected cases, limited drainage can be successful.[83]

Nonoperative therapy has been reported.[11, 20, 62, 68] In many of the reported cases, the antibiotic therapy was initiated to treat another infection, but later in the patient's course, the epidural infection was discovered and noted to be resolving.[11, 20] Planned nonoperative therapy has generally been used in patients who were poor surgical candidates because of their underlying medical conditions, as well as in patients who have extensive multilevel disease, those with minimal neurologic deficits that are nonprogressive, and those in whom there has been complete paralysis for more than 72 hours.[62] Antibiotic therapy is often used for eight to 10 weeks—longer than in patients treated operatively.

In summary, the outcome of the treatment of epidural abscess is affected by the time from admission to diagnosis and by the location of the abscess. Patients with ventral infection do better than those with dorsal infection. Recovery is related to the severity of the neurologic deficit before surgery. Many authors have noted that those with deficits persisting more than 36 hours have essentially no chance of recovery.[20, 45, 63, 79] In at least one reported case, however, a patient improved from quadriparesis 72 hours after loss of function.[24]

The outcome of an epidural abscess is reported to be adversely affected by steroid use.[20] The effects of age, underlying disease, and myelographic block are not definitive. Danner and Hartman believed that age and underlying disease were not important in the patient's overall outcome,[20] but Kaufman and associates found that the elderly, even those in good health, seemed prone to residual deficits and sometimes death from spinal epidural abscesses.[53]

When considering epidural abscesses, Heusner's statement remains as true today as in 1948. "Bad results are usually traceable to the mistaking of these disorders for a more everyday ailment until paralysis is complete and neurologic damage is irreversible."[45]

INTRAMEDULLARY ABSCESSES AND SUBDURAL EMPYEMA

Although once thought extremely rare, intramedullary spinal cord abscesses and spinal subdural empyemas are now more commonly diagnosed because of the availability and sensitivity of MRI scans.[15] Generally, these patients have histories of constitutional symptoms, including fever and leukocytosis. The clinical presentation frequently varies from that of patients with epidural abscesses, in that the spinal tenderness characteristic of epidural abscesses is usually absent.[88] Because subdural and intraspinal infections are less common than epidural abscesses, frequently the diagnosis is not made until neurologic dysfunction occurs.

Pathophysiology

Preceding or concurrent bacterial infection is commonly seen in both subdural empyemas and intramedullary abscesses.[23, 32] Congenital anomalies, especially dermal sinuses, have been implicated in the pathophysiology of abscess formation.[23] Other sources of infection are direct trauma and hematogenous spread from distant infectious foci, such as endocarditis, bronchopneumonia, bronchiectasis, lumbar puncture, middle ear infection, and mastoiditis.[23, 67] Spinal cord abscesses have been associated with ependymomas.[4] An experimental model of epidural abscess showed creation of a subdural empyema in animals that had inadvertent openings of the dura.[27]

Clinical Presentation

Signs of systemic involvement such as abdominal pain, fever, chills, and lymphocytosis are common but not always present. Progressive neurologic dysfunction is often the predominant clinical symptom.[15] Lumbar puncture often reveals evidence of meningitis or a parameningeal infection. In subdural empyemas, pleocytosis with elevated protein is frequently noted. The CSF glucose is frequently diminished.[32] With intramedullary abscesses, lumbar puncture results are often consistent with those of a parameningeal infection, with elevated protein and elevated white cell count with a lymphocytic predominance. Leukocytes and polymorphonuclear cells may predominate.[23, 70] The CSF findings are often abnormal but nondiagnostic.[67]

S. aureus is often the predominant organism, but there have been reports of tuberculomas,[17] as well as infections with streptococcal species and *L. monocytogenes*,[54, 67, 70, 76] *Candida albicans*,[64] and *Brucella*.[18] Abscesses related to congenital dermal sinuses commonly have mixed flora in which gram-negative organisms often predominate. A recent review by Bartels and coworkers[7] found that for intramedullary abscesses, the culture was sterile in 38.7 per cent of cases; positive culture grew staph A in 23.7 per cent of cases and strep species in 17 per cent of cases.

Diagnosis

The frequency of the diagnosis of these relatively rare entities has markedly increased with the use of MRI. As in the case of epidural abscesses, this could result in an improved overall outcome and lessening of permanent neurologic deficits. In an intramedullary spinal cord abscess, the characteristic myelographic finding is of a widened cord. A subdural empyema is diagnosed by an intradural extramedullary block. MRI diagnostic features include an intramedullary mass with spotty peripheral enhancement on T1 gadolinium-enhanced scans and an increased or isointense signal on T2 scans, similar to that of brain abscesses.[15]

Treatment

The treatment of subdural abscesses of the spinal cord as described in the literature is laminectomy with opening of the dura.[1, 32] The use of drains is variable in the cases reported. Treatment of intramedullary spinal abscesses includes laminectomy, opening of the dura, aspiration of the abscess cavity, and myelotomy to drain and débride.[15, 17, 67]

These infected patients need continued therapy with appropriate antibiotics based on culture or, in the rare case of a negative culture, clinical impression. The duration of antibiotics is not absolutely specific, but therapy is most commonly given for four to eight weeks. The outcome of intramedullary and subdural infections is usually related to the preoperative neurologic deficits and the length of time the deficits existed.[15, 17, 23, 32, 67, 70]

PEDIATRIC INTRASPINAL INFECTIONS

Spinal sepsis in children is even less common than in adults. Knowledge has been collected from case reports of epidural infections and intramedullary infections.[6, 10, 23, 66, 89, 94] The largest case review was published by Jacobsen and Sullivan in 1994 and includes two new cases plus 90 cases in the literature.[51] Because of an inability to articulate symptoms, the initial presentation of a child is usually nonspecific. The presenting symptoms are often fever and back pain. Spinal tenderness is often present, and the child may exhibit signs of rigidity.[82] Fever and nonspecific limp may be associated with a lumbar epidural abscess.[31] The diagnosis is commonly not made until definitive neurologic signs appear, as occurred in 76 per cent of Jacobsen and Sullivan's cases. In infants, fever and irritability are common.[80]

The pathologic process is similar to that found in adults. *S. aureus* is the most common organism found, although mixed flora are reportedly associated with dermal sinuses.[31] In addition to staphylococcosis, reported infections have included *Streptococcus* species (e.g., *S. pneumoniae*), *F. necrophorum*, and *Salmonella en-*

teritidis.[80] The posterior epidural space is involved 86 per cent of the time.[40, 47, 59, 80, 82, 91, 94]

Unique clinical circumstances associated with epidural abscesses in children have included spondylosis, dermal sinuses, serial lumbar punctures, and the Swenson procedure.[10, 82, 91, 94] Spinal epidural abscesses in children may present as an acute abdomen.[87]

Diagnostic studies are similar to those used in adults. Myelography has been used extensively, but MRI is most useful for the early evaluation and screening of patients with suspicious clinical findings and leads to earlier detection and treatment.

Treatment

As in adults, laminectomy is usually the treatment of choice, especially because few children have underlying medical conditions that increase surgical morbidity. Fisher and associates recommended that the spinal laminae be removed and replaced en bloc to decrease the risk of postoperative scoliosis.[31] Postoperative scoliosis has been reported in a few cases.[80] Good results have been seen when wounds are closed primarily and the patient is treated vigorously with appropriate antibiotics. If the wounds are closed primarily, drains are usually left in place if frank pus is present. The duration of antibiotic therapy is generally about four to six weeks.[31, 66, 94]

The outcome for young children is good, provided the neurologic deficits are recognized early enough. Children have an overall better prognosis for recovery than adults despite prolonged periods of paralysis.[66] Mortality between 12 and 17 per cent is reported, however, in the largest series. Mortality occurred at a high rate before 1980, in those presenting with paralysis, and in patients who were not treated surgically. Mortality was predominantly caused by sepsis.[51, 80]

References

1. Allen, M. B., Jr., and Beveridge, W.: Spinal epidural and subdural abscesses. *In* Wilkins, R. H., and Rengachary, S. S. (eds.): Neurosurgery. Vol. 3. New York, McGraw-Hill, 1985, pp. 1972–1975.
2. Allen, S. S., and Kahn, E. A.: Acute pyogenic infection of the spinal epidural space. JAMA 98:875–887, 1932.
3. Artz, P.: Abscess within the spinal cord. Arch. Neurol. Psych. 51:533–543, 1944.
4. Babu, R., Jafar, J. J., Huang, P. P., et al.: Intramedullary abscess associated with a spinal cord ependymoma: Case report. Neurosurgery 30:121–124, 1992.
5. Baker, A. S., Ojemann, R. G., Swartz, M. N., and Richardson, E. P., Jr.: Spinal epidural abscesses. N. Engl. J. Med. 293:463–468, 1975.
6. Baker, C. J.: Primary spinal epidural abscess. Am. J. Dis. Child. 121:338–339, 1971.
7. Bartels, R. H., deJong, T. R., and Grotenhuis, J. A.: Spinal subdural abscess: Case report. J. Neurosurg. 76:307–311, 1992.
8. Benson, C. A., and Harris, A. A.: Acute neurologic infections. Med. Clin. North Am. 70:990–1104, 1986.
9. Benzil, D. L., Epstein, M. H., and Knuckey, N. W.: Intramedullary epidermoid associated with an intramedullary spinal abscess secondary to a dermal sinus. Neurosurgery 30:118–121, 1992.
10. Bergman, I., Wald, E. R., Meyer, J. D., and Painter, M. J.: Epidural abscess and vertebral osteomyelitis following serial lumbar punctures. Pediatrics 72:476–480, 1983.
11. Bouchez, B., Arnott, G., and Delfosse, J. M.: Acute spinal epidural abscess. J. Neurol. 231:343–344, 1985.
12. Browder, J., and Meyers, R.: Pyogenic infections of the spinal epidural space. Surgery 10:296–308, 1941.
13. Buruma, O. J. S., Craane, H., and Kunst, M. W.: Vertebral osteomyelitis and epidural abscess due to mucormycosis. Clin. Neurol. Neurosurg. 81:39–44, 1979.
14. Byrd, B. F., III, Weiner, M. H., and McGee, Z. A.: *Aspergillus* spinal epidural abscess. JAMA 248:3138–3139, 1982.
15. Byrne, R. W., von Roenn, K. A., and Whisler, W. W.: Intramedullary abscess: A report of two cases and a review of the literature. Neurosurgery 35:321–326, 1994.
16. Campbell, M.: Pyogenic infections within the vertebral canal. Bull. Neurol. Inst. N. Y. 6:574, 1937.
17. Citow, J. S., and Ammirati, M.: Intramedullary tuberculoma of the spinal cord: Case report. Neurosurgery 35:327–330, 1994.
18. Cokca, F., Meco, O., Arasil, E., and Unla, A.: An intramedullary dermoid cyst abscess due to *Brucella abortus* biotype 3 at T11–L2 spinal levels. Infection 22:359–360, 1994.
19. Dandy, W. E.: Abscesses and inflammatory tumors in the spinal epidural space (so-called pachymeningitis externa). Arch. Surg. 13:477–494, 1926.
20. Danner, R. L., and Hartman, B. J.: Update of spinal epidural abscess: 35 cases and review of the literature. Rev. Infect. Dis. 9:265–274, 1987.
21. Darouiche, R. O., Hamill, R. J., Greenberg, S. B., et al.: Bacterial spinal epidural abscess: Review of 43 cases and literature survey. Medicine 71:369–385, 1992.
22. Del Curling, O., Jr., Gower, D. J., and McWhorter, J. M.: Changing concepts in spinal epidural abscess: A report of 29 cases. Neurosurgery 27:185–192, 1990.
23. DiTullio, M. V., Jr.: Intramedullary spinal abscess: A case report with a review of 53 previously described cases. Surg. Neurol. 7:351–354, 1977.
24. Durity, F., and Thompson, G. B.: Localized cervical extradural abscess. J. Neurosurg. 28:387–390, 1968.
25. Dus, V.: Spinal peripachymeningitis (epidural abscess). J. Neurosurg. 17:972–983, 1960.
26. Erntell, M., Holtas, S., Norlin, K., et al.: Magnetic resonance imaging in the diagnosis of spinal epidural abscess. Scand. J. Infect. Dis. 20:323–327, 1988.
27. Feldenzer, J. A., McKeever, P. E., Schaberg, D. R., et al.: Experimental spinal epidural abscess: A pathophysiological model in the rabbit. Neurosurgery 20:859–867, 1987.
28. Ferguson, J. F., and Krisch, W. M.: Epidural empyema following thoracic extradural block. J. Neurosurg. 41:762–764, 1974.
29. Fine, P. G., Hare, B. D., and Zahnisher, J.: Epidural abscess following epidural catheterization in a chronic pain patient: A diagnostic dilemma. Anesthesiology 69:422–424, 1988.
30. Firsching, R., Frowein, R. A., and Nittner, K.: Acute spinal epidural empyema. Acta Neurochir. 74:68–71, 1985.
31. Fisher, E. G., Greene, C. S., and Winston, K. R.: Spinal epidural abscess in children. Neurosurgery 9:257–260, 1981.
32. Fraser, R. A., Ratzan, K., Wolpert, S. M., and Weinstein, L.: Spinal subdural empyema. Arch. Neurol. 28:235–238, 1973.
33. Friedman, D. P., and Hills, J. R.: Cervical epidural spinal infection: MR imaging characteristics. AJR Am. J. Roentgenol. 163:699–704, 1994.
34. Garrido, E., and Rosenwasser, R.: Experience with the suction-irrigation technique in the management of spinal epidural infection. Neurosurgery 12:678–679, 1983.
35. Gelber, B. R., Peirson, E. W., and Birkmann, L. W.: Spinal epidural abscess. Nebr. Med. J. 66:10–15, 1981.
36. Ghosh, K., Duncan, R., and Kennedy, P.: Acute spinal epidural abscess caused by *Streptococcus milleri*. J. Infect. 16:303–304, 1988.
37. Gokalp, H. Z., and Ozkal, E.: Intradural tuberculomas of the spinal cord. J. Neurosurg. 55:289–292, 1981.
38. Grant, F.: Epidural spinal abscess. JAMA 128:509–512, 1965.
39. Grub, P., Freidrich, B., Mertens, H. G., and Bockhorn, J.: Purulent osteomyelitis of the cervical spine with epidural abscess. Clin. Neurol. Neurosurg. 79:57–61, 1977.
40. Guerrero, I. C., Slap, G. B., Macgregor, R. R., et al.: Anaerobic spinal epidural abscess. Neurosurgery 48:465, 1978.
41. Haid, R. W., Kaufman, H. H., Schochet, S. S., and Marano, G. D.: Epidural lipomatosis simulating an epidural abscess: Case report and literature review. Neurosurgery 21:744, 1987.

42. Hainline, B., Tuszynski, M. H., and Posner, J. B.: Ataxia in epidural spinal cord compression. Neurology 42:2193–2195, 1992.
43. Hardjasudarma, M., Willis, B., Black-Payne, C., and Edwards, R.: Pediatric spinal blastomycosis: Case report. Neurosurgery 37:534–536, 1995.
44. Hendrix, W. C., Arruda, L. K., Platts-Mills, T. A., et al.: *Aspergillus* epidural abscess and cord compression in a patient with aspergilloma and empyema: Survival and response to high dose systemic amphotericin therapy. Am. Rev. Respir. Dis. 145:1483–1486, 1992.
45. Heusner, A. P.: Nontuberculous spinal epidural infections. N. Engl. J. Med. 239:845–854, 1948.
46. Hlavin, M. L., Kaminski, H. J., Ross, J. S., and Ganz, E.: Spinal epidural abscess: A ten-year perspective. Neurosurgery 27:177–184, 1990.
47. Hulme, A.: Spinal epidural abscess. Br. Med. J. 1:64–68, 1954.
48. Hutton, P. W.: Acute osteomyelitis of cervical spine with epidural abscess. Br. Med. J. 1:153–154, 1956.
49. Iannettoni, M. D., Whyte, R. I., and Orringer, M. B.: Catastrophic complications of the cervical esophagogastric anastomosis. J. Thorac. Cardiovasc. Surg. 110:1493–1500, 1995.
50. Jabbari, B., and Pierce, J.: Spinal cord compression due to *Pseudomonas* in a heroin addict. Neurology 27:1034–1037, 1977.
51. Jacobsen, F. S., and Sullivan, B.: Spinal epidural abscesses in children. Orthopedics 17:1131–1138, 1994.
52. Jamison, M. H., Stanworth, P., and Maclennan, I.: An unusual rectal fistula: Extradural abscess discharging per rectum. Br. J. Surg. 71:651–652, 1984.
53. Kaufman, D. M., Kaplan, J. G., and Litman, N.: Infectious agents in spinal epidural abscesses. Neurology 30:844–850, 1980.
54. King, S. J., and Jeffree, M. A.: MRI of an abscess of the cervical spinal cord in a case of *Listeria* meningoencephalomyelitis. Neuroradiology 35:495–496, 1993.
55. Kirzner, H., Oh, Y. K., and Lee, S. H.: Intraspinal air: A CT finding of epidural abscess. AJR Am. J. Roentgenol. 151:1217–1218, 1988.
56. Kokes, F., Iplikcioglu, A. C., Camurdanoglu, M., et al.: Epidural spinal abscess containing gas: MRI demonstration. Neuroradiology 35:497–498, 1993.
57. Koppel, B. S., Tuchman, A. J., Mangiardi, J. R., et al.: Epidural spinal infection in intravenous drug abusers. Arch. Neurol. 45:1331, 1988.
58. Kricun, R., Shoemaker, E. I., Chovanes, G. I., and Stephens, H. W.: Epidural abscess of the cervical spine: MR findings in five cases. AJR Am. J. Roentgenol. 158:1145–1149, 1992.
59. Kuiters, R. F., Douma, G., and Hekster, R. E. M.: Spinal epidural abscess. Clin. Neurol. Neurosurg. 89:255–260, 1987.
60. Lagging, L. M., Breland, C. M., Kennedy, D. J., et al.: Delayed treatment of pulmonary blastomycosis causing vertebral osteomyelitis, paraspinal abscess, and spinal cord compression. Scand. J. Infect. Dis. 26:111–115, 1994.
61. LaRocca, H.: Spinal sepsis. *In* Rothman, R., and Simeone, F. (eds.): The Spine. Philadelphia, W. B. Saunders, Co., 1982, pp. 757–774.
62. Leys, D., Lesoin, F., Viaud, C., et al.: Decreased morbidity from acute bacterial spinal epidural abscesses using computed tomography and nonsurgical treatment in selected patients. Ann. Neurol. 17:350–355, 1985.
63. Liem, L. K., Rigamonti, D., Wolf, A. L., et al.: Thoracic epidural abscess. J. Spinal Disord. 7:449–454, 1994.
64. Lindner, A., Becker, G., Warmuth-Metz, M., et al.: Magnetic resonance image findings of spinal intramedullary abscess caused by *Candida albicans*: Case report. Neurosurgery 36:411–412, 1995.
65. Markham, J. W., Lynge, H. N., and Stahman, G.: The syndrome of spontaneous spinal epidural hematoma. J. Neurosurg. 26:334–342, 1967.
66. Marks, W., and Bodensteiner, J.: Anterior cervical epidural abscess with pneumococcus in an infant. J. Child Neurol. 3:25–29, 1988.
67. Menezes, A. H., Graf, C. J., and Perret, G. E.: Spinal cord abscess: A review. Surg. Neurol. 8:461–467, 1977.
68. Messer, H. D., Lenchner, G. S., Brust, J. C., and Resor, S.: Lumbar spinal abscess managed conservatively. J. Neurosurg. 46:825–829, 1977.
69. Mixter, W. J., and Smithwick, R.: Acute intraspinal epidural abscess. N. Engl. J. Med. 207:126–131, 1932.
70. Morrison, R., Brown, J., and Gooding, R. S.: Spinal cord abscess caused by *Listeria monocytogenes*. Arch. Neurol. 37:243–244, 1980.
71. Murr, M. M., and Metcalf, A. M.: Spinal epidural abscess complicating an ileal J-pouch-anal anastomosis: Report of a case. Dis. Colon Rectum 36:293–294, 1993.
72. Numaguchi, Y., Rigamonti, D., Rothman, M. I., et al.: Spinal epidural abscess: Evaluation with gadolinium-enhanced MR imaging. Radiographics 13:545–559, 1993.
73. Nussbaum, E. S., Rigamonti, D., Standiford, H., et al.: Spinal epidural abscess: A report of 40 cases and review. Surg. Neurol. 38:225–231, 1992.
74. Obrador, G. T., and Levenson, D. J.: Spinal epidural abscess in hemodialysis patients: Report of three cases and review of the literature. Am. J. Kidney Dis. 27:75–83, 1996.
75. Paz, J. F., Alvarez, F. J., Roda, J. M., et al.: Spinal epidural abscess caused by brucella: Case report. J. Neurosurg. Sci. 38:245–249, 1994.
76. Pfadenhauer, K., and Rossmanith, T.: Spinal manifestation of neurolisteriosis. J. Neurol. 242:53–156, 1995.
77. Rana, P., Raghunath, D., Parakkal, K., et al.: Spinal epidural abscess to *Salmonella* group C monophasic 1, 5. J. Neurosurg. 62:942–943, 1985.
78. Richmond, B. K., and Schmidt, J. H.: Seventeen level laminectomy for extensive spinal epidural abscess: Case report and review. W. V. Med. J. 90:468–471, 1994.
79. Rigamonti, D., Liem, L., Wolf, A. L., et al.: Epidural abscess in the cervical spine. Mt. Sinai J. Med. 61:357–362, 1994.
80. Rubin, G., Michowiz, S. D., Ashkenasi, A., et al.: Spinal epidural abscess in the pediatric age group: Case report and review of the literature. Pediatr. Infect. Dis. J. 12:1007–1011, 1993.
81. Sage, R. A., Miller, J. M., Stuck, R., and Pinzur, M.: The foot as a primary site for distant metastatic infection. J. Foot Ankle Surg. 33:567–571, 1994.
82. Salmon, J. H.: Intraspinal infections. *In* Pediatric Neurosurgery. New York, Grune & Stratton, 1982, pp. 587–590.
83. Sathi, S., Schwartz, M., Cortez, S., and Rossitch, E.: Spinal subdural abscess: Successful treatment with limited drainage and antibiotics in a patient with AIDS. Surg. Neurol. 42:424–427, 1994.
84. Scerpella, E. G., Wu, S., and Oefinger, P. E.: Case report of spinal epidural abscess caused by *Haemophilus paraphrophilus*. J. Clin. Microbiol. 32:563–564, 1994.
85. Schlossberg, D., and Shulman, J. A.: Spinal epidural abscess. South. Med. J. 70:669–673, 1977.
86. Schmutzard, E., Aichner, F., Dierchx, A., et al.: New perspectives in acute spinal epidural abscess. Acta Neurochir. 80:105–181, 1986.
87. Tyson, G. W., Grant, A., and Strachan, W. E.: Spinal epidural abscess presenting as acute abdomen in a child. Br. J. Surg. 66:3–4, 1979.
88. Verner, E. F., and Musher, D. M.: Spinal epidural abscess. Med. Clin. North Am. 69:375–384, 1985.
89. Villiers, J. C., and de V. Cluver, P. F.: Spinal epidural abscess in children. S. Afr. J. Surg. 16:149–155, 1978.
90. Wagner, D., Varkey, B., Sheth, N., and DaMert, G.: Epidural abscess, vertebral destruction, and paraplegia caused by extending infection from an aspergilloma. Am. J. Med. 78:518–522, 1988.
91. Watters, D. A., Moussa, S. A., and Buyukpamukcu, N.: Epidural abscess complicating Swenson procedure: A case report and a review of the literature. J. Pediatr. Surg. 9:218–220, 1984.
92. Watts, J. W., and Mixter, W. J.: Spinal epidural granulomas. N. Engl. J. Med. 204:1335–1344, 1931.
93. Wright, R. L.: Infections of the spine and spinal cord. *In* Youmans, R. (ed.): Neurological Surgery. Philadelphia, W. B. Saunders Co., 1982.
94. Yu, L., and Emans, J.: Epidural abscess associated with spondylosis. J. Bone Joint Surg. [Am.] 70:444–447, 1988.

45

Interventional Neuroradiology of the Spine

Robert C. Wallace, M.D.

Thomas J. Masaryk, M.D.

SPINAL VASCULAR ANATOMY

Thirty-one pairs of segmental arteries (or the regional equivalent, e.g., bronchial arteries) supply the spinal column and surrounding structures.[38, 42, 43, 117, 151, 195] The bone, muscle, and connective tissues at each vertebral level (with the exception of the spinal cord) receive blood from the bilateral segmental arteries or their equivalents at the same and/or adjacent levels.[38, 42, 43, 117, 151, 195] Branches of the segmental arteries extend posteriorly from the aorta, providing extraspinal arteries that supply muscle, bone (via the anterior central arteries), and nerve roots as well as intraspinal radicular branch arteries that supply bone and neural structures, including the meninges, epidural soft tissue structures, and spinal cord within the vertebral canal.[42, 43, 117, 151, 195] The radicular arteries are the first branches of the dorsal segmental arteries or their equivalent. They enter the intervertebral foramina (as either single or multiple vessels) accompanying the emerging veins and spinal nerves. At this point the radicular arteries on each side of the vertebrae may ultimately divide into a triad of vessels: the posterior central and prelaminar arteries (to supply the bony vertebral body and posterior elements and spinal cord, respectively) and, variably, a radiculomedullary artery to the anterior spinal cord.[38, 42, 43, 117, 151, 195] Radicular arteries have an ascending course with their segmental nerve roots whose obliquity increases from the cranial to caudal.[42, 43, 117] Therefore, the levels of spinal cord supply are frequently not the same as those of the bone served by the same segmental trunk.

The blood supply to the spinal cord itself is based on three rostracaudal arterial trunks, a single anterior spinal artery and paired posterior spinal arteries, which extend from the medulla oblongata to the conus medullaris, covering three major vascular territories or "zones":[38, 42, 43, 117, 119, 120] cervicothoracic, midthoracic, and thoracolumbar. Although these vertical arteries are usually continuous along the length of the cord, the anterior spinal artery is narrowest in the midthoracic region and widest in the cervical region.[52]

The number of anterior radiculomedullary arteries supplying the single *anterior spinal artery* rarely exceeds 9 but has been reported to vary from 2 to 17. The artery of Adamkiewicz is the largest anterior medullary feeder and supplies the thoracolumbar region. It occurs on the left side in 80 per cent of subjects and can arise anywhere between T5 and L4 (T9–L2 in 85 per cent, T9–T11 in 75 per cent, L1–L2 in 10 per cent, and T5–T8 in 15 per cent).[52] The anterior arterial trunk to the spinal cord is a centrifugal system formed by central arteries that arise from the anterior spinal artery, run horizontally in the central sulcus, and turn alternately to the right and to the left.[93, 197] This centrifugal system supplies the central gray matter and an adjacent mantle of central white matter that includes the corticospinal tracts.[197]

The posterior radiculomedullary feeders supplying the paired *posterior spinal arteries* are more numerous, varying from 10 to 23.[86, 102] The posterior spinal arteries run in the posterolateral sulcus and are also supplied by radicular arteries derived from segmental arteries or their regional equivalents (including the vertebral arteries and the posterior inferior cerebellar arteries). The posterior spinal vessels comprise an interconnected anastomotic plexus forming a centripetally oriented vascular territory with penetrating branches that supply one third to one half of the outer spinal cord.[65] In some cases the artery of Adamkiewicz supplies the entire lumbosacral cord, including the posterior spinal arteries.

VASCULAR MALFORMATIONS

In the past, vascular malformations of the spine and spinal cord have been categorized according to etiology and histologic configuration, angiographic pattern and relationship to the vascular supply of the spinal cord, and macroscopic appearance at the time of surgery.[4, 44, 185] Unfortunately, this diversity of classification criteria resulted in a wide variety of complex and confusing nomenclature for a group of relatively rare lesions. It is hoped that this section represents a distillation of the seminal features of each malformation that are important to its diagnosis and management. Readers interested in additional information are referred to the articles by Rosenblum and colleagues,[159] Heros and coworkers,[92] and Oldfield and Doppman.[146]

Technically, vascular malformations of the spine and spinal cord are analogous to similar malformations in the brain; such lesions may be further subdivided into (1) arteriovenous malformations (both dural and parenchymal), (2) cavernous angiomas (cavernous hemangiomas), and (3) capillary telangiectases. Exceptions to the analogy between the brain and spine vascular malformations are the venous angiomas, which represent a distinct entity in the brain. With respect to the spine, the term *venous angioma* has in the past been erroneously applied to the radiculomeningeal (dural) arteriovenous malformations; it is unclear as to whether venous angiomas exist as such in the spine and, if so, whether they are clinically significant or, like those in the brain, are normal variants of venous anatomy.

ARTERIOVENOUS MALFORMATIONS

The arteriovenous malformations (AVMs) may contain a complex network with multiple interconnecting channels called the "nidus," which is situated between an artery and vein; this may consist of a single direct connection between the feeding artery and draining vein known as a fistula. Lesions within the spinal cord containing a nidus are called spinal cord arteriovenous malformations (SCAVMs) or radiculomedullary AVMs. Those spinal cord lesions with fistulous connections may have single or sometimes multiple, direct, artery-to-vein connections that are usually located on the surface of the cord. Fistulas occurring outside of the neuraxis along the dural covering have vascular supply in common with the spinal cord but are separate lesions and in this location are called spinal dural fistulas (SDFs) or radiculomeningeal fistulas.[159]

Of paramount importance to the pathophysiology, presenting signs/symptoms, diagnosis, and treatment of these lesions is the location of the fistulous nidus with respect to the spinal cord and its vascular supply.[46] The presence of posterior or lateral cutaneous angiomas at the same segmental level as the AVM occurs in 12 to 21 per cent of such patients.[3, 41, 47] These are referred to as metameric malformations, indicating their common embryologic origin, and can, by simple inspection, be seen to denote the approximate level of the intraspinal portion of the malformation. In a retrospective review of their experience with 81 spinal vascular malformations, Rosenblum and associates found 67 per cent of cases to be intradural and in 33 per cent the nidus was located within the meninges; in other series SDFs are more common, with reports suggesting as many as 85 per cent of spinal vascular malformations may be dural.[145, 159]

Intradural (Radiculomedullary) Malformations: SCAVMs

Classification

Previous classifications of spinal cord arteriovenous malformations (SCAVMs) referred to intradural-intramedullary lesions as either "juvenile" or "glomus malformations" and intradural-extramedullary malformations as superficially placed direct pial AV fistulas involving a radiculomedullary feeding artery. Both lesions possess arterial supplies common to the spinal cord. Intramedullary (often with anterior radiculomedullary supply) lesions are embedded deep within the spinal cord and are extremely difficult to treat without grave risk of neurologic deficit. This is in contradistinction to lesions that have the nidus located more superficially, usually on the dorsal aspect of the cord. These more superficial lesions (commonly with posterior radiculomedullary supply) are more remedial to surgical resection.[45]

Diagnostic Evaluation

Magnetic resonance imaging (MRI) is the modality of choice for the initial evaluation of a vascular malformation in the spinal cord. Experiences of Doppman and colleagues[45] and DiChiro and coworkers[37] indicate that MRI may be useful in detecting such lesions by its ability to reveal low-signal feeding and draining vessels within the spinal cord by identifying flow voids most noticeable on T2-weighted images (Fig. 45–1). Additionally, sagittal and/or coronal T1-weighted images may further characterize the malformation by revealing the low-signal nidus and enlarged anterior spinal artery of intramedullary lesions.[37, 45] With this constellation of findings, MRI can distinguish such lesions from spinal hemangioblastomas—a task that may be difficult with myelography, computed tomography (CT), or even angiography.[37] It is also possible to document the response to therapy of such lesions with MRI by virtue of its ability to detect thrombosis through the absence of flow void.[45]

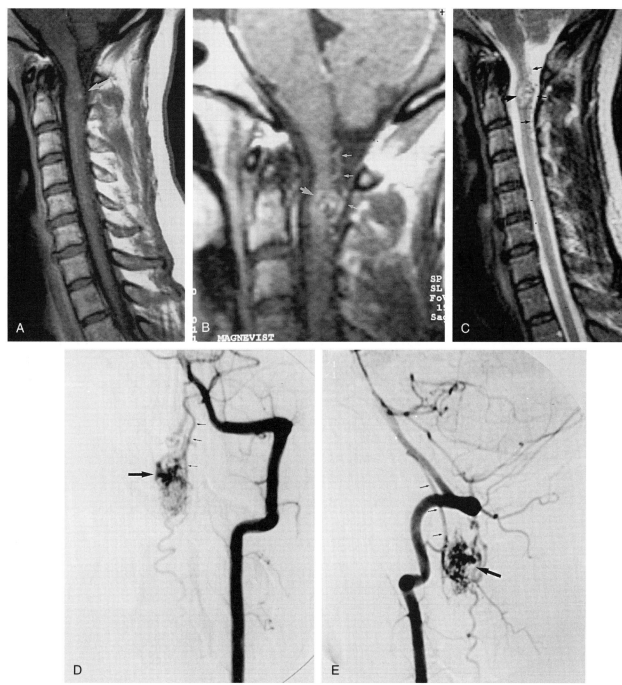

Figure 45–1. Cervical cord arteriovenous malformation (AVM). *A,* Sagittal noncontrast T1-weighted image shows mild cord expansion, mild heterogeneous signal, and tiny flow voids *(arrow)*. *B,* Magnified post-gadolinium T1-weighted sagittal image of the cervical spine demonstrates mild cord enlargement at the C2 level. There is enhancement following contrast administration within the nidus *(short arrow)* of the AVM and enhancement of several vessels dorsal to the cord *(small arrows)* at the C1–C2 level. *C,* Sagittal T2-weighted image shows focal flow voids dorsal to the cord *(small arrows)* and cord enlargement with heterogeneous signal within the cord *(short arrow)* at the site of the AVM nidus. Anteroposterior *(D)* and lateral *(E)* left vertebral angiogram run demonstrates the nidus of the AVM *(arrow)* centered within the cervical cord with arterial supply from the anterior spinal artery *(small arrows)*.

Angiography is critical in determining the relationship of the vascular anatomy of the lesion and the relation to the spinal cord vascular supply prior to embolization or surgical resection. Angiography will also provide the most accurate information about the location of feeding arteries, draining veins, and the nidus angioarchitecture (Fig. 45–2). Because of their high-flow state, such lesions may be accompanied by arterial aneurysms (44 per cent).[145] Angiography provides information about aneurysms on the feeding pedicle, intranidal aneurysms, or aneurysmal dilatation of the drainage vein (varix). All of these indicate the AVM or fistula has a higher risk of hemorrhage.

Natural History and Clinical Presentation

SCAVMs are congenital and are more commonly cervical or cervicothoracic, possessing a relatively large shunt volume fed by arteries that normally supply the cord.[92, 159] Consequently, these lesions generally present relatively early (before 50 years of age; in Rosenblum's series, mean age was 27 years) with symptoms of vascular steal (ischemia) or, more commonly, subarachnoid hemorrhage, and/or hematomyelia.[159] Among patients with intradural malformations (i.e., those fed by both anterior and posterior radiculomedullary vessels), there is an approximately equal distribution among both sexes.

Symptoms of SCAVMs at presentation range from back and radicular pain in 15 to 20 per cent to paresis in over 90 per cent of patients. Sensory as well as bowel and bladder dysfunction also is commonly seen in 75 to 80 per cent, respectively.[40, 159, 200] The most significant and most common complication is hemorrhage, which may result in neurologic deficit from intramedullary hemorrhage or result in a subarachnoid hemorrhage. The incidence of hemorrhage is higher for cervical than for thoracolumbar lesions, ranging from 57 to 78 per cent in the cervical region and 20 to 37 per cent in the thoracolumbar levels.[16, 40, 200] The overall mortality rate from hemorrhage is in the range of 18 per cent,[4] with significant morbidity occurring in the remaining patients. The natural history for SCAVM second hemorrhage is 10 per cent in the first month and 40 per cent in the first year.[4]

Rationale and Technical Aspects of Treatment

Because of the severe consequences of hemorrhage, patients presenting and diagnosed with SCAVMs should be treated with the primary goal of treatment being total obliteration by endovascular embolization and/or surgical resection. If complete obliteration cannot be obtained by one of these methods, the treatment should be directed toward endovascular occlusion of high-risk portions of the AVM—specifically aneurysms

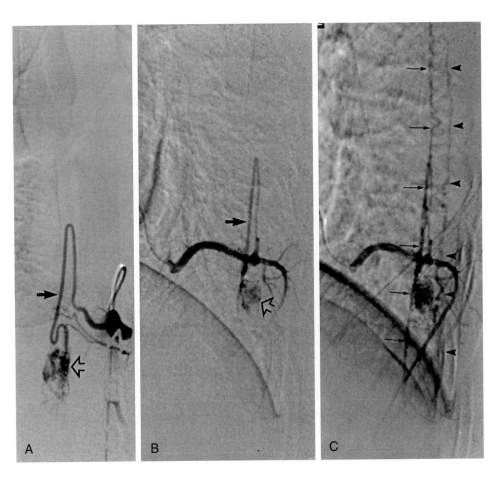

Figure 45–2. Thoracic cord AVM. Anteroposterior *(A)* and early phase lateral *(B)* spinal angiogram demonstrates supply from the anterior spinal artery *(arrow)* to the AVM nidus *(open arrow)* located in the lower thoracic cord. *C,* Lateral angiogram run later in the series demonstrates drainage into the veins surrounding the ventral *(arrows)* and dorsal *(arrowheads)* aspect of the spinal cord.

of the feeding pedicle, intranidal aneurysms, or varices that would be the likely source for hemorrhage. Second hemorrhages may occur in incompletely treated lesions.

Patients with permanent deficits may not improve with embolization; however, these lesions should be treated to prevent subsequent hemorrhage, which could be life-threatening. Cervical and upper thoracic cord lesions have potentially higher risk because of the proximity to the intracranial subarachnoid cisterns, where subarachnoid hemorrhage is likely to result in more severe neurologic impairment. Once a fixed deficit is present, the likelihood of making it worse is much less likely. Patients with associated cutaneous lesions (metameric AVMs) should be considered as having CNS and non-CNS components, with the CNS component treated as a SCAVM and the non-CNS component treated as necessary for preservation of function and cosmesis.

N-butyl-cyanoacrylate (NBCA) and PVA (polyvinyl alcohol) particles are the two most common embolic agents used for the treatment of SCAVMs. Because NBCA is a more permanent agent, it has advantages over particulate agents if durable cure is the goal of embolization. Complication rates from embolization have been reported as 11 per cent permanent and 11 per cent transient neurologic deficits.[16] While PVA has been described to be safer[128, 187] for palliative embolization, it may not provide a permanent cure.[80] However, PVA may be used for temporary devascularization prior to surgery.

Somatosensory evoked potential monitoring has been used to rapidly determine compromise in spinal cord blood flow during therapeutic embolization procedures.[17] Provocative testing can also be used prior to embolization to predict the likelihood of a resultant neurologic deficit. If the patient is awake, neurologic status can be compared before and after a superselective injection of 50 to 75 mg of amobarbital sodium (Amytal) from the catheter position to be used for embolization. Spinal electrophysiologic monitoring using somatosensory evoked potentials can be performed in conjunction with a superselective injection of Amytal in patients embolized while under general anesthesia.[16]

Radiculomeningeal Malformations: SDFs

Classification

Dural vascular malformations—long an enigmatic vascular spinal lesion—most frequently are recognized surgically and angiographically by the enlarged, arterialized, slow, draining coronal veins of the spinal cord. These lesions have previously been referred to as *angioma racemosum venosum, malformation retro-medulaire, venous angioma,* or *long dorsal arteriovenous malformations,* but are best referred to as spinal dural fistulas (SDFs). Unlike their high-flow medullary counterparts, these lesions are believed to be acquired and are typically present in the thoracic and thoracolumbar spine of

patients over age 50 (the large majority of whom are men).[4, 44, 145, 159]

Diagnostic Evaluation

Spinal angiography demonstrates direct shunting of contrast from the radiculomeningeal artery supply into the extensive and tortuous perimedullary system (Fig. 45–3*A*). Usually, the feeding artery arises from dural arterial supply, most commonly in the thoracolumbar region. Myelography may be used as a less invasive screening tool to demonstrate abnormal intradural vessels. These vessels represent the dilated coronal venous plexus along the dorsal surface of the spinal cord and are best seen on supine myelogram films.

Magnetic resonance is unlikely to replace myelography and angiography in the evaluation of such lesions; however, it is important to recognize the MRI findings (Fig. 45–3*B, C,* and *D*) in patients being evaluated for myelopathy because these lesions are potentially amenable to surgical relief. As are parenchymal AVMs of the spinal cord, draining vessels of these dural lesions are identified as serpentine areas of low signal within the spinal canal on sagittal T2-weighted images.[123] Axial T1- and T2-weighted images locate the low-signal dilated coronal veins in their expected peripheral and circumferential location about the spinal cord.[123] Occasionally higher-signal thrombi may be seen within these structures. It is possible to appreciate the spinal cord edema first described by Aminoff and coworkers[2] in the lower spinal cord segments as areas of low signal on T1-weighted images that progressively increase in signal with more T2-weighting, despite the fact that the actual nidus may be far removed from this region.[123] These intramedullary signal derangements may reverse following successful treatment. Furthermore, Terwey and associates[186] have described contrast enhancement within the ischemic segment of the distal cord (centrally) as well as more peripheral enhancement in the draining veins that was more conspicuous on delayed images (40 to 45 minutes) than on those acquired immediately after injection. Larsson and colleagues[116] have also described MRI findings in patients suspected of having sustained venous spinal cord infarction secondary to a dural AVM, although in these patients the degree of cord enhancement appeared to be much greater. Such findings may mimic an intramedullary neoplasm during the acute phase, when there is often cord enlargement with variable enhancement; chronic cases may demonstrate cord atrophy.

Natural History and Clinical Presentation

The mode of presentation is quite different from SCAVMs, commonly a slowly progressive myelopathy with (typically) lower extremity paraparesis and bowel or bladder symptoms[145, 159] that often are exacerbated by exertion; one report[110] even describes deterioration with menses. Rarely a sudden thrombophlebitis, the probable cause of a so-called Foix-Alajouanine syndrome, may produce rapid deterioration.[33, 196] Alterna-

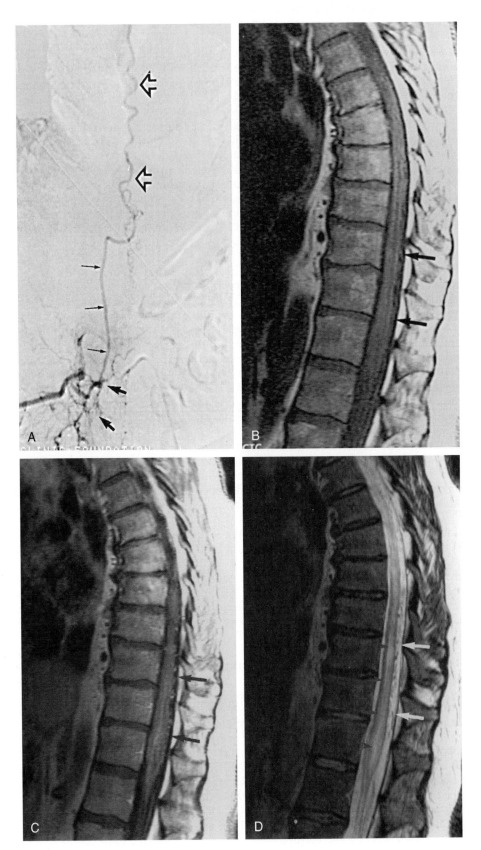

Figure 45–3. Spinal dural fistula. *A,* Diagnostic spinal angiogram demonstrates the spinal dural fistula *(short arrows)* with drainage through the radicular vein *(small arrows)* into the coronal plexus *(open arrows).* Sagittal noncontrast T1-weighted image *(B)* and sagittal post-gadolinium administration T1-weighted image *(C)* of the thoracic spine demonstrate vessels dorsal to the thoracic cord *(arrows).* These vessels are better seen after gadolinium contrast administration. *D,* T2-weighted sagittal thoracic MRI demonstrates flow voids dorsal to the cord in the same area as enhancement on T1-weighted image *(white arrows).* This corresponds to an abnormally engorged coronal venous plexus within the thoracic spine. There is also abnormal increased signal within the cord due to edema *(black arrowheads).*

tively, hemorrhage is not associated with SDFs unlike its intradural counterpart (SCAVMs). Rare exceptions may occur due to hemorrhage from an aneurysm on the feeding artery pedicle to a dural fistula. Originally termed *extramedullary*, these lesions came under serious scrutiny in 1974 when Aminoff and associates[2] argued that their myelopathic symptoms were the product of intramedullary edema and ischemia secondary to raised venous back pressure within the varicosed coronal veins of the spinal cord. The dural site of arteriovenous shunting, however, remained to be discovered by Kendall and Logue[109] in 1977. Interestingly, the edema appears to cause symptoms initially in the most distal (dependent) portion of the spinal cord regardless of the level of the dural nidus. Indeed, numerous reports[66, 153, 177, 198] describe lesions arising from feeding arteries in the internal iliac pedicles as well as cervicocerebral vessels, including posterior meningeal branches of the vertebral, middle meningeal, occipital, and ascending pharyngeal artery branches of the external carotid and dural vessels arising at the carotid siphon.

Rationale and Technical Aspects of Treatment

Both endovascular and conventional surgery for SDFs have minimal risk. Successful treatment is obtained by interrupting the venous drainage by coagulation or excision of the dura at the site of the fistula at surgery[135, 145, 180, 200] or by simply occluding the fistula by endovascular means.[16, 128] Obliteration of the fistula relieves the congestive myelopathy, usually resulting in clinical improvement, and in the remaining patients the progression of progressive myelopathy is stopped, arresting the progression of symptoms. The best clinical results will be seen in patients with the shortest time between onset of symptoms and treatment.[80, 128, 135]

A spinal dural AV fistula (SDF) is an indication for treatment because of relatively low treatment risk relative to the natural history. Because improvement in neurologic sequela is common, this also applies to patients with fixed neurologic deficits. In general, the principle of embolization is permanent occlusion of the fistula usually with NBCA.[16] Occlusion of the proximal portion of the draining vein ensures occlusion of the fistula. PVA particles will occlude the feeding pedicle proximal to the fistula with resultant collateral formation that will reconstitute the fistula and therefore should not be used.[16, 118] Contraindications to embolization include anterior spinal artery supply from the same pedicle as the SDAVF and patients in whom the anterior spinal artery is not identified and may arise or have collateral supply from the same pedicle.[129] However, conventional surgical treatment can be performed with excellent clinical results in these patients. Anticoagulation after treatment has been advocated in patients with large draining veins to reduce the likelihood of thrombosis until the vein is decreased in size due to the decreased flow. If no improvement is seen in 4 to 6 weeks, a repeat angiogram should be performed to confirm absence of the fistula.

Cavernous Hemangiomas

Cavernous hemangiomas are uncommon spinal vascular malformations. They are postcapillary malformations that consist of dilated endothelium-lined sinusoids separated by thin strands of fibrous tissue devoid of smooth muscle and elastic fibers.[106, 126, 165] They are histologically distinguished from capillary telangiectases by their abundance of hemosiderin and the paucity of intervening normal neural tissue.[106, 126, 165] Histologic parallels and the reported presence of both lesions in the central nervous system of a single patient suggest that they are, in fact, representatives of a single entity.[18, 85, 106, 125, 126, 165]

Cavernous angiomas, or cavernomas, may affect any part of the neural axis but are generally seen intracranially. Whereas they have been estimated to represent 5 to 12 per cent of all spinal vascular anomalies, most arise within the vertebral bodies and only occasionally extend into the extradural space.[106] Purely extradural or intradural extramedullary lesions have been reported, but strictly intramedullary lesions are rare.[76, 106, 151, 157] Grossly the intramedullary lesions are usually solitary and can be identified as a mulberry lesion or simply a discoloration of the cord substance. There are no abnormal leptomeningeal vessels. Cavernous angiomas are composed of multiple cysts containing old blood with dense fibrous walls and occasional calcification. The presence of a fibrous capsule may facilitate surgical excision.[203]

Diagnostic Evaluation

Fontaine and coworkers[59] have described the MRI appearance of intramedullary cavernous hemangiomas. These lesions typically have a peripheral area of low signal on T1- and T2-weighted spin-echo images thought to be secondary to the abundant hemosiderin contained within them[59] (Fig. 45–4). The central portion may have variable areas of increased and decreased signal secondary to the presence of calcifications and various forms of hemoglobin.[59] It should be remembered that the signal-intensity characteristics of hemoglobin and its breakdown products are variable depending on the concentration, magnetic field strength, and pulse sequence used.[51, 68]

Because of calcifications that are commonly present in these lesions, these malformations may be seen as punctate areas of increased density on CT. Mild cord enlargement may be appreciated on myelography depending on the size of the cavernous hemangioma. However, neither CT or myelography are routinely used for evaluation of these lesions. The imaging appearance of capillary telangiectasia of the spinal cord has yet to be reported.

Natural History and Presentation

Clinically the lesions may be asymptomatic, or may present with progressive paraparesis and sensory loss with pain that is difficult to distinguish from chronic

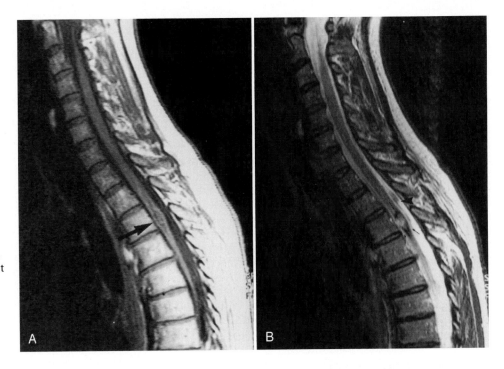

Figure 45–4. Cavernous malformation. *A,* Sagittal T1-weighted image at the cervicothoracic junction demonstrates a focal area of mild cord expansion and hypointense signal *(arrow)*. *B,* In the same area the T2-weighted image demonstrates a focal area of hyperintense signal surrounded by a rim of decreased signal intensity *(small black arrows)*. There is CSF flow artifact dorsal to the cord *(arrowhead)* but no flow in abnormal vessels. Decreased signal surrounding the margins of the lesion is consistent with hemosiderin or ferritin deposition from chronic hemorrhage.

progressive radiculomyelopathy or the Foix-Alajouanine syndrome.[31] Rarely a patient may present with acute subarachnoid hemorrhage or hematomyelia.[106] Surgical strategies are related to extirpation, with no current role for endovascular treatment.

Direct Vertebral Arteriovenous Fistulas

Classification

A separate type of fistula, called a direct vertebral arteriovenous fistula, may occur with a single direct communication between the vertebral artery and the immediately adjacent foraminal and/or intradural veins. Many of these lesions are spontaneous and relate to underlying vascular dysplasia such as fibromuscular dysplasia (FMD),[94] collagen vascular disorders (e.g., Ehlers-Danlos syndrome),[14] or neurofibromatosis Type I (NF I),[152] but in a trauma setting lesions are more commonly due to gunshot or knife-stab wounds.[79] Iatrogenic fistulas associated with anterior cervical diskectomy have also been reported.[32]

Diagnostic Evaluation

Diagnostic angiography will show a high-flow lesion with rapid shunting of contrast from the vertebral artery into the adjacent vein (Fig. 45–5). Evaluation of the contralateral vertebral artery usually demonstrates "steal" effect with retrograde flow down the distal

Figure 45–5. Vertebral artery fistula. *A,* Early AP projection angiogram shows the fistulous connection *(small arrows)* between the vertebral artery *(bold arrow)* and internal jugular vein *(open arrow)*. Retrograde flow into the intracranial system–sigmoid sinus *(arrowheads)* is seen early in the run. *B,* Slightly delayed view demonstrates retrograde flow through the left sigmoid and transverse sinus *(single arrowheads),* filling the contralateral transverse sinus *(double arrowheads)*. *C,* Right vertebral angiogram demonstrates retrograde flow in the distal left vertebral artery *(arrow)* filling the fistula *(small arrows)*. This creates a "steal" from the intracranial posterior circulation. *D,* Lateral external carotid angiogram demonstrates a fistulous connection between the occipital artery *(small arrows)* and early filling of the jugular vein *(open arrow)* and dural sinus *(arrowhead)* during the arterial phase. Trapping the vertebral artery fistula component would result in a residual occipital artery fistula. *E,* Transvenous catheter placement in the internal jugular vein *(open arrow)* for retrograde coil occlusion of the fistula. Initial coils are placed within the fistula *(small arrows)*. *F,* Posttreatment lateral angiogram of the external carotid artery shows no residual occipital artery supply. Because of reduced flow the size of the artery has decreased. Normal occipital artery *(small arrows)*. *G,* AP view of the right vertebral artery shows no reversal of flow in the distal left vertebral artery *(arrow)*. *H,* Lateral view of the left vertebral artery demonstrating a patent vertebral artery with a focal outpouching at the previous fistula site *(arrow)*. *I,* Posttherapeutic coil occlusion of the vertebral artery was performed at 6-month follow-up because of slight enlargement of the aneurysm (outpouching). Coils occlude the fistula site *(arrow)* and extend above and below that level. The patient tolerated the procedure without any difficulty.

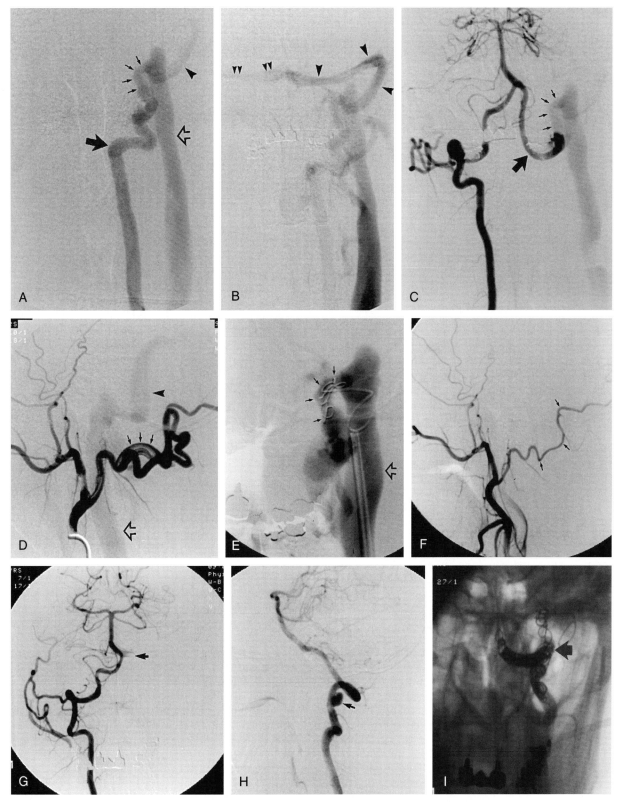

Figure 45–5 *See legend on opposite page*

aspect of the ipsilateral vertebral artery with early opacification of the veins (Fig. 45–5C). A "steal" from the cerebral circulation may also be demonstrated on carotid angiography. Angiography should include evaluation of the adjacent territories to determine additional fistulous sites (Fig. 45–5D), as well as an assessment of the venous drainage. Those draining superficially into the jugular system may present differently than those with common epidural or especially intradural spinal cord drainage. Arterial irregularity is commonly present in cases in which vascular dysplasias are the etiology.

Spin-echo MRI studies typically demonstrate a unilaterally enlarged vertebral artery with multiple lobulated areas of flow void intra- and extradurally at the approximate level of the fistulous communication. Gradient echo studies may identify these same vessels with high signal on the basis of flow-related enhancement. Intradural vessels may demonstrate significant mass effect on the cervical spinal cord. There is very little role for myelography or CT.

Natural History and Clinical Presentation

Patients may be asymptomatic or may present with direct or indirect symptoms related to the fistula. A bruit and pulsatile mass are common symptoms directly related to the high flow through the fistula and can give a general localization of the site of the fistula for angiographic evaluation. Indirect symptoms of vertebral fistulas are generally related to venous hypertension or arterial deprivation (vascular "steal").[118, 138, 155] Venous hypertension may be localized or widespread, depending on the venous outflow pattern from the fistula. Spinal cord ischemia may occur due to increased venous pressure in a similar manner to SDFs. Papilledema may also occur from pressure transmitted into the intracranial venous system. When intracranial cortical venous drainage is demonstrated, there is a risk of cerebral hemorrhage in a similar manner to intracranial dural fistulas. Local mass effect secondary to enlarged foraminal or intradural veins may cause radicular symptoms.[134]

Rationale and Technical Aspects of Treatment

Because of the arterial to venous pressure gradient favoring flow through the fistula, large fistulas may cause a significant "sump" effect resulting in vascular insufficiency to the normal arterial territory distal to the fistula—the posterior circulation of the brain. In these cases a hyperperfusion syndrome may occur once the fistula is occluded. This is the result of a sudden return to normal arterial pressure in a maximally vasodilated vascular system—the result of autoregulation from chronic vascular insufficiency. A staged occlusion should be considered, particularly in cases that are long standing.[78, 111] Associated fistulas involving the occipital artery, superficial temporal artery, or other surrounding vascular territories may also be involved. High flow through these fistulas and the continuing

hemodynamic stresses acting on the fistula, draining veins, and feeding arteries make spontaneous thrombosis a rare event. Therefore, the natural history of these fistulas is to increase in size. Because of the natural history and severe potential consequences, symptomatic and asymptomatic fistulas should be treated.

Embolization is usually best performed by occlusion of the fistula site with a balloon or coils in an attempt to maintain patency of the parent vessel.[72] The proximal draining vein is usually occluded to ensure the fistula remains closed and to keep embolic material from prolapsing into the parent artery (Fig. 45–5E). The vertebral artery may need to be sacrificed and in most cases can be occluded safely without concern of ischemia to the normal distal territory because of adaptation and collateral development due to the vertebral "steal" effect.[95, 191] However, in cases where there is an isolated vertebral artery without obvious collateral supply to the distal vertebral territory, a test balloon occlusion of the vertebral artery should be performed. Alternative measures in the case of a failed test occlusion might include a posterior circulation bypass procedure prior to parent vessel occlusion. When a parent vessel occlusion is performed, the fistula site should be incorporated in the occlusion. Simply "trapping" the fistula with proximal and distal occlusion (by endovascular or open surgical methods) has the potential to result in collateral arterial supply through muscular or spinal collaterals with reconstitution of the fistula. Subsequent treatment in this situation is much more difficult.

SPINAL TUMORS

The crux of the diagnostic imaging evaluation of spine tumors lies with their physical location vis-à-vis to the neural axis. In conjunction with such information as age and medical history, tumor location often enables the radiologist to predict a brief differential diagnosis and thus the mode of therapy and prognosis with a reasonable degree of confidence. Myelography was long the diagnostic mainstay in the evaluation of spinal neoplasms by providing an indirect image of the spinal cord and nerve roots from the foramen magnum to the sacrum. Visualization of the negative shadow margins of the cord and its coverings as well as direct assessment of the integrity of the bony canal frequently enables radiologists to predict the location of a mass lesion as intramedullary, extramedullary intradural, and extramedullary extradural.[171] In addition, the use of water-soluble intrathecal contrast material in conjunction with high-resolution CT provided a second imaging plane to define the suspected location and thus increase the specificity of the radiographic work-up.[6, 81, 139]

MRI combines the best of both modalities with few (if any) of the disadvantages. Many early reports[20, 37, 82, 83, 103, 113, 130–132, 143] documenting the utility of MRI in the spine commented on its ability to image the cord in multiple planes and thus accurately pinpoint neoplastic disease. Additionally, MRI characterizes lesions based on morphology and location not only with respect to the cord but also according to signal intensity characteristics that reflect tissue T1, T2, and spin density as well as paramagnetic or chemical shift effects and motion. The subsequent implementation of surface coil technology, cardiac gating, gradient refocusing, and paramagnetic contrast agents has done much to improve visualization of the spinal cord and surrounding tissues as well as increase both the sensitivity and the specificity of lesion diagnosis.[8, 22, 23, 25, 26, 39, 54, 55, 58, 70, 77, 114, 150, 161–163, 166, 170, 181–183, 190] Innovations in pulse-sequence design such as saturation pulses, gradient-echo imaging, and rapid acquisition with relaxation enhancement (RARE), also known as "fast spin-echo" and "turbo spin-echo" imaging, are likely to refine further the utility of MRI of spinal neoplasia.[50, 90, 108]

Spinal Vertebral Tumors

Extradural tumors consist of primary or metastatic, benign or malignant neoplasms involving the vertebrae, adjacent soft tissue, nerve roots, and dura. This section focuses specifically on tumors that may require devascularization by embolization.

Unlike plain film radiographs, myelography, and CT (which focus primarily on the bony architecture of the spinal canal and its adjacent soft tissues), magnetic resonance images the vertebral marrow space and its nearby soft tissues. To some extent, this puts MRI at a disadvantage when primary vertebral tumors (which are best known to radiologists on the basis of location, integrity of cortical bone, pattern of cancellous bone involvement, and the presence and type of calcified matrix) are evaluated. The terms osteolytic and osteoblastic have no meaning with MRI. Nonetheless, certain primary lesions involving the vertebrae have been noted to present a unique appearance with MRI. Vertebral lesions are usually well defined as low-intensity masses surrounded by the higher intensity of normal fat-containing marrow on short TR images.[13] Although often nonspecific, this finding has been determined[7, 60] to be more sensitive to marrow abnormalities than radionuclide bone scans. The typical MRI parameters for the sensitive detection of vertebral body lesions generally consist of T1-weighted spin-echo sequences.[13, 27, 34, 60, 168, 192] Occasionally marrow uninvolved by neoplasm will appear to have a low signal, especially in young patients, in whom the vertebral body marrow does not contain much fat or in patients with chronic disease.[34, 63, 168, 178, 192] Alternative acquisitions, such as T2-weighted spin-echo sequences, STIR sequences, or gradient-echo sequences, may help for further evaluation.[75, 179]

Enhancement by extradural neoplasms can vary to such a degree that the utility of paramagnetic contrast in evaluating extradural disease is reserved for particular clinical questions. Specifically, tumors can enhance markedly (to become hyperintense relative to normal marrow) or minimally (to remain hypointense). Most disturbing, however, are those that enhance modestly (to become isointense with normal marrow) and thus go undetected.[182] This variability of enhancement has

been reported to occur among different lesions within a single patient. Nevertheless, paramagnetic contrast administration may be useful for defining epidural tumor extension.[182]

Secondary (Metastatic) Extradural Tumors

Classification

Spinal metastases are the most frequently encountered symptomatic tumor in the spine, occurring frequently in neoplastic disease; 5 to 10 per cent of cancer patients develop spinal metastases with neurologic manifestations.[12, 64] Involvement of the spine or epidural soft tissues is most commonly seen with breast carcinoma, prostate and uterine carcinoma, lung carcinoma, myeloma, and lymphoma.[64] However, renal and thyroid carcinoma are the most common vascular metastases requiring endovascular treatment. Constans and co-workers[29] reviewed 600 cases of spinal metastases and classified the lesions as (1) purely intradural (1.16 per cent), (2) purely epidural (5.00 per cent), (3) purely osseous (10.34 per cent), and complex (83.50 per cent). Gilbert and colleagues[64] state that the site of epidural tumor is thoracic in approximately 68 per cent, lumbar or sacral in 16 per cent, and cervical in 15 per cent.

Diagnostic Evaluation

Although MRI is sensitive in detecting most primary or secondary extradural spinal neoplasms, their appearance is generally nonspecific.[27, 75, 121, 173, 194] Typically the lesions are recognized by their involvement with one or more vertebrae and the adjacent soft tissues. Most possess a long T1 relative to the fat normally present within the bone marrow and are thus recognized as focal areas of decreased signal on T1-weighted images within the bony spine. On T2-weighted studies the lesions demonstrate variably increased signal and consequently may be less conspicuous relative to the adjacent normal marrow than on T1-weighted studies. In adults the vast majority of such lesions are represented by metastatic foci that frequently involve the bony canal (e.g., lung, breast, prostate). Malignant lymphoma (Hodgkin's disease and reticulum cell sarcoma) may also manifest in this fashion; however, most of these cases have minimal vertebral body involvement compared with epidural and paravertebral disease.[61] Additional, more subtle findings of spinal malignancy include diffuse changes in marrow signal intensity that can cause the discs to have relatively high signal on T1-weighted images[28]; or tumor confined strictly to the vertebral canal may present only as a subtle interruption of normal epidural fat (i.e., the "fat-cap sign").[97]

The role of paramagnetic contrast in evaluating malignant extradural disease is less clearly defined than are the indications for its use with intradural mass lesions. The preliminary experience of Sze and associates[182] suggests that intravenous gadolinium-DTPA may actually mask osseous spinal implants by making them isointense with normal vertebral marrow. Contrast, however, may increase the specificity of MRI for extradural masses (e.g., distinguishing metastases from disc fragment) and aid in directing needle biopsy.[182]

Clinical Presentation

Whereas primary or metastatic tumors of the spine are evaluated in terms of their biologic activity, they are also (and possibly more urgently) evaluated with respect to the degree of mechanical compression they exert on the cord. Classically, the clinical manifestations of spinal cord compression have been divided into three stages:[147, 167] the first (neuralgic) stage is characterized by root pain and segmental sensory and motor loss. The second (transitional, or incomplete transsection) is heralded by the onset of a Brown-Séquard syndrome. In the third stage, or complete transsection, there is total deficit, usually beginning in the distal extremities and ascending as the lesion progresses. Unfortunately, it may be difficult to determine clinically what stage of compression a patient is experiencing at the time of presentation; and it is certainly impossible to predict the rate of progression from stage to stage (and thus the imminent risk of permanent neurologic deficit).

Historically, such clinical questions have been answered by myelography (occasionally aided by CT) and the complete obstruction to flow of contrast in the subarachnoid space was considered to be an indication for emergency therapy.[171] Unfortunately, CSF pressure shifts induced by lumbar puncture in the presence of complete subarachnoid block may lead to rapid neurologic deterioration in a significant percentage of these patients.[96] Other potential pitfalls include (1) puncture site hematoma, (2) inability to examine the entire spine in the presence of multiple compression sites, and (3) inability to demonstrate paravertebral disease.[122, 156, 158] In a prospective review of 70 patients with suspected epidural metastases and cord compression, Carmody and coworkers[27] found MRI to have a sensitivity of 0.92 and a specificity of 0.90 compared with 0.95 and 0.88 for myelography in the diagnosis of cord compression. For extradural masses and osseous metastases, MRI was found to be far superior to myelography; and because it is also noninvasive, it was considered the examination of choice in evaluating spinal metastases and possible cord compression. Additional, retrospective studies[61, 194] have reached similar conclusions. Frank and coworkers,[60] likewise, compared the sensitivities of spin-echo and inversion recovery MRI to technetium-99m scintigraphy in 106 patients with suspected spinal metastasis and found MRI statistically more sensitive.

The MRI examination may be tailored specifically to particular clinical questions. With respect to cord compression, obtaining a localizing sagittal T1 body coil image through the midline followed by rapid serial sagittal and axial studies over the length of the spinal cord may expeditiously detect "block." This is especially effective with a large field of view and additional K_y lines to improve spatial resolution and signal to noise.[5] New coil designs may permit rapid single-acquisition studies of the spine with quality comparable with that obtained by multiple surface coil studies.[201]

If tumor is found but the clinical question of a "complete block" lingers, it may be possible to perform a magnetic resonance version of the Queckenstedt test. More specifically, a nongated nonrefocused long TR/long TE sagittal image through a suspected compressive lesion will not demonstrate ghosting artifact secondary to CSF pulsation in the presence of complete block.[154] This will be more apparent when the phase-encoding direction is oriented perpendicular to the spine. Finally, several studies have attempted to define criteria for distinguishing between benign senile osteoporotic compression fractures and pathologic fractures resulting from underlying tumor. Although they implemented a variety of T1- and T2-weighted pulse sequences, these studies have generally stressed the complete replacement of normal high-signal marrow fat within the vertebral body only on T1-weighted images as a useful sign a malignancy, especially if the suspected lesion was subacute or chronic.[9, 202] However, even acute benign fractures will demonstrate some residual high signal within the affected body, and, additionally, paraspinal fat planes are usually undisturbed by a paraspinal mass (unlike some neoplastic fractures).

Rationale and Technical Aspects of Treatment

Because embolization of spinal tumors is most commonly employed to interrupt the vascular supply prior to surgery, lesions most likely to benefit are relatively vascular lesions. Vascularity may be predicted by prominent flow voids seen on MRI or a clinical history of a known primary that is vascular such as metastatic kidney or thyroid tumors. Diagnostic spinal angiography may be helpful to the surgeon for preoperative localization of the artery of Adamkiewicz when transthoracic operative approaches are used. Focused angiography in the region of the spinal column tumor is usually performed (Fig. 45–6). Additionally, segmental supply for tumors in the thoracic or lumbar region should include angiography at least two levels above and below the tumor to evaluate collateral blood supply and potential for adjacent normal cord vascular supply.[16, 117] As tumor grows outside of the confines of the spine it will recruit adjacent vascular supply, which also should be studied.

The choice of embolic agents for preoperative embolization is usually particulate material, specifically PVA (polyvinyl alcohol) most commonly in the range of 150 to 250 μm in size.[118] Once the tumor has been devascularized, proximal pedicle occlusion with a coil or Gelfoam can be obtained. This type of embolization will devascularize without devitalizing tissue and will be effective for several days prior to surgery. If surgery is not performed within this period of time, recanalization and collateral formation can occur over several weeks.[118] A more aggressive embolization is not neces-

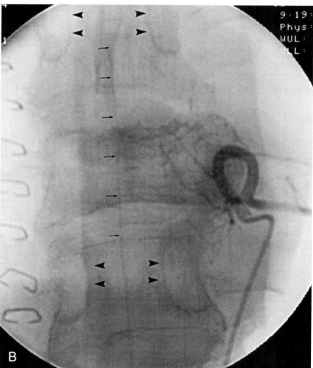

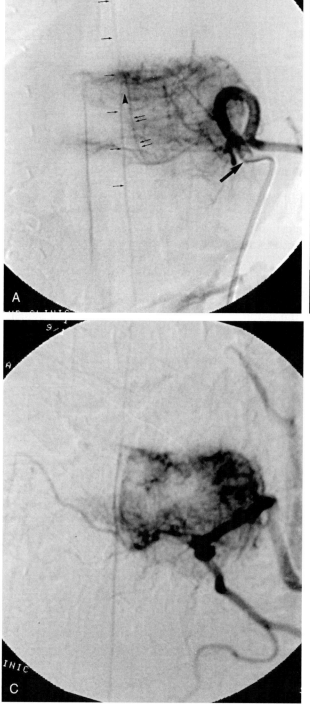

Figure 45–6.   Renal cell spinal vertebral metastasis. *A,* Digital subtraction angiogram demonstrates supply from the left L2 segmental artery *(arrow)* to the L2 vertebral body. Tumor blush involves the left half of the L2 vertebral body. The artery of Adamkiewicz *(small double arrows)* with its characteristic "hairpin" curve *(arrowhead)* supplies the anterior spinal artery *(small arrows). B,* Unsubtracted digital angiogram with bony structures visible. The pedicles *(double arrowheads)* define the lateral margin of the spinal canal. The anterior spinal artery *(small arrows)* runs superiorly and inferiorly along the anterior aspect of the spinal cord and is centered within the spinal canal. *C,* Late phase angiogram demonstrates prominent blush within the metastasis at L2.

sary unless the procedure is designed for palliation without surgery.[16] Palliative embolization with the intent of infarcting the tumor may be performed utilizing small-size PVA or Gelfoam powder (40 to 60 μm) or absolute alcohol.[118] Very selective catheter placement is crucial in these cases because this aggressive embolization will infarct any normal tissue supplied by the same vascular territory.

Vertebral Hemangiomas

Classification

The majority of spinal cavernous hemangiomas arise in the vertebral bodies with extension to the epidural space.[23] Vertebral hemangiomas are slow growing benign lesions that have been demonstrated in 11 per cent of spines at autopsy. Histologically, vertebral hemangiomas are collections of thin-walled blood vessels or sinuses lined by endothelium that are interspersed among bony trabeculae and abundant adipose tissue.[10] These lesions are postcapillary vascular malformations that occur in the vertebral elements, most commonly the vertebral body.

Diagnostic Evaluation

The lesions are commonly incidentally seen on imaging studies, particularly MRI, where they have a relatively distinctive appearance. On T1-weighted images the intraosseous portions appear mottled and of increased signal intensity secondary to the adipose tissue interspersed among thickened bony trabeculae. Extraosseous components often display lower (soft tissue) signal on T1-weighted images.[91] On T2-weighted images both intraosseous and extraosseous tumor demonstrates increased signal intensity, possibly related to more cellular components of the tumor.[91] Since these are low-flow lesions, flow voids are not a feature of cavernous malformations and if prominent surrounding vessels are present a high-flow lesion such as an AVM or fistula should be considered. Focal fat deposition within the spine may mimic a vertebral hemangioma on T1-weighted images but fail to have the same increased signal on T2-weighted studies. In the experience of Laredo and colleagues,[56] fatty vertebral hemangiomas may represent an inactive form, whereas the increased soft tissue content at CT and the low signal intensity on T1-weighted MRI images may indicate a more aggressive vascular lesion with the potential for spinal cord compression. Large lesions may weaken the vertebral structure, resulting in collapse and pain, or the hemangioma may break through the cortex and cause spinal canal compromise.

Clinical Presentation

The majority of vertebral hemangiomas are discovered incidentally[73, 90, 167] and are only rarely symptomatic.[22, 164, 175] Symptomatic lesions tend to occur in the thoracic region, usually presenting with localized pain and tenderness that often is associated with muscle spasm.[167] Radiculopathy may result from impingement on a nerve root. Myelopathic symptoms are frequently attributed to pathologic vertebral body collapse, epidural extension of tumor, epidural hematoma, or bony expansion resulting in cord compression.[73, 167]

Rationale and Technical Aspects of Treatment

Transarterial embolization has been shown to decrease the symptoms of cord compression related to these lesions,[69, 71, 88, 89] but the effect is transient. Blocking the arterial side of this postcapillary malformation does not permanently treat the lesion[48, 87]; therefore, this technique should be reserved for preoperative treatment. Embolization may decrease blood loss or even result in thrombosis of the lesion, making the surgical procedure more manageable.

More permanent ablation by use of direct embolization with methyl methacrylate has been described.[62, 141] However, a hard mass may result with methyl methacrylate embolization, and if extraosseous tumor is present, the mass may cause further cord compression. Permanent ablation has also been accomplished by directly puncturing the malformation and injecting absolute alcohol, which will sclerose the endothelial lining and has been shown to stimulate reossification.[48, 87] Percutaneous treatment with absolute ethanol can be performed with CT guidance, by directly puncturing the lesion with a spinal needle. Although sclerosis decreases lesion size after ethanol ablation, acute swelling of any extravertebral hemangioma component may occur. In this case, increased spinal cord compromise may result with potentially permanent consequences and decompressive surgery may be necessary. Pretreatment with steroids decreases the risk of significant swelling of the hemangioma. Pretreatment spinal angiography should be obtained to identify the normal spinal cord vascular supply, most notably the artery of Adamkiewicz. If arterial supply to the cord arises from the same segmental artery as the vertebral hemangioma, there is the potential of refluxing ethanol into normal spinal cord vasculature at the time of embolization with resultant spinal cord infarction. Because of intersegmental arterial collaterals, this potential also exists when normal spinal cord supply is within one or two vertebral levels from the target lesion.

Aneurysmal Bone Cyst

Classification

Aneurysmal bone cysts (ABCs) are benign osseous tumors representing only a small fraction (1.4 to 2.3 per cent) of primary bone neoplasms.[30, 36] ABCs consist of large anastomosing cavernous spaces or cysts filled with unclotted blood and contained by thinly calcified or noncalcified periosteal membranes.[11, 15, 74, 100, 193] Although most often arising de novo, in approximately a third of the cases, they have been reported to occur[19, 35, 176] with other bone lesions (giant cell tumor, chondroblastoma, chondromyxoid fibroma, fibrous dysplasia, and nonossifying fibroma).

The lesions affect the spine in up to 20 per cent of cases, more often involving the posterior elements than the vertebral bodies.[30, 35, 74, 84] Although thought to be benign, when anterior they have been reported[35, 84] to cross the intervertebral disc space and involve an adjacent vertebra. There may be an associated soft tissue mass. Of those located in the spine, an estimated 44 per cent occur in the lumbosacral region, 34 per cent in the thoracic spine, and 22 per cent in the cervical spine.

Diagnostic Evaluation

Plain films of the spine demonstrate an expanding, radiolucent, or lytic lesion usually involving the posterior elements with marked thinning of adjacent cortical bone.[84, 136] Lesions involving the vertebral body may be destructive and produce collapse.[84, 188] CT can confirm the geographic expansion of such lesions, delineate multicystic components with fluid-fluid levels, and define soft tissue extension.[15, 136, 193] As do vertebral hemangiomas, aneurysmal bone cysts have a somewhat unique MRI appearance. MRI typically demonstrates numerous well-defined cystic cavities that are surrounded by a rim of low signal intensity and may demonstrate multiple fluid-fluid levels.[15, 101, 204, 205] These cavities often show a wide range of signal intensities on both T1- and T2-weighted images depending on the various blood products present, their paramagnetic properties, and the field strength of the magnet utilized.[15, 101] Tsai and coworkers[189] have subsequently observed that other bony lesions can mimic this appearance of multiple blood-fluid levels on MRI, including telangiectatic osteosarcoma, chondroblastoma, and giant cell tumor of bone as well as fibrous dysplasia, simple bone cyst, recurrent malignant fibrous histiocytoma of bone, two "classic" osteosarcomas, and four "classic" aneurysmal bone cysts. The soft tissue tumors that they found mimicking aneurysmal bone cysts included soft tissue hemangioma and two synovial sarcomas.[189]

Spinal angiography is not commonly used in the evaluation of these tumors because the imaging findings are usually diagnostic. Spinal angiographic findings vary from mild vascularity to a rich vascular tumor supply.[16] Contrast material may collect within the cysts with late disappearance during the venous phase.

Clinical Presentation

Patients typically present in the first two decades of life and are equally divided between males and females.[19, 36, 84, 188] Presenting symptoms usually consist of localized pain and/or swelling.[19, 19, 84, 188] Large lesions may expand to compress the spinal cord, resulting in myelopathy.[84, 144] Giant cells present within the trabeculae of these lesions often lead to confusion with the tumor of the same name, but presentation of giant cell tumors is usually in patients older than 30 years of age.[19, 35, 74, 188] Transarterial devascularization may be

performed preoperatively or before biopsy to reduce the blood supply if a vascular lesion is suspected.

Giant Cell Tumor

Classification

Giant cell tumors comprise 4 to 5 per cent of all primary bone tumors and are typically seen after the second decade of life.[36, 105, 127] There is no sex predilection.[127] In Dahlin and Unnie's series,[36] they were the second most common benign spinal tumor, after vertebral hemangiomas. Additionally, they are the most common benign neoplasm involving the sacrum.[67] Local pain (occasionally with swelling) is the usual presentation.[1, 21, 67, 127]

Diagnostic Evaluation

Plain films show a geographically expansile lytic lesion, rarely with a sclerotic border.[127] CT may be useful in demonstrating any soft tissue mass.[1] With MRI, unenhanced short TR images demonstrate low-signal tumor within the higher-signal marrow space. The extraosseous extent of the lesion can be delineated with more T2-weighted images or, alternatively, the administration of contrast with T1-weighted images.[21] As noted, both the MRI and the histologic findings may be similar to those seen with aneurysmal bone cysts.[189] As with many spinal tumors, there is no pathognomonic angiographic pattern, but these lesions may be vascular.[130] Transarterial embolization may be performed to devascularize these lesions prior to biopsy or surgery.

Other Spinal Vertebral Tumors

The role of interventional neuroradiology is limited for other vertebral tumors. Lesions such as osteoid osteomas, osteoblastomas, and chordomas are usually well characterized with imaging. Angiography may be obtained if there is suspicion of increased vascularity, and if necessary, the lesion may be embolized prior to biopsy or surgery.

SPINAL CORD TUMORS

Angiographic evaluation and embolization of spinal cord tumors are primarily limited to hemangioblastomas. These are the only truly vascular tumors of the spinal cord. Meningiomas located in the spinal canal are dural based and may be vascular; but unlike intracranial meningiomas, they are generally hypovascular and do not require angiography or embolization.

Hemangioblastoma

Classification

Hemangioblastomas are uncommon. Frequent confusion with vascular malformations and other vascular tumors, as well as the lack of uniformity in classification, has in the past made assessment of their incidence relative to other spinal tumors difficult. In the review of Sloof and associates[172] of 1322 primary spinal canal tumors, there were 300 intramedullary lesions and only 4 of these were hemangioblastomas. They usually present in the third or fourth decade of life.[24, 172]

While they can occur as isolated masses, hemangioblastomas are frequently multiple and seen in association with posterior fossa tumors as part of the von Hippel–Lindau syndrome (VHL).[169] This autosomal dominant complex has been linked to a defect on chromosome 3 and features hemangioblastomas of the posterior fossa and spinal neuraxis; retinal angiomas; cysts or cystadenoma of the pancreas, adrenals, kidneys, and ovaries; pheochromocytoma; and renal cell carcinoma.[98, 99, 169, 199] Although previously thought to be relatively rare, spinal hemangioblastomas may be much more common in association with this disorder, are frequently asymptomatic, and can be either intramedullary or intradural-extramedullary in location.[104] It has been estimated[52, 98, 140] that approximately one in four patients with brain and spinal cord hemangioblastomas has underlying VHL and approximately a third of patients with known VHL have hemangioblastomas.

Hemangioblastomas are histologically similar to angioblastic meningiomas and apparently arise as small nodules from the pia.[199] They most often present as intramedullary cysts containing a vascular nodule; cyst formation is seen in up to 67 per cent of intramedullary spine lesions.[24, 107] Another unique feature of hemangioblastomas reported by Solomon and Stein[174] is the striking intramedullary edema seen with these relatively well-circumscribed lesions. Usually the thoracic cord is involved (51 per cent), followed by the cervical cord (41 per cent).[24, 53]

Diagnostic Evaluation

Because there are no significant external manifestations of the disease and no readily available genetic tests, imaging plays an important role in the screening and management of these patients.[52] Magnetic resonance is particularly well suited to the evaluation of these lesions because of its superior ability to image not only the spinal cord but also posterior fossa structures. Unenhanced MRI studies typically demonstrate extensive widening of the cord with or without associated cysts.[107, 174] Whereas the cord typically demonstrates prolongation of T1 and T2 relaxation times, the cysts may vary in signal intensity depending on their contents.[107] Signal characteristics can parallel those of CSF or may be of greater intensity as a result of increased protein content.[107, 164] Because these tumors are typically quite vascular, serpentine areas of signal void may be seen that represent feeding arteries or draining veins associated with the tumor nidus.[24, 53] The administration of paramagnetic contrast dramatically improves visualization of the tumor nidus, often allowing its differentiation from the adjacent edematous spinal cord.[39, 52, 107, 174, 182, 190]

Rationale and Technical Aspects of Treatment

Diagnostic angiography shows a hypervascular mass supplied by medullary arterial feeders. There is a solid stain with lucencies that can occur within the mass and likely represent cysts. Unlike spinal cord AVMs, there is no direct arteriovenous shunting and no individual vessels within the lesion that would be characteristic of the nidus of an AVM. These lesions occur more commonly along the dorsal spinal cord where they are supplied by the posterior spinal arteries. Those lesions supplied by the anterior spinal artery should not be embolized because of significant risks of cord infarction. However, for those supplied by the posterior spinal artery, superselective catheterization and embolization can be obtained prior to surgical removal.[16]

References

1. Aisen, A. M., Martel, W., Braunstein, E. M., et al.: MRI and CT evaluation of primary bone and soft tissue tumors. A. J. R. Am. J. Roentgenol. 146:749–756, 1986.
2. Aminoff, M. J., Barnard, R. O., and Logue, V.: The pathophysiology of spinal cord vascular malformations. J. Neurosci. 23:255–263, 1974.
3. Aminoff, M. J.: Associated lesions. In Aminoff, M. J. (ed.): Spinal Angiomas. Boston, Blackwell, 1976, pp. 18–27.
4. Aminoff, M. J.: Introduction: The nature of spinal angiomas. In Aminoff, M. J. (ed.): Spinal Angiomas. Boston, Blackwell, 1976, pp. 1–4.
5. Anderson, C. M., and Lee, R.: Large FOV spine screening with 512 matrix and body coil: Contrast to noise comparison with surface coil imaging. Presented at the 9th SMRM, 1990.
6. Aubin, M. L., Jardin, C., Bar, D., et al.: Computerized tomography in 32 cases of intraspinal tumor. J. Neuroradiol. 6:81–92, 1979.
7. Avrahami, E., Tadmor, R., Dally, O., et al.: Early MRI demonstration of spinal metastases in patients with normal radiographs and CT and radionuclide bone scans. J. Comput. Assist. Tomogr. 13:598–602, 1989.
8. Axel, L.: Surface coil magnetic resonance imaging. J. Comput. Assist. Tomogr. 8:381–384, 1984.
9. Baker, L. L., Goodman, S. B., Perkash ,I., et al.: Benign versus pathologic compression fractures of vertebral bodies: Assessment with conventional spin-echo, chemical shift, and STIR MRI imaging. Radiology 174:495–502, 1990.
10. Ball, M. J., and Dayan, A. D.: Pathogenesis of syringomyelia. Lancet 2:799–801, 1972.
11. Banna, M.: Clinical Radiology of the Spine and Spinal Cord. Rockville, MD, Aspen, 1985.
12. Barron, K. D., Hirano, A., Araki, S., et al.: Experiences with metastatic neoplasms involving the spinal cord. Neurology 9:91–106, 1959.
13. Beltram, J., Noto, A. M., Chakeres, D. W., and Christoforidis, A. J.: Tumors of the osseous spine: Staging with MRI imaging versus CT. Radiology 162:565–569, 1987.
14. Beltramello, A., Maschiao, A., Piovane, E., et al.: Spontaneous arteriovenous fistula of the vertebral artery: Diagnostic and therapeutic considerations. Eur. J. Radiol. 8:148–152, 1988.
15. Beltran, J., Simon, D. C., Levy, M., et al.: Aneurysmal bone cysts: MRI imaging at 1.5 T. Radiology 158:689–690, 1986.
16. Berenstein, A., and Lasjaunias, P.: Surgical neuroangiography. In Endovascular Treatment of Spine and Spinal Cord Lesions. Vol. 5. New York, Springer-Verlag, 1992.
17. Berenstein, A., Young, W., Ransohoff, J., et al.: Somatosensory evoked potentials during spinal angiography and therapeutic transvascular embolization. J. Neurosurg. 60:777–785, 1984.
18. Bicknell, J. M., Carlow, T. J., and Kornfield, M.: Familial cavernous angiomas. Arch. Neurol. 35:746–749, 1978.
19. Biescker, J. L., Marcove, R. C., Huvos, A. G., and Mike, V.:

Aneurysmal bone cyst: A clinical pathologic study of 66 cases. Cancer 26:615–625, 1970.

20. Bradley, W. G., Waluch, V., Yadley, R. A., and Wycoff, R. R.: Comparison of CT and MRI in 400 patients with suspected disease of the brain and cervical spinal cord. Radiology 152:695–702, 1984.

21. Brady, T. J., Gebhardt, M. C., and Pickett, I. L.: NMR imaging of forearms in healthy volunteers and patients with giant cell tumor. Radiology 144:549–552, 1982.

22. Brasch, R. C.: Contrast enhancement in NMR imaging. In Newton, T. H., and Potts, D. G. (eds.): Advanced Imaging Techniques: Moderate Neuroradiology. Vol. 2. San Anselmo, CA, Clavadel, 1983, pp. 63–79.

23. Breger, R. K., Williams, A. L., Daniels, D. L., et al.: Contrast enhancement in spinal MRI imaging. A. J. N. R. Am. J. Neuroradiol. 10:633–637, 1989.

24. Browne, T. R., Adams, R. D., and Roberson, G. H.: Hemangioblastoma of the spinal cord. Review and report of five cases. Arch. Neurol. 33:435–441, 1976.

25. Bydder, G. M., Brown, J., Niendorf, H. P., and Young, I. R.: Enhancement of cervical intraspinal tumors in MRI imaging with intravenous gadolinium-DTPA. J. Comput. Assist. Tomogr. 9:847–885, 1985.

26. Bydder, G. M., Kingsley, D. P., Brown, J., et al.: MRI imaging of meningiomas including studies with and without gadolinium-DTPA. J. Comput. Assist. Tomogr. 9:690–697, 1985.

27. Carmody, R. F., Yankg, D. J., et al.: Spinal cord compression due to metastatic disease: Diagnosis with MRI imaging versus myelography. Radiology 173:225–229, 1989.

28. Castillo, M., Malko, J. A., and Hoffman, J. C., Jr.: The bright intervertebral disk: An indirect sign of abnormal spinal bone marrow on T1-weighted MRI images. A. J. N. R. Am. J. Neuroradiol. 11:23–26, 1990.

29. Constans, J. P., de Divitiis, E., Donzelli, R., et al.: Spinal metastases with neurological manifestations. Review of 600 cases. J. Neurosurg. 59:111–118, 1983.

30. Cory, D. A., Fritsch, S. A., Cohen, M. D., et al.: Aneurysmal bone cysts: Imaging findings and embolotherapy. A. J. R. Am. J. Roentgenol. 153:369–373, 1989.

31. Cosgrove, G. R., Bertrand, G., Fontaine, S., et al.: Cavernous angiomas of the spinal cord. J. Neurosurg. 68:31–36, 1988.

32. Cosgrove, G. R., and Theron, J.: Vertebral arteriovenous fistula following anterior cervical spine surgery. Report of two cases. J. Neurosurg. 66:297–299, 1987.

33. Crissuolo, G. R., Oldfield, E. H., and Doppman, J. L.: Reversible acute and subacute myelopathy in patients with dural arteriovenous fistulas. Foix-Alajouanine syndrome reconsidered. J. Neurosurg. 70:354–359, 1989.

34. Daffner, R. H., Lupetin, A. R., Cash, N., et al.: MRI in the detection of malignant infiltration of bone marrow. A. J. R. Am. J. Roentgenol. 146:353–358, 1986.

35. Dahlin, D. C., and McLeon, R. A.: Aneursymal bone cyst and other non-neoplastic conditions. Skeletal Radiol. 8:243–250, 1982.

36. Dahlin, D. C., and Unni, K. K.: Bone Tumors: General Aspects and Data on 8,542 Cases. Springfield, IL, Charles C Thomas, 1986, pp. 62–69.

37. DiChiro, G., Doppman, J. L., Dwyer, A. J., et al.: Tumors and arteriovenous malformations of the spinal cord: Assessment using MRI. Radiology 156:689–697, 1985.

38. DiChiro, G.: Angiography of obstructive vascular disease of the spinal cord. Radiology 100:607–614, 1971.

39. Dillon, W. P., Norman, D., Newton, T. H., et al.: Intradural spinal cord lesions: Gd-DTPA–enhanced MRI imaging. Radiology 170:229–237,1989.

40. Djindjian, R.: Clinical symptomatology and natural history of arteriovenous malformations of the spinal cord: A study of the clinical aspects and prognosis, based on 150 cases. In Pia, H. W., and Djindjian, R. (eds.): Spinal Angiograms: Advances in Diagnosis and Therapy. Berlin, Springer-Verlag, 1978.

41. Djindjian, R.: Neuroradiological examination of spinal cord angiomas. In Vinken, P. J., and Bruyn, G. W. (eds.): Handbook of Clinical Neurology. Vol. 12. New York, Elsevier, North-Holland, 1972, pp. 631–643.

42. Dommisse, G. F.: The arteries, arterioles, and capillaries of the spinal cord. Surgical guidelines in the prevention of postoperative paraplegia. Ann. R. Coll. Surg. Engl. 62:369–376, 1980.

43. Dommisse, G. F.: The blood supply of the spinal cord. J. Bone Joint Surg. 56B:225–235, 1974.

44. Doppman, J., DiChiro, G., and Ommaya, A. K.: Arteriovenous malformations. In Doppman, J., DiChiro, G., and Ommaya, A. K. (eds.): Selective Arteriography of the Spinal Cord. St. Louis, Warren H. Green, 1969, pp. 59–124.

45. Doppman, J. L., DiChiro, G., Dwyer, A. J., et al.: Magnetic resonance imaging of spinal arteriovenous malformations. J. Neurosurg. 66:830–834, 1987.

46. Doppman, J. L., DiChiro, G., and Oldfield, E. H.: Origin of spinal arteriovenous malformation and normal cord vasculature from a common segmental artery: Angiographic and therapeutic considerations. Radiology 154:687–689, 1985.

47. Doppman, J. L., Wirth, F. P., Jr., DiChiro, G., et al.: Value of cutaneous angiomas in the arteriographic localization of spinal-cord arteriovenous malformations. N. Engl. J. Med. 281:1440–1444, 1969.

48. Doppman, J. L.: Percutaneous treatment of symptomatic vertebral hemangiomas by direct injection of alcohol. American Society of Interventional and Therapeutic Neuroradiology 1995 Course Syllabus, pp. 49–54.

49. Edelman, R. R., Atkinson, D. J., Silver, M. S., et al.: FRODO pulse sequences: A new means of eliminating motion, flow and wraparound artifacts. Radiology 166:231–236, 1988.

50. Edelman, R. R., Johnson, K., Buxton, R., et al.: MRI of hemorrhage: A new approach. A. J. N. R. Am. J. Neuroradiol. 7:751–756, 1986.

51. El-Toraei, I., and Juler, G.: Ischemic myelopathy. Angiology 30:81–94, 1979.

52. Elster, A. D.: Radiologic screening in the neurocutaneous syndromes: Strategies and controversies. A. J. N. R. Am. J. Neuroradiol. 13:1078–1082, 1982.

53. Enomoto, H., Shibata, T., Ito, A., et al.: Multiple hemangioblastomas accompanied by syringomyelia in the cerebellum and the spinal cord. Surg. Neurol. 22:197–203, 1984.

54. Enzman, D. R., Rubin, J. B., and Wright, A.: Cervical spine MRI imaging: Generating high signal CSF in sagittal and axial images. Radiology 163:233–238, 1987.

55. Enzman, D. R., Rubin, J. B., and Wright, A.: Use of cerebrospinal fluid gating to improve T$_2$ weighted images: I. The spinal cord. Radiology 162:763–767, 1987.

56. Epstein, F., and Epstein, N.: Intramedullary tumors of the spinal cord. In Shillito, J., Jr., and Matson, D. D. (eds.): Pediatric Neurosurgery of the Developing Nervous System. New York, Grune & Stratton, 1982, pp. 529–539.

57. Feuerman, T., Divan, P.S., Young, R. F.: Vertebrectomy for treatment of vertebral hemangioma without preoperative embolization. J. Neurosurg. 65:404–406, 1986.

58. Fisher, M. R., Barker, B., Amparo, E. G., et al.: MRI imaging using specialized coils. Radiology 157:443–447, 1985.

59. Fontaine, S., Melanson, D., Cosgrove, R., et al.: Cavernous hemangiomas of the spinal cord: MRI imaging. Radiology 166:839–841, 1988.

60. Frank, J. A., Ling, A., Patronas, N. J., et al.: Detection of malignant bone tumors: MRI imaging vs. scintigraphy. A. J. R. Am. J. Roentgenol. 155:1043–1048, 1990.

61. Friedman, M., Kim, T. H., and Panahon, A.: Spinal cord compression in malignant lymphoma. Cancer 37:1485–1491, 1976.

62. Gangi, A., Kastler, B., and Dieteman, J. L.: Percutaneous vertebroplasty guided by a combination of CT and fluoroscopy. A. J. N. R. Am. J. Neuroradiol. 15:83–86, 1994.

63. Geremia, G. K., McCluney, R., Adler, S. S., et al.: The magnetic resonance hypointense spine of AIDS. J. Comput. Assist. Tomogr. 14:785–789, 1990.

64. Gilbert, R. W., Kim, J. H., and Posner, J. B.: Epidural spinal cord compression from metastatic tumour. Diagnosis and treatment. Ann Neurol 3:40–51, 1978.

65. Gillilan, L.: The arterial blood supply of the human spinal cord. J. Comp. Neurol. 110:75–103, 1958.

66. Gobin, Y. P., Rogopoulos, A., Aymard, A., et al.: Endovascular treatment of intracranial dural arteriovenous fistulas with spinal perimedullary venous drainage. J. Neurosurg. 77:718–723, 1992.

67. Goldenberg, R. R., Campbell, C.J., and Bonfiglio, M.: Giant cell tumor of bone, an analysis of 218 cases. J. Bone Joint Surg. 52A:619–664, 1970.

68. Gomori, J. M., Grossman, R. I., Goldberg, R. I., et al.: Intracranial hematoma imaging by high-field MRI. Radiology 157:87–93, 1985.

69. Graham, J., and Yang, W.: Vertebral hemangioma with compression fracture and paraparesis treated with preoperative embolization and vertebral resection. Spine 9:97–101, 1984.

70. Greco, A., McNamara, M. T., Lanthiez, P., et al.: Gadodiamide injection: Nonionic gadolinium chelate for MRI imaging of the brain and spine—phase II-III clinical trial. Radiology 176:451–456, 1990.

71. Gross, C. E., Hodge, C. J., Binet, E. F., et al.: Relief of spinal block during embolization of vertebral body hemangioma. Case report. J. Neurosurg. 45:327–330, 1976.

72. Guglielmi, G., Vinuela, F., Duckwiler, G., et al.: High-flow, small-hole arteriovenous fistulas: Treatment with electrode-tachable coils. A. J. N. R. Am. J. Neuroradiol. 16(2):325–328, 1995.

73. Guidetti, B., Mercuri, S., and Vagnozzi, R.: Long term results of surgical treatment of 129 intramedullary spinal gliomas. J. Neurosurg. 54:323–330, 1981.

74. Gunterberg, B., Kindblom, L. G., and Laurin, S.: Giant cell tumor of bone and aneurysmal bone cyst. Skeletal Radiol. 2:65–74, 1977.

75. Gusnard, D. A., Grossman, R. I., and Hackney, D. B.: The differential utility of gradient-echo and spin-echo MRI of the abnormal spine. Presented at the Twenty-Sixth Annual Meeting of ASNR, Chicago, 1988, p. 15.

76. Guthkelch, A. N.: Hemangiomas involving the spinal epidural space. J. Neurol. Neurosurg. Psychiatr. 11:199–210, 1948.

77. Haacke, E. M., and Lenz, G. W.: Improving MRI image quality in the presence of motion by using rephasing gradients. A. J. R. Am. J. Roentgenol. 148:1251–1258, 1987.

78. Halbach, V. V., Higashida, R. T., and Hieshima, G. B.: Normal perfusion breakthrough occurring during treatment of carotid and vertebral fistulas. A. J. N. R. Am. J. Neuroradiol. 8:751–756, 1987.

79. Halbach, V. V., Higashida, R. T., and Hieshima, G. B.: Treatment of vertebral arteriovenous fistulas. A. J. N. R. Am. J. Neuroradiol. 8:1121, 1987.

80. Hall, W. A., Oldfield, E. H., and Doppman, J. L.: Recanalization of spinal cord arteriovenous malformations following embolization. J. Neurosurg. 27:530–540, 1989.

81. Hammerschlag, S. B., Wolpert, S. M., and Carter, B. L.: Computed tomography of the spinal canal. Radiology 121:361–367, 1976.

82. Han, J. S., Kaufman, B., El Yousef, S. J., et al.: NMR imaging of the spine. A. J. R. Am. J. Roentgenol. 141:1137–1145, 1983.

83. Haughton, V. M., Rimm, A. A., Sobocinski, K. A., et al.: A blinded clinical comparison of MRI imaging and CT in neuroradiology. Radiology 160:751–755, 1986.

84. Hay, M. C., Paterson, D., and Taylor, T. K.: Aneurysmal bone cysts of the spine. J. Bone Joint Surg. 60B:406–411, 1978.

85. Heffner, R. R., and Solitare, G. B.: Hereditary hemorrhagic telangiectasia: Neuropathological observations. J. Neurol. Neurosurg. Psychiatr. 32:604–608, 1969.

86. Hegedus, K., and Fekete, I.: Case report of infarction in the region of the posterior spinal arteries. Eur. Arch. Psychiatr. Neurol. Sci. 234:281–284, 1984.

87. Heiss, J. D., Doppman, J. L., and Oldfield, E. H.: Brief report: Relief of spinal cord compression from vertebral hemangioma by intralesional injection of absolute ethanol. N. Engl. J. Med. 25:508–511, 1994.

88. Hekster, R. E. M., Luyendijk, W., and Tan, T. I.: Spinal cord compression caused by vertebral hemangioma relieved by percutaneous catheter embolization. Neuroradiology 3:160–164, 1972.

89. Hemmy, D. C., McGee, D. M., Armbrust, F. H., et al.: Resection of vertebral hemangioma after preoperative embolization. Case report. J. Neurosurg. 47:282–285, 1977.

90. Hennig, J., Naureth, A., and Friedburg, H.: RARE imaging: A fast method for clinical MRI. Magn. Reson. Med. 3:823–833, 1986.

91. Henry, J. M., Heffner, R. R., and Easle, K. M.: Ganglioglioma of CNS: A clinicopathological study of 50 cases. J. Neuropathol. Exp. Neurol. 37:626, 1978.

92. Heros, R. C., Debrun, G. M., Ojemann, R. G., et al.: Direct spinal arteriovenous fistula: A new type of spinal AVM. J. Neurosurg. 64:134–139, 1986.

93. Herren, R. Y., and Alexander, L.: Sulcal and intrinsic blood vessels of human spinal cord. Arch. Neurol. Psychiatr. 41:678–687, 1939.

94. Hieshima, G. B., Cahan, L. D., Mehringer, C. M., and Bentson, J. R.: Spontaneous arteriovenous fistulas of cerebral vessels in association with fibromuscular dysplasia. Neurosurgery 18(4):454–458, 1986.

95. Higashida, R. T., Halbach, V. V., Tsai, F. Y., et al.: Interventional neurovascular treatment of traumatic carotid and vertebral artery lesions. Results in 234 cases. A. J. R. Am. J. Roentgenol. 153(3):577–582, 1989.

96. Hollis, P. M., Malis, L. I., and Zappulla, R. A.: Neurologic deterioration after lumbar puncture below complete spinal subarachnoid block. J. Neurosurg. 64:253–256, 1986.

97. Horner, N. B., and Pinto, R. S.: The fat-cap sign: An aid to MRI evaluation of extradural spinal tumors. A. J. N. R. Am. J. Neuroradiol. 10(5 Suppl.):S93, 1989.

98. Horton, W. A., Wong, V., and Eldridge, R.: Von Hippel–Lindau disease. Clinical and pathological manifestations in nine families with 50 affected members. Arch. Intern. Med. 136:769–777, 1976.

99. Hosoe, S., Brauch, H., Latif, F., et al.: Localization of von Hippel–Lindau disease to a small region of chromosome 3. Genomics 6:634–640, 1990.

100. Hudson, T. J: Fluid levels in aneurysmal bone cysts: A CT feature. A. J. R. Am. J. Roentgenol. 142:1001–1004, 1984.

101. Hudson, T. M., Hamlin, D. J., and Fitzsimmons, J. R.: Magnetic resonance imaging of fluid levels in an aneurysmal bone cyst and in anticoagulated human blood. Skeletal Radiol. 13:267–270, 1985.

102. Hughes, J. T.: Thrombosis of the posterior spinal arteries. A complication of an intrathecal injection of phenol. Neurology 20:659–664, 1970.

103. Hyman, R. A., Edwards, J. H., Vacirca, S. J., and Stein H. L.: 0.6 T MRI imaging of the cervical spine: Multislice and multiecho techniques. A. J. N. R. Am. J. Neuroradiol. 6:229–236, 1985.

104. Ismail, S. M., and Cole, G.: Von Hippel–Lindau syndrome with microscopic hemangioblastomas of the spinal nerve roots. J. Neurosurg. 60:1279–1281, 1984.

105. Jacobs, P.: The diagnosis of osteoclastoma (giant cell tumours): A radiological and pathological correlation. Br. J. Radiol. 45:121–136, 1972.

106. Jellinger, K.: Pathology of spinal vascular malformations and vascular tumors. In Pia, H. W., and Djindjian, R. (eds.): Spinal Angiomas: Advances in Diagnosis and Therapy. New York, Springer-Verlag, 1978, pp. 9–20.

107. Kaffenberger, D. A., Sah, C. P., Murtagh, F. R., et al.: MRI imaging of spinal cord hemangioblastoma associated with syringomyelia. J. Comput. Assist. Tomogr. 12:495–498, 1988.

108. Katz, B. H., Quencer, R. M., and Hinks, R. S.: Comparison of gradient-recalled-echo and T2 weighted spin-echo pulse sequences in intramedullary spinal lesions. A. J. N. R. Am. J. Neuroradiol. 10:815–822, 1989.

109. Kendall, B. E., and Logue, V.: Spinal epidural angiomatous malformations draining into intrathecal veins. Neuroradiology 13:181–189, 1977.

110. Kim, D.-I., Choi, I.-S., and Berenstein, A.: A sacral dural arteriovenous fistula presenting with an intermittent myelopathy aggravated by menstruation. J. Neurosurg. 75:947–949, 1991.

111. Kondoh, T., Tamaki, N., Takeda, N., et al.: Fatal intracranial hemorrhage after balloon occlusion of an extracranial vertebral arteriovenous fistula. Case report. J. Neurosurg. 69(6):945–948, 1988.

112. Krueger, E. G., Sobel, G. L., and Weinstein, C.: Vertebral hemangiomas: Radiologic evaluation. J. Neurosurg. 18:331–338, 1961.

113. Kucharczyk, W., Brant-Zawadzki, M., Sobel, D., et al.: Central nervous system tumors in children: Detection by magnetic resonance imaging. Radiology 155:131–136, 1985.

114. Kulkarni, M. V., Patton, J. A., and Price, R. R.: Technical considerations for the use of surface coils in MRI. A. J. R. Am. J. Roentgenol. *147*:373–378, 1986.
115. Laredo, J. D., Assouline, E., Gelbert, F., et al.: Vertebral hemangiomas: fat content as a sign of aggressiveness. Radiology *177*:467–472, 1990.
116. Larsson, E.-M., Desai, P., Hardin, C. W., et al.: Venous infarction of the spinal cord resulting from dural arteriovenous fistula: MRI imaging findings. A. J. N. R. Am. J. Neuroradiol. *12*:739–743, 1991.
117. Lasjaunias, P., and Berenstein, A.: Surgical neuroangiography. *In* Functional Vascular Anatomy of Brain, Spinal Cord and Spine. Vol. 3. New York, Springer-Verlag, 1990.
118. Lasjaunias, P., and Berenstein, A.: Surgical neuroangiography. *In* Endovascular Treatment of Craniofacial Lesions. Vol. 2. New York, Springer-Verlag, 1989.
119. Lazorthes, G., Gouaze, A., Zadeh, J. O., et al.: Arterial vascularization of the spinal cord. J. Neurosurg. *35*:253–269, 1971.
120. Lazorthes, G., Poulhes, J., Bastide, G., et al.: La vascularization arterielle de la moelle. Neurochirurgie *4*:3–19, 1958.
121. Lien, H. H., Blomlie, V., and Heimdal, K.: Magnetic resonance imaging of malignant extradural tumors with acute spinal cord compression. Acta Radiol. *31*:187–190, 1990.
122. Mapstone, T. B., Rekate, H. L., and Shurin, S. B.: Quadriplegia secondary to hematoma after lateral C1–2 puncture in a leukemic child. Neurosurgery *12*:230–231, 1983.
123. Masaryk, T. J., Ross, J. S., Modic, M. T., et al.: Radiculomeningeal vascular malformations of the spine: MRI imaging. Radiology *164*:845–849, 1987.
124. McAllister, V. L., Kendall, B. E., and Bull, J. W.: Symptomatic vertebral hemangiomas. Brain *98*:71–80, 1975.
125. McCormick, W. F., Hardman, J. M., and Boulter, T. R.: Vascular malformations ("angiomas") of the brain with special reference to those occurring in the posterior fossa. J. Neurosurg. *28*:241–251, 1968.
126. McCormick, W. F.: The pathology of vascular ("arteriovenous") malformations. J. Neurosurg. *24*:807–816, 1966.
127. McInerney, D. P., and Middlemiss, J. H.: Giant cell tumor of bone. Skeletal Radiol. *2*:195–204, 1978.
128. Merland, J. J., and Reizine, D.: Treatment of arteriovenous spinal cord malformations. Semin. Intervent. Radiol. *4*:281–290, 1987.
129. Merland, J. J., Riche, M. C., and Chires, J.: Intraspinal extramedullary arteriovenous fistulae draining into the medullary veins. J. Neuroradiol. *7*:271–320, 1980.
130. Modic, M. T., Hardy, R. W., Jr., Weinstein, M. A., et al.: Nuclear magnetic resonance of the spine: Clinical potential and limitation. Neurosurgery *15*:582–592, 1984.
131. Modic, M. T., Weinstein, M., Pavlicek, W., et al.: Magnetic resonance imaging of the cervical spine: Technical and clinical observations. A. J. R. Am. J. Roentgenol. *141*:1129–1136, 1983.
132. Modic, M. T., Weinstein, M., Pavlicek, W., et al.: Nuclear magnetic resonance imaging of the spine. Radiology *147*:757–762, 1983.
133. Mohan, V., Gupta, S. K., Tuli, S. M., and Sanyal, B.: Symptomatic vertebral hemangiomas. Clin. Radiol. *31*:575–579, 1980.
134. Morello, F., Moro, G., Tibaldo, M., et al.: Acute cervical radiculopathy due to vertebral A-V fistula. Ital. J. Neurolog. Sci. *13*(7):603–605, 1992.
135. Morgan, M. K., and Marsh, W. R.: Management of spinal dural arteriovenous malformations. J. Neurosurg. *70*:832–836, 1989.
136. Munk, P. L., Helms, C. A., Holt, R. G., et al.: MRI imaging of aneurysmal bone cysts. A. J. R. Am. J. Roentgenol. *153*:99–101, 1989.
137. Murray, R. O., and Jacobson, H. G.: Radiology of Skeletal Disorders. 2nd ed. New York, Churchill Livingstone, 1977, p. 578.
138. Nagashima, C., Iwasaki, T., Kawanuma, S., et al.: Traumatic arteriovenous fistula of the vertebral artery with spinal cord symptoms. Case report. J. Neurosurg. *46*(5):681–687, 1977.
139. Nakagawa, H., Haung, Y. P., Malis, L. I., et al.: Computed tomography of intraspinal and paraspinal neoplasm. J. Comput. Assist. Tomogr. *1*:377–390, 1977.
140. Neumann, H. P., Eggert, H. R., Weigel, K., et al.: Hemangioblastomas of the central nervous system: A 10 year study with special reference to von Hippel–Lindau syndrome. J. Neurosurg. *70*:24–30, 1989.
141. Nicola, N., and Lins, E.: Vertebral hemangioma, retrograde embolization-stabilization with methyl methacrylate. Surg. Neurol. *27*:481–486, 1987.
142. Nittner, K.: Spinal meningiomas, neurinomas and neurofibromas and hourglass tumors. *In* Vinken, P. J., and Bruyn, G. W. (eds.): Handbook of Clinical Neurology. Vol. 20. New York, Elsevier North-Holland, 1976, pp. 177–322.
143. Norman, D., Mills, C. M., Brant-Zawadzki M., et al.: Magnetic resonance imaging of the spinal cord and canal: Potentials and limitations. A. J. R. Am. J. Roentgenol. *141*:1147–1152, 1983.
144. Nosrat, O. A., Ameli, N. O., Abbassioun, K., et al.: Aneurysmal bone cysts of the spine. J. Neurosurg. *63*:685–690, 1985.
145. Oldfield, E. H., DiChiro, G., Quindlen, E. A., et al.: Successful treatment of a group of spinal cord arteriovenous malformations by interruption of dural fistula. J. Neurosurg. *59*:1019–1030, 1983.
146. Oldfield, E. H., and Doppman, J. L.: Spinal arteriovenous malformations. Clin. Neurosurg. *9*:161–183, 1961.
147. Oppenheim, H.: Lehrbuch der Nervenkrankheiten fur Arzte und Studierende. 6th ed. Berlin, S. Karger, 1923, vol. 1.
148. Padovani, R., Tognetti, F., Proietti, D., et al.: Extrathecal cavernous hemangioma. Surg. Neurol. *118*:475–476, 1982.
149. Paige, M. L., and Hemmati, M.: Spinal cord compression by vertebral hemangioma. Pediatr. Radiol. *6*:43–45, 1977.
150. Parizel, P. M., Baleriaux, D., Rodesch, G., et al.: Gd-DTPA–enhanced MRI imaging of spinal tumors. A. J. N. R. Am. J. Neuroradiol. *10*:249–258, 1989.
151. Parke, W. W.: Applied anatomy of the spine. *In* Rothman, R. H., and Simeone, F. A. (eds.): The Spine. 2nd ed. Philadelphia, W. B. Saunders Co., 1982, pp. 18–51.
152. Parkinson, D., and Hay, R.: Neurofibromatosis. Surg. Neurol. *25*(1):109–113, 1986.
153. Partington, M. D., Rufenacht, D. A., Marsh, W. R., and Piepgras, D. G.: Cranial and sacral dural arteriovenous fistulas as a cause of myelopathy. J. Neurosurg. *76*:615–622, 1992.
154. Quint, D. J., Patel, S. C., Sanders, W. P., et al.: Importance of absence of CSF pulsation artifacts in the MRI detection of significant myelographic block at 1.5 T. Am. J. Neuroradiol. *10*:1089–1095, 1989.
155. Reivich, M., Holling, H. E., Robert, B., et al.: N. Engl. J. Med. *265*:878–885, 1961.
156. Rengachary, S. S., and Murphy, D.: Subarachnoid hematoma following lumbar puncture causing compression of the cauda equina: Case report. J. Neurosurg. *41*:252–254, 1974.
157. Richardson, R. R., and Cerullo, L. J.: Spinal epidural cavernous hemangioma. Surg. Neurol. *12*:266–268, 1979.
158. Rogers, L. A.: Acute subdural hematoma and death following lateral cervical spinal puncture: Case report. J. Neurosurg. *58*:284–286, 1983.
159. Rosenblum, B., Oldfield, E. H., Doppman, J. L., and DiChiro, G.: Spinal arteriovenous malformations: A comparison of dural arteriovenous fistulas and intradural AVM's in 81 patients. J. Neurosurg. *67*:795–802, 1987.
160. Ross, J. S., Masaryk, T. J, Modic, M. T., et al.: Vertebral hemangiomas: MRI imaging. Radiology *165*:165–169, 1987.
161. Rubin, J. B., Enzman, D. R., and Wright, A.: CSF-gated MRI imaging of the spine: Theory and clinical implementation. Radiology *163*:784–792, 1987.
162. Rubin, J. B., and Enzman, D. R.: Harmonic modulation of proton MRI precessional phase by pulsative motion: Origin and spinal CSF flow phenomena. A. J. R. Am. J. Roentgenol. *148*:938–994, 1987.
163. Rubin, J. B., and Enzman, D. R.: Optimizing conventional MRI imaging of the spine. Radiology *163*:777–783, 1987.
164. Rubin, J. M., Aisen, A., and DiPietro, M. A.: Ambiguities in MRI imaging of tumoral cysts in the spinal cord. J. Comput. Assist. Tomogr. *10*:395–398, 1986.
165. Rubinstein, L. J.: Tumors and malformation of blood vessels. *In* Firminger, H. I. (ed.): Tumors of the Central Nervous System. Washington, DC, Armed Forces Institute of Pathology, 1985, pp. 235–256.
166. Runge, V. M., Bradley, W. G., Brant-Zawadzki, M. N., et al.: Clinical safety and efficacy of gadoteridol: A study in 411 patients with suspected intracranial and spinal disease. Radiology *181*:709–709, 1991.

167. Russell, D. S., and Rubinstein, L. J. (eds.): Pathology of Tumors of the Nervous System. Baltimore, Williams & Wilkins, 1989.

168. Ruzal-Shapiro, C., Berdon, W. E., Cohen, M. D., and Abramson, S. J.: MRI imaging of diffuse bone marrow replacement in pediatric patients with cancer. Radiology 181:587–589, 1991.

169. Sato, Y., Waziri, M., Smith W., et al.: Hippel-Lindau disease: MRI imaging. Radiology 166:241–246, 1988.

170. Schroth, G., Thron, A., Guhl, L., et al.: Magnetic resonance imaging of spinal meningiomas and neurinomas: Improvement of imaging by paramagnetic contrast enhancement. J. Neurosurg. 66:695–700, 1987.

171. Shapiro, R.: Tumors. In Shapiro, R. (ed.): Myelography. Chicago, Year Book Medical Publishers, 1984, pp. 345–421.

172. Sloof, J. L., Kernohan, J. W., and MacCarty, C. S.: Primary Intramedullary Tumors of the Spinal Cord and Filum Terminale. Philadelphia, W. B. Saunders Co., 1964.

173. Smoker, W. R. K., et al.: The role of MRI imaging in evaluating metastatic spinal disease. A. J. N. R. Am. J. Neuroradiol. 8:901–908, 1987.

174. Solomon, R. A., and Stein, B. M.: Unusual spinal cord enlargement related to intramedullary hemangioblastoma. J. Neurosurg. 68:550–553, 1988.

175. Sonneland, P. R., Scheithauer, B. W., and Onofrio, B. M.: Myxopapillary ependymoma, a clinicopathologic and immunocytochemical study of 77 cases. Cancer 56:883–893, 1985.

176. Spjut, H. J., and Ayala, A. G.: Skeletal Tumors in Childhood and Adolescence: Pathology of Neoplasia in Children and Adolescents. Philadelphia, W. B. Saunders Co., 1984.

177. Stein, S. C., Ommaya, A. K., Doppman, J. L., and DiChiro, G.: Arteriovenous malformation of the cauda equina with arterial supply from branches of the internal iliac arteries. J. Neurosurg. 36(5):649–651, 1972.

178. Steinbach, L. S., Tehranzadeh, J., Fleckenstein, J. L., et al.: Human immunodeficiency virus infection: Musculoskeletal manifestations. Radiology 186:833–838, 1993.

179. Stimac, G. K., Porter, B. A., Olson, D. O., et al.: Gadolinium-DTPA enhanced MRI imaging of spinal neoplasms: Preliminary investigation and comparison with unenhanced spin-echo and STIR sequences. A. J. N. R. Am. J. Neuroradiol. 9:839–846, 1988.

180. Symon, L., Kuyama, H., and Kendall, B.: Dural arteriovenous malformations of the spine: Clinical features and surgical results in 55 cases. J. Neurosurg. 60:238–247, 1984.

181. Sze, G., Abramson, A., Krol, G., et al.: Gadolinium-DTPA in the evaluation of intradural extra-medullary spinal disease. A. J. N. R. Am. J. Neuroradiol. 9:153–163, 1988.

182. Sze, G., Krol, G., Zimmerman, R. D., and Deck, M. D. F.: Intramedullary disease of the spine: Diagnosis using gadolinium-DTPA enhanced MRI imaging. A. J. N. R. Am. J. Neuroradiol. 9:847–858, 1988.

183. Sze, G., Stimac, G. K., Barlett, C., et al.: Multicenter study of gadopenetate dimeglumine as an MRI contrast agent: Evaluation in patients with spinal tumors. A. J. N. R. Am. J. Neuroradiol. 11:967–974, 1990.

184. Sze, G., Abramson, A., Krol, G., et al.: Gadolinium-DPTA: Malignant extradural spinal tumors. Radiology 167:217–233, 1988.

185. Teny, P., and Papatheodorou, C.: Myelography appearance of vascular anomalies of the spinal cord. Br. J. Radiol. 37:358–366, 1964.

186. Terwey, B., Becker, H., Thron, A. K., and Vahldiek, G.: Gadolinium-DTPA enhanced MRI imaging of spinal dural arteriovenous fistulas. J. Comput. Assist. Tomogr. 13(1):30–37, 1989.

187. Theron, J., Cosgrove, R., Melanson, D., and Ethier, R.: Spinal arteriovenous malformations: Advances in therapeutic embolization. Radiology 158:163–169, 1986.

188. Tillman, B. P., Dahlin, D. C., Lipscomb, P. R., and Stewart, J. R.: Aneurysmal bone cyst: An analysis of 95 cases. Mayo Clin. Proc. 43:478–495, 1968.

189. Tsai, J. C., Dalinka, M. K., Fallon, M. D., et al.: Fluid-fluid level: A nonspecific finding in tumors of bone and soft tissue. Radiology 175:779–782, 1990.

190. Valk, J.: Gadolinium-DTPA in MRI of spinal lesions. A. J. N. R. Am. J. Neuroradiol. 9:345–350, 1988.

191. Vinchon, M., Laurian, C., George, B., et al.: Vertebral arteriovenous fistulas: A study of 49 cases and review of the literature. Review. Cardiovasc. Surg. 2(3):359–369, 1994.

192. Vogler, J. B., and Murphy, W. A.: Bone marrow imaging. Radiology 168:679–693, 1988.

193. Wang, A., Lipson, S., Hay Kal, H. A., et al.: Computed tomography of aneurysmal bone cyst of the vertebral body. J. Comput. Assist. Tomogr. 8:1186–1189, 1984.

194. Williams, M. P., Cherryman, G. R., and Husband, J. E.: Magnetic resonance imaging in suspected metastatic spinal cord compression. Clin. Radiol. 40:286–290, 1989.

195. Willis, T. A.: Nutrient arteries of the vertebral bodies. J. Bone Joint Surg. 31A:538–541, 1949.

196. Wirth, F. P., Post, K. D., DiChiro, G., et al.: Foix-Alajouanine disease. Spontaneous thrombosis of a spinal cord arteriovenous malformation: A case report. Neurology 20:1114–1118, 1970.

197. Woollam, D. H., and Millen J. W.: The arterial supply of the spinal cord and its significance. J. Neurol. Neurosurg. Psychiatr. 18:97–102, 1955.

198. Wrobel, C. J., Oldfield, E. H., DiChiro, G., et al.: Myelopathy due to intracranial dural arteriovenous fistulas draining intrathecally into spinal medullary veins. J. Neurosurg. 69:934–939, 1988.

199. Wyburn Mason, R.: The Vascular Abnormalities and Tumors of the Spinal Cord and Its Membranes. London, Kimpton, 1943.

200. Yasirgil, M. G., Symon, L., and Teddy, P. G.: Arteriovenous malformations of the spinal cord. In Symon, L. (ed.): Advances in Technical Standards in Neurosurgery. Vol. 11. Wien, Springer, 1984, pp. 61–102.

201. Yousem, D. M., and Schnall, M. D.: MRI examination for spinal cord compression: Impact of a multicoil system on length of study. J. Comput. Assist. Tomogr. 15(4):598–604, 1991.

202. Yuh, W. T., Zachar C. K., Barloon T. J., et al.: Vertebral compression fractures: Distinction between benign and malignant causes with MRI imaging. Radiology 172:215–218, 1989.

203. Zabramski, J. M., Spetzler R. F., and Sonntag, V. K. H.: Treatment of spinal cavernous angiomas. J. Neurosurg. 69:476, 1988.

204. Zimmer, W. D., Berquist, T. H., McLeod, R. A., et al.: Bone tumors: Magnetic resonance imaging versus computed tomography. Radiology 155:709–718, 1985.

205. Zimmer, W. D., Berquist, T. H., Sim, F. H., et al.: Magnetic resonance imaging of aneurysmal bone cysts. Mayo Clin. Proc. 59:633–636, 1984.

46

Arteriovenous Malformations of the Spinal Cord

Paul C. McCormick, M.D.

Bennett M. Stein, M.D.

Vascular malformations are a rare cause of spinal cord or nerve root dysfunction. These heterogeneous lesions encompass a wide range of etiology, anatomy, pathophysiology, clinical features, and natural history. They occur throughout the spine and may affect any age group. Symptoms and signs result from ischemia, hemorrhage, or compression of the spinal cord. Most spinal vascular malformations are characterized by an abnormal arteriovenous communication, which may be located within the dura, on the spinal cord surface, or within the substance of the spinal cord. The communication may take the form of a simple direct arteriovenous fistula or of a more complex conglomeration (i.e., nidus) of dysmorphic arteries and veins that communicate directly without an intervening capillary bed. While the latter lesions are clearly congenital in nature, the more commonly occurring simple fistulas are probably acquired lesions.

The evaluation and management of spinal vascular malformations have evolved considerably in recent years primarily as a result of accumulating clinical experience and sensitive real-time dynamic visualization and characterization of these lesions with selective spinal angiography. A more fundamental understanding of the diverse anatomy and pathophysiology of these lesions, in conjunction with improved imaging sophistication, advances in endovascular catheter technology and embolization methods, and refined microsurgical techniques, has allowed definitive treatment of these lesions in most patients.

CLASSIFICATION

Spinal vascular malformations are broadly divided according to the presence, or absence, of an abnormal arteriovenous shunt (Table 46–1). Cavernous malformation, a malformation of capillary structure, appears to be the only clinically relevant vascular malformation in which abnormal arteriovenous shunting is not apparent.[19] Arteriovenous malformations (AVMs) are further classified into four types based on the form, location, and structure of the abnormal arteriovenous connection. Type I and IV AVMs represent simple direct arteriovenous fistulas that occur within the dural root sleeve (Type I) or on the spinal cord surface (Type IV). Type II AVMs are true congenital malformations—similar to their intracranial counterparts. Type III AVMs are also congenital but demonstrate extensive contiguous involvement of spinal and paraspinal tissues.

Table 46–1. CLASSIFICATION OF SPINAL VASCULAR MALFORMATIONS

Arteriovenous malformations
Type I (dural fistula)
Type II (glomus AVM)
Type III (juvenile AVM)
Type IV (intradural fistula)
Cavernous malformations

Type I

Type I AVMs are also referred to as a long dorsal AVM, single coiled vessel AVM, angioma racemosum venosum, and dural fistula.[1, 4, 14, 20, 23, 24, 26] The characterization and understanding of this lesion have evolved considerably. Wyburn-Mason,[26] for example, considered these lesions as pure venous malformations and referred to them as angioma racemosum venosum. With the introduction of selective spinal angiography in the 1960s, these lesions were reclassified as slow-flow AVMs. Early surgical treatment was directed at stripping this long dorsal vein off the dorsal spinal cord surface. It was assumed that tiny feeding vessels, too small to be visualized angiographically, supplied this vessel throughout its length. Stripping of this vessel was the only method of definitive treatment. While these treatments did stabilize or improve symptoms in some patients, the postoperative neurologic function worsened in others. It was not until 1977 that Kendall and Logue correctly recognized these lesions as simple arteriovenous fistulas located in a dural nerve root sleeve.[14] The entire intradural portion of the malformation, therefore, represents the enlarged spinal cord venous system that has been pathologically engorged from retrograde venous flow from the fistula into the spinal cord veins (Fig. 46-1). These malformations, therefore, are probably acquired in nature. They almost always arise at lower thoracic and thoracolumbar levels.

Type II

This lesion is considered a glomus or nidus type of malformation and is angiographically and operatively well visualized and defined. These lesions consist of distinct conglomeration, or nidus, of dysmorphic arteries and veins that communicate directly without an intervening capillary bed.[8, 10] The location of this nidus may be completely or partially intramedullary (Fig. 46-2). The nidus is rarely completely confined to the surface of the spinal cord within the epipial tissue (perimedullary). These perimedullary Type II glomus AVMs most commonly occur at the dorsal cervicomedullary junction (Fig. 46-3). Type II glomus AVMs occur throughout the spinal cord, although most arise from the cervical or lumbar enlargement or conus medullaris levels. Cervical AVMs typically demonstrate multiple feeding vessels from the anterior spinal artery and radiculomedullary vessels. Lower thoracic and conus malformations, however, are usually supplied through a single enlarged branch of the anterior spinal artery. Latent anastomotic channels invariably exist, however, and will appear after proximal surgical ligation or endovascular occlusion of the feeding vessel.

Type III

Type III AVMs (juvenile AVMs) are fortunately quite rare. Unlike glomus AVMs, these congenital malformations do not possess a discrete nidus but rather consist of diffuse arteriovenous shunts with variable degrees of involvement of the spinal cord, vertebral, and paraspinal tissues (Fig. 46-4). Associated skin and other metameric anomalies are commonly associated with these lesions.

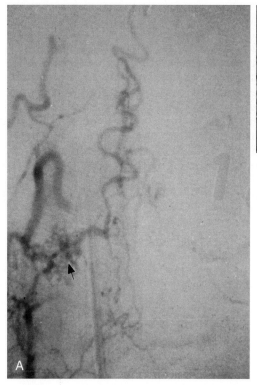
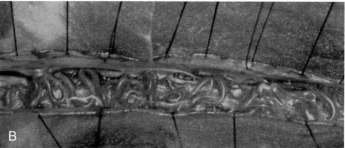

Figure 46-1. *A,* Anteroposterior view of selective spinal angiography of Type I dural fistula demonstrates fistula site *(arrow)* and the characteristic intradural draining vein that extends on the dorsal surface of the spinal cord over several rostral spinal segments. *B,* Surgical view of a Type I dural arteriovenous malformation (AVM) shows enlarged coiled vein on dorsal spinal cord surface. (From Youmans, J. R.: Neurological Surgery. 3rd ed. Philadelphia, W. B. Saunders Co., 1990.)

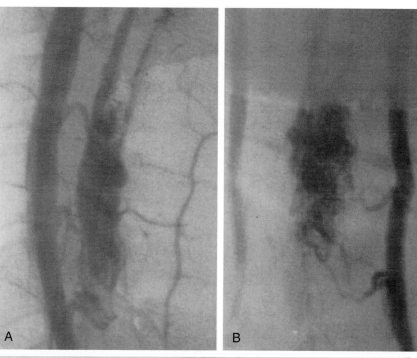

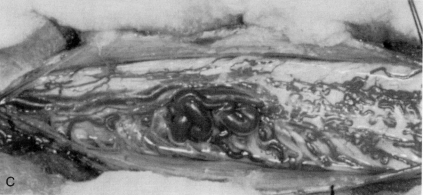

Figure 46–2. *A,* Vertebral arteriogram (lateral view) showing the central location of a midcervical AVM. *B,* Vertebral arteriogram (anteroposterior view) demonstrating the blood supply from the vertebral arteries and the central location of the lesion. *C,* Surgical view of the lesion shown by angiography. The lesion reaches the surface in the form of a large coiled arterialized vein but for the most part lies intramedullary. It was totally removed without additional neurologic deficit. (From Youmans, J. R.: Neurological Surgery. 3rd ed. Philadelphia, W. B. Saunders Co., 1990.)

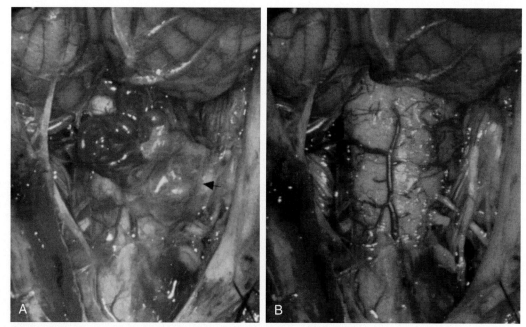

Figure 46–3. *A,* Surgical view of a malformation of the glomus type with associated partially thrombosed venous aneurysm *(arrow).* The lesion was at the dorsal aspect of the cervicomedullary junction. *B,* Complete removal along with the venous aneurysm. (From Youmans, J. R.: Neurological Surgery. 3rd ed. Philadelphia, W. B. Saunders Co., 1990.)

Type IV

Type IV AVMs are intradural fistulas.[4, 5, 22] Most occur in the thoracolumbar region as a fistula between the anterior spinal artery and vein on the ventral spinal cord surface. These perimedullary malformations have been further subdivided according to the complexity and appearance of the lesion.[4, 22] Type IV-A lesions are simple direct fistulas. Type IV-B lesions have one major

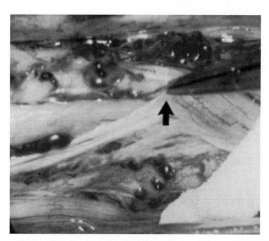

Figure 46–4. Surgical view of a juvenile or diffuse AVM. The spinal cord is rotated by grasping the dentate ligament *(arrow).* This demonstrates the dorsal, dorsolateral, and ventral location of this lesion, which permeates the spinal cord. Removal was impossible. (From Youmans, J. R.: Neurological Surgery. 3rd ed. Philadelphia, W. B. Saunders Co., 1990.)

anterior spinal artery feeder but also demonstrate smaller feeding vessels off the posterior spinal artery. Type IV-C lesions demonstrate several enlarged feeding anterior spinal artery and posterior spinal artery branches into a huge fistula. These subtypes may represent evolutionary changes resulting from venous outflow impairment, thrombosis, collateral vessel recruitment, or ischemia. These lesions occur sporadically and seem to be more likely acquired than congenital in nature. Males and females are affected equally. Symptoms may arise at any age, although most patients present in childhood and early to middle adult years.

SYMPTOMS AND SIGNS

The symptoms and signs of spinal vascular malformations are variable and related primarily to the specific type of malformation. These clinical features result from vascular derangements such as hemorrhage and/or ischemia, or from localized mass effect.

Type I dural malformations usually produce symptoms in middle and advanced adult years, as a result of progressive spinal cord ischemia.[2, 3, 17, 24] The mean age of symptom onset is about 50 years. Men are four to five times more commonly affected than women. Symptom onset is usually insidious with back and leg pain and mild sensory/motor dysfunction. These symptoms are often transiently worsened with activity, particularly exercise or walking. In the early stages functional impairment is minimal and often mimics the much more commonly occurring neurogenic claudication from spinal stenosis. Examination, however, will often show mixed upper and lower motor neuron paresis and patchy sensory loss, which are useful differentiating features from lumbar spinal stenosis. Left untreated, these symptoms inexorably progress and may be punctuated by episodes of acute worsening. In some patients, neurologic worsening may rapidly progress following months or even years of subtle or mildly advancing symptoms. Without treatment, most patients will be significantly disabled or wheelchair-bound within six months to three years following symptom onset.[23]

Most Type II glomus AVMs present in childhood and early adult years. An acute presentation from subarachnoid or intramedullary hemorrhage is most common.[24] Patients who harbor venous aneurysms seem to be more likely to experience a hemorrhagic event. Presumably, the site of the hemorrhage is the aneurysm. The acute onset of severe neck or back pain—approximating the level of the malformation—is typically the first symptom of a hemorrhagic event. The occurrence and progression of neurologic deficit are variable and depend on the location and severity of the hemorrhage. There is often no neurologic deficit if the hemorrhage is confined to the subarachnoid space. Instead, the patient may present with nonspecific localizing signs and symptoms of subarachnoid hemorrhage. One of our patients had such a hemorrhage, which was unassociated with definite localizing features of a spinal cord lesion. The presence of subhyoid hemorrhages, severe nuchal rigidity, and cerebral symptoms suggested rupture of an intracranial aneurysm. It was only after negative cerebral angiography and the findings of a plantar Babinski response and a level to pain perception over the thoracolumbar region that the origin of the hemorrhage was suspected in the spinal cord.[13] Subsequent angiography demonstrated a T12 glomus AVM (Fig. 46–5). Hemorrhage into the substance of the spinal cord usually results in an objective neurologic deficit. Typically these deficits evolve within a few minutes to hours after the initial hemorrhagic presentation. The severity of the deficit ranges from mild to complete. Some degree of recovery usually follows an incomplete lesion. A slowly progressive neurologic syndrome occurs less commonly as a result of vascular steal or rarely from mass effect of the enlarged coils of the malformation. Type III (juvenile AVMs) and Type IV (intradural fistula) present similarly with hemorrhage or progressive neurologic deficit from steal or mass effect.

PATHOPHYSIOLOGY

The pathophysiology of vascular malformations reflects localized derangements in the spinal cord blood flow. In Type I dural AVMs, for example, spinal cord ischemia results from venous hypertension.[1, 23, 24] Despite the relatively slow flow through the small fistula, intradural venous pressure becomes markedly elevated and may approach systemic mean arterial pressure. This reduces spinal cord perfusion pressure (e.g., spinal cord perfusion pressure = mean systemic arterial pres-

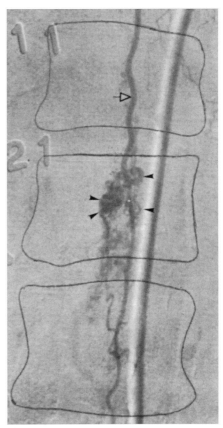

Figure 46–5. Spinal angiogram (anterior/posterior view) showing AVM of the spinal cord with a large draining *(open arrow)* and the nidus of the malformation *(small arrows)*. The lesion was at T12 and gave rise to diffuse hemorrhage mimicking a cerebral aneurysm rupture. (Reprinted by the permission of the publisher from Kasdon, D. L., Wolpert, S. M., and Stein, B. M.: Surgical and angiographic localization of spinal arteriovenous malformations. Surg. Neurol. 5:279–283, 1976. Copyright 1976, Elsevier Science Publishing Company, Inc.)

sure − venous pressure) and results in progressive spinal cord ischemia. Intraspinal venous pressure may be transiently elevated during activity and exercise, which accounts for the reversible exacerbation of ischemic symptoms during these activities. Venous hypertension may be more significantly impaired from structural intravascular changes such as vessel wall intimal thickening and hyalinization with progressive narrowing of the intradural veins chronically exposed to elevated intravascular pressures (Fig. 46–6). Episodic acute neurologic deterioration in these patients may occur as a result of venous thrombosis. In the early stages, these symptoms are often reversible. In untreated cases, however, progressive chronic ischemia ultimately leads to irreversible neuronal loss and infarction.

Progressive ischemia may also result from a high-flow lesion, which is demonstrated in Type II, III, and IV malformations. In these cases, the AVM nidus acts as a high-flow, low-resistance sump that siphons blood

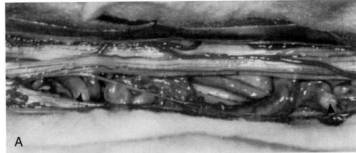

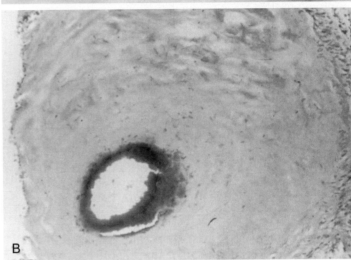

Figure 46–6. *A,* Surgical view of a spinal AVM located partially in the cauda equina. There are thrombosed vessels within this malformation *(arrow)*. *B,* Histologic specimen of vessel removed, showing hyalinization and endarteritis obliterans with a minimal lumen. (In Youmans, J. R.: Neurological Surgery. 3rd ed. Philadelphia, W. B. Saunders Co., 1990.)

flow from the surrounding normal spinal cord vascular system. Although vascular resistance in these systems is fairly low, the high pressure and flow characteristics through these dysmorphic vessels render them susceptible to hemorrhage. In most cases the hemorrhage occurs on the venous side of the malformation—commonly from a venous aneurysm. Progressive neurologic deficit may also result from localized mass effect of the lesion. Enlarged tortuous feeding vessels or draining veins can produce spinal nerve root or spinal cord compression with resultant radicular pain or progressive myelopathy, respectively.

RADIOLOGIC DIAGNOSIS

Although selective spinal angiography is the procedure of choice for a definitive diagnosis and characterization of spinal AVMs, its invasive nature precludes its use as a practical screening study. Fortunately, water-soluble myelography and magnetic resonance imaging (MRI) will sensitively identify or suggest a spinal AVM. Myelography remains particularly useful for identification of Type I dural fistulas. Although the site of the fistula is not identified, the characteristic serpentine filling defect on the dorsal spinal cord surface strongly suggests the diagnosis (Fig. 46–7). Occasionally, the filling defect may be seen extending toward a neural foramen, which may suggest the level and side of the dural fistula and direct subsequent selective angiography ac-

cordingly. This serpentine filling defect should be differentiated from the commonly seen filling defects that extend rostrally from a high-grade extradural stenotic block. These lumbar stenosis–associated defects arise from congested intradural vessels and redundant nerve roots.

MRI also sensitively identifies abnormal surface vascular abnormalities and is a useful screening study for spinal vascular malformations. In some cases, however, circular flow voids—erroneously suggesting a pathologically enlarged spinal vessel—may result from a differential CSF flow caused by arachnoid septations. MRI is particularly useful for identifying intramedullary vascular malformations and defines the relationship of the malformation to the spinal cord (Fig. 46–8). This latter feature is particularly useful for operative planning. Thus, MRI is complementary to spinal angiography. The definitive diagnosis and characteristics of a spinal AVM are achieved with selective spinal angiography. This study identifies the site of abnormal arteriovenous communication, defines flow characteristics, and locates critical spinal cord vessels (e.g., artery of Adamkiewicz) (Fig. 46–9).[5–8, 10, 11, 14, 16, 22, 25]

TREATMENT

Successful treatment of a spinal AVM requires total obliteration or excision of the abnormal AVM.[1, 4, 5, 11, 13, 15–18, 20, 21, 23, 25, 27] Procedures that only partially reduce the

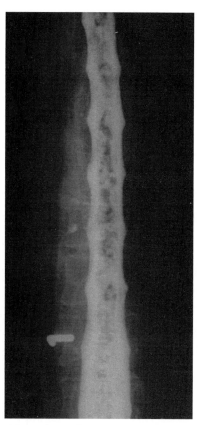

Figure 46–7. Thoracic myelogram anteroposterior view demonstrates a typical long serpentine filling defect, which is characteristic of a Type I dural AVM.

malformation such as embolization or proximal feeding vessel ligation may have temporary benefit, but their long-term efficacy has not been established.

Embolization

The role of embolization in the management of spinal vascular malformation continues to evolve. Early experience with particulate embolic agents (i.e., Gelfoam, pellets, polyvinyl alcohol [PVA]) were encouraging but short lived because of recanalization of the occluded vessels and/or recruitment of collateral channels. However, improvements in catheter technology, endovascular techniques, and embolic agents have significantly improved the safety and efficacy of these techniques, not only as a preoperative adjunct to surgery but also, in some cases, as an independent treatment modality.[12, 22] More precise delivery of rapidly polymerizing liquid adhesives (isobutyl-2-cyanoacrylate [IBCA]) directly into the interstices (i.e., nidus) of the malformation forms a cast that is less likely to recanalize. While embolization remains essentially a surgical adjunct for most intradural glomus AVMs and some fistulas, long-term endovascular repair is increasingly achieved for Type I dural fistulas using embolization as an independent treatment technique.

Operation

General Considerations

On the basis of an improved understanding of the anatomy and pathophysiology of spinal AVMs, surgeons have been able to use the operating microscope to develop better operative techniques aimed at obliteration, resection, or major occlusion of these lesions. The cornerstone of treatment has been microsurgery.

The axiom that the preoperative neurologic status is often related to the postoperative outcome is particularly pertinent in these lesions. Operation should be accomplished early in the disease rather than after waiting for the development of major neurologic deficits, since function is unlikely to improve in the presence of severe incapacity.

The patient is prepared with dexamethasone before operation and may be positioned in a number of ways. Malis prefers to use the sitting position for malformations in the upper thoracic, cervical, and cervicomedullary regions.[18] This position creates a certain degree of hypotension, which may be useful in the removal of the lesion. It also eliminates respiratory movement artifact. For malformations at the lower levels, he prefers an oblique position so as to limit respiratory excursions. Both of these positions preclude the effective use of an assistant during the operation, which we consider a major disadvantage, perhaps outweighing the disadvantage of having respiratory excursions interfere with the focus of the microscope. We prefer to operate on all these lesions with the patient in the prone position, leaving the abdomen and chest free for respiratory excursions.

The surgeon and assistant work together across the operating table. The laminectomy is centered over the extent of the lesion, as identified by myelography and spinal angiography. The laminectomy should be moderately wide and the dura opened widely with preservation of the arachnoid until the extent of the lesion is determined by visualization through the arachnoid. The operating microscope is always used from the time of dural opening. Malformations of the juvenile variety or those that penetrate the spinal cord will be easily identified by visualization of the dorsal, dorsolateral, and ventrolateral portions of the cord. Decisions as to what may be done intraoperatively with these lesions will be discussed under the relevant section. Lesions that have a primary intramedullary location may be identified by a local bulge of the spinal cord in association with draining veins extending over the dorsal surface of the spinal cord or even discoloration due to old hemorrhage or thrombosis within the lesion. As will be discussed, these are treated by myelotomy and techniques similar to operations for intramedullary tumors.

Usually the small bipolar cautery and occasionally the pinpoint type are used under constant irrigation during the occlusion of the AVM. Only the largest vessels are clipped, and from a practical point of view this means clipping no arteries or only one or two

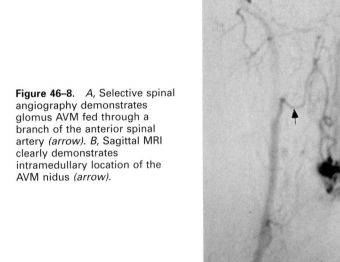
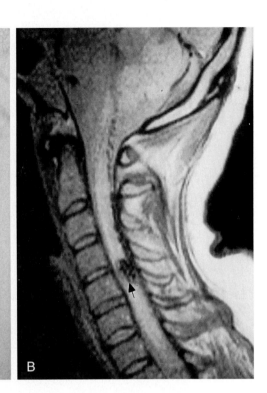

Figure 46–8. *A,* Selective spinal angiography demonstrates glomus AVM fed through a branch of the anterior spinal artery *(arrow)*. *B,* Sagittal MRI clearly demonstrates intramedullary location of the AVM nidus *(arrow)*.

during removal of the usual spinal malformation. It is extremely difficult to use standard metallic clips when removing an intramedullary lesion, and this is best accomplished by bipolar cautery. We prefer to approach the lesions from the arterial side first, while realizing that the venous flow, even though arterialized, is often slow and can be managed easily if rupture occurs on the venous side. We see no advantage to approaching the lesion primarily from the venous side if definite arterial contributions are easily visualized. The lesion is generally peeled away from the spinal cord while additional arterial contributions are coagulated and divided.

In general, malformations within the spinal cord are associated with large venous aneurysms that are often partially thrombosed. These are rather dangerous lesions and one should not rupture them by reducing the venous drainage of the aneurysm more than necessary for collapsing the malformation so that it may be removed safely from within the spinal cord.

Regardless of the location of the malformation, hemostasis is checked carefully after its removal. We have not used therapeutic hypotension during removal, especially in the patient who is in the sitting position. In the prone position, hypotension is not necessary because of the low flow in these malformations. Closure of the dura is highly desirable. If it cannot be accomplished, a covering of Gelfoam will create less scarring than if the dura is left open. In addition, the latter method makes it almost impossible to reoperate on the same site.

SPECIFIC CONSIDERATIONS

Type I Dural AVMs

Treatment of Type I dural AVMs (dural fistula) has been simplified in recent years. Stripping of the long dorsal vein off the spinal cord surface is no longer advocated. It is now recognized that this tedious procedure is not only unnecessary but also may exacerbate neurologic morbidity because of excision of normal, albeit pathologically enlarged, spinal cord venous drainage pathways. Currently, a much more limited procedure—either excision of the dural fistula or interruption of the intradural draining vein—is advocated (Fig. 46–10).[1–3] This can be easily accomplished through a two-level hemilaminectomy and partial medial facetectomy to expose the dural root sleeve and foramen. A paramedian longitudinal dural incision allows exposure of the intradural nerve root and initial segment of the associated draining vein of the malformation. Simple interruption of the draining vein is performed in circumstances in which the radicular vessel that supplies the AV fistula also provides a spinal cord medullary artery. This occurs in less than 10 per cent of cases. Excision of the fistula in these patients risks medullary artery occlusion and possible spinal cord infarction. If no such medullary vessel is present, fistula excision is preferred to prevent re-establishment of retrograde intradural venous drainage through collateral longitudinal extradural venous channels at adjacent radicular levels. To accomplish dural fistula excision, several millimeters of the feeding radicular artery and intradural

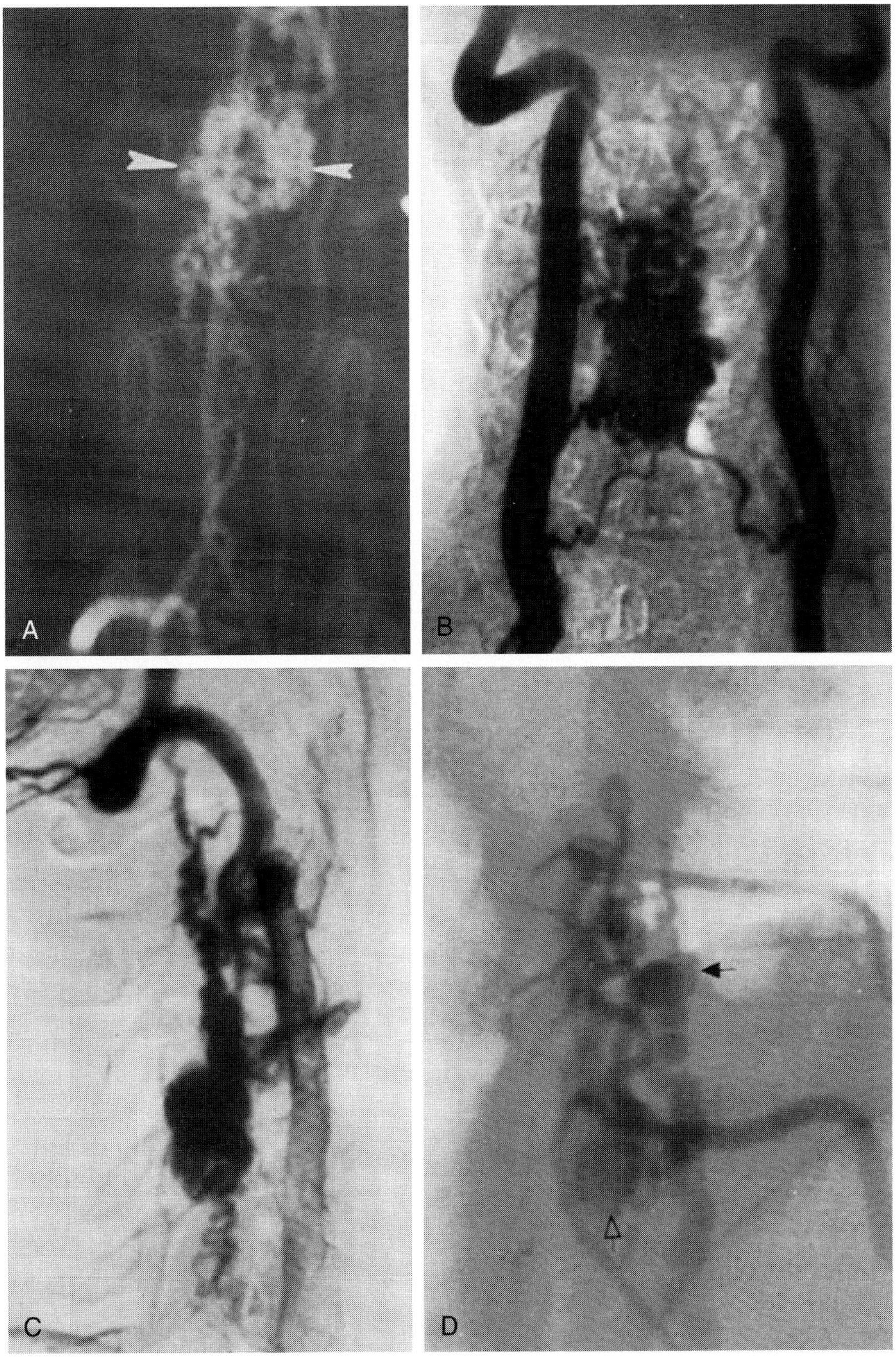

Figure 46–9. Spinal angiograms from various patients. *A,* Unobstructive views showing a prominent AVM at the T12 level with a nidus *(arrows),* draining veins, and feeding arteries. *B,* Bilateral vertebral arteriogram (anteroposterior) showing intramedullary AVM with vertebral artery feeding via the radicular arteries. *C,* Vertebral arteriogram (lateral view) showing the intramedullary location of the nidus of a large AVM. *D,* Spinal angiogram showing the typical configuration of an AVM partially intramedullary and partially extramedullary. Venous aneurysms are identified by arrows. (From Youmans, J. R.: Neurological Surgery. 3rd ed. Philadelphia, W. B. Saunders Co., 1990.)

draining vein are cauterized and divided and contiguously excised along with a small window of the dural root sleeve that contains the actual fistula. The dura can usually be repaired primarily with suture. The remainder of the wound is closed in layers.

Glomus Arteriovenous Malformation

The malformations in the form of a nidus or glomus are the easiest to understand and to treat. They produce symptoms from mass effect, hemorrhage, or venous thrombosis. Therefore, it is logical that they be circumscribed by the interruption of their feeding arteries at the exact margin of the glomus. This approach is preferable to interruption of the major venous drainage, since occlusion of the veins adds nothing to the operation and may jeopardize the outcome by creating intolerable intraluminal forces within the malformation that result in hemorrhage.

The situation is similar for malformations that are primarily intramedullary. They are glomus in configuration, although a rare abnormality is associated with

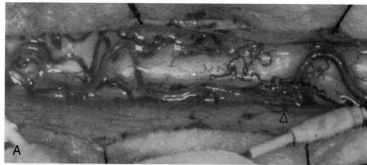
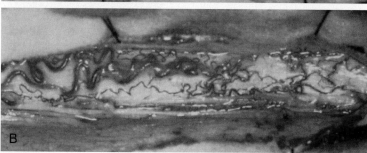

Figure 46–10. *A,* Dorsal arterialized venous malformation (Type I) with a distinct fistulous feeder at T7 *(arrow).* This feeder arterialized not only the dura but also a major portion of the malformation. *B,* Interruption of the feeder and removal of the primary artery to vein fistula. The dorsal surface of the spinal cord still shows some abnormalities but is much improved in appearance. The patient demonstrated a modest recovery after this procedure. (From Youmans, J. R.: Neurological Surgery. 3rd ed. Philadelphia, W. B. Saunders Co., 1990.)

a long dorsal type of malformation in conjunction with the primary intramedullary lesion. We have noted an unusually high incidence of intramedullary lesions in our patients (approximately 20 per cent of all AVMs of the spinal cord). They are managed in the same way as removing a glomus malformation from the dorsal or dorsolateral surface of the cord with the addition of procedures used in the removal of an intramedullary spinal cord tumor. The locus of the lesion is visualized as the cord is exposed. A myelotomy is then made in a longitudinal direction from the polar aspects of the lesion. This maneuver allows visualization of the rostral and caudal margins of the malformation. Dissection may be carried around the appropriate margin, depending on the anatomy of the venous drainage and arterial supply as determined from angiograms and intraoperative observations (Fig. 46–11). These lesions are preferably approached from the arterial side; bipolar cautery is used to interrupt the arterial feeders while the malformation is rolled toward the venous pedicle. Occasionally the venous pedicle is in direct relationship to the major blood supply from the anterior spinal artery. It should be possible to approach the lesion from the arterial side, and once the artery is interrupted the venous pedicle is easy to manage. Clips are rarely used.

Sharp dissection is always preferred when removing the lesion, as opposed to blunt or tearing types of dissection techniques. Frequently these lesions are associated with a large aneurysmal dilatation. The aneurysms may cause special problems, as they often are partially thrombosed but are still active and thin walled. These findings predispose the aneurysms to intraoperative hemorrhage secondary to excessive manipulation—a catastrophic event that should be avoided. Careful use of a broad bipolar cautery tip

under irrigation may be utilized to shrink these venous aneurysms, but care must be taken that the wall is not violated. In many cases, the intact aneurysm may be gently teased out of the cord. The aneurysm is often on the edge of the shunt component of the malformation. The cavity left by removal of these lesions is similar in size and configuration to that left by the total removal of a large intramedullary tumor. It is remarkable how thin the surrounding spinal cord structure can be and yet still result in an improving neurologic picture postoperatively, and eventually in a functional neurologic state.

Juvenile or Diffuse Arteriovenous Malformations

These lesions are the most difficult ones to treat. They penetrate the spinal cord, and histologic examination indicates violation of presumably functional cord tissue interspersed with vascular channels of the malformation. It is obvious that these malformations do not have well-defined margins permitting resection and that they comprehensively involve both the interior and the exterior of the spinal cord over many segments. Confirmation of these lesions must be left to operative exploration, as definitive knowledge of their presence, which would preclude intraoperative resection, cannot be obtained by the usual radiographic studies now available. Perhaps MRI will answer this question in the future. Although these are nonresectable lesions, in one instance we were able to clip a major radicular artery using evoked potential monitoring and witness significant clinical improvement in an individual who had been plagued by progressive deterioration of spinal cord function (Fig. 46–12). In most instances, these lesions can be treated with little more than a decom-

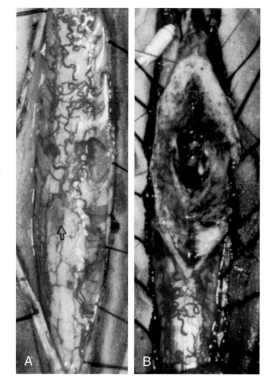

Figure 46–11. *A,* Surgical view of the large intramedullary AVM that is partially thrombosed. The arrow indicates the tip of the intramedullary, partially thrombosed venous aneurysm. *B,* Total extirpation by myelotomy of the malformation and partially thrombosed venous aneurysm. This patient showed remarkable improvement from the near total loss of spinal cord function at this level. (From Youmans, J. R.: Neurological Surgery. 3rd ed. Philadelphia, W. B. Saunders Co., 1990.)

pressive procedure and perhaps, in exceptional cases, with selective ligation of arteries under evoked potential monitoring. All of these maneuvers are of questionable benefit, however, and should not be performed if there is a hint that harm is being done to the patient.

Type IV AVMs

Management of Type IV AVMs is dependent on the size and complexity of the lesion.[5, 22] For small Type IV-A fistulas, surgical ligation of the fistula is definitive.

Adequate exposure of these ventral lesions often requires facetectomy and spinal cord rotation with suture retraction on a divided dentate ligament. For more complex, higher flow lesions, endovascular occlusion with liquid adhesive or detachable balloons is effectively utilized either as primary treatment or as a preoperative adjunct.[22]

Cavernous Malformations

The technique of cavernous malformation removal depends upon its intramedullary location. A circumscrib-

Figure 46–12. *A,* Interruption of two major feeders (Yasargil aneurysm clips) to a juvenile type of AVM. *B,* Identification of a single major arterial feeder *(arrows)* to an intramedullary conus and cauda equina AVM. The interruption of this single feeder led to marked clinical improvement without resection of any additional portion of the malformation. This was considered to be a diffuse or juvenile AVM. (In Youmans, J. R.: Neurological Surgery. 3rd ed. Philadelphia, W. B. Saunders Co., 1990.)

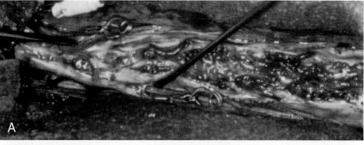
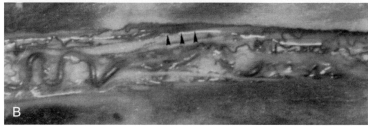

ing pial incision allows detachment of pial-based lesions to be delivered out of the substance of the spinal cord. Deep lesions are exposed through a midline myelotomy. These unencapsulated lesions are usually well circumscribed and present a clear surface plane for dissection.[19] Rarely, a more diffuse lesion permeates the spinal cord tissue and precludes surgical removal.

SUMMARY

Vascular malformations of the spinal cord are rare, and even in tertiary care centers that specialize in microsurgery and the treatment of such unusual lesions, the number of cases per year is small. Accordingly, there is still a lack of detailed information about the pathophysiology of these lesions, which is necessary to design appropriate operative therapy. However, the availability of sophisticated spinal angiography techniques and the enumeration of operative results have led to proposals concerning treatment that appear to have changed the course of the disease. These malformations produce a high rate of incapacity in a relatively young and productive group of patients. Other techniques that have been used to manage intracranial AVMs, such as radiotherapy, embolization, and partial ligation procedures, are less applicable to such malformations of the spinal cord.

The primary aim is obliteration or excision of the abnormal arteriovenous communication. This is now routinely achieved for most Type I dural AVMs, Type II glomus AVMs, and Type IV arteriovenous fistulas. Similarly, most cavernous malformations can be successfully excised with preservation of neurologic function. Although repeat endovascular techniques may significantly, albeit temporarily, palliate debilitating symptoms of juvenile AVMs, no definitive treatment exists for these lesions.

The operative mortality in our series has been zero, and the morbidity is usually related to additional temporary deficits that eventually clear and in most cases show improvement in the postoperative period. However, if the patient is in very poor condition prior to the operation because of the effects of the lesion, it is unlikely that much improvement can be expected even after a technically successful operation. Therefore, it is important to recognize these lesions in their early stages and institute proper diagnostic measures followed by operative obliteration by a neurosurgeon versed in the techniques of spinal, intramedullary, and vascular surgery.

References

1. Afshar, J. K. B., Doppmann, J. L., and Oldfield, E. H.: Surgical interruption of intradural draining vein as curative treatment of spinal dural arteriovenous fistulas. J. Neurosurg. 82:196–200, 1995.
2. Aminoff, M. J., and Logue, V.: Clinical features of spinal vascular malformations. Brain 97:197–210, 1974.
3. Aminoff, M. J., and Logue, V.: The prognosis of patients with spinal vascular malformations. Brain 97:211–218, 1974.
4. Anson, J. A., and Spetzler, R. F.: Classification of spinal arteriovenous malformations and implications for treatment. Barrow Neurol. Inst. Q. 8:2–8, 1992.
5. Barrow, D. L., Colohan, A. R. T., and Dawson, R.: Intradural perimedullary arteriovenous fistulas (Type IV spinal cord arteriovenous malformations). J. Neurosurg. 81:221–229, 1994.
6. Cogen, P., and Stein, B. M.: Spinal cord arteriovenous malformations with significant intramedullary components. J. Neurosurg. 59:471–478, 1983.
7. Djindjian, R.: Embolization of angiomas of the spinal cord. Surg. Neurol. 4:411–420, 1975.
8. Doppman, J. L.: The nidus concept of spinal cord arteriovenous malformations: A surgical recommendation based upon angiographic observations. Br. J. Radiol. 44:758–763, 1971.
9. Hall, W. A., Oldfield, E. H., and Doppman, J. L.: Recanalization of spinal arteriovenous malformation following embolization. J. Neurosurg. 70:714–720, 1989.
10. Houdart, R., Djindjian, R., and Hurth, M.: Vascular malformations of the spinal cord: The anatomic and therapeutic significance of arteriography. J. Neurosurg. 24:583–594, 1966.
11. Houdart, R., Djindjian, R., Hurth, M., et al.: Treatment of angiomas of the spinal cord. Surg. Neurol. 2:186–194, 1974.
12. Hurst, R. W., and Berenstein, A.: Endovascular treatment of spinal arteriovenous malformations. In Cohen, A. R., and Haines, S. J. (eds.): Minimally Invasive Techniques in Neurosurgery. Baltimore, Williams & Wilkins, 1995, pp. 185–198.
13. Kasdon, D. L., Wolpert, S. M., and Stein, B. M.: Surgical and angiographic localization of spinal arteriovenous malformations. Surg. Neurol. 5:279–283, 1976.
14. Kendall, B. E., and Logue, V.: Spinal epidural angiomatous malformations, draining into intrathecal veins. Neuroradiology 13:181–189, 1977.
15. Krayenbuhl, H., Yasargil, M. G., and McClintock, H. G.: Treatment of spinal cord vascular malformations by surgical excision. J. Neurosurg. 30:427–435, 1969.
16. Kunc, Z., and Bret, J.: Diagnosis and treatment of vascular malformations of the spinal cord. J. Neurosurg. 30:436–445, 1969.
17. Logue, V.: Angiomas of the spinal cord: Review of the pathogenesis, clinical features, and results of surgery. J. Neurol. Neurosurg. Psychiatr. 42:1–11, 1979.
18. Malis, L. I.: Microsurgery for spinal cord arteriovenous malformations. Clin. Neurosurg. 26:543–555, 1979.
19. McCormick, P. C., Michelsen, W. J., Post, K. D., et al.: Cavernous malformations of the spinal cord. Neurosurgery 23:459–463, 1988.
20. McCormick, P. C., and Stein, B. M.: Management of spinal vascular malformations. In Barnett, H. J. M., Mohr, J. P., Stein, B. M., and Yatsu, F. M. (eds.): Stroke: Pathophysiology, Diagnosis, and Management. 2nd ed. New York, Churchill Livingstone, 1992, pp. 1135–1143.
21. McCormick, P. C.: Vascular tumors and vascular malformations of the spine. In Vinken, P. J., and Bruyn, G. W. (eds.): Handbook of Clinical Neurology. Amsterdam, Elsevier, 1996.
22. Mourier, K. L., Gobin, Y. P., and George, B.: Intradural perimedullary arteriovenous fistulae: Results of surgical and endovascular treatment in a series of 35 cases. Neurosurgery 32:885–891, 1993.
23. Oldfield, E. H., Di Chiro, G., and Quindlen, E. A.: Successful treatment of a group of spinal cord arteriovenous malformations by interruption of dural fistula. J. Neurosurg. 59:1019–1030, 1983.
24. Rosenblum, B., Oldfield, E. H., and Doppmann, J. L.: Spinal arteriovenous malformations: A comparison of dural arteriovenous fistulas and intradural AVMs in 81 patients. J. Neurosurg. 67:795–802, 1987.
25. Stein, B. M.: Arteriovenous malformations of the brain and spinal cord. In Hoff, J. (ed.): Practice of Surgery. New York, Harper & Row, 1979.
26. Wyburn-Mason, R.: The Vascular Abnormalities and Tumours of the Spinal Cord and Its Membranes. London, Henry Kimpton, 1943.
27. Yasargil, M. G., DeLong, W. B., and Guarnaschelli, J. J.: Complete microsurgical excision of cervical extramedullary and intramedullary vascular malformations. Surg. Neurol. 4:211–224, 1975.

47

Medical Myelopathies

Joseph R. Berger, M.D.

Stephen J. Ryan, M.D., M.A.

Spinal cord disease may result from a variety of insults. A general classification of these various etiologies is provided in Table 47–1. The "medical" causes of spinal cord dysfunction are addressed in this chapter.

The natural history of these myelopathies and the physical findings resulting from them are dependent on the rapidity of onset of the lesion and its specific location in the spinal cord, particularly with respect to the spinal tracts involved. Typically, the chief complaints of patients presenting with these forms of myelopathy are lower extremity weakness and gait disturbance. A sense of stiffness of the legs is common. If the cervical spinal cord is involved, upper extremity weakness is to be expected. A loss of dexterity in the fingers and hands is often perceived by the patient. Not infrequently, the patient may complain of numbness and other sensory abnormalities. If the illness involves the posterior columns in the cervical region, the patient may demonstrate Lhermitte's phenomenon, characterized by a sense of lightning-like electric shocks that generally radiate down the spine and into the extremities on neck flexion. Variants of this phenomenon may occur, and other forms of head and neck movement may precipitate this fleeting discomfort. Spinal cord disease involving the posterior columns in the thoracic region may result in a disquieting bandlike or girdle-like sensation across the chest or abdomen. This phenomenon is a helpful localizing clue. Paresthesias of the distal extremities may also result from these lesions. Incontinence of bladder and bowel and sexual impotence are common.

Generally, but not invariably, a thorough neurologic examination allows the physician to distinguish spinal cord involvement from other causes of these neurologic complaints. The presence of concomitant neurologic illness attributable to disease of the cerebral hemispheres or brain stem, such as hemianopsia, ophthalmoplegia, or dysarthria, does not rule out the possibility of concomitant spinal cord disease, but it should suggest that the neurologic findings may be ascribed to single or multiple lesions higher in the neuraxis than the spinal cord. The physical examination of patients with spinal cord lesions that have developed gradually or who have acute lesions that have been present for several weeks typically reveals a spastic weakness of the involved extremities, with associated hyperreflexia and pathologic reflexes. The latter include Hoffmann's sign (palmar flexion of the thumb when the distal phalanx of the middle finger of the same hand is rapidly tapped) in the upper extremities and Babinski's sign (plantar extension of the hallux when the sole of the foot is stroked) in the lower extremities. Several variants of these signs have been described.[36] Superficial reflexes, such as abdominal and cremasteric reflexes, are absent.

In the early period of an acutely developing spinal cord lesion, "spinal shock" is typical, in which a flaccid weakness of the extremities predominates. Although this entity is more common with traumatic lesions of the spinal cord, it may result from infectious, vascular, or other insults. The presence of a flaccid weakness with areflexia or hyporeflexia may falsely lead to a

Table 47–1. ETIOLOGIES OF MYELOPATHY

Congenital and developmental defects
Trauma
Compromise of the spinal canal by degenerative spinal disease
  and disc herniation
Idiopathic acute or subacute transverse myelitis
Postinfectious and postvaccination myelitis
Multiple sclerosis
Adrenomyeloneuropathy
Infectious myelitis—viral, bacterial, fungal, parasitic
Epidural abscess
Arachnoiditis
Vascular disease of the spinal cord—atherosclerotic,
  arteriovenous malformation, epidural hematoma
Connective tissue diseases—rheumatoid arthritis, Sjögren's
  syndrome, systemic lupus erythematosus
Sarcoid myelopathy
Paraneoplastic myelopathy
Metabolic and nutritional disease of the spinal cord—vitamin
  B_{12} deficiency, chronic liver disease, hyperparathyroidism,
  hyperthyroidism
Toxin
Decompression illness
Electrical injury
Radiation therapy
Necrotic myelopathy of unknown etiology
Heredofamilial degeneration—hereditary spastic paraplegia,
  Friedreich's ataxia, others

diagnosis of an acute peripheral neuropathy, as may be observed with Guillain-Barré syndrome. A careful sensory examination is critical to distinguish between these possibilities. A sensory level is to be expected with a spinal cord lesion but is hardly an invariable finding. Guillain-Barré syndrome is predominantly a motor neuropathy, and when it results in sensory loss, a mild decrease in vibratory sensation in the distal extremities is usually observed. Although more severe forms of sensory loss may be seen with this and other causes of peripheral neuropathy, a sensory level is not present.

The appearance of a Brown-Séquard syndrome is pathognomonic of spinal cord disease. The latter results from injury to half of the spinal cord and is characterized by the presence of weakness and loss of position and vibratory sensory perception ipsilateral to the side of the lesion and the loss of pinprick and temperature sensory perception on the side of the body contralateral to the lesion.

ACUTE IDIOPATHIC TRANSVERSE MYELITIS

Acute idiopathic transverse myelitis most often presents with paresthesias of the feet, toes, or fingertips.[125] Gradually developing numbness and coincident weakness of the legs follow, with subsequent paralysis of the legs. The features of this illness usually evolve over one to three weeks, but it may develop abruptly. The initial symptoms may be predominantly unilateral, and asymmetric findings are not uncommon. As the illness progresses, upper extremity numbness and weakness

and bowel and bladder incontinence may ensue. In some patients, the posterior column is spared early but affected later (decreased vibration and position senses). Occasionally, back (interscapular) pain and, more rarely, calf, arm, or radicular pain may accompany the progressive myelopathy, suggesting other pathologic processes, such as an intraspinal neoplasm or epidural abscess. To be considered idiopathic, it should be unassociated with a known preceding or concomitant viral infection. The dominant pathologic feature in the spinal cord is demyelination. Treatment with adrenocorticotrophin (ACTH) or corticosteroids is advocated, but the response to this therapy is highly variable. Approximately one third of patients have a return of normal gait and bladder function.[125] When recovery to a normal or nearly normal level of function occurs, it does so within one year of the onset of the illness. Twenty-five per cent of affected patients are left wheelchair bound or bedridden, and the remainder have varying degrees of lesser disability.[125]

In some instances, the myelopathy develops abruptly. Frequently, a flaccid, areflexic paralysis of the affected limbs accompanies spinal shock. Loss of vision resulting from optic nerve inflammation may accompany this myelopathy. The combination of acute optic neuritis and transverse myelitis has been referred to as Devic's disease. Like the more slowly evolving idiopathic transverse myelitis, demyelination is a characteristic neuropathologic hallmark. The pathology has been described as a necrotizing hemorrhagic leukomyelitis. The prognosis of patients with this rapidly evolving myelopathy, particularly when it is accompanied by spinal shock, is worse than that for the more gradually developing transverse myelitis.[95]

The differential diagnosis of idiopathic transverse myelitis includes multiple sclerosis and postinfectious or postvaccination myelitis, which are quite similar clinically and pathologically. Multiple sclerosis may initially present as a transverse myelitis. The likelihood of transverse myelitis being the presenting manifestation of multiple sclerosis was previously placed at 5 to 15 per cent,[7, 16, 95, 125] but with the advent of more sensitive testing (magnetic resonance imaging), this likelihood has been estimated at 42 to 80 per cent.[50, 105, 108] A temporal association with a viral illness (see Table 47–3), signs and symptoms that develop over a few days, and a monophasic course should suggest the possibility of a viral myelitis.[3]

The diagnostic approach to a patient suspected of having acute transverse myelitis begins with a thorough history and physical examination. Evidence of a recent viral illness should be sought. A history of syphilis, connective tissue disease, or prior neurologic illness may prove essential in arriving at the correct diagnosis. Serologic studies should always include a serum VDRL and FTA-ABS for syphilis. Magnetic resonance imaging (MRI) of the involved area of the spinal cord is the single best radiographic study. The MRI may be normal or reveal cord swelling and/or hyperintense lesions on T2-weighted imaging intrinsic to the spinal cord. Miller and colleagues[104] found lesions on

MRI at the clinically expected level in 64 per cent of patients with a clinical syndrome suggestive of cervical involvement, but in only 28 per cent with a suspected thoracic or lumbar lesion. However, other investigators have found a higher correlation between spinal MRI findings and neurologic deficits.[135] Generally, MRI, if available, negates the need for myelography. If an MRI scan is not available, myelography should be done, with water-soluble contrast and computed tomography (CT) of the affected area. If pain is a significant component of the patient's illness, a CT scan of the appropriate area and a bone scan may be desirable to eliminate the possibility of an epidural abscess or neoplasm. Cerebrospinal fluid (CSF) examination typically reveals mononuclear pleocytosis, often with up to 100 to 200 cells, and increased protein. With necrotizing myelopathy, the spinal cord may swell enough to result in spinal block, with an abnormal Queckenstedt's test and an extremely high CSF protein (Froin's reaction). CSF VDRL, immunoglobulins, basic myelin protein, and viral cultures should be performed.

Somatosensory evoked potentials can be very helpful in the assessment of suspected cord lesions. The presence of abnormalities on brain stem (BAER) and optic (VEP) testing raises the suspicion of a multifocal disease (e.g., multiple sclerosis). Absent F waves on nerve conduction testing can also support evidence of a cord lesion.[144]

ADRENOMYELONEUROPATHY

Adrenomyeloneuropathy is a phenotypic variant of the genetic disorder adrenoleukodystrophy, in which myelin sheath abnormalities of the white matter are associated with adrenal insufficiency. Although adrenoleukodystrophy is a sex-linked disorder, it has variable expressions, including mild disease in heterozygous women. Pathologically, the white matter abnormality appears to be a diffuse myelinoclastic sclerosis, but it may occasionally appear as a dysmyelinating condition. The neurologic variants are explained by the degree of involvement of brain, spinal cord, and peripheral nerve. Biorefringent material in the adrenal glands and brain that is observed histopathologically has been demonstrated by sequential extraction methods to be cholesterol esters with high quantities of very long chain fatty acids. Moser and colleagues[109] measuring fatty acids in cultured skin fibroblasts from affected persons, demonstrated abnormally large amounts of very long chain fatty acids (C_{24}–C_{30}), as well as a high ratio of C_{26} to C_{22} fatty acids. The latter has become the preferred method of diagnosing the disorder.

In patients with the spinal-neuropathic form of this disorder, adrenal insufficiency is usually present since early childhood, and a progressive spastic paraparesis and relatively mild peripheral neuropathy develop in the third decade.[56] Other variants affecting the spinal cord have been observed, including a progressive myelopathy in adult males, a mild spastic paraparesis in females, and combined cerebral and spinal involvement in juveniles and young adult men. A positive family history is present in approximately 50 per cent of affected persons. The presence of Addison's disease also provides a strong clue to the diagnosis. Because of primary adrenal failure, Addison's disease is often accompanied by bronzing of the skin, owing to excessive secretion of melanocyte-stimulating hormone in association with adrenocorticotrophic hormone.

INFECTIOUS MYELOPATHIES

Viral Myelitis

HIV Infection

Between 40 and 60 per cent of all patients with AIDS develop neurologic complications,[13, 93, 140] and in 10 to 20 per cent of HIV-infected patients, neurologic disease heralds the infection.[13] In retrospective clinical series, spinal cord disease occurring in association with AIDS has been observed infrequently. Levy and colleagues[93] found a viral myelitis in 3 of 128 neurologically symptomatic AIDS patients, and the collective incidence of viral myelitis in AIDS, when data were pooled from three different hospital series of the neurologic complications of AIDS, was 1 per cent.[65] The most common form of myelopathy observed with HIV infection is a unique degeneration of the spinal cord first described by Petito and colleagues.[117] In pathologic series, it has been observed in 11 to 22 per cent of unselected cases.[37, 117] These pathologic series suggest that spinal cord disease occurring in association with HIV infection is common but clinically underrecognized.

The prototypic myelopathy observed with HIV infection is a unique degeneration of the spinal cord.[53, 117] Petito and colleagues[117] observed this myelopathy in 20 of 89 consecutively autopsied AIDS patients. Although the clinical presentation of this myelopathy may overlap with that of other myelopathies associated with HIV-1 infection, the pathologic appearance is quite distinct. Clinically, these patients complain of leg weakness, unsteadiness, and gait impairment. Incontinence of bladder and bowel often supervenes. In one study, incontinence was observed in 60 per cent of patients.[117] Patients with this disorder often complain of paresthesias and vague discomfort in their legs. Frequently, these complaints are attributed to the general debilitation of the patient, and the true nature of the illness remains undiagnosed until pathologic examination of the spinal cord at the time of autopsy. On physical examination, a spastic paraparesis is detected, with the degree of weakness exceeding that of spasticity. Rarely, marked asymmetry of leg weakness, monoparesis, or quadriparesis may be found. Gait ataxia is seen, and the heel-to-knee-to-toe test may reveal dysmetria and dyssynergy. On occasion, weakness is slight or absent on confrontation testing, but hyperreflexia of the lower extremities and extensor plantar responses are noted. Muscle stretch reflexes may also be diminished or absent in this disorder as a result of concomitant peripheral neuropathy. Sensory examination reveals that vibratory and position senses are disproportionately affected in comparison to pinprick, temperature, or light touch. A significant impairment of the latter modalities suggests the presence of a concomitant peripheral neuropathy. Electrophysiologic studies may reveal a prolonged latency of cortical evoked responses following tibial nerve stimulation. Typically, this myelopathy is seen late in the course of HIV-1 infection, but it has been described as the presenting manifestation of this viral infection.[71]

Gross examination of the spinal cord and dura is generally normal in HIV-associated myelopathy, except when the myelopathy is particularly severe.[117] The striking finding on histologic examination is the loss of myelin and spongy degeneration. The lateral and posterior columns are more severely affected than the anterior columns. A microvacuolization of the white matter of the spinal cord (Fig. 47–1), associated with lipid-laden macrophages, bears an uncanny resemblance to the pathology of subacute combined degeneration of the spinal cord. The vacuolization appears to result from intramyelin swelling. Axons are preserved, except in areas of marked vacuolization. Microglial nodules may be detected in the spinal cord gray matter, and 20 per cent of the patients in one series also exhibited central chromatolysis of the anterior horn motor cells.[117] Inflammation and intranuclear viral inclusions are generally not seen. Although HIV has been cultured from the spinal cord, the specific role of HIV in the cause of this illness is uncertain. Indeed, a similar clinicopathologic condition has been observed in patients with cancer or other immunosuppressive conditions in the absence of HIV infection.[80] The spinal cord pathology is most prominent in the middle and lower thoracic regions. The cord involvement may be asymmetric and does not appear to be confined to particular tracts.[117] However, Goldstick and colleagues[53] found that involvement of the posterior columns increased in intensity with rostral progression, whereas pyramidal tract involvement increased caudally. Petito and associates[117] were able to correlate the frequency and severity of symptoms to the degree of spinal cord pathology. Nutritional deficiency has been suggested as a potential cause of spinal cord pathology.[136] Clinically symptomatic vacuolar myelopathy is seldom observed in young children with AIDS, but pathologic abnormalities of the spinal cord are frequently seen at autopsy.[40] The most common abnormality appears to be a loss of both myelin and axons in the corticospinal tracts.

The diagnosis of this illness is one of exclusion. A number of other myelopathies have been observed in association with HIV infection. An acute myelopathy of uncertain pathogenesis has been noted at the time of seroconversion.[39] Other etiologies of spinal cord disease occurring in association with HIV are listed in Table 47–2.

The single most useful study is MRI of the spinal cord. We generally forgo myelography if MRI of the spinal cord reveals no evidence of mass lesion. The presence of unusual features, such as back pain or radicular findings, may dictate a more aggressive diagnostic approach. If the MRI is negative, the CSF is examined for the presence of HIV and other pathogens. The latter includes viral cultures, with specific emphasis on cytomegalovirus and herpes simplex types 1 and 2. Additionally, routine bacterial and fungal cultures and cryptococcal antigen are obtained. No treatment is known to be effective in this condition, although high-dose zidovudine ($\geq$1 g per day) and other antiretroviral regimens should be tried.

HTLV-I

Although thought to be rare in the United States, human T-cell lymphotropic virus type I (HTLV-I) has been observed with increasing frequency in certain subpopulations. A study of volunteer blood donors by the American Red Cross revealed a seropositivity rate of 0.025 per cent.[150] Intravenous drug abusers seem to be

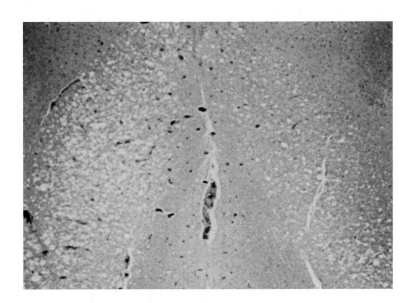

Figure 47–1. Microvacuolization of the posterior columns of the thoracic spinal cord in a patient with HIV-1–related myelopathy.

Table 47–2. POTENTIAL ETIOLOGIES OF MYELOPATHIES ASSOCIATED WITH HIV INFECTION

Infectious
  Viral
    HIV
      Acute transient myelopathy occurring at the time of seroconversion[39]
      Chronic progressive myelopathy (vacuolar)[117]
    HTLV-I[1, 101]
    Cytomegalovirus[145]
    Herpes simplex[21]
    Herpes zoster[100]
  Bacterial
    Epidural abscess
    Mycobacterium tuberculosis[41, 151]
    Treponema pallidum[11]
  Fungal
    Cryptococcus neoformans
    Other
  Parasites
    Toxoplasma gondii[68]
Noninfectious
  Multiple sclerosis–like illness[15]
  Tumors[148]
    Plasmacytoma
    Spinal cord astrocytoma
    Other
  Epidural hemorrhage secondary to thrombocytopenia
  Vascular injury secondary to vasculitis

at particularly high risk for infection with HTLV-I. Seroprevalence rates in this population have varied between 7 and 49 per cent.[124, 149] In a study of the seroprevalence among female prostitutes in eight areas of the United States, 6.7 per cent were seropositive for HTLV-I/II, with prevalence rates ranging from 0 in southern Nevada to 25.4 per cent in Newark, New Jersey.[84] A case of transmission of HTLV-I by blood transfusion associated with myelopathy has been confirmed.[81] In ten native-born patients in the United States, half had received blood transfusions, and six had had multiple sex partners.[133]

In addition to being associated with adult T-cell leukemia and lymphoma, HTLV-I is associated with a chronic progressive myelopathy.[52, 114] In population-based surveys[54, 75, 83] and a cohort study,[112] myelopathy was observed in 0.5 to 1.5 per cent of HTLV-I–infected persons. In a cohort of HTLV-I and HTLV-II blood donors, HTLV-associated myelopathy was seen in 2.4 per cent of HTLV-I–infected persons and 0.25 per cent of HTLV-II–infected persons.[111] The latter confirms the initial observation of Berger and colleagues[14] that HTLV-II may be associated with a myelopathy similar to that caused by HTLV-I. An association between the presence of seropositivity for HTLV-I and multiple sclerosis has also been suggested[90] but remains controversial.

The myelopathy that occurs with HTLV-I has been referred to as tropical spastic paraparesis (TSP) or HTLV-I–associated myelopathy (HAM). This myelopathy is characterized neuropathologically by chronic involvement of the pyramidal tracts, chiefly at the tho-

racic level, resulting in spastic lower extremity weakness and a spastic bladder. Paresthesias, pain, and sensory disturbances may also be observed. It is estimated that one in 250 individuals infected with HTLV-I will develop this progressive myelopathy.[147] The major pathologic features of HTLV-I myelopathy are long-tract degeneration and demyelination affecting the pyramidal, spinocerebellar, and spinothalamic tracts, associated with hyalinoid thickening of the media and adventitia of blood vessels in the brain, spinal cord, and subarachnoid space, with perivascular cuffing with leukocytes, astrocytic gliosis, and foamy macrophages.[6] These lesions may extend from the upper cervical cord to the lumbar regions. Vacuolization may be observed at the periphery of the lesions.

Enteroviruses

Enteroviruses, particularly poliovirus, can affect the spinal cord. Fortunately, effective vaccination has made this illness very rare in the Western world. In the United States, approximately 10 to 15 cases of polio are reported yearly; most of these are vaccine associated, although several are imported by immigrants. Paralytic poliomyelitis is a rare complication of poliovirus infection (1 to 2 per cent); most infections result in inapparent infection (90 to 95 per cent) or a minor illness with mild systemic symptoms (5 to 10 per cent). The poliovirus has a unique predilection for the anterior horn cells of the spinal cord and therefore causes a lower motor neuron type of weakness. This is characterized by a flaccid weakness with wasting, fasciculations, and areflexia. Sensory and sphincter functions are spared. Following infection, weakness may arise rapidly over a 48-hour period or occur in a delayed fashion over weeks. The risk of paralysis rises with age: infants are rarely paralyzed, adults experience paralysis much more frequently, and children's risks are in between. Other enteroviruses, including Coxsackie and echoviruses, may also result in a myelitis.

Herpesviruses

Varicella-zoster, herpes simplex type 2, and cytomegalovirus have been reported to cause myelopathy. Varicella-zoster is responsible for varicella (chickenpox) and causes shingles in adults. The virus remains latent within the dorsal root ganglia and spreads centrifugally along the corresponding nerves following reactivation, resulting in a severely painful, blistering dermatomal eruption. On rare occasions, when the thoracic dermatomes are involved, the virus may spread centripetally and result in a necrotizing myelopathy.[126]

In rare instances, usually with primary infection, herpes simplex type 2, the cause of genital herpes, may produce a sacral radiculitis[24] or an ascending myelitis.[88] Epstein-Barr virus,[58, 134] the etiologic agent of infectious mononucleosis, and cytomegalovirus[146] may also result in a transverse myelitis at the time of primary infection.

Table 47–3. VIRAL ETIOLOGIES OF MYELITIS

RNA Viruses	DNA Viruses
Nonenveloped	*Nonenveloped*
Picornaviruses	Hepatitis B
Coxsackie	*Enveloped*
Echo	Herpesviruses
Polio	Herpes simplex
Other enteroviruses	Varicella-zoster
Hepatitis A	Epstein-Barr virus
Encephalomyocarditis virus	Cytomegalovirus
Enveloped	Herpes simiae
Togaviruses	Poxviruses
Arbovirus	Vaccinia
Rubella	Variola
Tick-borne encephalitis virus	
Retroviruses	
Human immunodeficiency virus, type 1	
Human T-cell lymphotropic virus, type I	
Human T-cell lymphotropic virus, type II	
Orthomyxovirus	
Influenza	
Paramyxoviruses	
Measles	
Mumps	
Bunyaviruses	
California encephalitis virus	
Arenavirus	
Lymphocytic choriomeningitis	
Rhabdovirus	
Rabies	

Adapted from Tyler, K. L., Gross, R. A., and Cascino, G. D.: Unusual viral causes of transverse myelitis: Hepatitis A virus and cytomegalovirus. Neurology *36*:855, 1986.

Other Viruses

Many other viruses have been associated with transverse myelitis (Table 47–3). Twenty to 40 per cent of all patients with transverse myelitis have evidence of preceding or concurrent viral infection.[7, 16, 95, 115, 125] With the increasing availability and efficacy of antiviral therapy and improved diagnostic techniques, these percentages are likely to increase.

Myelopathies Resulting From Bacterial Disease

Syphilis

Central nervous system (CNS) invasion by *Treponema pallidum* generally occurs within the first year of syphilitic infection. Abnormal CSF results have been found with an incidence of 13.9 to 70 per cent in untreated patients with primary or secondary syphilis. Although CNS symptoms are infrequent at this stage of the infection, headache and meningismus can be observed during secondary syphilis, and acute meningitis complicates 1 to 2 per cent of secondary syphilis cases. If left untreated, about 5 per cent of syphilitics will develop clinical neurosyphilis.

The spinal cord is not immune to the ravages of this disease. Before the development of effective antibiotics,

it was believed that syphilis was the most frequent cause of spinal cord disease. Historically, tabes dorsalis has been the most frequent type, with an estimated frequency of 10 times that of other forms of spinal syphilis. Syphilitic meningomyelitis and spinal vascular syphilis were the second and third most common forms of spinal syphilis, respectively. Spinal syphilis rarely occurs in the absence of syphilitic involvement at other sites of the neuraxis. It has been estimated that the incidence of pure spinal syphilis is approximately one fifth the incidence of cerebrospinal syphilis.

Syphilis can affect the spinal cord in a variety of ways.[12] The pathology may be predominantly meningovascular or parenchymatous in nature. Gummas may grow within the substance of the cord or compress the cord by growth from the surrounding meninges. The clinical picture of spinal cord compression in syphilis may also arise as a result of hypertrophic pachymeningitis or vertebral lesions resulting from syphilitic osteitis. A classification based on pathology and modifying the one proposed by Adams and Merritt[2] is presented in Table 47–4.

Tabes Dorsalis

Tabes dorsalis is the prototypic spinal cord disorder associated with syphilis. It is characterized by incoordination, pain, anesthesia, and various visceral trophic abnormalities.[12] The earliest recognized descriptions of this disorder date from the mid-eighteenth century. By the turn of the twentieth century, tabes dorsalis was recognized with increased frequency and, according to Erb, was unequaled in frequency or importance by any other chronic disease of the spinal cord.

Currently, tabes dorsalis probably accounts for no more than 5 per cent of neurosyphilis. Approximately 65 per cent of patients recall a prior history of venereal disease. The latency from infection to the development of tabes averages 10 to 15 years, but it varies between 2 and 38 years. The average age of onset is 40 years, with the majority arising in the fourth and fifth decades. Tabes dorsalis is a rare complication of congenital syphilis. It exhibits an equal sex frequency, unlike

Table 47–4. SYPHILIS OF THE SPINAL CORD

Syphilitic meningomyelitis
Syphilitic spinal pachymeningitis
  Spinal cord gumma
  Syphilitic hypertrophic pachymeningitis
Spinal vascular syphilis
Syphilitic poliomyelitis
Tabes dorsalis
Miscellaneous
  Syringomyelia
  Syphilitic aortic aneurysm
  Syphilitic vertebral osteitis
  Charcot's vertebrae

Adapted from Adams, R. D., and Merritt, H. H.: Meningeal and vascular diseases of the spinal cord. Medicine *23*:181, 1944. © 1944 Williams & Wilkins.

adult tabes, in which the incidence in men exceeds that in women by 10 to 1.

The clinical course of tabes is typically divided into three phases. The initial phase is known as the "preataxic" phase or the "period of lightning pain." This phase is insidious in onset and may last months to decades, although it generally averages three years in duration. It is characterized by a variety of subjective complaints, the most classic being the "crisis," a severe lancinating pain. These lightning pains are absolutely characteristic of tabes dorsalis. They occur in 90 per cent of individuals and are the presenting manifestation in 70 per cent. Impotence and sphincter disturbances may also be early features. Physical examination reveals loss of muscle stretch reflexes, sensory loss, a positive Romberg's sign, and Argyll Robertson pupils. The latter is characterized by intact visual acuity, decreased pupillary light reaction, intact near response, miosis, and irregular pupils. It occurs in classic form in 50 per cent of tabetics. In early tabes, the tactile sense may be well preserved, but the pain sense is invariably disturbed. Hypalgesia, hyperalgesia, allochiria, pallesthesia, a delay in pain perception of up to 15 seconds following application of a stimulus, and an aftersensation lasting up to 30 seconds may all be detected. Loss of deep pain sensation, as evidenced by diminished sensation of pressure applied to the ulnar nerve (Biernacki's sign), the Achilles tendon (Abadie's sign), and the testicle (Pitres' sign), may occur in the absence of significant loss of superficial sensation.

The second stage of tabes is known as the "ataxic" phase. It has a variable duration of 2 to 10 years and is characterized by severe ataxia, chiefly affecting the legs. Generally, the tabetic pains worsen during this period. Arthropathy develops in 5 to 10 per cent of patients from recurrent traumatic injury resulting from loss of deep pain sensation. Proprioceptive loss that results in a slapping gait predisposes the knee joint to this injury. The tarsal joints, hip, ankle, spine, and other joints can be similarly involved.

The third stage is known as the "terminal" or "paralytic" stage. It, too, has an average duration of 2 to 10 years. In this phase of the illness, cachexia, leg stiffness and paralysis, and autonomic dysfunction, typified by obstinate constipation and bladder incontinence, are prominent. Sepsis from decubital infections and pyelonephritis is frequently the terminal event.

The classic signs of tabes dorsalis are absent in approximately 50 per cent of patients in the early stages of the disease. The most frequently observed findings in these patients are absent ankle jerks and impaired vibratory sensation. In as many as 10 per cent of cases, tabes dorsalis remains atypical throughout the course of the illness. Tabes may also be associated with other complications of neurosyphilis, such as general paresis, syphilitic meningomyelitis, and spinal cord gummas.

The pathology of tabes dorsalis is characterized by changes in the posterior spinal roots and posterior spinal columns (see Fig. 47–3). Shrinkage of the spinal cord may be apparent by gross inspection. Leptomeningitis is evidenced by round cell infiltration. The dorsal columns are demyelinated, particularly in the regions of the fasciculus gracilis, the root entry zone, and Lissauer's tract. Astrocytic proliferation in the posterior columns is accompanied by an increase in connective tissue and thickening of the blood vessel walls. The lower spinal cord bears the brunt of the damage. Nerve fibers in the posterior root are destroyed and replaced by fibrosis. Not infrequently, lesions are observed in the anterior horns, cranial nerves, and brain stem.

Syphilitic Meningomyelitis

This disorder occurs most commonly in individuals between the ages of 25 and 40 years, although it may arise in both younger and older age groups. In most series, males predominate. The latency from the onset of the infection to the onset of symptoms varies from 1 to 30 years, with the majority arising within 6 years of infection.[48]

Typically, the patient initially notices a heavy sensation or weakness in his legs. Rarely the symptoms are confined to a single leg. Paresthesias and fleeting pain may accompany the motor disturbance. The onset is slow and gradual, and the symptoms are indistinguishable from those of the myelopathy associated with cervical spondylosis. A variety of subjective complaints have been recorded, including sensations of lower extremity numbness, cold, and tingling and girdle tightness, but objective sensory disturbances are slight. Autonomic dysfunction is also observed. It is generally characterized by precipitate frequency, hesitancy, and impotence. The predominant finding on neurologic examination is a spastic weakness in the extremities, especially the lower extremities. Muscle bulk is preserved, and the muscle stretch reflexes are exaggerated, with positive Babinski's signs. Sensory loss is slight. Occasionally, a Brown-Séquard syndrome, significant amyotrophy, or a clinical picture of transverse myelitis may complicate syphilitic meningomyelitis.

Pathologic examination reveals thickened, inflamed meninges. The cervical region is believed to be the site where the lesions predominate. The pathologic changes prevail in the periphery of the spinal cord, often with a surprisingly symmetric involvement of the lateral columns. The spinal cord dysfunction results from granulomatous invasion, inflammation, and vascular changes. The latter is caused by Heubner's and Nissl-Alzheimer's endarteritis, medium and small vessel lesions that are characterized by plasma cell and lymphocytic perivascular cuffing.

Other Forms of Spinal Syphilis

Hypertrophic pachymeningitis[55] is an insidious, slowly progressive syphilitic process that results in spinal root and spinal cord dysfunction. A rare but well-recognized complication of tertiary syphilis is a gumma of the spinal cord. The clinical features of a spinal gumma are indistinguishable from an intramedullary glioma if it arises within the cord, or it may simulate the appearance of an extramedullary tumor if it arises from the meninges and compresses the spinal cord. Spinal cord infarction is a well-recognized complication of syphilis.

Another vascular complication of syphilis is aortitis, which may result in an aortic aneurysm and rarely in myelopathy by erosion of the vertebrae and ultimately compression of the spinal cord. Progressive spinal muscular atrophy (PSMA) has been observed in association with neurosyphilis, although the relationship may be coincidental. Occasionally, syphilitic caries may affect the vertebrae, particularly those of the cervical spine, resulting in pain, tenderness to palpation, loss of mobility, and an abnormal spinal curvature in the involved area. Radicular pains are observed in one third of patients. Compression of the spinal cord, though rare, has been reported.

As with other forms of neurosyphilis, the recommended treatment is 12 to 24 million units of aqueous penicillin daily in divided doses administered every four hours for 10 to 14 days.[26] Other treatment regimens using doxycycline, ceftriaxone, or erythromycin may be considered if the patient is intolerant of penicillin.[10] However, these treatment regimens are not well established in treating symptomatic neurosyphilis.

Tuberculosis

Neurologic complications of *Mycobacterium tuberculosis* remain common in some parts of the world but are rare in the developed countries of the Western world. Myelopathy occurring in association with tuberculosis is usually the consequence of tuberculous spondylitis (Pott's disease), which accounts for half of all skeletal tuberculosis. Typically, the anterior portion of the vertebral body is affected; the mycobacterial spread to the vertebrae is hematogenous, lymphatic, or by direct extension from the lung.[57] The characteristic roentgenographic defect is anterior wedging of two adjacent vertebrae, with loss of the intervening disc space. The spine is enveloped by pus extruding anteriorly from the affected vertebrae. Myelopathy typically results from pressure on the anterior spinal cord by caseous or granulating tissue, inflammatory thrombosis of the anterior spinal artery, or injury to the cord from spinal instability. The latter may lead to complete spinal cord transection.

Other Forms of Bacterial Myelopathy

A number of other bacterial infections have been associated with myelitis. On rare occasions, the spinal cord may be seeded by bacteria, leading to a suppurative myelitis with abscess formation. In a review by Dutton and Alexander,[43] direct spread from adjacent infections was most commonly observed, but hematogenous dissemination from endocarditis, pulmonary infections, and other sites was also frequently observed. Staphylococci, streptococci, *Escherichia coli,* and *Nocardia* are among the organisms that have been isolated in these cases.

More often, the myelopathies associated with bacterial infection are parainfectious in nature, similar clinicopathologically to those occurring after viral infection or vaccination. Among the potential causes are scarlet fever, pertussis, mycoplasma pneumonia, and pneumococcal pneumonia.[87, 106] A myelitis resulting in a Brown-Séquard syndrome has also been described with cat-scratch disease.[118] Lyme disease, the result of infection with *Borrelia burgdorferi,* a treponema, may also result in a myelopathy.[122]

Fungal Myelopathies

Fungal disease of the spinal cord is a rarity. Certain fungi (*Blastomyces, Coccidioides, Aspergillus*) may invade the spinal epidural space. Generally, the spinal cord is compromised by lesions arising from a vertebral osteomyelitic focus or by those extending through the intervertebral foramina. Certain fungi that result in granulomatous meningitis (e.g., *Cryptococcus neoformans*) may result in intraspinal or extradural granuloma. Alternatively, these organisms can lead to spinal cord infarction as a result of the associated meningovascular inflammation.

Parasitic Myelopathies

Among the most common parasitic infections that result in spinal cord disease is schistosomiasis, particularly schistosomiasis haematobia and schistosomiasis mansoni. These organisms are seen only in certain geographic regions, namely, the Far East, South America, and Africa. A history of travel to these regions and swimming or bathing in water contaminated with the cercariae that are released from certain aquatic snails may suggest the diagnosis.

Hydatid disease resulting from the larval form of the canine tapeworm, *Echinococcus granulosus,* may result in spinal intramedullary cysts or compress the spinal cord and roots as a consequence of bone invasion. The bone invasion by hydatid disease generally occurs in the lower thoracic region.

Cysticercosis, a particularly common disease in Mexico and in Central and South American countries, is the result of infection with the larval form of pork tapeworm, *Taenia solium.* Spinal cord involvement may complicate as many as 5 per cent of cases, although the brain is the preferred site in the CNS. Cysticercosis most frequently infiltrates the subarachnoid space, but intramedullary fluid-filled cysts are also observed. A slowly progressive myelopathy implicating a lesion in the cervical or thoracic spinal cord is the typical mode of presentation for these lesions. Therapy with albendazole may be effective in eradicating the live parasite.

Paragonimiasis, caused by a lung fluke acquired by eating undercooked freshwater crabs, occurs chiefly in China but may be seen in other parts of the world. Spinal cord disease results from extradural or, more rarely, intradural granuloma formation. In patients with AIDS, toxoplasmosis has been reported in rare instances to cause an abscess of the spinal cord.

EPIDURAL ABSCESS

Spinal epidural abscess may present as a surgical emergency evolving rapidly over several days or may arise more indolently. *Staphylococcus aureus* is the etiologic agent in over 50 per cent of acute spinal epidural abscesses, although a broad spectrum of other organisms may be implicated.[82] The spread of infection may occur directly from a focus of osteomyelitis or hematogenously from a distant site, such as skin furuncles or pulmonary infections. Trauma to the back, typically minor in nature, has been reported by as many as one third of individuals developing spinal epidural abscess.[9] A high degree of suspicion for spinal epidural abscess should be maintained when intravenous drug abusers present with fever and back pain.

ARACHNOIDITIS

Invasion or irritation of the spinal subarachnoid space, as occurs with subarachnoid hemorrhage, meningitis, myelography, spinal or epidural anesthesia, or spinal surgery, can result in arachnoiditis. Arachnoidal inflammation leads to connective tissue proliferation and ultimately to arachnoid thickening, opacification, and adhesion and obliteration of the subarachnoid space. In the most severe cases, nerve roots and the spinal cord itself may be compressed by bands of connective tissue or cystic loculations of CSF, resulting in a myeloradiculopathy. Patients present most frequently with slowly progressive paraparesis, sensory loss, and sphincter dysfunction. Radicular pain may also be present. On examination, weakness, hyporeflexia, and sensory deficits can be seen. Diagnosis is made by myelography or MRI. Although some patients, particularly those with mass lesions resulting in cord compression and myelopathic symptoms, may respond to decompression, surgical exploration with resection of adhesions has not proved to be of benefit in most patients.

VASCULAR DISEASE OF THE SPINAL CORD

Paired segmental arteries arising from the aorta and branches of the subclavian and internal iliac arteries supply blood to the spinal cord (Fig. 47–2).[67] The most important vascular supply to the cervical spinal cord arises from the vertebral artery, which provides the cephalad origin of the anterior median and posterior lateral spinal arteries. The blood supply to the thoracic and lumbar spinal cord arises from the aorta and internal iliac arteries and segmental branches of the lateral sacral arteries nourish the sacral spinal cord. The segmental branches that arise from the aorta divide into anterior and posterior rami. A branch of the posterior ramus (Fig. 47–3), the spinal artery, enters the vertebral foramen and branches at irregular intervals into anterior and posterior medullary arteries, which feed the anterior median spinal artery and the posterior spinal arteries, respectively. At regular intervals, the spinal artery also branches into the anterior and posterior radicular arteries, which supply the spinal ganglia and roots.

The chief blood supply to the spinal cord comes

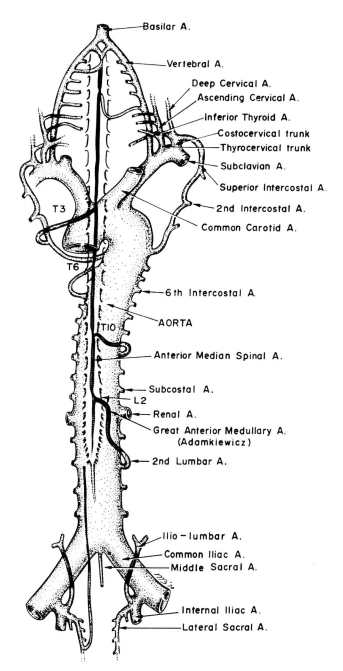

Figure 47–2. Anterior view of the spinal cord with its segmental blood supply from the aorta. (From Herrick, M., and Mills, P. E., Jr.: Infarction of spinal cord. Arch. Neurol. *24*:228, 1971. Copyright 1971, American Medical Association.)

from the six to eight anterior and 10 or more posterior medullary arteries that arise from the spinal arteries. The most important anterior medullary artery is the artery of Adamkiewicz, which usually approaches the cord on the left side between the T10 and L3 cord segments. Because of the variability of the vascular anatomy of the spinal cord, however, it is impossible to predict the deficits that will occur following occlusion of a specific artery.

Although an anastomosing vascular network can be

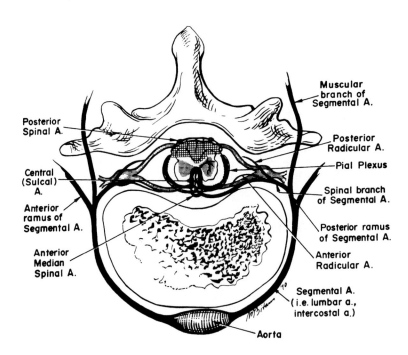

Figure 47–3. Representative cross section of the lumbar vertebrae and spinal cord with its blood supply. (From Herrick, M., and Mills, P. E., Jr.: Infarction of spinal cord. Arch. Neurol. *24*:228, 1971. Copyright 1971, American Medical Association.)

found over the surface of the spinal cord, the anterior median spinal artery is responsible for nourishing the anterior two thirds of the spinal cord. The territory in its distribution includes the anterior and lateral cortical spinal tracts and the lateral spinothalamic tracts, whereas the posterior columns (fasciculus gracilis and cuneatus) are supplied by the posterior spinal arteries.

Occlusion of a dominant medullary artery or, more rarely, the anterior median spinal artery results in an ischemic softening of a variable portion of the anterior two thirds of the spinal cord. This entity is referred to as an anterior spinal artery syndrome and may arise as the consequence of thrombotic atherosclerotic disease, aortic dissection, embolization, or vasculitis (particularly polyarteritis nodosa) or as a complication of aortic angiography.[85] Cross clamping of the aorta for more than 30 minutes during cardiac surgery may also result in an infarction in this territory. A clinical hallmark of this entity is a dissociated sensory loss in which position and vibratory sensory perception is maintained but a sensory level to pinprick is present. The latter is accompanied by paralysis below the level of the lesion, which typically presents in association with spinal shock. On rare occasions, anastomotic blood flow allows for the preservation of the white matter of the spinal cord, and the gray matter alone is infarcted. Painful segmental spasm and spinal myoclonus may be observed with this condition.[3]

Hemorrhage may occur wihin the epidural or subdural space or directly into the spinal cord. Trauma, hemorrhagic disorders, the administration of anticoagulant therapy, and bleeding from vascular malformations may lead to these complications. These events are usually apoplectic in nature, with rapidly developing paralysis and sensory loss. Immediate radiographic

demonstration of the region of the hemorrhage and surgical evacuation are indicated.

Another etiology of hemorrhage into or around the spinal cord is vascular malformations. One type of spinal cord vascular malformation is the venous angioma, which is found most often on the dorsal portion of the spinal cord. Middle-aged and elderly men are chiefly affected. The slow and temporally irregular development of symptoms resulting from this lesion is believed to be secondary to ischemic compromise and compression of the spinal cord. Another type of spinal cord vascular malformation is the arteriovenous malformation, which predominantly affects younger patients. It is most often located on the dorsal thoracic or upper lumbar spinal cord. Slowly progressive or suddenly appearing symptoms may occur with this lesion. The rapidly developing symptoms may result from occlusion of a key nutrient vessel or hemorrhage. The association of a cutaneous vascular nevus with a vascular malformation of the spinal cord has been referred to as the Klippel-Trénaunay-Weber syndrome. The syndrome of Foix-Alajouanine is a necrotic myelopathy resulting in a slowly evolving amyotrophic paraplegia in adult males that has been attributed to spinal venous thrombosis. Its exact nature remains controversial.

MYELOPATHY SECONDARY TO CONNECTIVE TISSUE DISEASES

Rheumatoid Arthritis

Rheumatoid arthritis may result in myriad complications involving the spinal cord. Among the major abnormalities of the spine and spinal cord in rheumatoid arthritis are vertebral body erosion,[96] discitis,[18] and spinal cord compression that may be secondary to pannus formation.[72] The most dramatic and frequent abnormality occurs at the atlantoaxial region.[131] Cervical subluxation may assume many forms in this disorder,[22, 131] including anterior subluxation, posterior subluxation, vertical subluxation with protrusion of the odontoid, and rotational atlantoaxial subluxation. Other abnormalities include ligamentous calcification, erosion, cystic changes, and spinous process erosion.[22] Cervical subluxation may be asymptomatic, although neck pain is common. Lower extremity weakness and spasticity, sensory loss, and sphincter disturbances are seen less frequently. Hyperextension of the cervical spine, such as may occur with endotracheal intubation, in the face of cervical instability secondary to rheumatoid arthritis may cause severe displacement with a rapidly evolving myelopathy. Unusual causes of myelopathy in rheumatoid arthritis patients include "epidural lipomatosis" in those on high-dose corticosteroid therapy[116] and progressive cervical osteomyelitis.[102] On rare occasions, these patients may develop pseudoaneurysm of the vertebral artery or anterior spinal artery occlusion secondary to compression. Marked C1–C2 abnormalities appear to be more frequent in young women with severe, long-standing, seropositive rheumatoid arthritis.[61] MRI may be useful in identifying pannus formation and craniovertebral involvement in rheumatoid arthritis.[130] Many patients stabilize with conservative therapy,[138] and the presence of cervical subluxation does not correlate with decreased survival from rheumatoid arthritis. Surgical craniocervical decompression can be helpful in early cases in which the patients remain ambulatory, but it is probably not helpful in advanced nonambulatory cases.[25]

Sjögren's Disease

Sjögren's disease is typically a disease of women that is characterized by dry eyes (xerophthalmia), dry mouth (xerostomia), and noninflammatory arthritis. Spinal involvement includes a progressive myelopathy, an acute transverse myelitis, and intraspinal hemorrhage.[49] One woman with Sjögren's disease and primary biliary cirrhosis had recurrent transverse myelitis that was characterized pathologically by angiitis and necrotizing myelitis.[127] Sjögren-related myelopathy can be associated with optic neuropathy or cutaneous vasculopathy.[63, 97] In one person with a Sjögren-related myelitis, improvement was noted after the institution of prednisone and plasma exchange.[89]

Systemic Lupus Erythematosus

Myelopathy is an uncommon manifestation of systemic lupus erythematosus (SLE).[44] Most patients have evidence of other systemic disease at the time of diagnosis. Typically, they complain of numbness and weakness of the lower extremities presenting in a subacute fashion. SLE-related myelopathy disables two thirds of those afflicted, but the other one third may recover significantly.[8] Aggressive treatment with intravenous high-dose steroids within a week of the onset of symptoms has been associated with better outcomes.[64] Subarachnoid spinal hemorrhage may occur in association with SLE.[49] As some cases of SLE-related myelopathy are associated with antiphospholipid antibodies, hypercoagulability or vasculopathy may be partly responsible for the pathogenesis of the disorder.[32]

Other Autoimmune Myelitides

A transverse myelitis occurring at any level of the spinal cord may complicate polyarteritis nodosa, a disease of small and medium-sized arteries. Cervical spine disease may also be seen with psoriatic arthritis. In 35 per cent of these cases, there is an ankylosing spondylosis with syndesmophytes and ligamentous ossifications. It may also result in atlantoaxial subluxation in a manner akin to that of rheumatoid arthritis.[19]

Acute transverse myelitis is also known to occur in mixed connective tissue disorders and ulcerative colitis.[107, 121]

SARCOID MYELOPATHY

Sarcoidosis is a chronic idiopathic granulomatous disease that may involve multiple organ systems. Bilateral hilar adenopathy and pulmonary infiltrates are the most common manifestations of the disease. Skin, eyes, heart, bone, and kidney may also be involved. Sarcoidosis involves the nervous system in only 5 per cent of patients. This may take the form of CNS mass lesions, hydrocephalus, recurrent aseptic meningitis, cranial neuropathies, myopathy, neuropathy, or mononeuropathy multiplex. Granulomatous infiltrates may appear in nearly any structure of the spine and cause arachnoiditis, cauda equina syndrome, intradural and extradural extramedullary granulomas, and intramedullary spinal sarcoidosis.

In the study of Junger and associates,[78] the patients were noted to have paraparesis, urinary bladder dysfunction, radiculopathies, chest wall numbness, gait problems, Brown-Séquard syndrome, or limb numbness or pain. The mean age at onset of neurologic symptoms was 35 years. Evaluation of the CSF revealed mild or moderate pleocytosis (1 to 200, mean 36) and elevated protein (52 to 568, mean 162).

Definitive diagnostic testing requires a biopsy showing noncaseating epithelioid granulomas. An intramedullary biopsy is rarely desirable, so biopsy material can be obtained from safer sites (e.g., the lungs) if available. MRI can be normal in some suspected cases of spinal sarcoidosis.[45] Observed changes in spinal sarcoidosis include gadolinium-enhancing nerve roots, gadolinium-enhancing parenchymal spinal cord masses,[94] diffuse spinal cord enlargement, spinal cord atrophy, or focal or diffuse areas of increased T2-weighted signals.[78] Gallium scanning may demonstrate uptake in the lungs and the parotid, salivary, or lacrimal glands. Systemic disease can be detected by raised serum angiotensin-converting enzyme (ACE) levels. It is not currently clear whether CSF measurements of ACE levels are helpful in diagnosing nervous system involvement. Serum ACE levels are not informative with respect to CNS involvement.

Spontaneous recovery over months or years can occur in 60 to 80 per cent of patients with isolated pulmonary disease, but little is known about the natural history of CNS disease. Most authorities proceed aggressively with steroids if neurologic involvement becomes symptomatic. If the sarcoidosis is refractory to corticosteroids, cyclosporine, cyclophosphamide, chlorambucil, methotrexate, and radiation therapy have been applied in combination with steroids with some success.[5, 28]

NUTRITIONAL MYELOPATHIES

Vitamin B_{12} deficiency may result from an inadequate dietary intake or as the result of an inability to absorb vitamin B_{12} from the small intestine because of a lack of intrinsic factor. The latter condition is referred to as pernicious anemia, although the effects of vitamin B_{12} deficiency on the CNS may occur in the absence of the characteristic megaloblastic anemia. Indeed, the neurologic disease may occur even in the absence of pathologically abnormal serum levels of B_{12}. Therefore, a Schilling test or measurements of methylmalonic acid are warranted when the illness is suspected clinically.

The brain, spinal cord, optic nerve, and peripheral nerves may be adversely affected by the absence of vitamin B_{12}. Typically, the patient comments on a sense of weakness and easy fatigability of the lower extremities that is accompanied by paresthesias. Occasionally, Lhermitte's phenomenon is noted. With progression of the disease, a spastic-ataxic gait and loss of vibratory and position sense ensue. The limbs are symmetrically affected. Cognitive and behavioral abnormalities, decreasing visual acuity, and a peripheral neuropathy may be superimposed on the spinal cord symptoms. Physical examination may reveal areas of vitiligo. Hyperpigmentation of the palms and soles is observed in blacks.

The myelopathy that results from vitamin B_{12} deficiency (subacute combined degeneration) is chiefly characterized neuropathologically by foci of demyelination in the posterior and lateral columns of the cervical and upper thoracic spinal cord. The earliest changes of demyelination are fusiform expansions of the myelin sheaths. Subsequently, the myelin degenerates, and if the process is uninterrupted, gliosis and involvement of the axons eventually ensue. Clinical remissions are anticipated when this myelopathy is treated expeditiously with hydroxocobalamin or cyanocobalamin. The mechanism by which vitamin B_{12} deficiency results in demyelination is unknown. It is a cofactor in choline synthesis and is important in the conversion of methylmalonyl-CoA to succinyl-CoA, both of which are important to the myelin sheath.[91] Fusiform expansion of the myelin sheaths is followed by myelin degeneration.[91, 139] If the process is uninterrupted, gliosis and involvement of the axons eventually ensue.[91]

Following effective therapy, the myelopathy of vitamin B_{12} deficiency may resolve not only clinically but also radiographically.

Pernicious anemia is treated by the intramuscular injection of cyanocobalamin 1000 μg daily for the first week, then one injection weekly for the next one to three months, and one injection monthly thereafter.

METABOLIC MYELOPATHIES

A progressive myelopathy has been observed in association with portosystemic shunting.[119] Although the illness generally accompanies alcoholic cirrhosis, it may arise secondary to other causes of portosystemic shunting. A selective demyelination predominates in the posterior and lateral funiculi of the spinal cord. Hepatic encephalopathy often accompanies the myelopathy, which is manifested by an insidiously developing spastic paraparesis and gait, with relative preservation of sensory and sphincter function.

Hyperparathyroidism and hyperthyroidism have been rarely associated with cervical myelopathies that remit when the endocrinologic derangement is removed.[69, 77, 103]

PARANEOPLASTIC MYELOPATHIES

Paraneoplastic syndromes are associated with underlying malignancies but are not caused by direct tumoral invasion or macroscopic metastatic disease. These remote effects of cancer are usually without identifiable etiology, although some syndromes are associated with circulating antibodies to nervous system tissue or are the result of a presumptive concomitant viral infection. In general, these syndromes are uncommon. Approximately 50 per cent of all paraneoplastic syndromes are associated with small cell carcinoma of the lung.[143] The prototypic paraneoplastic syndrome is subacute cerebellar degeneration, which is associated with loss of Purkinje's cells in the cerebellar cortex and a variety of circulating antibodies directed against these cells. Paraneoplastic myelopathy is quite rare[113]; it is much less common than myelopathy resulting from metastatic epidural spinal cord compression. Myelopathy occurring in association with malignancy can also be secondary to radiation therapy; the combined effects of radiation therapy and intrathecal chemotherapy, especially methotrexate chemotherapy[31, 51]; herpes zoster[110]; abscess; or hematoma. These myelopathies may occur in isolation or as part of a syndrome in which encephalomyelitis,[66] cerebellar degeneration, or peripheral radiculoneuropathies are also observed.

The most typical myelopathy is a necrotizing myelopathy. It is a rare entity, associated with lymphoma, leukemia, and small cell lung cancer. It may present before, concomitant with, or after the initial tumor presentation. Clinically, it is characterized by a rapidly ascending spinal cord dysfunction leading to a flaccid areflexic paraplegia. The myelopathy may present asymmetrically and often results in a Brown-Séquard syndrome,[62] but it eventually becomes bilateral and symmetric. The brain stem may also be involved. There is no effective treatment. One patient with Hodgkin's disease and a paraneoplastic myelopathy was believed to respond favorably to intrathecal corticosteroids.[34] The CSF usually shows elevated protein and a mild pleocytosis. Pathologically, there is widespread necrosis of the cord, mostly in the thoracic region.[120] Both gray and white matter are involved, and lesions may be identified elsewhere in the CNS. In two cases of "paraneoplastic" necrotizing myelopathy, immunohistochemical studies and electron microscopy revealed convincing evidence of infection with herpes simplex type 2.[73]

Other even less common syndromes include a subacute motor neuropathy associated with Hodgkin's disease and other malignant lymphomas.[129] It is typically diagnosed at a later stage and, at times, after radiation therapy. The motor weakness is clinically of the lower motor neuron type and involves the legs more than the arms. Sensory loss is mild. The course is benign and may stabilize or improve with specific therapy. Pathologically, it shows degeneration of the anterior horn cells and resembles an indolent poliomyelitis.[129]

A syndrome of paraneoplastic myelopathy with limbic encephalitis is associated with the antineuronal autoantibody anti-Hu.[33] This syndrome is almost always related to small cell lung cancer, and the presence of anti-Hu should lead to aggressive work-up for neoplasms. This antibody is also associated with a subacute generalized sensory neuronopathy.

MYELOPATHY SECONDARY TO RADIATION THERAPY

Myelopathy secondary to radiation therapy is an iatrogenic illness. Its incidence is affected by the total dose of radiation delivered, the dose per fraction, and the total volume of tissue irradiated.[38] In a large study by Kagen and coworkers,[79] it was determined that spinal cord injury could be avoided if the total dose delivered was kept to 6000 rads and given over a 30- to 70-day period at a rate not exceeding 200 rads per day or 900 rads per week.

Two pathophysiologic mechanisms are proposed for this myelopathy: direct damage to the nervous tissue of the spinal cord by irradiation, and damage to the vascular supply of the spinal cord. The effects of radiation take the form of an early delayed and late delayed myelopathy. There are no acute effects of radiation on the spinal cord.[38] The incidence of this complication is 2 to 3 per cent but is substantially higher when radiation therapy is combined with hyperthermia.[42]

The early delayed radiation myelopathy usually presents several weeks after radiation therapy as sensory symptoms and paresthesias. These symptoms may be exacerbated by neck flexion, and a typical Lhermitte's phenomenon may be detected. These symptoms are believed to be secondary to demyelination and depletion of oligodendrocytes.[3] The presence of this early delayed myelopathy does not predict the development of a late delayed radiation injury.[76]

The late delayed radiation myelopathy may evolve in two distinct forms: a progressive myelopathy that usually occurs 12 to 15 months after radiation therapy and never before 6 months, and a progressive lower motor neuron weakness that occurs from 3 to 14 months after radiation. The former is characterized by sensory symptoms similar to the early delayed myelopathy, but it is accompanied by an asymmetric weakness. Frequently, the initial picture is that of a Brown-Séquard syndrome that often progresses to a complete transverse myelopathy with spastic paraplegia, a truncal sensory level, and bowel, bladder, and sexual dysfunction. The CSF profile is unremarkable, except for the frequent presence of a slightly elevated protein. The pathologic changes include areas of necrosis that affect both gray and white matter, but white matter appears to be preferentially affected. The posterior columns and posterolateral column may be especially involved.[38]

There is no specific therapy, although steroids may slow the tempo of the illness. The differential diagnosis includes recurrent tumor or epidural spinal cord compression. The painless nature of the radiation damage is a useful diagnostic clue, particularly when MRI is indeterminate.

The progressive lower motor neuron weakness following radiation therapy is, not unexpectedly, accompanied by pathologic alterations in the anterior horn cells. There is an asymmetric atrophy with fasciculations and areflexia.[92, 128] However, no sensory or sphincter disturbances are noted. This peculiar myelopathy resembles a paraneoplastic subacute motor neuropathy described in patients with lymphoma.[129]

TOXINS

Several agents with industrial, pharmaceutical, and medical applications have been identified as toxins capable of producing myelopathy. Toxic iatrogenic causes of myelopathy include spinal anesthesia and exposure to myelographic and angiographic contrast agents. Epidural or intrathecal administration of local anesthetics has been reported to produce myelopathy. Although an extremely rare occurrence, the myelopathy following spinal anesthesia may be permanent and may include frank paraplegia, sensory loss, and loss of sphincter function. The mechanism of spinal anesthesia–induced myelopathy has not been well established and may include direct neurotoxicity of these agents, toxicity of drug diluents or contaminants, hypotension leading to spinal cord infarction, or exacerbation of an underlying process. Thus, cases of myelopathy following spinal anesthesia in the setting of spinal cord tumors or herniated discs have been reported.

Although both oil- and water-soluble myelographic contrast agents may induce arachnoiditis, which may lead to spinal cord dysfunction, these agents may themselves produce a toxic myelopathy. The use of modern contrast agents has essentially eliminated this complication, but nearly 6 per cent of patients had permanent myelopathic findings after myelography in early reports. Transient myelopathic symptoms lasting up to 24 hours have also been reported subsequent to the administration of water-soluble contrast agents.[87]

Myelopathy as a complication of spinal angiography has been well recognized. Although this complication is most often ascribed to the induction of vasospasm or embolic thrombosis of spinal vessels, resulting in ischemic infarction, a direct neurotoxic effect of the angiographic agents has been implicated in some instances.[85] Patients may develop pain and spasms immediately upon contrast injection, or this may be delayed by several hours. Subsequently, they progress to flaccid paraplegia with frequent sensory and sphincter dysfunction. Partial recovery occurs in about half the patients, and complete recovery occurs in about 20 per cent within weeks.[87] Many are left with a spastic paraplegia. Although it is an extremely safe agent when used according to recommendations, nitrous oxide can manifest neurotoxicity when it is abused or under conditions of chronic exposure. The resulting myeloneuropathic syndrome is usually long delayed after nitrous oxide exposure and may include sensory dysesthesias, leg weakness, spasticity, sphincter dysfunction, and ataxia. Thought to result from a nitrous oxide–induced inhibition of vitamin B_{12} utilization, the symptoms tend to resolve after exposure is discontinued.

Intrathecal administration of antineoplastic agents, such as methotrexate or cytosine arabinoside, has been reported to produce both transient and permanent myelopathy.[29, 60, 132] Intrathecal steroid administration may initiate an acute meningeal reaction, probably owing to polyethylene glycol detergent included in the preparation.[17, 98] Distinct from those problems caused by secondary arachnoiditis, this acute syndrome may result in back and leg pain, paresthesias, and sphincter dysfunction. Intravenous heroin administration may also cause an acute transverse myelitis. This syndrome may result from direct drug toxicity, a systemic reaction to the drug itself or to quinine or another drug diluent, a hypersensitivity reaction, or transient spinal cord ischemia.[123]

Iodochlorhydroxyquinoline, a drug used in the treatment of infectious diarrhea, has been reported to cause a syndrome of myeloneuropathy sometimes accompanied by optic atrophy.[141] Seen most frequently in Japan, this syndrome usually follows an episode of abdominal pain or diarrhea and therapy with the iodochlorhydroxyquinoline. Although apparently related to the total accumulated dose of the drug, this syndrome might also be related to an enteric virus associated with the initial abdominal symptoms. Patients initially complain of ascending numbness and paresthesias, which then develop into a profound sensory loss. Gait ataxia, leg weakness, and sphincter dysfunction are frequent concomitants; optic atrophy and visual loss are seen in about 25 per cent of patients. After discontinuing the drug, complete or near complete recovery is the rule.

Triorthocresyl phosphates, used as industrial lubricating oils and solvents, are highly neurotoxic. Although accidental occupational exposure is rare, patients are often exposed by ingesting triorthocresyl phosphates in lieu of ethanol or by ingesting cooking oils contaminated with these compounds. The most profound neurologic complication of triorthocresyl phosphate ingestion is acute peripheral neuritis, but clinical signs of spinal cord degeneration can be seen in those with persistent symptoms. Wallerian degeneration of the pyramidal tract and chromatolytic changes in both dorsal and ventral horn cells have been identified.[27, 137] In those patients developing myelopathic findings, the clinical syndrome is usually permanent.

A peculiar myelopathy seen in India and certain parts of Africa is believed to be the result of a neurotoxin (beta, N, oxalylaminoalanine) found in chickpeas (*Lathyrus sativus*). It is most often observed with prolonged consumption of flour made from chickpeas in times of famine, when other grains are scarce. The patients complain of the gradual onset of leg weakness, stiffness, and cramping. Paresthesias, formication, and numbness of the legs are frequent symptoms. Sphincter disturbances, impotence, and variable involvement of the arms and hands are observed. The prognosis for recovery is poor.

ELECTRICAL INJURY

Electrical injury of the nervous system results most frequently from accidental exposure to high-tension currents, although lightning and complications of electroshock therapy have also been reported to cause neurologic injury. Although current sufficient to cause damage to the nervous system is usually fatal, those who survive such injuries are subject to damage throughout the neuraxis.[87, 142] Acutely, patients may suffer neurologic symptoms referable to cerebral anoxia, secondary to cardiac arrhythmias or respiratory arrest. Neural tissue examined shortly after electrical injury shows petechial and perivascular hemorrhages and severe ganglion cell changes. Short-term survivors of this acute phase may demonstrate focal myelomalacia and mild gliosis upon autopsy. Although the pathophysiology is not fully understood, the injury most probably reflects a direct vascular injury to spinal cord vessels, an indirect vascular injury to spinal vasomotor nerves, or a direct effect of current on spinal cord tissue.

Following electrical injury, patients may initially complain of paresthesias, pain, urinary dysfunction, or impotence, but these tend to improve rapidly. Permanent neurologic manifestations of electrical injury are uncommon. A cervical myelopathy with atrophic quadriparesis is the most frequent complication; this myelopathy results from current passing from hand to hand.[46, 74] With low-voltage injuries (less than 1000 volts), muscular atrophy from anterior horn cell damage is most common; with higher voltages, more profound injuries occur to the lateral and posterior columns.[87] The deficits arising from these injuries tend to appear immediately and either remain static or slowly improve over a few months. Rarely, delayed neurologic deficits can appear after a latency of several months.[35, 70] The symptoms of delayed myelopathy following electrical injury are often permanent, but rapid recovery has been reported.[30]

BAROTRAUMA

Spinal cord injury following rapid changes in atmospheric pressure, as can occur in caisson work, scuba diving, and flying, has been well documented.[59, 86, 99] Spinal cord damage results from too rapid decompression following exposure to significant increases in atmospheric pressure. At higher atmospheric pressures, increasing amounts of gas are dissolved into tissue. The higher tissue concentration of oxygen is used in oxidative metabolism, whereas nitrogen gas, which is inert, remains dissolved only by virtue of the hyperbaric condition. With decompression, the nitrogen is released; when decompression is too rapid, nitrogen bubbles may form and occlude the spinal cord vasculature.

Symptoms tend to develop during or immediately after decompression. Patients frequently complain of interscapular pain, followed by lower extremity paresthesias, frank leg weakness, and sphincter disturbances within hours. Examination usually reveals a flaccid paraplegia with loss of pain and temperature sensation and frequent sparing of proprioceptive sensation. In most cases, the thoracic spinal cord is the major site of involvement; less commonly, combined lesions in the lower cervical and lumbar cord may occur. Pathologic examination of the cord demonstrates early white matter hemorrhages followed by perivascular demyelination. These changes tend to be most extensive in the posterior and lateral columns, and over time, secondary ascending and descending tract degeneration may be seen.

The therapy for decompression myelopathy is recompression followed by controlled slow decompression. If such treatment is instituted rapidly, complete recovery may be accomplished. If it is delayed more than a few hours, the chances of recovery are remote.[20, 99]

HEREDOFAMILIAL DEGENERATION

A large number of genetic neurodegenerative diseases can include spasticity attributable in whole or in part to spinal cord involvement in the complex of signs and symptoms, but in two disorders, spastic paraparesis is prominent. Hereditary spastic paraplegia appears in autosomal recessive, autosomal dominant, and X-linked forms. A locus for the autosomal recessive form has been found on chromosome 8q; loci for the dominant form are at 2p, 14q, and 15q, and for the X-linked form at Xq22. In one family with the X-linked form, this has been shown to be caused by a mutation in a proteolipoprotein.[47] There is spastic weakness in the legs, gait difficulties, hyperactive reflexes, and extensor plantar signs. The course is one of slow but relentless progression. There are rare variants with other associated degenerations, such as optic neuropathy. Diagno-

sis is made by family history and exclusion of any other causes.[3]

Patients with Friedreich's ataxia begin having problems in childhood. There is spastic quadriparesis owing to upper motor neuron degeneration, ataxia from cerebellar degeneration, numbness and foot deformity from neuropathy, nystagmus, tremor, and other problems. There is also degeneration of the posterior columns, corticospinal tracts, spinocerebellar tracts, dentate nuclei, cranial nerve nuclei, and myocardial muscle fibers. There is no treatment, and death occurs in young adulthood. It has recently been found that most cases of the illness are caused by trinucleotide repeat expansion in gene X25, which codes for a protein frataxin, on chromosome 9q13. A few cases are caused by point mutations in the same gene.[23]

References

1. Aboulafia, D. M., Saxton, E. H., Koga, H., et al.: A patient with progressive myelopathy and antibodies to human T-cell leukemia virus type I and human immunodeficiency virus type 1 in serum and cerebrospinal fluid. Arch. Neurol. 47:477, 1990.
2. Adams, R. D., and Merritt, H. H.: Meningeal and vascular diseases of the spinal cord. Medicine 23:181, 1944.
3. Adams, R. D., and Victor, M.: Diseases of the spinal cord. In Principles of Neurology. 5th ed. New York, McGraw-Hill, 1993, pp 1078–1116.
4. Adams, R. D., and Victor, M.: Viral infections of the nervous system. In Principles of Neurology. 5th ed. New York, McGraw-Hill, 1993, pp. 639–668.
5. Agbobu, B., Stern, B. J., Sewell, C., and Yang, G.: Therapeutic considerations in patients with refractory neurosarcoidosis. Arch. Neurol. 52:875, 1995.
6. Akizuki, S., Nakazato, O., Higuchi, Y., et al.: Necropsy findings in HTLV-I associated myelopathy (letter). Lancet 1:156, 1987.
7. Altrocchi, P. H.: Acute transverse myelopathy. Arch. Neurol. 9:111, 1963.
8. Andrianakos, A. A., Duffy, J., Suzuki, M., and Sharp, J. T.: Transverse myelopathy in systemic lupus erythematosus: Report of three cases and review of the literature. Ann. Intern. Med. 83:616, 1975.
9. Baker, A. S., Ojemann, R. G., Swartz, M. N., and Richardson, E. P., Jr.: Spinal epidural abscess. N. Engl. J. Med.293:463, 1975.
10. Berger, J. R.: Neurosyphilis. In Johnson, R. (ed.): Current Therapies in Neurology. 1990, Philadelphia, B. C. Dekker, 1990, pp. 143–148.
11. Berger, J. R.: Spinal cord syphilis associated with HIV infection: A treatable myelopathy. Am. J. Med. 92:101–103, 1992.
12. Berger, J. R.: Syphilis of the spinal cord. In Davidoff, R. A. (ed.): Handbook of the Spinal Cord. Vol. 5. New York, Marcel Dekker, 1987, pp. 491–538.
13. Berger, J. R., Moskowitz, L., Fischl, M., and Kelley, R. E.: Neurologic disease as the presenting manifestation of acquired immunodeficiency syndrome. S. Med. J. 80:683, 1987.
14. Berger, J. R., Raffanti, S., Svenningoson, A., and Resnick, L.: Tropical spastic paraparesis-like illness occurring in a dually infected individual with HIV-I and HTLV-II. Neurology 41:85–88, 1991.
15. Berger, J. R., Sheremata, W. A., Resnick, L., et al.: Multiple sclerosis–like illness occurring with human immunodeficiency virus infection. Neurology 39:324–328, 1989.
16. Berman, M., Feldman, S., Alter, M., et al.: Acute transverse myelitis: Incidence and etiologic considerations. Neurology 31:966, 1982.
17. Bernat, J. L.: Intraspinal steroid therapy. Neurology 31:168, 1981.
18. Blass, J. H.: Rheumatoid arthritis of the cervical spine. Bull. Rheum. Dis. 18:471, 1967.
19. Blau, E. H., and Kaufman, R. L.: Erosive and subluxing cervical spine disease in patients with psoriatic arthritis. J. Rheumatol. 14:111, 1987.

20. Bokerila, L. A., and Kobaneva, R. A.: Hyperbaric oxygenation in caisson disease. Klin. Med. (Mosk.) *51:*50, 1973.

21. Britton, C. B., Mesa-Tejada, R., Fenoglio, C. M., et al.: A new complication of AIDS: Thoracic myelitis caused by herpes simplex virus. Neurology *35:*1071, 1985.

22. Bundschuk, C., Modic, M. T., Kearney, F., et al.: Rheumatoid arthritis of the cervical spine: Surface-coil MR imaging. AJR Am. J. Roentgenol. *151:*181, 1988.

23. Campuzano, V., Montermini, L., Molto, M. D., et al.: Friedreich's ataxia: Autosomal recessive disease caused by an intronic GAA triplet repeat expansion. Science *271:*1374, 1996.

24. Caplan, L. R., Kleeman, F. J., and Berg, S.: Urinary retention probably secondary to herpes genitalis. N. Engl. J. Med. *297:*920, 1977.

25. Casey, A. T., Crockard, H. A., Bland, J. M., et al.: Surgery on the rheumatoid cervical spine for the non-ambulant myelopathic patient—too much, too late? Lancet *347:*984, 1996.

26. CDC: Syphilis: Recommended treatment schedules, 1976. Ann. Intern. Med. *85:*94, 1976.

27. Chaduri, R. N.: Paralytic disease caused by contamination with tricresyl phosphate. Trans. R. Soc. Trop. Med. Hyg. *59:*98, 1965.

28. Chapelon, C., Ziza, J. M., Piette, J. C., et al.: Neurosarcoidosis: Signs, course and treatment in 35 confirmed cases. Medicine *69:*261, 1990.

29. Clark, A. W., Cohen, S. R., Nissenblatt, M. J., and Wilson, S. K.: Paraplegia following intrathecal chemotherapy. Cancer *50:*42, 1982.

30. Clouston, P. D., and Sharpe, D.: Rapid recovery after delayed myelopathy from electrical burns (letter). J. Neurol. Neurosurg. Psychiatry *52:*1308, 1989.

31. Cohen, M. E., Duffner, P. K., and Terplan, K. L.: Myelopathy with severe structural derangement associated with combined modality therapy. Cancer *52:*1590, 1983.

32. Cordeiro, M. F., Lloyd, M. E., Spalton, D. J., and Hughes, G. R.: Ischaemic optic neuropathy, transverse myelitis, and epilepsy in an anti-phospholipid positive patient with systemic lupus erythematosus (letter). J. Neurol. Neurosurg. Psychiatry *57:*1142, 1994.

33. Dalmau, J., Graus, F., Rosenblum, M. K., and Posner, J. B.: Anti-Hu–associated paraneoplastic encephalomyelitis/sensory neuronopathy: A clinical study of 71 patients. Medicine *71:*59, 1992.

34. Dansey, R. D., Hammond-Tooke, G. D., Lai, K., and Bezwoda, W. R.: Subacute myelopathy: An unusual paraneoplastic complication of Hodgkin's disease. Med. Pediatr. Oncol. *16:*284, 1988.

35. Davidson, G. S., and Deck, J. H.: Delayed myelopathy following lightning strike: A demyelinating process. Acta Neuropathol. (Berl.) *77:*104, 1988.

36. DeJong, R. N.: Neurologic Examination. New York, Harper & Row, 1979.

37. de la Monte, S. M., Ho, D. D., Schooley, R. T., et al.: Subacute encephalomyelitis of AIDS and its relation to HTLV-III infection. Neurology *37:*562, 1987.

38. Delattre, J. -Y., and Posner, J. B.: Neurological complications of chemotherapy and radiation therapy. *In* Aminoff, M. (ed.): Neurology and General Medicine. 2nd ed. New York, Churchill Livingstone, 1995, pp. 421–445.

39. Denning, D. W., Anderson, J., Rudge, P., and Smith, H.: Acute myelopathy associated with primary infection with human immunodeficiency virus. Br. Med. J. *294:*143, 1987.

40. Dickson, D. W., Belman, A. L., Kim, T. S., et al.: Spinal cord pathology in pediatric acquired immunodeficiency syndrome. Neurology *39:*227, 1989.

41. Doll, D. C., Yarbro, J. W., Phillips, K., and Klott, C.: Mycobacterial spinal cord abscess with an ascending polyneuropathy (letter). Ann. Intern. Med. *106:*333, 1987.

42. Douglas, M. A., Parks, L. C., and Bebin, J.: Sudden myelopathy secondary to therapeutic total body hyperthermia after spinal cord irradiation. N. Engl. J. Med. *304:*583, 1981.

43. Dutton, J. E. M., and Alexander, G. L.: Intramedullary spinal abscess. J. Neurol. Neurosurg. Psychiatry *17:*303, 1954.

44. Ellis, S. G., and Verity, M. A.: Central nervous system involvement in systemic lupus erythematosus: A review of neuropatho-

logical findings in 57 cases, 1955–1977. Semin. Arthritis Rheum. *8:*212, 1979.

45. Endo, T., Koike, J., Kusama, Y., et al.: Spinal cord sarcoidosis. Neurology *43:*1059, 1993.

46. Farrel, D. F., and Starr, A.: Delayed neurological sequelae of electric injuries. Neurology *18:*601, 1968.

47. Fink, J. K., Heiman-Patterson, T., Bird, T., et al.: Hereditary spastic paraplegia: Advances in genetic research. Neurology *46:*1507, 1996.

48. Fisher, M., and Poser, C. M.: Syphilitic meningomyelitis. Arch. Neurol. *34:*785, 1977.

49. Fody, E. P., Netsky, M. G., and Mrak, R. E.: Subarachnoid spinal hemorrhage in a case of systemic lupus erythematosus. Arch. Neurol. *37:*173, 1980.

50. Ford, B., Tampieri, D., and Francis, G.: Long-term follow-up of acute partial transverse myelopathy. Neurology *42:*250–252, 1992.

51. Gagliano, R. G., and Castanzi, J. J.: Paraplegia following intrathecal methotrexate. Cancer *37:*1663, 1976.

52. Gessain, A., Vernant, J., Maurs, L., et al.: Antibodies to human T-lymphotropic virus type-I in patients with tropical spastic paraparesis. Lancet *2:*407, 1985.

53. Goldstick, L., Mandybur, T. I., and Bode, R.: Spinal cord degeneration in AIDS. Neurology *35:*103, 1985.

54. Goubau, P., Carton, H., Kazadi, K., et al.: HTLV seroepidemiology in a central African population with high incidence of tropical spastic paraparesis. Trans. R. Soc. Trop. Med. Hyg. *84:*577–579, 1990.

55. Gribble, L. D.: Syphilitic spinal pachymeningitis. S. Afr. Med. J. *46:*1326, 1972.

56. Griffin, J. W., Gorlin, E., Schaumburg, H., et al.: Adrenomyeloneuropathy: A probable variant of adrenoleukodystrophy. Neurology *27:*1107, 1977.

57. Griffiths, D. L.: Tuberculosis of the spine: A review. Adv. Tuberc. Res. *20:*92, 1980.

58. Grose, C., and Feorino, P. M.: Epstein-Barr virus and transverse myelitis. Lancet *1:*892, 1973.

59. Gwozdziewicz, J.: Changes in the spinal cord of divers connected with chronic forms of caisson disease. Biul. Ist. Med. Morsk. Gdansk *16:*171, 1965.

60. Hahn, A. F., Feasby, T. E., and Gilbert, J. J.: Paraparesis following intrathecal chemotherapy. Neurology *33:*1032, 1983.

61. Halla, J. T., Hardin, J. R., Jr.: The spectrum of atlantoaxial facet joint involvement in rheumatoid arthritis. Arthritis Rheum. *33:*325, 1990.

62. Handforth, A., Nag, S., Sharp, D., and Robertson, D. M.: Paraneoplastic subacute necrotic myelopathy. Can. J. Neurol. Sci. *10:*204, 1983.

63. Harada, T., Ohashi, T., Miyagishi, R., et al.: Optic neuropathy and acute transverse myelopathy in primary Sjögren's syndrome. Jpn. J. Ophthalmol. *39:*162, 1995.

64. Harisdangkul, V., Doorenbos, D., and Subramony, S. H.: Lupus transverse myelopathy: Better outcome with early recognition and aggressive high-dose intravenous corticosteroid pulse treatment. J. Neurol. *242:*326, 1995.

65. Helweg-Larsen, S., Jakobsen, J., Boesen, F., and Arlien-Soborg, P.: Neurological complications and concomitants of AIDS. Acta Neurol. Scand. *74:*467, 1986.

66. Henson, R. A., and Urich, H.: Cancer and the Nervous System. London, Blackwell Scientific Publications, 1982.

67. Herrick, M., and Mills, P. E., Jr.: Infarction of spinal cord. Arch. Neurol. *24:*228, 1971.

68. Herskovitz, S., Siegel, S. E., Schneider, A. T., et al.: Spinal cord toxoplasmosis in AIDS. Neurology *39:*1552, 1989.

69. Heyman, S. N., Michaeli, J., Brezis, M., et al.: Primary hyperparathyroidism presenting as cervical myelopathy. Am. J. Med. Sci. *291:*112, 1986.

70. Holbrook, L. A., Beach, F. X., and Silver, J. R.: Delayed myelopathy: A rare complication of severe electrical burns. Br. Med. J. *4:*659, 1970.

71. Honig, L. S., Vogel, H., and Horoupian, D. S.: Chronic myelopathy as a presenting symptom in HIV infection (abstract). Neurology *39* (suppl. 1):419, 1989.

72. Hopkins, J. S.: Lower cervical rheumatoid subluxation and tetraplegia. J. Bone Joint Surg. *49:*46, 1967.

73. Iwamasa, T., Utsumi, Y., Sakuda, H., et al.: Two cases of necrotizing myelopathy associated with malignancy caused by herpes simplex virus type 2. Acta Neuropathol. (Berl.) 78:252, 1989.

74. Jackson, F. E., Martin, R., and Davis, R.: Delayed quadriplegia following electrical burn. Mil. Med. 130:601, 1965.

75. Jeannel, D., Garin, B., Kazadi, K., et al.: The risk of tropical spastic paraparesis differs according to ethnic group among HTLV-I carriers in Indongo, Zaire. J. Acquir. Immune Defic. Syndr. 6:840–844, 1993.

76. Jones, A.: A transient radiation myelitis. Br. J. Radiol. 37:727, 1964.

77. Juchet, H., Ollier, S., Durroux, R., et al.: [Neurologic and psychiatric manifestations of primary hyperparathyroidism]. Rev. Med. Interne 14:123, 1993.

78. Junger, S. S., Stern, B. J., Levine, S. R., et al.: Intramedullary spinal stenosis: Clinical and magnetic resonance imaging characteristics. Neurology 43:333, 1993.

79. Kagen, R. A., Wollin, M., Gilbert, H. A., et al.: Comparison of the tolerance of the brain and spinal cord to injury by radiation. In Gilbert, H. A., and Kagan, R. A. (eds.): Radiation Damage to the Nervous System. New York, Raven Press, 1980.

80. Kamin, S. S., and Petito, C. K.: Idiopathic myelopathies with white matter vacuolation in non–acquired immunodeficiency syndrome patients. Hum. Pathol. 22:816–824, 1991.

81. Kaplan, J. E., Litchfield, B., Rouault, C., et al.: HTLV-I–associated myelopathy associated with blood transfusion in the United States: Epidemiologic and molecular evidence linking donor and recipient. Neurology 41:192, 1991.

82. Kaufman, D. M., Kaplan, J. G., and Litman, N.: Infectious agents in spinal epidural abscesses. Neurology 30:844, 1980.

83. Kayembe, K., Goubau, P., Desmyter, J., et al.: A clustover of HTLV-I associated tropical spastic paraparesis in Equateur (Zaire): Ethnic and familial distribution. J. Neurol. Neurosurg. Psychiatry 53:4–10, 1990.

84. Khabbaz, R. F., Darrow, W. W., Hartley, T. M., et al.: Seroprevalence and risk factors for HTLV-I/II infection among female prostitutes in the United States. JAMA 263:60, 1990.

85. Killen, D. A., and Foster, J. H.: Spinal cord injury as a complication of contrast angiography. Surgery 59:962, 1966.

86. Kim, S. W., Kim, R. C., Choi, B. H., and Gordon, S. K.: Nontraumatic ischaemic myelopathy: A review of 25 cases. Paraplegia 26:262, 1988.

87. Kincaid, J. C.: Myelitis and myelopathy. In Joynt, R. J. (ed.): Clinical Neurology, Vol III. Philadelphia, Lippincott–Raven, 1990, pp. 1–36.

88. Klastersky, J., Capperl, R., Snoeck, J. M., et al.: Ascending myelitis in association with herpes simplex virus. N. Engl. J. Med. 287:182, 1982.

89. Konttinen, Y. T., Kinneenen, E., von Bonsdorff, M., et al.: Acute transverse myelopathy successfully treated with plasmapheresis and prednisone in a patient with primary Sjögren's syndrome. Arthritis Rheum. 30:339, 1987.

90. Koprowski, H., DeFreitas, E., Harper, M. E., et al.: Multiple sclerosis and human T-cell lymphotropic retroviruses. Nature 318:154, 1985.

91. Kunze, K., and Leitenmaier, K.: Vitamin B$_{12}$ deficiency and subacute combined degeneration of the spinal cord (funicular spinal disease). In Vinken, P. J., and Bruyn, G. W. (eds.): Handbook of Neurology. Vol. 28. Amsterdam, Elsevier, 1976, pp. 141–198.

92. Laqueny, A., Aupy, M., Aupy, P., et al.: Syndrome de la corne anterieure postradiotherpique. Rev. Neurol. (Paris) 141:222, 1985.

93. Levy, R. M., Bredesen, D. E., and Rosenblum, M. L.: Neurological manifestations of the acquired immunodeficiency syndrome (AIDS): Experience of UCSF and review of the literature. J. Neurosurg. 62:475, 1985.

94. Lexa, F. J., and Grossman, R. I.: MR of sarcoidosis in the head and spine: Spectrum of manifestations and radiographic response to steroid therapy. AJNR Am. J. Neuroradiol. 15:973, 1994.

95. Lipton, H. L., and Teasdall, R. D.: Acute transverse myelopathy in adults. Arch. Neurol. 28:252, 1973.

96. Lorber, A., Pearson, C. M., and Rene, R. M.: Osteolytic vertebral lesions as a manifestation of rheumatoid arthritis and related disorders. Arthritis Rheum. 4:514, 1961.

97. Lyu, R. K., Chen, S. T., Tang, L. M., and Chen, T. C.: Acute transverse myelopathy and cutaneous vasculopathy in primary Sjögren's syndrome. Eur. Neurol. 35:359, 1995.

98. Mastaglia, F. L.: Iatrogenic (drug-induced) disorders of the nervous system. In Aminoff, M. (ed.): Neurology and General Medicine. 2nd ed. New York, Churchill Livingstone, 1989, pp. 587–614.

99. Mastaglia, F. L., McCallum, R. I., and Walder, D. N.: Myelopathy associated with decompression sickness: A report of six cases. Clin. Exp. Neurol. 19:54, 1983.

100. McArthur, J. C.: Neurologic manifestations of AIDS. Medicine 66:407, 1987.

101. McArthur, J. C., Griffin, J. W., Cornblath, D. R., et al.: Steroid-responsive myeloneuropathy in a man dually infected with HIV-1 and HTLV-I. Neurology 40:938, 1990.

102. McGrath, H. J., McCormick, C., and Carey, M. E.: Pyogenic cervical osteomyelitis presenting as a massive prevertebral abscess in a patient with rheumatoid arthritis. Am. J. Med. 84:363, 1988.

103. Melamed, E., Berman, M., and Lavy, S.: Posterolateral myelopathy associated with thyrotoxicosis (letter). N. Engl. J. Med. 293:778, 1975.

104. Miller, D. H., McDonald, W. I., Blumhardt, L. D., et al.: Magnetic resonance imaging in isolated noncompressive spinal cord disorders. Ann. Neurol. 22:714, 1987.

105. Miller, D. H., Ormerod, I. E., Rudge, P., et al.: The early risk of multiple sclerosis following isolated acute syndromes of the brainstem and spinal cord. Ann. Neurol. 26:635, 1989.

106. Miller, H. G., Stanton, J. B., and Gibbons, J. L.: Parainfectious encephalomyelitis and related syndromes: A critical review of the neurologic complications of certain specific fevers. J. Med. 25:427, 1956.

107. Mok, C. C., and Lau, C. S.: Transverse myelitis complicating mixed connective tissue disease. Clin. Neurol. Neurosurg. 97:259, 1995.

108. Morrissey, S. P., Miller, D. H., Kendall, B. E., et al.: The significance of brain magnetic resonance imaging abnormalities at presentation with clinically isolated syndromes suggestive of multiple sclerosis. Brain 116:135–146, 1993.

109. Moser, H., Moser, A., Kawamura, N., et al.: Adrenoleukodystrophy: Elevated C$_{26}$ fatty acid in cultured skin fibroblasts. Ann. Neurol. 7:542, 1980.

110. Muder, R. R., Lumish, R. M., and Corsello, G. R.: Myelopathy after herpes zoster. Arch. Neurol. 40:445, 1983.

111. Murphy, E. L., Fridey, J., Smith, J. W., et al.: HTLV-associated myelopathy in a cohort of HTLV-I and HTLV-II infected blood donors. Neurology 48:315–320, 1997.

112. Murphy, E. L., Wilks, R., Morgan, O. S., et al.: Health effects of human T-lymphotrophic virus type-I in a Jamaican cohort. Int. J. Epidemiol. 25:1090–1097, 1995.

113. Norris, F. H.: Remote effects of cancer on the spinal cord. In Vinken, P. J., and Bruyn, G. W. (eds.): Handbook of Clinical Neurology. Vol. 38. Amsterdam, North Holland Publishing, 1979, pp. 669–677.

114. Osame, M., Usuku, J., Izumo, S., et al.: HTLV-I associated myelopathy: A new clinical entity. Lancet 1:1031, 1986.

115. Paine, R. S., and Byers, R. K.: Transverse myelopathy in childhood. Am. J. Child. 85:151, 1953.

116. Perling, L. H., Laurent, J. P., and Cheek, W. R.: Epidural hibernoma as a complication of corticosteroid treatment: Case report. J. Neurosurg. 69:613, 1988.

117. Petito, C. K., Navia, B. A., Cho, E. S., et al.: Vacuolar myelopathy pathologically resembling subacute combined degeneration in patients with the acquired immunodeficiency syndrome. N. Engl. J. Med. 312:874, 1985.

118. Pickeritt, R. G., and Milder, J. E.: Transverse myelitis associated with cat-scratch disease in an adult. JAMA 246:2840, 1981.

119. Plum, F., and Hindfelt, B.: The neurological complication of liver disease. In Vinken, P. J., and Bruyn, G. W. (eds.): Handbook of Clinical Neurology. Vol. 27. Amsterdam, North Holland Publishing, 1976, pp. 349–377.

120. Posner, J. B.: Paraneoplastic syndromes involving the nervous

system. *In* Aminoff, M. (ed.): Neurology and General Medicine. 2nd ed. New York, Churchill Livingstone, 1989, pp. 401–420.

121. Ray, D. W., Bridger, J., Hawnaur, J., et al.: Transverse myelitis as the presentation of Jo-1 antibody syndrome (myositis and fibrosing alveolitis) in long-standing ulcerative colitis. Br. J. Rheumatol. *32:*1105, 1993.

122. Reik, L., Steere, A. C., Bartenhagen, N. H., et al.: Neurologic abnormalities of Lyme disease. Medicine *58:*281, 1979.

123. Richter, R. W.: Drug abuse. *In* Rowland, L. P. (ed.): Merritt's Textbook of Neurology. 8th ed. Philadelphia, Lea & Febiger, 1989, pp. 909–917.

124. Robert-Guroff, M., Weiss, S. H., Giron, J. A., et al.: Prevalence of antibodies to HTLV-I, -II, and -III in intravenous drug abusers from an AIDS endemic region. JAMA *255:*3133, 1986.

125. Ropper, A. H., and Poskanzer, D. C.: The prognosis of acute and subacute transverse myelopathy based on early signs and symptoms. Ann. Neurol. *4:*51, 1978.

126. Rose, F. C., Brett, E. M., and Burton, J.: Zoster encephalomyelitis. Arch. Neurol. *11:*155, 1964.

127. Rutan, G., Martinez, A. J., Fieshko, J. T., and Van Thiel, D. H.: Primary biliary cirrhosis, Sjögren's syndrome and transverse myelitis. Gastroenterology *90:*206, 1986.

128. Sadowsky, G. H., Sachs, E., and Ochoa, J.: Post radiation motor neuron syndrome. Arch. Neurol. *33:*786, 1976.

129. Schold, S. C., Cho, E. S., Somasundaram, M., and Posner, J. B. B.: Subacute motor neuropathy: A remote effect of lymphoma. Ann. Neurol. *5:*271, 1979.

130. Semple, E. L., Elster, A. D., Loeser, R. F., et al.: Magnetic resonance imaging of the craniovertebral junction in rheumatoid arthritis. J. Rheumatol. *15:*1367, 1988.

131. Shannon, K. M., and Goetz, C. G.: Connective tissue diseases and the nervous system. *In* Aminoff, M. (ed.): Neurology and General Medicine. 2nd ed. New York, Churchill Livingstone, 1989, pp. 447–471.

132. Shapiro, W. R., and Young, D. F.: Neurological complications of antineoplastic therapy. Acta Neurol. Scand. *70:*125, 1984.

133. Sheremata, W. A., Berger, J. R., Harrington, W. J., et al.: Human T lymphotrophic virus type I–associated myelopathy: A report of 10 patients born in the United States. Arch. Neurol. *49:*1113, 1992.

134. Silverstein, A.: Epstein-Barr virus infections of the nervous system. *In* Vinken, P. J., and Bruyn, G. W. (eds.): Infections of the Nervous System. Part II. Vol. 34. Amsterdam, North Holland Publishing, 1978, pp. 185–191.

135. Simnad, V. I., Pisani, D. E., and Rose, J. W.: Multiple sclerosis presenting as transverse myelopathy: Clinical and MRI features. Neurology *48:*65–73, 1997.

136. Singh, B. M., Levine, S., Yarrish, R. L., et al.: Spinal cord syn-dromes in the acquired immune deficiency syndrome. Acta Neurol. Scand. *73:*590, 1986.

137. Smith, H. V., and Spalding, J. M. K.: Outbreak of paralysis in Morocco due to orthocresyl phosphate poisoning. Lancet *2:*1019, 1959.

138. Smith, P. H., Benn, R. T., and Sharp, J.: Natural history of rheumatoid cervical luxations. Ann. Rheum. Dis. *31:*431, 1972.

139. Smith, W. T.: Nutritional deficiencies and disorders. *In* Blackwood, W., and Corsellis, J. A. N. (eds.): Greenfield's Neuropathology. London, Edward Arnold Publications, 1977.

140. Snider, W. D., Simpson, D. M., Nielsen, S., et al.: Neurological complications of the acquired immunodeficiency syndrome: Analysis of 50 patients. Ann. Neurol. *14:*403, 1983.

141. Sobue, I., Ando, K., Iida, M., et al.: Myeloneuropathy with abdominal disorders in Japan: A clinical study of 752 cases. Neurology *21:*178, 1971.

142. Sprofkin, B. E.: Electrical injuries. *In* Rowland, L. (ed.): Merritt's Textbook of Neurology. 7th ed. Philadelphia, Lea & Febiger, 1984.

143. Swash, M., and Schwartz, M. S.: Paraneoplastic syndromes. *In* Johnson, R. T. (ed.): Current Therapies in Neurologic Diseases—3. Philadelphia, B. C. Dekker, 1990, pp. 236–243.

144. Syme, J. A., and Kelly, J. J.: Absent F-waves early in a case of transverse myelitis. Muscle Nerve *17:*462, 1994.

145. Tucker, T., Dix, R. D., Katzen, C., et al.: Cytomegalovirus and herpes simplex virus ascending myelitis in a patient with acquired immune deficiency syndrome. Ann. Neurol. *18:*74, 1985.

146. Tyler, K. L., Gross, R. A., and Cascino, G. D.: Unusual viral causes of transverse myelitis: Hepatitis A virus and cytomegalovirus. Neurology *36:*855, 1986.

147. Vernant, J. C., Maurs, L., Gessain, A., et al.: Endemic tropical spastic paraparesis associated with human T-lymphotropic virus type I: A clinical and seroepidemiological study of 25 cases. Ann. Neurol. *21:*123, 1987.

148. Weill, O., Finaud, M., Bille, F., et al.: Gliome malin medullaire: Une nouvelle complication de l'infection par le HIV? (letter) Presse Med. *16:*1977, 1987.

149. Weiss, S. H., Ginzburg, S. H., Saxinger, W. C., et al.: Emerging high rates of human T-cell lymphotropic virus type I (HTLV-I) and HIV infections among US drug abusers. Abstract S.6.5. Washington, DC, III International Conference on AIDS, June 1987.

150. Williams, A. E., Fang, C. T., Slamon, D. J., et al.: Seroprevalence and epidemiological correlates of HTLV-I infection in US blood donors. Science *240:*643, 1988.

151. Woolsey, R. M., Chambers, T. J., Chung, H. K., and McGarry, J. D.: Mycobacterial meningomyelitis associated with human immunodeficiency virus infection. Arch. Neurol. *45:*691, 1988.

CHAPTER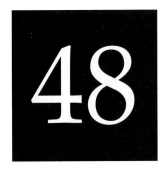

Syringomyelia

Parley W. Madsen, III, M.D., Ph.D.

Barth A. Green, M.D.

Brian C. Bowen, M.D., Ph.D.

Syringomyelia is defined by the *Oxford English Dictionary* as a "dilatation of the central canal of the spinal cord or formation of abnormal tubular cavities in its substance."[114] The classic clinical feature of syringomyelia can be described as segmental dissociative loss of sensory function in the upper extremities, which most commonly consists of the loss of distal sensation to pain and temperature and the preservation of proprioceptive sensation and light touch. Although cervical enlargement occurs most frequently, the clinical presentation is directly related to the involved spinal segments, and the affected areas can range from the conus to the midbrain. The disorder can be described as slowly progressive and ultimately involves the loss of lower motor function. If a syrinx extends to the medulla, the pathologic lesion is termed a syringobulbia, and compromise of brain stem function has been reported with this lesion. Extension of the more frequently encountered cervical syrinx has been implicated in syringobulbia formation.[2, 155, 173]

In the first monograph on syringomyelia, Schlesinger in 1902 stated that this condition ranks among the most common of spinal diseases, but Wilson cited admission statistics for the National Hospital from 1909 to 1925 to dispute this claim.[145, 187] There were only 115 cases of syringomyelia identified among the 6846 patients admitted. This group represented only 1.6 per cent of the total admissions, and the admissions for each of the following diagnoses were more frequent: tabes, syphilitic paraplegia, multiple sclerosis, subacute combined degeneration, and spinal tumor. Barnett and

colleagues reported that syringomyelia was diagnosed only 75 times out of 535,464 admissions over a 24-year period at the Toronto General Hospital.[17] Poser found only 18 cases of syringomyelia during a review of 1600 autopsies performed at the Neurological Institute of New York over a 20-year period.[127] The discrepancy between the early statistics reported in the German literature and the relatively later reports from England and the United States most likely reflects the slow course of the disorder, with the majority of patients dying at home, so that autopsies were not obtained.[187]

The most commonly reported age of clinical presentation of a symptomatic syrinx of the spinal cord is between 25 and 40 years. There is a slight predominance in males compared with females. Although syringomyelia had been described as a slowly progressive, degenerative disorder of insidious onset and with periods of quiescence, the natural history of the lesion has been reported to be extremely variable.[2, 4, 53]

Cavitation of the gray matter of the spinal cord, adjacent to or directly involving the central canal, and an inner layer of gliotic tissue were the most frequently reported pathologic features of syringomyelia (Fig. 48–1).[167, 174] Tumors, vascular anomalies, infective processes, and extramedullary compressive lesions have been reported in association with syrinx formation.[30, 37, 173] The presence of these associated pathologic lesions has contributed to the lively debate over the pathophysiologic basis of this disorder. No consensus has emerged, and the existing clinical and experimental data suggest that this disorder is not a single disease

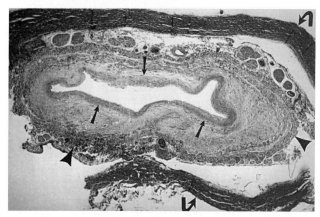

Figure 48–1. Posttraumatic cord cyst. A low-power (X1.25) microscopic section image of a posttraumatic syringomyelia in a 56-year-old man who expired five years after an upper thoracic gunshot wound. There is a large, centrally located syrinx in the parenchyma of the spinal cord, which is surrounded by a thick wall of reactive astrocytes *(arrows)*. The pia is thickened, and there are tissue changes that involve the spinal roots *(arrowheads)*. The dura is also thickened *(curved arrows)*. (From Madsen, P. W., Falcone, S., Bowen, B., and Green, B. A.: Post-traumatic syringomyelia. *In* Levine, A., Garfin, S., Eismont, F., and Zigler, J. (eds.): Spine Trauma. Philadelphia, W. B. Saunders Co. (in press).)

entity with a solitary cause. The evidence appears to be more consistent with the hypothesis that syringomyelia represents a syndrome of similar clinical entities with a diversity of pathologic changes that produce cavitation of the substance of the spinal cord. Adams and Victor used the term *syringomyelia* to refer directly to a "central cavitation of the spinal cord of undetermined cause" and *syringomyelic syndrome* to denote "the syndrome of segmental sensory dissociation with brachial amyotrophy."[2]

Treatment of syringomyelia is dependent on the practitioner's perception of the underlying pathologic derangement and should be modified for each individual patient. Considerable controversy continues regarding the preferred therapy for this disorder. As understanding of the pathophysiologic basis of syrinx formation has evolved, an alteration in therapeutic interventions has occurred to conform to the new information. This process has been impaired by the extremely variable clinical course of patients diagnosed with syringomyelia and necessitates following them for extended periods before efficacy of treatment can be accurately determined.[4, 8, 28, 60, 150, 177] Frazier and Rowe lamented the difficulty of objectively analyzing the late results of surgical treatment of syringomyelia because of the variability and complexity of the cases, as well as the lack of detail in the reports in the clinical literature.[58] Aschoff and associates reported that although more than 3000 operations have been reported for the treatment of syringes, there continues to be no optimal treatment for this disorder because of the variability in the types of syringes, the multiple procedures performed in individual cases, and the lack of long-term follow-up.[8]

The diagnosis of syringomyelia was a formidable task as recently as two decades ago, because there were no acceptable clinical or roentgenologic diagnostic criteria for the disorder.[41] Diagnostic techniques used before the advent of computed tomography (CT) and magnetic resonance imaging (MRI) were unreliable and exposed the patient to a significant risk of morbidity. Fortunately, it is no longer necessary to perform pneumoencephalography in the operating suite, with the patient prepared to undergo emergent ventriculostomy or craniotomy.[65, 69] Newer MRI techniques promise to facilitate the diagnosis of syringomyelia and to elucidate the pathophysiologic basis of its formation and progression (Fig. 48–2).[3, 46, 78, 120, 153, 162]

HISTORY

Syringomyelia, or cavitation within the substance of the spinal cord, has been recognized for more than three centuries as a pathologic entity. Finlayson credited Etienne in 1564 with the first published description of the disorder in *La Dissection du Corps Humain.*[53] The latter author reported a cystic lesion in the spinal cord that contained a "fluid, reddish, like the fluidity of that in the ventricles." Since this initial description, others, including Brunner in 1688, Morgagni in 1740, and Santorini, have published additional descriptions. Portal, in 1804, was the first to appreciate and report the relationship between clinical signs of motor paralysis and the observed pathologic changes.[187] Two decades later, Ollivier conceived the term *syringomyelia*, combining the Greek words for "tube or pipe" and "marrow," and applied it to any pathologic cavitation of the substance of the spinal cord, including the persistent central canal. He also documented a connection between the fourth ventricle and this cystic structure, which he believed to be a congenital anomaly.[12, 53, 55]

Following the description by Stilling in 1859 of a persistent dilatation of the central canal in an adult and the demonstration by Hallopeau in 1870 of pathologic cavitation that was anatomically separated from the central spinal canal, Simon proposed in 1875 that the term *syringomyelia* be reserved for the latter entity. Then-current medical opinion held that syringomyelia resulted from either myelitis or neoplastic growths. Those cavities that appeared to be pathologic dilatations of the central canal were termed *hydromyelia* by not only Simon but also other practitioners, including Virchow and Leyden. Other authors viewed hydromyelia, in which the central canal was dilated but preserved, and syringomyelia, with or without an obvious connection to the central canal, as stages of a common process. This view gained support and resulted in a unification of the terms into *syringohydromyelia* or *hydrosyringomyelia.*[12, 53, 78, 181]

Tamaki and Lubin credited Bruhl with the first description, during the late nineteenth century, of sensory dissociation and muscular atrophy with main en griffe as being diagnostic of syringomyelia.[161] Schultze in 1887 and Kahler in 1888, publishing in German, outlined the clinical features of syringomyelia essentially

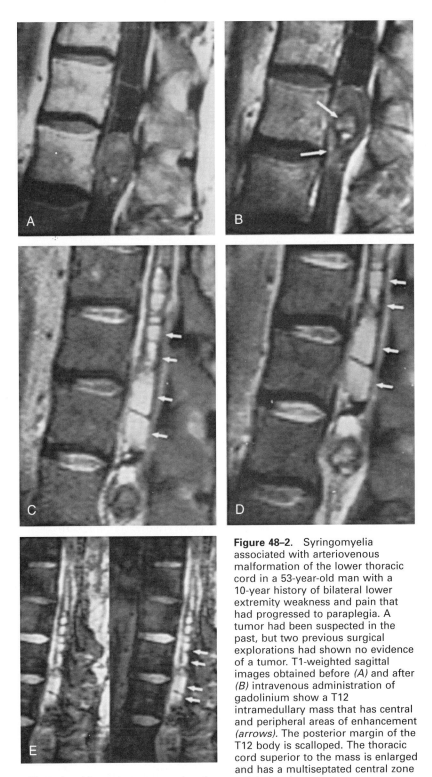

Figure 48–2. Syringomyelia associated with arteriovenous malformation of the lower thoracic cord in a 53-year-old man with a 10-year history of bilateral lower extremity weakness and pain that had progressed to paraplegia. A tumor had been suspected in the past, but two previous surgical explorations had shown no evidence of a tumor. T1-weighted sagittal images obtained before (A) and after (B) intravenous administration of gadolinium show a T12 intramedullary mass that has central and peripheral areas of enhancement (arrows). The posterior margin of the T12 body is scalloped. The thoracic cord superior to the mass is enlarged and has a multiseptated central zone of low signal intensity, representing the associated syrinx. T2-weighted images without (C) and with (D) flow compensation pulse sequences demonstrate an identical appearance of the loculated contents (short arrows) of the syrinx, indicating that there is no pulsatile flow of cerebrospinal fluid within the syrinx in this region. E, Two representative images from a cardiac-gated, gradient-echo acquisition at fixed sagittal position demonstrate no change in the signal properties of the syrinx (short arrows), again indicating no pulsatile flow of fluid in the thoracic portion of the syrinx.

as it is recognized today. The first American report was by Starr in 1888.[187] Hassin credited Thomas and Quercy with recognizing, in 1913, that syringomyelia was a syndrome of multiple causes.[76] Barnett, in the first English-language monograph on syringomyelia, published in 1973, proposed a classification based on a variety of clinical and experimental observations and studies.[16] This chapter uses a slight modification of that classification to organize the remaining discussion of the pathophysiology, diagnosis, and treatment of the syndrome:

1. Communicating syringomyelia (syringohydromyelia) (a) with associated developmental anomalies at the foramen magnum and of the posterior fossa contents or (b) associated with acquired abnormalities at the skull base
2. Syringomyelia as a sequel to arachnoiditis confined to the spinal canal
3. Syringomyelia associated with spinal cord tumors
4. Syringomyelia as a late sequel to trauma (post-traumatic cystic myelopathy)
5. Idiopathic syringomyelia

Although these categories are reasonable for a method of formal classification, Types 2, 4, 5 and the majority of Type 1 lesions can be grouped together in consideration of treatment. The exceptions are Type 1 lesions with the cyst in direct communication with the ventricular system. Type 3 lesions are adequately treated, in the majority of cases, by tumor removal.

Recent experimental and clinical work, including that by Oldfield and Milhorat and their colleagues, has helped clarify the pathophysiology and treatment of this syndrome.[107, 108, 110–113, 120] The latter group has proposed a classification and treatment algorism based on MRI findings (Fig. 48–3).[109]

Communicating Syringomyelia

Although the pathogenesis of syringomyelia has not yet been completely elucidated, the association of syringomyelia and congenital abnormalities was appreciated more than a century ago. Tamaki and Lubin credited Baumler in an 1887 paper with establishing this relationship, and Poser noted that Schlesinger's 1895 monograph stated that there was an associated congenital anomaly in fully one third of the cases of syringomyelia he had reviewed (Fig. 48–4).[127, 161]

MacKay and Favill credited Ollivier d'Angers with formulating the developmental theory of syringomyelia formation,[97] and Poser cited an 1876 publication by Leyden.[127] The latter author stated that syringomyelia must be considered a congenital disorder, and he believed that the syrinx was a result of incomplete occlusion of the primitive fold. However, this developmental theory was largely ignored until an 1894 report by Gerlach of a teratoma associated with a syrinx. A similar case by Bielschowsky in 1920 revived enthusiasm for the hypothesis. Proponents of this theory argued that improper fusion of the two folds of the primitive medullary groove allowed the groove to become lined with germinal cells, resulting in simple hydromyelia. A more significant malformation of the median dorsal septum caused not only proliferation of the glia in the region but also increased connective tissue in the lining of the cavity. Inclusion of mesodermal elements trapped during the defective closure was thought to be the cause, and this resulted in proliferation of blood vessels in the adjacent spinal cord substance. The cases of teratoma reported by Gerlach and Bielschowsky represented the worst-case scenarios according to this theory.[97] Kahler and Pick in 1879 theorized that the aberrant development of the spinal cord that led to syrinx formation was the result of chronic intrauterine inflammation, with resultant gliosis.[127]

Haener in 1910 speculated that birth trauma may arouse neural activity in the abnormally enclosed tissue, with resultant syrinx formation. Oppenheim in 1920 denied the need for a triggering mechanism and stated that this proliferation may occur spontaneously.[127] Hassin argued forcefully that although syringomyelia was a congenital lesion, the lesion was a developmental defect of the glia cells. He termed this defect an *abiotrophy*, which caused the glial tissue to break down; the abnormal glial tissue was separated from the substance of the cord by a connective tissue reaction.[76] Netsky postulated that congenital vascular anomalies were the pathophysiologic basis for syrinx formation. These abnormal vessels become occluded with aging, and the resultant ischemic tissue damage provides the initial cavitation. Reactive gliosis and connective tissue proliferation complete the syrinx formation and cause any observed extension of the mature cavitary lesion.[116]

In 1896, Chiari published an addition to an earlier (1891) work in which he described anomalies associated with congenital hydrocephalus. Included in the latter publication were a number of patients with hydromyelia. Turnbull and then Russel and Donald noted the association between hydromyelia and the Chiari malformation,[141, 165] and Gardner and Goodall found that 13 of 17 patients undergoing operation for symptomatic Arnold-Chiari malformation had a concurrent syringomyelia.[69] Gardner and coworkers demonstrated, at operation, communication between the syrinx of the upper cervical cord and the ventricles in patients undergoing suboccipital craniotomy and cervical laminectomy as treatment for symptomatic Arnold-Chiari malformation.[65] Indigo-carmine was injected into the patient's lateral ventricle via a burr hole craniotomy, and then dye-colored fluid was recovered by direct puncture of the cervical syrinx. The authors stated that in their experience, "a hydromyelic cyst always communicates with the fourth ventricle by a patent central canal," but they acknowledged that this communication was difficult to demonstrate in every case.

In a series of papers, W. J. Gardner expounded his hydrodynamic theory of the pathogenesis of syringomyelia.[61–64, 66, 67, 70] His contention was that syringomyelia resulted from a failure of the embryonic rhombic roof to fenestrate during a critical period of develop-

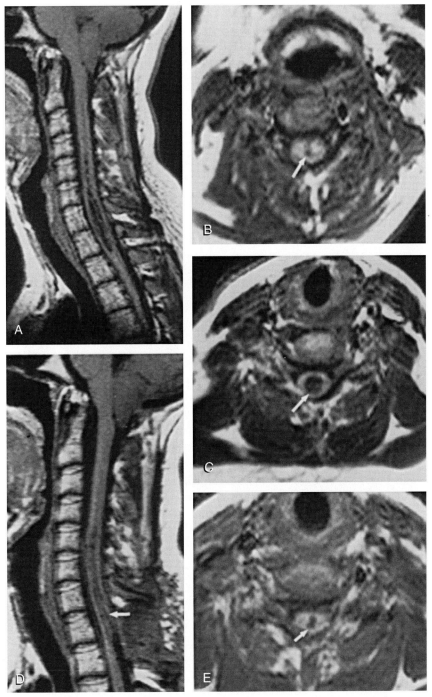

Figure 48–3. Communicating syringomyelia (syringohydromyelia) with associated Chiari I malformation. A 33-year-old woman presented with tingling and numbness of the left upper extremity. *A,* T1-weighted sagittal images show ectopia of the cerebellar tonsils and an intramedullary cystic cavity extending from C2 to T2. The T1-weighted axial images demonstrate the central location of the cyst *(arrow)* at C5 *(B)* and C7 *(C)*. The postshunting sagittal *(D)* and axial *(E)* images show a decrease in the size of the cyst at C7–T1. Comparison of the axial T1-weighted images at the C7 level before *(C)* and after *(E)* shunting best demonstrates the change in cyst size. The bilobed appearance of the central cord low signal in *(D)* is produced by the confluence of the residual cyst and the shunt tube entering the cyst dorsally *(arrow)*. The course of the shunt tube can be seen as a linear hypodensity *(arrow)* traversing the dorsal aspect of the cord in the sagittal image *(D)*.

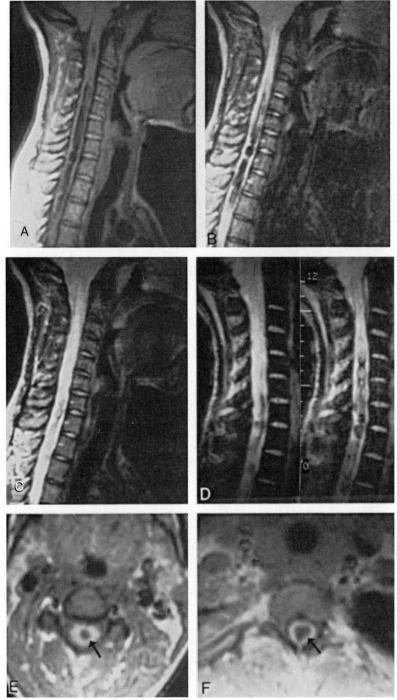

Figure 48–4. Communicating syringomyelia—demonstration of markedly diminished cerebrospinal fluid (CSF) flow within the central cavity after shunting. A 37-year-old woman with a Chiari I malformation presented with right upper extremity numbness and mild gait disturbance. The preoperative T1-weighted sagittal image *(A)* shows a cerebellar tonsil projecting below the foramen magnum and a large septated central cavity extending from C2 to T3–T4. The upper portion of the cavity is not well visualized because of partial volume averaging with cord tissue. The T2-weighted images without *(B)* and with *(C)* flow compensation show extensive and minimal low signal intensity within the cavity, respectively, indicating CSF flow within the cavity. A cardiac-gated, gradient-echo cine MRI study *(D)* confirms the presence of pulsatile flow within the cyst, as evidenced by the change in signal intensity within the cavity in sequential gated images. Axial T1-weighted images demonstrate the cavity *(arrow)* at C3 *(E)* and at T2 *(F)*.

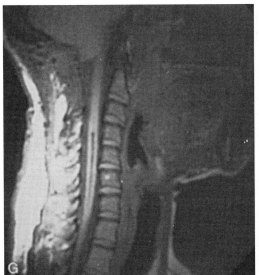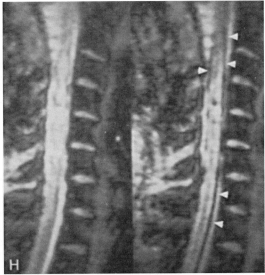

Figure 48–4 *Continued* After placement of a shunt tube from the thoracic subarachnoid space into the cyst, the central cavity has decreased in size. The T1-weighted sagittal image *(G)* shows the uniform diameter of the shunt tube within the collapsed cyst. A cine MRI study *(H)* obtained at the same time shows minimal change in signal intensity within the cavity in sequential gated images, indicating that there is minimal pulsatile CSF flow within the cyst (compare with *D*). The change in signal intensity *(arrowheads)* within the spinal canal ventral and dorsal to the cervical cord and ventral to the thoracic cord in the two gated images indicates pulsatile CSF flow in the subarachnoid space, as expected normally.

ment, and he cited a 1917 report by Weed of a study conducted on pig embryos as the experimental evidence for his hypothesis.[67] His contention was that the inability of cerebrospinal fluid (CSF) in the fourth ventricle to gain the usual access to the subarachnoid space during the sixth to eighth week of embryogenesis forced the hindbrain through the foramen magnum. A Chiari malformation was thereby created, and the failure of the CSF to expand the subarachnoid space resulted in communicating hydrocephalus. Gardner believed that the effect of the hindbrain malformation was to both increase the obstruction to outflow at the foramen of Magendie and deflect the pulse wave of CSF described by Bering onto the opening of the central spinal canal at the obex.[22, 63] This action of the CSF gradually either dilated the central canal or dissected the substance of the spinal cord around the canal and formed a syrinx. The experimental and clinical evidence Gardner cited to support his view of a direct communication from the syrinx to the ventricular system consisted of three observations[67]:

1. Dye injected into the ventricular system was recovered from the syrinx at operation.[65]
2. Fluid withdrawn from the syrinx at operation strongly resembled CSF found in the ventricular system.
3. Experimental hydrocephalus produced by obstruction of the normal outflow of CSF from the fourth ventricle resulted in the formation of syringomyelia that was in communication with the ventricular system.[104]

A spinal cord syrinx with a direct connection to the fourth ventricle through either the central canal or a developmental diverticulum was labeled a communicating syringomyelia by Williams in a 1969 publication.[172] However, Gardner objected to the term as misleading; he believed that it "confuse[d] thinking concerning [this] disease process" because the term implied the existence of noncommunicating syringes. From his perspective, a congenital hindbrain defect that obstructed the CSF outflow from the fourth ventricle to the subarachnoid space was the sine qua non of syringomyelia. Therefore, an asymptomatic, congenital anomaly must have existed in all patients who were found to have syringomyelia.[70] This included those cases associated with spinal "arachnoiditis" and trauma. Ellertsson and Greitz were able to demonstrate communication of syringes with the cerebrospinal spaces after intrathecal injection of fluorescein or a radioisotope in a series of patients,[43] but others, including West and Williams and Ball and Dayan, questioned the necessity of a direct connection to the fourth ventricle for production of a syrinx.[11, 170] Milhorat and colleagues demonstrated that the majority of syringes found in a large necropsy series did not communicate with the fourth ventricle and that the central canal was not patent in a majority of normal adult patients.[107, 111]

Williams proposed an alternative theory to explain syrinx formation and extension and speculated that a partial block of the spinal subarachnoid space produced a pressure differential between the ventricular system and the spinal subdural space during Valsalva-type maneuvers.[172] He implicated the venous distention associated with these maneuvers in producing an increased intracranial pressure that was not completely distributed to the lumbar subarachnoid space because of the complete or partial block. This pressure difference was labeled craniospinal pressure dissociation, and the lower pressure in the lumbar theca caused fluid to be drawn into the syrinx. This phenomenon was labeled "suck," and the author was able to demonstrate, with simultaneous pressure recordings at the cisterna magna and lumbar subarachnoid space, a particularly prominent effect after a cough or a Valsalva maneuver.[175] This theory underwent modification in a series of publications after its initial presentation.[149, 150, 170, 172–177, 179–182] The hypothesis was offered not to totally obviate acceptance of the pathophysiology mechanisms advocated by Gardner but rather to afford a parsimonious pathophysiologic basis for the development of syringomyelia in patients with either a congenital or an acquired foramen magnum abnormality or a spinal subarachnoid lesion.[63]

Williams and Ellertsson and Greitz disagreed with the arterial pulse mechanism proposed by Gardner to explain extension of the syrinx, especially in the rostral direction, thereby creating syringobulbia.[44, 174] Both groups of investigators reportedly found no evidence for the arterial pulsations in pressure recordings of the syrinx, ventricle, or spinal subarachnoid spaces, and both concluded that venous pressure changes were more important in syringomyelia formation.[180] Williams also believed that the cavity enlarged after its initial formation as the result of several forces, the most important of which was compression of the lower end of the cavity with the rapid filling of the epidural venous plexus during a cough or sneeze. The fluid in the syrinx was then propelled rostrally, dissecting the central canal or pericentral parenchyma of the spinal cord. Bertrand also thought that coughing, straining, and postural changes modified the size and extent of syringes in the three cases constituting his report, and Williams applied the term "slosh" to this phenomenon as a matter of economy.[24, 179] Martin invoked Laplace's theorem to explain syrinx expansion.[101, 102] Oldfield and associates used MRI with and without cardiac gating, intraoperative ultrasonography, and direct intraoperative observation of the exposed hindbrain and documented the downward movement of the cerebellar tonsils during systole.[120] This group interpreted the data collected as obviating the necessity of a direct connection with the fourth ventricle, as advocated by Gardner and McMurray,[70] and observed that the syringomyelic cord did not enlarge with the Valsalva maneuver unless the subarachnoid space around the hindbrain had been re-established by a decompressive procedure. The latter observation, coupled with the observations that the pulsatile movement of the enlarged cord segment was synchronous with the movement of the cerebellar tonsils and that the pulse waves of the abnormal cord ceased when the subarachnoid obstruction was cleared, led to the proposal that venous pressure had little to do with syrinx elongation. The authors proposed that the abnormal pulse waves in the spinal subarachnoid

space, caused by the partial obstruction by the hindbrain, placed relentless pressure on the spinal cord and dissected the central canal, causing the cyst to enlarge. Milhorat and colleagues proposed that normal CSF flow was from the spinal subarachnoid space through the parenchyma of the spinal cord into the central canal.[113] The CSF then flowed into the fourth ventricle outlet at the obex. By injecting kaolin into the central canal of rats, the resulting inflammatory reaction stenosed the proximal central canal, and a syrinx was formed. The syrinx was a dilated, yet isolated, segment of the spinal canal. The authors suggested that the disruption of normal CSF flow by the inflammatory stenosis caused the syrinx to form and was a model of syringes associated with the majority of hindbrain malformations that pressed on the proximal spinal cord, obstructing the central canal and blocking communication of the syrinx and the fourth ventricle. Stoodley and coworkers demonstrated that CSF in the spinal subarachnoid space is rapidly forced into the spinal cord central canal in normal rats and speculated that this one-way flow was a result of arterial pulsations.[159] This group supported the proposal of Milhorat and colleagues that disruption of the central canal outflow could cause an isolated central canal to be dilated into a syrinx without a disruption of the free flow of fluid in the subarachnoid space, as proposed by Williams.[113, 178]

Diagnosis of syringomyelia was based on clinical presentation and course in the late nineteenth and early twentieth centuries. This represented a formidable task to the attending physician, as the disorder had an insidious onset and a variable clinical course. Many of the earliest authors would have disputed the statement in a well-known neurology text that the "clinical neurologic picture is so characteristic that diagnosis is seldom in doubt."[2] Netsky commented that at the onset of symptoms, a syrinx may be particularly difficult to diagnose,[116] and Finlayson stated that intramedullary neoplasms were the most troublesome to differentiate from a syringomyelic process.[53] A careful interview and thorough examination of the patient have been, and will continue to be, the initial and most informative elements of any investigation. Adams and Victor emphasized the existence of certain clinical features of syringomyelia and stated that "the clinical diagnosis can hardly be made without them."[2] These features are segmental weakness and atrophy of the hands and arms, with loss of tendon reflexes and segmental anesthesia of the dissociated type. Honan and Williams, however, were able to find dissociated sensory loss in only 49 per cent of patients with documented syringomyelia.[80] Milhorat and colleagues demonstrated that a significant number of syringes had asymmetric involvement of the parenchyma of the spinal cord—a finding that could account for the clinical presentation.[107]

A lateral roentgenogram of the upper cervical spine was recommended by Finlayson as an initial ancillary examination to rule out cervical spondylosis and basilar impression of the skull.[53] These conditions have been confused clinically with syringomyelia and have also been reported to coexist with the lesion. Gardner and associates employed pneumoencephalography to diagnose syringomyelia and noted that the procedure was done in the operating suite only after preparations for an immediate surgical intervention were completed.[65] This rather dramatically underscores the risk that the diagnostic procedure posed to the patient.

The introduction of myelography allowed the presurgical diagnosis of syringomyelia. With the use of conventional myelography, one could not differentiate a cavitary lesion from an intramedullary tumor or a collapsed lesion from an atrophic cord.[158] Positive contrast myelography was used in the series reported by Foster and Hudgson, and in 14 per cent of the patients with syringomyelia, no evidence of any abnormality could be found with this test.[56] Conway reported that gas myelography was more sensitive than contrast myelography in detecting syringomyelia.[32] Even though Ellertsson credited gas myelography with being the first significantly useful diagnostic procedure, in his series, four of 34 patients known to have syringomyelia had normal gas myelograms.[41, 42]

Delayed CT following metrizamide myelography was the next significant advancement in the roentgenographic diagnostic technique.[36, 37] Although this test was more sensitive and resulted in less morbidity when compared with the earlier techniques, differentiation between a syrinx and an intramedullary tumor remained challenging.[158] Quencer demonstrated that percutaneous needle aspiration and endomyelography could be safely performed and that these procedures yielded important diagnostic information in the evaluation of spinal cystic lesions.[130, 132]

MRI assumed the role of the test of choice for the diagnosis of syringomyelia by the mid-1980s.[126] Although it is both accurate and noninvasive, some intramedullary tumors and areas of myelomalacia are difficult to differentiate from a syrinx.[152] Sherman and coworkers noted a loss of signal in the syrinx, thereby lending creditability to Williams's "slosh" theory of cavity extension.[152] Cine MRI has also been used, and although the initial experience suggested the possibility of a preoperative determination of the relative benefit of surgical intervention, subsequent clinical experience was not favorable.[128] The introduction of gadolinium-diethylenetriamine pentaacetic acid (Gd-DTPA) decreased the difficulty of differentiating a syrinx from a tumor.[153] Batzdorf has used MRI to demonstrate a decrease in syrinx size postoperatively, and this test has been reported to be a valuable method of monitoring the effectiveness of surgical decompression.[20, 147] Others have not found a correlation between the postoperative images and clinical outcome.[10, 150]

The treatment of syringomyelia continues to be controversial. There is no universally accepted method of intervention or consensus on the benefit of therapy (Fig. 48–5). Wechsler stated that "the treatment is symptomatic," and "although syringomyelia may show remissions, the prognosis is very unfavorable."[169] Wilson related the use of radiation therapy during his

training in 1902 and continued to advocate, in the second edition of his book, the use of either x-ray or radium radiation before consideration of surgical therapy.[187] In a case report, Putnam stated that "in every case, as soon as the diagnosis is made, roentgen radiation should be administered," and he advocated a trial of radiation as a "measure of prevention."[129] This recommendation was voiced despite the acknowledgment that morbidity was associated with radiation therapy and that his personal experience was not as favorable as the 60 per cent improvement reported in the then-current medical literature. Wechsler stated that "deep x-ray therapy to the spine at the level of the syrinx may have occasional good effect, if not on the progress, at least on the pains and trophic disturbances."[169] Conway related that there was no "unanimity of thought" as to the best therapy for treatment of syringomyelia and cited four studies in which radiation was the primary therapy.[33] Finlayson related that a total dosage as high as 10,540 rad was recommended.[53] The use of radiation therapy may seem extreme by current treatment standards, but it was rational therapy for those clinicians who believed that disordered gliosis was the underlying pathophysiologic disorder in syringomyelia that was not associated with an intramedullary neoplasm.

Radiation therapy was not without critics, and Netsky in 1953 noted the lack of controlled studies on the effects of radiation in the treatment of syringomyelia.[116] He questioned the value of radiation and cautioned that much of the benefit attributed to its use was related to subjective complaints. Gardner and Angel believed that positive results from radiation therapy were likely to occur in those patients with an ependymoma producing the syrinx.[66] Ballantine and associates agreed that the positive result was a consequence of treating an intramedullary neoplasm.[12] The latter authors assumed that Borysowicz's positive results from the use of nitrogen mustard in 1967 could be similarly rationalized. The study of Boman and Iivanainen demonstrated no effect of radiation on the progression of either the signs or the symptoms of patients with syringomyelia.[28] Currently, the use of radiation therapy should be restricted to the primary therapy of a known neoplasm or as an adjunct to its surgical excision.

The first report of successful surgical therapy of syringomyelia was by Abbe and Coley.[1] They performed a three-level laminectomy and opened the dura to expose the cyst. The authors described the cord as swollen to twice its normal size by a lemon-shaped cystic cavity from which was aspirated a clear fluid. The cyst collapsed with the aspiration of the fluid, but no CSF escaped on opening of the dura. This suggested that a subarachnoid block was present, but the authors reported finding only delicate adhesions of the cord to the meninges. This report was significant not because of any amelioration of the clinical symptoms but because it demonstrated that the spinal cord syrinx could be approached surgically without morbidity.

Elsberg recounted his report to the International Congress held in London in 1913 of an operation for

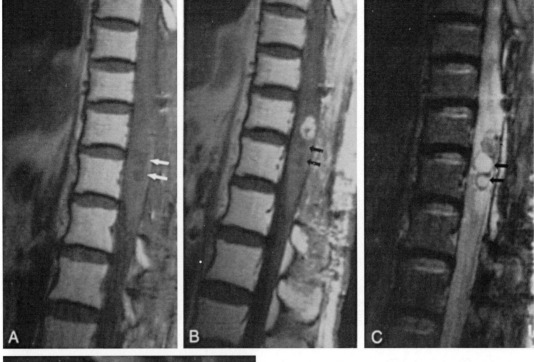

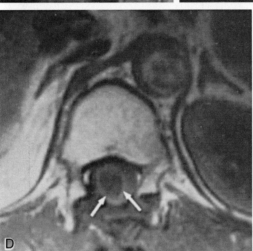

Figure 48–5. Syringomyelia associated with invasive ependymoma of the cord. A 43-year-old woman had had subtotal resection of an ependymoma of the conus and postoperative radiation one year earlier. T1-weighted sagittal images obtained before *(A)* and after *(B)* gadolinium administration demonstrate the isointense, enhancing intramedullary mass at T11. Immediately inferior to the mass is an associated cyst or cysts *(arrows).* The cord is enlarged. An intramedullary cyst extending from C3 to T7 is not shown. There had been previous laminectomies from T9 to T12. *C,* A T2-weighted sagittal image shows the high signal intensity of fluid within the cyst(s) *(arrows)* and the relatively low signal intensity of the tumor. *D,* A T1-weighted axial image shows the eccentrically located cystic cavity *(arrows),* containing low-signal-intensity fluid, within the enlarged cord.

drainage of the cystic cavity in cases of syringomyelia via a midline myelotomy.[45] Edgar and Quail credited Poussepp as well as Elsberg with the development of myelotomy for the treatment of spinal cord cysts and noted that this procedure was referred to as the "Elsberg-Poussepp operation."[40] Frazier was apparently unaware of previous reports when he stated that his case was the first report by an American author.[57] He also performed a laminectomy and, in spite of spontaneous cyst collapse, decided to perform a paramedian myelotomy. Unlike Elsberg, Frazier attempted to maintain patency of the opening to the subarachnoid space with "a thin strip of the finest percha tissue."[45, 57] The patient improved neurologically during the convalescent period, and the author found "this initial experience with the surgery of syringo-myelia . . . more than

pleasing." The author's enthusiasm had not diminished when he presented a review of selected cases of syringomyelia with several years of postoperative follow-up, even though the patient who was the subject of his previous case report had relapsed. At reoperation, no evidence of the previous myelotomy was initially visible because of dense adhesions. He suggested that the scarring was evidence of the glial proliferation theory and advocated repeated operative intervention when the patient deteriorated. In a later report, however, Frazier acknowledged that long-term follow-up was necessary before the effectiveness of a particular treatment could be assessed.[58] Adelstein collected reports of 120 patients who were subjected to laminectomy and myelotomy and was able to tabulate clinical data on 86 cases.[3] Of these, 76 per cent were reported improved, and 12 per cent had declined in neurologic function.[12] Pitts and Groff reported that 67 per cent of patients who underwent laminectomy improved,[125] and Love and Olafson reported that 72 per cent of their patients either stabilized or improved.[93] A recent review of the surgical treatment of syringomyelia as reported in the medical literature since the initial reports of Abbe and Cooley established that the reported effectiveness of surgical intervention has not changed with time; more recent series report the same rates of response to surgery that were reported in the initial 75 cases treated before 1940.[1, 9] Only the mortality rate had decreased—from 5 per cent in the initial series to 1 per cent in the most recent report period (1971–1989).

Gardner and Angel championed a new approach to the patient with a posterior fossa herniation (Chiari I malformation) based on their theory of syringomyelia formation previously reviewed.[66] The operation advocated was suboccipital craniectomy for decompression of the hernia and closure of the communication between the syrinx and the fourth ventricle by plugging the obex with a piece of muscle. Although there have been a number of variations of posterior fossa surgery for decompression of the hindbrain, a lively debate in the medical literature continues over the necessity or the advisability of using an obex plug.[9, 103, 124] Hoffman and colleagues presented data that documented an increase in favorable results when an obex plug was used,[78] and Pillay and coworkers reported that 182 Gardner procedures had been successfully performed without adverse complications.[124] Sahuquillo and associates noted that plugging of the obex has all but been abandoned during the last decade because of increased complications associated with this procedure and a paucity of evidence of therapeutic benefit.[142]

Rhoton did not plug the obex but rather stented the foramen of Magendie if dense scarring was found and performed a dorsal root entry zone myelotomy in the upper cervical cord.[135] Schlesinger and colleagues also reported that plugging of the obex was unnecessary and carried the risk of increased morbidity; they questioned the advisability of cervical myelotomy, however.[144] Logue and Edwards demonstrated that simple posterior fossa decompression was as effective as obstruction of the opening of the central canal, and they argued that clinical improvement following the operation was the result of relief of the mechanical compressive effect of the cerebellar tonsils on the medulla.[91] These authors advocated preservation of the arachnoid membrane and the use of syringostomy only if the syrinx did not respond to simple decompression.

Batzdorf outlined an approach to the patient with symptomatic syringomyelia associated with a Chiari I malformation and combined a suboccipital decompression with opening of the foramen of Magendie and a duraplasty to re-establish the subarachnoid path at the skull base.[20] He argued that a plug of the obex was not necessary and potentially blocked a drainage path for the syrinx when the obstruction to CSF flow at the skull base was resolved. Postoperative MRI scan confirmed drainage of the syringes, and the author has extended

his series to more than 20 patients.[21] Included in this series was one patient with coccidioidomycosis meningitis who required a second operation for placement of a shunt. The operative mortality in the series reported by Batzdorf was zero and represented a significant improvement over the 6 per cent reported by Ballantine and coworkers in a review of operative treatment of syringomyelia.[12, 20] Whereas Batzdorf advocated a limited suboccipital craniectomy to prevent downward herniation of the cerebellar tonsils postoperatively, Milhorat, in a comment that followed the report of Sahuquillo and associates, praised the authors for performing a large craniectomy in a subgroup of patients.[20, 142] The cisterna magna was restored in this subgroup, and the cerebellar tonsils actually ascended; in the subgroup that received smaller craniectomies, the majority of the tonsils paradoxically descended. Milhorat also noted that the syrinx associated with the Chiari malformation did not necessarily resolve with the former procedure and reported a shunting technique called syringocisternostomy to connect the syrinx to the posterior fossa cisterns.[109]

The high incidence of operative morbidity and mortality associated with decompression of the posterior fossa limited initial acceptance of the technique. Even the staunchest supporter of posterior fossa decompression reported a series of patients who had undergone resection of the filum terminale (terminal ventriculostomy) as an alternative therapy for symptomatic syringomyelia.[68] Williams and Fahy had little enthusiasm for the technique and thought that its use was based on faulty comprehension of the pathophysiologic basis of syrinx formation.[183] In their series, they did not achieve the improvement rate reported by the authors of the earlier series.

Barbaro and associates and Suzuki and coworkers reported 80 and 86 per cent favorable response rates with syringoperitoneal shunting.[13, 160] Tator and colleagues demonstrated that laminectomy with midline myelotomy continued to be a viable alternative to other surgical techniques and used silicone rubber ventricular catheter tubing to stint the myelotomy.[163] Padovani and coauthors reported a 90 per cent favorable response rate with this technique.[122] Milhorat and colleagues reported good short-term follow-up of patients treated with a syrinx–to–posterior fossa cistern shunt as the primary surgical procedure.[109] Sgouros and Williams reported that drainage procedures alone have a poor long-term prognosis and that only half the patients so treated continued to enjoy a favorable outcome 10 years after surgery.[149] They therefore recommended that drainage procedures be reserved for patients who do not respond to posterior fossa decompression. Milhorat and colleagues advocated a ventriculoperitoneal shunt for communicating syringes associated with hydrocephalus, as did Sgouros and Williams.[110, 149] Milhorat also treated syringes associated with Chiari II malformations with a ventriculoperitoneal shunt if there was an isolated fourth ventriculomegaly.[109]

Reports on the natural history of syringomyelia have

tempered the enthusiasm for surgical therapy without totally eliminating its use for the amelioration of symptomatic syringomyelia. Boman and Iivanainen documented the relatively favorable outcome of patients treated conservatively,[28] and Anderson and coworkers confirmed the earlier observation of Faulhauer and Loew that the long-term results of surgical therapy were less favorable than results reported after a limited postoperative observation period.[5] Gamache and Ducker also documented a significant decrease in the percentage of patients continuing to have favorable outcomes after extended periods of observation.[60]

As the majority of syringes associated with hindbrain malformation are not communicating but are isolated both rostrally and caudally by central spinal canal stenosis, a posterior decompression may not effectively treat the syringes, and a drainage procedure may be effective.[109, 134] Sgouros and Williams advocated posterior fossa decompression for all lesions involving the craniocervical junction, even for the majority in which communication with the fourth ventricle could not be established.[149, 150] Because there continues to be substantial differences among the reported methods advocated by groups treating syringomyelia, a multicenter clinical trial must be organized before optimal treatment can be established.[8]

Syringomyelia Associated With Arachnoiditis of the Spinal Canal

The report of Appleby and colleagues established that a "communicating" type of syringomyelia could be acquired from chronic arachnoiditis involving the basal cisterns and obstructing the outflow of CSF from the fourth ventricle.[7] Barnett correctly advised his readers that the term *arachnoiditis* was inaccurate, because all meningeal membranes were usually involved. He suggested that a more accurate terminology would be "pachymeningitis with a leptomeningitis."[14] He also noted that use of the term did not implicate an etiology and cited multiple reviews of the subject. Arachnoiditis has been reported with syphilis, tuberculosis, pyogenic meningitis, nontraumatic hemorrhage into the subarachnoid space, the use of spinal anesthetics, and a variety of intrathecally introduced agents. In a significant number of cases, no etiologic factor was identified.[14]

The association of spinal arachnoiditis and syringomyelia was reported by Vulpian in 1861 and by Charcot and Joffroy in 1869. MacKay reviewed a series of five patients with chronic adhesive spinal arachnoiditis and included two cases in which autopsies were conducted.[96] Syringomyelia was noted in the latter cases, and the author implicated occlusion of the blood vessels supplying the cord by the arachnoid scarring as the cause of the cavitation. Nelson also reported a patient with chronic arachnoiditis who subsequently developed an intramedullary cavitation; he believed that the underlying pathophysiologic process was interference with the spinal cord circulatory system.[115] Caplan and associates found occlusion of spinal feed-

ing arteries in one patient with syringomyelia and chronic arachnoiditis and suggested that this evidence supported ischemic damage as the initial event in the development of a cavitary lesion.[29]

Barnett reviewed the published reports of experimental ischemic spinal cord lesions, starting with the initial attempts by Tauber and Langworthy and including those of Woodard and Freeman and Wilson and colleagues.[15, 164, 186, 189] The experimental evidence supporting a role for ischemia in the formation of cavitary lesions in the spinal cord was unconvincing in the former author's opinion, because the majority of the cavitary lesions produced experimentally were microscopic in size. Williams implicated craniospinal pressure dissociation, secondary to obstruction of the subarachnoid space, as the factor responsible for cyst extension if not for its initial formation.[172] Cho and associates investigated the role of arachnoiditis in syringomyelia formation and demonstrated that an injury to the spinal cord was necessary for the production of the cavity.[31] The dense arachnoiditis produced by intrathecal injection of kaolin did not result in a syrinx, whereas a weight-drop lesion of the cord performed before or after the production of the arachnoid adhesions resulted in an enlarging cystic cavity.

Barnett reviewed the published reports of syringomyelia and determined that only seven cases appeared to have been related to arachnoiditis limited to the spinal canal.[14] To these he added seven cases. In his series, all patients were shown to have arachnoiditis on myelography, but only one patient was known to have a cavitary lesion prior to surgical exploration. The author stated that even retrospective review of the myelograms failed to demonstrate the cystic lesion. Arachnoid cysts were demonstrated in five of the 14 patients reviewed. The author considered syringomyelia to be of the "noncommunicating" type, because no connection between the cyst and the fourth ventricle could ever be demonstrated. Milhorat and colleagues found several cases of syrinx associated with arachnoid scarring and documented that there was no communication with the fourth ventricle.[107]

Barnett reported that management of his patients with arachnoiditis was unrewarding, whether medical or surgical therapy was attempted. He considered both steroids and lysis of adhesions to be ineffective in the treatment of the disorder. The author suggested surgery for exploratory laminectomy if the practitioner faced a "serious progression of the neurological deficit" in a patient known to have arachnoiditis. The recommended procedure was an exploratory laminotomy at the superior limit of the arachnoiditis, with placement of a Silastic catheter from the cyst into the superior subarachnoid space.[14] Sgouros and Williams agreed with Barnett that "dissecting adhesions [was] an unrewarding surgical task" and thought that placement of a permanent drain was of "questionable value."[14, 149, 150]

Syringoperitoneal and syringosubarachnoid shunting was reported as an effective therapy for syringomyelia.[13, 122, 160, 163] A small number of patients in each of the series was identified as having spinal arachnoiditis (10 with syringoperitoneal shunts and four with subarachnoid shunts).

Sgouros and Williams recommended that the management of syringes associated with areas of "meningeal fibrosis [or] arachnoiditis" concentrate on the reconstruction of an alternative subarachnoid pathway around the area of adhesion.[150] After a wide laminectomy, a surgical meningocele was created, and the dissection of adhesions was limited to the establishment of free communication of the meningocele with the inferior and superior subarachnoid space. The total number of patients with spinal arachnoiditis treated was small and the period of postoperative follow-up was limited, so the efficacy of the reported treatments could not be accurately assessed. All authors reported that diagnostic work-up included an MRI examination that revealed the presence of the lesion preoperatively.

Syringomyelia Associated With Spinal Cord Tumors

The association of syringomyelia and spinal cord tumors has been well established. Barnett and Rewcastle cited an 1875 paper by Simon as the first to address the simultaneous occurrence of syringomyelia and tumors.[19] The cited author speculated that the syringomyelic cavity might be formed by the softening of a glioma. Other early authors who reported patients diagnosed with both syringomyelia and spinal tumors included Langhans in 1881, Baumler in 1887, Dimitroff in 1897, and Schlesinger in 1902.[127, 145]

The discussion of the pathogenesis of syringomyelia presented by Bernstein and Horwitt reflected the early perception of syrinx formation.[23] They acknowledged that multiple processes could form cavitary lesions in the spinal cord but regarded the development of syringomyelia as the result of an unspecified but specific, progressive pathologic process. They identified gliosis as the "commonly accepted" primary lesion that had undergone cystic degeneration to form a syrinx. The primary lesion, which they called a "glial neoplasm," was formed by the previously described defect in neural tube closure. They rejected the proposal that glial proliferation was a secondary reaction to the presence of the cyst.

These authors would have concurred with Riley's conclusion that the high incidence of congenital anomalies associated with syringomyelia was suggestive of "some malignant controlling central agency" and that both resulted from the faulty closure process during the embryogenesis of the spinal cord.[136] The deranged closure resulted in the inclusion of undifferentiated spongioblasts within the substance of the cord, which remained dormant until "some pathological moment as yet unknown incites them to abnormal activity." Also unknown was the exact nature of the relationship of the syringomyelic cavity to the neoplasm, but a variety of opinions have been expressed in the medical literature.

The report of MacKay and Favill documented the association of syringomyelia and an intramedullary

ependymoblastoma.[97] In their opinion, both lesions were products of germinal cells of the medullary plate and were the divergent manifestations of the same proliferative process. Woods had earlier offered a similar explanation for the discovery of a syrinx and an ependymoma in a case that was surgically explored (Fig. 48–6).[190] Lichtenstein and Zeitlin thought that the syrinx was residuum from the degeneration of a tumor mass.[89]

Other authors have proposed a variety of pathophysiologic mechanisms for the creation of syringes associated with neoplasms, and all have been speculation based on the authors' interpretation of pathology specimens. Edema, blockage of the perivascular spaces with resultant tissue fluid stasis, cavitation secondary to disturbance in blood supply to the cord, and spontaneous hemorrhage into or autolysis of the mass have all been reported as the causal or sustaining events of syrinx formation.[51, 88, 140] Lohle and associates demonstrated that the predominant protein found in a cavitary lesion associated with an intramedullary ependymoma was of plasma origin and postulated that the syrinx was based on exudation secondary to disruption of the blood-brain barrier.[92]

The reviews by Peerless and Durward, Barnett and Rewcastle, Ferry and coworkers, Slooff and colleagues, and Poser all document the association of intramedullary spinal cord tumors and syringomyelia, and all the authors favor classification of the latter lesion as a true neoplastic growth.[19, 52, 123, 127, 154] The hydrodynamic theories discussed in the previous section on communicating syringomyelia were not entertained, and these cases were classified as noncommunicating syringomyelia. Barnett and Rewcastle tabulated the published series of extramedullary tumors associated with syringomyelia and identified only seven cases.[19] They suggested that these tumors may have interfered with the blood supply or venous drainage to form the syringomyelic cavity. Blaylock and Quencer and colleagues have reported additional cases of the simultaneous presentation of syringomyelia and an extramedullary tumor.[26, 131] Castillo and coworkers reported five cases in which postoperative development of syringomyelia was documented after excision of an extramedullary tumor.[30] The simultaneous occurrence of syringomyelia and an intracranial tumor was documented by Williams and Timperley.[185]

Kernohan and associates stated that "it can thus be seen that syringomyelia does not accompany any special type of tumor."[85] Barnett and Rewcastle also found no difference in histology between tumors associated with a syrinx and those without an association.[19] The latter authors tabulated the series of Poser, Slooff, and Ferry, to which they added their own series, and demonstrated that the tumors most often found with an accompanying cystic lesion were gliomas.[52, 127, 154] They also reported that intramedullary tumors were accompanied by syringomyelia in 25 to 58 per cent of cases and that autopsy studies of patients known to have syringomyelia revealed a concurrent tumor in 8 to 16 per cent. Slooff and colleagues reported that 50 per

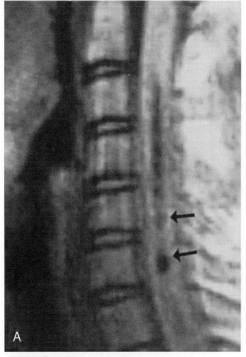

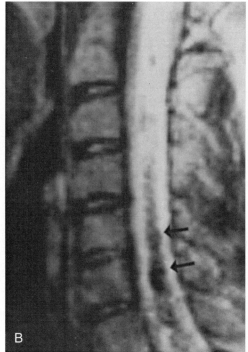

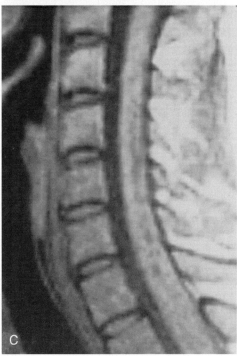

Figure 48–6. Hematosyringomyelia associated with hemangioblastoma of the cord. A 32-year-old man with acute onset of back pain and paralysis had an emergency myelogram that demonstrated an intramedullary mass and myelographic block at T9. Sagittal images show an intramedullary cavity with regions *(arrows)* that are approximately isointense to cerebrospinal fluid on T1-weighted scans *(A)* yet are markedly hypointense on T2-weighted scans *(B)*, representing acute hemorrhage. At surgery, an intramedullary hematoma was found cephalad to a hemangioblastoma of the cord at T9. *C,* One week following surgery and shunting of the syrinx, a sagittal T1-weighted image demonstrates decompression of the syrinx.

cent of ependymomas were associated with cavitary lesions of the spinal cord.[154]

Peerless and Durward recommended metrizamide myelography followed by delayed CT scan for the evaluation of patients clinically suspected of syringomyelia,[123] but a later paper by Slasky and coworkers presented evidence of the superiority of Gd-DTPA–enhanced MRI for the evaluation.[153] These authors reviewed recent advances in MRI techniques and equipment that have greatly improved its sensitivity and demonstrated the increased diagnostic accuracy of MRI after augmentation with Gd-DTPA. This enhanced diagnostic accuracy allowed improved differentiation of cystic areas within tumors from associated cavitary cord lesions.

A systemic approach to the diagnosis and treatment of a patient suspected of harboring a syrinx was outlined by Peerless and Durward.[123] They noted that preoperative drainage of the cyst may be accompanied by rapid neurologic improvement and that surgical removal of the tumor also may decompress the syrinx (Fig. 48–7). One must remain alert to the possibility of increased neurologic deficit secondary to delayed development of syringomyelia after spinal surgery.[133]

Syringomyelia Associated With Trauma

Although there were several early case reports of syringomyelia or cavitary lesions of the spinal cord preceded by a history of trauma, including Bastiam in 1876 and Strumpel in 1880, these publications were tainted by the lack of pathologic data to confirm the presumed diagnosis.[166] The lack of noninvasive diagnostic procedures and the reliance on exploratory laminectomy precluded the procurement of diagnostic evidence. Patients were accepted as suffering from syringomyelia based on the presence of clinical symptoms and supporting signs.[19] More neurologically sophisticated authors, including Charcot in 1892, Lloyd, and Cushing, reported cases in which spinal cord injury produced an immediate clinical picture with the symptoms of syringomyelia.[18, 34, 90] Although Tauber

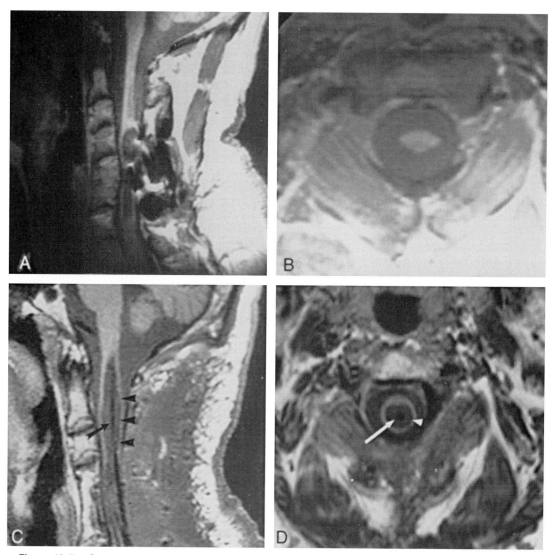

Figure 48–7. Syringomyelia associated with trauma. *A,* T1-weighted sagittal image shows an enlarged cord, with an intramedullary cyst, from C4 to C7 in this patient with C5 and C6 fractures. Ferromagnetic artifacts from wires placed during a previous posterior fusion partially obscure the dorsal aspect of the canal from C4 to C6. Superior to C3, the cord is narrowed, and no cyst is present. *B,* T1-weighted axial image at the C2 level confirms the narrowed anteroposterior diameter of the cord, secondary to dorsal tethering of the cord by scar tissue at C4. *C, D,* Following anterior cervical fusion of C4 through C6, release of dural adhesions, and shunting of the intramedullary cyst, another MRI study was performed. The T1-weighted sagittal image *(C)* and the axial image *(D)* at the C2 level show a shunt catheter *(arrow)* within an enlarged cyst *(arrowheads)* that extends from the foramen magnum to C7. Later, a second shunt catheter was placed, and the cyst was decompressed.

and Langworthy reported a case of syringomyelia that became symptomatic eight years after an episode of questionable trauma, no evidence was provided to substantiate the claim that a syrinx existed, except for clinical signs.[164] Trauma was eventually causally linked to the formation of cystic lesions in the spinal cord. Although late deterioration of residual neurologic function following spinal cord trauma was rarely reported prior to the 1950s, the improvement in longevity of paraplegic and quadriplegic patients allowed the complication to develop and become symptomatic.[17, 139]

Increased recognition of the disorder and improved diagnostic techniques resulted in clinical reports from a number of institutions that care for spinal injury patients, but a uniform terminology had not been established. Late deterioration of function following spinal cord injury has been reported as progressive myelopathy as a sequel to traumatic paraplegia, posttraumatic syringomyelia, ascending cystic degeneration of the cord, syndrome of chronic injury to the central cervical spinal cord, posttraumatic progressive myelopathy, and posttraumatic cystic myelopathy.[17, 71, 74, 94, 118, 119, 146, 148, 168] The latter term is favored by the current authors.

The reported overall incidence of the development of a posttraumatic cyst has ranged from 1.1 to greater than 50 per cent in more recent studies using MRI.[10, 82] The rate of syringomyelia reported in one of the later studies was challenged by Sgouros and Williams, because the study included small cysts at the injury site, which they referred to as primary cysts.[150] These were cavities of less than two vertebral segments in length at the injury site and did not constitute an enlarging cyst but rather were the result of spinal cord parenchymal damage that occurred at the time of the initial injury. Sgouros and Williams believed that these lesions did not need to be treated, as they were difficult to collapse and did not correlate with clinical signs of delayed neurologic deterioration.[150] A prospective study of 449 patients with spinal cord injury followed yearly for a six-year period found that 4.45 per cent developed a symptomatic syrinx.[147] Some groups reported that symptomatic syringes developed at a rate of 8 per cent in those patients suffering from a complete quadriplegic lesion but with a 9:1 ratio of paraplegia to quadriplegia in incompletely injured spinal cords.[74, 137] Sgouros and Williams and Backe and colleagues found no correlation between the location or severity of spinal cord injury and the development of a cavitary lesion in their respective series.[10, 150] The former group stated that their series and a review of the literature demonstrated that any degree of spinal injury, including rather trivial incidences, can be associated with the development of posttraumatic syringomyelia. Two autopsy series found that 20 and 17 per cent of spinal cord injured subjects had syringes identified.[156, 191] The range for the onset of symptoms has been reported to be as early as 2 months and as late as 33 years after injury.[77] Rossier and associates reported that the most common initial presentation in their series was a complaint of pain, which occurred in

89 per cent of their patients.[137] Vernon and coworkers documented an occurrence rate of 63 per cent in their series.[166] Pain was well established as the most frequent complaint upon initial presentation, but considerable disagreement existed regarding the frequency of the finding of motor weakness.[168] Although the former authors documented increased motor deficit in 63 per cent of symptomatic patients, the latter group reported a frequency of only 20 per cent in their series. Edgar and Quail found dissociated sensory loss in 87 per cent of the 600 patients with posttraumatic syringes in their report and motor loss in 80 per cent.[40]

The pathophysiologic basis for the formation and extension of syringes of the injured spinal cord remains the subject of considerable debate and published speculation. Studies conducted on animal models of syringomyelia have generated considerable information, but progress toward the final definition of the disorder has been impeded by the paucity of adequate experimental models of expanding cystic cavitation in the spinal cord parenchyma. This deficiency has also slowed the formation of a consensus regarding the relative contribution of the many factors implicated in the development of symptomatic syringomyelia. The diversity of these putative factors has also confused efforts to define the disorder and to unravel the conundrum of cyst formation and enlargement. The lack of a scientific method to test a hypothesis derived from a clinical observation has meant that a significant portion of the publications describing syringomyelia in general—and specifically those that developed after traumatic spinal cord injury—contains untested and perhaps untestable conclusions regarding the basic pathophysiologic mechanisms underlying the creation of these cavitary lesions in the spinal cord parenchyma. Relevant animal models would obviate this deficiency.

Gardner and McMurray asserted that all cases of syringomyelia were of the "communicating" variety, and therefore only those patients with the embryonic substrate would develop the disorder.[70] They cited the low incidence figures as evidence supporting their conjecture. Oakley and colleagues "unequivocally demonstrated a communication with the fourth ventricle through the cord parenchyma" in the subject of their case report.[119] A similar connection in another case of posttraumatic syringomyelia had been reported earlier by McLean and coworkers.[105] The necropsy study by Milhorat and colleagues demonstrated that syringes associated with trauma had distinctly different histopathologic findings and were associated with different clinical symptoms when compared with those lesions that were in communication with the fourth ventricle or those cavities that appeared to be isolated dilatations of the spinal cord central canal.[107] The syringes associated with spinal cord injury involved the parenchyma of the cord asymmetrically. They were not associated with the central canal and often extended to the pial surface. The authors found a good correlation between the presenting neurologic deficit and the location of the syrinx. Examination of pathologic specimens revealed nonreversible damage to spinal nuclei and tracts, including focal necrosis, central chromatolysis, and wallerian degeneration.

Williams and associates rejected Gardner's contention and stressed the fact that the majority of cases of traumatic syringomyelia had no evidence of posterior fossa abnormality.[184] Nurick and colleagues reported the absence of any anomalies of the posterior fossa in the two patients who were the subject of their report.[118] Barnett and coworkers and Williams and colleagues emphasized the temporal disparity between the onset of symptoms and the initial injury, as well as the spatial separation of that segment of the spinal cord from which the symptoms of deterioration arose and the segment affected initially.[17, 180]

The latter group was disposed to view the formation of syringomyelia after trauma as a two-staged process: the creation of the initial cyst and its extension by secondary factors. Although a clinically relevant experimental model of syringomyelia associated with trauma has not been developed, many reports of experimental studies of the effects of trauma on the spinal cord have been published.[98] Fehlings and Tator credited Schmasus in 1890 with being the first to experimentally produce spinal degeneration and cavitation in rabbits by direct application of blows to the backs of the animals.[50] Since this initial study, many other groups have confirmed that trauma can be a cause of cavitary spinal cord lesions.[27, 38, 117] The possible factors implicated in the production of the initial cystic lesions in posttraumatic spinal cords included ischemia secondary to arterial and/or venous obstruction, lysosomes and other intracellular enzymes, liquefaction of a prior hematoma, or mechanical damage from compression of the substance of the cord at the initial injury.[34, 47, 79, 83, 84, 100, 106, 188, 189] Yezierski and colleagues reported that neuronal degeneration and spinal cavitation were observed following the intraspinal injection of the excitatory amino acid (EAA) receptor agonist quisqualic acid.[192] It was proposed that in posttraumatic and postischemic spinal cord injury, excitotoxic cell death occurring secondary to elevated levels of EAAs initiated a pathologic process leading to the formation of spinal cavities. Rossier and coworkers rejected ischemia as the causal factor, because of the paucity of symptoms in the segments remote to the injury site at the time of the initial injury,[139] and this view was supported by the experimental work of Fairholm and Turnbull.[47] The latter authors demonstrated that the pathologic changes that accompany the development of a necrotic central lesion in experimental trauma of the spinal cord were more consistent with mechanical destruction than with disruption of the vasculature. This view was not shared by Koyanagi and associates, who demonstrated quite elegantly that microvascular changes accompanied the mechanical injury to the spinal cord.[86, 87]

The mechanism for the extension of the syringomyelia remains a matter of controversy, and several mechanisms have been proposed. Hughes felt strongly that the mechanism of both rostral and caudal extension of the syrinx, which produced the late neurologic symptoms, was a valvelike connection of the cavity to the subarachnoid space, but he admitted that evidence for an alteration of fluid dynamics was difficult to obtain.[81] Savoiardo and McLean and colleagues presented evidence of a syrinx-to-subarachnoid connection, and the latter authors agreed with Williams's explanation of altered fluid dynamics discussed previously.[105, 143, 172] Extensive subarachnoid adhesions have also been noted at operation in patients undergoing laminectomy for this disorder, and the resultant tethering of the spinal cord may have combined with the increased compensatory movement of the cervical spine to produce syrinx extension.[72, 81, 118, 121] The experimental model reported by Cho and coworkers documented that subarachnoid scarring induced by local intrathecal injection of kaolin or as a result of traumatic subarachnoid scarring could cause the development of syringomyelia in rabbits.[31] Local injection of kaolin into the subarachnoid space without an underlying injury to the spinal cord did not cause a lesion. This was also confirmed in the rat by Madsen and Marcillo.[99] These observations were consistent with the view of Williams that the development of a posttraumatic syringomyelia involved a two-staged process and that injury of the spinal cord must occur before expansion of the primary cyst can occur.[180] Although Cho and coworkers reported that their experimental animal work was a model of posttraumatic syringomyelia, there was no description of a delayed increasing neurologic deficit related to the cystic cavity development.[31] The rat model of Madsen and Marcillo showed tropic changes and neurologic deficits more consistent with those seen in human spinal cord injured patients who develop syringes.[99]

Both Haney and Andrews and their colleagues reported the association of arachnoid cysts with posttraumatic intramedullary cystic lesions, and the latter authors speculated that they may result from the same mechanism that was responsible for the formation of the intramedullary syringes.[5, 75] The theories of Aboulker were cited by Williams and associates and included venous stasis and fluid influx via the perivascular spaces.[184] The latter authors initially found little to suggest that these mechanisms were important in cyst extension, but in a later publication, the senior author of the group acknowledged that a connection to the fourth ventricle was not the most common finding in "communicating" syringomyelia and conceded that the syrinx cavity had to be in communication with the spinal subarachnoid space.[180] A recent study demonstrated in normal rats a rapid unidirectional flow of CSF from the subarachnoid space into the central canal of the spinal cord via the Virchow-Robin spaces.[159] The fact that solutes in the spinal subarachnoid space were in continuity with the intramedullary cavity of syringomyelia had been demonstrated both clinically and experimentally in the past, but this study demonstrated the flow of fluid from the subarachnoid space through the parenchyma of the spinal cord in normal rats.[11] Stoodley and associates and Milhorat and coworkers believed that this normal flow of fluid from the subarachnoid space through the parenchyma was an important factor in the extension and formation of syringomyelic cavities (Fig. 48–8).[112, 159]

The difficulties inherent in the diagnosis of syringomyelia of any cause (reviewed earlier) are responsible in large measure for the delay in diagnosing syringomyelia in spinal cord injured patients.[138] As with other types of syringomyelia, CT represented a major diagnostic advance but was pre-empted by the introduction of MRI.[40, 46, 94, 148] The use of cine MRI to identify pulsatile cystic lesions was reported by Post and colleagues.[128] The speculation was that this technique would allow the differentiation of cystic lesions amenable to surgical intervention from cases of microcystic degeneration without a significant cavity, as reported by MacDonald and coworkers.[95] However, a more recent study by Falcone and associates documented the necessity of intraoperative ultrasonography to make this differentiation (Figs. 48–9 and 48–10).[48]

Surgical intervention for a posttraumatic cyst was apparently first undertaken with good results by Freeman in 1955, and he advocated surgical drainage as the treatment for posttraumatic syringomyelia.[59] Others have reported favorable results from shunting procedures or from transection of the spinal cord in cases of complete lesions.[39, 40, 137, 139, 151] Although Hida and colleagues suggested that a syringosubarachnoid shunt was the first option,[77] Sgouros and Williams believed that drainage procedures should be subordinate to the reconstruction of the subarachnoid space with a surgical meningocele.[149, 150] Edgar and Quail recommended a syringosubarachnoid shunt in cysts of 4 to 20 cm length and a syringoperitoneal shunt for larger cysts.[40] They stated that a shunt failure rate of 10 to 15 per cent should be anticipated, even in experienced hands. Steinmetz and associates reported that 16 per cent of their patients treated with a shunt deteriorated and suggested that this was caused by iatrogenic tethering of the spinal cord to the dura.[157] The introduction of a foreign body in the form of a shunt tube and the surgical procedure may result in fixation of the cord to the dura by scar tissue (Fig. 48–11).

Rossier and associates believed that the risk of sudden development of tetraplegia was sufficient to be an absolute indication for operation in a symptomatic patient, and this group documented progression of symptoms in 18 of 19 patients who did not undergo operative intervention.[137, 139] Edgar and Quail listed documented progressive neurologic deterioration, severe progressive new somatic pain, the late onset of burning central pain, and a blocked shunt tube as indications for surgical intervention for the treatment of posttraumatic syringes.[40] Watson stated that although the symptoms reported by patients in his series were troublesome, he opted for conservative management because there was no significant motor loss.[168] The controversy over treatment was intensified by the case report of Foo and coworkers, in which radiologic evidence of cyst drainage was not accompanied by clinical improvement.[54] This observation has been reported by others, as discussed earlier.[10, 25] The optimal treatment and determination of the indications for surgery await further research with relevant experimental models and a well-designed, multicenter clinical trial.[8]

Idiopathic Syringomyelia

Barnett included this category in his classification system on the basis of the pathologic data available for review.[16] He asserted that some previously described cases of syringomyelia were not associated with any of the etiologic factors implicated in the other categories and arose for reasons as yet undefined. The author also stated that rational therapy for any of the other syringes might be inappropriate for this type. Groups led by Wiedemayer, Suzuki, Barbaro, and Tator classified syringes without hindbrain abnormalities, without evidence of arachnoiditis or tumor, or without a history of trauma as idiopathic and treated the lesions with a shunting procedure.[13, 160, 163, 171] Wiedemayer and colleagues did not identify communication of the syringes with the fourth ventricle in their 20 patients with idiopathic syringomyelia.[171] Following surgical treatment, no patient had full reversal of the presenting neurologic deficit, and four patients deteriorated significantly. Sherman and associates used MRI examination to identify tethered spinal cords in two of 10 cases classified as idiopathic syringomyelia.[152] We tend to place the majority of these cases in either the congenital or the posttraumatic group. In our experience, a history of significant trauma may be elicited by careful interrogation of the patient, and several cases of significant but nonparalyzing spinal trauma have been documented.[73]

THE CONTEMPORARY APPROACH TO THE DIAGNOSIS AND TREATMENT OF SPINAL CORD CYSTS

The initial evaluation of patients suspected of having a spinal cord syrinx or cyst includes a comprehensive history and physical and neurologic examinations. The neurologic examination always includes a detailed motor assessment using the standard 0–5 scale and a multimodality sensory evaluation, testing either pain or temperature for the anterolateral columns and either vibration or position sense for the dorsal columns. A rectal examination is carefully performed and includes an evaluation of volitional sphincter control and a multimodality sensory assessment of the perianal area. Reflexes are the least reliable part of a neurologic assessment, but side-to-side asymmetries or the presence of a pathologic reflex such as Babinski's response are important to document. Because some spinal cord cysts are continuous rostrally past the foramen magnum and go into the brain stem, a careful examination of cerebral, cerebellar, and cranial nerve function is part of the initial neurologic examination. Brain stem signs and symptoms are especially common in congenital syringomyelia and are often associated with Chiari malformations. These signs and symptoms may be at least partially caused by tonsillar and brain stem herni-

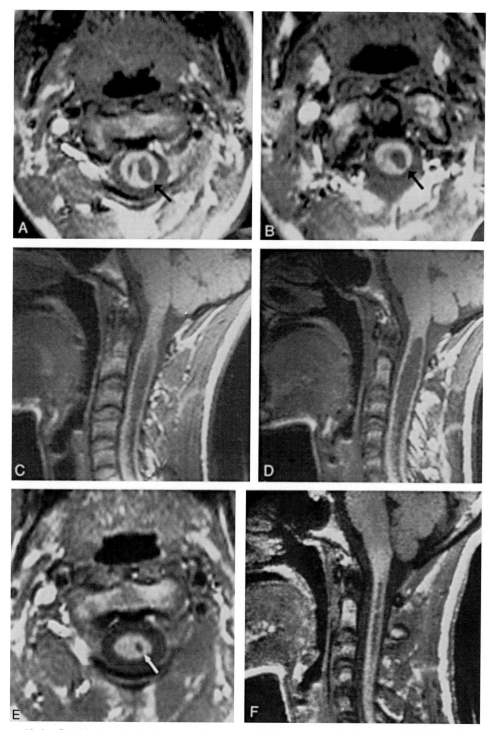

Figure 48–8. Double-barreled syringomyelia associated with trauma. *A, B,* T1-weighted axial images at the C2 level demonstrate a bilobed syrinx *(arrow)* with a larger left-sided component. T1-weighted right *(C)* and left *(D)* parasagittal images show that the left-sided component reaches a higher level (approximately C1) than the right-sided component. *E, F,* Placement of a shunt catheter into the left-sided component *(arrow)* decompressed both components. Compare the postshunt axial *(E)* and sagittal *(F)* images with the preshunt images *(A* and *D).*

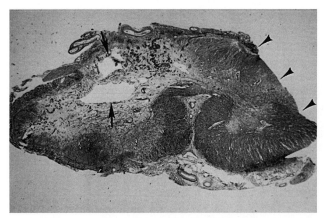

Figure 48–9. Low-power (X1.25) microscopic section showing microcystic myelomalacia in a 74-year-old man with anklylosing spondylitis who suffered a midcervical fracture-distraction injury and survived only four days. (From Madsen, P. W., Falcone, S., Bowen, B., and Green, B. A.: Post-traumatic syringomyelia. *In* Levine, A., Garfin, S., Eismont, F., and Zigler, J. (eds.): Spine Trauma. Philadelphia, W. B. Saunders Co. (in press).)

ation at the craniovertebral junction. In some cases of Chiari malformation, the syrinx may be located in the lower cervical or thoracic area and not at the craniovertebral junction.

Once a detailed history and physical and neurologic assessments are completed and documented, the information obtained guides the imaging studies. Imaging tests always include a plain radiographic series of the involved spinal levels and flexion and extension views

to rule out any bony instability. A high-resolution CT scan or conventional polytomography can aid in the detailed assessment of a particular level of bony spinal column components.

Currently, the most sensitive imaging test for soft tissue is the new-generation high-resolution MRI scan. The initial MRI examination includes, as a minimum, sagittal and transverse views of the lesion plus the adjacent spinal cord and/or brain stem tissue in T1 images. The addition of either T2 or mixed proton density scans can complement but not replace the T1 views, and special coronal or oblique views may be helpful in selected cases. Inclusion of the entire rostro-caudal extent of each cyst or cysts is important, and if a tumor is suspected, the addition of gadolinium-enhanced images must be considered an essential part of the diagnostic work-up. Gadolinium-enhanced images are also helpful in differentiating between scar or disc material associated with a syrinx, especially in postoperative or posttraumatic cases.

In addition to conventional MRI, a new generation of MRI software technology is currently available, including cine MRI, which is a real-time, motion picture–like analysis of spinal fluid flow dynamics in and around the spinal cord cyst. It has been our experience that cysts demonstrating pulsatile CSF contents are more often symptomatic and are more likely to require surgical intervention than cysts with nonpulsatile CSF flow.[72] Magnetic resonance angiography (MRA) represents another technologic advance that can be especially helpful in cases of syringomyelia associated with vascular lesions.

Although certain institutions continue to use air myelography or conventional myelography with delayed

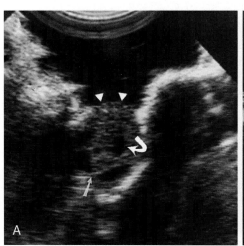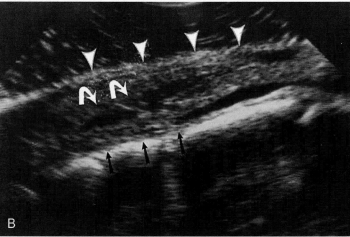

Figure 48–10. Microcystic myelomalacia in a 56-year-old with radicular pain and a history of spine trauma. Axial *(A)* and sagittal *(B)* intraoperative sonogram images during laminectomy at T6 show that the spinal cord is tethered to the dura both dorsally *(arrowheads)*, with loss of normal hypoechoic space, and ventrally *(arrows)*. As a result of the tethering, the spinal cord is enlarged. The echo pattern of the spinal cord parenchyma is heterogeneous, with absence of a normal central echo and presence of microcysts *(curved arrows)*. A confluent cyst was not present, and after the spinal cord was surgically untethered, the cysts collapsed. (From Madsen, P. W., Falcone, S., Bowen, B., and Green, B. A.: Post-traumatic syringomyelia: *In* Levine, A., Garfin, S., Eismont, F., and Zigler, J. (eds.): Spine Trauma. Philadelphia, W. B. Saunders Co. (in press).)

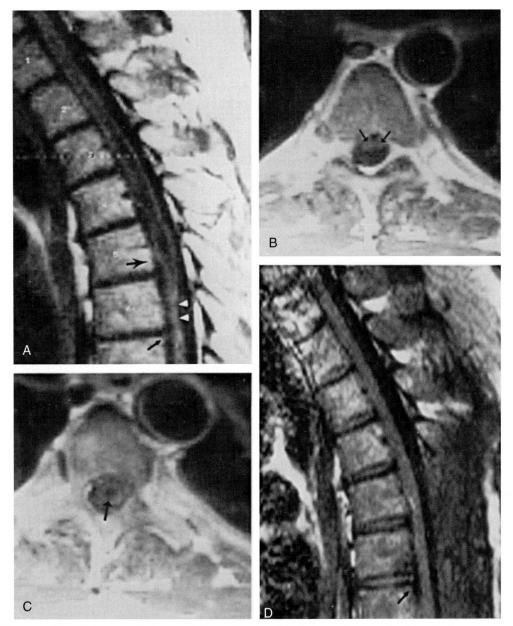

Figure 48–11. Syringomyelia in association with a herniated disc and subarachnoid cyst. *A,* Preoperative T1-weighted sagittal image shows the intramedullary cyst and widening of the thoracic cord superior to the T5–T6 level *(large arrow).* Other imaging sequences better demonstrate the herniated disc at T6–T7 *(small arrow).* There is a smooth, concave impression on the dorsal aspect of the cord at T6–T7 *(white arrowheads).* T1-weighted axial images at the level of T6 *(B)* and T5 *(C)* demonstrate the low signal intensity of the dorsal subarachnoid cyst, which is compressing the cord *(short arrows),* and the intramedullary cyst *(long arrow),* which is enlarging the cord. *D,* Postoperative T1-weighted sagittal image reveals successful decompression of both the subarachnoid and the intramedullary cysts following removal of the T6–T7 *(small arrow)* herniated disc and shunting of the subarachnoid cyst.

CT enhanced images, it is our opinion that MRI techniques are the tests of choice for both the initial evaluation and the postsurgical follow-up of cystic spinal cord lesions. The solitary exception to this generalization concerns cases in which metal wires, rods, plates, screws, or other instrumentation or bullet fragments degrade the MRI scan sufficiently to prevent adequate anatomic assessment. In these cases, a myelogram in combination with immediate and delayed high-resolution CT that cuts through the area of the syrinx is performed. The delayed CT scans are obtained anywhere from 4 to 24 hours after the initial tests in some institutions, but we find a 6- to 8-hour period to be adequate. Difficulty in differentiating myelomalacia from a confluent syrinx represents a significant limitation of this technique and may lead to unnecessary surgical intervention.

Myelography does, however, allow diagnosis of a fissure; the associated intramedullary cyst fills rapidly, compared with a cyst not associated with a fissure. The latter lesion depends on transependymal migration of the contrast agent over several hours before becoming visible. Patients with the former lesions typically develop symptoms from the cystic lesion within weeks of the initial trauma.

Real-time ultrasonography may be useful for postsurgical follow-up studies of patients undergoing laminectomy. This procedure is much more effective and feasible in young children or thin patients than in patients with a large soft tissue mass over the lesion. The evolution of MRI has severely restricted the use of ultrasonography for the postoperative evaluation of these patients. Multimodality neurophysiologic assessment includes an electromyographic study and both somatosensory and motor evoked responses for the evaluation of afferent and efferent spinal cord pathways plus the local H-reflex. A clinical intraoperative study of motor evoked potentials evoked by electrical cortical stimulation from scalp surface electrodes is currently under way in our institution under the direction of the senior author. Magnetic cortical stimulation may be more appropriate for awake patients, although this technique needs additional refinement before it is clinically useful. The combination of the physical and neurologic examination findings, the imaging studies, and the neurophysiologic assessment battery provides an important database for the clinician to consult when planning therapy.

Presentation of Progressive Posttraumatic Cystic Myelopathy

The senior author became acquainted with the syndrome of progressive posttraumatic myelopathy through a collaboration with Dr. Robert Edgar from the Craig-Swedish Medical Center in Englewood, Colorado. The syndrome consists of single or multiple spinal cord cysts that may be intramedullary, subarachnoid, or in both areas simultaneously and may be associated with a fissure. These cysts, like those associated with neoplasms or congenital lesions, may occur in various locations within or around the spinal cord. Cysts may have a variety of etiologies, ranging from a high-velocity injury from a penetrating missile causing quadriplegia or paraplegia to a relatively minor trauma characteristically associated with transient or minimal neurologic deficit. Postsurgical patients account for the second most common category of posttraumatic spinal cord cysts, and these patients typically have undergone a spinal procedure that results in local tethering of the spinal cord and/or subarachnoid space. Most of the senior author's patients in this group presented with a spinal canal mass—a meningioma or a neurofibroma or, less frequently, an intramedullary neoplasm.[72] Included in this group are patients who have undergone cordotomies or other spinal procedures involving the spinal cord parenchyma. Delayed formation of a cyst after surgical excision of a spinal mass that results in a progressive neurologic dysfunction must be differentiated from cysts that present primarily in association with intramedullary or extramedullary tumors. Less frequently observed presentations of posttraumatic cysts include patients with a history of herniated cervical or thoracic discs and individuals with a history of a therapeutic spinal puncture that results in the introduction of an irritative chemical substance into the thecal sac. This substance may cause a lumbar arachnoiditis that can ascend to involve the thoracic area and may be associated with subarachnoid and/or intramedullary syringes.

The onset of the signs and symptoms of progressive posttraumatic cystic myelopathy can range from as early as two to three months following the initial traumatic event to as long as 30 years after injury. The signs and symptoms are listed here in order of decreasing frequency:

1. Motor loss
2. Sensory loss
3. Local or radicular pain (not deafferentated, neurogenic, "burning" pain)
4. Increased spasticity and tone
5. Hyperhidrosis (above the level of lesion)
6. Autonomic dysreflexia
7. Sphincter loss or sexual dysfunction
8. Horner's syndrome (may be alternating)
9. Respiratory insufficiency (usually related to changes in position)

At presentation, the signs and symptoms may be unilateral or bilateral and may alternate from side to side with changes in position. They may also present as a solitary sign or symptom or in any combination. With the more frequent use of noninvasive MRI, more asymptomatic cases have been identified than with previously employed imaging techniques.[73]

Approximately 5 to 10 per cent of patients suffering a traumatic spinal cord injury experience progressive spinal cord dysfunction associated with an expanding syrinx. Symptoms are usually accompanied by rostral extension of the cyst from the lesion site, but they may also accompany caudal extension. In the majority of these patients, the spinal cord is tethered by either a soft tissue scar or a bony gibbus or a combination of both. The scar tissue tethering is most frequently dorsal in location, because the majority of these patients spend several days in the supine position, and the spinal cord assumes a dependent position abutting the dorsal dura. As the blood congeals and scar tissue forms, the pulped spinal cord is tethered to the dura. In the majority of cases in which a bony gibbus or herniated disc material tethers the cord locally, the ventral aspect of the spinal column is involved. A limited number of spinal cord injury patients present with the signs and symptoms of progressive posttraumatic cystic myelopathy without having a demonstrable confluent cyst. The symptoms are believed to be related to spinal cord tethering.

The pathogenesis of posttraumatic syringomyelia is not well defined, but contemporary imaging modalities suggest possible factors that may form the physiologic basis for these progressively destructive lesions. Most spinal cord injuries are associated with local hemorrhage and swelling of the spinal cord as a result of the initial trauma. Months and years later, these initial "bruises" of the spinal cord undergo multicystic degenerative changes and become myelomalacic. Although some of these injured cords remain multicystic and myelomalacic, in others, the microcysts evolve into a macroscopic confluent cyst.

If one uses serial MRI to follow symptomatic spinal cord cyst patients treated nonsurgically, it becomes apparent that a zone of myelomalacia almost always precedes an expanding confluent cyst. Our hypothesis is that the combination of the tethered cord and the pressure gradients arising from Valsalva maneuvers occurring during the course of normal activity creates a shearing effect that is responsible for the progressive expansion of the cystic lesions. Because most spinal injuries occur at the two most mobile levels of the spinal column, i.e., the mid to low cervical level and the thoracolumbar junction, the shearing effect of local tethering is exaggerated by the movement at these levels. This effect is particularly pronounced in quadriplegic patients whose head and neck movements are the only major voluntary motor functions that remain intact.

Although the majority of intramedullary cysts are localized in the dorsal central area of the spinal cord, i.e., the dorsal gray matter and adjacent white matter, a significant number present as eccentric unilateral cysts or even double- or triple-barreled lesions. These cysts may be connected at the rostral or caudal end of the lesion, although sometimes they remain totally independent of each other.

The subarachnoid cysts associated with posttraumatic cysts, in contrast to congenital subarachnoid cysts, have a thinner wall and contain the same clear CSF as is found in the adjacent subarachnoid space. They also are more firmly anchored to the adjacent dura and do not present with the same gallbladder or balloon-type configuration characteristic of congenital lesions. A rare variation of this lesion is a traumatic pseudomeningocele, which can create an epidural compressive lesion on the spinal cord and may be difficult to identify with routine MRI.

There is little consensus among clinicians regarding the surgical management of posttraumatic syringomyelia, and many neurosurgeons contend that there is no effective surgical treatment. These practitioners believe that patients should ultimately resign themselves to accepting their fate, i.e., a progressive neurologic deterioration to complete paralysis or even death. Less controversial is the doctrine that asymptomatic syringes should not be treated. The exception to this rule in the senior author's experience is traumatic spinal cord injury in which the cystic lesion typically extends at least several segments rostral and/or caudal to the injury site. The cyst may initially be asymptomatic, but it will enlarge to become symptomatic. Although the cyst may be effectively drained, the resultant neurologic deficit tends not to revert.

Our basic criterion for surgical treatment of posttraumatic cysts is the presence of one or more signs and symptoms of progressive posttraumatic cystic myelopathy. Normally, cysts less than 1 cm in rostrocaudal extent are not considered large enough for successful shunting and are therefore followed with serial MRIs and clinical observation.

Surgical management of a posttraumatic syrinx requires preoperative assessment of several factors, including the rostrocaudal extent of the cyst or cysts, the exact location in the spinal cord parenchyma, the relationship of associated intramedullary or subarachnoid cysts, and the presence of a fissure. An essential component of the surgery is the untethering of the spinal cord and nerve root adhesions, as well as reduction of any bony gibbus or soft tissue mass at the site of injury. This may first require a posterior approach for intradural exploration and untethering of the cord and root adhesions, followed by an anterior approach to remove any bony gibbus or soft tissue mass. The second essential component of a surgical treatment protocol is shunting of the spinal cord cyst or cysts to a communicating segment of the subarachnoid space. This is accomplished using illumination and magnification from either loupes and headlight or the operating microscope under real-time ultrasonography guidance.

Exploration and shunting of the intramedullary cyst should always proceed from the caudal end, with the tube being directed up toward the rostral extent of the cyst. If the tube will not traverse the entire length of the cyst, the possibility exists that the distal part of the cyst will become loculated and symptomatic. Some syringes extend from the conus up into the brain stem, and one shunt tube may not be adequate to drain the lesion. Passage of the shunt tube may be obstructed by the thoracic kyphosis. In this case, a single-level laminectomy is performed at the caudal end of the cyst, and a second laminectomy is performed just below the innervation of the hands, i.e., approximately T2. Cyst-to-subarachnoid shunts are performed via myelotomies at both levels, and the upper shunt is guided into the most rostral extent of the lesion.

A small 2-mm vertical myelotomy is usually performed in the midline, avoiding the loops of the dorsal central vein of the spinal cord. The myelotomy is usually performed with a number 11 blade, which, in our experience, is more accurate and less destructive than the microlaser. In the case of an eccentrically placed cyst, the myelotomy is placed in the dorsal root entry zone rather than in the midline. In patients with double-barreled or multiloculated cysts, more than one myelotomy and shunt tube may be required. The senior author has designed a series of shunt tubes that are Silastic and double headed (two tips), with holes at each end. These shunts are available in 7-, 15-, and 30-cm lengths.

If special spinal cord cyst shunt catheters are not available, a regular peritoneal shunt catheter can be modified by removing the pressure valve and cutting extra holes in the distal and proximal ends. A plain radiograph is mandatory intraoperatively to ascertain that the shunt tubing has not kinked or folded upon itself; it must therefore be radiopaque.

Whenever a syringosubarachnoid shunt is placed, several centimeters of shunt tubing should protrude from the myelotomy opening and into the distal subarachnoid space. If severe scarring with tethering of the spinal cord or obliteration of the subarachnoid space from a previous trauma or surgery is encountered, placement of a subarachnoid shunt tube in the conventional dorsal position is usually not adequate because of increased vulnerability to obstruction by scar tissue. When faced with this situation, one may place the shunt catheter into the ventral subarachnoid space by carefully passing the shunt tubing laterally and caudally between the nerve roots. Care must be taken to avoid pressure on the roots, as this may result in postoperative pain. The chance of inadvertent drainage of the subarachnoid space and the development of spinal headache syndrome makes syringoperitoneal or syringopleural shunting procedures less attractive alternatives. The incorporation of a freeze-dried dural heterograft or fascia lata autograph may be necessary to create a locally enlarged subarachnoid space and an environment that is less likely to scar and posteriorly tether the spinal cord. Syringosubarachnoid shunts appear to work best when oriented so that fluid drains dependently. The placement of a shunt tube from a cyst into the rostral subarachnoid space should be avoided.

The maintenance of meticulous hemostasis is important, as blood in the surgical site can result in accelerated scarring and obstruction of the Silastic shunt tubing postoperatively. Spinal cord bleeding is best managed with a piece of thrombin-soaked Gelfoam. Perioperative intravenous antibiotics and steroids are routinely used in our institution. Electromyographic monitoring complements intraoperative motor and somatosensory evoked response monitoring to warn of compromise of the spinal cord or nerve roots.

After the initial shunting procedure, it is essential to repeat real-time ultrasonography with sagittal and transverse images to ensure that the entire cystic cavity is collapsed and that the shunt tube is in a good position. This imaging technique is particularly useful to verify successful treatment of both parts of a confluent doubled-barreled cystic lesion when attempting to use a single catheter.

Although subarachnoid cysts may be adequately treated by resection and removal of the cyst wall, some cases require a subarachnoid cyst–to–subarachnoid space shunt tube for adequate drainage. Shunting of a subarachnoid cyst to the pleural or peritoneal space should be avoided because of the potential for severe headaches. Some patients with a combination of subarachnoid and intramedullary cysts connected by a fistula have been adequately treated with a wide removal of the subarachnoid cyst wall. In these cases, it is not necessary to stent the fissure, but when the fissure is less apparent, a syringosubarachnoid shunt needs to be placed.

In the future, the best therapy for posttraumatic syringomyelia may be bio-obliteration of the cyst via percutaneous injection of cellular implants. An adequate animal model of progressive posttraumatic cystic myelopathy is needed for the development of this and other potentially effective therapies.

Congenital "Communicating" Cysts

A congenital syrinx may present in association with other congenital anomalies and is most frequently located in the cervical or upper thoracic spinal cord. The spinal cord may be tethered by brain stem or cerebellar impaction in the upper cervical canal, by a congenital bony ridge splitting the canal (diastematomyelia), or by a lipoma. Patients with an associated Chiari malformation may have a cyst in continuity with the fourth ventricle. Occasionally, the entire length of the cord is involved, or the syrinx may be isolated to the distal spinal cord segments. The clinical presentation of congenital syringomyelia characteristically begins with a complaint of dysesthetic pain involving a hand and the ipsilateral upper extremity. This may subsequently extend to the other upper extremity. Upper extremity motor weakness and atrophy frequently develop. Sensory loss typically presents in a capelike distribution and is classically described as a suspended sensory level. The exact sensory findings are related to the location of the cyst cavity, which typically involves the dorsal or central parenchyma. The work-up of patients with congenital syringomyelia follows the process outlined in the previous section.

Although surgical treatment of these lesions has been disappointing in the past, recent advances in imaging and surgical technology have improved the prognosis. Today, patients with symptomatic congenital syringomyelia have an excellent response to surgical intervention, and they routinely have a much better outcome when compared with patients presenting with a posttraumatic syrinx. The paucity of associated scarring and tethering of the cord in the former group is responsible for this improvement.

The senior author's experience has been that a congenital syrinx is best treated with a cyst–to–

subarachnoid space shunt. The surgical complication rate and postoperative obstruction rate are minimal compared with the rates for posttraumatic lesions. Patients undergoing a shunting procedure commonly report a patchy sensory loss of dorsal column sensation that usually resolves in a few weeks or months. The improvement seen postoperatively is not as rapid or as dramatic as that which characteristically accompanies surgical treatment of patients with posttraumatic lesions. Our patients are told preoperatively that the surgery is to stop the progression of the neurologic deficit and that reversal of an established deficit is less likely. This difference may reflect the more chronic nature of both the congenital lesions and the changes in the spinal cord parenchyma. Postoperative MRI studies demonstrate a less complete collapse of congenital lesions when compared with posttraumatic syringes, and this finding may correlate with the less dramatic reversal of the neurologic deficit.

Patients with a Chiari malformation associated with a syringomyelia represent a therapeutic enigma, for it is difficult to distinguish which lesion is the cause of the symptoms. If the patient has neck pain of the occipital neuralgia type or signs of cranial nerve dysfunction, the hindbrain impaction is more likely to be the cause of the symptoms, and a posterior fossa decompression should be considered. If the primary complaint is local or radicular pain, the syrinx should be treated with a shunt. If there is evidence that both lesions are symptomatic, both procedures can be performed at a single anesthetic setting. The senior author treats these patients with a suboccipital craniectomy and C1 laminectomy and then employs real-time ultrasonography to determine whether there is adequate subarachnoid space ventral and dorsal to the brain stem and cerebellar tonsils. If ultrasonography reveals insufficient subarachnoid space, an expansile duraplasty is performed. A similar therapeutic dilemma occurs when patients with syringomyelia associated with diastematomyelia become symptomatic. The question of whether the syrinx or the tethering of the cord by the bony or cartilaginous spicule is causing the symptoms is rendered moot by addressing both lesions at a single setting. The surgical treatment for congenital syringomyelia has not been associated with significant complications in our patient series, and shunt obstruction is rarely encountered.[72]

Cysts Associated With Spinal Cord and Nerve Root Tumors

Spinal cord cysts are known to be commonly associated with certain types of intramedullary and extramedullary intradural spinal cord and nerve root tumors. The most common intramedullary tumors associated with intramedullary cysts include hemangioblastomas, ependymomas, and astrocytomas. Less frequently, intramedullary cysts present in association with an extramedullary neurofibroma or meningioma. The removal of the extramedullary lesion is commonly followed by a spontaneous collapse of the associated syrinx. This observation suggests that obstruction of the central canal is the most probable mechanism involved in the intramedullary cyst formation. When a smaller loculated cyst persists after removal of the tumor, the most appropriate management has not been established.

CONCLUSION

Although technologic advances in noninvasive imaging methods have improved the ability to diagnose syringomyelia, and the extent of the lesion can be quite accurately delineated preoperatively in the majority of cases, effective therapy for these lesions has not similarly evolved. The accumulated experience of surgical therapy for these lesions has affirmed that the use of a foreign body (the Silastic shunt tube) is not optimal and that reinsertion of the shunt or the lysis of adhesions frequently causes the production of additional scar tissue. An increased number of patients are being identified with spinal cord cysts because of improvements in imaging techniques and because of the improved longevity of persons suffering spinal cord injury and other paralytic disorders. The research laboratory holds the key to the ultimate solution for the problem of syringomyelia, and only experimental work with animal models offers hope for the final determination of the optimal therapy for spinal cord cysts.

References

1. Abbe, R., and Coley, W.: Syringo-myelia, operation—exploration of cord—withdrawal of fluid—exhibition of patient. J. Nerv. Ment. Dis. *19*:512, 1892.
2. Adams, R. D., and Victor, M.: Principles of Neurology. 4th ed. New York, McGraw-Hill, 1989, pp. 747–754.
3. Adelstein, L. J.: The surgical treatment of syringomyelia. Am. J. Surg. *40*:384, 1938.
4. Al-Mefty, O., Harkey, L. H., Middleton, T. H., et al.: Myelopathic cervical spondylitic lesions demonstrated by magnetic resonance imaging. J. Neurosurg. *68*:217, 1988.
5. Anderson, N. E., Willoughby, W. E., and Wrightson, P.: The natural history and the influence of surgical treatment in syringomyelia. Acta Neurol. Scand. *71*:472, 1985.
6. Andrews, B. T., Weinstein, P. R., Rosenblum, M. L., and Barbaro, N. M.: Intradural arachnoid cysts of the spinal canal associated with intramedullary cysts. J. Neurosurg. *68*:544, 1988.
7. Appleby, A., Bradley, W. G., Foster, J. B., et al.: Syringomyelia due to chronic arachnoiditis at the foramen magnum. J. Neurol. Sci. *8*:451, 1969.
8. Aschoff, A., Donauer, E., Huwel, N., et al.: Evaluation of syrinx-surgery: A critical comment on requirements for reliable follow-up-studies. Acta Neurochir. (Wien) *123*:224, 1993.
9. Aschoff, A., and Kunze, S.: 100 years of syrinx-surgery: A review. Acta Neurochir. (Wien) *123*:157, 1993.
10. Backe, H. A., Betz, R. R., Mesgarzadeh, M., et al.: Post-traumatic spinal cord cysts evaluated by magnetic resonance imaging. Paraplegia *29*:607, 1991.
11. Ball, M. J., and Dayan, A. D.: Pathogenesis of syringomyelia. Lancet *2*:799, 1972.
12. Ballantine, H. T., Ojemann, R. G., and Drew, J. H.: Syringomyelia. *In* Kraybuhl, H., Maspes, P. E., and Sweet, W. H. (eds.): Progress in Neurological Surgery. Vol. 4. New York, S. Karger, 1971, pp. 227–245.
13. Barbaro, N. M., Wilson, C. B., Gutin, P. H., and Edwards, M. S. B.: Surgical treatment of syringomyelia: Favorable results with syringoperitoneal shunting. J Neurosurg. *61*:531, 1984.

14. Barnett, H. J. M.: Syringomyelia associated with spinal arachnoiditis. *In* Barnett, H. J. M., Foster, J. B., and Hudgson, P. (eds.): Syringomyelia. London, W. B. Saunders Co., 1973, pp. 220–244.

15. Barnett, H. J. M.: The pathogenesis of syringomyelic cavitation associated with arachnoiditis localized to the spinal canal. *In* Barnett, H. J. M., Foster, J. B., and Hudgson, P. (eds.): Syringomyelia. London, W. B. Saunders Co., 1973, pp. 245–260.

16. Barnett, H. J. M.: The epilogue. *In* Barnett, H. J. M., Foster, J. B., and Hudgson, P. (eds.): Syringomyelia. London, W. B. Saunders Co., 1973, pp. 302–313.

17. Barnett, H. J. M., Botterell, E. H., Jousse, A. T., and Wynn-Jones, M.: Progressive myelopathy as a sequel to traumatic paraplegia. Brain 89:159, 1965.

18. Barnett, H. J. M., and Jousse, A. T.: Post-traumatic syringomyelia. *In* Vinken, P. J., and Bruyn, G. W. (eds.): Injuries of the Spine and Spinal Cord. Part II. Handbook of Clinical Neurology. Vol. 26. Amsterdam, North-Holland, 1976, pp. 113–157.

19. Barnett, H. J. M., and Rewcastle, N. B.: Syringomyelia and tumours of the nervous system. *In* Barnett, H. J. M., Foster, J. B., and Hudgson, P. (eds.): Syringomyelia. London, W. B. Saunders Co., 1973, pp. 261–301.

20. Batzdorf, U.: Chiari I malformation with syringomyelia: Evaluation of surgical therapy by magnetic resonance imaging. J. Neurosurg. 68:726, 1988.

21. Batzdorf, U.: Personal communication, 1990.

22. Bering, E. A.: Choroid plexus and arterial pulsation of cerebrospinal fluid: Demonstration of the choroid plexuses as a cerebrospinal fluid pump. AMA Arch. Neurol. Psychiatry 73:165, 1955.

23. Bernstein, E. P., and Horwitt, S.: Syringomyelia, with pathological findings. Med. Record (N. Y.) 84:698, 1913.

24. Bertrand, G.: Dynamic factors in the evolution of syringomyelia and syringobulbia. *In* Wilkins, R. H. (ed.): Clinical Neurosurgery. Vol. 20. Baltimore, Waverly Press, 1973, pp. 322–333.

25. Biyani, A., and El Masry, W. S.: Post-traumatic syringomyelia: A review of the literature. Paraplegia 32:723, 1994.

26. Blaylock, R. L.: Hydrosyringomyelia associated with a thoracic meningioma: Case report. J. Neurosurg. 54:822, 1981.

27. Blight, A. R.: Cellular morphology of chronic spinal cord injury in the cat: Analysis of myelinated axons by line sampling. Neuroscience 10:521, 1983.

28. Boman, K., and Iivanainen, M.: Prognosis of syringomyelia. Acta Neurol. Scand. 43:61, 1967.

29. Caplan, L. R., Morohna, A. B., and Amico, L. L.: Syringomyelia and arachnoiditis. J. Neurol. Neurosurg. Psychiatry 53:106, 1990.

30. Castillo, M., Quencer, R. M., Green, B. A., and Montalvo, B. M.: Syringomyelia as a consequence of compressive extramedullary lesions: Postoperative clinical and radiological manifestations. AJR Am. J. Roentgenol. 150:391, 1988.

31. Cho, K. H., Iwasaki, Y., Imamura, H., et al.: Experimental model of posttraumatic syringomyelia: The role of adhesive arachnoiditis in syrinx formation. J. Neurosurg. 80:133, 1994.

32. Conway, L. W.: Radiographic studies of syringomyelia: The hydrodynamics of the syrinx in relation to therapy. Trans. Am. Neurol. Assoc. 86:205, 1961.

33. Conway, L. W.: Hydrodynamic studies in syringomyelia. J. Neurosurg. 27:501, 1967.

34. Cushing, H. W.: Haematomyelia from gunshot wounds of the spine: A report of two cases, with recovery following symptoms of hemilesion of the cord. Am. J. Med. Sci. 115:654, 1898.

35. Davison, C., and Keschner, M.: Myelitic and myelopathic lesions VI: Cases with marked circulatory interference and a picture of syringomyelia. Arch. Neurol. Psychiatry 30:1074, 1933.

36. Di Chiro, G., Axelbaum, S. P., Schellinger, D., et al.: Computerized axial tomography in syringomyelia. N. Engl. J. Med 292:13, 1975.

37. Di Chiro, G., and Schellinger, D.: Computed tomography of spinal cord after lumber intrathecal introduction of metrizamide (computer assisted myelography). Radiology 120:101, 1976.

38. Ducker, T. B.: Experimental injury of the spinal cord. *In* Vinken, P. J., and Bruyn, G. W. (eds.): Injuries of the Spine and Spinal Cord. Part I. Handbook of Clinical Neurology. Vol. 25. Amsterdam, North-Holland, 1976, pp. 9–26.

39. Edgar, R. E.: Surgical management of spinal cord cysts. Paraplegia 14:21, 1976.

40. Edgar, R., and Quail, P.: Progressive post-traumatic cystic and non-cystic myelopathy. Br. J. Neurosurg. 8:7, 1994.

41. Ellertsson, A. B.: Semilogic diagnosis of syringomyelia related to roentgenologic findings. Acta Neurol. Scand. 45:385, 1969.

42. Ellertsson, A. B.: Syringomyelia and other cystic spinal cord lesions. Acta Neurol. Scand. 45:403, 1969.

43. Ellertsson, A. B., and Greitz, T.: Myelocystographic and fluorescein studies to demonstrate communication between intramedullary cysts and the cerebrospinal fluid space. Acta Neurol. Scand. 45:418, 1969.

44. Ellertsson, A. B., and Greitz, T.: The distending force in the production of communicating syringomyelia. Lancet 1:1234, 1970.

45. Elsberg, C. A.: Surgical Diseases of the Spinal Cord. New York, P. B. Hoeber, 1941, pp. 551–553.

46. Enzmann, D. R., O'Donohue, J., Rubin, J. B., et al.: CSF pulsations within nonneoplastic spinal cord cysts. AJR Am. J. Roentgenol. 149:149, 1987.

47. Fairholm, D. J., and Turnbull, I. M.: Microangiographic study of experimental spinal cord injuries. J. Neurosurg. 35:277, 1971.

48. Falcone, S., Quencer, R. M., Green, B. A., et al.: Progressive post-traumatic myelomalacic myelopathy (PPMM): Imaging and clinical features. AJNR Am. J. Neuroradiol. 15:747, 1994.

49. Faulhauer, K., and Loew, K.: The surgical treatment of syringomyelia: Long-term results. Acta Neurochir. (Wien) 44:215, 1978.

50. Fehlings, M. G., and Tator, C. H.: A review of models of acute experimental spinal cord injury. *In* Illis, L. S. (ed.): Spinal Cord Dysfunction: Assessment. Oxford, Oxford University Press, 1988, pp. 3–33.

51. Feigin, I., Ogayta, J., and Budzilovich, G.: Syringomyelia: The role of edema in its pathogenesis. J. Neuropathol. Exp. Neurol. 30:216, 1971.

52. Ferry, D. J., Hardman, J. M., and Earle, K. M.: Syringomyelia and intramedullary neoplasms. Med. Ann. (DC) 38:363, 1969.

53. Finlayson, A. I.: Syringomyelia and related conditions. *In* Joynt, R. J. (ed.): Clinical Neurology. Vol. 3. Philadelphia, J. B. Lippincott, 1989, pp. 1–17.

54. Foo, D., Bignami, A., and Rossier, A. B.: A case of post-traumatic syringomyelia: Neuropathological findings after 1 year of cystic drainage. Paraplegia 27:63, 1989.

55. Foster, J. B., and Hudgson, P.: Historical introduction. *In* Barnett, H. J. M., Foster, J. B., and Hudgson, P. (eds.): Syringomyelia. London, W. B. Saunders Co., 1973, pp. 3–10.

56. Foster, J. B., and Hudgson, P.: The radiology of communicating syringomyelia. *In* Barnett, H. J. M., Foster, J. B., and Hudgson, P. (eds.): Syringomyelia. London, W. B. Saunders Co., 1973, pp. 51–63.

57. Frazier, C. H.: Shall syringomyelia be added to the lesions appropriate for surgical intervention? JAMA 95:1911, 1930.

58. Frazier, C. H., and Rowe, S. N.: The surgical treatment of syringomyelia. Ann. Surg. 103:481, 1936.

59. Freeman, L. W.: Ascending spinal paralysis: Case presentation. J. Neurosurg. 16:120, 1959.

60. Gamache, F. W., and Ducker, T. W.: Syringomyelia: A neurological and surgical spectrum. J. Spinal Disord. 3:293, 1990.

61. Gardner, W. J.: Anatomic anomalies common to myelomeningocele of infancy and syringomyelia of adulthood suggest a common origin. Cleve. Clin. Q. 25:118, 1959.

62. Gardner, W. J.: Diastematomyelia and the Klippel-Feil syndrome. Cleve. Clin. Q. 31:19, 1964.

63. Gardner, W. J.: Hydrodynamic mechanism of syringomyelia: Its relationship to myelocele. J. Neurol. Neurosurg. Psychiatry 28:247, 1965.

64. Gardner, W. J.: Myelocele: Rupture of the neural tube? *In* Ojemann, R. G. (ed.): Clinical Neurosurgery. Vol. 15. Baltimore, Waverly Press, 1968, pp. 57–79.

65. Gardner, W. J., Abdullah, A. F., and McCormack, L. J.: The varying expressions of embryonal atresia of the fourth ventricle in adults: Arnold-Chiari malformation, Dandy-Walker syndrome, "arachnoid" cyst of the cerebellum, and syringomyelia. J. Neurosurg. 14:591, 1957.

66. Gardner, W. J., and Angel, J.: The cause of syringomyelia and its surgical treatment. Cleve. Clin. Q. 25:4, 1958.

67. Gardner, W. J., and Angel, J.: The mechanism of syringomyelia

and its surgical correction. *In* Fisher, R. G. (ed.): Clinical Neurosurgery. Vol. 6. Baltimore, Waverly Press, 1959, pp. 131–140.

68. Gardner, W. J., Bell, H. S., Poolos, P. N., et al.: Terminal ventriculostomy for syringomyelia. J. Neurosurg. *46*:609, 1977.

69. Gardner, W. J., and Goodall, R. J.: The surgical treatment of Arnold-Chiari malformation in adults. J. Neurosurg. *7*:199, 1950.

70. Gardner, W. J., and McMurray, F. G.: "Non-communicating" syringomyelia: A non-existent entity. Surg. Neurol. *6*:251, 1976.

71. Gebarski, S. S., Maynard, F. W., Gabrielsen, T. O., et al.: Posttraumatic progressive myelopathy: Clinical and radiologic correlation employing MR imaging, delayed CT metrizamide myelography, and intraoperative sonography. Radiology *157*:379, 1985.

72. Green, B. A.: Unpublished personal observations, 1990.

73. Green, B. A., Quencer, R. M., Post, M. J. D., et al.: A review of 100 patients surgically treated for progressive post-traumatic cystic myelopathy. J. Neurosurg. *72*:353A, 1990.

74. Griffiths, E. R., and McCormick, C. C.: Post-traumatic syringomyelia (cystic myelopathy). Paraplegia *19*:81, 1981.

75. Haney, A., Stiller, J., Zelnik, N., and Goodwin, L.: Association of post-traumatic spinal arachnoid cyst and syringomyelia. J. Comput. Assist. Tomogr. *9*:137, 1985.

76. Hassin, G. B.: A contribution to the histopathology and histogenesis of syringomyelia. Arch. Neurol. Psychiatry *3*:130, 1920.

77. Hida, K., Iwasaki, Y., Imamura, H., and Abe, H.: Posttraumatic syringomyelia: Its characteristic magnetic resonance imaging findings and surgical management. Neurosurgery *35*:886, 1994.

78. Hoffman, H. J., Neill, J., Crone, K. R., et al.: Hydrosyringomyelia and its management in childhood. Neurosurgery *21*:347, 1987.

79. Holmes, G.: The Goulstonian lectures on spinal injuries of warfare: Part I. The pathology of acute spinal injury. Br. Med. J. *2*:769, 1915.

80. Honan, W. P., and Williams, B.: Sensory loss in syringomyelia: Not necessarily dissociated. J. R. Soc. Med. *86*:519, 1993.

81. Hughes, J. T.: Pathological changes after spinal cord injury. *In* Illis, L. S. (ed.): Spinal Cord Dysfunction: Assessment. Oxford, Oxford University Press, 1988, pp. 34–40.

82. Hussey, R. W., Ha, C. Y., Vijay, M., et al.: Prospective study of the occurrence rate of post-traumatic cystic degeneration of the spinal cord utilizing magnetic resonance imaging. (Abstract.) J. Am. Paraplegia Soc. *13*:16, 1990.

83. Kao, C. C., and Chang, L. W.: The mechanism of spinal cord cavitation following spinal cord transection: Part 1: A correlated histochemical study. J. Neurosurg. *46*:197, 1977.

84. Kao, C. C., Chang, L. W., and Bloodworth, J. M. B.: The mechanism of spinal cord cavitation following spinal cord transection: Part 2: Electron microscope observation. J. Neuropathol. Exp. Neurol. *36*:140, 1977.

85. Kernohan, J. W., Woltman, H. W., and Adson, A. W.: Intramedullary tumors of the spinal cord: A review of fifty-one cases, with an attempt at histologic classification. Arch. Neurol. Psychiatry *25*:679, 1931.

86. Koyanagi, I., Tator, C. H., and Lea, P. J.: Three-dimensional analysis of the vascular system in the rat spinal cord with scanning electron microscopy of vascular corrosion casts. Part 2: Acute spinal cord injury. Neurosurgery *33*:285, 1993.

87. Koyanagi, I., Tator, C. H., and Theriault, E.: Silicone rubber microangiography of acute spinal cord injury in the rat. Neurosurgery *32*:260, 1993.

88. Liber, A. F., and Lisa, J. R.: Rosenthal fibers in non-neoplastic syringomyelia: A note on the pathogenesis of syringomyelia. J. Nerv. Ment. Dis. *86*:549, 1937.

89. Lichtenstein, B. W., and Zeitlin, H.: Ganglioglioneuroma of the spinal cord associated with pseudosyringomyelia: A histologic study. Arch. Neurol. Psychiatry *37*:1356, 1937.

90. Lloyd, J. H.: Traumatic affections of the cervical region of the spinal cord, simulating syringomyelia. J. Nerv. Ment. Dis. *21*:345, 1894.

91. Logue, V., and Edwards, M. R.: Syringomyelia and its surgical treatment: An analysis of 75 patients. J. Neurol. Neurosurg. Psychiatry *44*:273, 1981.

92. Lohle, P. M. N., Wurzer, H. A. L., Hoogland, P. H., et al.: The pathogenesis of syringomyelia in spinal cord ependymoma. Clin. Neurol. Neurosurg. *96*:323, 1994.

93. Love, G. J., and Olafson, R. A.: Syringomyelia: A look at surgical therapy. J. Neurosurg. *24*:714, 1966.

94. Lyons, B. M., Brown, D. J., Calvert, J. M., et al.: The diagnosis and management of post traumatic syringomyelia. Paraplegia *25*:340, 1987.

95. MacDonald, R. L., Findlay, J. M., and Tator, C. H.: Microcytic spinal cord degeneration causing post-traumatic myelopathy. J. Neurosurg. *68*:466, 1988.

96. MacKay, R. P.: Chronic adhesive spinal arachnoiditis. JAMA *112*:802, 1939.

97. MacKay, R. P., and Favill, J.: Syringomyelia and intramedullary tumor of the spinal cord. Arch. Neurol. Psychiatry *33*:1255, 1935.

98. Madsen, P. W., Holets, V., and Yezierski, R. P.: Syringomyelia: Clinical observations and experimental studies. J. Neurotrauma *11*:241, 1994.

99. Madsen, P. W., and Marcillo, A.: Unpublished data.

100. Mair, W. P. G., and Druckman, R.: The pathology of spinal cord lesions and their relation to the clinical features in protrusion of cervical intervertebral discs. Brain *76*:70, 1953.

101. Martin, G.: Syringomyelia, an hypothesis and proposed method of treatment. (Letter.) J. Neurol. Neurosurg. Psychiatry *46*:365, 1983.

102. Martin, G.: Syringomyelia, an hypothesis and proposed method of treatment. (Letter.) J. Neurol. Neurosurg. Psychiatry *48*:193, 1985.

103. Matsumoto, T., and Symon, L.: Surgical management of syringomyelia: Current results. Surg. Neurol. *32*:258, 1989.

104. McLaurin, R. L., Bailey, O. T., Schurr, P. H., and Ingraham, F. D.: Myelomalacia and multiple cavitations of spinal cord secondary to adhesive arachnoiditis. Arch. Pathol. *57*:138, 1954.

105. McLean, D. R., Miller, J. D. R., Allen, P. B. R., and Ezzeddin, S. A.: Posttraumatic syringomyelia. J. Neurosurg. *39*:485, 1973.

106. McVeigh, J. F.: Experimental cord crushes: With especial reference to the mechanical factors involved and subsequent changes in the areas of the cord affected. Arch. Surg. *7*:573, 1923.

107. Milhorat, T. H., Capocelli, A. L., Anzil, A. P., et al.: Pathological basis of spinal cord cavitation in syringomyelia: Analysis of 105 autopsy cases. J. Neurosurg. *82*:802, 1995.

108. Milhorat, T. H., Johnson, W. D., and Milhorat, R. H., et al.: Clinicopathological correlations in syringomyelia using axial magnetic resonance imaging. Neurosurgery *37*:206, 1995.

109. Milhorat, T. H., Johnson, W. D., and Miller, J. I.: Syrinx shunt to posterior fossa cisterns (syringocisternostomy) for bypassing obstructions of the upper cervical theca. J. Neurosurg. *77*:871, 1992.

110. Milhorat, T. H., Johnson, W. D., Miller, J. I., et al.: Surgical treatment of syringomyelia based on magnetic resonance imaging criteria. Neurosurgery *31*:231, 1992.

111. Milhorat, T. H., Kotzen, R. M., and Anzil, A. P.: Stenosis of central canal of spinal cord in man: Incidence and pathological findings in 232 autopsy cases. J. Neurosurg. *80*:716, 1994.

112. Milhorat, T. H., Miller, J. I., Johnson, W. D., et al.: Anatomical basis of syringomyelia occurring with hindbrain lesions. Neurosurgery *32*:748, 1993.

113. Milhorat, T. H., Nobandegani, F., Miller, J. I., and Rao, C.: Noncommunicating syringomyelia following occlusion of central canal in rats: Experimental model and histological findings. J. Neurosurg. *78*:274, 1993.

114. Murray, J. A. H., Bradley, H., Craigie, W. A., and Onions, C. T. (eds.): The Oxford English Dictionary: Being a Corrected Reissue With an Introduction, Supplement, and Bibliography of a New English Dictionary on Historical Principles. Vol. 10. Oxford, Oxford University Press, 1933, p. 391.

115. Nelson, J.: Intramedullary cavitation resulting from adhesive spinal arachnoiditis. AMA Arch. Neurol. Psychiatry *50*:1, 1943.

116. Netsky, M. G.: Syringomyelia: A clinicopathologic study. AMA Arch. Neurol. Psychiatry *70*:741, 1953.

117. Noble, L. J., and Wrathall, J. R.: Correlative analysis of lesion development and functional status after graded spinal cord contusive injuries in the rat. Exp. Neurol. *103*:34–40, 1989.

118. Nurick, S., Russell, J. A., and Deck, M. D. F.: Cystic degeneration of the spinal cord following spinal cord injury. Brain *93*:211, 1970.

119. Oakley, J. C., Ojemann, G. A., and Alvord, E. C.: Post-traumatic syringomyelia: Case report. J. Neurosurg. *55*:276, 1981.

120. Oldfield, E. H., Muraszko, K., Shawker, T. H., and Patronas, N. J.: Pathophysiology of syringomyelia associated with Chiari I malformation of the cerebellar tonsils. J. Neurosurg. *80*:3, 1994.

121. Osborne, D. R. S., Vavoulis, G., Nashold, B. S., et al.: Late sequelae of spinal cord trauma: Myelographic and surgical correlation. J. Neurosurg. *57*:18, 1982.

122. Padovani, R., Cavallo, M., and Gaist, G.: Surgical treatment of syringomyelia: Favorable results with syringosubarachnoid shunting. Surg. Neurol. *32*:173, 1989.

123. Peerless, S. J., and Durward, Q. J.: Management of syringomyelia: A pathophysiological approach. *In* Weiss, M. H. (ed.): Clinical Neurosurgery. Vol. 30. Baltimore, Williams & Wilkins, 1983, pp. 531–576.

124. Pillay, P. K., Awad, I. A., Little, J. R., and Hahn, J. F.: Symptomatic Chiari malformation in adults: A new classification based on magnetic resonance imaging with clinical and prognostic significance. Neurosurgery *28*:639, 1991.

125. Pitts, F. W., and Groff, R. A.: Syringomyelia: Current status of surgical therapy. Surgery *56*:806, 1964.

126. Pojunas, K., Williams, A. L., Daniels, K. L., and Haughton, V. M.: Syringomyelia and hydromyelia: Magnetic resonance evaluation. Radiology *153*:679, 1984.

127. Poser, C. M.: The Relationship Between Syringomyelia and Neoplasm. Springfield, IL, Charles C Thomas, 1956.

128. Post, M. J. D., Quencer, R. M., Hinks, R. S., and Green, B. A.: Spinal CSF flow dynamics: Qualitative and quantitative evaluation by cine MRI. Presented at the annual meeting of the American Society of Neuroradiology, Orlando, FL, March 24, 1989.

129. Putnam, T. J.: Syringomyelia—diagnosis and treatment. Med. Clin. North Am. *19*:1571, 1936.

130. Quencer, R. M.: Needle aspiration of intramedullary and intradural extramedullary masses of the spinal canal. Radiology *134*:115, 1980.

131. Quencer, R. M., El Gammal, T., and Cohen, G.: Syringomyelia associated with intradural extramedullary masses of the spinal canal. AJNR Am. J. Neuroradiol. 7:143, 1986.

132. Quencer, R. M., Green, B. A., and Eismont, F. J.: Post traumatic spinal cysts: Clinical features and characterization with metrizamide computed tomography. Radiology *146*:415, 1983.

133. Quencer, R. M., Morse, B. M., Green, B. A., et al.: Intraoperative spinal sonography adjunct to metrizamide CT in the assessment and surgical decompression of post-traumatic spinal cord cysts. AJNR Am. J. Neuroradiol. *5*:71, 1984.

134. Rascher, K., and Donauer, E.: Experimental models of syringomyelia: Personal observations and a brief look at earlier reports. Acta Neurochir. (Wien) *123*:166, 1993.

135. Rhoton, A. L.: Microsurgery of Arnold-Chiari malformation in adults with and without hydromyelia. J. Neurosurg. *45*:473, 1976.

136. Riley, H. A.: Syringomyelia or myelodysplasia. J. Nerv. Ment. Dis. *72*:1, 1930.

137. Rossier, A. B., Foo, D., Shillito, J., and Dyro, F. M.: Posttraumatic cervical syringomyelia: Incidence, clinical presentation, electrophysiological studies, syrinx protein and results of conservative and operative treatment. Brain *108*:439, 1985.

138. Rossier, A. B., Foo, D., Shillito, J., et al.: Progressive late posttraumatic syringomyelia. Paraplegia *19*:96, 1981.

139. Rossier, A. B., Werner, A., Wildi, E., and Berney, J.: Contribution to the study of late cervical syringomyelic syndromes after dorsal or lumbar traumatic paraplegia. J. Neurol. Neurosurg. Psychiatry *31*:99, 1968.

140. Russel, D. S.: Capillary haemangeioma of spinal cord associated with syringomyelia. J. Pathol. Bacteriol. *35*:103, 1932.

141. Russel, D. S., and Donald, C.: Mechanism of internal hydrocephalus in spinal bifida. Brain *58*:203, 1935.

142. Sahuquillo, J., Rubio, E., Poca, M., et al.: Posterior fossa reconstruction: A surgical technique for the treatment of Chiari I malformation and Chiari I/syringomyelia complex—preliminary results and magnetic resonance imaging quantitative assessment of hindbrain migration. Neurosurgery *35*:874, 1994.

143. Savoiardo, M.: Syringomyelia associated with postmeningitic spinal arachnoiditis: Filling of the syrinx through a communication with the subarachnoid space. Neurology *26*:551, 1976.

144. Schlesinger, E. B., Antunes, J. L., Michelsen, W. J., and Louis, K. M.: Hydromyelia: Clinical presentation and comparison of modalities of treatment. Neurosurgery *9*:356, 1981.

145. Schlesinger, H.: Die Syringomyelie. Leipzig, Deuticke, 1902, as cited in Wilson (see reference 187).

146. Schneider, R. C., and Knighton, R.: Chronic neurological sequelae of acute trauma to the spine and spinal cord: Part III: The syndrome of chronic injury to the cervical spinal cord in the region of the central canal. J. Bone Joint Surg. Am. *41*:905, 1954.

147. Schurch, B., Wichmann, W., and Rossier, A. B.: Post-traumatic syringomyelia (cystic myelopathy): A prospective study of 449 patients with spinal cord injury. J. Neurol. Neurosurg. Psychiatry *60*:61, 1996.

148. Seibert, C. E., Dreisbach, J. N., Swanson, W. B., et al.: Progressive posttraumatic cystic myelopathy: Neuroradiologic evaluation. AJR Am. J. Roentgenol. *136*:1161, 1981.

149. Sgouros, S., and Williams, B.: A critical appraisal of drainage in syringomyelia. J. Neurosurg. *82*:1, 1995.

150. Sgouros, S., and Williams, B.: Management and outcome of posttraumatic syringomyelia. J. Neurosurg. *85*:197, 1996.

151. Shannon, N., Symon, L., Logue, V., et al.: Clinical features, investigation and treatment of post-traumatic syringomyelia. J. Neurol. Neurosurg. Psychiatry *44*:35, 1981.

152. Sherman, J. L., Farkovich, A. J., and Citrin, C. M.: The MR appearance of syringomyelia: New observations. AJR Am. J. Roentgenol. *148*:381, 1987.

153. Slasky, B. S., Bydder, G. M., Niendorf, H. P., and Young, I. R.: MR imaging with gadolinium-DTPA in the differentiation of tumor, syrinx, and cyst of the spinal cord. J. Comput. Assist. Tomogr. *11*:845, 1987.

154. Slooff, J. L., Kernohan, J. W., and MacCarty, C. S.: Primary Intramedullary Tumors of the Spinal Cord and Filum Terminale. Philadelphia, W. B. Saunders Co., 1964.

155. Spiller, W. G.: Syringomyelia. Br. Med. J. *2*:1017, 1906.

156. Squier, M. V., and Lehr, R. P.: Post-traumatic syringomyelia. J. Neurol. Neurosurg. Psychiatry *57*:1095, 1994.

157. Steinmetz, A., Aschoff, A., and Kunze, S.: The iatrogenic tethering of the cord. Acta Neurochir. (Wien) *123*:219, 1993.

158. Stoaniemi, K. A., Pyhtinen, J., and Myllyla, V. V.: Computed tomography in the diagnosis of syringomyelia. Acta Neurol. Scand. *68*:121, 1983.

159. Stoodley, M. A., Jones, N. R., and Brown, C. J.: Evidence for rapid fluid flow from the subarachnoid space into the spinal cord central canal in the rat. Brain Res. *707*:155, 1996.

160. Suzuki, M., Davis, C., Symon, L., and Gentili, F.: Syringoperitoneal shunt for treatment of cord cavitation. J. Neurol. Neurosurg. Psychiatry *48*:620, 1985.

161. Tamaki, K., and Lubin, A. J.: Pathogenesis of syringomyelia: Case illustrating the process of cavity formation from embryonic cell rests. Arch. Neurol. Psychiatry *40*:748, 1938.

162. Tanghe, H. L. J.: Magnetic resonance imaging (MRI) in syringomyelia. Acta Neurochir. (Wein) *134*:93, 1995.

163. Tator, C. H., Meguro, K., and Rowed, D. W.: Favorable results with syringosubarachnoid shunts for treatment of syringomyelia. J. Neurosurg. *56*:517, 1982.

164. Tauber, E. S., and Langworthy, O. R.: A study of syringomyelia and the formation of cavities in the spinal cord. J. Nerv. Ment. Dis. *81*:245, 1935.

165. Turnbull, F. A.: Syringomyelic complications of spina bifida. Brain *56*:204, 1933.

166. Vernon, J. D., Silver, J. R., and Ohry, A.: Post-traumatic syringomyelia. Paraplegia *20*:339, 1982.

167. Walshe, F. M. R.: Developmental anomalies: Syringomyelia and syringobulbia (status dysraphicus). *In* Diseases of the Nervous System. 11th ed. Baltimore, Williams & Wilkins, 1970, pp. 267–272.

168. Watson, N.: Ascending cystic degeneration of the cord after spinal cord injury. Paraplegia *19*:89, 1981.

169. Wechsler, I. S.: Syringomyelia (including spinal gliosis). *In* A Textbook of Clinical Neurology. Philadelphia, W. B. Saunders Co., 1927, pp. 159–164.

170. West, R. J., and Williams, B.: Radiographic studies of the ventricles in syringomyelia. Neuroradiology *20*:5, 1980.

171. Wiedemayer, H., Nau, H. E., Rauhut, F., et al.: Operative treatment and prognosis of syringomyelia. Neurosurg. Rev. *17*:37, 1994.

172. Williams, B.: The distending force in the production of "communicating syringomyelia." Lancet 2:189, 1969.

173. Williams, B.: Current concepts of syringomyelia. Br. J. Hosp. Med. *4*:331, 1970.

174. Williams, B.: The distending force in the production of communicating syringomyelia. Lancet 1:41, 1970.

175. Williams, B.: Cerebrospinal fluid pressure changes in response to coughing. Brain *99*:331, 1976.

176. Williams, B.: Difficult labour as a cause of communicating syringomyelia. Lancet 2:51, 1977.

177. Williams, B.: A critical appraisal of posterior fossa surgery for communicating syringomyelia. Brain *101*:223, 1978.

178. Williams, B.: Experimental communicating syringomyelia in dogs after cisternal kaolin injection: Part 1. Pressure studies. J. Neurol. Sci. *48*:109, 1980.

179. Williams, B.: On the pathogenesis of syringomyelia: A review. J. R. Soc. Med. *73*:798, 1980.

180. Williams, B.: Simultaneous cerebral and spinal fluid pressure recordings: 2. Cerebrospinal dissociation with lesions at the foramen magnum. Acta Neurochir. *59*:123, 1981.

181. Williams, B.: Progress in syringomyelia. Neurol. Res. *8*:130, 1986.

182. Williams, B.: Pathogenesis of syringomyelia. Acta Neurochir. *123*:159, 1993.

183. Williams, B., and Fahy, G.: A critical appraisal of "terminal ventriculostomy" for the treatment of syringomyelia. J. Neurosurg. *58*:188, 1983.

184. Williams, B., Terry, A. F., Jones, H. W. F., and McSweeney, T.: Syringomyelia as a sequel to traumatic paraplegia. Paraplegia *19*:67, 1981.

185. Williams, B., and Timperley, W. R.: Three cases of communicating syringomyelia secondary to midbrain gliomas. J. Neurol. Neurosurg. Psychiatry *40*:80, 1976.

186. Wilson, C. B., Bertan, V., Norrell, H. A., and Hukuda, S.: Experimental cervical myelopathy: II. Acute ischemic myelopathy. Arch. Neurol. *21*:571, 1969.

187. Wilson, S. A. K.: Syringomyelia: Syringobulbia. *In* Bruce, A. N. (ed.): Neurology. Vol. 2. Baltimore, Williams & Wilkins, 1955, pp. 1187–1202.

188. Wolman, L.: The disturbance of circulation in traumatic paraplegia in acute and late stages: A pathological study. Paraplegia *2*:213, 1965.

189. Woodard, J. S., and Freeman, L. W.: Ischemia of the spinal cord: An experimental study. J. Neurosurg. *13*:63, 1956.

190. Woods, A. H.: Removal of a tumor from the spinal cord in syringomyelia: Its histology and relationship with the ependyma. Arch. Neurol. Psychiatry *20*:1258, 1928.

191. Wozniewicz, B., Filipowicz, K., Swiderska, S. K., and Deraka, K.: Pathophysiological mechanism of traumatic cavitation of the spinal cord. Paraplegia *21*:312, 1983.

192. Yezierski, R. P., Santana, M., Park, S., and Madsen, P. W.: Intraspinal injections of quisqualic acid in the adult rat: An experimental model of neurotoxicity and syringomyelia. J. Neurotrauma *10*:445–456, 1993.

Principles and Techniques of Spinal Surgery

CHAPTER 49

Surgical Approaches to the Spine

Rollin M. Johnson, M.D.

Michael J. Murphy, M.D.

Wayne O. Southwick, M.D.

Function and Surgical Anatomy of the Neck

FUNCTION OF THE NECK

The musculoskeletal portion of the neck is an extraordinarily versatile link between the head and body that is uniquely suited to three vital functions: it houses the spinal cord and protects it from injury; like a universal joint, it offers great flexibility in three planes; and it acts as a shock absorber to protect the brain from the rougher movements of the rest of the body. Figure 49–1 (see color plate) demonstrates all of the organs of the neck at the level of C6 in addition to the skeletal elements. The normal neck moves as much as 130 degrees in flexion and extension,[9, 13] 75 degrees in lateral bending, and 160 degrees in rotation. Under normal conditions, the ligaments and bony elements of the vertebrae protect the spinal cord and nerve roots even in these extremes of motion. Because the head accounts for only 7 per cent of body weight,[18, 20] the neck is not required to support large forces; rather, it serves as a flexible link, providing the movement needed to use the senses of sight, smell, and hearing.

In the developing embryo, the spinal axis forms a large "C" curve, as shown in Figure 49–2. However, as the spine matures, it becomes a double "S" curve, as viewed in the sagittal plane, with two segments of the curve convex to the front and two convex posteriorly. This double "S" shape appears to act as a springlike shock absorber, an effect that is enhanced by the cushioning of the intervertebral articulations. The posterior convex curves, at the thorax and sacrum, are the most rigid areas of the spine, whereas the lordotic curves of the cervical and lumbar levels are more flexible, accounting for a greater proportion of the spine's motion. This difference in flexibility appears to predispose the more mobile segments to the effects of injury and degeneration. The most common sites of disc degeneration occur in the lower cervical and lower lumbar segments, just above the more rigid thoracic and sacral levels. In the lower cervical spine, the C5–C6 articulation has the greatest range of sagittal plane motion, and this is the cervical level that is subject to the highest incidence of spinal injury and disc degeneration.[1]

The cervical spine has six degrees of freedom of motion. The traditionally appreciated motions are flexion and extension (sagittal plane), lateral bending (frontal plane), and rotation. In addition, the spine may distract or compress along the longitudinal axis, translate anteriorly or posteriorly along the sagittal plane, or move laterally along the frontal plane. As demonstrated by Fielding[2] and White,[21] these latter motions are fine movements that occur in conjunction with normal flexion and extension. However, in clinical practice, roentgenograms are required to appreciate these small degrees of "coupled" motion (Fig. 49–3). For example, in normal flexion the facets of the upper vertebra glide forward and superiorly, producing rotation of the upper vertebra in the sagittal plane, longitudinal distraction of the posterior elements, compression of the disc space anteriorly, and anterior displacement of the upper vertebra. Thus, flexion is the result of "coupled" motion in three planes. The phenomenon of

Figure 49–2. The spine begins as a "C" curve in the embryo and develops a double "S" curve by adulthood. The cervical and lumbar curves are convex anteriorly and are more mobile, accounting for the principal movements of the vertebrae. The lower cervical intervertebral discs are angled obliquely forward. (From Robinson, R. A., and Southwick, W. O.: Surgical Approaches to the Cervical Spine. *In* the American Academy of Orthopaedic Surgeons: Instructional Course Lectures, Vol. XVII. St. Louis, The C. V. Mosby Co., 1960.)

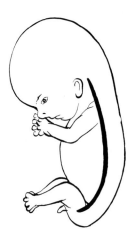
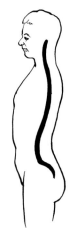
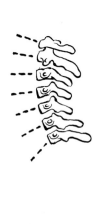

"coupling" one motion with another has been extensively studied in the thoracic, cadaver, bone–ligament construct by Panjabi and coworkers[15] and White.[21]

Sagittal plane motion at the individual intervertebral articulations has been studied in the normal young adult (Table 49–1). The greatest flexion and extension are found at the occipitoatlantal joint (25 degrees, mean) and in the lower cervical segments between the fifth and sixth cervical vertebrae (21 degrees). The least flexion and extension are found between the second and third cervical vertebrae and at the transition between the lowest cervical and first thoracic segment. Overall, the range of flexion from the neutral position almost equals that of extension. However, at the occipitoatlantal joint, the range of extension is significantly greater than that of flexion, whereas in the lower cervical segments, relatively more flexion is observed.

Accurate measurements of lateral bending and rotation at the individual segmental levels have been hampered by inadequate methods of measuring these motions clinically. Hohl[9] found on cineroentgenographic studies that no rotation or lateral bending occurred at the occipitoatlantal joint and that approximately half of the normal cervical rotation occurs at the atlantoaxial joint. Lysell[13] studied motion in human cadaver spines

and found that a total of 90 degrees of rotation was permitted in the lower cervical spine, coupled with 48 degrees of lateral bending. He also found that a total of 98 degrees of lateral bending was permitted in the lower cervical spine, coupled with 56 degrees of rotation. The obligate coupling of lateral bending with rotation is because of the 45-degree oblique relationship of the facet joints in the sagittal plane. In rotation, one superior facet glides forward and superiorly, and the other glides posteriorly and inferiorly (see Fig. 49–3C). Thus, as one vertebral body rotates on the other, it also tilts in the frontal plane to produce lateral bending.

In summary, all the cervical vertebral articulations contribute to flexion and extension. One half of the total rotation occurs at the atlantoaxial joint, and the other half occurs in the lower five articulations. Lateral bending occurs primarily in the lower cervical segments, from the second to the seventh vertebrae.

SURGICAL ANATOMY OF THE NECK

Triangles and Surface Anatomy of the Neck

For convenience of description, the neck is divided into two large triangles by the prominent sternomastoid muscle (Fig. 49–4). These are subdivided by the digastric and omohyoid muscles into several smaller triangles, which take their names from local anatomic features, such as the digastric, carotid, and subclavian triangles.

Certain surface landmarks are useful surgically in localizing the levels of the vertebrae. The third cervical vertebra is at the level of the hyoid bone, the fourth is opposite the upper border of the thyroid cartilage, and the sixth lies opposite the cricoid cartilage, a prominent ring palpable just below the thyroid cartilage. Posteriorly, the first prominence below the occiput is the second cervical spinous process. This is a large, bifid structure, which is ordinarily buried between the paracervical muscles but may be felt with firm pressure

Table 49–1. SAGITTAL PLANE FLEXION-EXTENSION OF THE NORMAL ADULT CERVICAL SPINE 20 TO 40 YEARS OF AGE AT EACH SEGMENTAL LEVEL

Cervical Level	Mean	± 2 S.D.*	Low	High
Occiput-C1	25.5	± 11.2	15	41
C1–C2	15.6	± 8.8	4	25
C2–C3	12.0	± 5.1	6	19
C3–C4	17.5	± 6.7	10	25
C4–C5	19.5	± 6.4	10	26
C5–C6	20.8	± 7.3	13	29
C6–C7	20.5	± 6.9	13	29
C7–T1	11.9	± 6.1	4	19

*± 2 standard deviations of the mean.

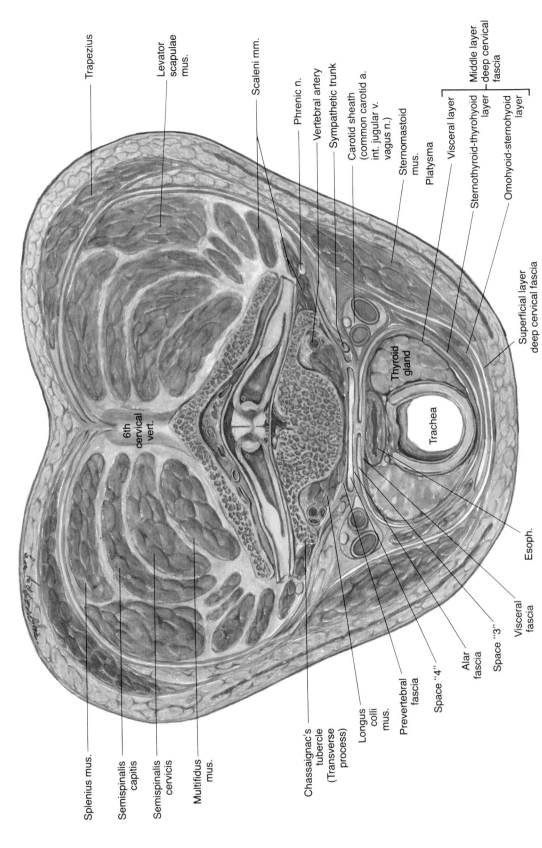

Trapezius

Levator
scapulae
mus.

Scaleni mm.

Phrenic n.

Vertebral artery

Sympathetic trunk

Carotid sheath
(common carotid a.
int. jugular v.
vagus n.)

Sternomastoid
mus.

Platysma

Visceral layer

Sternothyroid-thyrohyoid
layer

Omohyoid-sternohyoid
layer

Middle layer
deep cervical
fascia

Superficial layer
deep cervical fascia

Thyroid
gland

Trachea

6th
cervical
vert.

Splenius mus.

Semispinalis
capitis

Semispinalis
cervicis

Multifidus
mus.

Chassaignac's
tubercle
(Transverse
process)

Longus
colli
mus.

Prevertebral
fascia

Space "4"

Space "3"

Visceral
fascia

Alar
fascia

Esoph.

Figure 49–1. Transaxial section of the neck at C6 showing the fascial layers, muscles, spinal cord, nerve roots, and other structures useful for comparison with computed axial tomography and magnetic resonance imaging.

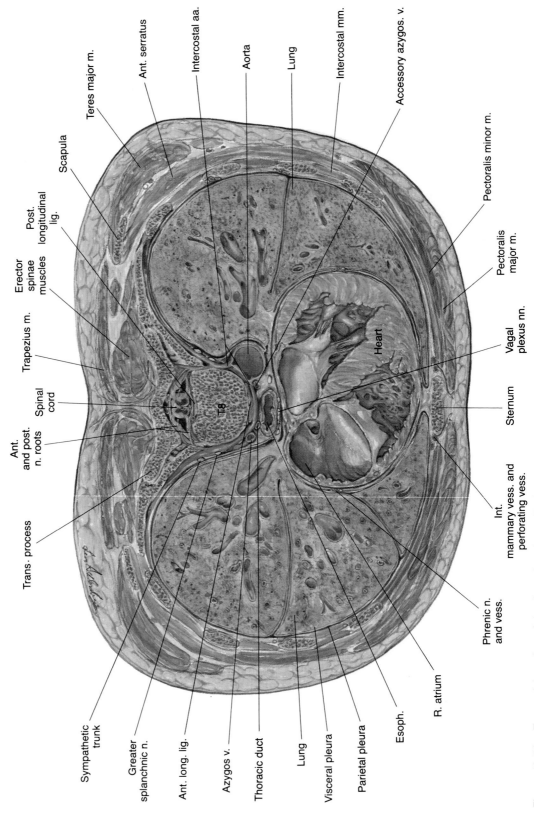

Sympathetic trunk

Greater splanchnic n.

Ant. long. lig.

Azygos v.

Thoracic duct

Lung

Visceral pleura

Parietal pleura

Esoph.

R. atrium

Phrenic n. and vess.

Int. mammary vess. and perforating vess.

Sternum

Vagal plexus nn.

Heart

Pectoralis major m.

Pectoralis minor m.

Accessory azygos. v.

Intercostal mm.

Lung

Aorta

Intercostal aa.

Ant. serratus

Teres major m.

Scapula

Post. longitudinal lig.

Erector spinae muscles

Trapezius m.

Spinal cord

Ant. and post. n. roots

Trans. process

T8

Figure 49–70. Transaxial section of the thoracic spine at T8 for comparison with computed axial tomography and magnetic resonance imaging.

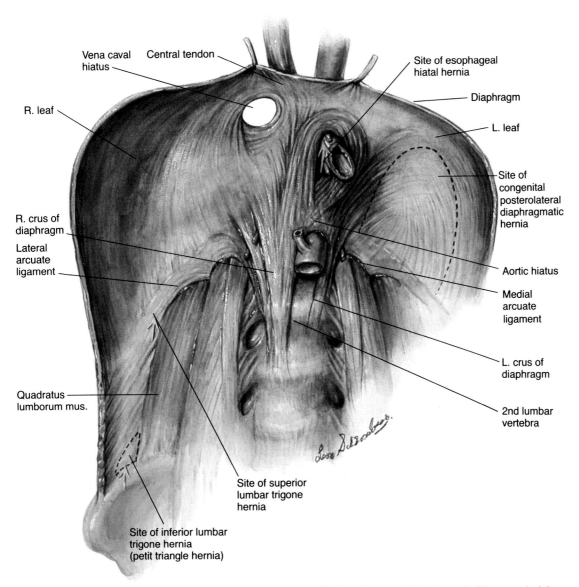

Vena caval
hiatus

Central tendon

Site of esophageal
hiatal hernia

Diaphragm

R. leaf

L. leaf

Site of
congenital
posterolateral
diaphragmatic
hernia

R. crus of
diaphragm

Lateral
arcuate
ligament

Aortic hiatus

Medial
arcuate
ligament

L. crus of
diaphragm

Quadratus
lumborum mus.

2nd lumbar
vertebra

Site of superior
lumbar trigone
hernia

Site of inferior lumbar
trigone hernia
(petit triangle hernia)

Figure 49–82. Diaphragm seen from below. (From Zuidema, G. D. (ed.), and Schlossberg, L. (illustrator): Atlas of Human Functional Anatomy, 3rd ed. Baltimore, Johns Hopkins University Press, 1985.)

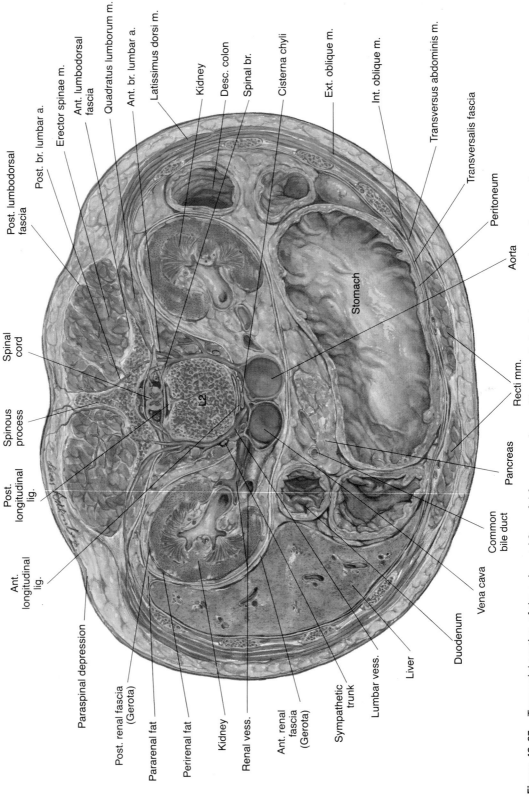

Figure 49–97. Transaxial section of the spine at L2, useful for comparison with computed axial tomography and magnetic resonance imaging. Note the fascial planes, especially important in the posterolateral approach.

Post. lumbodorsal fascia

Post. br. lumbar a.

Erector spinae m.

Ant. lumbodorsal fascia

Quadratus lumborum m.

Ant. br. lumbar a.

Latissimus dorsi m.

Kidney

Desc. colon

Spinal br.

Cisterna chyli

Ext. oblique m.

Int. oblique m.

Transversus abdominis m.

Transversalis fascia

Peritoneum

Aorta

Stomach

Spinal cord

Recti mm.

Pancreas

Spinous process

Common bile duct

L2

Vena cava

Post. longitudinal lig.

Duodenum

Liver

Lumbar vess.

Ant. longitudinal lig.

Sympathetic trunk

Ant. renal fascia (Gerota)

Paraspinal depression

Renal vess.

Kidney

Perirenal fat

Pararenal fat

Post. renal fascia (Gerota)

over the midline. Below this the sixth cervical spinous process is often palpable, and the seventh is most prominent.

Laterally, the transverse processes may be palpated through the sternomastoid muscle in the upper neck. The transverse process of the atlas is the most promi- nent transverse process and is found just below and somewhat anterior to the mastoid process. To clearly separate this from the skull, it may be necessary to rotate the neck. With rotation, the atlas appears to move independently from the skull. By following a gentle curve anteriorly and down, one can palpate all

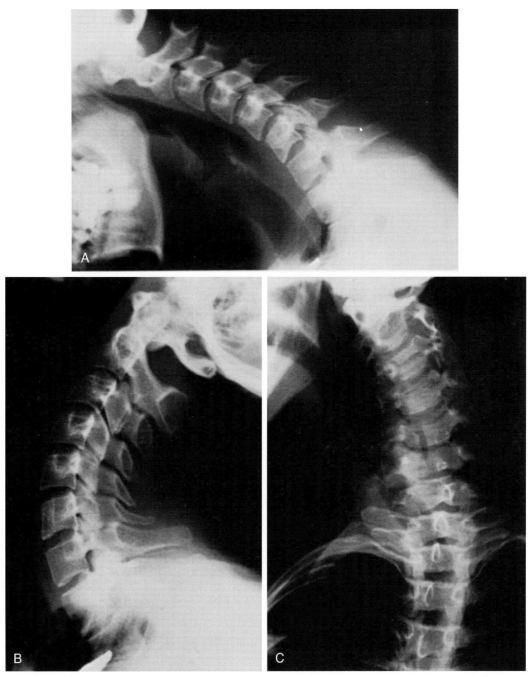

Figure 49–3. Radiographs of the cervical spine in maximal flexion *(A)*, extension *(B)*, and rotation to the right *(C)*. In flexion *(A)*, the facets glide anteriorly and superiorly on the facets below, resulting in rotation of the vertebra in the sagittal plane. Concomitantly, the posterior elements separate, the intervertebral disc is compressed anteriorly, and one vertebra moves forward horizontally on the vertebra below. In extension *(B)*, the reverse occurs, with distraction at the intervertebral disc anteriorly. In rotation *(C)*, there is obligate coupling of lateral bending with rotation, as the facet on one side moves forward and superiorly while the opposite facet moves posteriorly and inferiorly.

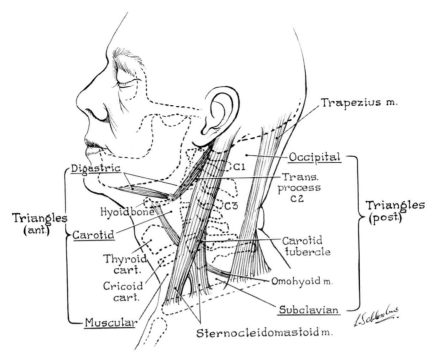

Figure 49–4. Triangles and surface anatomy of the neck. The transverse process of the first cervical vertebra is palpable below the mastoid process deep to the sternomastoid muscle. The hyoid bone is at the level of the third cervical vertebra, the thyroid cartilage opposite the fourth vertebra, and the cricoid cartilage opposite the sixth cervical vertebra. (From Robinson, R. A., and Southwick, S. O.: Surgical Approaches to the Cervical Spine. *In* the American Academy of Orthopaedic Surgeons: Instructional Course Lectures, Vol. XVII. St. Louis, The C. V. Mosby Co., 1960.)

the transverse processes of the neck. Ordinarily, these are so similar and their margins so obscure that one cannot accurately identify the vertebral level below the atlas from the lateral side of the neck.

Skin, Platysma, Superficial Nerves, and Veins

Anteriorly, the skin of the neck is mobile, soft, and thin and has an excellent blood supply. The anterior skin creases are transverse in the lower neck but tend to run obliquely upward near the mandible. Incisions in the anterior neck should follow these skin creases because these will heal more easily with a less noticeable scar than incisions that traverse these planes. The skin, subcutaneous fascia, and platysma muscle are mobile, allowing significant distortion with retraction. The skin of the back of the neck is much thicker and less mobile than the front, and longitudinal incisions here tend to heal with prominent scars that may spread because of tension from the trapezius muscle.

Just beneath the skin is a thin layer of superficial fascia that contains the platysma muscles anteriorly. The platysma muscles are rhomboid in shape and extend from the mandible to the superficial fascia over the chest and from the midline to the lateral border of the sternomastoid muscle. Their motor nerve supply is derived from the cervical branch of the facial nerve,

and the anterior cutaneous nerves of the neck pierce them to innervate the skin. In anterior surgical exposures, the platysma layer should be identified and its muscle fibers cut transversely or split longitudinally. These should be closed as a separate layer to avoid separation with healing and an ugly scar.

Beneath the platysma and embedded within the superficial layers of the deep cervical fascia are four superficial nerves of the neck, which emerge behind the posterior border of the sternomastoid muscle at its midpoint (Fig. 49–5). These nerves fan out radially and carry sensory fibers to the posterior occiput, the front and sides of the neck, and the cape over the clavicle and upper chest. The lesser occipital nerve is derived from the second cervical root and supplies the skin over the lateral occipital region. The great auricular nerve arises from the second and third cervical roots and appears slightly lower, behind the sternomastoid muscle. It then arches over this muscle, running parallel with the external jugular vein, and supplies the area over the parotid gland and the skin about the ear. The anterior cervical cutaneous nerve, arising from the second and third cervical roots, runs anteriorly across the sternomastoid muscle, supplying the region around the hyoid bone. The supraclavicular nerve arises from the third and fourth cervical roots and has three main branches, supplying the skin over the clavicle and anterior trapezius.

Short transverse incisions in the anterior cervical

triangle rarely transect these major cutaneous nerve trunks or cause permanent numbness, but longitudinal incisions in the anterior triangle or transverse incisions posterior to the sternomastoid muscle may divide these nerves. The greater and lesser occipital nerves and the great auricular nerve arise from the second cervical nerve root. This root passes between the ring of the atlas and lamina of the axis as it emerges from the spinal canal. With fractures of the posterior arch of the atlas, odontoid process, or neural arch of the axis, this second root may be irritated, causing pain over the back of the head, behind the ear, or over the parotid gland. This may be a valuable diagnostic symptom that should arouse suspicion in patients having a history of injury and pain in these locations.

Beneath the platysma and in the same plane as the superficial nerves lies the external jugular vein (see Fig. 49–5). It is formed by the posterior auricular vein and a branch of the posterior facial vein, which unite below the ear lobe to run vertically caudad. The external jugular vein crosses the sternomastoid muscle at its midpoint, passing into the posterior triangle of the neck, where it pierces the superficial layer of the deep cervical fascia posterior and lateral to the clavicular head of the sternomastoid muscle. The anterior jugular vein is formed by several small veins in the region of the protuberance of the mandible and descends just

lateral to the midline to enter the suprasternal space. Just above the sternum it crosses laterally and deep to the sternomastoid muscle to terminate either in the external jugular or in the subclavian vein. Communicating veins, between the anterior and external jugular veins, pass through the suprasternal space by means of a separate reflection of the superficial layer of the deep fascia.

Fasciae of the Neck

The fascial layers of the neck surround many major anatomic structures and separate these into discrete compartments. These fascial planes may be used as landmarks or paths to guide the surgeon on a safe and simple course through the front of the neck to the vertebral bodies beneath. The fascial layers enclose certain vital structures, such as those of the carotid sheath, and protect the contents from injury during surgical dissection. In addition, the natural cleavage planes between these fascial layers provide pathways for safe dissection between these complex structures. For example, in the anterior approach to the cervical vertebral bodies, the recurrent laryngeal nerve lies in potential jeopardy. This nerve lies deep to the visceral layer of the deep cervical fascia, however. By dissecting within the natural cleavage plane between the alar and vis-

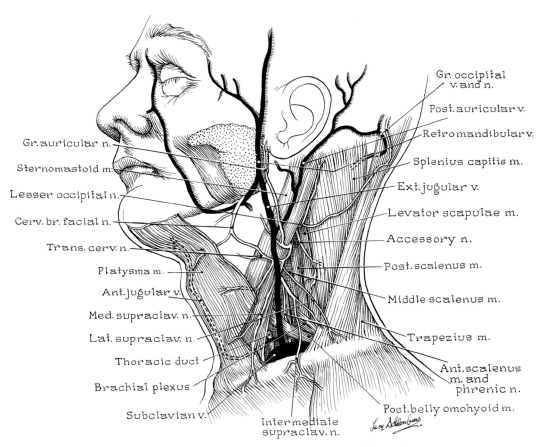

Figure 49–5. Superficial veins and nerves of the neck.

ceral fasciae and not within the visceral fascial envelope, this nerve may be safely bypassed and there is no need to identify it. Similar protection is provided by the alar fascia surrounding the carotid structures and the prevertebral fascia protecting the phrenic nerve. However, it is important to know the relationship of these fascial layers, using the natural cleavage planes, and not violate the integrity of certain fascial sheaths. Grodinsky and Holyoke[5] described these fascial layers in their classic article.

The cervical fascia is divided into one superficial and four deep layers (Figs. 49–6 and 49–7). The superficial fascia is a continuous plane that surrounds the neck in the subcutaneous tissue and envelops the platysma in its deep portion. The superficial layer of the deep cervical fascia surrounds the neck and en-

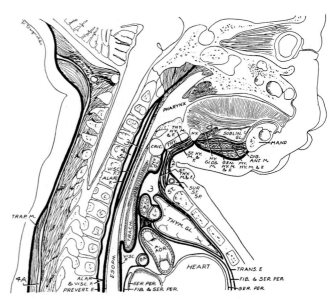

Figure 49–7. Fascial compartments of the neck in the sagittal plane. Note that space "4" between the prevertebral and alar fasciae is continuous with the posterior mediastinum. (From Grodinsky, M., and Holyoke, E. A.: Fasciae and fascial spaces of head, neck, and adjacent regions. Am. J. Anat. *63*:367, 1938. Copyright © 1938. Reprinted by permission of Wiley-Liss, Inc., a division of John Wiley and Sons, Inc.)

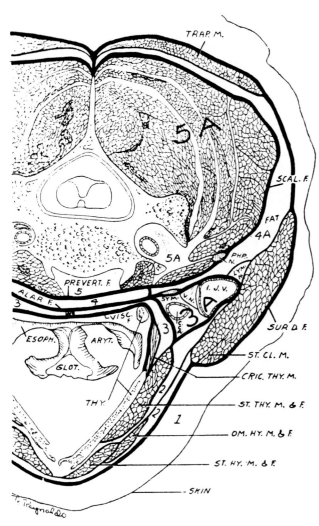

Figure 49–6. Cross section of the fascial compartments of the neck at the level of the thyroid cartilage. Alar F., alar fascia; Prevert. F., prevertebral fascia; Scal. F., scalenus fascia; Sup. D. F., superficial layer of deep fascia; Visc. F., visceral fascia. (From Grodinsky, M., and Holyoke, E. A.: Fasciae and fascial spaces of head, neck and adjacent regions. Am. J. Anat. *63*:367, 1938. Copyright © 1938. Reprinted by permission of Wiley-Liss, Inc., a division of John Wiley and Sons, Inc.)

closes the sternomastoid and trapezius muscles. The middle layers of the deep cervical fascia enclose the strap muscles and omohyoid in the anterior cervical region and extend as far laterally as the scapula. The deepest component of this middle layer is the visceral fascia, which surrounds the larynx, trachea, esophagus, and thyroid. The alar fascia spreads like two wings behind the esophagus and surrounds the carotid sheath structures laterally. The deepest layer is the prevertebral fascia, which surrounds the vertebrae and paraspinal muscles, enclosing structures such as the phrenic nerve and scalene muscles.

The superficial fascia is a continuous subcutaneous sheet that surrounds the neck and extends from the head into the thorax. This fascial plane is relatively loose in the front of the neck and contains the platysma in its deeper portion. The next fascial layer is the thicker superficial layer of the deep fascia, which surrounds the neck, fusing with the intermuscular septum posteriorly and the spinous processes of the vertebrae. It splits to surround the sternomastoid and trapezius muscles. Just above the sternum it divides to form the suprasternal or Burns' space, inserting on the anterior and posterior margins of the sternum, and laterally it fuses with the clavicle, acromion, and scapular spine. The superficial nerves and the anterior and external jugular veins are partially contained within the superficial fibers of this plane. Superiorly, at the hyoid, the superficial layer of the deep fascia fuses with the middle layers of fascia. These extend beyond the hyoid as one common layer of fascia to cover the muscles of the submental triangle and then split to form the capsules of the maxillary and parotid glands.

The suprasternal or Burns' space is a useful landmark for transecting the insertions of the sternomastoid muscle above the sternum and clavicle. Henry[8] and Nanson[14] described an approach to the lower cervical and upper thoracic spine through the clavicular head of the sternomastoid muscle (see "Anterior Cervical Approaches" in this chapter). The subclavian and internal jugular veins lie immediately behind this structure and may be injured unless carefully protected. The potential space between the two layers of fascia may be developed by blunt dissection, and the muscle may be transected with a finger, protecting these structures beneath (Fig. 49–8).

The middle layer of the deep cervical fascia is divided into three parts. The first of these is called the omohyoid-sternohyoid layer and forms a sheath around these muscles. Superiorly it attaches to the hyoid, inferiorly to the posterior border of the sternum and clavicle, and laterally it fuses with the deep surface of the sternomastoid sheath, a portion of the superficial layer of the deep fascia. Over the midportion of the omohyoid muscle, this fascia becomes thicker, forming a pulley for the omohyoid, which allows this muscle to change dissections as it proceeds laterally to the scapula, holding the central section of this muscle down. The second part of the middle cervical fascia is the relatively thin sternothyroid-thyrohyoid layer, which surrounds these muscles. It too inserts superiorly on the hyoid, inferiorly on the sternum and clavicle, and laterally fuses with the deep surface of the sternomastoid sheath. The third portion of the middle layer of the cervical fascia is the visceral fascia, which surrounds the trachea, esophagus, and thyroid. Posterior to the pharynx, it ascends to the base of the skull, and anteriorly it attaches to the thyroid cartilage and hyoid. Posteriorly and in the upper thorax, it fuses with the alar fascia, surrounds the intrathoracic portion of the trachea and esophagus, and is continuous with the fibrous pericardium. The visceral layer is important because it protects the recurrent laryngeal nerves and esophagus from injury during anterior exposures of the cervical spine.

The alar fascia lies behind the esophagus and spreads laterally as a sheet to surround the carotid structures like two wings. The alar fascia fuses with the prevertebral fascia beneath, over the transverse processes of the vertebrae. This tends to limit the lateral spread of a midline infection within this potential space. Between the alar and prevertebral fascial planes lies a loose potential space that extends from the atlas to the posterior mediastinum deep within the thorax. This space "4" of Grodinsky and Holyoke[5] is often

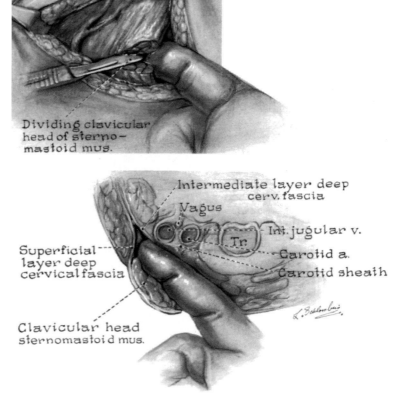

Figure 49–8. Blunt dissection within Burns' space to protect the structures within the carotid sheath and subclavian vein. The subclavian and internal jugular veins and the carotid artery lie beneath the sternomastoid muscle and can be injured during division of the sternomastoid in approaches through this structure. The potential space between two layers of the deep cervical fascia is developed by blunt dissection, and the muscle is transected with the finger protecting these structures beneath.

referred to as the "danger space," because retropharyngeal or prevertebral infections may extend through it into the posterior mediastinum.

The prevertebral fascia surrounds the vertebral bodies, the scalene and paravertebral muscles, and the phrenic nerves. Posteriorly this fascia fuses with the intermuscular septum and inserts on the vertebral spinous processes. Inferiorly it is continuous with the lumbodorsal fascia.

In approaching the middle and lower cervical vertebrae from the front (described later in this chapter), one divides the superficial fascia and the platysma muscle. The next layer is the well-developed superficial layer of the deep cervical fascia, which is divided longitudinally by sharp dissection at the anterior margin of the sternomastoid muscle. Beneath, the two thin muscular layers of the middle cervical fascia may be divided by finger dissection, medial to the carotid sheath. The plane of dissection then follows the natural cleavage plane between the visceral and alar fasciae to the midline, behind the esophagus and over the vertebral bodies. This dissection is made easier if these sheaths are left intact, protecting the esophagus and recurrent laryngeal nerves within the visceral fascia from injury. Finally, the alar and prevertebral layers must be divided by sharp, longitudinal dissection to expose the vertebral bodies beneath.

An understanding of the fascial planes of the neck also helps in localizing the source of cervical infections.

The prevertebral and alar fascial sheaths are fused laterally over the transverse processes and not in the midline. Therefore, an infection of vertebral origin usually occurs in the midline, spreading laterally to either side. If this infection then breaks through the prevertebral fascia, it may spread inferiorly into the posterior mediastinum through the space between the alar and prevertebral layers. Conversely, the visceral fascia is usually fused to the alar fascia in the midline, so that abscesses of pharyngeal origin tend to occur on one side lateral to the midline. Therefore, retropharyngeal abscesses that occupy a central position are often of vertebral origin, whereas those that are eccentric to one side more commonly arise from the pharynx, limited by these fascial connections.

Anterior Neck Muscles

The superficial muscles of the anterior triangle of the neck are divided by the hyoid bone (Fig. 49–9). Those above the hyoid in the digastric triangle are the stylohyoid, the anterior and posterior belly of the digastric, which is attached to the hyoid bone by a sling at its midportion, and the mylohyoid arising from the mandible. These are innervated by the hypoglossal nerve, which swings downward along the carotid sheath and dives deep to the stylohyoid and posterior belly of the digastric in company with the lingual artery. These structures are not normally encountered

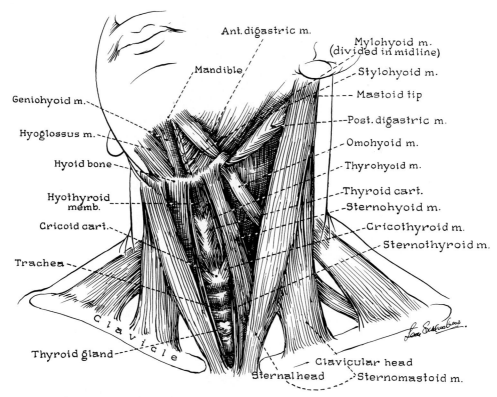

Figure 49–9. Superficial muscles of the anterior neck. The sternomastoid divides the neck into the anterior and posterior triangles, and the hyoid presents a natural division between the muscles of the digastric triangle and the infrahyoid or strap muscles.

except in anterior exposures to the upper cervical vertebrae.

Below the hyoid are the strap muscles, which are attached to the hyoid, thyroid cartilage, and sternum. The strap muscles are found in two layers: The superficial layer includes the sternohyoid and omohyoid, and the deep layer includes the thyrohyoid and sternothyroid muscles. These infrahyoid muscles are innervated by the ansa hypoglossi as it proceeds along the carotid sheath. Branches from the ansa arch forward to the muscles in the upper neck and can be retracted forward with care in exposures of the middle and lower neck. However, these branches will be stretched or divided in exposures to the upper cervical vertebrae medial to the carotid sheath.

The sternomastoid muscle is the most prominent muscle of the neck and divides the neck into its anterior and posterior triangles. It arises by two heads, the medial one from the manubrium of the sternum and the lateral one from the clavicle. The muscle inserts on the mastoid process in the lateral half of the superior nuchal line of the occipital bone. It is innervated by the spinal accessory nerve, which reaches the upper third of this muscle along its deep surface. The accessory nerve then emerges from behind the midportion of the sternomastoid and descends beneath the superficial layer of deep fascia to innervate the trapezius. This nerve should be identified and protected in approaches through the posterior triangle of the neck. Immediately subjacent to the sternomastoid muscle is the carotid sheath, surrounded by its alar fascia. Henry[8] and Whitesides and Kelly[23] described an approach in which the sternomastoid muscle is everted to expose structures of surgical importance in the lateral cervical spine, including the brachial plexus and vertebral artery. The accessory nerve must be identified and protected during this eversion, as described in the second section of this chapter.

The deepest muscles lie along the anterior surface of the vertebrae, covering the lateral aspect of the vertebral bodies and filling the hollow between the bodies and adjacent transverse processes (Fig. 49–10). The longus colli is the most central of these muscles, extending from the atlas to the third thoracic vertebra. It does not cover the centers of the vertebral bodies, except at the atlas. The longus capitis lies just lateral to the longus colli and is primarily a flexor of the head.

The sympathetic trunk lies directly over the longus colli and capitis in a loose reflection of alar fascia at the carotid sheath. Ordinarily, the sympathetic trunk is easily dissected from the carotid sheath and remains with the longus colli and capitis muscles when the carotid structures are displaced anteriorly. The sympathetic trunk and the superior cervical sympathetic ganglion should be protected in dissections of this area to prevent the development of Horner's syndrome.

Deep to the longus capitis and connecting the transverse processes at each level are the intertransverse muscles (Fig. 49–11). The anterior intertransverse muscles connect the anterior aspects of each gutter-like transverse process, one to the next, and the posterior

component connects the transverse processes posteriorly, behind the nerve roots. Over the upper spine two specialized muscles perform a similar function, lateral bending of the head and neck (see Fig. 49–10). The rectus capitis anterior covers the atlanto-occipital joint, extending from the lateral mass of the atlas to the occipital bone. The rectus capitis lateralis extends from the transverse process of the atlas to the jugular process of the occipital bone. The scaleni and levators, which also arise from the transverse processes, are described later.

All the capital cervical muscles are innervated by the ventral rami of the segmental cervical nerves close to their level of origin. Perry and Nickel[17] note that all these muscles contribute to stability of the cervical spine. When these are paralyzed, the major deficits are an inability to move the head, to maintain normal posture, and to support pharyngeal or respiratory function without external support; however, the intrinsic bond between vertebrae is not lost.

The Cervical Vertebrae

The upper two cervical vertebrae and articulations are very different from those of the middle or lower cervical spine. The first cervical vertebra, or atlas, is shaped like a ring with long transverse processes extending laterally from the anterior half of this ring and a short, truncated tubercle extending from the midline posteriorly (Fig. 49–12). Unlike any of the other cervical vertebrae, the atlas has no true spinous process or body, and the bone around the ring is small and delicate in cross section. The transverse processes of the atlas extend farther laterally than any of the other cervical vertebrae, a fact that may be used to identify this vertebra in palpating the lateral sides of the neck. The occipitoatlantal joint is a shallow ball-and-socket joint that is elongated front to back. The occipital condyles protrude downward to form two truncated balls, which fit into the shallow and elliptic cups of the atlas (see Fig. 49–12). The lateral wall of this cup is higher than the medial wall, which effectively limits lateral displacements. The ball-and-socket shape provides great overall stability but does permit the largest range of flexion and extension of any cervical articulation (25 degrees).

The vertebral artery leaves the transverse foramen of the atlas and curves abruptly back adjacent to the articular condyles of the atlas (Figs. 49–12 and 49–13). It then takes another sharp turn medially over the top of the first cervical ring behind the condyles. It follows a shallow groove on the surface of this ring to a point about 2 cm from the midline and dives into a hole in the posterior atlanto-occipital ligament, disappearing from view. In posterior fusions involving the atlas, it should be remembered that this artery and its accompanying venous plexus are less than 2 cm from the midline.

The second cervical vertebra, or axis, serves as a transition between the upper and lower cervical segments. The lower articulations are similar to those of

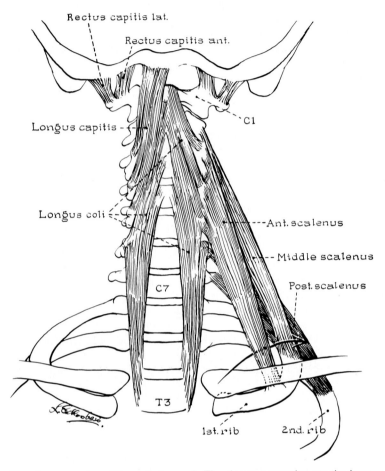

Figure 49–10. The deep muscles of the anterior neck. The deepest muscles are the longus colli and capitis, which lie along the lateral aspect of the vertebrae, filling the hollow between the bodies and adjacent transverse processes. The longus colli is a flexor of the neck and has three components: an inferior oblique part, which arises from the first three thoracic bodies and inserts on the anterior tubercles of the fifth and sixth cervical transverse process; the superior oblique component, which arises from the third through fifth transverse processes and inserts through a tendon on the anterior tubercle of the atlas in the midline; and the vertical component, which arises from the lower cervical and upper thoracic bodies and inserts on the upper cervical bodies from the second to the fourth vertebrae. The longus capitis lies lateral to the longus colli and is a flexor of the head. It arises from the anterior tubercles of the third through sixth cervical transverse processes and inserts on the basilar portion of the occiput. The scalene muscles arise from the tubercles of the cervical transverse processes and insert on the first and second ribs. The scalenus anterior is separated from the scalenus medius and scalenus posterior by the brachial plexus and subclavian artery. The scalenus anterior arises from the anterior tubercles of the third through the sixth vertebrae, and inserts on the first rib between the subclavian artery and vein and beneath the sternomastoid and prevertebral fascia. The scalenus medius arises from the posterior tubercles of the second through sixth cervical vertebrae and inserts on the first rib. The scalenus posterior is often a subdivision of the medius, which inserts on the second rib.

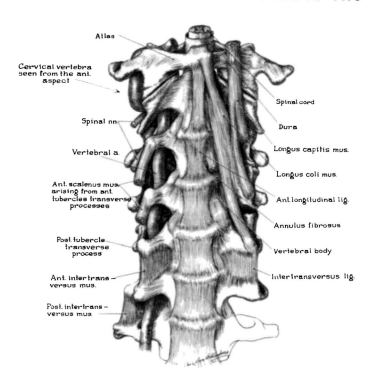

Figure 49–11. Cervical spine, ligaments, and intrinsic muscles seen from the front. Note that the vertebral artery ascends within the costotransverse foramina anterior to the nerve roots. (From Johnson, R. M., et al.: Some new observations on the functional anatomy of the lower cervical spine. Clin. Orthop. *3*:192–200, 1975.)

the middle and lower cervical spine, but the superior articulations are unique. The odontoid extends upward from the second vertebral body, articulates with the anterior ring of the first vertebra, and through its ligamentous connections provides a major bond among the atlas, the first cervical ring, and the occiput. The odontoid serves as a pivot between the first and second vertebrae, permitting almost 45 degrees of rotation to each side. Because this joint is hinged at the odontoid, in front of the spinal canal, rotations in excess of this will narrow the canal and sever the cord.

The atlantoaxial articulations sit like sloping shoulders on the lateral masses. Each opposing surface is relatively convex, which reduces the frictional resistance at this joint, increases the range of rotation in the longitudinal axis, and permits over 15 degrees of flexion and extension and small amounts of lateral bending.

The upper two cervical nerve roots are surrounded by bone on three sides as they leave the spinal canal. The first cervical nerve root divides into a large dorsal and smaller ventral ramus before it leaves the spinal canal. These emerge from a hole in the atlanto-occipital ligament just posterior to the articular condyles between the occiput and ring of the first vertebra. The dorsal ramus proceeds beneath the vertebral artery and laterally to enter and supply the muscles of the suboccipital triangle. The smaller ventral ramus proceeds anteriorly, medial to the vertebral artery and over the transverse process. The second cervical nerve root emerges behind the atlantoaxial facet. It supplies the posterior capitocervical muscles and terminates in three major branches, the greater and lesser occipital nerves and the great auricular nerve. Irritation or

trauma to this root or nerve trunks produces pain, headache, or hyperesthesia in their dermal distribution over the occiput and about the ear.

The lower five cervical vertebrae and articulations are similar to one another. The upper pole of the vertebral body is shaped like a cup and appears to cradle the vertebral body above (Fig. 49–14). This effect is created by the joints of Luschka, which articulate with the posterolateral aspect of the vertebral body above. The transverse processes extend laterally from the posterior half of the vertebral body. These are shaped like a gutter and support the nerve roots as they leave the neural foramina. Each of the transverse processes from the first through the sixth vertebrae contains a foramen through which the vertebral arteries ascend into the head (see Fig. 49–11). The transverse processes terminate in an anterior and posterior tubercle from which many of the capitocervical muscles arise. The most prominent tubercle is usually found at the sixth vertebra and is known as the carotid or Chassaignac's tubercle. Although this may be a useful landmark to determine the segmental level at surgery, there is enough anatomic variation that roentgenographic confirmation is recommended in the operating room.

The pedicles project posteriorly and laterally to the prominent pillars of the facets behind. The facet joints are angled obliquely at a 45-degree plane, front to back; in the lower cervical spine the angle of obliquity increases to a more vertical plane. The facet joints permit a gliding motion between their articular surfaces of 4 to 6 mm with the superior facet gliding forward and up, or backward and down with respect to the lower face. With rotation or lateral bending, the facet on one side moves forward and up and the

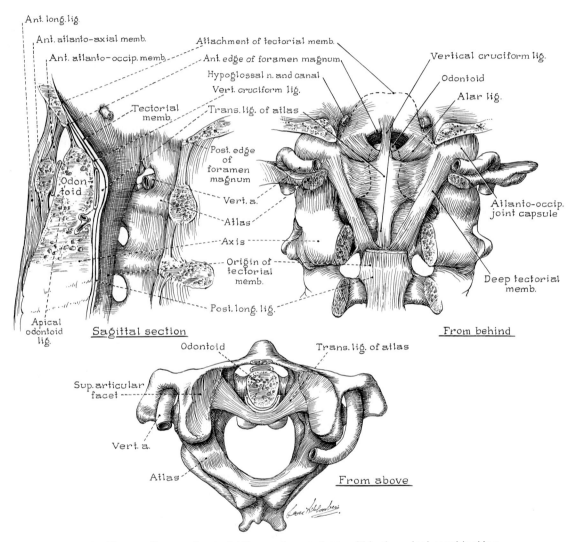

Figure 49–12. The cruciform and tectorial ligaments seen from within the spinal canal looking anteriorly, in sagittal section and from above. The cruciform ligament holds the odontoid in a sling to the anterior ring of the atlas. It is composed of a superior arm, which inserts on the basiocciput; an inferior arm, which reinforces the base of the dens; and two lateral arms, the transverse ligament. The transverse ligament inserts on the ring of the atlas and is one of the primary stabilizers of the atlantoaxial joint. This is reinforced by the tectorial and deep tectorial membranes or ligaments. The odontoid is fixed to the base of the skull through the apical odontoid and alar ligaments.

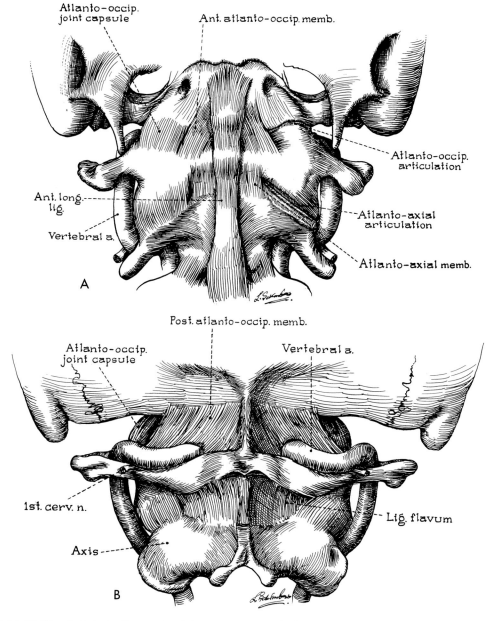

Figure 49–13. *A,* Anterior ligaments of the upper two cervical vertebrae from the basiocciput to the axis. *B,* Posterior ligaments of the upper cervical vertebrae from the occiput to the axis.

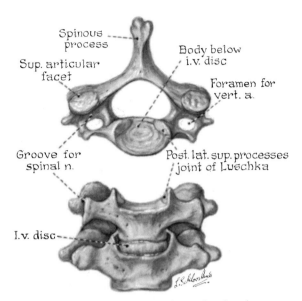

Figure 49–14. Lower cervical vertebrae, showing the relationships of the discs, facets, vertebral foramina, and joints of Luschka. (From Robinson, R. A., and Southwick, W. O.: Surgical Approaches to the Cervical Spine. *In* the American Academy of Orthopaedic Surgeons: Instructional Course Lectures, Vol. XVII. St. Louis, The C. V. Mosby Co., 1960.)

contralateral facet moves in the opposite direction, accounting for the "coupling" of rotation with lateral bending.

The laminae close the spinal canal posteriorly, ending in the spinous processes behind. All of these from the second to the sixth vertebrae are normally bifid. The seventh spinous process is the most prominent projection and is usually single and not bifid.

The intervertebral neural foramina between the second and seventh cervical vertebrae are posterior and lateral to the vertebral body and anterior to the facet pillars. The superior and inferior walls of the foramen are formed by the pedicles of the two adjacent vertebrae. The posterior wall is primarily formed by the superior facet pillar. The anterior wall is formed by the vertebral body, the joint of Luschka, and the vertebral artery and vein and their investing fascia. The transverse processes extend laterally and slightly anterior from the foramina and are shaped like a trough, holding the nerve roots, ganglia, and accompanying vessels. The cervical intervertebral foramina may be visualized roentgenographically with oblique views. The right neuroforamina are outlined with a left posterior oblique roentgenogram, and the left are outlined with a right posterior oblique view.

The lower six cervical nerve roots are surrounded by bone and the intervertebral articulations as they leave the spinal canal. With degeneration of the intervertebral disc, the facet joint, or joints of Luschka, osteophytes may develop, which decrease the size of the foramina. Osteophytes or extravasated disc material may impinge directly on the nerve roots, as demonstrated by Hadley,[6] or they may irritate adjacent soft

tissues, which react with edema and secondarily compress or irritate the nerve roots.

Ligaments of the Upper Cervical Spine

The vertebrae and articulations of the upper two cervical vertebrae are morphologically and functionally very different from those of the lower cervical elements. The anterior longitudinal ligament is the superior extension of this same ligament in the lower spine. It narrows appreciably over the body of the second cervical vertebra, is attached to the anterior tubercle of the first cervical ring, and inserts on the basiocciput (see Fig. 49–13A). Beneath this is the anterior atlanto-occipital membrane or ligament, which joins the superior ring of the first vertebra to the basiocciput. At the next lower level, the anterior atlantoaxial ligament joins the inferior ring of the atlas to the upper body of the axis. Both of these are broad, dense bands of fibrous tissue that extend laterally to the capsular ligaments.

The capsular ligaments are short but thick ligaments that essentially surround the occipitoatlantal and atlantoaxial articulations. The individual ligament fibers lie perpendicular to the plane of the facet, permitting maximal laxity of the ligament when the facets are in a neutral or fully opposed position. The capsular ligaments of the atlantoaxial joint are remarkably lax and normally permit almost 45 degrees of rotation from the neutral position in either direction.

Within the spinal canal and posterior to the dens, there are a number of ligaments that firmly bond the odontoid to the anterior ring of the atlas and occiput (see Fig. 49–12). These are primarily responsible for stability between the occiput and the first and second vertebrae. The cruciform ligament has an upper vertical arm, which inserts on the posterior aspect of the basiocciput. Two transverse arms, the transverse ligament, extend from the dens to the ring of the atlas and hold the dens firmly in a sling to the anterior arch of the atlas. The cross is completed by a vertical inferior arm, which extends down the posterior aspect of the dens to the body of the second vertebra, reinforcing the base of the dens and limiting anterior displacement following fracture at the base of the dens in many cases. The lateral alar odontoid ligaments are fibrous bands that join the superolateral aspect of the dens to the medial aspect of the occipital condyles. Finally, the apical odontoid ligament joins the tip of the dens to the posterior tip of the basiocciput beneath the vertical cruciform ligament.

The tectorial membrane is an extension of the posterior longitudinal ligament and covers the cruciform ligament as a broad band. The tectorial membrane inserts on the basilar groove of the basiocciput. It has an accessory or deep portion laterally, which joins the anterolateral ring of the atlas to the posterior body of the axis.

Posteriorly, the occiput is joined to the posterior ring of the atlas by a broad but thin and elastic posterior atlanto-occipital ligament (see Fig. 49–13B). The posterior ring of the atlas is joined to the lamina of the axis by the analogous ligamentum flavum.

The dens forms a pivotal position within the atlantoaxial joint. The majority of the atlantoaxial ligaments are lax, permitting almost 90 degrees of rotation to both sides and 15 degrees of flexion and extension. The dens and its integral ligaments, particularly the transverse ligament, are primarily responsible for stability at this joint. The intact dens limits posterior displacement of the ring of the atlas, and the ligaments limit anterior and lateral displacements as well as rotation. In our clinical experience, the dens ordinarily fractures before its ligaments give way. Rheumatoid degeneration or pure shearing injuries, such as a violent blow to the back of the head, can produce pure ligament injuries at this joint without fractures.[4]

Fractures of the ring of the atlas may be reasonably stable as long as the transverse ligament remains intact.[10] When the transverse ligament has ruptured, the ring may spread laterally, and atlantoaxial stability may be impaired. This can be identified on open-mouth, anteroposterior roentgenograms of the odontoid. Spence and colleagues[19] note that when the transverse measurement of the atlas is 7 mm wider than the axis, rupture of the transverse ligament should be suspected.

Ligaments of the Lower Cervical Spine

The lower five cervical articulations between the second and seventh cervical vertebrae are similar anatomically. We studied the ligaments of the lower cervical spine in 15 fresh cadaver spines, 19 to 73 years of age.[12] Eight intervertebral ligaments were found, four anterior to the spinal canal and four posterior to it.

The anterior longitudinal ligament is a thin, translucent structure, closely adherent to the midportion of the vertebral bodies (see Fig. 49–11). The ligament is thickest and widest in the frontal plane over the disc spaces and blends intimately with the underlying annulus fibrosus.

The annulus fibrosus is a dense, fibrous structure firmly bonded to the cartilaginous end plates. It blends completely with the anterior and posterior longitudinal ligaments. In none of the specimens dissected was a discrete nucleus pulposus found. The whole of the intervertebral disc was occupied by dense ligament, the largest ligament of the cervical spine.

The posterior longitudinal ligament is a thick band of dense, fibrous tissue running over the posterior vertebral bodies (Figs. 49–15*B* and *C* and 49–16) that is considerably thicker than its anterior counterpart. It is firmly attached to the posterior lips of the vertebral bodies and blends intimately with the fibers of the

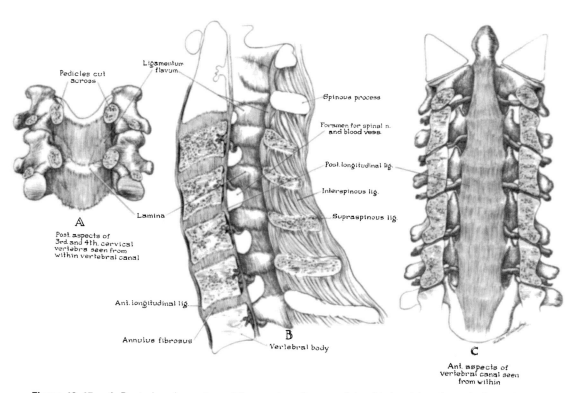

Figure 49–15. *A,* Posterior elements and ligamentum flavum of the third and fourth cervical vertebrae viewed from within the spinal canal looking posteriorly. *B,* Longitudinal cross section of the cervical spine. *C,* Posterior longitudinal ligament viewed from within the spinal canal looking anteriorly. Note the nutrient vessels entering the space beneath the ligament from the sides. (From Johnson, R. M., et al.: Some new observations on the functional anatomy of the lower cervical spine. Clin. Orthop. *3:*192–200, 1975.)

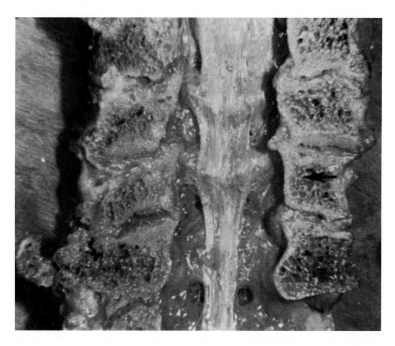

Figure 49–16. Posterior longitudinal ligament viewed from within the spinal canal looking anteriorly. The spine has been divided longitudinally through the pillars of the facets in the lower cervical and upper thoracic spine. The arrow is at the level of the seventh cervical vertebra. Note that the posterior longitudinal ligament narrows significantly in the lower cervical and upper thoracic spine.

annulus. In most cases, it is not attached to the concave midportion of the vertebral bodies, leaving a space between the bone and ligament. The nutrient vessels enter this space from the side and disappear into the small nutrient foramina at the midportion of the vertebral bodies. The ligament appears as an undulating band, widest at the disc spaces and narrowest at the midportion of the vertebral body. The ligament is widest in the frontal plane in the upper cervical spine and becomes progressively narrower but thicker in the lower cervical and upper thoracic spine (see Fig. 49–16).

Running longitudinally between adjacent costotransverse processes is a thin, fibrous septum that joins the anterior lips of one transverse process to the next (see Fig. 49–11). This thin, translucent septum lies beneath the overlying intertransverse muscles and is just anterior to the vertebral artery.

The ligamentum nuchae is a fibrous midline intermuscular septum, attached to the spinous processes and paracervical muscles. In humans it has relatively few elastic fibers and appears to provide little intrinsic structural support, although in bovines it is most prominent and contains many elastic fibers.[3]

The supraspinous and interspinous ligaments connect the spinous processes of the cervical vertebrae (Figs. 49–17 and 49–18). As Halliday and coworkers[7] found, these structures are often poorly defined or incomplete in the upper cervical spine. In the lower levels, they become better and more consistently developed. The supraspinous ligaments are a continuation of the ligamentum nuchae. They overlap and cross at midline, are attached to the bifid spinous processes, and blend with the interspinous ligaments anteriorly. The interspinous ligaments join the inferior aspect of one vertebral spine to the superior aspect of the subja-

cent spine. The fibers tend to run obliquely from the upper vertebrae, posteriorly to the next lower spine.

The ligamentum flavum joins the lamina of one vertebra to the lamina of the next (see Fig. 49–15A). It is a thick, orange-yellow ligament that is grossly elastic.

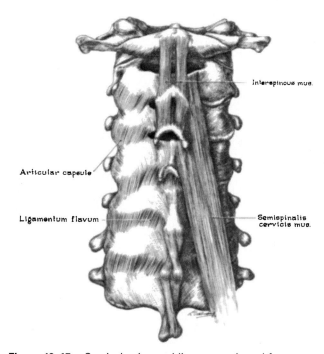

Figure 49–17. Cervical spine and ligaments viewed from behind. The supraspinous ligaments are attached to the bifid spinous processes and cross one another at the midline. (From Johnson, R. M., et al.: Some new observations on the functional anatomy of the lower cervical spine. Clin. Orthop. *3*:192–200, 1975.)

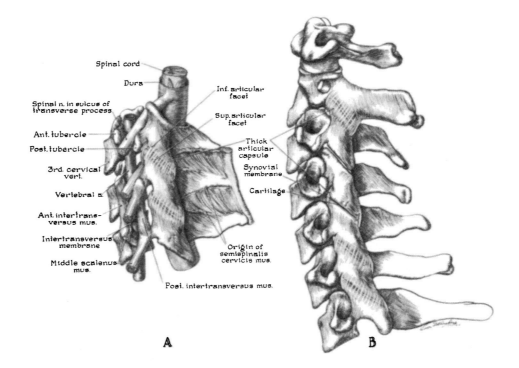

Figure 49–18. *A, B,* Cervical spine, facets, and capsular ligaments viewed from the side. (From Johnson, R. M., et al.: Some new observations on the functional anatomy of the lower cervical spine. Clin. Orthop. *3:*192–200, 1975.)

It connects the anterior and inferior aspects of the upper lamina with the superior aspect of the subjacent lamina. Most of this ligament is contained within the spinal canal.

The facet joints are covered with a thin layer of cartilage. Between the facets and beneath the capsular ligament is a thin band of synovial tissue that appears to surround the joint and is loosely attached to the capsule. The capsular ligaments bind the facets together, beginning anterolaterally at the transverse process and extending posteromedially, in a 180-degree arc, to the lamina (see Fig. 49–18). The capsular ligaments are short but thick fibrous structures. The fibers of the ligament are arranged at a 90-degree angle to the plane of the facet joint and are firmly bound to the bony prominence above and below the facet, extending a total length of only 5 to 7 mm.

The anterior longitudinal ligament, although thin and translucent, appears on the basis of our biomechanical studies to effectively limit extension of the spine.[11, 16, 22] The annulus fibrosus is a thick, dense structure that is more firmly attached to the outer perimeter of the vertebral body than the central cartilaginous plate. Its fibers are arranged in circumferential lamellae, with one layer running 60 degrees obliquely to the next. This arrangement, plus its size, effectively limits shear movements between the vertebrae, for shear displacement in any direction increases the tension along at least a portion of its fibers. With age and degeneration, hemorrhages, tears, and fissures appear in the ligament, which reduces its functional strength. Ultimately, the disc space narrows, and bony osteophytes may bridge the gap between vertebral bodies, increasing strength at the expense of mobility.

The posterior longitudinal ligament appears to limit flexion as well as intervertebral distraction.[11] It is thick and wide and appears to protect the spinal cord at the cervical level from posterior protrusion of disc material. Laterally, the nerve roots are not similarly protected, and disc material may protrude into the neuroforamina and irritate the roots. As long as the posterior longitudinal ligament remains intact, the spinal cord may be protected during anterior surgical dissections of the disc or body, but the nerve roots laterally are not similarly protected.

Halliday and associates[7] report that the supraspinous and interspinous ligaments are often poorly defined or incomplete in the upper cervical spine, whereas in the lower cervical levels they become better and more consistently developed. Our gross anatomic observations were similar; however, biomechanical trials indicated that the ligaments did consistently limit flexion and anterior horizontal displacement.[11, 16, 22] We must conclude that although the supraspinous and interspinous ligaments are not well defined anatomically, they are active functionally and should be spared, if possible, in posterior surgical approaches.

The capsular ligaments have been described as "thin and lax," contributing little to the strength of the spine. In our study, they consistently appeared thick and dense but did permit considerable motion within well-defined limits. This controlled motion appears to be related to the orientation of the ligament fibers perpendicular to the plane of the facet. When the facet is in a neutral or fully opposed position, the capsular ligament is most lax. As the facet glides forward or back from midposition, the capsular fibers progressively tighten, effectively limiting motion of more than 2 to 3 mm from the neutral position (Fig. 49–19A). The 45-degree plane of the facets appears to contribute to flexion of the cervical vertebrae and stabilizes the vertebrae by limiting anterior displacements. When the facets were removed, flexion was consistently decreased, but anterior horizontal displacement increased.[11] Because of this stabilizing effect, the facets and capsular ligaments should be spared, if possible, in posterior surgical approaches to the spine.

A large volume of the ligamentum flavum is found within the posterior spinal canal. Because of its inherent elasticity, the ligament normally contracts on itself when the neck is extended. With age or degeneration, however, this elasticity may be lost, and the ligament may bulge with neck extension and may protrude into the spinal canal and cord (Fig. 49–19B).

Deep Anterior Vessels and Nerves

The vertebral artery is the first branch of the subclavian artery. It passes directly to the costotransverse foramen of the sixth cervical vertebra, ascending through successive vertebral foramina (see Fig. 49–11) to the first vertebra. At the atlas it leaves the costotransverse foramen and curves posteriorly and medially over the posterior ring of the first vertebra, penetrates the posterior atlanto-occipital ligament, and ascends through the foramen magnum. Here it joins the artery from the opposite side to form the basilar artery, which leads to the circle of Willis at the base of the brain. The vertebral

vein draining the suboccipital region enters the transverse process at the first vertebra and descends through the costotransverse foramina in company with the artery. A portion of the sympathetic chain also accompanies the artery and vein through these foramina. Care is required prior to blind ligation of the vertebral artery because the nerve root passes directly behind the artery and could be traumatized during this maneuver. Unilateral ligation of the vertebral artery is ordinarily safe in younger individuals. In older individuals, such ligation may result in basilar artery insufficiency and receptive blindness owing to ischemia of the calcarine fissure. The left vertebral artery is ordinarily dominant, but there is enough anatomic variation that preoperative angiography is recommended. If there is a discrepancy in size, the larger vertebral artery should be considered dominant and spared if possible. Hadley[6] pointed out that spurs arising from the facets or joints of Luschka may impinge on the vertebral arteries (Fig. 49–20). The vertebral artery may be exposed through the anterolateral approach described by Henry,[8] discussed in "Anterior Cervical Approaches" later in this chapter. The longus capitis and colli muscles are reflected anteriorly, and the anterior portion of the transverse process over the foramen is removed using rongeurs to expose the artery beneath.

The cervical sympathetic chain is a deep structure, closely associated with the longus capitis and colli muscles. It lies in a loose reflection of the carotid sheath along the anterior surface of the lateral masses and

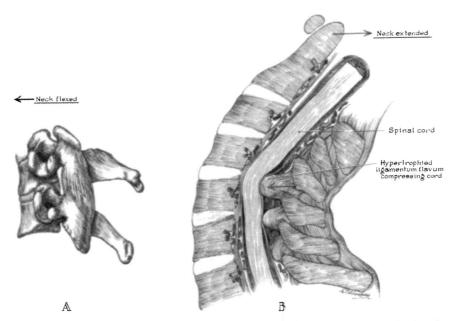

Figure 49–19. *A,* Two cervical vertebrae viewed from the side in flexion. Note that in flexion the spinous processes separate, the superior facet glides forward and anteriorly on its subjacent facet, and the disc space separates posteriorly and approximates anteriorly. The fibers of the capsular ligaments are no longer aligned perpendicular to the plane of the facets. They are oriented obliquely and are taut, limiting further gliding anteriorly. *B,* Longitudinal cross section of the cervical spine in extension illustrating a hypertrophied and relatively inelastic ligamentum flavum protruding into the spinal cord. (From Johnson, R. M., et al.: Some new observations on the functional anatomy of the lower cervical spine. Clin. Orthop. *3:*192–200, 1975.)

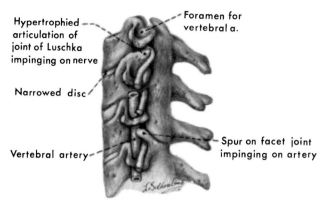

Figure 49–20. Encroachment of the neural foramen and vertebral artery by hypertrophic osteoarthritic spurs. (From Robinson, R. A., and Southwick, W. O.: Surgical Approaches to the Cervical Spine. *In* the American Academy of Orthopaedic Surgeons: Instructional Course Lectures, Vol. XVII. St. Louis, The C. V. Mosby Co., 1960.)

prevertebral muscles. It extends from the second cervical vertebra downward and has three ganglionic enlargements: the superior ganglion, beside the second and third cervical vertebrae; the middle ganglion (sometimes lacking), beside the sixth; and the inferior ganglion. The inferior ganglion is frequently fused with the first thoracic vertebra just below the seventh cervical vertebra to form the stellate ganglion. A simple and effective method of blocking the stellate ganglion is to

retract the carotid sheath with a finger at the level of the sixth cervical vertebra and infiltrate a local anesthetic into the space between the prevertebral and alar fasciae (see Fig. 49–6), with the patient sitting up. A block is usually effective in a few minutes, when the anesthetic solution rolls down between these fascial layers, and may be recognized by pupillary constriction on the affected side.

The hypoglossal nerve (Fig. 49–21) courses anteriorly over the carotid artery just above the greater horn of the hyoid bone. It rests on the hypoglossus muscle and bends upward under the posterior belly of the digastric. It is usually slightly superior and superficial to the lingual artery, a branch of the external carotid, and is usually not exposed unless one is approaching the upper two cervical vertebrae anteriorly. In this approach it should be identified and protected.

The ansa hypoglossi is a nerve loop derived from the first, second, and third cervical nerve roots and travels as two separate limbs into the neck, the upper root anteriorly and the lower root located more posteriorly on the carotid sheath. The upper root, or descendens hypoglossi, travels with the hypoglossal nerve. It separates from the hypoglossal nerve at the angle of the mandible and descends over the carotid sheath, giving off branches to the omohyoid, sternothyroid, and sternohyoid muscles. The branches to these muscles are given off in the midcervical region and are not usually disturbed in anterior approaches to the middle and lower neck, as the plane of dissection is between these and the carotid sheath. However, in exposures to

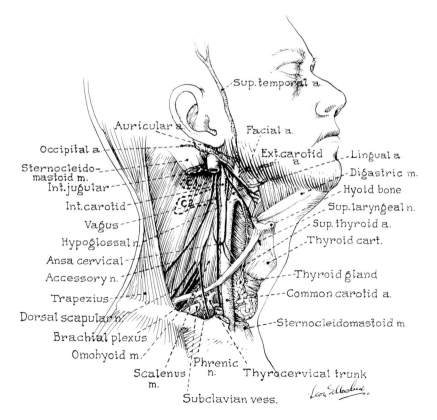

Figure 49–21. Deep structures of the anterior and posterior triangles of the neck. (From Robinson, R. A., and Southwick, W. O.: Surgical Approaches to the Cervical Spine. *In* the American Academy of Orthopaedic Surgeons: Instructional Course Lectures, Vol. XVII. St. Louis, The C. V. Mosby Co., 1960.)

the upper vertebrae, anterior and medial to the carotid, these may be stretched or injured. Another smaller branch of the descendens hypoglossi travels with the hypoglossal nerve anteriorly and supplies the geniohyoid and thyrohyoid muscles high in the neck. The upper root of the ansa cervicalis loops posteriorly in the lower neck and joins the lower root of the ansa, which emerges from behind the jugular vein and crosses the carotid artery.

The internal jugular vein and common carotid arteries are buried beneath the sternomastoid muscle within the carotid sheath. The sheath and its contents may be identified by the pulsations of the carotid artery. The carotid divides at the upper border of the thyroid cartilage into the internal and external carotid arteries. The internal carotid remains within the carotid sheath and yields no branches within the neck. The external carotid gives off one branch below the hyoid bone, the superior thyroid artery, which loops conveniently upward before descending to give off its hyoid and superior laryngeal branches. Inferior to this loop, the carotid sheath may be separated from the visceral fascia (containing the trachea and esophagus) to expose the cervical vertebral bodies without ligating a single artery.

The pharyngeal and superior laryngeal branches of the vagus nerve lie deep to the carotid and superior thyroid arteries and supply the trachea, the muscles of the posterior pharynx, and the cricothyroid and pro-

vide sensory innervation to the larynx. Because they run in a longitudinal, oblique course, they are not damaged by retraction except in exposures of the upper spine anterior to the carotid sheath. The recurrent laryngeal nerve on the right (Fig. 49–22) arises from the vagus at the level of the subclavian artery, loops beneath the subclavian artery, and ascends between the trachea and esophagus, protected by the visceral fascia. The left recurrent nerve arises at the level of the aortic arch within the thorax and loops beneath the arch to ascend between the trachea and esophagus. Excessive retraction has caused temporary paralysis of the recurrent nerve following the anterior cervical approaches. Because the right recurrent laryngeal nerve can recur above the level of the subclavian artery, it may be injured in a right anterolateral approach. For this reason, we prefer to approach the neck to the left of the midline.

Structures of the Posterior Triangle

Deep to the superficial layer of the deep fascia, the spinal accessory and third and fourth cervical nerves emerge from the posterior border of the sternomastoid to innervate the trapezius muscle. The posterior belly of the omohyoid is one or two finger breadths above the clavicle and is covered by a thin, additional layer of fascia, the omohyoid-sternohyoid fascia, which

Figure 49–22. Arteries and nerves at the base of the neck on the right side. The right recurrent laryngeal nerve arises from the vagus at the level of the subclavian artery, loops beneath the subclavian artery, and ascends between the trachea and esophagus. The right recurrent laryngeal nerve can recur above the level of the subclavian artery and could be injured in an approach to the middle cervical spine to the right of the midline.

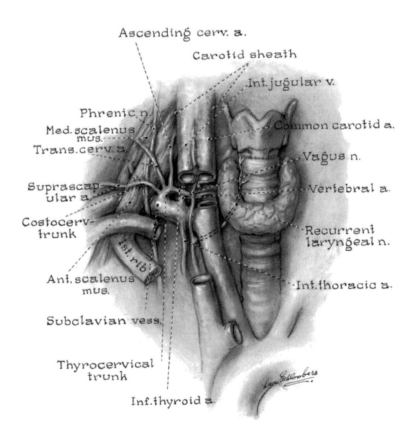

forms its sling. The external jugular vein crosses the sternomastoid at the midpoint of the posterior triangle.

The floor of the posterior triangle (see Figs. 49–5 and 49–21) is formed by several muscles, the most central being the levator scapulae deep to the spinal accessory nerve. It inserts on the vertebral border of the scapula and originates from the transverse processes of the first four cervical vertebrae. Superior to the levator scapulae is the splenius capitis, and inferior to the levator are the scaleni (see Fig. 49–10). The scalene muscles arise from the tubercles of the cervical transverse processes and insert on the first and second ribs. The scalenus anterior is separated from the scalenus medius and posterior by the brachial plexus and subclavian artery. The brachial plexus lies deep to the prevertebral or scalenus fascia. Its cords are covered by a sheath of prevertebral fascia as they descend into the axilla. The plexus is formed from the anterior rami of the fifth cervical to the first thoracic nerve.

The scalenus anterior is occasionally thought to encroach upon the subclavian artery and brachial plexus, particularly in the presence of a cervical rib, and may be sectioned surgically for the relief of pain. This exposure is described later with the Nanson anterolateral approach to the lower cervical vertebrae. The phrenic nerve crosses the midportion of the scalenus anterior, beneath the prevertebral fascia, and should be identified prior to scalenus section. It arises from the anterior ramus of the fourth cervical root, receives twigs from the third and fifth roots, crosses the first part of the subclavian artery, and enters the thorax to innervate the diaphragm. The thoracic duct is found at the base of the neck on the left, between the phrenic nerve and carotid sheath. It loops over the subclavian artery at the level of the first thoracic vertebra anterior to the scalenus anterior and phrenic nerve and enters the subclavian vein.

The Back of the Neck

The structures of this area are described in the order in which they are encountered surgically, from superficial to deep. Stretching in the midline from the external occipital protuberance to the spinous process of the seventh cervical vertebra is a fibrous intermuscular septum known as the ligamentum nuchae. Lateral to this and deep to the superficial fascia is the trapezius muscle. This is attached to the ligamentum nuchae, the dorsal vertebrae, and the medial border of the superior nuchal line and inserts into the scapula and clavicle. Just lateral to its superior border lies the great occipital nerve and the occipital artery. In the lower part of the neck, the rhomboid minor and serratus posterior superior muscles attach to the ligamentum nuchae and the seventh cervical spinous process to run obliquely downward toward the scapula and ribs. The next deeper muscle encountered is the splenius capitis (Fig. 49–23), arising from the lower half of the ligamentum nuchae and the upper six thoracic vertebrae to attach deep to the sternomastoid on the occiput. The splenius cervicis arises from the upper six thoracic vertebrae,

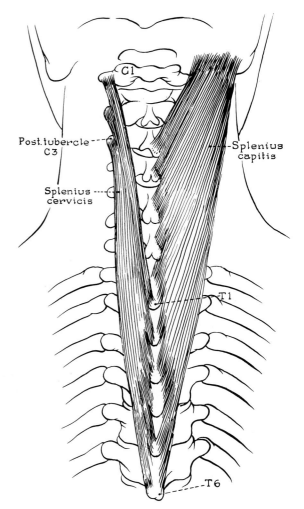

Figure 49–23. Deep muscles of the back of the neck, the splenius capitis and cervicis. These act as extensors of the head and neck, respectively.

passes deep to the levator scapulae, and inserts on the posterior tubercles of the first, second, and third cervical vertebrae. Deep to the splenius is the semispinalis capitis and cervicis (Fig. 49–24), a long muscle group that originates through a series of tendinous slips from the articular processes of the fourth, fifth, and sixth cervical vertebrae and from the transverse processes of the upper five or six thoracic vertebrae. It has a thick insertion on the occipital bone and is pierced by the greater occipital nerve. The deeper muscles of this group, the iliocostalis and longissimus cervicis, are rarely separated in the usual surgical approaches to the back of the neck (Fig. 49–25).

There are a group of small head extensors, including the rectus capitis posterior major and minor and the superior and inferior capitis obliques, all attaching to the spinous or transverse processes of the axis (see Fig. 49–24). These muscles must be mobilized in posterior approaches to the atlas and axis. The inferior oblique muscle has been implicated as a cause of entrapment of the greater occipital nerve as this nerve emerges from beneath this muscle belly.

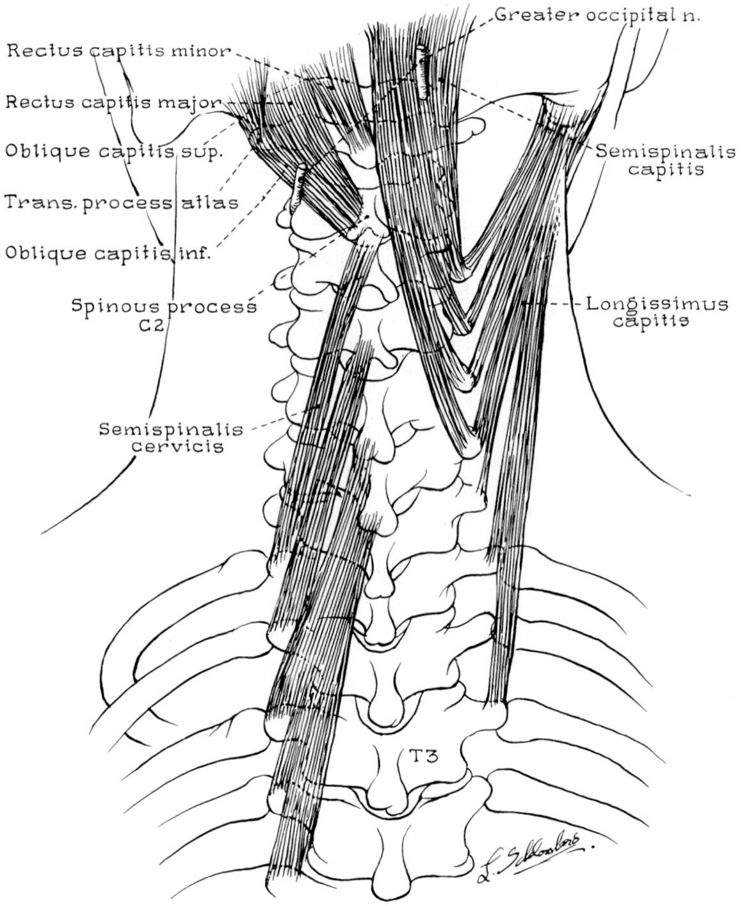

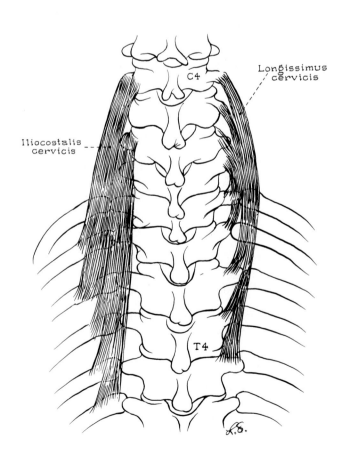

Figure 49–24. Deep muscles of the back of the neck, the semispinalis and short-head extensors.

Figure 49–25. The deepest muscles of the back of the neck, the iliocostalis cervicis and longissimus cervicis.

References

1. Bosch, A., Stauffer, E. S., and Nickel, V. L.: Incomplete traumatic quadriplegia: A ten year review. Final report, Regional Spinal Cord Injury Rehabilitation Center, Rancho Los Amigos Hospital, Giii–Gv, 1972.
2. Fielding, J. W.: Normal and abnormal motion of the cervical spine from C2 to C7, cineroentgenography. J. Bone Joint Surg. [Am.] 46:1779–1782, 1964.
3. Fielding, J. W., Burstein, A. H., and Frankel, V. H.: The nuchal ligament. Spine 1:3–14, 1976.
4. Fielding, J. W., Cochran, G. V. B., Lawsing, J. F., and Hohl, M.: Tears of the transverse ligament of the atlas. J. Bone Joint Surg. [Am.] 56:1683–1691, 1974.
5. Grodinsky, M., and Holyoke, E. A.: The fasciae and facial spaces of the head, neck, and adjacent regions. Am. J. Anat. 63:367–408, 1938.
6. Hadley, L. A.: Covertebral articulations and cervical foramen encroachment. J. Bone Joint Surg. [Am.] 39:910–920, 1957.
7. Halliday, D. R., Sullivan, C. R., Hollinshead, W. H., and Bahn, R. C.: Torn cervical ligaments: Necropsy examination of normal cervical region. J. Trauma 4:219–232, 1964.
8. Henry, A. K.: Extensile Exposure. 2nd ed. Edinburgh, Essex, Longman Group Ltd., 1970, pp. 53–80.
9. Hohl, M.: Normal motions in the upper portion of the cervical spine. J. Bone Joint Surg. [Am.] 46:1777–1779, 1964.
10. Jefferson, G.: Fracture of the atlas vertebra. Report of four cases, and a review of those previously recorded. Br. J. Surg. 7:407–422, 1920.
11. Johnson, R. M.: Biomechanical stability of the lower cervical spine. Thesis, Yale University School of Medicine, Section of Orthopaedic Surgery, 1973, pp. 1–58.
12. Johnson, R. M., Crelin, E. S., White, A. A., et al.: Some new observations on the functional anatomy of the lower cervical spine. Clin. Orthop. 3:192–200, 1975.
13. Lysell, E.: Motion in the cervical spine. Acta Orthop. Scand. Suppl. 123:1–61, 1969.
14. Nanson, E. M.: The anterior approach to upper dorsal sympathectomy. Surg. Gynecol. Obstet. 104:118–120, 1957.
15. Panjabi, M. M., Brand, R. A., and White, A. A.: Mechanical properties of the human thoracic spine. J. Bone Joint Surg. [Am.] 58:642–652, 1976.
16. Panjabi, M. M., White, A. A., and Johnson, R. M.: Cervical spine mechanics as a function of transection of components. J. Biomech. 8:327–336, 1975.
17. Perry, J., and Nickel, V. L.: Total cervical spine fusion for neck paralysis. J. Bone Joint Surg. [Am.] 41:37–60, 1959.
18. Ruff, S.: Brief acceleration: Less than one second. German Aviation Medicine, World War II. Vol. 1, p. 584, 1950. The Surgeon General.
19. Spence, K. F., Decker, S., and Sell, K. W.: Bursting atlantal fracture associated with rupture of the transverse ligament. J. Bone Joint Surg. [Am.] 52:543–549, 1970.
20. Verbiest, H.: Anterolateral operation for fractures and dislocations in the middle and lower parts of the cervical spine. J. Bone Joint Surg. [Am.] 51:1489–1530, 1969.
21. White, A. A.: Analysis of the mechanics of the thoracic spine in man. An experimental study in autopsy specimens. Thesis. Acta Orthop. Scand. (Suppl.) 127:1–105, 1969.
22. White, A. A., Johnson, R. M., Panjabi, M. M., and Southwick, W. O.: Biomechanical analysis of clinical stability in the cervical spine. Clin. Orthop. 109:85–96, 1975.
23. Whitesides, T. E., Jr., and Kelly, R. P.: Lateral approach to the upper cervical spine for anterior fusion. South. Med. J. 59:879–883, 1966.

Surgical Approaches to the Cervical Spine

APPROACHES TO THE CERVICAL SPINE

Anterior Versus Posterior

Under most circumstances, the choice of approach to the cervical spine should be dictated by the site of the primary pathologic condition. For example, to biopsy a tumor of the vertebral body, the most direct approach is anterior. There are, however, certain indications for and limitations to each approach.

Anterior

The anterior approach provides the most direct access to the vertebral body, vertebral artery, and transverse processes. The anterior approach is the most direct means of removing an osteophyte on the posterior wall of the vertebral body that is protruding into the spinal canal or nerve roots. It is also the most appropriate route to decompress the spinal cord when a vertebral body is fractured and displaced posteriorly into the canal (Fig. 49–26). In this situation, the spinal cord may be tethered to or tented over these fragments and may not be adequately relieved by laminectomy alone, and attempts to remove these bony fragments around the cord may only cause further neurologic damage.

The major limitation to anterior exposures is that most fusion techniques from the front do not add to spinal stability immediately after surgery, and in some cases stability is removed. This is particularly true when the primary injury occurs over the posterior elements and the last threads of remaining stability are in the front.[62] In these conditions, anterior fusion removes these last elements of continuity and creates a precarious situation. Figure 49–27A is the preoperative lateral roentgenogram illustrating a fracture through the body of C5. This was wired and fused anteriorly in an attempt to improve stability, but despite this, progressive anterior displacement occurred (Fig. 49–27B). Stabilization was ultimately provided with interspinous wiring and fusion. Figure 49–28A and B are the roentgenograms taken at the time of and immediately after surgery of an unstable spine fused anteriorly between the fourth and fifth cervical vertebral bodies. Because of this posterior instability, the fourth vertebra continued to migrate anteriorly on the fifth (Fig. 49–28C). Posterior interspinous wiring and fusion were required to stop this progressive anterior displacement. Figure 49–29A is an example of what may happen following anterior fusion when the graft is not properly fixed or "keyed" into the adjacent vertebrae and there is associated posterior instability. This 20-year-old man

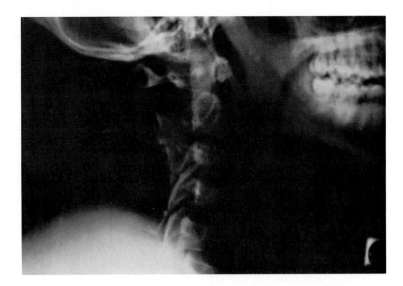

Figure 49–26. Traumatic fracture and posterior displacement of the fifth cervical vertebral body with associated quadriplegia.

was struck by a car and sustained a fracture-dislocation of the fifth cervical vertebra with posterior displacement of the vertebral body into the spinal canal and incomplete spinal cord injury. The vertebral body was excised to decompress the spinal canal, and the body was replaced with a fibular strut graft wedged between the adjacent vertebrae. Shortly after surgery the graft

moved posteriorly and to the right into the spinal canal, and all function of the fifth and sixth cervical nerve roots on the right was lost (Fig. 49–29B). Nine weeks later the fibular graft was removed and replaced with an iliac graft using keys (see Fig. 49–66A) to secure the graft to the upper and lower vertebral body. Because of the extensive injury to the posterior liga-

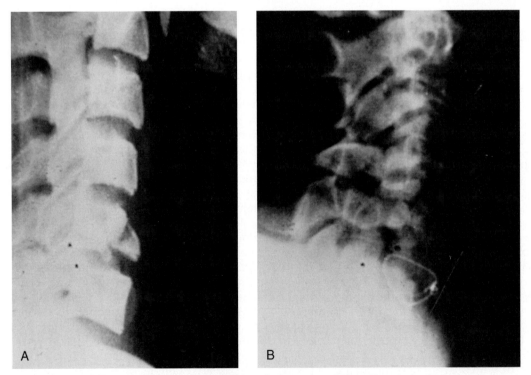

Figure 49–27. *A,* Traumatic fracture of the fifth cervical vertebra. *B,* Despite anterior fusion and wire stabilization, the fifth vertebral body continued to migrate anteriorly on the sixth beneath. Note the position of the marks on the posterior aspect of the fifth and sixth vertebral bodies *(A)* and the subsequent position in *(B)* after anterior subluxation.

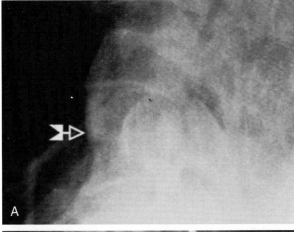

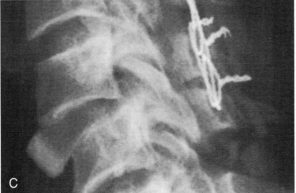

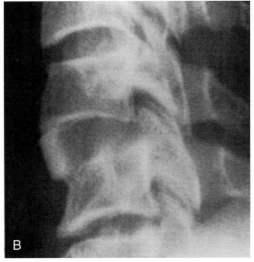

Figure 49–28. Anterior stabilization and fusion at C4–C5 for flexion injury at this level with posterior instability. Radiographs taken of the graft during surgery *(A)* and postoperatively *(B)*. *C,* Despite external stabilization with a brace, the graft and fourth vertebra continued to migrate anteriorly, requiring posterior interspinous wiring and fusion.

ments, posterior wiring and fusion were performed to increase the immediate stability and to speed rehabilitation without the use of a halo-cast (see Fig. 49–66*B* and *C*). Twenty-four months after this procedure, the patient has regained a significant return of motor and sensory function and is walking with crutches and a short leg brace on the left leg.

Posterior

The posterior approach provides the most direct access to the spinous processes, laminae, and facets. In addition, the spinal canal may be explored and decompressed over a large area with less loss of stability than equivalent anterior decompression would afford. Laminectomy does remove some intrinsic stability, but the immediate integrity of the spine is not usually jeopardized. Conversely, resection of one or more vertebral bodies creates an obvious problem, and these bodies must be replaced, and the spine must be rigidly supported until fusion is established.

Certain posterior fusion techniques using wire through the spinous processes or facets offer increased strength immediately after surgery through internal stabilization. The anterior elements do not offer similar vantage points for internal fixation, and the surrounding structures, such as the esophagus, may be injured by wires, plates, or screws. Therefore, in very

unstable situations where improved strength through internal fixation may be needed, posterior wiring and bone graft offer the advantage of increased immediate strength, whereas most anterior fusion techniques do not. Once osseous union is complete, however, there does not appear to be any advantage of posterior over anterior methods of fusion.

Selection of Approach and Level of Involvement

The posterior approach through a midline longitudinal incision provides access to the posterior elements at all levels of the cervical spine. The standard anterior approach through a transverse incision provides adequate access from the third through seventh cervical vertebrae. However, the upper and lower anterior cervical elements have to be approached more selectively because of certain anatomic restrictions.

Anterior

The basiocciput may be reached anteriorly through the pharynx by dividing the soft palate and part of the hard palate.[1, 59] This introduces the element of contamination by pharyngeal organisms and restricted working area but provides direct local access, suitable for

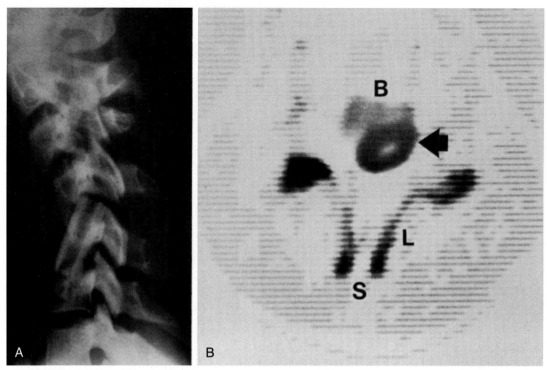

Figure 49–29. Posterior displacement of a vertebral body graft into the spinal canal with associated neural injury. This 20-year-old man was struck by a car and sustained a fracture-dislocation of the fifth cervical vertebra with posterior displacement of the vertebral body into the spinal canal and incomplete spinal cord injury. The vertebral body was excised to decompress the spinal canal, and the body was replaced with a fibular strut graft wedged between adjacent vertebrae. Shortly after surgery, the upper pole of the graft moved posteriorly and to the right into the spinal canal, and all function of the fifth and sixth cervical nerve roots on the right was lost. A, Lateral roentgenogram revealing the upper pole of the fibular vertebral body graft displaced posteriorly into the spinal canal and the posterior separation of the spinous processes suggesting associated posterior instability. B, Computed axial tomogram at the upper level of the fifth cervical vertebra and fibular graft. B, vertebral body; L, lamina; and S, spinous process of the fifth cervical vertebra. The arrow points to the fibular graft, which is displaced posteriorly and to the right into the spinal canal. Note the central lucency over the intramedullary canal of the fibular graft. (From Light, T. R., Wagner, F. C., Johnson, R. M., and Southwick, W. D.: Correlation of spinal instability and recovery of neurologic loss following cervical body replacement—A case report. Spine 5:392–394, 1980.)

biopsy, drainage, or limited resection. DeAndrade and MacNab[12] described an effective extraoral approach to this region through an oblique incision (Fig. 49–30A) parallel to the anterior border of the sternomastoid and medial to the carotid sheath. This requires retraction or division of certain laryngeal nerves that cross the neck anteriorly and may result in minor but persistent hoarseness.

The first and second cervical vertebrae may be reached directly anteriorly via the pharynx or antero-laterally through the approach described by Henry[22] and Whitesides and Kelly,[69] posterior to the carotid sheath. The transcutaneous anterolateral approach is made via an oblique incision at the anterior margin of the sternomastoid (Fig. 49–30B). The sternomastoid muscle is everted at its origin on the mastoid process, and the anterior elements of the spine are approached posterior to the carotid sheath. Because the internal carotid artery, jugular vein, and vagus and hypoglossal nerves are tethered to their foramina at the base of the skull and may not be retracted anteriorly with safety,

the upper limit of dissection is restricted to the anterior ring of the first vertebra, and the basiocciput cannot be reached.

The anterior bodies of the third through seventh cervical vertebrae are easily exposed via the anterior approach described by Robinson and Southwick,[48, 49] with dissection anterior and medial to the carotid sheath (Fig. 49–30C). The lower cervical and upper thoracic spine, as well as structures of the thoracic inlet, may be reached through the transverse supraclavicular approach (Fig. 49–30D) described by Nanson.[39] This approach provides limited exposure through the thoracic inlet, in many cases as far as the body of the third thoracic vertebra.

McAfee and colleagues[35] described a method of high anterior exposure for resection to the basiocciput. It is an extension of the original approach requiring considerable dissection of the upper fascia, which is adequate for resection of anterior tumors or other lesions that cross the midline in the upper anterior neck, described later in this section.

Posterior

Satisfactory access to all levels of the posterior cervical spine is afforded by the midline longitudinal incision made over the spinous processes. The incision is extended superiorly over the occiput for occipitocervical fusions and fusions of the atlas and axis.

Occipitocervical fusion is reserved for atlanto-occipital instability or if the ring of C1 is fractured and stability between the odontoid and anterior ring of the first vertebra is lost. It may also be required after extensive resection of the posterior ring of C1 or the anterior elements of the atlas and axis. Fractures of the base of the odontoid and ruptures of the transverse ligament with atlantoaxial dislocation are usually treated with the Brooks' circumlaminar wiring and bone graft at C1–C2 (see later in this chapter).

Fusion techniques below the level of the first cervical vertebra are selected dependent upon the amount of bone remaining in the posterior elements. If the spinous processes are intact, a simple interspinous wiring and fusion are performed. If the spinous processes and laminae have been sacrificed for the sake of decompression, the facets are wired and fused. If the laminae and facets are missing, a strut of cortical bone is bridged across the posterior defect and wired to the first intact spinous processes or facets, but additional anterior interbody fusions may be required to provide long-term stabilization in these cases.

Posterior laminectomy is ordinarily sufficient to ex-

pose and decompress the cervical cord posteriorly. Occasionally, part or all of a facet must also be removed to decompress a nerve root. If only one nerve root needs to be decompressed through the posterior approach, the laminotomy-foraminotomy exposure described by Scoville[54, 55] should be considered (described later in this chapter). This exposure is primarily indicated to excise a soft disc protruding into the neural foramen or causing unilateral single nerve root irritation.

PREOPERATIVE PREPARATIONS

Intraoperative Stabilization

Most surgical procedures of the cervical spine require some form of traction stabilization intraoperatively. The type of stabilization should be selected on the basis of the spinal instability present before surgery and the amount anticipated in the early postoperative period. The obviously unstable spine with associated paraplegia is controlled well with skull tongs of the Gardner-Wells type. These may be used before, during, or after surgery, but a turning frame or bed is required until healing is complete and internal stabilization is established. If a more rigid external support is required, which frees the patient from a turning frame and allows him or her to get out of bed, a halo-vest should be considered. Traction may be applied to the halo

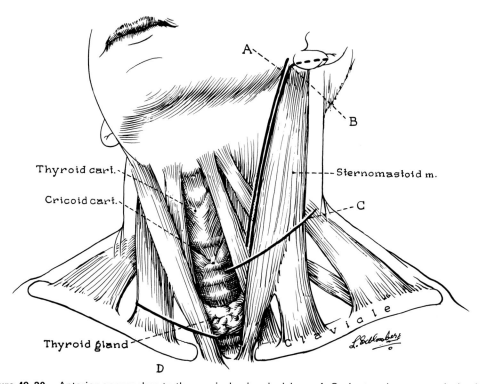

Figure 49–30. Anterior approaches to the cervical spine; incisions. *A,* Occiput and upper cervical spine medial to the carotid sheath. *B,* Anterior approach to the first and second vertebrae lateral to the carotid sheath. *C,* Anterior approach to the middle and lower cervical vertebrae medial to the carotid sheath. *D,* Anterior approach to the lower cervical and upper thoracic vertebrae.

before or during surgery, and the halo may be fixed to a body jacket following surgery to mobilize the patient out of bed. Most surgical approaches to the neck may be performed with the halo and body jacket in place, but they cause inconvenience to the surgeon.

In some circumstances, traction is only required intraoperatively. Posterior cervical wiring and fusion techniques often add enough immediate stability that simple braces are sufficient to protect the spine postoperatively. For most posterior approaches, we prefer a three-point pin headrest with countertraction applied to the shoulders to maintain position and alignment during surgery. With uncomplicated anterior interbody fusion, minimal external support as well as a short period of longitudinal distraction is needed. We use a simple head halter with 5 to 10 pounds of weight and increase the distraction briefly during graft insertion.

Head-Halter Traction. In an elective case in which there is no cervical instability, head traction is set up after endotracheal intubation is completed (see Fig. 49–50). A disposable halter is applied to the chin and occiput, using a spreader to align the halter ropes surrounding the ears. Then a rope is attached to the spreader bar, which passes over the ether screen (in a position of about 40 degrees of flexion to hold the head in neutral position). One or two rolled surgical towels are placed underneath the middle of the back of the neck to maintain the normal lordotic position during surgery. This position is important in maintaining an open disc space while tapping in the iliac bone graft. The shoulders are gently pulled distally, using 3-in adhesive tape going from the spine of the scapula over the lateral clavicle and deltoid down to attach to the side rail of the operating table to provide countertraction. This makes it possible to depress the shoulders to obtain lateral cervical spine radiographs of the lower vertebra during the operation. A soft, padded doughnut headrest is positioned under the occiput to

prevent pressure on the head. The position of the head should be rotated slightly (about 20 degrees). The neck should be in neutral position with the shoulders out of the way, but not stretching the anterior muscle or anterior fascia unduly. The operating table should be in mild, 20 degrees reversed Trendelenburg position to reduce pressure on the jugular system. This reduces the bleeding during the procedure. A normal disc excision should result in the loss of less than 1 to 2 oz of blood.

Crutchfield Tongs. The skull traction devices designed by Crutchfield and Vinke have been largely replaced in major U.S. hospital centers by Gardner-Wells tongs. However, because many of the Crutchfield and Vinke devices are still being used, the description of their insertion is included. These older tongs have the disadvantage of requiring more instrumentation, the use of drills, and a need for shaving a portion of the head to make small incisions for drilling. The Gardner-Wells system eliminates these additional preparations. A large area over the top of the head is shaved and surgically prepared. Using sterile marking solution, a line is drawn across the top of the head along the plane of the external auditory meatus. A cross mark is made at the vertex of the skull. The Crutchfield tongs themselves are used as a guide for making the drill holes. The points of the tongs approach the skull at right angles to the plane of the skull. The tongs should be opened to three fourths of their maximal width, with 10 to 11 cm separating the tips of the tongs (Fig. 49–31). If the tongs are not opened wide enough, the points will not satisfactorily penetrate the outer table and may pull out. If they are spread too far, the points of the tongs will approach the skull at an angle almost parallel with the direction of traction and also may pull out.

Using a sterile marking pen, cross marks are made at the points of insertion into the skull. Local anesthetic solution is infiltrated into the skin, subcutaneous tissues, and periosteum. A longitudinal incision is made

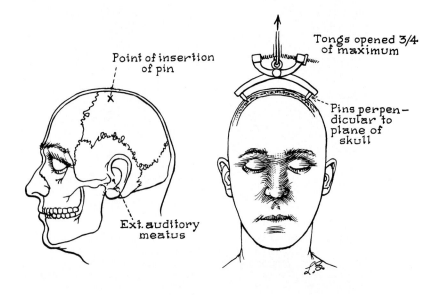

Figure 49–31. Crutchfield tongs are applied to the crown of the skull along the plane of the external auditory meatus. The points of the tongs should be perpendicular to the plane of the skull and are opened approximately three quarters of their maximal width.

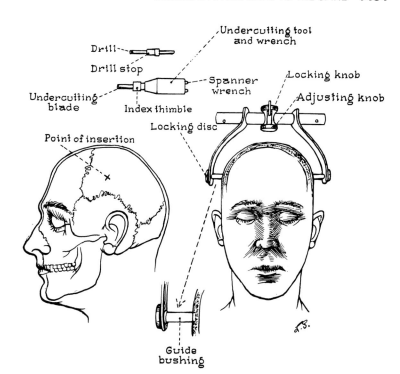

Figure 49–32. Vinke tongs are applied to the widest portion of the skull above the ears. Special tools are provided, such as a drill with a stop to prevent penetration of the inner table of the skull and an undercutting tool to cut the bone between the outer and inner tables of the skull. The points of the tongs are equipped with a flat eccentric metal table, which expands within the space cut between the outer and inner tables and locks the tongs to the skull.

to the bone with a small scalpel over the points of insertion. A special drill with safety flanges is used to drill the skull, permitting penetration through the outer table only. The drill depth is 3 mm in children and 4 mm in adults. The opened tongs are held by an assistant adjacent to the skin wounds and are used as a guide to proper placement and angle of the drill holes. The points of the tongs are inserted into the drill holes, and the tongs are tightened snugly and locked in place. Traction is applied to the ring at the center of the tongs. The wounds are dressed with small, cut gauze flaps and sealed with collodion.

The tongs should be checked daily and tightened only if loose. If the tongs are tightened too aggressively, they tend to penetrate the inner table. To flex or extend the neck, the traction pulley is placed anterior or posterior to the midsagittal plane. The tongs may be inserted anterior or posterior to the external auditory meatus to encourage flexion or extension, but this procedure limits later adjustments and changes in alignment.

Crutchfield[11] recommends traction weights according to the level of cervical involvement as outlined in Table 49–2. Traction should be applied within these limits, depending on the size and muscular development of the patient, the amount of paraspinal muscle spasm, and the type of injury. Traction weights exceeding these limits may be required temporarily to reduce a fracture-dislocation or locked facet. However, serial roentgenograms and frequent neurologic examinations should be performed when these limits are exceeded, and the patient should be constantly attended. Initially, roentgenograms should be made every day to check that no level of the cervical spine becomes excessively distracted as the paraspinal mus-

cle spasm subsides. Excessive distraction may impair satisfactory healing or may irritate the spinal cord or nerve roots.

Vinke Tongs. The Vinke tongs are somewhat easier to apply correctly than Crutchfield tongs, and there is less risk of them pulling out or penetrating the inner table of the skull. Because the pins of these tongs are larger and more elaborate, there is, in our experience, a higher incidence of local irritation or pin-tract infection than with Crutchfield tongs. The Vinke tongs fit over the horizontal aspect of the skull about the temporal ridge rather than at the apex (Fig. 49–32). Thus, the traction forces are applied at right angles to the longitudinal axis of the skull and body. The points of the tongs are equipped with a flat, eccentric metal table, which is locked into the space between the outer and inner tables of the skull. This prevents penetration through the inner table and reduces the risk of the tongs pulling out. Included with the tongs is a drill

Table 43–2. CERVICAL TRACTION WEIGHTS

Level of Injury	Minimum Weight in Pounds	Maximum Weight in Pounds
C1	5	10
C2	6	12
C3	8	15
C4	10	20
C5	12	25
C6	15	30
C7	18	35

that limits the depth of penetration into the bone. In addition, a tool is provided to undercut the bone between the outer and inner tables.

The tongs are inserted in the plane of the external auditory meatus about the temporal ridge. The skin is shaved locally and prepared surgically over the intended drill holes. Marks are made using sterile marking solution, and local anesthetic is infiltrated into the skin, subcutaneous tissue, and periosteum. A short longitudinal incision is made to the bone over the skin marks, using a small scalpel. The periosteum is elevated slightly, anteriorly and posteriorly, to allow the guide bushing to fit directly against the bone of the skull. The traction frame is closed against the skull and held by an assistant. The special drill is inserted through the guide bushing, and drilling is continued until the drill stop reaches the outer surface of the guide frame to ensure that a hole of sufficient depth is made. It is important to remove all bone chips from the drilled hole, and repeated clearing of the drill or saline irrigations are recommended. The undercutting blade is inserted through the guide bushing into the drill hole with the blade retracted into position 1. The index thimble is progressively advanced to position 5, and the blade is rotated clockwise at least one full revolution to complete the undercut. The undercutting tool is returned to position 1 and removed. The locking pins are inserted through the guide bushing into the skull, with the locks retracted. The locks are extended between the tables of the skull by turning the locking discs 180 degrees in either direction and are then snapped in place. At this point, the tongs are locked securely to the skull. The side frames are adjusted so the patient feels no pressure laterally. The side frames are locked into position with the locking knob, and the knob is tightened using the spanner wrench on the

handle of the undercutting tool. The wounds are dressed, and traction is applied to the traction bail or ring on the center bar.

Gardner-Wells Tongs. These tongs (Fig. 49–33) have largely replaced Crutchfield and Vinke tongs in most U.S. hospitals because they can be applied without removing hair and without drilling a hole in the outer table of the skull. They also provide more stable fixation that is less likely to slip out of place. The Gardner-Wells tongs consist of a C-shaped rectangular rod with an S-shaped link welded to its center, to which one can add the traction rope and weights. Also welded to this link are the directions for their use. At each end of the C that arches over the head are threaded bolts with sharp, pin-pointed ends. These sharp points are simply screwed in place. The points must be needle sharp. The entire apparatus should be sterilized prior to use. On one pin there is a spring device, which produces sufficient pressure to hold the pins in place by the pins penetrating the outer table of the skull when the indicator protrudes 1 mm.

With the head in neutral position, stabilized by sandbags if needed, the hair is combed and maintained vertically. An aerosol antiseptic, an organic iodine, or other type of antiseptic solution is rubbed into the area above each ear, in the plane of the external auditory meatus. With an assistant holding the Gardner-Wells tongs midline in the longitudinal axis, it is simple to visualize the exact insertion location for the points. As an assistant holds the tongs in position at the exact site for the pin insertion, the operator instills 5 ml of one half per cent lidocaine into the skin, subcutaneous tissue, scalp, and periosteum. At the same level on the opposite side, a similar anesthetic solution is instilled. Then the pins are twisted into place by hand twisting

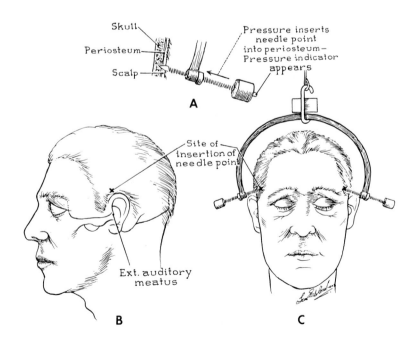

Figure 49–33. Gardner-Wells tongs may be applied without removing the patient's hair. The areas over the ears are thoroughly prepped with a sterilizing solution, and a local anesthesia is instilled into the skin, subcutaneous tissue, and the periosteum. Once the device is properly aligned, the screws are tightened until the pressure indicator appears.

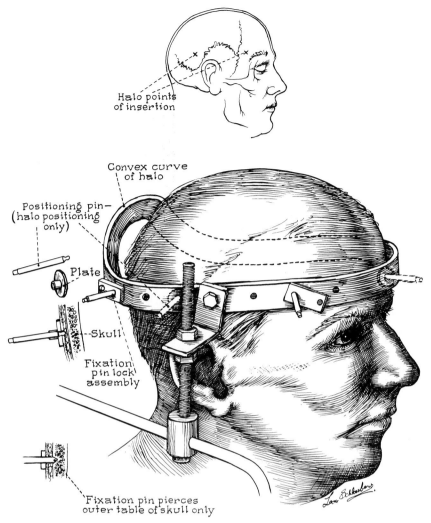

Figure 49–34. The halo-brace provides four-point skeletal fixation using pins that pierce the outer table of the skull. These pins are attached by threads to a circumferential steel ring. The pins are locked to the steel ring with a rectangular metal device with Allen screw lock. Traction may be applied to the ring, or the ring may be fixed to the torso through threaded steel uprights. The halo is placed just above the ears and eyebrows and is temporarily held in position with four positioning pins and plates that fit firmly against the skin. The skull pins are inserted just behind the eyebrows and ears and pierce the skin without an incision. These are tightened two at a time on opposite sides of the head using two torque screwdrivers. Torques should not exceed 5 in/lb in children or 6 in/lb in adults.

of the knurled knobs in this exact area without making any incision in the skin or drilling into the skull. The knurled handles of the pins are twisted with the fingers until the spring device pushes out 1 mm on the spring side of the Gardner-Wells tongs. At this point, the operator tilts the tongs back and forth to set the pins. Traction can then be applied. There are nuts on the threaded pins to fix the position depth exactly, and these should be tightened and left in place. Within 12 to 24 hours, a slight tightening should be tried; after this, the pins should not be disturbed.

Halo Traction.   The halo provides four-point skeletal fixation through a circumferential steel ring (Fig. 49–34). This rigidly controls the head and, when attached

to a body jacket with steel uprights (Fig. 49–35), permits mobilization of the patient without sacrificing control of the head and neck.[13, 28, 41, 42] The halo may be used with dynamic traction intraoperatively, or surgery may be performed between the steel uprights of the halo-body assembly. There is a cosmetic objection to the frontal pin placement in the forehead. However, these pin wounds ordinarily heal with a visible but small scar that is not cosmetically objectionable.

The skull pins have a thin, sharp point that pierces the outer table of the calvarium. These points are fragile and are easily blunted with repeated use. To improve fixation to the skull and to avoid the complication of these pins pulling out, new pins should be used with each application. Physiologic traction to 35

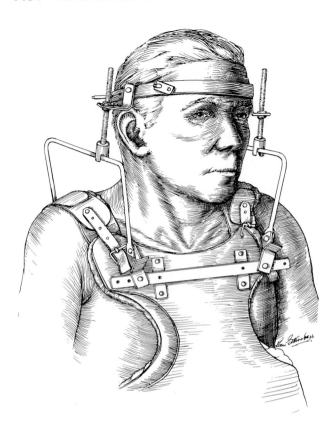

time, using torque screwdrivers, with the surgeon and assistant working simultaneously on diametrically opposed pins to prevent displacement of the ring. The same torques should be registered by the surgeon and assistant. Torques should not exceed 5 in/lb in children or 6 in/lb in adults. The pins enter the outer table. The most reliable indication of satisfactory pin placement is a gradually increasing bony resistance.[28] A sudden decrease in this resistance is a warning that the pin is entering the space between the tables of the skull. When the halo is secure, the pins are locked in place with a pin-lock assembly.

Traction may be applied to the ring, or the ring may be attached to the torso with a plastic vest (see Fig. 49–32), plaster of Paris body cast, or pins through the pelvis. For the first few days after the halo is applied, the pins should be checked and tightened with a torque screwdriver. Ordinarily, irritation about a pin tract is caused by loosening, and this may be easily corrected by tightening the pin to 5 or 6 in/lb. If a pin must be removed for any reason, a new pin is inserted in a hole adjacent to the unsatisfactory pin, and the old pin is removed.

There are a number of newer varieties of halo devices on the market. We favor the one recently designed by Krag (Figs. 49–36 and 49–37), because it

Figure 49–35. The halo-ring may be attached to a plastic vest, plaster of Paris body cast, or pins through the pelvis through rigid steel uprights. This rigidly controls the head and neck and allows the patient with an unstable spine to transfer or ambulate, speeding the course of rehabilitation and avoiding the morbidity associated with prolonged bed rest and traction.

pounds may be applied without difficulty; however, larger loads, as may be required to reduce locked facets, are not recommended, because the pins are not designed for large forces and may pull out of the skull.

A halo-ring is selected that is almost 4 cm larger than the head circumference. This permits a gap between the ring and skull of almost 1.5 cm. The raised portion of the ring is located over the occiput, with the convex curve directed superiorly (see Fig. 49–34). The lower rim of the ring should be placed at the level of the eyebrows just above the ear. The skull pins pierce the skin without an incision and should enter the skull perpendicular to its surface. The anterior skull pins are directed at the frontal bone 1 cm above the eyebrows and 1 cm anterior to the temporal ridge. The posterior pins enter the skull above and 1 cm behind the ear. These positions usually correspond to the middle hole in each of the three-hole sets about the ring.

The patient's head is prepared with surgical scrub about the pin sites. The halo is positioned around the skull using the positioning pins and plates (see Fig. 49–34). The skin is marked with sterile surgical dye over the sites of intended pin fixation, and local anesthetic is infiltrated into the skin and periosteum over these marks. The skull pins are advanced two at a

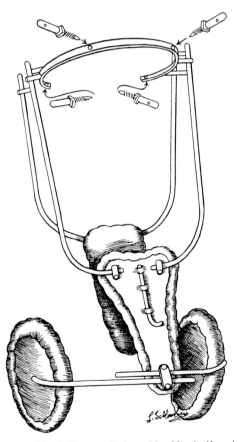

Figure 49–36. The halo-vest designed by Martin Krag largely avoids motion produced by the shoulders. The incomplete halo-ring in the occipital area makes lying supine much less uncomfortable.

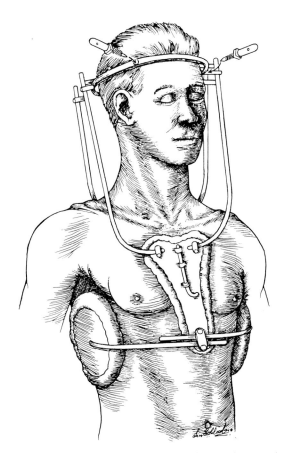

Figure 49–37. The Krag halo-vest aligns the head to the thorax with four pads. The anterior pad can be quickly opened in case of a cardiac emergency.

reduces the large motion and forces on the cervical spine by avoiding pressure from the shoulders, and it is lighter and more comfortable. As with other newer models, it has graphite supports, which allow radiographic study from any direction without interference. The pad and trunk design allows shoulder movement without producing axial traction and compression on the neck vertebrae. It is also rather simply installed on a firm stretcher. Another advantage of the Krag device is that the halo-rings are not complete circles, leaving the occiput free and allowing more comfortable use of a pillow.

When a patient enters the emergency room in jeopardy from cervical instability and lying on a stretcher in the supine position (often with a cervical collar and other support), it is important to maintain this position while applying the halo-ring or halo-arch. If the bed or stretcher surface is firm, the patient may not need to be moved. If there is a soft surface, some additional support may be needed to protect the head-thoracic relationship.

Halo devices come in many sizes, and the right one should clear the skull between 1 and 1.5 cm and should not touch the patient's head or the top of the ears. The ring should be placed 0.5 to 1 cm above the lobe of the

ears and at equal heights over the eyebrows. This is the point of the largest circumference of the skull. As with other devices, the head is prepped and surgically scrubbed. At the proposed pin sites, a sterile marking pencil is used to identify the fixation sites and a local anesthetic is instilled. A torque screwdriver is used as described previously. Skull pins are advanced two at a time with a torque screwdriver, with the operator and an assistant working simultaneously. Torque should not exceed 5 in/lb in children and 6 in/lb in adults. After they have been applied, they should be tested again at about 20 minutes and then again at 24 to 48 hours. It is not necessary to shave the head.

Three-Point Pin Headrest.   The three-point pin headrest is fixed to the operating table and provides rigid immobilization and distraction of the cervical spine during surgery. We generally employ the pin headrest for posterior cervical fusions in which we anticipate adding enough immediate strength that simple braces are sufficient to protect the spine postoperatively. The pin headrest is composed of a U-shaped frame that is adjustable in width (Fig. 49–38). Two pins are fixed to a hinged yoke on one side of the frame, and the third pin is fixed to the opposite side. The frame is attached to the operating table through a universal joint that permits a wide variety of positions. The pin headrest is generally applied with the patient supine, and the patient is then turned to the prone position. To avoid confusion when using this assembly for the first time, we recommend a mock placement on a cooperative volunteer.

The patient is anesthetized on a stretcher in the supine position using a noncollapsible endotracheal tube. The hair is not shaved but is scrubbed with Betadine. The pins and headrest are sterilized, and the pins are inserted into the frame. The frame is centered over the patient's head, and the surgeon holds the cross bar of the frame in one hand with the back of his or her fingers resting on the patient's forehead (Fig. 49–39). This ensures that the frame does not rest on the patient's skin. The single pin is centered just above the ear, and the double pins are placed at the same level on the opposite side. The frame is closed firmly using the turning knob until fixation is satisfactory.

The surgeon holds and applies traction to the frame with one hand and supports the neck with the second hand. The patient is then rolled like a log onto the operating table, with the surgeon controlling the head and neck and directing the other members of the team. An assistant then secures the frame to the operating table while the surgeon maintains traction until the neck is satisfactorily positioned and stabilized (Fig. 49–40). Countertraction is applied by taping the shoulders to the distal end of the operating table. A lateral roentgenogram is then obtained to check vertebral alignment. In children or adults with a narrow head, pediatric pins should be used (see Fig. 49–38*A*). These have a longer shank, which decreases the distance between pins and allows secure fixation even when the skull is narrow.

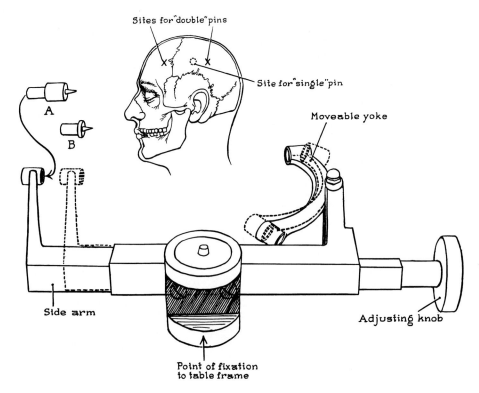

Figure 49–38. The three-point pin headrest is a U-shaped frame that is adjustable in width. Two pins are fixed to a hinged yoke on one side of the frame, and a third pin is fixed to the opposite side. These are placed just above the ear of the patient at the widest point of the skull. Pediatric pins *(A)* are available that have a longer shank and should be used in children or adults with a narrow head. These decrease the distance between the pins and provide satisfactory fixation even when the skull is narrow.

ANTERIOR CERVICAL APPROACHES

Transoral Pharyngeal Approach to the Upper Cervical Spine

The bodies of the upper three cervical vertebrae are separated from the posterior pharynx by four thin layers of tissue and are readily palpable through this posterior pharyngeal wall. Despite this apparent acces-

sibility, the pharyngeal approach to these vertebrae has not been very popular because of the risk of infection by pharyngeal flora and the confined working area.

Since antiquity, posterior pharyngeal abscesses have been drained through the mouth by local stab incisions. Thomson and Negus[64] reported the use of the transoral approach to evacuate retropharyngeal abscesses. Crowe and Johnson resected a large osteoma of the second and third cervical vertebrae through this ap-

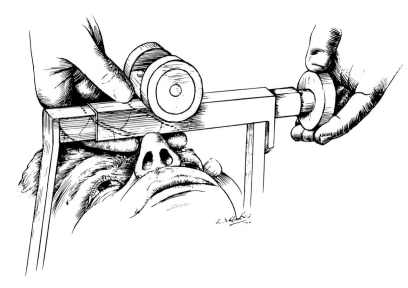

Figure 49–39. To place the pin headrest on the patient, the surgeon holds the center of the frame in one hand with his or her fingers resting on the patient's forehead. This ensures that the frame does not press against the patient's skin. The pins are placed just above the ear at the widest portion of the skull, and the frame is closed firmly using the turning knob until the pins are well seated in the outer table of the skull. The frame should be moved to check that all of the pins are well fixed to bone and do not move within the soft tissues.

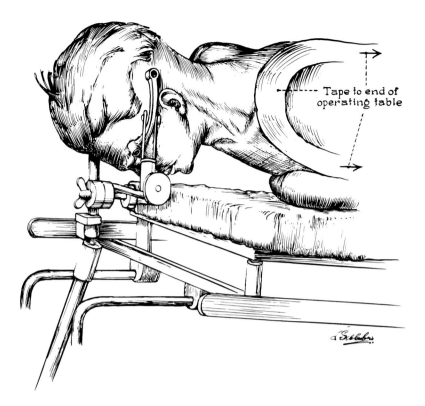

Figure 49–40. The patient is turned onto the operating table with the surgeon controlling the head and neck by holding the pin headrest. The surgeon places the head and neck in the desired position, and an assistant secures the frame to the operating table. Countertraction is then applied to the neck by taping the shoulders to the distal end of the operating table, and a lateral roentgenogram is made to verify that the vertebrae are properly aligned. (From Griswold, D. M., et al.: Atlantoaxial fusion for instability. J. Bone Joint Surg. *60A*:285–292, 1978.)

proach in 1944,[59] and Alonso and coworkers[1] reported on the resection of a chordoma of the clivus (basiocciput) through a transoral-transpalatal approach.

Fang and Ong[16] described six cases in which a fairly extensive vertebral body resection and bone grafting were attempted through the mouth. These authors recommend this approach to reduce and fuse chronic atlantoaxial fracture-dislocations that cannot be reduced with skeletal traction. In this series, four of the six patients developed wound infections, and one of these four died of septic encephalomeningitis. Two of the six developed significant intraoperative hemorrhage from tears of the vertebral artery. These were immediately controlled with Gelfoam packing. In another two cases, the surgeons had difficulty closing the wound, owing to inadequate reduction of the vertebrae and the extra volume of the bone graft.

Our experience with this approach has been less morbid, but we have restricted our procedures to biopsy, incision and drainage, or limited resection and have not attempted more extensive open reductions and bone grafting. Because of the risk of infection and the relatively confined working area through the mouth, we recommend this route primarily for limited or direct procedures, such as drainage, biopsy, excision, or even resection of the odontoid.

The approach is suitable to expose the basiocciput and the vertebral bodies to the third cervical level. The ring of the first cervical vertebra lies above the soft palate, and considerable retraction or division of the soft palate may be necessary to gain suitable direct vision at this level or above. The third cervical body is

at the level of the epiglottis, and the tongue must be firmly depressed to gain proper access to this level or below. The approach is ideally suited to lesions of the body of the second vertebra, which is directly visible through the mouth.

Technique

Parenteral prophylactic antibiotics are given, based on preoperative nasopharyngeal culture and sensitivity studies. Anesthesia is administered by endotracheal intubation using a noncollapsible tube and cuff. If extensive dissection is anticipated, tracheostomy is advisable. Despite the use of a cuffed endotracheal tube, the patient should be placed in the Trendelenburg position to prevent aspiration of blood and debris. A mouth gag of the Davis-Crowe type is placed in the mouth to maintain retraction (Fig. 49–41). The operating surgeon wears a head lamp to light the operative field. The hypopharynx is packed, and often the soft palate is folded back on itself and temporarily sutured to the junction of the hard and soft palates to expose the upper cervical vertebrae. The soft palate may be divided in the midline, and the posterior hard palate may be resected to expose the clivus or basiocciput.[1] The vertebral bodies should be identified by palpation. The ring of the first vertebra has a midline anterior tubercle, and the disc between the second and third vertebrae is prominent and provides another localizing landmark. The eustachian tube orifices are at the level of the basiocciput.

A longitudinal incision is made in the midline of the

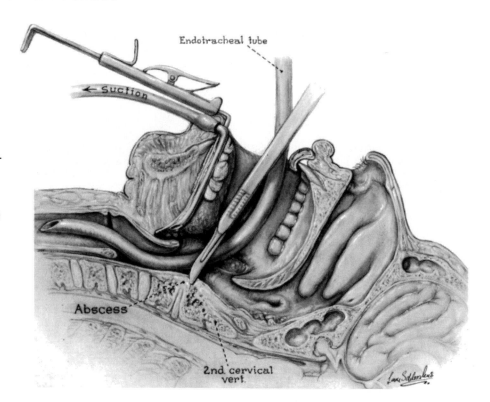

Figure 49–41. Transoral pharyngeal approach to the upper cervical spine. At this level there are only four thin layers: the pharyngeal mucosa, the pharyngeal constrictor muscles, the buccopharyngeal fascia, and the anterior longitudinal ligament. (From Southwick, W. O., and Robinson, R. A.: Surgical approaches to the vertebral bodies in the cervical and lumbar regions. J. Bone Joint Surg. *39A*:631, 1957.)

posterior pharynx over the desired level (see Fig. 49–41). The incision is carried down through the mucous membrane and soft tissues to bone. The incision should be long enough to provide adequate exposure. Although the midpharynx is relatively avascular, small bleeders will be encountered, which should be clamped and cauterized. Soft tissues may be stripped laterally by subperiosteal dissection as far as the lateral masses of the axis. The soft tissue flaps may be retracted using long stay sutures. Following the procedure, the wound and hypopharynx should be carefully irrigated, and all debris and fluid should be removed. The wound is closed loosely with interrupted absorbable sutures. Drainage may be provided through a small rubber drain attached to heavy silk, which is then passed through the nose and taped to the cheek. Packs are removed, and the pharynx and hypopharynx are inspected to ensure that all loose material is removed. Parenteral antibiotics are given prophylactically for a total of at least three days.

This exposure may be augmented by creating an inferiorly based horseshoe-shaped flap of nasopharyngeal and oropharyngeal mucosa and muscle. This is best suited to exposures of the basiocciput and ring of the first cervical vertebra, because the posterior nasopharyngeal soft tissues are thicker and more redundant at this level than below.

Complications

Many problems may be encountered. Children with lymphoid proliferation tend to bleed actively. If an atlantoaxial fracture-dislocation is reduced by manipulation, the vertebral arteries may be injured, with life-threatening hemorrhage or basilar artery ischemia, particularly in the elderly. Infection is always a potential problem. The risk of infection increases with the extent of resection and the application of a bone graft. Opening or exposing the dura is hazardous because of the risk of direct contamination and septic encephalomeningitis. For this reason, prophylactic, broad-spectrum antibiotics are given parenterally for at least 72 hours postoperatively and are selected on the basis of preoperative nasopharyngeal culture and sensitivity studies.

Wound closure may be a problem, particularly if the incision is extended low on the third cervical body, where the overlying soft tissues are thin, adherent to the underlying bone, and less redundant. Flaps may be created laterally to provide the tissue length necessary for closure, and bone grafts should be recessed within the vertebral body so they do not protrude beyond the anterior margin.

The airway is of prime concern, and for this reason the patient should be placed in the Trendelenburg position even when the trachea is presumably sealed with an endotracheal tube and cuff. Prior to extubation, the pharynx should be carefully irrigated and inspected. Following surgery, the airway remains at risk because of edema, hemorrhage, or continued drainage. For this reason, tracheostomy should be seriously considered if the surgical dissection is extensive or if significant postoperative drainage is anticipated.

Anterior Approach to the Occiput and Upper Cervical Spine, Medial to the Carotid Sheath

DeAndrade and MacNab[12] described an approach to the basiocciput and upper cervical spine that is an extension of the approach described by Southwick and Robinson[59] and Bailey and Badgley,[5] entering anterior to the sternomastoid and carotid sheath. The working area is somewhat limited by the mandible and subglottic structures, particularly in patients with short and muscular necks, and one has to accept the risk of injuring the superior laryngeal nerves.

McAfee[35] and a number of others from the Johns Hopkins cervical spine group reported 17 cases using a superior extension of the anterior approach originally described by Southwick and Robinson in 1957 for anterior cervical spine fusion in the middle and lower neck. This upper approach provides an anterior access to the neural elements from the clivus to the body of the third cervical vertebra, without the need for posterior dissection of the carotid sheath and the foramina for the tenth nerve. This approach is primarily used for extensive removal of tumors and replacement of the anterior bodies of C2 and C3 and the arches of C1 and the dens for certain decompression procedures in which infection could be a problem with the anterior retropharyngeal approach.

Technique

Somatosensory evoked potentials are needed for monitoring spinal cord function. The Gardner-Wells skull tongs using 4.5 kg (10 lb) of traction are used routinely. The skull tongs should be put in place with the patient awake as an aid to transferring to the operating table. With this fragile group of patients, fiberoptic nasotracheal intubation is carried out under local anesthesia to prevent movement of the neck and to keep the mouth free of all tubes. No esophageal stethoscopes or other tubes in the esophagus are used, so that nothing limits the operative site or opens the mandible. With the patient awake, the neck is carefully extended while monitoring neurologic symptoms and watching the evoked potentials. In some early cases tracheostomy was needed, but this should be necessary only rarely with the recent advances in anesthesia, whereby endotracheal intubation can be maintained for several days postoperatively.

A transverse submandibular incision is used on either side, depending on the presence of tumor mass. If need be, the incision can be converted to a longitudinal incision along the sternomastoid, but this is usually not necessary or desirable (Fig. 49–42). This exposure is a superior extension of the standard anterolateral exposure of the midpart of the cervical spine and requires familiarity with the fascial planes. They consist of (1) the superficial fascia containing the platysma; (2) the superficial layer of the deep fascia surrounding the sternomastoid muscle; (3) the middle layer of deep fascia enclosing the omohyoid, sternohyoid, sternothy-roid, and thyrohyoid muscles and visceral fascia enclosing the trachea, esophagus, and recurrent nerve; and (4) the deep layer of cervical fascia, which is divided into the alar fascia connecting the two carotid sheaths and fused midline to the visceral fascia, and the prevertebral fascia covering the longus colli and scaleni muscles. This high extrapharyngeal exposure of the atlas and axis is sufficiently superior to the right recurrent laryngeal nerve that there should be no increased risk of damage to the nerve with a right-sided exposure.

Deep to the skin, the submandibular incision continues through the platysma and superficial fascia. As this layer is mobilized in the subplatysmal plane, the marginal mandibular branch of the fascial nerve is found with the aid of a nerve stimulator. It is also necessary to dissect out and ligate the retromandibular veins and other superficial jugular veins that appear at this level (see Figs. 49–42 and 49–5). The common facial vein is continuous with the retromandibular vein, and the branches of the mandibular nerve usually cross the lateral veins superficially and superiorly. By ligating the retromandibular vein as it joins the internal jugular vein and keeping the dissection deep and inferior to the vein as the exposure is extended superiorly to the mandible, the superficial branch of the facial nerves is protected.

At this point, the anterior border of the sternomastoid is mobilized by incising the superficial layer of the deep cervical fascia that surrounds the muscle belly around its anterior border, thus exposing the middle layer of deep fascia. This allows localization of the carotid sheath by palpation of the carotid arterial pulse. The salivary gland is now resected, and the salivary duct sutured to prevent a salivary fistula. The lymph nodes from the submandibular and carotid triangles can be resected and sent for frozen section if needed. The posterior belly of the digastric muscle and the stylohyoidal muscle are identified, and the digastric tendon divided and tagged for further repair (see Fig. 49–42). Excessive superior traction at the base of the origin of the stylohyoid muscle may cause injury to the facial nerve as it exits from the skull. The hyoid bone may be mobilized now by dividing the digastric and stylohyoid muscles, which allows better traction and helps avoid exposure and injury or perforation of the nasopharynx, hypopharynx, and esophagus, which contain a high concentration of anaerobic bacteria.

The hypoglossal nerve that is identified with a nerve stimulator is then completely mobilized from the base of the skull to the anterior border of the hypoglossal muscle. It is retracted superiorly throughout the remainder of the procedure (Fig. 49–43).

The dissection then proceeds into the retropharyngeal space between the contents of the carotid sheath laterally and the visceral fascia containing the larynx and pharynx anteromedially. Ligation and section of the tethering branches of the carotid artery and jugular veins superiorly are needed to improve the exposure at this point. Beginning inferiorly and progressing superiorly, ligation of the superior thyroid artery and vein, lingual artery and vein, ascending pharyngeal

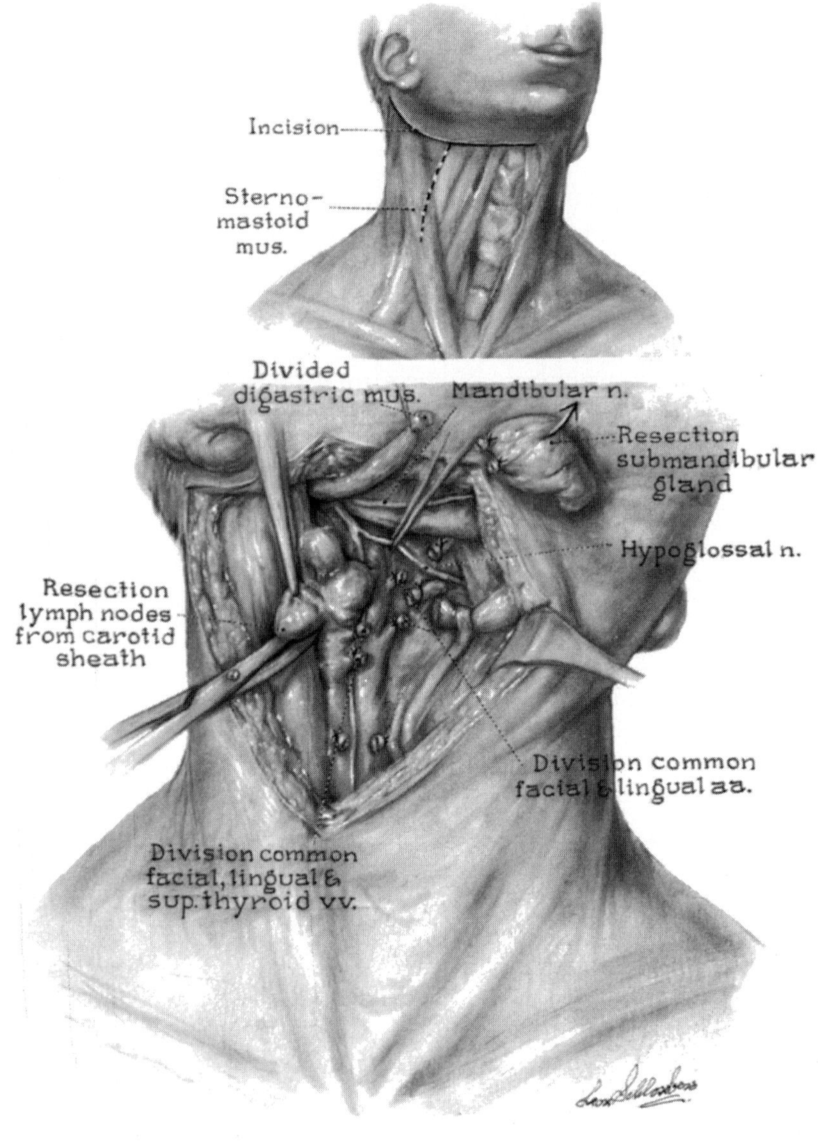

Figure 49–42. The anterolateral approach to the atlas and axis is usually made through a submandibular incision. The submandibular gland and the digastric tendon are divided. Rarely, if a more extensive dissection is required in the lower neck, the incision can be made into a "T." However, this tends to heal poorly and often leaves an unattractive scar. (From McAfee, P. C., Bohlman, H. H., Riley, L. H., et al.: The anterior retropharyngeal approach to the upper part of the cervical spine. J. Bone Joint Surg. *69A*:1374–1383, 1987.)

artery and vein, and facial artery and vein helps mobilize the carotid sheath laterally. The superior laryngeal nerve is also identified with the help of a nerve stimulator as it is mobilized from its origin near the nodose ganglion to its entrance into the larynx (see Fig. 49–43). The external branch of the superior laryngeal nerve is closely associated with the superior thyroid artery. This nerve is often compromised in this dissection, because of its small size and its location.

At this point, the alar and prevertebral fasciae are palpated and incised longitudinally along the anterior longitudinal ligament of the midline of the upper cervical vertebrae. The attachments of the longus colli muscle converge at the atlas, which is directly midline. Their orientation defines the amount of head rotation. It is important to have the exact orientation to the position of the head and the midline of the upper cervical vertebrae, so that one can excise exactly the middle portion of the vertebral body and basiocciput.

Four cranial nerves (the hypoglossal, glossopharyngeal, vagus, and accessory nerves), as well as the internal carotid artery and jugular vein, are tethered to the occiput as they leave their foramina and may be injured by vigorous retraction or dissection (Fig. 49–44). The hypoglossal nerve leaves the occiput from the anterior condyloid foramen just lateral to the midportion of the occipital condyle, and the jugular vein and carotid artery enter the skull just lateral to this. This leaves only 2 cm of working area from the midline to these structures laterally at the base of the skull. The pharyngeal and laryngeal branches of the vagus nerve arise shortly below this level and are stretched by anterior retraction of the pharynx. The longus colli and longus capitis muscles lie over the transverse processes and bodies of the first and second cervical vertebrae. The longus colli meets in midline at the anterior tubercle of C1. Beneath is the anterior longitudinal ligament and its extension to the skull. To minimize bleeding

Figure 49–43. After the superficial layer of the deep cervical fascia is incised along the anterior border of the sternocleidomastoid muscle, the superior thyroid artery and vein are divided. The hypoglossal and superior laryngeal nerves are mobilized. Additional branches of the carotid artery and internal jugular vein are ligated to allow mobilization of the contents of the carotid sheath laterally as the hypopharynx is mobilized medially. (From McAfee, P. C., Bohlman, H. H., Riley, L. H., et al.: The anterior retropharyngeal approach to the upper part of the cervical spine. J. Bone Joint Surg. *69A*:1374–1383, 1987.)

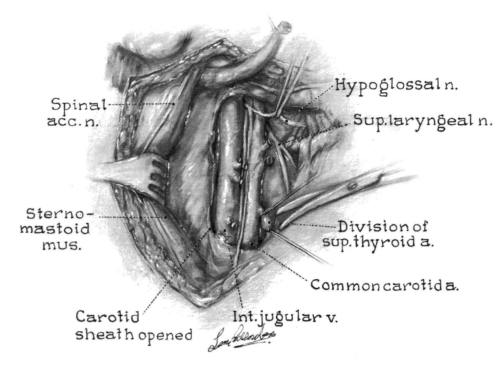

Figure 49–44. The first step of the anterior spinal decompression is a meticulous removal of the disc between the second and third cervical vertebrae. The longus colli muscle is dissected in a lateral direction, exposing the second cervical vertebral body and the anterior arch of the atlas. Removal of the body of the second cervical vertebra can then be performed with a high-speed burr. (From McAfee, P. C., Bohlman, H. H., Riley, L. H., et al.: The anterior retropharyngeal approach to the upper part of the cervical spine. J. Bone Joint Surgery. *69A*:1374–1383, 1987.)

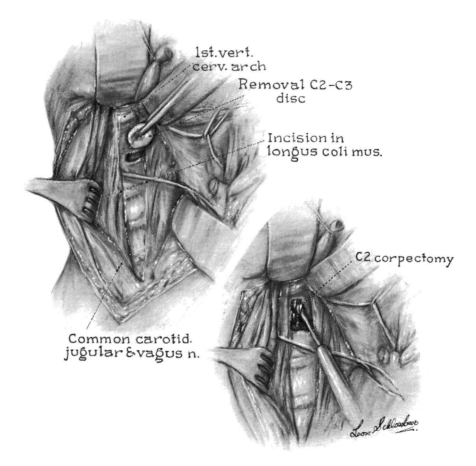

from the profuse plexus of veins within the longus colli and capitis muscles, a longitudinal incision is made to the bone in the midline over the first and second vertebrae and basiocciput. The ligament and muscle are dissected subperiosteally and laterally to expose the bone.

Decompression is best begun through the disc spaces as described for the lower neck (see Fig. 49–44). Some typical cases from the series of McAfee and associates are seen in Figure 49–45. The technique of bone grafting is identical to the previously described methods in this section.

Postoperative management requires frequent neurologic examination and, on occasion, continued study of the spinal cord monitoring, along with careful management of the airway. All this is carried out in the intensive care unit, often with continued head traction to maintain alignment. Also, a halo-vest or accompanying posterior fusion wired to threaded rods or cortical struts may be used for stabilization. The head and trunk need to be elevated about 30 degrees to prevent early postoperative edema. The nasal intubation is often used for the first 48 hours.

Complications

Airway obstruction caused by edema of the pharynx and larynx or bulging of bone graft into the posterior pharynx is the most immediate threat. One should consider tracheostomy either preoperatively or postoperatively, although in the series of McAfee and others[35] it was often not needed.

Laryngeal and pharyngeal dysfunction may be anticipated in the immediate postoperative period, secondary to retraction of the laryngeal nerves, even if none has been transected. Patients should be advised to expect difficulty with phonation and swallowing, especially in the early postoperative course. Persistent but minor problems will arise if the external branch of the superior laryngeal nerve has been transected. DeAndrade and MacNab[12] reported persistent postoperative hoarseness, laryngeal fatigue, and an inability to produce high tones in three of five cases in their study.

Shifting of the bone grafts can also be a problem, along with problems with halo fixation.

Other potential complications include injury to the medulla or upper cervical spinal cord. Hemorrhage from the carotid artery, the jugular vein, or their tributaries may be difficult to control without cerebral ischemia or possible air embolism. Because of these many dangers, this approach probably should be reserved for situations that permit no alternative route.

Anterolateral Approach to the Upper Cervical Spine, Lateral to the Carotid Sheath

Whitesides and Kelly[69] reported on their experience with the anterolateral approach to the atlantoaxial ver-

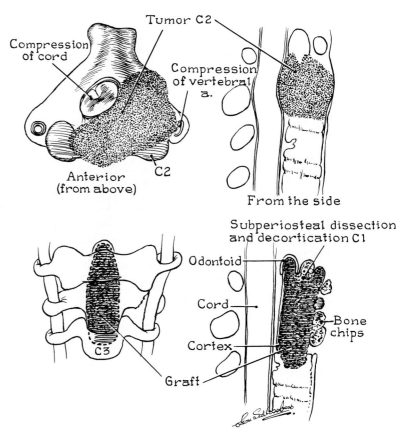

Figure 49–45. Typical tumors in the second cervical vertebral body from the series of McAfee and associates (aneurysmal bone cyst, chordoma, or metastasis). The anterior and posterior columns of spinal stability may be affected and the spinal cord compressed from an anterior direction; the vertebral artery is occasionally involved laterally. The lower figures show the use of a clothespin-shaped strut graft wedged below the anterior arch of the atlas after subperiosteal dissection and decortication. (From McAfee, P. C., Bohlman, H. H., Riley, L. H., et al.: The anterior retropharyngeal approach to the upper part of the cervical spine. J. Bone Joint Surg. *69A*:1374–1383, 1987.)

tebral bodies originally described by Henry[22] for exposing the vertebral artery. This approach partially transects the sternomastoid and goes lateral and posterior to the carotid sheath. The major branches of the external carotid artery and laryngeal nerves are thus not disturbed. The upper end of the exposure is limited to the ring of the first cervical vertebra. The basiocciput cannot be reached safely through this route lateral and posterior to the carotid sheath without the risk of injuring the internal carotid artery, jugular vein, and vagus, accessory, and hypoglossal nerves. These structures are effectively tethered to the skull posterior to the basiocciput and would be injured if retracted sufficiently to fully expose the basiocciput. The anterolateral approach is excellent for one-sided lesions high in the neck.

This approach is ideally suited to reach the anterior aspect of the first and second cervical vertebrae without risk of bacterial contamination by nasopharyngeal flora. It also permits direct distal extension to the first thoracic vertebra without permanently affecting laryngeal function.

Because of the many potential hazards, this approach should be restricted to those circumstances that require anterior and lateral exploration at this level, such as biopsy and curettage of tumor or infection or resecting the odontoid. Anterior fusion of the first three cervical vertebrae is possible through this exposure but probably should be considered only in situations in which posterior fusions are impractical, such as following extensive posterior laminectomy or in the presence of a fixed flexion deformity.

In summary, if an extrapharyngeal exposure as high as the basiocciput is needed, the approach should be medial to the carotid sheath, accepting the risk of injuring the superior laryngeal nerves and causing postoperative hoarseness. If access only as high as the first cervical ring is necessary, this route lateral and posterior to the carotid sheath is available, and the superior laryngeal nerves can be spared. However, it is important to remember that the carotid sheath should be retracted forward gently because of the threat of avulsing these vessels as well as certain cranial nerves from the base of the skull.

Technique

Because of potential postoperative edema and airway obstruction, either preoperative or postoperative tracheostomy should be considered, although with new techniques of nasotracheal anesthesia this is rarely necessary. If the spine is unstable or if extensive surgical dissection is planned, skull traction with tongs or halo may be needed. A longitudinal incision is made along the anterior margin of the sternomastoid muscle (Fig. 49–46). At the superior end, the incision is carried transversely and back over the mastoid prominence. Deep to the platysma is the broad sheath of the superficial layer of the deep cervical fascia. Embedded within this at the superior pole of the incision is the external jugular vein (see Fig. 49–5), which crosses the

anterior margin of the sternomastoid muscle. This must be ligated and divided. Posterior to the external jugular vein and running parallel with it in the same tissue plane is the great auricular nerve, which usually divides into its terminal branches at the anterior border of the sternomastoid, providing sensation over the parotid gland and around the ear. Some of these anterior branches may need to be divided. The sternomastoid muscle is divided at its mastoid origin, and the splenius capitis muscle beneath may be partially sectioned if necessary. The superficial layer of the deep cervical fascia is opened anterior to the sternomastoid, and this muscle is mobilized by sharp and blunt dissection. The spinal accessory nerve courses downward, anterior and deep to the sternomastoid muscle, and enters this muscle at its upper third (Fig. 49–47). The accessory nerve should be identified and separated from the jugular vein to provide greater mobility and should be protected throughout the procedure. The sternomastoid branch of the occipital artery is inferior to the accessory nerve but travels in the same plane and should be ligated.

Dissection then proceeds lateral and posterior to the carotid sheath, separating the carotid sheath from the sternomastoid (Fig. 49–48). The sternomastoid muscle and accessory nerve are retracted posteriorly, and the carotid sheath is retracted anteriorly. The transverse processes of all the cervical vertebrae are palpable within this space. Using sharp and finger dissection, the plane between the alar and prevertebral fasciae is developed along the anterior aspect of the transverse processes to the vertebral bodies. The dissection plane is anterior to the longus colli and capitis muscles as well as the overlying sympathetic trunk and superior cervical ganglion. The sympathetic trunk tends to remain with the longus capitis muscle during this dissection and is not usually disturbed. The ring of the first cervical vertebra and its anterior tubercle may be identified by palpation. Below this, the next major prominence is at the disc space between the second and third vertebrae (Fig. 49–49). When the vertebral level is accurately identified, a longitudinal incision is made to the bone over the middle of the vertebra through the anterior longitudinal ligament. The ligament and overlying muscles are dissected subperiosteally and laterally.

The upper cervical vertebrae may be visualized through this approach, and by extending the incision distally, the vertebral bodies of the middle and lower spine may be reached in continuity. The basiocciput, clivus, and sphenoid may be palpated but are poorly seen. Biopsy, curettage, or anterior fusion using corticocancellous strips in a longitudinal trough is possible. The retropharyngeal space should be drained to prevent excessive retropharyngeal hematoma, and the wound should be closed. If stability is in doubt, external stabilization in a brace is recommended until fusion is established roentgenographically.

An alternative approach within the retropharyngeal space is to separate the longus colli and capitis muscles from their bony insertions on the transverse processes

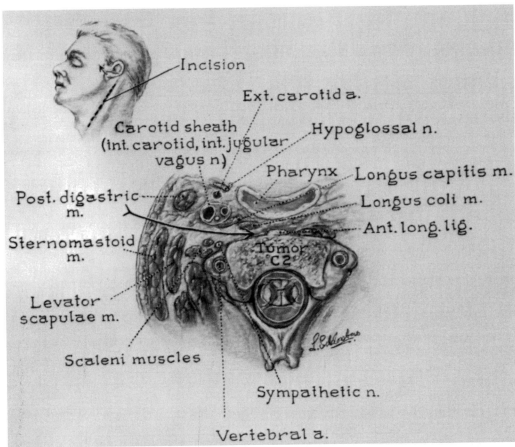

Figure 49–46. For the Henry-Whitesides approach, the incision needs to begin along the anterior border of the sternomastoid muscle, passing across its mastoid attachment under the ear. The arrow shows how the approach to the anterior longitudinal ligament passes posterior to the carotid sheath. This approach to the upper cervical spine gives direct lateral and anterior access to C1–C2–C3 posterior to the carotid sheath, avoiding dissection of the facial hypoglossal, superior, and inferior laryngeal nerves. However, it is important to avoid stretching of the carotid sheath structures.

and retract these muscles anteriorly. This provides direct exposure of the nerve roots, transverse processes, and vertebral artery but disturbs the sympathetic rami communicantes and may cause Horner's syndrome.

Complications

Airway obstruction and difficulty with swallowing owing to retropharyngeal edema or hematoma are the most immediate threats. We recommend nasotracheal intubation preoperatively and postoperatively to reduce the risk of airway obstruction, intensive care nursing, and the provision of a high-humidity tent or a mask for a few days after surgery to reduce pharyngeal edema. Intravenous feeding may be required for five to seven days because of dysphagia.

The long, oblique skin incision tends to leave an area of hypoesthesia around it and the ear. This is more pronounced than one sees around short, transverse incisions in the lower neck but is rarely a problem. The spinal accessory nerve should be carefully identified and protected throughout the procedure to prevent

weakness of the sternomastoid and trapezius muscles. The sympathetic trunk and superior cervical ganglion lying over the longus capitis muscle and opposite the second and third cervical vertebrae should be preserved to prevent Horner's syndrome. Prolonged or excessive retraction of the carotid sheath medially can interfere with function of the vagus and recurrent laryngeal nerves on that side.

Hemorrhage can occur from a variety of sources. The vertebral artery is reasonably well protected in its course through the costotransverse foramina, but it may be injured in the interval between transverse processes. Ordinarily, the right vertebral artery is not dominant, but injury to the left or dominant vertebral artery can cause receptive blindness with infarction of the calcarine fissure.

Anterior Approach to the Middle and Lower Cervical Vertebrae, Below C2, Medial to the Carotid Sheath

This approach has been clearly described by Southwick and Robinson[59, 60] and Bailey and Badgley.[5] Although

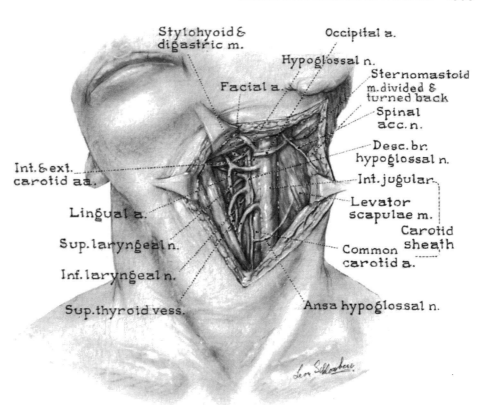

Figure 49–47. Structures that lie anteromedial and posterolateral to the carotid sheath in the high cervical approach. Only the occipital artery needs to be ligated when the dissection proceeds posterolateral to the carotid sheath high in the neck.

Figure 49–48. The sectioned belly of the sternomastoid could be retracted posterolaterally and the carotid sheath retracted anteromedially to this extreme in order to show the deep structures that could be accessed through this approach. However, this incision along the anterior edge of the sternomastoid is cosmetically objectionable, and would be rarely used for surgery low in the neck. Below C3, the standard anterior approach is commonly used (see Fig. 49–51).

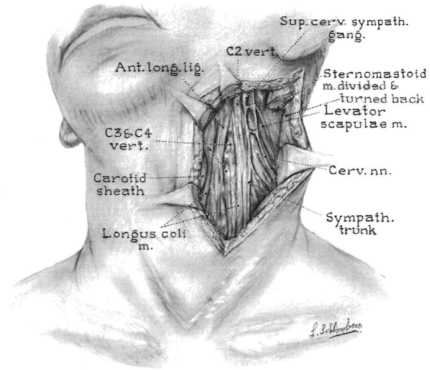

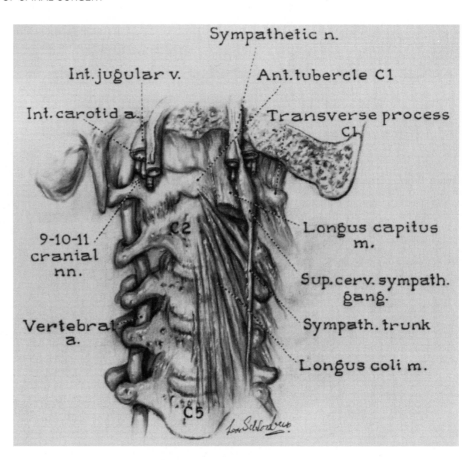

Figure 49–49. Deep structures of the upper neck. The anterior tubercle of C1 is usually prominent, and usually one may palpate the anterior longitudinal ligament between the muscles (the longus colli and longus capitis). Note the close relationship of the carotid sheath structures and the ninth, tenth, and eleventh cranial nerves, and the sympathetic trunk to the lateral masses of the upper vertebrae. It is of extreme importance to have positive identification of the midline prior to bony resection.

its origin is unknown, Lahey and Warren[30] described a similar approach to excise diverticula of the esophagus. Robinson and Smith[47] successfully used the exposure in a series of anterior interbody arthrodeses of the cervical vertebrae, and it has subsequently gained wide popular acceptance as an approach to the spine. Because of the abundance of vital structures in the neck, a thorough knowledge of the anatomic landmarks is a basic requirement for the safety of the patient. The plane of dissection is beneath the vascular leash of the superior thyroid vessels, the external branch of the superior laryngeal nerve, and through certain natural cleavage planes. The landmarks are well defined, and a relatively safe and straightforward route to the vertebral bodies unfolds without dividing any major structure or vessel.

This approach provides direct access to the bodies of the vertebrae from the third through the first thoracic levels. It may be used to biopsy or excise a lesion of the anterior vertebral body or to drain an abscess. Vertebral bodies may be excised and replaced with bone graft; the disc space may be cureted, and posterior osteophytes compressing the nerve roots or spinal cord may be removed, and the resultant defect may be filled with bone graft.

Technique

Although local anesthesia could be used, general endotracheal anesthesia is routinely employed in our center to maintain an unobstructed airway. Head-halter traction (10 to 15 lbs) is generally required, especially for interbody fusion. Countertraction is applied by securing the shoulders with tape to the distal end of the operating table. The head is in neutral position, slightly rotated to the right, and a folded towel is placed under the middle of the neck to support it during dissection and graft insertion. The skin and muscles of the neck should not be under tension, but the chin needs to be slightly to the right side (or left, if the incision is to be made on the right). The traction using a head halter is applied as illustrated in Figure 49–50.

The area from the mandible to the upper thorax is prepared, and the neck is draped free. If a bone graft is to be used, the anterior iliac crest is also prepared. A short, transverse incision is made within a skin crease two to four finger breadths above the clavicle (Fig. 49–51), depending on the level of exposure required. It is a good idea to place a metal marker such as a paper clip over the proposed incision level and check by taking a lateral radiograph if one is uncertain of landmarks. Although the incision may be made on either side, an incision to the left of the midline is less likely to injure an aberrant recurrent laryngeal nerve on the right.

The incision is begun at the midline and is extended over the belly of the sternomastoid muscle laterally. The platysma is divided in the same line as the skin incision. Skin flaps are developed superiorly and inferi-

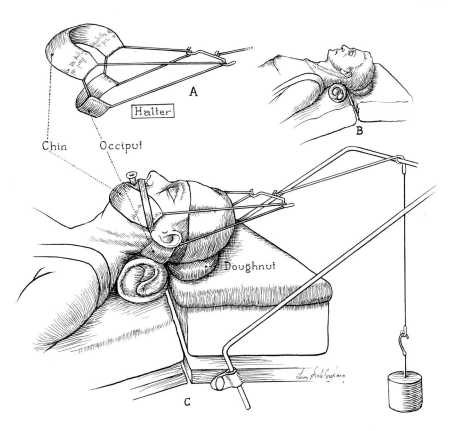

Figure 49–50. *A–C,* Head-halter traction for anterior neck surgery. Note the 20-degree reverse Trendelenburg angle of traction to reduce venous pressure, the support for the midneck to permit safe and stable insertion of bone grafts, the use of the anesthesia screen to maintain a neutral position of the head, and the taping of the shoulders to give counter traction and to obtain lateral x-rays of the lower cervical spine.

orly beneath the platysma but superficial to the subjacent deep fascia. The superficial layer of the deep fascia overlying the strap and sternomastoid muscles is incised longitudinally. The margin between the strap muscles medially and the sternomastoid muscle later-

ally is identified and developed. A plane is then created medial to the carotid sheath and lateral to the thyroid through the thin intermediate layers of the deep cervical fascia (Fig. 49–52) using a combination of sharp and blunt dissection. The carotid artery is easily identified

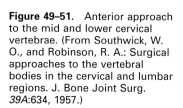

Figure 49–51. Anterior approach to the mid and lower cervical vertebrae. (From Southwick, W. O., and Robinson, R. A.: Surgical approaches to the vertebral bodies in the cervical and lumbar regions. J. Bone Joint Surg. *39A*:634, 1957.)

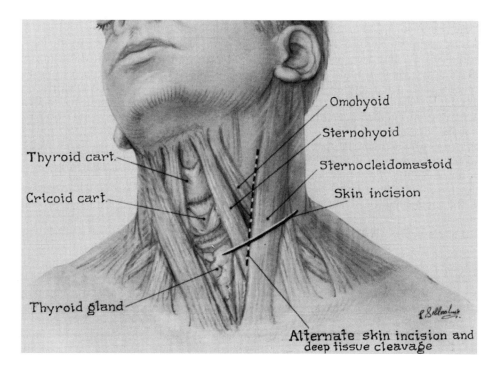

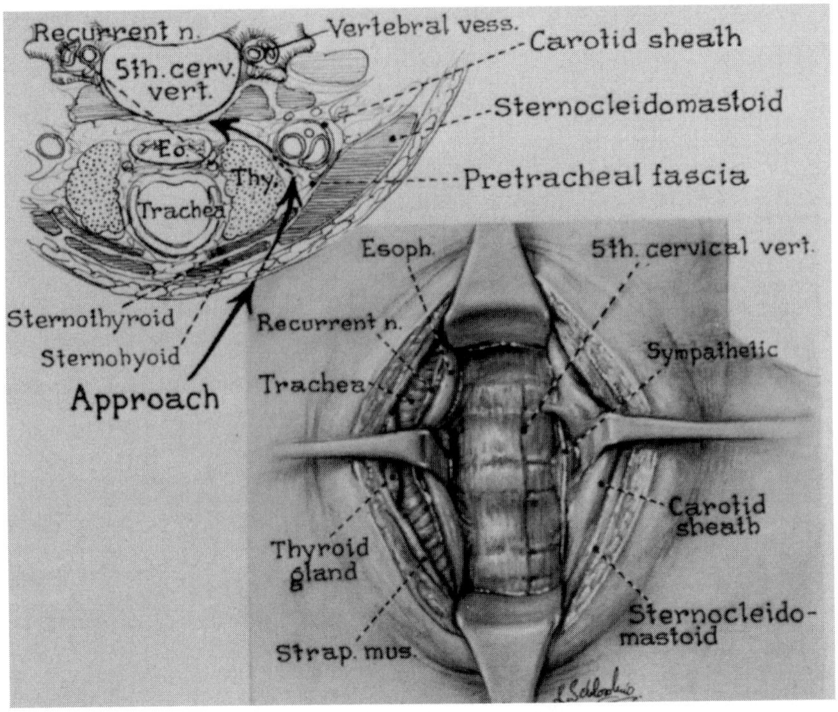

Figure 49–52. Anterior approach to the mid and lower cervical vertebrae, deep dissection. (From Southwick, W. O., and Robinson, R. A.: Surgical approaches to the vertebral bodies in the cervical and lumbar regions. J. Bone Joint Surg. *39A*:634, 1957.)

by its pulsations, and the carotid sheath is retracted laterally with a finger to protect it from injury. The dissection then proceeds within the natural cleavage plane between the alar and visceral fasciae behind the esophagus to the anterior aspect of the vertebral bodies. This is best performed with blunt finger dissection, preserving the integrity of these fascial sheaths. The alar fascia surrounds the carotid sheath structures, the visceral fascia, the esophagus, and recurrent laryngeal nerves. If these sheaths are left intact, there is less likelihood of entering or injuring these structures. The plane between the alar and visceral fasciae should be extended inferiorly and superiorly along the vertebral bodies to allow adequate exposure. The trachea and esophagus are retracted medially, and the carotid sheath is retracted laterally, using smooth deep blade retractors. Care is required to properly identify the smooth-walled esophagus and to protect it during retraction. The vertebral bodies are palpable through the alar and prevertebral fasciae. The disc spaces may be identified as they protrude above the level of the vertebral bodies; the vertebral bodies themselves are slightly concave. A longitudinal incision is made with scissors in the prevertebral fascia over the midline of the vertebral bodies, and the fascia is separated laterally by blunt dissection. The thin translucent anterior longitudinal ligament covers the anterior aspect of the vertebrae. Laterally, the longus colli fibers crowd the vertebral bodies and cover the transverse processes. The sympathetic nerves lie over the longus capitis muscles laterally and should not be disturbed.

In order to identify the proper vertebral level, it is recommended that a lateral roentgenogram be obtained in the operating room with a radiopaque marker placed in the disc at the level desired. Other aids to localization are the cricoid cartilage, which is opposite the body of the sixth cervical vertebra, and the carotid (Chassaignac's tubercle), which is the prominent, anterior, transverse process of the sixth cervical vertebra. When osteoarthritic spurs are present along the anterior bodies of the vertebrae, they are usually palpable and may be an aid to localization.

For exposures of the lower cervical vertebrae below C5, the skin incision should be located about two finger breadths above the clavicle, and dissection should proceed beneath the omohyoid muscle. For higher levels of exposure, the skin incision should be located above this, and dissection may proceed above the omohyoid muscle. A common mistake is to locate the skin incision too inferiorly. For example, to approach the C4–C5 interspace, an incision above the cricoid cartilage and at least three finger breadths above the clavicle is required.

Complications

There are a number of potential complications associated with this procedure. Perforation of the esophagus may occur directly if the visceral fascia is opened or if the esophagus is not properly identified. The esophagus is a soft, smooth-walled structure, and if its location is in doubt, a soft rubber nasogastric tube may be inserted by the anesthetist and the lumen can be identified. The nasogastric tube should be removed before the esophagus is retracted and the vertebrae are exposed. The esophagus may be injured by vigorous retraction or by the use of retractors with sharp blades, teeth, or self-retaining features. Hand-held retractors with smooth blades are, therefore, recommended. If the esophagus is perforated, it should be repaired immediately with sutures, and bone grafting should be delayed until healing has occurred. Perforations that are overlooked usually result in retroesophageal abscesses with attendant fever, swelling, and dysphagia. The diagnosis may be established by fluoroscopy using a water-soluble, radiopaque dye swallow. Retroesophageal abscesses require prompt drainage and débridement with repair of the defect, if possible, and prolonged nasogastric intubation until continuity and healing are established.

The recurrent laryngeal nerve is ordinarily protected by the visceral fascia, but it may be injured in this approach by harsh dissection or retraction. On the left side, the recurrent laryngeal nerve descends into the thorax within the carotid sheath. It leaves the vagus nerve and carotid sheath within the thorax, loops under the aortic arch, beneath the ligamentum arteriosum, and ascends into the neck beside the trachea and esophagus. On the right side, the course of the recurrent laryngeal nerve is not so constant. Usually, it descends within the carotid sheath and loops beneath the subclavian artery, ascending into the neck between the trachea and esophagus (see Fig. 49–22). The recurrent nerve on the right may leave the carotid sheath at a higher level, however, crossing anteriorly behind the thyroid. For this reason, we select the left rather than the right anterior approach to avoid direct injury to an aberrant recurrent nerve.

Horner's syndrome will occur if the sympathetic nerve fibers are irritated or damaged in their course from the stellate ganglion over the longus capitis muscles and the transverse processes. This may be avoided if these muscles are not disturbed or if they are retracted only slightly and subperiosteally from the midline.

The vertebral artery may be injured as it ascends within the costotransverse foramina from one vertebra to the next. Usually, bleeding may be controlled with Gelfoam pack, and no adverse cerebral effects should result if the injury is unilateral.

The superior thyroid artery is the second branch of the external carotid artery and crosses anterior and inferior to the superior pole of the thyroid at the level of the third cervical vertebra. This artery should be protected in dissections of the upper cervical vertebrae. The external laryngeal nerve courses across the neck adjacent and superior to the superior thyroid artery. This nerve innervates the cricothyroid muscle and, when injured, produces hoarseness and laryngeal fatigue. For this reason, it should be identified and protected in dissections of the upper cervical vertebrae.

The inferior thyroid artery, a small branch of the subclavian artery, also crosses the neck and enters the inferior pole of the thyroid gland and should be identified and ligated in dissections of the lower cervical vertebrae.

The thoracic duct ascends from the thorax just lateral to the esophagus, lying on the prevertebral fascia. It loops over the subclavian artery at the level of the

first thoracic vertebral body, anterior to the scalenus anterior and phrenic nerve, and enters the subclavian vein (see Fig. 49–5). In anterior approaches to the lower cervical and upper thoracic spine, the duct should be protected, or a surgical approach to the right of the midline should be employed.

Postoperative hoarseness or laryngeal edema is occasionally a problem caused by irritation of the trachea or larynx by retraction or endotracheal intubation. This may be minimized by placing the patient in a high-humidity tent for 24 to 36 hours after surgery.

Anterior Approach to the Lower Cervical and Upper Thoracic Vertebrae

Nanson[39] described an approach to the lower cervical and upper thoracic vertebrae through the thoracic inlet. This approach was designed to provide access to the upper thoracic sympathetic ganglia, but the approach may also be used for scalene node dissection, section of the scalenus anterior muscle, and exploration of the soft tissues at the base of the neck. In addition, it provides excellent exposure of the lower cervical vertebral bodies and more limited exposure of the upper thoracic vertebral bodies.

Access within the thorax is dependent upon several variables: the diameter of the thoracic inlet, the height of the clavicles and manubrium anteriorly, and the extent of cervicothoracic kyphos. Preoperatively, the upper margin of the clavicles and manubrium should be compared with the vertebral body level on a standard lateral roentgenogram of the upper thoracic spine. In some patients, the manubrium and thoracic inlet ride high to the level of the first or second thoracic vertebra, and exposures within the thorax below this level will be limited and impractical. In others, a lower-riding manubrium may permit access as far as the third or fourth thoracic level. In patients with a narrow anteroposterior chest diameter or significant cervicothoracic kyphos, the intrathoracic exposure will be restricted.

The approach may be made to either side of the midline, although we prefer the right side to avoid the thoracic duct on the left. The recurrent laryngeal nerve on the right should be identified and protected as it loops beneath the subclavian artery (see Fig. 49–22). Proximal extension via this exposure along the cervical spine is hampered by the subclavian vessels and recurrent nerve. The subclavian vessels effectively tether the carotid artery and internal jugular vein so that proximal extension lateral to the carotid sheath is impractical. Dissection medial to the carotid sheath jeopardizes the recurrent laryngeal nerve. However, the recurrent nerve may be identified and mobilized sufficiently to permit retraction of the esophagus, trachea, and thyroid and to reach the spine as high as the fifth cervical level without extending the skin incision.

Technique

A towel is placed beneath the scapulae to extend the neck, the head is rotated away from the proposed incision, and the arm on the side of the incision is pulled down to open the supraclavicular space. A transverse incision at least 8 cm in length is made parallel to and 1 cm above the right clavicle (see Fig. 49–53A, inset). The incision extends from the midline to the lateral margin of the sternomastoid muscle. The platysma muscle is divided transversely in line with the incision. The external jugular vein and medial supraclavicular nerve, a cutaneous nerve to the anterior chest, are located within the superficial fascia just lateral to the platysma and sternomastoid and should be spared if possible (see Fig. 49–53A). The clavicular head of the sternomastoid is separated from its manubrial head by blunt dissection in line with the muscle fibers.

The internal jugular and subclavian veins lie behind the sternomastoid muscle and are separated from it by the deep cervical fascia and a potential space (known as Burns' space) between two layers of fascia. To protect these major vessels from injury, the operator should bluntly dissect with a finger behind the clavicular head of the sternomastoid within this potential space (Fig. 49–53B). The clavicular head of the sterno-

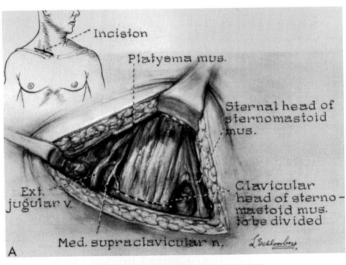

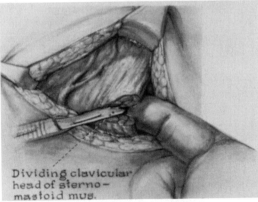

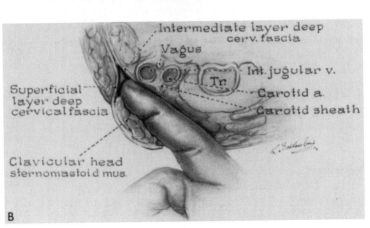

Figure 49–53. Anterior approach to the lower cervical and upper thoracic vertebrae. *A,* Incision. *Inset,* line of incision across the clavicular head of the sternomastoid muscle. *B,* Dissection within Burns' space behind the sternomastoid muscle. A finger is placed within this space to protect the internal jugular and subclavian veins as well as the carotid artery from injury during the division of the clavicular head of the sternomastoid.

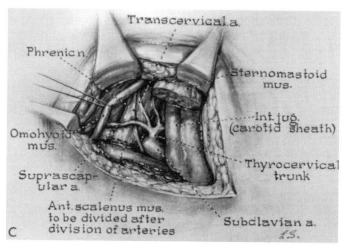

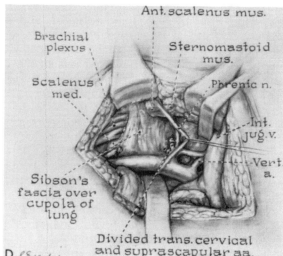

Figure 49–53 *Continued C*, Arteries and phrenic nerve crossing the scalenus anterior muscle. The omohyoid muscle is retracted upward and laterally. The subclavian vein lies anterior to the scalenus anterior muscle at the bottom of the wound. *D*, The scalenus anterior muscle is divided, exposing Sibson's fascia and the subclavian artery. The dome of the lung lies beneath this thin layer of Sibson's fascia. *E*, The visceral pleura and lung have been retracted laterally and downward and are protected with a moist pad. The posterior thorax, stellate ganglion, and upper thoracic vertebral bodies are now visible looking from above downward through the thoracic inlet.

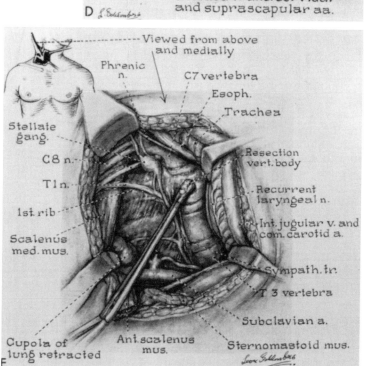

mastoid is then divided transversely, close to its clavicular insertion, with a finger behind the muscle, protecting these vessels.

Beneath the sternomastoid is the intermediate layer of deep fascia. The omohyoid muscle is invested in this fascia and crosses the field descending obliquely from medial to lateral. At its midportion, it is tendinous and is invested in a well-developed fascial expansion of the intermediate layers of fascia. This fascial expansion serves as a pulley, which permits the muscle to change directions from its oblique descent within the neck to a more lateral course extending to the shoulder. This middle layer of deep fascia is divided transversely, and the omohyoid is released from its pulley and retracted superiorly and laterally. Beneath is a fairly dense fat pad with small lymph nodes overlying the scalenus anterior muscle. This fat pad effectively hides the thyrocervical arterial trunk, phrenic nerve, and scalene muscle and should be cleared to visualize the structures beneath (Fig. 49–53C). By blunt finger dissection, the internal jugular vein and contents of the carotid sheath can be separated from the prevertebral fascia and retracted medially away from the scalenus anterior muscle. Two large arteries cross the field: the suprascapular artery, which crosses low and transversely, and the transverse cervical artery, which crosses obliquely high in the field (see Fig. 49–53C). These arteries or the thyrocervical trunk from which they arise should be doubly ligated and divided. The phrenic nerve crosses the scalenus anterior muscle from lateral to medial. It should be carefully mobilized along its entire length within the wound and should be retracted medially.

Both margins of the scalenus anterior muscle are defined, and a right-angle clamp is passed behind this muscle. The muscle is divided sharply by cutting onto this right-angle clamp 1 cm proximal to the muscle's insertion. Often a small branch of the subclavian artery is found entering this muscle, and this should be ligated. Beneath the scalenus anterior muscle is a thin, often translucent layer of fascia (Fig. 49–53D) that covers the dome of the lung known as Sibson's fascia. This is a continuation of the prevertebral fascia lining the intrathoracic surfaces of the ribs. It passes over the dome of the lung and down the anterior side of the pleura and fuses with the lateral wall of the alar fascia at the carotid sheath. Sibson's fascia is opened transversely using scissors, and the visceral pleura and lung beneath are dissected free using a finger. The visceral pleura may be bluntly dissected to the neck of the third rib, and the pleura and lung may be retracted inferiorly and laterally using a moist pad (Fig. 49–53E). Care is required to avoid injuring the pleura, causing a pneumothorax. The stellate ganglion is visible over the neck of the first rib, and the vertebrae are medial to this. The first thoracic nerve root is seen climbing out of the thorax over the first rib and should be protected. The vertebral level may be identified in reference to the first rib. The first rib articulates with the seventh cervical and first thoracic vertebral bodies and intervening discs. However, lateral roentgenograms

should be obtained in the operating room with a radiopaque marker fixed to the vertebra in question to verify the level.

Through this approach, exposures of the seventh cervical and first thoracic vertebrae are usually adequate, but exposures distal to this may be limited by the size and position of the anterior thorax. The distal extent of the exposure may be predicted with preoperative lateral roentgenograms of the upper thoracic spine as discussed earlier. Proximal extension along the cervical spine is hampered by the recurrent laryngeal nerve on the right, but this nerve usually may be mobilized and retracted sufficiently to provide access to the fifth cervical vertebral body. Biopsy, curettage, disc excision, or bone grafting is possible through this approach.

The wound should be flooded with saline before closure, and the lungs should be inflated to check for possible air leak. The scalenus anterior muscle and clavicular head of the sternomastoid muscle may be repaired, and the platysma and skin should be approximated. We recommend inserting a drain through the wound to the dome of the lung to prevent the accumulation of fluid and blood, which might otherwise compromise chest expansion. Prior to extubation, a chest roentgenogram should be obtained in the operating room to check for pneumothorax, and a chest tube should be inserted if one is present.

Complications

All the complications discussed in the section on anterior approaches to the middle and lower cervical vertebrae are possible. In addition, the pleura should be inspected carefully for tears, and these should be repaired if present. The inferior thyroid artery should be identified and ligated if necessary. If the approach is to the left of the midline, the thoracic duct should be identified and ligated if injured. A troublesome chylous effusion may occur if perforations are not identified. The thoracic duct may be divided without incident, as collateral pathways will develop with time, but it should be doubly ligated both proximally and distally.[33] It should be noted that although the thoracic duct usually arises in the thoracic inlet to the left of the midline, it may bifurcate or ramify within the thorax and present to the right or on both sides of the midline.

The phrenic and recurrent laryngeal nerves may be injured during retraction, and temporary paralysis of the involved diaphragm or vocal cord can occur. Because of this, special care is required to protect these structures during their mobilization and retraction, and some assistance with ventilation may be required following surgery. The right recurrent laryngeal nerve normally arises below the subclavian artery and crosses the neck anterior to the thyroid gland and trachea (see Fig. 49–22). The right recurrent nerve can arise higher in the neck and cross the larynx at almost any level. Therefore, it is important to identify this nerve, particularly when proximal extension along the cervical spine is planned.

Fluid may accumulate postoperatively above the dome of the lung and may depress the lung and thus limit the tidal volume of ventilation. For this reason, it is wise to drain this space and check that collapse of the upper lobe does not occur on follow-up chest roentgenograms.

Biopsy, Curettage, and Drainage Through the Anterior Approach to the Cervical Spine

The most direct and effective means of diagnosing a lesion of the anterior cervical spine is via the transoral, pharyngeal approach or through one of the anterolateral exposures. The operative approach is dictated by the cervical level and the extent of the proposed dissection. On reaching the vertebral body, a needle should be inserted into the suspected area, and roentgenograms should be made on the operating table to verify the level and position of the lesion. Often the lesion is grossly evident, and a direct biopsy specimen can be obtained using a drill and curets. Large sterile defects should be grafted primarily.

Osteomyelitis of the vertebral body or disc space infections can be effectively cureted and drained through these anterior exposures. The curettage should be thorough to remove as much diseased bone and divitalized tissue as possible. If the spine is made unstable, the patient should be protected with traction or a halo-cast, and posterior interspinous wiring and fusion should be performed at a later date. If a large anterior defect persists, anterior grafting may ultimately be required to fill this defect. A tuberculous abscess may be drained anteriorly and at the time of drainage and curettage should be grafted primarily with antibiotic coverage. Direct surgical exposure of a suspect lesion offers the best chance to identify the pathologic condition and treat the disease process primarily.

Excision of Intervertebral Discs, Osteophytes, and Interbody Fusion Anteriorly

Herniated intervertebral discs compressing the spinal cord or nerve roots may be treated expeditiously through the anterior approach. In addition, osteophytes of the posterior lip of the vertebral body impinging on the cord or nerve roots may be removed through this approach.

The radicular pain associated with cervical spondylosis is often caused by compression of the nerve root by herniated disc material or osteophytes. Disc excision, osteophyte excision, or both and interbody fusion will effectively improve persistent symptoms if the involvement is restricted to one or two levels and if there is objective neurologic and myelographic evidence of nerve root impingement. The incidence of successful fusion and satisfactory clinical results tends to decrease with each additional level fused.[67, 70]

Despite these optimistic statements about surgery,

the authors still feel that the *primary* treatment of most cervical spondylotic or discogenic problems is conservative, using anti-inflammatory drugs, orthoses, or traction for an extended period of time. In most cases, symptoms will be significantly improved. Only if these conservative measures fail should surgery be considered.

The rationale for surgery is to remove the disc and posterior osteophyte to relieve the pressure on the spinal cord or nerve root. The disc space is then filled with a bone graft, which distracts the disc space and effectively enlarges the neural foramina. We suspect that small but pathologic motion between vertebrae is responsible for the development of posterior osteophytes. Fusion is performed to maintain the height of the disc space and to eliminate this motion and recurrent osteophyte formation. Fusion alone without osteophyte excision is often sufficient to relieve radicular symptoms, for after osseous union is complete, the osteophytes usually resorb in nine to 12 months' time and symptoms subside. However, in order to provide immediate relief of symptoms, offending osteophytes may be removed at the time of anterior interbody fusion.

Anterior fusion should be restricted to those levels that are producing clinical symptoms and objective signs. Often, multiple levels appear to be involved radiographically, and the myelogram may demonstrate obliteration of the nerve root sleeves at levels that do not appear to be involved clinically. In these situations, we recommend fusing only those levels that are involved clinically. When there is a discrepancy between the myelographic and clinical findings, we advocate fusing only those levels that are involved clinically.

Fusion may also be used effectively to relieve discogenic symptoms in which the pain is localized to the neck and in which there is no radicular component. The problem here is to accurately localize the source of symptoms at a single or perhaps two intervertebral segments, because any of the eight cervical articulations can produce symptoms. Local neck pain may be caused by degeneration of the disc with posterior protrusion of disc material into the posterior longitudinal ligament. This distorts the posterior longitudinal ligament and may irritate local nerve fibers within the ligament. Pain may also be produced by arthritic degeneration of the facet joints. It is hard to differentiate between these causes, although plane roentgenograms may reveal degeneration of the disc and loss of disc space height or narrowing of the articular space between the facets and local spurs or osteophytes. Unfortunately, these are only presumptive pieces of evidence and do not prove that these are the levels of involvement or sources of symptoms. Injection of the disc space or involved facet joints with saline, lidocaine (Xylocaine), or steroids may improve the localization, but these techniques are potentially dangerous and are only sometimes helpful. Motion of the neck may aggravate these symptoms, with flexion or rotation of the neck irritating the facets and extension placing increased stress on the posterior disc and ligament.

Because of the difficulties in accurately localizing the source of local symptoms, we advocate a very cautious approach to the treatment of discogenic pain. Conservative measures, such as anti-inflammatory drugs, traction, collars, and braces, should be tried for an extended period of time and often yield satisfactory results. Only if these measures fail and if satisfactory localization is possible should surgical fusion be considered.

Many patients may present with pain radiating up the back of the neck to the occiput above and behind the ear. This pain may be caused by irritation of the greater occipital nerve at the atlantoaxial level. Anterior fusions at a lower cervical level cannot improve this symptom.

Technique

The vertebral bodies and interspaces are reached through one of the anterolateral approaches, depending on the level of the spine involved. A needle is placed in the involved disc space, and a control lateral roentgenogram is obtained to verify the level. A rectangular window may be cut in the anterior longitudinal ligament over the interspace. An alternative approach is to develop a flap in the anterior longitudinal ligament over the midvertebral body, which may be replaced after surgery. The bulk of the annulus fibrosus is removed from the disc space using curets and pituitary rongeurs (Fig. 49–54A). The cartilaginous end plate is removed with angled curets, but the subchondral cortical end plate is left intact. It is important to remember that the cervical disc space is angled superiorly and that dissection should proceed along this plane, to prevent inadvertent injury of the cortical end plate. The anterior cortical lip of the vertebra is also spared,

unless a significant osteophyte is present, and this anterior lip is later used to lock the bone graft in place. The whole of the annulus is removed to the posterior longitudinal ligament. In the cervical spine the posterior longitudinal ligament is a broad, dense ligament, which effectively protects the cord during this phase of the dissection. However, the posterior longitudinal ligament does not extend laterally over the neural foramina, so the nerve roots are not similarly protected.

To remove a posterior osteophyte, a drill with a small round burr may be used to create a transverse trough in the cortical end plate adjacent to the posterior edge of the vertebra. This weakens the bone around the osteophyte. A small, angled curet is then used to reach behind the osteophyte, break it off, and deliver it into the wound (Fig. 49–54B). This maneuver is repeated until the osteophyte is completely removed and the cord and nerve root are free of impingement (Fig. 49–54C). The osteophyte may also be removed directly using a very fine, 60-degree angled rongeur with a cup diameter of only 2 mm. The rongeur is introduced into the disc space using two hands, and the terminal end of the rongeur blade is carefully placed posterior to the osteophyte. The rongeur is pulled firmly against the osteophyte, and the blades are closed to prevent the rongeur from moving posteriorly into the cord or nerve roots. This maneuver is repeated until the osteophyte or transverse bar is completely removed.

The defect in the intervertebral disc space is then measured using a flexible probe. This defect usually measures 15 by 15 by 8 mm, and a graft that is 10 to 12 mm in depth, 15 mm wide, and 8 mm in height usually fills this defect adequately. To obtain the bone graft, a short incision is made over the anterior iliac crest. Two parallel cuts are made in the ilium through both cortical tables using osteotomes or an oscillating

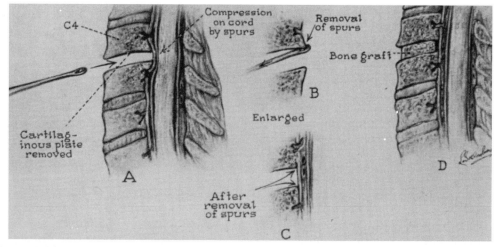

Figure 49–54. Anterior cervical interbody fusion and posterior osteophyte excision. *A*, The annulus fibrosus and cartilage end plates are removed with curets and pituitary rongeurs. The subchondral cortical end plate is left intact. *B* and *C*, The posterior osteophyte is removed. *D*, A horseshoe-shaped plug of iliac bone is tamped into the intervertebral defect. (From White, A. A., Southwick, W. O., DePonte, R. J., et al.: Relief of pain by anterior cervical spine fusion for spondylosis. J. Bone Joint Surg. *55A*:525, 1973.)

saw with two parallel blades set 8 to 10 mm apart. A horseshoe-shaped plug of bone with cortex on three margins is removed. The bone graft is then shaped to fit the defect in the disc space. The height of the graft should be somewhat greater than the height of the disc space so that it will fit snugly under compression. The anteroposterior dimension of the graft should be at least 5 mm less than the depth of the vertebra, so that when the graft is recessed behind the lips of the vertebra, it will not compress the cord posteriorly.

A small transverse trough is cut at the front of the end plate of the upper vertebra to lock the graft in place anteriorly. The neck is carefully extended by the anesthetist, and about 20 lb of head-halter traction is applied. The graft is gently tamped into position with a metal punch and mallet. The anterior aspect of the graft should be recessed behind the anterior cortical lip of the vertebra and locked into the transverse trough previously created. This is done to hold the graft and to prevent it from sliding forward into the esophagus (see Fig. 49–28). On release of traction, the graft should fit snugly and should be compressed by the remaining cervical ligaments and muscles. A lateral roentgenogram should be obtained to check position and alignment and to verify that the graft is not protruding into the spinal canal posteriorly.

The wound is irrigated, the superficial layer of the deep fascia is repaired loosely, and the platysma is closed with interrupted inverting sutures to prevent a wide scar. The skin is closed, and a narrow, cosmetically pleasing transverse scar that is concealed by adjacent skin folds should result in 10 to 12 weeks. The neck should be protected with external support to prevent hyperextension until bony fusion is established in three to six months.

Although all of the hyaline cartilage plate is removed, the bony cortical end plates of the vertebral bodies are spared throughout the dissection. The graft is inserted so that the horseshoe of cortical bone abuts with the end plate, effectively distracting the vertebrae. The end plates are spared to provide as much support for the graft as possible and to minimize postoperative compression of the disc space. This distraction creates significant enlargement of the nerve root foramina and reduces nerve root impingement. Although some settling of the graft will occur with time, a satisfactory and permanent enlargement of the foramina can be obtained.

Case Report

P. D., a 45-year-old woman, was involved in a motor vehicle accident eight years previously and sustained a fracture of the odontoid. She was successfully treated with an atlantoaxial posterior fusion using the Brooks technique (see "Posterior Cervical Approaches"). Six years later she developed pain in the right shoulder radiating to her right arm. Conservative treatment with intermittent traction, a cervical collar, and aspirin did not provide lasting relief. After two years of such treatment, she was admitted to the hospital for myelogra-

phy. At this time, a slight sensory deficit in the right C5 and C6 nerve root distribution was noted. There was objective weakness of the right biceps and brachioradialis muscles and an asymmetric deficit in these reflexes.

A myelogram revealed blunting of the C5 and C6 nerve root sleeves and, on lateral views, vertebral body osteophytes indenting the dye column were seen. With extension of the neck, a posterior defect in the dye column over the ligamentum flavum was also noted (Fig. 49–55A). We concluded that this defect in the posterior dye column was caused by hypertrophy or loss of the normal elasticity of the ligamentum flavum. With neck extension, the redundant ligamentum flavum protruded anteriorly, effectively reducing the anteroposterior dimension of the canal, forcing the spinal cord against the vertebral bodies and osteophytes.

The therapeutic options were to perform a wide posterior decompressive laminectomy at multiple levels and to fuse the spine. We thought that a simpler and functionally less debilitating approach was to enter the spine anteriorly, remove the osteophytes, relieve the nerve root compression, and fuse the spine to prevent further osteophyte formation. If this was not completely effective, a posterior approach could be performed at a later date.

Decompression and fusion at two levels anteriorly, C4–C5 and C5–C6, were accomplished. Postoperative roentgenograms revealed that the posterior osteophytes were satisfactorily excised (Fig. 49–55B and C) and the foramina were considerably enlarged, particularly at the C4–C5 level (Fig. 49–55D and E). The patient enjoyed complete improvement of her preoperative symptoms and neurologic deficit and established a stable fusion in four months. The nerve root foramina remain open, as demonstrated radiographically, seven years following fusion, and there is no evidence of collapse of the grafts.

Excision of Vertebral Body and Replacement With Bone Graft Through the Anterior Approach

Complete excision of one or more vertebral bodies may be required when the body is extensively involved with infection or tumor or when the body is fractured and displaced posteriorly into the spinal canal. In many of these cases the body should be replaced with bone graft to maintain vertebral height and alignment and to provide stability when osseous union is complete. Bone graft replacement should be considered even when the spinal cord is completely and irreversibly damaged, to prevent progressive ascending neurologic damage.

Fractures of the cervical vertebral bodies with posterior displacement and spinal cord injury are most often associated with hyperflexion-compression injuries, such as diving accidents.[6] In these injuries, the body is often severely comminuted with some fragments displaced posteriorly into the spinal canal, or the fracture occurs at the pedicles, with the vertebral body as

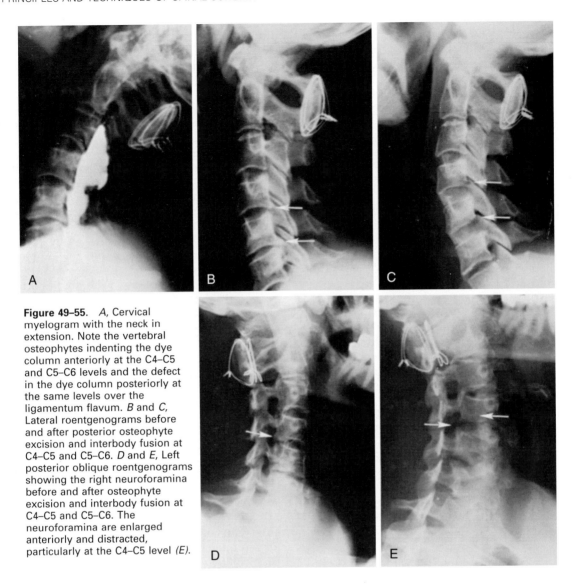

Figure 49–55. *A,* Cervical myelogram with the neck in extension. Note the vertebral osteophytes indenting the dye column anteriorly at the C4–C5 and C5–C6 levels and the defect in the dye column posteriorly at the same levels over the ligamentum flavum. *B* and *C,* Lateral roentgenograms before and after posterior osteophyte excision and interbody fusion at C4–C5 and C5–C6. *D* and *E,* Left posterior oblique roentgenograms showing the right neuroforamina before and after osteophyte excision and interbody fusion at C4–C5 and C5–C6. The neuroforamina are enlarged anteriorly and distracted, particularly at the C4–C5 level *(E).*

a whole displaced posteriorly. The spinal cord may be compressed and draped over these fragments. Posterior laminectomy may effectively decompress the canal; however, the cord may still be draped over the fragments and may continue to be irritated or damaged. Furthermore, it is almost impossible to remove a cervical vertebral body through the posterior approach without injuring the cord more extensively. Finally, posterior laminectomy will remove the last threads of spinal stability remaining and will compound the structural problems present. For these reasons, we prefer to treat vertebral body fractures that are displaced posteriorly and in which there is incomplete or progressive neurologic deficit with anterior decompression and fusion.

Anterior fusion techniques rarely add any stability in the immediate postoperative period, and vertebral body resection may seriously contribute to any pre-existing instability, even when the body is replaced by

a bone graft. A number of authors have advocated notching the graft,[68] recessing the graft behind the anterior cortical margin of the vertebra,[4, 5, 46, 65] or using sutures, screws, or plates to improve fixation. We advocate carving keys on either end of the graft and fitting these into troughs burred into the end plates of the upper and lower vertebrae. These prevent anteroposterior displacement of the graft into the spinal cord or esophagus. Without these keys, catastrophic displacements can occur (see Fig. 49–29).[32] Despite this, the spine may remain unstable, particularly in flexion or against shear forces between vertebrae. Stauffer and Kelly[62] demonstrated that instability is most prevalent following anterior fusion when there is coexistent damage of the posterior elements. For this reason, traction, a halo-cast, or subsequent posterior interspinous wiring and fusion may be required to maintain vertebral alignment until anterior osseous union is complete. Of these three, we much prefer posterior spinal wiring.

Technique

Endotracheal anesthesia and skeletal traction are ordinarily required for this procedure. The involved vertebral body is exposed through one of the anterior approaches as dictated by the level of involvement (see Fig. 49–30). The involved vertebra is carefully resected using rongeurs and curets (Fig. 49–56). As the dissection proceeds posteriorly, care is required to prevent further injury to the spinal cord. Most often the posterior longitudinal ligament is torn or frayed and does not present a natural barrier between the vertebral body and the canal. The body is extremely vascular, and considerable hemorrhage is usually encountered. For this reason, it is recommended that as the dissection approaches the canal, the lateral side of the body that is least involved be resected first. The joint of Luschka is removed laterally, and the nerve root is identified. Using this landmark, the dissection should proceed medially, following the nerve root to the dura. In this manner, the neural elements may be spared.

The intervening annulus fibrosus and cartilaginous end plates on either side of the involved body should be resected, but the subchondral, cortical end plates of the adjacent vertebrae should be spared (Fig. 49–57A and B). These will provide support for the bone graft and will prevent collapse of the graft into the softer cancellous portion of the body. The dura and nerve roots should be carefully inspected to ensure that the decompression is adequate.

The bone graft is usually obtained from the anterior ilium. A long plug that has three cortical surfaces and that includes the inner and outer tables of the ilium is removed. The defect is measured, and the graft is fashioned so that it will fit the defect tightly. Keys are shaped at either end of the graft, as illustrated in Figure 49–57C and D. The keys are fitted into transverse troughs in the end plates of the adjacent vertebrae to prevent anterior or posterior migration of the graft.

Transverse troughs are cut into the end plates of the adjacent vertebrae, as illustrated in Figure 49–57C and D and Figure 49–58. These are fashioned so that the graft may slide into the trough from one lateral side. The cervical spine is slightly extended, and longitudinal traction is increased. The graft is tamped into place, and control lateral roentgenograms are obtained to ensure that placement is satisfactory and that there is no protrusion of the graft into the canal. A corticocancellous spike of bone may be inserted into the trough and driven into the soft, cancellous vertebral body to lock the graft in place and prevent it from slipping laterally. The wound is carefully irrigated, and the deeper layers are closed loosely to permit drainage. A subcutaneous drain may be used to prevent compressive hematoma and subsequent airway obstruction.

The troughs in the vertebrae and keys in the graft are fashioned to prevent graft migration posteriorly into the spinal canal or anteriorly into the esophagus. These do not prevent distraction, anteroposterior shear displacements, or flexion if the posterior elements are damaged. Therefore, some form of external stabilization, such as longitudinal skeletal traction, a halo-brace, or a halo-cast, is required following this procedure until fusion is established. Anterior bone grafting provides little or no immediate postoperative stabilization; however, when osseous union is established, the stability is excellent.

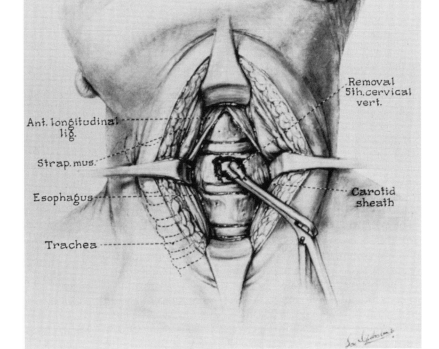

Figure 49–56. Resection of cervical vertebral body through the anterior approach.

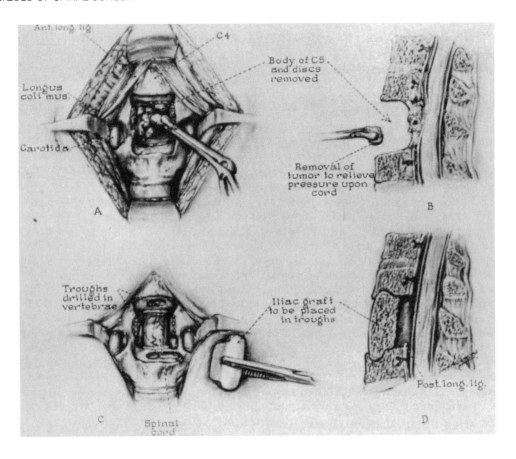

Figure 49–57. *A*, The involved vertebra is resected using rongeurs and curets. *B*, The annulus fibrosus and cartilaginous end plates are resected on either side of the involved vertebra, and the cord is decompressed. The subchondral cortical end plates of the uninvolved vertebrae are left intact to support the graft. *C*, Troughs are drilled in the adjacent vertebrae, and an iliac graft is fashioned with keys at either end. *D*, Sagittal section with iliac graft in place.

POSTERIOR APPROACHES TO THE CERVICAL SPINE

Posterior Occipitocervical Fusion

Although occipitocervical fusions are rarely required, there are certain situations in which fusion of the occiput to the upper cervical spine is necessary. Bursting fractures of the ring of the first cervical vertebra[23] with associated rupture of the transverse ligament[61] may make the cervical spine extremely unstable. Not only is the posterior ring of the first vertebra separated from the front, but the stability provided by the transverse ligament between the odontoid and anterior ring of the atlas is lost as well. Fusion may be required to bridge the occiput to the second or third vertebra. Extensive resection of the anterior atlantoaxial elements also creates instability, which may be controlled by occipitocervical fusion. Fractures of the odontoid or ruptures of the transverse ligament at the atlas with atlantoaxial subluxation do not ordinarily require occipitocervical fusion unless the posterior arch of the first or second vertebra is compromised. Generally, these may be adequately stabilized with a posterior atlantoaxial fusion of the Brooks' type, to be described in the next section.

The fusion technique described using corticocancellous struts of bone wired to the involved vertebrae adds immediately to the stability of the atlanto-occipital articulation and upper cervical vertebrae. Ordinarily, sufficient strength is provided so that the patient

may be mobilized in a cervicothoracic brace, and traction or a halo-brace is not required in the postoperative regimen. Nevertheless, if a significant kyphos or flexion deformity is present at this level, a posteriorly placed graft will be situated under tension and might attenu-

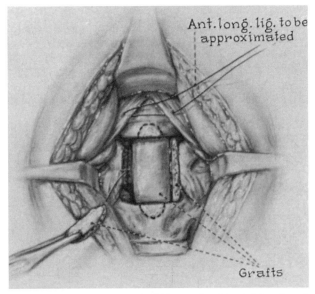

Figure 49–58. Anterior view of iliac graft with additional graft material being placed on either side.

ate with time. In this condition, a posterior fusion may be used to provide immediate postoperative stability, and a second-stage anterior fusion may be added to provide long-term support.

Technique

Endotracheal anesthesia is required to maintain the airway. The three-point pin headrest (see Figs. 49–38 and 49–39) is applied to the skull under aseptic conditions, and the patient is turned to the prone position while maintaining cervical traction through the pin headrest. The pin headrest is attached to the operating table with the spine distracted to maintain stability intraoperatively (see Fig. 49–40). Countertraction is recommended by taping the shoulders to the distal end of the operating table. A lateral roentgenogram of the cervical spine is taken to verify that the vertebrae are properly aligned.

A longitudinal midline incision is made, extending from the occipital protuberance to the lower cervical spine (Fig. 49–59A). The incision is extended deeply within the relatively avascular midline structures, the intermuscular septum. Deviation from the midline may result in troublesome hemorrhage. The spinous processes, posterior tubercle of the atlas, and median nuchal line of the occiput are palpated. The incision is carried down to these midline bony prominences using a scalpel. The laminae of the second and third cervical vertebrae are dissected subperiosteally and laterally to the facets, but the capsular ligaments of the facets should be preserved to maintain stability. The posterior ring of the first vertebra is cleared of soft tissues by subperiosteal dissection. Care is required to avoid injuring the vertebral arteries and vertebral venous plexus, which lie on the superior aspect of the first cervical ring less than 2 cm from midline. The posterior occiput is dissected laterally by sharp subperiosteal dissection to the level of the external occipital protuberance. The posterior lip of the foramen magnum is

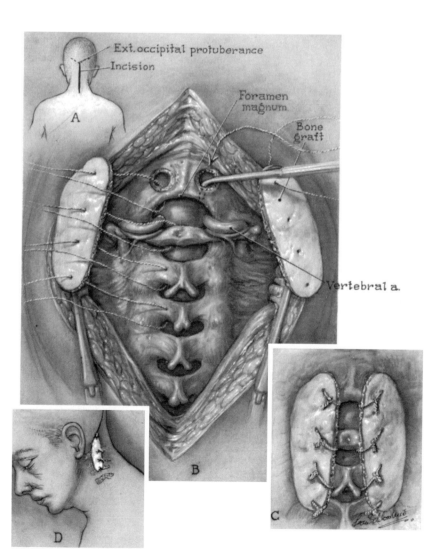

Figure 49–59. *A–D,* Occipitocervical fusion. (From Robinson, R. A., and Southwick, W. O.: Surgical approaches to the cervical spine. *In* the American Academy of Orthopaedic Surgeons: Instructional Course Lectures, Vol. XVII. St. Louis, The C. V. Mosby Co., 1960.)

visible, and the vertebral arteries may be palpated as they enter the atlanto-occipital ligament on their course to the foramen magnum. Two burr holes are made in the posterior occiput about 7 mm from the foramen magnum and 10 mm lateral to midline (Fig. 49–59*B*). The dura is exposed and depressed from the inner table by gentle, blunt dissection with a right-angled dissector. The posterior atlanto-occipital ligament is separated from the posterior lip of the foramen magnum using fine curets and an elevator. The epidural space between the burr holes and foramen magnum is connected. A twisted wire is passed from the burr holes through the epidural space and out the foramen magnum, using a right-angled Mixter clamp and nerve protector.

The ring of the first vertebra is cleared of ligament using straight and angled fine curets. The dura is depressed using a right-angled dissector, and twisted wire is passed around the posterior ring about 1 cm lateral to midline. The grafts may also be secured to the spinous processes of the second and third cervical vertebrae. Holes are drilled in the outer table of the spinous processes, on either side, adjacent to the laminae (Fig. 49–60*A*). These holes are connected with a "sweetheart" or towel clip, and two strands of twisted wire are passed through these (Fig. 49–60*B* and *C*).

A long, ovoid graft of corticocancellous bone is taken from the iliac crest. Holes are made in the graft at appropriate intervals to accept the twisted wires. Wires are passed through these holes so that the cancellous surface of the graft will lie against the spinous processes, laminae, and occiput. The graft is settled

snugly against the laminae, and the wires are tightened and twisted to hold the graft firmly in place. This procedure is duplicated on the opposite side, and the grafts are manipulated to ensure that satisfactory stabilization is achieved (see Fig. 49–59*B* and *D*). Long, thin strips of cancellous iliac bone are laid about the cortical grafts to stimulate osseous fusion.

The grafts and wires should be inspected to ensure that they do not impinge on the dura or vertebral arteries. The wound is copiously irrigated with saline and is closed in multiple layers using interrupted absorbable sutures, approximating the intermuscular septum and ligamentum nuchae. The skin is closed cosmetically, the wound is dressed, and the head and neck are splinted to protect the neck during turning, extubation, and transfer to bed. Some form of external support is strongly recommended until fusion is established to prevent motion in all planes. The type of immobilization needed depends on the degree of primary instability, but ordinarily a cervicothoracic brace will suffice.

For immediate stability, one of us (M.J.M.) devised a method of fixation using the identical technique just described, except that instead of using iliac corticocancellous bone grafts to maintain alignment, a threaded Harrington compression rod is used (Fig. 49–61). The rod or a 5/32-inch threaded Steinmann pin is bent to fit along the facet joints and occiput in a horseshoe-shaped configuration. The wires can be twisted around the threaded rod and do not slip. Cancellous bone grafts are laid in place, and the construct can usually give sufficient stability to eliminate the need

Figure 49–60. Posterior interspinous fusion. *A,* Holes are drilled in the outer cortex of the spinous process adjacent to the laminae. *B,* The drill holes are connected with a towel clip. *C,* Wires are passed through the holes in adjacent vertebrae and are twisted in place. *D,* One additional wire is passed to surround all the vertebrae involved in the area of intended fusion. *E,* Corticocancellous strips of bone graft are laid down about the posterior elements in the area of intended fusion.

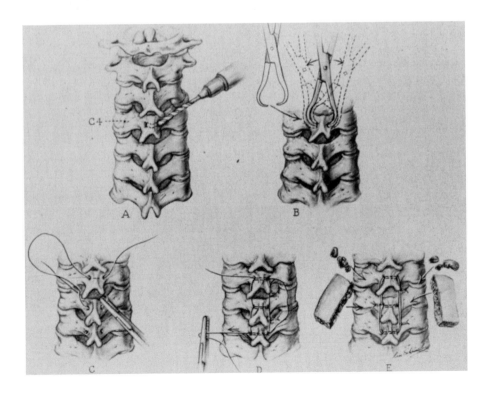

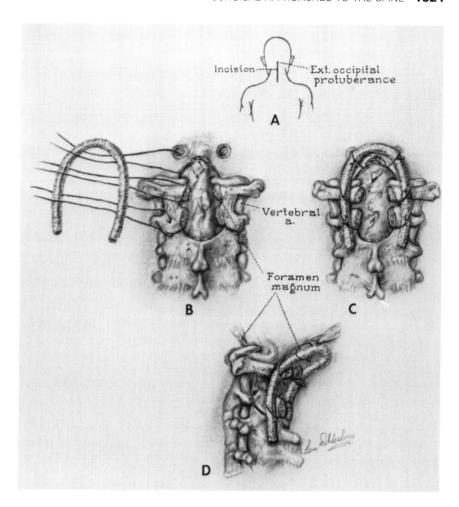

Figure 49–61. *A–D,* Bent Harrington compression rods or bent 5/32-inch Steinmann pins fixed accurately to the facet joints offer immediate stability of extensive laminectomy.

for collars and braces. This construct is especially useful in the management of tumors and in debilitated individuals.

Complications

Care is required in passing the wires to prevent injury to the brain stem or spinal cord. Posterior fusion without decompressive laminectomy tends to constrict the spinal canal. Following trauma to the spine, a certain amount of edema and hemorrhage of the cord and adjacent structures is anticipated. Three weeks following trauma, the swelling begins to subside. Because of this, we recommend a delay of three to six weeks following trauma before fusion without associated laminectomy is attempted. This will help minimize any compromise of cord or nerve root function that surgery might add immediately following trauma.

The vertebral artery and associated venous plexus should be identified and spared throughout the dissection. The venous plexus, which is closely related to the vertebral artery, can cause particularly troublesome hemorrhage if it is disturbed.

Brooks' Posterior Atlantoaxial Fusion

Fractures of the base of the odontoid (Type II)[2] or disruptions of the transverse ligament with atlantoaxial

dislocation generally heal poorly. When fractures at the base of the odontoid are treated conservatively, nonunion rates of 5 to 64 per cent are reported.[2, 3, 44, 53] Because of the high incidence of nonunion, recurrent dislocation, and the ever-present threat of sudden death with insignificant trauma, the treatment of choice in most clinics is early reduction and fusion.

A review of our experience with this lesion by Griswold and associates[20] revealed a 63 per cent nonunion rate after "satisfactory" conservative treatment. Over half of these were symptomatic and required surgical fusion at a later date. Patients with fractures that united satisfactorily were all younger than 21 years of age. Because of the high incidence of nonunion, conservative treatment is probably indicated only in patients younger than 21 years of age or in those too old or debilitated to withstand the rigors of a major surgical procedure.

In 1910, Mixter and Osgood reported on posterior stabilization of the first two cervical vertebrae using a fascial loop. Gallie[18] and others revised this technique, using a wire loop for immediate stabilization and bone graft to induce fusion. The atlantoaxial joint permits more physiologic motion than any other vertebral articulation. Fusion at this level should prevent flexion, extension, and rotation as well as horizontal displacements. The simple posterior wiring technique described by Gallie prevents flexion and anterior horizontal displacement but does not restrict extension, rotation, and posterior or lateral horizontal displacements. For this reason, we have adapted a method described to us by Dr. Arthur Brooks of Vanderbilt University.[7] Two prism-shaped pieces of corticocancellous iliac graft are secured to the posterior laminae on either side of the midline. The apex of the cancellous portion of the graft fits between the laminae. Each graft is held firmly in position with two loops of twisted wire surrounding the laminae and graft. The wedge-shaped graft functions like a brake shoe, effectively preventing flexion, rotation, and translation. This fusion technique provides enough immediate stability that in most cases a simple cervicothoracic brace is sufficient to protect the spine until osseous union is established. In our experience, the ultimate rate of stable fusion has improved from 67 per cent using other fusion techniques to 97 per cent using the Brooks approach.

Fielding and coworkers[17] described a modification of the Gallie fusion technique using a single butterfly or U-shaped corticocancellous graft secured to the posterior elements of the atlas and axis with a wire loop. They obtained a very high rate of fusion using this technique but protect their patients with traction or a Minerva jacket for the first six weeks following surgery. Leider and Ferlic[31] reported the use of the halo-cast to treat fractures of the base of the odontoid and obtained a union rate of 90 per cent using this technique in 20 patients. The halo-cast appears to offer a significant improvement in the incidence of union compared with other conservative measures; however, additional experience is required to verify this.

Technique

The patient is anesthetized on a stretcher next to the operating table using endotracheal intubation and a noncollapsible tube. Care is required during intubation to prevent flexion or extension of the head and neck. The three-point pin headrest is applied to the parietal portion of the skull to provide rigid control of the neck intraoperatively (see Figs. 49–38 and 49–39). The patient is rolled like a log onto the operating table. During this maneuver, the surgeon controls the head and neck by holding the pin headrest with one hand, applying firm, longitudinal traction. The surgeon uses his or her second hand to support the neck and directs the other members of the team in turning the patient. The pin headrest is attached to the table with the neck in a neutral position and the head slightly flexed. The head is flexed by rotating the skull and mandible anteriorly in a military posture, separating the occiput from the posterior ring of the atlas and providing more room for dissection about the atlas. The neck is distracted gently with the pin headrest, and countertraction is applied by taping the shoulders to the distal end of the operating table (see Fig. 49–40). A lateral roentgeno-gram of the cervical spine is obtained to ensure that the vertebrae are properly reduced.

After the skin is prepared, a wide operative field is draped from the occiput to the lower cervical spine. Bleeding may be reduced by infiltrating the midline structures with 10 ml of a 1:200,000 solution of epinephrine. A midline incision is made from the lower occipital region to the level of the fourth cervical spinous process. The incision is extended deeply within one of the relatively avascular midline structures, the intermuscular septum or ligamentum nuchae. The spinous processes and posterior tubercle of the atlas are palpated, and the incision is carried down to these midline bony prominences using a scalpel. The ligaments and muscles are dissected from the spinous processes and laminae of the first and second cervical vertebrae by subperiosteal dissection. The small muscular attachments to the bifid spinous process of C2 (see Fig. 49–24) can be removed with a curet while holding the vertebra with a Kocher clamp to prevent gross motion. Care is required in dissecting laterally over the atlas to prevent injury to the vertebral arteries and vertebral venous plexus. These lie on the superior aspect of the ring, less than 2 cm lateral to the midline. We have found that this dissection is facilitated by making a transverse incision through the periosteum along the posterior ring of the atlas. The periosteum is raised using a Joseph elevator, and the vertebral vessels are mobilized in continuity with the periosteum. This maneuver protects the vertebral vessels from injury as they are separated from the plane of dissection by an intact layer of tissue. The occiput should not be exposed, to avoid inadvertent fusion to the base of the skull. Using right-angled curets and elevators, the first and second cervical laminae are exposed circumferentially. Two strands of 24-gauge stainless steel wire are twisted on themselves in a drill. This increases the strength of the wire while not adding greatly to its stiffness. Two separate wires are passed on each side of the midline beneath the laminae of the first and second vertebrae, using a small right-angled Mixter clamp or aneurysm needle (Fig. 49–62A–E). Great care is required during this maneuver to prevent injury to the dura or cord.

The bone graft is taken from the posterior iliac crest superficial to the sacroiliac joint where the ilium is thick. Ordinarily, there is a longitudinal prominence in this area that parallels the posterior margin of the ilium. A rectangle about 2 by 4 cm in size is marked in the ilium, centered over this ridge, and a prism-shaped piece of corticocancellous bone is removed from the outer table, as shown in Figure 49–62F. This is divided into two segments, 1.5 by 2.0 cm in length. The wedge-shaped cancellous apex of the graft is tailored to fit between the laminae of the upper two vertebrae without impinging on the spinal canal or vertebral artery. Notches are fashioned in the upper and lower cortical surfaces to hold the circumferential wires and prevent them from slipping. The grafts are placed snugly against the denuded laminae, and the two wires are tightened and twisted on each side (Fig.

49–62G and H). The wires should be separated so that they encompass the lateral and medial sides of the graft and do not cluster toward the midline. The ring of the atlas is carefully manipulated to ensure that stabilization is satisfactory. The wires and grafts are inspected to verify that they do not impinge on the dura or the vertebral arteries.

The wound is copiously irrigated with saline and closed in multiple layers with interrupted absorbable sutures approximating the intermuscular septum. The skin is closed cosmetically, and the wound is dressed. The head and neck are splinted during turning, extubation, and transfer of the patient to bed. External support is recommended until fusion is established in three to six months (five months average in our series). Skeletal tongs or a halo-brace may be used initially, but a simple cervicothoracic brace provides enough support in most cases.

Complications

In the series reviewed by Griswold and colleagues,[20] there were several complications. Two patients developed recurrent anterior atlantoaxial subluxation in the early postoperative period. Two developed spontaneous extension of the fusion, one to the third and one to the fourth cervical vertebra. One resulted in an inadequate fusion to the posterior ring of the atlas. This patient had two previous failures of fusion by other techniques and a marginal vascular supply to the posterior ring of the atlas. The early recurrent subluxation could have been prevented by more adequate external bracing in the early postoperative period. We would recommend the SOMI brace to prevent this problem based on our functional studies of cervical orthoses.[26] Spontaneous extension of fusion is a minor problem that may be minimized by careful dissection confined to the areas of intended fusion. All patients ultimately developed stability, and none acquired any neurologic embarrassment.

We are aware of several instances in which the spinal cord has been injured during this procedure, resulting in some permanent neurologic deficit. This presumably occurred while passing the wires about the lamina, and for this reason, care is required during this maneuver. Posterior fusion without decompressive laminectomy tends to constrict the spinal cord. Because of this, we recommend a delay of three to six weeks following trauma before fusion is attempted. This permits the hemorrhage and edema of trauma to subside before constrictive fusion is attempted.

The vertebral artery and associated venous plexus should be identified and spared throughout the dissection. The vertebral venous plexus ordinarily lies superficial to the vertebral artery and can cause particularly troublesome hemorrhage if disturbed.

In our experience, fusion of the atlantoaxial joint results in a loss of almost half of normal cervical rotation, and patients should be advised of this prior to surgery. Many of our patients have noticed this restriction when driving a motor vehicle but have been able

to accommodate for this easily. It is possible that the successful treatment of odontoid fractures using a halo-cast may not affect rotation of the atlantoaxial joint as significantly as does fusion, and this factor should be examined in future clinical studies.

Posterior Interspinous Wiring and Fusion of the Lower Cervical Spine, From C2 to the Thorax

Two areas are available for wiring and fusion posteriorly: the spinous processes and facets. The authors have found that in most cases wiring and fusion of the spinous processes is a less complex technique and provides almost as much immediate stabilization as facet posterolateral fusion. For these reasons, we recommend interspinous wiring and fusion and reserve the more complex fusion techniques for those situations in which the spinous processes, laminae, or facets are deficient or have been removed.

We have found that in many circumstances interspinous wiring and fusion provides effective immediate stabilization and that in most cases a precariously unstable spine may be converted to one in which only a simple cervicothoracic brace is required for protection until osseous fusion is established. In biomechanical studies performed on human cadaver spines, we have found that a mean of 284 newtons may be added to the strength of the spine by this wiring technique alone.[27] If the facet joints have not been disturbed, this wiring will effectively restrict flexion and anterior horizontal translation but will not control extension. Therefore, interspinous wiring and fusion should provide the most effective stabilization of flexion injuries of the neck with primary involvement of the posterior ligaments. However, interspinous wiring provides little control over extension injuries in which the anterior stabilizing ligaments have been destroyed. In these situations, additional internal fixation such as threaded rods (see Figs. 49–61 and 49–64) or external support using a halo-cast may be required. When the facet joints have been fractured or removed, interspinous wiring provides little control over anterior horizontal shear displacements, and interfacet wiring may be required to provide satisfactory immediate stabilization.

Technique

The authors prefer an interspinous fusion technique similar to the method described by Rogers.[51, 52] The patient is anesthetized on a stretcher next to the operating table, using endotracheal intubation and a non-collapsing tube. The three-point pin headrest is applied to the skull (see Figs. 49–38, 49–39, and 49–40). The patient is turned onto the operating table, and the headrest is fixed to the operating table in moderate distraction. Countertraction is applied by taping the shoulders to the distal end of the operating table, and a control lateral roentgenogram is obtained to verify that the vertebrae are in proper alignment.

The skin over the back of the head and neck is

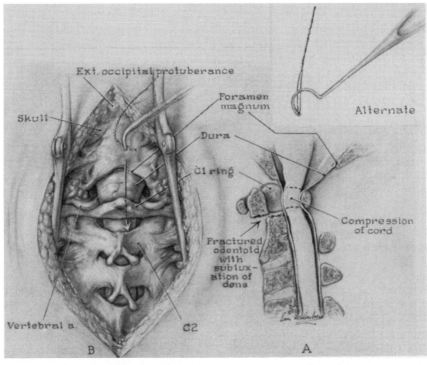

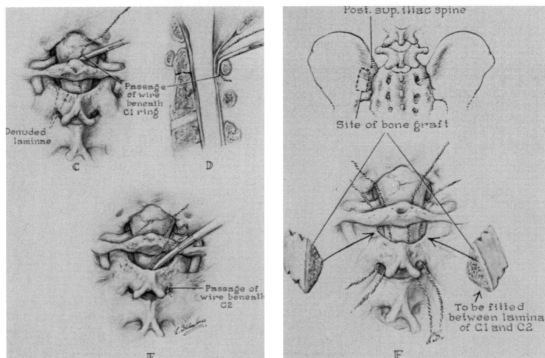

Figure 49–62 *See legend on opposite page*

shaved, surgically prepared, and draped from the occiput to the upper thoracic spine. Bleeding may be reduced by infiltrating the midline structures with 10 to 15 ml of a 1:200,000 solution of epinephrine. A generous midline incision is made over the area of intended fusion and is extended deeply to the spinous processes, through the relatively avascular midline structures. Deviation to either side into the paraspinal muscles will produce troublesome hemorrhage. Throughout this dissection, the spinous processes are palpated to verify their position and level. Scalpel dissection should be used only over these bony prominences and not within the interspinous ligaments or over a suspected spina bifida. The bifid spinous processes are grasped with a

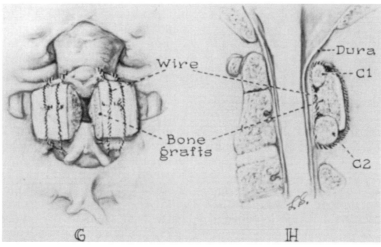

Figure 49–62. *A* and *B*, Brooks' atlantoaxial fusion. *A*, The odontoid should be reduced and its position should be checked with a lateral roentgenogram made in the operating room prior to preparing or draping the patient. This must be done before dissecting around the posterior elements or passing wires to prevent injury to the spinal cord or medulla. *B*, The posterior ring of the atlas and lamina of the axis are cleared of soft tissue by gentle subperiosteal dissection. The base of the occiput is not dissected free as shown to avoid inadvertent fusion to the skull. Twisted 24-gauge stainless steel wires are passed beneath the ring of the atlas and lamina of the axis using a right-angled clamp. An alternative method is to pass an aneurysm needle around the lamina of the axis from above. A heavy silk suture is threaded into the eye of the aneurysm needle, the needle is withdrawn upward, and the suture is retrieved. The silk suture is passed in a similar manner beneath the posterior ring of the atlas. The wires then may be attached to the silk suture and passed atraumatically beneath both posterior rings. *C, D,* and *E,* Two 24-gauge twisted wires are passed beneath the posterior atlantoaxial rings, two on each side of the midline to hold the grafts in place. *F,* A rectangle of bone graft 2 × 4 cm in size is taken from the posterior ilium superficial to the sacroiliac joint and includes only the outer cortex. This rectangle is centered over the longitudinal ridge, normally present over the posterior ilium. The graft is divided into two prism-shaped pieces, 1.5 × 2.0 cm in length and 1 cm deep. The deep surface should be carved to create a triangle, the apex of which will fit snugly between the posterior vertebral rings. The grafts are notched at their upper and lower ends to hold the wires and to keep them from slipping. *G* and *H,* The two wires on either side are separated as far as possible without injuring the vertebral vessels. The wires are then tightened and twisted to wedge the grafts in place between the vertebral rings. This creates a secure bone block, which effectively limits motion in all planes. (From Griswold, D. M., et al.: Atlantoaxial fusion for instability. J. Bone Joint Surg. *60A:*285–292, 1978.)

Kocher clamp to prevent gross motion or injury during this dissection and are cleared of muscle and tendon insertions using a sharp periosteal elevator. Dissection is extended laterally to the lamina but not to the capsular ligaments and facets. The capsular ligaments surrounding the facets contribute significantly to stability of the spine and should be spared if possible.

Holes are made in the outer cortex of the spinous processes adjacent to the lamina using a 4-mm drill (see Fig. 49–60A). These holes should be centered over the midportion of the spinous processes to prevent the stabilizing wires from cutting out above or below. Drill holes are made on either side of the spinous processes through the outer cortical surface and are connected, using a towel clip or "sweetheart" clamp in a rotary motion, as illustrated in Figure 49–60B. The drill holes or towel clip should not enter the spinal canal or injure the dura. Two strands of 24-gauge stainless steel wire are twisted on themselves in a drill. The twisted wires are passed through these holes in adjacent vertebrae (see Fig. 49–60C) and are secured by twisting either end of the wire on itself in a clockwise direction. The twisted wires are passed through these holes and adja-

cent vertebrae (see Fig. 49–60C) and are secured by twisting either end of the wire on itself in a clockwise direction. By taking a 50-cm strand of 24-gauge wire and folding it in half and then twisting the ends from this midpoint in a clockwise direction, one has a smooth end to pass through the holes in the bone. The smooth end makes it much less difficult to pass through drill holes in the lamina. Similar loops of wire go between adjacent spinous processes. If all 24-gauge wires have been twisted clockwise about three times per centimeter, they have more flexibility and more tensile strength. When they are tied in simple loops and also twisted clockwise, they are much less likely to break than is straight wire. However, the technique of using twisted wire needs to be learned hands-on from someone familiar with this technique. In this manner, adjacent spinous processes are secured in pairs to each other. One additional wire is used to surround all the vertebrae within the area of intended fusion (see Fig. 49–60D). Ordinarily, if instability is confined to one level, three vertebrae are wired together, two surrounding the lesion and one below. If a larger area is involved, the general rule is to fuse one vertebra above and two below the area of involvement. The wiring of one additional segment below the area of involvement provides supplementary strength, which may be useful in certain unstable situations. We have found that when this fusion fails, either clinically or experimentally, the wire usually pulls out of the lower spinous process. By adding this extra level, one can improve the protection of the unstable segment.

The vertebrae are manipulated to ensure that the wires are contributing to stability. The wiring should be examined, and a control lateral roentgenogram should be obtained to verify that the wires are not too tight and that the vertebrae are not held in hyperextension. Hyperextension may compromise the spinal canal or neural foramina; the wires should be loosened if this is present.

Corticocancellous strips of bone are taken from the posterior iliac crest and are laid down around the posterior elements in the area of intended fusion (see Fig. 49–60E). The wound is carefully irrigated, and the intermuscular septum is closed in multiple layers with interrupted absorbable suture material. The subcutaneous tissue and skin are closed cosmetically, the wound is dressed, and the neck is splinted. The patient is turned onto his or her bed, the headrest is removed, and the patient is extubated. External support with a cervicothoracic brace is recommended to prevent extremes of motion until the fusion is established radiographically in four to six months.

Complications

Wound complications are somewhat more common in our experience with the posterior approaches than with anterior approaches. Most problems, however, are encountered after long procedures in which decompression by one surgical team is combined with fusion by another.

Care is required in making the drill holes and in passing the wires to prevent injury to the spinal cord or dura. Posterior fusion without decompressive laminectomy tends to constrict the spinal canal. Because of this we recommend a delay of three to six weeks following trauma before fusion is attempted. This permits the hemorrhage and edema of trauma to subside before constrictive fusion is attempted.

Laminectomy and Facet Fusion

Cervical laminectomy is generally used to decompress the spinal canal posteriorly. It is indicated primarily to relieve the spinal cord and nerve roots from pressure or encroachment arising from the posterior elements, as may occur with certain fractures, dislocation, tumor, infection, and degenerative joint disease. Although laminectomy is not frequently indicated, it is useful to decompress multiple spinal levels and to provide wide surgical exposure, and it may be helpful when the level of the pathologic condition is not well localized. Laminectomy also provides effective decompression of the stenotic spinal canal, which is narrowed in the

anteroposterior plane at multiple levels.[8] On the other hand, laminectomy is less effective when the focus of compression is anterior to the spinal cord or nerve roots. In these situations, anterior decompression and fusion yield equal if not better results, with less surgical morbidity.[10, 14, 19, 34]

In the traumatized cervical spine with fractures, dislocations, and associated complete quadriplegia, there is little hope of recovery if no clinical improvement has occurred within 24 hours. Decompressive laminectomy under these circumstances rarely improves neurologic function and often adds to the patient's pre-existing instability. However, decompression may be considered when there is an incomplete neurologic deficit, particularly when there is evidence of progressive neurologic deterioration. A salvage attempt at decompression may be justified under these circumstances, but the decompression should be directed at the primary focus of impingement. For example, if the vertebral body is displaced posteriorly into the canal, anterior vertebral body resection and fusion would be indicated, whereas if the posterior elements are primarily involved, laminectomy could be useful.

Although cervical laminectomy may not cause obvious immediate instability, progressive deformity can occur and has been reported both clinically[5, 9, 15, 21, 34, 37, 57, 63] and experimentally.[25, 38, 40, 66] In a review by Callahan and colleagues,[8] the authors found that three groups of patients appeared to have a high risk of developing deformity following wide laminectomy. These were children and adults younger than 25 years of age; patients whose stability was already compromised by fracture-dislocation with primary involvement of the intervertebral ligaments; and those who had foraminotomy or extensive resection of the facets. Fusion is indicated in these higher-risk groups at the time of laminectomy. We as well as others[14, 24, 50, 55] have found that older patients with spondylosis and advanced degenerative changes have a lower incidence of acquired structural complications, but fusion may be beneficial in these patients to eliminate motion, continuing nerve root irritation, and associated spondylotic changes. Although laminectomy at multiple levels does influence the amount of deformity, the extent of resection at any one level appears to be of primary importance, and stabilization should be considered whether one or more segments have been resected.[8]

Fusion can be performed lateral to the area of laminectomy by passing wires through drill holes in the facets and binding two longitudinal struts of corticocancellous iliac bone graft to the facet pillars at each segment. This technique provides a secure fusion that may be performed at the same time as laminectomy, does not interfere with decompression, adds significantly to the strength of the spine, and allows early mobilization of the patient with external support. When the procedure is performed correctly, it yields a high rate of fusion (96 per cent) and provides long-term structural stability without the development of progressive deformity.[8] On the other hand, facet fusion is a complicated surgical technique, and the risks of complications are great. For this reason, we reserve this procedure for situations in which the spinous processes and lamina are deficient or have been removed and use the simpler interspinous wiring and fusion techniques when the spinous processes are available.

The authors have found that in most cases facet fusion adds enough immediate strength that a precariously unstable spine may be converted to a stable one in which only a simple cervicothoracic brace is required for protection until the fusion is established. Biomechanical studies of this facet fusion technique performed on human cadaver spines in the laboratory have demonstrated that a mean of 467 newtons is added to the strength of the spine by the bone struts and wires.[27] The strength of the construct appears to be proportional to the strength of the graft material and not to the wires or drill holes in the facet pillars. Therefore, in very unstable situations, the choice of a strong bone graft, such as the iliac crest with its outer and inner tables, tibia, or fibula, might be preferable to corticocancellous struts of iliac crest, using a single cortex.

Facet fusion is only one of many means of stabilizing the spine following laminectomy. A number of posterior fusion techniques, such as strut grafts,[57] H-grafts,[15] and check-rein fusions,[49] have been reported, but each has inherent limitations. In most cases, anterior fusions provide an optimal bed for bone grafting, are rapidly incorporated with fewer surgical complications, and may be used in addition to posterior fusion when stability is uncertain. The major disadvantage to the anterior techniques is that no immediate strength is added by the graft, and some may be lost, as Stauffer and Kelly[62] have reported. Casts, traction, or a halobrace may be required in very unstable situations until the anterior fusion is established. Facet fusion, on the other hand, adds immediate strength and serves as a posterior hinge to prevent horizontal movement between vertebrae.

Technique

Decompressive laminectomy and facet fusion may be performed in one surgical procedure using a neurosurgical and orthopedic team. The patient is anesthetized using endotracheal anesthesia, and the spine is stabilized intraoperatively with a three-point pin headrest (see Figs. 49–38, 49–39, and 49–40). The spine is approached posteriorly, through a generous midlongitudinal incision. The posterior elements are cleared of soft tissues by subperiosteal dissection, including the capsular ligaments over the facets. The spinous processes and laminae are removed over the area of intended decompression and exploration. To do this, the ligamentum flavum is cleared from the superior surface of the lamina below with a sharp curet. The free end is retracted upward with a clamp, and a cottonoid patty is inserted between the lamina and dura to protect the dura during further dissection. Oblique or right-angled punch rongeurs are used to resect the lamina from the facet pillar on one side to the facet on the other. The

spinous processes, lamina, and ligamentum flavum are resected until the cord and dura are fully exposed and decompressed. The cord itself may be exposed through a longitudinal incision in the dura, but the dura should be closed with fine sutures in a nonconstrictive fashion. At this time, the nerve roots may also be unroofed as they enter the neural foramina by removing the medial side of the superior articular facet. To do this, a significant portion of the inferior articular facet must also be removed. The nerve root is located at the level of this articulation and should be protected with a cottonoid patty inserted into the foramen anterior to the superior facet. Bone is carefully removed from the overlying facets using a high-speed burr or angled rongeur until the nerve root is clearly visible and free of encroachment.

After exploration and decompression are complete, fusion is performed posterolaterally at the level of the facets, using the technique described by Robinson and Southwick[48, 49] and Callahan and colleagues.[8] The facet surfaces are fused from the upper level of laminectomy to the first intact spinous process below, using corticocancellous bone graft wired to the facets at each level. The soft tissues and capsular ligaments are stripped from the facets and posterior pillars, and the facet joints are pried open using a small, curved elevator. The elevator is rotated to open the joint, and the articular cartilage is removed using a small angled curet. Drill holes 3 mm in diameter are made in the posterior pillars (Fig. 49–63A and B) at a right angle to the plane of the facet joints. These holes are made somewhat eccentrically toward the midline, so that the grafts may rest on a large area of the posterior pillar. A flat elevator is held within the facet joint to protect the facet below and the vertebral artery and nerve roots in front. Two strands of 24-gauge wire are twisted together using a hand drill. The twisted wire is inserted into each hole, and the tip of the wire is grasped within the joint space, using a fine, curved clamp. One clamp is used to feed the wire into the hole in the posterior pillar, while a second clamp is simultaneously used to advance the wire from the facet joint space. Wires are placed at each level of intended fusion bilaterally.

A bone graft that is curved in two planes and is long enough to cover the entire area of intended fusion is taken from the posterior iliac crest (Fig. 49–63C and D). This double curve conforms with the normal cervical lordosis and prevents the graft from impinging on the exposed dura and spinal cord. The graft is composed of the outer table of the iliac crest and subjacent cancellous bone, but to increase its strength, the superior cortical surface of the iliac crest is included. Two biconcave corticocancellous struts are obtained and applied to the facets with the cancellous surfaces facing the facet pillars (Fig. 49–63E and F). Notches are made in the lateral sides of the graft for the wires at the upper and lower ends of the fusion to improve fixation of the wires to the graft. The wires at each facet are then passed around the graft and tightened by twisting the wire at each segmental level. This is ordinarily started at the midpoint of the fusion so the graft may

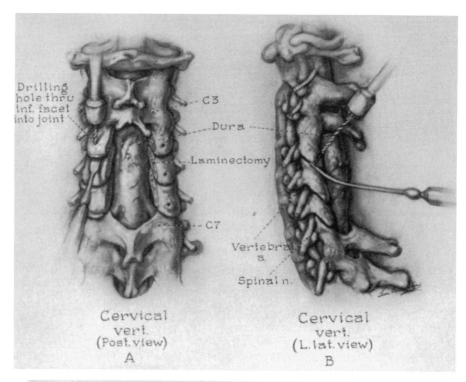

Cervical vert. (Post. view)
A

Cervical vert. (L. lat. view)
B

Figure 49–63 *See legend on opposite page.*

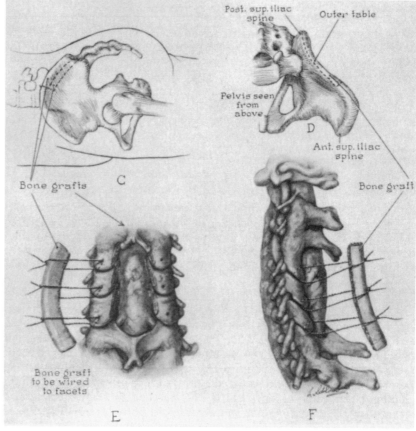

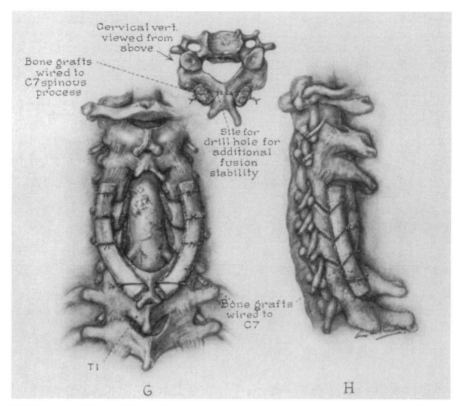

Figure 49–63. *A* and *B*, Facet fusion: The soft tissues and capsular ligaments are cleared from the facets and posterior pillars, and the facet joints are pried open using a small curved elevator. Drill holes are made in the posterior pillars, using a 3-mm drill, at a right angle to the plane of the facet joints *(B)*. These holes are made eccentrically toward the midline so that the grafts ultimately may rest on a large area of the posterior pillar. During the drilling, a flat elevator is left between the facets to protect the facet below and the vertebral artery and nerve roots to the front.
C and *D*, Bone graft that is curved in two planes is taken from the posterior iliac crest. The posterior ilium is normally curved in two planes. One of these curves *(C* and *E)* keeps the graft from impinging on the exposed dura and spinal cord; the other *(D* and *F)* conforms with the normal cervical lordosis. Two biconcave grafts are taken from the outer table of the ilium. These are notched laterally at their upper and lower poles to keep the wires from slipping off the grafts. *E* and *F*, Twisted 24-gauge stainless steel wire is then inserted into each hole, and the tip of the wire is grasped within the joint space using a fine, curved clamp. Wires are placed at each level of intended fusion bilaterally. The grafts are then placed along the posterior facet pillars, and the wires are tightened and twisted around the grafts. This is usually started at the midpoint of the fusion so the graft will rest snugly against the apex of the lordotic curve. The wire that extends through the hole in the facet pillar is passed medially about the graft *(E)*, while the wire that emerges from the facet joint is passed laterally. This prevents the graft from drifting medially toward the exposed spinal canal.
G and *H*, To secure the graft to the spinous process below the laminectomy, a 4-mm hole is drilled in the outer cortex on either side of the base of the spinous process at its junction with the lamina. These holes are connected using a towel clip or sharp bone clamp, and two additional twisted wires are passed through this hole. The wires are passed around each bone graft and twisted on the lateral aspect of each graft, first on one side and then on the other *(G)*. By using two separate wires, they may be twisted around one graft and then advanced through the hole in the spinous process to bring this graft in close apposition with the posterior elements. The other graft is then secured by twisting the wires on its lateral side. The fusion should extend cranially to the inferior articular processes at the upper end of the laminectomy. If there is doubt about stability at this level, the fusion should be extended further to the spinous process of the vertebra above. Distally, the fusion should extend to the spinous process of the first intact vertebra below the laminectomy. Interspinous wiring to the thoracic vertebrae is indicated only when the stability at the cervicothoracic junction is in doubt or if there is a significant kyphosis at this level. (From Callahan, R. A., Johnson, R. M., Margolis, R. N., et al.: Cervical facet fusion for control of instability following laminectomy. J. Bone Joint Surg. *59A*:991–1002, 1977.)

be closely applied to the facet at the apex of the lordotic curve. The wire that extends through the hole in the facet pillar is passed medially about the graft (Fig. 49–63E), while the wire that emerges from the facet joint is passed laterally. This prevents the graft from drifting medially toward the exposed spinal cord.

To secure the graft to the spinous process, a 4-mm hole is drilled in the outer cortex on either side of the base of the spinous process at its junction with the lamina (Fig. 49–63G and H). These holes are connected with a towel clip or sharp bone clamp, and two twisted wires are passed through this hole. These two wires are passed around the bone graft and twisted laterally to secure the graft, first on one side and then the other (Fig. 49–63G). By using two separate strands, the wires may be twisted around one graft and advanced through the spinous process to bring the graft in close apposition with the posterior elements. The second side is then secured by twisting the wires laterally on the opposite side.

The fusion should extend cranially to the facet at the upper level of the laminectomy (Fig. 49–63H). If there is any doubt about stability at this level, the fusion should be extended further, to the facet or spi-

nous process of the intact vertebra above. Distally, the fusion should extend to the first intact spinous process below the laminectomy. Interspinous wiring to the thoracic vertebrae is indicated only when the stability at these segments is in doubt.

The wound is irrigated and closed, approximating the intermuscular septum, in multiple layers to eliminate dead space and strengthen the closure. A drain is inserted in the deep subcutaneous layer and removed 48 hours postoperatively. The patient is nursed supine for several days until pain and muscular spasm have subsided. The patient is then mobilized, and the neck is protected with a cervicothoracic brace for six to 12 months until fusion is well established radiographically along the facet pillars and there is no motion across the fused segments on flexion-extension roentgenograms. Fusion was established in our series at a mean of 6.5 months.[8]

Recently we have used compression rods or threaded Steinmann pins as internal struts instead of pelvic corticocancellous bone grafts for most patients who need stabilization after radical laminectomy (Fig. 49–64). The procedure for facet wiring is identical to the method described here. However, one must bend

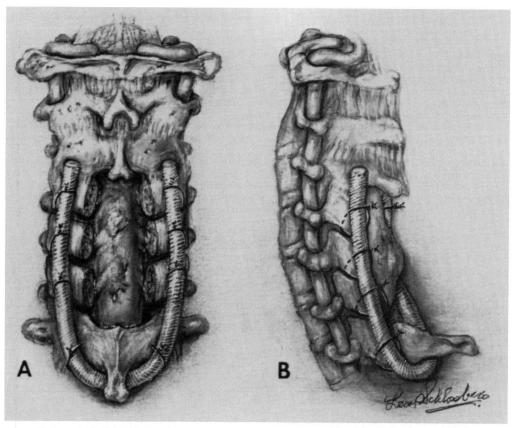

Figure 49–64. *A, B,* Technique of facet fusion using a bent rod. Usually a compression rod from the Harrington set, or a 5/32-inch Steinmann pin, cut to length and shaped with plate benders and a plier, conforms exactly to the facet surfaces. Lower cervical spine stability is improved by placing the rod around the lowest intact spinous process, leaving the interspinous ligament intact. This construct offers immediate stability and is particularly useful in severe osteoporosis, arthritis, and malignancy. Various sizes of threaded rods and pins have been used.

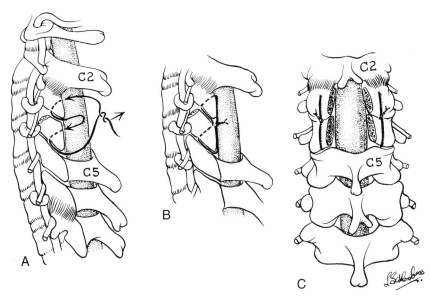

Figure 49–65. Drill holes are made in the posterior pillars of the involved facets using a 3-mm drill directed at right angles to the plane of the facet joint. A curved elevator is placed within the facet joint to protect the lower facet and the vertebral artery and nerve roots to the front. Holes are made in the facets at the level of instability and the facet below. A single strand of 18-gauge wire is passed through the hole in the upper facet pillar *(A)* and is retrieved within the joint using a fine-angled clamp. The wire is advanced by a combination of pushing the wire into the hole within the facet pillar with one hand while pulling the wire from the facet joint with a clamp. When sufficient wire has been retrieved, the free end is introduced into the hole within the next lower facet pillar, and the wire is retrieved from that joint. The wire is pulled snugly, and the facet joints are reduced in a fully apposed position *(B and C)*. The wire is then tightened and twisted. A lateral roentgenogram is obtained in the operating room to insure that satisfactory stabilization is provided and that there is not too much extension or posterior overriding of the facets. Excessive overriding will compromise the spinal canal and the neural foramina. The wire that leaves the facet joint and is then passed posteriorly to the next lower facet pillar provides a horizontal buttress *(B)* that effectively prevents anterior translation of one vertebra forward on the next.

these rods to fit the facet joints and the cervical curve exactly. The threads prevent migration of the wires. The rod should be looped under the inferior intact spinous process for greater stability.

Complications

We have experienced a number of surgical complications, but all but four of these were minor or temporary and did not result in a permanent deficit.[8] Wound complications, such as hematoma, seroma, dehiscence, or infection, were encountered, particularly in association with long procedures involving multiple surgical teams. We have found that prolonged retraction of soft tissues leads to ischemia of the paraspinal muscles and adjacent soft tissues. For this reason, we recommend releasing the retraction of these structures periodically throughout the procedure to permit vascular filling. The intermuscular septum should be closed carefully to prevent wound separation or dehiscence when the shoulders are flexed or when the trapezius muscles contract.

Care is required throughout dissection about the dura and spinal cord to prevent injury to these structures. The wires should be passed carefully to avoid

inadvertent puncture of the dura or cord. Although posterolateral facet fusion adds considerable stability to the spine in the immediate postoperative period, extremes of motion may dislodge the bone graft or fixation wires. For this reason, we recommend protection with a cervicothoracic brace until the fusion is well established radiographically. When this procedure is performed correctly and the grafts have been wired at each involved segmental level, facet fusion yields a high rate of fusion with long-term structural stability.

Interfacet Wiring

We have found that stabilization of the injured spine may be particularly troublesome when the facet joints are damaged or when they have been removed. In these situations, the standard posterior fusion techniques, such as interspinous wiring or facet fusion, have often failed to prevent anterior horizontal displacements, and progressive drifting of one vertebral body forward on another has occurred. To control this problem, we have tried a number of technical modifications but have found that a simple wiring technique between the facets is most effective (Figs. 49–65 and 49–66). To date, we have used this technique on eight

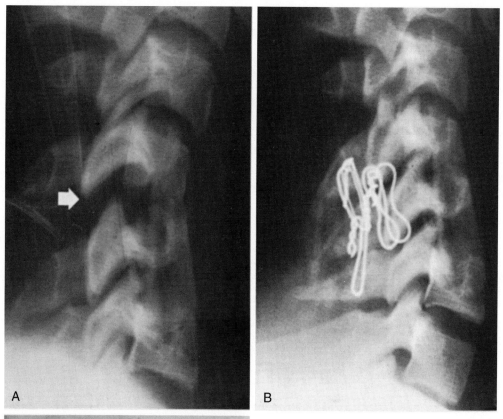

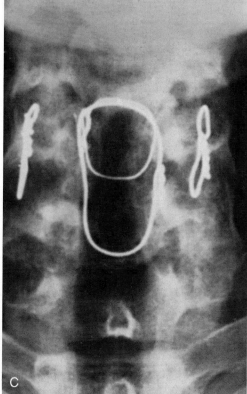

Figure 49–66. Twenty-year-old man with posterior displacement of a fibular graft into the spinal canal, presented in Figure 49–29. The fibular graft was removed and replaced with a graft taken from the iliac crest, which was "keyed" in place (see Fig. 49–57). *A,* Note the wide separation of the spinous processes and facet joints posteriorly, suggesting extensive injury to the posterior ligaments. Because of this posterior instability, interfacet as well as interspinous wiring and fusion was performed *(B* and *C)* to increase the immediate strength of the spine and to speed this patient's rehabilitation without a halo-cast. The interfacet wires are seen in front of the interspinous wires on the lateral roentgenogram *(B)* and are seen laterally on the anteroposterior roentgenogram *(C).*

patients with instability and deficiencies of the facet joints and have found that it controlled anterior horizontal displacements well in most cases. This technique has proved to be effective in controlling shear instability caused by fractures through the facets or the instability that occurs following bilateral facet dislocation when the superior articular facets have been removed to facilitate reduction. Because of the importance of recognizing fractures through the facet surfaces and controlling the resultant instability, we now obtain lateral laminagrams, which cut through the plane of the facets, in all patients with serious spinal injury to clearly visualize these structures. In addition to identifying facet fractures, these studies may also localize fragments of bone driven forward into the neural foramen compressing the nerve root (Fig. 49–67). These fragments may be removed at the time of stabilization. In several such cases we have been able to gain functional return of the involved nerve root with significant improvement in the patient's level of rehabilitative function.

In previous biomechanical studies on human cadaver spines,[25, 40] we found that the facets contribute to the angular rotation of the spine in flexion. When the facet joints were removed experimentally, a significant drop in angular rotation was observed in flexion. In addition, the facets were found to limit anterior horizontal translation of one vertebral body on the other, and when the facets were removed, a large increase in horizontal displacement was observed. We have also tested the interfacet wiring technique in human cadaver spines[27] and have found that a mean of 753 newtons is added to the strength of the spine when tested in flexion. This technique provides the greatest strength of any wiring method tested in flexion.

Technique

Interfacet wiring is normally performed as an adjunct to other posterior fusion techniques. The posterior elements of the spine are approached through a longitudinal midline incision, and the soft tissues are cleared laterally to expose the facets by subperiosteal dissection. The capsular ligaments are removed from the facet surfaces, and the involved facet joints are pried open using a curved Joseph periosteal elevator. At this point, resection of bone fragments or the superior facet, foraminotomy, or reduction of a locked dislocation may be performed. Drill holes are then made in the posterior pillars of the involved facets using a 3-mm drill directed at right angles to the plane of the facet joint (see Fig. 49–63A and B). A flat elevator is placed within the facet to protect the opposing surface from injury when the drill enters the joint. Holes are made in the facets at the level of instability and at the facet below. A single strand of 18-gauge wire is passed through the hole in the upper facet pillar (see Fig. 49–65A) and is retrieved within the joint using a fine-angled clamp. The wire is advanced by a combination of pushing the wire into the hole within the facet pillar with one hand while pulling the wire from the facet joint with a

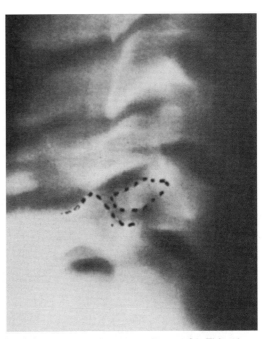

Figure 49–67. Lateral laminagram C6 and C7: This 19-year-old college student was in an automobile accident while vacationing in the West and sustained a bilateral facet dislocation of the sixth on seventh cervical vertebra. He had complete spinal cord injury at this level, with almost complete loss of his triceps muscle function. He was treated acutely with closed reduction and maintained in skeletal traction. He was transferred to the East three weeks later, at which time continued anterior subluxation of the sixth vertebra on the seventh was noted, despite continued traction. Lateral laminagrams revealed bilateral fractures of the superior articular processes of the facets with these fragments driven forward into the neural foramina. These fractures, as well as the associated ligamentous injury at this level, created a remarkably unstable situation and left almost no support against shear forces forward. As a result, the spine continued to sublux forward and could not be adequately held with any form of external support, including a halo-cast. It was hoped that we could stabilize these segments surgically and provide enough immediate strength to prevent this forward drift. In addition, we thought that by removing the fragments driven into the seventh nerve root, we might improve the function of his triceps and increase his overall level of function. The spine was explored posteriorly and the bone fragments were removed, which appeared to alleviate the pressure on the nerve roots. Interfacet wires and bone grafts were installed. This provided enough immediate strength that we could mobilize this patient in a cervicothoracic brace four days after surgery and could begin his therapy in an erect position. The patient has ultimately acquired antigravity strength of his triceps and has been able to use this effectively in his transfers. He has returned to college in a wheelchair without residual vertebral deformity.

clamp. When sufficient wire has been retrieved, this free end is introduced into the hole in the next lower facet pillar, and the wire is retrieved from that joint. The wire is pulled snugly, and the facet joints are reduced in a fully apposed position (see Fig. 49–65B and C). The wire is then tightened and twisted using a Shifrin wire tightener. The twisted end is cut short and turned into the bone to prevent irritation of adjacent

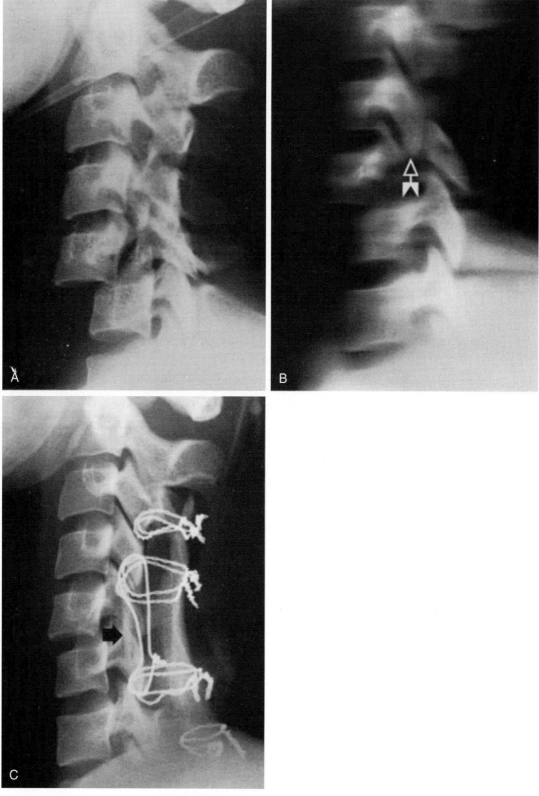

Figure 49–68. *See legend on opposite page*

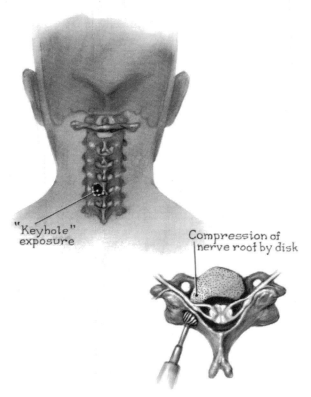

riding of the facets has not occurred. Excessive overriding will compromise the spinal canal and neural foramina and should therefore be avoided.

The wire that leaves the facet joint and is then passed posteriorly to the next lower facet pillar provides a horizontal buttress (see Fig. 49–65B), which effectively prevents anterior translation of one vertebra forward on the next. This buttress is effective even when the superior articular surface or part of the upper facet is missing and has been used to control shear displacements when an entire facet pillar has been lost (Fig. 49–68A, B, and C).

Posterior Laminotomy-Foraminotomy

Nerve root decompression may be performed through the posterior laminotomy-foraminotomy approach described by Scoville.[54, 55] This "key-hole" exposure of the neural foramen is most conserving of the bone of the posterior elements and facets (Fig. 49–69). The exposure is limited but is most useful to excise a soft disc protruding into the neural foramen, causing unilateral, single nerve root irritation. A hole is burred at the junction of the lamina and facet, and a portion of the superior facet is removed. This decompresses the entrance to the neural foramen by removing its posterior wall without jeopardizing the integrity of the posterior ring or the facet joint.

Technique

Scoville[56] describes the procedure performed under local anesthetic block with the patient sitting upright to reduce venous bleeding. The exposure is through a midlongitudinal incision, and the posterior elements on the involved side are stripped of soft tissues by subperiosteal dissection as far laterally as the facets. A lateral roentgenogram should be obtained with a towel clip fixed to the appropriate spinous process to verify the correct segmental level. A hand-held Meyerding or

Figure 49–69. Posterior laminotomy-foraminotomy exposure of the cervical nerve root. (From Robinson, R. A., and Southwick, W. O.: Surgical Approaches to the Cervical Spine. *In* the American Academy of Orthopaedic Surgeons: Instructional Course Lectures, Vol. XVII. St. Louis, 1960, The C. V. Mosby Co.: drawing modified after "keyhole" exposure of Scoville, W. B.: Discussion. J. Neurosurg. *15*:614, 1958.)

soft tissues. When completed, the wiring should be inspected, and a lateral roentgenogram should be obtained to ensure that satisfactory stabilization is provided and that too much extension or posterior over-

Figure 49–68. This 28-year-old woman was a passenger in the front seat of a car involved in a head-on collision. She sustained a bilateral facet dislocation of the fifth on the sixth cervical vertebra *(A)* with complete spinal cord injury at this level. Laminagrams *(B)* revealed a fracture through the middle of the facets. This was easily reduced with longitudinal traction, but there was no resistance against shear displacements anteriorly. As a result, she continued to drift forward at the C5–C6 level. It has been our experience that no external support, including the halo-brace, will prevent these kinds of shear displacement. Therefore, surgical stabilization was attempted to provide enough integral strength so that rehabilitation could be started out of bed and fusion could be performed to prevent late deformity. At surgery, the whole posterior neural arch of the fifth vertebra was found floating freely. This was removed to protect the spinal canal. As a result, the whole posterior pillar of the facets on one side was missing, and even with reduction, she tended to angulate backward. To correct this, a longitudinal graft *(C, arrow)* was made to replace this facet pillar and was notched into the fourth and sixth facets. This provided a fulcrum that helped to maintain the longitudinal alignment of the vertebrae. An interfacet wire was then installed between the fourth and sixth facets *(C)*, bridging the fifth vertebra but forcing the facet pillar graft forward and snugly into its notches. This was supplemented by two struts of corticocancellous iliac bone, which were wired to the intact facets on either side as described in Facet fusion (see Fig. 49–63). This technique provided enough immediate rigidity that we were able to mobilize this patient shortly after surgery in a cervicothoracic brace. She went on to fuse without significant deformity in four and one half months.

self-retaining blade and hook retractor are inserted. The posterior wall of the neural foramen is opened lateral to the dural sleeve at the junction of the lamina and facet using a large burr on a low-speed drill. A diamond burr on a high-speed drill and Cloward oblique rongeurs are used to complete the exposure. The nerve root and epidural vein ventral to the root are packed off and protected until the exposure through the bone is completed. Hemostasis of the epidural vessels is obtained by packing with Gelfoam or with the use of "bipolar" coagulation forceps. The exposure may be extended medially by resecting a portion of the lamina with angled rongeurs and excising a part of the ligamentum flavum.

The sensory and motor nerve roots are seen within their separate dural sleeves as they enter the neural foramen. The motor nerve root is one fourth the size of the sensory root and is located anterior and caudal to the larger sensory root. Both roots are freed of adherent tissue and the protruding disc and are retracted carefully upward. The extruded disc is then excised with fine pituitary rongeurs and is teased out from beneath the roots with the assistance of a dental spatula.

Scoville[56] reports a large series with few complications, although the upright position has been implicated as an occasional cause of air embolism. On completing the procedure, the spinal column should be tested for stability. If stability is in doubt or if an entire facet has been removed, we recommend interfacet wiring and fusion to avoid the complication of late spinal deformity. Care is required in removing bone around the nerve roots to protect them from injury. The use of a diamond burr or angled rongeurs reduces this risk.

References

1. Alonso, W.A., Black, P., Connor, G. H., and Vematsu, S.: Transoral, transpalatal approach for resection of clival chordoma. Laryngoscope 81:1626–1631, 1971.
2. Anderson, L. D., and D'Alonzo, R. T.: Fractures of the odontoid process of the axis. J. Bone Joint Surg. [Am.] 56:1663–1674, 1974.
3. Aymes, E. W., and Anderson, F. M.: Fracture of the odontoid process. Arch. Surg. 72:377–393, 1956.
4. Bailey, R. W.: Surgical techniques. In Bailey, R. W. (ed.): The Cervical Spine. Philadelphia, Lea & Febiger, 1974, pp. 146–156.
5. Bailey, R. W., and Badgley, C. E.: Stabilization of the cervical spine by anterior fusion. J. Bone Joint Surg. [Am.] 42:565–594, 1960.
6. Braakman, R., and Penning, L.: Injuries of the Cervical Spine. Amsterdam, Excerpta Medica, 1971, pp. 193–213.
7. Brooks, A. L., and Jenkins, E. B.: Atlanto-axial arthrodesis by the wedge compression method. J. Bone Joint Surg. [Am.] 60:279–284, 1978.
8. Callahan, R. A., Johnson, R. M., Margolis, R. N., et al.: Cervical facet fusion for control of instability following laminectomy. J. Bone Joint Surg. [Am.] 59:991–1002, 1977.
9. Cattell, H. S., and Clark, G. L.: Cervical kyphosis and instability following multiple laminectomies in children. J. Bone Joint Surg. [Am.] 49:713–720, 1967.
10. Crandall, P. H., and Batzdorf, U.: Cervical spondylotic myelopathy. J. Neurosurg. 25:57–66, 1966.
11. Crutchfield, W. G.: Skeletal traction in the treatment of injuries to the cervical spine. JAMA 155:29–32, 1954.
12. DeAndrade, J. R., and MacNab, I.: Anterior occipitocervical fu-

13. DeWald, R. L.: Halo traction systems. In American Academy of Orthopaedic Surgeons: Atlas of Orthotics, Biomechanical Principles and Application. St. Louis, C. V. Mosby Co., 1975, pp. 407–417.
14. Fager, C. A.: Results of adequate posterior decompression in the relief of spondylotic cervical myelopathy. J. Neurosurg. 38:684–692, 1973.
15. Fairbank, T. J.: Spinal fusion after laminectomy for cervical myelopathy. Proc. R. Soc. Med. 64:634–636, 1971.
16. Fang, H. S. Y., and Ong, G. B.: Direct anterior approach to the upper cervical spine. J. Bone Joint Surg. [Am.] 44:1588–1604, 1962.
17. Fielding, J. W., Hawkins, R. J., and Ratzan, S. A.: Spine fusion for atlanto-axial instability. J. Bone Joint Surg. [Am.] 58:400–407, 1976.
18. Gallie, W. E.: Skeletal traction in the treatment of fractures and dislocations of the cervical spine. Ann. Surg. 106:770–776, 1937.
19. Gregorius, F. K., Estrin, T., and Crandall, P. H.: Cervical spondylotic radiculopathy and myelopathy, a long term follow-up study. Arch. Neurol. 33:618–625, 1976.
20. Griswold, D. M., Albright, J. A., Schiffman, E., et al.: Atlanto-axial fusion for instability. J. Bone Joint Surg. [Am.] 60:285–292, 1978.
21. Hall, J. E., Denis, F., and Murray, J.: Exposure of the upper cervical spine for spinal decompression. J. Bone Joint Surg. [Am.] 59:121–123, 1977.
22. Henry, A. K.: Extensile Exposure. 2nd ed. Edinburgh, E. and S. Livingstone, Ltd., 1957, pp. 53–80.
23. Jefferson, G.: Fracture of the atlas vertebra. Report of four cases, and a review of those previously recorded. Br. J. Surg. 7:407–422, 1920.
24. Jenkins, D. H. R.: Extensive cervical laminectomy. Br. J. Surg. 60:852–854, 1973.
25. Johnson, R. M.: Biomechanical stability of the lower cervical spine. Thesis, Yale University School of Medicine, Section of Orthopaedic Surgery, 1973, pp. 1–58.
26. Johnson, R. M., Hart, D. L., Simmons, E. F., et al.: Cervical orthoses: A study in normal subjects comparing their effectiveness in restricting cervical motion. J. Bone Joint Surg. [Am.] 59:332–339, 1977.
27. Johnson, R. M., Owen, J. R., Panjabi, M. M., et al.: Immediate strength of certain cervical fusion techniques. Orthop. Trans. 4:42, 1980.
28. Kopits, S. E., and Steingass, M. H.: Experience with the "halo-cast" in small children. Surg. Clin. North Am. 50:935–943, 1970.
29. Krag, M. H., and Beynnon, B. D.: A new halo-vest: Rationale, design and biomechanical comparison to standard halo-vest designs. Spine 13:228–235, 1988.
30. Lahey, F. H., and Warren, K. W.: Esophageal diverticula. Surg. Gynecol. Obstet. 98:1–28, 1954.
31. Leider, L. L., and Ferlic, F.: Odontoid fractures treated by halo cast immobilization. Presented at the American Academy of Orthopaedic Surgeons annual meeting, Las Vegas, 1977.
32. Light, T. R., Wagner, F. C., Johnson, R. M., and Southwick, W. O.: Correction of spinal instability and recovery of neurologic loss following cervical vertebral body replacement: Case report. Spine 5:392–394, 1980.
33. Lindskog, G. E., Liebow, A. A., and Glenn, W. W. L.: Thoracic and Cardiovascular Surgery With Related Pathology. New York, Appleton-Century-Crofts, 1962, pp. 439–440.
34. Mayfield, F. H.: Cervical spondylosis: A comparison of the anterior and posterior approaches. Clin. Neurosurg. 13:181–188, 1966.
35. McAfee, P. C., Bohlman, H. H., Riley, L. H., et al.: The anterior retropharyngeal approach to the upper part of the cervical spine. J. Bone Joint Surg. [Am.] 69:1371–1383, 1987.
36. Mixter, S. J., and Osgood, R. B.: Traumatic lesions of the atlas and axis. Ann. Surg. 51:193–207, 1910.
37. Morgan, R. C., Brown, J. C., and Bonnett, C. A.: The effect of laminectomy on the pediatric spinal cord injured patient. J. Bone Joint Surg. [Am.] 57:1025–1026, 1975.
38. Munechika, Y.: Influence of laminectomy on stability of the spine. J. Jpn. Orthop. Assoc. 47:111–126, 1973.
39. Nanson, E. M.: The anterior approach to upper dorsal sympathectomy. Surg. Gynecol. Obstet. 104:118–120, 1957.

40. Panjabi, M. M., White, A. A., and Johnson, R. M.: Cervical spine mechanics as a function of transection of components. J. Biomech. 8:327–336, 1975.
41. Perry, J.: The halo in spinal abnormalities, practical factors and avoidance of complications. Orthop. Clin. North Am. 3:69–80, 1972.
42. Perry, J., and Nickel, V. L.: Total cervical spine fusion for neck paralysis. J. Bone Joint Surg. [Am.] 41:37–60, 1959.
43. Riley, L. H.: Surgical approaches to the anterior structures of the cervical spine. Clin. Orthop. 91:16–20, 1973.
44. Roberts, A., and Wickstrom, J.: Prognosis of odontoid fractures. In Proceedings of the American Academy of Orthopaedic Surgeons. J. Bone Joint Surg. [Am.] 54:1353, 1972.
45. Robinson, R. A.: Fusions of the cervical spine. J. Bone Joint Surg. [Am.] 41:1–6, 1959.
46. Robinson, R. A., and Riley, L. H.: Techniques of exposure and fusion of the cervical spine. Clin. Orthop. 109:78–84, 1975.
47. Robinson, R. A., and Smith, G. W.: Anterolateral cervical disc removal and interbody fusion for cervical disc syndrome. Bull. Johns Hopkins Hosp. 96:223–224, 1955.
48. Robinson, R. A., and Southwick, W. O.: Indications and technics for early stabilization of the neck in some fracture dislocations of the cervical spine. South. Med. J. 53:565–579, 1960.
49. Robinson, R. A., and Southwick, W. O.: Surgical approaches to the cervical spine. Instructional course lectures. American Academy of Orthopaedic Surgeons. Vol. 17. St. Louis, C. V. Mosby Co., 1960, pp. 299–330.
50. Rogers, L.: The surgical treatment for cervical spondylotic myelopathy. J. Bone Joint Surg. [Br.] 43:3–6, 1961.
51. Rogers, W. A.: Treatment of fracture dislocation of the cervical spine. J. Bone Joint Surg. 24:245–258, 1942.
52. Rogers, W. A.: Fractures and dislocations of the cervical spine. An end result study. J. Bone Joint Surg. [Am.] 39:341–376, 1957.
53. Schatzker, J., Rorabeck, C. H., and Waddell, J. P.: Fractures of the dens (odontoid process), an analysis of thirty-seven cases. J. Bone Joint Surg. [Br.] 53:392–405, 1971.
54. Scoville, W. B.: Discussion. J. Neurosurg. 15:615, 1958.
55. Scoville, W. B.: Cervical spondylosis—operative treatment. J. Neurosurg. 18:423–428, 1961.
56. Scoville, W. B.: Cervical disc lesions treated by posterior operations. In Rob, C., Smith, R., and Logue, V. (eds.): Operative Surgery, Neurosurgery, 2nd ed. Vol. 14. Philadelphia, J. B. Lippincott Co., 1971, pp. 250–258.
57. Sim, F. H., Svien, H. J., Bickel, W. H., and Janes, J. M.: Swanneck deformity following extensive cervical laminectomy. J. Bone Joint Surg. [Am.] 56:564–580, 1974.
58. Smith, G. W., and Robinson, R. A.: The treatment of certain cervical spine disorders by anterior removal of the intervertebral disc and interbody fusion. J. Bone Joint Surg. [Am.] 40:607–624, 1958.
59. Southwick, W. O., and Robinson, R. A.: Surgical approaches to the vertebral bodies in the cervical and lumbar regions. J. Bone Joint Surg. [Am.] 39:631–644, 1957.
60. Southwick, W. O., and Robinson, R. A.: Recent advances in surgery of the cervical spine. Surg. Clin. North Am. 41:1661–1683, 1961.
61. Spence, K. F., Decker, S., and Sell, K. W.: Bursting atlantal fracture associated with rupture of the transverse ligament. J. Bone Joint Surg. [Am.] 52:543–549, 1970.
62. Stauffer, E. S., and Kelly, E. G.: Fracture-dislocations of the cervical spine. Instability and recurrent deformity following treatment by anterior interbody fusion. J. Bone Joint Surg. [Am.] 59:45–48, 1977.
63. Tachdjian, M. O., and Matson, D. D.: Orthopaedic aspects of intraspinal tumors in infants and children. J. Bone Joint Surg. [Am.] 47:223–248, 1965.
64. Thomson, S. C., and Negus, V. E.: Diseases of the Nose and Throat. A Textbook for Students and Practitioners. 5th ed. London, Cassell and Co., Ltd., 1947, pp. 489–509.
65. Verbiest, H.: Anterolateral operations for fractures and dislocations in the middle and lower parts of the cervical spine. J. Bone Joint Surg. [Am.] 51:1489–1530, 1969.
66. White, A. A., Johnson, R. M., Panjabi, M. M., and Southwick, W. O.: Biomechanical analysis of clinical stability in the cervical spine. Clin. Orthop. 109:85–96, 1975.
67. White, A. A., Southwick, W. O., DePonte, R. J., et al.: Relief of pain by anterior cervical spine fusion for spondylosis: a report of sixty-five patients. J. Bone Joint Surg. [Am.] 55:525–534, 1973.
68. Whitecloud, T. S., and LaRocca, H.: Fibular strut graft in reconstructive surgery of the cervical spine. Spine 1:33–43, 1976.
69. Whitesides, T. E., Jr., and Kelly, R. P.: Lateral approach to the upper cervical spine for anterior fusion. South. Med. J. 59:879–883, 1966.
70. Williams, J. L., Allen, M. B. Jr., and Harkess, J. W.: Late results of cervical discectomy and interbody fusion: Some factors influencing the results. J. Bone Joint Surg. [Am.] 50:277–286, 1968.

Surgical Approaches to the Thoracic Spine

As an aid to the understanding of cross-sectional anatomic relationships and the interpretation of computerized axial tomography and magnetic resonance imaging we have added three color plates, Figures 49–1, 49–70, and 49–97. Figure 49–70 illustrates a transaxial section of the thoracic spine at T8.

CHOICE OF APPROACH TO THE THORACIC SPINE

Under most circumstances, the choice of approach to the thoracic spine should be dictated by the site of the primary pathologic condition. Disease or deformity that primarily involves the vertebral bodies anteriorly may be approached directly through the chest or through a posterolateral costotransversectomy, whereas lesions of the posterior elements may be readily reached through the posterior exposures. There are,

however, certain indications for and limitations to each approach.

Anterior

The anterior transthoracic approach provides direct access to most of the thoracic vertebral bodies. It should be considered for extensive resection, débridement, and fusion of the vertebral bodies, particularly when multiple levels are involved. The disadvantages to thoracotomy are that it presents a greater operative risk than any of the posterior approaches incur, and it does not yield an effective exposure at the extreme upper and lower levels of the thoracic spine.

The anterior transthoracic approach should be considered in certain specific circumstances. Severe, rigid kyphosis of the thoracic spine is often best controlled by anterior interbody fusion, as posterior fusions tend to attenuate over a severe kyphos.[19, 31] Scoliosis with associated absence of the posterior elements or severe anterior deformity may be effectively treated with anterior instrumentation and fusion.[12, 13, 27] Spinal cord compression caused by lesions of the vertebral bodies protruding posteriorly into the canal should be decompressed anteriorly in most cases.

Posterolateral

Posterolateral costotransversectomy provides direct access to the transverse processes and pedicles of the thoracic spine and limited access to the vertebral bodies. Exposure at all levels of the thoracic spine is possible without restriction about the thoracic inlet or diaphragm. Costotransversectomy should be considered for simple biopsy or local débridement. However, it does not provide the operative working area or length of exposure to the thoracic vertebral bodies that thoracotomy affords.

Posterior

The midlongitudinal posterior approach provides direct access to the posterior elements of the thoracic spine at all levels. It should be considered for biopsy or débridement of lesions of the posterior elements, decompressive laminectomy, or posterior fusion. Spinal cord compression caused by lesions of the posterior elements impinging on the cord is rare but may be relieved by laminectomy. However, cord compression caused by lesions arising from the anterior elements is rarely improved with laminectomy alone.[4, 9, 17, 31] Idiopathic scoliosis may be corrected and fused posteriorly with satisfactory results, and the injured spine may be stabilized and fused with rods or wires through this exposure.

SELECTION OF APPROACH BASED ON VERTEBRAL LEVEL OF INVOLVEMENT

The posterior and posterolateral approaches provide direct access to the posterior elements and limited access to the vertebral bodies at all levels of the thoracic spine. The anterior approaches may be required to provide wide access to the vertebral bodies at multiple levels. However, the exposure is restricted anteriorly at the upper and lower extremes of the thoracic spine by the thoracic inlet and diaphragm. Therefore, modifications in the anterior approach must be made at these levels.

Upper Thoracic Level

The most direct access to the lower cervical and upper thoracic vertebral bodies is provided by the supraclavicular approach described previously. This approach provides access as low as the level of the third thoracic vertebral body in some patients. The exposure is reasonably unencumbered to the first and often the second thoracic vertebrae, but the working area to the third vertebral body becomes restricted by the thoracic inlet.

An alternative approach to the upper thoracic spine is via a left posterolateral thoracotomy at a level as high as the third rib. This requires resection of the dorsal scapular muscles and elevation of the scapula. Working area is limited by the converging rib cage and thoracic inlet. In addition, reversal of the thoracic kyphos in the upper thoracic spine makes resection of the vertebral bodies technically more difficult. Thoracotomy above the level of the third rib is impractical, as the shorter first and second ribs limit the scope of the incision, and the scapula interferes with the exposure posteriorly.

Hodgson and colleagues[17, 18] discuss the sternum-splitting approach to the upper thoracic anterior elements first described by Cauchoix and Binet.[7] Theoretically, this provides direct access to the vertebral bodies and continuity of exposure from the cervical to the thoracic vertebrae. In fact, Hodgson found this to be an unusually complex procedure, with a high operative mortality (40 per cent in 10 cases). The thymus, great vessels, trachea, and esophagus need to be retracted, and the spine appears at the bottom of a deep hole with limited operative working area. The restricted working area over the vertebral bodies is complicated by the fact that one must dissect directly back, toward the spinal canal, from the anterior aspect of the vertebral bodies and not from the side. In Hodgson's opinion, this increases the risk of injuring the spinal cord during decompression. Hodgson found that resection and bone grafting of the upper thoracic spine were easier through a thoracotomy at the level of the third rib than through this sternum-splitting approach.

Lower Thoracic Level

A left posterolateral thoracotomy provides access to the lower thoracic vertebral bodies as far as the twelfth vertebra. As one approaches the diaphragm, the working area becomes more restricted, so that exposures of the twelfth and sometimes the eleventh vertebral bodies become difficult without dividing the medial diaphragmatic insertion. To provide wide exposure across the lower thoracic and upper lumbar vertebral bodies in continuity, a transdiaphragmatic, thoracoabdominal approach is required. This significantly increases the operative risk and should be considered only in reasonably healthy candidates. Limited access to the lower thoracic vertebrae in continuity with the lumbar spine is possible via the retroperitoneal approach through a left flank incision. The operative morbidity is lower with this retroperitoneal approach than with the thoracoabdominal exposure, but the visibility and working area within the thorax are restricted.

Anterior Transthoracic Approach to the Thoracic Spine

The transthoracic approach to the spine has become widely used only in the past 20 years and had to await the development of the sophisticated techniques and support systems required to reduce the risks of thoracic surgery. There were reports of successful thoracotomy in the early literature,[25, 28] but these were attended by high risks. In 1933, Reinhoff[26] reported on two successful pneumonectomies, beginning the era of reliable intrathoracic surgery. However, it was not until Hodgson and associates[15–17] demonstrated the effectiveness of the transthoracic approach to the spine that thoracotomy was accepted as an exposure to the vertebral bodies. Since their first report in 1956, thoracotomy has been used with increasing frequency in treating diseases that primarily involve the thoracic vertebral bodies.

Hodgson and Stock first used thoracotomy to débride and bone graft tuberculous abscesses of the spine.[16] In 1960, they noted that tuberculosis of the spine usually involved the anterior elements and that the involvement was often more extensive than was apparent radiographically. They found that the best results of treatment occurred after extensive and complete débridement of all involved tissue and that spinal canal decompression and stabilizing fusion were often required. Such extensive procedures are hard to perform effectively through the more limited exposure offered by posterolateral costotransversectomy; therefore, Hodgson and coworkers[17] recommended the transthoracic approach. They reported a relatively low complication rate and an operative mortality of only 2.9 per cent in a large series.

The anterior approach to the spine is useful in resecting tumors of the vertebral bodies and in providing bone graft replacement. It may be used to débride osteomyelitis of the vertebral bodies or disc space infections. It has been used to correct certain scoliotic deformities,[12, 13, 27] particularly when the posterior elements of the spine are deficient, as in myelomeningocele. It has been used to resect certain fixed anterior deformities and to correct severe, fixed kyphoses.

Winter and associates[31] found that fixed thoracic kyphoses measuring over 50 degrees in patients older than 3 years of age often require correction and stabilization through the chest. In these situations, osteotomy may be necessary, and if there is associated neurologic involvement, decompression may be performed effectively from the front. Anteriorly placed bone grafts across a kyphos have a higher incidence of stable fusion than posterior grafts.[31] Johnson and Robinson[19] pointed out that anterior grafts are subject to compressive forces in the thoracic spine and are fixed to the large area of corticocancellous bone between the vertebral bodies. These factors appear to increase the incidence of stable fusion. Conversely, they noted that posterior grafts are subject to tensile forces and may attenuate with time. They illustrated the resorption of a posterior graft across a kyphos in one case.

A major indication for the transthoracic approach is to decompress the spinal canal in those conditions in which the cord is compromised by lesions protruding from the anterior elements. These include tumor or infection of the anterior spine extending into the spinal canal, fixed thoracic kyphosis with associated neuro-

logic involvement, and fractures of the vertebral body with fragments displaced posteriorly into the spinal canal. In all these situations, the cord may be tethered to or tented over these lesions and may have to traverse a longer arc. Laminectomy only decompresses the spinal canal but cannot remove the source of irritation, whereas anterior resection can do both effectively. In these conditions, anterior decompression has proved to be more effective than laminectomy[4, 9, 15–17, 19, 23, 31] and does not remove any remaining support provided by the posterior elements.

Posterolateral costotransversectomy permits effective decompression of the anterior spinal canal; however, the exposure is limited, control of bleeding may be difficult, and application of a large anterior bone graft may be impossible. The transthoracic approach adds a significant operative risk and is certainly more hazardous than posterior or even posterolateral approaches. In most cases, however, the increased operative risk of thoracotomy must be weighed against the more limited exposure provided by alternative routes.

The transthoracic approach to the spine provides direct access to the vertebral bodies from the second to the twelfth thoracic segments. The midthoracic vertebral bodies are best exposed, whereas the upper and lower extremes yield a more limited view. In general, we recommend an approach through a left posterolateral thoracotomy incision. Some surgeons prefer a right thoracotomy for approaches to the upper thoracic spine to avoid the subclavian and carotid arteries in the left superior mediastinum. In our experience, these vessels arise far enough anterior to the vertebral bodies to not affect dissection over the vertebrae. In the lower thoracic spine, a left thoracotomy is definitely preferred. The heart, on the left, may be retracted anteriorly with ease, whereas the liver, on the right, may present a significant obstacle to exposure. The level of the incision should be varied to meet the level of exposure required. We recommend directing the incision as far posteriorly as possible and resecting the rib just beyond its posterior angle to improve the vertebral body exposure. Ordinarily, an intercostal space is selected at or just above the involved segment. When only one segment is involved, the rib at that level should be removed. If multiple levels are involved, however, the rib at the upper level of the proposed dissection should be removed. Because of the natural thoracic kyphosis, dissection is easier from above downward for most surgeons. Although resection of a rib is not always necessary, it does improve the intrathoracic exposure and provides a suitable bone graft for fusion.

Technique

The patient is placed on the operating table in a lateral decubitus position. The arm on the operated side is fixed above the head, and an axillary pad is placed in the dependent axilla to prevent neurovascular damage of the dependent extremity. A curvilinear incision is made from the anterior axillary line to the border of the paraspinal muscles, posteriorly over the rib to be resected (Fig. 49–71, inset). The latissimus dorsi muscle

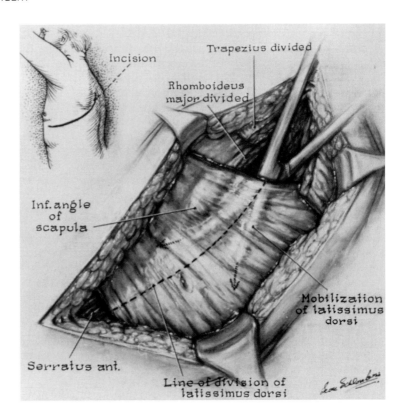

Figure 49–71. A curvilinear incision is made from the anterior axillary line to the paraspinal muscles posteriorly over the rib to be resected *(inset)*. The latissimus dorsi muscle is mobilized from the subjacent serratus anterior muscle and is transected. In approaches through the upper thorax, the lateral margin of the trapezius and rhomboid major may be divided as well.

is mobilized by blunt dissection and transected over the line of the incision (Fig. 49–71). The posterior border of the subjacent serratus anterior muscle is mobilized, and the space between the serratus anterior muscle and the underlying rib cage is developed (Fig. 49–72). The lateral margin of the trapezius muscle is identified and transected, if necessary. Approaches as high as the third rib may be required to reach the upper thoracic spine. In such cases, the trapezius and rhomboid major and minor muscles may be sectioned adjacent to their scapular insertions to mobilize and elevate the scapula.

The appropriate rib level is selected, and the fibers of the overlying serratus anterior muscle are severed

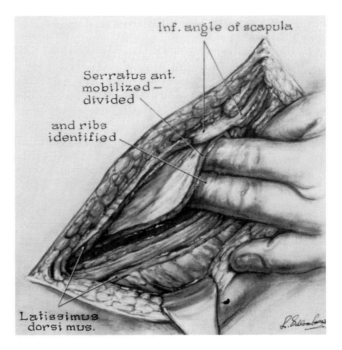

Figure 49–72. The serratus anterior muscle is mobilized and opened in line with its fibers. The surgeon may palpate superiorly within the space between the serratus anterior and the rib cage. The second rib is the uppermost rib, which may be reached within this plane and may be used to identify the level of the incision.

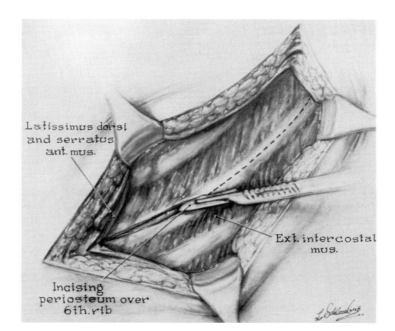

Figure 49–73. The periosteum over the anterior surface of the rib is incised sharply to the bone.

(see Fig. 49–72). To verify the correct rib level, the surgeon may palpate superiorly within this space between the serratus anterior muscle and the rib cage. The second rib is the uppermost rib that may be reached within this plane. The periosteum over the anterior surface of the rib is incised longitudinally (Fig. 49–73) and elevated, using curved periosteal elevators. Care is required to avoid injury to the neurovascular bundle lying within the subcostal groove on the inferior surface of the rib (Fig. 49–74). The subjacent endo-

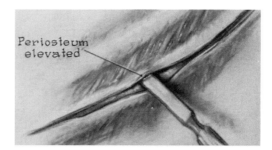

Figure 49–74. The periosteum is elevated from the rib circumferentially using straight and curved elevators. Note the neurovascular bundle lying within the subcostal groove on the deep and inferior surface of the rib. This should be elevated freely along with the periosteum.

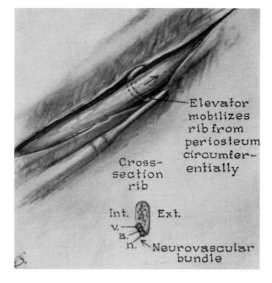

thoracic fascia and parietal pleura are left intact. The rib should be resected from the costochondral junction anteriorly to the angle of the rib posteriorly, using rib cutters (Fig. 49–75). The paraspinal muscles should be retracted to visualize the posterior angle of the rib during its resection. The rib is removed or rotated upward, and the parietal pleura is opened using scissors. The ribs are spread using a large, self-retaining thoracotomy retractor. The lung is then manually deflated and retracted anteriorly with padded retractors to expose the aorta and vertebral bodies behind (Fig. 49–76A). Adhesions between the visceral and parietal pleura ordinarily yield to gentle finger dissection, but sharp dissection occasionally may be required. Unless grossly diseased, the vertebral bodies are covered by the glistening parietal pleura. The intervertebral discs protrude prominently, and the vertebral bodies between are relatively concave. The aortic arch reaches to the level of the fourth thoracic vertebra and is closely applied to the anterior aspect of the vertebral bodies to the left of midline. Above the level of the aortic arch, the esophagus, thoracic duct, and subclavian artery are in close proximity to the vertebral body in this order, posterior to anterior. In the lower thorax, the aorta lies to the left of midline and the azygos vein and thoracic duct to the right of midline, immediately anterior to the vertebral bodies (Fig. 49–77). The aorta leaves the thorax at the level of the twelfth thoracic vertebra. The aorta and azygos system are tethered to the vertebral

bodies by the intercostal vessels. These are draped over the vertebral bodies between the disc spaces (see Fig. 49–76B) and join the intercostal nerve lateral to the sympathetic trunk. Together they proceed to the costal groove on the undersurface of the rib.

The correct vertebral level may be identified within the thorax by counting downward from the thoracic inlet. The first rib articulates with the superior aspect of the first thoracic vertebral body, and the second rib articulates with the first and second vertebrae. Because the thoracic vertebrae are so similar, we recommend radiographic confirmation of the vertebral level in the operating room, using a radiopaque marker fixed at the level of intended dissection.

An incision is made through the parietal pleura over the posterior rib and is extended to the lateral aspect of the vertebral body (see Fig. 49–76B). The pleura is cleared by blunt dissection, sparing the intercostal bundle and sympathetic trunk. A generous space is cleared over the involved vertebra and costovertebral articulations. The intercostal vessels may be ligated and transected to permit greater exposure or to mobilize the aorta. We have found that the intercostal vessels may be easily ligated using metal vascular clips and a long-handled holder. The segmental blood supply to the lower thoracic spinal cord is sparse, and for this reason we recommend that the intercostal arteries be spared when possible.

The transthoracic approach provides a generous ex-

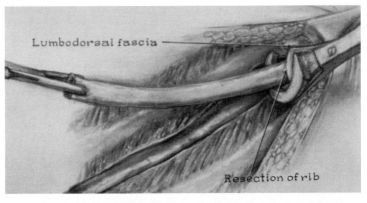
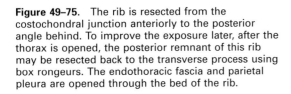
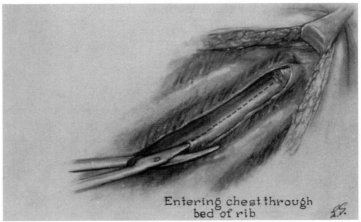

Figure 49–75. The rib is resected from the costochondral junction anteriorly to the posterior angle behind. To improve the exposure later, after the thorax is opened, the posterior remnant of this rib may be resected back to the transverse process using box rongeurs. The endothoracic fascia and parietal pleura are opened through the bed of the rib.

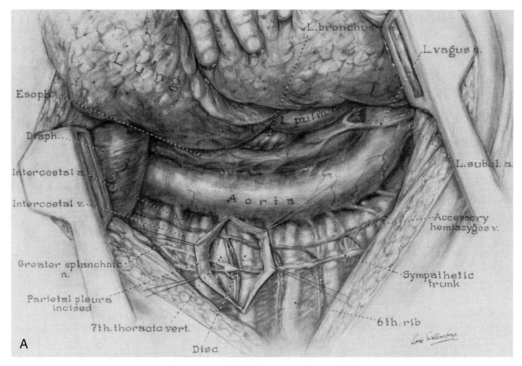

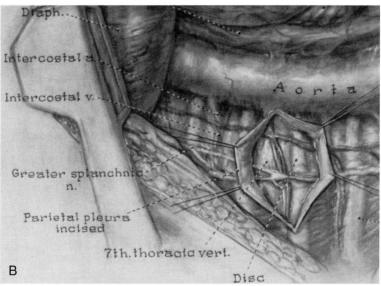

Figure 49–76. *A,* The lung is manually deflated and retracted anteriorly, revealing the aorta lying over the vertebral bodies. The vertebrae are covered by the normally translucent parietal pleura. Note that the intervertebral discs protrude prominently, and the vertebral bodies are relatively concave. The sympathetic trunk lies over the costovertebral articulations. *B,* Detail of the segmental vessels draped over the waist or midportion of the concave vertebral bodies. Lateral to the sympathetic trunk, these are joined by the intercostal nerve, and together they proceed to the subcostal groove on the lower surface of the rib.

posure to the vertebral bodies anteriorly. It permits complete excisional biopsy of the bodies and bone grafting at multiple levels. The intrathoracic correction of scoliotic deformities has been well perfected, and the spinal cord may be effectively decompressed even when the body and posterior longitudinal ligament are destroyed. In these situations, the segmental nerve is

identified and is followed into the canal, and only the bone and ligament anterior to it are removed. In this way, the dura and cord are protected from injury.

The vertebral bodies protrude prominently within the thoracic cavity and are not encumbered laterally by the transverse processes, as they are at the cervical levels. This facilitates keying or locking an anterior

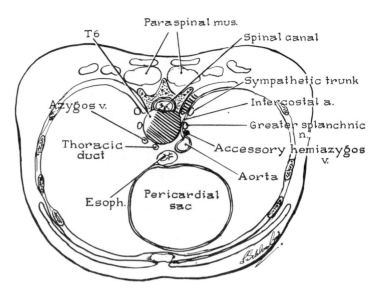

Figure 49–77. Cross section of the thorax at the level of the sixth thoracic vertebra, showing the relationship of the most significant perivertebral structures. See also Figure 49–70 (color plate).

intervertebral graft in place, as troughs may be prepared and the graft may be inserted from the side (Fig. 49–78).

Chest tubes are inserted to evacuate blood and air. Ordinarily, these are placed one or two intercostal spaces above and below the incision, and the tubes are tunneled beneath the skin to create an air seal and to prevent leakage about the tube (Fig. 49–79). One tube is directed superiorly within the thorax toward the apex of the lung to collect air, and the other is placed below, at the posterior corner of the diaphragm, to evacuate blood. A purse-string suture is installed in the skin around each tube and is then tied to the tube to hold it in place during turning or transfer of the patient. The ribs are reapproximated and held in place with heavy absorbable sutures (see Fig. 49–79). The periosteum and intercostal muscles are approximated, using a running suture, to effect an airtight closure. The serratus anterior, trapezius, latissimus dorsi, and

rhomboid muscles are approximated in separate layers (Fig. 49–80). The subcutaneous tissue and skin are closed (Fig. 49–81), and the chest tubes are attached to water-seal, constant suction.

Anterior exposures of the upper thoracic vertebral

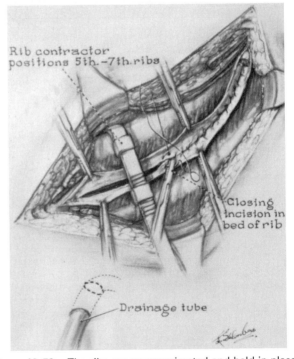

Figure 49–79. The ribs are reapproximated and held in place with heavy absorbable pericostal sutures placed around the ribs above and below the thoracotomy site. The intercostal muscles and periosteum are closed with a running suture to create an airtight closure. Prior to closure, chest tubes are placed at the apex of the lung to collect air and at the posterior base of the thoracic cavity to evacuate blood. The tubes are placed one or two intercostal spaces away from the incision and are tunneled beneath the skin to create an air seal.

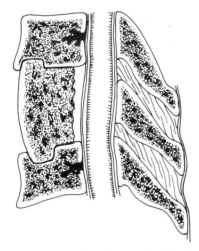

Figure 49–78. Sagittal section of a vertebral body replacement graft.

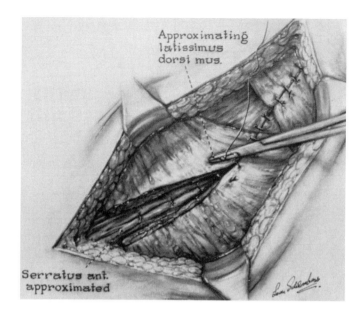

Figure 49–80. Closure of the serratus anterior, trapezius, and latissimus dorsi muscles.

bodies pose one of the great surgical challenges. Ordinarily, the third rib is the highest level through which effective intrathoracic exposure can be gained, as the first and second ribs are too short to provide reasonable room within the chest. To expose the upper thoracic vertebrae through the bed of the third rib, the scapula must be mobilized and retracted laterally and superiorly. To do this, the rhomboid muscles may be detached from their insertion on the vertebral border of the scapula. This may be done by subperiosteally stripping them from the scapula, leaving a layer of periosteum and tendon for later repair. At closure, holes may be made in the scapula, sutures are inserted through these holes, and the rhomboids are repaired through this periosteal-tendon sheath.

If spinal stability is in doubt, plaster of Paris or fiberglass plastic turning shells, similar to a bivalved body cast, are made for the patient, extending from the upper thorax to the pelvis. The front and back components are secured with a circumferential binder or Velcro straps, and the patient is transferred to a bed or turning frame.

The patient is nursed supine but is rolled like a log from side to side at two-hour intervals. When drainage of air and blood has stopped, the chest tubes are removed, and when the patient's condition has stabilized and the wounds are healed, a body cast or brace is made to protect the spine. Ordinarily, we use a hyperextension body cast made on a fracture table using Goldthwait irons. The cast is padded over the entire posterior thorax and pelvis with a single large sheet of felt, and additional pads are placed anteriorly over the manubrium, lower ribs, iliac crests, and pubic symphysis. The cast extends from the manubrium to the pubic symphysis and is well molded about the pelvis and thorax. A hole is made in the front of the cast about 10 cm high and 15 cm wide over the upper abdomen just below the rib cage to facilitate respiration.

If the patient has insensate skin, we avoid using circumferential plaster and usually employ a molded plastic body brace. This is similar to a body cast but has separate front and back components and is made of a "high-temperature," lightweight plastic. The front and back components are connected with Velcro closures and may be removed to inspect the skin. If the level of instability is in the upper thorax, above the sixth vertebra, we add a chin-occiput extension, or if the instability extends into the lumbar spine, we add a hip spica to the thigh to improve external control. The patient is then mobilized, and roentgenograms are obtained with the patient erect to ensure that appropriate control of the spine is maintained and that the vertebrae remain well aligned. Roentgenograms are made at regular intervals until osseous fusion is established, and the patient is then weaned from the brace or cast.

Complications

The transthoracic approach to the spine adds the considerable risk of thoracotomy to the risks of spinal surgery. Postoperatively, these patients require intensive nursing care and close supervision by the surgical team. Many of these patients are debilitated, are poor operative risks, and require heroic efforts to carry them through their postoperative course.

All the complications of major thoracic surgery may occur, such as atelectasis, pneumonia, and airway obstruction. Congestive heart failure and pulmonary edema may occur if fluid replacement is excessive and if venous pressures are not closely monitored.

On resecting the vertebral bodies, considerable bleeding may be encountered from the posterior nutrient vessels. These must be controlled with bone wax, Gelfoam, and thrombin, as it is often unsafe to cauterize these vessels adjacent to the dura.

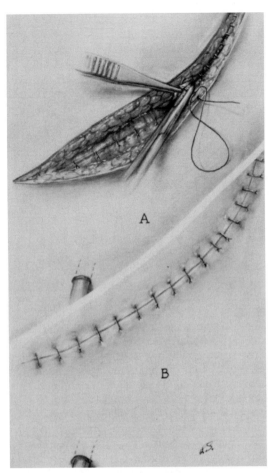

Figure 49–81. Closure of the subcutaneous layer *(A)* and skin *(B)*. Note the chest tubes tunneled beneath the skin away from the incision to create an air seal.

Injury to the spinal cord is always possible, particularly with extensive anterior decompression, if the operative field is covered with blood or if the normal landmarks are distorted by disease. For this reason, we recommend meticulous control of hemorrhage. When the anatomic landmarks are severely distorted, one can identify a nerve root and follow it centrally until the dura and cord are safely identified. An alternative approach is to initiate the decompression over an uninvolved area and proceed to the involved area following the plane of the dura. Perhaps the greatest neurologic threat is associated with correction of a severe fixed kyphos by osteotomy, and because of this, patients and their families should be advised preoperatively that paraplegia may complicate this procedure.

Spinal cord ischemia secondary to ligation of the segmental intercostal vessels is a potential threat. Anterior spinal artery syndromes with paraplegia, loss of pain and temperature sense, and sphincter disturbance have occasionally been reported following scoliosis correction[10, 21] or circumferential spinal osteotomy.[11] Conversely, no complications have been reported by a number of authors following unilateral resection of multiple segmental vessels in the lower thoracic spine.[5, 8, 9, 17, 31] Burrington and colleagues[5] recommend that the segmental arteries be ligated close to the aorta on one side only, maintaining the collateral circulation through the intercostals described by Lazorthes and coworkers.[22]

Although pseudarthrosis following anterior fusion is rare, it has been reported.[31] Wound infections are rare but do occur, and pressure sores have been a problem, particularly over a prominent gibbus. Hodgson and coworkers[17] reported the development of a cerebrospinal fluid fistula into the pleural cavity in four cases following resection of a tuberculous spinal abscess, one of which resulted in death.

Thoracoabdominal Approach to the Lower Thoracic and Upper Lumbar Vertebral Bodies

It is occasionally necessary to expose the lower thoracic and upper lumbar vertebral bodies in continuity. This presents a problem in exposure because of the presence of the diaphragm and adds to the risk of surgery if two major body cavities are opened. A number of different approaches are available, beginning from above with a posterolateral thoracotomy at the left seventh intercostal space and dividing the diaphragm peripherally within the thorax. At the inferior extreme, the thorax may be left intact and the vertebrae may be approached through a long, oblique flank incision made below the rib cage, and the diaphragm may be detached posteriorly and medially from below. The approach selected should depend upon the level of vertebral involvement and the patient's ability to tolerate major surgery. Ordinarily, thoracic lesions should be approached through the chest, whereas lesions that involve primarily the upper lumbar vertebrae may be approached through a flank incision with less operative risk.

The diaphragm is a dome-shaped organ that is muscular around its periphery and tendinous centrally (Fig. 49–82, see color plate). Anteriorly and laterally, it originates from the cartilaginous ends of the lower six ribs and xiphoid. Posteriorly, it originates from the upper lumbar vertebrae through the crura, the aponeurotic arcuate ligaments, and the twelfth ribs. The crura are musculotendinous structures that arise from the anterior longitudinal ligament of the lumbar vertebrae and extend superiorly to surround the aortic and esophageal hiatus. The medial arcuate ligaments arise from the crura on their respective sides, cross over the psoas muscles like a bridge, and insert on the transverse processes of the first lumbar vertebra. The lateral arcuate ligaments arise from the transverse process of the first lumbar vertebra and extend over the quadratus lumborum muscles to the tips of the twelfth ribs.

The diaphragm is innervated by the phrenic nerve, which descends through the thorax on the pericardium. The phrenic nerve joins the diaphragm adjacent to the fibrous pericardium, dividing into three major branches that extend peripherally in an anterior, lateral, and posterior direction. In addition, there are numerous interconnections that loop between these branches.[29] Cutting many of these major branches or intercommunications interferes with diaphragmatic function and reduces respiratory reserves. An incision around the periphery of the diaphragm interferes least with diaphragmatic function and is recommended for thoracoabdominal approaches to the spine. A short, radiate incision through the central tendon spares most major nerve fibers but does not provide direct access to the vertebral bodies posteriorly. To provide wide exposure of the thoracic and lumbar vertebrae in continuity, an incision is made through the periphery of the diaphragm, extending posteriorly through the lateral arcuate ligament. A second incision is then required through the insertions of the medial and lateral arcuate ligaments adjacent to the first lumbar transverse process to open the diaphragm posteriorly and to provide continuity of exposure between the thoracic and lumbar spine.

The eleventh and twelfth thoracic vertebrae may be approached from above or below the diaphragm, but each route provides certain advantages and limitations. For example, in the subdiaphragmatic approach, the surgeon may reflect the left aortic crus and divide the arcuate ligament insertion but leave the muscular diaphragm intact. In addition, he or she may avoid entering the pleural cavity by limiting the dissection to the retropleural plane around the vertebral bodies. This yields an excellent view of the upper lumbar vertebrae but allows a more limited exposure as high as the eleventh thoracic vertebral body. Conversely, the transthoracic route through the diaphragm offers a much larger working area over the lower thoracic vertebrae but obligates a more extensive dissection, opening two major body cavities.

Most general surgical approaches to the abdominal viscera are directed anteriorly and laterally. Because the vertebral bodies are posterior to the abdominal viscera, the approach should be modified in a posterolateral direction to bring the vertebrae as close to the incision as possible and to reduce the depth of the wound. We recommend an approach to the left of midline, as the vena cava on the right may complicate surgery with troublesome hemorrhage, and the liver may be hard to retract.

The anterior approaches are required only when extensive resection and bone grafts are planned. Simple excisional biopsy, drainage, or débridement of the vertebral bodies may be effectively handled through a posterolateral costotransversectomy (see next section) with less operative morbidity.

Technique

To approach the lower thoracic spine through the chest, the patient is positioned on the operating table in a lateral decubitus position. An axillary pad is placed in the dependent axilla, and the left arm is fixed above the head. A left lateral or posterolateral incision is made at the level of the seventh to eleventh ribs, de-

pending upon the desired level of dissection (Fig. 49–83). The incision extends from the paraspinal muscles posteriorly to the anterior margin of the rib cage. The incision is deepened through the subcutaneous tissues to the thoracic musculature. The latissimus dorsi muscle is transected across the plane of its fibers, and the serratus anterior muscle is divided and spread over the intended rib level. The external and internal intercostal muscles are divided in the intercostal space using scalpel dissection. The endothoracic fascia and parietal pleura are opened, the ribs are spread with a large self-retaining rib retractor, and the lung is deflated and retracted anteriorly. If bone grafting is planned, the rib may be removed. A circumferential incision is made in the muscular portion of the diaphragm adjacent to the costal margin (see Fig. 49–83) and extended posteriorly to the lateral arcuate ligament. This incision is extended through the peritoneal reflection of the diaphragm, and the spleen and contents of the left upper quadrant of the abdomen are exposed. The retroperitoneal space is opened either by blunt dissection of the peritoneum at the level of the diaphragmatic incision or through a separate incision adjacent to the spleen (Fig. 49–84). The retroperitoneal space is developed by blunt dissection posterior to the renal fascia. The spleen, kidney, and stomach are gently retracted medially, using a broad, padded Deaver retractor. The psoas muscle, vertebral bodies, and aorta are exposed. The aorta is carefully mobilized by a combination of sharp and blunt dissection, and the segmental vessels are ligated with metal vascular clips and divided at only those levels required for satisfactory exposure. The sympathetic trunk extends over the anterolateral aspect of the vertebral bodies adjacent to the psoas muscle. It is recognized by its periodic ganglionic enlargements and should be spared. The left crus of the diaphragm is dissected from the anterior longitudinal ligament over the upper lumbar vertebral bodies (Fig. 49–85A). The insertion of the arcuate ligament is divided at the first lumbar transverse process. The incision in the diaphragm is extended through the lateral arcuate ligament, providing continuity of exposure from the thoracic to the lumbar vertebrae. A longitudinal incision is made in the anterior longitudinal ligament, and the ligament is reflected laterally to expose the vertebral bodies (Fig. 49–85B). At this point, drainage, resection of a lesion, osteotomy, decompression, or bone grafting may be performed with excellent visibility throughout the thoracic and upper lumbar spine. Fusion and inlay bone grafting in a trough created in the twelfth thoracic and first two lumbar vertebrae are illustrated in Figure 49–86A and B.

The anterior longitudinal ligament may be repaired over the vertebral bodies. The diaphragmatic crus is sutured to the anterior longitudinal ligament to close the defect in the aortic hiatus. The arcuate ligament is repaired at the transverse process of the first lumbar vertebra. The diaphragm is closed with interrupted sutures in an airtight fashion (Fig. 49–87). Chest tubes are inserted for drainage of fluid and air, and the ribs are reapproximated. The pleura and intercostal muscles

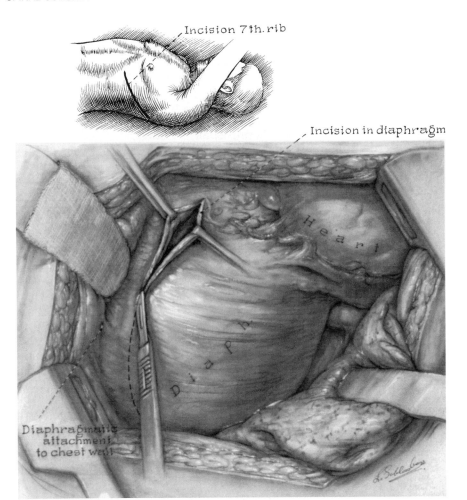

Figure 49–83. Thoracotomy incision *(inset).* Circumferential incision in the muscular portion of the diaphragm adjacent to the costal margin.

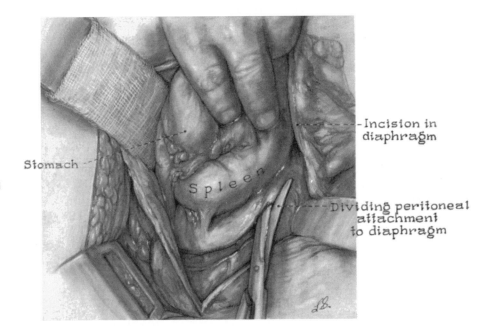

Figure 49–84. The abdominal contents are retracted medially and inferiorly, and the retroperitoneal space is opened through a peritoneal incision adjacent to the diaphragm.

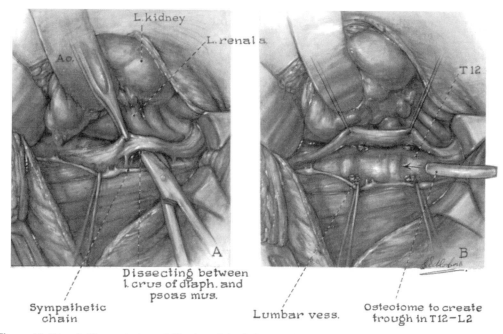

Figure 49–85. *A,* The aorta is mobilized, and the left crus of the diaphragm is dissected from the anterior longitudinal ligament over the vertebral bodies. *B,* A longitudinal incision is made in the anterior longitudinal ligament, and the vertebral bodies are exposed.

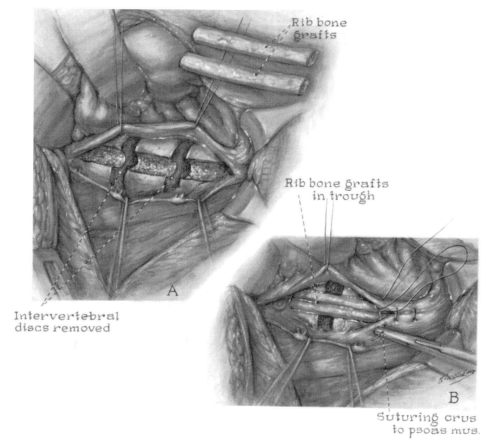

Figure 49–86. *A,* A trough is created in the twelfth thoracic and upper two lumbar vertebrae, and the intervertebral disc spaces are excised. *B,* Bone plugs are installed in the disc spaces, rib grafts are laid in the trough, and the anterior longitudinal ligament and left crus are repaired.

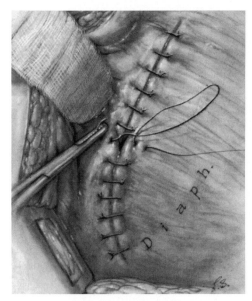

Figure 49–87. The diaphragm is closed in an airtight fashion.

are repaired with running absorbable suture material, and the serratus anterior and latissimus dorsi muscles are reapproximated with separate layers of running suture. The subcutaneous tissue and skin are closed, and the chest tubes are attached to water-seal suction.

Postoperatively, the patient is usually nursed in plaster of Paris shells or a turning frame to protect the integrity of the spine. At about two weeks following surgery, the patient may be placed in a localizer cast or brace, depending upon the intrinsic stability of the spine (see previous section).

Complications

The thoracoabdominal exposure of the thoracic and lumbar spine adds significantly to the risks of surgery, as two major body cavities are exposed. The specific complications encountered are similar to those of thoracotomy alone, as described in the previous section. In addition, injury to the spleen, kidney, or ureters may occur without gentle retraction or cautious dissection. Gastrointestinal complications such as prolonged ileus may be anticipated. Injury to the sympathetic chain may induce a sympathectomy effect with asymmetric warmth of the involved extremity, but this is rarely a problem. The peritoneum and diaphragm should be closed carefully to restore their continuity and to prevent herniation of visceral structures.

As a rule, these patients are exceedingly sick in the first week postoperatively and require intensive nursing care for much of this period. For this reason, the combined thoracoabdominal exposure should be reserved for those patients with satisfactory cardiopulmonary reserves who are likely to tolerate such surgical risks. In the case of a poor operative risk, the exposure through the flank with retroperitoneal dissection

should be considered if limited exposure over the thoracic vertebrae is acceptable.

Posterolateral Approaches to the Thoracic Spine

There is only one commonly used posterolateral approach, the costotransversectomy approach. There are extensions and variations of the approach that remove more than one rib. The routine approach is described in the section on costotransversectomy.

Posterolateral Costotransversectomy Approach to the Thoracic Vertebral Bodies

The costotransversectomy approach provides access to the anterior and lateral elements of the thoracic vertebrae through a posterolateral incision. With careful dissection in the retropleural space, the vertebral bodies may be reached without entering the pleural cavity. The approach is ideally suited to a poor-risk or elderly patient who cannot tolerate formal thoracotomy and provides access for biopsy, drainage of an abscess, and limited resection of the vertebral bodies. In addition, the spinal cord may be decompressed anterolaterally, and a limited anterior fusion may be performed. The posterolateral approach is a less extensive procedure and affords less operative risk than formal thoracotomy imposes. On the other hand, costotransversectomy provides less satisfactory exposure of the midthoracic vertebral bodies, and extensive vertebral resection or fusion at multiple levels may not be technically feasible.

Costotransversectomy was first used by Haidenhaim and described by Menard in 1894.[24] As originally described, it provides limited exposure of the lateral vertebral bodies through a midline posterior longitudinal incision. The transverse process of the vertebra and medial 2 inches of rib are resected at one of several levels. The vertebral bodies can be palpated within the retropleural space, but because the incision is made in midline and only a short segment of rib is removed, visualization of the vertebral body is limited, and the anterior aspect cannot be reached directly.

Seddon[30] augmented this exposure by approaching the spine through a more lateral, curvilinear incision. He recommended resecting longer segments of rib over at least three levels, permitting more extensive exposure and direct visualization of the anterolateral aspect of the vertebral bodies. In 1933, Capener (reported in 1954) made a major addition to this approach by including anterolateral decompression of the cord.[6] He referred to this as lateral rhachotomy. The spine is approached through a curvilinear incision lateral to the midline. The trapezius muscle is detached medially and retracted laterally, and the paraspinal muscles are divided transversely. The transverse processes of the vertebrae and a generous length of rib are resected at several levels. The cord is decompressed laterally and anteriorly by resecting the pedicles and posterior aspect of the vertebral bodies. Until Hodgson popularized transthoracic resection and decompression of the tuberculous spine, this approach was frequently used to resect tuberculous lesions of the thoracic spine.[20]

The authors use a minor modification of this approach through a straight, longitudinal incision lateral to the paraspinal muscle mass. The paraspinal muscles are retracted medially, and the transverse process and a generous section of rib are removed. Through this exposure, biopsy or drainage of an abscess, limited resection, anterolateral decompression, and fusion are possible, and it may be the safest approach to excise a herniated intervertebral disc at the thoracic level.[2] When a kyphos is present, exposure of the vertebral body is improved and may be increased by removing the ribs and transverse processes at three or four levels, but visualization of the anterior aspect of the vertebral bodies remains limited. Some surgeons have successfully performed extensive decompression and fusion using this exposure,[3] but we have found this approach more limiting and prefer thoracotomy when extensive resection and grafting are planned at multiple levels. We have also been reluctant to remove more than four

ribs posteriorly for fear of removing the lateral stability they provide and allowing a scoliosis to develop.

Anatomic Considerations

Certain superficial muscles of the posterior thorax must be divided in the costotransversectomy approach, lateral to the paraspinal muscle mass. The trapezius muscle (Fig. 49–88) extends from the head to the twelfth thoracic spinous process, its fibers running obliquely and laterally to the scapular spine. Beneath this lie the rhomboid muscles, arising from the spinous processes of the seventh cervical and upper five thoracic vertebrae. In the lower thorax, the latissimus dorsi muscle arises beneath the trapezius muscle from the lower six thoracic vertebrae and extends as a broad sheet across the back to the axilla. The serratus posterior inferior muscle is the most characteristic muscle found in the lower thorax beneath the latissimus. It arises as separate, short muscular bundles from the lower four ribs, becomes tendinous, and descends obliquely downward to insert on the lumbar fascia. In posterolateral approaches to the upper five thoracic vertebrae, the trape-

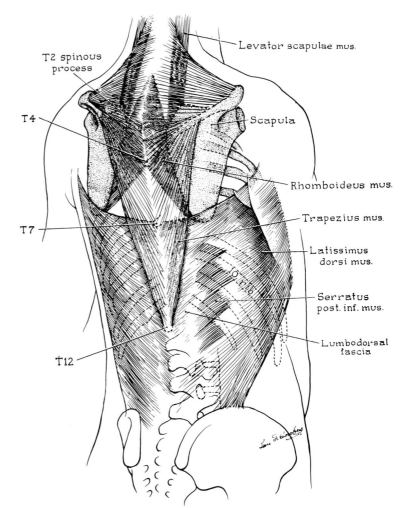

Figure 49–88. Superficial muscles of the posterior thorax. In costotransversectomy approaches lateral to the paraspinal muscle mass and over the upper thorax, the trapezius and rhomboid muscles must be divided. Over the lower thorax, the latissimus dorsi must be transected and the serratus posterior inferior is found about the lowest thoracic vertebrae.

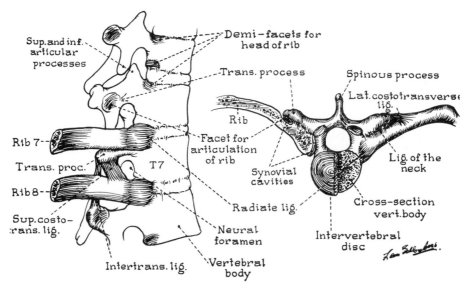

Figure 49–89. Extrinsic ligaments of the thoracic spine and detail of the thoracic vertebrae. Unique to the thoracic spine are a group of ligaments that bind the ribs to the vertebral bodies and transverse processes. This ligament system is additional to the intrinsic ligaments between vertebrae and increases the inherent stability of the thoracic spine.

zius and rhomboid muscles must be divided. These may be sectioned medially about their tendinous origins. Over the lower thorax, the latissimus dorsi as well as the trapezius muscles must be sectioned, and the serratus posterior inferior muscle is found over the lowest three vertebrae.

Extrinsic Ligaments

Unique to the thoracic spine is a group of ligaments that bind the ribs to their respective transverse processes and the vertebral bodies. This is an additional ligament system that through the ribs increases the stability over the thoracic spine. These must be divided in a costotransversectomy exposure before the posterior and medial aspect of the ribs can be mobilized and removed.

The costotransverse ligaments are divided into a number of named individual components. The most significant of these is the superior costotransverse ligament (Fig. 49–89), which extends from the inferior aspect of one transverse process to the superior aspect of the rib beneath. Medial to this ligament is a space through which the dorsal rami of the segmental nerves and vessels course posteriorly toward the erector spinae muscle mass (see Fig. 49–93, inset). In dissections beneath the transverse processes, these vessels should be identified and ligated to prevent persistent hemorrhage. The posterior costotransverse ligament extends from the inferior aspect of the base of the transverse process to the superior aspect of the rib beneath.

Anterior to the transverse process is the capsular ligament, which secures the neck of the rib to the front of the transverse process. Laterally, the lateral costotransverse ligaments extend from the tip of the

transverse process to the posterior tubercle of the same rib (see Fig. 49–89). Finally, the costovertebral or radiate ligaments bind the head of each rib to its respective vertebral body articulations. The sympathetic trunk courses over the heads of the ribs within the thorax just lateral to the radiate ligament insertions on the ribs (see Fig. 49–93).

The transverse processes extend like wings from the upper and lateral aspects of the laminae, arching superiorly and posteriorly in their lateral course (see Fig. 49–89). Laterally, these widen into a prominent tubercle, which articulates with the rib at the same level on its anterior surface. The pedicle lies directly in front of the base of each transverse process, a fact that is helpful in locating the pedicle and avoiding the nerve root, which emerges from the foramina beneath, during costotransversectomy.

Technique

Endotracheal anesthesia is recommended to provide positive-pressure ventilation in case the pleura is opened during the surgical dissection. The patient is placed on the operating table, either in a lateral position with an axillary pad in the dependent axilla or in the prone position with chest rolls on either side of the thorax.

A straight, longitudinal incision is made about 2.5 inches lateral to the spinous processes, centered over the level of the desired vertebral dissection (Fig. 49–90). At this location a slight depression is palpable between the dorsal paraspinal muscle mass and the prominent posterior angle of the rib (Fig. 49–91). The incision should be centered over this groove, lateral to the spinous processes. The incision is extended deeply

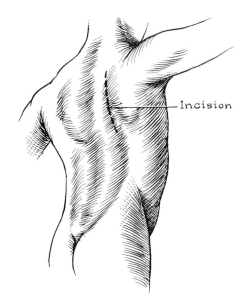

Figure 49–90. A longitudinal incision is made lateral to the paraspinal muscle mass over the posterior angle of the ribs. A depression is normally visible here, and the prominent posterior angles can be palpated beneath this depression.

through the subcutaneous tissues; the trapezius and latissimus dorsi muscles (see Fig. 49–88), as well as the lumbodorsal fascia, are divided longitudinally. The paraspinal muscles are dissected sharply from their insertions on the ribs and transverse processes and are retracted medially. In a muscular patient, it may be impossible to effectively retract these muscles medially, and one may need to divide the paraspinal muscles transversely; however, subsequent closure may be difficult.

If simple drainage of a small abscess or biopsy of a lesion of the pedicle or vertebral body is contemplated, the rib and transverse process are resected at one or two levels only. Roentgenographic control films should be taken in the operating room with a needle or towel clip attached to the vertebra in question to ensure that the proper spinal level is selected. The costotransverse ligaments (see Fig. 49–89) are divided sharply, and the transverse process is generously resected at its junction with the lamina (see Fig. 49–91) using bone rongeurs or osteotomes. An incision is made through the periosteum into the rib, from the costovertebral articulation to the angle of the rib. The rib is exposed by careful subperiosteal dissection, leaving the pleura and intercostal neurovascular bundles intact (Fig. 49–92). The rib is transected with rib cutters about 3.5 inches lateral to the vertebra at its prominent posterior angle. The cut end of the rib is grasped with a clamp and rotated with one hand while the costovertebral ligaments are separated with a sharp periosteal elevator, dissecting along the rib toward the vertebral articulation. If a porotic rib breaks at its neck, the medial end should be resected cleanly with rongeurs.

Anterior to the stump of the amputated transverse process is the vertebral pedicle, and above and below the pedicle lie the neural foramina (Figs. 49–89 and 49–93). The nerve roots emerge from the inferior pole of the foramina, giving off a dorsal and a ventral ramus. The dorsal ramus sweeps posteriorly, with its accompanying vessels, below the transverse process and medial to the superior costotransverse ligaments (see Fig. 49–93, inset). The artery and veins should be identified and ligated, or they will bleed continually throughout the procedure. The ventral ramus becomes the intercostal nerve and is joined by the intercostal vessels. These travel laterally and meet the ribs at their

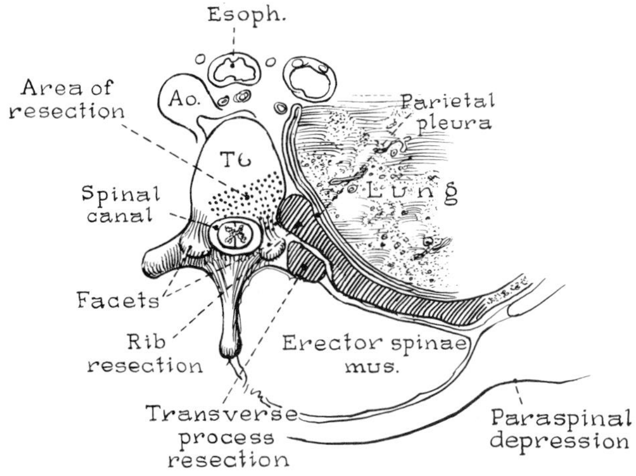

Figure 49–91. Cross section of the thoracic vertebrae and ribs. The hatched area indicates the bony structures that are normally removed to provide adequate exposure. The stippled area over the vertebral body and pedicle may be removed to decompress the spinal canal.

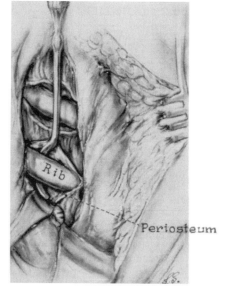

Figure 49–92. The rib is exposed by circumferential subperiosteal dissection from its posterior angle to the transverse process of the vertebra.

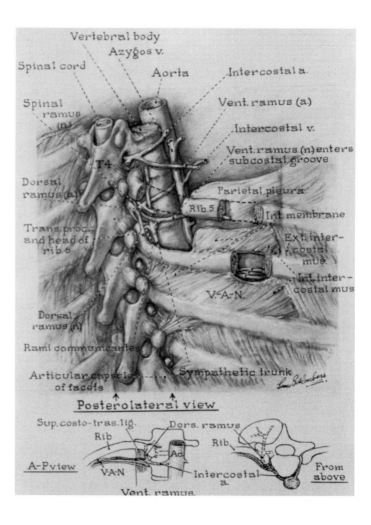

Figure 49–93. Anatomic detail of the deep structures of the posterior thorax showing the relationship of the dorsal and ventral neurovascular structures. *Inset,* The dorsal nerve and artery course beneath the transverse processes and medial to the superior costotransverse ligament. These vessels should be identified and ligated in approaches through the transverse processes.

posterior angle and then enter the subcostal groove. Anteriorly, the intercostal vessels sweep around the waist or midportion of the vertebral body before dividing into the ventral and dorsal branches at the outlet of the neural foramen (see Fig. 49–93).

Once the pedicles, neural foramina, and these neuro-vascular structures have been identified, the dissection should proceed directly anteriorly, on the pedicle, to the vertebral body along a path that is relatively free of major vessels or nerves (Fig. 49–94). We generally use a Cobb elevator beginning at the pedicle, raising the sympathetic trunk and parietal pleura before it and

Figure 49–94. The pedicles lie directly in front of the transverse processes. To expose the vertebral body, the dissection should proceed anterior to the stump of the transected transverse process, along the pedicles, to the vertebral body. By restricting the dissection to this plane, one can avoid the nerve roots leaving their foramina above and below the pedicles as well as the segmental vessels draped over the midportion of the vertebral body. We find that a 0.5-in Cobb periosteal elevator is most useful for this part of the dissection. Once an initial path has been cleared, dissection can proceed inferiorly and superiorly along the vertebral body to widen the exposure, using the periosteal elevator to raise these tissues.

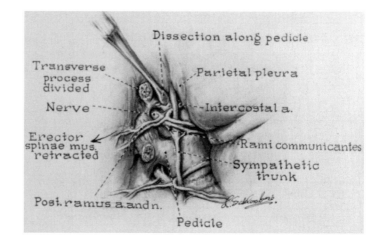

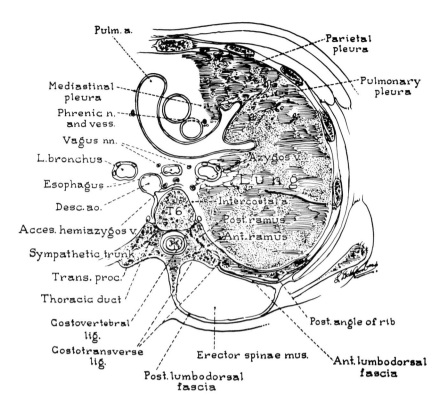

Figure 49–95. Cross section of the thorax at the level of the sixth thoracic vertebra. See also Figure 49–70 (color plate).

advancing forward to the anterolateral aspect of the body (Fig. 49–95). Once this path is clear, we extend the dissection inferiorly and superiorly along the vertebral body and disc space, being careful not to injure the segmental vessels draped over the vertebral body. The parietal pleura is then teased from the vertebral body by gentle finger dissection. If the pleura is perforated, the defect should be sealed and repaired.

At this stage, an abscess may be drained, and necrotic debris may be removed over a limited area. If a biopsy of the vertebral body is planned, the pleura is retracted, using a padded Deaver retractor, and the vertebral body is biopsied, using curets or rongeurs. If the exposure is not adequate, the transverse processes and ribs should be resected at one or two additional levels.

If a relatively extensive resection, decompression, and bone grafting are planned, at least three and no more than four transverse processes and ribs should be resected. Ordinarily, the intercostal vessels may be retracted sufficiently to provide adequate exposure; however, the vessels may be ligated and divided if necessary. The intercostal nerves are isolated from adjacent tissue, and the pleura is depressed, leaving the nerves suspended across the wound (Fig. 49–96).

If decompression is required, the pedicles and posterior aspect of the vertebral bodies may be removed (see Figs. 49–91 and 49–96). Decompression is started at the pedicles adjacent to a nerve root in an area that is least involved with disease. The nerve root is followed centrally as a guide, and the dura and spinal cord are identified and protected. Bone is removed using

rongeurs and a high-speed drill and diamond burr to remove dense cortical bone. One should be able to see the dura throughout the procedure, and the dura should be used as a guide to protect the cord as bone is resected around the spinal canal. The pedicles may be removed anterior to the facets, but the facets should be left intact to maintain anterior and lateral stability.

If decompression of a kyphos is required, resection of relatively large amounts of the posterior vertebral body may be necessary. The posterior longitudinal ligament and the posterior aspect of the vertebral body may be removed. An alternative method is to enter the cancellous bone anterior to the posterior cortex of the vertebral body. Sufficient bone is removed to provide effective decompression. Using a flat elevator, the posterior cortex is broken and depressed anteriorly, relieving the spinal obstruction. This leaves the posterior longitudinal ligament and a veneer of cortical bone between the spinal cord and any sharp subcortical bone fragments. Following this, the cord should be inspected to ensure that it is well decompressed and that there are no sharp projections into the canal. Throughout this dissection, it is best to avoid traction or manipulation of the dura or cord.

At the time of closure, the wound is filled with saline, and the lungs are inflated to check for air leaks. The paraspinal muscles, lumbodorsal fascia, and trapezius and latissimus dorsi muscles are repaired in separate layers. The wound is closed with a drain at the lower pole to prevent hematoma collection. The patient is generally nursed in plaster of Paris body shells or a

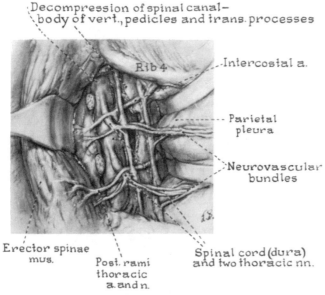

Decompression of spinal canal—
body of vert., pedicles and trans. processes

Rib 4

Intercostal a.

Parietal
pleura

Neurovascular
bundles

Erector spinae
mus.

Post. rami
thoracic
a. and n.

Spinal cord (dura)
and two thoracic nn.

Figure 49–96. For relatively extensive decompression and bone grafting, three or four ribs and transverse processes may be transected, leaving the neurovascular structures at each level suspended across the wound. The spinal canal may then be decompressed laterally and anteriorly by removing the pedicles to the side and a portion of the vertebral bodies in front of the spinal canal. The parietal pleura is retracted away from the vertebra with handheld retractors.

turning frame until a body cast or brace may be applied (see previous section on thoracotomy).

Complications

Although costotransversectomy is a less formidable approach than thoracotomy, there are significant surgical risks. Decompression of the spinal canal is potentially hazardous, and neurologic complications have occurred. Tears in the dura should be identified and repaired to prevent cerebrospinal fluid fistula. Throughout the procedure, bleeding should be meticulously controlled so the operative field is not obscured and the spinal cord is not inadvertently injured. Bleeding about the open vertebral body may be troublesome and can be controlled by cautery away from the cord or by packing and bone wax. Prior to closure, the pleura should be inspected for air leaks, and repairs should be made as required. If a pneumothorax is suspected, roentgenograms of the chest should be obtained in the operating room prior to extubation, and a chest tube should be installed in the upper anterior thorax.

Extensive decompression may induce significant spinal instability. Stability should be assessed at surgery by manipulation of the vertebral elements. If there is any doubt about spinal stability, instrumentation of fusion should be performed, and the spine should be carefully protected postoperatively with traction, a brace, or a cast until fusion is established.

Midline Posterior Approaches to the Thoracic Spine

This is apparently the oldest and most common approach to the spine, probably first used in orthopedics by Hibbs[14] and Albee[1] for spinal fusions for tuberculosis. They both published their separate methods in 1911. This approach is used for laminectomy and posterior spinal fusion, as well as spinal fixation for scoliosis, fractures, tumors, and so forth. A midline approach is generally considered very simple, because one need only identify the midline spinous processes and strip sharply or subperiosteally the erector spinae muscle mass from the lamina and interspinous ligaments to the transverse processes. However, the technique of separation may vary from clean atraumatic separation with minimal hemorrhage and cautery to extensive damage to the muscle mass and bone because of ragged, crude technique. The skin incision should be midline and straight, because many young patients are very sensitive to the cosmetic effects of surgery. We often scratch an orientation mark for the skin incision after the patient has been positioned face down, using a straight edge such as an x-ray film, to minimize asymmetry of the incision. The anatomic and surgical details of this approach are described elsewhere in this text.

References

1. Albee, F. H.: Transplantation of a portion of the tibia into the spine for Potts disease: A preliminary report. JAMA 57:885, 1911.
2. Benson, M. K. D., and Byrnes, D. P.: The clinical syndromes and surgical treatment of thoracic intervertebral disc prolapse. J. Bone Joint Surg. [Br.] 57:471–477, 1975.
3. Bohlman, H. H.: Late, progressive paralysis and pain following fractures of the thoracolumbar spine. J. Bone Joint Surg. [Am.] 58:728, 1976.
4. Brice, J., and McKissock, W.: Surgical treatment of malignant extradural spinal tumors. Br. Med. J. 1:1341–1344, 1965.
5. Burrington, J. D., Brown, C., Wayne, E. R., and Odom, J.: Anterior approach to the thoracolumbar spine—technical considerations. Arch. Surg. 111:456–463, 1976.
6. Capener, N.: The evolution of lateral rhachotomy. J. Bone Joint Surg. [Br.] 36:173–179, 1954.
7. Cauchoix, J., and Binet, J.: Anterior surgical approaches to spine. Ann. R. Coll. Surg. Engl. 27:237–243, 1957.
8. Chou, S. N., and Seljeskog, E. L.: Alternative surgical approaches to the thoracic spine. Clin. Neurosurg. 20:306–321, 1973.
9. Cook, W. A.: Trans-thoracic vertebral surgery. Ann. Thorac. Surg. 12:54–68, 1971.
10. Dommisse, G. F.: The blood supply of the spinal cord. A critical vascular zone in spinal surgery. J. Bone Joint Surg. [Br.] 56:225–235, 1974.
11. Dommisse, G. F., and Enslin, T. E.: Hodgson's circumferential osteotomy in the correction of spinal deformities. J. Bone Joint Surg. [Br.] 52:778, 1970.
12. Dwyer, A. F.: Experience of anterior correction of scoliosis. Clin. Orthop. 93:191–206, 1973.
13. Dwyer, A. F., and Schafer, M. F.: Anterior approach to scoliosis: Results of treatment in fifty-one cases. J. Bone Joint Surg. [Br.] 56:218–224, 1974.
14. Hibbs, R. A.: An operation for progressive spinal deformities. N. Y. State Med. J. 93:1013, 1911.
15. Hodgson, A. R.: Correction of fixed spinal curves. A preliminary communication. J. Bone Joint Surg. [Am.] 47:1221–1227, 1965.
16. Hodgson, A. R., and Stock, F. E.: Anterior spinal fusion, a preliminary communication on the radical treatment of Pott's disease and Pott's paraplegia. Br. J. Surg. 44:266–275, 1956.

17. Hodgson, A. R., Stock, F. E., Fang, H. S. Y., and Ong, G. B.: Anterior spinal fusion: The operative approach and pathologic findings in 412 patients with Pott's disease of the spine. Br. J. Surg. *48*:172–178, 1960.
18. Hodgson, A. R., and Yao, A. C. M. C.: Anterior approaches to the spinal column. *In* Apley, A. G. (ed.): Recent advances in orthopaedics. London, Longman Group, 1969, pp. 289–323.
19. Johnson, J. T. H., and Robinson, R. A.: Anterior strut grafts for severe kyphosis. Clin. Orthop. *56*:25–36, 1968.
20. Johnson, R. W., Jr., Hillman, J. W., and Southwick, W. O.: The importance of direct surgical attack upon lesions of the vertebral bodies, particularly in Pott's disease. J. Bone Joint Surg. [Am.] *35*:17–25, 1953.
21. Kiem, H. A., and Sadek, K. H.: Spinal angiography in scoliosis patients. J. Bone Joint Surg. [Am.] *53*:904–912, 1971.
22. Lazorthes, G., Gouaze, A., Zadeh, J. O., et al.: Arterial vascularization of the spinal cord: Recent studies of the anastomotic substitution pathways. J. Neurosurg. *35*:253–262, 1970.
23. Martin, N. S., and Williamson, J.: The role of surgery in the treatment of malignant tumors of the spine. J. Bone Joint Surg. [Br.] *52*:227–237, 1970.
24. Menard, V.: Causes de la paraplegie dans le mal de Pott. Rev. Orthop. *5*:47–64, 1894.
25. Nissen, R.: Exstirpation eines ganzen Lungenflügels. Zentralbl. Chir. *58*:3003–3006, 1931.
26. Reinhoff, W. J.: Pneumonectomy. Preliminary report of the operative technique in two successful cases. Bull. Johns Hopkins Hosp. *53*:390–393, 1933.
27. Riseborough, E. J.: The anterior approach to the spine for the correction of deformities of the axial skeleton. Clin. Orthop. *93*:207–214, 1973.
28. Robinson, S.: The surgery of bronchiectasis: Including a report of five complete resections of the lower lobe of the lung with one death. Surg. Gynecol. Obstet. *24*:194–215, 1917.
29. Scott, R.: Innervation of the diaphragm and its practical aspects in surgery. Thorax *20*:357–361, 1965.
30. Seddon, H. J.: Pott's paraplegia. *In* Platt, H. (ed.): Modern Trends in Orthopaedics. London, Butterworth and Co., Ltd., 1956, pp. 220–245.
31. Winter, R. B., Moe, J. H., and Wang, J. F.: Congenital kyphosis, its natural history and treatment as observed in a study of 130 patients. J. Bone Joint Surg. [Am.] *55*:223–256, 1973.

Surgical Approaches to the Lumbosacral Spine

SELECTION OF APPROACH TO THE LUMBAR SPINE, ANTERIOR VERSUS POSTERIOR

Under most circumstances, the choice of approach to the lumbar spine should be dictated by the site of the primary pathologic condition. Disease or deformity that primarily involves the vertebral bodies may be approached directly through the abdomen or flank. The posterior elements may be approached directly through a vertical, posterior incision in midline. The spinous processes, laminae, and facets are directly accessible through this approach, and the transverse processes and pedicles may be reached with somewhat more difficulty. The posterolateral approach provides direct access to the transverse processes and pedicles, as well as limited exposure of the vertebral bodies themselves.

Anterior

The anterolateral approach to the lumbar vertebral bodies through a long, oblique flank incision provides direct access to all the upper lumbar vertebral bodies in continuity. It should be considered for extensive resection, débridement, or grafting at multiple levels. If access to the lower lumbar vertebrae is desired, the incision may be directed more anteriorly and inferiorly, beginning midway between the symphysis pubis and iliac crest. This incision is extended laterally and obliquely along the iliac crest to the midflank.[21] A short, transverse flank incision may be used to provide less extensive exposure of the midlumbar spine.[34] Longitudinal left paramedian incisions with retroperitoneal or transperitoneal dissections have also been used.[43, 46] The

theoretic advantage of the transperitoneal approach is that the abdominal viscera may be more easily retracted than with a retroperitoneal dissection; however, the viscera and the hypogastric nerve plexus are more vulnerable in this line of dissection from the front.

Posterior

The posterior approach through a posterior longitudinal incision in midline provides direct access to the spinous processes, laminae, and facets at all levels of the lumbar spine. The transverse processes and even the pedicles may be reached with some difficulty by retracting the paraspinal muscles laterally. The posterior aspect of the vertebral body and disc space over the lower lumbar levels may be reached following laminectomy by retracting the dura, but the exposure is limited.

Posterolateral

The posterolateral approach through a longitudinal paraspinal incision, retracting the erector spinae muscles medially, provides direct access to the transverse processes and the mamillary processes of the facets (Fig. 49–97, color plate).[49, 50] This area provides an excellent bed for posterolateral lumbosacral fusion even in the face of pre-existing pseudarthrosis, laminar defects, or spondylolisthesis. Through this approach, the transverse process may be removed, and the pedicle and vertebral body may be exposed in a limited fashion, as described later in this section. Wiltsie and colleagues[53] described a similar approach, dividing the erector spinae muscles using a muscle-splitting dissection. They note that with this approach there is less muscle mass to retract medially, that the facets are more directly reached, and that operative hemorrhage may be less significant.

ANTERIOR AND ANTEROLATERAL APPROACHES

Anterolateral Approach to the Bodies of the Lumbar Vertebrae

The anterolateral approach to the lumbar vertebrae is an extension of the standard flank incision used by general surgeons for years for lumbar sympathectomy.[34, 41, 42] The transverse flank approach to the sympathetics provides limited access to the bodies of the lower three lumbar vertebrae. By extending this exposure through a long oblique incision from the twelfth rib posteriorly to the lower abdomen in front, broad access to all the lumbar vertebrae in continuity and particularly the upper lumbar levels is gained.[15, 33] The lateral half of the twelfth rib is resected subperiosteally, and the anterior abdominal muscles are divided. The major dissection is behind the kidney in the potential space between the renal or Gerota's fascia and the quadratus lumborum and psoas muscles. A chest retractor is used, which provides direct exposure of most lumbar vertebral bodies and allows sufficient room for extensive excision and bone grafting.

This approach to the lumbar spine is useful for drainage of a psoas abscess on the operated side. It provides exposure for complete débridement and reconstructive bone grafting over the upper four lumbar vertebral bodies and should be considered when extensive resection or grafting at these levels is planned. By

dividing the insertion of the arcuate ligaments on the first lumbar transverse process (see Fig. 49–82), limited access as high as the eleventh thoracic vertebral body may be gained. The working area within the thorax is restricted, however, and if extensive resection or grafting is planned over the eleventh thoracic vertebral body, we recommend considering the thoracoabdominal approach. To provide access to the lower lumbar vertebral bodies and sacrum, alternative anterior exposures are available, which are discussed later.

The authors recommend the left lateral approach if all other considerations are equal and if the pathologic condition is not asymmetric. The liver, on the right side, is large and difficult to retract. The vena cava, also on the right, is a capricious structure that, in the presence of infection, may be hard to locate. In addition, the vena cava is injured easily, and bleeding from it may be hard to control. The spleen, on the left, is fragile but smaller than the liver and is more easily retracted. The aorta, owing to its pulsations, is easier to locate than the vena cava, is less susceptible to injury, and bleeding from it is easier to control.

Technique

The patient is placed on the operating table with the side to be operated upon tilted upward, at an angle of 60 degrees, by supporting the shoulder and hip on sandbags. This tends to shift the abdominal and retroperitoneal contents toward the nonoperated side and facilitates retraction. The arm on the operated side is held across the chest and supported.

The incision is begun over the lateral half of the twelfth rib and extends obliquely downward and ante-

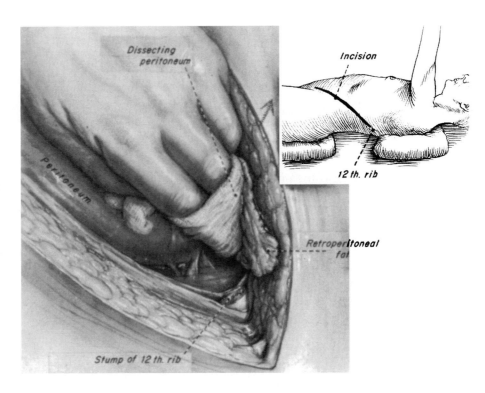

Figure 49–98. Anterolateral approach to the bodies of the lumbar vertebrae. The peritoneum is exposed through an oblique flank incision beginning over the twelfth rib. (From Southwick, W. O., and Robinson, R. A.: Surgical approaches to the vertebral bodies in the cervical and lumbar regions. J. Bone Joint Surg. *39A*:638, 1957.)

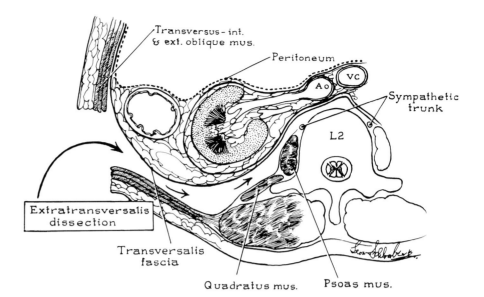

Figure 49–99. Transverse section through L2 illustrates the plane of dissection to the vertebral bodies posterior to the transversalis fascia and anterior to the quadratus and psoas muscles.

riorly to the lateral margin of the rectus fascia, at the level of the anterosuperior iliac spine (Fig. 49–98). The lateral and inferior fibers of the latissimus dorsi and serratus posterior inferior muscles lie over the medial aspect of the twelfth rib and may be partially transected. The distal half of the twelfth rib is resected subperiosteally, and the external oblique muscle is split in line with its fibers to the lower pole of the incision, at the lateral border of the rectus fascia. The internal oblique and transversus abdominis muscles are cut across their fibers in the same oblique line as the skin incision.

Deep to the transversus abdominis muscle is the peritoneum. Continuous with the peritoneum and extending posteriorly behind the kidney is the transversalis fascia (Fig. 49–99). This fascia surrounds the kidney, ureters, adrenals, and peritoneal fat and is loosely applied to the quadratus lumborum and psoas muscles posteriorly. This layer blends loosely with the psoas fascia and is attached to the vertebral column, anterior to the medial margin of the psoas. Dissection proceeds along the peritoneum and renal fascia posterior to the kidney. This is best accomplished by finger dissection, as there is a natural plane of cleavage immediately posterior to the fascia. A common mistake is to dissect within or posterior to the fat pad, which lies behind the renal fascia. This leads to a blind space posterior to the quadratus lumborum and psoas muscles. The anterior surfaces of the quadratus lumborum and psoas muscles are fully exposed (Fig. 49–100). A self-retaining chest retractor is used to open the wound longitudinally. A padded Deaver retractor is used to retract the kidney and peritoneal contents medially. Care should be taken not to tract hard on the aorta and vena cava, which lie immediately anterior to the vertebral bodies.

The lumbar veins and arteries effectively tether the aorta and vena cava to the vertebrae. In order to provide access to the anterior aspect of the vertebral bod-

ies, these should be isolated, ligated, or clipped with silver clips and cut at the level of the desired dissection.

All the lumbar vertebral bodies are easily palpated, and the anterolateral aspects of the third, fourth, and fifth vertebral bodies are easily seen. The left diaphragmatic crus extends to the second vertebral body, and if exposure at this level or above is desired, the left crus may be separated from the anterior longitudinal ligament. If exposures of the lower thoracic vertebrae in continuity are desired, the arcuate ligament insertions on the first lumbar transverse process may be divided (see Fig. 49–82), and the arcuate ligaments may be retracted upward, anteriorly. Working beneath the diaphragm and by blunt dissection, the posterior parietal pleura is elevated from the vertebral bodies and posterior ribs. Ordinarily, this may be done without violating the integrity of the parietal pleura or entering the pleural cavity. In this way, limited exposure as high as the eleventh thoracic vertebral body is possible. The working area from below is limited, however, and if extensive resection or grafting is planned within the thorax, we recommend considering the thoracoabdominal approach described later.

Two nerves are in close proximity with this level of the dissection and should be spared. The genitofemoral nerve is a small-caliber, white structure lying on the muscle belly of the psoas. The sympathetic chain is closely applied to the vertebral bodies medial to the psoas muscle. It may be distinguished by its yellow-white color and periodic ganglionic enlargements. The sympathetic chain and psoas may be displaced posteriorly by careful blunt dissection to reveal the lateral aspect of the vertebral bodies.

The bodies of the vertebrae, unless grossly diseased, are covered in front by the thick, anterior longitudinal ligament and small slips of the psoas muscle laterally. The intervertebral bodies between are relatively concave. The fifth lumbar vertebra is usually most promi-

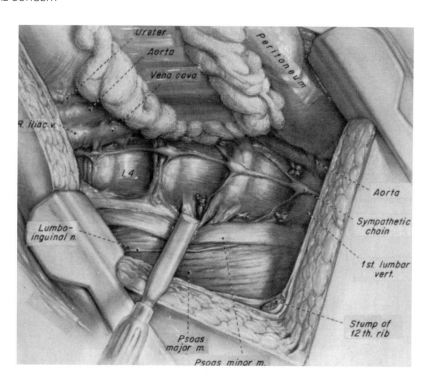

Figure 49–100. A chest retractor opens the wound longitudinally. The peritoneal contents are retracted medially, exposing the vertebral bodies. (From Southwick, W. O., and Robinson, R. A.: Surgical approaches to the vertebral bodies in the cervical and lumbar regions. J. Bone Joint Surg. *39A*:639, 1957. *Reproduced with permission.*)

nent, and using this as a reference point, the vertebral level may be accurately identified. Despite this, we strongly recommend obtaining a lateral roentgenogram of the spine on the operating table, with a radiopaque marker embedded at the desired level to verify anatomic position.

The anterior longitudinal ligament may be elevated from the midportion of the vertebral body at the desired level, and the vertebral body may be entered with drills, probes, or curets as the clinical situation dictates. This flap of ligament may be restored anatomically with sutures after a limited resection to provide continuity and stability.

Anterior Approach to the Lumbar Spine Through a Transverse Flank Incision

The anterolateral approach to the lumbar vertebral bodies just described is best suited to expose the upper and midlumbar vertebral bodies. A long, oblique incision is used, two abdominal wall muscle layers are divided across their fibers, and considerable dissection behind the renal fascia is needed. Such an extensive exposure may not be required for relatively direct biopsy or drainage procedures and may not be tolerated by the elderly or critically ill patient. In addition, in the presence of overt sepsis or when draining an abscess, there may be an advantage to limiting the dissection, using muscle-splitting techniques, rather than dividing muscle groups. The transverse flank approach used for lumbar sympathectomy may be ideally suited for this kind of limited exposure, particularly in the high-risk patient.

This approach has been used for years by general and vascular surgeons for lumbar sympathectomy.[34, 41, 42] It employs a muscle-splitting dissection and provides limited but direct access to the third and fourth lumbar vertebral bodies, as well as the sympathetic chain and psoas muscle on one side. The upper lumbar vertebrae and the lumbosacral junction can be reached by extending the dissection behind the renal or Gerota's fascia, but the working area is small and crowded. In addition to unilateral lumbar sympathectomy, it is ideally suited to drain a psoas abscess on one side, as the approach is direct and the dissection is limited, so there is less chance of spreading an infection. The muscle-splitting approach through the three layers of the abdominal wall tends to reduce the incidence of wound dehiscence or herniations, as the three layers tend to close on themselves.

An incision 12 to 15 cm in length is made over the lateral flank, midway between the iliac crest and the lower ribs. The first layer of the abdominal wall, the external oblique muscle, is divided in line with its fibers, obliquely downward and medially. The internal oblique fibers course at right angles to the external oblique fibers and are opened in a muscle-splitting fashion. The deepest layer, the transversus abdominis, is directed medially and laterally and is spread in line with its fibers. Retractors are placed in the wound, and the peritoneum is identified. By blunt dissection, the peritoneum and the renal fascia behind it are separated from the abdominal wall. The dissection proceeds below the kidney, behind the ureter, along the quadratus lumborum and psoas muscles to the vertebral bodies (see Fig. 49–99). The genitofemoral and sympathetic nerves should be identified, and the vertebral bodies should be exposed as described in the preceding section. The third and fourth lumbar vertebral bodies are directly accessible within the base of the wound. The upper lumbar vertebrae and lumbosacral junction can be reached but are relatively distant, and the working area is confined.

Anterior Approach to the Lower Lumbar and Lumbosacral Spine Through an Anterior Oblique Incision

This approach is identical to the anterolateral exposure described first; however, the incision is directed more anteriorly and inferiorly over the lower lumbar elements.[21] The incision begins in the lower abdomen lateral to the rectus muscle and extends laterally and superiorly above the iliac crest to the midflank. The external oblique muscle is divided in line with its fibers, and the internal oblique and transversus abdominis muscles are divided across their fibers in line with the incision. Dissection proceeds posterior to the renal fascia, below the kidney and behind the ureter, to the vertebral bodies, as described before.

Through this route, broad exposure of the lower lumbar vertebrae and upper sacrum is obtained. This is suitable for extensive resection and bone grafting as well as anterior lumbosacral fusion. The aorta, iliac vessels, and hypogastric nerve plexus lie anterior to the vertebral bodies and are not in direct line with the dissection. These may be elevated in a block away from the anterior vertebral bodies with less likelihood of disturbing genitourinary function (see "Urogenital Complications").

Anterior Approach to the Lumbosacral Spine Through a Paramedian Incision Around the Rectus Muscle

The paramedian approach provides direct access to the anterior elements of the lumbosacral spine in continuity with the upper lumbar segments. Once the initial exposure is made through the anterior abdominal wall, the vertebrae may be reached through a transperitoneal or retroperitoneal route. The advantage to the transperitoneal route is that somewhat more extensive exposure is provided, and the abdominal viscera may be packed neatly away from the spine. The disadvantage is that one approaches the spine directly from the front, and one has to mobilize the great vessels and hypogastric nerve plexus before the spine can be reached. This introduces potential urogenital complications, particularly in the male. These may be avoided by careful dissection about the aortic bifurcation, described later, or by approaching the spine from the side, behind these structures.

A paramedian incision is made over the lower abdomen, extending from the umbilicus to the pubis. The rectus fascia beneath is identified and opened longitudinally in line with the incision. The rectus muscle is mobilized laterally, taking care to isolate and ligate these segmental vessels, which reach it from behind. The rectus abdominis muscle is retracted medially, and

the posterior rectus fascia is opened longitudinally. On closing the wound, this provides a two-layer fascial closure with an intervening muscle layer between. At this stage, the peritoneum may be opened, or dissection may proceed around it laterally, depending upon the surgeon's needs.

Transperitoneal

In the transperitoneal approach, the peritoneum is opened longitudinally in line with the skin incision, protecting the bowel beneath from injury. The intra-abdominal contents are packed away from the incision to expose the posterior peritoneal layer, draped over the great vessels and vertebral bodies.

The superior hypogastric plexus provides the sympathetic innervation of the urogenital system. It is a direct extension of the thoracolumbar sympathetic chain (Fig. 49–101), which ramifies about the inferior mesenteric artery at the level of the third and fourth lumbar vertebrae. Caudal to this, these fibers ramify as a fine and extensive network that lies primarily anterior to the aorta on the left side. These extend across the left iliac vessels, the fifth lumbar vertebral body, and the lumbosacral junction and will be injured unless special precautions are taken in the dissection. To avoid this sympathetic, superior hypogastric plexus, Duncan and Jonck[13] recommend an approach through this plane eccentric to the right side to avoid the majority of these hypogastric fibers.

A longitudinal incision is made in the posterior peritoneum in the midline about the aortic bifurcation. This peritoneal incision is extended distally and to the right, along the right common iliac artery to its bifurcation at the external and internal iliac arteries. At this point, the right ureter should be identified, crossing the right external iliac artery, and the incision should be curved medially to avoid this structure. The dissection proceeds at the lower pole of the posterior peritoneal incision, directly posteriorly, through the prevertebral tissues to the right and lateral side of the sacrum. This is extended superiorly to the lateral edge of the fifth lumbar vertebra by spreading the tissues longitudinally away from this plane. Dissection continues on to the anterior longitudinal ligament of the spine. By continued blunt dissection along the spine, the iliac vessels and aorta may be mobilized from the vertebrae. In this way, the left side of the peritoneum and all the structures subjacent to it (including the prevertebral tissues, vessels, and hypogastric plexus) may be mobilized as a block away from the vertebrae, anteriorly and to the left. By displacing these structures from the side and en bloc and not dissecting through them, there is less risk of injuring the hypogastric nerve fibers, particularly those on the left side, which are responsible for normal urogenital function.

The middle sacral artery may be adherent to the vertebral bodies, and some difficulties may be encountered in mobilizing it. Vascular clips may be used to ligate this artery while sparing the hypogastric plexus. If cautery is to be used in this area, we recommend the

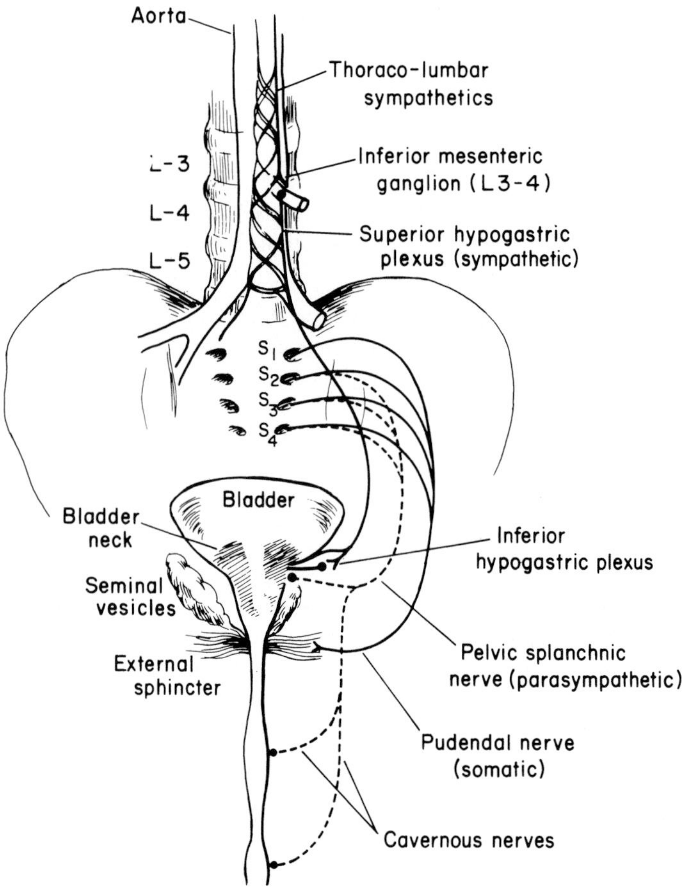

Figure 49–101. Innervation of the urogenital system. Sympathetic via the superior hypogastric plexus, parasympathetic via the pelvic splanchnic nerve, and somatic via the pudendal nerve. (From Johnson, R. M., and McGuire, E. J.: Urogenital complications of anterior approaches to the lumbar spine. Clin. Orthop. *154*:114–118, 1981.)

bipolar rather than the unipolar machine, as the spark gap or area of thermal injury is confined to the space between the bipolar cautery forceps tips, and there is less likelihood of injuring these nerves with a propagated current or thermal burn.

Retroperitoneal

As mentioned previously, once the exposure through the anterior abdominal wall is complete, the spine may be approached using a retroperitoneal plane of dissection. This should proceed laterally, and we prefer dissection to the left side, posteriorly along the renal fascial plane behind the ureter. The hypogastric nerve plexus lies anterior to the great vessels. This and the vessels may be mobilized from the side and behind, en bloc, sparing the ramifying fibers of the hypogastric plexus over the spine. The retroperitoneal dissection provides a less direct route to the spine, but if the tissue planes are well developed by blunt dissection and if the abdominal contents are packed away, satisfactory exposure is obtained with less risk to the viscera and hypogastric nerve plexus.

Anterior Lumbosacral Fusion

Anterior fusion at the lumbosacral junction is useful in certain specific conditions, such as in myelodysplasia,

when the posterior elements are deficient, or when the posterior elements have been extensively removed to decompress a stenotic spinal canal. Some authors have found the anterior route useful for the treatment of spondylolisthesis[6, 23, 38, 43, 45] and to reduce and stabilize severe spondylolisthetic displacements.[4] A number have used this route for intervertebral disc excision and interbody fusion, either as a primary treatment modality or as a salvage procedure after failure of previous posterior approaches.[17–19, 22, 30, 43, 46]

The authors have found that anterior lumbosacral fusion is rarely required. The posterolateral fusion technique described by Watkins,[49, 50] in which cancellous bone grafts are laid over the facets and transverse processes, is so effective, if done properly, that the anterior route is rarely needed. Furthermore, there is no evidence available that anterior lumbosacral fusions are more reliable or that they have a higher incidence of fusion or better overall clinical results. In fact, Stauffer and Coventry,[46, 47] in their articles contrasting their experience with anterior and posterolateral fusions, found that anterior fusions had a lower incidence of stable fusion and a less satisfactory clinical outcome. Despite this, a few circumstances remain in which anterior lumbosacral fusion is needed. Instability with associated deficiency or absence of the posterior elements, or pathologic conditions of the vertebral bodies anteriorly requiring resection and grafting, are best served using anterior approaches. In addition, infection or extensive scarring posteriorly may make posterior or posterolateral approaches impractical.

Technique

The fusion techniques at the lumbosacral junction are similar to those used elsewhere in the spine and vary from simple disc excision and interbody fusion to an extensive resection and replacement grafting. The only modification is that because of the size of the vertebrae and forces across these, larger or duplicate grafts are usually required with cortical margins around their periphery. The intervertebral lumbosacral disc is excised using rongeurs and curets. We favor leaving the vertebral end plates intact to support the graft and to prevent subsequent collapse of the disc space, which could occur if the softer cancellous portion of the body is entered. Two or more horseshoe-shaped plugs of bone are obtained from the iliac crest, which have their cortical margins intact on three sides (as described for anterior cervical interbody fusion). These should be thick enough to completely fill the defect and should be under a significant compressive force, holding the graft in place. The disc space is distracted with an intervertebral spreader, and the first graft is tamped in place. The second graft is turned around 180 degrees from the orientation of the first and is tamped in place. Additional graft material is added to fill the defect, and control roentgenograms are obtained to be certain that the grafts are not displaced posteriorly into the spinal canal. The grafts are tested for stability, and if they are satisfactory, the soft tissues are repaired about the vertebrae. Postoperatively, when the patient's condition is fully stabilized, we prefer to protect the spine and limit lumbosacral motion using a body cast until the fusion is established roentgenographically. Thereafter, we use a Norton-Brown lumbosacral brace for an additional three to six months. We prefer the Norton-Brown brace,[40] as this appears to control lumbosacral motion best of any of the conventional and readily available orthoses and is well tolerated by most patients.

In some circumstances, more extensive resection and grafting are required. Longer struts of cortical or corticocancellous graft material may be used. We recommend supporting these on the vertebral body end plates to limit collapse of vertebral height. These struts should be locked into slots previously made in the vertebrae, above and below the levels of intended fusion, to prevent displacement of the grafts. The grafts may be driven in from the lateral side of the vertebral body.

If extensive resection and bone grafts are required over the lumbosacral spine, special care is required to protect the spine in the postoperative period until osseous fusion is established to prevent collapse of the vertebrae and loss of longitudinal height. These patients may be nursed on a turning frame, or the spine may be protected with plaster of Paris turning shells.

Most often when the wounds have healed, a plaster of Paris body cast is required. Occasionally, supplementary stabilization using Harrington or Knodt rods and hooks or a sacral bar may be required to protect the lumbosacral vertebrae from the large forces and torque across them.

Complications

Perforation of the vena cava or iliac veins may produce dangerous hemorrhage that is difficult to control. Openings into the peritoneal cavity should be avoided, especially in the presence of infection. Irritation of the crus of the diaphragm was considered the cause of prolonged hiccups in one patient. Postoperative ileus is relatively common, but none has been severe or prolonged.

Because one or more major anterior abdominal wall muscles are divided, wound dehiscence or herniation is a potential problem. For this reason, when drainage of an abscess of the lower vertebral bodies is anticipated, the muscle-splitting sympathectomy approach, leaving the peritoneum intact, should be considered.

Two rare but potential complications of anterior approaches to the thoracolumbar and lumbosacral spine have been reported. These are (1) the anterior spinal artery ischemic syndrome following extensive dissections about the thoracolumbar spine or scoliosis correction, and (2) the urogenital complications, particularly sterility in males, which may follow anterior exposures of the lumbosacral spine. Some controversy remains as to whether these complications do occur, how they are produced, and how they may be avoided. Because of this, both of these potential complications are discussed in greater detail, and the information currently available in the literature is summarized.

Anterior Spinal Artery Ischemic Syndrome

Anterior spinal artery ischemic syndromes with paraplegia, loss of pain and temperature sense, and sphincter disturbance have been reported, particularly following resection and grafting of the aorta. This syndrome has been reported to occur with a frequency as high as 4 per cent when the aorta is cross-clamped proximal to the renal vessels.[28] It has also been reported occasionally following spinal surgery for scoliosis correction[11, 28] or circumferential spinal osteotomy.[12] However, no complications have been reported by a number of authors following unilateral ligation of multiple segmental vessels over the lower thoracic spine.[7–9, 20, 55]

The blood supply of the spinal column is derived from segmental vessels at most levels of the spine. These supply two general networks: an outer network, which feeds the bony elements of the vertebrae, the paraspinal muscles, and the extradural space, and an inner network, which nourishes the spinal cord itself.

The segmental arteries of the thoracic and lumbar spine hug the vertebral bodies, giving off a main dorsal branch as they approach the neural foramina. This main dorsal branch continues posteriorly beneath the transverse process and supplies the bone of the posterior elements and paraspinal muscles. Shortly after its origin, the dorsal branch gives off one or more intraspinal branches, which enter the spinal canal through the neural foramina and feed the nerve roots, vertebral bodies, and dura. This outer network is fed by segmental vessels at most levels of the spine and has extensive anastomotic communications within itself and with the extraspinal system.[16, 52]

At certain segmental levels, separate branches that feed the anterior two thirds of the spinal cord arise from the dorsal segmental artery. These are known as the anterior segmental medullary arteries. These most commonly occur over the upper and lower cervical levels, the upper thoracic spine, and one at the lower thoracic or upper lumbar level. The latter is known as the great anterior medullary artery and is one of the larger and better-known segmental feeders. The anterior medullary arteries normally join the anterior median spinal artery directly without branching. The anterior median spinal artery usually occurs as a single channel that meanders along the anterior median fissure of the spinal cord. This varies considerably in size along its course but becomes narrowest over the midthoracic spine and only widens after it is joined by the great anterior medullary artery around the thoracolumbar level. The anterior median spinal artery gives off numerous central perforating arteries, which supply the anterior two thirds of the spinal cord. Although there are extensive anastomotic communications in the outer network and about the cord, the arterioles and capillaries within the spinal cord appear to function as end arteries with few significant collateral channels.[16] This leaves the spinal cord, particularly its anterior two thirds, vulnerable to ischemia.

The posterior third of the spinal cord is supplied by two posterior spinal arteries and appears to be less vulnerable to vascular ischemia. In part, this is because of the rather extensive anastomoses between the posterior spinal arteries and a well-developed arterial plexus posteriorly. In addition, the posterior segmental medullary feeders are relatively large and numerous (10 to 20 per spine).[11]

The source of the great anterior medullary artery is variously described by different authors,[11, 16, 28, 31, 32] but there is a consensus that it most frequently arises on the left side over the lower thoracic or upper lumbar spine. Occasionally, the great anterior medullary artery originates on the right side, and less frequently no single dominant feeder is present and a number of smaller vessels are found. When present, the great anterior medullary artery enters the spinal canal through the neural foramen and courses proximally along the nerve root. It then divides into a small ascending branch and turns at an acute angle to descend as the anterior median spinal artery, which suddenly enlarges. When the great anterior medullary artery is present, it supplies a significant volume of blood to the anterior two thirds of the lower spinal cord.

There is evidence that the functional integrity of the lower spinal cord is not solely dependent upon the great anterior medullary artery. No complications have been reported by several authors following unilateral resection of multiple segmental vessels in the lower thoracic spine.[7–9, 20, 55] DiChiro and colleagues[10] ligated the great anterior medullary artery in a number of rhesus monkeys without complication, but when the anterior spinal artery was ligated distal to this, paraplegia occurred. This suggests that the anterior median spinal artery and its collaterals are more important than any single feeder, including the great anterior medullary artery.

Lazorthes and others[32] found extensive anastomotic pathways within the segmental arterial system, such as through the dorsal muscular branches and through the nutrient arteries within the vertebral bodies. This would provide collateral pathways from one side to the other or from above or below when an artery at one level was ligated. They concluded that the closer to the aorta and the further from the spinal cord an artery was interrupted, the greater the possibility of collateral flow through these anastomoses. This prompted Burrington and others[7] to recommend that the segmental artery be ligated close to the aorta to protect this collateral circulation to the cord.

The one factor that appears instrumental in jeopardizing the blood supply to the lower thoracic spinal cord is interruption or compromise of the anterior median spinal artery. This could be interrupted by ligating the great anterior medullary artery as well as a number of smaller medullary feeders, but collateral pathways could maintain the circulation to the cord. Aggressive correction of scoliotic or kyphotic deformities could stretch and narrow the anterior spinal artery and compromise it, even though none of the segmental medullary arteries were injured. This would account for the reports of anterior spinal artery syndromes occurring after scoliosis correction,[11, 28] even when no major segmental arteries were ligated.

It would seem that the most hazardous manipulation of the circulation to the lower spinal cord includes a combination of ligating the medullary feeders and stretching the spinal artery by aggressive correction of spinal deformity. Therefore, in anterior approaches to the lower thoracic and upper lumbar spine, it seems prudent to ligate as few intercostal or segmental arteries as possible, to restrict ligation to one side only, and to ligate these arteries as close to the aorta as possible. If bilateral ligation is absolutely necessary, particularly at multiple levels, correction of spinal deformity should be minimized. On the other hand, if correction of deformity is primarily required, the segmental arteries should be spared, and the surgeon should be prepared to reduce this correction if there is evidence of spinal ischemia in the early postoperative period.

Urogenital Complications and Sterility in Males Following Anterior Exposures of the Lumbosacral Spine

Sexual impotence or sterility has been reported following anterior surgical approaches to the lumbosacral spine in males.[13, 17, 43, 46] These reports are rare, and there is uncertainty as to whether the problem seen is a physiologic failure of normal penile erection, a failure of normal ejaculation, or a psychologically based problem.

The anatomic nerve supply to the urogenital system has been known for many years, but the function of these nerve systems remains controversial. Most of our current knowledge about the neurophysiology of the urogenital system is derived from clinical studies of patients with specific nerve damage following spinal cord and cauda equina injuries or following surgical dissections about the pelvis and lower lumbar spine.[26, 35, 37] These have been reinforced by a number of neurophysiologic laboratory studies using animal models.[1, 3, 48]

The urogenital system is innervated by three basic nerve complexes—the sympathetic, parasympathetic, and somatic—through the pudendal nerve. Sexual function is directly influenced by these systems. In the normal male, sperm are continuously created in the testes and are passed on to the epididymis, where the sperm flagella become mobile and are then referred to as spermatozoa. These spermatozoa are carried along the vas deferens via peristaltic action to the seminal vesicles, where they are stored and where certain essential nutrients are added, such as fructose. With ejaculation, the smooth muscle of the seminal vesicles contracts, delivering a bolus of sperm into the prostatic urethra. At the same time, the bladder neck closes by reflex, directing the spermatozoa out the tip of the penis.[26]

Sympathetic. The sympathetic nerve supply to the urogenital system is a direct continuation of the thoracolumbar sympathetic nerves,[13, 14, 29] coursing along the anterolateral aspects of the lumbar vertebral bodies (see Fig. 49–101). At the level of the third and fourth lumbar vertebrae, these ramify about the inferior mesenteric artery at the inferior mesenteric ganglion. Almost 80 per cent of these ramifications occur on the left side of the aorta; the remainder are found centrally or to the right. Once ramified, these fibers are referred to as the superior hypogastric plexus as they course distally. Most commonly, the superior hypogastric fibers are found within the retroperitoneal space lying along the left side of the aorta. These cross the left common iliac artery and vein and below this are closely applied to the fifth lumbar vertebral body and lumbosacral disc space within the prevertebral tissues. At the level of the pelvic brim, the plexus normally separates into two complexes, one on the right, the other on the left, each extending distally to reach the bladder, vas deferens, and seminal vesicles.

The sympathetic nervous system, through the superior hypogastric plexus, appears to have a direct effect upon normal ejaculation. The sympathetic nerves control the transfer of spermatozoa from the epididymis to the seminal vesicles by affecting the motility of the vas deferens. They appear to affect seminal function by controlling the storage of sperm and secretion of seminal fluid. With ejaculation, they control the emission of spermatozoa and properly direct the delivery

of sperm by closing the bladder neck, where a specialized area rich in alpha receptors is found.[26]

Parasympathetic. The parasympathetic innervation of the urogenital system is derived from the second, third, and fourth sacral segments.[5] These leave the anterior foramina of the sacrum (see Fig. 49–101) well below the pelvic brim and course along the side of the rectum as the pelvic splanchnic nerve.[54] These fibers ramify at the inferior hypogastric plexus and extend to the prostate, posterior bladder, and base of the penis as the cavernous nerves.

The parasympathetic system, through the pelvic splanchnic nerves, appears to influence penile erection by regulating the venous plexus at the base of the penis. In addition, with voiding, these nerves contract the bladder and open the urethra through an intrinsic reflux.

Somatic. The somatic innervation of the urogenital system is through the pudendal nerves (see Fig. 49–101). These are derived from the first, second, third, and fourth sacral segments below the pelvic brim and provide both motor and sensory innervation of the pelvic floor and external genitalia. The pudendal nerves control the external urethral sphincter and the muscles of the pelvic floor. With ejaculation, the muscles of the pelvic floor contract, providing the force to emit a bolus of spermatozoa under pressure. In addition, the pudendal nerves provide sensation over the urethra and penis.

Complications. In anterior exposures of the lower lumbar spine, it appears that the only nerve complex to the urogenital system that is normally at risk is the sympathetic (superior hypogastric plexus). Only if the dissection is carried well below the pelvic brim could the parasympathetic (pelvic splanchnic nerve) or the pudendal nerve be injured. Therefore, if the surgical dissection is restricted to the lumbar spine above the pelvic brim, one should see only impairment of sympathetically mediated urogenital function.

Theoretically, if the superior hypogastric plexus is completely divided at the pelvic brim, a normal male could develop sterility, through the loss of normal spermatozoal transport from the testicles and retrograde ejaculation into the bladder. Sterility would occur because of the loss of normal spermatozoal transport along the vas deferens to the seminal vesicles and failure of the seminal vesicles to store spermatozoa or secrete seminal fluid. Dry or retrograde ejaculation would occur because the seminal vesicles would fail to contract, and any spermatozoa delivered to the prostatic urethra would be misdirected in a retrograde manner to the bladder, as the bladder neck would not close as part of its normal reflex.

Following dissections about the pelvic brim, dry or retrograde ejaculation is more likely to occur than sterility, as the control of muscle contraction at the bladder neck and seminal vesicles appears to be more sensitive to denervation.[25] Furthermore, retrograde ejaculation is most difficult to correct, whereas sterility caused by the loss of normal spermatozoal transport along the vas deferens or storage within the seminal vesicles may be reversed by certain alpha-adrenergic agents.[27, 36]

In general, one would not expect failure of penile erection or impotence to follow sympathectomy at any level in normal males. On the contrary, there is evidence that suggests that the normal, young male may be afflicted with prolonged penile erection or priapism as the normal sympathetic control of the arteriovenous sphincter complex at the penis would be lost, leaving the parasympathetic control of venous egress unopposed.[2] Although this is true in young and otherwise healthy males, in older males with advanced peripheral vascular disease, erectile impotence has been reported following extensive lumbar sympathectomy.[51]

In women there is a possibility that sympathectomy would affect normal bladder control, resulting in inappropriate urine leakage owing to the loss of the normal smooth muscle control at the internal urethral sphincter. Clinically, this is more likely to occur in patients subjected to radical pelvic surgery, in which a more complete sympathetic neural transection could occur than with surgery at the pelvic brim. Females do not have a genital sphincter, so the influence of sympathectomy on genital function is less striking.

Surgical Approach. Because the superior hypogastric plexus is situated directly anterior to the fifth lumbar vertebral body and lumbosacral disc space, it lies in jeopardy in midline exposures to the lumbosacral spine from the front. To avoid injuring this plexus, the vertebral bodies may be exposed from the side using a retroperitoneal dissection or by careful dissection from the right side as described earlier.[13]

POSTEROLATERAL APPROACH TO THE LUMBAR SPINE

Posterolateral Approach to the Lumbar Vertebral Bodies

The posterolateral approach to the lumbar vertebrae was developed as a means of providing direct access through the transverse processes to the pedicles and vertebral bodies with less extensive surgical dissection and operative risk than the anterior approaches require.[44] It is an extension of the costotransversectomy approach to the thoracic vertebrae described in the preceding section and in the Watkins[49, 50] posterolateral approach to the lumbosacral spine. The posterolateral approach provides limited exposure of the lumbar vertebral bodies and is suitable for open surgical biopsy or drainage of small lesions. It is ideally suited for high-risk surgical candidates who could not tolerate more extensive procedures.

The direct posterior approach to the lumbar vertebrae through a midline incision provides direct access to the posterior elements but is limited in exposing the pedicles or vertebral bodies. The vertebral bodies may be approached around the posterior elements, but this requires retraction of the erector spinae muscles laterally, which may be difficult in obese or muscular individuals. Laminectomy provides access to the posterior vertebral body and disc through a confined working area. It does not permit thorough inspection or curettage, particularly of the anterior and lateral aspects of the vertebral bodies. In addition, there is always the risk of injuring the dura, inducing hemorrhage from the epidural vessels, or spreading infection from the anterior elements into the spinal canal.

Open biopsy has been demonstrated to improve the accuracy of diagnosis in obscure lesions of the spine.[24, 39] The direct surgical approach may be safer than needle biopsy even under fluoroscopic control and provides more material for culture and pathologic examination. In addition, open biopsy may provide an opportunity to remove a small tumor or focus of infection and maintain drainage. The posterolateral approach provides limited access to the vertebral bodies and is primarily useful for biopsy, curettage, and débridement of small lesions. The anterior approach provides more direct access to the anterior vertebral bodies and may be required for more extensive resection and grafting.

Technique

General endotracheal anesthesia is recommended for this procedure. The patient is placed on the operating table in a lateral decubitus position with an axillary pad in the dependent axilla or in the prone position with chest rolls on either side of the thorax to protect ventilation. A roentgenogram cassette holder should be placed beneath the patient so that localizing roentgenograms may be made during surgery in the anteroposterior and lateral planes. A control roentgenogram is obtained with a radiopaque skin marker at the proposed level to verify position and standardize radiographic technique.

A 4- to 6-inch longitudinal incision is made at the lateral border of the erector spinae muscles centered over the vertebral level to be biopsied (Fig. 49–102, inset). The incision is extended through the lumbar fascia, and the erector spinae muscles are identified. The lateral border of the erector spinae is found, and dissection proceeds between these muscles and the anterior layer of the lumbar fascia to the transverse processes of the vertebrae (Figs. 49–102 and 49–103). The paraspinal muscles are retracted medially, the transverse process at the desired level is tagged with a radiopaque marker, and roentgenograms are made to confirm the vertebral level. The transverse process is divided with an osteotome and is retracted laterally with its musculotendinous attachments. The vertebral pedicle is palpated, and the lumbar nerves are identified and protected as they leave their foramina above and below the pedicle (Fig. 49–104). The psoas muscle is carefully separated from the vertebra using a periosteal elevator. The lumbar vessels lie on the waist or midportion of the vertebral body posterior to the psoas

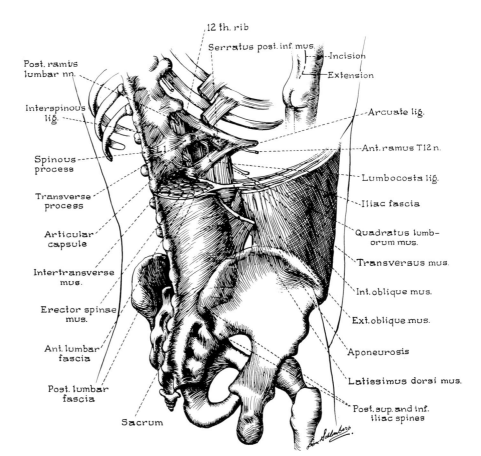

Figure 49–102. *Inset,* Longitudinal skin incision over the lateral border of the erector spinae muscles. Anatomy of the lumbosacral spine and paraspinal muscles viewed from the side and posteriorly.

12 th. rib
Serratus post. inf. mus.
Incision
Extension
Arcuate lig.
Ant. ramus T12 n.
Lumbocosta lig.
Iliac fascia
Quadratus lumborum mus.
Transversus mus.
Int. oblique mus.
Ext. oblique mus.
Aponeurosis
Latissimus dorsi mus.
Post. sup. and inf. iliac spines

Post. ramus lumbar nn.
Interspinous lig.
Spinous process
Transverse process
Articular capsule
Intertransverse mus.
Erector spinae mus.
Ant. lumbar fascia
Post. lumbar fascia
Sacrum

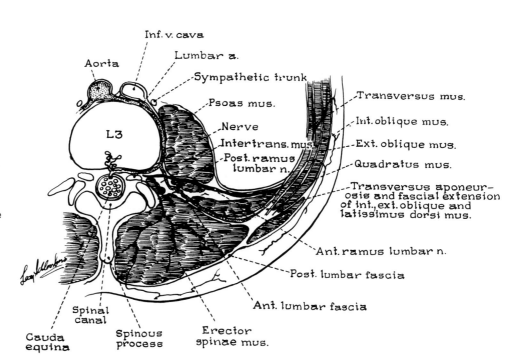

Figure 49–103. Cross section of the lumbar spine and paraspinal structures at the level of the third lumbar vertebra. Compare with Figure 49–97.

Inf. v. cava
Aorta
Lumbar a.
Sympathetic trunk
Psoas mus.
Nerve
Intertrans. mus.
Post. ramus lumbar n.
Transversus mus.
Int. oblique mus.
Ext. oblique mus.
Quadratus mus.
Transversus aponeurosis and fascial extension of int., ext. oblique and latissimus dorsi mus.
Ant. ramus lumbar n.
Post. lumbar fascia
Ant. lumbar fascia
L3
Cauda equina
Spinal canal
Spinous process
Erector spinae mus.

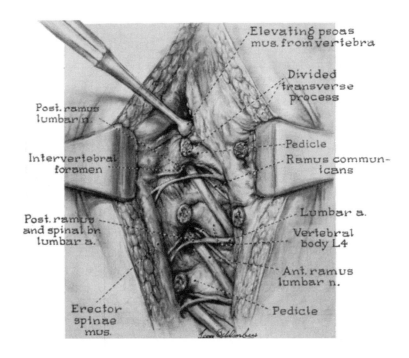

Figure 49–104. Lumbar vertebrae as viewed from the posterolateral approach. The transverse processes have been divided at their junctions with the pedicles and retracted laterally. The dissection proceeds directly anterior to the stump of the transverse process, along the pedicle, to the vertebral body in front. Note the lumbar segmental vessels draped over the waist or midportion of the vertebral bodies. By dissecting directly anterior to the pedicles, one can avoid these vessels as well as the lumbar nerves leaving the neural foramina below the pedicles.

muscle and should be separated from the body during this portion of the dissection. They may be clamped and cauterized if necessary. An opening may be made in the lateral aspect of the vertebral body anterior to the pedicle, using a curet or drill (Fig. 49–105). The lesion may be identified grossly at this time but should be verified radiographically with a curet placed within the lesion.

Through this approach, specimens may be obtained from the lateral, central, or anterior aspect of the vertebral body or pedicle. The lesion may be cureted, and small chips of cancellous bone graft may be installed to stimulate osteogenesis within a sterile defect. The wound is copiously irrigated with saline and inspected for hemorrhage. The margins are allowed to fall together, and the lumbar fascia is closed with interrupted

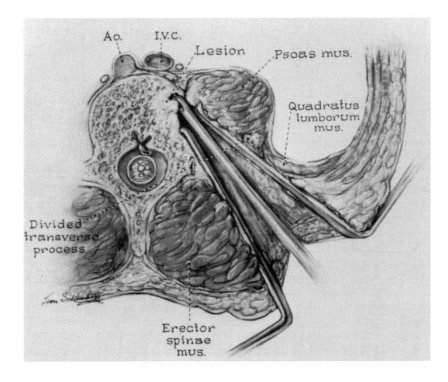

Figure 49–105. Posterolateral approach to the lumbar vertebrae, lateral to the erector spinae muscle mass and behind the psoas. The transverse process is divided and retracted laterally with its musculotendinous insertions to gain access to the lateral aspect of the vertebral body.

sutures. The skin is repaired, and the patient is nursed with some form of external spinal support, depending upon the postoperative stability of the spine.

If wider exposure is required, two transverse processes may be divided, and the intervening nerve root may be retracted. If the lower lumbar vertebrae are to be approached, the distal end of the skin incision should be curved medially over the posterior crest of the ilium to the sacrum. The iliac attachment of the sacrospinalis may be released by dividing the superior aspect of the posterior ilium with an osteotome, separating the remaining attachments with a periosteal elevator. In this fashion, the posterior sacrum may be exposed in continuity with the lumbar vertebrae, and the transverse process of the fifth lumbar vertebra may be more easily approached.

Complications

In our experience there have been few serious complications. Some of the most likely potential complications are injury to the lumbar nerves or vessels with ensuing troublesome hemorrhage. Dissection within the anterior aspect of the vertebral body is often performed under limited direct vision. Care is required to prevent injury to the inferior vena cava or aorta immediately anterior to the vertebral body. To ensure that the spinal lesion is accurately identified, control roentgenograms are required with a radiopaque marker within the lesion.

POSTERIOR APPROACH TO THE LUMBAR SPINE

The midline approach is the common laminectomy and spinal fusion approach described elsewhere. Essentially a midline incision is made between the spinous processes of the levels to be exposed, and the erector spinae muscles are dissected from the bony elements (spinous processes, interspinous ligaments, laminal joints, and transverse processes) as needed for the levels that must be visualized, using electrocautery or sharp dissection. Care should be taken not to injure the facet joint capsules in areas where motion will be expected following the operation.

With the advent of pedicle screw fixation for the lumbar vertebrae, there are now several additional anatomic relationships that are of importance at the level of the posterior bony elements.

The location of the pedicles is identified by anatomic landmarks and by radiography or image-intensification fluoroscopy in the operating room. For this type of surgery, special imagery with radiolucent table construction is essential.

In the lumbar region, the center of the pedicles is usually at the inferolateral edge of the facet joint, on an imaginary transverse line bisecting the transverse processes (Fig. 49–106). In the lumbar region from this point one may start a drill point, with a 20-degree medial inclination at L5, 10 degrees at L4, 5 degrees at L3 and L2, and no inclination at L1 (Fig. 49–107). One may follow the progress of the drill point by feeling inside the pedicle with a small curet and by checking

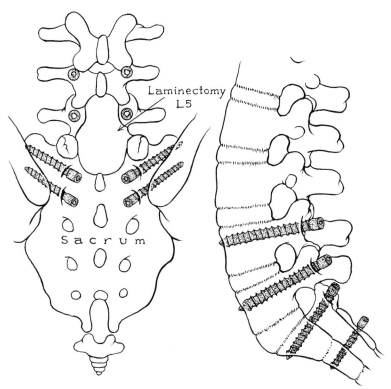

Figure 49–106. Anteroposterior and lateral positions for pedicle screws.

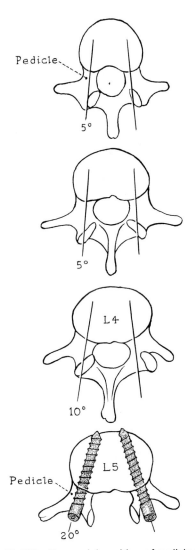

Figure 49–107. Transaxial position of pedicle screws.

with the image intensifier or by radiographs. In the lateral view, this drill should be parallel to the disc space.

In the sacrum, the pedicles or dense bone is somewhat more difficult to identify. At S1, the pedicle location is halfway between the lumbosacral facet and the posterior first sacral neuroforamen, medial from the neuroforamen about one third the distance of the neuroforamen to the midline (see Fig. 49–106). Sacral screws should be oriented at an angle of about 30 degrees from the angle of the lumbar screws as seen from a lateral radiograph and about 30 degrees away from the midline to reach into the lateral ala of the sacrum. Because all the pedicle screws have a potential danger of causing a neurovascular injury, it is very important that these techniques be learned from an experienced surgeon and not solely from books.

References

1. Albert, N. E., Sparks, F. C., and McGuire, E. J.: Effect of pelvic and retroperitoneal surgery on the urethral pressure profile and perineal floor electromyogram in dogs. Invest. Urol. *15*:140–142, 1977.
2. Appell, R. A., Shield, D. E., and McGuire, E. J.: Thioridazine induced priapism. Br. J. Urol. *49*:160, 1977.
3. Awad, S. A., and Downie, J. W.: The effect of adrenergic drugs and hypogastric nerve stimulation on the canine urethra. A radiologic and urethral pressure study. Invest. Urol. *13*:298, 1976.
4. Bradford, D. S.: Management of severe spondylolisthesis by the combined anterior and posterior approach. Presented at University of Miami symposium, Surgery of the Spine—Indications and Techniques, April 1979.
5. Bradley, W. E., Timm, G. W., and Scott, F. B.: Innervation of the detrusor muscle and urethra. Urol. Clin. North Am. *1*:3, 1974.
6. Burns, B. H.: An operation for spondylolisthesis. Lancet *1*:1233, 1933.
7. Burrington, J. O., Brown, C., Wayne, E. R., and Odom, J.: Anterior approach to the thoracolumbar spine—technical considerations. Arch. Surg. *111*:456–463, 1976.
8. Chou, S. N., and Seljeskog, E. L.: Alternative surgical approaches to the thoracic spine. Clin. Neurosurg. *20*:306–321, 1973.
9. Cook, W. A.: Trans-thoracic vertebral surgery. Ann. Thorac. Surg. *12*:54–68, 1971.
10. DiChiro, G., Fried, L. C., and Doppman, J. L.: Experimental spinal cord angiograph. Br. J. Radiol. *43*:19, 1970.
11. Dommisse, G. F.: The blood supply of the spinal cord. A critical vascular zone in spinal surgery. J. Bone Joint Surg. [Br.] *56*:225–235, 1974.
12. Dommisse, G. F., and Enslin, T. E.: Hodgson's circumferential osteotomy in the correction of spinal deformity. J. Bone Joint Surg. [Br.] *52*:778, 1970.
13. Duncan, H. J. M., and Jonck, L. M.: The presacral plexus in anterior fusion of the lumbar spine. Suid-Afrikaanse Tydskrif Vir Chirurgie *3*:93–96, 1965.
14. Elaut, L.: The surgical anatomy of the so called presacral nerve. Surg. Gynecol. Obstet. *53*:581–589, 1932.
15. Francioli, P.: Voies d'acces dans les sympathectomies lumbaire et lumbothoracique. Helv. Chir. Acta *18*:536–543, 1951.
16. Gillilan, L. A.: The arterial blood supply of the human spinal cord. J. Comp. Neurol. *110*:75–103, 1958.
17. Goldner, J. L., McCollum, D. E., and Urbaniak, J. R.: Anterior disc excision and interbody spine fusion for chronic low back pain. *In* American Academy of Orthopaedic Surgeons, Symposium on the Spine. St. Louis, C. V. Mosby Co., 1969, pp. 111–131.
18. Harmon, P. H.: The removal of lower lumbar intervertebral discs by the transabdominal extraperitoneal route. Permanente Found. Med. Bull. *6*:169, 1948.
19. Harmon, P. H.: Anterior excision and vertebral body fusion operation for intervertebral disc syndromes of the lower lumbar spine: Three to five year results in 244 cases. Clin. Orthop. *26*:107–127, 1963.
20. Hodgson, A. R., Stock, F. E., Fang, H. S. Y., and Ong, G. B.: Anterior spinal fusion: The operative approach and pathologic findings in 412 patients with Pott's disease of the spine. Br. J. Surg. *48*:172–178, 1960.
21. Hodgson, M. B., and Wong, S. K.: A description of a technic and evaluation of results in anterior spinal fusion for deranged intervertebral disc and spondylolisthesis. Clin. Orthop. *56*:133–162, 1968.
22. Humphries, A. W., Hawk, W. A., and Berndt, A. L.: Anterior interbody fusion of lumbar vertebrae: Surgical technique. Surg. Clin. North Am. *41*:1685–1700, 1961.
23. Jenkins, J. A.: Spondylolisthesis. Br. J. Surg. *24*:80–85, 1936.
24. Johnson, R. W., Jr., Hillman, J. W., and Southwick, W. O.: The importance of direct surgical attack upon lesions of the vertebral bodies, particularly in Pott's disease. J. Bone Joint Surg. [Am.] *35*:17–24, 1953.
25. Johnson, R. M., and McGuire, E. J.: Urogenital complications of anterior approaches to the lumbar spine. Clin. Orthop. *154*:114–118, 1981.
26. Kedia, K. R., Markland, C., and Fraley, E. E.: Sexual function following high retroperitoneal lymphadenectomy. J. Urol. *114*:237, 1975.
27. Kelly, M. E., and Needle, M. A.: Imipramine for aspermia after lymphadenectomy. Urology *13*:414, 1979.

28. Kiem, H. A., and Sadek, K. H.: Spinal angiography in scoliosis patients. J. Bone Joint Surg. [Am.] *53*:904–912, 1971.
29. LaBate, J. S.: The surgical anatomy of the superior hypogastric plexus—"presacral nerve." Surg. Gynecol. Obstet. *67*:199–211, 1938.
30. Lane, J. D., Jr., and Moore, E. S., Jr.: Transperitoneal approach to the intervertebral disc in the lumbar area. Ann. Surg. *127*:537–551, 1948.
31. Lazorthes, G., Bastide, G., and Chancholle, A.: Etude anatomique de l'artere du renflement lombaire. C. R. Ass. Anat. *120*:883–885, 1964.
32. Lazorthes, G., Gouaze, A., Zadeh, J. O., et al.: Arterial vascularization of the spinal cord: Recent studies of the anastomotic substitution pathways. J. Neurosurg. *35*:253–262, 1971.
33. Lilly, G. D., Smith, D. W., and Biggane, C. F.: An evaluation of "high" lumbar sympathectomy in arteriosclerotic circulatory insufficiency of the lower extremities. Surgery *35*:1–8, 1954.
34. Madden, J. L.: Atlas of Techniques in Surgery. 2nd ed. New York, Appleton-Century-Crofts, 1964, pp. 398–405.
35. McGuire, E. J.: Urodynamic observations after abdominoperineal resection and lumbar intervertebral disc herniation. Urology *6*:63, 1975.
36. McGuire, E. J.: Neurogenic male incontinence. Urol. Clin. North Am. *5*:335, 1978.
37. McGuire, E. J., Wagner, F. C., and Diddel, G.: Balanced bladder function in spinal cord injury. J. Urol. *118*:626, 1977.
38. Mercer, W.: Spondylolisthesis, with a description of a new method of operative treatment and notes on ten cases. Edin. Med. J. *43*:545–572, 1936.
39. Nagel, D. A., Albright, J. A., Keggi, K. J., and Southwick, W. O.: A closer look at spinal lesions. Open biopsy of vertebral lesions. JAMA *191*:975–978, 1965.
40. Norton, P. L., and Brown, T.: The immobilizing efficiency of back braces. J. Bone Joint Surg. [Am.] *39*:111–138, 1957.
41. Pearl, F. L.: Muscle splitting extraperitoneal lumbar ganglionectomy. Surg. Gynecol. Obstet. *65*:107–112, 1937.
42. Royle, N. D.: The treatment of spastic paralysis by sympathetic rami-section. Surg. Gynecol. Obstet. *39*:701–720, 1924.
43. Sacks, S.: Anterior interbody fusion of the lumbar spine. Indications and results in 200 cases. Clin. Orthop. *44*:163–170, 1966.
44. Southwick, W. O., and Robinson, R. A.: Surgical approaches to the vertebral bodies in the cervical and lumbar regions. J. Bone Joint Surg. [Am.] *39*:631–643, 1957.
45. Speed, K.: Spondylolisthesis: Treatment by anterior bone graft. Arch. Surg. *37*:175–189, 1938.
46. Stauffer, R. N., and Coventry, M. B.: Anterior interbody lumbar spine fusion, analysis of Mayo Clinic series. J. Bone Joint Surg. [Am.] *54*:756–768, 1972.
47. Stauffer, R. N., and Coventry, M. B.: Posterolateral lumbar-spine fusion. Analysis of Mayo Clinic series. J. Bone Joint Surg. [Am.] *54*:1195–1204, 1972.
48. Tulloch, A. G. S.: Sympathetic activity of internal urethral sphincter. Urology *5*:353, 1975.
49. Watkins, M. B.: Posterolateral fusion of the lumbar and lumbosacral spine. J. Bone Joint Surg. [Am.] *35*:1014–1018, 1953.
50. Watkins, M. B.: Posterolateral bone grafting for fusion of the lumbar and lumbosacral spine. J. Bone Joint Surg. [Am.] *41*:388–396, 1959.
51. Whitelaw, G. P., and Smithwick, R. H.: Some secondary effects of sympathectomy with particular reference to disturbance of sexual function. N. Engl. J. Med. *245*:121, 1951.
52. Wiley, A. M., and Trueta, J.: The vascular anatomy of the spine and its relationship to pyogenic vertebral osteomyelitis. J. Bone Joint Surg. [Br.] *41*:796–809, 1959.
53. Wiltsie, L. L., Bateman, J. G., Hutchinson, R. H., and Nelson, W. E.: Paraspinal sacrospinalis-splitting approach to the lumbar spine. J. Bone Joint Surg. [Am.] *50*:919–926, 1968.
54. Winkler, G.: Contribucion al estudio de la inervacion de las visceras pelvianas. Archivos Espanoles de Urologia *20*:295, 1967.
55. Winter, R. B., Moe, J. H., and Wang, J. F.: Congenital kyphosis, its natural history and treatment as observed in a study of 130 patients. J. Bone Joint Surg. [Am.] *55*:223–256, 1973.

C H A P T E R

Spinal Fusion

Principles of Bone Fusion

George F. Muschler, M.D.

Joseph M. Lane, M.D.

Spinal fusion may be defined as a bony union between two vertebrae spaces following surgical manipulation. Spinal fusion was first reported in 1911 for treatment of Pott's disease. The mechanical stability provided by fusion was intended to inhibit progressive deformity and the spread of the tuberculous infection.[1] Following early successes, fusion surgery was later used to treat a variety of spinal deformities and diseases, including scoliosis, kyphosis, fracture, dislocation, spondylolisthesis, and intervertebral disc disease.

Much has changed since the pioneering efforts of Albee[1] and Hibbs[2] in the early part of this century. Specialized techniques and surgical approaches have been developed for internal fixation and fusion of every part of the spine. Additionally, there have been significant advances in diagnostic techniques, intraoperative monitoring, and bone graft materials. These advances have allowed for the aggressive correction of many severe spinal deformities with relative safety and predictability. Furthermore, the biologic principles on which these procedures are based have become increasingly better understood and used.

All fusion surgery involves the surgical preparation of the site of intended fusion and some attempt to stimulate the formation of bone in a defined tissue volume. The stimulus for the bone healing response, commonly referred to as the "bone graft," may be autologous or homologous bone (also called allograft bone) or an increasing number of synthetic materials or bioactive substances. As the graft is incorporated, bone tissue is formed. Union is accomplished when the

newly synthesized bone matrix becomes mechanically contiguous with the local host bone and has mineralized and remodeled sufficiently to bear physiologic loads without injury. Failure of bone formation, matrix union, and remodeling results in pseudarthrosis, the incidence of which ranges from 5 to 34 per cent in large adult series[3-6] and is lower in idiopathic scoliosis procedures.

The fundamental requirements for a successful spinal fusion are adequate osteogenic, osteoinductive, and osteoconductive activity within the grafted volume; adequate local blood supply to support a bone healing response; and a local mechanical environment suitable for bone formation. The following is a discussion of these fundamental concepts and principles, as well as a review of contemporary and future bone grafting materials, as they pertain to spinal fusion. Each is examined in the context of the fusion site as it is prepared by the surgeon, the graft material, systemic factors, and local factors.

FUSION SITE

The bone growth between vertebrae in a spinal fusion, as in all bone healing, is a cellular process, and the fusion site itself is the primary source of viable cells. The other potential source of living cells is the graft material. However, in the case of autogenous bone grafts, few of the transplanted cells survive.[7-9] Consequently, preparation of the fusion site and handling of the tissue bed are of paramount importance for a successful arthrodesis. The components of the tissue bed that contribute most to the healing process are its blood supply, cells of the inflammatory response, and cells responsible for osteogenesis and subsequent re-modeling. Because the basic tissue elements of the graft bed are generally constant regardless of the area of the spine, the quality of the local tissue bed is determined by the surgeon to a large degree.

The quality of the blood supply at the fusion site is an important feature of bone healing. The surgeon should therefore attempt to minimize trauma to the host tissue bed and remove any avascular, nonviable, or heavily traumatized tissue. The local blood supply's role in any fusion attempt cannot be understated and is manyfold: (1) as a source of oxygen and nutrients to the healing tissue, as well as control of local pH; (2) as a vehicle for endocrine stimulation; (3) as a conduction pathway for the recruitment of inflammatory cells, which produce paracrine factors that may mediate the early proliferation of osteoblastic progenitor cells as well as reduce the potential for infection; (4) as a source of endothelial cells, which produce paracrine factors that may enhance osteoblastic differentiation;[10] and (5) as a potential source of osteoblastic progenitors in the form of the vascular pericyte.[11]

The effect of the postoperative hematoma on the success of a fusion attempt is uncertain. On the one hand, it has been suggested that spinal fusion wounds should not be drained, because the fibrin-rich local hematoma may provide an osteoconductive scaffold or matrix that may facilitate some of the initial phases of bone healing. Additionally, the trapped platelets in the hematoma release platelet-derived growth factor (PDGF), transforming growth factor beta (TGF-β), and other growth factors that play a critical role during the repair process (see later).[12] On the other hand, the presence of a hematoma may displace some of the vascular tissue surrounding the graft site away from the graft, slowing the vascularization of the graft site.

The inflammatory response in the wound site and the grafted bed represents a critical event in the healing process. This response involves the removal of necrotic tissue debris, lysis of the local fibrin clot, establishment and re-establishment of a vascular supply to the graft and host tissue, and synthesis of an early matrix that is rich in hyaluronic acid.[13–17] After the surgical procedure, polymorphonuclear cells, lymphocytes, monocytes, and macrophages migrate to the fusion site and perform their various functions. Among these, and possibly most important in terms of effecting vascular endothelial cells and osteoblastic progenitors in the graft site, is the local production of paracrine signals: cytokines, kinins, and prostaglandins. These messages act as chemotactic signals and growth factors, affecting the migration, differentiation, and activity of a variety of cells, including modulation of local blood flow and angiogenic response of local endothelial cells. In this way, the inflammatory response establishes the local environment in which the early events of the bone healing response occur. Indeed, known modifiers of the inflammatory response have been shown to alter

the process of bone healing. Administration of the non-steroidal anti-inflammatory agent indomethacin, which inhibits PGE$_2$ synthesis, has been shown to delay the onset of mineralization if given in the first six days of healing.[18] Other anti-inflammatory drugs may have similar effects in the clinical setting.[19–21]

In addition to the influence of the local blood supply and the inflammatory response, host bone itself is known to have a profound effect on the healing process in spinal fusions. When properly prepared by the surgeon, local bone serves as a reservoir of osteogenic cells and osteoinductive proteins, as an osteoconductive surface for graft incorporation, and as part of the local blood supply to the graft site. Thus the goal of surgical preparation of local bone is to minimize cellular and mechanical damage to the host bone while maximizing the availability of osteoprogenitor cells and osteoinductive matrix proteins. This is achieved by decorticating the fusion site. In this regard, some debate has taken place regarding the use of a power burr, with its risk of thermal necrosis, versus the use of an osteotome or rongeur. Continuous irrigation and short periods of contact between host bone and the cutting tip of power tools can reduce the risk of thermal damage. To date, no known study has shown the advantage of one method over another.

The surface area of cancellous bone exposed during decortication is another factor thought to affect the success of a spinal fusion. Increasing the available surface area also increases the number of exposed osteogenic cells at the fusion site, which should have a positive effect on the rate of graft incorporation. Additionally, an increase in the osteoconductive surface area available should lead to greater mechanical stability of the bony union, owing to an increase in the area of contact between the osteogenic host bone and the graft material. This may account for the greater success of allografts in anterior fusions[22] as compared with posterior fusions, which generally rely on a smaller area of decorticated bone per fusion segment. Similarly, this may contribute to the low fusion rates seen in myelomeningocele, along with the difficult fixation and increased infection rates.[23, 24]

The fusion site must contain osteogenic cells if a graft is to be successful. Osteogenic cells are defined as cells capable of producing bone or differentiating into a bone-forming cell. Several authors have conceptually divided osteogenic cells into two groups: determined osteogenic precursor cells (DOPCs) and inducible osteogenic precursor cells (IOPCs).[25–29] The DOPCs are likely to be cells that have already begun the differentiation process, beginning as undifferentiated pluripotential cells. They are capable of proliferation but have committed reversibly or irreversibly to express a bone phenotype at maturity, without further induction. DOPCs can be found primarily in marrow stroma and on bone surfaces. In contrast, IOPCs are probably a more immature population of cells, including early-stage progenitors and nonproliferating or resting pluripotential connective tissue stem cells. These cells are capable of differentiation along two or more pathways.

The least mature connective tissue stem cells have the capacity to produce progeny that express a phenotype characteristic of bone, cartilage, adipocyte, fibroblast, or smooth muscle cell at maturity. The IOPCs must be acted on by an osteoinductive stimulus, such as bone morphogenic proteins (BMPs), in order to become bone-producing cells. IOPCs are found primarily in bone marrow, periosteum, and perhaps in the circulating blood.[30, 31] Vascular pericytes in local soft tissues surrounding the graft site may also serve as a source of IOPCs.[11]

By decorticating the fusion site, both determined and inducible osteoblastic progenitors may be stimulated to differentiate as osteogenic cells. In theory, then, any exposure of local bone marrow cavities to the graft bed that does not excessively weaken the mechanical strength of local bone should increase the number of osteoblastic progenitors with access to the graft site. Methods of actively recruiting progenitor cells or enhancing the number of progenitors in a grafted site are active areas of research. Some of these issues are discussed later in this chapter.

BONE GRAFT

Bone grafting is performed to accelerate, augment, or substitute for the normal regenerative capacity of bone. In an ideal graft, the graft material possesses osteogenic, osteoinductive, and osteoconductive properties.[32] (Table 50–1 summarizes these properties as they relate to current clinical and experimental graft material.)

The osteogenic potential of a graft is derived from progenitor cells that are transplanted as part of the graft, both DOPCs and IOPCs. Osteoinductive activity refers to the capacity of some proteins to stimulate the cascade of events leading to bone formation by inducing progenitors to undergo osteoblastic differentiation. This activity is defined specifically as a property of the matrix-derived BMPs. However, other matrix-bound growth factors likely contribute to this process, including TGF-β, insulin-like growth factors I and II (IGF-I and IGF-II), and basic fibroblast growth factor (bFGF). In addition to growth factors within the matrix, other autocrine and paracrine stimuli may originate from DOPCs, IOPCs, and other viable cells in the graft. As a result, the concept of osteoinduction is generally broadened to included the stimulatory activities of the other growth factors that mediate osteoblastic differentiation.

In contrast to osteoinduction, osteoconduction is the result of the structural and surface features of a graft matrix. Osteoconductivity refers to the capacity of a graft matrix to facilitate or enhance the attachment, migration, proliferation, and differentiation of endothelial cells and osteoblastic progenitors. The result is the distribution of a bone healing response throughout the graft volume. Osteoconductivity is a function of surface shape, texture, roughness, porosity, free energy, and the degradation properties of the given substrate. In addition, the presence of cell adhesion molecules and other proteins in or bound to the surface of a matrix is likely to have a profound effect on osteoconductive activity. Molecules that may be involved in this process include collagens, fibronectin, osteonectin, laminin, vitronectin, hyaluronan, and various proteoglycans. The extracellular matrix of an allograft is a prototype for an osteoconductive scaffolding that facilitates the distribution of a bone healing process throughout a graft site. Many of the current and future options for bone graft materials are discussed later.

Autologous Cancellous Bone

Autologous cancellous bone is, by most measures, the most effective graft material for spinal fusion.[33–36] An autogenous cancellous graft transplants osteogenic bone and marrow cells—an osteoconductive matrix of collagen, mineral, and matrix proteins, which also contains osteoinductive proteins.

There are, however, several disadvantages and limitations to the use of cancellous bone. Graft harvest adds operative time, pain, blood loss, and increased risk of infection and cutaneous nerve damage. The incidence of major complications associated with the harvest of iliac crest bone graft has been reported to be 5 to 10 per cent.[37, 38] Increased blood loss results in increased exposure to blood products, along with associated risks of transfusion reaction and the much lower

Table 50–1. PROPERTIES OF CLINICAL AND EXPERIMENTAL GRAFT MATERIALS

Material	Osteogenic	Osteoinductive	Osteoconductive
Autogenous cancellous bone	+	+	+
Autogenous cortical bone	+	+	+
Vascularized autograft	+	+	+
Allograft		±	+
Deproteinated xenograft			+
Bone marrow	+	±	+
DBM		+	+
Collagen			+
Ceramics			+
BMP		+ +	

DBM, demineralized bone matrix; BMP, bone morphogenic protein.

risk of inoculation with hepatitis and human immuno-deficiency viruses. Furthermore, the amount of autogenous bone is limited and may be insufficient, particularly in children undergoing arthrodesis over multiple segments.

Autologous Cortical Bone

Cortical bone grafts are generally less successful than cancellous grafts[36] as a result of several factors. Cortical bone contains fewer osteoblasts and osteoblastic progenitors than trabecular bone. Furthermore, those cells that are present are less likely to survive, because a larger fraction of cells is buried within the matrix, where diffusion is insufficient to provide adequate nutrients to support viability. The absence of nonosteogenic marrow cells and endothelial cells further limits the biologic potential of a cortical graft. In comparison to trabecular bone, cortical grafts have a much lower available surface area per unit volume. This reduces the potential surface for new bone formation (and therefore osteoconductive potential) and also reduces the bioavailability of osteoinductive factors buried in the matrix. The marked reduction in porosity of cortical bone also represents a barrier to vascular ingrowth and bony remodeling, both of which are critical to bone healing and the development of optimal mechanical strength.

The only advantage of cortical bone versus cancellous bone and other graft materials stems from its superior mechanical strength and the availability of cortical segments of sufficient size to fill virtually any skeletal defect. The ability to provide immediate mechanical strength at the time of implantation is a critical advantage in many situations,[30] particularly in anterior interbody fusions. However, the mechanical strength of a cortical graft is not constant. Allograft bone is remodeled by the process of creeping substitution, resulting in increased porosity and progressive loss of strength during the first 12 to 24 months after implantation, before remodeling and new bone formation reconstitute the mechanical properties of the grafted segment.[14] This is associated with increased risk of graft failure and collapse during the first 24 months after implantation.

Combined grafts of intact cortical and cancellous bone from the iliac crest are common and readily available, with good mechanical properties and biologic properties of incorporation. The mechanical strength of these grafts is variable, however. Grafts from the anterior crest exhibit greater mechanical compressive strength than grafts from the posterior crest.[40]

Vascularized Autologous Grafts

Vascularized grafts are now used extensively in many centers for musculoskeletal reconstructive procedures. High rates of vascular patency can be achieved by experienced microsurgeons. Many studies have shown clear advantages to using vascularized grafts in a number of settings.[41–44] In anterior spinal fusions, donor vessels are available to support the vascularized graft. Suitable grafts with good mechanical strength are available from the anterior iliac crest, posterior iliac crest,[45] fibula,[46] or rib.[47] In addition, an iliac graft pedicle flap on the quadratus lumborum has been described.[48] In intrathoracic procedures, a vascularized rib graft may be mobilized on its intercostal pedicle, with limited additional morbidity and in much less time than a free vascularized graft.[49, 50] However, a rib graft provides less mechanical strength when compared with the iliac crest or fibula[51] and therefore must be mechanically supplemented by additional cortical bone or internal fixation.

Although routine use of vascular grafts is limited by the increased operative time, technical difficulty, and added morbidity, the improved incorporation of these grafts may make them highly desirable in some settings where incorporation of avascular grafts may be compromised—for example, in areas of radiation-induced fibrosis or previous infection.

Autologous Bone Marrow

Bone marrow is a valuable and accessible source of osteogenic cells that is probably underutilized in contemporary clinical practice. The osteogenic potential of transplanted bone marrow was first documented by Goujon in 1869,[52] and later by Senn in 1889.[53] Studies by Burwell in the 1960s concluded that the formation of new bone following autografting resulted from the differentiation of osteogenic precursor cells contained within the marrow, in addition to osteoblasts on the surface of the graft material itself.[54] Burwell postulated that following transplantation, these reticular cells free themselves from the sinusoidal walls to become primitive migratory cells; they then differentiate into osteogenic cells when they are exposed to osteoinductive substances released from the necrotic portion of the graft,[55] or perhaps from osteoinductive materials contained within or secreted by the marrow itself.

Many studies have demonstrated the ability of marrow cells to form bone intramuscularly,[56, 57] subcutaneously,[25] interperitoneally,[27, 58, 59] in the anterior chamber of the eye,[60] and orthotopically. Using a suspension of marrow cells in diffusion chambers, Friedenstein showed that hematopoietic cells die following transplantation, whereas fibroblasts and other stromal elements proliferate to produce immature bone, suggesting the presence of an undifferentiated precursor cell in postnatal marrow.[25–28] As previously described, many investigators have suggested the presence of two types of osteogenic precursor cells: DOPCs and IOPCs.[25, 61, 62] The DOPC is a stem cell for the osteoblast alone and is located on bone surfaces and in peritrabecular marrow stroma. The IOPC, conversely, is a pluripotent stem cell capable of differentiation into an osteoblast, but only in the presence of an appropriate inducing agent. Precisely which inducing agent (or agents) is responsible for differentiation of the IOPC remains uncertain, although many cytokines appear to be involved.

Maniatopoulos and coworkers,[63] Lian and Stein,[64] and others have shown that osteoblastic differentiation proceeds in a series of steps, which can be divided conceptually. An initial proliferative phase is characterized by expression of H4 histone, c-fos, and c-jun. A matrix synthesis phase is characterized by a reduction in proliferation and up-regulation of gene products for Type I collagen, osteopontin, osteonectin, and alkaline phosphatase. Finally, a matrix mineralization phase culminates in an osteoblastic phenotype characterized by expression of osteocalcin, bone sialoprotein, and responsiveness to 1,25-dihydroxy vitamin D and parathyroid hormone. A conceptual summary of the large body of literature related to osteoblastic differentiation is presented in Figure 50–1.

The value of bone marrow as a bone graft, used alone or as a component in a composite bone graft material, has been supported by numerous studies in rats and rabbits.[65–77] Lane and colleagues[78] demonstrated the efficacy of autogenous bone marrow grafting in a 5-mm rat femoral defect and showed that the efficacy of bone marrow grafts was dependent on transplantation of viable cells. Yasko and associates[79] also showed that bone marrow enhanced the performance of an effective synthetic BMP-2 material in rats. However, in contrast to clinical practice, almost all these studies in rodents used bone marrow obtained by open harvesting of bone and/or irrigation of bone explants rather than by aspiration.

Some evaluation of bone marrow grafting has been carried out in larger nonrodent models. Johnson and coworkers[80] found canine bone marrow much less osteogenic than rabbit marrow when transplanted in different fusion chambers. Using a canine tibial model, Tiedeman and colleagues[77] found that the percutaneous injection of marrow mixed with demineralized bone matrix powder produced overall results comparable to those of open cancellous grafting.

A few uncontrolled clinical series also imply that aspirated bone marrow has value.[55, 81–84] Connolly reported successful treatment of 18 of 20 nonunions treated with casting or intramedullary nails plus percutaneous marrow injection. Healy and associates[71] reported healing in five of eight delayed unions or nonunions of allograft host junction sites using marrow injection alone.

Recognizing the potential biologic value, many surgeons currently use bone marrow as an adjuvant to allograft bone grafts. This can be supported by available data, only because the risk and morbidity of bone marrow aspiration from the iliac crest are very low; no prospective trials have documented the value or limitations of bone marrow grafting. If bone marrow grafting is to be performed, data reported by Muschler and coworkers[85] provide some guidance for the surgeon wishing to optimize the biologic potential of a graft. They showed that a mean of approximately 2100 osteoblastic progenitors (CFU-Os) could be harvested in a 2-cc aspirate of human bone marrow from the iliac crest, and that the mean prevalence of CFU-Os among nucleated marrow cells was approximately 1 in 37,000 cells. They further documented that the yield of CFU-Os dropped rapidly as the volume of bone marrow aspirated was increased, owing to contamination with peripheral blood. Based on these findings, they recommended that aspiration of marrow be limited to 2 cc from each aspiration site in order to maximize the concentration of CFU-Os in the marrow graft. Further studies will be necessary to answer several important questions regarding bone marrow grafting: Does bone marrow grafting improve the results of contemporary allograft and synthetic bone grafts? What are the optimal characteristics for a carrier matrix for bone marrow grafts? Is the efficacy of a bone marrow graft determined by the number of osteoblastic progenitors transplanted? (In fact, data from Connolly and associates already suggest that the biologic efficacy of bone marrow grafts can be improved by processing to concentrate the number of osteoblastic progenitors.[86]) Are all patients suitable bone marrow donors, or are there limitations imposed on the availability of these cells or their biologic potential by aging, disease, or health habits (e.g., smoking). Unpublished data from Muschler and colleagues indicate that the number of osteoblastic progenitors in bone marrow declines significantly with age and that patients younger than 40 who smoke have reduced number of progenitors when compared with nonsmokers.

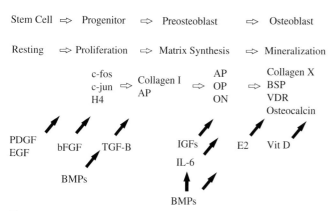

Figure 50–1. The osteoblastic pathway. A schematic illustration of the stages of osteoblastic differentiation, the predominant activity of the differentiation cell at each stage, some of the characteristic genes expressed at each stage, and the approximate site of principal action for some of the principal osteotropic growth factors and hormones. H4, H4 histone; AP, alkaline phosphatase; OP, osteopontin; ON, osteonectin; BSP, bone sialoprotein; VDR, vitamin D receptor; PDGF, platelet-derived growth factor; EGF, epithelial growth factor; bFGF, basic fibroblast growth factor; BMPs, BMP family members; TGF-β, transforming growth factor–beta; IGFs, insulin-like growth factors I and II; IL-6, interleukin-6; E2, estradiol; Vit D, vitamin D₃.

Allografts

Use of allograft bone has been well characterized over the last 30 years. Although fresh osteochondral shell allografts have been used in the hip and knee, fresh allografting does not have a role in spinal surgery, where only frozen or freeze-dried bone is used. There are three principal advantages of an allograft. First, it eliminates the morbidity of harvesting autologous bone. Second, there is access to essentially an unlimited volume of graft material in settings where the quantity of available autograft bone is insufficient. Third, because cortical allografts can be selected from any bone (not just the iliac crest or tibial hemicortex), they provide the surgeon with access to grafts that have mechanical strength that is superior to any autograft site. Currently, whole bone segments of the fibula, humerus, and femur are readily available from regional bone banks. Also available are blocks, chips, and powder prepared from cortical and/or cancellous bone, which can be selected to match the requirements of a specific clinical setting.

The method of sterilization and preparation of allograft tissue has a significant impact on osteoconductive, osteoinductive, and mechanical properties, as well as immunogenicity.[87] Donor cells and cell fragments are the most immunogenic material in allogenic bone. Processing of allograft bone therefore includes steps that attempt to remove as many cells as possible from the graft. Immunogenicity is further reduced, although not eliminated, by freezing to $-20°C$.[88–96] Freeze-drying is even more effective at reducing the immunogenicity of allogenic bone, but at the price of reducing mechanical strength by 50 per cent.[88, 97]

With the use of contemporary processing and storage techniques, clinical evidence of overt immunologic reaction against the graft is rare. Even so, histologic evidence of a low-grade inflammatory reaction can be found around essentially all allografts. This reaction probably slows the incorporation of many allografts and may contribute to the failure of some, as suggested by several canine studies that documented improved biologic behavior in antigen-matched allografts.[97–100] Antigen matching is not currently being considered, however. The relatively high success rates for allografts makes the large cost of antigen matching unfeasible and probably unwarranted in general practice.[101]

Sterility of frozen allografts is ensured through expedient postmortem harvesting using sterile surgical technique and careful monitoring using surface cultures and polymerase chain reaction (PCR) screening for bacterial and viral genome fragments. The current risk of disease transmission via a musculoskeletal allograft is approximately 1 in 1,667,000.[102] A variety of secondary sterilization procedures have been designed and may be used, depending on the source of the allograft. Ethylene oxide sterilization was evaluated by Cornell and coworkers, who found a 70 per cent decrease in bone induction by demineralized bone powder in rats.[103] Other authors have reported variable changes in inductive capacity of ethylene oxide–sterilized matrix.[104–106] Heating or autoclaving bone tissue is generally avoided, owing to the disruption of matrix proteins. Some processing techniques may not only affect the biologic potential of bone matrix, reducing bone formation and lowering union rates, but also

alter the mechanical properties of the graft. For example, irradiation to 2.5 megarads or freeze-dried processing may reduce the torsional strength of the cortical allograft by as much as 50 per cent.[107]

Results from other clinical and experimental studies using allograft bone in spinal fusions have been mixed. Some investigators found allograft to be significantly inferior to autogenous bone grafting,[22, 23, 108–118] whereas others found little or no difference between them.[22, 49, 119–133] Allograft bone is particularly valuable in settings that require the graft to serve a significant mechanical function, such as struts for anterior interbody fusions or bone-wire fixation constructs in the upper cervical spine.[134] Autografts from rib, fibula, tricortical iliac crest, and tibial hemicortex have all been used in these settings, but each can result in significant donor site morbidity, a problem eliminated by the use of allograft bone. Use of banked bone also frequently allows the surgeon to select a graft of better size and/ or better mechanical properties than the available autograft. This can be a critical factor in the mechanical success of a graft. Furthermore, biologic success of allograft bone grafts in these settings compared with autograft bone can be similar, particularly if autogenous cancellous bone or bone marrow[39, 81, 82, 108, 134] is used to supplement the allograft at the fusion site.

Demineralized Allograft Bone Matrix

Demineralization is one means by which the biologic activity of allograft bone can be modified. In settings where mechanical properties are not critical to the graft application, demineralization may enhance the osteoinductive activity of the allograft matrix by making growth factors embedded in the matrix more available. Several preparations of demineralized bone matrix are available.

The history of demineralization as a means to enhance allograft performance is richly linked to many of the recent biologic insights into bone biology and bone healing. It was over a century ago, in 1889, that Senn reported the repair of long bone and cranial defects in patients with chronic osteomyelitis using hydrochloric acid–treated decalcified heterologous bone implants.[53] Although his primary motive was to promote antisepsis within the bone cavities, Senn observed rapid substitution of the demineralized tissue by ossification invading from the perimeter of the defects. However, several of Senn's contemporaries obtained equivocal results, and clinical efforts over the next 70 years were minimal.[135–138]

Reddi and Huggins revived this concept when they reported on their observation of a matrix-induced bone induction phenomenon in rats.[139, 140] Urist went on to demonstrate bone induction using a variety of demineralized matrix preparations in muscular pouches of rabbits, rats, mice, and guinea pigs.[141] Subsequently, matrix-induced heterotopic bone formation was documented at many soft tissue sites, including muscle, tendon, and fascia,[133, 140, 142–146] as well as in thymus[25] and in the soft connective tissue of visceral organs.[147]

Nathanson also observed the differentiation of neonatal embryonic skeletal tissue into cartilage when cultured on demineralized bone matrix substratum and suggested that the tissue transformation of bone induction was analogous to embryonic bone tissue differentiation.[148, 149]

Reddi subsequently characterized the inductive phenomenon of bone matrix as a cascade of events parallel to those occurring in endochondral ossification and postulated that the process was the result of stimulation by a series of soluble matrix factors that potentiated events along the cascade.[150–152] In this paradigm, activation of a matrix chemotactic factor stimulates stem cell migration, activation of a mitogenic factor promotes cell proliferation, and activation of an inductive factor potentiates cell differentiation. Matrix proteins that were chemotactic for mesenchymal cells were eluted from bone matrix extracts by gel filtration, as were matrix-derived growth-promoting factors.[153, 154]

Sato and Urist showed that demineralized bone matrix was both inductive and synergistic with bone marrow in the healing of rat femoral defects.[155] Urist went on to provide a clinical outlet for these discoveries with the development of chemosterilized, autolyzed, antigen-extracted allogenic bone (AAA), a procedure that included chloroform-methanol extraction, 0.6 N hydrochloric acid extraction of soluble proteins with partial demineralization, and neutral phosphate autodigestion.[142–144, 146] This preparation appeared to reduce the immunogenicity of the allograft matrix without loss of inductive properties. Using this preparation, Urist and Dawson reported on 40 patients undergoing posterolateral lumbar spinal fusion with an 80 per cent success rate and a pseudarthrosis rate of 12 per cent.[156]

Demineralized bone prepared by a variety of methods has been used effectively by a number of investigators. Glowacki and associates were among the first to report successful repair of craniofacial defects.[157–159] Tiedeman and colleagues[77] and Wilkins and Stringer[160] reported clinical efficacy in long bone defects. Other clinical reports showed efficacy for demineralized bone matrix. Some studies reported a benefit of adding demineralized bone matrix to autograft or ceramic matrices in animal spine fusion models.[161–166] There are as yet no reports describing the clinical efficacy of demineralized bone matrix grafts in spinal fusion.

Because demineralized bone preparations do not have mechanical properties that will resist external forces, the use of these materials is restricted primarily to grafting of contained defects or graft sites protected by rigid internal fixation.

Deproteinated Heterologous Bone

In contrast to allograft bone, heterologous bone (xenograft) fails to induce osseous repair owing to its high level of antigenicity. Partially deproteinated and partially defatted heterologous bone (Kiel bone or Oswestry bone) does exhibit greatly reduced antigenicity and therefore evokes a minimal immune response.[167] The denaturing process, however, also destroys osteoinduc-

tive matrix proteins. Accordingly, implantation of such materials in bone defects and muscular compartments has failed to generate bone formation.[81]

The impregnation of this material with cells capable of osteogenic activity, however, has been studied. Salama and colleagues[81] and Plank and colleagues[168] demonstrated that deproteinated xenograft bone supplemented with autologous marrow facilitated osteogenesis in both experimental animals and humans. Deproteinated bone, in these experiments, serves as an osteoconductive scaffolding, providing a stable mechanical environment for revascularization and differentiating osteoblastic cells. Salama and Weissman[82] reported satisfactory results in clinical attempts to use composite xenograft/autograft (Kiel bone/marrow) in a variety of bone defects. Recently, Rawlinson reported poor results using bovine-derived Cloward grafts.[169] Owing to the wide availability of more effective allograft matrix materials in the United States at similar cost, xenograft materials are not currently used.

SYNTHETIC BONE GRAFT MATERIALS

Recent years have seen an explosion of new information about cellular and molecular events that occur in bone grafts and as part of a bone healing response. Purified human recombinant growth factors are readily available. Many are active in multiple events in the bone healing process and are therefore potential therapeutic agents. In addition, rapid developments in ceramic engineering and bioerodable polymers allow us to design customized matrix materials. Given these converging events, we are now producing an army of first-generation and second-generation biosynthetic bone grafting materials. It is beyond the scope of this chapter to comprehensively review any of these areas. The following is intended as an introduction and overview of some of the ongoing developments in this area—specifically, the application of growth factors, collagen matrices, and ceramics in synthetic bone grafting materials.

Bone Morphogenic Proteins

A major advance occurred in 1978, when Urist and associates reported the isolation of a hydrophobic, low-molecular-weight osteoinductive protein from insoluble bone matrix gelatin.[170] Further characterization of this inductive factor, BMP, was made possible by quantitative extraction accomplished by differential precipitation in a buffer containing 4 M guanidine hydrochloride.[171] Lovell and Dawson went on to report the success of a partly purified BMP preparation on polylactic acid strips in a canine segmental spinal fusion model.[172]

After an extensive search for the protein responsible for the inductive activity of bone matrix extract, in 1988, Wozney and coworkers identified and characterized three proteins isolated from a highly purified preparation from bovine bone, each capable of induc-

Synonyms

BMP-1	Procollagen C-Proteinase [244]
BMP-2	BMP-2a
BMP-3	Osteogenin
BMP-4	BMP-2b
BMP-5	
BMP-6	
BMP-7	OP-1
BMP-8	OP-2
BMP-9	
BMP-10	
BMP-11	
BMP-12	
BMP-13	

Figure 50–2. The BMP family of proteins: the known members of the BMP family and some of the corresponding names that identify the same protein.

ing bone formation in a rat subcutaneous bioassay.[173] Human cDNA clones for each peptide were isolated and expressed as recombinant human proteins. Two of the encoded proteins were homologous and were described as members of the TGF-β supergene family, whereas the third appeared to be a novel polypeptide (BMP-1). BMP-1 has turned out not to be a growth factor at all. Rather, this molecule has been characterized as a procollagen c-proteinase that may have a biologic function in the activation of TGF-β-like molecules, including the BMPs.[174, 175]

The BMP story has developed rapidly in recent years. At the time this chapter was written, a total of 12 members of the BMP family had been identified. BMP-2 through BMP-13 are homologous proteins (molecular weight 12–14 kD) that are post-transcriptionally modified by glycosylation and are secreted as homo- or heterodimers linked by one disulfide bond (molecular weight ≡30 kD).[176, 177] The currently known proteins are listed in Figure 50–2, along with synonyms or alternative names that are now or have been used for some of these molecules. Figure 50–3 illustrates the per cent

RNA sequence homology within and between subgroups of the BMP family.

Each of these proteins can interact with one or more of a family of cell surface receptors. Some of these interactions are illustrated in Figure 50–4. Cells must express both Type I and Type II receptors in order to be responsive to BMPs. Formation of a complex of BMP and the Type I and Type II receptor results in phosphorylation of the Type I receptor, initiating the signal transduction mechanism that results in the cells' response.

Among the homodimers that are most active in bone induction are BMP-2, BMP-3 (osteogenin), and BMP-7 (osteogenic protein-1, or OP-1). Each is currently being developed for potential applications in bone grafting and skeletal reconstruction. A growing number of animal studies have demonstrated the great promise for these proteins as powerful stimulants of a local bone healing response in rodents, canines, and nonhuman primates, using various carrier matrices and a dosage range of 100 to 10,000 µg/ml. Available data suggest that in young animals with uncompromised tissue beds, BMPs delivered in an acellular matrix are capable of reliably uniting bone defects and inducing spinal arthrodesis. Schimandle and colleagues[178] reported 100 per cent union in an uninstrumented posterolateral intertransverse fusion model in the rabbit using BMP-2 delivered in a collagen carrier, compared with only 42 per cent fusion with autogenous corticocancellous iliac crest bone. Muschler and associates,[179] using an instrumented posterior canine spinal fusion model, found that BMP-2 delivered in a degradable polymer carrier (PLGA) had equal efficacy to 100 per cent autogenous cancellous bone. Cook and coworkers[180] found similar results in a canine spine model using OP-1 (BMP-7). Several other promising reports using noninstrumented lumbar intertransverse fusions in

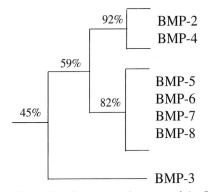

Figure 50–3. Homology between subgroups of the BMP family. Illustration of the per cent homology in the active protein within and between subgroups of the BMP family.

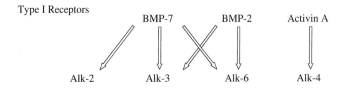

Type I receptors are phosphorylated by Type II receptors after binding.

Figure 50–4. The BMP receptor family. BMPs act on cells through interaction with a family of membrane-bound cell surface receptors. Cells must express one or more of these receptors in order to be responsive to BMPs. Some of the cross reactivity between BMP-7, BMP-4, and another TGF-β superfamily member, Activin A, is illustrated. BMPs bind first to a Type I receptor, including Alk-2, Alk-3, Alk-4, and Alk-6. The BMP–Type I receptor complex is then phosphorylated by a Type II receptor protein to activate the signal transduction mechanism in the cell, which results in the BMP induced response.

rabbits and a nonhuman primate are available only in abstract form.[176, 181–185] At the time this chapter was written, several FDA-approved prospective clinical trials were under way for the treatment of fractures. Clinical trials to establish the safety and efficacy of these proteins for human spinal fusion are pending.

To date, no animal studies have evaluated the efficacy of these proteins in animals with advanced age or in tissue beds compromised by trauma, scar tissue, previous surgery, or radiation. In these situations, the efficacy of these proteins may be compromised by the relative lack of osteoblastic progenitor cells, the presumed principal target cell for BMP activity. However, Yasko and colleagues showed that the efficacy of BMP-2 can be enhanced by combining a BMP-2 graft with bone marrow. The strategy of combined grafts using marrow and BMPs may prove to be important, particularly when these materials are used in settings where the local osteoblastic progenitor population may be reduced or functionally compromised.[79]

Other Growth Factors

A large number of peptide growth factors and hormones are known to have important effects on the recruitment, proliferation, and differentiation of osteoblastic progenitors, which may have potential therapeutic importance. Only some of the examples of candidate growth factors can be listed here. Epidermal growth factor (EGF) and PDGF are both capable of inducing colony formation by osteoblastic progenitors in vitro.[12] Basic FGF increases proliferation of human osteoblastic progenitors and reversibly inhibits the expression of alkaline phosphatase and matrix synthesis, in addition to its known potent angiogenic effects. TGF-β1 increases matrix synthesis and decreases alkaline phosphatase expression. However, Joyce and associates[186] showed that subperiosteal injection of TGF-β can produce a marked periosteal response, resulting in rapid formation of a cartilage tissue mass and bone formation via endochondral ossification. IGF-I and IGF-II potentiate a mature osteoblastic phenotype in culture.[32, 187–189] Each of these proteins is under investigation as a potential component in future composite synthetic bone graft materials.

In addition to factors that may have direct effects on osteoblastic differentiation, factors that enhance or modulate angiogenesis may have a role in future bone grafting materials. Folkman recently published an excellent review of angiogenesis and the potential therapeutic application of angiogenic and antiangiogenic factors.[190]

Collagen

The major components of organic matrix of bone are Type I collagen (90 per cent dry weight), a large number of noncollagenous matrix proteins, at least two proteoglycans (biglycan and decorin), and several minor collagens (mostly Types III and X). These proteins contribute an osteoconductive substrate for cell attach-

ment and migration and are necessary elements of new bone formation and mineralization. The precise contribution of each element of organic bone matrix is not yet known. Nor is it understood how the structural organization of the various components within the matrix influences the biologic function of these proteins. This makes purposeful engineering of synthetic matrices difficult.

Collagen is the obvious focus of most matrix engineering. Most of the noncollagenous proteins in bone matrix can be solubilized using 4 M guanidine. However, the majority of Type I collagen in bone matrix is heavily interconnected by covalent pyridinum cross links. This makes native collagen I insoluble and virtually impossible to manipulate as a reagent to create new structures. Unfortunately, demineralized Gm extracted matrix is only modestly effective as osteoconductive material by itself, mostly in small rodent defect models. It has, however, been used effectively as a delivery vehicle for purified proteins and extracts of bone matrix. In contrast, fibrillar collagen (uncrosslinked collagen) is soluble and can be extracted from bone and skin. Fibrillar collagen can be engineered to produce a variety of matrices, such as gels, sponges, and filaments. These are often secondarily cross-linked to stabilize their structure using a variety of chemical methods. Collagen matrices generated in this way make up the majority of the new matrices currently being developed. However, few of these engineered collagen matrices are effective by themselves in strongly promoting bone formation. Lane and coworkers studied the efficacy of commercially prepared soluble fibrillar collagen for healing bone defects.[191] Using a rat femoral defect model, they demonstrated that fibrillar collagen as a soluble gel or a sponge combined with bone marrow was more effective than cancellous bone in bridging large segmental defects in rats, and that marrow plus collagen was superior to marrow alone. In the absence of marrow supplementation, however, the collagen implants were inferior to cancellous bone histologically, biomechanically, and radiographically. These studies illustrate the value of collagen as an osteoconductive substrate, but it is not effective as a graft without the addition of osteogenic cells and/or osteoinductive stimuli. Therefore, most new collagen matrices focus on composites of collagen with ceramics, growth factors, or exogenous osteogenic cells.

Noncollagenous Matrix Proteins

Bone matrix contains many proteins other than collagens and growth factors. These proteins may serve a role in the organization of the collagenous matrix and other proteins into higher-ordered structures, attachment sites for cells, or binding sites for growth factors. Some may play a role in the initiation and organization of mineralization.

Osteonectin, for example, has been shown to be a promoter of hydroxyapatite crystal deposition in vitro when in complex with collagen.[192] Bone and dentin phosphoproteins have independently been shown to cause in vitro hydroxyapatite formation.[193, 194] Proteolipids and calcium–acidic phospholipid phosphate complexes isolated from mineralizing collagenous matrices have been shown to facilitate hydroxyapatite deposition.[195] Bone sialoprotein has also been shown to be strongly associated with the ability of a matrix to mineralize.[196]

In addition to these matrix proteins associated with mineralization, other matrix proteins appear to provide significant contributions to the osteoconductive nature of the extracellular matrix. Fibronectin, a matrix and cell-membrane protein produced by platelets, myofibroblasts, and fibroblasts, is thought to serve as an attachment site for mesenchymal cells in their attachment to the matrix.[197] Osteoblasts and osteoblastic cell lines appear to express integrins that bind selectively to both fibronectin and vitronectin.[198–200] Osteocalcin, a low-molecular-weight carboxylated matrix protein, one of the most abundant noncollagenous proteins in bone matrix, has been associated with increased bone turnover.[201] Osteocalcin appears to be chemotactic for osteoclasts and monocytes,[202] critical elements of normal bone remodeling. No specific structural or binding role has been identified for this bone/dentin specific protein in the bone formation process.

Ceramics

Calcium phosphate biomaterials fused at their crystal grain boundaries into polycrystalline ceramics by high-temperature sintering confer stability to these minerals and reduce bioresorbability.[203] A variety of ceramics are currently being evaluated, most of which are composed of either hydroxyapatite (HA) or tricalcium phosphate (TCP). Ceramics may be prepared as porous three-dimensional implants, dense block implants, granular particles (usually 0.5 to 2 mm in size), or thin surface coatings. Almost all calcium phosphate ceramics have a high degree of biocompatibility,[204, 205] and some have already been extensively used in dentistry and maxillofacial surgery.[167, 168, 197, 201–208]

Studies by Klawitter and Hulbert indicated that the minimal macropore size in porous ceramics needed for effective ingrowth of bone is 100 m.[209] Most porous ceramics currently being manufactured contain interconnecting macropores ranging from 100 to 400 m. The various calcium phosphate ceramics generally differ with regard to their bioresorbability characteristics. A number of investigators have reported that ceramic HA does not exhibit extensive bioresorption and is essentially inert.[203, 205, 210] Conversely, there is unequivocal evidence that ceramic TCP undergoes biodegradation.[203–205, 210–212] In addition, implants with a large surface area tend to exhibit more rapid degradation.[204]

Early studies of ceramics suggested that they might be capable of osteogenic stimulation.[213] In fact, one can often find new bone formation in an HA ceramic implant placed at heterotopic sites in the absence of other stimuli. This occurs only after several months and would not be likely to contribute to the early success of a bone graft. The role of ceramics, therefore, is primarily that of osteoconduction. One possible mechanism for this apparent late osteoinductive property of HA ceramics is that an HA implant selectively binds proteins to its surface based on their relative affinity to HA. This may result in the accumulation of some protein growth factors such as BMPs, TGF-βs, and insulin-like binding protein-5 (IGFBP-5), which have strong affinity to HA. Accumulation of these low-abundance proteins, and their presentation on a stable surface, may secondarily create a local growth factor environment on the ceramic surface that is capable of recruiting local osteoblastic progenitors and inducing bone formation. This affinity of many osteotropic growth factors for the highly charged surface of HA may make HA ceramics an effective delivery system for growth factors as composite synthetic bone grafting materials are developed.

The stability of the bone-ceramic interface and preparation of local bone are also important. Cameron and associates demonstrated that ceramic implants placed against intact bony cortex do not exhibit bone ingrowth and simply resorb over time.[214] However, when they are placed subperiosteally and immobilized on a scarified cortex, bone ingrowth readily takes place. The requirement of stability and the rigidity of ceramic material may limit their application to settings in which mechanical micromotion can be well controlled. In the presence of micromotion, the mechanical strain in the tissue at the surface of a rigid ceramic block or in the tissue between adjoining ceramic granules may be magnified to create an environment where bone formation is inhibited.

Another drawback of ceramic implants is that they are brittle and have low impact and fracture resistance.[215] Furthermore, the limited solubility and remodeling capacity of highly crystalline HA ceramics may retard late stages of bone healing and remodeling and compromise late mechanical properties of the bone formed in a fusion site.[203] This concern has been reduced by the work of Ohgushi and colleagues,[216] which showed that ceramic combined with bone marrow exhibited greater biomechanical properties following implantation with marrow cells as a result of new bone formation in the implant. In addition, Muschler and coworkers[217, 218] performed a series of spinal fusion experiments evaluating composites of collagen and ceramic granules (60 per cent HA, 40 per cent TCP). Although these studies found that all composites tested had a significantly higher nonunion rate than autogenous cancellous bone graft, the mechanical properties of successful unions achieved with the collagen ceramic composites were comparable to the mechanical properties of unions resulting from autogenous bone graft, despite the presence of unresorbed granules in the fusion mass.

Ceramic blocks have been evaluated in a goat anterior cervical fusion model. These studies reported a 50 to 70 per cent fusion rate.[219, 220] An injectable ceramic preparation that will crystallize at body temperature has also been described, which may both provide mechanical fixation for acute fractures and have utility as a delivery system for bioactive proteins.[221]

SYSTEMIC FACTORS INFLUENCING SPINAL FUSION

Many systemic factors have been shown to influence bone healing in the laboratory. Clinically, however, it is unlikely that any of these factors result in significant alterations of fracture or defect healing. Nevertheless, the surgeon should at least attempt to optimize each factor, whenever possible. A list of systemic factors and their relative effects on bone healing appears in Table 50–2.

Nutritional status has been shown to impact the clinical outcome of surgical procedures generally[222] and bone healing specifically.[223] Identification of a nutritional deficit using anthropomorphic measurements, serum albumin levels, lymphocyte count, skin antigen testing, and nitrogen balance studies can be important in selected patients. Recent weight loss, anergy to skin testing, serum albumin levels less than 3.4 mg/dl, or a total lymphocyte count of less than 1500 should be strong signals indicating the need for a careful nutritional evaluation and a possible need for nutritional support.[224] Lenke and associates[225] documented that patients undergoing multiple-level spinal fusion procedures may take 6 to 12 weeks to recover from the perioperative nutritional insult and suggest more aggressive nutritional assessment in these patients.

Because most evidence suggests that the critical period in determining the success of a fusion attempt is the first three to seven days of healing, manipulation of systemic factors should be carefully controlled during this period, especially the administration of radiation,[226] chemotherapeutic agents[227] and corticosteroids, and smoking or systemic nicotine.[228]

LOCAL FACTORS INFLUENCING SPINAL FUSION

Many local factors also influence bone healing, and a partial list appears in Table 50–3. Osteoporosis is generally assumed to be an undesirable factor in fracture healing, but there is no direct scientific evidence. It is difficult to separate bone mass as an independent variable from age and other factors. The quality of internal fixation, for example, is significantly affected by bone mass and is an important variable in the outcome of spinal fusions. Furthermore, the quality of the local bone marrow and the number and proliferative capacity of osteogenic stem cells are reduced in elderly patients. These changes may or may not be related to the pathophysiology of osteoporosis but will likely have a negative impact on the biology of a graft site for spinal arthrodesis.

The mechanical stability of the graft site is one factor in the surgeon's control. Good internal fixation clearly increases the chances of achieving union by decreasing motion in the grafted segment. The anatomic site, the patient's weight, the patient's activity level, and the use of external immobilization are all important factors. The increased union rates seen in patients with spinal muscular atrophy[229] and Duchenne muscular dystrophy[230, 231] may be the result of decreased voluntary motion and improved local mechanics.

Local tumor invasion weakens bone and replaces normal marrow, and the tumor may directly invade the fusion site. These problems may be partly overcome by the use of special fixation techniques[232] and appropriate radiation and chemotherapy, depending on the individual tumor. Use of autologous bone or bone marrow is desirable, but harvest must be performed in a separate surgical field to prevent tumor seeding in the donor site.

Marrow-packing disorders such as thalassemia major may decrease the osteogenic potential of marrow by the overgrowth of normal marrow, altering the marrow growth factor environment and/or crowding out osteogenic stem cells. Similarly, local bone disease, such as Paget's disease or fibrous dysplasia, can replace the bone in a successful fusion with bone that is structurally inferior.

Table 50–2. SYSTEMIC FACTORS INFLUENCING BONE HEALING

Positive Factors	Negative Factors
Insulin	Corticosteroids
IGF and other somatomedins	Vitamin A intoxication
Testosterone	Vitamin D deficiency
Estrogen	Vitamin D intoxication
Growth hormone	Anemia; iron deficiency
Thyroxine	Negative nitrogen balance
PTH	Calcium deficiency
Calcitonin	NSAIDs
Vitamin A	Adriamycin
Vitamin D	Methotrexate
Anabolic steroids	Rheumatoid arthritis
Vitamin C	Sepsis
	Syndrome of inappropriate ADH
	Castration
	Tobacco

IGF, insulin-like growth factor; PTH, parathyroid hormone; NSAIDs, nonsteroidal anti-inflammatory drugs; ADH, antidiuretic hormone.

Table 50–3. LOCAL FACTORS INFLUENCING BONE HEALING

Positive Factors	Negative Factors
Increased surface area	Osteoporosis
Local bone marrow	Radiation scar
Electrical stimulation	Radiation
Mechanical stability	Denervation
Mechanical loading	Tumor
Bone morphogenic protein	Marrow-packing disorder
Factors promoting angiogenesis	Infection
Factors promoting induction recruitment, and proliferation	Local bone disease
	Mechanical motion
	Bone wax

Radiation is an adverse factor, especially when administered perioperatively. This may be a function of its direct cytotoxic effects on proliferating cells or the intense vasculitis induced by radiation injury. Long after the acute phase, radiation-induced osteonecrosis and the dense hypovascular scar left in the radiation bed may leave a poor environment for fusion. In some cases, therefore, it may be advantageous to use free vascularized grafts and donor vessels outside the area of previous radiation to enhance the vascular supply of local tissues and the likelihood of a successful fusion. Emery and colleagues[233–235] showed that the timing of radiation after a spinal fusion procedure has a significant effect on outcome, and that radiation has the least adverse effect if given three weeks after grafting. Radiation was best timed to be performed either preoperatively or in the late postoperative period, avoiding the early postoperative period when vascular invasion of the graft site and proliferation of osteoblastic progenitors would be most vulnerable.

Electrical stimulation has been shown to be of benefit in the treatment of nonunions,[236, 237] failed arthrodeses,[238, 239] and congenital pseudarthroses.[240] There is some evidence that it may also be useful in spinal fusions. In one study,[241] 13 patients with failed posterior interlumbar spinal fusions (at least 18 months postoperatively) were treated in an uncontrolled fashion with pulsating electromagnetic fields (PEMF). The investigators found that 10 of these patients (77 per cent) went on to fuse. Kahanovitz and colleagues[242] found accelerated bone formation with PEMF at four, six, and nine weeks postoperatively using an instrumented segmental canine spinal fusion model; no difference was found at 12 and 15 weeks. Constant current electrical stimulation has also been shown to enhance bone formation.[243]

FUTURE CONSIDERATIONS

The potential for advancements in the area of spinal fusions is tremendous. Advances in bone graft research, diagnostic modalities, methods of clinical evaluation, and surgical techniques (including advancements in fixation, anesthesia, and instrumentation) will offer surgeons even greater success in fusion and other forms of bone repair. In the next decade, the role of electrical stimulation will be more clearly defined, and our knowledge and ability to manipulate and augment the bone healing response using systemic hormones and local growth factors will be greatly advanced. The clinical availability of effective materials composed in part of purified recombinantly manufactured protein growth factors appears imminent. However, clinical trials of these materials require prudence, caution, and a detailed understanding of the biologic processes that are being manipulated. A large body of work remains to define the safety and efficacy of such materials in the wide variety of clinical settings in which they may be valuable.

Optimal grafting materials are likely to be formulated as composites of an osteoconductive matrix used as a delivery system plus selected growth factors and/or osteogenic cells harvested from bone marrow. Over the next several decades, these technologies and materials promise to significantly improve the reliability of spinal arthrodesis and reduce the frequency with which autogenous bone is used as a graft material. Elimination of the need to harvest cortical or cancellous bone autografts in a large fraction of patients will significantly reduce the morbidity and cost of spinal arthrodesis. Moreover, the availability of customized graft materials, and materials suitable for injection, will facilitate the development and increased use of percutaneous and arthroscopic spinal fusion techniques. Additionally, ex vivo manipulation of osteoprogenitor cells to concentrate these cells in a bone graft in the operating room or to expand the number of these cells in the laboratory may allow for more rapid and more successful grafting, particularly in settings where the local tissue bed or host is compromised with respect to the size or function of the osteoblastic progenitor population.

References

1. Albee, F. H.: Transplantation of a portion of the tibia into the spine for Pott's disease. JAMA 57:885–886, 1911.
2. Hibbs, R. A.: A report of fifty-nine cases of scoliosis treated by the fusion operation. J. Bone Joint Surg. 6:3, 1924.
3. Eie, N., Solgaard T., and Kleppe H.: The knee-elbow position in lumbar disc surgery: A review of complications. Spine 8:897–900, 1983.
4. Lehman, T. R., and La Rocca H. S.: Repeat lumbar surgery: A review of patients with failure from previous lumbar surgery treated by spinal canal exploration and lumbar spinal fusion, 1981.
5. De Palma, A. F.: The nature of pseudoarthrosis. Clin. Orthop. 59:113–118, 1968.
6. Zdeblick, T. A.: A prospective, randomized study of lumbar fusion. Preliminary results. Spine 18:983–991, 1993.
7. Burwell, R. G.: The fate of bone grafts. In Apley, G. A. (ed.): Recent Advances in Orthopaedics. London, Churchill, 1969, pp. 115–207.
8. Bos, G. D., Goldberg, V. M., Gordon, N. H., et al.: The long term fate of fresh and frozen orthotopic bone allografts in genetically defined rats. Clin. Orthop. Rel. Res. 197:245–254, 1985.
9. Urist, M. R.: Bone and bone transplants. In Urist, M. R. (ed.): Fundamental and Clinical Physiology of Bone. Philadelphia, W.B. Saunders, 1980, p. 131.
10. Villanueva, J. E., and Nimni, M. E.: Promotion of calvarial cell osteogenesis by endothelial cells. J. Bone Min. Res. 5:733–739, 1990.
11. Brighton, C. T., Lorich, D. G., Kupcha, R., et al.: The pericyte as a possible osteoblast progenitor cell. Clin. Orthop. Rel. Res. 275:287–299, 1992.
12. Gronthos, S., and Simmons, P. J.: The growth factor requirements of STRO-1 positive human bone marrow stromal precursors under serum-deprived conditions in vitro. Blood 85:929–940, 1995.
13. Simmons, D. J.: Fracture healing perspective. Clin. Orthop. 200:100–113, 1985.
14. Bone injury, regeneration, and repair (Chapter 7). In Simon, S. R. (ed.): Orthopaedic Basic Science. Rosemont, IL, American Academy of Orthopaedic Surgeons, 1995, p. 284.
15. Cruess, R. L.: Healing of bone, tendon, and ligament. In Rockwood, C. A., and Green, D. P. (eds.): Fractures. Philadelphia, J. B. Lippincott, 1984, p. 153.
16. Urist, M. R.: Bone and bone transplants. In Urist, M.R. (ed.):

Fundamental and Clinical Physiology of Bone. Philadelphia, J.B. Lippincott, 1980, p. 131.

17. Prolo, D. J., and Rodrigo, J. J.: Contemporary bone graft physiology and surgery. Clin. Orthop. 200:322–342, 1985.

18. Nilsson, O. S., Bauer, H. C. F., Brosjo, O., and Tornkvist, H.: Influence of indomethacin on heterotopic bone formation in rats: Importance of length of treatment and age. Clin. Orthop. 207:239–245, 1986.

19. Keller, J. C., Trancik, T. M., Young, F. A., et al.: Effects of indomethacin on bone ingrowth. J. Orthop. Res. 7:28, 1989.

20. McLaren, A. C.: Prophylaxis with indomethacin for heterotopic bone. After open reduction of fracture of the acetabulum. J. Bone Joint Surg. [Am.] 72:245, 1990.

21. Nilsson, O. S., Bauer, H. C. F., Brosjo, O., et al.: Influence of indomethicin on heterotopic bone formation in rats. Importance of length of treatment and of age. Clin. Orthop. 207:239, 1986.

22. Brown, M. D., Malinin, T. I., and Davis, P. B.: A roentgenographic evaluation of frozen allografts versus autografts in anterior cervical fusion. Clin. Orthop. 119:231–236, 1976.

23. Curtis, B. H.: Orthopaedic management of muscular dystrophy and related disorders. A.A.O.S. Instr. Course Lect. 19:78–89, 1970.

24. Allen, B. L., and Ferguson, R. L.: The operative treatment of myelomenigocele spinal deformity. Orthop. Clin. North Am. 10:845–862, 1979.

25. Friedenstein, A. J.: Determined and inducible osteogenic precursor cells. In Sognaes, R., and Vaughan, J. (eds.): Hard Tissue Growth, Repair, and Remineralization. Ciba Foundation Symposium II. New York, Elsevier, 1973, p. 169.

26. Friedenstein, A. J.: Precursor cells of mechanocytes. Int. Rev. Cytol. 47:327, 1976.

27. Friedenstein, A. J., Chailakhyan, R. K., Latsinik, N. V., et al.: Stromal cells responsible for transferring the microenvironment of the hematopoietic tissues. Transplantation 17:331, 1974.

28. Friedenstein, A. J., Petrakova, K. V., Kurolesova, A. I., and Frolova, G. P.: Heterotopic transplants of bone marrow: Analysis of precursor cells for osteogenic and hematopoietic tissues. Transplantation 6:230, 1968.

29. Beresford, N. J.: Osteogenic stem cells and the stromal system of bone marrow. Clin. Orthop. Rel. Res. 240:270–280, 1989.

30. Chalmers, J., Grey, D. H., and Bush, J.: Observations on the induction of bone in soft tissues. J. Bone Joint Surg. 57B:36, 1975.

31. Urist, M. R., Hay, P. H., Dubuc, F., et al.: Osteogenic competence. Clin. Orthop. 64:194, 1969.

32. Muschler, G. F., and Lane, J. M.: Clinical applications of bone grafts in orthopaedic surgery. In Habal, M. B., and Reddi, R. H. (eds.): Bone Grafts and Bone Substitutes, Philadelphia. W.B. Saunders Co., 1992.

33. Heiple, K. G., Chase S. W., and Herndon, C. H.: A comparative study of the healing process following different types of bone transplantation. J. Bone Joint Surg. 45A:1592, 1963.

34. Oikarinen, J., and Korkonen, L. K.: The bone induction capacity of various bone matrix and deep-frozen allogeneic bone in rabbits. Clin. Orthop. 40:208, 1979.

35. Tuli, S. M.: Bridging of bone defects by massive bone grafts in tumorous conditions and in osteomyelitis. Clin. Orthop. 87:60, 1972.

36. Wilson, P. D., and Lance, E. M.: Surgical reconstruction of the skeleton following segmental resection of bone tumors. J. Bone Joint Surg. 47A:1629, 1965.

37. Younger, E. M., and Chapman, M. W.: Morbidity at bone graft donor sites. J. Orthop. Trauma 3:192–195, 1989.

38. Hu, R. W., and Bohlman H: Fracture at the iliac bone graft harvest site after fusion of the spine. Clin. Orthop. Rel. Res. 309:208–213, 1994.

39. Epersen, J. O., Buhl, M., Eriksen, E. F., et al.: Treatment of cervical disc disease using Cloward's technique: General results, effect of different operative methods and complications in 1,106 patients. Acta Neurochir. 70:97–114, 1984.

40. Takeda, M.: Experience in posterior lumbar interbody fusion: Unicortical versus bicortical autogenous grafts. Clin. Orthop. 193:120–126, 1985.

41. Weiland, A. J., Moore, J. R., and Daniel, R. K.: Vascularized bone autografts: Experience with 41 cases. Clin. Orthop. 174:87–95, 1983.

42. Dell, P. C., Burchardt, H., and Glowczewskie, F. P.: A roentgenographic, biomechanical, and histological evaluation of vascularized and non-vascularized segmental fibular canine autografts. J. Bone Joint Surg. 67A:105–112, 1985.

43. Shaffer, J. W., Field, G. A., Goldberg, V. M., and Davy, D. T.: Fate of vascularized and non-vascularized autografts. Clin. Orthop. 197:32–43, 1985.

44. Weiland, A. J., Phillips, T. W., and Randolph, M. A.: Bone grafts: A radiologic, histologic, and biomechanical model comparing autografts, allografts, and free vascularized bone grafts. Plast. Reconstr. Surg. 74:368–379, 1984.

45. Hayashi, A., Maruyama, Y., Okajima, Y., and Motegi, M.: Vascularized iliac bone graft based on a pedicle of upper lumbar vessels for anterior fusion of the thoraco-lumbar spine. Br. J. Plastic Surg. 47:425–430, 1994.

46. Hubbard, L. F., Herndon, J. H., and Buonanno, A. R.: Free vascularized fibula transfer for stabilization of the thoracolumbar spine: A case report. Spine 10:891–893, 1985.

47. Lascombes, P., Grosdidier, G., Orly, R., and Thomas, C.: Anatomical basis of the anterior vertebral graft using pediculated rib. Surg. Radiol. Anat. 13:259–263, 1991.

48. Hartmen, J. T., McCarron, R. F., and Robertson, W. W.: A pedicle bone grafting procedure for failed lumbosacral spinal fusion. Clin. Orthop. 178:223–227, 1983.

49. McBride, G. G., and Bradford, D. S.: Vertebral body replacement with femoral neck allograft and vascularized rib strut graft. A technique for treating post-traumatic kyphosis with neurologic deficit. Spine 8:406–415, 1983.

50. Rose, G. K., Owen, R., and Sanderson, J. M.: Transposition of rib with blood supply for the stabilization of spinal kyphosis. J. Bone Joint Surg. 57B:112, 1975.

51. Bradford, D. S.: Anterior vascular pedicle bone grafting for the treatment of kyphosis. Spine 5:328, 1980.

52. Goujon, E.: Researches experimentales sur les proprietes physiologiques de la moelle des os. Journal de l'Anatomie et de Physiologie Normales et Pathologiques de l'Homme et des Animaux 6:399, 1869.

53. Senn, N.: On the healing of aseptic cavities by implantation of antiseptic decalcified bone. Am. J. Med. Sci. 98:219, 1889.

54. Burwell, R. G.: Studies in the transplantation of bone: VII. The fresh composite homograft-autograft of cancellous bone. An analysis of factors leading to osteogenesis in marrow transplants and in marrow-containing bone grafts. J. Bone Joint Surg. 46B:110, 1964.

55. Burwell, R. G.: The function of bone marrow in the incorporation of a bone graft. Clin. Orthop. 200:125, 1985.

56. Nade, S.: Osteogenesis after bone and bone marrow transplantation: II. The initial cellular events following transplantation of decalcified allografts of cancellous bone. Acta Orthop. Scand. 48:572, 1977.

57. Nade, S.: Clinical implications of cell function in osteogenesis. A re-appraisal of bone graft surgery. Ann. R. Coll. Surg. Engl. 61:189, 1979.

58. Ashton, B. A., Allen, T. D., Howlet, C. R., et al.: Formation of bone and cartilage by marrow stromal cells in diffusion chambers in vivo. Clin. Orthop. 151:294, 1980.

59. Budenz, R. W., and Bernard, G. W.: Osteogenesis and leukopoiesis within diffusion chamber implants of isolated bone marrow subpopulations. Am. J. Anat. 159:455, 1980.

60. Pfeiffer, C. A.: Development of bone from transplanted marrow in mice. Anat. Rec. 102:225, 1948.

61. Owen, M.: The origin of bone cells in the post natal organism. Arthritis Rheum. 23:1074, 1980.

62. Vaughan, J.: Osteogenesis and hematopoiesis. Lancet 2:133, 1981.

63. Maniatopoulos, C., Sodek, J., Melcher, A. H.: Bone formation in vitro by stromal cells obtained from bone marrow of young adult rats. Cell Tissue Res. 254:317–330, 1988.

64. Lian, J. B., Stein, G. S.: Concepts of osteoblast growth and differentiation: Basis for modulation of bone cell development and tissue formation. Crit. Rev. Oral Biol. Med. 3:269–305, 1992.

65. Burwell, R. G.: The function of bone marrow in the incorporation of bone graft. Clin. Orthop. Rel. Res. 200:125–141, 1985.

66. Connolly, J., Guse, R., Lippiello, L., and Dehne, R.: Development

of an osteogenic bone-marrow preparation. J. Bone Joint Surg. *71A*:684–691, 1989.

67. Connolly, J. F., Guse, R., Tiedeman, J., and Dehne, R.: Autologous marrow injection as a substitute for operative grafting of tibial nonunions. Clin. Orthop. Rel. Res. *266*:259–270, 1991.

68. Friedenstein, A. J.: Determined and inducible osteogenic precursor cells. *In* Sognaes, R., and Vaughan, J. (eds.): Hard Tissue Growth, Repair, and Remineralization. New York Ciba Foundation Symposium II, Elsevier, 1973, p. 169.

69. Friedenstein, A. J.: Precursor cells of mechanocytes. Int. Rev. Cytol. *47*:327, 1976.

70. Friedenstein, A. J., Chailakhyan, R. K., Latsinik, N. V., et al.: Stromal cells responsible for transferring the microenvironment of the haemopoietic tissues. Transplantation *17*:331, 1974.

71. Healey, J. H., Zimmerman, P. A., McDonnell, J. M., and Lane, J. M.: Percutaneous bone marrow grafting of delayed union and nonunion in cancer patients. Clin. Orthop. Rel. Res. *256*:280–285, 1990.

72. Paley, D., and Young, M. C.: Percutaneous bone marrow grafting of fractures and bony defects. An experimental study in rabbits. Clin. Orthop. *208*:300–312, 1986.

73. Pfeiffer, C. A.: Development of bone from transplanted marrow in mice. Anat. Rec. *102*:225, 1948.

74. Ragni, P., Lindholm, T. S., and Lindholm, T. C.: Vertebral fusion dynamics in the thoracic and lumbar spine inducted by allogenic demineralized bone matrix combined with autogenous bone marrow. An experimental study in rabbits. Ital. J. Orthop. Traumatol. *13*:241–251, 1987.

75. Takagi, K., and Urist, M. R.: The role of bone marrow in bone morphogenetic protein induced repair of femoral massive diaphyseal defects. Clin. Orthop. Rel. Res. *171*:224–231, 1982.

76. Tiedeman, J. J., Walter, W. W., Connolly, J. F., and Strates, B. S.: Healing of a large nonossifying fibroma after grafting with bone matrix and marrow. Clin. Orthop. Rel. Res. *265*:302–305, 1991.

77. Tiedeman, J. J., Connolly, J. F., Strates, B. S., and Lippiello, L.: Treatment of nonunion by percutaneous injection of bone marrow and demineralized bone matrix. Clin. Orthop. Rel. Res. *268*:294–302, 1991.

78. Lane, J. M., Muschler, G. F., Werntz, J., et al.: The use of composite bone graft materials in a segmental femoral defect model in the rat. J. Orthop. Trauma *2*:57–58, 1988.

79. Yasko, A. W., Lane, J. M., Fellinger, E. J., et al.: The healing of segmental bone defects, induced by recombinant bone morphogenetic protein (rhBMP-2). A radiographic, histological, and biomechanical study in rats. J. Bone Joint Surg. *74A*:659–670, 1992.

80. Johnson, K. A., Howlett, C. R., Bellenger, C. R., and Armati-Gulson, P.: Osteogenesis by canine and rabbit bone marrow in diffusion chambers. Calci. Tissue Int. *42*:113, 1988.

81. Salama, R., Burwell, R. G., and Dickson, I. R.: Recombined grafts of bone and marrow. J. Bone Joint Surg. *55B*:402, 1973.

82. Salama, R., and Weissman, S. L.: The clinical use of combined xenografts of bone and autologous red marrow. J. Bone Joint Surg. *60B*:111, 1978.

83. Garg, N. K., and Gaur, S.: Percutaneous autogenous bone-marrow grafting in congenital tibial pseudarthrosis. J. Bone Joint Surg. [Br.] *77*:830–831, 1995.

84. Garg, N. K., Gaur, S., and Sharma, S.: Percutaneous autogenous bone marrow grafting in 20 cases of ununited fracture. Acta Orthop. Scand. *64*:671–672, 1993.

85. Muschler, G. F., Boehm, C., and Easley, K.: The harvest of osteoblastic progenitors from human bone marrow by aspiration: The influence of aspiration volume. J. Bone Joint Surg. [Am.]. (In review.)

86. Connolly, J., Guse, R., Lippielo, L., et al.: Development of an osteogenic bone marrow preparation. J. Bone Joint Surg. *71A*:684–691, 1989.

87. Tomford, W. W., Starkweather, R. J., and Goldman, M. H.: A study of the incidence of infection in the use of banked allograft bone. J. Bone Joint Surg. *63A*:244–248, 1981.

88. Friedlander, G. E., and Mankin, H. J.: Bone banking: Current methods and suggested guidelines. A.A.O.S. Instr. Course Lect. *30*:36–55, 1981.

89. Bos, G. D., Goldberg, V. M., Zika, J. M., et al.: Immune response

of rats to frozen bone allografts. J. Bone Joint Surg. *65A*:239–246, 1983.

90. Chalmers, J.: Transplantation immunity in bone homografting. J. Bone Joint Surg. *41B*:160–179, 1959.

91. Friedlander, G. E., Strong, D. M., and Sell, K. W.: Studies in antigenicity of bone. I. Freeze-dried and deep frozen allografts in rabbits. J. Bone Joint Surg. *58A*:854–858, 1976.

92. Halloran, P. F., Lee, E. H., Ziv, I., et al.: Orthotopic bone transplantation in mice. II. Studies of the alloantibody response. Transplantation *27*:420–426, 1979.

93. Langer, F., Czitrom, A., Pritzker, K. P., and Gross, A. E.: The immunogenicity of fresh and frozen allograft bone. J. Bone Joint Surg. *57A*:216–220, 1975.

94. Muscolo, D. L., Kawai, S., and Ray, R. D.: Cellular and humoral immune response analysis of bone-allografted rats. J. Bone Joint Surg. *58A*:826–832, 1976.

95. Friedlander, G. E., Strong, D. M., and Sell, K. W.: Studies of the antigenicity of bone. II. Donor-specific anti-HLA antibodies in human recipients of freeze-dried allografts. J. Bone Joint Surg. *66A*:107–112, 1984.

96. Lee, E. H., Langer, F., Halloran, P., et al.: The immunology of osteochondral and massive allografts. Trans. Orthop. Res. Soc. *4*:61, 1979.

97. Pelker, R. R., Friedlander, G. E., and Markham, T. C.: Biomechanical properties of bone allografts. Clin. Orthop. *174*:54–57, 1983.

98. Stevenson, S.: The immune response to osteochondral allografts in dogs. J. Bone Joint Surg. *69A*:573, 1987.

99. Bos, G. D., Goldberg, V. M., Powell, A. E., et al.: The effect of histocompatibility matching on canine frozen bone allografts. J. Bone Joint Surg. *65A*:89–96, 1983.

100. Stevenson, S., Hohn, R. B., and Templeton, J. W.: Effects of tissue antigen matching on the healing of fresh cancellous allografts in dogs. Am. J. Vet. Res. *44*:201–206, 1983.

101. Muscolo, D. L., Caletti, E., Schajowicz, F., et al.: Tissue typing in human massive allografts of frozen bone. J. Bone Joint Surg. *69A*:583, 1987.

102. Fideler, B. M., Vongsness, C. T., Moore, T., et al.: Effects of gamma radiation on the human immunodeficiency virus. A study in frozen human bone-patellar-ligament-bone grafts obtained from infected cadavers. J. Bone Joint Surg. [Am.] *76*:1032–1035, 1994.

103. Cornell, C. N., Lane, J. M., Nottebaert, M., et al.: The effect of ethylene oxide sterilization upon the bone inductive properties of demineralized bone matrix. Orth. Transactions *11*:1, 74, 1987.

104. Doherty, M. J., Mollan, R. A., and Wilson, D. J.: Effect of ethylene oxide sterilization on human demineralized bone. Biomaterials *14*:994–998, 1993.

105. Thoren, K., and Aspenberg, P.: Ethylene oxide sterilization impairs allograft incorporation in a conduction chamber. Clin. Orthop. Rel. Res. *318*:259–264, 1995.

106. Ijiri S., Yamamuro, T., Nakamura, T., et al.: Effect of sterilization on bone morphogenetic protein. J. Orthop. Res. *12*:628–636, 1994.

107. Pelker, R. R., Friedlaender, G. E., and Markham, T. C.: Biomechanical properties of bone allografts. Clin. Orthop. Rel. Res. *174*:54–57, 1983.

108. Oikarinen, J.: Experimental spinal fusion with decalcified bone matrix and deep-frozen allogeneic bone in rabbits. Clin. Orthop. *162*:210–218, 1982.

109. Bowen, J. R., Angus, P. D., Huxster, R. R., and MacEwen, G. D.: Posterior spinal fusion without blood replacement in Jehovah's Witnesses. Clin. Orthop. *198*:284–288, 1985.

110. Stabler, C. L., Eismont, F. J., Brown, M. D., et al.: Failure of posterior cervical fusions using cadaveric bone graft in children. J. Bone Joint Surg. *67A*:371–375, 1985.

111. Zdeblick, T. A., Cooke, M. E., Wilson, D., et al.: Anterior cervical discectomy, fusion, and plating. A comparative animal study. Spine *18*:1974–1983, 1993.

112. Kozak, J. A., Heilman, A. E., and O'Brien, J. P.: Anterior lumbar fusion options. Technique and graft materials. (Review.) Clin. Orthop. Rel. Res. *300*:45–51, 1994.

113. Nugent, P. J., and Dawson, E. G.: Intertransverse process lumbar arthrodesis with allogeneic fresh-frozen bone graft. Clin. Orthop. Rel. Res. *287*:107–111, 1993.

114. Brantigan, J. W.: Pseudarthrosis rate after allograft posterior lumbar interbody fusion with pedicle screw and plate fixation. Spine 19:1271–1279, 1994.

115. Fernyhough, J. C., White, J. I., and LaRocca, H.: Fusion rates in multilevel cervical spondylosis comparing allograft fibula with autograft fibula in 126 patients. Spine 16:S561–S564, 1991.

116. Jorgenson, S. S., Lowe, T. G., France, J., and Sabin, J.: A prospective analysis of autograft versus allograft in posterolateral lumbar fusion in the same patient. A minimum of 1-year follow-up in 144 patients. Spine 19:2048–2053, 1994.

117. Zdeblick, T. A., and Ducker, T. B.: The use of freeze-dried allograft bone for anterior cervical fusions. Spine 16:726–729, 1991.

118. Wetzel, F. T., Hoffman, M. A., and Arcieri, R. R.: Freeze-dried fibular allograft in anterior spinal surgery: Cervical and lumbar applications. Yale J. Biol. Med. 66:263–275, 1995.

119. Collis, J. S.: Total disc replacement: A modified posterior lumbar interbody fusion: Report of 750 cases. Clin. Orthop. 193:64–67, 1985.

120. Aurori, B. F., Weierman, R. J., Lowell, H. A., et al.: Pseudoarthrosis after spinal fusion for scoliosis. A comparison of autogenic and allogeneic bone grafts. Clin. Orthop. 199:153–158, 1985.

121. McCarthy, R. E., Peek, R. D., Morrissy, R. T., and Hough, A. J.: Allograft bone in spinal fusion for paralytic scoliosis. J. Bone Joint Surg. 68A:370–375, 1986.

122. Malinin, T. I., Rosomoff, H. L., and Sutton, C. H.: Human cadaver femoral head homografts for anterior cervical spine fusions. Surg. Neurol. 7:249–251, 1977.

123. Schneider, J. R., and Bright, R. W.: Anterior cervical fusion using preserved bone allografts. Transplant. Proc. 8 (Suppl. 1): 73–76, 1976.

124. Gepstein, R., Nakamura, K., Latta, M., et al.: Posterior spinal fusion with various types of bone grafts. Trans. Orthop. Res. Soc. 11:203, 1986.

125. Nasca, R. J., and Whelchel, J. D.: Use of cryopreserved bone in spinal surgery. Spine 12:222–227, 1987.

126. Savolainen, S., Usenius, J. P., and Hersenesniemi, J.: Iliac crest versus artificial bone grafts in 250 cervical fusions. Acta Neurochir. 129:54–57, 1994.

127. Fabry, G.: Allograft versus autograft bone in idiopathic scoliosis surgery: A multivariate statistical analysis. J. Ped. Orthop. 11:465–468, 1991.

128. Young, W. F., and Rosenwasser, R. H.: An early comparative analysis of the use of fibular allograft versus autologous iliac crest graft for interbody fusion after anterior cervical discectomy. Spine 18:1123–1124, 1993.

129. Bridwell, K. H., O'Brien, M. F., Lenke, L. G., et al.: Posterior spinal fusion supplemented with only allograft bone in paralytic scoliosis. Does it work? Spine 19:2658–2666, 1994.

130. Grossman, W., Peppelman, W. C., Baum, J. A., and Kraus, D. R.: The use of freeze-dried fibular allograft in anterior cervical fusion. Spine 17:565–569, 1992.

131. Bridwell, K. H., Lenke, L. G., McEnery, K. W., et al.: Anterior fresh frozen structural allografts in the thoracic and lumbar spine. Do they work if combined with posterior fusion and instrumentation in adult patients with kyphosis or anterior column defects? Spine 20:1410–1418, 1995.

132. Tiedeman, J. J., Garvin, K. L., Kile, T. A., and Connolly, J. F.: The role of a composite, demineralized bone matrix and bone marrow in the treatment of osseous defects. Orthopedics 18:1153–1158, 1995.

133. Whitehill, R., Wilhelm, C. E., Moskal, et al.: Posterior strut fusions to enhance immediate postoperative cervical stability. Spine 11:6–13, 1986.

134. Deaver, J. B.: Secondary bone implantation by a modification of Senn's method. Med. News 55:714, 1889.

135. Bradford, D. S.: Instrumentation of the lumbar spine. An overview. Clin. Orthop. 203:209–218, 1986.

136. Mackie, W.: Clinical observations of the healing of aseptic bone cavities by Senn's method of implantation of antiseptic decalcified bone. Med. News 57:202, 1890.

137. Miller, A. C.: A case of bone grafting with decalcified bone chips. Lancet 2:618, 1890.

138. Weir, R. F.: Antiseptic irrigation for synovitis of the bone: Im-

plantation of mucous membrane in traumatic structure of the urethra. Implantation of bone. Med. News 56:125, 1890.

139. Reddi, A. H.: Bone matrix in the solid state geometric influence on differentiation of fibroblasts. In Lawrence, J. H., and Gotman, J. W. (eds.): Advances in Biological Medical Physics. Vol. 15. New York, Academic Press, 1973, p. 1.

140. Reddi, A. H., and Huggins, C. B.: Biochemical sequences on the transformation of normal fibroblasts in adolescent rats. Proc. Natl. Acad. Sci. U.S.A. 69:1601, 1972.

141. Urist, M. R.: Bone: Formation by autoinduction. Science 150:893, 1965.

142. Urist, M. R., Hay, P. H., Dubuc, F., et al.: Osteogenic competence. Clin. Orthop. 64:194, 1969.

143. Urist, M. R., Iwata, H., Cecottie, P. L., et al.: Bone morphogenesis in implants of insoluble bone gelatin. Proc. Natl. Acad. Sci. U.S.A. 70:3571, 1973.

144. Urist, M. R., Nakagawa, M., Nakata, N., et al.: Experimental myosistis ossificans. Arch. Pathol. Lab. Med. 102:312, 1978.

145. Urist, M. R., Silverman, B. F., Buring, K., et al.: The bone induction principle. Clin. Orthop. 53:243, 1967.

146. Van de Putte, K. A., and Urist, M. R.: Osteogenesis in the interior of intramuscular implants of decalcified bone matrix. Clin. Orthop. 43:257, 1966.

147. Chalmers, J., Grey, D. H., and Bush, J.: Observations on the induction of bone in soft tissues. J. Bone Joint Surg. 57B:36, 1975.

148. Nathanson, M. A.: Analysis of cartilage differentiation from skeletal muscle grown on bone matrix: III. Environmental regulation of glycosaminoglycan and proteoglycan synthesis. Dev. Biol. 96:46, 1983.

149. Nathanson, M. A., and Hay, E. D.: Analysis of cartilage differentiation from skeletal muscle grown on bone matrix: I. Ultrastructural aspects. Dev. Biol. 78:332, 1980.

150. Reddi, A. H.: Cell biology and biochemistry of endochondral bone development. Coll. Relat. Res. 1:209, 1981.

151. Reddi, A. H.: Extracellular bone matrix dependent local induction of cartilage and bone. J. Rheumatol. 11:67, 1983.

152. Muthukumaran, N., and Reddi, A. H.: Bone matrix–induced local bone induction. Clin. Orthop. 200:159, 1985.

153. Somerman, M., Hewitt, A. T., Varner, H. H., et al.: Identification of a bone matrix derived chemotactic factor. Calcif. Tissue Int. 35:41, 1983.

154. Sampath, T. R., DeSimone, R., and Reddi, A. H.: Extracellular bone matrix–derived growth factor. Exp. Cell Res. 142:460, 1982.

155. Sato, K., and Urist, M. R.: Induced regeneration of calvaria by bone morphogenic protein (BMP) in dogs. Clin. Orthop. 197:301, 1985.

156. Urist, M. R., and Dawson, E.: Intertransverse process fusion with the aid of chemosterilized autolyzed allogeneic (AAA) bone. Clin. Orthop. 154:97–113, 1981.

157. Glowacki, J., Altobelli, D., and Mulliken, J. B.: Fate of mineralized and demineralized osseous implants in cranial defects. Calcif. Tissue Int. 30:71, 1981.

158. Glowacki, J., Kaban, L. B., Murray, J. E., et al.: Application of the biological principle of induced osteogenesis for craniofacial defects. Lancet 93:959, 1981.

159. Kaban, L. B., Mulliken, J. B., and Glowacki, J.: Treatment of jaw defects with demineralized bone implants. J. Oral Maxillofac. Surg. 40:623, 1982.

160. Wilkins, R. M., and Stringer, E. A.: Demineralized bone powder: Use in grafting space-occupying lesions of bone. Internat. Orthop. 2:71–78, 1994.

161. Flatley, T. J., Lynch, K. L., and Benson, M. D.: Tissue response to implants of calcium phosphate ceramic in rabbit spine. Clin. Orthop. Rel. Res. 179:246, 1983.

162. Lindholm, T. S., Ragni, P., and Lindholm, T. C.: Response of bone marrow stroma cells to demineralized cortical bone matrix in experimental spinal fusion in rabbits. Clin. Orthop. Rel. Res. 230:296–302, 1988.

163. Lynch, K. L., Ladwig, D. A., Skrade, D. A., and Flatley, T. J.: Evaluation of collagen/ceramic bone graft substitutes in dogs with spinal fixation. Trans. Soc. Biomaterials 13:196, 1990.

164. Ragni, P., Lindholm, T. S., and Lindholm, T. C.: Vertebral fusion dynamics in the thoracic and lumbar spine inducted by allogenic demineralized bone matrix combined with autogenous bone

marrow. An experimental study in rabbits. Ital. J. Orthop. Traumatol. 13:241–251, 1987.

165. Zerwekh, J. E., Kourosh, S., Scheinberg, R., et al.: Fibrillar collagen-biphasic calcium phosphate composite as a bone graft substitute for spinal fusion. J. Orthop. Res. 10:562–572, 1992.

166. Frenkel, S. R., Moskovich, R., Spivak, J., et al.: Demineralized bone matrix. Enhancement of spinal fusion. Spine 18:1634–1639, 1993.

167. Elves, M. W., and Salama, R.: A study of the development of cytotoxic antibodies produced in recipients of xenografts (heterografts) of iliac bone. J. Bone Joint Surg. 56B:331, 1974.

168. Plank, H., Hollman, K., and Wilfert, K. H.: Experimental bridging of osseous defects in rats by the implantation of Kiel bone containing fresh autologous marrow. J. Bone Joint Surg. 54B:735, 1972.

169. Rawlinson, J. N.: Morbidity after anterior cervical decompression and fusion. The influence of the donor site on recovery, and the results of a trial of surgibone compared to autologous bone. Acta Neurochir. 131:106–118, 1994.

170. Urist, M. R., Mikulski, A., and Leitz, A.: Solubilized and insolubilized bone morphogenetic protein. Proc. Natl. Acad. Sci. U.S.A. 76:1828, 1978.

171. Urist, M. R., Lietz, A., Mizutani, H., et al.: A bovine low molecular weight bone morphogenic protein (BMP) fraction. Clin. Orthop. 162:219, 1982.

172. Lovell, T., and Dawson, E. G.: BMP augmentation of experimental spinal fusion. Proceedings of the Orthopaedic Research Society, 1986.

173. Wozney, J. M., Rosen, V., et al.: Novel regulators of bone formation: Molecular clones and regulators. Science 242:1528, 1988.

174. Reddi, A. H.: BMP-1: Resurrection as procollagen C-proteinase. Science 271:463, 1996.

175. Kessler, K., Takahara, L., Biniaminov, M., et al.: Bone morphogenetic protein–1: The type I procollagen C-proteinase. Science 271:360–362, 1996.

176. Wozney, J. M.: The bone morphogenetic protein family and osteogenesis. (Review.) Mol. Reprod. Devel. 32:160–167, 1992.

177. Wozney, J. M., Rosen, V., Celeste, A. J., et al.: Novel regulators of bone formation: Molecular clones and activities. Science 242:1528–1534, 1988.

178. Schimandle, J. H., Boden, S. D., and Hutton, W. C.: Experimental spinal fusion with recombinant human bone morphogenetic protein–2. Spine 20:1326–1327, 1995.

179. Muschler, G. F., Hyodo, A., Manning, T., et al.: Evaluation of human bone morphogenetic protein 2 in a canine fusion model. Clin. Orthop. Rel. Res. 308:229–240, 1994.

180. Cook, S. D., Dalton, J. E., Tan, E. H., et al.: In vivo evaluation of recombinant human osteogenic protein (rhOP-1) implants as a bone graft substitute for spinal fusions. Spine 19:1655–1663, 1994.

181. Sandhu, H. S., Kanim, L. E. A., Kabo, J. M., et al.: Effective doses of recombinant bone morphogenetic protein in experimental spinal fusion. Transactions of the 42nd Annual Meeting of the Orthopaedic Research Society, Atlanta, February 18–22, 1996, p. 116.

182. Cunningham, B. W., Kanayama, M., Parker, L. M., et al.: Osteogenic protein versus autologous fusion in the sheep thoracic spine. A comparative endoscopic study using the BAK interbody fusion device. Transactions of the 42nd Annual Meeting of the Orthopaedic Research Society, Atlanta, February 18–22, 1996, p. 117.

183. Boden, S. D., Schimandle, J. H., and Hutton, W. C.: Lumbar intertransverse-process spinal arthrodesis with use of a bovine bone-derived osteoinductive protein. J. Bone Joint Surg. 77A:1404–1417, 1994.

184. Boden, S. D., Schimandle, J. H., and Hutton, W. C.: Evaluation of a bovine-derived osteoinductive bone protein in a non-human primate model of lumbar spinal fusion. Transactions of the 42nd Annual Meeting of the Orthopaedic Research Society, Atlanta, February 18–22, 1996, p. 118.

185. David, S. M., Gruber, H. E., Murakami, T., et al.: Lumbar spinal fusion using recombinant human bone morphogenetic protein (rhBMP-2): A randomized, blinded and controlled study. Transactions of the 42nd Annual Meeting of the Orthopaedic Research Society, Atlanta, February 18–22, 1996, p. 119–120.

186. Joyce, M. E., Roberts, A. B., Sporn, M. B., and Bolander, M. E.: Transforming growth factor–beta and the initiation of chondrogenesis and osteogenesis in the rat femur. J. Cell Biol. 110:2195–2207, 1990.

187. Baylink, D. J., Finkelman, R. D., and Mohan, S.: Growth factors to stimulate bone formation. (Review.) J. Bone Min. Res. 8:S565–S572, 1993.

188. Delany, A. M., Pash, J. M., and Canalis, E.: Cellular and clinical perspectives on skeletal insulin-like growth factor I. (Review.) J. Cell. Biochem. 55:328–333, 1994.

189. Canalis, E.: The hormonal and local regulation of bone formation. Endocr. Rev. 42:62, 1983.

190. Folkman, J: Clinical applications of research on angiogenesis. New Engl. J. Med. 333:1757–1763, 1995.

191. Lane, J. M., Muschler, G. F., Werntz, J., et al.: The use of composite bone graft materials in a segmental defect model in the rat. J. Orthop. Trauma 2:51–58, 1988.

192. Termine, J. D., Kleinman, H. K., Whitson, S. W. K., et al.: Osteonectin: A bone-specific protein linking mineral to collagen. Cell 26:99, 1981.

193. Nawrot, C. F., Campbell, D. J., Schroeder, J. K., et al.: Dental phosphoprotein-induced formation of hydroxyapatite during in vitro synthesis of amorphous calcium phosphate. Biochemistry 15:3445, 1976.

194. Veis, A.: The role of acidic proteins in biological mineralization. Ions in macromolecular and biological systems. In Everett, D. H., and Vicent, B. (eds.): Colston Paper 29. Bristol, Society Technics, 1978, pp. 259–272.

195. Bovan-Salvars, B. D., and Boskey, A. L.: Relationship between proteolipids and calcium phospholipid phosphate complexes in calcification. Calcif. Tissue Int. 30:167, 1980.

196. Stanford, C. M., Jacobson, P. A., Eanes, E. D., et al.: Rapidly forming apatitic mineral in an osteoblastic cell line (UMR-106-01 BSP). J. Biol. Chem. 16:9420–9428, 1995.

197. Weiss, R. E., and Reddi, A. H.: Rose of fibronectin in collagenous matrix induced mesenchymal cell proliferation and differentiation in vivo. Exp. Cell Res. 133:243, 1981.

198. Howlett, C. R., Evans, M. D., Walsh, W. R., et al.: Mechanism of initial attachment of cells derived from human bone to commonly used prosthetic materials during cell culture. Biomaterials 15:213–222, 1994.

199. Hughes, D. E., Salter, D. M., Dedhar, S., and Simpson, R.: Integrin expression in human bone. J. Bone Min. Res. 8:527–533, 1993.

200. Salto, T., Albeida, S. M., and Brighton, C. T.: Identification of integrin receptors on cultured human bone cells. J. Orthop. Res. 12:384–394, 1994.

201. Canalis, E.: Effect of growth factors on bone cell replication and differentiation. Clin. Orthop. 193:246, 1985.

202. Mundy. G. R., and Poser, J. W.: Chemotactic activity of the carboxyglutamic acid containing protein in bone. Calcif. Tissue Int. 35:164, 1983.

203. Jarcho, M.: Calcium phosphate ceramics as hard tissue prosthetics. Clin. Orthop. 157:259, 1981.

204. Flatley, T. J., Lynch, K. L., and Kenson, M. D.: Tissue response to implants of calcium phosphate ceramic in rabbit spine. Clin. Orthop. 179:246, 1983.

205. Jarcho, M., Kay, J. F., Gumaer, K. I., et al.: Tissue cellular and subcellular events at bone-ceramic hydroxylapatite interface. J. Bioengineering 1:79, 1977.

206. Dennison, H. W., and de Groot, K.: Immediate dental root implants from synthetic dense calcium hydroxyapatite. J. Prosthet. Dent. 42:511, 1979.

207. Dennison, H. W., de Groot, K., Kakkas, P., et al.: Animal and human studies of sintered hydroxyapatite as a material for tooth root implants. (Abstract.) Presented at the First World Biomaterial Congress, Baden, Austria, 1980.

208. Kent, J., James, R., Finger, I., et al.: Augmentation of deficient edentulous alveolar ridges with dense polycrystalline hydroxyapatite. (Abstract.) Presented at the First World Biomaterial Congress, Baden, Austria, 1980.

209. Klawitter, J. J., and Hulbert, S. F.: Application of porous ceramics for the attachment of load bearing orthopaedic applications. J. Biomed. Mater. Res. 2:161, 1971.

210. Hoogendoorn, H. A., Renooij, W., Akkerman, L. M. A., et al.: Long-term study of large ceramic implants (porous hydroxyapatite in dog femorae). Clin. Orthop. *187*:281, 1984.
211. Rejda, B. V., Peelan, J. G. J., and de Groot, K.: Tricalcium phosphate as a bone substitute. J. Bioeng. *1*:93, 1977.
212. Grower, M. F., Haron, M., Miller, R., et al.: Bone inductive potential of biodegradable ceramic in millipore filter chambers. J. Dent. Res. *52*:160, 1973.
213. Ragni, P., and Lindholm, T. S.: Interaction of allogeneic demineralized bone matrix and porous hydroxyapatite bioceramics in lumbar interbody fusion in rabbits. Clin. Orthop. Rel. Res. *272*:292–299, 1991.
214. Cameron, H. U., MacNab, I., and Piliar, R. M.: Evaluation of biodegradable ceramic. J. Biomed. Mater. Res. *11*:179–186, 1977.
215. Bhaskar, S. N., Brady, J. M., Getter, L., et al.: Biodegradable ceramic implants in bone. Oral Surg. *32*:294, 1980.
216. Ohgushi, H., Goldberg, V. M., and Caplan, A. L.: Heterotopic osteogenesis in porous ceramics induced by marrow cells. J. Orthop. Res. *7*:568–578, 1989.
217. Muschler, G. F., Huber, B., Ullman, T., et al.: Evaluation of bone-grafting materials in a new canine segmental spinal fusion model. J. Orthop. Res. *11*:514–524, 1993.
218. Muschler, G. M., Negami, S., Hyodo, A., et al.: Evaluation of collagen/ceramic composite bone graft materials in a spinal fusion model. Clin. Orthop. Rel. Res. (in press).
219. Zdeblick, T. A., Cooke, M. E., Kunz, D. N., et al.: Anterior cervical discectomy and fusion using a porous hydroxyapatite bone graft substitute. (Review.) Spine *19*:2348–2357, 1994.
220. Pintar, F. A., Maiman, D. J., Hollowell, J. P., et al.: Fusion rate and biomechanical stiffness of hydroxylapatite versus autogenous bone grafts for anterior discectomy. An in vivo animal study. Spine *19*:2524–2528, 1994.
221. Constantz, B. R., Ison, I. C., Fulmer, M. T., et al.: Skeletal repair by in situ formation of the mineral phase of bone. Science *267*:1796–1799, 1995.
222. Einhorn, T. A., Bonnarens, F., and Burstein, A. H.: The contributions of dietary protein and mineral to the healing of experimental fractures. J. Bone Joint Surg. *68A*:1389–1395, 1986.
223. Dickhaut, S., DeLee, J. C., and Page, C. P.: Nutritional status: Importance in predicting wound-healing after amputation. J. Bone Joint Surg. *66A*:71–75, 1984.
224. Jensen, J. E., Jensen, T. G., Smith, T. K., et al.: Nutrition in orthopaedic surgery. J. Bone Joint Surg. *64A*:1263–1272, 1982.
225. Lenke, L. G., Bridwell, K. H., Blanke, K., and Baldus, C.: Prospective analysis of nutritional status normalization after spinal reconstructive surgery. Spine *20*:1359–1367, 1995.
226. Coventry, M. B., and Scanlon, P. W.: The use of radiation to discourage ectopic bone: A nine year study in surgery about the hip. J. Bone Joint Surg. *63A*:201, 1981.
227. Nilsson, O. S., Bauer, H. C. F., and Brostrom, L. A.: Methotrexate effects on heterotopic bone in rats. Acta Orthop. Scand. *58*:47–53, 1987.
228. Silcox, D. H., Daftari D., Boden, S. D., et al.: The effect of nicotine on spinal fusion. Spine *20*:1549–1553, 1995.
229. Aprin, H., Bowen, J. R., MacEwen, G. D., and Hall, J. E.: Spinal fusion in patients with spinal muscular atrophy. J. Bone Joint Surg. *64A*:1179–1187, 1982.
230. Swank, S., Brown, J. C., and Perry, R. E.: Spinal fusion in Duchenne's muscular dystrophy. Spine *7*:484–491, 1982.
231. Bunch, W. H.: Muscular dystrophy. *In* Hardy, J. H. (ed.): Spinal Deformity in Neurological and Muscular Disorders. St. Louis, C. V. Mosby, 1974, pp. 92–110.
232. Clark, C. R., Keggi, K. J., and Panjabi, M. M.: Methylmethacrylate stabilization of the cervical spine. J. Bone Joint Surg. *66A*:40–46, 1984.
233. Emery, S. E., Hughes, S. S., Junglas, W. A., et al.: The fate of anterior vertebral bone grafts in patients irradiated for neoplasm. Clin. Orthop. Rel. Res. *300*:207–212, 1994.
234. Emery, S. E., Brazinski, M. S., Koka, A., et al.: The biological and biomechanical effects of irradiation on anterior spinal bone grafts in a canine model. J. Bone Joint Surg. [Am.] *76*:540–548, 1994.
235. Bouchard, J. A., Koka, A., Bensusan, J. S., et al.: Effects of irradiation on posterior spinal fusions. A rabbit model. Spine *19*:1836–1841, 1994.
236. Bassett, C. A. L., Mitchell, S. N., and Gaston, S. R.: Treatment of ununited tibial diaphyseal fractures with pulsing electromagnetic fields. J. Bone Joint Surg. *63A*:511, 1981.
237. Paterson, D.: Treatment of nonunion with constant direct current: A totally implantable system. Orthop. Clin. North Am. *15*:47–59, 1984.
238. Bassett, C. A. L., Mitchell, S. N., and Gaston, S. R.: Pulsing electromagnetic field treatment in ununited fractures and failed arthrodeses. JAMA *247*:263, 1982.
239. Bassett, C.: The development and application of pulsed electromagnetic fields (PEMFs) for ununited fractures and arthrodeses. Orthop. Clin. North Am. *15*:61–87, 1984.
240. Bassett, C. A., Pilla, A. A., and Pawluk, R. J.: A non-operative salvage of surgically resistant pseudoarthrosis and non-union by pulsing electromagnetic fields. Clin. Orthop. *124*:128, 1977.
241. Simmons, J. W.: Treatment of failed posterior lumbar interbody fusion (PLIF) of the spine with pulsing electromagnetic fields. Clin. Orthop. *193*:127–132, 1985.
242. Kahanovitz, N., Arnoczky, S. P., Hulse, D., and Shires, P. K.: The effect of postoperative electromagnetic pulsing on canine posterior spinal fusions. Spine *9*:273–279, 1984.
243. Nerubay, J., Marganit, B., Bubis, J. J., et al.: Stimulation of bone formation by electrocurrent on spinal fusion. Spine *11*:167–169, 1986.
244. Shore, E. M., Cook, A. L., Hahn, G. V., et al.: BMP-1 sublocalization on human chromosome 8. Molecular anatomy and orthopaedic implications. Clin. Orthop. Rel. Res. *311*:199–209, 1995.

Techniques and Complications of Bone Graft Harvesting

Lawrence T. Kurz, M.D.

L. Carl Samberg, M.D.

Harry N. Herkowitz, M.D.

In conjunction with surgery of the spine, harvesting autogenous bone graft is performed with reasonable frequency. Autogenous bone grafts may be used for arthrodesis of the posterior or anterior spine at any level (sacral, lumbar, thoracic, cervical). Although many sites are available for removal of autogenous graft (ilium, proximal tibia, fibular shaft, and greater trochanter), most commonly the ilium is used. Both anterior and posterior ilium sites are discussed, along with advantages and disadvantages of each. Techniques are also offered to avoid complications of the procedure.

POSTERIOR ILIAC CREST

Although there are numerous methods of harvesting autogenous bone graft from the posterior ilium, many of them (oblique sectioning of the crest,[31] cortical sub-

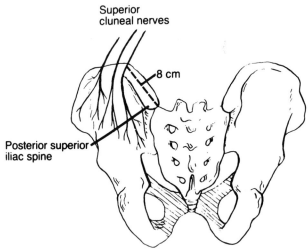

Figure 50–5. Posteroanterior view of the pelvis showing the superior cluneal nerves as they cross over the posterior iliac crest beginning 8 cm lateral to the posterior superior iliac spine.

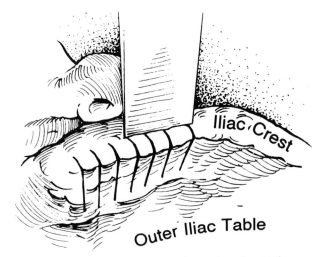

Figure 50–7. A straight osteotome is used to elevate the corticocancellous strips off the outer table.

crestal windows, and trapdoors) render only a portion of the cancellous bone available for harvest. The ideal method renders the maximum amount of nonstructural cancellous and corticocancellous bone available to the surgeon from a posterior approach. Gouges tend to provide uneven chips and strips of bone that may not be suitable for the first layer in contact with the transverse processes in the fusion bed. Curets have a similar disadvantage, as they may provide only small chips of bone that can be used as "filler" pieces. An osteotome works well by providing consistency in the size of pieces for bridging across the transverse processes. The osteotome should yield the desired pieces:

ideally, at least 6 cm in length, 5 to 7 mm in width, and a cancellous thickness of 5 to 10 mm.

Bone graft harvest is begun by accessing the posterior iliac crest through a separate skin incision (Fig. 50–5). Alternatively, if the laminectomy skin incision is long enough and distal enough, subcutaneous dissection may be possible, thereby avoiding a separate skin incision. In any case, the iliac crest periosteum is incised, and then subperiosteal stripping of the outer table muscles of the posterior ilium is performed, using a Cobb elevator in conjunction with electrocoagulation. After the muscles are stripped, a Taylor retractor is placed deep in the wound and oriented vertically, in order to avoid penetrating the sciatic notch. A sterile gauze or chain is then hung from the handle of the retractor, thereby suspending a small weight (usually

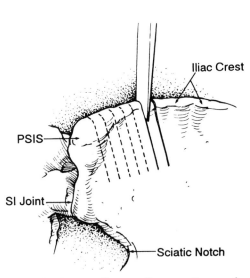

Figure 50–6. Corticocancellous and/or cancellous grafts may be removed from the outer table of the iliac crest (see also Figs. 50–7 through 50–9). Longitudinal cuts are made in the outer table of the iliac crest with a 1/2-inch straight osteotome.

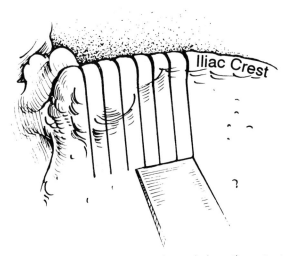

Figure 50–8. A curved osteotome is used along the outer table of the iliac crest, along the inferior border of the previously made longitudinal osteotomies.

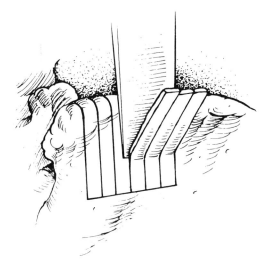

Figure 50–9. The bone graft harvesting is completed by removal of the corticocancellous strips.

5 pounds) and leaving both of the surgeon's hands free. The graft harvesting begins with a 1/2-inch straight osteotome malleted from the crestal edge in a ventral direction (Fig. 50–6). Only half of the osteotome's distal edge should project into the intramedullary cavity; the other half should project out of the outer table (see Fig. 50–6). This prevents excessive thickness of the cancellous layer attached to the undersurface of a corticocancellous piece. Successive vertical cuts of equal length are made approximately 7 mm apart. A 1-inch osteotome is then used to connect the cuts on top of the crest (Fig. 50–7) and at the most ventral extent of the vertical cuts (Fig. 50–8). Then, with the surgeon beginning at the top of the crest, the curved osteotome is malleted ventrally between the inner and outer tables of the ilium, thereby connecting the previous vertical cuts (Fig. 50–9). The surgeon removes the corticocancellous strips, and this leaves the entire cancellous

intramedullary cavity available for removal with gouges. Curets may then be used to remove whatever cancellous bone (in the form of chips and scrapings) is left.

ANTERIOR ILIAC CREST

A number of methods of harvesting autogenous bone graft are more suited to the anterior iliac crest, because they render only a portion of the cancellous bone available for harvest. However, these methods do have other uses.

Trephine curettage is a method of harvesting bone graft from either the anterior or the posterior ilium. It usually yields only cancellous bone, and usually in the form of curetings. A small incision is made over either the posterior superior iliac spine or the iliac tubercle, which is 5 cm posterolateral along the crest from the anterior superior iliac spine. The incision is carried down through the skin and subcutaneous tissue, and the periosteum over the iliac crest is incised. The outer and inner table muscles are stripped just slightly over the edge of the iliac crest. A rectangular window is fashioned in the iliac crest itself, with a 1/4-inch curved osteotome, by removing the cortex. This allows access to the medullary cavity of the iliac wing, and curets are used to remove scrapings of cancellous bone. The crest is much thicker anteriorly than posteriorly, but the area beneath the iliac tubercle is the thickest portion of the anterior iliac wing available for harvest. Appropriate size curets are used to remove all the cancellous bone available in the medullary cavity.

The trapdoor method of harvesting bone graft (Fig. 50–10) is best suited to the anterior ilium. A skin incision is made over the anterior iliac crest, and an incision is made into the periosteum overlying the outer aspect of the iliac crest. A 3/4-inch straight osteotome is used in a horizontal fashion, beginning at the outer periosteal incision, to make a cut in the cortex of the iliac crest through both tables. The periosteum and

Figure 50–10. Coronal section of the ilium indicating the trapdoor method of harvesting bone graft. The periosteum and fascial attachments of the iliacus and abdominal wall muscles remain intact on the inner edge of the horizontal cut through the iliac crest, thus allowing the crest to be "hinged back" like a trapdoor.

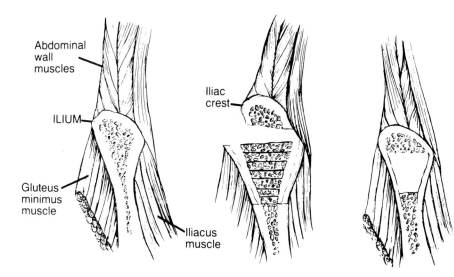

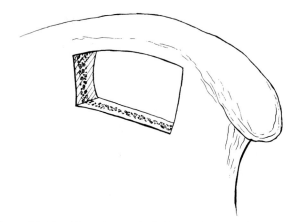

Figure 50–11. The subcrestal window technique of harvesting bone graft. The iliac crest is left completely intact.

fascial attachments of the iliacus and abdominal wall muscles must remain intact on the inner edge of the horizontal cut, thereby allowing the crest to be "hinged back" like a trapdoor. The medullary cavity is then available for harvest in any manner, and the gluteal and abdominal wall fasciae are reapproximated following harvest. This allows minimal, if any, altering of the contour of the iliac crest. This method renders cancellous strips and chips of bone available for harvest.

The subcrestal window technique (Fig. 50–11) of harvesting bone grafts is performed by making a skin incision over the anterior iliac crest, preferably near the iliac tubercle. The outer and inner table muscles are stripped subperiosteally from the ilium, and a small straight osteotome is used to fashion out the desired shape of bicortical ilium. This bone block can be of any size or shape, provided there is enough available in the ilium itself. Care must be taken with the osteotome not to penetrate through the iliacus muscle.

On occasion, full-thickness grafts may be harvested from the anterior ilium. When this is desired, both the inner and outer table muscles must be subperiosteally stripped. A skin incision is made just distal or proximal to the anterior iliac crest. Alternatively, if a retroperitoneal or thoracoabdominal approach to the lumbar spine has been performed, subcutaneous dissection over the iliac crest but superficial to the abdominal musculature avoids a separate skin incision. The periosteum is then incised overlying the anterior iliac crest, thus releasing the abdominal wall muscles from their insertion on the iliac crest itself. Stripping of the outer (tensor fascia lata and gluteus medius) and inner (iliacus) table muscles can be accomplished, thereby exposing the entire thickness of the ilium for harvest. Full-thickness grafts may then be taken using an oscillating saw or an osteotome.

FIBULA

Although the fibula is not as commonly used for bone grafting procedures as is the ilium, its harvest is no less important. Because of its location in the lower leg, the harvest must be meticulous to avoid interfering with ambulation. The harvest of the fibula is begun by exsanguinating the leg through elevation or use of a

Figure 50–12. Axial view of the lower leg depicting the fibro-osseous compartments, as well as the neurovascular structures.

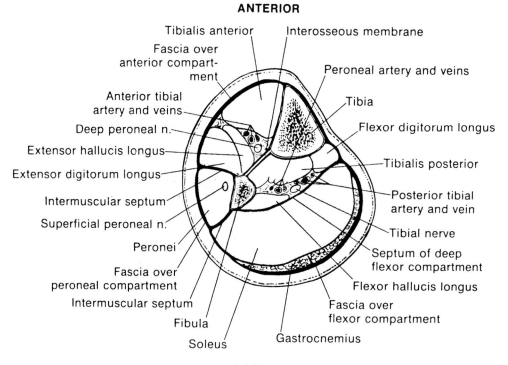

ANTERIOR

Tibialis anterior
Fascia over anterior compartment
Anterior tibial artery and veins
Deep peroneal n.
Extensor hallucis longus
Extensor digitorum longus
Intermuscular septum
Superficial peroneal n.
Peronei
Fascia over peroneal compartment
Intermuscular septum
Fibula
Soleus

Interosseous membrane
Peroneal artery and veins
Tibia
Flexor digitorum longus
Tibialis posterior
Posterior tibial artery and vein
Tibial nerve
Septum of deep flexor compartment
Flexor hallucis longus
Fascia over flexor compartment
Gastrocnemius

POSTERIOR

compression bandage. A tourniquet is inflated, and a skin incision parallels the posterior border of the fibula and should be centered at the junction of the middle and distal thirds of the fibular shaft. The incision is carried down through the intermuscular septum onto the fibular bone itself. Strict subperiosteal dissection elevates the peroneal muscles located on the anterolateral surface of the bone, the extensor digitorum longus muscle from the anterior surface, the tibialis posterior muscle from the anteromedial surface, the flexor hallucis longus muscle from the posteromedial surface, and the soleus from the posterior surface (Fig. 50–12). Although these muscles may not be individually recognizable, it is essential to stay subperiosteal when circumferentially stripping the fibula. After the bone is completely stripped, a graft may be harvested with either a Gigli or an oscillating saw.

RIB

Ribs are harvested almost exclusively for use during thoracoabdominal or transthoracic approaches to the spine. In fact, frequently a rib is removed as part of the exposure. Dissection through the latissimus dorsi and trapezius muscles brings the rib into view and allows for harvest. The periosteum over the rib is incised, either with the use of electrocautery or sharply with a scalpel (Fig. 50–13). Subsequently, a periosteal elevator is used to subperiosteally strip the superficial portion of the rib. A rib-stripper is then used to completely subperiosteally strip the pleural surface of the rib. This maneuver is performed all the way to the vertebral and sternal ends of the ribs. A rib-cutter is then used

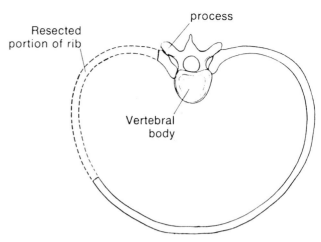

Figure 50–14. Axial view of the thoracic cage showing the region of resection of the rib.

to excise the rib at its costochondral and costovertebral junctions (Fig. 50–14).

COMPLICATIONS OF BONE GRAFT HARVEST

Ilium

Documented complications occurring at the iliac donor site include arterial injury, nerve injury, cosmetic deformity, gait disturbance, infection, hematoma, pain, fracture, peritoneal perforation, sacroiliac joint injury, hernia, and ureteral injury.

Arterial Injury

The superior gluteal artery exits the pelvis after it branches off the internal iliac artery. It subsequently enters the gluteal region through the most proximal portion of the sciatic notch, supplying the bulk of the gluteal muscle mass (Fig. 50–15). An arteriovenous fistula of the superior gluteal vessels has been reported[13] and documented by an arteriogram two weeks following surgical injury. The fistula was caused by penetration of the sharp tip of a Taylor retractor into the sciatic notch, which was used for exposure during the harvesting. Massive hemorrhage deep in the sciatic notch has been seen owing to errant penetration by an osteotome or gouge during harvest from the posterior ilium. In these cases, the injured superior gluteal artery usually retracts proximally into the pelvis. Although successful control of bleeding may necessitate removal of bone from the sciatic notch to expose the injured and retracted vessel, on occasion, a separate retroperitoneal approach may be necessary to gain access to the vessel for ligation.

Three major arterial structures that traverse the anterior surface of the iliacus muscle are the iliolumbar artery, the fourth lumbar artery, and the deep circumflex iliac artery (Fig. 50–16). Frequently, they anasto-

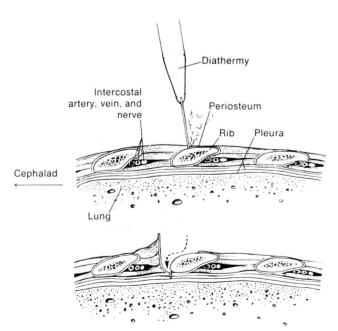

Figure 50–13. The pleura is entered from above the rib to avoid damage to the intercostal neurovascular bundle, which courses along the rib's posteroinferior border.

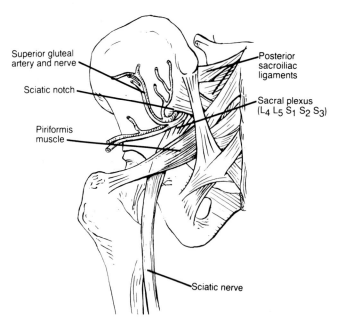

Figure 50–15. Posteroanterior view of the pelvis showing the neurovascular structures in the sciatic notch. Note that the sciatic nerve may still be present as individual components of the sacral plexus for 1 to 5 cm below the superior border of the notch. The superior gluteal artery and nerve course together and are the superiormost structures in the notch.

mose with one another and provide an extensive blood supply to the quadratus lumborum, psoas, and iliacus muscles. This vast network of blood vessels may be easily damaged during harvesting of bone grafts from the inner table of the anterior ilium. Blood loss can be minimized by paying strict attention to stripping the iliacus muscles subperiosteally.

Nerve Injury

There are seven nerves that may be injured during the harvesting of bone graft from the ilium: sciatic, superior cluneal, superior gluteal, lateral femoral cutaneous, ilioinguinal, iliohypogastric, and femoral.

Sciatic Nerve

The sciatic nerve is actually a condensation of the sacral plexus (L4–S3) and enters the gluteal region through the sciatic notch after exiting the pelvis (see Fig. 50–15). It subsequently courses down the posterior thigh. Because of its proximity to the sciatic notch, this nerve is prone to injury. Our cadaver dissections show that the sciatic nerve is frequently still present as five components of the sacral plexus for a distance as far as 5 cm distal to the proximal border of the sciatic notch (see Fig. 50–15). Therefore, an injury to the nerve near the notch may actually mimic a lumbosacral nerve root injury rather than a complete sciatic nerve injury.

Superior Cluneal Nerves

The superior cluneal nerves supply sensation to the largest area of the skin over the buttock (Fig. 50–17). These nerves are cutaneous branches that arise from the proximal three lumbar nerves. They cross the posterior iliac crest lateral to a point 8 cm lateral to the posterior superior iliac spine, after piercing the lumbodorsal fascia just proximal to the crest (see Fig. 50–5). Postoperative numbness over the buttock is usually a minor complaint because of significant cross innervation. However, we have encountered a number of patients whose painful neuromas were refractory to localized injections of steroids and subsequently required surgical excision for relief of symptoms. These nerves may be spared from injury by limiting the surgical field to within 8 cm of the posterior superior iliac spine during the posterior approach to the iliac crest.

Figure 50–16. Anteroposterior view of the lower abdomen and pelvis showing the course of the neurovascular structures of the iliac fossa; the femoral nerve; and the deep circumflex iliac, iliolumbar, and fourth lumbar arteries.

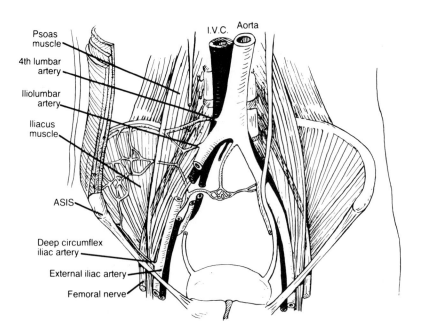

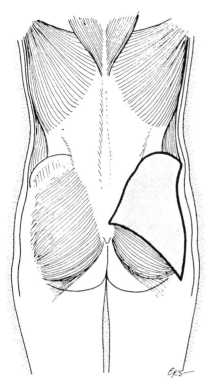

Figure 50–17. Posteroanterior view of the back. The dotted area depicts the cutaneous innervation of the superior cluneal nerves.

Superior Gluteal Nerve

Along with the superior gluteal artery, the superior gluteal nerve courses through the sciatic notch and supplies motor branches to the gluteus minimus and medius and tensor fascia lata muscles (see Fig. 50–15). Weakness of hip abduction may be the only manifestation of significant injury to this nerve in the region of the sciatic notch.

Lateral Femoral Cutaneous Nerve

Sensation to the lateral aspect of the thigh is provided by the lateral femoral cutaneous nerve (Fig. 50–18). It first traverses the psoas muscle and subsequently crosses the anterior surface of the iliacus muscle before passing into the thigh, near the anterior superior iliac spine. Normally, the nerve courses underneath the inguinal ligament and sartorius muscle, both of which attach to the anterior superior iliac spine (Fig. 50–19). In up to 10 per cent of cases, however, a normal anatomic variant causes the nerve to cross over the anterior iliac crest at a point up to 2 cm lateral to the anterior superior iliac spine (Fig. 50–20).[16] In this case, the nerve is subject to injury when harvesting bone from the anterior crest.

Pain, numbness, or paresthesias in the distribution of the nerve are manifestations of injury to the lateral femoral cutaneous nerve. This may present as classic "meralgia paresthetica."[17] Symptoms usually resolve within three months of injury when caused by a neura-

praxia owing to retraction of the nerve. However, sometimes the injury is secondary to inadvertent crushing or severing of the nerve during its course over the anterior iliac crest. In that case, numbness is frequently permanent. Local nerve blocks may sometimes successfully treat unresolved pain or paresthesias.

Ilioinguinal Nerve

The ilioinguinal nerve is a branch of the first lumbar nerve and subsequently crosses the psoas muscle and winds laterally around and over the iliacus and quadratus lumborum muscles (Fig. 50–21). At the level of the anterior iliac crest, it traverses the internal oblique and transversus abdominis muscles and supplies their lowermost portions with motor fibers. It then courses under the external oblique muscle, enters the inguinal canal, and descends to supply sensory fibers to parts of the penis, proximal and medial thigh, scrotum, and adjacent abdomen (Figs. 50–21 and 50–22). Two cases of ilioinguinal neuralgia have been reported following harvesting of bone graft from the inner table of the anterior ilium.[29] Traction on the nerve from vigorous retraction of the abdominal wall and iliacus muscles was probably the cause. Despite the fact that treatment with local nerve blocks was successful in both cases, prevention is preferable. Gentle retraction of the iliacus and abdominal wall muscles may help avoid injury to this nerve.

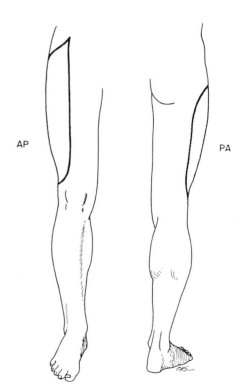

Figure 50–18. Anteroposterior and posteroanterior views of the leg. The dotted area depicts the cutaneous innervation of the lateral femoral cutaneous nerve.

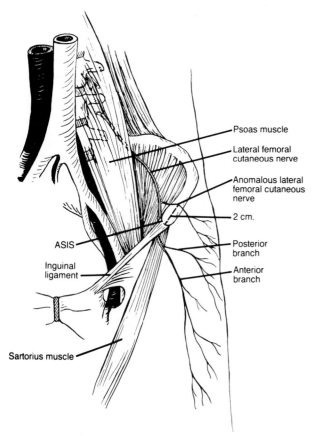

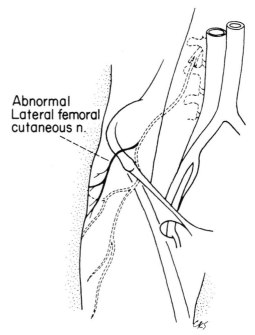

Figure 50–20. Anteroposterior view of the right hemipelvis showing an anomalous course that the lateral femoral cutaneous nerve may take. It may course over the iliac crest up to 2 cm lateral to the anterior superior iliac spine.

Figure 50–19. Anteroposterior view of the right hemipelvis showing the normal course of the lateral femoral cutaneous nerve.

site rarely occurs. However, problems may arise after harvesting full-thickness grafts from the anterior ilium that alter the contour of the iliac crest, leaving an unsightly deformity. The subcrestal window method

Iliohypogastric Nerve

The iliohypogastric nerve courses slightly proximal to the ilioinguinal nerve (see Fig. 50–21), supplies motor fibers to the lower portion of the abdominal wall, and supplies sensation to the skin surrounding the anterior two thirds of the iliac crest (see Fig. 50–22). Iliohypogastric neuralgia may arise from the same causes as those of ilioinguinal neuralgia.

Femoral Nerve

The femoral nerve (L2, L3, L4) passes behind the psoas muscle, courses over the iliacus muscle, and enters the thigh underneath the inguinal ligament (see Fig. 50–16). It supplies motor branches to the muscles of the anterior compartment of the thigh and sensation to the medial lower leg and foot and anteromedial thigh (see Fig. 50–22). The femoral nerve is vulnerable to injury in its location in the iliac fossa, and avoiding injury requires careful retraction and dissection during harvesting of bone from the inner table of the anterior ilium.

Cosmetic Deformity

After removing unicortical bone grafts or cancellous strips from the ilium, cosmetic deformity of the donor

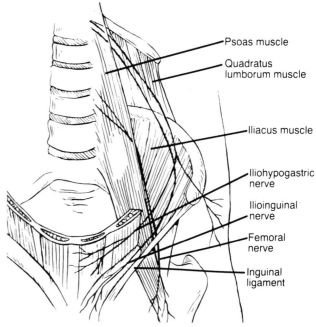

Figure 50–21. Anterposterior view showing the normal course of the ilioinguinal and iliohypogastric nerves.

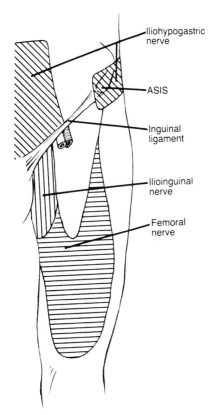

Figure 50–22. Anteroposterior view indicating the cutaneous innervation of the ilioinguinal, femoral, and iliohypogastric nerves.

(see Fig. 50–11) completely avoids the iliac crest. In addition, the trapdoor method (see Fig. 50–10) reconstitutes the crest and renders an excellent cosmetic result. In some patients, iliac crests may partially remodel following harvest.

Gait Disturbance

Some patients have difficulty climbing stairs or getting up from a sitting position following removal of bone graft from the posterior ilium.[2, 7] This is probably caused by weakness of the gluteus maximus muscle following subperiosteal stripping. Gait studies have shown that after having bone graft harvested from the anterior iliac crest, some patients have a dragging limp or an abductor lurch, which has been described as a gluteal gait. This is probably caused by extensive stripping of the outer table muscles, leading to weakness of the hip abductor muscles (primarily the gluteus medius). These gait disturbances can usually be prevented by securely reapproximating the gluteal fascia to the iliac crest periosteum.

Infection

Infection is no more likely at the donor site of iliac bone graft harvest than at sites of other orthopedic procedures. Deep wound infections are treated similarly with incision, drainage, and appropriate antibiotic therapy. During bone grafting of an infected recipient site, cross-contamination of the donor site must be avoided. Use of separate surgical instruments, as well as fresh gowns and gloves, should prevent this occurrence.

Hematoma

Bleeding from the cancellous bone of the harvested bed can be profuse, because the ilium is endowed with a rich vascular supply. The incidence of hematoma formation has been reported to be as high as 10 per cent in patients whose donor site wounds were not closed over suction drainage.[11, 27, 30] It has been demonstrated that hematomas occur less frequently in posterior sites than in anterior sites. This is probably because of the hemostatic effect of pressure on posterior wounds in the supine position.[12] The anterior iliac crest is very superficial, and local hemostasis from pressure tamponade is difficult.

There are many methods for hemostasis of the donor site. Microcrystalline collagen,[6, 23] bone wax,[1, 3] thrombin-soaked gelatin foam,[28] and injection of an epinephrine and saline solution[18] have all been used with varying success. Closed suction drainage for one to two days has decreased our incidence of donor site hematomas to less than 1 per cent. Although, theoretically, the exposed bone could continue bleeding indefinitely under suction drainage, we have never observed this in clinical practice, and we routinely drain all donor site wounds.

Pain

Pain is presented here as a complication because it is the most common complaint of patients who have undergone harvesting of autogenous bone graft from the ilium. It has been found that donor site pain can persist for a long time following harvesting.[14] A number of investigators[10] have found that as many as 15 per cent of patients have persistent pain at the iliac donor site more than three months after surgery. Although similar rates of pain have been seen in both posterior and anterior harvest sites,[3] the exact cause of the persistence of the pain is not known. Hypotheses such as the rich blood supply and innervation, degree of responsibility for weight bearing, and extent of periosteal dissection all fall short in their ability to explain this phenomenon. Common sense mandates that periosteal stripping and dissection be minimized in order to decrease the incidence of this complication.

Fracture

Although stress fractures of the ilium have been reported following bone graft harvest,[19] they occur rarely, and only after removal of full-thickness grafts from the anterior ilium. It is important to leave a wide margin of bone from the anterior superior iliac spine to prevent

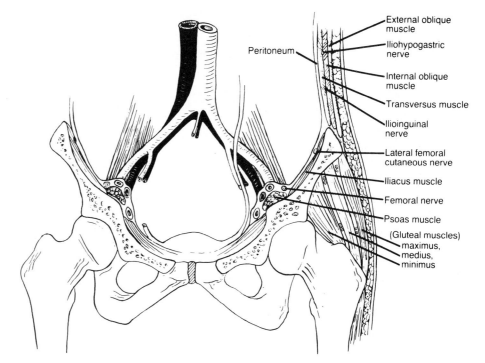

Figure 50–23. Coronal section of the lower abdomen and pelvis showing the neural structures in the iliac fossa and abdominal wall. The peritoneum is closely applied to the inner surface of the abdominal wall and iliacus muscles.

stress fracture owing to the downward pole of the sartorius and rectus femoris muscles. It is also important that the distal bone graft cut does not deviate anteromedially, in order to avoid breaking through the ilium anteroinferior to the anterior inferior iliac spine.

Peritoneal Perforation

Harvesting bone graft from the inner table of the ilium poses a threat to the integrity of the peritoneum, because it is closely applied to the inner surface of the abdominal wall and iliacus muscles (Fig. 50–23). Peritoneal perforation may occur after exuberant stripping of the periosteum on the iliac crest if one deviates into the abdominal wall and iliacus muscles during exposure of the inner table.

Sacroiliac Joint Injury

Most of the stability of the sacroiliac joint arises from its strong posterior ligamentous complex (Fig. 50–24). The complex is composed of deep interosseous ligaments that are continuous with the posterior capsule, and short and long sacroiliac ligaments more superficially (Fig. 50–25). During harvesting of full-thickness grafts from the posterior superior iliac spine, these ligaments may be injured or disrupted. Sacroiliac joint instability may manifest itself as joint subluxation and dislocation,[8, 21, 30] as well as mechanical and intermittent pain.

Hernia

Normally, the abdominal contents are prevented from herniating over the iliac crest because the abdominal

wall muscles are firmly attached to the periosteum (see Fig. 50–23). The broad iliacus muscle usually prevents herniation through defects in the ilium, because it lines the entire inner table of the iliac wing. During routine exposure of the inner table, however, the abdominal wall and iliacus fascial and muscular attachments to the crest are detached. This can lead to weakening of this "retaining wall." Herniation of abdominal contents has been reported only after harvesting of full-thickness grafts that include the iliac crest.[4, 5, 9, 15, 20, 22, 24–26] It has not been reported with subcrestal windows. Although the best treatment is prevention, numerous methods have been reported for repairing these defects. Strict attention should be paid to securely reapproximating the fascial and periosteal attachments, using heavy sutures and drill holes if necessary.

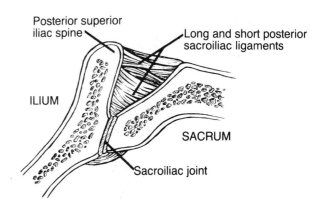

Figure 50–24. Horizontal section of the sacroiliac joint showing the posterior ligamentous complex.

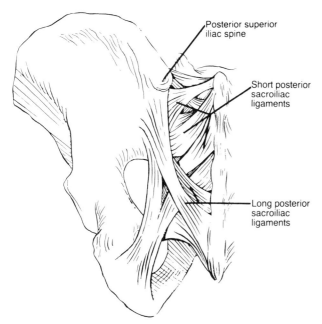

Figure 50–25. Posteroanterior view showing the posterior sacroiliac ligaments and their proximity to the posterior superior iliac spine.

Ureteral Injury

As it descends in the retroperitoneum, the ureter makes a sharp posterior angle at the sciatic notch (Fig. 50–26), just anterolateral to the gluteal vessels as they enter the sciatic notch. The ureter's proximity to these blood vessels renders it prone to damage coincident with an injury to these vessels. Postoperative hematuria, fever, hydronephrosis, and ileus have been reported in a patient following harvesting of bone graft from the posterior ilium.[13] Extensive electrocoagulation was necessary deep in the sciatic notch to control massive bleeding from an injury to the superior gluteal vessels. It was determined that the patient had a fulguration injury to the ureter, which resolved within five months without any treatment. It is obviously important to avoid the sciatic notch, because the ureter lies in close proximity to it.

Fibula

Injuries to the ankle joint or neurovascular structures may occur as complications of fibular harvest.

Common Peroneal Nerve Injury

The common peroneal nerve courses over the fibular neck, within the substance of the peroneus longus muscle, and then divides into superficial and deep branches. If dissection or resection of the fibula is carried out too proximally, this nerve may be injured.

Damage to Deep Neurovascular Bundles

There are two deep neurovascular bundles surrounding the fibular shaft that must be avoided. One contains the tibial/peroneal artery/vein and lies medial to the fibula (see Fig. 50–12). This bundle may be injured during stripping of the tibialis posterior muscle from the anteromedial surface of the fibular shaft. The second bundle contains the deep peroneal nerve/anterior tibial artery/vein and lies anteromedial to the fibular shaft, on the interosseous membrane (see Fig. 50–12). This bundle may be damaged if, after stripping the extensor digitorum longus and the extensor hallucis longus muscles, the surgeon strays anteromedially along the interosseous membrane.

Ankle Joint Injury

Fibular harvest should be carried out at the junction of the middle and distal thirds of the fibular shaft. Because the syndesmosis of the ankle joint ends about 10 cm proximal to the ankle joint itself, harvest should approach no closer than this 10-cm margin. Symptoms of instability of the ankle joint may arise from disruption of this syndesmosis.

Rib

Lung damage, intercostal neurovascular injury, and pain may arise as complications from harvesting rib as bone graft.

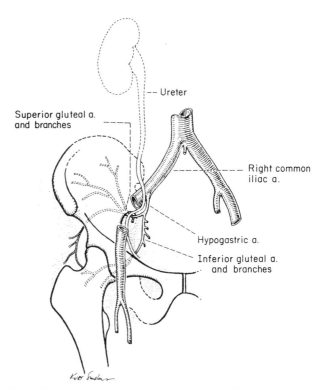

Figure 50–26. Anteroposterior view showing the course of the ureter. The sharp posterior angle it makes in the pelvis brings it in close proximity to the sciatic notch.

Lung Damage

Lung damage, if it occurs, is usually in the form of a direct fulguration injury. Although usually only minor problems arise from these burns, the lung should be inspected prior to closure, especially to detect any overt bleeding.

Intercostal Neurovascular Injury

The intercostal neurovascular bundle is usually injured from errant periosteal stripping of the rib. This vascular bundle, which is located in a groove on the posteroinferior edge of each rib (see Fig. 50–13), must be tied off or coagulated if hemorrhage occurs from an injury.

Pain

Severe intercostal pain may result from rib harvest. This pain tends to be incisional and to radiate from the costovertebral end of the resected rib. Shallow respirations and diminished clearance of secretions may result in the postoperative period, because patients frequently splint from the pain. Although pneumonia can occur, long-term problems are unusual. A nerve block at the costovertebral junction with a long-acting anesthetic may reduce the incidence of intercostal pain and its possible sequela of pneumonia. The block is usually performed before wound closure and can easily be repeated percutaneously in the early postoperative period.

CLINICAL RECOMMENDATIONS

Ilium

The sciatic notch should be avoided, because the superior gluteal nerve and artery, the ureter and the sciatic nerve lie close to this structure (see Figs. 50–15 and 50–26). When approaching the posterior ilium, a limited incision within 8 cm of the posterior superior iliac spine should avoid injury to the superior cluneal nerves and prevent formation of painful neuromas (see Fig. 50–5). In addition, an attempt should be made to preserve as much of the ligamentous structures as possible to avoid sacroiliac joint instability when taking full-thickness bone grafts from the posterior ilium (see Figs. 50–24 and 50–25).

Secure reapproximation of the gluteal fascia may help prevent the occurrence of a gluteal gait. When taking bone graft from the outer table, one should avoid penetrating the inner table to prevent injury to the neurovascular structures that are present in the iliac fossa overlying the iliacus muscle; these include the deep circumflex iliac, iliolumbar, and fourth lumbar arteries and the lateral femoral cutaneous, ilioinguinal, and femoral nerves (see Figs. 50–16 and 50–23). When approaching the outer table of the anterior ilium, the incision should remain within 2 cm lateral to the anterior superior iliac spine, in order to avoid the lateral femoral cutaneous nerve, the inguinal ligament, and

the sartorius muscle, which attach there, and to avoid fracture of the ilium (Fig. 50–27).

Secure closure of the fascia of the abdominal wall muscles may decrease the risk of herniation of abdominal contents through defects in the iliac crest. When the inner table of the anterior ilium is approached, careful retraction of the iliacus and abdominal wall muscles may prevent injury to the nerves that overly the iliacus muscle, including the ilioinguinal, femoral, and lateral femoral cutaneous nerves, as well as the peritoneum (see Fig. 50–23).

Strict attention to subperiosteal dissection may minimize bleeding and hematoma formation, because all the muscles involved have an extensive blood supply. Anteriorly, this includes attention to the iliolumbar, fourth lumbar, and deep circumflex iliac arteries (see Fig. 50–16); posteriorly, this includes attention to the superior gluteal artery (see Fig. 50–15). Suction drainage has been shown to decrease the incidence of significant hematoma formation.

Fibula

In order to avoid injury to the neurovascular bundles (see Fig. 50–12), one must remain strictly subperiosteal when harvesting fibular grafts. By resecting the fibula no closer than 10 cm proximal to the ankle joint, and thereby avoiding the syndesmosis, one may prevent instability of the ankle joint.

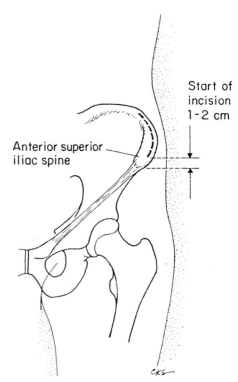

Figure 50–27. Approach to the anterior iliac crest. The skin incision should be at least 2 cm lateral to the anterior superior iliac spine.

Rib

Injecting long-acting anesthetic near the costovertebral junction before closing the wound may minimize postoperative pain and splinting. In order to avoid and most common complications of injury to the intercostal neurovascular bundle (see Fig. 50–13) and the lung, one should stay strictly subperiosteal when harvesting rib grafts.

SUMMARY

Strict attention to specific technical details of harvesting autogenous bone grafts, knowledge of the anatomic considerations, and an awareness of the possible complications should help the surgeon in planning the approach and in minimizing the risk.

References

1. Abbott, L. C.: The use of iliac bone in the treatment of ununited fractures. AAOS Instructional Course Lectures. St. Louis, C.V. Mosby, 1944, Vol. 2, pp. 13–22.
2. Abbott, L. C., Schottstaedt, E. R., Saunders, J. B., and Bost, F. C.: The evaluation of cortical and cancellous bone as grafting material. J. Bone Joint Surg. 29:381–414, 1947.
3. Bloomquist, D. S., and Feldman, G. R.: The posterior ilium as a donor site for maxillo-facial bone grafting. J. Maxillofac. Surg. 8:60–64, 1980.
4. Bosworth, D.: Repair of hernias through iliac crest defects. J. Bone Joint Surg. 37A:1069–1073, 1955.
5. Challis, J. H., Lyttle, J. A., and Stuart, A. E.: Strangulated lumbar hernia and volvulus following removal of iliac crest bone graft. Acta Orthop. Scand. 46:230–233, 1975.
6. Cobden, R. H., Thrasher, E. L., and Harris, W. H.: Topical hemostatic agents to reduce bleeding from cancellous bone. J. Bone Joint Surg. 58A:70–73, 1976.
7. Converse, J. M., and Campbell, R. M.: Bone grafts in surgery of the face. Surg. Clin. North Am. 34:375–401, 1954.
8. Coventry, M. B., and Topper, E. M.: Pelvic instability. A consequence of removing iliac bone for grafting. J. Bone Joint Surg. 54A:83–101, 1972.
9. Cowley, S. P., and Anderson, L. D.: Hernias through donor sites for iliac bone grafts. J. Bone Joint Surg. 54A:1023–1025, 1983.
10. Dawson, E. G., Lotysch, M., III, and Urist, M. R.: Intertransverse process lumbar arthrodesis with autogenous bone graft. Clin. Orthop. 154:90–96, 1981.
11. De Palma, A., Rothman, R., Lewinnek, G., et al.: Anterior interbody fusion for severe cervical disc degeneration. Surg. Gynecol. Obstet. 134:755–758, 1972.
12. Dick, I. L.: Iliac-bone transplantation. J. Bone Joint Surg. 28:1–14, 1946.
13. Escalas, F., and De Wald, R. L.: Combined traumatic arteriovenous fistula and ureteral injury: A complication of iliac bone grafting. J. Bone Joint Surg. 59A:270–271, 1977.
14. Flint, M. Chip bone grafting of the mandible. Br. J. Plast. Surg. 17:184–188, 1964.
15. Froimson, A. I., and Cummings, A. G., Jr.: Iliac hernia following hip arthrodesis. Clin. Orthop. 80:89–91, 1971.
16. Ghent, W.B.: Further studies on meralgia paresthetica. Can. Med. Assoc. J. 85:871–875, 1961.
17. Goldner, J.L., McCollum, D.E., and Urbaniak, J.R.: Anterior disc excision and interbody spine fusion for chronic low back pain. In American Academy of Orthopaedic Surgeons: Symposium on the Spine. St. Louis, C.V. Mosby, 1969, pp. 111–131.
18. Goldstein, L.A., and Dickerson, R.C. (eds.): Pelvis. In Atlas of Orthopaedic Surgery. New York, C.V. Mosby, 1974, pp. 450–453.
19. Guha, S.C., and Poole, M.D.: Stress fracture of the iliac bone with subfascial femoral neuropathy: Unusual complications at a bone graft donor site: Case report. Br. J. Plast. Surg. 36:305–306, 1983.
20. Lewin, M.L., and Bradley, E.T.: Traumatic iliac hernia with extensive soft tissue loss. Surgery 26:601–607, 1949.
21. Lichtblau, S.: Dislocation of the sacroiliac joint. A complication of bone grafting. J. Bone Joint Surg. 44A:193–198, 1962.
22. Lotem, M., Moor, P., Haimoff, H., et al: Lumbar hernia at an iliac bone graft donor site. Clin. Orthop. 80:130–132, 1971.
23. Mrazik, J., Amato, C., Leban, S., et al: The ilium as a source of autogenous bone for grafting: Clinical considerations. J. Oral Surg. 38:29–32, 1980.
24. Oldfield, M.C.: Iliac hernia after bone grafting. Lancet 248:810–812, 1945.
25. Pyrtek, L.J., and Kelly, C.C.: Management of herniation through large iliac bone defects. Ann. Surg. 152:998–1003, 1960.
26. Reid, R.L.: Hernia through an iliac bone graft donor site. J. Bone Joint Surg. 50A:757–760, 1968.
27. Sacks, S.: Anterior interbody fusion of the lumbar spine. J. Bone Joint Surg. 47B:211–223, 1965.
28. Scott, W., Petersen, R.C., and Grant, S.: A method of procuring iliac bone by trephine curettage. J. Bone Joint Surg. 31A:860, 1949.
29. Smith, S.E., De Lee, J.C., and Ramamurthy, S.: Ilioinguinal neuralgia following iliac bone grafting. Report of two cases and review of the literature. J. Bone Joint Surg. 66A:1306–1308, 1984.
30. Stauffer, R.N., and Coventry, M.B.: Posterolateral lumbar spine fusion. J. Bone Joint Surg. 54A:1195–1204, 1972.
31. Wolfe, S.A., and Kawamoto, H.K.: Taking the iliac bone graft. A new technique. J. Bone Joint Surg. 60A:411, 1978.

Augmenters and Alternatives to Autogenous Bone Graft

Allograft Bone in Spinal Surgery

Gray C. Stahlman, M.D.

Edward N. Hanley, M.D.

Eric Phillips, M.D.

Bone grafting is a common orthopedic procedure; approximately 200,000 of these adjunct procedures are performed annually in the United States. Most of these are autografts, but the use of allograft for bone grafting is becoming an accepted substitute for autogenous graft, particularly in spinal procedures.[13, 23, 29] The concept of bone preservation was considered as early as 1867 by Ollier.[26] It was not until 1942, however, that the first effort to store bone for use in elective surgery was undertaken.[19] Advances have been made in developing guidelines for donor selection, procurement, testing, preservation, and storage.[7, 14, 21, 30] Increased utilization has resulted from improved confidence in allograft performance, due in part to improved infectious disease screening, advances in storage methods, and the growing number of reports of successful clinical experiences. The desire to avoid complications at the donor site and technical advances in major reconstructive surgery, as well as patient request, have also influenced the increase in allograft usage.

Clinical and laboratory studies have confirmed that in many instances allograft bone has appropriate biologic and mechanical properties and can be used successfully in surgery.[11, 13]

BIOLOGY OF BONE GRAFT INCORPORATION

Material for bone grafting, no matter its form, should emulate as closely as possible the properties of host bone. Fresh autogenous bone is osteogenic, osteoconductive, and, at least to some degree, osteoinductive. The available materials for allografting generally lack one or more of these properties, which alters its incorporation (Table 50–4).

The process of incorporation of autogenous cancellous bone graft, like that of fracture healing and remodeling, begins with an inflammatory phase and organization of a fibrous clot, followed by clot absorption and marrow necrosis in one to two weeks. By two weeks, a fibrous tissue union is usually present, followed over the next few weeks by organization, callus formation, and osteochondral bridging. By three months, there should be new bone throughout the matrix, and marrow elements are mature; union is generally by bridging bone. Remodeling follows with cortical consolidation and retubulization. Incorporation of cortical bone follows a similar pathway but is markedly slower, given the more compact nature of the substrate, the fewer osteogenic cells and proteins, and slower revascularization.

The incorporation of allograft can take three biologic paths. The first, rejection, is of importance only if fresh allograft is used, because of the significant antigenic prosperity response to this material. The desired path is complete incorporation with no difference from the result seen in autograft. The last and most common path is often delayed but usually complete incorpora-

Table 50–4. PROPERTIES OF AVAILABLE GRAFT MATERIALS

	Osteo-inductive	Osteo-conductive	Osteo-genic
Autograft	Yes	Yes	Yes
Allograft			
Fresh	Yes	Yes	Yes
Frozen	?	Yes	No
Deep-frozen	?	Yes	No
Freeze-dried	No	Yes	No
Bone marrow	?	No	Yes
Ceramic	No	Yes	No
DEM	Yes	Yes	Yes

DBM, demineralized bone matrix.

tion. Allograft, particularly cortical allograft, has been shown to have a higher nonunion rate than that of autograft, owing to less internal repair by creeping substitution.[15]

DONOR SELECTION AND PROCUREMENT OF OSSEOUS ALLOGRAFTS

Safety, mechanical integrity, and convenience of use are important issues when choosing allograft over autograft. In 1979, the Musculoskeletal Council of the American Association of Tissue Banks published a review of bone banking and the clinical application of allograft bone. This review suggested that certain standards should be applied to ensure a safe supply of musculoskeletal allografts.

Of paramount importance in the selection and procurement of donor grafts is the exclusion of all possible infectious donor tissue. Transmissible diseases, particularly viral diseases such as hepatitis and the human immunodeficiency virus (HIV), are of most concern.[34] There are documented reports of fatal illnesses transmitted to the recipients of donor musculoskeletal tissue, including four cases of transmission of HIV, although there are 26 known cases of nontransmission from an HIV-infected donor.[8, 31] Buck and colleagues estimated in 1989 that the chance of obtaining a bone allograft from an HIV-infected donor who failed to be excluded by current HIV screening was well over one in a million.[6]

A comprehensive medical history of any potential donor must be obtained,[13, 14, 18] including previous hospitalizations, blood transfusions, risk factors such as intravenous drug use or high-risk sexual behavior, and cause of death. Systemic infection, malignant disease, and metabolic disorders that might compromise the quality of bone harvested must also be considered. Once a potential donor is identified, laboratory testing for bacterial, fungal, and viral microorganisms, as well as other diseases, must be carried out. Specific serologic testing must be performed for syphilis, anti-HIV, anti-HCV (hepatitis C or non-A, non-B hepatitis), and HbsAg (hepatitis B surface antigen). Retesting for HIV should be performed 90 to 180 days after harvest in order to exclude donors who may have been in the latency window at the time of donation.[2, 27] An unrestricted autopsy must be performed on every cadaver donor.[13, 14, 18]

Strict documentation of donor-related information is vital. A comprehensive medical history, laboratory and microbiologic test results, and description of the grafts (particularly of larger structural grafts such as the femur or tibia) with radiographs of the bone are important. Recipient information should be kept as well. Such painstaking record keeping is crucial, as it relates directly to quality control, continued tissue availability, and safe use of donor tissue.

If any one of the screening studies is abnormal, the donor should be rejected. If the screening studies are unremarkable, then bone harvest is performed under

Table 50–5. THE EFFECTS OF PRESERVATION ON ALLOGRAFT

	Fresh	Frozen	Deep-Frozen	Freeze-Dried
Antigenicity	+ + +	+ +	+ +	+
Strength				
Axial	+ + +	+ + + +	+ + + +	+ + +
Torsion	+ + +	+ + +	+ + +	+
Bending	+ + +	+ + +	+ + +	+
Longevity	+	+ +	+ +	+ + +
Cost	+ +	+ +	+ +	+ + +

sterile conditions, generally within the first 24 hours after death. Clean harvest with later sterilization is possible, but not preferred. Multiple bacterial and viral cultures must be obtained of each specimen at the time of harvest.

The harvest of allograft bone in a sterile manner is time- and labor-intensive and requires the use of an operating facility. Sterile harvesting obviates the need for secondary sterilization (by ethylene oxide [ETO] or high-dose radiation), which has been shown to degrade the biologic and mechanical properties of the bone. Treatment of allograft bone with antibiotics is not indicated, particularly because of concern for potential allergic response in the recipient.

Once it is processed and preserved (freezing or freeze-drying, in most cases), and once all the laboratory studies have been verified as negative (including the hepatitis core antigen and HIV), the bone is made available for clinical use.

PROCESSING, PRESERVATION, AND STORAGE

Bone grafts are generally preserved by freezing or freeze-drying. Fresh allograft is not generally used, because of significant antigenicity and high risk of disease transmission. Treatment with ETO or high-dose radiation has been employed but has been shown to substantially degrade both the biologic and the mechanical qualities of the preserved bone. Freezing is accomplished in several ways, including conventional mechanical freezing at $-15°$ C to $-30°$ C, deep freezing at $-60°$ C to $-80°$ C, or freezing with liquid nitrogen at $-160°$ C to $-180°$ C. Liquid nitrogen, however, requires periodic replenishment. Freezing renders the bone inert but does not compromise its clinical usefulness. Temperatures of $-80°$ C have been shown to preserve the enzymes in most human tissues without affecting the mechanical properties. If the bone is allowed to thaw prematurely, however, enzymatic degradation will occur.[11] Maintaining frozen allograft bone at a constant temperature requires refrigeration equipment with backup power supplies. Although the length of safe storage for allograft bone preserved by freezing is unknown, three years has been considered the accepted limit.[13, 14, 33]

To be freeze-dried, tissues must first be frozen, then sublimated and maintained in a vacuum. Freeze-dried bone may be shipped and stored at room temperature indefinitely if the vacuum containers are not violated. These grafts must be reconstituted with immersion in sterile physiologic solution.[21]

Freezing also decreases the antigenicity of bone tissue. There is some question whether freezing can eradicate viruses such as hepatitis or HIV.[13, 14, 31, 33] Freeze-drying decreases the antigenicity of bone and is thought to inactivate viral agents. While the structural architecture is maintained, bending and torsional stiffness are reduced (Table 50–5). Most modern experience with allografts in spinal surgery has been with frozen or freeze-dried bone.

CLINICAL RESULTS OF ALLOGRAFT BONE IN SPINAL SURGERY

Allograft bone is attractive to spine surgeons because its use negates donor site morbidity and because of the wide variety of shapes and sizes and the availability of an unlimited quantity of grafts. Autograft is the comparison standard material for bone grafting, with a higher healing rate and no risk for disease transmission.[17, 23] Autograft, however, is not always available in sufficient quantity, quality, or form for particular surgical procedures.

Donor site morbidity includes the potential for infection, persistent donor site pain, and functional impairment. Younger and Chapman noted an overall donor site morbidity rate of 8.6 per cent for major complications and 20.6 per cent for minor ones.[39] They concluded that this level of morbidity was justification enough for the use of synthetic or allograft bone if it was found to be of equal or greater effectiveness. Whitecloud, in a review of the literature up to 1978, found an overall donor site complication rate of 20 per cent.[37] This was compared with a 0.2 per cent complication rate associated with the operative site. Complications included hematoma, superficial and deep infection, and lateral femoral cutaneous nerve injury. Gore and Sepic reviewed their experience with anterior cervical fusions in 1987 and reported a 13 per cent incidence of donor site complications.[16]

Significantly less blood loss and shorter operative times have been demonstrated with the use of allograft.[3, 17] In addition, postoperative hospital stay was reported to decrease by 50 per cent (average 4.7 days with autograft versus 2.3 days with allograft).[17]

Clinical Results of Allograft in Fusion of the Cervical Spine

The most extensive experience with the use of allograft bone in the spine comes from anterior cervical fusion procedures. Brown and associates in 1976 reported the use of frozen allograft in anterior cervical fusion using the Smith-Robinson technique.[5] Fifty-three patients who had 76 cervical interspaces fused with frozen allograft were compared with 45 patients who had 63 interspaces fused with autograft iliac crest bone. They found a 94 per cent fusion rate in the allograft group, which was nearly identical to that of the autograft group, but noted that the allograft bone was subject to greater graft collapse than was autograft. Similarly, Rish and colleagues in 1976 reported their experience with freeze-dried allograft using the Smith-Robinson technique.[28] They found no difference in the clinical or radiographic outcomes between freeze-dried allograft and autograft bone. They had an 80 per cent fusion rate of allograft, compared with 82 per cent fusion of autograft. Similar results were reported by Schneider and Bright.[29] Cloward reported on 28 patients who received 50 gas-sterilized allografts after anterior cervical discectomy.[9] All had clinical improvement, and there was a 100 per cent fusion rate. He did note settling of grafts in two patients. More recently, 87 patients undergoing Smith-Robinson anterior cervical discectomy and fusion with either allograft or autograft tricortical iliac crest showed a 5 per cent nonunion rate with either graft at one year.[40] If multiple levels were fused, however, the nonunion rate at one year jumped to 17 per cent for autograft and 63 per cent for allograft. Graft collapse was seen in 30 per cent of allograft levels, and only 5 per cent of autograft fusions. The clinical outcome was equal.

Hanley and coworkers found that the form of the allograft bone affected the degree of graft collapse.[17] Allograft fibula averaged a 10 to 15 per cent rate of collapse, whereas tricortical cancellous grafts showed a collapse rate of 40 to 60 per cent. A retrospective review in 1991 of 126 multilevel cervical fusions with allograft or autograft fibular strut showed a high nonunion rate in both graft types.[12] Twenty-seven per cent of autografts and 41 per cent of allografts did not heal. Again, these rates increased as the number of levels fused increased. Young and Rosenwasser in 1993 described their 23 cases of cervical fusion with fibular allograft after discectomy.[38] Hospital stay was significantly reduced (5.4 days versus 7.25 days) when compared with that of patients with autograft fusion, postoperative pain was less, and there was a 92 per cent radiographic fusion rate at the last follow-up in the allograft patients.

The effectiveness of allograft bone for posterior cervical fusion is less well supported. Stabler and associates in 1985 reported poor results in posterior cervical fusion in children.[32] None of the seven patients achieved bony union. Four went on to bony fusion when reoperated on with autograft augmentation. Malinin and Brown commented in 1981 that freeze-dried allografts placed under tension posterior to the axis of rotation of the spine do not perform as well as those grafts placed under compression anteriorly.[23]

Freeze-dried fibular allograft bone may be the best grafting material, other than autograft, for interbody fusions of the cervical spine (Fig. 50–28). Fusion rates are universally good, nearing those of autogenous bone. The bone is easily shaped and is generally mechanically stable until healing occurs. The graft, whether allogeneic or autogenous, is merely acting as a spacer upon which new bone is formed.

Clinical Results in the Thoracic and Lumbar Spine

Use of allograft bone in the lumbar spine is an attractive alternative when the surgeon is faced with salvage reconstruction after major bone loss, as in replacement of vertebral bodies lost to infection, tumor (Fig. 50–29), or trauma (Fig. 50–30) or in the correction of congenital deformity. Autograft bone, particularly of the structural strength required in such cases, is generally not available in the quantities needed. Thus, allograft bone is often the best reconstructive option. Malinin and Brown argue that the rate of union of freeze-dried allograft placed in compression is comparable to that of autograft; thus allograft bone in anterior lumbar reconstruction should behave well.[23] Corticocancellous matchstick graft used on the tension side, however, showed significant graft resorption in their hands. Knapp and Jones in 1988 made the point that use of allograft in posterior lumbar fusion is probably appro-

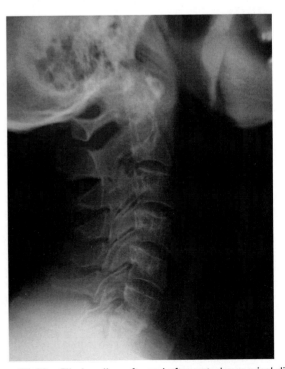

Figure 50–28. Fibular allograft used after anterior cervical disc excision.

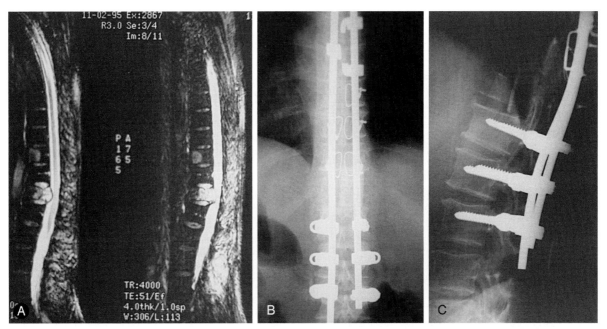

Figure 50–29. *A,* MRI of metastatic neoplasm at the thoracolumbar junction. Anteroposterior *(B)* and lateral *(C)* radiograph following posterior instrumentation combined with anterior reconstruction with allograft bone.

priate if strict attention is paid to the details of preparing the fusion bed and well-planned instrumentation is used.[20] Eleven patients with thoracic or lumbar fractures were treated with posterior spinal fusion with corticocancellous allograft and a variety of instrumentation. All went on to fusion. Kumar and associates reported on 32 patients undergoing anterior lumbar fusion with femoral strut allograft; 66 per cent showed radiographic union with flexion-extension radiographs, 12 per cent had an obvious nonunion with instability,

and graft subsidence averaging 4 mm occurred in 61 per cent of patients.[22] A "functional arthrodesis" was obtained in 88 per cent, however. Urist and Dawson found that chemosterilized, autolyzed antigenic-extracted allogeneic bone gave comparable results to autograft for posterolateral spinal fusion for degenerative conditions.[35] Wetzel and colleagues found that fibular strut allograft gave a 68 per cent clinical and 58 per cent radiographic success rate, as compared with an 87 per cent clinical and 65 per cent radiographic success

Figure 50–30. L1 burst fracture with comminution of the vertebral body and intrusion of bone into the canal, with neurologic deficit. *A,* Anterior decompression and fusion. *B,* Anterior fixation is supplemented with cortical allograft and cancellous autograft.

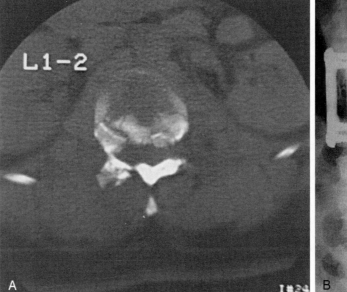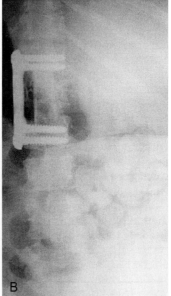

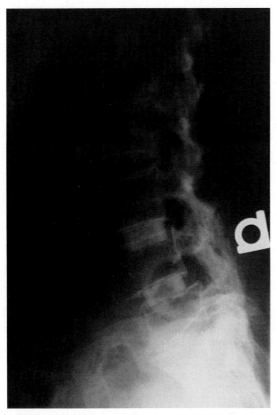

Figure 50–31. Anterior interbody fusion at L3–L4 and L4–L5 for treatment of pseudarthrosis of previous posterior decompression. Tibial cortical allograft rings are used. The inside of the allograft is filled with cancellous autograft from the patient's iliac crest. The allograft provides the structural support, and the autograft enhances healing potential.

rate of fibular allograft used in anterior cervical fusion.[36] The authors cautioned against using fibular strut allograft in the lumbar spine.

There are several reports of allograft bone used in fusion for scoliosis, particularly in cases of myelodysplasia. Surgery in these patients is fraught with a high rate of pseudarthrosis, and adequate autograft quantity may be limited. May and Mauck explored pseudarthroses after posterior fusion for scoliosis of several causes, and at six months found a 36 per cent pseudarthrosis rate with autograft and a 66 per cent rate when allograft bone was used.[24] The McCarthy, Dodd, and Bridwell groups, however, had good results with allograft, with little or no difference in fusion rates when compared with autograft used for posterior spinal fusion for neuromuscular scoliosis.[4, 10, 25] Aurori and colleagues found similar results when allograft bone was used in fusion for adolescent idiopathic scoliosis.[3]

Available scientific reports thus support the concept that allograft bone can be used with confidence in anterior lumbar or thoracic spinal surgery (Fig. 50–31). As in surgery of the cervical spine, allograft bone cannot be recommended in posterior lumbar spinal fusion alone. If adequate instrumentation is used, however, good results can be obtained. Again, patient factors such as bone quality, along with the quantity of bone needed, will dictate whether autograft bone will be adequate or must be augmented or replaced with allograft bone.

CONCLUSIONS

Allograft bone is a versatile and reasonable alternative to autograft for spinal fusion. Available scientific evidence supports the use of allograft in anterior spinal fusion in both the cervical and the lumbar spine. Its use in posterior spinal fusion, although less reliable than anteriorly, may be appropriate in limited circumstances but cannot be supported for the majority of situations.

To ensure continued availability of a safe and plentiful supply of allograft bone material, careful attention should be paid to proper methods of procurement and storage. A thorough knowledge of the characteristics of allograft as a substitute for autograft is essential to maximize surgical outcomes.

References

1. American Association of Tissue Banks: Standard for Tissue Banking. Arlington, VA, 1984, p. 27.
2. American Association of Tissue Banks: 180-day quarantine for HCV and HIV for living donors effective April 1, 1991. AATB Newsletter, 13:1, 1990.
3. Aurori, B. F., Weierman, R. J., Lowell, H. A., et al.: Pseudarthrosis after spinal fusion for scoliosis: A comparison of autogenic and allogeneic bone grafts. Clin. Orthop. 199:153–158, 1985.
4. Bridwell, K. H., O'Brien, M. F., Lenke, L. G., et al.: Posterior spinal fusion supplemented with only allograft bone in paralytic scoliosis. Does it work? Spine 19:2658–2666, 1994.
5. Brown, M. D., Malinin, T. I., and Davis, P. B.: A roentgenographic evaluation of frozen allografts versus autografts in anterior cervical fusions. Clin. Orthop. 119:231–236, 1976.
6. Buck, B. E., Malinin, T. I., and Brown, M. D.: Bone transplantation and human immunodeficiency virus: An estimate of risk of acquired immune deficiency syndrome (AIDS). Clin. Orthop. 240:129–136, 1989.
7. Burchardt, H., and Enneking, W. F.: Transplantation of bone. Surg. Clin. North Am. 58:403–427, 1978.
8. Centers for Disease Control: Transmission of HIV through bone transplantation: Case report and public health recommendations. MMWR 37:597–599, 1988.
9. Cloward, R. B.: Gas-sterilized cadaver bone grafts for spinal fusion operations. Spine 5:4–10, 1980.
10. Dodd, C. A., Fergusson, C. M., Freedman, L., et al.: Allograft versus autograft bone in scoliosis surgery. J. Bone Joint Surg. 70B:431–434, 1988.
11. Ehrlich, M. G., Lorenz, J. R., and Tomford, W. W.: Collagenase activity in banked bone. Trans. Orthop. Res. Soc. 8:166, 1983.
12. Fernyhough, J. C., White, J. I., and LaRocca, H.: Fusion rates in multilevel cervical spondylosis comparing allograft fibula with autograft fibula in 126 patients. Spine 16(10 Suppl.):S561–S564, 1991.
13. Friedlander, G. E., and Mankin, H. J.: Bone banking: Current methods and suggested guidelines. AAOS Instr. Course Lect. 30:36–55, 1979.
14. Friedlander, G. E., and Mankin, H. J.: Guidelines for the banking of musculoskeletal tissues. AATB Newsletter 3:2–4, 1979.
15. Goldberg, V. M., Stevenson, S., and Shaffer, J. W.: Biology of Autografts and Allografts in Bone and Cartilage Allografts: Biology and Clinical Applications. AAOS, 1991, pp. 3–13.
16. Gore, D. R., and Sepic, S. B.: Anterior cervical fusion for degenerated or protruded discs: A review of 146 patients. Spine 9:667–671, 1984.

17. Hanley, E. N., Harvell, J. C., Shapiro, D. E., and Kraus, D. R.: Use of allograft bone in cervical spine surgery. Semin. Spine Surg. *1*:262–270, 1989.
18. Hyatt, G. W., and Butler, M. C.: Bone grafting. The procurement, storage, and clinical use of bone homografts. AAOS Instr. Course Lect. *14*:343–373, 1957.
19. Inclan, A.: The use of preserved bone graft in orthopaedic surgery. J. Bone Joint Surg. *24*:81–92, 1992.
20. Knapp, D. R., and Jones, E. T.: Use of cortical cancellous allograft for posterior spinal fusion. Clin. Orthop. *229*:99–106, 1988.
21. Kreuz, F. P., Hyatt, G. W., Turner, T. C., and Bassett, A. L.: The preservation and clinical use of freeze-dried bone. J. Bone Joint Surg. *33A*:863–872, 1951.
22. Kumar, A., Kozak, J. A., Doherty, B. J., and Dickson, J. H.: Interspace distraction and graft subsidence after anterior lumbar fusion with femoral strut allograft. Spine *18*:2393–2400, 1993.
23. Malinin, T. I., and Brown, M. D.: Bone allografts in spinal surgery. Clin. Orthop. *154*:68–73, 1981.
24. May, V. R., and Mauck, W. R.: Exploration of the spine for pseudarthrosis following spinal fusion in the treatment of scoliosis. Clin. Orthop. *53*:115, 1967.
25. McCarthy, R. E., Peek, R. D., Morrissy, R. T., and Hough, A. J.: Allograft bone in spinal fusion for paralytic scoliosis. J. Bone Joint Surg. *68A*:370–375, 1986.
26. Ollier, L: Traité experimental et clinique de la regeneration des os et de la production artificielle du tissue osseuz. Paris, Masson, 1867.
27. Rank, A., Krohn, M., Allain, J. P., et al.: Long latency precedes overt seroconversion in sexually transmitted human immunodeficiency virus infection. Lancet *2*:589–593, 1987.
28. Rish, B. L., McFadden, J. T., and Penix, J. O.: Anterior cervical fusion using homologous bone grafts: A comparative study. Surg. Neurol. *5*:119–121, 1976.
29. Schneider, J. R., and Bright, R. W.: Anterior cervical fusion using preserved bone allografts. Transplant Proc. *8*(Suppl. 1):73–76, 1976.
30. Sell, K., and Friedlander, G.: Tissue Banking for Transplantation. New York, Grune & Stratton, 1976.
31. Simonds, R. J.: HIV transmission by organ and tissue transplantation. AIDS *7*(Suppl. 2):S35–S38, 1993.
32. Stabler, C. L., Eismont, F. J., Brown, M. D., et al.: Failure of posterior cervical fusions using cadaveric bone graft in children. J. Bone Joint Surg. *67A*:370–374, 1985.
33. Tomford, W. W., Ploetz, J. P., and Mankin, H. J.: Bone allografts of femoral heads: Procurement and storage. J. Bone Joint Surg. *68A*:534–537, 1986.
34. Tomford, W. W., Starkweather, R. J., and Goldman, M. H.: A study of the clinical incidence of infection in the use of banked allograft bone. J. Bone Joint Surg. *63A*:244–248, 1981.
35. Urist, M. F., and Dawson, E.: Intertransverse process fusion with the aid of chemosterilized autolyzed antigen-extracted allogeneic (AAA) bone. Clin. Orthop. *154*:97–113, 1981.
36. Wetzel, F. T., Hoffman, M. A., and Arcieri, R. R.: Freeze-dried fibular allograft in anterior spinal surgery: Cervical and lumbar applications. Yale J. Biol. Med. *66*:263–275, 1993.
37. Whitecloud, T. S.: Complications of anterior cervical fusion. AAOS Instr. Course Lect. *27*:223–227, 1976.
38. Young, W. F., and Rosenwasser, R. H.: An early comparative analysis of the use of fibular allograft versus autologous iliac crest graft for interbody fusion after anterior cervical discectomy. Spine *18*:1123–1124, 1993.
39. Younger, E. W., III, and Chapman, M. W.: Morbidity at bone graft donor sites. Orthop. Trans. *10*:494, 1986.
40. Zdeblick, T. A., and Ducker, T. B.: The use of freeze-dried allograft bone for anterior cervical fusions. Spine *16*:726–729, 1991.

Electricity

Neil Kahanovitz, M.D.

The use of electricity to promote osteogenesis began in the mid-1950s when Yasuda and colleagues first demonstrated increased callus formation at the site of a cathode or negative electrode experimentally placed in the long bone in an animal model.[21] Since this early interest, several hundred studies have been published on the experimental and clinical use of electricity to enhance primary fracture healing and pseudarthrosis repair. Electrical stimulation has now become an accepted treatment adjunct in patients with established pseudarthrosis of the long bones.

As the number of basic research and clinical studies examining the use of electrical stimulation to improve the success of spinal fusion increases, the acceptance and popularity of electrical stimulation to enhance the healing of spinal fusions continue to grow. Both direct-current electrical stimulation and pulsed electromagnetic fields are currently in use and have been shown to be safe and, for specific indications, efficacious in promoting improved osteogenesis over nonstimulated spinal fusions.

BASIC RESEARCH

Most in vitro and animal studies have examined the effects of electricity on long bones. Although the process is not completely understood, the effects of stress and, therefore, fracture healing produce electrical signals. The addition of externally applied electricity appears to enhance this normal process of osteogenesis and bone repair. An applied direct current between 5 and 20 microamperes appears to result in the maximal amount of bone formation typically present around the cathode or negative electrode.[20]

Many in vitro and experimental animal studies have been performed, examining the effects of electrical stimulation on the musculoskeletal system.[1] Fewer experimental studies have directly examined the primary effects of electrical stimulation on spinal fusion in a controlled experimental setting.

In 1984, Kahanovitz and associates examined the effects of electromagnetic pulsing on canine lumbar spinal fusions.[7] The spinal fusions were performed posteriorly with standard midline and facet fusion augmented by Harrington distraction-type internal fixation. The initial histologic and radiographic studies showed an accelerated osteogenic response in the stimulated animals at six and nine weeks. However, by 12 and 15 weeks, both the stimulated and nonstimulated groups had solid bony fusion and were radiographically and histologically indistinguishable.

In 1986, Nerubay and colleagues reported the results of direct-current electrical stimulation on lumbar spinal fusion in young swine.[15] At one month postoperatively, there were no statistical differences in the histologic or radiographic appearance of the fusions. However, by two months there was a statistically significant improvement in the quality of the fusion mass in stimulated compared with nonstimulated controls.

Similar good results were found in a later experimental study reported in 1990 by Kahanovitz and Arnoczky on the efficacy of direct-current electrical stimulation (DCES) to enhance canine spinal fusions.[6] Lumbar facet fusions were performed in adult mongrel dogs. An electrode was placed across each facet fusion, but only half of the electrodes were functioning and delivered 5 microamperes of direct current to the fusion site. At two, four, and six weeks, there were no demonstrable radiographic or histologic differences between the stimulated and control specimens. However, by 12 weeks, every stimulated facet fusion showed radiographic and histologic evidence of solid bony fusion, whereas none of the control specimens showed evidence of solid fusion.

Using the same experimental animal model, Kahanovitz and Arnoczky attempted to improve the rate and quality of fusion by increasing the direct-current density delivered to the fusion mass.[5] Although all direct-current-stimulated specimens had solid fusions by 12 weeks, a five- and 15-fold increase in current density resulted in significantly improved fusion quality at six and nine weeks over the previously tested and proven direct-current stimulator. Not only did direct-current stimulation result in solid arthrodesis, but increasing the current density improved both the quality and the rapidity of fusion, without any detectable deleterious effects on the adjacent bony or soft tissues.

After the initial attempt to improve fusion success with a pulsing electromagnetic field (PEMF) failed, in 1994 Kahanovitz and associates changed the PEMF from the previously used bone healing signal to a fresh fracture healing signal.[8] Unfortunately, as with the bone healing signal, the fresh fracture healing signal failed to provide any improvement in the stimulated group compared with the control group. Thus neither the bone healing signal nor the fresh fracture healing signal was able to improve the success of primary posterior spinal fusions in a controlled experimental canine model.

One other study examining the use of PEMF as an adjunct to posterolateral spinal fusion in canines reported an initial improved response to healing in the stimulated group, but by the final follow-up at 24 weeks, there was no apparent difference between the stimulated and control groups' rates of successful fusion.[4]

Although the number of experimental studies examining the effects of either DCES or PEMF on the healing of posterior spinal fusions is small, there are no studies examining the usefulness of either DCES or PEMF in an anterior spinal fusion model. In posterior and posterolateral spinal fusions, the experimental results of electromagnetic pulsing seem to indicate an improved early osteogenic response compared with nonstimulated controls. However, the long-term benefits did not appear to be beneficial in studies utilizing PEMF to improve the success of posterior or posterolateral spinal fusion in a controlled experimental setting. Conversely, all studies observing the effects of direct current on lumbar spinal fusion showed conclusive experimental evidence supporting the use of implantable DCES to enhance lumbar spinal fusion.

DIRECT-CURRENT STIMULATION

The first clinical study examining the results of DCES was reported by Dwyer and associates in 1974.[3] Forty of 47 patients (85 per cent) were found to have solid fusion after stimulation. This compared favorably to an unpublished but extensive review by Evans of 31 papers examining lumbosacral fusions in 3383 patients presented at the International Society for the Study of the Lumbar Spine in 1981. The overall success rate was reported to be 74 per cent.

In 1982, a nonrandomized multicenter study examining results of direct-current stimulation in 84 patients was reported.[11] Eighty per cent of these patients had previous spinal surgery, and 55 per cent had pseudarthrosis. Although both previous surgery and established pseudarthrosis are well known to decrease the expected rate of fusion, 91 per cent of the patients were found to have a solid fusion at final follow-up. An age- and sex-matched control group had a significantly lower success rate of only 81 per cent.

In 1988, Kane reported a randomized prospective study consisting of 59 patients considered at high risk for pseudarthrosis formation.[10] These patients included those with previous failed fusions, Grade II or worse spondylolisthesis, or multiple-level fusions. The fusion rate at follow-up for the 20 control patients was 54 per cent, and the fusion rate for the 31 stimulation patients was 81 per cent. Kane also reported a nonrandom multicenter group of 116 patients treated with electrical stimulation to enhance the rate of spinal fusion.[10] The overall rate of fusion was 93 per cent. Of the 29 patients in this group with previous fusion attempts, the success rate was 87 per cent.

More recent studies involving the use of DCES to enhance posterolateral spinal fusions have reported results similar to those reported previously. In a retrospective study, Pettine found an overall success rate of 89 per cent in patients undergoing posterolateral spinal fusions augmented with DCES.[16] Tejano and coworkers examined the effects of DCES on 143 patients undergoing noninstrumented multilevel posterolateral spinal fusions.[19] The overall success rate was 91 per cent in the stimulated groups at five-year follow-up.

The only study examining the results of adjunctive DCES to improve the outcome of anterior spinal fusion found similar success rates.[13] Patients undergoing anterior interbody fusion either by an anterior interbody approach or by a posterior lumbar interbody approach were found to have a 93 per cent fusion success rate. This was significantly higher than in those patients surgically treated in a similar manner but without DCES.

The DCES device appears to be safe. There have been no reports of any early or late complications associated with its use. Both the basic science and the clinical studies show a rather clear-cut advantage for the use of DCES to enhance lumbar spinal fusion, particularly in those patients believed to be at high risk for developing pseudarthrosis.

Technique

Implantation of the device is simple and requires little additional operative time. After preparation of the fusion site, a thin layer of corticocancellous bone graft is placed between the transverse processes or ala to be fused. The single electrode is then coiled to take advantage of the increase in contact surface area. The electrode is placed in the fusion area, extending from the distal to the proximal extent of the fusion. This is done bilaterally. The generator pack is placed subcutaneously, and the surgical wound is closed in a routine manner. At nine months postoperatively, the stimulator may be removed under local anesthesia at the discretion of the surgeon. Normally, portions of the electrode remain encased in the fusion mass. There have been no reports of morbidity due to these retained electrodes after long-term follow-up.

There is no contraindication to using DCES in the presence of internal fixation devices, as long as the electrode is not in contact with the exposed metal. In fact, a recent study examining the cost-effectiveness of DCES in a large group of patients found that less money and less time were spent following the initial hospitalization for fusion when both DCES and internal fixation were used at the time of the primary fusion.[9]

PULSING ELECTROMAGNETIC FIELDS

The use of PEMFs to enhance spinal fusion in high-risk patients has not gained as wide acceptance as the direct-current method. Although it is not invasive, its success is dependent solely on patient acceptance and compliance. The device is normally worn eight to 10 hours per day for six to eight months. The external placement of the device and the length of daily treatment are often not well accepted by the patient, adversely affecting the compliance level. In addition, the laboratory data do not compare favorably with the success found in the basic research data examining direct-current stimulation as an adjunct to posterior spinal fusion.[7, 8]

Despite these apparent drawbacks, several clinical studies have reported varying results with electromagnetic pulsing to enhance posterior spinal fusion healing. In 1985, Simmons reported a 77 per cent success rate in achieving solid interbody fusion in 13 patients with previous failed posterior lumbar interbody fusions.[17] Brodsky and Khalil reported a 36 per cent success rate of fusion in 30 patients with established lumbar spinal pseudarthrosis.[2]

Mooney reported a large multicenter study examining the results of the immediate postoperative use of an external PEMF to enhance the healing of either anterior lumbar interbody fusions or posterior lumbar interbody fusions in 195 patients.[14] None of the patients in the study underwent posterior fusions. The results were similar to those reported for direct-current-stimulated posterior fusions, with a 92 per cent success rate.

In 1989, Lee reported a 67 per cent success rate of posterior pseudarthrosis repair utilizing a PEMF.[12] These results fell short of Simmons's 77 per cent success rate for pseudarthrosis repair anteriorly. In the same year, Simmons and colleagues reported the results of using PEMF as an adjunct to attempted posterolateral fusion.[18] Successful fusion was found in only 71 per cent of patients. This was significantly lower than the 92 per cent success rate reported by Mooney using a PEMF in anterior interbody fusions or the rate of success in posterior spinal fusions augmented with direct-current stimulation.[10, 14]

The use of PEMF as an adjunct to enhance posterior and posterolateral spinal fusions does not have the favorable basic science or clinical validation that DCES has. However, there is clinical evidence that PEMF is useful in improving the rate of healing of anterior interbody fusions.[16] As opposed to PEMF, it does appear that DCES is a reliable treatment adjunct in patients undergoing either posterior or anterior spinal fusion.

References

1. Black, J.: Electrical Stimulation, Its Role in Repair and Remodeling of the Musculoskeletal System. New York, Praeger, 1987, pp. 103–144.
2. Brodksy, A. E., and Khalil, M. A.: Preliminary report on the use of EBI. Pulsing electromagnetic field therapy for treatment of pseudarthrosis of lumbar spine fusion. Presented at the North American Spine Society, Banff, Canada, June 28, 1987.
3. Dwyer, A. F., Yau, A. C., and Jeffcoat, K. W.: Use of direct current in spinal fusion. J. Bone Joint Surg. 56A:442, 1974.
4. Ito, M., Fay, Y., Edwards, W. T., and Yuan, H. A.: The effect of pulsed electromagnetic fields on posterolateral fusions and device related osteopenia. Poster presented at ISSLS, Seattle, 1994.
5. Kahanovitz, N., and Arnoczky, S. P.: The effect of varied direct current electrical densities on the healing of posterior spinal fusion in dogs. Presented at the American Academy of Orthopaedic Surgeons, Atlanta, February 1996.
6. Kahanovitz, N., and Arnoczky, S. P.: The efficacy of direct current electrical stimulation to enhance canine spinal fusions. Clin. Orthop. 251:295–299, 1990.
7. Kahanovitz, N., Arnoczky, S. P., Hulse, D., and Shires, P. K.: The effect of postoperative electromagnetic pulsing on canine posterior spinal fusions. Spine 9:273–279, 1984.
8. Kahanovitz, N., Arnoczky, S. P., Nemzek, J., and Shores, A.: The effect of electromagnetic pulsing on posterior lumbar spinal fusions in dogs. Spine 19:705–709, 1994.
9. Kahanovitz, N., and Pashos, C. L.: The role of implantable direct current stimulation in the critical pathway for lumbar spinal fusion. Presented at the North American Spine Society Annual Meeting, Vancouver, October 1996.
10. Kane, W.J.: Direct current electrical bone growth stimulation for spinal fusion. Spine 13:363–365, 1988.
11. Kane, W. J., Lunceford, E. M., and Dyer, A. R.: An analysis of the utility of implantable bone growth stimulators in lumbar fusions. Orthop. Trans. 6:464, 1982.
12. Lee, K.: Clinical investigation of the spinal stem system, open trial phase: Pseudarthrosis stratum. Presented at the annual meeting of the AAOS, Las Vegas, 1989.
13. Meril, A. J.: Direct current (DC) stimulation of allograft in anterior and posterior lumbar interbody fusions. Spine 19:2393–2397, 1994.
14. Mooney, V.: A randomized double-blind prospective study of the efficacy of pulsed electromagnetic fields for interbody lumbar fusions. Spine 15:708–712, 1990.
15. Nerubay, J., Marganit, B., Bubis, J. J., et al.: Stimulation of bone

formation by electrical current on spinal fusion. Spine *11:*167–169, 1986.
16. Pettine, K. A.: A retrospective controlled study of implantable direct current stimulation in lumbar spinal fusion. Presented at the North American Spine Society Annual Meeting, Washington, DC, October 1995.
17. Simmons, J. W.: Treatment of failed posterior lumbar interbody fusion (PLIF) with pulsing electromagnetic fields. Clin. Orthop. *183:*127–132, 1985.
18. Simmons, J. W., Hayes, M. A.; Christensen, D. K., et al.: The effect of postoperative pulsing electromagnetic fields on lumbar

fusion: An open trial phase study. Presented at the North American Spine Society, Quebec, Canada, June 1989.
19. Tejano, N. A., Puno, R., and Ignacio, J. M. F.: The use of implantable direct current stimulation in multi-level spinal fusion without instrumentation: A prospective clinical and radiographic evaluation with long term follow-up. Spine. (In press.)
20. Treharne, R. W., Brighton, C. T., Korostoff, E., et al.: An in vitro study of electrical osteogenesis using direct and pulsating currents. Clin. Orthop. *145:*300–306, 1979.
21. Yasuda, I., Noguchi, K., and Sata, T.: Dynamic callus and electric callus. J. Bone Joint Surg. *37A:*1292–1993, 1955.

Bone Grafts and Bone Graft Substitutes for Spinal Fusion

Jeffrey H. Schimandle, M.D.

Scott D. Boden, M.D.

One of the most commonly performed procedures in the field of spinal surgery is spinal fusion, which can be defined as the elimination of movement across an intervertebral motion segment by bony union. The concept of spinal fusion surgery was first reported in 1911 by Albee,[1] who performed spinal fusions in an attempt to inhibit tuberculous spread in Pott's disease by providing mechanical support and stability to involved vertebrae. In the same year, Hibbs[87] reported the use of spinal fusion surgery to halt the progression of scoliotic deformity. Since then, the spinal fusion process has been extensively studied, and its success has been shown to be dependent on myriad factors, including local and systemic biologic factors (blood supply, graft bed preparation, hormones, drugs, smoking), local biomechanical factors (instability, loading), and bone graft factors (source, type, quantity, osteoinductive vs. osteoconductive properties).

Recent advances in surgical techniques and in our knowledge regarding the spinal fusion process, as well as in the potential for biologic manipulation of bone formation, make it timely to re-examine our understanding of the relationship between bone grafts, graft adjuncts, and bone graft substitutes and the spinal fusion process. This chapter briefly reviews the multiplicity of local and systemic factors affecting spinal fusion and discusses the properties and use of various graft materials. Results from studies using animal models to study graft materials and data from limited clinical studies are presented. Lastly, gaps in our existing knowledge are identified and future areas of research discussed. An understanding of the biology and properties of bone graft materials, including adjuncts and substitutes, will enable the clinician to apply sound principles when seeking solutions to the current problems associated with achieving a successful spinal fusion.

THE BIOLOGY OF SPINAL FUSION

The outcome of a spinal fusion is dependent on a complex process influenced primarily by the type of graft material used and the many local and systemic factors that affect the fusion healing response. These factors may have positive or negative effects on graft healing[26, 27] and are listed in Table 50–6.

Table 50–6. LOCAL AND SYSTEMIC FACTORS AFFECTING BONE HEALING

Local		Systemic	
Positive	*Negative*	*Positive*	*Negative*
Good vascular supply	Radiation	Growth hormone/somatomedins	Osteoporosis
Large surface area	Tumor	Thyroid hormone	Corticosteroids
Mechanical stability	Local bone disease	Vitamin A	Vitamin D deficiency
Growth factors	Infection	Vitamin D	Methotrexate
BMF	Mechanical instability	Insulin	Adriamycin
Electrical stimulation	Bone wax	PTH	NSAIDs
Mechanical loading	Denervation	Calcitonin	Smoking
		Anabolic steroids	Anemia
			Rheumatoid arthritis
			Sepsis
			Diabetes
			SIADH
			Malnutrition
			Sickle cell disease
			Thalassemia major

BMP, bone morphongenic protein; PTH, parathyroid hormone; NSAIDs, nonsteroidal anti-inflammatory drugs; SIADH, syndrome of inappropriate antidiuretic hormone.

Local Factors

Soft Tissue Bed

The characteristics of the host tissue bed into which the bone graft material is to be placed are of foremost importance. The entire fusion process is dependent on the ingress of osteoprogenitor and inflammatory cells from the recipient bed, as well as the few surviving bone cells transplanted when autogenous bone is used. The tissue bed must therefore be able to suppport the complex processes involved in bone graft healing. These processes are greatly affected by the adequacy of the local blood supply, the efficacy of the inflammatory response, and the availability of osteoprogenitor cells.

An adequate blood supply to the fusion bed is critical for fusion healing. Host bed tissue should not be traumatized, and any avascular (nonviable) or traumatized tissue should be debrided before implantation of the graft material. The fusion bed vascularity is a source of nutrients to the healing fusion, a vehicle for endocrine stimuli, and a pathway for the recruitment of inflammatory and osteoprogenitor cells, which are essential for the successful incorporation of graft material.

Hurley and colleagues,[97] using a dog posterior spinal fusion model, evaluated the role played by overlying soft tissues during the spinal fusion process. Thirty-seven animals underwent one of the following procedures: (1) a modified Hibbs fusion as the control procedure, (2) a Hibbs fusion with nylon-reinforced sheets of millipore (plastic membrane filter permeable to tissue fluids but impermeable to cells) interposed between the fusion site and overlying muscle mass, or (3) a Hibbs fusion with Silastic sheets (silicone rubber impermeable to both tissue fluids and cells). All 10 L5–L6 fusions with interposed Silastic sheets resulted in nonunion, and all 12 L5–L6 fusions with interposed millipore filters resulted in a solid union. These results supported the role of the adjacent soft tissues in providing a source of nutrition for migrating osteoprogenitor cells and possibly a source of diffusible growth factors during the spinal fusion process.

Graft Site Preparation

There are several methods of preparing the bony surfaces onto which the graft material is placed, and they include the use of a power burr, rongeurs, curets, and osteotomes. Regardless of the technique used, the goal is to maximize the area of exposed and viable vascular bone. In general, the larger the surface area decorticated for fusion, the greater the availability of potential osteogenic cells and the greater the contact area exposed to support a bony bridge large enough to carry a mechanical load. Decreased surface area may be responsible for the lower fusion rates seen in patients with myelomeningocele,[3] although other factors may also contribute (e.g., increased infection rate, difficulty of fixation).

Mechanical Stability

The mechanical stability of the spinal segments to be fused will affect the rate of fusion.[76, 126–128, 144, 228] Several studies have shown higher union rates when internal fixation is used to decrease motion in the fusion segment,[19, 76, 121, 126, 127, 227, 228] but when device loosening occurs, nonunion is more likely to occur.[8] Patients with muscular dystrophy or spinal muscular atrophy have higher than average fusion rates, which may be the result of decreased spinal segment motion and improved mechanics from decreased voluntary motion.[6, 200] The level of fusion (L4–L5 vs. L5–S1), the number of segments fused, the patient's weight and activity level, and the use of postoperative external mobilization (bracing)[190] are all important mechanical factors that may influence the rate of fusion.

In studying the effects of spinal instrumentation and biomechanical stability on the spine, most research has focused on the acute or short-term in vitro biomechanical properties of the system under study.[74, 75, 100, 129, 222] Extrapolation of these laboratory findings to the clinical application of spinal instrumentation in spinal fusion surgery has been predicated on the information derived from this "bench-top" biomechanical testing rather than on studies of the long-term in vivo biologic effects on the fusion mass or vertebral bone. The common shortcoming of these bench-top studies is that the interaction between the biology of the spinal fusion process and the instrumentation is not taken into account. It is therefore critical to use appropriate in vivo animal models to study the relationship between spinal instrumentation and the long-term biologic effects on spinal fusion.

McAfee and colleagues created a dog instability model to study the effect of spinal instrumentation on achieving a successful fusion[76, 126, 228] and the radiographic incidence of spinal fusion with respect to spinal stability.[76, 126–128] Radiographic assessment of trabecular bridging six months after surgery revealed a greater probability of achieving a successful spinal fusion if instrumentation was used. Nondestructive mechanical testing showed the instrumented fusions to be significantly more rigid.[76, 126, 127] In 1991, Zdeblick and associates[228] reported a model using the coon hound to simulate an unstable L5 burst fracture. Use of anterior instrumentation resulted in an increased fusion rate radiographically and a more rigid fusion when biomechanically tested. Shirado and coworkers,[194] using this model, replicated these results. Overall, the dog spinal instability and corpectomy model has proved useful in studying the in vivo response to spinal instrumentation and stabilization.

The mechanical stresses (e.g., load, torque) imparted to the graft material itself also affect the fusion rate.[60] For example, 80 per cent of the mechanical load of a motion segment is sustained by the intervertebral disc; thus, graft material placed into an intervertebral body location will be subjected to compressive loading. These compressive forces act on the graft and promote fusion by stimulating the ingrowth of vascular buds and proliferating mesenchymal cells from the cancellous host bone into the donor graft. In contrast, graft placed posteriorly and, to a lesser extent, in the intertransverse process area experiences tensile forces, and healing will be less favorable mechanically and more dependent on biologic factors (e.g., osteogenic cells, osteoinductive factors).

Radiation

Irradiation to a healing spinal fusion has an adverse effect on fusion rate and is especially detrimental within the first few weeks after fusion.[16, 58] This effect may be caused by direct cytotoxic effects on the migrating, proliferating, and differentiating mesenchymal cells,[44] or it may be related to the alteration in vascularity from both the intense vasculitis induced by the radiation injury and the inhibition of angiogenesis. After the acute injury phase, radiation-induced osteonecrosis and dense hypovascular scar in the area of radiation make the fusion bed a poor biologic environment to support the spinal fusion process; the use of vascularized grafts anastomosed to unirradiated vessels may increase the chance of successful fusion in this situation.

Tumor and Bone Disease

Local tumor or bone disease (e.g., Paget's disease, fibrous dysplasia) may directly permeate the fusion area and replace normal marrow, structurally weakening the recipient bone and the developing fusion mass. These obstacles can be partly overcome by using specific fixation techniques[82, 110] and by the appropriate use of local radiation and/or systemic chemotherapy. Use of autograft bone is desirable if the prognosis is favorable, but the harvest site must be maintained as a separate surgical field to prevent tumor seeding to the donor site.

Growth Factors

Several local growth factors are known to stimulate the migration, differentiation, and activity of potential bone-forming mesenchymal cells.[34–36] Bone morphogenic proteins (BMPs) are the most widely investigated of these substances and are discussed in several reviews.[212, 224] In addition to BMPs, other growth factors that influence these processes have been extracted from bone matrix and other tissues (e.g., transforming growth factor-beta [TGF-β], insulin-like growth factor). Several of these proteins are already available through recombinant genetic technology. As the roles of these biologic mediators are further elucidated, they will become an important clinical means of biologically manipulating the complex cascade of cellular events essential to the fusion process.

Electrical Stimulation

Several animal and clinical studies have documented the osteogenic effect of direct-current stimulation or pulsed electromagnetic fields on bone repair.[65, 83, 197, 225] Most studies, however, have centered on long bone delayed unions or nonunions[20, 84, 159, 160, 230] and congenital pseudarthrosis of the tibia.[115, 161]

Electrical stimulation has been shown to enhance the rate of spinal fusion in various animal studies[103–105, 147] and human clinical trials.[53, 54, 72, 78, 107, 134, 138, 146] Several mechanisms of action have been proposed; all appear to act directly or indirectly at the cellular level. Optimal biologic currents appear to be between 5 and 25 microamperes and can be delivered directly or via pulsed electromagnetic fields (PEMFs).

Systemic Factors

Osteoporosis

Osteoporosis is the most prevalent metabolic bone disease in the United States, affecting 25 million individuals. It is commonly assumed to be a negative factor in bone healing. Although decreased bone mass is the hallmark of osteoporosis, alterations in bone marrow quality and the rate of bone turnover may also be present. The number of osteogenic stem cells may be deficient in elderly patients and may actually be more important than absolute bone mass. In performing a spinal fusion in an osteoporotic patient, the vertebrae are weak and difficult to adequately stabilize with or without internal fixation, especially across the mobile lumbosacral junction. All these factors adversely affect the spinal fusion rate.

Hormones

Over the last decade, a considerable amount of knowledge has been gained about the control of bone formation by hormones.[34] These chemical messengers have complex direct and indirect effects on bone formation and may influence spinal fusion healing both positively and negatively.

Thyroid hormones are necessary for normal growth and development. They are required for the synthesis of somatomedins by the liver[186] and have a direct stimulatory effect on cartilage growth and maturation[28, 209] and thus a positive effect on bone healing. Thyroid hormones act synergistically with growth hormone.[209]

Growth hormone has no direct effects on cartilage or bone formation but exerts its stimulatory effects through somatomedins.[167, 168] In vivo, growth hormone stimulates bone healing by increasing intestinal absorption of calcium, bone formation, and bone mineralization.[136, 209]

In both experimental and clinical situations, corticosteroids have been shown to have deleterious effects on bone healing as a result of increased bone resorption and decreased formation.[77, 102] Corticosteroids have been shown to both inhibit and promote the differentiation of osteoblasts from mesenchymal cells[7, 196] and to decrease the synthesis rates of the major components of bone matrix necessary for bone healing.[45]

Estrogens and androgens (testosterone) are considered important in the skeletal maturation of growing individuals and in the prevention of the bone loss associated with aging. The in vivo effects of these hormones on bone healing, however, are controversial. Although some studies indicate that they may stimulate bone formation,[10] most do not support this possibility.[111, 177] In vitro studies have shown that neither estrogens nor androgens affect bone collagen synthesis,[37] but estrogens may increase bone mineralization by increasing serum PTH and 1,25-(OH)$_2$D3 concentrations.[68]

Nutrition

Nutritional status has been shown to affect bone healing in orthopedic patients.[56, 99] If nutritional deficiencies are suspected, they can be identified using serum albumin and transferrin levels, total lymphocyte count, skin antigen testing, anthropometric measurements, and nitrogen balance studies. These studies can be useful in assessing the nutritional status of patients undergoing spinal fusion to determine the need for nutritional support.

Drugs

Various drugs taken during the perioperative period can inhibit or delay bone formation. Chemotherapeutic agents, such as methotrexate and adriamycin, inhibit bone formation and healing if administered early in the postoperative period.[30, 67, 152, 166] Nonsteroidal anti-inflammatory drugs (e.g., ibuprofen) suppress the inflammatory response and may inhibit bone formation and spinal fusion.[116]

Smoking

Cigarette smoking interferes with bone metabolism, retards osteogenesis, and inhibits bone graft revascularization. Extracts from tobacco smoke have been reported to induce calcitonin resistance,[88] increase bone resorption at fracture ends,[113] and interfere with osteoblastic function.[49] In a rabbit model, nicotine has been shown to decrease the vascular ingrowth into autogenous iliac crest cancellous bone graft implanted in an orthotopic location (anterior eye chamber, distal femur).[47, 176] Clinically, the rate of nonunion in smokers

after spinal fusion has been shown to be higher than that in nonsmokers.[11, 21, 79, 132, 227]

Recently, in a validated animal model for spinal fusion,[12] a direct relationship between the development of a spinal fusion nonunion and the presence of systemic nicotine was established. Silcox and colleagues[195] performed single-level lumbar posterolateral intertransverse process fusions at L5–L6 in 28 New Zealand white rabbits using autogenous iliac crest bone graft. Animals were randomly assigned to receive pumps delivering either systemic nicotine at a level comparable to that in a human smoking one to one and a half packs of cigarettes per day or placebo infusions of normal saline solution. Five weeks after surgery, the animals were killed, and manual, radiographic, and biomechanical testing of the fusion mass was performed. Fifty-six per cent of the control animals were judged to have solid fusions; no solid fusions were seen in the nicotine group (p = 0.02). Biomechanically, the mean relative fusion strength and stiffness in the control group were greater than in the nicotine group (p = 0.09 and p = 0.08, respectively).

PROPERTIES OF GRAFT MATERIALS

In addition to local and systemic factors, the choice of graft material influences the outcome of a spinal fusion. Graft materials participate in the fusion process in different ways, depending on the properties they possess (Table 50–7).[112, 171] Ideally, bone graft materials should possess four properties: (1) an osteoconductive matrix that is a nonviable scaffolding conducive to bone ingrowth; (2) osteogenic cells that have the potential to differentiate and facilitate the various stages of bone regeneration; (3) osteoinductive factors, which are the biochemical substances that stimulate osteoprogenitor cells to differentiate into osteogenic cells (osteoblasts); and (4) structural integrity.

Osteoconduction

Osteoconductivity is the physical property of a graft material that allows the ingrowth of neovasculature and the infiltration of osteogenic precursor cells during the process known as creeping substitution. A graft material that is only osteoconductive transfers neither osteogenic cells nor inductive stimuli, but acts as a

Table 50–7. PROPERTIES OF GRAFT MATERIALS

Graft Material	Osteogenic Potential	Osteoinduction	Osteoconduction
Autogenous bone	X	±	X
Bone marrow cells	X		
Allograft bone		?	X
Xenograft bone		?	X
DBM		X	X
BMP		X	
Ceramics			X

DBM, demineralized bone matrix; BMP, bone morphogenic protein.

nonviable scaffold or trellis that supports the bone healing response. Materials that are osteoconductive include autogenous and allograft bone, bone matrix, collagen, and calcium phosphate ($CaPO_4$) ceramics.

Osteogenic Potential

The osteogenic potential of a graft is derived from its cellular content. Osteogenic graft materials contain viable cells that possess the ability to form bone (determined osteogenic precursor cells) or the potential to differentiate into bone-forming cells (inducible osteogenic precursor cells). These cells participate in the early stages of the healing process to unite the graft to the host bone and must be protected during the grafting procedure to ensure viability. This potential to produce bone is characteristic only of fresh autogenous bone and bone marrow cells.

Osteoinduction

Bone induction is the process by which some factor or substance stimulates an undetermined osteoprogenitor stem cell to differentiate into an osteogenic cell type, and it is mediated by numerous growth factors provided by the bone matrix itself. This concept was introduced by Urist and coworkers in the 1960s after his initial studies on the osteoinductive properties of demineralized bone matrix (DBM) and BMP.[210, 216] In addition to these materials, autogenous bone and allograft are known to possess osteoinductive properties.

Structural Integrity

Biomechanical strength is important when the graft material will experience compressive loads. Specific graft materials (e.g., cancellous bone) begin with no structural integrity but change as a result of fusion mass augmentation and union (osteointegration) with pre-existing osseous structures. The bone strength increases as the bone mass accumulates and the construct is remodeled along the lines of stress. Other graft material (e.g., cortical bone) initially conveys structural strength, but as it undergoes remodeling and osteointegration, it can lose up to one third of its strength.[59]

GRAFT MATERIALS

Autograft

Autogenous bone is considered the most successful bone graft material available.[59, 85, 95, 153, 171, 207, 223] Complications with its use, however, may occur in as many as 25 per cent of patients.[9, 114, 226] Graft harvest disadvantages include increased surgical morbidity from an additional operative site, chronic donor site pain,[61, 175] increased operative time, increased blood loss and risk of transfusion, and additional cost.[171] The quantity of bone available to harvest may be insufficient for a long, multisegment fusion or in a patient with previous graft harvests. These problems have stimulated the investi-

gation of growth factors (DBM and BMP) and bone graft substitutes (allograft or xenograft bone, $CaPO_4$ ceramics, composite grafts) to achieve spinal fusion.

Autogenous cancellous bone is currently the most successful grafting material available for achieving a spinal fusion. Inherent in this material are three of the ideal transplant properties: osteoconductivity, osteogenic potential, and osteoinductivity. These properties are present by virtue of bone mineral and collagen, surviving bone cells, and bone matrix proteins. Additionally, a large trabecular surface area is available that can be incorporated through new bone formation, a property called "connectivity."

Autogenous cortical bone is used as a graft material when structural support is needed at the graft site. Except for the advantage of mechanical strength, cortical bone is less desirable than cancellous bone for a number of reasons. Fewer osteogenic cells are present in cortical bone because of the absence of marrow. The cells that are present are less likely to survive, because they are embedded in the more compact cortical matrix and shielded from the diffusion of nutrients. Cortical bone has less surface area per unit weight than cancellous bone, limiting the area into which new bone can form and from which osteoinductive proteins can pass. Lastly, cortical bone is more resistant to vascular ingrowth and remodeling, both of which are necessary for bone healing and the development of mechanical strength. Cortical bone initially possesses biomechanical strength, but then it undergoes a remodeling phase whereby nonviable bone is removed by osteoclast tunneling and resorption, which can last from six to 18 months and result in a significant loss of strength. Cancellous grafts tend to be completely remodeled in time, but cortical grafts remain as admixtures of viable and necrotic bone throughout the life of the individual.

Vascularized grafts of autogenous fibula, iliac crest, or rib have many advantages[17, 50, 130, 181, 191, 221] and are used in selected cases of anterior spinal fusion. When free vascularized grafts are used, the bone does not undergo significant cell necrosis and remains viable through its arterial and venous anastomoses, avoiding some of the problems of nonvascularized cortical bone. The improved incorporation of these grafts makes their use desirable in cases in which avascular graft healing is poor, such as in areas of radiation-induced fibrosis or when radiation and/or chemotherapy is to be given in the perioperative period. Vascularized grafts are clearly superior to nonvascularized grafts when the area to be spanned is more than 12 cm. Reported stress-fracture rates for this distance when nonvascularized cortical bone is used approach 50 per cent, whereas the fracture rate for vascularized grafts is less than 25 per cent.[69]

Allograft

The use of allograft bone as a graft material has been expanded in recent years as a result of improved methods of procurement, preparation, and storage; technical advances in surgical methods; and the desire to avoid the donor site complications associated with using autogenous bone. Although bone allografts are versatile and widely used in spinal surgery, concerns exist regarding their ability to consistently achieve a successful fusion and the possibility of infectious disease transmission.[25, 38, 46, 131, 204] Thus, knowledge regarding the methods of graft procurement, testing, processing, and storage is necessary for its efficient and safe use.[66] The ultimate decision to use allograft bone in a particular spinal procedure depends on the underlying disease or pathology, the region of the spine where the graft is to be placed, the types of graft available, the surgical goals, and the preferences of the patient and surgeon.

Allograft bone from living and cadaver donors is acceptable, but it requires meticulous attention to donor selection criteria. A comprehensive sociomedical history must be obtained, the cause of death determined, and serologic and other laboratory testing performed. If screening is normal, the allograft bone is sterilely harvested within 12 to 24 hours of death, multiply cultured, and processed for preservation and storage.

Immunogenicity and the maintenance of the osteoinductive and osteoconductive properties of the allograft bone are related to the method of graft processing and preservation. Preservation of allograft bone is generally accomplished by freezing or freeze-drying carried out as soon after harvest as possible. These methods diminish allograft degradation by enzymes, are effective in decreasing the immunogenicity of the graft, preserve biomechanical properties, and allow the graft to be stored for an extended period of time. Allograft bone that meets the criteria for use (i.e., negative screen) is processed by deep-freezing at $-70°$ C or in liquid nitrogen at $-196°$ C.[46] Despite being preserved in an inert, nonviable state, the mechanical properties of the bone are not affected.[163–165] The shelf-life of frozen allograft bone stored at $-70°$ C is five years.[46] Alternatively, allograft bone may be processed by freeze-drying (lyophilization). This method involves the removal of water from the frozen tissue, and it is more effective in decreasing immunogenicity and inactivating viral agents. It does not affect the limited osteoinductive properties but may result in a reduction in mechanical strength of the graft.[163–165] Freeze-dried allograft bone must be dehydrated under vacuum conditions and preserved in a sealed vacuum container, but it can be stored at room temperature and, as long as the vacuum is retained, has an indefinite shelf-life. In both freezing and freeze-drying, the osteoconductive properties are retained in terms of their cancellous and cortical structure, the osteoprogenitor cells are destroyed, and the limited osteoinductive substances present in the graft are partially retained.

Sterilization of allograft bone is not a substitute for meticulous screening and sterile harvesting, but it can be an additional safety measure against infection. The methods most commonly used are gas sterilization with ethylene oxide (450 to 1500 mg/L at 30 to 60 per cent humidity and 21° C) and high-dose gamma irradiation (1.5 to 2.5 megarads).[46, 204] Although effective, these methods interfere with either the biologic properties (decreased osteoinduction) or the mechanical integrity of the allograft bone.[163] Other methods of graft sterilization such as heating or autoclaving are destructive to matrix proteins and are generally not used.

Bone Marrow Cells

Bone marrow is osteogenic[31, 32, 36, 143, 154, 201] and has been used clinically as an adjunctive graft material for spinal fusion. Osteogenic precursor cells exist in bone marrow on the order of 1 per 50,000 nucleated cells and result in bone formation when transplanted to heterotopic sites (e.g., muscle, subcutaneous tissue). This bone-forming ability can be sustained or augmented in combination with bone[183, 184] or with bone extracts containing BMP.[201] Although the clinical use of bone marrow has had only limited reporting, it offers the ability to augment all the allografts and synthetic graft substitutes that are currently used for spinal fusion.

Xenograft

Xenogeneic graft materials have been used extensively in orthopedic surgery and have included ivory, cow horn, and bovine bone. Despite processing, xenografts evoke an immune response by the host and may become encapsulated, resulting in obstruction of microanastomoses between vessels of the recipient tissue and graft. Owing to their resistance to incorporation into host bone, ivory and cow horn are currently not used as graft materials. Freeze-dried[5, 81, 86, 169] and deproteinized[133, 175, 182] bovine xenografts, both weakly antigenic, have been used in spinal fusion surgery but have had mixed success in achieving a solid bony fusion and are not recommended as graft material.

Demineralized Bone Matrix and Bone Morphogenetic Protein

DBM is a less immunogenic form of allograft bone.[73] The general technique of DBM preparation involves removal of all soft tissue and bone marrow from diaphyseal bone. The bone is then extracted with ethanol followed by ethyl ether to remove surface lipids and dehydrate the bone. The bone is pulverized in liquid nitrogen, sieved to a particle size of 74 to 420 μm, and extracted with dilute acid (0.5 N or 0.6 N HCl) to extract the acid-soluble proteins and demineralize the bone matrix, leaving the collagen, noncollagenous proteins, and bone growth factors as a composite material.[106] Currently, DBM is prepared by bone banks and is available freeze-dried as a powder, as crushed granules, and in chip form. A chemically processed form is produced commercially under the name Grafton (Osteotech, Shrewsbury, NJ) and is supplied in gel form.

Since the initial studies performed by Urist and coworkers,[210, 216] the osteoinductive capacity of DBM has been well established.[39, 48, 57, 70, 71, 73, 96, 120, 140, 156, 201, 208, 213, 218, 219] The primary active osteoinductive components of DBM are a series of low-molecular-weight glycoproteins including BMP. This BMP constitutes only 0.1 per cent of all bone protein by weight and is most abundant in diaphyseal cortical bone. BMP exists in the extracellular bone matrix[215] and remains inactive until the matrix has been demineralized by acid extraction.[52, 216, 217] Once exposed, BMP induces the formation of cartilage and bone in vivo and stimulates a cascade of processes not unlike that seen in fracture repair. Chemotaxis, proliferation, and differentiation of pluripotential mesenchymal cells result in the transient formation of cartilage and the subsequent production of mature bone with hematopoietic marrow.[224] Additionally, demineralization of bone matrix by acid extraction destroys the highly antigenic cell membranes and soluble glycopeptides, thereby minimizing the host versus graft immune response.[73]

Bone matrix contains a number of other growth factors in addition to the BMPs. TGF-β is produced and secreted by bone and other cells and is stored in bone matrix and platelets. Numerous experimental findings indicate that TGF-β is of primary importance in controlling the proliferation and expression of the differentiated phenotype of several types of cells specific to the skeleton—among them the mesenchymal precursor cells for chondrocytes, osteoblasts, and osteoclasts—and in regulating bone metabolism.[27, 55, 137, 199] Other growth factors found in bone matrix include insulin-like growth factors I and II, acidic and basic fibroblast growth factors, platelet-derived growth factors, interleukins, granulocyte-colony stimulating factors, and granulocyte-macrophage colony stimulating factors. The role of these individual factors in spinal fusion healing is difficult to determine, owing to the large number of proteins involved in osteogenesis and osteoinduction. The interaction between these various factors is an area for future study.

The enhanced osteoinductive capability of DBM is afforded most notably by the BMP that is present, although the amount of BMP is far lower than that used to achieve spinal fusion in published studies. In addition to the low amounts of BMP present in DBM, there are many variables involved in the preparation of DBM and the purification of BMPs that may affect the osteoinductive activity of these substances. The Food and Drug Administration requires sterilization of the DBM prepared by bone banks, which may decrease the viability of the available BMP. The commercially prepared Grafton bone matrix is processed by means of a permeation treatment that does not expose tissue to ethylene oxide or gamma radiation, which may protect more of the BMP from inactivation.[69]

Ceramics

In recent years, a number of biodegradable osteoconductive $CaPO_4$ ceramic bone graft substitutes have received attention as alternatives to autogenous bone. They have been used solely as osteoconductive bone graft matrices, but because they are biodegradable, they have the advantage of being compatible with the

new bone remodeling process required to attain optimal mechanical strength. A nonresorbable graft material may hinder remodeling and prolong the strength deficiency of new bone, as well as leave permanent stress risers in the fusion mass.[98] The majority of $CaPO_4$ ceramics being used in spine surgery are synthetic and are composed of hydroxyapatite (HA), tricalcium phosphate (TCP), or a combination of the two.[24] These biomaterials are produced commercially as porous or nonporous implants and granular particles with pores and are created with the use of a high-temperature process called sintering, along with high-pressure compaction techniques.

For synthetic implants to be useful in vivo, they must have certain properties: (1) compatibility with surrounding tissues, (2) chemical stability in body fluids, (3) compatibility of mechanical and physical properties, (4) ability to be fabricated into functional shapes, (5) ability to withstand the sterilization process, (6) reasonable cost of manufacturing, and (7) reliable quality control. $CaPO_4$ ceramics possess these properties[63, 98, 157] and have been used successfully as bone graft substitutes in dentistry and maxillofacial surgery,[43, 51, 98, 108, 117, 118, 135, 148–151, 179, 198, 220] in animal bone defect models,[89–91, 93, 94, 139, 162, 193] and in humans, to a limited extent.[23, 24, 89, 158, 180, 192]

Hydroxyapatite and tricalcium phosphate ceramics are brittle materials with low fracture resistance and vary in their chemical and structural (crystalline) composition.[171] Different preparative methods lead to either a compact or a porous material with interconnective macropores that is the structural and spatial equivalent of cancellous bone. The optimal osteoconductive pore size for ceramics appears to be between 150 and 500 μm. In a biologic system, greater crystalline formation and material density result in greater mechanical strength and resistance to dissolution and promote long-lasting stability (e.g., hydroxyapatite). In contrast, an amorphous ultrastructure and greater porosity enhance interface activity and bone ingrowth, but also result in faster biodegradation of the implant (e.g., tricalcium phosphate).[98] Commercially available HA is resorbed very slowly, if at all, under normal physiologic conditions,[92, 94, 98] whereas TCP undergoes biologic degradation 10 to 20 times faster and is generally resorbed by six weeks after implantation.[62, 98] The resorbing cell for HA is the foreign body giant cell, which stops its degradation after resorbing 2 to 10 μm of HA.[69] Thus, large segments of HA may remain in the body for up to 10 years.

Ceramics, being brittle, have very little tensile strength. Use of ceramics in applications requiring significant impact, torsional, bending, or shear stress is presently impractical. The mechanical properties of porous calcium phosphate materials, however, are comparable to those of cancellous bone once they have been incorporated and remodeled. Ceramics must be shielded from loading forces until bone ingrowth has occurred; they tolerate minimal bending and torque loads before failing.

Replamineform ceramics are porous HA materials

derived from the calcium carbonate skeletal structure of sea coral. They are produced from a marine coral specimen using a hydrothermal exchange method that replaces the original carbonate of the coral with calcium phosphate replicas. In contrast to the random pore structure created in synthetic ceramics, the pore structure of the coralline calcium phosphate ceramics is highly organized and is similar to that of human cancellous bone. The pore size of these materials is determined by the genus of the coral used. Coralline HA derived from the genus *Goniopora* has large pores measuring from 500 to 600 μm in diameter, with interconnections measuring 220 to 260 μm. The coral genus *Porites* has a microstructure that appears similar to that of interstitial bone, with its smaller pore diameter of 230 μm, its parallel channels interconnected by 190-μm fenestrations, and its void volume (porosity) of 66 per cent.[24] It exhibits only 2.2 per cent of the ultimate strength of human femoral cortical bone. Coralline HAs are available commercially as Pro Osteon Implant 500 and Pro Osteon Implant 200 (Interpore Orthopaedics, Irvine, CA), with average pore sizes of 500 and 200 μm, respectively.

ANIMAL STUDIES OF GROWTH FACTORS AND BONE GRAFT SUBSTITUTES

Owing to the many uncontrollable variables in clinical studies of spinal fusion, animal investigations have played a significant role in evaluating bone graft materials. Several animal models, including the rabbit, dog, rat, and rhesus monkey, have been used to study the various osteoinductive growth factors (DBM and BMPs) and bone graft substitutes (allograft bone, HA, TCP) in spinal fusions. Different types of spinal fusions have been studied, including laminar/facet, spinous process, anterior or posterior interbody, and posterolateral intertransverse process fusion methods. Most animal experiments have compared only fusion quality and characteristics using these materials to the results obtained using autogenous bone graft in the same model.

In evaluating the ability of DBM to achieve or enhance spinal fusion (Table 50–8), many studies have used a rabbit posterior spinal fusion model.[119, 120, 155, 173, 174] Most studies have shown that DBM combined with bone marrow cells, which are osteogenic themselves,[31, 32, 36, 143, 154, 201] was a more successful inducer of spinal fusion than either DBM or marrow cells alone, but it was not as good as autograft bone with or without marrow cells.[119, 120, 155, 174] Oikarinen performed posterior L3–L4 fusions in 29 rabbits and showed DBM to be a better substitute for autogenous bone than deep-frozen allograft.[155] In a posterior thoracic and lumbar spinal fusion model in rats, Guizzardi and colleagues[73] showed that the osteoinductive effect of heterologous powdered DBM was comparable to that of autograft, as determined by similar fusion callus development seen on histologic sections of the fusion mass. In a dog posterior thoracic spinal fusion model,

Frenkel and associates[64] used DBM gel to enhance spinal fusion. DBM gel in combination with autogenous bone graft produced the most vigorous osteoinductive response histologically, but the development of a solid fusion was not assessed biomechanically. More recently, Cook and coworkers[41] evaluated the efficacy of DBM as a bone graft substitute for posterior lumbar fusions in mongrel dogs. Unilateral arthrodeses were performed at four levels in each of nine subjects to compare DBM alone, DBM with allograft, allograft bone alone, and autograft in the same dog. The results of radiographic, biomechanical, and histologic evaluation showed DBM alone or with allograft bone to be ineffective in achieving solid posterior spinal fusion. Results from this study, however, are difficult to interpret, because multiple interventions in the same animal were performed. In addition, separate control animals were not used, and fusions were seen at the end point of their study in all control levels arthrodesed using autogenous bone graft.

Several recent animal studies have investigated the application of osteoinductive growth factors in achieving spinal fusion (Table 50–9). To evaluate the action of bovine BMP compared with local bone graft in the spine, Lovell and colleagues[122] used a dog posterior spinal fusion model. Four different fusion methods were used in the thoracic spine of each dog, including one BMP level. The fusions were examined by radiographs and histology, which showed the BMP/autograft level to have two to three times more new bone than comparison levels and a 71 per cent fusion rate compared with 0, 14, and 29 per cent in the three comparison levels. Cook and associates[42] reported their results evaluating recombinant human osteogenic protein (BMP-7; rhOP-1, Creative BioMolecules, Inc., Hopkinton, MA) as a bone graft substitute for spinal fusion in a canine posterior lumbar fusion model. Unilateral arthrodeses were performed at four levels in each of nine mongrel dogs, comparing four different implants in the same animal. As in the Cook study on DBM reported earlier,[41] results from this study are difficult to interpret. Schimandle and coworkers[189] were the first to report results using recombinant bone morphogenetic protein-2 (rhBMP-2) in a posterolateral intertransverse process spinal fusion model. Spinal arthrodeses were performed at L5–L6 in 56 rabbits using rhBMP-2/collagen carrier, autogenous bone graft, or carrier alone. Inspection, manual palpation, radiography, histology, and biomechanical testing were used to assess the fusion mass. All rabbits implanted with rhBMP-2 achieved solid spinal fusion by manual palpation and were fused radiographically, whereas only 42 per cent of the autograft control fusions and none of the collagen carrier fusions were solid (p = 0.01). Fusions achieved with rhBMP-2 were biomechanically stronger (p = 0.05) and stiffer (p = 0.03) than fusions achieved using autogenous bone graft. Boden and coworkers[13] evaluated the use of a bovine-derived osteoinductive protein extract as a bone graft substitute in a validated rabbit model of intertransverse process arthrodesis of the lumbar spine. Arthrodeses were performed at

Table 50–8. ANIMAL SPINAL FUSION MODELS USING DEMINERALIZED BONE MATRIX

Year[Ref]	Purpose	Animal	N	Fusion Type	Graft Material	Histology	X-ray	Biomechanical Testing	Miscellaneous
1982[155]	To compare DBM vs. allograft vs. autograft cancellous bone	Rabbit	29	• Posterior spinous process • L3–L4	• DBM • Allograft • Autograft (iliac)	H	R	—	• DBM much better than allograft • DBM and autograft had comparable results
1982[119]	Pilot study using DBM and BM in spinal fusions	Rabbit	12	• Posterior spinous process and lamina • T and L spine	• Autograft BM • DBM • DBM + BM • Iliac crest ± BM • Tibial periosteum	H	—	—	• DBM + BM > BM = iliac crest < iliac crest and BM
1987[174]	To examine capability of DBM/BM to enhance T + L spine fusions	Rabbit	13	• Posterior plus intertransverse	• DBM/BM	H	R	—	• DBM/BM a sound alternative to using autograft bone
1988[120]	To study BM ± DBM as a graft material	Rabbit	23	• Posterior • T3–T4 and T7–T8	• DBM • BM • DBM/BM	H	R	—	• BM alone insignificant • DBM/BM better than DBM alone
1989[173]	To assess the fusion time after spinal fusion with DBM and whether static changes develop after symmetric or asymmetric fusion	Rabbit	20	• Posterior plus intertransverse • T spine	• DBM • Autograft (iliac)	H		—	• 67% of fusion late at 3 mons. using DBM and 100% at 5 mos.
1992[73]	To test osteoinductive effect of DBM	Rat	20	• Posterolateral • Lumbar	• Right side DBM • Left side autograft	H			• DBM with similar osteoinductive effect and callus development to autograft
1992[?]			12	• Posterolateral • T and L spine	• Local autograft in T spine • DBM bilateral in L spine	SEM	—	—	• Endochondral ossification
1993[64]	To determine ability of DBM gel to act as an osteoconductive/ inductive material	Dog	7	• Posterolateral • Thoracic	• DBM gel • Local autograft	HM	R		• 4 fusion procedures in each dog • DBM gel may be a valuable means of enhancing spinal fusion
1995[41]	To determine efficacy of DBM	Dog	9	• Posterior laminar unilateral fusions • T13–L7/4 sites	• DBM • DBM + allograft • Allograft • Autograft	H	R	+	• Autograft fused • Allograft DBM did not fuse

DBM, demineralized bone matrix; BM, autograft bone marrow cells; T, thoracic; L, lumbar; H, routine histology; HM, histomorphometry; SEM, scanning electron microscopy; R, plain radiographs.

Table 50–9. ANIMAL SPINAL FUSION MODELS USING BONE MORPHOGENIC PROTEIN

Year[Ref]	Purpose	Animal	N	Fusion Type	Graft Material	Histology	X-ray	Bio-mechanical Testing	Miscellaneous
1989[122]	To investigate action of BMP on local bone graft	Dog	13	• Posterior laminar • Thoracic	• Local autograft ± BMP	H	R RM MR	−	• 4 fusion procedures in each dog • BMP: 1 new bone, ↑ fusion
1994[42]	To determine efficacy of rhOP-1	Dog	9	• Posterior laminar unilateral fusions • T13–L7/4 sites	• rhOP-1/collagen • Carrier alone • Autograft • No implant	H	R	+	• OP-1 fused by 12 weeks • Autograft fused by 24 weeks
1994[142]	To determine efficacy of rhBMP-2/PLGA	Dog	11	• Posterior laminar lumbar fusion/3 sites	• rhBMP-2/PLGA • PLGA alone • Autograft	H	R	+	• rhBMP-2/PLGA and autograft were equal: 73–82% fusion rate at 12 weeks
1995[189]	To determine efficacy of rhBMP-2/collagen	Rabbit	56	• Intertransverse process fusion L5–L6	• rhBMP-2/collagen • Carrier alone • Autograft • rhBMP-2/autograft	H	R	+	• 100% fusion rhBMP-2 • 42% fusion autograft • 4-week end point
1995[13]	To determine efficacy of bovine BMP extract	Rabbit	45	• Intertransverse process fusion L5–L6	• Bovine BMP/DBM • DBM alone • Autograft	H	R	+	• 100% fusion BMP • 62% fusion autograft • 17% fusion DBM • 5-week end point
1995[14]	To determine effect of dose, carrier, and species on bovine BMP extract	Rabbit	115	• Intertransverse process fusion L5–L6	• Bovine BMP/DBM • bBMP/biocoral • bBMP/autograft	H	R	+	• 100% fusion when at least 150 μg used per site • Coral and autograft also good carriers
1995[14]		Monkey	10	• Intertransverse process fusion L4–L5	• Bovine BMP/DBM • DBM alone	H	R	−	• Much higher BMP dose needed in primate
1995[185]	To determine efficacy of rhBMP-2/OPLA	Dog	14	• Posterior plus intertransverse L4–L5	• rhBMP-2/OPLA • OPLA alone • Autograft	H	R	+	• 100% rhBMP-2 fused by 3 mos. • No autograft fusions

DBM, demineralized bone matrix; BM, autograft bone marrow cells; BMP, bone morphogenic protein; H, routine histology; HM, histomorphometry; R, plain radiographs; MR, microradiography; RM, radiomorphometry.

L5–L6 in 45 adult rabbits using one of three bone graft materials: autogenous iliac crest bone, osteoinductive protein delivered in a DBM/collagen carrier, or carrier alone. Fusion was assessed by inspection, manual palpation, radiography, biomechanical testing, and light microscopy. Of the 35 rabbits that were examined at five weeks, all 10 in the group that had received osteoinductive bone protein had a solid fusion, but the rate of fusion was significantly less in the other two groups: 8 of 13 rabbits (p = 0.05) in the group that had received autogenous bone graft, and 2 of 12 rabbits (p = 0.0001) in the group that had received DBM/collagen carrier alone. The use of osteoinductive bone protein resulted in stronger (p = 0.02) and stiffer (p = 0.005) fusions compared with those obtained with autogenous bone graft. Sandhu and associates[185] performed posterolateral transverse process arthrodeses at L4–L5 in 14 beagles using rhBMP-2/open-cell polylactic acid polymer (OPLA) carrier, autogenous bone graft, and carrier alone. All six rhBMP-2 implanted sites had solid transverse process fusions by three months, whereas no autograft fusions were solid at that time. In a recent multifaceted study by Boden and colleagues,[14] posterolateral intertransverse process lumbar arthrodeses were performed in 115 rabbits and 10 rhesus monkeys to evaluate different doses and carrier materials for a bovine-derived osteoinductive bone protein extract. Successful fusions were achieved in the rabbit model using the osteoinductive growth factor with three different carriers: autogenous bone graft, DBM, and natural coral (Figs. 50–32 through 50–34). A dose-dependent response to the growth factor in the rabbit was noted, indicating that a dose threshold must be overcome before bone formation is induced. The methodology for biologic enhancement of spinal fusion developed in the rabbit model was successfully transferred to the rhesus monkey, where use of the osteoinductive growth factor with a DBM carrier resulted in radiographic spinal fusion masses at 12 weeks. Continued work is needed with growth factors such as BMP both in the naturally extracted form and with the various recombinant proteins such as BMP-2 and OP-1 (BMP-7) in an effort to evaluate the technology of biologic enhancement of spinal fusion in humans.

The use of allograft bone can minimize many of the limitations seen with autogenous bone graft. Allograft bone, however, is less osteogenic, carries a small but finite risk of disease transmission,[25, 38, 46, 131, 204] and may elicit an immune response that can impair graft incorporation into the host.[29, 63] A study comparing autograft and allograft for anterior interbody and posterior fusions in a dog model showed a slower fusion rate, greater resorption of the graft material, and an increased infection rate in the dogs with allograft.[206] These problems have led many to use allograft clinically as a graft expander rather than as a graft substitute.

The ability of $CaPO_4$ ceramics to act as bone graft substitutes for spinal fusion has been studied in dog and rabbit spinal fusion models (Table 50–10). Flatley

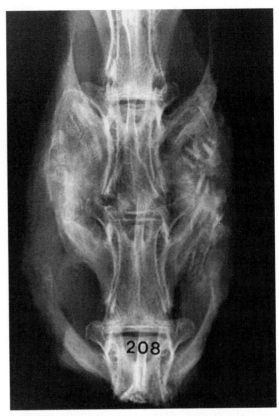

Figure 50–32. Radiograph of a rabbit posterolateral intertransverse process fusion five weeks after implantation of an osteoinductive growth factor with autogenous bone graft as the carrier. (From Boden, S. D., Schimandle, J. H., and Hutton, W. C.: 1995 Volvo Award in Basic Sciences. The use of an osteoinductive growth factor for lumbar spinal fusion. Part II: Study of dose, carrier, and species. Spine *20*:2633–2644, 1995.)

and coworkers[63] used porous ceramic blocks of a 1:1 ratio of calcium HA and TCP to perform posterolateral vertebral body fusions across the intervertebral disc space in 21 rabbits. At 12 weeks, histologic sections showed bone ingrowth reaching the central portion of the ceramic block, with no fibrous tissue barrier noted between the new bone and ceramic residue. Holmes and associates,[89] using coralline HA in a canine posterior facet spinal fusion model, showed no solid fusions, even at six months, using this ceramic, but the distribution of new bone ingrowth was similar in the ceramic and autograft fusion masses. In a goat model for anterior discectomy and fusion (ADF), Pintar and colleagues[170] evaluated the fusion rate and biomechanical stiffness for 56 fusion segments in 14 animals who underwent ADF in the cervical and lumbar spine using HA or autogenous bone graft. Radiography, biomechanical testing, and histologic analysis were used to assess the fusion. In the cervical spine, the fusion rate was 30 per cent for HA and 40 per cent for autograft fusions, whereas the fusion rates in the lumbar spine were equal (70 per cent). The overall fusion rate at 12 and 24 weeks was 50 for the HA and 55 per cent for the autograft fusions. Fused levels demonstrated no statistical difference in biomechanical stiffness between the HA and autograft fusions. Their results indicated that HA used as a bone graft substitute performed as well as autogenous bone graft for anterior interbody fusions of the cervical and lumbar spine in this animal model. Toth and associates[205] performed a similar study in goats comparing the efficacy of a 50-50 HA-TCP ceramic of 30, 50, or 70 per cent porosity with that of autogenous bone graft in promoting anterior cervical interbody fusion. Upon evaluation, all ceramic fusions had better radiographic fusion scores than did autograft. No statistically significant differences were found between autograft and the porous ceramics with biomechanical testing and peri-implant bone mineral density values, as measured by dual-energy x-ray absorptiometry. At six months, the histologic union rate was 67 per cent for the ceramic and 50 per cent for the autograft fusions.

Ceramic composites consist of the osteoconductive ceramic combined with an osteoinductive agent such as collagen, DBM, autograft bone, extracted bone matrix proteins, or recombinant BMP.[139, 202, 214] They have also been investigated as bone graft substitutes in ani-

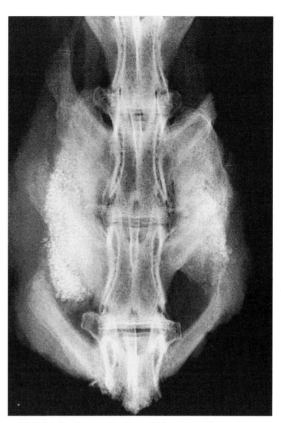

Figure 50–34. Radiograph of a rabbit posterolateral intertransverse process fusion five weeks after implantation with an osteoinductive growth factor with natural coral as the carrier. (From Boden, S. D., Schimandle, J. H., and Hutton, W. C.: 1995 Volvo Award in Basic Sciences. The use of an osteoinductive growth factor for lumbar spinal fusion. Part II: Study of dose, carrier, and species. Spine *20*:2633–2644, 1995.)

mal spinal fusion models.[141, 172, 229] Ragni and Lindholm[172] used an experimental rabbit model of interbody fusion in which the incorporation of a porous HA block was enhanced by the addition of DBM. The animals implanted with the HA/DBM composite showed significantly earlier fusion consolidation than the animals implanted with DBM alone, HA alone, or autograft. By six months, however, the results were comparable to those attained using autograft bone. Zerwekh and colleagues[229] compared the efficacy of a collagen/ceramic (HA-TCP)/autograft composite with that of autograft bone alone in a dog L2–L4 posterior spinal fusion model. At 12 months, histologic quantitation of bone ingrowth and results from biomechanical testing were similar in both groups. Muschler and colleagues,[141] in two experiments using a dog segmental posterior spinal fusion model, compared posterior fusions attained using autograft, collagen/ceramic (HA-TCP) composite, collagen/ceramic (HA-TCP)/autograft composite, collagen/ceramic (HA-TCP)/bone matrix protein composite, and no graft material (control). Autograft bone was the most effective material tested and had a statistically superior union score. Results using the ceramic composite alone were no better

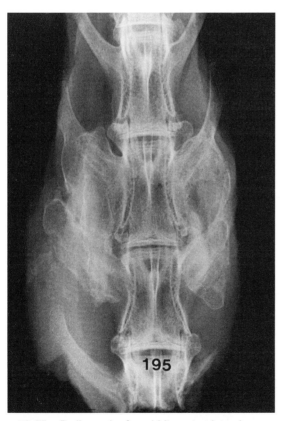

Figure 50–33. Radiograph of a rabbit posterolateral intertransverse process fusion five weeks after implantation with an osteoinductive growth factor with rabbit demineralized bone matrix as the carrier. (From Boden, S. D., Schimandle, J. H., and Hutton, W. C.: 1995 Volvo Award in Basic Sciences. The use of an osteoinductive growth factor for lumbar spinal fusion. Part II: Study of dose, carrier, and species. Spine *20*:2633–2644, 1995.)

Table 50–10. ANIMAL SPINAL FUSION MODELS USING CERAMIC BONE GRAFT SUBSTITUTES

Year[Ref]	Purpose	Animal	N	Fusion Type	Graft Material	Histology	X-ray	Bio-mechanical Testing	Miscellaneous
1983[63]	To study the use of $CaPO_2$ ceramic as a bone graft substitute	Rabbit	26	• Posterolateral vertebral body	• $CaPO_4$ ceramic	H	R MR	—	• Evaluated bony ingrowth into ceramic
1984[89]	To evaluate coralline HA as a bone graft substitute	Dog	16	• Posterior • L3–L6	• Coralline HA on one side/ local autograft on other	H	R	—	• No solid fusions at 24 mos. • Bone incorporation similar on both sides
1994[170]	To evaluate HA as a bone graft substitute	Goat	14	• Anterior interbody • 2 levels	• $CaPO_4$ ceramic	H	R	+	• 55% autograft fused • 50% HA fused
Ceramic Composites									
1991[172]	To evaluate HA/DBM as a bone graft substitute	Rabbit	26	• Anterior interbody • L4–L5 and L5–L6	• DBM • HA/DBM • HA • Autograft	H HM	R DR	—	• HA/DBM similar to autograft • HA/DBM facilitates earlier stabilization of the fusion
1992[229]	To assess osteoconductive capacity of HA/TCP/ collagen composite as a bone graft "filler"	Dog	12	• Posterior • L2–L4 c̄ wire/pin	• Composite/autograft • Autograft (iliac)	H SEM	R	+	• All fused with host bone • Composite/autograft is a suitable alternative to autograft alone • 2 experiments done
1993[141]	To describe a canine segmental spinal fusion model for comparison of bone grafting materials	Dog	26	• Posterior • Lumbar c̄ wire/ PMMA	• Autograft • TCP/HA/collagen composite • Composite/autograft • Composite/matrix protein	H	—	+	• Autograft best (12 of 13 fused) • Composite was a good carrier and graft expander • Composite alone not effective • Cell count/viability measured

DBM, demineralized bone matrix; HA, hydroxyapatite; TCP, tricalcium phosphate; PMMA, polymethyl methacrylate; H, routine histology; HM, histomorphometry; SEM, scanning electron microscopy; R, plain radiographs; MR, microradiography; DR, dynamic radiography.

than those with no graft material. The addition of a bone matrix protein extract to the composite, however, significantly improved the union score, making it comparable to that obtained using composite plus autograft bone.

These animal studies suggest that the use of ceramics and ceramic composites in spinal fusion surgery holds promise as a viable alternative to autogenous bone grafting, either as a graft replacement or for graft augmentation.[24, 33, 98, 135] These findings need to be confirmed in primate studies and ultimately in human clinical trials.

CLINICAL STUDIES USING BONE GRAFT SUBSTITUTES

The use of allograft bone as a graft material has expanded in recent years and appears to be a reasonable alternative to autogenous bone in meeting the need for supplemental or primary graft material for spinal fusion. Although there are many animal studies evaluating allograft, few clinical studies of adequate design have been reported. In general, allograft has compared favorably with autogenous bone in interbody fusions (cervical, anterior/posterior lumbar),[11, 18, 22, 40, 80, 124, 130, 178] but the results have not been reliable when it has been used posteriorly in the lumbar spine.[4, 101, 123] Thus, allograft seems to be more successful when placed in the anterior column under compression, as opposed to posteriorly under tension.

In 1981, Malinin and Brown[123] described the use of freeze-dried allograft bone in posterior lumbar spinal fusions. They observed a high incidence of graft resorption leading to nonunion using cortical strips of allograft wired to the facets, as well as with posterolateral intertransverse process fusions using corticocancellous matchsticks. Urist and Dawson[211] used antigen-extracted allograft bone with local autogenous bone to perform posterior thoracolumbar and lumbosacral intertransverse process fusions for a variety of diagnoses in 40 patients. Radiographic evidence of fusion was noted in 88 per cent of patients. In 1987, Nasca and Whelchel[145] reported their series of consecutive spinal fusions performed using a wide variety of anterior and posterior procedures. In posterior thoracolumbar and lumbosacral fusions using cryopreserved allograft, the fusion rate was 90 per cent (65 of 72), whereas in those fusions using autogenous bone, the fusion rate was 86 per cent (32 of 37). Knapp and Jones[109] in 1988 reported the results of a retrospective review of 50 consecutive patients in whom allograft was used in instrumented posterior spinal fusions. Thirty-seven patients were fused for spinal deformity, and 13 for fractures. Using freeze-dried corticocancellous allograft, the fusion rate was 98 per cent (49 of 50); the only nonunion occurred in the deformity group. The authors felt that the graft material used was not as important as the fusion technique and that the use of allograft was justified. In 1995, An and colleagues[4] reported their results comparing frozen allografts, freeze-dried allografts, autograft, and a mixture of allograft and autograft in the same

patient undergoing an instrumented posterolateral lumbar fusion. Twenty patients underwent lumbar fusion with pedicle screw instrumentation, with an autogenous bone graft being placed on one side in each patient and an allograft on the contralateral side. Bone fusion quality and density were graded radiographically at nine months. The results of this study indicated that autogenous bone grafts were superior to freeze-dried grafts, frozen allografts, or mixed grafts in providing higher fusion quality radiographically and significantly greater bone density in the fusion masses of adult patients undergoing an instrumented posterolateral fusion of the lumbar spine.

Many published reports on allograft have addressed its use in fusions for spinal deformity. In 1967, May and Mauck[125] performed fusion mass explorations for nonunion in patients fused for scoliosis. The nonunion rate at six months in patients fused with autoclaved or frozen allograft was 66 per cent (12 of 18), whereas in those fused with autogenous bone, the nonunion rate was 36 per cent (10 of 28). Aurori and coworkers[8] reviewed the records of 208 patients with adolescent idiopathic scoliosis treated surgically with Harrington instrumentation and posterior fusion with autogenous bone or frozen allograft. In all patients with suspected nonunion, the fusion mass was explored. Nonunion was confirmed in 5 of 94 patients (5.3 per cent) when allograft was used and in 5 of 114 patients (4.4 per cent) when autogenous bone was used. The difference in nonunion rates was not statistically significant. In 1986, McCarthy and associates[131] used fresh frozen allograft exclusively in 32 patients undergoing instrumented posterior fusions for paralytic scoliosis. At 12 months, there were no nonunions, and all patients had well-marginated fusion masses with distinct trabecular markings radiographically. Bridwell and colleagues[18] performed a prospective study of 24 adult patients with kyphosis or anterior column spinal defects treated with anterior fresh frozen allograft and posterior instrumentation and autogenous bone grafting. Upright radiographs were analyzed to assess maintenance of correction and success of anterior fusion. Twenty-two of 24 patients maintained correction of their deformity and experienced no graft collapse. At least 18 patients (range, 18 to 21) were graded radiographically as having fusions that were solid with remodeling and trabeculae noted, thus supporting the effectiveness of anterior structural allografting when combined with posterior instrumentation and autogenous bone grafting.

The clinical efficacy of ceramics as a graft material or as a component in a composite graft for spinal fusion has not been clearly established. In a study of 12 patients with severe scoliosis, Passuti and associates[158] used internal fixation and blocks of HA-TCP (3:2) alone or mixed with autogenous cancellous bone to stabilize the spine and fuse the facet joints. Clinical and radiographic assessment of the fusions was performed, and in two cases, biopsies of the graft material were obtained. At an average follow-up of 15 months, all patients exhibited complete radiographic fusions. Histologic examinations of the biopsy specimens revealed the formation of new bone that was directly bonded to the ceramic implant surface and inside the macropores. Although these results are favorable, they must be interpreted with consideration of the limitations of the study (small number of patients, average age of 14 years, limited diagnoses).

KNOWLEDGE GAPS AND FUTURE RESEARCH DIRECTIONS

Despite the large amount of knowledge gleaned from previous animal and clinical studies on spinal fusion, there is a void in our basic understanding of this multifactorial process. As a result, several critical questions deserve consideration.

What type of healing occurs during fusion consolidation? Although much is known about the sequence of bone repair in fracture healing, little is known about spinal fusion. Is fusion occurring through membranous bone formation, endochondral ossification, or both? Few previous studies described the sequential histology during the spinal fusion process, and the existing reports are conflicting and inconsistent.[174] Some studies reported cartilage as part of the early fusion mass,[89, 104, 155, 203] whereas others suggested that endochondral ossification is *not* part of the healing process[2, 97] Boden and coworkers[15] qualitatively and quantitatively analyzed the sequential histology of spinal fusion in a validated rabbit model for posterolateral intertransverse process fusion. Three distinct phases of healing were identified—inflammatory, reparative, and remodeling—and they occurred in sequence but in a delayed fashion in the central zone of the fusion mass compared with the outer transverse process zones. Membranous bone formation, evident first at the ends of the fusion emanating from the decorticated transverse processes, was the predominant mechanism of healing. The central zone of the fusion mass exhibited a period of endochondral bone formation in the middle phase of the fusion healing sequence. Understanding this process at a histologic level in humans can be the first step in preventing nonunions and predicting biologic interventions that will enhance union.

What is the ideal rigidity required for the fastest healing and strongest fusion mass? Biomechanical studies have focused on the effects of rigid instrumentation and resultant osteopenia. No study has determined what degree of rigidity is sufficient and whether too much rigidity is detrimental.

The molecular biology of the spinal fusion process is also a topic about which little knowledge exists. What triggers bone induction in this setting, and what is the sequence of gene expression occurring in the fusion healing process? Because the tissue and mechanical environment is different from that in fractures and long bone defects, we cannot assume that the biology is the same. Studies on gene expression in early fusion mass specimens would allow the characterization on a molecular level of the temporal sequence of bone formation and quantitation of specific osteoinductive proteins at various stages of fusion.

In attempting to answer any question relevant to spinal fusion, it is important that if an animal model is used, it be carefully considered in order to be a good analogue and to prevent the waste of excessive animal lives as well as the time, effort, and funding of the researcher.[188] The first requirement of any model used to study the spinal fusion process is the ability to replicate the surgical technique in the animal chosen. The second basic model requirement is the replication of an outcome similar to that seen in humans—that is, a similar nonunion rate. Despite optimal planning, experimental design, and equipment, selection of an inappropriate animal model will lead to useless, irrelevant, or possibly misleading information. Determination of the appropriateness of an animal model, however, can be the most difficult and time-consuming aspect of the study design.[187]

The particular aspect of the fusion process to be studied must be carefully considered. Will the study focus on mechanical or biologic questions? If biomechanics or spinal instrumentation is of interest, the larger, more expensive animals may be more suitable, as they more closely approximate the size and bony anatomy of the human spine. Although larger animals provide advantages for studies involving biomechanics, they offer little advantage for investigating biologic questions. Smaller, skeletally mature animals are useful in studying biologic questions, and by virtue of their lower cost and faster healing, they provide a larger data pool on which to base results.

Experimental design should follow valid scientific principles and replicate the specific clinical situation being modeled. Ideally, only one intervention should be studied in each animal and only one level fused with the same technique on each side. For any valid fusion model, concurrent autograft controls should be established, optimal study lengths and observation intervals must be carefully determined, and evaluation or assessment techniques must be validated. The development and refinement of a valid animal model to investigate these growth factors would prove useful in realizing this potential and would allow the further study and characterization of the multitude of factors affecting this complex process.[12]

With the discovery, isolation, and availability of extractable and recombinant osteoinductive bone matrix proteins, we have entered a new era of biologic manipulation and enhancement of bone formation. Whereas previous bone graft substitutes have strived only to equal the results of autograft, the use of osteoinductive proteins may result in a more rapid, more reliable, and more biomechanically sound fusion than the autograft gold standard. After appropriate animal studies are performed, prospective, blinded, and randomized clinical trials must carefully validate any potential bone graft substitute in each spinal application for which it will be used. The ultimate goal is that fusion nonunion will no longer be of clinical concern.

References

1. Albee, F. H.: Transplantation of a portion of the tibia into the spine for Pott's disease. JAMA 57:885–886, 1911.

2. Albee, F. H.: An experimental study of bone growth and the spinal bone transplant. JAMA *60:*1044–1049, 1913.

3. Allen, B. L., and Ferguson, R. L.: The operative treatment of myelomeningocele spinal deformity—1979. Orthop. Clin. North Am. *10:*845–862, 1979.

4. An, H. S., Lynch, K., and Toth, J.: Prospective comparison of autograft vs. allograft for adult posterolateral lumbar spine fusion: Differences among freeze-dried, frozen, and mixed grafts. J. Spinal Disord. *8:*131–135, 1995.

5. Anderson, K. J., LeCocq, J. F., and Mooney, J. G.: Clinical evaluation of processed heterologous bone transplants. Clin. Orthop. *29:*248–263, 1963.

6. Aprin, H., Bowen, J. R., MacEwen, G. D., and Hall, J.: Spine fusion in patients with spinal muscular atrophy. J. Bone Joint Surg. *64:*1179–1187, 1982.

7. Aronow, M. A., Gerstenfeld, L. C., Owen, T. A., et al.: Factors that promote progressive development of the osteoblast phenotype in cultured rat calvarial cells. J. Cell. Physiol. *143:*213–221, 1990.

8. Aurori, B. F., Weierman, R. J., Lowell, H. A., et al.: Pseudarthrosis after spinal fusion for scoliosis: A comparison of autogeneic and allogeneic bone grafts. Clin. Orthop. *199:*153–158, 1985.

9. Banwart, J. C., Asher, M. A., and Hassanein, R. S.: Iliac crest bone graft harvest donor site morbidity: A statistical evaluation. Spine *20:*1055–1060, 1995.

10. Baran, D. T., Bergfeld, M. A., Teitelbaum, S. L., and Avioli, L. V.: Effect of testosterone therapy on bone formation in an osteoporotic hypogonadal male. Calcif. Tissue Res. *26:*103–106, 1978.

11. Blumenthal, S. L., Baker, J., Dossett, A., and Selby, D. K.: The role of anterior lumbar fusion for internal disc disruption. Spine *13:*566–569, 1988.

12. Boden, S. D., Schimandle, J. H., and Hutton, W. C.: An experimental lumbar intertransverse process spinal fusion model: Radiographic, histologic, and biomechanical healing characteristics. Spine *20:*412–420, 1995.

13. Boden, S. D., Schimandle, J. H., and Hutton, W. C.: Lumbar intertransverse process spine arthrodesis using a bovine-derived osteoinductive bone protein. J. Bone Joint Surg. Am. *77:*1404–1417, 1995.

14. Boden, S. D., Schimandle, J. H., and Hutton, W. C.: 1995 Volvo Award in Basic Sciences. The use of an osteoinductive growth factor for lumbar spinal fusion. Part II: Study of dose, carrier, and species. Spine *20:*2633–2644, 1995.

15. Boden, S. D., Schimandle, J. H., Hutton, W. C., and Chen, M. I.: 1995 Volvo Award in Basic Sciences. The use of an osteoinductive growth factor for lumbar spinal fusion. Part I: The biology of spinal fusion. Spine *20:*2626–2632, 1995.

16. Bouchard, J. A., Koka, A., Bensusan, J. S., and Stevenson, S.: Effect of radiation on posterior spinal fusions: A rabbit model. (Abstract.) American Academy of Orthopaedic Surgeons annual meeting, 1994, p. 229.

17. Bradford, D. S.: Anterior vascular pedicle bone grafting for the treatment of kyphosis. Spine *5:*318–323, 1980.

18. Bridwell, K. H., Lenke, L. G., McEnery, K. W., et al.: Anterior fresh frozen structural allografts in the thoracic and lumbar spine. Spine *20:*1410–1418, 1995.

19. Bridwell, K. H., Sedgewick, T. A., O'Brien, M. F., et al.: The role of fusion and instrumentation in the treatment of degenerative spondylolisthesis with spinal stenosis. J. Spinal Disord. *6:*461–472, 1993.

20. Brighton, C. T.: The treatment of non-unions with electricity. J. Bone Joint Surg. Am. *63:*847–851, 1981.

21. Brown, C. W., Orme, T. J., and Richardson, H. D.: The rate of pseudarthrosis (surgical nonunion) in patients who are smokers and patients who are nonsmokers: A comparison study. Spine *11:*942–943, 1986.

22. Brown, M. D., Malinin, T. I., and Davis, P. B.: A roentgenographic evaluation of frozen allografts versus autografts in anterior cervical spine fusions. Clin. Orthop. *119:*231–236, 1976.

23. Bucholz, R. W.: Clinical experience with bone graft substitutes. J. Orthop. Trauma *1:*260–262, 1987.

24. Bucholz, R. W., Carlton, A., and Holmes, R. E.: Hydroxyapatite and tricalcium phosphate bone graft substitutes. Orthop. Clin. North Am. *18:*323–334, 1987.

25. Buck, B. E., Malinin, T. I., and Brown, M. D.: Bone transplantation and human immunodeficiency virus. Clin. Orthop. *240:*129–136, 1989.

26. Buckwalter, J. A., and Cruess, R. L.: Healing of the musculoskeletal tissues. *In* Rockwood, C. A., and Green, D. P. (eds.): Fractures in Adults. 3rd ed. Philadelphia, J. B. Lippincott Co., 1991, pp. 181–222.

27. Buckwalter, J. A., Glimcher, M. J., Cooper, R. R., and Recker, R.: Bone biology. Part II: Formation, form, modeling, remodeling, and regulation of cell function. J. Bone Joint Surg. Am. *77:*1276–1289, 1995.

28. Burch, W. M., and Lebovitz, H. E.: Triiodothyronine stimulation of in vitro growth and maturation of embryonic chick cartilage. Endocrinology *111:*462–468, 1982.

29. Burchardt, H., and Enneking, W. F.: Transplantation of bone. Surg. Clin. North Am. *58:*403–427, 1978.

30. Burchardt, H., Glowczewskie, F. P., and Enneking, W. F.: The effect of adriamycin and methotrexate on the repair of segmental cortical autografts in dogs. J. Bone Joint Surg. *65:*103–108, 1983.

31. Burwell, R. G.: Studies in the transplantation of bone. VII. The fresh composite homograft-autograft of cancellous bone. An analysis of factors leading to osteogenesis in marrow transplants and in marrow-containing bone grafts. J. Bone Joint Surg. Br. *46:*110–140, 1964.

32. Burwell, R. G.: The function of bone marrow in the incorporation of a bone graft. Clin. Orthop. *200:*125–141, 1985.

33. Cameron, H. U., Macnab, I., and Pilliar, R. M.: Evaluation of a biodegradable ceramic. J. Biomed. Mater. Res. *11:*179–186, 1977.

34. Canalis, E.: The hormonal and local regulation of bone formation. Endocr. Rev. *4:*62–77, 1983.

35. Canalis, E.: Effect of growth factors on bone cell replication and differentiation. Clin. Orthop. *193:*246–263, 1985.

36. Canalis, E., McCarthy, T., and Centrella, M.: Growth factors and the regulation of bone remodeling. J. Clin. Invest. *81:*277–281, 1988.

37. Canalis, E., and Raisz, L. G.: Effect of sex steroids on bone collagen synthesis in vitro. Calcif. Tissue Res. *25:*105–110, 1978.

38. CDC: Transmission of HIV through bone transplantation: Case report and public health recommendations. JAMA *260:*2487–2488, 1988.

39. Chalmers, J., Gray, D. H., and Rush, J.: Observations on the induction of bone in soft tissues. J. Bone Joint Surg. Br. *57:*36–45, 1975.

40. Cloward, R. B.: Gas-sterilized cadaver bone grafts for spinal fusion operations: A simplified bone bank. Spine *5:*4–10, 1980.

41. Cook, S. D., Dalton, J. E., Prewett, A. B., and Whitecloud, T. S.: In vivo evaluation of demineralized bone matrix as a bone graft substitute for posterior spinal fusion. Spine *20:*877–886, 1995.

42. Cook, S. D., Dalton, J. E., Tan, E. H., et al.: In vivo evaluation of recombinant human osteogenic protein (rhOP-1) implants as a bone graft substitute for spinal fusions. Spine *19:*1655–1663, 1994.

43. Coviello, J., and Brilliant, J. D.: A preliminary clinical study on the use of tricalcium phosphate as an apical barrier. J. Endocrinol. *5:*6–13, 1979.

44. Craven, P. L., and Urist, M. R.: Osteogenesis by radioisotope labelled cell populations in implants of bone matrix under the influence of ionizing radiation. Clin. Orthop. *76:*231–243, 1971.

45. Cruess, R. L., and Sakai, T.: Effect of cortisone upon synthesis rates of some components of rat matrix. Clin. Orthop. *86:*253–259, 1972.

46. Czitrom, A. A.: Principles and techniques of tissue banking. *In* Heckman, J. D. (ed.): American Academy of Orthopaedic Surgeons Instructional Course Lectures. 42nd ed. Rosemont: American Academy of Orthopaedic Surgeons, 1993, pp. 359–362.

47. Daftari, T. K., Whitesides, T. E., Heller, J. G., et al.: Nicotine on the revascularization of bone graft: An experimental study in rabbits. Spine *19:*904–911, 1994.

48. Dahners, L. E., and Jacobs, R. R.: Long bone defects treated with demineralized bone. South. Med. J. *78:*933–934, 1985.

49. de Vernejoul, M. C., Bielakoff, J., Herve, M., et al.: Evidence for

defective osteoblastic function: A role for alcohol and tobacco consumption in osteoporosis in middle-aged men. Clin. Orthop. *179*:107–115, 1983.

50. Dell, P. C., Burchardt, H., and Glowczewskie, F. P.: A roentgenographic, biomechanical, and histological evaluation of vascularized and non-vascularized segmental fibular canine autografts. J. Bone Joint Surg. *67*:105–112, 1985.

51. Denissen, H. W., and de Groot, K.: Immediate dental root implants from synthetic dense calcium hydroxylapatite. J. Prosthet. Dent. *42*:551–556, 1979.

52. Dubuc, F. L., and Urist, M. R.: The accessibility of the bone induction principle in surface-decalcified bone implants. Clin. Orthop. *55*:217–223, 1967.

53. Dwyer, A. F.: The use of electrical current stimulation in spinal fusion. Orthop. Clin. North Am. *6*:265–279, 1975.

54. Dwyer, A. F., and Wickham, G. G.: Direct current stimulation in spinal fusion. Med. J. Aust. *1*:73–75, 1974.

55. Einhorn, T. A.: Current concepts review: Enhancement of fracture-healing. J. Bone Joint Surg. Am. *77*:940–956, 1995.

56. Einhorn, T. A., Bonnarens, F., and Burstein, A. H.: The contributions of dietary protein and mineral to the healing of experimental fractures: A biomechanical study. J. Bone Joint Surg. Am. *68*:1389–1395, 1986.

57. Einhorn, T. A., Lane, J. M., Burstein, A. H., et al.: The healing of segmental bone defects induced by demineralized bone matrix: A radiographic and biomechanical study. J. Bone Joint Surg. Am. *66*:274–279, 1984.

58. Emery, S. E., Brazinski, M. S., Koka, A., et al.: The biological and biomechanical effects of irradiation on anterior spinal bone grafts: A canine model. J. Bone Joint Surg. Am. *76*:540–548, 1994.

59. Enneking, W. F., Burchardt, H., Puhl, J. J., and Piotrowski, G.: Physical and biological aspects of repair in dog cortical bone transplants. J. Bone Joint Surg. Am. *57*:237–252, 1975.

60. Evans, J. H.: Biomechanics of lumbar fusion. Clin. Orthop. *193*:38–46, 1985.

61. Fernyhough, J. C., Schimandle, J. H., Weigel, M. C., et al.: Chronic donor site pain complicating bone graft harvesting from the posterior iliac crest for spinal fusion. Spine *17*:1474–1480, 1992.

62. Ferraro, J. W.: Experimental evaluation of ceramic calcium phosphate as a substitute for bone grafts. Plast. Reconstr. Surg. *63*:634–640, 1979.

63. Flatley, T. J., Lynch, K. L., and Benson, M.: Tissue response to implants of calcium phosphate ceramic in the rabbit spine. Clin. Orthop. *179*:246–252, 1983.

64. Frenkel, S. R., Moskovitch, R., Spivak, J., et al.: Demineralized bone matrix: Enhancement of spinal fusion. Spine *18*:1634–1639, 1993.

65. Friedenberg, Z. B., and Brighton, C. T.: Bioelectric potentials in bone. J. Bone Joint Surg. Am. *48*:915–923, 1966.

66. Friedlaender, G. E.: Current concepts review: Bone-banking. J. Bone Joint Surg. *64*:307–311, 1982.

67. Friedlaender, G. E., Tross, R. B., Doganis, A. C., et al.: Effects of chemotherapeutic agents on bone: I. Short-term methotrexate and doxorubicin (Adriamycin) treatment in a rat model. J. Bone Joint Surg. *66*:602–607, 1984.

68. Gallagher, J. C., Riggs, B. L., and DeLuca, H. F.: Effect of estrogen on calcium absorption and serum vitamin D metabolites in postmenopausal osteoporosis. J. Clin. Endocrinol. Metab. *51*:1359–1364, 1980.

69. Gazdag, A. R., Lane, J. M., Glaser, D., and Forster, R. A.: Alternatives to autogenous bone graft: Efficacy and indications. J. Am. Acad. Orthop. Surg. *3*:1–8, 1995.

70. Gepstein, R., Weiss, R. E., Saba, K., and Hallel, T.: Bridging large defects in bone by demineralized bone matrix in the form of a powder. J. Bone Joint Surg. Am. *69*:984–992, 1987.

71. Glowacki, J., Murray, J. E., Kaban, L. B., et al.: Application of the biological principle of induced osteogenesis for craniofacial defects. Lancet *1*:959–963, 1981.

72. Goldberg, V., Sloss, A., and Powell, A.: Survival of bone marrow in irradiated rats receiving composite marrow/bone allografts. (Abstract.) Trans. Orthop. Res. Soc. *31*:107, 1985.

73. Guizzardi, S., Di Silvestre, M., Scandroglio, R., et al.: Implants of heterologous demineralized bone matrix for induction of posterior spinal fusion in rats. Spine *17*:701–707, 1992.

74. Gurr, K. R., McAfee, P. C., and Shih, C.: Biomechanical analysis of anterior and posterior instrumentation systems after corpectomy: A calf spine model. J. Bone Joint Surg. Am. *70*:1182–1191, 1988.

75. Gurr, K. R., McAfee, P. C., and Shih, C.: Biomechanical analysis of posterior instrumentation systems after decompressive laminectomy. J. Bone Joint Surg. Am. *70*:680–691, 1988.

76. Gurr, K. R., McAfee, P. C., Warden, K. E., and Shih, C.: Roentgenographic and biomechanical analysis of lumbar fusions: A canine model. J. Orthop. Res. *7*:838–848, 1989.

77. Hahn, T. J.: Corticosteroid-induced osteopenia. Arch. Intern. Med. *138*:882–885, 1978.

78. Ham, A., and Gordon, S.: The origin of bone that forms in association with cancellous chips transplanted into muscle. Br. J. Plast. Surg. *5*:154–160, 1952.

79. Hanley, E. N., and Levy, J. A.: Surgical treatment of isthmic lumbosacral spondylolisthesis: Analysis of variables affecting results. Spine *14*:48–50, 1989.

80. Hanley, E. N., Jr., Harvell, J. C., Shapiro, D. E., and Kraus, D. R.: Use of allograft bone in cervical spine surgery. Semin. Spine Surg. *1*:262–270, 1989.

81. Harmon, P.: Processed heterologous bone implants (Boplant, Squibb) as grafts in spinal surgery. Acta Orthop. Scand. *35*:98–116, 1964.

82. Harrington, K. D.: Metastatic tumors of the spine: Diagnosis and treatment. J. Am. Acad. Orthop. Surg. *1*:76–86, 1993.

83. Hartshorne, E.: On the causes and treatment of pseudarthrosis, and especially of the form of it sometimes called supernumerary joint. Am. J. Med. Sci. *1*:121–156, 1841.

84. Heckman, J. D., Ingram, A. J., Loyd, R. D., et al.: Nonunion treatment with pulsed electromagnetic fields. Clin. Orthop. *161*:58–66, 1981.

85. Heiple, K. G., Chase, S. W., and Herndon, C. H.: A comparative study of the healing process following different types of bone transplantation. J. Bone Joint Surg. *45*:1593–1616, 1963.

86. Heiple, K. G., Kendrick, R. E., Herndon, C. H., and Chase, S. W.: A critical evaluation of processed calf bone. J. Bone Joint Surg. *49*:1119–1127, 1967.

87. Hibbs, R. A.: An operation for progressive spinal deformities: A preliminary report of three cases from the service of the Orthopaedic Hospital. N. Y. State J. Med. *93*:1013–1016, 1911.

88. Hollo, I., Gergely, I., and Boross, M.: Smoking results in calcitonin resistance. JAMA *237*:2470, 1977.

89. Holmes, R., Mooney, V., Bucholz, R., and Tencer, A.: A coralline hydroxyapatite bone graft substitute. Clin. Orthop. *188*:252–262, 1984.

90. Holmes, R. E.: Bone regeneration within a coralline hydroxyapatite implant. Plast. Reconstr. Surg. *63*:626–633, 1979.

91. Holmes, R. E., Bucholz, R. W., and Mooney, V.: Porous hydroxyapatite as a bone substitute in metaphyseal defects. J. Bone Joint Surg. Am. *68*:904–911, 1986.

92. Holmes, R. E., Bucholz, R. W., and Mooney, V.: Porous hydroxyapatite as a bone graft substitute in diaphyseal defects: A histometric study. J. Orthop. Res. *5*:114–121, 1987.

93. Holmes, R. E., and Salyer, K. E.: Bone regeneration in a coralline hydroxyapatite implant. Surg. For. *29*:611–612, 1978.

94. Hoogendoorn, H. A., Renooij, W., Akkermans, L. M. A., et al.: Long-term study of large ceramic implants (porous hydroxyapatite) in dog femora. Clin. Orthop. *187*:281–288, 1984.

95. Hopp, S. G., Dahners, L. E., and Gilbert, J. A.: A study of the mechanical strength of long bone defects treated with various bone autograft substitutes: An experimental investigation in the rabbit. J. Orthop. Res. *7*:579–584, 1989.

96. Hulth, A., Johnell, O., and Henricson, A.: The implantation of demineralized fracture matrix yields more new bone formation than does intact matrix. Clin. Orthop. *234*:235–249, 1988.

97. Hurley, L. A., Stinchfield, F. E., Bassett, A. L., and Lyon, W. H.: The role of soft tissues in osteogenesis: An experimental study of canine spine fusions. J. Bone Joint Surg. Am. *41*:1243–1254, 1959.

98. Jarcho, M.: Calcium phosphate ceramics as hard tissue prosthetics. Clin. Orthop. *157*:259–278, 1981.

99. Jensen, J. E., Jensen, T. G., Smith, T. K., et al.: Nutrition in orthopaedic surgery. J. Bone Joint Surg. *64*:1263–1272, 1982.

100. Johnston, C. E., Ashman, R. B., Sherman, M. C., et al.: Mechanical consequences of rod contouring and residual scoliosis in sublaminar segmental instrumentation. J. Orthop. Res. 5:206–216, 1987.

101. Jorgenson, S. S., Lowe, T. G., France, J., and Sabin, J.: A prospective analysis of autograft versus allograft in posterolateral lumbar fusion in the same patient: A minimum of 1 year follow-up in 144 patients. Spine 19:2048–2053, 1994.

102. Jowsey, J., and Riggs, B. L.: Bone formation in hypercortisonism. Acta Endocrinol. (Copenh.) 63:21–28, 1970.

103. Kahanovitz, N., and Arnoczky, S. P.: The efficacy of direct current electrical stimulation to enhance canine spinal fusions. Clin. Orthop. 251:295–299, 1990.

104. Kahanovitz, N., Arnoczky, S. P., Hulse, D., and Shires, P. K.: The effect of postoperative electromagnetic pulsing on canine posterior spinal fusions. Spine 9:273–279, 1984.

105. Kahanovitz, N., Arnoczky, S. P., Nemzek, J., and Shores, A.: The effect of electromagnetic pulsing on posterior lumbar spinal fusions in dogs. Spine 19:705–709, 1994.

106. Kale, A. A., and DiCesare, P. E.: Osteoinductive agents: Basic science and clinical applications. Am. J. Orthop. 24:752–761, 1995.

107. Kane, W. J.: Direct current electrical bone growth stimulation for spinal fusion. Spine 13:363–365, 1988.

108. Kent, J. K., Quinn, J. H., Zide, M. F., et al.: Alveolar ridge augmentation using nonresorbable hydroxylapatite with or without autogenous cancellous bone. J. Oral Maxillofac. Surg. 41:629–642, 1983.

109. Knapp, D. R., and Jones, E. T.: Use of cortical cancellous allograft for posterior spinal fusion. Clin. Orthop. 229:99–106, 1988.

110. Kostuik, J. P., Errico, T. J., Gleason, T. F., and Errico, C. C.: Spinal stabilization of vertebral column tumors. Spine 3:250–256, 1988.

111. Lafferty, F. W., Spencer, G. E., and Pearson, O. H.: Effects of androgens, estrogens, and high calcium intakes on bone formation and resorption in osteoporosis. Am. J. Med. 36:514–528, 1964.

112. Lane, J. M., and Sandhu, H. S.: Current approaches to experimental bone grafting. Orthop. Clin. North Am. 18:213–225, 1987.

113. Lau, G. C., Luck, J. V., Marshall, G. J., and Griffith, G.: The effect of cigarette smoking on fracture healing: An animal model. Clin. Res. 37:132A, 1989.

114. Laurie, S. W. S., Kaban, L. B., Mulliken, J. B., and Murray, J. E.: Donor-site morbidity after harvesting rib and iliac bone. Plast. Reconstr. Surg. 73:933–938, 1984.

115. Lavine, L. S., Lustrin, I., and Shamos, M. H.: Treatment of congenital pseudarthrosis of the tibia with direct current. Clin. Orthop. 124:69–74, 1977.

116. Lebwohl, N. H., Starr, J. K., Milne, E. L., et al.: Inhibitory effect of ibuprofen on spinal fusion in rabbits. (Abstract.) American Academy of Orthopaedic Surgeons annual meeting, 1994, p. 278.

117. Levin, M. P., Getter, L., Adrian, J., and Cutright, D. E.: Healing of periodontal defects with ceramic implants. J. Clin. Periodontol. 1:197–205, 1974.

118. Levin, M. P., Getter, L., and Cutright, D. E.: A comparison of iliac marrow and biodegradable ceramic in periodontal defects. J. Biomed. Mater. Res. 9:183–195, 1975.

119. Lindholm, T. S., Nilsson, O. S., and Lindholm, T. C.: Extraskeletal and intraskeletal new bone formation induced by demineralized bone matrix combined with bone marrow cells. Clin. Orthop. 171:251–255, 1982.

120. Lindholm, T. S., Ragni, P., and Lindholm, T. C.:Response of bone marrow stroma cells to demineralized cortical bone matrix in experimental spinal fusion in rabbits. Clin. Orthop. 230:296–302, 1988.

121. Lorenz, M., Zindrick, M., Schwaegler, P., et al.: A comparison of single-level fusions with and without hardware. Spine 16:S455–S458, 1991.

122. Lovell, T. P., Dawson, E. G., Nilsson, O. S., and Urist, M. R.: Augmentation of spinal fusion with bone morphogenetic protein in dogs. Clin. Orthop. 243:266–274, 1989.

123. Malinin, T. I., and Brown, M. D.: Bone allografts in spinal surgery. Clin. Orthop. 154:68–73, 1981.

124. Malinin, T. I., Rosomoff, H. L., and Sutton, C. H.: Human cadaver femoral head homografts for anterior cervical spine fusions. Surg. Neurol. 7:249–251, 1977.

125. May, V. R., and Mauck, W. R.: Exploration of the spine for pseudarthrosis following spinal fusion in the treatment of scoliosis. Clin. Orthop. 53:115–122, 1967.

126. McAfee, P. C., Farey, I. D., Sutterlin, C. E., et al.: Device-related osteoporosis with spinal instrumentation. Spine 14:919–926, 1989.

127. McAfee, P. C., Farey, I. D., Sutterlin, C. E., et al.: The effect of spinal implant rigidity on vertebral bone density: A canine model. Spine 16:S190–S197, 1991.

128. McAfee, P. C., Regan, J. J., Farey, I. D., et al.: The biomechanical and histomorphometric properties of anterior lumbar fusions: A canine model. J. Spinal Disord. 1:101–110, 1988.

129. McAfee, P. C., Werner, F. W., and Glisson, R. R.: A biomechanical analysis of spinal instrumentation systems in thoracolumbar fractures: Comparison of traditional Harrington distraction instrumentation with segmental spinal instrumentation. Spine 10:204–217, 1985.

130. McBride, G. G., and Bradford, D. S.: Vertebral body replacement with femoral neck allograft and vascularized rib strut graft: A technique for treating post-traumatic kyphosis with neurologic deficit. Spine 8:406–415, 1983.

131. McCarthy, R. E., Peek, R. D., Morrissy, R. T., and Hough, A. J.: Allograft bone in spinal fusion for paralytic scoliosis. J. Bone Joint Surg. Am. 68:370–375, 1986.

132. McGuire, R. A., and Amundson, G. M.: The use of primary internal fixation in spondylolisthesis. Spine 18:1662–1672, 1993.

133. McMurray, G. N.: The evaluation of Kiel bone in spinal fusions. J. Bone Joint Surg. Br. 64:101–104, 1982.

134. Meril, A. J.: Direct current stimulation of allograft in anterior and posterior lumbar interbody fusions. Spine 19:2393–2398, 1994.

135. Metsger, D. S., Driskell, T. D., and Paulsrud, J. R.: Tricalcium phosphate ceramic—a resorbable bone implant: Review and current status. J. Am. Dent. Assoc. 105:1035–1038, 1982.

136. Misol, S., Samaan, N., and Ponseti, I. V.: Growth hormone in delayed fracture union. Clin. Orthop. 74:206–208, 1971.

137. Mohan, S., and Baylink, D. J.: Bone growth factors. Clin. Orthop. 263:30–48, 1991.

138. Mooney, V.: A randomized double-blind prospective study of the efficacy of pulsed electromagnetic fields for interbody lumbar fusions. Spine 15:708–712, 1990.

139. Moore, D. C., Chapman, M. W., and Manske, D.: The evaluation of a biphasic calcium phosphate ceramic for use in grafting long-bone diaphyseal defects. J. Orthop. Res. 5:356–365, 1987.

140. Mulliken, J. B., Glowacki, J., Kaban, L. B., et al.: Use of demineralized allogeneic bone implants for the correction of maxillocraniofacial deformities. Ann. Surg. 194:366–372, 1981.

141. Muschler, G. F., Huber, B., Ullman, T., et al.: Evaluation of bone grafting materials in a new canine segmental spinal fusion model. J. Orthop. Res. 11:514–524, 1993.

142. Muschler, G. F., Hyodo, A., Manning, T., et al.: Evaluation of human bone morphogenetic protein 2 in a canine spinal fusion model. Clin. Orthop. 308:229–240, 1994.

143. Nade, S., Armstrong, L., McCartney, E., and Baggaley, B.: Osteogenesis after bone and bone marrow transplantation. Clin. Orthop. 181:255–263, 1983.

144. Nagel, D. A., Kramers, P. C., Rahn, B. A., et al.: A paradigm of delayed union and nonunion in the lumbosacral joint: A study of motion and bone grafting of the lumbosacral spine in sheep. Spine 16:553–559, 1991.

145. Nasca, R. J., and Whelchel, J. D.: Use of cryopreserved bone in spinal surgery. Spine 12:222–227, 1987.

146. Nerubay, J., and Katznelson, A.: Clinical evaluation of an electrical current stimulator in spinal fusions. Int. Orthop. 7:239–242, 1984.

147. Nerubay, J., Margant, B., Bubis, J. J., et al.: Stimulation of bone formation by electrical current on spinal fusion. Spine 11:167–169, 1986.

148. Nery, E. B., and Lynch, K. L.: Preliminary clinical studies of bioceramic in periodontal osseous defects. J. Periodontol. 49:523–527, 1978.

149. Nery, E. B., Lynch, K. L., Hirthe, W. M., and Mueller, K. H.:

Bioceramic implants in surgically produced infrabony defects. J. Periodontol. *46:*328–347, 1975.

150. Nery, E. B., Lynch, K. L., and Rooney, G. E.: Alveolar ridge augmentation with tricalcium phosphate ceramic. J. Prosthet. Dent. *40:*668–675, 1978.

151. Nery, E. B., Pflughoeft, F. A., Lynch, K. L., and Rooney, G. E.: Functional loading of bioceramic augmented alveolar ridge: A pilot study. J. Prosthet. Dent. *43:*338–343, 1980.

152. Nilsson, O. S., Bauer, H. C. F., and Brostrom, L.: Methotrexate effects on heterotopic bone in rats. Acta Orthop. Scand. *58:*47–53, 1987.

153. Nisbet, N. W.: Antigenicity of bone. J. Bone Joint Surg. Br. *59:*263–266, 1977.

154. Ohgushi, H., Goldberg, V. M., and Caplan, A. I.: Heterotopic osteogenesis in porous ceramics induced by marrow cells. J. Orthop. Res. *7:*568–579, 1989.

155. Oikarinen, J.: Experimental spinal fusion with decalcified bone matrix and deep-frozen allogeneic bone in rabbits. Clin. Orthop. *162:*210–218, 1982.

156. Oikarinen, J., and Korhonen, L. K.: The bone inductive capacity of various bone transplanting materials used for treatment of experimental bone defects. Clin. Orthop. *140:*208–215, 1979.

157. Osborn, J. F., and Newesely, H.: The material science of calcium phosphate ceramics. Biomaterials *1:*108–111, 1980.

158. Passuti, N., Daculsi, G., Rogez, J. M., et al.: Macroporous calcium phosphate ceramic performance in human spine fusion. Clin. Orthop. *248:*169–176, 1989.

159. Paterson, D. C., Carter R. F., Maxwell, G. M., et al.: Electrical bone growth stimulation in an experimental model of delayed union. Lancet *1:*1278–1281, 1977.

160. Paterson, D. C., Lewis, G. N., and Cass, C. A.: Treatment of delayed union and nonunion with an implanted direct current stimulator. Clin. Orthop. *148:*117–128, 1980.

161. Paterson, D. C., Lewis, G. N., and Cass, C. A.: Treatment of congenital pseudarthrosis of the tibia with direct current stimulation. Clin. Orthop. *148:*129–135, 1980.

162. Patka, P., den Otter, G., de Groot, K., and Driessen, A. A.: Reconstruction of large bone defects with calcium phosphate ceramics—an experimental study. Neth. J. Surg. *37:*38–44, 1985.

163. Pelker, R. R., and Friedlaender, G. E.: Biomechanical aspects of bone autografts and allografts. Orthop. Clin. North Am. *18:*235–239, 1987.

164. Pelker, R. R., Friedlaender, G. E., and Markham, T. C.: Biomechanical properties of bone allografts. Clin. Orthop. *174:*54–57, 1983.

165. Pelker, R. R., Friedlaender, G. E., Markham, T. C., et al.: Effects of freezing and freeze-drying on the biomechanical properties of rat bone. J. Orthop. Res. *1:*405–411, 1984.

166. Pelker, R. R., Friedlaender, G. E., Panjabi, M. M., et al.: Chemotherapy-induced alterations in the biomechanics of rat bone. J. Orthop. Res. *3:*91–95, 1985.

167. Phillips, L. S., and Vassilopoulou-Sellin, R.: Somatomedins: Part II. N. Engl. J. Med. *302:*438–446, 1980.

168. Phillips, L. S., and Vassilopoulou-Sellin, R.: Somatomedins: Part I. N. Engl. J. Med. *302:*371–380, 1980.

169. Pieron, A. P., Bigelow, D., and Hamonic, M.: Bone grafting with Boplant: Results in thirty-three cases. J. Bone Joint Surg. *50:*364–368, 1968.

170. Pintar, F. A., Maiman, D. J., Hollowell, J. P., et al. Fusion rate and biomechanical stiffness of hydroxylapatite versus autogenous bone grafts for anterior discectomy: An in vivo animal study. Spine *19:*2524–2528, 1994.

171. Prolo, D. J., and Rodrigo, J. J.: Contemporary bone graft physiology and surgery. Clin. Orthop. *200:*322–342, 1985.

172. Ragni, P., and Lindholm, S.: Interaction of allogeneic demineralized bone matrix and porous hydroxyapatite bioceramics in lumbar interbody fusion in rabbits. Clin. Orthop. *272:*292–299, 1991.

173. Ragni, P. C., and Lindholm, T. S.: Bone formation and static changes in the thoracic spine at uni- or bilateral experimental spondylodesis with demineralized bone matrix (DBM). Ital. J. Orthop. Traumatol. *15:*237–252, 1989.

174. Ragni, P. C., Lindholm, T. S., and Lindholm, T. C.: Vertebral fusion dynamics in the thoracic and lumbar spine induced by allogenic demineralized bone matrix combined with autogenous bone marrow: An experimental study in rabbits. Ital. J. Orthop. Traumatol. *13:*241–251, 1987.

175. Rawlinson, J. N.: Morbidity after anterior cervical decompression and fusion: The influence of the donor site on recovery, and the results of a trial of surgibone compared to autologous bone. Acta Neurochir. *131:*106–118, 1994.

176. Riebel, G. D., Boden, S. D., Whitesides, T. E., and Hutton, W. C.: The effect of nicotine on incorporation of cancellous bone graft in an animal model. Spine *20:*2198–2202, 1995.

177. Riggs, B. L., Jowsey, J., Goldsmith, R. S., et al.: Short- and long-term effects of estrogen and synthetic anabolic hormone in postmenopausal osteoporosis. J. Clin. Invest. *51:*1659–1663, 1972.

178. Rish, B. L., McFadden, J. T., and Penix, J. O.: Anterior cervical fusion using homologous bone grafts: A comparative study. Surg. Neurol. *5:*119–121, 1976.

179. Roberts, S. C., and Brilliant, J. D.: Tricalcium phosphate as an adjunct to apical closure in pulpless permanent teeth. J. Endocrinol. *1:*263–269, 1975.

180. Rokkanen, P., Vainionpaa, S., Tormala, P., et al.: Biodegradable implants in fracture fixation: Early results of treatment of fractures of the ankle. Lancet *1:*1422–1424, 1985.

181. Rose, G. K., Owen, R., and Sanderson, J. M.: Transposition of rib with blood supply for the stabilisation of a spinal kyphos. J. Bone Joint Surg. Br. *57:*112, 1975.

182. Salama, R.: Xenogeneic bone grafting in humans. Clin. Orthop. *174:*113–121, 1983.

183. Salama, R., Burwell, R. G., and Dickson, I. R.: Recombined grafts of bone and marrow: The beneficial effect upon osteogenesis of impregnating xenograft (heterograft) bone with autologous red marrow. J. Bone Joint Surg. Br. *55:*402–417, 1973.

184. Salama, R., and Weissman, S. L.: The clinical use of combined xenografts of bone and autologous red marrow: A preliminary report. J. Bone Joint Surg. Br. *60:*111–115, 1978.

185. Sandhu, H. S., Kanim, L. E. A., Kabo, J. M., et al.: Evaluation of rhBMP-2 with an OPLA carrier in a canine posterolateral (transverse process) spinal fusion model. Spine *20:*2669–2682, 1995.

186. Schalch, D. S., Heinrich, U. E., Draznin, B., et al.: Role of the liver in regulating somatomedin activity: Hormonal effects on the synthesis and release of insulin-like growth factor and its carrier protein by the isolated perfused rat liver. Endocrinology *104:*1143–1151, 1979.

187. Schimandle, J. H., and Boden, S. D.: The use of animal models to study spinal fusion. Spine *19:*1998–2006, 1994.

188. Schimandle, J. H., and Boden, S. D.: Animal use in spinal research. Spine *19:*2474–2477, 1994.

189. Schimandle, J. H., Boden, S. D., and Hutton, W. C.: Experimental spinal fusion with recombinant human bone morphogenetic protein-2 (rhBMP-2). Spine *20:*1326–1337, 1995.

190. Schimandle, J. H., Weigel, M., and Edwards, C. C.: Indications for thigh cuff bracing following instrumented lumbosacral fusions. (Abstract.) North American Spine Society annual meeting, 1993, pp. 41–42.

191. Shaffer, J. W., Field, G. A., Goldberg, V. M., and Davy, D. T.: Fate of vascularized and nonvascularized autografts. Clin Orthop. *197:*32–43, 1985.

192. Shima, T., Keller, J. T., Alvira, M. M., et al.: Anterior cervical discectomy and interbody fusion. J. Neurosurg. *51:*533–538, 1979.

193. Shimazaki, K., and Mooney, V.: Comparative study of porous hydroxyapatite and tricalcium phosphate as bone substitute. J. Orthop. Res. *3:*301–310, 1985.

194. Shirado, O., Zdeblick, T. A., McAfee, P. C., et al.: Quantitative histologic study of the influence of anterior spinal instrumentation and biodegradable polymer on lumbar interbody fusion after corpectomy. Spine *17:*795–803, 1992.

195. Silcox, D. H., Daftari, T., Boden, S. D., et al.: The effect of nicotine on spinal fusion. Spine *20:*1549–1553, 1995.

196. Simmons, D. J., and Kunin, A. S.: Autoradiographic and biochemical investigations of the effect of cortisone on the bones of the rat. Clin. Orthop. *55:*201–215, 1967.

197. Spadaro, J. A.: Electrically stimulated bone growth in animals and man: Review of the literature. Clin. Orthop. *122:*325–332, 1977.

198. Strub, J. R., Gaberthuel, T. W., and Firestone, A. R.: Comparison of tricalcium phosphate and frozen allogenic bone implants in man. J. Periodontol. *50*:624–629, 1979.
199. Sumner, D. R., Turner, T. M., Purchio, A. F., et al.: Enhancement of bone ingrowth by transforming growth factor beta. J. Bone Joint Surg. Am. *77*:1135–1147, 1995.
200. Swank, S. M., Brown, J. C., and Perry, R. E.: Spinal fusion in Duchenne's muscular dystrophy. Spine *7*:484–491, 1982.
201. Takagi, K., and Urist, M. R.: The role of bone marrow in bone morphogenetic protein induced repair of femoral massive diaphyseal defects. Clin. Orthop. *171*:224–231, 1982.
202. Takaoka, K., Nakahara, H., Yoshikawa, H., et al.: Ectopic bone induction on and in porous hydroxyapatite combined with collagen and bone morphogenetic protein. Clin. Orthop. *234*:250–254, 1988.
203. Thomas, I., Kirkaldy-Willis, W. H., Singh, S., and Paine, K. W. E.: Experimental spinal fusion in guinea pigs and dogs: The effect of immobilization. Clin. Orthop. *112*:363–375, 1975.
204. Tomford, W. W.: Current concepts review: Transmission of disease through transplantation of musculoskeletal allografts. J. Bone Joint Surg. Am. *77*:1742–1754, 1995.
205. Toth, J. M., An, H. S., Lim, T., et al.: Evaluation of porous biphasic calcium phosphate ceramics for anterior cervical interbody fusion in a caprine model. Spine *20*:2203–2210, 1995.
206. Tsuang, Y. H., Yang, R. S., Chen, P. Q., and Liu, T. K.: Experimental allograft in spinal fusion in dogs. J. Formos. Med. Assoc. *88*:989–994, 1989.
207. Tuli, S. M.: Bridging of bone defects by massive bone grafts in tumorous conditions and in osteomyelitis. Clin. Orthop. *87*:60–73, 1972.
208. Tuli, S. M., and Singh, A. D.: The osteoinductive property of decalcified bone matrix: An experimental study. J. Bone Joint Surg. Br. *60*:116–123, 1978.
209. Udupa, K. N., and Gupta, L. P.: The effect of growth hormone and thyroxine in healing of fracture. Indian J. Med. Res. *53*:623–628, 1965.
210. Urist, M. R.: Bone: Formation by autoinduction. Science *150*:893–899, 1965.
211. Urist, M. R., and Dawson, E.: Intertransverse process fusion with the aid of chemosterilized autolyzed antigen-extracted allogeneic (AAA) bone. Clin. Orthop. *154*:97–113, 1981.
212. Urist, M. R., DeLange, R. J., and Finerman, G. A. M.: Bone cell differentiation and growth factors. Science *220*:680–686, 1983.
213. Urist, M. R., Dowell, T. A., Hay, P. H., and Strates, B. S.: Inductive substrates for bone formation. Clin. Orthop. *59*:59–96, 1968.
214. Urist, M. R., Lietze, A., and Dawson, E.: Beta-tricalcium phosphate delivery system for bone morphogenetic protein. Clin. Orthop. *187*:277–280, 1984.
215. Urist, M. R., Lietze, A., Mizutani, H., et al.: A bovine low molecular weight bone morphogenetic protein (BMP) fraction. Clin. Orthop. *162*:219–232, 1982.
216. Urist, M. R., Silverman, B. F., Buring, K., et al.: The bone induction principle. Clin. Orthop. *53*:243–283, 1967.
217. Urist, M. R., and Strates, B. S.: Bone formation in implants of partially and wholly demineralized bone matrix. Including observations on acetone-fixed intra and extracellular proteins. Clin. Orthop. *71*:271–278, 1970.
218. Van de Putte, K. A., and Urist, M. R.: Osteogenesis of the interior of intramuscular implants of decalcified bone matrix. Clin. Orthop. *43*:257–270, 1965.
219. Volpon, J. B., Xavier, C. A. M., and Concalves, R. P.: The use of decalcified granulated homologous cortical bone matrix in the correction of diaphyseal bone defect: An experimental study in rabbits. Arch. Orthop. Trauma Surg. *99*:199–207, 1982.
220. Walter, C., and Brunt, P. B.: Tricalciumphosphate as an implant material: Preliminary report. Br. J. Plast. Surg. *35*:510–516, 1982.
221. Weiland, A. J., Phillips, T. W., and Randolph, M. A.: Bone grafts: A radiologic, histologic, and biomechanical model comparing autografts, allografts, and free vascularized bone grafts. Plast. Reconstr. Surg. *74*:368–379, 1984.
222. Wenger, D. R., Carollo, J. J., Wilkerson, J. A., et al.: Laboratory testing of segmental spinal instrumentation versus traditional Harrington instrumentation for scoliosis treatment. Spine *7*:265–269, 1982.
223. Wilson, P. D.,and Lance, E. M.: Surgical reconstruction of the skeleton following segmental resection for bone tumors. J. Bone Joint Surg. Am. *47*:1629–1656, 1965.
224. Wozney, J. M.: Bone morphogenetic proteins. Prog. Growth Factor Res. *1*:267–280, 1989.
225. Yasuda, I., Noguchi, K., and Sata, T.: Dynamic callus and electric callus. J. Bone Joint Surg. Am. *37*:1292–1293, 1955.
226. Younger, E. M., and Chapman, M. W.: Morbidity at bone graft donor sites. J. Orthop. Trauma *3*:192–195, 1989.

Lumbar Pseudarthrosis: Diagnosis and Treatment

H. Ulrich Bueff, M.D.

David S. Bradford, M.D.

Pseudarthrosis is defined as the failure of an attempted spinal fusion to fuse by one year after surgery.[43] The reported incidence of pseudarthrosis after posterolateral lumbar fusion surgery varies from 3 to 25 per cent.[5] Jackson and colleagues reviewed 129 patients who had had low back fusion surgery and found a pseudarthrosis rate of 13 per cent.[20] Kiviluoto and associates studied 80 consecutive patients who had undergone posterolateral spinal fusion and found a 3 per cent nonunion rate.[24] Anterior lumbar interbody fusions have an incidence of nonunion ranging from 4 to 68 per cent.[46] Zucherman and coworkers reviewed the literature and found a 6 to 27 per cent pseudarthrosis rate in posterior lumbar interbody fusions.[51] Fusion rates can be significantly enhanced with rigid internal fixation, as shown by Zdeblick in a prospective study.[48]

Although asymptomatic nonunions are common, pseudarthrosis is the main reason for reoperation in up to 78 per cent of patients, as shown in a long-term follow-up study of 205 patients after lumbar fusion surgery.[14] The successful repair of a nonunion and the achievement of fusion after an initial surgery remain major challenges.

ETIOLOGY OF PSEUDARTHROSIS

Spinal fusion has been studied extensively in animal models, yet its complex, multifactorial mechanism remains poorly understood.[39] Many factors affect the formation of a solid fusion. A significant inhibition of bone formation was observed after dexamethasone and diclofenac sodium administration in mice.[30, 33] Similarly, the pseudarthrosis rate in lumbar fusions appears to be increased in patients who use nonsteroidal anti-inflammatory drugs.[19] Several studies have shown the negative influence of smoking on spinal fusion rates. Brown and colleagues retrospectively reviewed 100 patients one to two years after two-level laminectomy and fusion of the lumbar spine. Forty per cent of the smokers developed a pseudarthrosis, compared with only 8 per cent of the nonsmokers. The authors showed lower oxygen saturation levels in smokers and hypothesized that this may be an important factor in nonunion.[7] Smoking has also been demonstrated to inhibit the revascularization of bone graft because of its vasoconstrictive action on the microvasculature.[11] Silcox and associates demonstrated a significant decrease in the rate and strength of lumbar fusions after systemic administration of nicotine in a rabbit model.[41]

Schofferman and coworkers evaluated 47 patients with lumbar pseudarthrosis and found that metabolic bone disease did not play a frequent or significant causative role.[40] Nevertheless, clinical experience shows that it is more difficult to achieve a solid fusion in patients with severe osteoporosis or osteomalacia.[22] Patients treated for spinal fractures who suffer from inflammatory disorders such as ankylosing spondylitis have an increased nonunion rate if their underlying disease has not been recognized.[13, 18, 23, 37] Deep wound infections can often lead to pseudarthrosis as well.[37]

In addition to these biologic factors, pseudarthrosis can be caused by mechanical failure owing to inadequate surgical technique. Excessive motion at the fusion site, poor fixation, and failure to neutralize shear stresses can lead to nonunion. Distraction forces at the fusion site (for example, forces created by Knodt rods) increase the rate of pseudarthrosis. A fusion mass must stabilize and mature in compression in order to achieve a successful outcome. Thus, external immobilization is mandatory in the absence of internal fixation. Technical errors such as soft tissue interposition, inadequate decortication, an avascular graft bed, and postoperative hematoma and seroma may also lead ultimately to failed fusion.

Numerous studies deal with the use of allograft versus autograft. The pseudarthrosis rate is clearly increased when allograft is used.[1, 17] However, in select patients with paralysis in whom autogenous harvesting is not feasible, allograft bone graft is a suitable substitute.[4] The method of sterilization of banked bone graft influences the outcome of a fusion. At our institution, we use fresh-frozen bone with excellent results. Herron and Newman showed nonunion rates of up to 79 per cent with the use of ethylene oxide gas–sterilized freeze-dried bank bone graft. They concluded that graft in this form is inferior to autogenous bone graft or bank bone graft preserved and/or sterilized by other methods.[17] Its use in thoracic or lumbar posterior or posterolateral fusion cannot be recommended. An and colleagues compared autografts, frozen allografts, freeze-dried allografts, and a mixture of allograft and autograft in a prospective study of patients undergoing instrumented posterolateral lumbar fusion. The fusion rate with autograft was highest (80 per cent). All fusion attempts with freeze-dried graft resulted in nonunion. Bone densitometry results showed that autograft sites had significantly greater bone density, followed by sites using a mixture of frozen allograft and freeze-dried allograft.[1]

The search for a suitable bone graft substitute continues. Experience with biomaterials such as coral hydroxyapatite shows that fusions can be achieved with these materials; the fusion rate, however, is lower than that obtained with autograft or fresh-frozen allograft.[49]

NATURAL HISTORY

The presence of a pseudarthrosis does not necessarily imply pain. Watkins and Bragg studied 14 patients with posterior lumbar pseudarthrosis and found 43 per cent to be asymptomatic.[45] However, the majority of patients with documented nonunion of a lumbar fusion do complain of pain. They may also develop an increase in deformity. Loss of correction in a failed lumbar fusion can lead to spondylolisthesis with subsequent stenosis and neurologic deficit. Failure of the implant is strongly indicative of a pseudarthrosis.

CLASSIFICATION

Heggeness evaluated imaging studies and operative records of 55 patients who underwent repair of a lumbar pseudarthrosis. He distinguished among four distinct morphologic categories of pseudarthrosis: atrophic, transverse, shingle, and complex. Atrophic pseudarthrosis, the most severe type, exhibits gross atrophy and resorption of bone graft. Transverse pseudarthrosis, the most common variety, involves a significant mass of remodeled bone with horizontal discontinuity. The shingle type involves a substantial mass of bone graft but has a defect in the fusion. The fourth and least common type of pseudarthrosis is the complex type, which has more than one type of defect in the fusion mass.[15]

Biopsy specimens from 35 patients undergoing pseudarthrosis repair after failed posterior spinal fusions showed predominantly fibrous tissue; in many cases, this was accompanied by signs of local fibrocartilaginous metaplasia. Multiple microtrabecular fractures with appositional new bone formation and subchondral bony sclerosis with cartilage fissuring were consistent features.[16]

DIAGNOSIS

It is important to detect a failed spinal fusion at an early stage and to develop a diagnostic and therapeutic strategy. The earlier a revision surgery is performed, the better the chances for an ultimate solid fusion. Pain and failure of instrumentation with loss of correction are relatively late findings.

The most reliable method of determining solidity of a fusion is surgical exploration, which is obviously impractical on a routine basis. Brodsky removed internal fixation devices or implantable batteries after low back fusions in 175 patients, enabling him to assess the fusions intraoperatively. The preoperative radiologic studies (plain roentgenographs, polytomography, bending films, and computed tomography [CT] scans) were then compared with the surgical findings. A significant percentage of inaccuracy was found in all radiologic modalities used. CT scanning produced the lowest percentage of inaccuracy (22 per cent); bending films had the highest percentage (27 per cent).[6]

Nevertheless, since routine exploration is not feasible, surgeons must rely on diagnostic imaging studies. Such studies fall into two major categories: structural imaging studies, which demonstrate the defect in the fusion mass, and functional imaging studies, which can show motion at the nonunion site. Plain radiography, tomography, CT, magnetic resonance imaging (MRI), and technetium bone scanning are imaging studies that provide information on the structural integrity of a fusion mass. Functional studies include stress radiography (lateral flexion-extension radiographs), stereophotogrammetry, and discography.

Anteroposterior, lateral, and Ferguson view radiographs of the spine are obtained at follow-up evaluation. Early resorption of the bone graft and lack of continuous trabeculation of the fusion mass are indicative of the development of a nonunion. If instability is suspected, additional studies can be obtained, including oblique views and lateral flexion-extension films. (Abnormal segmental motion is defined as 4 mm of horizontal translation or 10 degrees of angular rotation.) However, these lateral motion studies are difficult to interpret in the presence of spinal instrumentation. On plain radiography, the presence of a halo around a pedicle screw is indicative of loosening and nonunion. Conventional tomography is helpful in detecting an occult spinal nonunion. Linear and trispiral techniques have shown 96 per cent correlation with intraoperative findings. Although the availability of tomography has decreased in many hospitals,[9] we have found this technique to be one of the most useful.

CT provides excellent information on the solidity of a fusion mass. Axial images can show bony masses detached from the vertebral segment as well as open facet joints, both of which indicate failed fusion (Fig. 51–1). Sagittal reformatting and three-dimensional scans enhance the accuracy in assessing spinal fusions. Lang and colleagues studied three-dimensional (3D) surface reconstructions and multiplanar CT reformations in 30 patients with clinically suspected spinal fusion pseudarthrosis.[27] They found that sagittal, planar, and curved coronal two-dimensional (2D) reformations were more useful than axial CT scans in the detection of bony nonunion. The amount of bone stock available for pseudarthrosis repair at the fusion site could also be easily assessed.

Three-dimensional CT proved to be useful as an adjunctive imaging method in the evaluation of patients with suspected pseudarthrosis of a posterior lumbar fusion.[27] Zinreich and associates compared direct axial, 2D multiplanar, and 3D CT images in 100 consecutive patients with postsurgical "failed back" syndrome. Three-dimensional imaging provided additional information, as compared with direct axial and 2D imaging, in 56 of 100 patients with failed fusion and in 76 of 100 patients with fusion.[50] Lin evaluated interbody fusions with CT scans and found that the formation of a peripheral cortical ring 9 to 12 months after surgery was indicative of a solid fusion.[29] CT seems to be the best method of demonstrating fragmentation or hairline pseudarthrosis in patients after low back fusion surgery.[25]

The role of MRI in assessing fusions is unclear. Vertebral MR signal intensity in solid lumbar fusions is related to marrow composition changes resulting from decreased biomechanical stress; the vertebral signal intensities in patients with unstable fusions are related to reparative granulation tissue, inflammation, edema, and hyperemic changes. These findings have not been correlated with intraoperative findings. MRI can determine clinically important functional instability when CT and conventional radiography are inconclusive.[26] Unstable fusions reveal subchondral bands of low signal intensity adjacent to vertebral end plates on T1-weighted images, whereas solid fusions show subchondral bands with increased signal intensity on T1-weighted images.[12]

The specificity of technetium bone scans in detecting spinal pseudarthrosis used to be low. McMaster and Merrick found a pseudarthrosis in only 50 per cent of those posterior spinal fusions in which a localized increased uptake of the radionuclide had been demonstrated.[31] Since the advent of single photon emission computed tomography (SPECT), however, both the sensitivity and the specificity of bone scanning in detecting nonunion have significantly increased. In one clinical study comparing flexion and extension radiographs with SPECT scans after lumbar fusion, scintigraphy had a sensitivity of 0.78 and a specificity of 0.83, whereas radiography had a sensitivity of 0.43 and a specificity of 0.50. The authors concluded that bone scintigraphy with SPECT is of significant value in detecting painful pseudarthrosis in patients who remain symptomatic after lumbar spinal fusion.[42]

Other rarely used imaging modalities include biplanar roentgenographic techniques and stereophotogrammetry. Pearcy and Burrough used a biplanar roentgenographic technique to evaluate lumbar interbody fusions. Segmental motion of 2 degrees can be detected with this technique. Analysis of biplanar radiographs requires a sophisticated computerized digitizing program.[36] Stereophotogrammetry of the lumbar spine requires implantation of 0.5-mm cobalt chromium balls into the posterior elements. Using this technique in 50 patients, Morris and coworkers were able to show early pseudarthrosis in four patients.[34]

Discography has been used to confirm painful pseudarthrosis of the lumbar spine in 19 of 24 patients.[21] However, it is doubtful that this invasive test is necessary, as other techniques provide the surgeon with basically the same information,[35] and in fact, the results may be misleading.

In summary, despite the advances in imaging pseudarthroses, diagnosing a nonunion and correlating the clinical findings with the imaging results remain major challenges.

INDICATIONS FOR SURGERY

The most common reasons for repairing pseudarthrosis are pain, increasing deformity, and neurologic deficit (Fig. 51–2). Paraparesis related to a nonunion can occur several years after a posterior spinal fusion. Savini and associates reported on three cases in which the spinal cord was either stretched in a progressive kyphosis or compressed by bony overgrowth owing to local instability.[38] Before deciding on a specific treatment plan, the surgeon must identify the factors that caused the pseudarthrosis and should seek to correct any contributing health risks, including smoking, endocrinopathy, or anemia, prior to nonunion repair.

TECHNIQUES

Pseudarthrosis after an anterior procedure is usually repaired with a posterior fusion (Fig. 51–3). A failed posterior fusion may require not only a posterior approach but a combined anterior fusion as well. The fusion should always be under compression, not distraction. Pseudarthroses that are associated with significant or progressive deformity generally require a combined approach.

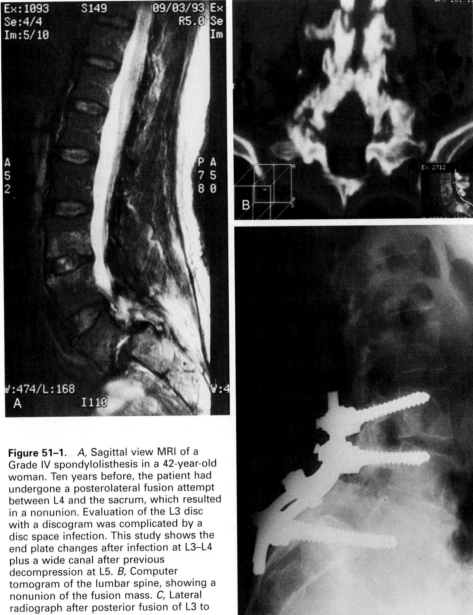

Figure 51–1. *A,* Sagittal view MRI of a Grade IV spondylolisthesis in a 42-year-old woman. Ten years before, the patient had undergone a posterolateral fusion attempt between L4 and the sacrum, which resulted in a nonunion. Evaluation of the L3 disc with a discogram was complicated by a disc space infection. This study shows the end plate changes after infection at L3–L4 plus a wide canal after previous decompression at L5. *B,* Computer tomogram of the lumbar spine, showing a nonunion of the fusion mass. *C,* Lateral radiograph after posterior fusion of L3 to the sacrum.

Illustration continued on opposite page

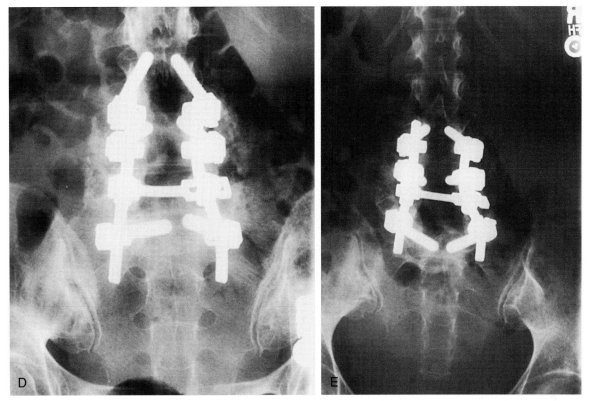

Figure 51–1 *Continued.* *D,* Ferguson view of the lumbar spine allows evaluation of the fusion mass between L5 and the sacrum. *E,* Anteroposterior radiograph after posterior fusion of L3 to the sacrum.

Repair of a spinal pseudarthrosis requires thorough preparation of the fusion bed. Avascular scar and muscle have to be excised, followed by extensive decortication. Autograft has proved to be superior to allograft or other bone substitutes such as coral or hydroxyapatite for posterior lumbar fusions.[1, 3, 17] The authors' preferred technique for anterior lumbar fusions involves the placement of fresh-frozen femoral allograft rings with cancellous autograft in the center of the ring. The structural integrity of the femoral ring prevents disc space collapse, and the autologous central portion facilitates graft incorporation and fusion. Tricortical autograft tends to collapse after axial loading and does not maintain disc height. New cage technologies have shown promising early results. The cages can be placed through an open approach or via laparoscopy.[52] One should be cautious in using anterior implants in the presence of a failed posterior fusion, as the structural integrity of the bone anteriorly is compromised secondary to disuse osteoporosis (stress shielding).

Loose posterior implants are a source of pain and have to be removed. Consideration must be given to rigid internal fixation if the previous fusion attempt was done without instrumentation. Zdeblick's prospective study demonstrated a significantly increased posterior lumbar fusion rate when rigid instrumentation was used.[48] Correction of any deformity, especially in the sagittal and coronal planes, is mandatory for future success. Sagittal imbalance, such as flatback syndrome, should be evaluated preoperatively using long films of the spine with the patient in a standing position.

Although controversial, there are supplemental modalities for the treatment of pseudarthrosis. These include direct or indirect electrical stimulation. One study demonstrated significantly higher overall fusion rates in stimulated patients (93 vs. 75 per cent). Lumbar interbody fusion rates have been improved by direct current treatment.[32] Another supplemental modality, bone morphogenic protein (BMP-2), has significantly enhanced lumbar fusion rates in animal models.[2, 39] Application of recombinant human BMP-2 or other osteoinductive growth factors may become the preferred method of treating spinal nonunion in the future. Clinical studies are currently in progress to evaluate the efficacy of BMP in augmenting spinal fusions in humans. Osteoinductive materials, such as demineralized bone matrix, have been disappointing in achieving stable posterior spinal fusions.[10]

RESULTS

Results of pseudarthrosis repair in the lumbar spine are variable. Frequently, a combined anterior and posterior procedure is necessary to achieve a successful arthrodesis. Thalgott and colleagues reviewed 45 patients after repair of a lumbar nonunion. Eighty per cent had a solid fusion after posterior instrumentation and fusion with autologous graft alone, but 20 per cent

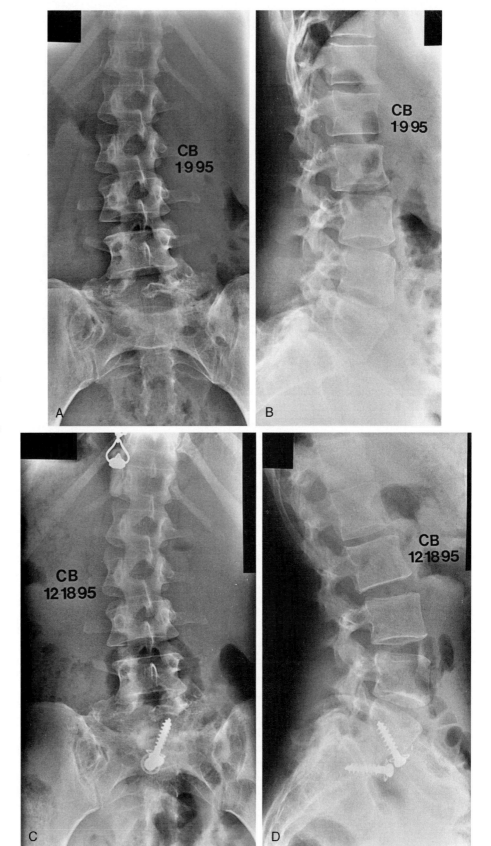

Figure 51–2. *A,* Anteroposterior radiograph of a pseudarthrosis after attempted posterior lumbar fusion of a Grade I spondylolisthesis in a 30-year-old woman. *B,* Lateral radiograph of the same patient. *C,* Anteroposterior radiograph of the patient after anterior fusion for chronic low back pain and leg pain. *D,* Lateral radiograph showing a solid anterior fusion.

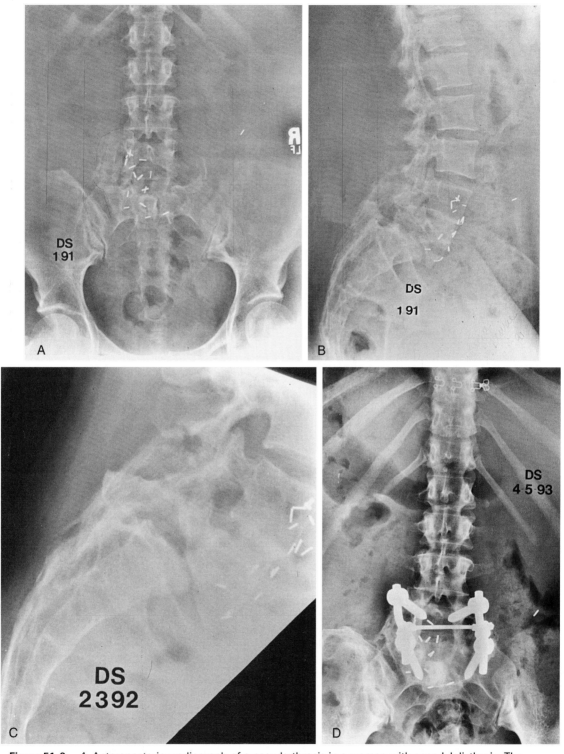

Figure 51–3. *A,* Anteroposterior radiograph of a pseudarthrosis in a woman with spondylolisthesis. The patient developed a nonunion after a combined anterior and posterior fusion attempt. *B, C,* Lateral radiographs of the same patient. *D,* Anteroposterior radiograph of the patient, who required a posterior refusion of L4 to the sacrum with pedicle screw fixation and autologous bone graft. An autogenous fibula graft was advanced from the sacrum into L5.

Illustration continued on following page

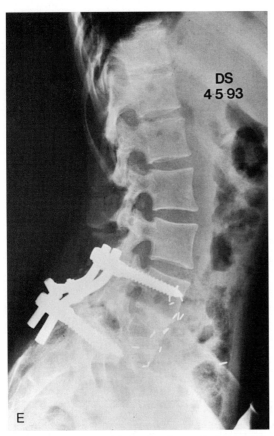

Figure 51–3 *Continued.* *E*, Lateral radiograph after revision of the fusion.

required an additional anterior interbody fusion. The highest rate of graft resorption and implant failure was seen in 12 patients with an attempted three-level fusion.[44]

Lauerman and coworkers reviewed 40 patients after repair of lumbar pseudarthrosis. Solid fusion was achieved in 49 per cent of cases. Eighty-six per cent of patients continued to have low back pain. Sublaminar wires, Harrington compression rods, and variable pedicle screw–plate constructs were used.[28] West and associates reported a 65 per cent fusion rate after repair of lumbar pseudarthrosis with pedicle screw fixation.[47]

Combined surgery has the highest chance of achieving a union after pseudarthrosis repair. Buttermann and colleagues found a 3 per cent pseudarthrosis rate with anterior allograft and a 6 per cent pseudarthrosis rate with anterior autograft.[8]

CONCLUSION

The diagnosis and treatment of lumbar pseudarthrosis remain a challenge. Contributing factors need to be identified and corrected preoperatively. Combined anterior and posterior procedures have the highest chance of achieving solid fusion. Preoperative complaints of leg pain will improve if a compressive lesion can be identified and decompressed.

References

1. An, H. S., Lynch, K., and Toth, J.: Prospective comparison of autograft vs. allograft for adult posterolateral lumbar spine fusion: Differences among freeze-dried, frozen, and mixed grafts. J. Spinal Disord. *8*:131–135, 1995.
2. Boden, S. D., Schimandle, J. H., and Hutton, W. C.: An experimental lumbar intertransverse process spinal fusion model: Radiographic, histologic, and biomechanical healing characteristics. Spine *20*:412–420, 1995.
3. Brantigan, J. W.: Pseudarthrosis rate after allograft posterior lumbar interbody fusion with pedicle screw and plate fixation. Spine *19*:1271–1279, 1994.
4. Bridwell, K. H., O'Brien, M. F., Lenke, L. G., et al.: Posterior spinal fusion supplemented with only allograft bone in paralytic scoliosis: Does it work? Spine *19*:2658–2666, 1994.
5. Brodsky, A. E., Hendricks, R. L., Khalil, M. A., et al.: Segmental ("floating") lumbar spine fusions. Spine *14*:447–450, 1989.
6. Brodsky, A. E., Kovalsky, E. S., and Khalil, M. A.: Correlation of radiologic assessment of lumbar spine fusions with surgical exploration. Spine *16*:261–265, 1991.
7. Brown, C. W., Orme, T. J., and Richardson, H. D.: The rate of pseudarthrosis (surgical nonunion) in patients who are smokers and patients who are nonsmokers: A comparison study. Spine *11*:942–943, 1986.
8. Buttermann, G. R., Glazer, P. A., Hu, S. S., and Bradford, D. S.: Revision of failed lumbar fusions: A comparison of anterior autograft versus allograft. Spine (in press).
9. Clader, T. J., Dawson, E. G., and Bassett, L. W.: The role of tomography in the evaluation of postoperative spinal fusion. Spine *9*:686–689, 1984.
10. Cook, S. D., Dalton, J. E., Prewett, A. B., and Whitecloud, T. S., 3rd.: In vivo evaluation of demineralized bone matrix as a bone graft substitute for posterior spinal fusion. Spine *20*:877–886, 1995.
11. Daftari, T. K., Whitesides, T. E., Jr., Heller, J. G., et al.: Nicotine on the revascularization of bone graft: An experimental study in rabbits. Spine *19*:904–911, 1994.
12. Djukic, S., Lang, P., Morris, J., et al.: The postoperative spine: Magnetic resonance imaging. Orthop. Clin. North Am. *21*:603–624, 1990.
13. Fang, D., Leong, J. C., Ho, E. K., et al.: Spinal pseudarthrosis in ankylosing spondylitis: Clinicopathological correlation and the results of anterior spinal fusion. J. Bone Joint Surg. [Br.] *70*:443–447, 1988.
14. Frymoyer, J. W., Metteri, J. D., Hanley, E. N., et al.: Failed lumbar disc surgery requiring a second operation: A long-term follow-up study. Spine *3*:7–11, 1978.
15. Heggeness, M. H., and Esses, S. I.: Classification of pseudarthroses of the lumbar spine. Spine *16*:449–454, 1991.
16. Heggeness, M. H., Esses, S. I., and Mody, D. R.: A histologic study of lumbar pseudarthrosis. Spine *18*:1016–1020, 1993.
17. Herron, L. D., and Newman, M. H.: The failure of ethylene oxide gas–sterilized freeze-dried bone graft for thoracic and lumbar spinal fusion [see comments]. Spine *14*:496–500, 1989.
18. Ho, E., Chan, F. L., and Leong, J. C.: Migrating spinal pseudarthrosis in the spine affected by ankylosing spondylitis. Spine *14*:546–548, 1989.
19. Huo, M. H., Troiano, N. W., Pelker, R. R., et al.: The influence of ibuprofen on fracture repair: Biomechanical, biochemical, histologic, and histomorphometric parameters in rats. J. Orthop. Res. *9*:383–390, 1991.
20. Jackson, R. K., Boston, D. A., and Edge, A. J.: Lateral mass fusion: A prospective study of a consecutive series with long-term follow-up. Spine *10*:828–832, 1985.
21. Johnson, R. G., and Macnab, I.: Localization of symptomatic lumbar pseudarthroses by use of discography. Clin. Orthop. *197*:164–170, 1985.
22. Kahanovitz, N.: Osteoporosis and fusion. Instr. Course Lect. *41*:231–233, 1992.
23. Karlstrom, G., and Olerud, S.: Spinal pseudarthrosis with paraplegia in ankylosing spondylitis: A case report. Arch. Orthop. Trauma Surg. *98*:297–300, 1981.
24. Kiviluoto, O., Santavirta, S., Salenius, P., et al.: Posterolateral

spine fusion: A 1–4-year follow-up of 80 consecutive patients. Acta Orthop. Scand. *56*:152–154, 1985.

25. Laasonen, E. M., and Soini, J.: Low-back pain after lumbar fusion: Surgical and computed tomographic analysis. Spine *14*:210–213, 1989.

26. Lang, P., Chafetz, N., Genant, H. K., and Morris, J. M.: Lumbar spinal fusion: Assessment of functional stability with magnetic resonance imaging. Spine *15*:581–588, 1990.

27. Lang, P., Genant, H. K., Chafetz, N., et al.: Three-dimensional computed tomography and multiplanar reformations in the assessment of pseudarthrosis in posterior lumbar fusion patients. Spine *13*:69–75, 1988.

28. Lauerman, W. C., Bradford, D. S., Ogilvie, J. W., and Transfeldt, E. E.: Results of lumbar pseudarthrosis repair. J. Spinal Disord. *5*:149–157, 1992.

29. Lin, P. M.: Radiographic evidence of posterior lumbar interbody fusion with an emphasis on computed tomographic scanning. Clin. Orthop. *242*:158–163, 1989.

30. Lindholm, T. S., and Tornkvist, H.: Inhibitory effect on bone formation and calcification exerted by the anti-inflammatory drug ibuprofen: An experimental study on adult rat with fracture. Scand. J. Rheumatol. *10*:38–42, 1981.

31. McMaster, M. J., and Merrick, M. V.: The scintigraphic assessment of the scoliotic spine after fusion. J. Bone Joint Surg. [Br.] *62*:65–72, 1980.

32. Meril, A. J.: Direct current stimulation of allograft in anterior and posterior lumbar interbody fusions. Spine *19*:2393–2398, 1994.

33. Mizuno, H., Liang, R. F., and Kawabata, A.: Effects of oral administration of various non-steroidal anti-inflammatory drugs on bone growth and bone wound healing in mice. Meikai Daigaku Shigaku Zasshi *19*:234–250, 1990.

34. Morris, J., Chafetz, N., Baumrind, S., et al.: Stereophotogrammetry of the lumbar spine: A technique for the detection of pseudarthrosis. Spine *10*:368–375, 1985.

35. Nachemson, A.: Lumbar discography—where are we today? [see comments]. Spine *14*:555–557, 1989.

36. Pearcy, M., and Burrough, S.: Assessment of bony union after interbody fusion of the lumbar spine using a biplanar radiographic technique. J. Bone Joint Surg. [Br.] *64*:228–232, 1982.

37. Richards, B. S.: Delayed infections following posterior spinal instrumentation for the treatment of idiopathic scoliosis. J. Bone Joint Surg. [Am.] *77*:524–529, 1995.

38. Savini, R., Di, S. M., and Gargiulo, G.: Late paraparesis due to pseudarthrosis after posterior spinal fusion. J. Spinal Disord. *3*:427–432, 1990.

39. Schimandle, J. H., Boden, S. D., and Hutton, W. C.: Experimental spinal fusion with recombinant human bone morphogenetic protein-2. Spine *20*:1326–1337, 1995.

40. Schofferman, J., Schofferman, L., Zucherman, J., et al.: Metabolic bone disease in lumbar pseudarthrosis. Spine *15*:687–689, 1990.

41. Silcox, D. H., 3rd, Dafarti, T., Boden, S. D., et al.: The effect of nicotine on spinal fusion. Spine *20*:1549–1553, 1995.

42. Slizofski, W. J., Collier, B. D., Flatley, T. J., et al.: Painful pseudarthrosis following lumbar spinal fusion: Detection by combined SPECT and planar bone scintigraphy. Skeletal Radiol. *16*:136–141, 1987.

43. Stauffer, R. N., and Coventry, M. B.: Anterior interbody lumbar spine fusion. J. Bone Joint Surg. [Am.] *54*:756–768, 1972.

44. Thalgott, J., La Rocca, H., Gardner, V., et al.: Reconstruction of failed lumbar surgery with narrow AO DCP plates for spinal arthrodesis. Spine *16*:S170–175, 1991.

45. Watkins, M. B., and Bragg, C.: Lumbosacral fusion: Results with early ambulation. Surg. Gynecol. Obstet. *102*:604, 1956.

46. Watkins, R. G.: Results of anterior interbody fusions. *In* White, A. H., Rothman, R. H., and Day, R. C. (eds.): Lumbar Spine Surgery. St. Louis, Mosby, 1987.

47. West, J., Bradford, D. S., and Ogilvie, J. W.: Results of spinal arthrodesis with pedicle screw-plate fixation. J. Bone Joint Surg. [Am.] *73*:1179–1184, 1991.

48. Zdeblick, T. A.: A prospective, randomized study of lumbar fusion: Preliminary results [see comments]. Spine *18*:983–991, 1993.

49. Zdeblick, T. A., Cooke, M. E., Kunz, D. N., et al.: Anterior cervical discectomy and fusion using a porous hydroxyapatite bone graft substitute. Spine *19*:2348–2357, 1994.

50. Zinreich, S. J., Long, D. M., Davis, R., et al.: Three-dimensional CT imaging in postsurgical "failed back" syndrome. J. Comput. Assist. Tomogr. *14*:574–580, 1990.

51. Zucherman, J. F., Selby, D., and DeLong, W. B.: Failed posterior lumbar interbody fusions. *In* White, A. H., Rothman, R. H., and Day, R. C. (eds.): Lumbar Spine Surgery. St. Louis, Mosby, 1987.

52. Zucherman, J. F., Zdeblick, T. A., Bailey, S. A., et al.: Instrumented laparoscopic spinal fusion: Preliminary results. Spine *20*:2029–2034, 1995.

CHAPTER 52

Spinal Instrumentation

Todd J. Albert, M.D.

Alexander M. Jones, M.D.

Richard A. Balderston, M.D.

Alexander R. Vaccaro, M.D.

Spinal instrumentation is perhaps the most quickly changing and expanding field for students of the spine to master. A discussion of the philosophy, indications, and techniques for all presently developed instrumentation systems would encompass a major textbook in itself. Therefore, the goals of this chapter are to enable practitioners and residents to better understand the more commonly used spinal instrumentation systems and to build a framework on which to evaluate new instrumentation systems as they are developed for the more common spinal deformities and afflictions.

To accomplish this goal, we present the history and evolution of spinal instrumentation systems and the mechanics of a few commonly used systems. A discussion of the biomechanics of spinal instrumentation enables the reader to better evaluate and understand the indications for and the goals of the various systems. We then evaluate a few systems employing these biomechanical principles. A discussion of the goals of instrumentation should remind us that the armamentarium of instrumentation available to us is only as useful as our knowledge of the diseases we treat and of the indications for and philosophy behind the particular system we choose.

HISTORICAL DEVELOPMENT OF SPINAL INSTRUMENTATION

Although two surgeons in New York reported successful fusion technique in 1911,[5, 63] Hadra[53] of Galveston had used wires to stabilize a fracture-dislocation of the cervical spine 20 years earlier. Hadra apparently learned this technique from Dr. W. Wilkins, who had performed the same operation at the thoracolumbar junction. Lang[80] from Munich reported the first attempts to stabilize the spine with a true instrumentation system in 1909. He used rigid celluloid (later changing to steel) rods affixed to either side of the spinous processes with silk threads and steel wires. Lang's construct is similar to that developed by Eduardo Luque in Mexico in the 1970s.[86]

The Harrington Rod

The evolution of the present-day Harrington rod system began in 1953, when Dr. Paul Harrington in Houston assumed the care of children with progressive neuromuscular scoliosis secondary to polio, which was epidemic at the time.[56, 58] Given the unacceptably high complication rates of Stagnara-type casting and spinal fusion procedures (the accepted treatment modalities of the day), Harrington embarked on the development of the ratcheted rod and hook system available today.

Harrington's initial attempt at surgical intervention in this population was an operation in which facet screws were placed through the vertebral bodies in the corrected position. Although initially satisfying, the result deteriorated relatively quickly postoperatively, leading to the abandonment of the facet screw fixation concept. After the failure of facet screw fixation, correction was obtained with a threaded rod and hook system that could be used in a compression or distraction mode and was hand-made on the night before surgery. Two important concepts became apparent from the failures of this early work. First, dynamic correction without fusion augmentation was untenable owing to hook disengagement, rod failure,[65] and the subsequent recurrence of deformity. Second, redesign for greater durability was necessary, because it was estimated that the instrumentation would need to withstand 7 million cycles of loading before fatigue failure. This figure was double the estimated cycles for a one-year period, assuming 10,000 cycles per day. The necessary changes were accomplished by doubling the hardness and changing the fillet design of the ratchets. Widespread use of the current Harrington system began after presentation of the modified construct at the American Orthopaedic Association meeting in 1960.[55] Over 47 changes or steps have taken place since the original facet screw fixation system to create the modern Harrington rod system.[58] Over a 30-year period, the Harrington rod-hook system has been the gold standard for instrumentation systems, not only for scoliosis but also for the treatment of the fractured spine (particularly at the thoracolumbar junction).

Post–Harrington Rod Devleopment

As clinical indications for Harrington rod instrumentation expanded, modifications were made to improve stability, capability, and adaptability. These modifications included Moe's squaring of the end of the rod and distal hook, thus achieving greater rotational control (Fig. 52–1).[30, 98] Moe also modified the system for subcutaneous distraction,[97] which is helpful in infantile or juvenile scoliosis patients with significant residual growth potential. Problems with hook dislodgement were handled variously by employing a tongue to lock the sublaminar hook[66–68] or by using two upper hooks[4] (Fig. 52–2). The use of the double-hook model theoretically decreases individual hook-site stress by 50 per cent.[101] These modifications all employ Harrington's original design.

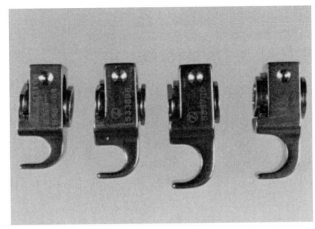

Figure 52–2. Bobechko hooks are designed to allow placement of double hooks at the ends of the construct and linearly decrease hook-site stresses.

Luque instrumentation, developed in the 1970s by Dr. Eduardo Luque in Mexico City, is a tribute to necessity as the mother of invention. His scoliosis patients were poor, and they traveled great distances for treatment. This made follow-up difficult and the postoperative bracing necessary with the Harrington system impossible.[86, 87] The Luque system employs smooth 3/16-inch or 1/4-inch rods that can be configured into different shapes and fixed segmentally with sublaminar wires (Fig. 52–3), providing immediate stability and obviating the need for postoperative bracing in many cases.

As with the Harrington system, the Luque system has been modified for particular needs. To address the need for fixation for lumbosacral arthrodesis, Allen and Ferguson developed the Galveston technique, which entails driving the lower part of the Luque rod between the tables of the wings of the ilia bilaterally,[6, 7] thereby effecting substantial mechanical purchase. To simultaneously overcome shortcomings of both the Harrington

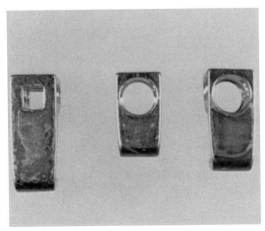

Figure 52–1. Squaring of the aperture of the Moe hook *(left)* renders greater rotational control than the round aperture of the Harrington hooks *(Middle and right).*

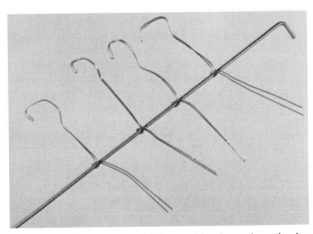

Figure 52–3. Luque L-rod with four sublaminar wires, tips bent in a configuration for sublaminar passage.

(lack of rotational control) and the Luque (lack of axial stability) systems, Winter and associates employed a hybrid consisting of the Harrington distraction rod with the Moe square-ended hook, combined with segmental wiring.[140]

To answer concerns about potential neurologic complications with intracanal passage of sublaminar wires,[49, 137, 143] Drummond developed the Wisconsin wiring technique using a square-ended Harrington distraction rod; a contoured, C-shaped Luque rod; and 18-gauge wires (Fig. 52–4) with a metallic button.[33, 34] The wires are passed in pairs through the base of the spinous processes, effectively gaining purchase on the posterior elements. Success rates with this system parallel that obtained with Luque and Harrington systems with regard to curve correction. As with the Luque system, postoperative bracing is not necessary.

In the early 1980s, Cotrel and Dubousset in Paris developed a "universal" spinal instrumentation system[26] with particular application to scoliotic deformity. Realizing the biplanar nature of scoliotic curves, the C-D system was designed to restore sagittal curvature while correcting the obvious coronal abnormality.

Combining features of the Luque system, a group at the Texas Scottish Rite Hospital (TSRH) in Dallas have added flexibility in cross linking the rods, distal sacral fixation, and a simplified hook application procedure to the biplanar corrective capabilities of the C-D system.[24]

Edwards developed a modular spinal instrumentation system employing rods, hooks, pedicle screws, pedicle connectors, and rod sleeves to effect compression, neutralization, distraction, lordosis, posterior translation, lateral loading, and derotation.[35, 36] The modularity of the system (Fig. 52–5) allows the combination of these corrective forces to treat a variety of spinal disorders, including acute or late traumatic deformity, spondylolisthesis, scoliosis, and kyphosis. The hook and rod design attempted to improve fixation from Harrington devices and to allow for convenient

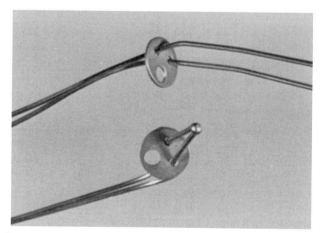

Figure 52–4. Eighteen-gauge wires connected to metallic buttons are employed for the Wisconsin spinous process wiring technique.

alteration in forces employed, depending on the deformity. Early experience with this system, especially in treating traumatic deformity, appears favorable. Although some surgeons still use this type of instrumentation for lumbar disorders and corrective surgery, Edwards' instrumentation has largely been replaced with some of the newer instrumentation systems that exhibit easier linkage between rod and screws or rod and hooks.

The C-D and TSRH systems represented the first generation of modular spinal fixation in which multiple hooks and screws could be attached on a single rod. This allowed greater corrective capabilities, as well as the concept of rod rotation. Since these revolutionary systems were developed, we have seen further refinement in modular spinal fixation, including a variable angle to the screw attachment, top loading for hook systems, and a trend toward smaller rods. Additionally, Asher introduced the concept of adding sublaminar and subpars wires with the Isola system to connect the spine to the rod rather than exclusively forcing the rod to the spine.[9, 11] All these developments have made deformity surgery more surgeon-friendly. It remains to be seen whether overall spinal alignment is improved with the power of the new systems.

Transpedicular Fixation

Transpedicular fixation was originally described by Michele and Krueger in 1949,[96] but the popularity of this technique has blossomed only in the last 10 to 15 years. Systems employing pedicular fixation had been simultaneously developed in Ohio,[124] Vermont,[78] Gothenburg,[107] and Davos.[31] These systems all share the advantage of simultaneously controlling all three mechanical columns of the spine and limiting the number of normal motion segments requiring immobilization. The *fixateur interne*[3, 31] evolved from the external fixator for the spine developed by Dick and Aebi.[90] Using Schanz pins, a steel rod, and a clamp system, this instrument allows reduction of fractures and restoration of vertebral body height. It is difficult to contour and can maximally span three or four disc spaces. Some investigators report utility with the external fixator in predicting response to fusion for back pain.[105, 107] The Swedish[107] and Vermont[78] fixators are similar to the *fixateur interne* with regard to indications, advantages, and shortcomings. Roy-Camille and colleagues[117] and Steffee and colleagues[124–126] each developed transpedicular systems that derive from the AO plate and screw systems for the appendicular skeleton (Fig. 52–6) and that allow contouring to retain sagittal plane curvature.[37] Neither system allows significant distractive or compressive forces to be applied. Luque and Rapp[89] and Guyer and associates (including Wiltse)[51] also developed transpedicular systems. Wiltse's includes a malleable rod, allowing greater flexibility in screw placement. Since the initial development of pedicular systems, many changes have occurred in all systems, allowing greater variability in screw placement and rod linkage, which leads to easier application.

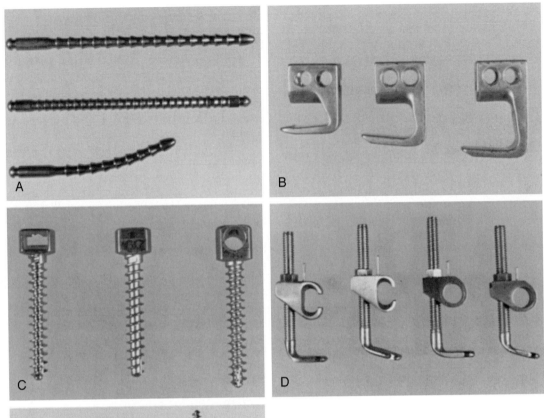

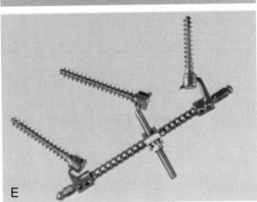

Figure 52–5. The Edwards modular spinal instrumentation system. *A,* Rod design variations. *B,* Various hook designs for better purchase and lower cut-out rate. *C,* Pedicle screws allow rod, connector, or hook attachment *D.* Connectors with open and closed and rod attachments allow improved sagittal plane correction and fixation. *E,* Example of one Edwards modular configuration.

The problems of screw breakage as a result of the design of the early screws forced redesign of pedicle screw systems. Thickening of the core diameter of the screw and a gentler tapering of the screw head have led to a significant decrease in screw breakage.

Food and Drug Administration (FDA) classification of pedicle screws became a significant issue in 1993. Bone screws were to be labeled for investigational use only. Down-classification of the screws was analyzed. The FDA oversaw a study in conjunction with the spine societies. This study essentially demonstrated that for the diagnosis of degenerative spondylolisthesis and spinal fracture, bone screws used in the pedicle increased the fusion rate without significantly increasing risk to the patient.[145] At the time of this writing, bone screws remain labeled as Class III devices for use in the spine. The technology of pedicle screws has improved in terms of ease of application, with variability and top-loading capabilities, variable-angle screws, and polyaxial screws being developed over the last few years.

Cage Technology

The last few years have seen a rapid growth in the use of interbody cages and cages for vertebral body replacement. Cages for vertebral body replacement usually employ a titanium cylinder that is filled with morselized autogenous bone and serves as a strut reconstruction for resected vertebral bodies. Interbody cages are screw-in devices with hollow interiors, usually filled with autogenous bone (Fig. 52–7). They are indicated for painful disc degeneration, postlaminectomy syndrome, and Grade I degenerative spondylo-

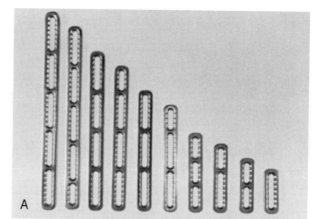

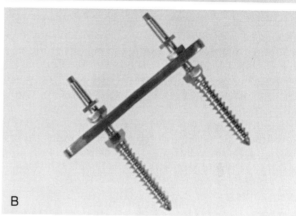

Figure 52–6. The Steffee variable spinal plating (VSP) system. *A,* Plates are available in a variety of lengths and screw-hole configurations and can be contoured depending on the length and sagittal contour of the construct. *B,* Example of one VSP construct. Plate and nuts need to be tightened, and the projecting screw above the plate must be cut. Screws come in varying lengths and thread diameters.

listhesis without severe central canal stenosis. Early reports, including the report submitted to the FDA for approval of the BAK device (Spinetech, Minneapolis, MN), were encouraging in terms of fusion rate and radiographic and functional success. These cages have been used extensively in one- and two-level fusions. It is preferable to do it at one level rather than two. As an additional advantage, these cages can be placed laparoscopically in experienced hands.

Cervical Spine

Posterior cervical instrumentation has historically been limited to wire and wire–bone graft constructs. The

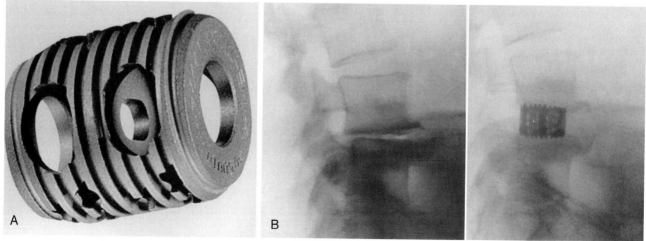

Figure 52–7. The BAK device *(A),* a hollow threaded titanium cage, is typically filled with autogenous bone and *(B)* implanted with a distraction technique.

original method described by Rogers[113] in 1942 involved a simple wire interspinous loop. Although there is no need to decorticate or supply additional bone graft in the pediatric population, most authors advocate posterior laminar decortication and autogenous bone grafting in adults. Bohlman and colleagues described a triple-wire technique (Fig. 52–8) in which two additional smaller wires are passed around the spinous process above and below, respectively.[16, 94] These smaller wires are then used to tie down the corticocancellous bone graft through which they have been passed.

Alternative posterior cervical instrumentation methods, including the Dabb plate[17, 75] and the Halifax interlaminar clamp,[28, 64] have been proposed. The Dabb plate is a malleable plate that is impacted onto the spinous processes and does not seem to hold any obvious advantage over conventional wiring techniques. The Dabb plate has also been used for thoracolumbar spinal fusions.[17] The Halifax clamp (Fig. 52–9), a posterior cervical sublaminar hook and screw system, is reportedly easy and quick to apply, but it requires the introduction of metal into the spinal canal. Long-term follow-up is as yet unavailable to determine the utility of the construct. Early experience suggests that rigid fixation is not ideally attained with this construct.

Roy-Camille and Saillant described posterior cervical plate fixation with screws placed into the articular processes.[116] Uhlrich and colleagues (including Magerl), potentially limiting posterior cervical fusion to one functional unit, employed the AO hook plate (Fig. 52–10). Although these are stable constructs, they both require posterior-to-anterior placement of screws in close proximity to the vertebral artery and exiting nerve root, with attendant risks to these neurovascular structures.

The use of lateral mass fixation in the cervical spine has become increasingly popular in the last few years (Fig. 52–11). Significant work has been done in the analysis of the anatomic structure of the lateral mass and the appropriate trajectory to use when placing lateral mass screws. Both An and Heller have analyzed the Magerl versus the Roy-Camille techniques for safety when placing lateral mass screws. They have delineated safe and appropriate pathways for lateral mass screws with a starting point approximately 1 mm medial to the middle of the lateral mass pointing proximally at 17 degrees and laterally at 33 degrees. Fixation with lateral mass screws has been found to be a significant improvement over wiring techniques.[8, 61] Bicortical fixation is superior to unicortical lateral mass fixation.[62] We have demonstrated the utility of C7 pedi-

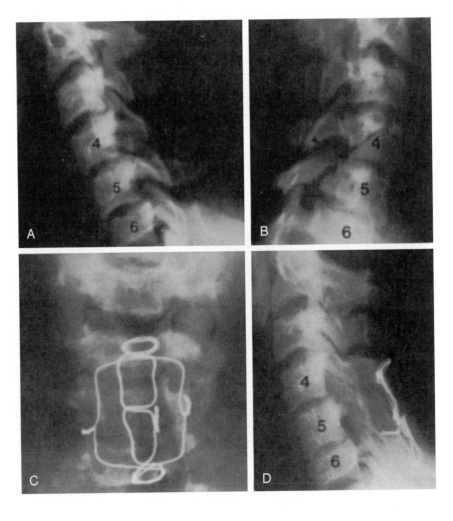

Figure 52–8. *A–D,* The Bohlman triple-wire technique renders posterior stability to this flexion-distraction cervical injury, does not invade the canal with wire passage, and does incorporate two corticocancellous grafts into the wiring technique. (Reproduced with permission from Bohlman, H. H.: Cervical spine and cord trauma. *In* Fitzgerald, R. H., Jr., Coleman, S., Gustilo, R. B., et al. [eds.]: American Academy of Orthopaedic Surgeons. Orthopaedic Knowledge Update 2: Homestudy Syllabus. Park Ridge, IL. American Academy of Orthopaedic Surgeons, 1987, p. 275.)

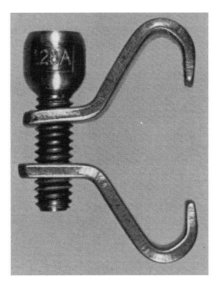

Figure 52–9. The Halifax clamp introduces metal hooks into the cervical canal, and compresses the hooks with a screw.

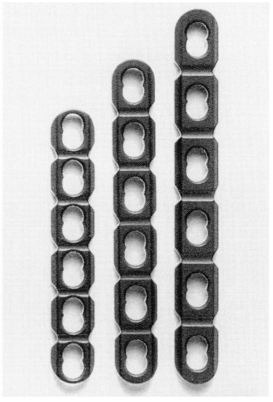

Figure 52–11. Typical lateral mass plate with the ability to aim screws for lateral mass fixation or pedicle fixation.

cle screws when performing long constructs in the cervical spine ending at or below C7. Because of the vertebral artery's location just lateral to the pedicle and the small size of the pedicle, blind placement of pedicle screws with only fluorography or placement with foraminotomy and palpation is probably not safe above C7. Likewise, when placing lateral mass screws, great appreciation for the anatomy of the adjacent vertebral artery and exiting nerve root must be maintained. This form of fixation is an excellent addition to the spine surgeon's armamentarium for any situation requiring rigid fixation for fusion in the cervical spine. Thorough anatomic knowledge and respect for adjacent vital structures are paramount to avoid complications.

For atlantoaxial fusions, variable rates of nonunion have been reported with Gallie's fusion method, which uses a bone block placed posteriorly between the arches of C1 and C2 and secured with a sublaminar wire at C1 passed around the base of C2 and around the graft.[44] Although Fried[40] reported an 80 per cent failure rate, Fielding and associates[39] reported only one

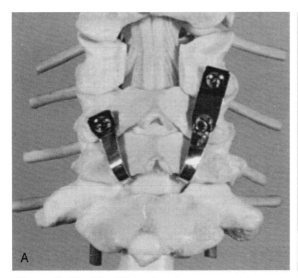

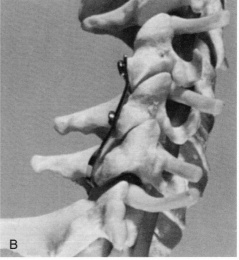

Figure 52–10. The AO hook plate, a very stable construct, requires an intracanal hook and posterior-to-anterior screw placement. *A,* Posterior view. *B,* Lateral view.

nonunion out of 46 Gallie C1–C2 fusions. The Brooks wedge compression fusion, developed to enhance postoperative stability and subsequent fusion rate, requires the passage of sublaminar wires beneath both C1 and C2 to secure two separate wedges of bone graft placed between the posterior lamina of C1 and C2 off the midline (Fig. 52–12).[21] Although there is a higher risk of neurologic complication with the Brooks technique, it has a high rate of fusion and may not require a halo-brace, as is recommended after a Gallie fusion.

Both Brooks and Gallie fusions can now be performed with the use of cable systems. Both titanium and stainless steel cables are available. One must be cautious when using braided titanium cables, as the potential for unwinding and fraying is significant. However, passage of the soft cable system is easier than passage of the standard 18- or 20-gauge traditional wires.

Transarticular screw fixation at C1–C2, first described by Magerl, has become increasingly popular (Fig. 52–13). The added stability in both rotation and flexion-extension moments has been well documented.[91] Minimal orthotic management is needed, and a high rate of fusion is obtained when bone graft is added posteriorly with a Gallie or Brooks technique in addition to the Magerl fusion. One must balance the added fixation capabilities and decreased orthotic requirements with the increased risk of vertebral artery injury when passing a screw from the lamina of C2 into the transarticular process of C1. A preoperative thin-cut computed tomography (CT) scan with reconstruction to evaluate the course of the vertebral artery in C2 is essential before performing this technique.

Anterior instrumentation and fixation techniques are demanding and generally have a higher complication rate than posterior systems. Interfragmentary screw fixation of odontoid fractures[46, 84] requiring an anterior cervical approach through the body of C2, close to major vascular, neural, and alimentary structures, should be reserved for those expert with this technique.

Whereas the original proponents of anterior odon-

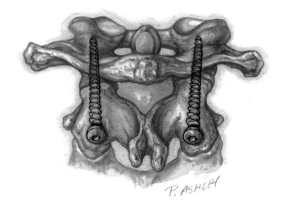

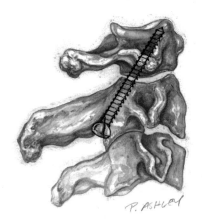

Figure 52–13. Magerl technique for C1–C2 transarticular screws.

toid screws suggested two screws, more recent reports have shown that one 4.0 or 4.5 screw in the odontoid may provide adequate fixation for healing. This technique is contraindicated if there is an atrophic nonunion of the odontoid and is better for fractures in which good interdigitation and healing can be expected. Anterior screw-plate constructs[15, 129] are used primarily to effect an arthrodesis after complete vertebrectomy for tumor, but they have been used for cervical fractures[115] and after anterior disc excision and grafting.[45] Technical difficulty exists in the need to drill and screw from anterior to posterior directly toward the neutral elements.

Newer locking screw mechanisms developed first by Synthes (Paoli, PA) and blocking screws by Sofamor Danek (Memphis, TN) have allowed the safer use of plate constructs employing shorter unicortical screws (Fig. 52–14). More widespread use of anterior plates has not been associated with a significant number of new complications as yet. If anterior plates do fail, however, esophageal injury can ensue. Advantages of plate fixation in degenerative disease include decreased postoperative orthotic requirements and quicker func-

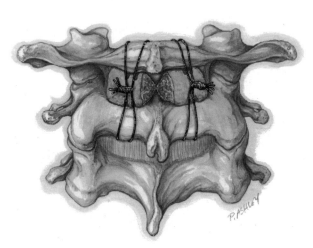

Figure 52–12. Brooks fusion, C1–C2.

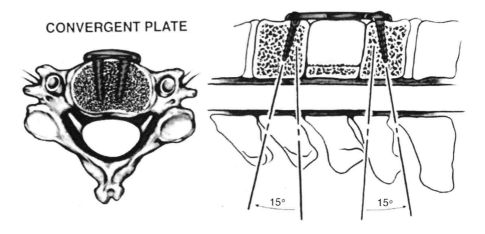

CONVERGENT PLATE

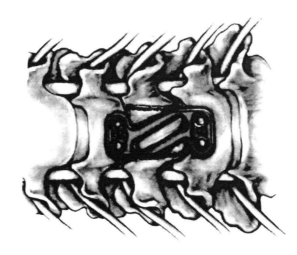

Figure 52–14. ORION blocking plate for anterior fixation. Note that screws converge mediolaterally and diverge craniocaudally.

tional restoration. The addition of anterior plates has not yet been shown to improve the fusion rate for one-, two-, or three-level anterior cervical discectomy and fusions. However, these plates have decreased the incidence of graft extrusion and decreased orthotic requirements.

Lumbosacral Spine

Instrumentation for anterior fixation of the lumbosacral spine has a controversial history. The development of anterior devices paralleled the rapid proliferation of posterior instrumentation in the 1970s and 1980s. For treatment of scoliosis with single thoracolumbar and lumbar curves, Dwyer and Zielke systems have proved useful. Both systems require retroperitoneal approaches to the thoracolumbar spine and the placement of transvertebral coronal plane screws in adjacent vertebrae to be derotated. Screws are connected with a fully threaded compression rod in the Zielke system[54] and by a flexible steel cable in the Dwyer system.[130] Although both constructs can effect compression, only the Zielke system (Fig. 52–15) allows rotational control and anterior displacement of the spine by an outrigger

device, thus avoiding the strong tendency toward kyphosis.

New systems such as the TSRH anterior system, the Isola anterior system, and the Moss-Miami system have allowed for better rod contouring and better rod rotation. The technique of placing the screws is similar. The ability to top-load the screws and the capability of rod rotation have made the operation somewhat less demanding.[132] Meticulous surgical technique (described later in this chapter) is still mandatory for success of anterior instrumentation. Choosing patients without underlying kyphosis is also mandatory, as all the anterior systems tend to be kyphosing rather than lordosing.

The anterior Kostuik-Harrington system, employing Harrington distraction-type ratcheted instrumentation secured by screws in adjacent vertebral bodies, allows the surgeon to obtain distraction.[77]

New thoracolumbar plate systems have been developed, allowing the surgeon to limit some operations to an anterior fixation alone and to correct the spine deformed by burst fractures, tumors, and neglected fractures with late kyphosis (Fig. 52–16). We have been particularly satisfied with the ability to obtain good

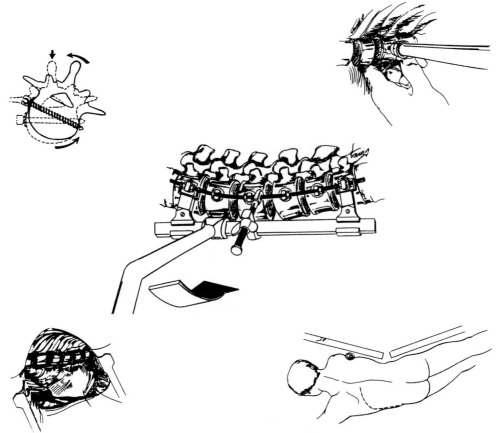

Figure 52–15. The Zielke anterior instrumentation system for the lumbosacral spine requires a retroperitoneal approach, employs an outrigger for anterior displacement, and allows derotation. (From Hammerberg, K. W., Rodts, M. F., and DeWald, R. L.: Zielke Instrumentation. Orthopedics 11:1368, 1988.)

fixation and restore segmental alignment at the level above and below fractures or tumors.[47, 146] These new plating systems are contraindicated in osteopenia and in the face of infection. As the plates are placed quite laterally on the spine, we have not yet seen problems with the great vessels.

For short segment instrumentation, present-day plating techniques represent an evolution. Most techniques involve screw and plate systems such as the Yuan I-plate,[144] the Kaneda screw plate system, and a low-profile, multihole plate that is applied anterolaterally.[14, 22] Although anterior systems offer the advantage of providing an anterior buttress or strut to a kyphotic deformity, a significant disadvantage involves the

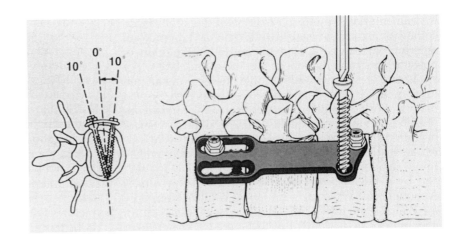

Figure 52–16. The Z-plate, a new thoracolumbar plate, has the ability to compress and distract through the vertebral body screws.

placement of instrumentation at the level of the adjacent great vessels,[70] along with other complications associated with the anterior approach.

INDIVIDUAL INSTRUMENTATION SYSTEMS

Harrington Instrumentation

The components of the system include multiple numbered hooks (Fig. 52–17), usually inserted under the lamina and occasionally inserted under the upper transverse processes in compression modes in the thoracic spine. Distraction rods are ¼ inch, and compression rods are ⅛ inch and ³⁄₁₆ inch in diameter.

After exposure of the necessary spinal segments, hook site preparation, and fusion site preparation, the hooks are placed. The Harrington outrigger device can be used to effect distraction by inserting it directly into the hooks or, preferably, into special clamps that attach to the hooks and leave the hook holes open. After distraction, facet excision, and fusion, the distraction rod is placed. The Harrington spreader device is used to gain final distraction by placing it against a hook and into a ratchet site for leverage. The distraction rod often needs to be contoured to fit the individual features of the spine. For scoliosis, distraction in the concavity lengthens the curve and moves the apex toward the midline. Compression rods on the convexity help stabilize the instrumentation and decrease the rib-hump deformity, particularly in thoracic curves with increased kyphosis. In the lumbar spine, compression rods help preserve lordosis.[41] Compression rods are not indicated with thoracic lordosis or in thoracic curves greater than 90 degrees, because thoracic lordosis worsens with compression of the posterior column. Compression rods in thoracic curves greater than 90 degrees limit the total correction possible by the distraction instrumentation.[25, 55, 99, 130, 140] Compression and distraction rods can be coupled with a device for transverse traction (DTT) or a 16-gauge wire, further drawing the convexity of the curve toward the concavity. Patients

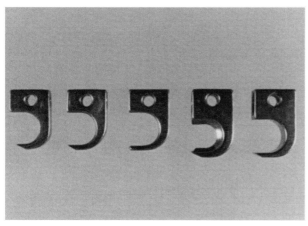

Figure 52–17. Harrington hooks.

usually require up to six months of postoperative external immobilization after Harrington construct implantation. Very few, if any, North American surgeons use Harrington instrumentation anymore.

Luque Instrumentation

This system uses ¼- and ³⁄₁₆-inch rods and 16- or 18-gauge wires (see Fig. 52–3). Rod configurations include rectangles,[32, 86, 130] rhomboids, and squares. After midline exposure of the spine, a window of ligamentum flavum is removed at each level to be fused, as well as one level above and below the extent of the fusion. The single segmental wires are then passed through the canal, with double wires passed beneath each end vertebral lamina. The following rules should be followed in passing wires:[49]

1. Do not pass wires laterally.
2. In curving the wire, the radius of curvature should be less than the laminar width.
3. The bend of the wire tip should be no greater than 45 degrees.
4. Additional removal of bony lamina is not necessary.
5. Remove spinous processes before direct midline passage.

In contouring the rods, thoracic kyphosis and lumbar lordosis should be preserved or created. For scoliosis, rods should be bent to 10 degrees less than the corrected curve on preoperative bending stretch radiographs. After placement of rods, wires are tightened. The "L" portion of the rod is placed between the spinous processes at the ends of the construct to prevent migration. No postoperative cast or brace is required. Principal uses for Luque instrumentation are in neuromuscular scoliosis and in fractures of pathologic bone.

Harrington Rods With Sublaminar Wires

Harrington instrumentation with sublaminar wires is used primarily in scoliosis and fracture stabilization. Square-ended, Moe-type Harrington instrumentation should be used to control rotation, and rods may be contoured in the coronal and sagittal planes. Sixteen-gauge wires should be used for more secure fixation. For scoliosis, minimal wire placement would entail an apical wire for transverse force application, and end vertebral placement for stabilization of distraction hooks.[99, 130, 140] The reader should be aware that this construct is potentially dangerous, and its use should be discouraged with compression instrumentation. There have been reports of spinal injury from compression hooks penetrating into the spinal canal after wire tightening. Many surgeons protect their patients with bracing postoperatively when using this construct, especially if using a minimal number of wires.

Wisconsin Instrumentation

This system is reportedly effective in the treatment of scoliosis, neuromuscular disorders, and thoracolumbar

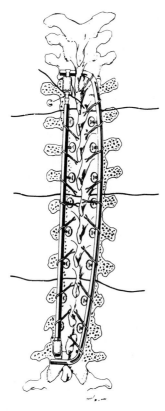

Figure 52–18. Wisconsin instrumentation construct with square-ended distraction rod, hooks, C-shaped Luque rod (³/₁₆ inch), and wire/button units (as shown in Fig. 52–4). (From Drummond, D. S., and Keene, J. S.: Spinous process segmental spinal instrumentation. Orthopedics 11:1405, 1988.)

fractures.[33, 34] The components of the Drummond system consist of the following (see Figs. 52–4 and 52–18):

1. A contoured, square-ended distraction rod and C-shaped Luque rod (³/₁₆ inch).
2. A bifid upper pedicular hook and a lower hook to accommodate a square rod.
3. Eighteen-gauge wire with a button attached. The button has a hole to accommodate the bead from a companion wire passed through it.

The spinal segments for fusion are approached and hook sites are prepared in a standard fashion, with the exception that spinous processes are preserved during preparation. Wires with buttons are inserted through the bases of the spinous processes in pairs, except at the top and bottom of the fusion segment, where single wires are passed. After facet fusion and decortication (of lamina and transverse processes lateral to buttons), Moe-modified Harrington distraction rods with contouring that preserves thoracic kyphosis and lumbar lordosis are placed. Luque rods are contoured for sagittal plane control and to span the hook sites of the Harrington rod. The ends of the Luque rod should be cephalad under the upper hook and caudad adjacent to the lower hook. The spinous process wires are then tightened around the Luque rod. If the Luque rod is

being used for correction, wires should not be tightened to bring the spine to meet the rod. Rather, an assistant should press the rod against the spine during wire tightening to prevent wire breakage. After wires are tightened around the Harrington rod, the two rods are coupled. Postoperative external bracing is needed only if considerable osteopenia is present or the spine is instrumented to L4–L5.

Cotrel-Dubousset Instrumentation

This versatile instrumentation system has reported indications including scoliosis, trauma, tumors, and spondylolisthesis.[26, 50, 122] The parts include:

I. Rods: 7-mm adult size and 5-mm pediatric rod, both with rough surfaces (Fig. 52–19)
II. Bone-metal interface elements:
   A. Hooks (Fig. 52–20)
      1. Closed (for ends)
      2. Open (for intermediate area)
      3. Laterally open (for end of short segment instrumentation of kyphosis)
         a. Pedicle—thoracic spine
         b. Lamina—all other areas of spine (many blade designs)
   B. Screws: not for distraction or compression, but to control the sagittal plane and protect hooks from pull-out
      1. Vertebral—open or closed for lumbar spine
      2. Sacral
III. Hook blocker: converts open to closed hook
IV. C-ring: placed on rod to fix hook position during rotation
V. DTT: coupler placed at ends to rigidly fix construct, especially in torsion

The application for scoliosis is described, because the concepts of use can be extrapolated for other indications if the principles are understood. The hook sites are carefully planned and marked on a standing spinal radiograph for type of hook (laminar or pedicle, open or closed). Decortication and preparation of the fusion area are completed after hook placement. A malleable rod is contoured to fit the first side to be instrumented

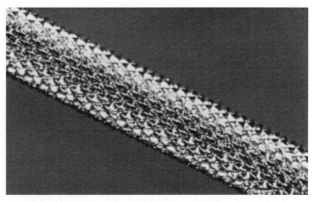

Figure 52–19. Cotrel-Dubousset rough-surfaced rod.

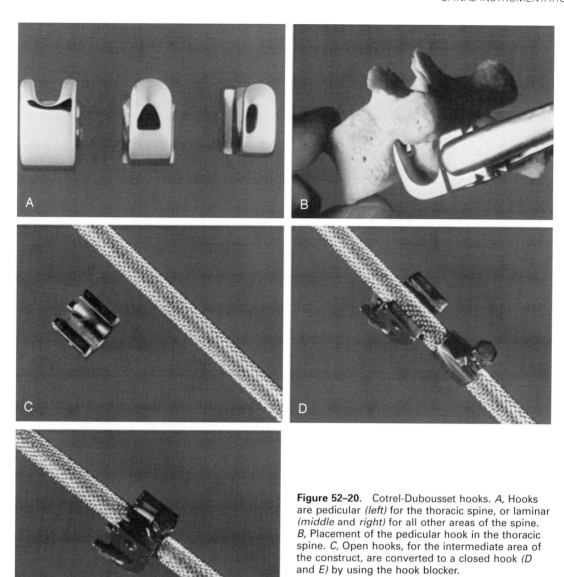

Figure 52–20. Cotrel-Dubousset hooks. *A,* Hooks are pedicular *(left)* for the thoracic spine, or laminar *(middle* and *right)* for all other areas of the spine. *B,* Placement of the pedicular hook in the thoracic spine. *C,* Open hooks, for the intermediate area of the construct, are converted to a closed hook *(D* and *E)* by using the hook blocker.

(the concavity in the thoracic area, and the convexity in the lumbar area). The rod is contoured to fit the residual scoliosis, and sight distraction (concavity) or compression (convexity) is applied to "set" the hooks. This distraction is not of the same magnitude as Harrington distraction, because the rod is difficult to rotate if the initial level of longitudinal correction is too great. The C-rings are placed to hold tension on the hooks while allowing rotation of the rod within the hooks. The rotation converts scoliosis to appropriate thoracic kyphosis and lumbar lordosis. After rotation, the set screws are tightened onto each hook, but the heads are not twisted off, in case there is a need for later adjustment. The second rod is then contoured in a sagittal plane and inserted with little further correction. Usually, two DTT rods are connected. Patients generally do not need braces postoperatively.

Pedicle screws are available in open or closed varieties and are useful in cases of necessary decompression, deficient posterior elements, degenerative curves, tumors, and spondylolisthesis. For rigid curves, less rotation of the initially placed concave rod is possible; in curves greater than 75 degrees, contouring of the rod into the desired sagittal position is difficult.

A newer model of the conventional C-D system is called the CD-Horizon (Fig. 52–21). The manufacturers have added top loading, myriad hook designs, and smaller rods. There are also useful instruments for persuading the rod into the hooks to help correct the spine to the rod. Top loading and the ability to remove the set screw if a problem occurs are additional advantages to this system. Likewise, the Isola system (Acromed Corporation, Cleveland, OH) allows for top loading with open and closed hooks, the use of

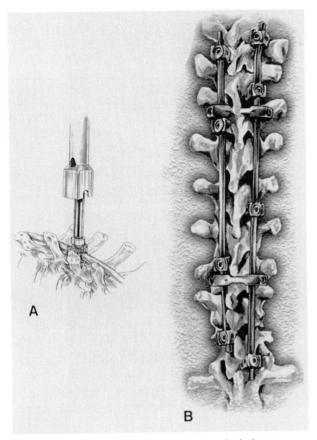

Figure 52–21. *A, B,* The CD-Horizon system includes top-loading, the ability to loosen locking screws after breakage, smaller rods (5.5), and easier placement of rods into hooks and screws.

supplemental screws and offset connectors, and the ability to place subpars or sublaminar wires for better correction of the spine through translation.

Anterior Instrumentation

The Zielke system was a modification of Dwyer instrumentation, using the same principles with less chance of instrumentation kyphosis. Newer instrumentation systems (TSRH, ISOLA) utilize the same principles. The primary indication for this instrumentation is single-curve pattern scoliosis.[54, 130, 132] The fusion length, or instrumentation levels, should extend from the neutral vertebra at the upper end of the bending film to the inferior vertebra with less than 10 degrees of rotation and 15 degrees obliquity from the horizontal on bending radiographs opposite to the convexity of the curve. A thoracolumbar approach is recommended with the patient in the lateral decubitus position and the convexity of the curve up (see Fig. 52–15). The table is flexed to increase the working space. A rib is resected one level above the highest instrumented vertebra. The segmental vessels are identified and ligated near the midline. Care is taken to avoid the great vessels, ureter, and intra-abdominal contents. After exposure of the

necessary levels, a thorough discectomy is undertaken at each interspace within the instrumented levels. The disc space is cleaned to the posterior longitudinal ligament to decrease the kyphosing tendency. The annulus is taken down. Screws are place at the end vertebra and at the intermediate vertebrae in a line to allow rotational correction. The transverse diameter of the vertebral body is measured, and a screw is chosen that is 5 mm longer than this diameter. The surgeon places a finger around the vertebral body and tightens the screw toward the pulp of the index finger, penetrating the second cortex. A preoperative CT scan helps plan the length of the screw. The rod is placed into the screw heads after contouring. The derotation device is applied and lordoses and derotates the spine. Rib graft in approximately 2.4-cm lengths is placed into the intervertebral disc spaces anterior to the axial compression line, further enhancing the lordosis effect. A postoperative brace or support is recommended by most authors until fusion is solid. Although this system is more rigid than Zielke, pseudarthrosis can still occur.

PEDICLE SCREW PLATE SYSTEMS

Because a variety of systems have been described,[51, 85, 89, 117, 124] techniques common to most systems and to placement of pedicular screws are discussed. Indications and contraindications are listed in Figure 52–22. Most authors recommend a midline approach, especially with a decompression, but some have suggested that screw placement below L3 is easier with the paraspinal approach.[51, 78, 124, 147] The pedicular landmark is described by the bisection of a vertical line through the facet joints and a horizontal line through the transverse processes. The entrance point to the pedicle is made with an awl, burr, or 00 curet and should be just lateral to the superior articular process.

For S2, the pedicular landmark is midway between the first and second sacral foramina.[9] The cancellous

PRINCIPAL INDICATIONS
Existing painful spinal instability:
    Post-laminectomy spondylolisthesis
    Painful pseudarthrosis
Potential instability:
    Spinal stenosis
    Degenerative scoliosis
Unstable fractures.
Augmenting anterior strut grafting:
    Tumor
    Infection
Stabilizing spinal osteotomies.

CONTRAINDICATIONS
Recent infection.
Laminectomies that will not cause instability.
Fusions which are normally successful without fixation.

Figure 52–22. Indications for and contraindications to posterior plate-screw fixation of the spine. (From Guyer, D. W., Wiltse, L. E., and Peek, R. D.: The Wiltse pedicle screw fixation system. *Orthopedics 11:*1458, 1988.)

bone within the cortical tube of the pedicle is sounded with a probe, such as a "joystick." The probe and subsequent screw should be aimed medially, except at S2. Although investigators differ slightly on the medial angulation of the pedicular cortical tube,[51, 78, 147] most surgeons add 5 degrees of medial angulation for every lumbar vertebra below L1, so that

L1 = 5 degrees medially
L2 = 10 degrees medially
L3 = 15 degrees medially
L4 = 20 degrees medially
L5 = 25 degrees medially
S1 = 25 degrees medially
S2 = 40 to 50 degrees laterally and 10 to 15 degrees cephalad

Steffe and Sitkowski believe that a second screw can be placed at S2 at 45 degrees.[126] After the pedicles are sounded, place Steinmann pins or drill bits into the pedicles, and check their placement radiographically. When positioning is verified, tap the pedicles. Some surgeons have turned to triggered electromyographic monitoring to test for violation of the pedicle (a "breech").[23] A Penfield is used to check that the threads are not "cut out" of the pedicle. Screw and tap sizes vary slightly from system to system. In general, the diameter of screws ranges from 4.5 to 7 mm. Zindrick and associates showed the increasing transverse diameter of the pedicles in the lower lumbar spine (Fig. 52–23).[147] Krag and associates demonstrated that most

pedicles below T10 are greater than 7 mm in diameter, and most below L1 are greater than 8 mm in diameter.[78] Screws are then placed after tapping. After decorticating the lamina and transverse processes, the plates are bent to preserve or restore lordosis. Every effort should be made to keep the plate away from the superior unfused facet. Adding bone graft and securing the rods complete the fusion. Authors disagree on the necessity of postoperative bracing. Although newer system designs do not change the technique with which pedicle screws are placed, many of the new polyaxial systems and systems with great modularity make it easier to place pedicle screws on multiple levels and hook them to their longitudinal members (Fig. 52–24).

BIOMECHANICS OF SPINAL INSTRUMENTATION

An understanding of the biomechanical principles and tests used in evaluating instrumentation enables spine surgeons to critically appraise the literature and make informed choices regarding the particular instrumentation systems. The goal of this section is to acquaint readers with a few necessary biomechanical concepts, as well as to provide a framework for evaluation of the literature on the different instrumentation systems.

The goal is not to review every biomechanical paper published in the last 10 years regarding spinal instrumentation. Rather, we would like readers to understand the different testing mechanisms and have an

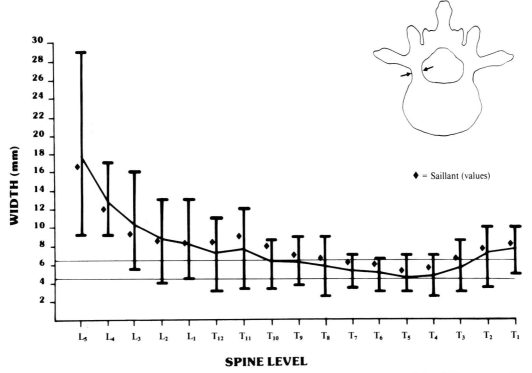

Figure 52–23. The width of the pedicles increases in the lower lumbar spine. Pedicle widths average 7 to 16 mm from L1 to L5. (From Zindrick, M. R., et al.: A biomechanical study of interpedicular screw fixation of the lumbosacral spine. Clin. Orthop. *203*:99, 1986.)

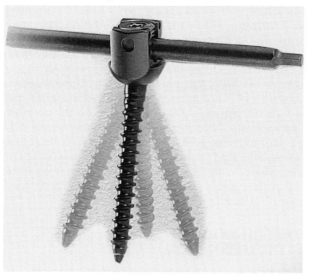

Figure 52–24. New polyaxial screw systems make rod-screw mating technically easier.

ability to discern whether individual literature evaluations are clinically relevant to their particular practice.

An understanding of instrumentation biomechanics demands an understanding of materials testing and spinal biomechanics. The tested entity is called a construct, which usually involves an appropriately injured and instrumented specimen. Because it is not economically feasible to exhaustively test constructs in vivo, the current tests usually employ an instrumented cadaveric spine. When evaluating the testing of different constructs, it is important to ask what type of specimen was used (animal vs. human, fresh vs. frozen vs. preserved, young vs. old, and the species used).

One must also understand the different types of testing and their implications. Destructive tests impart loads to the construct that are large enough to cause failure. Historically, this type of test, measuring the ultimate strength of implant systems, was popular because it was assumed that high ultimate strength could be equated with good implant stability. A stable construct would not require postoperative immobilization. The logic of this testing was flawed, in that spinal constructs rarely fail catastrophically, but rather fail through fatigue. Fatigue failure occurs from repeated loading within the metal device or, more commonly, at the bone-metal interface. For failure testing, nondestructive cyclic loading is more directly related to what happens clinically when a construct fails before solid fusion or fracture healing occurs. This type of testing in the laboratory was found to be impractical, however, because of the time and number of slow loading cycles required. To simulate average time to fusion, it is generally accepted that 1 to 4 million cycles should be performed. Most cyclic studies do not go beyond 10,000 cycles.[12] Another problem with destructive testing is that too few load types can be tested, because the construct can be used only once. Load-deformation

testing has partially obviated the need for destructive cyclic testing. In this type of testing, implants are instrumented with strain gauges (measuring a change in unit angle or length in response to load), and the tensile stress (the component of stress that produces fatigue failure in metals) is calculated for the instrumented site. By calculating the tensile stresses and knowing the endurance limit (the stress below which metal will not fail, even if cycled indefinitely), the implant's susceptibility to fatigue can be determined at the site of stress analysis without having to cyclically load the implant to failure.[121] One must always keep in mind that one of the major goals of spinal instrumentation is to stabilize the spine until a fusion matures. There is no substitute for a solid fusion, and no instrumentation system has been developed yet that can stabilize an unfused spine or correct a deformity indefinitely without a solid fusion.[19, 110, 111]

As Panjabi described, there are three biomechanical tests in evaluating spinal instrumentation: strength, fatigue, and instability. Strength, as described earlier, is destructively tested. An applied load is increased until failure occurs. This test identities the construct's load-carrying capability and its failure mechanism. Stability is tested with physiologic loads nondestructively. Therefore, multiple loading modes can test the rigidity of the construct and the potential for healing or fusion. In Panjabi's proposal for standardization of biomechanical testing of instrumentation, stability testing is equivalent to rigidity and inversely related to flexibility or instability. Stability or rigidity can be described by the load applied to the spine divided by the intervertebral motion produced. In a three-dimensional coordinate system (X, Y, Z), complex loading patterns can be broken down into one-dimensional loads (Fig. 52–25). These consist of six forces along the positive and negative directions of each axis and six moments, a positive and a negative, along the three axes. The motion of the loaded vertebrae can be defined by degrees of freedom, defined as the number of independent movements of a body. A vertebra has six degrees of freedom, translating in an anteroposterior, left-right lateral, and inferosuperior plane. It can also rotate in sagittal, horizontal, and frontal planes. Awareness of these concepts of mechanical testing is necessary in the evaluation of any instrumentation system.

Bone-Metal Interface

Although failure of spinal constructs can occur through failure of the metal components of instrumentation, constructs more commonly fail at the bone-metal interface with hooks, wires, or screws. This situation obviously would destabilize the construct and inhibit fusion. Factors that affect the stability of the bone-metal interface for all systems mentioned include bone quality, technique of implantation, and properties of the device. Individual interface stresses are decreased when the load is shared. For example, for a single Harrington distraction rod in scoliosis, significant axial and distractive stresses are placed on the upper and

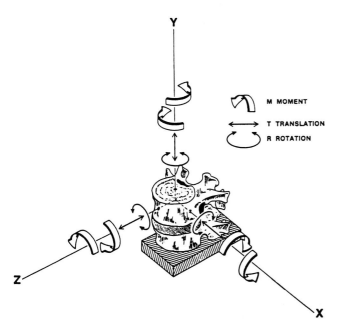

Figure 52–25. The loads acting on a vertebral body employing a three-dimensional coordinate system. See text for explanation. (From Panjabi, M. M.: Biomechanical evaluation of spinal fixation devices: A conceptual framework. Spine *13*:1129–1134, 1988.)

lower laminar hooks. These hook stresses could be lowered by the addition of more hooks to share the load. Likewise, less load is placed on individual sublaminar wires in a construct with six pairs of wires than in a construct with only three pairs of wires.

Screw-bone interface failure could conceivably occur by pull-out (a shear stress) or cut-out (medial-lateral stress). Of course, screws can fatigue or undergo metal-metal interface failure.[78, 81, 147] The results of screw studies show bone quality to be the most important factor. Tremendous variability in the quality of bone among specimens in these studies makes these data somewhat difficult to interpret. Larger screw diameter and deeper penetration, when in the high-quality bone of the pedicles, increase screw fixation. In evaluating the screw-bone interface, screw design considerations are extremely important. Major and minor screw diameter (determining thread depth), thread pitch, and length of thread on the screw are important variables in determining interface strength. Anterior cortical penetration may increase fixation,[147] but clinical data suggest that the added risk to the anterior structures is not warranted.[124-126] Zindrick and colleagues[147] demonstrated no significant difference in the pull-out strength between 4.5-mm and 6.5-mm fully threaded cancellous screws when the cortex was penetrated. However, with only 50 per cent vertebral body penetration or placement to but not through the cortex, the 6.5-mm screws had a significantly higher pull-out strength. Krag and associates[78] demonstrated that cut-out, or twisting failure, occurred at higher loads with greater depth of penetration, although the study did not test the effect

of cortical penetration. In the same study, screw pull-out strength varied with minor diameter and pitch for smaller (6-mm) but not for larger (7-mm) screws. Although pull-out and cut-out data serve a valuable purpose, the theoretic and practical primary mode of screw failure is by bending moments. Therefore, larger major diameter will probably remain the most important variable for screw failure, regardless of other design features. For the failed pedicular screw, methyl methacrylate seems to improve pull-out strength and stability under cyclic loading,[147] and it may provide a salvage technique in selected circumstances. Screw-plate constructs in the spine appear to have a stress shielding effect on the surrounding cancellous vertebral bodies.[48] Higher stresses are seen in the cortical pedicle regions and may contribute to screw loosening over time. These constructs, like all others, ultimately cannot last without a solid fusion.

The modern-day spine surgeon's choice of a specific instrumentation system in a given clinical situation should be based on a sound knowledge of biomechanical studies, as well as on clinical data that further define the indications, strengths, and weaknesses of the instrumentation. Although the wealth of biomechanical data helps clarify the indications for and choices of the various instrumentation systems available, further standardization and rigor in materials testing over the next decade will help surgeons choose the right instrument for the job. As stated previously, the goal of spinal instrumentation is fixation until solid fusion is obtained. This goal can be achieved only with meticulous surgical fusion technique and proper use of the available instrumentation systems. It is our hope that a basic understanding of biomechanical testing will help readers make appropriate choices regarding instrumentation.

References

1. Abumi, Y. C.: A biomechanical study on the stability of the injured thoracolumbar spine fixed with spinal instrumentation. J. Jpn. Orthop. Assoc. *62*:205–216, 1988.
2. Aebi, M.: Correction of degenerative scoliosis of the lumbar spine: A preliminary report. Clin. Orthop. 232:80–86, 1988.
3. Aebi, M., Etter, C., Kehl, T., and Thalgot, T. J.: The internal skeletal fixation system: A new treatment of thoracolumbar fractures and other spinal disorders. Clin. Orthop. 227:30, 1988.
4. Akeson, J., and Bobechko, W. P.: Treatment of scoliosis by instrumentation with double upper hooks and posterior fusion. Orthop. Trans. *10*:35, 1986.
5. Albee, F. H.: Transplantation of a portion of the tibia for Potts disease. JAMA 57:885–886, 1911.
6. Allen, B. L., Jr., and Ferguson, R. J.: The Galveston technique of pelvic fixation with L rod instrumentation of the spine. Spine 9:388–394, 1984.
7. Allen, B. L., Jr., and Ferguson, R. J.: Neurologic injuries with the Galveston technique of L rod instrumentation for scoliosis. Spine 11:14–17, 1986.
8. An, H. S., Gordin, R., and Renner, K.: Anatomic considerations for plate-screw fixation of the cervical spine. Spine *16*:S548–S551, 1991.
9. Asher, M., Carson, W. L., Heinig, C., et al.: A modular spinal rod linkage system to provide rotational stability. Spine *13*:272–277, 1988.
10. Asher, M. A., and Strippgen, W. E.: Anthropometric studies of

the human sacrum relating to dorsal trans sacral implant designs. Clin. Orthop. *203*:58, 1986.

11. Asher, M. A., Strippgen, W. E., Heinig, C. F., et al.: Isola Spine Implant System: Principles and Practice. Cleveland, Acro Med, 1991.

12. Ashman, R. B., Birch, J. G., Bone, L. B., et al.: Mechanical testing of spinal instrumentation. Clin. Orthop. *227*:113, 1988.

13. Bauer, R., Mostegl, A., and Eichenauer, M.: An analysis of the results of Dwyer and Zielke instrumentation in the treatment of scoliosis. Arch. Orthop. Trauma Surg. *105*:302–309, 1986.

14. Black, R. C., Gardner, V. O., Armstrong, G. W. D., et al.: A contoured anterior spinal fixation plate. Clin. Orthop. *227*:135, 1988.

15. Bohler, J., and Gandernack, T.: Anterior plate stabilization for fracture dislocations of the lower cervical spine. J. Trauma *20*:203–205, 1980.

16. Bohlman, H. H.: Cervical spine and cord trauma: Operative techniques. *In* Orthopaedic Knowledge Update II: Homestudy Syllabus. Park Ridge, IL, American Academy of Orthopaedic Surgeons, 1987, pp. 275–276.

17. Boostman, O., Myllynen, P., and Riska, E. B.: Posterior spinal fusion using internal fixation with Daab plate. Acta Orthop. Scand. *55*:310–314, 1984.

18. Bowen, J. R., and Ferrer, J.: Spinal stenosis caused by Harrington hook and neuromuscular disease: A case report. Clin. Orthop. *180*:179–181, 1983.

19. Bradford, D. S.: Instrumentation of the lumbar spine. Clin. Orthop. *203*:209, 1986.

20. Bradford, D. S., and Iza, J.: Repair of the defect in spondylolysis or minimal degrees of spondylolisthesis by segmental wire fixation and bone grafting. Spine *10*:673–679, 1985.

21. Brooks, A. L., and Jenkins, E. B.: Atlantloaxial arthrodesis by the wedge compression method. J. Bone Joint Surg. Am. *60*:279–284, 1978.

22. Buck, R. E.: Direct repair of the defect in spondylolisthesis. J. Bone Joint Surg. Br. *52*:432, 1952.

23. Calancie, B., Madsen, P., Lebwohl, N., et al.: Stimulus evoked EMG monitoring during transpedicular lumbosacral spine instrumentation. Spine *19*:2780–2786, 1994.

24. Camp, J. E., Birch, J. G., Corin, J. D., et al.: Rotational stability of various pedicle hook designs—an in vitro analysis. Proceedings of the combined meeting of the Scoliosis Research Society and European Spinal Deformities Society, Amsterdam, Netherlands, September 1989.

25. Cotler, J. M., Vernace, J. V., and Michalski, J. A.: The use of Harrington rods in thoracolumbar fractures. Orthop. Clin. North Am. *17*:87–103, 1986.

26. Cotrel, J., Dubousset, J., and Guillaumat, M.: A new universal instrumentation in spinal surgery. Clin. Orthop. *227*:10–23, 1988.

27. Cusick, J. F., Yoganandan, N., Pintar, F., et al.: Biomechanics of cervical spine facetectomy and fixation techniques. Spine *13*:808–812, 1988.

28. Cybulski, G. R., Stone, J. L., Crowel, R. M., et al.: Use of Halifax interlaminar clamps for posterior C1-2 arthrodesis. Neurosurgery *22*:429–431, 1988.

29. Denis, F.: Spinal instability as defined by the three column spinal concept in acute spinal trauma. Clin. Orthop. *189*:65–76, 1984.

30. Denis, F., Ruiz, H., and Searls, K.: Comparison between square ended distraction rods and standard round ended distraction rods in the treatment of thoracolumbar spinal injuries: A statistical analysis. Clin. Orthop. *189*:162–167, 1984.

31. Dick, W.: The fixateur interne as a versatile implant for spinal surgery. Spine *12*:882–900, 1987.

32. Dove, J.: Internal fixation of the lumbar spine: The Hartshill rectangle. Clin. Orthop. *203*:135, 1986.

33. Drummond, D. S.: Harrington instrumentation with spinous process wiring for idiopathic scoliosis. Orthop. Clin. North Am. *19*:281–289, 1988.

34. Drummond, D. S., and Keene, J. S.: Spinous process segmental spinal instrumentation. Orthopedics *11*:1403, 1988.

35. Edwards, C. L., Griffith, P. H., Levine, A. M., et al.: Early results using spinal rod-sleeves in thoracolumbar injuries. Orthop. Trans. *6*:345–346, 1982.

36. Edwards, C. L., and Levine, A. M.: Early rod-sleeve stabilization of the injured thoracic and lumbar spine. Orthop. Clin. North Am. *17*:121–145, 1986.

37. Esses, S. I., and Bednar, D. A.: The spinal pedicle screw: Techniques and systems. Orthop. Rev. *18*:676–682, 1989.

38. Fidler, M. W.: Posterior instrumentation of the spine: An experimental comparison of various possible techniques. Spine *11*:367–372, 1986.

39. Fielding, J. W., Hawkins, R. J., and Ratzau, S. A.: Spine fusion for atlantoaxial instability. J. Bone Joint Surg. Am. *58*:400, 1976.

40. Fried, L. C.: Atlanto-axial fracture-dislocations: Failure of posterior C1 to C2 fusion. J. Bone Joint Surg. Br. *55*:490–496, 1973.

41. Gaines, R. W., and Leatherman, K. D.: Benefits of the Harrington compression system in lumbar and thoracolumbar idiopathic scoliosis in adolescents and adults. Spine *6*:483–488, 1981.

42. Gaines, R. W., Breedlove, R. F., and Munson, G.: Stabilization of thoracic and thoracolumbar fracture dislocations with Harrington rods and sublaminar wires. Clin. Orthop. *189*:195–203, 1984.

43. Gaines, R. W., Jr., and Abernathie, D. L.: Mercilene tapes as a substitute for wire in segmental spinal instrumentation for children. Spine *11*:907–913, 1986.

44. Gallie, W. E.: Fractures and dislocations of the cervical spine. Am. J. Surg. *46*:495, 1939.

45. Gassman, J., and Zeligson, D.: The anterior cervical plate. Spine *8*:700–707, 1983.

46. Geisler, F. H., Cheng, C., Poka, A., and Brumback, R. J.: Anterior screw fixation of posteriorly displaced type II odontoid fractures. Neurosurgery *25*:30, 1989.

47. Ghanayem, A., and Zdeblick, T.: Anterior instrumentation in the management of thoracolumbar burst fractures. Clin. Orthop. *335*:89–100, 1997.

48. Goel, V. K., Kim, Y. E., Lim, T. H., and Weinstein, J. N.: An analytical investigation of the mechanics of spinal instrumentation. Spine *13*:1003–1011, 1988.

49. Goll, S. R., Balderston, R. A., Stambough, J. L., et al.: Depth of intraspinal wire penetration during passage of sublaminar wires. Spine *13*:503–509, 1988.

50. Gurr, K. R., and McAfee, P. C.: Cotrel-Dubousset instrumentation in adults: A preliminary report. Spine *13*:510–520, 1988.

51. Guyer, D. W., Wiltse, L. E., and Peek, R. D.: The Wiltse pedicle screw fixation system. Orthopaedics *11*:1455, 1988.

52. Hacker, R. J.: Comparison of interbody fusion approaches for disabling low back pain. Spine *22*:660–666, 1997.

53. Hadra, B. E.: Wearing of the spinous process in Potts disease. Trans. Am. Orthop. Assoc. *4*:206, 1891.

54. Hammerberg, K. W., Rodts, M. F., and DeWald, R. L.: Zielke instrumentation. Orthopedics *11*:1365, 1988.

55. Harrington, P. R.: Surgical instrumentation for management of scoliosis. J. Bone Joint Surg. Am. *42*:1448, 1960.

56. Harrington, P. R.: The history and development of Harrington instrumentation. Clin. Orthop. *227*:3, 1988.

57. Harrington, P. R., and Tullos, H. S.: Spondylolisthesis in children. Clin. Orthop. *79*:75, 1971.

58. Harrington, P. R., and Dixon, J. H.: An eleven year clinical investigation of Harrington instrumentation: A preliminary report on 578 cases. Clin. Orthop. *93*:113–130, 1973.

59. Harrington, P. R., and Dickson, J. H.: Spinal instrumentation in treatment of severe spondylolisthesis. Clin. Orthop. *117*:157, 1976.

60. Hasday, C. A., Pasoff, T. L., and Perry, J.: Gait abnormalities arising from iatrogenic loss of lumbar lordosis secondary to Harrington instrumentation and lumbar fractures. Spine *8*:501–511, 1983.

61. Heller, J. G., Carlson, G. D., Abitol, J. J., and Garfin, S. R.: Anatomic considerations of the Roy-Camille and Magerl techniques for screw placement in the lower cervical spine. Spine *16*:S552–S557, 1991.

62. Heller, J. G., Estes, B. T., Zaouali, M., and Diop, A.: Biomechanical study of screws in the lateral mass: Variables affecting pullout resistance. J. Bone Joint Surg. *78*:1315–1321, 1996.

63. Hibbs, R. A.: An operation for progressive spinal deformities. N. Y. State J. Med. *93*:1013–1016, 1911.

64. Holness, R. O., Huestis, W. S., Howes, W. J., and Langille, R.

A.: Posterior stabilization with an interlaminar clamp in cervical injuries: Technical note and review of the long-term experience with the method. Neurosurgery *14*:318–322, 1984.

65. Irwin, W. D., Dixon, J. H., and Harrington, P. R.: Clinical review of patients with broken Harrington rods. J. Bone Joint Surg. Am. *62*:1302–1307, 1980.

66. Jacobs, R. R., Dahners, L. E., Gertzbeine, S. D., et al.: A locking hook spinal rod: Current status of development. Paraplegia *21*:197–200, 1983.

67. Jacobs, R. R., Schlaepfer, F., Mathes, R., Jr., et al.: A locking hook spinal rod system for stabilization of fracture dislocations and correction of deformities of the dorsal lumbar spine: A biomechanical evaluation. Clin. Orthop. *189*:168–177, 1984.

68. Jacobs, R. R., and Montesano, P. X.: Development of the locking hook spinal rod system. Orthopaedics *11*:1415, 1988.

69. Jarvis, J. G., Ashman, R. B., Johnston, C. E., and Herring, J. A.: The posterior tether in scoliosis. Clin. Orthop. *227*:126–134, 1988.

70. Jendrisak, M. D.: Spontaneous abdominal aortic rupture from erosion by a lumbar spine fixation device: A case report. Surgery *99*:631–633, 1986.

71. Judet, R.: Osteosyntheses: Material, techniques, complications, actualities. De Chirugie Orthopedique de L'Hopital Raymond Pain Care *7*:196, 1970.

72. Kandea, K.: Personal communication, 1990.

73. King, D.: Internal fixation for lumbosacral fusion. Am. J. Surg. *66*:357, 1944.

74. Knodt, T. H. E., and Larrick, R.: Distraction fusion of the lumbar spine. Ohio Med. *12*:140, 1964.

75. Korkala, O., and Kytoomaa, J.: Reduction and fixation of late diagnosed lower cervical spine dislocations using the Daab plate: A report of two cases. Arch. Orthop. Trauma Surg. *103*:353–355, 1984.

76. Kornblatt, M. D., Casey, M. P., and Jacobs, R. R.: Internal fixation in the lumbosacral spine fusion: A biomechanical and clinical study. Clin. Orthop. *203*:141, 1986.

77. Kostuik, J. P.: Anterior Kostuik Harrington distraction systems. Orthopedics *11*:1379, 1988.

78. Krag, M. H., Beynnon, B. D., Pope, M. H., et al.: An internal fixator for posterior application to short segments of the thoracic, lumbar, or lumbosacral spine: Design and testing. Clin. Orthop. *203*:75–98, 1986.

79. Kramer, D. L., Ludwig, S. C., Balderston, R. A., et al.: Morphometry of the subaxial pedicles: Anatomical considerations related to three techniques of pedicle screw insertion. Presented at the CSRS, Palm Beach, FL, 1996.

80. Lang, E.: Support of the spondylitic spine by means of varied steel bars attached to the vertebra. Am. J. Orthop. Surg. *8*:344, 1910.

81. Lavaste, F.: Biomechanical experimental study on the thoracic and lumbar spine [in French]. Thesis, "Ingenuer" Ecole Nationale des Arts et Metiers, Paris, 1979.

82. Lee, C. K., and DeBarri, A.: Lumbosacral spinal fusion with Knodt distraction rods. Spine *11*:373–375, 1986.

83. Leong, J. C., Wilding, K., Mok, C. K., et al.: Surgical treatment of scoliosis following poliomyelitis: A review of 110 cases. J. Bone Joint Surg. Am. *63*:726–740, 1981.

84. Lesion, F., Autricque, A., Franz, K., et al.: Transcervical approach in screw fixation for upper cervical spine pathology. Surg. Neurol. *27*:459–465, 1987.

85. Louis, R.: Fusion of the lumbar and sacral spines by internal fixation with screw plates. Clin. Orthop. *203*:18–33, 1986.

86. Luque, E. R.: The anatomic basis and development of segmental spinal instrumentation. Spine *7*:256–259, 1982.

87. Luque, E. R.: Paralytic scoliosis in growing children. Clin. Orthop. *163*:202–209, 1982.

88. Luque, E. R.: Interpeduncular segmental screw fixation. Clin. Orthop. *203*:20, 1986.

89. Luque, E. R., and Rapp, G. F.: A new semi-rigid method for interpedicular fixation of the spine. Orthopaedics *11*:1445–1450, 1988.

90. Magerl, F.: External Skeletal Fixation of the Lower Thoracic and Lumbar Spine. Current Concepts of External Fixation of Fractures. Berlin, Springer-Verlag, 1982.

91. Magerl, F., and Seeman, P.: Stable posterior fusion of the atlas

and axis by transarticular screw fixation. *In* Kehr, P., and Weidner, A. (eds.): Cervical Spine. Vol. 1. New York, Springer-Verlag, 1987, p. 322.

92. McAfee, P. C., and Bohlman, H. H.: Complications following Harrington instrumentation for fracture of the thoracolumbar spine. J. Bone Joint Surg. Am. *67*:672–686, 1985.

93. McAfee, P. C., Bohlman, H. H., Ducker, T., and Eismont, F. J.: Failure of stabilization of the spine with methyl methacrylate: A retrospective analysis of twenty-four cases. J. Bone Joint Surg. Am. *68*:1145–1157, 1986.

94. McAfee, P. C., Bohlman, H. H., and Wilson, W. L.: The triple wire fixation technique for stabilization of acute cervical fracture dislocation: A biomechanical analysis. Orthop. Trans. *9*:142, 1985.

95. McAfee, P. C., Lubicky, J. P., and Werner, F. W.: The use of segmental spinal instrumentation to preserve longitudinal spinal growth: An experimental study. J. Bone Joint Surg. Am. *65*:935–942, 1983.

96. Michele, A. A., and Krueger, F. J.: Surgical approach to the vertebral body. J. Bone Joint Surg. Am. *31*:873–878, 1949.

97. Moe, J. H., Cummine, J. L., Winter, R. B., et al.: Harrington instrumentation without fusion combined with the Milwaukee brace for difficult scoliosis problems in young children. Orthop. Trans. *3*:59, 1979.

98. Moe, J. H., and Denis, F.: The iatrogenic loss of lumbar lordosis. Orthop. Trans. *1*:131, 1977.

99. Moe, J. H., Winter, R. B., Bradford, D. S., et al.: Scoliosis and Other Spinal Deformities. Philadelphia, W. B. Saunders Co., 1978.

100. Montesano, P. X., Magerl, F., Jacobs, R. R., et al.: Translaminar facet joint screws. Orthopedics *11*:1393, 1988.

101. Nasca, R. J., and Johnson, J. P.: Harrington-Bobechko instrumentation in the treatment of scoliosis: A preliminary report. Spine *13*:246–249, 1988.

102. Nicol, R. D., and Scott, J. H.: Lytic spondylolisthesis: Repair by wiring. Spine *11*:1027–1030, 1986.

103. O'Brien, J. P., Stevens, M. M., and Prickett, C. F.: Nylon sublaminar straps in segmental instrumentation for spinal disorders. Clin. Orthop. *203*:168–171, 1986.

104. Ogilvie, J. W., and Millar, E. A.: Comparison of segmental spinal instrumentation in the correction of scoliosis. Spine *8*:416–419, 1983.

105. Olerud, S., and Hamberg, M.: External fixation as a test for instability after spinal fusion L4–S1; A case report. Orthopedics *9*:547–549, 1986.

106. Olerud, S., Karlstrom, G., and Sjostrom, L.: Transpedicular fixation of thoracolumbar vertebral fractures. Clin. Orthop. *227*:44, 1988.

107. Olerud, S., Sjostrom, L., Karlstrom, G., and Hamberg, M.: Spontaneous effect of increased stability on the lower lumbar spine in cases of severe chronic back pain: The answer of an external transpedicular fixation test. Clin. Orthop. *203*:67–74, 1986.

108. Olson, S. A., and Gaines, R. W., Jr.: Removal of sublaminar wires after spinal fusion. J. Bone Joint Surg. Am. *69*:1419–1423, 1987.

109. Padua, S., Aulissa, L., and Fieri, C.: The progression of idiopathic scoliosis after removal of Harrington instrumentation following spinal fusion. Int. Orthop. *7*:85–89, 1983.

110. Panjabi, M. M.: Biomechanical evaluation of spinal fixation devices: I. A conceptual framework. Spine *13*:1129–1134, 1988.

111. Panjabi, M. M., Abumi, K., Duranceau, J., and Crisco, J. J.: Biomechanical evaluation of spinal fixation devices: II. Stability provided by eight internal fixation devices. Spine *13*:1135–1140, 1988.

112. Phillips, W. A., and Hensinger, R. N.: Wisconsin and other instrumentation for posterior spinal fusion. Clin. Orthop. *229*:41–51, 1988.

113. Rogers, W. A.: Treatment of fracture dislocation of the cervical spine. J. Bone Joint Surg. Am. *24*:254–258, 1942.

114. Romana, C., Michel, C. R., Dimnet, J., et al.: The Armstrong procedure in scoliosis surgery: Clinical, biomechanical and tridimensional study [translation]. Rev. Chir. Orthop. *71*:111–118, 1985.

115. Roseweig, N.: "The get up and go" treatment of acute unstable injuries of the middle and lower cervical spine. J. Bone Joint Surg. Br. *56*:392, 1974.

116. Roy-Camille, R., and Saillant, G.: Fracture complexes du rachis cervical inferieure. Tretraplegies. Nouv. Presse Med. *40*:2707–2711, 1972.
117. Roy-Camille, R., Saillant, G., and Mazel, C.: Internal fixation of the lumbar spine with pedicle screw plating. Clin. Orthop. *203*:18–33, 1986.
118. Ryan, M. D., Taylor, T. K., and Sherwood, A. A.: Bolt plate fixation for anterior spinal fusion. Clin. Orthop. *203*:196–202, 1986.
119. Saraste, H., and Ostman, A.: The effect of a device for transverse traction on vertebral rotation in surgery for scoliosis as studied by x-ray stereophotogrammetry. Int. Orthop. *10*:131–133, 1986.
120. Selby, D.: Internal fixation with Knodt's rods. Clin. Orthop. *203*:179, 1986.
121. Shigley, J. E., and Mitchell, L. D.: Mechanical Engineering Design. New York, McGraw-Hill, 1983, pp. 2070–277.
122. Shufflebarger, H. L., and Clark, C. E.: Cotrel-Dubousset instrumentation. Orthopedics *111*435, 1988.
123. Simmons, E. H., and Capicotto, W. N.: Posterior transpedicular Zielke instrumentation of the lumbar spine. Clin. Orthop. *236*:180–191, 1988.
124. Steffee, A. D., Biscup, R. S., and Sitkowski, D. J.: Segmental spine plates with pedicle screw fixation: A new internal fixation device for disorders of the lumbar and thoracolumbar spine. Clin. Orthop. *203*:45–53, 1986.
125. Steffee, A. D., and Sitkowski, D. J.: Reduction and stabilization of grade IV spondylolisthesis. Clin. Orthop. 227:82, 1982.
126. Steffee, A. D., and Sitkowski, D. J.: Posterior lumbar interbody fusion and plates. Clin. Orthop. 227:99, 1988.
127. Sullivan, J. A.: Sublaminar wiring of Harrington distraction rods for unstable thoracolumbar spine fractures. Clin. Orthop. *189*:178–185, 1984.
128. Thalgott, J. S., Aebi, M., and LaRocca, H.: Internal spinal skeletal fixation system. Orthopedics *11*:1465, 1988.
129. Tippets, R. H., and Apfelbaum, R. I.: Anterior cervical fusion with the Caspar instrumentation system. Neurosurgery 22:1008–1013, 1988.
130. Tolo, V.: Surgical treatment of adolescent scoliosis. Instr. Course Lect. *38*:143–156, 1989.
131. Tometz, J. G., and Emans, J. B.: A comparison between spinous processes and sublaminar wiring combined with Harrington distraction instrumentation on the management of adolescent idiopathic scoliosis. J. Pediatr. Orthop. *8*:129–132, 1988.
132. Turi, M., Johnston, C. E., II, and Richards, B. S.: Anterior correction of idiopathic scoliosis using TSRH instrumentation. Spine *18*:417–422, 1993.
133. Vanable, C. S., and Stuck, W. G.: Electrolysis controlling factor in the use of metals and treating fracture. JAMA 3:349, 1939.
134. White, A. H., Zucherman, J. F., and Hsu, K.: Lumbosacral fusions with Harrington rods and intersegmental wiring. Clin. Orthop. *203*:185, 1986.
135. Whitehill, R., Cicoria, A. D., Hooper, W. E., et al.: Posterior cervical reconstruction with methylmethacrylate and wire: A clinical review. J. Neurosurg. *68*:584, 1988.
136. Whitehill, R., Stowers, S. F., Fechner, R. E., et al.: Posterior cervical fusions using cerclage wires, methylmethacrylate cement and autogenous bone graft: An experimental study of a canine model. Spine *12*:12–22, 1987.
137. Wilber, R. G., Thompson, G. H., Shaffer, J. W., et al.: Postoperative neurologic deficit in segmental spinal instrumentation: A study using spinal cord monitoring. J. Bone Joint Surg. Am. *66*:1178–1187, 1984.
138. Wilkinson, H. A.: Stabilization of acrylic vertebral body replacement. Surg. Neurol. *24*:83–86, 1985.
139. Wilson, P. D., and Straub, L. R.: American Academy of Orthopaedic Surgeons Instructional Course Lecture. Vol. 9. Ann Arbor, MI, 1952.
140. Winter, R. B., Lonstein, J. E., Vandenbrink, K., et al.: Harrington rod with sublaminar wires in the treatment of adolescent idiopathic thoracic scoliosis: A study of sagittal plane correction. Orthop. Trans. *11*:89, 1987.
141. Wong, K. C., Webster, L. R., Coleman, S. S., and Dunn, H. K.: Hemodilution and induced hypotension for insertion of a Harrington rod in a Jehovah's Witness patient. Clin. Orthop. *152*:237–240, 1980.
142. Wu, Z. K.: Posterior vertebral instrumentation for correction of scoliosis. Clin. Orthop. *215*:40–46, 1987.
143. Yngve, D. A., Burke, S. W., Price, C. T., and Riddick, M. F.: Sublaminar wiring. J. Pediatr. Orthop. *6*:605–608, 1986.
144. Yuan, H., Mann, K., Found, E., at al.: Treatment of thoracic and lumber burst fractures using anterior stabilization: Clinical and experimental study. Orthop. Trans. *13*:50, 1988.
145. Yuan, H. A., Garfin, S. R., Dickman, C. A., and Mardjetko, S. M.: A historical cohort study of pedicle screw fixation in thoracic, lumbar and sacral spinal fusions. Spine *19*:2279S–2296S, 1994.
146. Zdeblick, T. A., Shirado, D., McAfee, P. C., et al.: Anterior spinal fixation after lumbar corpectomy: A study in dogs. J. Bone Joint Surg. Am. *72*:527–534, 1991.
147. Zindrick, M. R., Wiltse, L. L., Widell, E. H., et al.: A biomechanical study of intrapeduncular screw fixation of the lumbosacral spine. Clin. Orthop. *203*:99, 1986.
148. Zucherman, J., Hsu, K., White, A., and Wynne, G.: Early results of spinal fusion using variable spine plating system. Spine *13*:570–579, 1988.

CHAPTER

53

Intraoperative Neurophysiologic Monitoring of the Spinal Cord

Eric B. Geller, M.D.

Imad M. Najm, M.D.

This chapter provides an introduction to the uses of intraoperative monitoring of spinal cord function. We outline the neurophysiologic basis of monitoring and cover commonly used methods and their utility. Detailed protocols are beyond the scope of this chapter, and the interested reader is referred to the references for more details.

The purpose of intraoperative neurophysiologic monitoring is to provide feedback to the surgeon about possible iatrogenic injury to the nervous system. Such feedback may allow a change in procedure that prevents or limits injury, may provide prognostic information, or may help identify detrimental surgical techniques that would otherwise be unrecognized as part of a long operation.[11, 14, 17, 34] Animal studies have shown that somatosensory evoked potentials (SEPs) are affected by several mechanisms of spinal cord injury: cord compression, ischemia, systemic hypotension, and distraction.[14] Changes may be reversible if the mechanism of injury is relieved quickly enough. Thus, monitoring may allow the surgeon to correct potential injuries intraoperatively, preventing neurologic deficits. Monitoring should be performed by physicians and technologists who are experienced in clinical neurophysiology and trained in intraoperative techniques.[2, 34]

Spinal monitoring techniques may be useful in a variety of surgical procedures, such as for scoliosis, intramedullary and extramedullary spinal cord tumors, arteriovenous malformations of the spinal cord, and sometimes aortic aneurysm repair.[11, 17] The efficacy of monitoring procedures is discussed later. Neurophysio-

logic techniques have largely replaced the wake-up test as a means of preventing neurologic deficits in spine surgery.[22, 34]

Evoked potentials are electrical fields generated by a nervous structure in response to a stimulus. A basic principle of evoked potential monitoring is that the area at risk must lie in a pathway between the stimulus and the response. Although this seems obvious, it points out the need for an understanding of neuroanatomy and neurophysiology in order to design an effective monitoring strategy.

NEUROANATOMY OF THE SPINAL CORD

The spinal cord is made up of a central core of gray matter containing neuronal cell bodies, surrounded by white matter tracts made up of sensory axons ascending to the brain or upper motor axons descending to synapse with motor neurons. The tracts that can be monitored are the dorsal columns (somatosensory) and the lateral corticospinal tracts (motor). The lateral spinothalamic sensory tracts, spinocerebellar tracts, and extrapyramidal descending tracts do not contribute significantly to the evoked potentials that are typically monitored.

The dorsal columns carry information from mostly large, myelinated fibers in the periphery that subserve position sense, vibration, and fine touch discrimination. An axon from the dorsal root ganglion enters the spinal cord and ascends without synapsing until it reaches the cuneate (cervical region) or gracile (lumbar region) nuclei. Secondary axons decussate in the medulla and ascend the brain stem in the medial lemniscus, synapsing in upper brain stem structures and the ventrolateral nuclei of the thalamus. Thalamic neurons project onto the primary somatosensory cortex, located in the postcentral gyrus. This region is somatotopically organized, with representation of the face inferiorly near the sylvian fissure, the hand and arm over the lateral convexity, and the leg and foot at the vertex and in the interhemispheric fissure.

SOMATOSENSORY EVOKED POTENTIALS

SEPs are responses to repetitive electrical stimulation of a peripheral nerve. Such responses are of very low amplitude (microvolts) and are small compared with other brain activities, ECG, and the electrical noise that can be problematic in an operating room. In order to record SEPs, many responses must be recorded digitally and averaged by computer to reduce the unwanted noise and amplify the signal of interest. SEPs appear as positive or negative peaks that can be identified. Measurements of interest include absolute latency from onset of the stimulus to the peak, interpeak latencies, and peak amplitudes. Interpeak latencies represent central conduction time and should be independent of peripheral nerve problems.

There are two types of responses that can be recorded: near field and far field. Near-field responses are potentials that are detectable only if the recording electrode is located near the generating structure. Far-field responses can be detected by electrodes distant from the generator. By comparing the electrical potential in electrodes at different locations, specific responses can best be identified. The arrangement of different electrode pairs on different channels of the evoked potential machine is called a montage.

Although a number of peripheral nerves can be monitored, the median nerve and the posterior tibial nerve are most commonly used, as they have robust responses with well-characterized peaks. The ulnar nerve is sometimes used if the area at risk is in the cervical cord below the entry zone for the median nerve.

Several different structures generate SEPs. Table 53–1 summarizes the identifiable peaks and their generators. Figure 53–1 shows examples of normal SEP waveforms. The generators of the median and posterior tibial responses are analogous. A peripheral nerve response is the traveling action potential passing under the electrode and is useful in verifying that the stimulus actually entered the nervous system (see Fig. 53–1). Postsynaptic potentials from the central gray matter of the spinal cord may be seen, although these are usually not used in operative monitoring. Far-field potentials are generated by postsynaptic activity in the lower brain stem and upper brain stem/thalamus. These can be quite useful, as they are relatively resistant to anesthetic agents. Near-field cortical responses are seen over the somatotopic representation in the postcentral cortex. Cortical potentials may be depressed by anesthesia or hypothermia.[11] Later cortical potentials may be seen but are not used diagnostically. We should note that there are many different terms in the literature referring to the same SEP peaks. The terminology used in this chapter conforms to the standardized nomenclature of the American Electroencephalographic Society guidelines.[2]

Methods of SEP Monitoring

A number of different methods of SEP monitoring have been described, of varying invasiveness. All methods require stimulation across the area at risk of injury. Because the operating room is an electrically hostile environment with many sources of electrical artifact, artifact must be reduced as much as possible. Modern evoked potential equipment generally has automated artifact rejection, which excludes amplitudes above a preset cut-off. Filtering the signal also reduces artifact, but excessive filtering may alter the SEP latency and amplitude.[2, 11]

Table 53–1. SOMATOSENSORY EVOKED POTENTIAL PEAKS AND GENERATORS

Generator	Type	Median Nerve	Recording Montage	Posterior Tibial Nerve	Recording Montage
Peripheral nerve action potential	Near field	Erb's point (EP)	Erb's point	Popliteal fossa (PF)	Popliteal fossa
Spinal cord gray matter postsynaptic potential	Near field	N13	C5S–Erb's point or anterior cervical	N20	T12–iliac crest (IC)
Lower brain stem postsynaptic potentials	Far field	P14	Fz–C5S	P31	Fz–C5S
Upper brain stem/thalamus postsynaptic potentials	Far field	N18	Fz–C5S	N34	Fz–C5S
Cortical postsynaptic potentials	Near field	N20	CPc–CPi	P37	CPz or CPi–Fz

C5S, fifth cervical spinous process; T12, twelfth thoracic spinous process; Fz, midline frontal; CP, centroparietal (CPc, contralateral; CPi, ipsilateral; CPz, midline).

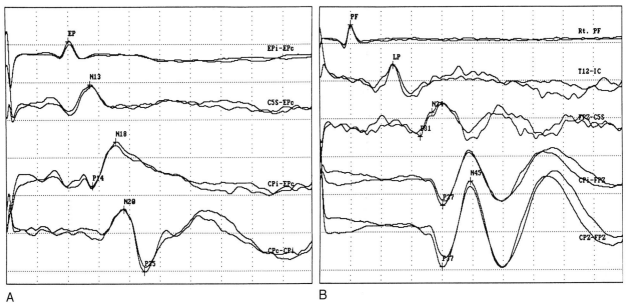

Figure 53–1. *A,* Median nerve SEPs. Time scale = 5 msec/division. *B,* Posterior tibial SEPs. Time scale = 10 msec/division. See text and Table 53–1 for explanation of montages and peaks.

Noninvasive SEPs

These techniques are similar to those used in outpatient SEP recording. They are the simplest to perform and the most commonly used.[11, 17, 34] Electrical stimulation is applied to one limb at a time. Responses are recorded below the level of surgery, often at the peripheral nerve (popliteal fossa or Erb's point), to ensure appropriate stimulation, and from subcortical and cortical sites. Although many published reports used only the scalp (cortical) potential, we agree with those who advocate monitoring several different sites simultaneously.[14, 15] Using several sites prevents technical problems with a single recording site from interfering with monitoring. Changes at a single site may not be significant if other sites are not affected. In particular, cortical potentials may be affected by anesthesia, hypotension, or hypothermia, and recording subcortical potentials may allow continuation of monitoring.[11, 17, 38]

Stimulation is given via a needle electrode either to the posterior tibial or peroneal nerve in the leg or to the median or ulnar nerve in the arm. Because the patient is anesthetized, high levels of stimulation can be given, producing more easily recordable responses. Although some authors have used bilateral simultaneous stimulation to achieve a more robust SEP, most centers stimulate one limb at a time.[34] The stimulation rate must balance the need of rapid acquisition for feedback during surgery against the loss of SEP amplitude with high stimulation rates, particularly under anesthesia.[11] A compromise rate of about 5 Hz is useful.

Recordings can be made from peripheral nerve and from subcortical and cortical areas. Electrode montages are described in Table 53–1. Recommended filter settings are 1 to 30 Hz and 250 to 3000 Hz.[2] Filter settings should be kept constant during the procedure, as changes will cause alteration of waveforms. Several hundred or more trials may be necessary to obtain a clear response.

Invasive Techniques

Subarachnoid. Tamaki and associates described recordings from the subarachnoid space.[42] This is the most invasive method. A recording electrode is introduced into the subarachnoid space via a Tuohy needle at the low lumbar level and advanced to the level of the conus medullaris. The recording electrode is referred to an indifferent electrode at the gluteal muscle. The spinal cord is stimulated extradurally via an electrode at the upper thoracic level, using rectangular impulses of 0.3 msec duration at 30 to 50 Hz frequency and an intensity of 30 to 120 V. An initial spike is followed by a multiphasic waveform. Changes were detected in four of 60 patients, with corrective action taken and no neurologic deficit in three and a transient deficit in one. Although this method has the advantage of robust recordings, there is concern about possible injury to the spinal cord.[14]

Epidural. This method is less invasive than subarachnoid recording and has been used by a number of groups.[43] Electrodes are inserted percutaneously using a Tuohy needle or under direct vision at surgery. Epidural stimulation is given at 50 Hz or greater at an intensity producing muscle twitching in the paravertebral muscles, 2 to 100 V, duration 0.1 to 0.3 msec. Recordings are made either rostral or caudal to the site of stimulation via epidural electrodes. Two negative peaks are seen. A number of studies have used the epidural technique and have reported detection of changes that were reversible when corrective action was taken by the surgeon. Koyanagi and colleagues[26] used epidural recordings during surgery for spinal cord tumors in 20 patients. Six patients had significant changes, five of whom had postoperative deficits. However, these authors had four false-negative cases, suggesting that epidural potentials should be used in conjunction with other monitoring modalities in such cases.

Spinous Process. Kirschner wires are inserted into the vertebral spinous processes.[9] The amplitude of responses recorded in this way are approximately half that of the epidurally recorded responses, making this technique less popular.[14]

Interspinous Ligament. Needles are inserted into the interspinous ligaments at levels above and below the operative site, using two to four different sites, with stimulation of the posterior tibial or median nerve as in the noninvasive technique.[21, 25, 30] Subcortical and cortical responses are also recorded.

Comparison of Techniques

The advantages of noninvasive recordings are the relative simplicity of the technique and the well-characterized responses. The disadvantage is that a variety of non-neurologic factors can affect the responses and potentially cause false-positive reports. For these reasons, invasive techniques have been developed to record responses directly from the spinal cord. Such responses are more resistant to anesthesia but are less well characterized, and placement of electrodes is more time-consuming.[14, 15, 17] At our center, we currently use noninvasive SEP recording for most cases.

Factors Affecting SEPs

A number of factors besides neurologic injury can affect SEPs.[11, 44] Such factors may be remediable by the surgeon or anesthesiologist. Increased peak latency or amplitude reduction, particularly of the cortical potentials, can occur because of anesthesia, especially inhalation agents.[17] Unfortunately, the needs of the surgeon, the anesthesiologist, and the neurophysiologist may conflict at times, and compromises must be made.[17] Subcortical and spinal responses are much less affected by anesthesia and can permit continued monitoring.[17, 38]

SEPs can be affected by systemic hypotension or hypothermia, and they may recover with increased blood pressure or body temperature.[44] Cool irrigation in the operative field may reduce or delay SEPs, with warm fluid causing recovery of potentials fairly rapidly.

Scoliosis alone does not seem to affect SEPs. Brinker and associates[8] found no difference in SEP latencies between patients with idiopathic scoliosis and normal controls. In contrast, Owen and associates[36] studied patients with neuromuscular causes of scoliosis and found that 27 per cent of such patients did not have useful cortical SEPs, compared with 2 per cent of patients with idiopathic scoliosis. Those with neuromuscular scoliosis also had a smaller intraoperative amplitude of the cortical SEP compared with the preoperative baseline than did those with idiopathic scoliosis. The authors found that recording both subcortical and motor responses rather than just cortical responses allowed monitoring to be useful.

Significant Changes in SEPs

Given the various factors that can affect SEPs, what are significant changes that should be reported to the surgeon? Different studies have used different cut-offs for defining a significant change. In a large multicenter survey, Nuwer and colleagues[34] found that most centers use the criterion of a 50 per cent or greater decrement in amplitude or a 5 to 10 per cent or greater increase in peak latency as abnormal. These numbers have support from animal research[14] and from clinical studies as criteria that predict neurologic deficits that may be reversible.

The concept of the false-positive test should be clarified. Although the meanings of false-negative, true-negative, and true-positive are clear in relation to SEP abnormalities predicting neurologic deficit, false-positive is more difficult. Because the surgeon may take action to correct a potential problem when warned by the neurophysiologist, a neurologic deficit that otherwise would have occurred may be averted, resulting in a false-positive result.[34] Although false-positive reports to the surgeon may prolong the operation needlessly, there is no absolute way to know whether the SEP changes truly reflect damage to the spinal cord. Thus the neurophysiology team should take great care to identify and correct any non-neurologic causes of SEP changes. Monitoring of subcortical as well as cortical responses may help avoid false-positive results by providing confirmation of a change in multiple peaks.

Clinical Efficacy of SEP Monitoring

For monitoring to be useful, it should be able to cost-effectively alter operative morbidity, not merely predict it.[3] Ethical considerations prevent the use of randomized, prospective trials of the effect of SEP monitoring on surgical outcome.[18] Therefore, case series and historic controls must be used to assess the value of SEP monitoring. There are few large studies in which to assess efficacy.

The largest study to date is that of Nuwer and colleagues,[34] which was a large multicenter survey of U.S. members of the Scoliosis Research Society (SRS). They questioned the surgeons about morbidity and the use of monitoring. The neurophysiologists involved were also questioned about monitoring techniques and criteria for significant SEP changes. One hundred fifty-three surgeons and 90 neurophysiologists responded. Results were compared with those of the MacEwen survey of 1967–71, which included many of the same surgeons.[31]

Monitoring was performed in 51,263 cases of spine surgery (53 per cent of 97,586 total cases), the majority of which were for scoliosis (60 per cent). Compared with the historic data, the neurologic deficit rate dropped from 0.72 to 0.55 per cent. Persistent deficits fell from 0.46 to 0.31 per cent. An even greater drop was seen in major neurologic deficits (paraparesis or paraplegia) from 0.61 to 0.24 per cent. These changes were statistically significant (p < .001). Using regression techniques, they found that the primary predictor of neurologic deficits was the years of experience with SEP monitoring, followed by the surgeon's years in practice. Teams with the least experience (100 cases or fewer) had deficit rates more than twice as high as teams with the most experience (300 cases or more). The false-negative rate was 0.127 per cent and the false-positive rate 1.51 per cent. The negative predictive value was 99.93 per cent, indicating that monitoring is highly likely to be correct when SEPs remain stable. The positive predictive value was relatively low (42 per cent), reflecting a tendency to false alarms. It must be noted that the false-positive rate may not be truly false, as the surgeon may have been able to avert a deficit based on the monitoring information. Based on these data, Nuwer and colleagues estimated that the cost of preventing one neurologic deficit for every 200 cases monitored was approximately $120,000. Although this is a large amount, it is less than the lifetime cost of medical care for a young paraplegic, suggesting that SEP monitoring is indeed cost-effective.

Studies of SEP monitoring during nonscoliosis spine surgeries have also shown efficacy. Epstein and associates[16] compared 100 consecutive cases of cervical surgery monitored by median and posterior tibial nerve SEPs with 218 unmonitored historic controls at the same center. The controls had a 3.7 per cent incidence of quadriparesis and a 0.5 per cent mortality. Among the monitored patients, only one incurred a deficit, and this patient did not have posterior tibial monitoring the entire time. Using the Ranawat grades to compare the patients' neurologic status pre- and postoperatively, the two groups had similar preoperative grades. Postoperatively, 70 per cent of unmonitored patients and 85 per cent of monitored patients had a good to excellent outcome, with the most severely impaired group dropping from 7 per cent (unmonitored) to 1 per cent (monitored).

Fisher and coworkers,[18] in reviewing the efficacy of intraoperative neurophysiologic monitoring, found SEP monitoring to be useful in resection or embolization of spinal dural arteriovenous malformations, surgery for cord tumors, repair of mechanical instability of the vertebral column, and surgery for syringomyelia.

MOTOR EVOKED POTENTIALS

SEPs travel within the dorsal columns but do not traverse any synapses within the spinal cord proper. Although SEPs proved useful for predicting the integrity of dorsal columns during surgery, they were not always accurate at predicting damage to the motor path-

ways.[14, 20, 27, 41] This is because the main descending motor tracts within the spinal cord are in the dorsolateral funiculus and are thus separate from the posterior columns. Moreover, the vascular supply of the dorsal columns is different from that of the anterior pathways and therefore does not accurately represent the vascular state of the cord. In addition, it is hypothesized that impulse transmission through axons is less affected by ischemia than is synaptic transmission.[6] It is therefore possible for the SEPs to be preserved despite ischemia that abolishes synaptic transmission within the cord.

Because preservation of motor function is the primary goal, investigators began to consider ways to monitor the motor system directly through the study of motor evoked potentials (MEPs). MEPs refer to electrical signals induced in a motor axon by stimulation of the nervous system. MEP techniques assess the integrity of the motor descending pathways at various levels. Current MEP techniques require activation of the motor pathways proximal to the surgical site, with recording of motor responses distally at various levels (spine, peripheral nerve, or muscle).

Methods of MEP Monitoring

The motor pathways may be stimulated by electrical stimulation of the cerebral cortex or brain stem[7, 28, 33, 39] or the spinal cord,[29, 32] or by magnetic stimulation of the cerebral cortex.[5] Techniques that involve transcranial stimulation of the motor cortex are minimally invasive and allow surveillance of the entire motor neuraxis.

Electrical Stimulation Techniques

Electrical activation of the motor cortex or brain stem is performed in various ways. Electroencephalograph (EEG) scalp electrodes[7, 33] or electrode plates placed adjacent to the scalp and hard palate[28] were previously used to stimulate the cortex. Stimulation rates may range from 0.2 Hz up to 17 Hz.[7, 28] In one study, the current level varied from 11 to 80 mA, and levels between 30 and 60 mA were usually needed to produce an MEP.[28] Transcranial electrical activation is not recommended in patients with a history of seizures or an abnormal EEG that shows epileptic discharges, because of the theoretic possibility of provoking seizures (seizure kindling effect). Moreover, its use is discouraged in patients with skull fractures or implanted intracranial metallic devices (such as aneurysm clips). Because of the pain generated by electrical stimulation, the use of this technique in awake patients is not indicated.

The motor system can also be activated by stimulating the spinal cord directly[29] or through epidural electrodes.[32, 35] The electrodes are placed in the midline to avoid unilateral stimulation that might lead to failure in the identification of spinal cord integrity. With spinal cord stimulation techniques, relatively higher stimulation repetition rates can be used (4 to 6 Hz),[32] permitting rapid acquisition of good averaged responses.

Transcranial Magnetic Stimulation Technique

In 1985, Barker and collaborators were the first to successfully record muscle action potentials in response to transcranial magnetic stimulation (TMS) of the brain.[4, 5] TMS involves generation of a rapidly changing magnetic field that induces an electric current in nearby conductors. A typical magnetic stimulator consists of a power supply, a storage capacitor, solid-state switching elements, and a magnetic stimulating coil.[10] TMS induces a magnetic field that passes through the scalp and skull without significant attenuation and produces an electric current in underlying cerebral tissues, leading to discharges in motor neurons.[19] The large current flow in the coil produces a local magnetic field that can reach 2 Tesla and has a peak intensity of approximately 150 microseconds.[6] Because the magnetic field does not stimulate nociceptive afferents in the scalp, magnetic stimulation is better tolerated than electrical stimulation in awake patients. TMS is not indicated in patients with skull defects, implantable metallic or electronic devices, cochlear implants, intracranial metallic devices, epilepsy, or cardiac pacemakers.

Motor Evoked Response Recordings

Once the motor cortex is stimulated, a propagated potential travels down the corticospinal tract, activates the anterior horn cells of the spinal cord gray matter, and then travels along the peripheral nerve, traverses the neuromuscular junction, and activates the muscle, leading to muscular contraction. Therefore, motor evoked responses can be recorded at the spinal levels using epidural electrodes[7, 28, 29] from peripheral nerves or from muscles[19, 28] (Fig. 53–2).

The most direct way to record motor stimulation evoked responses is by recording compound motor action potentials (CMAPs) that result from muscle depolarization using needle electrodes. CMAPs are large enough (200 to 2400 μV) and do not require signal averaging. CMAP recording is severely affected by the use of neuromuscular blocking agents. If transmission across the neuromuscular junction is pharmacologically blocked, recording electrodes can be placed over the peripheral motor nerves in order to record nerve action potentials. Nerve action potentials are much smaller in amplitude than CMAPs (up to 20 μV) and therefore need averaging (between 100 and 500 stimuli). MEP recordings from the spinal cord yield two types of waves: D or direct waves, and I or indirect waves. D waves are of short latency (0.6 msec), originate in the corticofugal fibers directly at the region of the axon hillock, and can be induced by direct stimulation of subcortical white matter. D waves are less affected by anesthesia. The I waves are of longer latency, occur in series, and are secondary to synaptic depolarization of the pyramidal tract neurons within the cortical gray matter. These waves are severely affected by halogenated anesthetics.[37]

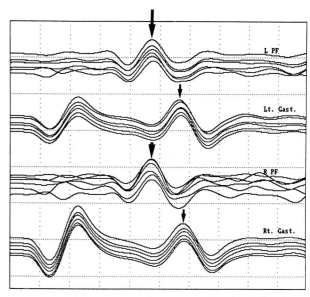

Figure 53–2. Motor evoked potentials. The spinal cord was stimulated by epidural electrodes. Responses were recorded from the peripheral nerve at the popliteal fossa (PF) and in the gastrocnemius muscle (Gast) on the left (upper two tracings) and right (lower two tracings). Arrows mark the nerve action potential (PF channels) and muscle potential (Gast channel). Time scale = 4 msec/division.

Comparison of Techniques

Electrical and magnetic stimulation techniques differ in a number of ways. One of the major advantages of TMS over electrical stimulation is that it is painless and consequently can be used in awake unanesthetized patients. Other differences include the fact that stimulation using magnetic techniques is less accurate and therefore less reproducible with the equipment currently available. Moreover, responses obtained with TMS are highly dependent on the direction of the current flow within the magnetic coil. Another important difference between the two techniques is related to the latency of the electromyogram (EMG) response.[1, 12, 24] TMS produces an EMG response with a latency slightly greater than that seen with electrical stimulation. This could be because electrical and magnetic stimulations activate the corticospinal tract at different anatomic loci,[1, 12, 24, 40] with electrical stimulation activating the corticospinal tract at deeper level. Other possibilities include a TMS recruitment of a population of neurons of slower conduction than is recruited with electrical stimulation, or a difference in the orientation and direction of induced current flow in the brain.[24, 40]

Factors Affecting MEPs

Numerous anesthetic agents and muscle relaxants directly affect the recording of MEPs. The composition of the monitored neural circuit represents the single most important factor regarding the anesthetic action on evoked potentials. The inclusion of cortical neurons and synapses in the circuit increases the probability of anesthetic interference. Transcranial electrical MEPs are less likely to be affected by anesthetics than are transcranial magnetic MEPs, because the sensitive cortical structures are not monitored in the former.

Neuromuscular blocking agents may affect EMG monitoring. However, MEPs from limb muscles after TMS can generally be recorded even in the presence of clinically near complete neuromuscular blockade.[13, 23] This is possible because of the temporal and spatial summation of the motor action potentials at the spinal level (D and I waves). It is therefore recommended that the amplitude of the peripheral nerve stimulated EMG be maintained at approximately one fifth of the pretreatment amplitude.

Clinical Applications of MEPs

In the operating room, MEPs have yet to be applied as widely as SEPs. Levy studied 98 patients undergoing electrical stimulation.[28] He concluded that the use of this technique may help warn the surgeon of potentially avoidable problems. Moreover, false-negative recordings are rare using transcranial electrical stimulation (none occurred in 148 patients monitored by Levy[28] or in those by Zentner[45]), but false-positives may be more common.[45] Although magnetic stimulation has been widely used in a variety of clinical settings, there is relatively little experience with the technique in regard to intraoperative monitoring. Motor stimulation techniques remain to be studied as thoroughly as SEP techniques for intraoperative monitoring.

CONCLUSIONS

Neurophysiologic monitoring can be useful in preventing intraoperative damage to the spinal cord. By alerting the surgeon to potential problems at the time they occur, reversible damage may be avoided. SEP monitoring is the most widely used and proven technique, but it monitors only the dorsal columns. Motor tract stimulation may increase monitoring sensitivity for deficits in the anterior cord, but techniques are not as standardized as for SEPs, and efficacy remains to be proved. Optimizing conditions for monitoring requires cooperation among and sometimes compromises from the neurophysiologist, surgeon, and anesthesiologist.

References

1. Amassian, V. E., Quirk, G. J., and Stewart, M.: Magnetic coil versus electrical stimulation of monkey motor cortex. J. Physiol. *394*:119P, 1987.
2. American Electroencephalographic Society: Guidelines for intraoperative monitoring of sensory evoked potentials. J. Clin. Neurophysiol. *11*:77–87, 1994.
3. Aminoff, M. J.: Intraoperative monitoring by evoked potentials for spinal cord surgery: The cons. Electroencephalogr. Clin. Neurophysiol. *73*:378–380, 1989.
4. Barker, A. T., Freeston, I. L., Jalinous, R., et al.: Magnetic stimulation of the human brain. J. Physiol. *369*:3P, 1985.
5. Barker, A. T., Jalinous, R., and Freeston, I. L.: Non-invasive magnetic stimulation of the human motor cortex. Lancet *2*:1106–1107, 1985.
6. Borges, L. F.: Motor evoked potentials. (Review.) Int. Anesthesiol. Clin. *28*:170–173, 1990.
7. Boyd, S. G., Rothwell, J. C., Cowan, J. M. A., et al.: A method of monitoring function in corticospinal pathways during scoliosis surgery with a note on motor conduction velocities. J. Neurol. Neurosurg. Psychiat *49*:251–257, 1986.
8. Brinker, M. R., Willis, J. K., Cook, S. D., et al.: Neurologic testing with somatosensory evoked potentials in idiopathic scoliosis. Spine *17*:277–279, 1992.
9. Brown, J. C., Axelgaard, J., and Rowe, D. E.: Monitoring of the human spinal cord. (Abstract.) Orthop. Trans. *3*:123, 1979.
10. Burgess, R. C.: Magnetic stimulators. J. Clin. Neurophysiol. *8*:121–129, 1991.
11. Daube, J. R.: Spinal cord monitoring. *In* Daube, J. R. (ed.): Clinical Neurophysiology. Philadelphia, F. A. Davis, 1996, pp. 457–463.
12. Day, B. L., Dick, J. P. R., Marsden, C. D., and Thompson, P. D.: Differences between electrical and magnetic stimulation of the human brain. J. Physiol. *378*:36P, 1986.
13. Deletis, V.: Intraoperative monitoring of the functional integrity of the motor pathways. *In* Devinsky, O., Beric, A., and Dogali, M. (eds.): Electrical and Magnetic Stimulation of the Brain: Advances in Neurology. Vol. 63. New York, Raven Press, 1993, pp. 201–214.
14. Dinner, D. S., Luders, H., Lesser, R. P., and Morris, H. H.: Invasive methods of somatosensory evoked potential monitoring. J. Clin. Neurophysiol. *3*:113–130, 1986.
15. Dinner, D. S., Lüders, H., Lesser, R. P., et al.: Intraoperative spinal somatosensory evoked potential monitoring. J. Neurosurg. *65*:807–814, 1986.
16. Epstein, N. E., Danto, J., and Nardi, D.: Evaluation of intraoperative somatosensory-evoked potential monitoring during 100 cervical operations. Spine *18*:737–747, 1993.
17. Erwin, C. W., and Erwin, A. C.: Up and down the spinal cord: Intraoperative monitoring of sensory and motor spinal cord pathways. J. Clin. Neurophysiol. *10*:425–436, 1993.
18. Fisher, R. S., Raudzens, P., and Nunemacher, M.: Efficacy of intraoperative neurophysiologic monitoring. J. Clin. Neurophysiol. *12*:97–109, 1995.
19. Follett, K. A.: Intraoperative electrophysiologic spinal cord monitoring. *In* Loftus, C. M., and Traynellis, V. C. (eds.): Intraoperative Monitoring Techniqes in Neurosurgery. New York, McGraw-Hill, 1994, pp. 321–238.
20. Ginsberg, H., Shetter, A., and Raudzens, P.: Postoperative paraplegia with preserved intraoperative somatosensory evoked potentials: Case report. J. Neurosurg. *63*:293–300, 1985.
21. Hahn, J., Lesser, R. P., Klem, G., and Lueders, H.: Simple technique for monitoring intraoperative spinal cord function. J. Neurosurg. *9*:692–695, 1981.
22. Hall, J. E., Levine, C. R., and Sudhir, K. G.: Intraoperative awakening to monitor spinal cord function during Harrington instrumentation and spine fusion. J. Bone Joint Surg. [Am.] *60*:533–536, 1978.
23. Herdmann, J., Deletis, V., Edmonds, H. L., and Morota, N.: Spine update: Spinal cord and nerve root monitoring in spine surgery and related procedures. Spine *7*:879–885, 1996.
24. Hess, C. W., Mills, K. R., and Murray, N. M. F.: Percutaneous stimulation of the human brain: A comparison of electrical and magnetic stimuli. (Abstract.) J. Physiol. *378*:35P, 1986.
25. Klem, G., Andrish, J., Gurd, A., et al.: Spinal cord potentials recorded from ligamentum interspinalis. Electroencephalogr. Clin. Neurophysiol. *50*:221, 1980.
26. Koyanagi, I., Iwasaki, Y., Isu, T., et al.: Spinal cord evoked potential monitoring after spinal cord stimulation during surgery of spinal cord tumors. Neurosurgery *33*:451–460, 1993.
27. Lesser, R., Raudzens, P., Luders, H., et al.: Postoperative neurological deficits may occur despite unchanged intraoperative somatosensory evoked potentials. Ann. Neurol. *19*:22–25, 1986.
28. Levy, W. J., Jr.: Clinical experience with motor and cerebellar evoked potential monitoring. Neurosurgery *20*:169–182, 1987.
29. Levy, W. J., Jr., and York, D. H.: Evoked potentials from the motor tract in humans. Neurosurgery *12*:422–429, 1983.
30. Lueders, H., Gurd, A., Hahn, J., et al.: A new technique for intraoperative monitoring of spinal cord function. Spine *7*:110–115, 1982.

31. MacEwen, G. D., Bunnell, W. P., and Sriram, K.: Acute neurological complications in the treatment of scoliosis. J. Bone Joint Surg. [Am.] 57:404–408, 1975.

32. Machida, M., Weinstein, S. L., Yamada, T., and Kimura, J.: Spinal cord monitoring—electrophysiological measures of sensory and motor function during spinal surgery. Spine 10:407–413, 1985.

33. Merton, P. A., and Morton, H. B.: Stimulation of the cerebral cortex in the intact human brain. Nature 285:277, 1980.

34. Nuwer, M. R., Dawson, E. G., Carlson, L. G., et al.: Somatosensory evoked potential spinal cord monitoring reduces neurologic deficits after scoliosis surgery: Results of a large multicenter survey. Electroencephalogr. Clin. Neurophysiol. 96:6–11, 1995.

35. Owen, J. H., Laschinger, J., Bridwell, K., et al.: Sensitivity and specificity of somatosensory and neurogenic motor evoked potentials in animals and humans. Spine 13:1111–1118, 1988.

36. Owen, J. H., Sponseller, P. D., Szymanski, J., and Hurdle, M.: Efficacy of multimodality spinal cord monitoring during surgery for neuromuscular scoliosis. Spine 20:1480–1488, 1995.

37. Patton, H. D., and Amassian, V. E.: Single and multiple unit analysis of cortical stage of pyramidal tract stimulation. J. Neurophysiol. 17:345–357, 1954.

38. Perlik, S. J., VanEgeren, R., and Fisher, M. A.: Somatosensory evoked potential surgical monitoring: Observations during combined isoflurane–nitrous oxide anesthesia. Spine 17:273–276, 1992.

39. Rossini, P. M., Gigli, G. L., Marciani, M. G., et al.: Non-invasive evaluation of input-output characteristics of sensorimotor cerebral areas in healthy humans. Electroencephalogr. Clin. Neurophysiol. 68:88–100, 1987.

40. Rothwell, J. C.: Physiological studies of electric and magnetic stimulation of the human brain. In Levy, W. J., Gracco, R. Q., Barker, A. T., and Rothwell, J. (eds.): Magnetic Motor Stimulation: Basic Principles and Clinical Experience (EEG Suppl. 43). New York, Elsevier, 1991, pp. 29–35.

41. Takaki, O., and Okumura, F.: Application and limitation of somatosensory evoked potential monitoring during thoracic aortic aneurysm surgery: A case report. Anesthesiology 63:700–703, 1985.

42. Tamaki, T., Tsuji, H., Inoue, S., and Kobayashi, H.: The prevention of iatrogenic spinal cord injury utilizing the evoked spinal cord potential. Int. Orthop. 4:313–317, 1981.

43. Tsuyama, N., Tsuzuki, N., Kurokawa, T., and Imai, T.: Clinical application of spinal cord action potential movement. Int. Orthop. 2:39–46, 1978.

44. York, D. H., Chabot, R. J., and Gaines, R. W.: Response variability of somatosensory evoked potentials during scoliosis surgery. Spine 12:864–876, 1987.

45. Zentner, J.: Noninvasive motor evoked potential monitoring during neurosurgical operations on the spinal cord. Neurosurgery. 24:709–712, 1989.

Complications

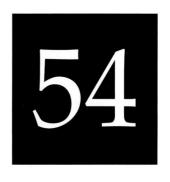

Complications of Spinal Surgery

Postoperative Infections of the Spine

John G. Heller, M.D.

Marc J. Levine, M.D.

Prior to the work of Joseph Lister (1827–1912), surgery existed in an era of "laudable pus." Many surgeons of that period believed that the formation of pus was part of the natural healing process. Before Lister, the term "hospitalism" was synonymous with the postoperative infections so commonly seen in surgical patients. The development of "listerism," or antiseptic surgery, was most profoundly based on Lister's ability to embrace the work of Louis Pasteur, who had shown a germ theory for disease. In 1867 Lister published his paper "On the Antiseptic Principle in the Practice of Surgery." Acceptance of Lister's work was not immediate, because many of his methods were considered time-consuming and expensive. However, with proponents such as William S. Halsted, Lister's principles slowly gained acceptance. In the years following Lister's initial work, the incidence of postoperative infections dropped dramatically.[33]

The inherent nature of microorganisms to rapidly mutate ensures a constant struggle against the emergence of resistant strains. By their very nature, surgical procedures violate some of the body's primary defense mechanisms against infection. Therefore, the most expertly conceived and executed surgical procedure can be ruined by an infection. In elective procedures, the surgeon must look past the radiographs and evaluate the entire patient to determine the risk of infection and whether this, as well as other risk, is justified. With respect to infection in the perioperative period, there are three basic tenets: *minimize, recognize, and treat.* This section helps to identify preoperative risk factors inher-

ent to the surgical procedure and patient. In addition, emphasis is placed on surgical prophylaxis, infection diagnosis, and treatment options.

INCIDENCE

Technical advances in orthopedic surgery continue to challenge the limits of antimicrobial therapy. Specifically, patients undergoing a spinal fusion represent a subset of individuals at an increased risk for developing an infection.[45, 54, 71, 91, 96, 131, 135, 158, 179] Because of the multitude of procedures performed on a diverse patient population for varying pathologies, the incidence of infection cannot be generalized.

Conventional lumbar discectomies in conjunction with prophylactic antibiotics continue to have a low incidence of infection. Most large series report an overall rate of less than 1 per cent.[45, 54, 71, 91, 96, 131, 135, 158, 179] Some authors report a higher rate of infection with microdiscectomies.[91, 158] Although the controversy regarding the efficacy of percutaneous lumbar discectomies continues, initial reports suggest a slightly lower rate of infection. Bonaldi and colleagues,[17] in a review of 237 patients, reported one infection; Schafer and Kambin's[147] report of 100 patients was without infection. These somewhat encouraging rates of infection should be kept in perspective. Conventional lumbar discectomies have an infection rate that reflects hundreds of thousands of surgical procedures, compared with the relatively small number of posterolateral percutaneous lumbar discectomies performed and reported.

Intuitively, the incidence of postoperative infections should increase with the addition of fusions and instrumentation. In fact, this has been borne out in the literature. Fusion procedures with or without instrumentation involve more extensive soft tissue dissection, longer operative times, greater blood loss, greater dead space, and increased soft tissue damage from poor vascularity. Each of these factors adds to the risk of infection. Wright showed an increase in infection rate from 3 to 8 per cent when a fusion was added to a discectomy.[179] Similarly, Horwitz and Curtin saw a 6 per cent incidence of infection in patients who underwent a discectomy and fusion, compared with a 1 per cent rate for discectomies alone.[71]

The introduction of metal implants into a wound may further increase the risk of infection. The incrementally higher infection risk of an extended surgical procedure is independent of the implant. The implants themselves may be a source of inoculation on rare occasions. Their principal contribution to infection risk is by acting as a *locus minoris resistentiae*. The increased rate of infection with the use of spinal instrumentation is well supported in the literature but varies by patient and disease.[3, 24, 48, 59, 62, 77, 83, 85, 93, 100, 108, 114, 144, 160, 162, 164, 176] Overall, most surgeons agree that the risk of infection following a conventional lumbar discectomy is less than or equal to 1 per cent which increases to roughly 2 per cent with the addition of a fusion. When instrumentation is used, the rate has been reported as high as 5 or 6 per cent.

Although most spine infection studies focus on complications of thoracic and lumbar surgery, one should not forget the risks associated with cervical spine surgery. Reported rates have generally been less but range from 0.1 and 0.3 per cent to as high 3 per cent.[13, 112, 163] Most studies state an incidence between 1 and 2 per cent.[163] Bertalanffy and Eggert reported a wound infection rate of 1.6 per cent in 450 consecutively performed anterior discectomies without fusion.[13]

PREVENTION

The probability of a successful outcome after surgical intervention is largely dependent on the surgeon's ability to choose the correct surgical procedure for a patient with the appropriate indications. Pre-existing morbidities and risk factors should be recognized and addressed during patient selection and preoperative planning. As in all surgical procedures, the potential benefits of surgery need to outweigh the potential risks of the surgery. It is the responsibility of the physician to present these patient-specific issues to surgical candidates.

Diabetes, particularly when poorly controlled, is well recognized as a predisposing condition. Roughly 3 to 4 per cent of the population suffers from diabetes, and about 50 per cent of these individuals will undergo a surgical procedure during their lifetime.[7, 63] It is estimated that 17 per cent of this population will have

some type of postoperative complication, two thirds of which will be of an infectious nature.[57] The comorbid conditions associated with diabetes, such as cardiovascular disease, hypertension, and renal disease, are of greater consequence than simply the presentation of well-controlled diabetes.[88] In general, patients with diabetes have been shown to have inferior results following lumbar spine surgery and a higher incidence of infections.[155]

The emergent nature of some spinal procedures often prevents the surgeon from properly addressing the various risk factors. However, in a nonemergent setting, risks such as nicotine usage and malnutrition, including both obesity and cachexia, should be recognized. The increased risk of infection in malnourished patients has been shown using a number of different indices.[73, 92, 103, 156] In one review of 19 spine infections, all but three were in malnourished patients with total lymphocyte counts of less than 2000.[156] In another study, Jensen and coworkers observed that 27 of 31 patients with postoperative infections were malnourished.[73] They suggested a number of criteria to screen patients preoperatively and incorporated them into an algorithm. A history of recent weight loss greater than 10 pounds, serum albumin less than 3.4 g/dL, total lymphocyte count less than 1500 cells/mL, skin test anergy, or arm muscle circumference less than 80 per cent of normal should lead to a consultation for nutritional repletion. Other criteria that can be useful to gauge a patient's nutritional status include transferrin levels, creatinine height indices, height to weight ratios, and skin fold thickness.[73, 181] The catabolic state of a patient postoperatively may be compounded in traumatic settings. Therefore, careful attention should be paid to the postoperative nutritional needs of a patient.

Obesity, which is recognized as the most common form of malnutrition in the United States, has also been shown to be a risk factor.[76] A number of different mechanisms may account for the increased rate of infection in obese patients. The poor vascularity and relatively decreased immune defenses of excess adipose tissue represent an excellent culture media for bacteria, particularly in the face of fat necrosis. Technically more challenging, surgery in an obese patient often requires more lengthy surgical times, possibly adding to the increased risk of infection in this group of individuals. If possible (though often not realistic), obese patients should be directed to proper medical personnel to undergo a supervised weight loss program.

The adverse effects of nicotine usage on the outcome of spinal fusions have been well documented in the literature.[153] The increased rate of postoperative infections expected among nicotine users has been shown with statistical significance.[76] Many surgeons find it prudent to recommend elimination of nicotine use prior to elective procedures and to check for patient compliance with a urinalysis.

A thorough evaluation of a patient's past medical history may reveal concomitant conditions that increase the risk of postoperative infection. Although these conditions cannot be reversed or eliminated before surgery, it is imperative to appreciate their presence, properly counsel patients preoperatively, and anticipate potential problems postoperatively. Both rheumatoid arthritis and chronic steroid therapy have been cited as risk factors.[27, 67] Attention to soft tissue management intraoperatively and postoperatively can decrease the incidence of infection. Acute steroid usage may be indicated in patients with neurologic deficits. When steroids are used, gastrointestinal prophylaxis is helpful. A history of previous infection or coexisting infection, as well as neoplasm, has been implicated in an increased infection rate.[156] In one study, a previous spine infection was associated with a 22 per cent risk of postoperative spine infection.[83] An attempt should be made to eradicate remote infections when possible, such as urinary tract infections or colonization, dysvascular or pressure ulcers, pneumonia, and so forth. A number of different disease entities, such as AIDS, as well as chemotherapeutic agents may lead to immunosuppression. When possible, surgery should be delayed until host defenses can be maximized.

Factors suspected of increasing infection risk, but not proved, include radiation therapy, adrenocortical insufficiency, and a pre-existing neoplasm.[132] In a review of 100 consecutive spinal tumor cases that included both anterior and posterior operative approaches and various stabilization techniques, the reported infection rate was 4 per cent. This rate is comparable to that reported for spinal fusions with instrumentation in nontumorous cases.[84] It is advisable to wait two to three weeks following surgery to begin radiation therapy, because of poor wound healing. If radiation therapy is performed initially, a waiting period of 6 to 12 weeks is preferred before elective incision into previously irradiated tissue. The increased risk of wound infection and dehiscence should be discussed with both the patient and the family preoperatively. In particularly high-risk patients, primary flap closure of the wound should be considered at the time of surgery or shortly thereafter as an intended second stage.

SURGICAL PLANNING AND EXECUTION

The length of preoperative hospitalization increases the rate of wound infection.[35, 117, 122, 132, 133] Cruse and Foord reported an infection rate of 1.1 per cent for those admitted within one day of surgery.[35] The rate doubled for each additional week.[35] It is likely that hospital flora adversely affect postoperative infection rates. Within two weeks of admission to an intensive care unit, patients are colonized with hospital pathogens.[124] Exposure to antibiotics may complicate matters further by promoting the emergence of resistant strains. Archer and Tanenbaum found that 54 per cent of postoperative cardiac surgery patients grew methicillin-resistant *Staphylococcus epidermidis* from their skin, whereas only 4 per cent of these patients grew such resistant strains preoperatively.[6]

If a surgical procedure can be done electively, the surgeon should consider discharging the patient for a period of time to allow normal skin flora to be reestablished. Often, however, this is not possible. Therefore, hospital epidemiology data, as well as a list of the antibiotics previously employed, should guide the choice of an appropriate prophylactic regimen.

With each surgical procedure comes a number of decisions that need to be made in the operative and perioperative periods. Each of these decisions can have a different impact on the risk of infection. As mentioned previously, the addition of instrumentation to a fusion has been shown to increase the rate of infection. In a review of 163 uninstrumented and 127 instrumented posterior spinal fusions for congenital scoliosis in patients between the ages of 5 and 19, Winter and associates found no infections in the uninstrumented group but reported four wound infections in the instrumented group.[177] These orthopedists also suggested an increased risk for infection in scoliosis surgery performed on patients older than 20 years of age.[100] Reconstructive scoliosis surgery in patients with myelodysplastic deformities represents a subset of surgeries at an even greater risk for infection, presumably owing to hygienic issues and/or colonized urinary tracts.[9, 100, 165]

The decision of whether to approach the spine anteriorly or perform combined anterior and posterior procedures in a single or staged fashion can affect the risk of infection. As thoracoscopic techniques develop, their use may one day be based on improved infection rates when compared with conventional open procedures. In preparation for an anterior-posterior spinal reconstruction that is performed in either one or two stages, a heightened awareness of the nutritional needs of the patient may help minimize the incidence of postoperative infections. The incidence of malnutrition in either of these two groups has been shown to be high and is associated with an increased rate of infection postoperatively. In one review of 11 staged and 13 combined anterior-posterior procedures, the malnutrition rate was over 50 per cent in both groups.[40]

Surgical adjuncts, including hemostatic agents, methyl methacrylate, and bone substitutes, may each have an effect on the incidence of spine infections. Methyl methacrylate has been shown to have a negative effect on the function of polymorphonuclear leukocytes.[129, 130] Its use in salvage and oncologic procedures in patients with less than one year of life expectancy is still advocated.[107] Interestingly, one literature review of anterior reconstructions using methyl methacrylate was without a reported infection.[12, 107] The goals of surgery in the terminally ill differ from those in patients with a normal life expectancy. Use of materials such as methyl methacrylate can be helpful in filling defects from tumor débridement but do not provide a substance that will incorporate into the host bone. However, the rapid fixation and stability that it provides with an apparently low infection rate make it a valuable resource in this population. Postoperatively, decisions of when to begin radiation therapy can be made independent of concerns about bone grafts.

Spine reconstruction can be among the most challenging of orthopedic surgical procedures. A surgeon must recognize his or her areas of expertise to avoid unwarranted and lengthy operative times. Although not statistically shown, some have suggested that surgical times greater than five hours may increase the risk of postoperative infection.[76, 117, 127, 157]

INTRAOPERATIVE PREVENTION

The host's ability to resist infection is influenced by the intraoperative techniques and decisions of the surgeon. Reduction of this incidence of infection can be accomplished many ways intraoperatively. Establishment of a wound infection is a function of three variables: the inoculum, the surgical wound, and the use of prophylactic antibiotics. The surgeon, who is responsible for coordinating care from the preoperative through the postoperative period, can have a profound influence on each of these factors.

Inoculum

The surgeon, in conjunction with other operating room personnel, can drastically decrease the bacterial exposure risk to surgical patients. Inocula generally arise from either the patient or the operative team and not necessarily from the operative suite. As demonstrated by Ritter, there are an average of 13 colony-forming units per cubic foot per hour in an empty operating suite. The presence of five surgical personnel increases this number to 447 colony-forming units per cubic foot per hour.[140] The potential benefit of minimizing traffic in the operating room is obvious. To further illustrate the benefit of restricting surgical suite access to the surgical team, consider that under normal circumstances, people shed slightly less than 1000 bacteria per minute into the environment. But there is a subset of individuals who shed more than 1000 bacteria per minute.[14, 100]

Operating room personnel should be properly gowned and gloved.[33, 64, 90, 111, 133] New shoe covers should be considered for each case.[33, 133] Proper scrubbing technique with commercially available antibacterial solutions must be performed before each case.[33, 35, 133] Many suggest that two pairs of gloves be worn in orthopedic cases for the protection of both patient and surgeon owing to a high rate of glove penetration.[33, 87, 121, 133] It is also advisable to change the outer pair of gloves during lengthy procedures and those involving metallic implants. Messengers may best serve patient care by calling into the room, as opposed to entering it.

Filtered air should be exchanged at a rate of 25 times per hour.[33, 122, 133] The value of laminar air flow systems has perhaps been best described in the total joint arthroplasty literature but may play a role in spine surgery, particularly in high-risk patients. It is generally prudent to avoid scheduling a clean procedure to follow an infected procedure.

Hair removal and antiseptic cleansing may be performed in the holding area to avoid contaminating the operative suite. Hair clipping just before surgery tends to impose less risk than shaving the night before surgery.[33, 35, 122, 133] The need for hair removal is somewhat controversial. Cruse and Foord found that unshaved patients had a 0.9 per cent infection rate, whereas those who were shaved had a 2.3 per cent infection rate.[35] The use of a depilatory was associated with the lowest rate of infection, 0.6 per cent.

The preparation of the patient's skin is a critical factor in reducing local bacterial exposure. When possible, the skin should be bathed with antiseptic soap on the night before surgery.[33, 122, 133] This process may be repeated on the morning of surgery. In the operating room, a large and generous field should be prepped. It is far better to prepare a larger area than needed than to violate an unprepared surface area after a surgical case has begun. Tincture of dichlorhexidine, iodophor, or tincture of iodine is recommended for preparing the operative site. Plain soaps, alcohol, or hexachlorophene is not to be used as a single agent but may be used preceding the aforementioned products as a matter of surgeon preference.[33, 133] Attention to patient allergies may dictate the choice of agent.

Draping of the proposed surgical site should be generous so as not to preclude any surgical options. Because patient-shed bacteria can penetrate cotton fabrics, especially when wet,[14] the use of barrier drapes made of water-resistant synthetic fibers is recommended.[122] The advantages of iodophor-impregnated adherent films are supported in the literature.[74]

Surgical Wound

All surgical wounds create a potential environment for bacterial colonization. Negligent soft tissue handling can promote tissue necrosis, which favors bacterial growth. Attention to the time-honored teachings of Halsted may reduce the postoperative risk of infection. Tissues should be handled gently to minimize necrosis. Necrotic and devitalized tissue should be débrided prior to closure. The use of excess cautery and ligature to achieve hemostasis needs to be weighed against the potential increase risk of infection that each carries. Intermittent release of retractors should not be neglected, particularly in long cases. Prolonged tissue retraction, because of increased pressure, leads to tissue ischemia, which may promote infection.[176]

The presence of a hematoma increases the risk of infection by undermining local defense mechanisms.[89] Accordingly, all appropriate measures should be taken to avoid hematoma formation. Ligatures and electrocoagulation are mainstays in this effort, but they leave foreign material and necrotic tissue within the wound. Other hemostatic products are available for local application. The choice of which agent to use, when to use it, and whether or not it should be left within the wound should be based on an understanding of how these materials affect bleeding, wound infection rates, scar formation, and bone healing.[5] Hematoma formation is further reduced by proper wound closure. Layered closure and obliteration of dead space are helpful.

An obese patient is particularly prone to trouble in this regard. Consideration should be given to the use of retention sutures tied over rubber bolsters, as in abdominal closure in the morbidly obese.

Meticulous sterile draping of equipment and wound coverage during imaging followed by irrigation can help prevent bacterial seeding of surgical sites. Care must be taken to maintain the sterile field during the procedure. Use of image intensification is a common occasion for breaks in sterile technique, but it is often desirable in spinal surgery.

Antibiotics

The use of perioperative antibiotics has had the most significant impact on decreasing the rate of postoperative spine infections.[178] Several large retrospective studies have shown a decreased incidence of postoperative infections with the use of preoperative antibiotics. Lonstein and colleagues reported an overall decrease in infections from 4.4 to 1.2 per cent in a series of patients comprised mostly of posterior instrumentations and fusions.[100] The most dramatic impact was seen in patients with idiopathic scoliosis, where the infection rate dropped to 0.1 per cent. Another large series reviewed over 500 lumbar disc surgeries and found a decrease in the infection rate from 9.3 to 1.0 per cent with the institution of antibiotic prophylaxis. Further analysis of the treated group revealed a rate of 0.6 per cent if the drugs were administered preoperatively, versus 2.7 per cent if they were not administered until after surgery.[71] More recently, Rubinstein and associates showed with a randomized double-blinded study the efficacy of preoperative cefazolin administration in reducing infection. Of 141 patients, those who received cefazolin preoperatively had an infection rate of 4.3 per cent, and those who received a placebo had a rate of 12.7 per cent.[146]

As pointed out by Rimoldi and Haye, the rationale for the use of prophylactic antibiotics is to prevent a naturally occurring organism from infecting a sterile surgical site.[139] Therapeutic doses of antibiotics should be circulating prior to the incision, as supported by the work of Horwitz and Curtin.[71] A first-generation cephalosporin should be administered 30 to 60 minutes before the incision is made for prophylaxis of clean lumbar procedures. Additional dosing is required for longer procedures and for those with significant blood loss.[4] Postoperatively, parenteral prophylactic antibiotics should be continued for 24 hours. Old traditions die hard. The axiom of "continuing the antibiotics until the drains come out" lives on but is scientifically unsubstantiated. It is still uncertain whether postoperative antibiotics provide a significant benefit. Administration for periods longer than 48 hours may be harmful. Longer regimens adversely influence not only the rates of infection but also the virulence of the organisms by selecting out resistant strains.[119] Rubinstein and associates demonstrated that postoperative infections in patients who had received proper antibiotic prophylaxis were of a more resistant nature than those postoperative infections in patients who had received placebo.[146]

Produced by the fungus *Cephalosporium acreminium*, cephalosporins were first discovered in 1945.[139] Cephalosporins are bactericidal by a mechanism that inhibits bacterial cell wall synthesis. They are metabolized by the kidneys via active tubular secretion and glomerular filtration. First-generation cephalosporins are most effective against gram-positive organisms such as *Staphylococcus* sp., with limited action on gram-negative organisms. Second- and third-generation cephalosporins generally have greater action against gram-negative organisms but decreased effectiveness against *Staphylococcus* sp. As most commonly isolated postoperative infections are gram-positive *Staphylococcus* sp., first-generation cephalosporins have gained wide acceptance as the prophylactic antibiotic of choice for elective spine procedures. Certain groups of individuals such as intravenous drug abusers, the immunocompromised, and those with sickle cell anemia require further attention to gram-negative organisms and warrant the addition of an aminoglycoside for adequate coverage. The same can be said for those likely to be colonized with hospital flora.

All cephalosporins reach therapeutic tissue levels in humans in both bone and tissue. It is prudent to remember, however, that first-generation cephalosporins are unable to cross the blood-brain barrier and therefore are unable to protect against potential cerebrospinal fluid infections. First-generation cephalosporins appear to achieve greater concentrations in muscle, bone, and hematoma when compared with second- and third-generation cephalosporins.[76] Of the first-generation cephalosporins, cefazolin has been shown to have the greatest peak serum level (188 uC/mL) and the longest half-life (1.9 hours).[136]

Penetration of antibiotics into disc spaces may vary with patient age.[139] The disc space is believed to be largely avascular after the age of 20. Penetration into the disc space occurs by passive diffusion through the vertebral end plates and annulus fibrosus. As discs degenerate, their vascularity increases, allowing a second route of access for circulating antibiotics. Currier and colleagues' work suggested that agents differ in their ability to reach the nucleus pulposus.[36] In a rabbit model, clindamyin and tobramycin were shown to to reach the disc space in the greatest concentrations. Overall, cefazolin has been shown to be a cost-effective perioperative prophylactic antibiotic in patients without allergies. Each patient's treatment must be individualized, as coexisting morbidities may alter the selection of antibiotic. In addition, a surgeon must be aware of the microbial environment in which he or she works and consider the risk from resistant organisms. In the future, the evolution of resistant strains of bacteria may change the currently accepted dogma regarding prophylactic antibiotics.

Antibiotic prophylaxis is not limited to IV administration. Antibiotic-impregnated methyl methacrylate and antibiotic irrigants are adjuncts employed by some surgeons. Topical irrigants should meet a number of criteria: efficacy against commonly found organisms, low tissue toxicity, low systemic absorption, and cost-effectiveness. A number of studies in both the orthopedic and nonorthopedic literature have shown the benefits of topical antibiotic irrigants.[41, 143] In vitro studies by Scherr and Dodd suggested that a mixture of neomycin, 5 per cent solution; bacitracin, 25,000 units/L; and polymixin, 25 mg/L, was sufficient to eradicate 19 commonly found strains of gram-negative and gram-positive orthopedically relevant pathogens.[148] Whether this applies to spinal wounds is a matter of conjecture. One must also consider whether the topical solution may be used when employing intraoperative red blood cell salvage techniques.

DIAGNOSIS AND TREATMENT

A certain incidence of infection is inevitable, despite the best efforts of the patient and the surgeon. Treatment of postoperative infections begins with their recognition. The clinical presentation varies considerably with the site of infection and possibly with the organisms involved.

Wound Infections

Wound infections in spinal surgery are relatively infrequent but may be a formidable problem. Gepstein and Eismont,[58] among others,[84, 93, 108, 159, 176] carefully distinguish between superficial and deep infections. Infections confined to the dermis and subcutaneous tissue are defined as superficial. Those occurring beneath the lumbodorsal fascia are deep. This dichotomy can be useful in distinguishing modes of presentation; however, it does not always hold true clinically. Many patients have infection in both planes at once.

The superficial infection is generally evident to inspection.[38] Erythema, swelling, and fluctuance accompany the patient's complaints of pain and tenderness. Fevers are usually low grade but may be quite high. Leukocytosis is mild, if present. The erythrocyte sedimentation rate (ESR) is elevated. Drainage may occur spontaneously. Gram's stain and culture of the drainage or an aspirate confirm the diagnosis. Treatment should not await culture results. Keep in mind that the presence of a superficial infection does not preclude the likelihood of a deep infection. They often coexist.

The typical deep infection may prove difficult to diagnose. Keller and Pappas noted that the average interval from surgery to diagnosis was 11 days (range, 7 to 16 days).[77] As in patients with postoperative discitis, the wound may appear deceptively normal.[58, 77] Patients may complain of more pain than would be anticipated at a given time postoperatively. They may seem less energetic than expected and tend to have a sense of ill-being. Temperature, white blood cell count (WBC), and ESR are generally higher than with superficial infection. Although somewhat unusual, we have treated one adult patient with a fever of 105°F, disorientation, and shock owing to a polymicrobial infection.

Diagnostic modalities such as WBC, ESR, C-reactive protein (CRP), and imaging techniques may be used to help supplement the clinical diagnosis of a postoperative wound infection. A normal WBC does not exclude the diagnosis. In one review of 19 wound infections, the average WBC was 9.1.[156] The usefulness of the ESR requires an appreciation of the normal rise of this value following spine procedures. Jonsson and colleagues measured the ESR and WBC in 110 patients who underwent lumbar spine surgery.[75] The peak ESR was reported on day four for spinal fusions, with a mean value of 102; the mean value for disc surgery on this day was 75. A steady decline of ESR values occurred, with normalization about two weeks after surgery. The usefulness of this test during the initial postoperative period is uncertain. However, comparison of repeated ESRs may be helpful in suggesting improvement or progression of a possible infection. Unlike ESR values, CRP levels decrease rapidly in the postoperative period. Thelander and Larsson prospectively measured CRP and ESR following four types of surgery: lumbar microdiscetomy, conventional lumbar discectomy, anterior lumbar fusion, and posterolateral interbody fusion.[166] Peak ESR values were found up to five days after surgery. A gradual resumption to normal levels then required 21 to 42 days. Alternatively, peak CRP levels were found within three days of surgery. This was followed by a dramatic decrease and normalization of values within 10 to 14 days. This differential rate of normalization implies that CRP levels may be more informative diagnostically than ESRs in the immediate postoperative period.

Diagnostic imaging modalities are of limited value in the immediate postoperative period. This is especially true if metallic implants have been employed, because of their inherent imaging artifact. Although titanium devices produce less artifact, they can still obscure the necessary information in a study. In the absence of such artifact, magnetic resonance imaging (MRI) remains the modality of choice for evaluating postoperative spine infections. When performed with and without gadolinium-DTPA, MRI is highly sensitive and specific for most postoperative infections, including intervertebral discitis, osteomyelitis, and epidural abscesses. Typical MRI changes associated with osteomyelitis, as outlined by Djukic and associates, include (1) confluent areas of hypointensity of involved vertebral bodies and disc spaces on T1-weighted images, (2) hyperintensity of involved bone and disc on T2-weighted images, (3) loss of distinction of adjacently involved vertebral bodies and discs, and (4) abnormal disc appearance (Fig. 54–1).[42] Some infectious processes yield isointense signals that cannot be distinguished from normal epidural or paraspinal tissues. In such cases, the diagnostic yield is increased with the post-gadolinium sequences, because vascularized inflammatory tissue enhances on T1-weighted images after gadolinium-DTPA.[42]

Computerized axial tomography–guided needle biopsies may be used to obtain deep cultures. However, the value of dry aspirations or negative Gram's stains and cultures should be viewed with skepticism. Pres-

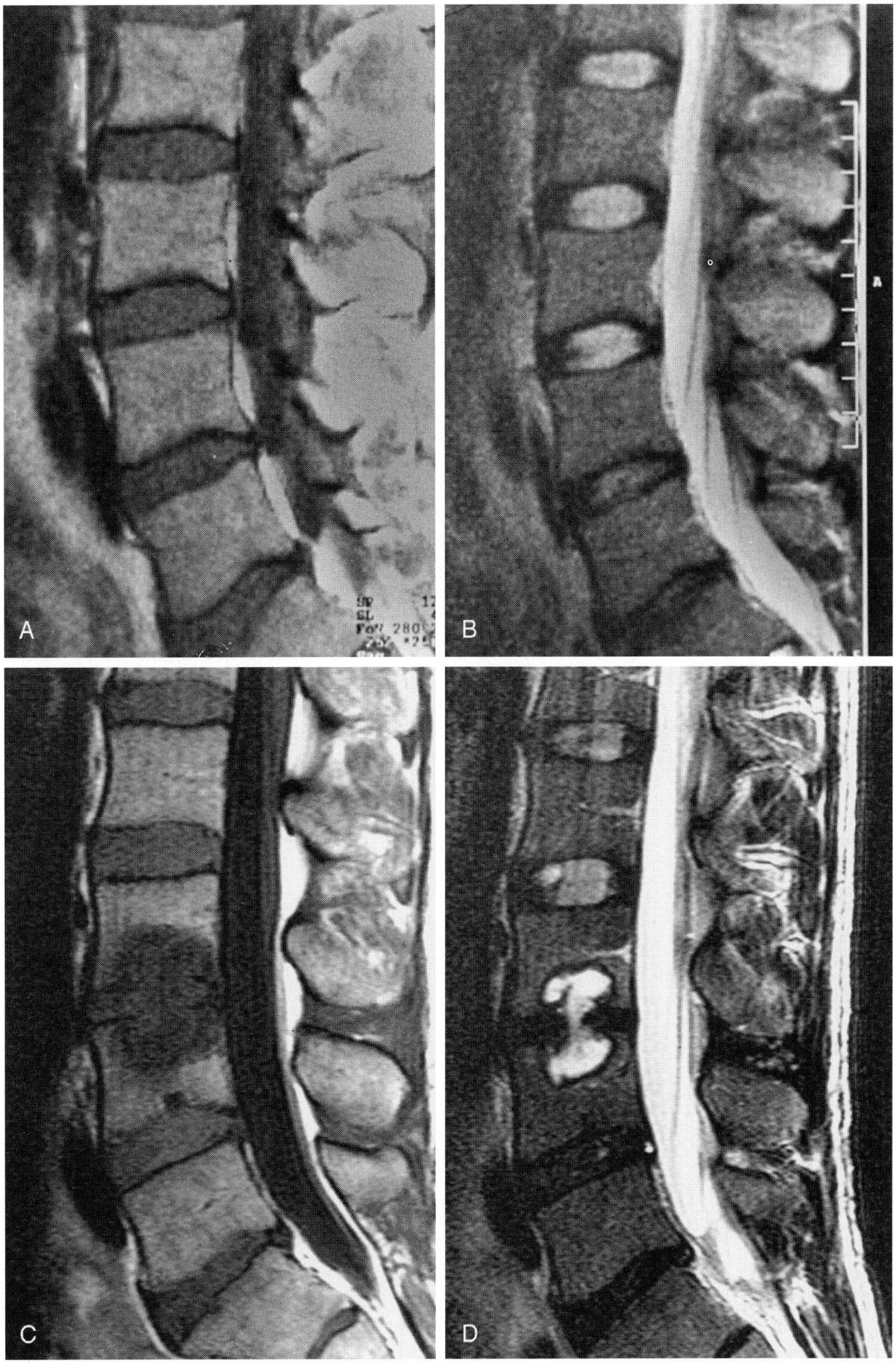

Figure 54–1. In an attempt to diagnose and treat a patient with refractory debilitating low back pain, a discogram was ordered. The levels injected included the two that appeared abnormal by MRI (L4–L5 and L5–S1), as well as a "control" level (L3–L4). Shown are the T1- and (A) T2-weighted (B) images prior to the discogram. The diminshed signal intensity within the discs, height loss, and posterior annular protrusion are readily appreciable at L4–L5 and L5–S1. The patient complained of increasing, relentless pain in the days following the discogram. These symptoms were accompanied by low-grade fevers and diaphoresis. A follow-up MRI clearly demonstrates an intervertebral discitis at the L3–L4 level. Note the loss of disc space defintition and peridiscal hypointensity on the T1 image (C), as well as the hyperintense signal on the T2 images (D). The latter also demonstrates the degree of intraosseous extension of the process.

ently there is no clear substitute for exploring a wound suspected of infection. Newer techniques, including diagnosis with the use of molecular genetics (i. e., polymerase chain reaction assays), are currently being used in total joint arthroplasty and may play a role in the detection of infection in spine surgery.[94, 104] The most commonly found pathogens are *Staphylococcus aureus* and *S. epidermidis*.[107]

The diagnosis of postoperative wound infection, superficial or deep, requires aggressive management.[100] Both superficial and deep wound infections require immediate attention and may be equally ominous. Measures such as local débridement, removal of sutures, and administration of antibiotics are generally insufficient. Such a casual strategy should be abandoned in favor of surgical intervention. On the basis of extensive clinical experience, Lonstein and coworkers believe that "treatment by antibiotics alone, the removal of a few sutures . . . or other similar halfhearted measures are mentioned only to be strongly condemned."[100]

A surgical approach to the wound reverses the manner in which it was closed and is performed in a stepwise approach. The dermal margins are excised, with tissue submitted for culture. If the process is superficial, a cavity of purulent material will be encountered in the subcutaneous plane. Fluid samples are cultured, as well as pieces of tissue débrided from the cavity walls. Before opening the fascial layer, the dermis and subcutaneous layers are thoroughly débrided to viable tissue, then irrigated generously with a pulse-lavage device. This layer should be surgically "clean" before proceeding. The fascia is opened so that the depth of the wound can be explored. Samples of the deep tissue and fluid are sent for culture. Only in this way can the presence of a deep infection be confirmed or refuted. Radical débridement of all devitalized soft tissues is mandatory. If either a fat graft or Gelfoam has been left over the exposed dura, it is carefully removed and cultured separately. Only those pieces of bone graft that are loosened in the lavage process or that appear engulfed in purulent material should be removed.[56, 58, 100, 114] Bone graft rarely if ever has to be removed, particularly during the first incision and drainage procedure. As before, this layer is thoroughly irrigated. The débridement is not complete until all areas of the wound appear healthy and viable. In the face of a pseudarthrosis, eradication of infection should precede further reinstrumentation and fusion repair. In late wound infections, instrumentation may be removed to better evaluate fusion masses.

Primary closure of wounds is favored.[39, 56] Open packing of wounds and delayed primary closures should be avoided whenever possible. This reduces protein losses and the risk of superinfection. Surgical closure of a débrided wound is done in layers as closed suction drains are placed within each layer. Irrigation-suction systems with initially high flow rates are advocated by some for the first three to four days in the face of apparently aggressive infections.[165] However, the benefit of these more labor-intensive systems is controversial.[67] Drains are generally removed after three to five days. Sequential re-exploration and débridement may be required every 48 hours in patients not responding clinically or if the drain effluent continues to grow organisms. The authors generally prefer a routine second-look procedure on the second postoperative day to culture, débride, and irrigate the wound again. The route of administration and duration of antibiotics must be individualized for each patient. Infections that involve vertebral bone and/or bone grafts and implants should be treated as presumptive osteomyelitis. Those infections involving only soft tissues may require shorter courses of treatment. Consultation with an infectious disease specialist is encouraged.

Soft tissue coverage may be a problem in the multiply operated or irradiated spine, both of which are at increased risk for postoperative infection. The utility of muscle flaps has been well described.[81] Musculocutaneous flaps provide important vascularized tissue to help facilitate healing and eliminate bacteria. The superiority of musculocutaneous flaps as compared with random and fasciocutaneous flaps is well documented in the literature.[24, 47] Commonly used muscle for upper, middle, and lower spine flaps include the trapezius, latissimus dorsi, and gluteus maximus.[145] An interdisciplinary approach with a plastic surgeon may help eliminate or prevent postoperative spine infections.

An obese patient not only poses an increased risk of infection but also makes wound closure difficult in the presence of infection. With débridement of all necrotic fat, the surgeon is usually confronted with a large volume of dead space that cannot be approximated by ordinary suture techniques. In this circumstance, a lesson can be borrowed from general surgery. Large retention sutures (No. 2 nylon) tied over rubber bolsters will adequately obliterate dead space and reinforce a conventional closure. Layered closed-suction drainage remains essential. Alternatively, if this method fails or appears unworkable, the surgeon should perform a tight fascial closure over drains with interrupted, nonabsorbable monofilament suture. The subcutaneous layer is then packed open. When adequate wound granulation has occurred and the wound appears clean, delayed primary closure is performed. This technique has been shown to reduce rates of abdominal wound infection in the obese.[172]

The status of metallic implants should be determined at the time of débridement. Although foreign bodies generally represent a *locus minoris resistentiae* for infection, their function in providing stability is clinically important. If well anchored, implants should be left in place.[28, 48, 58, 77, 93, 100, 114] Occasionally, drainage will persist until these devices are removed.[48, 108] However, if one can temporize until the fusion has consolidated, it will be to the advantage of patient and surgeon alike.

The effect of wound infections on pseudarthrosis rates is noteworthy. In a series of over 700 patients, Lonstein noted a pseudarthrosis rate of 11.5 per cent. Among the 64 patients with wound infections, the pseudarthrosis rate was 29.7 per cent.[97, 98, 100] Tamborino and colleagues similarly noted pseudarthrosis rates of 9 per cent without infection and 29 per cent in patients with infection.[162] Keller and Pappas felt that these data strengthened the argument to leave implants in place.[77] These statistics should alert the surgeon to carefully rule out pseudarthroses following wound infection. Their management is simplified if undertaken prior to implant failure. The choice of posterior or anterior technique must be individualized (Fig. 54–2). Occasionally, appropriate management requires a combination of anterior and posterior procedures (Fig. 54–3).

Postoperative Discitis

Disc space infections following lumbar discectomy surely have occurred since 1934, when Mixter and Barr

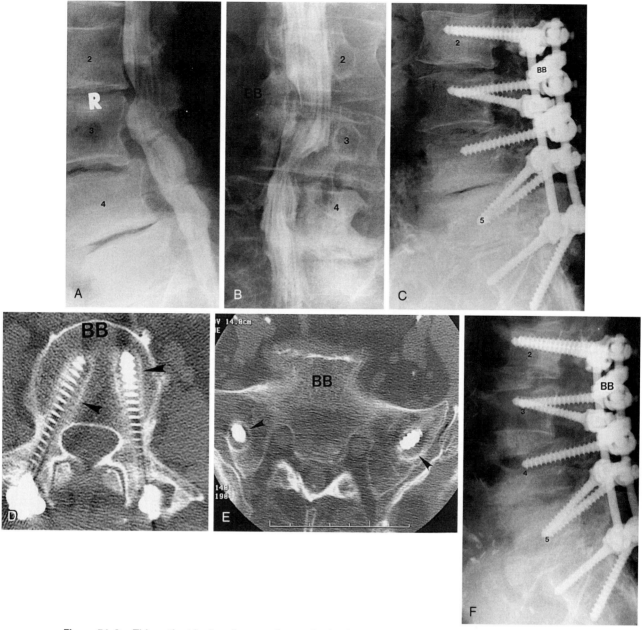

Figure 54–2.   This patient had undergone three prior lumbar laminectomy-discectomy procedures over two decades. He presented with recurrent severe neurogenic claudication after an extended interval of good relief. His preoperative images demonstrate multilevel stenosis with a combination of degenerative scoliosis and spondylolisthesis (*A* and *B*). His surgeon attempted a multilevel revision decompression, instrumentation, and fusion *(C)*. This was complicated by a deep wound infection that persisted for months with chronic drainage. The infection was eradicated with repeated surgical débridement, antibiotics, and delayed primary closure with local muscle flaps. Recurrence of leg pain and the evolution of profound lumbar pain heralded the presence of a symptomatic nonunion. CT images confirmed the failure of his intertransverse fusion. Note the "lucent zones" around the pedicle screws, which are indirect evidence of a failed fusion (*D* and *E, arrowheads*). Anterior interbody fusions were performed from L2 to the sacrum as a salvage procedure *(F)*.

first described the herniated lumbar disc and its surgical treatment. The difficulty in recognizing this entity is attested to by the fact that the first reported cases did not appear in the literature for two decades.[169]

The key to diagnosing this complication rests in a thorough understanding of its presentation. The pre-

sentation of discitis often consists of a lengthy period of pain relief after disc surgery followed by increasing low back pain that may or may not be associated with leg pain. The pain may be out of proportion to physical signs. Rarely, a patient demonstrates a septic course shortly after surgery.[86] Discitis has also been reported

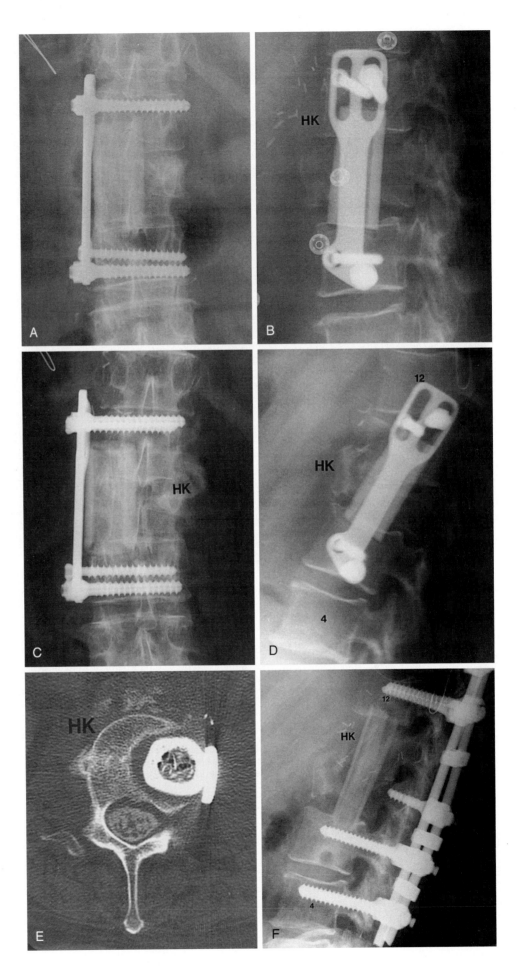

Figure 54–3. A 58-year-old woman sustained an L2 burst fracture with an incomplete neurologic deficit in a motor vehicle accident. She was treated with an anterior corpectomy and reconstruction using a tibial diaphyseal allograft and anterior instrumentation. Anteroposterior (A) and lateral (B) radiographs illustrate the appearance of the surgical reconstruction shortly after the procedure. She developed fevers and increasing back pain postoperatively, which were attributed to pneumonia. Despite a course of antibiotic therapy, her illness persisted and her pain escalated. Subsequent radiographs, when compared with the original postoperative films, demonstrated subsidence of the screws through the superior end plate of L1 and settling of the allograft with a lucent zone around it (C and D). Subsequent CT images (E) confirmed the nonunion by the lucency around the allograft, as well as suggesting the presence of a deep wound infection. Note the abnormally widened paraspinal soft tissue. Aspiration of the lucent zone yielded cultures positive for *Staphylococcus aureus*. Eradication of the infection and spinal reconstruction required a combination of anterior and posterior procedures (F).

to occur after discography, with a rate of 1.3 per cent per disc space, as well as following chymopapain injections (see Fig. 54–1).[55] Intradiscal use of antibiotics in discography has led to a decrease in the incidence of discitis. Patients may report fever, chills, or sweats and nocturnal pain. The pain severity is often disproportionate to other physical signs. The physician is also well advised to remember that epidural abscesses may further complicate a postoperative discitis.

Inspection of the wound site is usually unremarkable, but palpation or percussion may provoke pain. Paralumbar spasm may be present without the presence of a fluid collection. Sciatic or femoral stretch signs can elicit back pain without leg pain. In the face of concomitant leg pain on the straight leg raising test, the physician should be suspicious of an epidural abscess. New neurologic deficits are unusual. Their presence should raise the suspicion of an impending cauda equina syndrome owing to either massive recurrent disc herniation or an epidural abscess.

Screening laboratory tests should include WBC, ESR, and/or CRP levels. WBCs are usually normal, whereas the ESR and CRP are elevated.[15] Guidelines for the utilization of ESR and CRP values are as discussed earlier. A recent report suggested that discitis is probably present when the ESR is greater than 45 and the CRP level is more than 2.5 on the fifth or sixth day.[151]

The value of plain radiographs is variable. Within days to weeks of surgery, plain radiographs show little evidence of intervertebral discitis. There may be some decrease in disc height; however, this frequently accompanies discectomies. With the passage of weeks to months, the cardinal features of intervertebral discitis appear. Blurring of the vertebral end plates is followed by end plate erosion. Reactive bone formation occurs in the adjacent vertebral metaphyses (Fig. 54–4). Advanced cases show evidence of osteomyelitis with local osteolysis, collapse, and possible paravertebral abscess formation. These findings are best demonstrated by

computed tomography (CT) scans.[137] Obliteration of the disc space and bridging trabecular bone may be seen with healing.

Diagnosis should not await plain radiographic changes. Radionuclide imaging techniques are of limited help. Bone scans are frequently positive after discectomy. Furthermore, there is a significant incidence of false-negative studies in documented cases of postoperative discitis.[135, 161] Sequential technetium 99 (Tc-99) and gallium 67 (Ga-67) scans raise the diagnostic accuracy but require 48 to 72 hours to perform. Indium 111–labeled white blood cell scans have met with mixed results.[50] These tests may delay diagnosis and are of limited value in patients receiving antibiotics.

MRI is the imaging modality of choice for evaluating postoperative discitis. Pathognomonic anatomic changes include disc images that are hypointense on T1-weighted images and hyperintense on T2-weighted images. The normal definition between the disc space and vertebral body is lost. Sagittal sections are helpful for interpretation of the disc space and vertebral body, whereas axial sections may provide useful information regarding epidural or paravertebral soft tissue extension.[61] In comparing plain radiography, Tc-99 scanning, combined Tc-99 and Ga-67 scanning, and MRI, Modic and associates demonstrated the superiority of MRI.[113] Although the overall accuracy of Tc-99/Ga-67 and MRI were each 94 per cent, they favored the latter. MRI can be done quickly, allowing rapid diagnosis and initiation of treatment. MRI findings appear within three to five days of the onset of infection. According to some investigators, the term "discitis" may be a misnomer when used to describe a disc space infection following discectomy.[151] It is suggested that a retrodiscal infection may lead to discitis if not treated promptly. Clinically, a retrodiscal infection may cause pain earlier and might be more commonly associated with leg pain. MRI may be helpful in distinguishing these two entities, if they are indeed distinct diagnoses.[151]

Figure 54–4. This patient underwent a laminotomy and discectomy for persistent sciatica. Although his leg pain was relieved immediately, he complained of increasingly severe low back pain and muscle spasm. His problems went untreated for 10 weeks, at which time he was referred for evaluation. Comparison of his immediate postoperative lateral radiograph *(A)* with one obtained 10 weeks later *(B)* illustrates the plain radiographic features of intervertebral discitis: disc space height loss, loss of end plate definition, bone erosion, and surrounding reactive bone formation.

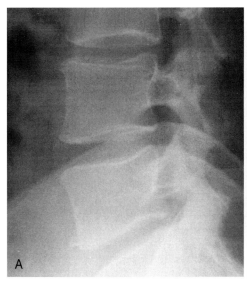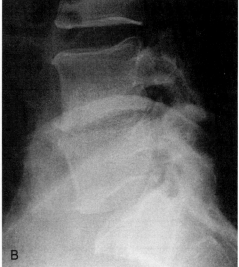

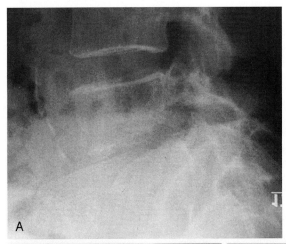

A

Figure 54–5. This patient is a 65-year-old, morbidly obese diabetic. Her surgeon performed an L5–S1 laminotomy and discectomy for sciatica. She returned shortly thereafter with fever, increasing pain, and an erythematous, draining wound. Treatment was attempted with local drainage and antibiotics. Because of increasing symptoms and impairment, she was ultimately referred for evaluation. By that time, her lateral radiograph demonstrated advanced disc space destruction with surrounding osteomyelitis and bone destruction *(A)*. Initially she underwent radical anterior débridement and reconstruction, combined with posterior débridement, segmental instrumentation, and grafting *(B)*. The quality of her remaining sacral bone proved insufficient, as she fractured the anterior portion of the sacrum and displaced her graft *(C)*. A more difficult and hazardous combination of procedures was required for salvage *(D)*.

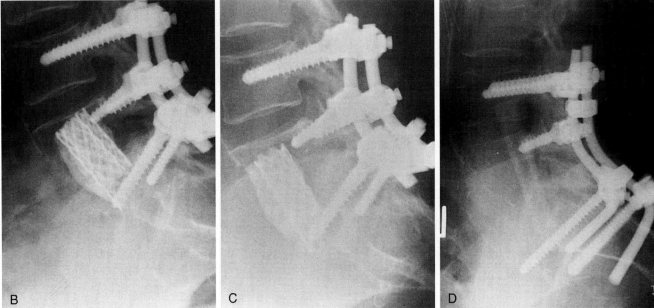

B   C   D

In the absence of neurologic deficits, sepsis, or epidural abscesses, the cornerstone of treatment remains antibiotic therapy and bed rest. Biopsy by either open or percutaneous techniques helps guide the choice of antibiotic therapy. When possible, initiation of antibiotic therapy should follow a successful biopsy. Parenteral therapy should continue for two to six weeks and may be followed by an additional period of oral antibiotics.[67] Culture-negative cases should be treated as presumed gram-positive infections, as the most commonly identified pathogen is *Staphylococcus*. Refractory cases may be caused by anaerobic organisms or fungal species (the latter is rare). Consultation with an infectious disease specialist is advised.

There are some strong indications for surgery. Postoperative sepsis associated with disc space infection warrants emergent surgical exploration and débridement. A cauda equina syndrome or an advancing neurologic deficit with an epidural abscess requires emergent surgery. Failure of nonsurgical treatment necessitates operative intervention. Severe or intractable pain is a relative indication for surgery. It is also wise to note that untoward delay or insufficient surgical intervention may lead to a much more formidable problem (Fig. 54–5).

The surgical approach varies with each patient. If the patient presents soon after discectomy, re-exploration through a posterior approach may suffice. The disc space must be thoroughly débrided and irrigated. In doing so, the surgeon should exercise due care in manipulation of the neural tissues, because they are inflamed and susceptible to injury. A dural tear might result in a persistent cerebrospinal fluid leak and/or meningitis. An anterior approach for disc space débridement and grafting is frequently necessary in chronic cases with significant bone involvement, with ventral compression of the thecal sac, or in the presence of a paraspinal abscess. Regardless of the chosen approach, thorough débridement is essential. All wounds should be drained appropriately.

The prognosis for patients with postoperative discitis is often favorable. The infection is readily managed with appropriate means; however, different authors report variable success in returning patients to work. Puranen and coworkers reported that seven of eight patients (88 per cent) returned to work,[135] whereas Pilgaard[131] and Lindholm and Pylkkanen[96] reported only 67 and 39 per cent of patients returning to work, respectively. There are more factors at work here than the presence of absence of infection. The extended duration of their illness and treatment may be partially responsible for this worse prognosis for return to function.

Epidural Abscess

An epidural abscess occurring in isolation after spinal surgery is a rare event. In their series, Baker and coworkers found that 16 per cent of epidural abscesses were caused by postoperative infection.[8] Overall, large tertiary care centers report an incidence of roughly 1 per 10,000 admissions per year.[8] The typical progression of symptoms is back pain followed by radicular pain and weakness and finally paralysis. Meningeal signs and nuchal rigidity may be present. In a recent review of 43 cases of bacterial epidural abscesses, presenting symptoms included backache (72 per cent), radicular pain (42 per cent), weakness (35 per cent), sensory deficit (23 per cent), bowel or bladder dysfunction (30 per cent), and frank paralysis (21 per cent).[38]

Patients usually present with a fever and leukocytosis. One should also expect to find an elevated ESR and CRP level. Cultures of the abscess are positive in 90 per cent of cases. *Staphylococcus aureus* is the most commonly found pathogen, although gram-negative organisms are found with higher frequency in intravenous drug abusers.[37, 126] Blood cultures are positive in 60 per cent of cases, and lumbar punctures are positive in 17 per cent of cases.[64]

MRI with and without gadolinium is the imaging modality of choice for evaluating a suspected epidural abscess. The abscess appears as a well-defined mass of variable size. Classically, it is isointense with the spinal cord on T1-weighted images and hyperintense on T2-weighted images.[42] Gadolinium increases the accuracy and sensitivity by enhancing and defining the epidural abscess. CT-myelography may show the degree of mechanical compression and block. The lumbar puncture should be performed at a distance from the suspected infection to avoid seeding of the cerebrospinal fluid.

Emergent surgical decompression and drainage is the accepted standard for the management of most epidural abscesses. The choice of surgical approach depends on the location of the compressive pathology. In the absence of vertebral destruction and osteomyelitis, dorsal and lateral abscesses can be approached through a laminectomy. If the vertebral bodies are involved, spinal reconstruction is necessary, because a laminectomy will destabilize the spine. A ventral abscess is best approached anteriorly to ensure thorough decompression without retraction of the neural elements. Involved vertebral bodies should be resected, and reconstruction is accomplished with appropriate grafting techniques. However, if the abscess surrounds the spinal cord or cauda equina, emergency laminectomy, decompression, and débridement of the canal can be considered and performed, followed later by the anterior, more definitive débridement and fusion.

The prognosis following an epidural abscess is largely dependent on the neurologic symptoms at presentation and the expediency of surgical management. Recovery from paraplegia, as pointed out by Watridge, is the exception rather than the rule.[174] Untreated, an epidural abscess is often fatal.[171]

Nosocomial Infection

A final subgroup of patients with spinal infections warrants mention. Occasionally, patients develop spinal infections associated with diagnostic or therapeutic procedures. These nosocomial spinal infections are known to occur after lumbar puncture, epidural injection or catheter insertion, intradiscal injections, and the like. The clinical presentation can vary across the spectrum from epidural abscess to intervertebral discitis to vertebral osteomyelitis. A history of such procedures should alert the physician to these possibilities, so that diagnosis and treatment are accomplished in a timely fashion.

SUMMARY

The economic impact of a postoperative infection is significant. Generalized cost predictions are confounded by the multifactorial nature of postoperative infections. However, in one review of 724 adult spinal fusions with an infection rate of 4 per cent, of which 11 were deep infections, an analysis was performed to estimate this cost. Based on data collected from two inner-city hospitals and one county hospital, it was shown that the average billing for treatment of a postoperative infection was in excess of $100,000, as compared with $27,000 for a lumbar fusion. Also of interest was that nonprofessional and hospital fees represented 90 per cent of the $100,000 cost.[23]

The need to pay meticulous attention to perioperative infection prophylaxis cannot be overemphasized. However, despite even the best of intentions, postoperative infections may arise. Early recognition and aggressive treatment can minimize the morbidity associated with this difficult postoperative complication.

References

1. Alexander, J. W.: Surgical infections and choice of antibiotics. *In* Sabiston, D. C. (ed.): Textbook of Surgery: The Biological Basis of Modern Surgical Practice. 13th ed. Philadelphia, W. B. Saunders Co., 1986, pp. 259–283.
2. Alexander, J. W., and Alexander, N. S.: The influence of route of administration on wound fluid concentration of prophylactic antibiotics. J. Trauma 16:488–495, 1976.
3. Allen, B. L., and Ferguson, R. L.: The Galveston experience with L-rod instrumentation for adolescent idiopathic scoliosis. Clin. Orthop. 229:59–69, 1988.

4. Antimicrobial prophylaxis for surgery. Med. Lett. *23*:77–80, 1981.
5. Arand, A. G., and Sawaya, R.: Intraoperative chemical hemostasis in neurosurgery. Neurosurgery *18*:223–233, 1986.
6. Archer, G. L., and Tanenbaum, M. J.: Antibiotic-resistant *S. epidermidis* in patients undergoing cardiac surgery. Antimicrob. Agents Chemother. *17*:269, 1980.
7. Babineau, T. J., and Bothe, A.: General surgery considerations in the diabetic patient. Infect. Dis. Clin. North Am. *9*:183–193, 1995.
8. Baker, A. S., Ojemann, R. G., Swartz, M. N., et al.: Spinal epidural abscess. N. Engl. J. Med. *293*:463–468, 1975.
9. Banta, J. V.: Combined anterior and posterior fusion for spinal deformity in myelomeningocele. Spine *15*:946–952, 1990.
10. Batson, O. V.: The vertebral vein system. AJR Am. J. Roentgenol. *78*:195–212, 1957.
11. Belthazar, E. R., Colt, J. D., and Nichols, R. L.: Preoperative hair removal: A random prospective study of shaving versus clipping. South. Med. J. *75*:799–801, 1982.
12. Berchuck, M., Garfin, S. R., Bauman, T., and Abitol, J. J.: Complications of anterior intervertebral grafting. Clin. Orthop. *284*:54–62, 1992.
13. Bertalanffy, H., and Eggert, H. R.: Complications of anterior cervical discectomy without fusion in 450 consecutive patients. Acta Neurochir. (Wien) *99*:41–50, 1989.
14. Bethune, D. W., Blowers, R., Parker, M., et al.: Dispersal of *Staphylococcus aureus* by patients and surgical staff. Lancet *1*:480–483, 1976.
15. Bircher, M. D., Tasker, T., Crawshaw, C., et al.: Discitis following lumbar surgery. Spine *13*:98–102, 1988.
16. Blumenthal, S., and Gill, K.: Complications of the Wiltse pedicle screw fixation system. Spine *18*:1867–1871, 1993.
17. Bonaldi, G., Belloni, G., Prosetti, D., and Moschini, L.: Percutaneous discectomy using Onik's method: 3 years experience. Neuroradiology *33*:516–519, 1991.
18. Boyd, R. J., Burke, J. F., and Colton, T.: A double-blind clinical trial of prophylactic antibiotics in hip fractures. J. Bone Joint Surg. Am. *55*:1251–1258, 1973.
19. Brown, H. P.: Management of spinal deformity in myelomeningocele. Orthop. Clin. North Am. *9*:391–403, 1978.
20. Bruschwein, D. A., Brown, M. L., and McLeod, R. A.: Gallium scintigraphy in the evaluation of disk-space infections: Concise communication. J. Nucl. Med. *21*:925–927, 1980.
21. Burke, J. F.: Identification of the sources of staphylococci contaminating the surgical wound during operation. Ann. Surg. *158*:898–904, 1963.
22. Burke, J. F.: The effective period of preventive antibiotic action in experimental incisions and dermal lesions. Surgery *50*:161–168, 1961.
23. Calderone, R. R., Garland, D. E., Capen, D. A., and Oster, H.: Cost of medical care for postoperative spinal infections. Orthop. Clin. North Am. *27*:171–182, 1996.
24. Chang, K. W., and McAfee, P. C.: Degenerative spondylolisthesis and degenerative scoliosis treated with a combination sequential rod-plate and transpedicular screw instrumentation system: A preliminary report. J. Spinal Dis. *1*:247–256, 1988.
25. Chang, N., and Mathes, S.: Comparison of the effect of bacterial inoculation in musculocutaneous and random-pattern skin flaps. Plast. Reconstr. Surg. *70*:1–10, 1982.
26. Chung-Hua Wai Ko Tsa Chih: Wound infection after spinal surgery. Chin. J. Surg. *29*:484–486, 524–525, 1991.
27. Clark, C. R., Goetz, D. D., and Menezes, A. H.: Arthrodesis of the cervical spine in rheumatoid arthritis. J. Bone Joint Surg. Am. *71*:381–391, 1989.
28. Cloward, R. B: Gas-sterilized cadaver bone grafts for spinal fusion operations: A simplified bone bank. Spine *5*:4–10, 1980.
29. Conte, J. E., Cohen, S. N., Roe, B. B., et al.: Antibiotic prophylaxis and cardiac surgery: A prospective double-blind comparison of single-dose versus multiple-dose regimens. Ann. Intern. Med. *76*:943–949, 1972.
30. Cooney, W. P., Fitzgerald, R. H., Jr., Dobyns, J. H., and Washington, J. A.: Quantitative wound cultures in upper extremity trauma. J. Trauma *22*:112–117, 1982.
31. Cosgrove, E. H. A., and Millard, F. J. C.: The radiological changes in infections of the spine and their diagnostic value. Clin. Radiol. *29*:31–40, 1978.
32. Coventry, M. B., Ghormley, R. K., Kernohan, J. W., et al.: The intervertebral disc: Its microscopic anatomy and pathology. Part I. Anatomy, development and physiology. J. Bone Joint Surg. *27*:105–112, 1945.
33. Cox, C. E.: Principles of operative surgery: Antisepsis technique, sutures, and drains. In Sabiston, D.C. (ed.): Textbook of Surgery: The Biological Basis of Modern Surgical Practice. 13th ed. Philadelphia, W. B. Saunders Co., 1986, pp. 244–258.
34. Craig, F. S.: Vertebral-body biopsy. J. Bone Joint Surg. Am. *38*:93–102, 1956.
35. Cruse, P. J. E., and Foord, R.: A five-year prospective study of 23,649 surgical wounds. Arch. Surg. *107*:206–209, 1973.
36. Currier, B. L., Banovac, K., and Eismont, F. J.: Gentamicin penetration into normal rabbit nucleus pulposus. Presented at Cervical Spine Research Society meeting, New Orleans, December 1989.
37. Danner, R. L., and Hartman, B. J.: Update of spinal epidural abscess: 35 cases and review of the literature. Rev. Infect. Dis. *9*:265–274, 1987.
38. Darouiche, A. O., Hamill, A. J., Greenberg, S. B., et al.: Bacterial spinal epidural abscess. Review of 43 cases and literature survey. Medicine *71*:369–385, 1992.
39. Dernbach, P. D., Gomez, H., and Hahn, J.: Primary closure of infected spinal wounds. Neurosurgery *26*:707–709, 1990.
40. Dick, J., Boachie-Adjei, O., and Wilson, M.: One-stage versus two-stage anterior and posterior spinal reconstruction in adults. Spine *17*:S310–S316, 1992.
41. Dirschl, D. R., and Wilson, F. C.: Topical antibiotic irrigation in the prophylaxis of operative wound infections in orthopaedic surgery. Orthop. Clin. North Am. *22*:419–426, 1991.
42. Djukic, S., Lang, P., Morris, J., et al.: The postoperative spine. Orthop. Clin. North Am. *21*:603–624, 1990.
43. Eismont, F. J., and Kitchel, S. H.: Pyogenic infections of the spine. In Evarts, C. M. (ed.): Surgery of the Musculoskeletal System. 2nd ed. New York, Churchill Livingstone, 1990, pp. 2277–2297.
44. Eismont, F. J., Bohlman, H. H., Soni, P. L., et al.: Pyogenic and fungal vertebral osteomyelitis with paralysis. J. Bone Joint Surg. Am. *65*:19–29, 1983.
45. El-Gindi, S., Aref, S., Salama, M., et al.: Infection of intervetebral discs after operation. J. Bone Joint Surg. Br. *58*:114–116, 1976.
46. Emery, S. L., Chan, D. P. K., and Woodard, H. R.: Treatment of hematogenous pyogenic vertebral osteomyelitis with anterior débridement and primary bone grafting. Spine *14*:284–291, 1989.
47. Eshima, I., Mathes, S., and Paty, P.: Comparison of the intracellular bacterial killing activity of leukocytes in musculocutaneous and random pattern flaps. Plast. Reconstr. Surg. *86*:541–547, 1990.
48. Esses, S. I.: The AO spinal internal fixator. Spine *14*:373–378, 1989.
49. Fernand, R., and Lee, C. K.: Postlaminectomy disc space infection: A review of the literature and a report of three cases. Clin. Orthop. *209*:215–218, 1986.
50. Fernandez-Ulloa, M., Vasavada, P. J., Hanslits, M. L., et al.: Diagnosis of vertebral osteomyelitis: Clinical, radiological and scintigraphic features. Orthopedics *8*:1144–1150, 1985.
51. Fitzgerald, R. H., and Thompson, R. L.: Current concepts review: Cephalosporin antibiotics in the prevention and treatment of musculoskeletal sepsis. J. Bone Joint Surg. Am. *65*:1201–1205, 1983.
52. Fogelberg, E. V., Zitzman, E. K., and Stinchfield, F. E.: Prophylactic penicillin in orthopaedic surgery. J. Bone Joint Surg. Am. *52*:95–98, 1970.
53. Ford, L. T., and Key, J. A.: Postoperative wound infection: A controlled study of the increased duration of hospital stay and direct cost of hospitalization. Ann. Surg. *185*:264–268, 1977.
54. Ford, L. T., and Key, J. A.: Postoperative infection of intervertebral disc space. South. Med. J. *48*:1295–1303, 1995.
55. Fraser, R. D., Osti, O. L., and Vernon-Roberts, B.: Discitis after discography. J. Bone Joint Surg. Br. *69*:26–35, 1987.
56. Gaines, D. L., Moe, J. H., and Bocklage, J.: Management of wound infections following Harrington instrumentation and spine fusion. J. Bone Joint Surg. Am. *52*:404–405, 1970.
57. Galloway, J. A., and Shuman, C. R.: Diabetes and surgery: A study of 667 cases. Am. J. Med. *34*:177–191, 1963.

58. Gepstein, R., and Eismont, F. J.: Postoperative spine infections. *In* Garfin, S. R. (ed.): Complications of Spine Surgery. Baltimore, Williams & Wilkins, 1989, pp. 302–322.

59. Goldstein, L. A.: Treatment of idiopathic scoliosis by Harrington instrumentation and fusion with fresh autogenous iliac bone grafts. J. Bone Joint Surg. Am. *51*:209–222, 1969.

60. Green, B.: Discussion on disc space infection. J. Spinal Dis. *1*:321–322, 1988.

61. Green, J. W., and Wenzel, R. P.: Postoperative wound infection: A controlled study of the increased duration of hospital stay and direct cost of hospitalization. Ann. Surg. *185*:264–268, 1977.

62. Gurr, K. R., and McAfee, P. C.: Cotrel-Dubousset instrumentation in adults: A preliminary report. Spine *13*:510–520, 1988.

63. Gusberg, R, J., and Moley, J.: Diabetes and abdominal surgery: The mutual risks. Yale J. Biol. Med. *56*:285–291, 1983.

64. Ha'eri, G. B., and Wiley, A. M.: The efficacy of standard surgical face masks: An investigation using "tracer particles." Clin. Orthop. *148*:160–162, 1980.

65. Hancock, D. O.: A study of 49 patients with acute spinal extradural abscesses. Paraplegia *10*:285–288, 1973.

66. Hanley, E. N., and Shapiro, D. P.: The development of low-back pain after excision of a lumbar disc. J. Bone Joint Surg. Am. *71*:719–721, 1989.

67. Heller, J. G.: Postoperative infections of the spine. *In* Rothman, R. H., and Simeone, F. A. (eds.): The Spine. 3rd. ed. Philadelphia, W. B. Saunders, Co., 1992, p. 1817.

68. Herron, L. D., and Newman, M. H.: The failure of ethylene oxide gas-sterilized freeze-dried bone graft for thoracic and lumbar spinal fusion. Spine *14*:496–498, 1989.

69. Hoffer, F. A., Strand, R. D., and Gebhardt, M. C.: Percutaneous biopsy of pyogenic infection of the spine in children. J. Pediatr. Orthop. *8*:442–444, 1988.

70. Horton, W. C.: Personal communication, 1990.

71. Horwitz, N. H., and Curtin, J. A.: Prophylactic antibiotics and wound infections following laminectomy for lumbar disc herniation: A retrospective study. J. Neurosurg. *43*:727–731, 1975.

72. Howe, C. W.: Experimental studies on determinants of wound infection. Surg. Gynecol. Obstet. *123*:507–514, 1966.

73. Jensen, J. E., Jensen, T. G., Smith, T. K., et al.: Nutrition in orthopaedic surgery. J. Bone Joint Surg. Am. *64*:1263–1272, 1982.

74. Johnston, D. H., Fairclough, J. A., Brown, E. M., et al.: Rate of bacterial recolonization of the skin after preparation: Four methods compared. Br. J. Surg. *74*:64, 1987.

75. Jonsson, B., Soderholm, R., and Stromqvist, B.: Erythrocyte sedimentation rate after lumbar spine surgery. Spine *16*:1049–1050, 1991.

76. Kayvanfar, J. F., Capen, D. A., Thomas, J. C., et al.: Wound infections after instrumented posterolateral adult lumbar spine fusions. Presented at the 1995 American Academy of Orthopaedic Surgeons annual meeting, Orlando, FL.

77. Keller, R. B., and Pappas, A. M.: Infections after spinal fusion using internal fixation instrumentation. Orthop. Clin. North Am. *3*:99–111, 1972.

78. Kemp, H. B. S., Jackson, J. W., Jeremiah, J. D., et al.: Anterior fusion of the spine for infective lesions in adults. J. Bone Joint Surg. Br. *55*:715–734, 1973.

79. Kemp, H. B. S., Jackson, J. W., Jeremiah, J. D., et al.: Pyogenic infections occurring primarily in intervertebral discs. J. Bone Joint Surg. Br. *55*:698–714, 1973.

80. Keusch, G. T., Douglas, S. D., Hammer, G., et al.: Antibacterial functions of macrophages in experimental protein-calorie malnutrition. II. Cellular and humoral factors for chemotaxis, phagocytosis, and intracellular bactericidal activity. J. Infect. Dis. *138*:134–142, 1978.

81. Kink, B. K., Thurman, R. T., Wittpenn, G. P., et al.: Muscle flap closure for salvage of complex back wounds. Spine *19*:1467–1470, 1994.

82. Kitchel, S., Eismont, F. J., and Green, B. A.: Closed subarachnoid drainage for management of cerebrospinal fluid leakage after an operation on the spine. J. Bone Joint Surg. Am. *71*:984–987, 1989.

83. Knapp, D. R., and Jones, E. T.: Use of cortical cancellous allograft for posterior spinal fusion. Clin. Orthop. *229*:99–106, 1988.

84. Kostuik, J.P., Errico, T. J., Gleason, T. F., and Errico, C. C.: Spinal stabilization of vertebral column tumors. Spine *13*:250–256, 1988.

85. Kostuik, J. P., Israel, J., and Hall, J. E.: Scoliosis surgery in adults. Clin. Orthop. *93*:225–234, 1973.

86. Lang, E. F.: Postoperative infection of the intervertebral disk space. Surg. Clin. North Am. *48*:649–660, 1968.

87. Lavernia, C. J., Bache, H., and Godin, M.: The incidence of unknown perforations of gloves during routine surgical procedures. (Abstract.) Presented at the Western Orthopaedic Association meeting, Anaheim, CA, October 1989.

88. Lawrie, G. M., Morris, G. C., and Glaser, D. H.: Influence of diabetes mellitus on the results of coronary bypass surgery: Followup of 212 patients 10–15 years after surgery. JAMA *256*:2967–2971, 1986.

89. Lee, J. T., Jr., Ahrenholz, D. H., Nelson, R. D., et al.: Mechanisms of the adjuvant effect of hemoglobin in experimental peritonitis: V. The significance of the coordinated iron component. Surgery *86*:41–47, 1979.

90. Letts, R. M., and Doermer, E.: Conversation in the operating theater as a cause of airborne bacterial contamination. J. Bone Joint Surg. Am. *65*:357–362, 1983.

91. Leung, P. C.: Complications in the first 40 cases of microdiscectomy. J. Spinal Dis. *1*:306–310, 1988.

92. Leventhal, M. R.: Surgical approaches in the treatment of spinal infections. Spine: State of the Art Reviews *3*:419–436, 1989.

93. Levine, D. B., Wilson, R. L., and Doherty, J. H.: Operative management of idiopathic scoliosis: A critical analysis of sixty-seven cases. J. Bone Joint Surg. Am. *52*:408, 1970.

94. Levine, M. J., Mariani, B. D., Tuan, R. S., and Booth, R. E.: Molecular genetic diagnosis of infected total joint arthroplasty. A case report. J. Arthroplasty *10*:93–94, 1995.

95. Lidwell, O. M., Lowbury, E. J., Whyte, W., et al.: Effect of ultraclean air in operating rooms on deep sepsis in the joint after a total hip replacement: A randomized study. BMJ *285*:10–14, 1982.

96. Lindholm, T. S., and Pylkkanen, P.: Discitis following removal of intervertebral disc. Spine *7*:618–622, 1982.

97. Lonstein, J. E.: Diagnosis and treatment of postoperative spinal infections. Surg. Rounds Orthop. *3*:25–32, 1989.

98. Lonstein, J. E.: Management of postoperative spine infections. *In* Gustilo, R. B. (ed.): Current Concepts in Management of Musculoskeletal Infections. Philadelphia, W. B. Saunders Co., 1989, pp. 243–249.

99. Lonstein, J. E., and Akbarnia, B. A.: Operative treatment of spinal deformities in patients with cerebral palsy or mental retardation. J. Bone Joint Surg. Am. *65*:43–55, 1983.

100. Lonstein, J., Winter, R., Moe, J., et al.: Wound infection with Harrington instrumentation and spine fusion for scoliosis. Clin. Orthop. *96*:222–223, 1973.

101. Mader, J. T., and Cierny, G.: The principles of the use of preventive antibiotics. Clin. Orthop. *190*:72–75, 1984.

102. Malinin, T. I., and Brown, M. D.: Bone allografts in spinal surgery. Clin. Orthop. *154*:68–73, 1981.

103. Mandelbaum, B. R., Tolo, V. T., McAfee, P. C., and Burest, P.: Nutritional deficiencies after staged anterior and posterior spinal reconstructive surgery. Clin. Orthop. *234*:5–11, 1988.

104. Mariani, B. D., Levine, M. J., Booth, R. E., and Tuan, R. S.: Development of a novel rapid processing protocol for polymerase chain reaction–based detection of bacterial infections in synovial fluids. J. Mol. Biotechn. (in press).

105. Marshall, K. A., Edgerton, M. T., Rodeheaver, G. T., et al.: Quantitative microbiology: Its application to hand injuries. Am. J. Surg. *131*:730–733, 1976.

106. Massie, J. B., Heller, J. G., and Abitol, J.J.: Postoperative posterior spinal wound infections. Clin. Orthop. *284*:99–108, 1992.

107. McAfee, P. C., Bohlman, H. H., Ducker, T., and Eismont, F. J.: Failure of stabilization of the spine with methylmethacrylate. J. Bone Joint Surg. Am. *67*:1145–1157, 1986.

108. McCarthy, R. E., Peek, R. D., Morrissy, R. T., et al.: Allograft bone in spinal fusion for paralytic scoliosis. J. Bone Joint Surg. Am. *68*:370–375, 1986.

109. McMurray, G. N.: The evaluation of Kiel bone in spinal fusions. J. Bone Joint Surg. Br. *64*:101–104, 1982.

110. Merkel, K. D., Fitzgerald, R. H., and Brown, M. L.: Scintigraphic evaluation in musculoskeletal sepsis. Orthop. Clin. North Am. *15*:401–416, 1984.

111. Mitchell, N. J., and Gamble, D. R.: Clothing design for operating-room personnel. Lancet 2:1133–1136, 1974.

112. Modal, C.: Cervical osteochondrosis and disc herniation. Eighteen years' use of interbody fusion by Cloward's technique in 755 cases. Acta Neurochir. 70:207–255, 1984.

113. Modic, M. T., Feiglin, D. H., Piraino, D. W., et al.: Vertebral osteomyelitis: Assessment using MR. Radiology 157:157–166, 1985.

114. Moe, J. H.: Complications of scoliosis treatment. Clin. Orthop. 53:21–30, 1967.

115. Moe, J. H., and Gustilo, R. B.: Treatment of scoliosis. J. Bone Joint Surg. Am. 46:293–312, 1964.

116. Monson, T. P., and Nelson, C. L.: Microbiology for orthopaedic surgeons: Selected aspects. Clin. Orthop. 190:14–22, 1984.

117. National Academy of Sciences–National Research Council: Postoperative wound infections: The influence of ultraviolet irradiation of the operating room and of various other factors. Ann. Surg. 160 (Suppl.):1–125, 1964.

118. Nauheim, K. S., Barnett, M. G., Crandall, D. G., et al.: Anterior exposure of the thoracic spine. Ann. Thorac. Surg. 57:1436–1439, 1994.

119. Nelson, C. L., Green, T. G., Porter, R. A., et al.: One day versus seven days of preventive antibiotic therapy in orthopaedic surgery. Clin. Orthop. 176:258–263, 1983.

120. Neu, H. C.: Cephalosporin antibiotics as applied in surgery of bones and joints. Clin. Orthop. 190:50–64, 1984.

121. Nichols, R. L.: Postoperative infections and antimicrobial prophylaxis. In Mandel, G. L., Douglas, R. G., and Bennett, J. E. (eds.): Principles and Practice of Infectious Diseases. 2nd ed. New York, Churchill Livingstone, 1988, pp. 1637–1644.

122. Nichols, R. L.: Techniques known to prevent postoperative wound infection. Infect. Control 3:34–37, 1982.

123. Nora, P. F., Vanecko, R. M., and Bransfield, J. J.: Prophylactic abdominal drains. Arch. Surg. 105:173–176, 1972.

124. Northey, D., Adess, M. L., Hartsuck, J. M., et al.: Microbial surveillance in a surgical intensive care unit. Surg. Gynecol. Obstet. 139:321–326, 1974.

125. Ottolenghi, C. E.: Aspiration biopsy of the spine: Technique for the thoracic spine and results of twenty-eight biopsies in this region and overall results of 1050 biopsies of other spinal segments. J. Bone Joint Surg. Am. 51:1531–1544, 1969.

126. Ozuna, R. M., and Delamarter, R. B.: Pyogenic vertebral osteomyelitis and postsurgical disc space infections. Orthop. Clin. North Am. 27:87–94, 1996.

127. Pavel, A., Smioth, R. L., Ballard, A., et al.: Prophylactic antibiotics in clean orthopaedic surgery. J. Bone Joint Surg. Am. 56:777–782, 1974.

128. Pavon, S. J., and Manning, C.: Posterior spinal fusion for scoliosis due to anterior poliomyelitis. J. Bone Joint Surg. Br. 52:420–431, 1970.

129. Petty, W.: The effect of methylmethacrylate on bacterial phagocytosis and killing by human polymorphonuclear leukocytes. J. Bone Joint Surg. Am. 60:752–757, 1978.

130. Petty, W.: The effect of methylmethacrylate on chemotaxis of polymorphonuclear leukocytes. J. Bone Joint Surg. Am. 60:492–498, 1978.

131. Pilgaard, S.: Discitis (closed space infection) following removal of lumbar intervertebral disc. J. Bone Joint Surg. Am. 51:713–716, 1969.

132. Polk, H. C., Jr.: Principles of preoperative preparation of the surgical patient. In Sabiston, D. C. (ed.): Textbook of Surgery: The Biological Basis of Modern Surgical Practice. 13th ed. Philadelphia, W. B. Saunders Co., 1988, pp. 87–98.

133. Polk, H. C., Jr., Simpson, C. J., Simmons, B. P., and Alexander, J. W.: Guidelines for prevention of surgical wound infection. Arch. Surg. 118:1213–1217, 1983.

134. Polk, H. C., Trachtenberg, L., and Finn, M. P.: Antibiotic activity in surgical incisions: The basis for prophylaxis in selected operations. JAMA 244:1353–1354, 1980.

135. Puranen, J., Makela, J., and Lahde, S.: Postoperative intervertebral discitis. Acta Orthop. Scand. 55:461–465, 1984.

136. Quintiliani, R., and Nightingale, C.: Principles of antibiotic usage. Clin. Orthop. 190:21–35, 1984.

137. Raininko, R. K., Aho, A. J., and Laine, M. O.: Computed tomography in spondylitis: CT versus other radiographic methods. Acta Orthop. Scand. 56:372–377, 1984.

138. Reddy, S., Leite, C. C., and Jinkins, J. R.: Imaging of infectious disease of the spine. Spine: State of the Art Reviews 9:119–140, 1995.

139. Rimoldi, R. L., and Haye, W.: The use of antibiotics for wound prophylaxis in spinal surgery. Orthop. Clin. North Am. 27:47–52, 1996.

140. Ritter, M. A.: Surgical wound environment. Clin. Orthop. 190:11–13, 1984.

141. Ritter, M. A., Eitzen, H. E., Hart, J. B., et al.: The surgeon's garb. Clin. Orthop. 153:204–209, 1980.

142. Robson, M. C., Duke, W. F., and Krizek, T. J.: Rapid bacterial screening in the treatment of civilian wounds. J. Surg. Res. 14:426–430, 1973.

143. Rosenstein, B. D., Wilson, F. C., and Funderbark, C. H.: The use of bacitracin irrigation to prevent infection in postoperative skeletal wounds. J. Bone Joint Surg. Am. 71:427–430, 1989.

144. Roy-Camille, R., Saillant, G., and Mazel, C.: Internal fixation of the lumbar spine with pedicle screw plating. Clin. Orthop. 203:7–17, 1986.

145. Rubayi, S.: Wound management in spinal infection. Orthop. Clin. North Am. 27:137–153, 1996.

146. Rubinstein, E., Findler, G., Amit, P., et al.: Perioperative prophylactic cephazolin in spine surgery. J. Bone Joint Surg. Br. 76:99–102, 1994.

147. Schaffer, J. L., and Kambin, P.: Percutaneous posterolateral lumbar discectomy and decompression with a 6.9-millimeter cannula. Analysis of operative failures and complications. J. Bone Joint Surg. 73:822–831, 1991.

148. Scherr, D. D., and Dodd, T. A.: In vitro bacteriological evaluation of the effectiveness of antimicrobial irritating solutions. J. Bone Joint Surg. Am. 58:119–122, 1976.

149. Schofferman, L., Schofferman, J., Zucherman, J., et al.: Occult infections causing persistent low-back pain. Spine 14:417–419, 1989.

150. Schonholtz, G. J., Borgia, C. A., and Blair, J. D.: Wound sepsis in orthopaedic surgery. J. Bone Joint Surg. Am. 44:1548–1552, 1962.

151. Schulitz, K. P., and Assheuer, J.: Discitis after procedures on the intervertebral disc. Spine 19:1172–1177, 1994.

152. Shapiro, M., Townsend, T. R., Rosner, B., et al.: Use of antimicrobial drugs in general hospitals: Patterns of prophylaxis. N. Engl. J. Med. 301:351–355, 1979.

153. Silcox, D. H., 3rd, Daftari, T., Boden, S. D., et al.: The effect of nicotine on spinal fusion. Spine 20:1549–1553, 1995.

154. Simchen, E., Stein, H., Sacks, T. G., et al.: Multivariate analysis of determinants of postoperative wound infection in orthopaedic patients. J. Hosp. Infect. 5:137–146, 1984.

155. Simpson, J. M., Silveri, C. P., Balderston, R. A., et al.: The results of operations on the lumbar spine in patients who have diabetes mellitus. J. Bone Joint Surg. Am. 75:1823–1829, 1993.

156. Stambough, J. L., and Beringer, D.: Postoperative wound infections complicating adult spine surgery. J. Spinal Disord. 5:277–285, 1992.

157. Stevens, D. B.: Postoperative orthopaedic infections. J. Bone Joint Surg. Am. 46:96–102, 1964.

158. Stolke, D., Solimann, W. P., and Seifert, V.: Intra and postoperative complications in lumbar disc surgery. Spine 14:56–59, 1989.

159. Swank, S. M., Cohen, D. S., and Brown, J. C.: Spine fusion in cerebral palsy with L-rod segmental spinal instrumentation: A comparison of single and two-stage combined approach with Zielke instrumentation. Spine 14:750–759, 1979.

160. Swank, S. M., Lonstein, J. E., Moe, J. H., et al.: Surgical treatment of adult scoliosis. J. Bone Joint Surg. Am. 63:268–287, 1981.

161. Szypryt, E. P., Hardy, J. G., Hinton, C. E., et al.: A comparison between magnetic resonance imaging and scintigraphic bone imaging in the diagnosis of disc space infection in an animal model. Spine 13:1042–1048, 1988.

162. Tamborino, J. M., Armbruss, E. N., and Moe, J. H.: Harrington instrumentation in correction of scoliosis. J. Bone Joint Surg. Am. 46:313–323, 1964.

163. Tew, J. M., and Mayfield, F. H.: Complications of surgery of the anterior cervical spine. Clin. Neurosurg. 23:424–434, 1976.

164. Thalgott, J. S., LaRocca, H., Aebi, M., et al.: Reconstruction of the lumbar spine using AO DCP plate internal fixation. Spine *14*:91–95, 1989.

165. Theiss, S. M., Lonstein, J. E., and Winter, R. B.: Wound infections in reconstructive spine surgery. Orthop. Clin. North Am. *27*:105–110, 1996.

166. Thelander, U., and Larsson, S.: Quantification of C-reactive protein levels and erythrocyte sedimentation rate after spinal surgery. Spine *17*:400–404, 1992.

167. Thibodeau, A. A.: Closed space infection following removal of lumbar intervertebral disc. J. Bone Joint Surg. Am. *50*:400–410, 1968.

168. Tomford, W. W., Starkweather, R. J., and Goldman, M. H.: A study of the clinical incidence of infection in the use of banked allograft bone. J. Bone Joint Surg. Am. *63*:244–248, 1981.

169. Turnbull, F.: Postoperative inflammatory disease of lumbar discs. J. Neurosurg. *10*:469, 1953.

170. Urist, M. R., and Dawson, E.: Intertransverse process fusion with the aid of chemosterilized autolyzed antigen-extracted allogenic (AAA) bone. Clin. Orthop. *154*:97–113, 1981.

171. Verner, E. F., and Musher, D. M.: Spinal epidural abscesses. Med. Clin. North Am. *69*:375–384, 1985.

172. Verrier, E. D., Bossart, K. J., and Heer, W. F.: Reduction of infection rates in abdominal incisions by delayed wound closure techniques. Am. J. Surg. *1380*:22–28, 1979.

173. Veterans Administration ad hoc Interdisciplinary Committee on Antimicrobial Drug Usage: Prophylaxis in surgery. JAMA *237*:1003–1008, 1977.

174. Watridge, C. B.: Surgical infections of the spinal canal. Spine: State of the Art Reviews *3*:437–451, 1989.

175. White, J. J., and Duncan, A.: The comparative effectiveness of iodophor and hexachlorophene surgical scrub solutions. Surg. Gynecol. Obstet. *135*:890–892, 1972.

176. Whitecloud, T. S., Butler, J. C., Cohen, J. L., et al.: Complications with the variable spinal plating system. Spine *14*:472–476, 1989.

177. Winter, R. B., Moe, J. H., and Lonstein, J. E.: Posterior spinal arthrodesis for congenital scoliosis. An analysis of the cases of two hundred and ninety patients five to 19 years old. J. Bone Joint Surg. Am. *66*:1188–1197, 1984.

178. Wisneski, R. J.: Infectious disease of the spine. Diagnostic and treatment considerations. Orthop. Clin. North Am. *22*:491–501, 1991.

179. Wright, R. L.: Septic Complications of Neurosurgical Spinal Procedures. Springfield, IL, Charles C Thomas, 1970.

180. Zdeblick, T. A., and Ducker, T. B.: The use of freeze-dried allograft bone for anterior cervical fusions. Presented at Cervical Spine Research Society meeting, New Orleans, December 1989.

181. Zoma, R. D., Sturrock, R. D., Fisher, W. D., et al.: Surgical stabilization of the rheumatoid spine. A review of indications and results. J. Bone Joint Surg. Br. *69*:8–12, 1987.

Postlaminectomy Kyphosis of the Cervical Spine

Thomas S. Whitecloud III, M.D.

James C. Butler, M.D.

Cervical laminectomy for decompression of the spinal cord and neural structures is a widely accepted surgical procedure. With the advent of anterior procedures of the cervical spine in the mid-1950s, the frequency of posterior cervical surgery diminished. Posterior cervical laminectomy afforded surgeons the ability to perform an extensile decompression of the spine. Indications are to remove external compressive forces on the spinal cord and nerve roots caused by a variety of conditions, including neoplasm, infection, degenerative disease, and degenerative disease with or without myelopathy. Although indicated rarely, decompression of fracture-dislocations can be done posteriorly.[17]

There is an unusually high incidence of instability and deformity following cervical laminectomy in the immature skeleton.[2, 5, 7, 11, 30, 49, 57] Lonstein noted a 49 per cent incidence of postlaminectomy kyphosis in a large series of children treated for spinal cord tumors.[31] In contrast, it is unusual for a kyphotic deformity or instability to result after multilevel laminectomy in the adult cervical spine.[1] Instability was previously believed to result if there had been a violation of facet joints during the laminectomy procedure, but Bailey showed that instability could be created by either bony deficiency or muscular imbalance.[3, 9, 27, 41, 51] White and coworkers suggested that instability can occur when the load-bearing capabilities of either the anterior or the posterior structures of the spinal motion segment are compromised.[54]

The biomechanical effects of multiple-level cervical laminectomy on spinal stability are beginning to be defined. Controversy exists over the relative incidence of instability following posterior cervical decompressive procedures. This controversy exists because of a lack of uniformity with regard to the surgical procedure performed, the extent of surgical decompression, and the patient population, particularly with respect to age groups.[29] Johnson and colleagues demonstrated that although cervical laminectomy alone diminished spinal stability by 20 per cent, disruption of the facet joints caused a 60 per cent increase in spinal instability.[28]

IATROGENIC CERVICAL KYPHOSIS IN CHILDREN

In the past, cervical laminectomy was performed in the immature spine primarily for treatment of spinal cord tumors. The difficulty in calculating the true incidence of postlaminectomy kyphosis in these patients has been attributed largely to the high morbidity associated with the disease itself. Haft and associates reported on 30 children ranging in age from 3 months to 15 years who underwent laminectomy for intradural and extradural tumors.[22] Of those who survived, 10 of 17 developed kyphoscoliosis. Bette and Engelhardt described three young patients in whom a dislocation occurred following laminectomy of the cervical spine.[7] Cattell and Clark reported severe kyphosis, anterior subluxation, and instability in the cervical spine in three children following multiple laminectomies.[12] They concluded that the causes of instability might include skeletal and ligamentous deficiencies, neuromuscular imbalance, and progressive osseous deformities consequent to bone growth. Lonstein and colleagues reviewed 32 patients younger than 20 years of age who had laminectomies, 19 of them for spinal cord tumors.[33] All patients developed a spinal deformity in the area of the laminectomy. In 26 of these patients, the kyphotic deformity averaged 82 degrees. In 1965, Tachdjian and Matson, in an evaluation of intraspinal tumors in infants and children, cited 17 cases of late kyphotic deformities of the cervical spine in 24 patients undergoing laminectomy.[50]

Other studies indicate an extremely high incidence of deformity following cervical laminectomy in children.[8, 18, 22] Sim and colleagues, in a report of 21 patients with postlaminectomy deformity, described five patients younger than 18 years of age who developed kyphosis following cervical laminectomy.[45] In addition to the surgical procedure, each of these five patients had an underlying neurologic disease that produced significant neuromuscular imbalance, which may have contributed to the development of the kyphotic deformity. Sim theorized that the instability caused by laminectomy, combined with weakness of the cervical muscles further aggravated by immobilization, caused the subluxation and deformity that subsequently developed.

Surgical compromise of the articular facet joints and their capsules has been implicated as a possible cause of postsurgical kyphosis.[28, 31, 32] The importance of the articular facet joint with regard to spinal stability has been demonstrated in both animal and cadaver experiments.[36, 38] However, Yasouka and coworkers were able to demonstrate postlaminectomy kyphotic deformity in several patients in whom the articular facet joints were not damaged.[56] They theorized that changes in spinal biomechanics caused by laminectomy alone increased compressive forces placed on the anterior vertebral body, leading to a wedging deformity of its cartilaginous portions and, later, alterations in vertebral body ossification. This, combined with an already acknowledged increased viscoelasticity of ligaments in children, could lead to a kyphotic deformity with intact posterior facet joints.

POSTLAMINECTOMY KYPHOSIS IN ADULTS

The development of kyphotic deformities following laminectomy in adult patients is less predictable when compared with the uniformly high rate in children and adolescents. Whereas the primary indication for laminectomy in children is for neoplastic disease, cervical laminectomy in the adult population is commonly performed for the treatment of degenerative disorders of the spine resulting in cervical radiculopathy, myelopathy, or a combination of both. Panjabi and colleagues, in a study of cervical spine biomechanics, experimentally demonstrated a progressively increasing degree of cervical instability to flexion loads with sequential removal of posterior supporting elements of

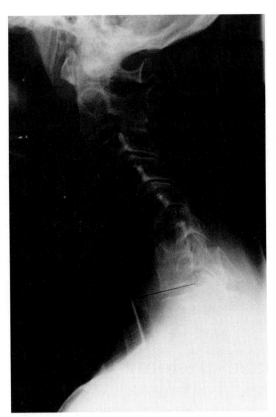

Figure 54–6. Adult postlaminectomy kyphosis that developed despite subsequent spontaneous anterior fusion.

the cervical spine (Fig. 54–6).[38] They noted that the most significant loss of stability occurred with removal of the posterior articular facet joints in the spine model with flexion loads placed on it. Saito and associates, in a finite element analysis of normal and postlaminectomy models, revealed that the primary cause of deformity was the removal of posterior ligaments and spinous processes from the cervical spine.[43] In the postlaminectomy model, tension was found to be transferred to the articular facet joints, with the resultant muscular imbalance subsequently leading to increased stresses on the vertebral bodies and a resultant wedging deformity. They also found that the development of kyphosis was related to the gravitational center of the head. When the center of gravity was located anterior to the midline, a kyphotic deformity occurred.

Rogers was one of the earliest advocates of wide cervical laminectomy in the treatment of cervical spondylotic myelopathy.[41] He noted successful results in 33 patients ranging in age from 38 to 72 years. He failed to specifically address late spinal deformity as a complication of this procedure. Jenkins followed five adults for 12 to 17 years after extensive cervical laminectomy for the treatment of cervical spondylotic myelopathy.[27] This long-term follow-up failed to demonstrate the development of postlaminectomy deformity in the patients studied. Scoville, in a study of patients treated with laminectomy and bilateral facetectomy for cervical spondylosis, thought that there was no risk of anterior dislocation of the cervical spine in older patients.[44] He therefore advocated bilateral multilevel total facetectomies when indicated. This assumption by Scoville has subsequently been proved wrong. Herkowitz, in a comparison of treatment modalities for multilevel spondylotic radiculopathy, noted that three of 12 patients with an average age of 64 years developed kyphotic deformities within two years following cervical laminectomy combined with partial bilateral facetectomies.[25] The contribution of the articular facet joints to posterior stability is now better appreciated. Nowinski and coworkers, in a biomechanical comparison of cervical laminoplasty and laminectomy with progressive facetectomy, found that kyphosis could be created by removal of as little as 25 per cent of the articular facet joint.[37] This is further elaborated in the discussion of the prevention of kyphotic deformities.

Mikawa and associates evaluated 64 patients who had undergone multilevel cervical laminectomy for both cervical spondylosis and ossification of the posterior longitudinal ligament syndrome (OPLL).[34] Eleven per cent of patients undergoing cervical laminectomy for OPLL developed postoperative kyphotic deformities; however, kyphosis did not develop in any patient with pre-existing cervical spondylosis. This study, therefore, supported the theory that adults with cervical spondylosis demonstrate some inherent instability of the spine owing to degenerative changes in the anterior spinal column (Fig. 54–7). This study also refuted the theory that pre-existing ossification foci prevent postlaminectomy cervical instability.

PREVENTION OF POSTLAMINECTOMY KYPHOSIS OF THE CERVICAL SPINE

In view of the profoundly high incidence of postlaminectomy kyphosis in the immature skeleton, children should be followed up routinely with repeat roentgenograms by both a neurosurgeon and an orthopedic surgeon.[7, 12, 31, 50] If it is recognized that a kyphotic deformity is developing, stabilization of that motion segment is warranted. Although it is possible to perform a posterior fusion following laminectomy in a growing child, it may be technically difficult, depending on the amount of bone removed and the amount of posterior bony surface area remaining. As in any case of cervical kyphosis, these patients are best treated initially by having traction applied in an attempt to reduce the deformity prior to stabilization. There are no data to suggest that external orthoses are effective in preventing the development of a deformity in the immature spine.

In the adult cervical spine, postlaminectomy kyphotic deformity occurs less frequently than in the immature spine. In adults with no preoperative spinal instability and reasonably normal spinal alignment, laminectomy alone rarely causes clinically symptomatic cervical kyphosis.[20, 32, 44, 59] What appears to be the most critical factor with regard to the late occurrence of postlaminectomy kyphosis in the cervical spine is the maintenance of the integrity of the articular facet joints and their capsules. Surgical compromise of the articular facet joints and their capsules has been impli-

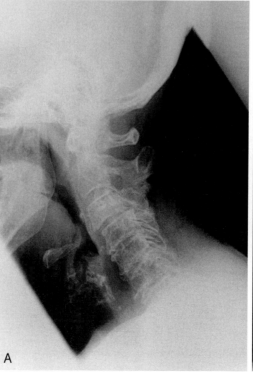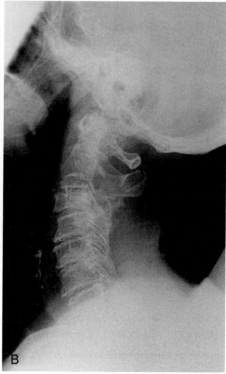

Figure 54–7. Lateral radiographs of an 80-year-old patient six years after laminectomy. *A,* Dynamic flexion views show no significant instability with active motion. *B,* Dynamic extension views show no significant instability with active motion.

cated as a cause of postsurgical kyphosis, and their importance with regard to spinal stability has been demonstrated in both animal and cadaver experiments.[27, 39, 44, 59] Munechica attempted to assess the importance of the articular facets and posterior laminae with regard to spinal stability in monkeys.[36] Laminectomy alone did not lead to deformity when fewer than five laminae were removed; however, a kyphotic deformity was noted to develop when laminectomy was associated with the resection of only one facet joint. Epstein, in an effort to stress the importance of the articular facet joint for postoperative stability, cautioned that no more than one third of the articular facet should be removed when performing a foramina decompression.[19] Zdeblick studied the effects of facet capsule resection and the progressive facetectomy with respect to cervical stability.[59, 60] In both cases, biomechanical testing was performed on specimens following progressive excision of the articular capsules or following progressively increasing facetectomies. These biomechanical tests demonstrated that greater than 50 per cent capsular resection led to a significant loss in spinal stability. Similarly, when 50 per cent or more of the articular facets were removed, a significant loss of spinal stability followed. However, the integrity of the articular facet joint and its capsule is not the only determining factor in the development of postlaminectomy deformity. Yonenobu and colleagues, in a study comparing subtotal carpectomy to laminoplasty in the treatment of cervical spondylotic myelopathy, found that 10 per cent of the laminoplasty patients later developed kyphosis when the articular facets and their capsules were left intact.[58]

SURGICAL TREATMENT FOR POSTLAMINECTOMY CERVICAL KYPHOSIS

When it becomes necessary to surgically stabilize a cervical spine with an established or progressing kyphotic deformity, it is necessary to achieve a solid arthrodesis of the unstable motion segments. The surgeon should decide whether an anterior or posterior procedure is indicated. A period of preoperative skeletal traction using either a halo device or skull tongs is suggested for significant kyphotic deformities, in an attempt to achieve maximum passive correction prior to surgery. Improvement of the kyphotic deformity before surgery usually makes the operative procedure technically easier and lessens the chance of neurologic injury caused by spinal manipulation of an anesthetized patient. Some kyphotic deformities may be relatively rigid, demonstrating little reversal with preoperative traction, and may require fusion in situ. Minor degrees of deformity usually do not require skeletal traction before the actual operative procedure.

Anterior Procedures for Stabilizing the Kyphotic Cervical Spine

Anterior spinal reconstruction and stabilization afford the surgeon the ability to directly decompress neural elements if neurologic compromise occurs as a result of postlaminectomy kyphosis. Preoperative assessment should include flexion and extension roentgenograms to determine whether the deformity is passively correctable. If radiographs demonstrate that a significant reversal of the kyphosis can be achieved and that the deformity is not rigid, a period of preoperative skeletal traction may not be necessary. A successful multilevel anterior cervical fusion must be achieved even for patients without neurologic compromise. Several techniques have been developed that allow stabilization by an anterior interbody fusion technique.[4, 13, 46, 47] One distinct disadvantage of either the Smith-Robinson or the Cloward technique is that it provides no immediate spinal stabilization. These techniques should not be used when more than two motion segments require fusion anteriorly, because of the increased risk of pseudarthrosis and graft extrusion.[14, 16, 48, 53]

The development of surgical techniques that use cortical bone obtained from the fibula provides a graft material that can span multiple segments and resist compressive forces without fracturing (Fig. 54–8).[6, 55] Initially, the use of fibula for graft material was advocated by Stauffer and Kelly for stabilization following fractures, and subsequently by Whitecloud and LaRocca when anterior decompression for multiple segments was required for the relief of cervical myelopathy.[48, 55] These and other authors reported a high rate of union using either autogenous or allograft fibula as

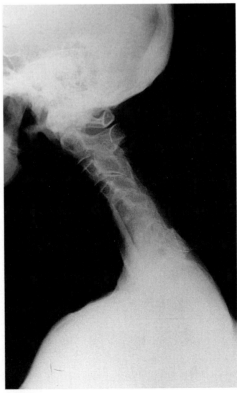

Figure 54–8. Anterior arthrodesis using fibular graft for postlaminectomy kyphosis. Excellent graft incorporation is noted two years after surgery.

graft material, and essentially no incidence of graft failure. Successful fusions have been achieved over as many as five cervical segments. Other authors have described techniques of utilizing corticocancellous iliac crest grafts when spanning multiple spinal segments.[4, 14] It is not believed that the constructs are strong enough to resist compressive forces if more than two motion segments are to be stabilized, however. Graft subsidence and recurrence of deformity are concerns regardless of the graft composition.

In the presence of neurologic compromise, direct anterior neural decompression must be performed in association with the reconstructive procedure. Subtotal carpectomies allow adequate spinal decompression. The reconstructive portion of the procedure with either interbody grafts for short segments or fibula grafts for reconstructions spanning three or more disc space levels may then be performed. Anterior reconstruction for postlaminectomy kyphosis as described does not provide immediate spinal stability, and the incidence of nonunion is increased in the presence of compromise of the posterior bony structures, as seen following cervical laminectomy with or without facetectomy. Adjunctive immobilization, therefore, should be considered. External immobilization using either a rigid orthosis or a halo-vest is recommended.

The development of anterior cervical plating systems may afford a degree of immediate spinal stability that alleviates the need for external immobilization following surgery. The exact indications for anterior cervical plating require further definition. Anterior plate fixation produces immediate rigidity and anterior column support for the reconstruction. The anterior column may be reconstructed using iliac crest, autogenous or allograft fibula, or a prosthetic cage (Fig. 54–9). Herman and Sonntag reported on 20 patients with symptomatic postlaminectomy kyphosis treated with anterior decompression, bone grafting, and anterior cervical plating.[26] All 20 patients exhibited anterior compressive pathology requiring spinal cord decompression in addition to spinal reconstruction. No patient had correction of kyphosis or improved enough neurologically with preoperative skeletal traction to be considered a candidate for a posterior stabilization procedure. These authors reported a 100 per cent union rate utilizing plates that span an average of 3.8 levels. These patients were noted to have on average a 16-degree residual kyphosis, with 65 per cent of neurologic symptoms either resolved or improved long term.[26]

Heller and Silcox suggest that anterior reconstruction followed by posterior segmental instrumentation and fusion may be considered as an alternative to anterior reconstruction and plating.[24] Biomechanical data suggest that such posterior fixation is more stable than anterior fixation. The extensive nature of this approach may exclude the elderly and patients with significant medical problems; however, it may be indicated in individuals considered to be high risks for nonunion, such as in the presence of osteoporosis or long-term steroid use.

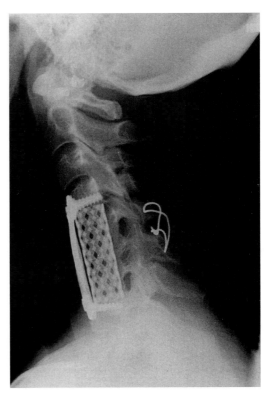

Figure 54–9. The most recent developments allowing anterior column reconstruction involve the use of a titanium prosthetic cage to reconstruct the anterior column. Bone graft material is placed within the cage. Plate fixation affords immediate stability to the construct.

When postlaminectomy cervical kyphosis is found to be fixed and not passively correctable by preoperative skeletal traction, or when it is suggested by flexion and extension lateral cervical radiographs, one must determine whether symptomatic neurologic compression exists. In the absence of neurologic compression, the objective is achieving a successful arthrodesis. One must decide whether the deformity requires only stabilization and fusion in situ or whether the deformity requires correction. Neurologic compression in the presence of postlaminectomy cervical kyphosis obviously requires anterior decompression, regardless of whether the surgeon undertakes the task of attempting to correct the deformity. Reduction of kyphosis may be a secondary goal in such cases, because the attempted reduction carries substantial intraoperative risks for neurologic injury.

Stabilization of the Cervical Spine by Posterior Fusion

Surgical techniques for posterior cervical fusion following cervical laminectomy were developed primarily to be performed immediately following the laminectomy procedure. Several technical problems exist when attempting a posterior stabilization procedure following cervical laminectomy, and these problems are only enhanced by postoperative scar formation in the presence of exposed dura and neural elements. Following an extensive cervical laminectomy, very little bony surface area may be available to achieve a solid arthrodesis. This problem is compounded by the presence of a previous aggressive partial or complete facetectomy. In the presence of segmental instability, posterior on-lay bone grafts are exposed to tensile rather than compressive forces, which increase the risk for pseudoarthrosis. The widely exposed dura is also at risk for injury during the operative procedure. If attempted reduction or improvement of the kyphosis is intended, spinal alignment is maintained during the procedure via skeletal traction using a halo-ring or cranial tongs. Some form of internal fixation, whether facet wires or rigid plate fixation, is usually advised. If a basic on-lay fusion technique is chosen, external immobilization in a halo-vest is recommended postoperatively.

Robinson and Southwick described a technique of facet wiring that can be used following laminectomy.[40] This procedure involves the passage of wires through the articular facet joints at all involved segments. Two longitudinal struts of corticocancellous bone may be attached to the facet wires. A variation of this procedure involves attachment of the wires to either a Luque rectangle or bent Steinmann pins (Fig. 54–10). This is particularly useful when immediate fixation is necessary or when the bone grafts are mechanically deficient. Sim and colleagues presented three cases of postlaminectomy kyphotic deformity stabilized using a tibial strut graft in which the graft was secured by means of wire sutures through the first intact spinous

process above and below the laminectomy.[45] The laminectomy defect itself was thus spanned. Fairbank described a posterior fusion technique using a long, H-shaped corticocancellous iliac graft.[21] This technique, however, resulted in only three of five patients obtaining a solid fusion. When the Southwick technique is modified by the implementation of internal fixation pins or a Luque rectangle, the bone graft is applied as an on-lay graft procedure. In any of the above-mentioned constructs, postoperative immobilization is recommended.[10]

As an alternative to facet wiring, more recent developments using posterior plates and lateral mass or pedicle screws may be considered. Presently, studies are relatively short and few. These procedures require a great deal of technical expertise, and the risk for neurologic or vascular injury is a concern. Roy-Camille and colleagues were the first to develop a screw-plate system for posterior osteosynthesis of the cervical spine.[42] Biomechanical studies have demonstrated the advantage of these constructs when compared with standard wiring configurations.[15, 35, 52] Biomechanical tests have found posterior plates to be equivalent or superior to anterior plating systems.

The lateral mass screw and plating technique is now beginning to gain acceptance. Reports, results, and complications using this system are now being reported. Heller and associates attempted to define the risk of posterior lateral mass screw insertion by comparing the Roy-Camille and Magerl screw techniques.[23] Their cadaveric study found a 2 per cent rate of nerve root injury using the Roy-Camille insertional tech-

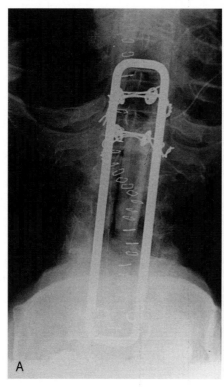
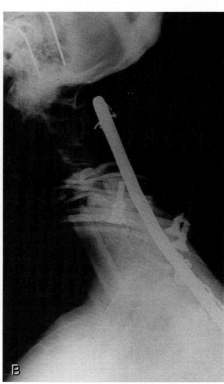

Figure 54–10. A combined anterior fibular strut graft with posterior Luque rectangle fixation was used to stabilize a postlaminectomy kyphotic deformity. *A,* Anterior radiograph. *B,* Lateral radiograph. More advanced techniques involving either anterior or posterior plate fixation have now replaced this procedure.

nique, as compared with a 6 per cent rate using the Magerl technique. In addition to nerve root or vertebral artery injury, other complications such as hardware failure or loosening, pseudarthrosis, and infection are presently being assessed.

References

 1. Aronson, D. D., Filtzer, D. K., and Bagan, M.: Anterior cervical fusion by the Smith-Robinson approach. J. Neurosurg. 29:397–404, 1968.
 2. Aronson, D. D., Kahn, R. J., and Canady, A.: Cervical spine instability following suboccipital decompression and cervical laminectomy for Arnold-Chiari syndrome. (Abstract.) Presented at the 56th annual meeting of the American Academy of Orthopaedic Surgeons, Las Vegas, 1989.
 3. Bailey, R. W.: Dislocation of the cervical spine. In Bailey, R. W., Sherk, H. H., Dunn, E. J., et al. (eds.): The Cervical Spine. Philadelphia, J. B. Lippincott Co., 1983, pp. 362–387.
 4. Bailey, R. W., and Badgley, C. E.: Stabilization of the cervical spine and anterior fusion. J. Bone Joint Surg. Am. 42:565–594, 1960.
 5. Bell, D. F., Walker, J. L., O'Connor, G., and Tibshirani, R.: Spinal deformity after multiple-level cervical laminectomy in children. Spine 4:406–411, 1994.
 6. Bernard, T. N., and Whitecloud, T. S.: Cervical spondylotic myelopathy and myeloradiculopathy: Anterior decompression and stabilization with autogenous fibula strut graft. Clin. Orthop. 221:149–160, 1987.
 7. Bette, H., and Engelhardt, H.: Folgezustande von Laminektomien an der Halswerbelsaule. Z. Orthop. 85:564–573, 1955.
 8. Boersma, G.: Curvatures of the Spine Following Laminectomies in Children. Amsterdam, Born, 1969.
 9. Braun, W.: Chirurgische Therapie. In Lewandowsky, M. (ed.): Handbuch der Neurologie. Vol. 1. All-gemeine Neurologie. Berlin, J. Springer, 1910, pp. 1251–1292.
10. Callahan, R. A., Johnson, R. M., Margolis, R. N., et al.: Cervical facet fusion for control of instability following laminectomy. J. Bone Joint Surg. Am. 59:991–1002, 1977.
11. Caspar, W.: Anterior stabilization with the trapezial osteosynthetic plate technique in cervical spine injuries. In Kehr, P., and Weidner, A. (eds.): Cervical Spine 1. New York, Springer Verlag, 1987, pp. 198–204.
12. Cattell, H. S., and Clark, G. L., Jr.: Cervical kyphosis and instability following multiple laminectomies in children. J. Bone Joint Surg. Am. 59:991–1002, 1977.
13. Cloward, R. B.: The anterior approach for removal of ruptured cervical discs. J. Neurosurg. 15:602–617, 1958.
14. Cloward, R. B.: Treatment of acute fractures and fracture dislocations of the cervical spine by vertebral body fusion. A report of eleven cases. J. Neurosurg. 18:201–209, 1961.
15. Coe, J. D., Warden, K. E., Sutterlin, C. E., and McAfee, P. C.: Biomechanical evaluation of cervical spinal stabilization methods in a human cadaveric model. Spine 14:1123–1131, 1989.
16. Connolly, E., Seymour, R., and Adams, J.: Clinical evaluation of anterior cervical fusions for degenerative cervical disc disease. J. Neurosurg. 23:431–437, 1965.
17. Cooper, O. R., and Ransohoff, J.: Injuries of the cervical cord—surgical treatment. In Bailey, R. W., Sherk, H. H., Dunn, E. J., et al. (eds.): The Cervical Spine. Philadelphia, J. B. Lippincott Co., 1983, pp. 305–317.
18. Dubousset, J., Buillamant, J., and Mechin, J. F.: Les Compressions Medullaires non Traumatiques de l'Infant. Paris, Masson, 1973.
19. Epstein, J. A.: The surgical management of cervical spinal stenosis, spondylosis, and myeloradiculopathy by means of the posterior approach. Spine 13:864–869, 1988.
20. Fager, C. A.: Results of adequate posterior decompression in the relief of spondylotic cervical myelopathy. J. Neurosurg. 38:684–692, 1973.
21. Fairbank, T. J.: Spinal fusion after laminectomy for cervical myelopathy. Proc. R. Soc. Med. 64:634–636, 1971.
22. Haft, H., Ransohoff, J., and Carter, S.: Spinal cord tumors in children. Pediatrics 23:1152–1159, 1959.
23. Heller, J. G., Carlson, G. D., Abitbol, J. J., and Garfin, S. R.: Anatomic comparison of the Roy-Camille and Magerl techniques for screw placement in the lower cervical spine. Spine 16(S):552–557, 1991.
24. Heller, J. G., and Silcox, D. H.: Postlaminectomy instability of the cervical spine. In Frymoyer, J. W., Ducker, T. B., Hadler, N. M., et al. (eds.): The Adult Spine: Principles and Practice. 2nd ed. Philadelphia, Lippincott-Raven, 1997, pp. 1413–1434.
25. Herkowitz, H. N.: A comparison of anterior cervical fusion, cervical laminectomy, and cervical laminoplasty for the surgical management of multiple level spondylotic radiculopathy. Spine 13:774–780, 1988.
26. Herman, J. M., and Sonntag, V. K. H.: Cervical carpectomy and plate fixation for postlaminectomy kyphosis. J. Neurosurg. 80:963–970, 1994.
27. Jenkins, D. H. R.: Extensive cervical laminectomy: Long term results. Br. J. Surg. 60:852–854, 1973.
28. Johnson, R. M., Owen, J. R., Panjabi, M. M., et al.: Biomechanical stability of the cervical spine using a human cadaver model. Orthop. Trans. 4:46, 1980.
29. Katsumi, Y., Honma, T., and Nakamura, T.: Analysis of cervical instability resulting from laminectomies for removal of spinal cord tumor. Spine 14:1171–1176, 1989.
30. LaRocca, S. H.: Personal communication, 1989.
31. Lonstein, J. E.: Postlaminectomy kyphosis. Clin. Orthop. 128:93–100, 1977.
32. Lonstein, J. E.: Postlaminectomy kyphosis. In Chou, S. N., and Seljeskog, E. L. (eds.): Spinal Deformities and Neurological Dysfunction. New York, Raven Press, 1978, pp. 53–63.
33. Lonstein, J. E., Winter, R. B., Bradford, D. B., et al.: Postlaminectomy spine deformity. J. Bone Joint Surg. Am. 58:727, 1976.
34. Mikawa, Y., Shikata, J., and Yamamuro, T.: Spinal deformity and instability after multi-level cervical laminectomy. Spine 12:6–11, 1987.
35. Montesano, P. X., Juach, E. C., Anderson, P. A., et al.: Biomechanics of cervical spine internal fixation. Spine 16(S):11–16, 1991.
36. Munechica, Y.: Influence of laminectomy on the stability of the spine: An experimental study with special reference to the extent of laminectomy and the resection of the intervertebral joint. J. Jpn. Orthop. Assoc. 47:111–126, 1973.
37. Nowinski, G. P., Visarious, H., Nolte, L. P., and Herkowitz, H. N.: A biomechanical comparison of cervical laminoplasty and cervical laminectomy with progressive facetectomy. Spine 18:1995–2004, 1993.
38. Panjabi, M. M., White, A. A., and Johnson, R. M.: Cervical spine biomechanics as a function of transection of components. J. Biomech. 8:327–336, 1975.
39. Raynor, R. B., Pugh, J., and Shapiro, I.: Cervical facetectomy and its effect on spine strength. J. Neurosurg. 63:278–282, 1985.
40. Robinson, R. A., and Southwick, W. O.: Indications and technics for early stabilization of the neck in some fracture dislocations of the cervical spine. South. Med. J. 53:565–579, 1960.
41. Rogers, L.: The surgical treatment of cervical spondylotic myelopathy: Mobilization of the complete cervical cord into an enlarged canal. J. Bone Joint Surg. Br. 43:3–6. 1961.
42. Roy-Camille, R., Mazel, C. H., and Soullant, G: Treatment of cervical spine injuries by a posterior osteosynthesis with plates and screws. In Kehr, P., and Weidner, A. (eds.): Cervical Spine I. New York, Springer Verlag, 1987, pp. 163–174.
43. Saito, T., Yamamuro, T., Shikata, J., et al.: Analysis and prevention of spinal column deformity following cervical laminectomy. I. Pathogenic analysis of postlaminectomy deformities. Spine 16:494–502, 1991.
44. Scoville, W. B.: Cervical spondylosis treated by bilateral facetectomy and laminectomy. J. Neurosurg. 18:423–428, 1961.
45. Sim, F. H., Suien, H. J., Bickel, W. H., and Janes, J. M.: Swanneck deformity following extensive cervical laminectomy. J. Bone Joint Surg. Am. 56:564–580, 1974.
46. Simmons, E. H., and Bhalla, S. K.: Anterior cervical discectomy and fusion: A clinical and biomechanical study with eight year follow-up. J. Bone Joint Surg. Br. 51:225–237, 1969.
47. Smith, G. W., and Robinson, R. A.: The treatment of certain cervical spine disorders by anterior removal of intervertebral disc and interbody fusion. J. Bone Joint Surg. Am. 40:607–624, 1958.

48. Stauffer, E. S., and Kelly, E.G.: Fracture-dislocations of the cervical spine. Instability and recurrent deformity following treatment by anterior interbody fusion. J. Bone Joint Surg. Am. *59*:45–48, 1977.
49. Stuck, R. M.: Anterior cervical disc excision and fusion: Report of 200 consecutive cases. Rocky Mountain Med. J. *60*:25–30, 1963.
50. Tachdjian, M. O., and Matson, D. D.: Orthopaedic aspects of intraspinal tumors in infants and children. J. Bone Joint Surg. Am. *47*:223–248, 1965.
51. Teng, P.: Spondylosis of the cervical spine with compression of the spinal cord and nerve roots. J. Bone Joint Surg. Am. *42*:392–407, 1960.
52. Ulrich, C., Woersdoerfer, O., Claes, L., and Magerl, F.: Comparative study of the stability of anterior and posterior cervical spine fixation procedures. Arch. Orthop. Trauma Surg. *106*:226–231, 1987.
53. White, A. A., III, Southwick, W. O., DePonte, R. J., et al.: Relief of pain by anterior cervical spine fusion for spondylosis: A report of sixty-five cases. J. Bone Joint Surg. Am. *55*:525–534, 1973.
54. White, A. A., Panjabi, M. M., and Thomas, C. L.: The clinical biomechanics of kyphotic deformities. Clin. Orthop. *128*:8–17, 1977.
55. Whitecloud, T. S., and LaRocca, H.: Fibular strut graft in reconstructive surgery of the cervical spine. Spine *1*:33–43, 1976.
56. Yasouka, S., Paterson, H. A., Laws, E. R., and MacCarty, C. S.: Pathogenesis and prophylaxis of postlaminectomy deformity of the spine after multiple level laminectomy: Difference between children and adults. Neurosurgery *9*:145–152, 1981.
57. Yasouka, S., Peterson, H. A., and MacCarty, C. S.: Incidence of spinal deformity after multi-level laminectomy: Difference between children and adults. Neurosurgery *9*:145–152, 1982.
58. Yonenobu, K., Hosono, N., Iwasaki, M., et al.: Laminoplasty versus subtotal carpectomy: A comparative study of results in multi segmental cervical spondylotic myelopathy. Spine *17*:1281–1284, 1992.
59. Zdeblick, T. A., Zou, D., Warden, K. E., et al.: Cervical stability after foraminotomy: A biomechanical in vitro analysis. J. Bone Joint Surg. *74*:22–27, 1992.
60. Zdeblick, T. A., Abitol, J. J., Kunz, D. N., et al.: Cervical stability after sequential capsule resection. Spine *18*:2005–2008, 1993.

Complications Associated With Posterior Spinal Instrumentation

Patrick J. Connolly, M.D.

Bruce E. Fredrickson, M.D.

Hansen A. Yuan, M.D.

Instrumentation of the spine is often used by spine surgeons. Currently there are a number of instrumentation systems available. These systems vary on the basis of their location of application, rigidity, or segmental characteristics. Selection of a particular posterior spinal system is dependent on the diagnosis, the specific requirements of the patient, and the surgeon's experience. In general, rigid implants do not rely on the ligaments or articulations of the spine for their support. To some degree, semirigid implants are load sharing and obtain some of their stability from the articulations and ligamentous attachments of the individual motion segments. Systems that are segmental allow attachment of the device to each individual vertebra. The method of attachment may be rigid (pedicle screw) or semirigid (hooks or wires).

Posterior spinal instrumentation is used effectively for two reasons: to change the spacial relationships of the vertebrae (i.e., to reduce the fracture), and to maintain the position of the vertebrae to enhance fusion. Without bone grafting, posterior spinal instrumentation is rarely used in the adult population. A solid fusion is required in all cases of instrumentation, or the device will ultimately fail.

HISTORY

The first use of internal fixation in the spine was by Hadra in 1891.[48] He used a wire to fix a cervical fracture-dislocation posteriorly. Following this introduction, the history of internal fixation of the spine has maintained an association with the history of spinal fusion.[3, 51, 124] Lange[69] was the first to implant a metal rod in an attempt to increase spinal stability. In 1936,

Jenkins[55] of New Zealand used a peg of tibia to fix L5–S1 anteriorly in a case of spondylolisthesis. Mercer[90] in 1936 and Speed[106] in 1938 described similar procedures involving the use of bone peg as a form of internal fixation at the L5–S1 junction for spondylolisthesis.

The first extensive use of posterior internal fixation was by King[59] in 1948. He used screws placed across the facet joints to increase the fusion rate in lumbosacral fusions. Boucher in 1959[11] and Andrews in 1986[4] described a similar procedure. Wilson and colleagues in 1952 described the use of a metal plate held to the spinous processes by a series of bolts.[123] They listed four specific objectives in their use of internal fixation: (1) to provide absolute immobilization of the operative area while fusion was occurring, (2) to shorten the period of postoperative recovery, (3) to reduce postoperative discomfort, and (4) to reduce the number of failed fusions.

The report of Harrington in 1962[49, 124] marked the beginning of the application of current techniques of internal fixation of the lumbar spine. His device relied on hooks placed around the lamina for purchase of the spine. Fixation was not segmental, and the construct was classified as semirigid. Modifications of the Harrington device have been made by several investigators.[103, 104] A distraction rod was specifically developed for the lumbar spine by Knodt and reported on by Beattie.[7] Their system was for use over one or two segments and formed a semirigid construct. Jacobs and colleagues reported on a stronger threaded device with a proximal locking hook in an attempt to decrease the incidence of hook dislodgement and rod breakage.[54] White and coworkers,[120] Selby,[102] and Lee and De Bari[71] reported on their results using the Knodt device. Kaneda and coworkers[57] reported on a similar device supplemented with compression hooks to help attain stability. Edwards and Levine[27] increased the torsional stability of the basic Harrington rods by the addition of polyethylene rod sleeves.

Segmental posterior systems were introduced to North American orthopedists by Luque.[76-81] Fixation was by sublaminar wires twisted to solid contoured rods. The technique is segmental, but only semirigid. Segmental techniques involving purchase by transpedicle screws were initially developed in Europe by Roy-Camille and associates[97-99] and later popularized by Louis.[74] An external pedicle fixation system was introduced by Magerl,[84, 85] modified by Dick,[21, 22] and reported by Aebi and colleagues.[2] Pedicle systems are segmental and provide rigid immobilization, with the exception of the Edwards system, which is semirigid. The initial systems using the transpedicle techniques in North America included those developed by Steffee and colleagues,[107] Edwards,[26, 27, 29] Wiltse,[47] Krag,[66] and Luque.[78] Today, numerous systems are available that rely on pedicle screw fixation.

OVERVIEW OF COMPLICATIONS

The surgical complications associated with posterior spinal instrumentation can be divided into three broad categories: (1) complications associated with all spine surgery, (2) complications associated with posterior fusion, and (3) specific complications associated with posterior instrumentation.[6, 9, 19, 28, 30, 35, 40, 42, 50, 87, 95, 96, 101, 110, 113, 114, 117, 118]

As in all surgical procedures, the avoidance of complications in spine surgery starts with the initial patient assessment and attention to detail. Kostuik and others have described the "three W's" of surgical failure: the wrong patient, the wrong diagnosis, and the wrong surgery.[61] Patients with strong psychosocial pathology are less likely to have a successful surgical outcome. Performing the right operation at the wrong level, or performing an inadequate operation at the right level, obviously contributes to a less successful surgical outcome.

As in all surgeries, the anesthesiologist plays an important role in the avoidance of surgical complications. Perioperative fluid and airway management are of utmost importance in the avoidance of pulmonary complications.[40] Posterior spinal instrumentation is generally performed in the prone position, and patient positioning is of utmost importance. Superficial skin irritation and transient ulnar neuritis are the most common position-associated complications.[40, 117] Other rare complications secondary to poor positioning and distribution of pressure are central retinal artery occlusion leading to blindness, carotid artery kinking leading to cerebral vascular accident, and femoral artery occlusion leading to lower extremity compartment syndrome.

The majority of patients who require posterior spinal fusion supplemented by posterior spinal instrumentation have an additional requirement for autologous bone harvested from the posterior ilium. Up to 15 per cent of patients have significant pain lasting longer than three months from the bone graft donor site.[39] Obtaining meticulous hemostasis and suction drainage to minimize hematoma formation, as well as careful closure of the gluteal musculature after periosteal stripping, are surgical principles that will help decrease the pain from the posterior bone graft donor site.

Difficulties associated with posterior spinal instrumentation can be broadly categorized into problems associated with poor implant placement, inadequate fixation, and pseudarthrosis.[6, 9, 19, 28, 30, 35, 40, 42, 50, 87, 89, 94-96, 101, 110-114, 117, 118] Spinal implants should not be used unless the surgeon has an excellent working knowledge of spinal anatomy.[19, 32, 34, 91, 100] Complications are significantly decreased when the surgeon has a thorough understanding of the biomechanics of posterior spinal fixation and does not expect the instrumentation to perform a role beyond its capabilities.[18, 72, 73, 116, 121, 127] Finally, pseudarthrosis will eventually lead to implant fracture or loosening. The surgeon must pay attention to the technical details of the spinal fusion. The spinal implants are an aid to the fusion, not a substitute.

COMPLICATIONS SECONDARY TO POSTERIOR SPINAL INSTRUMENTATION

Accelerated Degeneration Above or Below the Fusion (Fig. 54–15)

Accelerated degenerative change in motion segments above or below a spinal fusion has been a concern of spine surgeons for many years. Recent reports suggest an accelerated breakdown in patients with rigid metal fixation compared with those with no fixation.[53, 65] Whether the etiology of this accelerated degenerative change is secondary to implant rigidity or implant-induced facet impingement is unknown. To avoid creating further problems for a patient with accelerated degenerative changes, the surgeon must carefully plan the levels that require instrumentation and fusion. In general, spinal fusion should not end at an area of spinal stenosis, spondylolisthesis, rotatory subluxation, or posterior column deficiency.[12] If possible, fusion should stop at a level where the disc is "normal" above or below the level of fusion.

Pseudarthrosis (Fig. 54–13)

The rate of pseudarthrosis following posterior spinal fusion varies from 0 to 30 per cent.[5, 9, 15, 52, 118, 119] The criteria and the technique to diagnose pseudarthrosis have not been fully defined. Imaging studies are obscured by posterior spinal implants. Although pain is often associated with pseudarthrosis following spinal surgery, not all patients with pseudarthrosis have pain, and not all patients with pain have pseudarthrosis. The more commonly used criteria for determining pseudarthrosis on plain radiographs are movement of greater

Text continued on page 1700

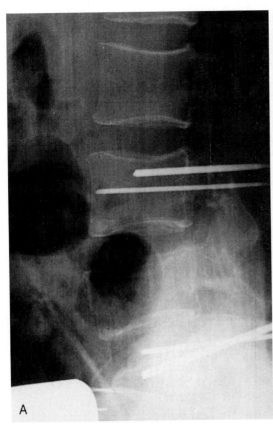

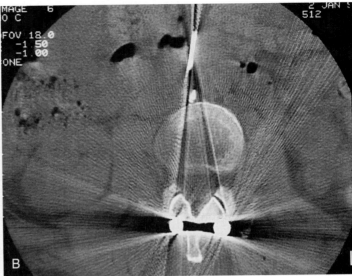

Figure 54–11. Intraoperative radiographs with guide pins are occasionally used to confirm pedicle hole placement before pedicle screw placement *(A)*. These pins must be long enough for retrieval prior to screw placement. The CT scan (B) demonstrates a guide pin that was short and dropped into the abdominal cavity. The patient required a laparotomy for pin retrieval.

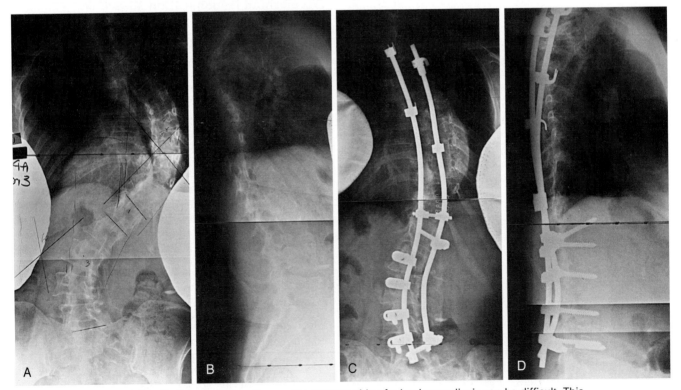

Figure 54–12. Pedicle screw insertion on the concave side of a lumbar scoliosis can be difficult. This patient required an anterior and posterior fusion for a painful progressive scoliosis *(A, B)*. At two-year follow-up, the patient was pain-free, with a solid fusion despite one broken screw at L5 on the concave side *(C, D)*. Having only one screw at L5 on the concave side of a significant curve may be biomechanically unrealistic, and the cause of the screw breakage was overstress of the screw at the time of application.

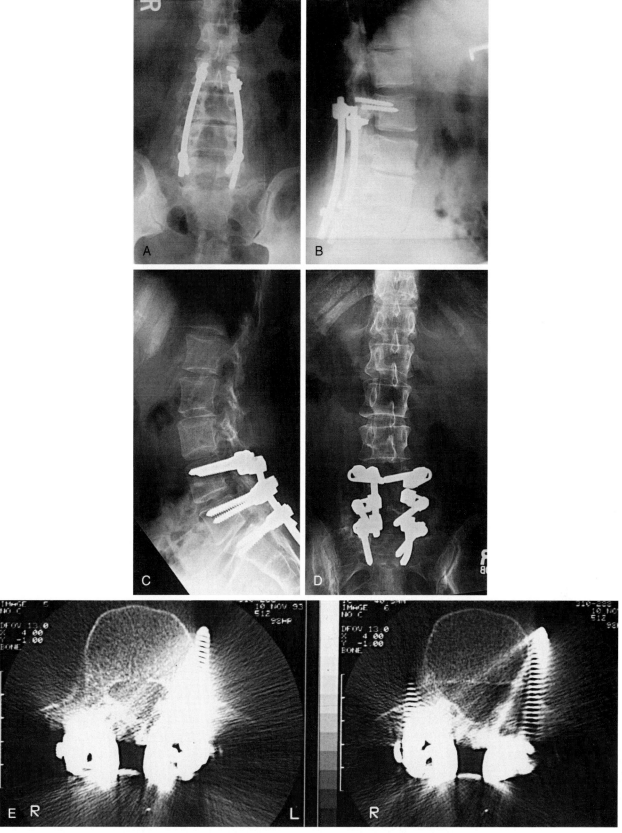

Figure 54–13. Pedicle screw instrumentation of the lumbar spine for degenerative disease may fail secondary to problems associated with the screw *(A, B)*, the rod or plate, the screw-rod connection *(C, D)*, or the bone-screw fixation. Despite excellent fixation, lumbar instrumentation will fail if the patient does not obtain a solid arthrodesis. *A* and *B* show bilateral fracture of the superior screws of a three-level fusion, with probable pseudarthrosis. *C* and *D* demonstrate a failure of the rod-screw. In *E*, a CT scan verifies lateral placement of the pedicle screw. This poorly placed pedicle screw will not provide adequate bone-screw fixation.

Figure 54–14. Lateral radiograph demonstrates a significant decrease in lumbar lordosis associated with uncontoured posterior spinal instrumentation to the lower lumbar spine. Clinically, patients present with a flat-back syndrome, and if they are significantly disabled, they require anterior-posterior osteotomy to re-establish lumbar lordosis.

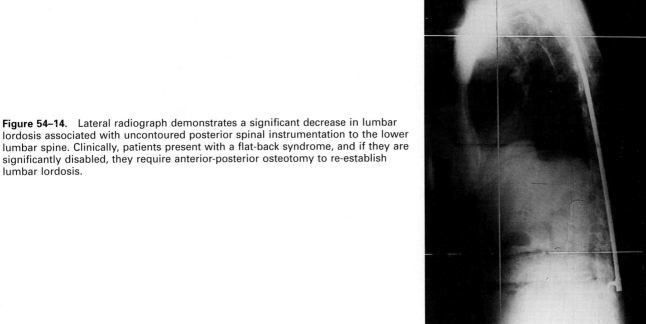

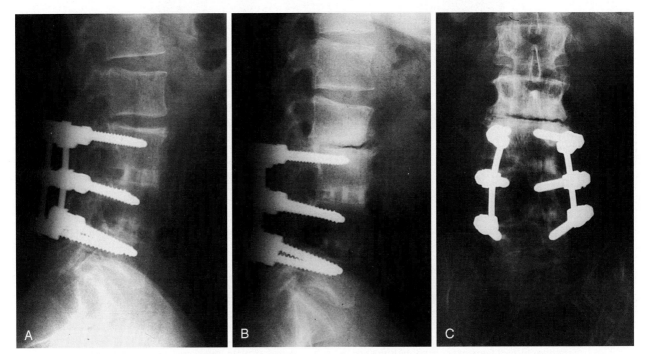

Figure 54–15. Accelerated degenerative change of motion segments above or below spinal fusion has been a concern of spine surgeons for many years. This patient initially had an anterior and posterior fusion from L3 to L5 for disabling back and leg pain (A). The patient was essentially pain-free for approximately three years, until he returned with a recurrence of significant low back pain. Radiographs demonstrated an accelerated degeneration of the L2-L3 motion segment (B, C). Ultimately, the patient's pain was controlled without further surgery.

Figure 54–16. Dural tears are known complications associated with revision spine surgery, with or without posterior spinal instrumentation. Tears may be related to misdirected screws, hooks, or sublaminar wire. The CSF leak needs to be controlled to avoid pseudomeningocele or fistula formation. This patient developed a pseudomeningocele following a revision posterior lumbar fusion. An additional procedure was required to directly repair the dural tear.

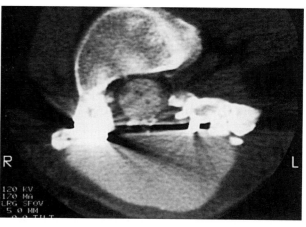

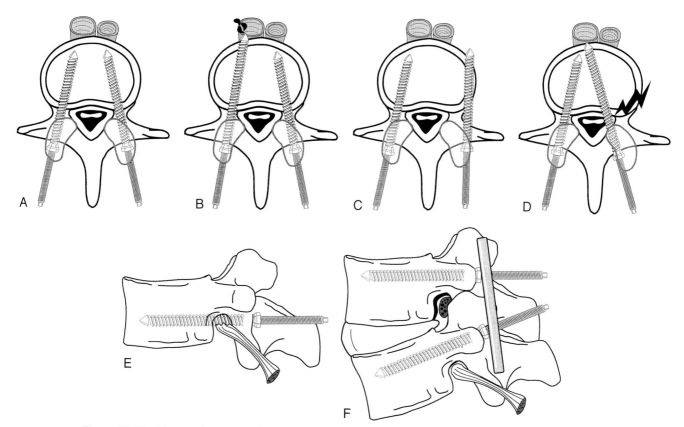

Figure 54–17. Proper placement of pedicle screws is essential to avoid loss of fixation on injury to closely related anatomic structures *(A)*. A screw that is too long can potentially injure the great vessels on the anterior surface of the spine *(B)*. A screw that has an entry point that results in lateral placement outside the pedicle will not provide optimal fixation *(C)*. A medially placed screw in the spinal canal may cause a dural tear and/or neurologic injury *(D)*. An inferiorly placed screw will cause foraminal encroachment and possible nerve root injury or irritation *(E)*. An excessive increase in lumbar lordosis via segmental fixation can cause a secondary foraminal stenosis and nerve root impingement through the facet joints *(F)*.

than 5 degrees on flexion-extension films, screw lucency, and implant fracture.

Meticulous decortication of the transverse process and sacral ala and placement of copious amounts of autologous bone graft prior to the placement of posterior spinal implants are techniques that are important in enhancing the fusion rate.

Iatrogenic Deformity (Fig. 54–14)

The problems of spinal alignment following posterior spinal instrumentation generally fall into the area of loss of correction or overcorrection.[1, 20, 36, 62, 107] In retrospective evaluation of iatrogenic deformity, the etiology is most often secondary to either poor application of spinal instrumentation or poor implant selection. Loss of stabilization and subsequent deformity are potential complications following reduction, instrumentation, and fusion for spine fracture. Hook dislodgement is the most frequently reported complication of posterior Harrington rod instrumentation following spine trauma.[8, 16, 27, 37, 44] The rate of hook dislodgement is dependent on the location of the distal hook and varies from 5 per cent at L4, up to 20 per cent at S1.[44, 115] This complication can be significantly decreased by selection of a more rigid segmental system of fixation.[28] Pedicle screw fracture and subsequent loss of correction of severe lumbar spondylolisthesis have been reported[10, 107] (Fig. 54–12). This complication can be decreased by increasing the number of screws placed in the sacrum and/or adding anterior column support following the initial reduction.[64, 107]

Flat-back syndrome is associated with loss of the normal lumbar lordosis.[1, 62, 63, 92] The most common cause of this syndrome is distraction instrumentation of the lumbar spine that ends caudally at the L5 or S1 level. This complication is best avoided by careful attention to sagittal alignment of the lumbar spine, utilizing contoured segmental fixation, and avoiding overdistraction. As surgeons, we have become more aware of the importance of lumbar lordosis and segmental fixation. A new iatrogenic entity has been introduced that is secondary to increased lumbar lordosis from segmental fixation, causing secondary foraminal stenosis and nerve root impingement.[107] The treatment of these iatrogenic deformities can be quite a challenge; they are therefore best avoided. If an iatrogenic deformity is diagnosed early, it can often be treated by a return to the operating room and subsequent realignment and fusion. In treating delayed complications of iatrogenic deformity, the source of the patient's pain must be identified preoperatively, and the treatment may consist of pseudoarthrosis repair, spinal osteotomy, or further nerve root decompression.

Implant Alternatives

In deciding on the method of posterior instrumentation, the surgeon's armamentarium consists of a multitude of systems and techniques using wire alone or in combination with rods, screws alone or in combination with plates or rods, hooks in combination with rods, rods with sleeves, or additional forms of segmental fixation.[103, 104] In the selection process, the surgeon must determine whether the patient's requirement is for a rigid or a semirigid system, and whether the particular surgical anatomy is best served with or allows the use of hook, wire, or screw fixation.

The Harrington system was one of the first effective implants introduced for spinal deformity as well as trauma of the spine.[1, 23, 49] Because the rods are held posteriorly to the lamina by hooks, they fail to provide the necessary lordosis or rotational control in the thoracolumbar or lumbar spine. Supplemental segmental wiring can be utilized with Harrington rods to improve rotational stability and fixation to the spine, and the rods can be contoured to preserve lumbar lordosis.[1, 103, 104, 124, 125] Despite these adjustments, Harrington rod fixation remains less than ideal in the thoracolumbar and lumbar spine.[21, 22, 44]

The Edwards-Rod sleeve distraction system was designed to provide superior lordosis and rotational control by use of a three-point system of fixation.[27, 29] Although this system has been utilized effectively by many authors, it does not truly rely on segmental fixation and remains semirigid in its fixation characteristics.

Segmental sublaminar wires connected to contoured L-shaped paravertebral rods were first introduced by Eduardo Luque in the early 1970s.[76–81] Although this system provides segmental fixation, it requires the passage of sublaminar wires, has minimal distractive reduction capabilities, and has little or no axial control.[58, 113, 115] For this reason, the Luque rod-wire technique remains a poor choice for burst fractures that require axial correction and control, but it is an excellent choice in the treatment of neuromuscular deformity.[13, 41, 43, 109]

Translaminar screws[84] can provide for immediate stabilization of facet joints, but because of their semirigid nature, they cannot be effective unless they are used with a stable anterior or middle column.

Transpedicle fixation of the spine was popularized by Roy-Camille in the early 1970s.[97–99] It was not until the introduction of the Steffe system in the 1980s that pedicle fixation gained popularity in the United States.[107] Today, pedicle fixation can provide both rigid and semirigid fixation. It allows for excellent distraction, compression, and rotational control. The system of fixation is largely dependent on the pedicle morphometry of the patient and the skill of the surgeon.[128, 131, 132] In the right hands and with proper application, it is an excellent technique of spinal fixation. In inexperienced hands or with the wrong application, it has the potential for complications.

SPECIFIC COMPLICATIONS ASSOCIATED WITH TYPES OF POSTERIOR INSTRUMENTATION

Hook-Rod Fixation

Systems that employ rods and hooks for posterior spinal reconstruction may fail secondary to the hook pulling out of its proper position, the hook disengaging from the rod, failure at the hook-bone interface secondary to lamina or pedicle fracture, or fracture of the rod.[28, 30] Edwards and associates,[30] in a review of hook dislodgement, noted four factors that account for most hook dislodgement: rigidity of fixation, anatomic level, hook design, and rod clearance. Lamina fracture is associated with excessive distraction, overaggressive laminotomy, or poor-quality bone. Rod fracture typically occurs months after the initial surgery and is secondary to an incomplete posterior fusion and the inevitable failure of the metal rod secondary to repetitive loading.

Most often, the hook-rod system fails in the distraction mode. Patient flexion and rotation may initiate the hook pulling out from underneath the lamina. The initial straight Harrington rod-hook system was a semirigid system that was often associated with hook dislodgement. Because of the semirigid nature of the Harrington rod construct, when the rod projected less than 1 cm above the hook, there was the potential for the tip of the rod to enter the hook body during flexion, causing dislodgement when the patient returned toward extension. Keeping more than 1 cm of rod extending beyond the hooks helps decrease this problem.

The development of segmental fixation with multiple hook, as well as changing the design of the lamina hooks to a more anatomic configuration, has significantly decreased the incidence of hook dislodgement.[17] With the development of segmental fixation and the technique of claw-hook configuration, the incidence of hooks disengaging from the rod has decreased. The rod-hook interface, however, may continue to fail if the screw locking mechanism is not properly tightened, thus allowing continued micromotion at the rod-hook interface.

Initially, the increased mobility of the lumbar spine in relationship to the thoracic spine, as well as the lordosis of the lumbar spine, contributed to a higher rate of hook dislodgement when instrumentation extended into the lower lumbar spine.[44, 115] With the development of contoured rods, claw-hook techniques, and pedicle fixation, the rate of dislodgement when extending instrumentation into the lower lumbar spine has significantly decreased.[8, 21, 22, 28]

Fracture of the lamina and/or pedicle can occur secondary to inadequate bone stock (i.e., osteoporosis), excessive stress at the bone-hook interface, or iatrogenic weakening of the lamina secondary to laminotomy or decortication. Minimizing the amount of bone removed during the laminotomy for hook placement, and proper placement of the hook under and not through the lamina, helps decrease the incidence of laminar fracture. The development of anatomic laminar hooks provides for better stress distribution, thereby decreasing stress-related laminar resorption and delayed fracture.[8, 28, 30]

Finally, the risk of neurologic injury secondary to hook placement overall is quite low. The reported incidence of a major neurologic injury secondary to segmental hook placement is 0.2 per cent, with a 1.7 per cent incidence of minor neurologic deficit.[28, 82] Despite this low clinical rate of neurologic injury, the theoretic increased risk of neurologic complications still exists whenever hooks are placed within the spinal canal.[14]

Sublaminar Wire

The utilization of sublaminar wire to achieve segmental fixation was popularized in the 1970s by Luque.[76–81] The complications associated with sublaminar wire are neurologic injury and loss of fixation.[58, 113, 115, 122, 125, 129, 130] Luque rods with sublaminar wiring provide semirigid segmental fixation. This method of fixation is inadequate to resist axial load and potentially allows rod pistoning, thereby minimizing axial control and distraction capabilities. The passage of sublaminar wires may cause neurologic deficit. Fortunately, many of the changes are electrophysiologic and not clinically significant. Although this complication decreases significantly with the experience of the operating surgeon, the rate of neurologic injury remains significantly higher than that associated with other techniques.[13, 46, 50, 129, 130] Regardless of the surgeon's experience, extreme caution should be used when passing a wire at the extreme kyphotic or lordotic portion of the deformity. Although neurologic injury is most often associated with the passage of sublaminar wires, it has been reported to occur in a delayed fashion[56] or when sublaminar wires must be removed secondary to sepsis, implant failure, or hardware prominence.[75]

Pedicle Screw Fixation

Posterior spinal instrumentation using pedicle screws has been utilized to treat spinal trauma, degenerative disc disease, lumbar spondylolisthesis, tumors, and spinal deformity. Even though spinal surgeons have used pedicle fixation for over 20 years, it remains controversial outside of spine surgery communities.[35, 38, 118, 119, 127] The potential complications of pedicle screw fixation are numerous but are usually avoidable.[20, 45, 70, 83, 93, 105, 108] Lonstein and coworkers[73] reported on their experience involving 405 patients with a total of 1999 pedicle screw insertions. The vast majority of these screws were placed in the lumbar spine, and 99 per cent of the screws were inserted without complication. A total of four screws (0.02 per cent) were found to cause nerve root irritation and required reoperation. A total of 18 screws (0.9 per cent) were broken at the time of follow-up. The results of this study support the belief that with an experienced surgeon, pedicle screw fixation is a safe method of rigid fixation of the lumbar spine.

Pedicle screws may potentially injure the dura, spinal cord, nerve root, great vessels, or bowels (Fig. 54–17). Screws can fracture the pedicle upon insertion, and they can potentially loosen, pull out, or break.[32, 33, 42, 67, 73, 74, 97–101] Proper placement of pedicle screws is important to decrease the risk of loss of fixation or injury to closely related anatomic structures.[45] A screw that has an entry point resulting in lateral placement outside the pedicle does not provide optimal fixation. A screw placed medially in the spinal canal may cause a dural tear and/or neurologic injury. A screw placed inferiorly may cause foraminal encroachment and possible nerve root injury or irritation. A screw that is too long can injure the great vessels on the anterior surface of the spinal column. A shorter screw poses less risk to the great vessels, but a screw that is too short risks pulling out. A larger-diameter screw has greater pull-out strength when placed in the lumbar pedicle, but if a screw is too large, it is at higher risk for cortical perforation and pedicle blowout[126, 131, 132] (Fig. 54–11).

In summary, avoidance of complications with pedicle screw fixation is somewhat dependent on the surgeon's experience and attention to the details of screw placement and the patient's particular pedicle morphometry.

Translaminar Lumbar Screws

Translaminar screws or facet screws have been used to promote posterior spinal fusion for many years.[59, 84] Their reported complication rate is low, but improper technique can allow violation of the spinal canal and/or nerve root injury. It is important that the screws are placed after the facet joint has been decorticated and packed with cancellous bone, to avoid a nonunion of the facet joint.

Dural Tears (Fig. 54–16)

Dural tears are known complications associated with revision spine surgery with or without posterior spinal instrumentation. Tears may be related to misdirected screws, hooks, or sublaminar wire. The cerebrospinal fluid leak needs to be controlled in order to avoid pseudomeningocele or fistula formation. The optimal treatment for a dural tear is direct surgical repair.[31] If this is not possible, or if the repair is less than ideal, a lumbar drain placed at the time of surgery has been shown to be effective in preventing the complications of persistent cerebrospinal fluid leak.[60]

Hardware Removal

In general, the vast majority of patients tolerate their posterior spinal instrumentation and do not request implant removal. There are some patients who, because of either their physical habitus or excessively prominent hardware, develop problems with skin irritation, pressure sores, facet impingement on the adjacent unfused segments, or painful bursitis over the hardware. In addition, there is a small group of patients who have persistent discomfort secondary to metal sensitivity and/or allergic reaction. In these instances, removal of the implant may benefit the patient.

SUMMARY

Ultimately, if enough surgery is performed, complications will occur. If posterior spinal instrumentation is used, complications secondary to their use will de-velop. A thorough knowledge of the instrumentation being used, familiarity with the patient's particular morphometry, and an honest assessment of one's own surgical skill and experience will help minimize the chance of instrument-related complications.

References

1. Aaro, S., and Ohlen, G: The effect of Harrington instrumentation on the sagittal configuration and mobility of the spine in scoliosis. Spine 8:570–575, 1983.
2. Aebi, M., Etter, C. H. R., Keh, T. H., and Thalgott, J.: The internal skeletal fixation system. Clin. Orthop. 227:30–43, 1988.
3. Albee, F. H.: Transplantation of portions of the tibia into the spine for Pott's disease. JAMA 57:885, 1911.
4. Andrew, T. A., Brooks, S., Piggott, H., et al.: Long-term follow-up evaluation of screw and graft fusion of the lumbar spine. Clin. Orthop. 203:113–119, 1986.
5. Axelsson, P., Johnsson, R., Stromqvist, B., et al.: Posterolateral lumbar fusion: Outcome of 71 consecutive operations after 4 years. Acta Orthop. Scand. 65:309–314, 1994.
6. Balderston, R. A.: Spinal cord injury. In Garfin, S. (ed.): Complications of Spine Surgery. Baltimore, Williams & Wilkins, 1989, pp. 144–151.
7. Beattie, F. C.: Distraction rod fusion. Clin. Orthop. 62:218–222, 1969.
8. Benzel, E. C., Kesterson, L., and Marchand, E. P.: Texas Scottish Rite Hospital rod instrumentation for thoracic and lumbar spree trauma. J. Neurosurg. 75:382–387, 1991.
9. Blumenthal, S., and Gill, K.: Complications of the Wiltse pedicle screw fixation system. Spine 18:1867–1871, 1993.
10. Boos, N., Marchesi, D., Zuber, K., and Aebi, M.: Treatment of severe spondylolisthesis by reduction and pedicular fixation. Spine 18:1655–1661, 1993.
11. Boucher, H. H.: A method of spinal fusion. J. Bone Joint Surg. Br. 41:248–259, 1959.
12. Bridwell, K. H.: Where to stop the fusion distally in adult scoliosis? AAOS Instr. Course Lect. 45:101–107, 1996.
13. Broom, M. J., Banter, J. V., and Renshaw, T. S.: Spinal fusion augmented by Luque rod segmental instrumentation for neuromuscular scoliosis. J. Bone Joint Surg. Am. 71:32–44, 1989.
14. Coe, J. D., Becker, P. S., and McAfee, P. C.: Neuropathology with spinal instrumentation. J. Orthop. Res. 7:359–370, 1989.
15. Colter, H. B., Colter, J. M., Stoloff, A., et al.: The use of autografts for vertebral body replacement of the thoracic and lumbar spine. Spine 10:748, 1985.
16. Colter, J. M., Vernace, J. V., and Michalski, J. A.: The use of Harrington rods in thoracolumbar fractures. Orthop. Clin. North Am. 17:87, 1986.
17. Cotrel, Y., Dubousset, J., and Guillaumat, M.: New universal instrumentation in spinal surgery. Clin. Orthop. 227:10–23, 1988.
18. Cunningham, B., Sefter, J., Shono, Y., and McAfee, P.: Static and cyclical biomechanical analysis of pedicle screw spinal constructs. Spine 18:1677–1688, 1993.
19. Davne, S. H., and Myers, D. L.: Complications of lumbar spinal fusion with transpedicular instrumentation. Spine 17(S):S184–S189, 1992.
20. Devlin, V., Boachie-Adjei, O., Bradford, D., et al.: Treatment of adult spinal deformity with fusion to the sacrum using CD instrumentation. J. Spinal Disord. 4:1–14, 1991.
21. Dick, W.: The "fixateur interne" as a versatile implant for spine surgery. Spine 12:882–900, 1987.
22. Dick, W., Kluger, P., Magerl, F., et al.: A new device for internal fixation of thoracolumbar and lumbar spine fractures: The "fixateur interne." Paraplegia 23:225–232, 1985.
23. Dickson, J. H., Harrington, P. R., and Irwin, W. D.: Results of reduction and stabilization of the severely fractured thoracic and lumbar spine. J. Bone Joint Surg. Am. 60:799, 1978.
24. Drummond, D. S., Guardagni, J., Kenne, J. S. et al.: Interspinous process segmental spinal instrumentation. J. Pediatr. Orthop. 4:397–404, 1984.
25. Dunham, W. K., Langford, K. H., and Ostrowsky, D. M.: The management of unstable fractures and dislocations of the thoracic and lumbar spine. Ala. J. Med. Sci. 21:194, 1984.

26. Edwards, C. C.: Sacral fixation device: Design and preliminary results. Proc. Scoliosis Research Society 6:135, 1984.
27. Edwards, C. C., and Levine, A. M.: Early rod-sleeve stabilization of the injured thoracic and lumbar spine. Orthop. Clin. North Am. 17: 121, 1986.
28. Edwards, C. C., and Levine, A. M.: Complications associated with posterior instrumentation in the treatment of thoracic and lumbar injuries. In Garfin, S. (ed.): Complications of Spine Surgery. Baltimore, Williams & Wilkins, 1989, pp. 164–199.
29. Edwards, C. C., and Levine, A. M.: Early rod-sleeve stabilization of the injured thoracic and lumbar spine. Orthop. Clin. North Am. 17:121–145, 1986.
30. Edwards, C. C., York, J. J., Levine, A. M., et al.: Determinants of spinal dislodgement. Orthop. Trans. 10:8, 1986.
31. Eismont, F. J., Wiesel, S. W., and Rothman, R. H.: Treatment of dural tears associated with spinal surgery. J. Bone Joint Surg. Am. 63:1132–1136, 1982.
32. Errico, T. J., and Dryer, J. W.: Pedicle screws. Curr. Opin. Orthop. 6:55–60, 1995.
33. Esses, S. I., and Bednar, D. A.: The spine pedicle screw: Technique and systems. Orthop. Rev. 18:676–682, 1989.
34. Esses, S. I., Botsford, D. J., Hulter, R. J., and Rauschning, W.: Surgical anatomy of the sacrum: A guide for rational screw fixation. Spine 16:S283–S288, 1991.
35. Esses, S. I., and Sachs, B. L.: Complications of pedicle screw fixation. Orthop. Trans. 12:160–161, 1992.
36. Fernyhough, J. C., Schimandle, J. H., and Levine, A. M.: Iatrogenic spondylolysis complicating distal laminar hook placement. Spine 16:849–850, 1991.
37. Flesch, J. R., Leider, L. L., Erickson, O. L., et al.: Harrington instrumentation and spine fusions for unstable fractures and fracture-dislocations of the thoracic and lumbar spine. J. Bone Joint Surg. Am. 59:143, 1977.
38. Garfin, S.: Editorial. Spine 19:2300–2305, 1994.
39. Garfin, S. R., and Amundson, G.: Minimizing blood loss during spine surgery. In Garfin, S. (ed.): Complications of Spine Surgery. Baltimore, Williams & Wilkins, 1989, pp. 29–52.
40. Garfin, S. R., Kurtz, L. T., and Booth, R. E.: Iliac bone grafting: Techniques and complications of harvesting. In Garfin, S. (ed.): Complications of Spine Surgery. Baltimore, Williams & Wilkins, 1989, pp. 323–342.
41. Gau, Y. L., Lonstein, J. L., Winter, R. B., et al.: Luque-Galveston procedure for correction and stabilization of neuromuscular scoliosis and pelvic obliquity: A review of 68 patients. J. Spinal Disord. 4:339–410, 1991.
42. Georgis, T., Rydevik, B., Weinstein, J. N., and Garfin, S. R.: Complications of pedicle screw fixation. In Garfin, S. (ed.): Complications of Spine Surgery. Baltimore, Williams & Wilkins, 1989, pp. 200–210.
43. Gersoff, W. K., and Renshaw, J. S.: The treatment of scoliosis in cerebral palsy by posterior spine fusion with Luque-rod segmental instrumentation. J. Bone Joint Surg. Am. 70:41, 1988.
44. Gertzbein, S. D., MacMichael, D., and Tile, M.: Harrington instrumentation as a method of fixation in fractures of the spine: A critical analysis of deficiencies. J. Bone Joint Surg. Br. 64:526, 1982.
45. Gertzbein, S., and Robbins, S.: Accuracy of pedicle screw placement in vivo. Spine 15:4–11, 1990.
46. Goll, S. R., Balderston, R. A., Stambough, J. L., et al.: Depth of intraspinal wire penetration during passage of sublaminar wires. Spine 13:503–509, 1988.
47. Guyer, D. W., Wiltse, L. L., and Peck, R. D.: The Wiltse pedicle screw fixation system. Orthopedics 11:1455–1460, 1988.
48. Hadra, B. E.: Wiring of the spinous process in Pott's disease. Trans. Am. Orthop. Assoc. 4:206, 1891.
49. Harrington, P. R.: Technical details in relation to the successful use of instrumentation in scoliosis. Orthop. Clin. North Am. 3:49, 1972.
50. Herring, J. A., and Wenger, D. R.: Segmental spinal instrumentation: A preliminary report of 40 consecutive cases. Spine 7:285–298, 1982.
51. Hibbs, R. A.: An operation for progressive spinal deformities. N. Y. Med. J. 93:1013, 1911.
52. Horowitch, A., Peck, R. D., Thomas, J. C., Jr., et al.: The Wiltse pedicle screw fixation: Early clinical results. Spine 14:461–467, 1989.
53. Hsu, K. Y., and Zucherman, J. F.: The long term effect of lumbar spinal fusion: Deterioration of adjacent motion segments. In Yonenobu, K., Ono, K., and Takemitsu, Y. (eds.): Lumbar Spinal Fusion and Stabilization. Berlin, Springer-Verlag, 1993, pp. 54–64.
54. Jacobs, R. R., Schlaepfer, F., Mathys, R., et al.: A locking hook spinal rod system for stabilization of fracture-dislocations and correction of deformity of the dorsolumbar spine. Clin. Orthop. 189:168–177, 1985.
55. Jenkins, J. A.: Spondylolisthesis. Br. J. Surg. 24: 80–85, 1936.
56. Johnson, C. E., Norris, R., Burke, S. W., et al.: Delayed paraplegia following segmental spinal instrumentation. Presented at the annual meeting of the Scoliosis Research Society, Orlando, FL, September 1984.
57. Kaneda, K., Kazama, H., Satoh, Y., et al.: Distraction rod instrumentation with posterolateral fusion in isthmic spondylolisthesis. Spine 10:383–389, 1985.
58. King, A. G.: Complications in segmental spinal instrumentation. In Luque, E. (ed.): Segmental Spinal Instrumentation. Thorofare, NJ, Slack, 1984, pp. 301–330.
59. King, D.: Internal fixation for lumbosacral fusions. J. Bone Joint Surg. 30:560–565, 1948.
60. Kitchel, S. H., Eismont, F. J., and Green, B. A.: Management of post-operative CSF leakage by closed subarachnoid drainage. Abstracts of the International Society for the Study of the Lumbar Spine meeting, Miami, April 1988, p. 38.
61. Kostuik, J. P.: Failures in spine surgery. Curr. Opin. Orthop. Surg. 4:160–169, 1993.
62. Kostuik, J. P., and Hall, B. B.: Spinal fusions to the sacrum in adults with scoliosis. Spine 8:489, 1983.
63. Kostuik, J. P., Israel, J., and Hall, J. E.: Scoliosis surgery in adults. Clin. Orthop. 93:225, 1973.
64. Kostuik, J., Munting, E., Esses, S., and Valdevit, A.: Biomechanical analysis of screw load sharing in pedicle fixation of the lumbar spine. Proceedings of the 29th annual meeting of the Scoliosis Research Society, Portland, OR, 1994, p. 159.
65. Krag, M. H.: Biomechanics of transpedicle spinal fixation. In Weinstein, J. N., and Weisel, S. (eds.): The Lumbar Spine. Philadelphia, W. B. Saunders Co., 1990, pp. 916–940.
66. Krag, M. H., Beynnon, D. D., Pope, M. H., et al.: An internal fixator for posterior application to short segments of the thoracic, lumbar, or lumbosacral spine. Clin. Orthop. 203:75–98, 1986.
67. Krag, M. H., Beynnon, B. D., and Pope, M. H.: Depth of insertion of transpedicular vertebral screws into human vertebrae: Effect upon screw vertebra interface strength. J. Spinal Disord. 1:287–294, 1988.
68. Krag, M. H., Weaver, D. L., Beynnon, B. D., and Haugh, L. D.: Morphometry of the thoracic and lumbar surgical spine fixation. Spine 13:27–32, 1988.
69. Lange, F.: Support for the spondylitic spine by means of buried steel bars attached to the vertebrae. Am. J. Orthop. Surg. 8:344, 1910.
70. Law, M., Tencer, A., and Anderson, P.: Caudo-cephalad loading of pedicle screws: Mechanisms of loosening and methods of augmentation. Spine 18:2438–2443, 1993.
71. Lee, C. K., and De Bari, A.: Lumbosacral fusion with Knodt distraction rods. Spine 11:373–375, 1986.
72. Levine, A. M., and Edwards, C. C.: Complications in the treatment of acute spinal injury. Orthop. Clin. North Am. 17:183–203, 1986.
73. Lonstein, J., Denis, F., Perra, J., et al.: Complications of pedicle screws. Proceedings of the 29th annual meeting of the Scoliosis Research Society. Portland, OR, 1994, p. 213.
74. Louis, R.: Fusion of the lumbar and sacral spine by internal fixation with screw plates. Clin. Orthop. 203:18–33, 1986.
75. Lowe, T.: The morbidity and mortality report. Read at the 21st annual meeting of the Scoliosis Research Society, Bermuda, June 1986.
76. Luque, E. R.: Sequential correction of scoliosis with rigid internal fixation. Orthop. Trans. 1:136, 1977.
77. Luque, E. R.: The anatomic basis development of segmental spinal instrumentation. Spine 7:256–259, 1982.

78. Luque, E. R.: Interpeduncular segmental fixation. Clin. Orthop. *203*:54–57, 1986.

79. Luque, E. R.: Segmental spinal instrumentation of the lumbar spine. Clin. Orthop. *203*:126–134, 1986.

80. Luque, E. R., and Cardoso, A.: A treatment of scoliosis without arthrodesis or external support: Preliminary report. Orthop. Trans. *1*:37, 1977.

81. Luque, E. R., and Cassis, N.: Segmental spinal instrumentation in the treatment of fractures of the thoracolumbar spine. Spine *7*:312, 1982.

82. MacEwen, D. G., Bunnell, W. P., and Sriram, K.: Acute neurological complications in the treatment of scoliosis. J. Bone Joint Surg. Am. *57*:404, 1975.

83. MacMillian, M., Cooper, R., and Haid, R.: Lumbar and lumbosacral fusions using Cotrel-Dubousset pedicle screws and rods. Spine *19*:430–434, 1994.

84. Magerl, F. P.: Stabilization of the lower thoracic and lumbar spine with external skeletal fixation. Clin. Orthop. *1989*:125–149, 1984.

85. Magerl, F.: External Skeletal Fixation of the Lower Thoracic and Upper Lumbar Spine: Current Concepts of External Fixation of Fractures. Berlin, Springer-Verlag, 1982.

86. May, V. R., and Mauck, W. R.: Exploration of the spine for pseudarthrosis following spinal fusion in the treatment of scoliosis. Clin. Orthop. *53*:115–122, 1967.

87. McAfee, P. C., and Bohlman, H. H.: Complications following Harrington instrumentation for fractures of the thoracolumbar spine. J. Bone Joint Surg. Am. *67*:672, 1985.

88. McAfee, P. C., Weiland, D. J., and Carlow, J. J.: Survivorship analysis of pedicle spinal instrumentation. Spine *16*:S422–S427, 1991.

90. Mercer, W.: Spondylolisthesis. Edinburgh Med. J. *43*:545–572, 1936.

91. Mirkovic, S., Abitbol, J. J., Steinman, J., et al.: Anatomic consideration for sacral screw placement. Spine *16*:S289–S294.

92. Moe, J. H., and Denis, F: The iatrogenic loss of lumbar lordosis. Orthop. Trans. *1*:131, 1977.

93. Pashman, R., Hu, S., Schendel, M., and Bradford, D.: Sacral screw loads in lumbosacral fixation for spinal deformity. Spine *18*:2465–2470, 1993.

94. Pfeifer, B., Krag, M., and Johnson C.: Repair of failed transpedicle fixation. Spine *19*:350–353, 1994.

95. Pinto, M. R.: Complications of pedicle screw fixation. *In* Arnold, D. M., and Lonstein, J. E. (eds.): State of the Art Review: Spine: Pedicle Fixation of the Lumbar Spine. Philadelphia, Hanley and Belfus, 1992.

96. Pinto, W. C.: Complications of surgical treatment of scoliosis. Isr. J. Med. Sci. *9*:837, 1973.

97. Roy-Camille, R., Saillant, G., Berteaux, D., and Salgado, V.: Osteosynthesis or thoraco-lumbar spine fractures with metal plates screwed through the vertebral pedicles. Reconstr. Surg. Traumatol. *15*:2–15, 1976.

98. Roy-Camille, R., Saillant, G., Bertreaux, D., and Salgado, V.: Osteosynthesis of thoracolumbar spine fractures with metal plates screwed through the vertebral pedicles. Reconstr. Surg. Traumatol. *15*:2–16, 1976.

99. Roy-Camille, R., Saillant, G., and Mazel, C: Internal fixation of the lumbar spine with pedicle screw plating. Clin. Orthop. *203*:7–17, 1986.

100. Saillant, G.: Anatomical study of vertebral pedicles. Surgical application (in French). Res. Chirurg. Orthop. *62*:157, 1976.

101. Sande, E., Witsoe, E., Lundbom, J., et al.: Vascular complications of lumbar disk surgery. Eur. J Surg. *157*:141–143, 1991.

102. Selby, D.: Internal fixation with Knodt's rods. Clin. Orthop. *203*:179–184, 1986.

103. Silverman, B. J., and Greenbarg, P. E.: Idiopathic scoliosis posterior spine fusion with Harrington rod and sublaminar wiring. Orthop. Clin. North Am. *19*:269–279, 1988.

104. Silverman, B. J., and Greenbarg, P. E.: Internal fixation of the spine for idiopathic scoliosis using square ended distraction rods and lamina wiring (Harrington-Luque technique). Bull. Hosp. Jt. Dis. Orthop. Inst. *44*, 1984.

105. Soshi, S., Shiba, R., Kondo, H., and Murota, K.: An experimental study of transpedicular screw fixation in relation to osteoporosis in the lumbar spine. Spine *16*:1335–1341, 1991.

106. Speed, K.: Spondylolisthesis: Treatment by anterior bone graft. Arch. Surg. *37*:175–189, 1938.

107. Steffe, A. D., Biscup, R. S., and Sitkowski D. J.: Segmental spine plates with pedicle screw fixation. Clin. Orthop. *203*:45, 1986.

108. Steinmann, J., Herkowitz, H., El-Kommos, H., and Wesolowski, P.: Spinal pedicle fixation: Confirmation of an image based technique for screw placement. Spine *18*:1856–1861, 1993.

109. Sullivan, J. A., and Conner, S. B.: Comparison of Harrington instrumentation in the management of neuro-muscular spinal deformity. Spine *7*:299–304, 1982.

110. Thompson, G. H., Wilber, R. B., Shaffer, J. W., et al: Complications of segmental spinal instrumentation in spinal deformities. Orthop. Trans. *9*:123, 1985.

111. Turner, J. A.: Surgery for lumbar spinal stenosis: Attempted meta-analysis of the literature. Spine *17*:1–8, 1992.

112. Turner, J. A.: Patient outcomes after lumbar spinal fusions. JAMA *268*:907–911, 1992.

113. Turner, P. L., Mason, S. A., and Webb, J. K.: Neurologic complications with segmental spinal instrumentation. Orthop. Trans. *10*:14, 1986.

114. Villano, M., Cantatore, G., Santilli, N. N., and Cerillo, B. A.: Vascular injury related to lumbar disk surgery. Neurochirurgia *35*:57–59, 1992.

115. Weber, S. C., and Benson, D. R.: A comparison of segmental fixation and Harrington instrumentation in the management of unstable thoracolumbar spine fractures. Orthop. Trans. *9*:36, 1985.

116. Weinstein, J. N., Spratt, K. F., Spengler, D., and Brick, C.: Spinal pedicle fixation: Reliability and validity of roentgenogram based assessment and surgical factors on successful screw placement. Spine *13*:1012, 1988.

117. Wenger, D. R., and Mubarak, S. J.: Managing complications of posterior spinal instrumentation and fusion. *In* Garfin, S. (ed.): Complications of Spine Surgery. Baltimore, Williams & Wilkins, 1989, pp. 127–143.

118. West, J. L., III, Ogilvie, J. W., and Bradford, D. S.: Complications of the variable screw plate pedicle screw fixator. Spine *16*:576–579, 1991.

119. West, J. L., Bradford, D. S., and Ogilvie, J. W.: Results of spinal arthrodesis with pedicle screw-plate fixation. J. Bone Joint Surg. Am. *73*:1179–1184, 1992.

120. White, A., Wynne, G., and Taylor, L. W.: Knodt rod distraction lumbar fusion. Spine *8*:434–437, 1983.

121. Whitecloud, T. S., III, Butter, J. C., Cohen, J. L., and Candelara, P. D.: Complications with the variable spinal plating system. Spine *16*:472–476, 1989.

122. Wilber, S. R., Thompson, S. H., Shaffer, J. W., et al.: Postoperative neurological deficits in segmental instrumentation. J. Bone Joint Surg. *66*:1178–1187, 1984.

123. Wilson, P. D., Straub, L., and Ramsay, M. D.: Lumbosacral fusion with metallic-plate fixation. AAOS Instr. Course Lect. *9*:53–65, 1952.

124. Wiltse, L. L.: History of spinal disorders. *In* Frymoyer, J. W. (ed.): The Adult Spine: Principles and Practices. Vol. 1. New York, Raven Press, 1991, pp. 3–41.

125. Winter, R. W.: Thoracic lordoscoliosis in neurofibromatosis: Treatment by Harrington rods with sublaminar wiring. J. Bone Joint Surg. Am. *66*:1102–1106, 1984.

126. Wittenberg, R., Kyu-Sung, L., Shea, M., et al.: Effect of screw diameter, insertion technique and bond cement augmentation of pedicle screw fixation strength. Clin. Orthop. *296*:278–287, 1993.

127. Yuan, S., Garfin, S., Dickman, C., and Mardjetko, S.: A historical cohort study of pedicle screw fixation in thoracic, lumbar, and sacral spine fusions. *19*:22795–22965, 1994.

128. Zdeblick, T., Kunz, D., Cooke, M., and McCabe, R.: Pedicle screw pull-out strength: Correlation with insertional torque. Spine *18*:1673–1676, 1993.

129. Zindrick, M. R., Knight, G., Bunch, W., et al: The depth of penetration of intra-segmental wire in the neural canal at insertion. Orthop. Trans. *10*:6, 1986.

130. Zindrick, M. R., Knight, G. W., and Bunch, W. H.: Factors influencing the penetration of wires into the neural canal during segmental wiring. J. Bone Joint Surg. *71*:742, 1989.

131. Zindrick, M. R., Wiltse, L. L., Doornick, A., et al: Analysis of the morphometric characteristics of the thoracic and lumbar pedicles. Spine *12*:160, 1987.

132. Zindrick, M. R., Wiltse, L. L., Widell, E. H., et al: A biomechanical study of intrapedicular screw fixation in the lumbosacral spine. Clin. Orthop. *203*:99, 1986.

Adhesive Arachnoiditis

Gabrielle F. Morris, M.D.

Adhesive arachnoiditis (AA) refers to a pathologic inflammation of the pia-arachnoid membrane surrounding the spinal cord, cauda equina, nerve roots, or a combination. It occurs most commonly in the lumbar region. Disease involvement is along a continuum, from mild membrane thickening through progressively more scarring. In its most severe form, it results in a blockage of cerebrospinal fluid (CSF) flow. Although once thought to represent a sequel to spinal infections, arachnoiditis is now recognized as a chronic syndrome of variable etiology. Patients suffer from persistent pain that may be compounded by neurologic deficits, resulting in pain and disability. This is a cause of failed back surgery and is one of the complications encountered after routine lumbar operative procedures.[6, 13, 54, 74]

ETIOLOGIES

Both the known and the suspected causes of arachnoiditis encompass a broad range of substances and factors. All tend to share a common mechanism leading to dysfunction. The intrathecal contents first must be exposed to an offending agent. An inflammatory reaction then ensues in which the leptomeninges become scarred and adherent to the neural elements, resulting in symptoms. These agents can broadly be classified as myelographic contrast materials, chemical irritants, and blood products. The process can also be triggered by surgical procedures or by infections. The following discussion provides a brief overview.

Myelographic Contrast Agents

Of all implicated causes of AA, the evidence is most clear in oil-based intrathecal radiographic contrast materials. Iophendylate, popularly known as Pantopaque or Myodil, was developed in the 1940s and was the preferred contrast material for over 30 years. This contrast was believed to be well tolerated, until the significant late pathology became widely appreciated.[13, 63, 73, 76] It is now accepted that iophendylate myelography causes arachnoiditis in a significant proportion of exposed patients. Risk is increased with repeated or traumatic myelograms,[12] particularly in the presence of spinal stenosis or previous spinal surgery.[51]

The development of water-soluble contrast agents has superseded the need for those based in oil. Iohexol, one of the most commonly used, has lower toxicity and a greater safety margin in both humans and primate models.[39, 87]

Postoperative

When arachnoiditis is present, it may result in persistent pain and dysfunction. In patients who have had surgical infections or intradural hemorrhage, this finding is common. Arachnoiditis is more frequent in patients who have had extensive procedures, repeated lumbar procedures, or bilateral procedures.[73, 104] There is a high correlation of AA with failed back surgery syndrome, in which poor clinical results are seen despite wide decompressions.[14, 52]

One must be cognizant of the fact that AA can be a postoperative complication of any spine surgery, including procedures for disc disease.[16, 75] Lumbar stenosis can be a cause of or coexist with arachnoiditis.[42] Other procedures that have been reported to cause arachnoiditis include direct trauma during puncture or catheter insertion for epidural and/or intraspinal anesthetics[55, 66] and after prophylactic blood patch application through a catheter.[2]

Chemical Irritants

Under physiologic circumstances, the central nervous system is protected from noxious substances by the blood-brain barrier. Any violation allows infiltration of foreign material and has the potential to incite arachnoiditis. In the course of management for certain medical conditions, therapy may be intentionally rendered intrathecally. This is an expected and perhaps acceptable risk when the pharmacologic agents are chemotherapeutic, attempting to control or treat malignancies. The deleterious effects of these medications have been well described.[4, 68]

Anesthetic agents, instilled either intrathecally or epidurally, also may be the initial insult that subsequently produces arachnoiditis. This diagnosis should be considered in patients presenting with back and leg pain syndromes after anesthetics.[38, 66, 89] Rarely, AA has been reported with epidural steroid injections, but usually only with multiple injections over a prolonged period.[1] Neurotoxicity can be a direct effect of the drug, one of its metabolites, or the preservatives in the solution. Alternatively, it can be indirect, related to the drug's concentration, duration of intrathecal exposure, or method of administration. Arachnoiditis may also be triggered by trauma.[55] Symptoms can result from underlying latent cord ischemia or from the aggravation of previously silent pathologies such as arteriovenous malformations.[34]

Infectious Diseases

Intraspinal bacterial infections incite scarring and result in arachnoiditis. This was formerly believed to be one of the only causes. These infections are most often postoperative in nature. However, other infectious causes merit discussion.

Spinal symptoms are rare in the common acute meningitides, whether bacterial or viral, community or hospital acquired. When such symptoms are encountered, suspicion should increase for the less common organisms. In the current era, mycobacterial infections are increasing in frequency and severity. Multiple drug-resistant strains have emerged. Many reports describe the clinical syndromes and radiographic findings seen as a complication of tuberculous meningitis.[19, 24, 49, 71] *Cryptococcus neoformans* can produce arachnoiditis and direct nerve root involvement.[99, 106] *Listeria monocytogenes* is an acute bacterial meningitis that has been reported to result in spinal complications.[70] Neurosyphilis can occasionally present in this manner.[31] The majority of these diseases will respond favorably to appropriate antimicrobial therapy.

Neurosarcoidosis, although inflammatory and not truly infectious, has also been reported to result in spinal arachnoiditis.[22]

Miscellaneous

Numerous other agents causing arachnoiditis have been reported with less frequency. These include familial forms; blood products; subarachnoid hemorrhage; benign neural tumors such as dermoid cysts, lipomas, and schwannomas; complications of the management of relatively common neurosurgical diseases; lumbo-peritoneal shunting; and myelomeningocele repair. It can also be seen as a late complication in penetrating spine wounds.[1, 5, 31, 37, 56, 64, 70, 80, 86, 96, 98]

NATURAL HISTORY

The course of clinical disease in patients with arachnoiditis is predominated by pain and its attendant preclusion from resuming premorbid activities. However, the majority of patients are relatively stable and rarely exhibit neurologic deterioration.[37]

Guyer and colleagues described the long-term follow-up (10 to 21 years) of 50 patients suffering from arachnoiditis. Their overall conclusions stressed that although arachnoiditis is disabling, it is usually not progressive. Increased neurologic deficits were more frequently caused by surgical intervention than by the natural course of the disease itself. There was a moderate incidence of late urinary symptoms.[37]

PATHOPHYSIOLOGY

Arachnoiditis leads to a soft tissue proliferation that ranges from filmy adhesions to a dense fibrous matrix. The term itself is somewhat of a misnomer, as usually only unimpressive inflammatory changes are seen microscopically. The exception is in the presence of trapped Pantopaque droplets, where islands of foreign body reaction may be seen.[104] The full pathologic mechanisms have not yet been elucidated, despite some suggestive evidence in the literature.

Experimental animal studies demonstrate that the severity and persistence of arachnoiditis and neural degeneration directly corresponded to the magnitude of the inflammation and wound healing processes.[108] Fibrosis and scarring are seen in response to nucleus pulposus, but not to lactic acid, chondroitin sulfate, or synovial fluid.[40]

Based on their study of nerve root vasculature, Parke and Watanabe concluded that arachnoiditis interferes with both the blood supply and nerve root nutrition.[65] The vascular supply of nerve roots within the subarachnoid space is more tenuous than that of the peripheral nerves, and the roots are dependent in part on the circulation of spinal fluid for nutritional support.[65] Venous obstruction and dilatation can result in endothelial damage, fibrin deposition, and intravascular thromboses, predisposing the initiation of neural fibrosis.[43]

Multiple reports in humans as well as experimental models relate arachnoiditis to the formation of a spinal cord syrinx.[10, 20, 30, 32, 48, 59] Caplan and associates proposed a mechanism by which this may occur. Scar formation from arachnoiditis alters the dynamics of CSF flow, and the associated obliteration of the spinal vasculature results in ischemia. Regions of myelomalacia become cystic, eventually coalescing to form cavities.[15]

Arachnoiditis itself may alter endogenous polypeptide concentrations, as suggested by animal studies. Lipman and Haughton showed significant elevations of brain beta-endorphin content in mice with arachnoiditis.[53] Beyer and coworkers corroborated this finding in a mouse experimental model that suggested that arachnoiditis was associated with a decreased pain threshold.[9]

There are case reports of arachnoid cysts and ossified arachnoiditis coexisting with AA, but the clinical significance of these is unclear.[62, 88, 95, 97]

CLINICAL PRESENTATION

There is not a set pattern, nor a distinct entity, that defines arachnoiditis. Rather, it is associated with a nonspecific, sometimes confusing clinical picture. Patients' complaints tend to emphasize pain. This may be of varying degrees, affecting one or both legs, the back, or a combination thereof. Pain is often burning in character, it can be constant or intermittent, and it may be aggravated by activity or prolonged sitting. Physical examination often has a positive tension sign, such as restricted straight leg raising. Neurologic status may be altered. Symptoms and signs can actually be the same as those that the patient presented with initially.[13, 33, 46, 58, 101, 104]

DIAGNOSIS (Figs. 54–18 and 54–19)

With modern neuroimaging, arachnoiditis can be demonstrated fairly easily. Its presence on radiographs must be evaluated in the context of the patient's clinical status. These radiographic pathoanatomic findings can occur in asymptomatic cases. Arachnoiditis tends to coexist with additional pathology. This is important to recognize, because entities such as recurrent disc herniation or instability may be amenable to treatment, and therapeutic planning needs to balance these components.

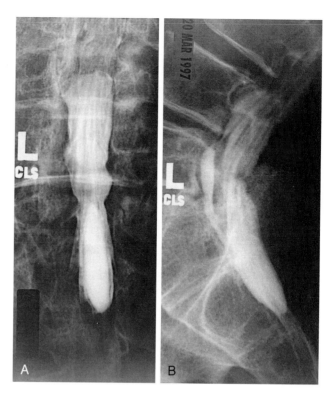

Figure 54–18. *A* and *B*, Anteroposterior and lateral radiographic images of this myelogram demonstrate the aggregation of contrast in the distal thecal sac. Here, the clumped nerve roots demonstrate the characteristic adherence of arachnoiditis.

Today, magnetic resonance imaging (MRI) is the primary imaging modality for arachnoiditis, allowing improved differentiation between other causes of failed back syndrome by identifying scar, infection, lateral recess stenosis, and retained or recurrent disc herniation. With the addition of paramagnetic contrast agents, MRI is able to distinguish between these entities with a greater degree of confidence than can other imaging modalities. It has replaced CT-myelography (CTM) as the first diagnostic study.[25, 27, 82, 85, 90, 91] Delamarter and colleagues compared these two radiographic modalities in the diagnosis of AA and found

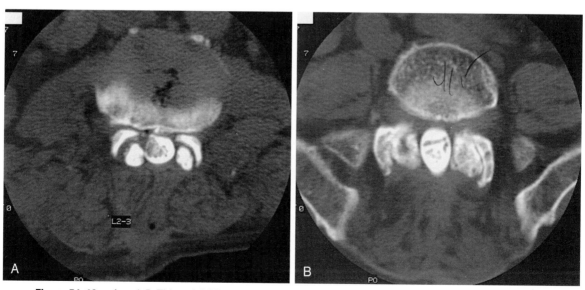

Figure 54–19. *A* and *B*, This axial CT scan was performed post-myelography. At L2-L3, central adherence of the entire cauda equina is seen. More distally, at L4-L5, only the anteriormost nerve roots adhere together; the posterior roots appear to float freely in cerebrospinal fluid.

that MRI had an excellent correlation with CTM.[25] In patients with suspected AA and a normal MRI, there is still occasionally a role for CTM to delineate the intrathecal nerve root anatomy. It may be a better modality in patients who have limited areas involved with arachnoiditis.[3, 41]

Radiographic findings consistent with a diagnosis of arachnoiditis on MRI include abnormal morphology and position of the nerve roots, with either central clumping or peripheral adhesions or marked thecal sac distortion. Axial T2-weighted images appear to be the most useful for this disease process.[83, 85] Myelographic features also depend on the severity of the pathologic changes and can show varying degrees of nerve root fusion, ranging to radiographic block.[84, 107]

Recently, there have been reports of diagnosing arachnoiditis by myeloscopy.[67] Given the procedure's invasive nature, this has not yet gained widespread popularity as strictly a diagnostic modality.

CLASSIFICATION

Two classification schemes have been described for arachnoiditis. These were devised to form a basis by which therapies and diagnostics could be compared. The original classification of Wilkinson incorporated both pathologic and myelographic data. Type I is associated with scarring confined to one nerve root exit site, causing nerve root blunting on myelography and largely monoradicular symptoms. Type II arachnoiditis is a circumferential type in which nerve roots become adherent to the arachnoid and dura around the circumference of a still patent central spinal fluid–filled space. Type III is a total transverse or annular obliteration of the subarachnoid space, usually at one or two segments—levels that most often are associated with either the diagnosis or the surgical treatment of "lumbar disc disease."[11, 45, 103, 104]

Comparatively, Delamarter and colleagues based their classification on radiographic data, which could be either CTM or MRI. Their scheme is as follows: Group 1—conglomerations of adherent nerve roots residing centrally within the thecal sac; Group 2—nerve roots adherent peripherally to the meninges, giving rise to an "empty sac" appearance; Group 3—a soft tissue mass replaces the subarachnoid space.[25]

TREATMENT

General

Overall, arachnoiditis responds poorly to treatment. Instead, it is best to focus on the prevention of its formation. Oil-based radiographic contrast agents that cause arachnoiditis have been replaced by water-based agents. Anesthetic techniques incorporate basic safety rules, such as using only preservative-free solutions, minimizing the quantity and duration of intrathecal or epidural contact with pharmacologic agents, and emphasizing technique. In the operating room, meticulous attention to surgical techniques can minimize leptomeningeal in-sults. This can be accomplished by delicate dissection, appropriate hemostasis, and limiting dural and intrathecal exposure to foreign bodies.[12, 39, 51, 63, 73, 76, 87]

Conservative Care

The mainstay of therapy is the control of symptoms. This can be accomplished by traditional measures such as the use of nonsteroidal anti-inflammatory medications, patient education, and/or modification of activities. Second-tier therapy is medical and includes the use of a variety of agents. Short-term use of muscle relaxants occasionally diminishes pain. Caution must be exercised if benzodiazepines are used, owing to their addictive potential. Elavil, a tricyclic customarily used in the treatment of depression, is used in low doses as a beneficial adjunct in analgesia. For intractable pain, membrane stabilizing agents such as phenytoin and carbamazepine can be considered.[55, 72]

Alternatives

Although not proved scientifically, the use of transcutaneous electrical nerve stimulation (TENS) units and dorsal column stimulators may be helpful in the management of arachnoiditis. These modalities work best for postoperative AA when the pain is predominantly confined to one lower extremity. They have, however, also shown some promise in patients with chronic back pain and the failed back surgery syndrome. The drawbacks of these therapies relate predominantly to the potential for mechanical failure as well as clinical failure. This is especially true for implantable units.[50, 52, 57, 69]

In some selected patients, continuous infusion of intrathecal morphine has allowed satisfactory management. This has been facilitated by the increased availability of implantable pump devices. They remain labor intensive for the patient and the family, requiring periodic refilling in the physician's office.[26, 100]

For cases refractory to traditional management, some authors have suggested the use of epidural steroids or more aggressive surgical pain procedures such as cingulotomy or deep brain stimulation.[26]

Surgery

Traditionally, arachnoiditis was thought to be an untreatable, intractable disease, not warranting direct invasive attempts. Several authors caution against surgical treatment, suggesting that operations rarely provide significant pain relief and may in fact exacerbate symptoms by further damaging the neural elements.[23, 74] Surgery is not warranted on an exploratory basis, nor in the absence of progressive neurologic deficit, nor in patients whose pain is readily controlled.[46, 102]

A review of different authors' personal surgical series reveals variable surgical results, mostly unfavorable, particularly in higher-grade cases of arachnoiditis or in those who manifested preoperative dysesthesias.[28, 44, 77, 79, 104, 105]

Wilkinson selected patients for surgery only if they

manifested crescendo pain and neurologic deficits. The operative goal was extensive microsurgical dissection and lysis of arachnoidal scarring and re-establishment of the subarachnoid fluid pathways, with concurrent decompression of the neural elements. Initial good improvement was seen in 75 to 80 per cent of his patients but was maintained by only 50 per cent of those at one-year follow-up.[7, 44, 66, 103, 104]

The role of operative resection of arachnoidal scar remains controversial and may be clarified in the future.

Miscellaneous

In light of the lack of a beneficial treatment modality in this disease, it is not surprising that multiple new therapeutic concepts are emerging. None of these has, to date, shown clear-cut clinical utility; they are mentioned only for the sake of completeness. Currently, animal studies are being performed to evaluate the role of synthetic interposition materials to diminish arachnoiditis formation.[36, 78] Urokinase has been preliminarily investigated and reported in rodents.[18] D-Penicillamine showed no benefit overall in a double-blind trial.[35] The use of intrathecal Depo-Medrol has resulted in controversy for over 20 years, and its role still remains inconclusive.[8, 17, 21, 29, 60, 61, 92, 103]

PROGNOSIS

Arachnoiditis is associated with a persistence of symptoms and, only rarely, with a progression of pain and increased functional impairment. The presence of arachnoiditis and its attendant disability adversely affects quality of life. Patients have a diminished ability to return to full-time occupation. The majority depend on daily narcotic analgesics, some with substance abuse and suicidal tendencies.[37]

CONCLUSION

Adhesive arachnoiditis is a spinal process that is frustrating for both patients and physicians alike. It appears to result in discomfort and often disability, although symptoms and imaging studies are not always consistent or concordant. None of today's treatments are satisfactory for reversal of the disease or resolution of the symptoms. Emphasis must be on a better understanding of the pathophysiology involved. This will delineate specific interventions that can reduce or prevent the development of arachnoiditis and identify that subgroup of patients at high risk for aquiring it. Neuroimaging is important to rule out other causes for the clinical findings. In particular, treatable lesions must be sought and addressed as indicated.

References

1. Abram, S. E., and O'Connor, T. C.: Complications associated with epidural steroid injections. Reg. Anesth. 21:149–162, 1996.
2. Aldrete, J. A., and Brown, T. L.: Intrathecal hematoma and arachnoiditis after prophylactic blood patch through a catheter. Anesth. Analg. 84:233–241, 1997.
3. Aprill, C. N., III: Myelography. In Frymoyer, J. W. (ed.): The Adult Spine: Principle and Practice. New York, Raven Press, 1991.
4. Arky, R.: Physicians' Desk Reference, 51st ed. Officers of Medical Economics, 1997.
5. Augustin, P., Vanneste, J., and Davies, G.: Chronic spinal arachnoiditis following intracranial subarachnoid haemorrhage. Clin. Neurol. Neurosurg. 91:347–350, 1989.
6. Bay, J. W.: Other causes of low back pain in sciatica: Lumbar disc disease. In Hardy, R. W. (ed.): Seminars in Neurological Surgery. New York, Raven Press, 1932, p. 203.
7. Benoist, M., Ficat, C., Baraf, P., and Cauchoix, J.: Postoperative lumbar epiduro-arachnoiditis: Diagnostic and therapeutic aspects. Spine 5:432–436, 1980.
8. Bernat, J. L., Sadowsky, C. H., Vincent, F. M., et al.: Sclerosing spinal pachymeningitis associated with intrathecal methylprednisolone acetate administration for multiple sclerosis. Neurology 26:351–352, 1976.
9. Beyer, G. A., Lipman, B. T., Haughton, V. M., and Ho, K. C.: Effect of arachnoiditis on pain threshold. Invest. Radiol. 22:781–785, 1987.
10. Brammah, T. B., and Jayson, M. I.: Syringomyelia as a complication of spinal arachnoiditis. Spine, 19:2603–2605, 1994.
11. Brodsky, A. E.: Cauda equina arachnoiditis: A correlative clinical and roentgenologic study. Spine 3:51–60, 1978.
12. Brodsky, A. E.: Post laminectomy and post fusion stenosis of the lumbar spine. Clin. Orthop. 115:130, 1976.
13. Burton, C. V.: Lumbar arachnoiditis. Spine 3:24–30, 1978.
14. Burton, C. V., Kirkaldy-Willis, W. H., Yong-Hing, K., and Heithoff, K. B.: Causes of failure of sugery on the lumbar spine. Clin. Orthop. 157:191–199, 1981.
15. Caplan, L. R., Norohna, A. B., and Amico, L. L.: Syringomyelia and arachnoiditis. J. Neurol. Neurosurg. Psychiatry 53:106–113, 1990.
16. Carroll, S. E., and Wiesel, S. W.: Neurologic complications and lumbar laminectomy: A standardized approach to the multiply-operated lumbar spine. Clin. Orthop. 284:14–23, 1992.
17. Carron, H., and Toomey, T. C.: Epidural steroid therapy for low back pain. In Stanton-Hicks, M., and Boas, R. (eds.): Chronic Low Back Pain. Philadelphia, Grune & Stratton, 1982, pp. 193–198.
18. Ceviz, A., Arslan, A., Ak, H. E., and Inaloz, S.: The effect of urokinase in preventing the formation of epidural fibrosis and/or leptomeningeal arachnoiditis. Surg. Neurol. 47:124–127, 1997.
19. Chang, K. H., Han, M. H., Choi, Y. W., et al.: Tuberculous arachnoiditis of the spine findings on myelography, CT, and MR imaging. AJNR Am. J. Neuroradiol. 10:1255–1262, 1989.
20. Cho, K. H., Iwasaki, Y., Imamura, H., et al.: Experimental model of posttraumatic syringomyelia: The role of adhesive arachnoiditis in syrinx formation. J. Neurosurg. 80:133–139, 1994.
21. Cohen, F. L.: Conus medullaris syndrome following multiple intrathecal corticosteroid injections. Arch. Neurol 36:228–230, 1979.
22. Cooper, S. D., Brady, M. B., Williams, J. P., et al.: Neurosarcoidosis: Evaluation using computed tomography and magnetic resonance imaging. J. Comput. Tomogr. 12:96–99, 1988.
23. Coventry, M. B., and Stauffer, R. N.: The multiply operated back. In American Academy of Orthopaedic Surgeons: Symposium on the Spine. St. Louis, C. V. Mosby, 1969, pp. 132–142.
24. de La Blanchardiete, A., Stern, J. B., Molina, J. M., et al.: Spinal tuberculous arachnoiditis. Presse Med. 25:1333–1335, 1996.
25. Delamarter, R. B., Ross, J. S., Masaryk, T. J., et al.: Diagnosis of lumbar arachnoiditis by magnetic resonance imaging. Spine 15:304–310, 1990.
26. DeLaPorte, C., and Siegfield, J.: Lumbosacral spinal fibrosis (spinal arachnoiditis): Its diagnosis and treatment by spinal cord stimulation. Spine 8:593–603, 1983.
27. Djukic, S., Lang, P., and Morris, J.: The postoperative spine: Magnetic resonance imaging. Orthop. Clin. North Am. 21:603–624, 1990.
28. Dolan, R. A.: Spinal adhesive arachnoiditis. Surg. Neurol. 39:479–484, 1993.

29. Duchesneau, P. M., Wesistein, M. A., and Wesolowski, D. P.: Long-term effects of intrathecal Depo-Medrol. Neuroradiology 15:224, 1978.

30. Eismont, F. I., Green, B. A., and Quencer, B. M.: Posttraumatic spinal cord cyst. J. Bone Joint Surg. Am. 66:614–618, 1984.

31. Ellenbogen, K. A.: Empty sella syndrome caused by syphilitic arachnoiditis. JAMA 255:1882, 1986.

32. Errea, J. M., Ara, J. R., Alberdi, J., et al.: Syringomyelia due to arachnoiditis. Clinical-radiological description of 5 patients. Neurologia 8: 226–230, 1993.

33. Frymoyer, J. W.: The Adult Spine: Principles and Practice. New York, Raven Press, 1991.

34. Gemma, M., Bricchi, M., Grisoli, M., et al.: Neurologic symptoms after epidural anaesthesia: Report of three cases. Acta Anaesthesiol. Scand. 38:742–743, 1994.

35. Grahame, R., Clark, B., Watson, M., and Polkey, C.: Toward a rational therapeutic strategy for arachnoiditis: A possible role for D-penicillamine. Spine 16:172–175, 1991.

36. Griffet, J., Bastiani, F., Hofman, P., and Argenson, C.: Prevention of scar formation by polyglactin 910 (Vicryl) mesh after lumbar laminectomy in the rat. Rev. Chir. Orthop. Reparatrice Appar. Mot. 78:365–371, 1992.

37. Guyer, D. W., Wiltse, L. L., Eskay, M. L., and Guyer, B. H.: The long-range prognosis of arachnoiditis. Spine 14:1332–1341, 1989.

38. Haisa, T., Todo, T., Mitsui, I., and Kondo, T.: Lumbar adhesive arachnoiditis following attempted epidural anesthesia--case report. Neurol. Med. Chir. (Tokyo) 35:107–109, 1995.

39. Haughton, V. M.: Intrathecal toxicity of iohexol versus metrizamide: Survey and current state. Invest. Radiol. 20 (1 Suppl.): S14–S17, 1985.

40. Haughton, V. M., Nguyen, C. M., and Ho, K. C.: The etiology of focal spinal arachnoiditis: An experimental study. Spine 18:1193–1198, 1993.

41. Hueftle, M. G., Modic, M. T., Ross, J. S., et al.: Lumbar spine: Postoperative MR imaging with gadolinium-DTPA. Radiology 167:817–824, 1988.

42. Jackson, A., and Isherwood, I.: Does degenerative disease of the lumbar spine cause arachnoiditis: A magnetic resonance study and review of the literature. Br. J. Radiol. 67:840–847, 1994.

43. Jayson, M. I.: Vascular damage, fibrosis, and chronic inflammation in mechanical back pain problems. Semin. Arthritis Rheum. 18(4 Suppl. 2):73–76, 1989.

44. Johnston, J. D., and Matheny, J. B.: Microscopic lysis of lumbar adhesive arachnoiditis. Spine 3:36–39, 1978.

45. Jorgensen, J., Hansen, P. H., Steenskow, V., and Ovesen, N.: A clinical and radiological study of chronic lower spinal arachnoiditis. Neuroradiology 9: 139–144, 1975.

46. Kaiser, M. C., and Ramos, L.: MRI of the Spine, A Guide to Clinical Applications. New York, Georg Thieme Verlag, 1990.

47. Kawauchi, Y., Yone, K., and Sakou, T.: Myeloscopic observation of adhesive arachnoiditis in patients with lumbar spinal canal stenosis. Spinal Cord 334: 403–410, 1996.

48. Klekamp, J., Batzdorf, U., and Samii Bothe, H. W.: Treatment of syringomyelia associated with arachnoid scarring caused by arachnoiditis or trauma. J. Neurosurg. 86:233–240, 1997.

49. Kumar, A., Montanera, W., Willinsky, R., et al.: MR features of tuberculous arachnoiditis. J. Comput. Assist. Tomogr. 17:127–130, 1993.

50. Kumar, K., Nath, R., and Wyant, G. M.: Treatment of chronic pain by epidural spinal cord stimulation: A 10 year experience. J. Neurosurg. 75:402–407, 1991.

51. Laitt, R., Hackson, A., and Isherwood, I.: Patterns of chronic adhesive arachnoiditis following Myodil myelography: The significance of spinal canal stenosis and previous surgery. Br. J. Radiol. 69:693–698, 1996.

52. Laus, M., Alfonso, C., Tigani, D., et al.: Failed back syndrome: A study on 95 patients submitted to reintervention after lumbar nerve root decompression for the treatment of spondylotic lesions. Chirurgia Degli Organi di Movimento 79:119–126, 1994.

53. Lipman, B. T., and Haughton, V. M.: Brain beta-endorphin and spinal-cord enkephalin concentrations in experimental arachnoiditis. Invest. Radiol. 22:197–200, 1987.

54. Long, D.: Chronic adhesive spinal arachnoiditis: Pathogenesis, prognosis, and treatment. Neurosurg. Q. 2:296, 1992.

55. Malinovsky, J. M., and Pinaud, M.: Neurotoxicity of intrathecally administered agents. Ann. Fr. Anesth. Reanim. 15:647–658, 1996.

56. McIvor, J., Krajbich, J. I., and Hoffman, H.: Orthopaedic complications of lumboperitoneal shunts. J. Pediatr. Orthop. 8:687–689, 1988.

57. Meilman, P. W., Leibrock, L. F., and Leong, F. T.: Outcome of implanted spinal cord stimulation in the treatment of chronic pain: Arachnoiditis versus single nerve root injury and mononeuropathy. Clin. J. Pain 5:189–193, 1989.

58. Menezes, A. H., and Sonntag, V. K. H.: Principles of Spinal Surgery. New York, McGraw-Hill, 1996.

59. Nainkin, L.: Arachnoiditis ossificans: Report of a case. Spine 3:83–86, 1978.

60. Nelson, D. A.: Complications from intrathecal steroid therapy in patients with multiple sclerosis. Acta Neurol. Scand. 49:176–188, 1973.

61. Nelson, D. A.: Dangers from methylprednisolone acetate therapy by intraspinal injection. Arch. Neurol. 45:84–86, 1988.

62. Ng, P., Lorentz, I., and Soo, Y. S.: Arachnoiditis ossificans of the cauda equina demonstrated on computed tomography scanogram: A case report. Spine 21:2504–2507, 1996.

63. Odin, M., Runstrom, G., and Lindblom, A.: Iodized oils as an aid to the diagnosis of lesions of the spinal cord and a contribution to the knowledge of adhesive circumscribed meningitis. Acta Radiol. Suppl. 7:1–86, 1929.

64. Ohry, A., Azaria, M., and Zeilig, G.: Long term follow up of patients with cauda equina syndrome due to intraspinal lipoma. Paraplegia 30:366–369, 1992.

65. Parke, W. W., and Watanabe, R.: The intrinsic vasculature of the lumbosacral spinal nerve roots. Spine 10:508–515, 1985.

66. Parnass, S. M., and Schmidt, K. J.: Adverse effects of spinal and epidural anaesthesia. Drug Saf. 5:179–194, 1990.

67. Peek, R. D., Thomas, J. C., Jr., and Wiltse, L. L.: Diagnosis of lumbar arachnoiditis by myeloscopy. Spine 18:2286–2289, 1993.

68. Pence, D. M., Kim, T. H., and Levitt, S. H.: Aneurysm, arachnoiditis and intrathecal Au (gold). Int. J. Radiat. Oncol. Biol. Phys. 18:1001–1004, 1990.

69. Penn, R. D., and Paice, J. A.: Chronic intrathecal morphine for intractable pain. J. Neurosurg. 67:182–186, 1987.

70. Pfadenhauer, K., and Rossmanith, T.: Spinal manifestation of neurolisteriosis. J. Neurol. 242:153–156, 1995.

71. Phadke, R. V., Kohli, A., Jain, V. K., et al.: Tuberculous radiculomyelitis (arachnoiditis): Myelographic and CT appearances. Australas. Radiol. 38:10–16, 1994.

72. PLIF complications. In Frymoyer, J. W. (ed.): The Adult Spine: Principles and Practice. New York, Raven Press, 1991, p. 1896.

73. Preacher, W. B., and Roberston, R. C.: Pantopaque myelography: Results, comparison of contrast media, and spinal fluid reaction. J. Neurosurg. 2:220–231, 1945.

74. Quiles, M., Machisello, P. J., and Tsairis, P.: Lumbar adhesive arachnoiditis: Etiologic and pathologic aspects. Spine 3:45–50, 1978.

75. Ramirez, L. F., and Thisted, R.: Complications and demographic characteristics of patients undergoing lumbar discectomy in community hospitals. Neurosurgery 25:226–231, 1989.

76. Ramsey, G. H., French, J. D., and Strain, W. H.: Iodinated organic compounds as contrast media for radiographic diagnoses: Pantopaque myelography. Radiology 43:236–240, 1944.

77. Ray, C. D.: Percutaneous peripheral nerve and spinal cord stimulation for pain. In Youmans, J. (ed.): Neurological Surgery. 3rd ed. Philadelphia, W. B. Saunders Co., 1990, pp. 3984–4006.

78. Reigel, D. H., Bazmi, B., Shih, S. R., and Marquardt, M. D.: A pilot investigation of poloxamer 407 for the prevention of leptomeningeal adhesions in the rabbit. Pediatr. Neurosurg. 19:250–255, 1993.

79. Roca, J., Moreta, D., Ubierna, M. T., et al.: The results of surgical treatment of lumbar arachnoiditis. Int. Orthop. 17:77–81, 1993.

80. Roeder, M. B., Bazan, C., and Jinkins, J. R.: Ruptured spinal dermoid cyst with chemical arachnoiditis and disseminated intracranial lipid droplets. Neuroradiology 37:146–147, 1995.

81. Romanick, P. C., and Smith, T. K.: Infection about the spine associated with low-velocity-missile injury to the abdomen. J. Bone Joint Surg. Am. 67:1105–1201, 1985.

82. Ross, J. S.: Magnetic resonance assessment of the postoperative spine: Degenerative disc disease. Radiol. Clin. North Am. 29:793–808, 1991.
83. Ross, J. S., Masaryk, T. J., Modic, M. T., et al.: Lumbar spine: Postoperative assessment with surface-coil MR imaging. Radiology 164:851–860, 1987.
84. Ross, J. S., Masaryk, T. J., Modic, M. T., et al.: MR imaging of lumbar arachnoiditis. AJNR Am. J. Neuroradiol. 8:855, 1987.
85. Ross, J. S., Masaryk, T. J., Modic, M. T., et al.: MR imaging of lumbar arachnoiditis. AJR Am. J. Roentgenol. 149:1025–1032, 1987.
86. Seppala, M. T., Haltia, M. J., Sankila, R. J., et al.: Long-term outcome after removal of spinal schwannoma: A clinicopathological study of 187 cases. J. Neurosurg. 83:621–626, 1995.
87. Shaw, D. D., and Potts, D. G.: Toxicology of iohexol. Invest. Radiol. 20 (1 Suppl.): S10–S13, 1985.
88. Shiraishi, T., Crock, H. V., and Reynolds, A.: Spinal arachnoiditis ossificans: Observations on its investigation and treatment. Eur. Spine J. 4: 60–63, 1995.
89. Sklar, E. M., Quencer, R. M., Green, B. A., et al.: Complications of epidural anesthesia: MR appearance of abnormalities. Radiology 181:549–554, 1991.
90. Smith, A. S., and Blaser, S. I.: Infectious and inflammatory processes of the spine. Radiol. Clin. North Am. 29:809–827, 1991.
91. Smith, A. S., and Blaser, S. I.: MR of infectious and inflammatory diseases of the spine. Crit. Rev. Diagn. Imaging 32:165–189, 1991.
92. Stanton-Hicks, M.: Therapeutic caudal or epidural block for lower back or sciatic pain. JAMA 243:369–370, 1980.
93. Sze, G.: Gadolinium-DTPA in spinal disease. Radiol. Clin. North Am. 26:1009, 1988.
94. Tator, C. H.: Pathophysiology and pathology of spinal cord injury. In Wilkins, R. H., and Rengachary, S. S., (eds.): Neurosurgery. 2d ed. New York, McGraw-Hill, 1994, p. 281.
95. Tetsworth, K. D., and Ferguson, R. L.: Arachnoiditis ossificans of the cauda equina: A case report. Spine 11:765–766, 1986.
96. Tjandra, J. J., Varma, T. R., and Weeks, R. D.: Spinal arachnoiditis following subarachnoid haemorrhage. Aust. N. Z. J. Surg. 59:84–87, 1989.
97. Toribatake, Y., Baba Maezawa, Y., Umeda, S., and Tomita, K.: Symptomatic arachnoiditis ossificans of the thoracic spine: Case report. Paraplegia 33: 224–227, 1995.
98. Venes, J. L.: Surgical considerations in the initial repair of meningomyelocele and the introduction of a technical modification. Neurosurgery 17:111–113, 1985.
99. Wan, C. L., Chang, C. S., Wei, C. P., et al.: Cryptococcal infection presenting with lumbosacral polyradiculopathy: Report of a case. J. Formos. Med. Assoc. 90:1218–1221, 1991.
100. Wester, K.: Dorsal column stimulation in pain treatment. Acta Neurol. Scand. 75:151–155, 1987.
101. Wiesel, S.: The Lumbar Spine. 2nd. ed. Philadelphia, W. B. Saunders Co., 1996.
102. Wiesel, S. W.: The multiply operated lumbar spine. Instr. Course Lect. 34:68–77, 1985.
103. Wilkinson, H. A.: The Failed Back Syndrome: Etiology and Therapy. Philadelphia, Harper and Rowe, 1983.
104. Wilkinson, H. A.: Lumbar adhesive arachnoiditis. In Long, D. M. (ed.): Current Therapy in Neurological Surgery. Philadelphia, B. C. Decker, 1985, pp. 198–200.
105. Wilkinson, H. A., and Schuman, N.: Results of surgical lysis of lumbar adhesive arachnoiditis. Neurosurgery 4:401–409, 1979.
106. Woodall, W. C., III, Bertorini, T. E., Bakhtian, B. J., and Gelfand, M. S.: Spinal arachnoiditis with Cryptococcus neoformans in a nonimmunocompromised child. Pediatr. Neurol. 6:206–208, 1990.
107. Wright, M. G.: Lumbo-sacral adhesive arachnoiditis. J. R. Soc. Med. 83:673, 1990.
108. Yamagami, T., Matsui, H., Tsuji, H., et al.: Effects of laminectomy and retained extradural foreign body on cauda equina adhesion. Spine 18:1774–1781, 1993.

Vascular Complications in Spine Surgery

Jeffery L. Stambough, M.D.

Frederick A. Simeone, M.D.

Vascular complications in spine surgery are, fortunately, rare. The exact incidence is difficult to determine and depends on one's exact definition of a vascular complication. For example, if significant bleeding from a decorticated vertebral end plate during an anterior discectomy is considered a vascular complication, the incidence would be high. For our purposes, a vascular complication is defined as an injury to a blood vessel and its sequelae that result directly or indirectly from a surgical approach, procedure, or operative technique.

Vascular complications carry potentially dire consequences, including death. As with any complication, the best treatment is prevention. However, if one does occur, prompt recognition and management are critical. Prevention of vascular complication is facilitated by (1) knowledge of the vascular anatomy and common variants,[49, 104] (2) knowledge of the blood vessel/bone relations,[88, 101] (3) gentle intraoperative techniques with appropriate illumination and magnification, and (4) proper preoperative planning. This chapter stresses the relations of vascular anatomy to the spine and emphasizes techniques of prevention and early recognition of vascular injuries.

In general, vascular complications in spine surgery have two implications: (1) the consequences and sequelae of brisk, prohibitive bleeding (i.e., hemorrhagic shock), or simply the inability to complete the case on a timely basis owing to impaired visualization; or (2) interruption of vascular supply to vital organs such as the spinal cord or the brain stem. These complications vary, depending on the area of the spine involved and the surgical approach used.[7] These are not necessarily mutually exclusive and are often seen in combination. The former category is self-explanatory, resulting from injury to or disruption of major vessels adjacent to the vertebral bodies. In the latter category, complete neurologic dysfunction can occur, but is poorly understood. Each of these categories has serious and perhaps permanent sequelae.

CERVICAL SPINE

Vascular complications in the cervical spine can be a result of improper and excessive retraction or inadvertent laceration with a scalpel or other surgical instrument.[5, 10, 11, 13, 15, 17, 18, 28, 62, 78, 107, 113, 116, 133–135] The exact incidence of vascular injuries from anterior cervical spine surgery is not known but is probably underreported. In a review of complications of anterior spine surgery involving over 500 cases, Tew and Mayfield found no vascular complications,[125] and neither did Bertalanffy and Eggert in their review of 450 cases.[7] Hohf reported four cases of carotid artery injury from anterior spinal fusion, three involving laceration and the other involving division of the carotid artery.[56] (No permanent neurologic sequelae occurred from these vascular injuries, and all were repaired primarily.) He also found 12 additional hearsay cases of carotid artery injury. Phillips emphasized that the vessels of the carotid sheath were at "some risk" from the self-retaining retractor but reported no cases of injury in his series.[99] Rizzoli reported one case of vertebral artery laceration during anterior discectomy and fusion from a pituitary rongeur.[103] Bleeding in this case was controlled by packing with oxidized regenerated cellulose. No complications or sequelae developed. Schweighofer and colleagues reported one vertebral artery injury occurring in 175 cases of interbody fusion.[108] The artery was sacrificed, and there were no adverse consequences for the patient. The authors are aware of two unreported cases of vertebral artery injury during anterior cervical disc surgery. Both resulted in no permanent injury, although one case had a pseudoaneurysm detected by a postoperative MRI. Golfinos and associates reported four cases of vertebral artery injuries in 2015 anterior cervical spine cases, for an incidence of 0.3 per cent.[46]

Exposure of the anterior cervical spine most commonly uses an approach medial to the sternocleidomastoid muscle and carotid sheath.[104] Other approaches may dissect medial to the sternocleidomastoid muscle but lateral to the carotid sheath or lateral to both.[33, 128, 131] These approaches risk direct injury to the external jugular vein. The internal jugular vein is of little clinical significance, except in regard to hemorrhage. It may be sacrificed and ligated with impunity. Laceration of a large vein may be of significance if the patient is positioned with the head higher than the heart. This creates a negative pressure, which may case air to be "sucked" into the lumen of the vessel and then into the heart, resulting in an air embolism in the heart, with disastrous consequences or even death.[8, 32] Zeidman and Ducker[134] reviewed their experience with the posterior approach to cervical radiculopathy. In their 172 cases done in the sitting position, four patients had air embolisms without clinical sequelae. Lacerations of the carotid sheath vessels should be repaired if possible, although the internal jugular vein may be ligated if necessary.[10]

The common carotid artery is at risk as one develops the dissection plane and during retraction for the deep anterior cervical spine exposure. Identification of the carotid artery by palpation and gentle finger dissection helps to minimize injury of this major vessel. Proper placement of self-retaining retractors requires mobilization of the longus colli muscles along the anterolateral aspect of the vertebral bodies. The blades of the retractor must be under these muscles, and the retractor

should apply only enough tension to retract these muscles away from the disc space margins. During the surgery, the anesthesiologist monitors the superficial temporal artery pulse for possible carotid artery occlusion secondary to excessive retraction.[94] Two cases of stroke believed to be caused by overzealous retraction of the carotid artery using hand-held Richardson retractors are known to us, resulting in left hemiplegia. One patient improved, but the other did not. This complication is more likely in an older patient with atherosclerotic disease requiring extensive exposure and dissection (e.g., multiple carpectomy).[20] If the carotid artery has been compromised, the chance of nervous system complications is great.[20, 45, 46]

The vertebral artery and vein are at risk from both anterior and posterior exposures of the cervical spine (Fig. 54–20) During anterior exposure, the vertebral arteries are at risk of injury by dissection lateral to the longus colli muscles and during anterior discectomy along the lateral margins of the disc.[51, 116] Rarely, the anterior dissection is off the midline and risks injury of the vessels as well. Prevention of vertebral vascular injuries requires careful dissection of the longus colli muscles. Coagulation of the medial edge of the muscles and use of a blunt, medium-sized periosteal elevator to mobilize laterally are recommended. (The periosteal elevator is never directed posteriorly.) Furthermore, use of the operative microscope and microinstruments within the disc space has been advocated to help decrease the risk of vertebral artery injury laterally.[31, 50] In the 2015-case series of Golfinos and coworkers, verte-

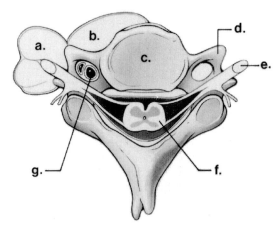

Figure 54–20. Cervical spine anatomic relationships. This schematic illustration represents a cross section of the cervical spine at C5. The anterior scalenus muscle (A), the longus colli muscle (B), the vertebral body (C), and the transverse foramina (D) are noted. The cervical nerve root (E) and the spinal cord (F) are seen relative to the anterior vertebral body (C) and musculature (A, B). The vertebral artery (G) is noted within the transverse foramina. The vertebral body enters the sixth cervical foramina and extends to the right of the C1 posteriorly, to become the basilar artery. Injury to the vertebral artery may occur when releasing or dissecting the longus colli muscles. It may also be injured in discectomies that involve dissection in the lateral aspect of the disc near the uncovertebral joint (not shown).

bral artery injuries were caused by decompression laterally in two, screw tapping in one, and soft tissue retraction in one.

The inferior and superior thyroid arteries, between the sternocleidomastoid muscle and the carotid sheath, are at risk for injury in the anterior approaches. Avoiding injury to these vessels is important not only for the sake of bleeding but also because each has a significant nerve accompanying it. If necessary, the vessels themselves may be divided and ligated for additional exposure.[10, 31] Jenis and LeClair reported an unusual case of an inferior thyroid artery pseudoaneurysm nine days after a routine anterior cervical discectomy and fusion.[62] Embolization without revision surgery corrected the complication.

The anterior spinal artery system is essentially an independent vascular system in the upper cervical segments and is dependent on contributions from the radicular arteries in the middle and lower segments.[16] The anterior spinal artery can be compressed by cervical spondylosis. Excision of the posterior longitudinal ligament protects against epidural bleeding and possible injury of the anterior spinal artery. The avoidance of unipolar coagulation around the posterior longitudinal ligament or the dura is to be emphasized.[14] Inadvertent coagulation of the anterior spinal artery could result in quadriplegia from ischemia of the cervical spinal cord.

Traumatic iatrogenic arteriovenous fistula between the vertebral artery and the surrounding venous plexus is a rare complication of anterior cervical discectomy.[26] It may complicate anterior cervical discectomy at or above the C5–C6 level because the vertebral artery runs just lateral to the disc space at these levels. The presence of a cervical bruit following surgery suggests fistulous communication and necessitates angiographic investigation. Minimally invasive endovascular occlusion of the fistula with interventional techniques is now the therapeutic procedure of choice.[7]

Treatment of vascular injuries during anterior cervical spine exposure involves recognition, control of bleeding, and repair or ligation when indicated. Primary repair of the vertebral artery and common carotid artery is indicated. If the vertebral artery is lacerated during the anterior dissection, the bleeding point must be tamponaded, and the dissection must then be carried laterally by mobilizing or dividing the longus colli muscles. The costotransverse lamellae can be removed with a high-speed drill, a diamond burr, and a Kerrison rongeur to allow for adequate exposure for primary vascular repair (Fig. 54–21A).[27, 33] The artery should first be exposed proximal to the laceration. Once the artery is exposed, vessel loops can be used for occlusion (Fig. 54–21B). The nerve roots should be identified and protected. Once the artery is exposed and controlled, the laceration can be repaired, if possible, with 7-0 polypropylene interrupted sutures (Fig. 54–21C).[27] It is the opinion of the authors that a laceration of the vertebral artery should be repaired primarily if at all possible. This is supported by recent studies by Golfinos and Pfeifer and colleagues.[46, 98] Others advocate ligating the vertebral artery if it is lacerated during the

anterior approach to the cervical spine.[8] If the vertebral artery is to be sacrificed, under ideal circumstances, it should first be studied radiographically by intraoperative angiography to ensure that the anatomy of the patient's vertebral system is likely to permit such a maneuver.[36, 58] The ability of the patient to tolerate unilateral occlusion of the vertebral artery is supported by a study of nine patients with traumatic occlusion of the vertebral artery.[111, 115] Only two developed neurologic deficits, and these were transient.[30] Neurologic deficit secondary to vertebral artery injuries depends in part on the collateralization of the circle of Willis and the status of the opposite vertebral artery and the basilar artery.[4, 7, 11, 34] However, Smith and associates reported that three out of seven cases of vertebral artery ligation developed symptomatic vertebral-basilar ischemic signs and symptoms.[116] These vertebral-basilar symptoms include syncope, drop attacks, dizziness, nystagmus, and the Wallenberg syndrome. Smith and associates favor repair if it can be accomplished, but it was not possible in their series.[116] Causgrove reported an arteriovenous fistula of the vertebral artery following anterior cervical discectomy.[120, 121] This patient presented with an audible bruit about two months after successful anterior cervical discectomy and fusion. Revision surgery was not necessary. The authors are aware of two other cases.

The vertebral artery and venous plexus are the only major vessels that course posterior to the lamina in the spinal column (Fig. 54–22) The vessels are at risk of injury in the upper cervical spine or during cervical spine or posterior fossa surgery.[32] Fortunately, the incidence of posterior vertebral artery injury is rare. Rizzoli reported three cases of vertebral artery injury, all of which were secondary to laceration from the bovie; two were ligated without neurologic deficits, and the other was repaired primarily.[29, 103] Hohf reported one case of vertebral artery injury during posterior cervical spine surgery, but the details of the injury were not given.[56] We are aware of two cases of vertebral artery injury during exposure of C1 for an occipital cervical fusion. Both of these cases resulted from vigorous subperiosteal dissection with a periosteal elevator. Both were managed by packing to control bleeding with absorbable gelatin sponge or oxidized regenerated cellulose left in situ. Fortunately, no neurologic sequelae developed in either case. Blood loss was profuse, approaching a liter. Cranial base surgery continues to offer significant challenges and limitations owing to the unpredictable nature of this region's cerebrovascular anatomy and physiology.[96]

Prevention of vertebral vascular injuries during posterior exposure of the upper cervical spine starts with identifying the posterior tubercle of the atlas and limiting lateral dissection to less than 1.5 cm in adults and 1 cm in children.[32] The vertebral artery is vulnerable, as it passes between the C1–C2 transverse foramina laterally. Here, lateral dissection should stop when one encounters the dorsal ramus of C2. Injury to the vertebral vasculature is controlled initially by packing and by administering antithrombotic agents. If possible and

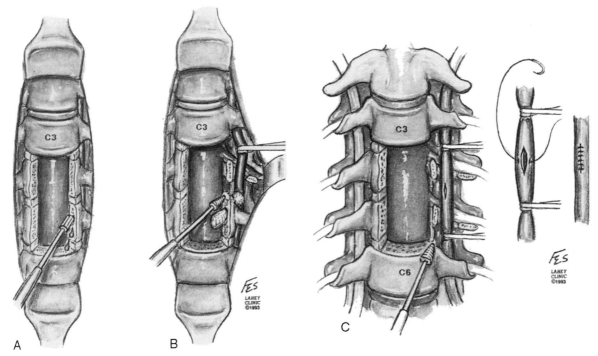

Figure 54–21. *A,* The surgical technique of repair of the vertebral artery. The trough has been cut in the C4–C5 bodies. The drill is tilted to get slightly more exposure. The bleeding area has been tamponaded. The bone anterior to the transverse foramen is drilled away to expose the vertebral artery. The C4, C5, and C6 nerve roots are exposed and protected. *B,* Elastic loops have been placed around the vertebral artery proximal and distal to the laceration. *C,* The laceration is repaired with interrupted sutures of 7-0 polypropylene. (From Pfeifer et al: Spine *19*(13):14, 71–74, 1994.)

technically feasible, posterior artery injury is repaired primarily to preserve brain stem flow. With the recent introduction of lateral mass plating (C2–C7), malpositioning of the lateral mass screw may injure the vertebral artery within the transverse foramen (Fig. 54–23).[47] Prevention includes knowledge of the bony landmarks and choosing appropriate screw lengths and angles of insertion.

THORACIC SPINE

Anterior exposure to the thoracic spine is well established, with ever-increasing applications.[12, 15, 32, 70, 91] Potential vascular-related complications involve injury to the major vessels and their branches, and the consequences of the interruption of the blood supply to the thoracic spinal cord (Fig. 54–24). The incidence of paraplegia secondary to unilateral vascular interrup-

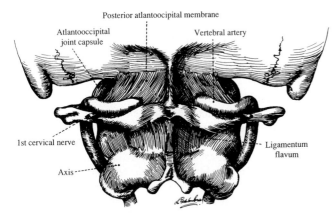

Figure 54–22. Diagram showing the vertebral arteries coursing over the posterior arch of C1. The medial extent is usually approximately 1 1/2 to 2 cm from the midline.

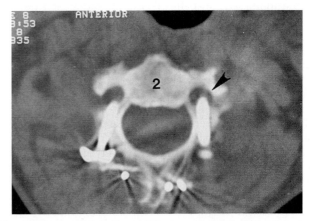

Figure 54–23. Malpostioned C2 screw violating the vertebral artery, fortunately without ill effects or vascular sequelae.

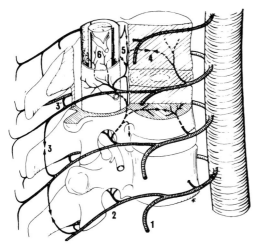

Figure 54–24. Diagram showing anastomoses of the dorsal branches of the spinal artery. *1*, intercostal artery; *2*, dorsal branches of spinal artery; *3* and *3'*, posterior anastomosis; *4*, vertebral anastomosis; *5*, retrovertebral anastomosis; *6*, perimedullar anastomosis. Segmental vessels are shown exiting from the posterior aspect of the aorta. The vessels lie along the thoracic spine, across the midportion of the vertebral bodies. (From Lazorthes, G., Gouaze, A., Zadeh, J. O., et al.: Arterial vascularization of the spinal cord: Recent studies of the anastomotic substitution pathways. *J. Neurosurg.* *35*:253–262, 1971.)

tion of the thoracic segmental vessels is almost nil. Bilateral disruption of the segmental blood supply, as in aortic surgery or dissecting aortic aneurysms, is not as forgiving.[37, 93, 110, 123] Other procedures associated with spinal cord infarction include bilateral sympathectomies,[109] aortic grafting,[54, 127] major chest surgery involving lobectomy,[110] anterior surgery for tuberculosis,[16, 52] anterior scoliosis surgery,[87] and angiography, most commonly using the abdominal aorta.[35, 36, 66]

The exact incidence of spinal cord infarction and paraplegia caused by vascular occlusion is now known. Statistics from the Scoliosis Research Society describe an incidence of 1 percent paraplegia in over 10,000 deformity cases.[87, 89] Paraplegia rates are higher in adult patients and patients treated for severe deformities, kyphosis, or kyphoscoliosis.[84, 87, 130] Vascular disruptions leading to paraplegia have been reported in 6 percent of one-stage circumferential spinal osteotomies.[32] Of these four were permanent and one recovered completely. In this series of circumferential osteotomies, there were 55 adult scoliotics, and all cases resulting in paraplegia were at the T5–T9 level. Hodgson reported one case of vascular-induced paraplegia in over 400 cases of anterior spine surgery for tuberculosis. He warned to be careful at the T10 level on the left.[54] Riseborough,[102] Micheli and Hall,[86] Dwyer and Schafer,[33] and Winter and colleagues,[131] reported a cumulative total of over 100 extensive anterior dissections and unilateral ligation of thoracic segmental arteries without any cases of paraplegia.

The transthoracic approach to the anterior thoracic spine usually requires direct mobilization of segmental arteries and veins over several vertebral levels.[63, 64, 114] A right-sided approach is recommended to avoid the pericardial structures. In cases of deformity, however, it is most advantageous to approach the convexity of the deformity, regardless of the side involved. To gain access to the thoracic segmental and intercostal arteries, the parietal pleura must be divided.[27] The authors begin the dissection over the disc space, where there are no vessels. The individual vessels are identified and isolated with a right-angle hemostat and ligated. About 1 cm of segmental vessel is maintained from the thoracic aorta to avoid cutting this vessel too close to the aorta, thereby creating a hole in the side of the aorta. Lazorthes has shown that better collateralization and anastomotic substitution can occur as these vessels are ligated or disrupted closer to the aorta.[69] Inadvertent laceration or avulsion of the segmental vessels from the aorta can result in brisk bleeding.[112] Should this occur, bleeding can be controlled by direct pressure proximal and distal to the defect. Repair of the aorta should be assisted by a surgeon experienced in vascular surgery. Mack and colleagues reported on 100 cases of video-assisted thoracoscopy (VAT) for a variety of thoracic spine conditions. A singular case of profound epidural bleeding occurred, but no incidence of segmental artery, aorta, or azygos vein injury was noted.[79, 80]

Great controversy exists over the relative importance of individual blood vessels that supply the spinal cord.[42] In 1939, Suh and Alexander noted that "much of what has been written in the past forty years about the circulation of the spinal cord is either inaccurate or incomplete."[123] In the same year, Bolton determined that the segmental vessels that supply the spinal cord are indeed end-arteries, and there are no anastomoses between the capillary beds.[11] Individually, vessels that travel with the spinal nerve into the spinal canal do not seem to be important, as evidenced by Dwyer's ligation of 3 to 16 ipsilateral segmental arteries in a single patient without neurologic loss.[33] Great attention was given in the past to the artery of Adamkiewicz (arteria radicularis or arteria magna), which is the largest of the feeders to the thoracolumbar spinal cord (Fig. 54–25).[85] It occurs on the left side in 80 per cent of patients between T7 and L4, with the greatest incidence between T9 and T11. It usually enters the spinal canal with at least one additional feeder. DiChiro and coworkers in 1970 noted that this artery could be tied in a rhesus monkey without complications, but paraplegia would follow when the anterior spinal artery (arterial median longitudinal artery) was simultaneously ligated.[30] Further evidence of the importance of disruption of this segmental vessel is the high incidence of paraplegia in thoracic aortic surgery involving cross clamping of the thoracic aorta or in cases in which dissection aneurysms occlude the segmental vessels bilaterally.[93, 98, 123] However, paraparesis or paraplegia as a result of unilateral ligation of thoracic, thoracolumbar, or lumbar segmental arteries is very rare.

Dommisse and Enslin noted four cases of permanent paraplegia in their series of 68 spinal procedures

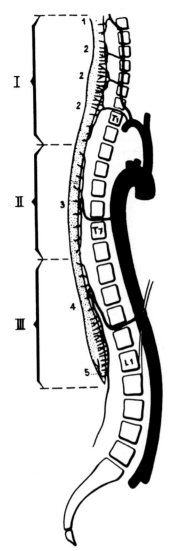

Figure 54–25. Major arterial vessels supplying the spinal cord through the anterior spinal artery are depicted. *4* is the area where the artery of Adamkiewicz is usually found. *I*, superior or cervicothoracic area; *II*, intermediate or midthoracic area; *III*, lower or thoracolumbar area. *1*, anterior spinal artery; *2*, artery of the cervical enlargement; *3*, posterior spinal artery; *4*, artery of the lumbar enlargement; *5*, anastomotic loop of the conus medullaris. (From Lazorthes, G., Gouaze, A., Zadeh, J. O., et al.: Arterial vascularization of the spinal cord: Recent studies of the anastomotic substitution pathways. *J. Neurosurg.* 35:253–262, 1971.)

(mostly for scoliosis), three of which occurred between T5 and T9; the other occurred with surgery below T10.[32] These authors emphasized a "critical zone of the spinal cord" that extends from T4 to T9. In the study by Lazorthes and coworkers, the artery of Adamkiewicz appeared between T9 and T12 in 75 per cent of cases, at the L1–L2 level in 10 per cent of cases, and at the T5 to T8 level in 15 per cent of cases.[69] When the artery of Adamkiewicz appeared in the midthoracic level, there was a supplemental artery that they referred to as the arteria conus medullaris supplying the thoracolumbar cord (see Fig. 54–24). The thoracolumbar spinal cord

has a very rich anastomotic blood supply formed by both the anterior and the posterior spinal arteries. The anterior spinal artery in the region of T4 to T9, however, is quite small and can be incomplete, as shown by Lazorthes.[69] In his excellent study, Dommisse demonstrated that the spinal canal was also narrow in this region, and this could predispose to surgical complications, particularly in the face of a chronic low reserve state of spinal fluid circulation.[31]

Actual case reports of spinal cord infarction with permanent paraplegia following anterior spinal surgery are rare. It is likely, in fact, that many individual thoracic and lumbar segmental arteries are expendable, as has been experienced by most thoracic, orthopedic, and neurologic surgeons. Even the artery of Adamkiewicz, which is substantially larger than the others, can be occluded under most circumstances. It is not uncommon in some scoliosis procedures to have an extensive ipsilateral sacrifice of these feeding arteries without significant sequelae.[33] Winter and associates reported 1197 consecutive anterior spinal cases with only two cases of paraparesis or paraplegia related to the ligation of sequential vessels unilaterally. These cases were unusual, in that both involved an unusual syndrome with congenital abnormalities (hypoplastic thoracic pedicles), suggesting a pre-existing vascular or spinal cord anomaly.[131, 132]

Posterior midline thoracic surgery endangers no major vessels.[19, 25] In contrast, the posterolateral approach or costotransversectomy (lateral rachitomy of Menard) has definite potential vascular complications, although major vascular injury is quite rare.[15] This approach requires mobilization of the neurovascular structures, which serve as a guide to the spinal canal. Injury to the intercostal vessels can result in profuse bleeding. These vessels can be ligated without a problem. Retrograde thrombosis of the left eleventh intercostal vessels from a left rib transthoracoabdominal approach during sympathectomy for hypertension was reported to cause paraplegia in one case.[109] In this regard, a right-sided approach is used, unless the pathologic process dictates a preference for a side. We have had to re-explore a case in the early postoperative period for hemothorax resulting from intercostal artery bleeding. Chan has warned of potential aortic perforation during a costotransversectomy for tuberculosis owing to the weakening of the vessel from the tuberculous inflammatory process.[18] Injury to the major vessels during a costotransversectomy requires packing off the bleeder in the depths of the wound, covering the wound, starting volume expanders, and preparing for immediate thoracotomy and repair of the thoracic vessels. Prevention of injury to the major vessels anteriorly during the costotransversectomy procedure is facilitated by careful blunt dissection of the pleura off the lateral border of the vertebral bodies.[25] No instrument should be placed in the depths of the wound unless visual identification of the position of this instrument can be verified. Once the parietal pleura has been mobilized, the segmentals can be further dissected away from the vertebral body, thereby allowing access to the disc and bone.

LUMBAR SPINE

Anterior exposure of the lumbar and lumbosacral spine can be accomplished by a lateral retroperitoneal approach,[65, 67, 97] a transperitoneal approach,[39, 105, 106] or a hypogastric "small incision" approach. Both approaches directly address the vasculature of the anterior lumbar spine. Vascular injuries and complications in these approaches are not commonly reported, because most surgeons understand that mobilization, dissection, and retraction of the great vessels can result in profuse bleeding and are prepared to deal with it. Therefore, an accurate incidence of the vascular injuries from anterior lumbar spine surgery is not known. Depending on the spine surgeon's level of expertise, a collaborative effort with a surgeon experienced in vascular surgical techniques is often helpful and necessary, especially in revision cases.[59]

Vascular injuries and complications rarely result in serious sequelae, unless the injury results in total disruption of the vascular channels to the lower extremity or other important viscera.[53] Recognition and repair remain the standard of care. In lumbar spine anterior approaches, the authors prefer to approach the spine from the left if all other factors are equal, because the aorta is more resilient than the vena cava. The retroperitoneal approach as described by Fey is a modified sympathectomy approach.[97] This is different from the thoracic spine. Here, in the lumbar spine, instrumentation should be placed on the right to avoid the potential late erosion or perforation of the pulsatile aortic due to irritation or prominence of the vertebral body implant.

The psoas major can be relaxed by flexing the hip and knee, making vascular dissection safer and easier. Incisions are placed according to the vertebral level of major interest, and the approach is carried to the retroperitoneal space. The psoas major is the most important landmark to guide the deep dissection. Each vessel is independently isolated with a right-angle hemostat and clipped or ligated. Double ligation is preferred toward the midline, leaving at least 1 cm of lumbar segmental vessel to prevent making a hole in the aorta or the vena cava. The use of clips versus suture ties is largely dependent on surgeon preference. Ligation of the segmental vessels should be over the middle or anterior half of the vertebral body. By staying away from posterior ligation of the segmental vessels, the risk of interference with foraminal or collateral blood flow is reduced. In addition, it is technically easier to control the vessels in this anatomic location. Ligation too close to the aorta or vena cava should also be avoided so as not to be left with a vessel stump that is too short. If the ligation, suture, or clip should tear or dislodge, the major vessel may end up with a large hole in its side wall.

Major hemorrhage can occur if the segmental lumbar vessels, aorta, or vena cava is lacerated or torn

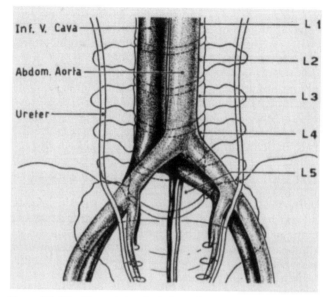

Figure 54–26. Transabdominal view of the *abdominal aorta* and *inferior vena cava.* The vertebral column is posterior to the vessels. The aorta lies to the left of the vena cava. (From Montorsi, W., and Ghiringhelli, C.: Genesis: Diagnosis and treatment of vascular complications after intervertebral disc surgery. *Int. Surg. 58*:233–235, 1973.)

(Fig. 54–26). The left common iliac vein is the vessel most at risk in lower left-sided retroperitoneal spinal dissections. Bleeding is first controlled by direct pressure. Ligation of the segmental vessels is facilitated by carefully compressing the aorta and vena cava medially to identify the bleeder. Repair of the abdominal aorta and especially the vena cava requires expertise in vascular surgery. If the surgeon lacks this, the bleeding should be controlled by direct pressure until help can arrive. Exposure of the lumbar spine anteriorly may require extensive dissection and mobilization of the segmental vessels. Cases of major vascular injury from anterior lumbar spine surgery are very uncommon. Dwyer and Schafer averaged 1800 ml blood loss in their 51 cases, but no major vascular injuries were reported using the Dwyer cable.[33]

Baker and associates reviewed 102 consecutive cases of anterior lumbar spinal surgery performed for a wide variety of lumbar spinal conditions (L3–S1), all assisted by fellowship-trained vascular surgeons.[5] The overall incidence of vascular injury was 15.6 per cent (16 cases). All the injuries involved the venous structures: 11 common iliac vein injuries, 4 inferior vena cava injuries, and 1 iliolumbar vein injury. All were identified and repaired primarily (5-0 or 6-0 Prolene suture) without any reported clinical significance. The incidence of venous injury differed by the extent of surgical approach. The hypogastric "mini-incision" muscle-splitting approach was associated with 14 of the 76 exposures (18.4 per cent), compared with 2 of the 26 (7.7 per cent) anterolateral muscle-dividing retroperitoneal exposures. This study emphasizes the relatively common association of vascular injury with anterior lumbar spinal cases, which is undoubtedly underreported in the literature. Primary repair is the standard of care. Successful repair did not result in any ill effects in this series, other than one case of deep vein thrombosis requiring vena cava filter placement.

Hohf found three cases of major arterial injuries from anterior lumbar spine surgery—two from disc excision, and the other from an anterior vertebral body exploration.[56] In 1986, Louis reported a series of 440 cases involving anterior lumbar surgery over a 10-year period.[76] Two vascular complications occurred in this group: one common iliac vein laceration, and one inferior vena cava thrombosis. The case involving laceration of the common iliac vein was repaired primarily and did not have any serious sequelae, despite severe hemorrhage. Other authors have reported large series of anterior interbody fusions of the lumbar spine for degenerative disc disease and spondylolisthesis without major vascular injuries.[22–24, 28, 39, 41, 42, 44, 48, 60, 105, 106, 117]

Delayed aortic erosion, laceration, and retroperitoneal hemorrhage have been reported in three cases in which the Dunn device was used anteriorly for thoracolumbar spine burst fractures. In 1985, Brown and associates reported three cases out of a total of 22.[14] Blood loss varied from 8000 to 15,000 ml and manifested itself 21 days to 9 months postoperatively. All these devices were placed on the left side, and a sharp edge on the device was implicated as the cause of the delayed aortic rupture. The current recommendation is to remove all Dunn devices placed on the left side of the spine as soon as clinically indicated. A similar experience with the Dwyer cable, Zielke instrumentation, and other anterior systems has not been encountered.[33, 90, 102]

The transperitoneal approach, described by Lane and Moore, offers direct access to the lumbosacral area.[67] The surgeon must work at the bifurcation of the abdominal aorta and the formation of the inferior vena cava from the common iliac veins (see Fig. 54–26). The middle sacral vessels have to be retracted or ligated. The left common iliac vein, as it passes dorsal to the aortic bifurcation, becoming ventral and inferior to the left common iliac artery, is vulnerable to laceration and tearing. Should the bifurcation of the major vessels be more caudal at the L5–S1 disc level, or should exposure above the L4–L5 disc level be desired, mobilization of the vessels would be necessary. If this approach is chosen, it is wise to perform preoperative digital subtraction angiography or abdominal ultrasonography to confirm the level of the anterior vasculature. Bleeding may be profuse and difficult to localize in this region of the retroperitoneum. The use of electrocautery in this area should be limited because of the risk of injury to the sympathetic nervous system. Saline can be used to infiltrate the retroperitoneal space to allow gentle dissection, decrease bleeding, and preserve the parasympathetic and sympathetic nerves.[122]

Vascular injuries as a consequence of percutaneous or limited-exposure video-assisted laparoscopy have been reported. This technology is only in its developmental stages for thoracolumbar and lumbosacral spine surgery but holds great promise for the future. However, major vascular structures are at risk for injury from either trocar insertion or direct laceration. The learning curve appears steep in this regard. Nordestgaard and colleagues reported several major vascular injuries during laparoscopy, reporting five new cases and about 20 more from a literature review.[95] These injuries characteristically involved the distal aorta, distal vena cava, iliac arteries, or iliac veins. Interestingly, four of the injuries were not recognized immediately, and three of these led to death from exsanguination and hypovolemic shock. McAfee and coworkers reported a single common iliac vein laceration during their first 100 endoscopically assisted anterior thoracolumbar spinal reconstruction procedures.[83] This case required an open repair. The authors routinely set up for such an occurrence, emphasizing the need for preparation and early treatment of large vessel injuries.

Kozak and associates reported two venous injuries in a recent series of 45 open anterior lumbosacral spinal reconstructions.[65] One involved the iliolumbar vein, with 1500 ml of blood loss; the other involved 200 ml of blood loss due to a 3-mm vena cava tear. Both were recognized primarily and either reported (iliolumbar vein) or repaired (vena cava) without sequelae. These authors also reported a rare vascular complication in which a rectus sheath hematoma developed for an inferior epigastric artery tear caused by violent coughing in a patient three days postoperatively. Drainage of the hematoma and ligation of the vessel were required.

Vascular complications in posterior lumbar spine surgery are almost always associated with lumbar discectomy (Fig. 54–27).[57] The exact incidence of lumbar vascular complications associated with lumbar discectomy is not known (see Figs. 54–26 and 54–27). In 1945, about a decade after the first discectomy, Linton and White reported a case of arteriovenous fistula formation between the right common iliac artery and the inferior vena cava after an L4–L5 discectomy.[21, 74] Three years later, Horschler reported another case of arteriovenous fistula formation after an L4–L5 discectomy and stated that he knew of five more cases that had occurred over the previous five years.[57] Hohf surveyed over 3500 orthopedists with a 33 per cent response rate about arterial injuries from orthopedic surgery.[56] He found 58 well-documented cases of major vascular injury secondary to disc surgery. Seventeen of these cases resulted in death. Disc surgery clearly was the most common procedure resulting in major vascular injury and death. DeSaussure surveyed 739 neurosurgeons and 2228 orthopedic surgeons and found 106 cases of major vascular injury secondary to disc surgery.[29] Mortality rates varied from 16 to 100 per cent, depending on the timing of surgery and the type of vascular injuries. Arteriovenous fistula formation is the most common vascular injury secondary to disc surgery. In 1976, Jarster and Rich reviewed 68 cases of arteriovenous fistula formation and added five more cases.[61] Sporadic reports continued to appear, but the

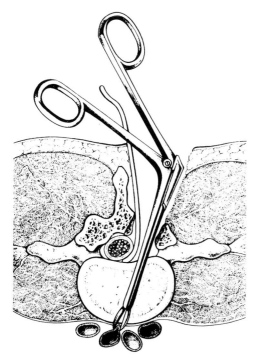

Figure 54–27. Diagram of a pituitary rongeur transgressing the anterior annulus and anterior longitudinal ligament, creating an injury to the anterior vascular structures. (From Montorsi, W., and Ghiringhelli, C.: Genesis: Diagnosis and treatment of vascular complications after intervertebral disc surgery. *Int. Surg. 58*:233–235, 1973.)

serious vascular complications secondary to disc surgery appeared to be decreasing.[82, 83, 91, 92, 108]

Vascular injury secondary to discectomy occurs most commonly from L4–L5 discectomy, followed by L5–S1 and other higher lumbar levels (Figs. 54–28 and 54–29). To some extent, this incidence reflects the frequency of symptomatic disc herniations in the lower two disc levels; however, the vascular anatomy at the anterior L4–L5 disc level directly contributes to this higher incidence. The most common instrument implicated in these injuries is the pituitary rongeur, followed by a cure. Freeman stated that "the pituitary rongeur is the primary instrument of destruction."[44] Partial or total discectomy in DeSaussure's series did not affect the incidence of vascular complications.[29] Another contributing factor is the failure to appreciate disruption of the anterior annulus fibrosus.[9, 69–72] Lindblum, in a cadaveric study, found 7 per cent anterior and 6 per cent lateral radial annular tears in a series of 916 lumbar spine specimens, 393 of which actually had annular tears.[73, 75] Bolesta reported an injury to the left common iliac vein in an obese male with prior surgery.[10] The significance of peridiscal fibrosis was emphasized as a risk factor in this case.

Recognition and prompt treatment of lumbar vascular injuries are essential. Recognition intraoperatively or perioperatively depends on (1) brisk bleeding or blood welling up in the disc space, (2) hypotension with associated tachycardia, and/or (3) abdominal ri-

gidity or a palpable mass. There are no pathognomonic findings. Less than 50 per cent of reported cases have bleeding from the disc space. Furthermore, less than 50 per cent in DeSaussure's series were recognized early.[29] Intraoperative hypotension unexplained by anesthetic effect is the most sensitive and early diagnostic measure. Should bleeding occur intraoperatively from the disc space in association with hypotension, the interspace should be packed, the wound covered with a sterile dressing, volume expanders or blood started immediately, a vascular or general surgeon called emergently, and the patient turned to the supine position and the abdomen prepped and draped for laparotomy. Not infrequently, these injuries go undetected during the procedure but are noted in the recovery room. Acute unexplained hypotension should alert one to the possibility of this complication.

Arteriovenous fistula formation is the most common type of late vascular injury from lumbar disc surgery and has been recognized from 24 hours to over 12 months postoperatively.[74] After discectomy, arteriovenous fistula formation most commonly occurs between the right common iliac artery and the right common iliac vein (29.1 per cent), followed by the left common iliac artery and the left common iliac vein (25.5 per cent), the right common iliac artery and the inferior vena cava (21.8 per cent), the right common iliac artery and the left common iliac vein (12.7 per cent), and others (10.7 per cent). High-output cardiac failure with cardiomegaly is the most common presenting problem, found in 27 of 73 cases reported by Jarster and Rich.[61] Cardiomegaly and/or bruits over the abdomen after disc surgery should raise the level of suspicion, especially in a patient younger than 45 years of age. A variety of other presenting symptoms have been described, including lower extremity pulse abnormalities (two cases), thrombophlebitis (five), abdominal pain (five), disc space hemorrhage (three), leg pain (two), lower extremity edema (two), lower extremity varicosities (one), inguinal pain (one), and pulmonary embolus (one).[8]

Lumbar vascular injuries from disc surgery can be minimized by patient positioning, careful surgical technique, and adequate visualization (see Fig. 54–25). A modified kneeling position helps avoid this complication.[121, 126] The patient rests in a three-point position—on both knees and on pads under the chest and axillae. The abdomen is allowed to hang free, minimizing epidural venous distention and allowing the major vessels to fall slightly away from the spine.[125, 129] Care should be used to avoid orbital or periorbital pressure in the prone (or facedown) position. Vascular complications involving the eye can and do occur. These ophthalmologic complications include ischemia of the optic nerve, central retinal artery occlusion, air embolism, and occipital lobe infarct. Retinal artery occlusion leading to irreversible blindness has been reported.[119, 121, 123]

Operations are performed with adequate illumination and magnification (2.5 to 3.5× loupes or operative microscope). We perform limited or subtotal discectomies in all cases.[6, 118] Our experience and the experience

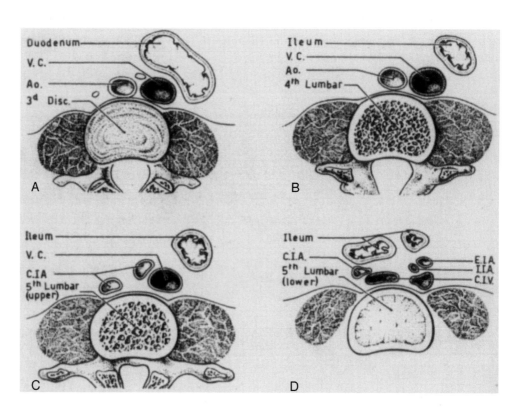

Figure 54–28. Schematic representation of anatomic structures in the immediate vicinity, anteriorly, of the lower lumbar spine. *A*, L3–L4 disc space; *B*, L4 vertebral body; *C*, L5 vertebral body; *D*, inferior end plate of L5. (From Montorsi, W., and Ghiringhelli, C.: Genesis: Diagnosis and treatment of vascular complications after intervertebral disc surgery. *Int. Surg.* 58:233–235, 1973.)

of others confirm that this gives satisfactory long-term results, with a success rate of 95 per cent. In contrast, DeSaussure commented on a series reported by Semmes involving radial discectomy with vascular injuries occurring in 1 out of 6000 cases.[29] Only those disc

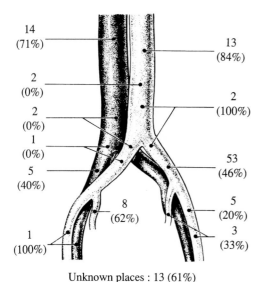

Unknown places : 13 (61%)
Total: 122 (53%)

Figure 54–29. Cases of arterial venous fistulas reported by Morisi and Terragni, as modified by Montorsi and Ghirnghelli. (From Montorsi, W., and Ghirnghelli, C.: Genesis: Diagnosis and treatment of vascular complications after intervertebral disc surgery. *Int. Surg.* 58:233–235, 1973.)

fragments that are loose should be removed. If not torn already, the posterolateral annulus is excised with a scalpel blade, which is inserted no more than 4 to 5 mm deep. The pituitary rongeur is inserted only under direct vision and is limited to less than 2 cm deep in most cases. The goal of surgery is to relieve tension and/or compression of the nerve root, not to perform a total or subtotal discectomy per se. Using these principles, vascular complications from routine discectomy and "recurrent disc herniation" can be kept to a minimum.

Horschler emphasized several other important considerations for disc surgery.[57] He emphasized that the surgery should be performed only for precise indications with adequate anesthesia, good exposure, and meticulous hemostasis. He suggested that the instruments not be inserted more than 2.5 to 3.75 cm below the posterior margin of the vertebral body at L2–L3 through L4–L5 and not more than 4 cm below the vertebral margin at L5–S1. Marking scales on instruments can facilitate this safety maneuver. Finally, he warned to remove the disc slowly and not to extirpate the disc substance forcefully.

Vascular injuries from spine surgery are serious complications. Mortality rates are variable and depend on the type of injury.[106] Early recognition and repair do not guarantee survival, especially in lumbar vascular injuries. Birkeland and Taylor give mortality rates from arterial and venous injuries of 78 and 89 per cent, respectively.[8, 9] These complications tend to manifest early and require emergency attention. Mortality from arteriovenous fistula formation ranges from 9 to 11 per cent. DeSaussure reported mortality rates from 16 to 100 per cent, depending on the nature of the vascular injury and the temporal relationship between recognition and treatment.[29]

Thromboembolic disease in patients undergoing spinal surgery is increasingly being recognized as a clinical problem. Once believed to be extremely rare, recent studies have established an incidence of 1 to 6 per cent in patients undergoing routine posterior lumbosacral surgery[38, 39, 116] and 6.5 per cent in patients undergoing complex, sometimes two-staged, anterior and posterior spinal reconstruction.[130] Pulmonary embolism can occur as well and may be seen with negative venous Doppler ultrasonography of the lower extremity. There are no studies to establish the incidence of deep vein thrombosis or pulmonary emboli in patients undergoing cervical spinal surgery. Risk factors for deep vein thrombosis and pulmonary emboli clearly are the type of surgery and the length of surgery. Patients undergoing anterior spinal reconstructive surgery have a higher incidence of lower extremity thrombus formation, as well as pulmonary emboli. West and Anderson established a 14 per cent incidence of thromboembolic disease as it relates to the length of surgery in their retrospective review.[129] Prothero and associates identified several factors that heighten the risk of thrombophlebitis and/or pulmonary embolism. These include inactivity or recumbency, increasing age, anterior spinal procedures, and iliac crest donor site. The authors found that two thirds of the lower extremity deep vein thromboses occurred on the same side as the bone graft.[100]

Marsicano and coworkers reported a rare case of thrombotic occlusion of the left common iliac artery in a 59-year-old man with peripheral vascular occlusive disease following anterior spinal surgery.[81] Iliac-iliac open revision bypass grafting was required, with resolution of the patient's postoperative radiculopathy. Vascular insufficiency of the patient's left leg following the left lateral retroperitoneal exposure was noted postoperatively.

The prevention of thromboembolic disease, including deep vein thrombosis of the lower extremity and pulmonary embolism, in patients undergoing spinal surgery is a two-edged sword. Traditional antithrombotic agents such as heparin, low-molecular-weight heparin, or warfarin are contraindicated owing to the high risk of bleeding with or without epidural hematoma.[16, 38, 39, 117] This risk extends well into the postoperative period—up to two to four weeks following the initial surgery.[16, 38, 39, 117] Most authors recommend intermittent pneumatic compression sleeves with or without elastic stockings as the primary mode of prophylaxis of thromboembolic disease in patients undergoing spinal surgery. There is no clear consensus on the use of aspirin as an antiplatelet agent. Patients with proven lower extremity thromboembolic disease or patients with symptomatic pulmonary emboli are best managed by insertion of a vena cava filter.[130] Patients undergoing complex anterior spinal reconstruction who have one or more of the routine risk factors, such as obesity, sedentary lifestyle, or history of prior deep vein throm-

bosis or pulmonary embolus, are potential candidates for consideration of a prophylactic vena cava filter before embarking on spinal reconstructive surgery.

CONCLUSION

Vascular complications during spinal surgery are usually few in number, if careful surgical planning and execution are employed. Knowledge of the vascular anatomy is another preventive key. In the neck, the internal and common carotid and vertebral arteries should be primarily repaired if injured. In the chest, the artery of Adamkiewicz should be spared, when possible. The keys to the management of vascular complications of spine surgery are prevention and advance preparation. The important aspects of retractor placement, dissection planes, operative technique, and cooperation between the vascular surgeon and spine surgeon have been stressed to further aid in the prevention and treatment of these serious complications. Finally, in the lumbar spine, injury to the aorta, vena cava, and their primary branches must be avoided or repaired immediately, if possible.

References

1. Adams, H. D., and Vangeertruyden, H. H.: Neurologic complications of aortic surgery. Ann. Surg. *144*:574–610, 1956.
2. Albert, T. J., Balderston, R. A., Heller, J. G., et al.: Upper lumbar disk herniations. J. Spinal Disord. *6*: 351–359, 1993.
3. An, H. S., Vaccaro, A., Simeone, F. A., et al.: Herniated lumbar disc in patients over the age of 50. J. Spinal Disord. *3*:143–146, 1990.
4. Argenson, C., Francke, T. P., Sylla, S., et al.: The vertebral arteries. Anat. Clin. *2*:29–42, 1979.
5. Baker, J. B., Reardon, P. R., Reardon, M. J., and Heggeness, M. H.: Vascular injury in anterior lumbar surgery. Spine *18*:2227–2230, 1993.
6. Balderston, R. A., Gilyard, G. G., Jones, A. A., et al.: The treatment of lumbar disk herniation: Simple fragment excision versus disk space curettage. J. Spinal Disord. *4*:22–25, 1991.
7. Bertalanffy, H., and Eggert, H. R.: Complications of anterior cervical discectomy without fusion in 450 consecutive patients. Acta Neurochir. *99*:41–50, 1989.
8. Birkelan, I. W., and Taylor, T. K. F.: Major vascular injuries in lumbar disc surgery. J. Bone Joint Surg. Br. *51*:41–49, 1969.
9. Birkeland, I. W., and Taylor, T. K. F.: Bowel injuries coincident to lumbar disc surgery: A report of four cases and review of literature. J. Trauma *10*:163–168, 1970.
10. Bolesta, M.: Vascular injury during lumbar diskectomy associated with peridiscal fibrosis: Case report and literature review. J. Spinal Disorders *8*:224–227, 1995.
11. Bolton, B.: The blood supply of the human spinal cord. J. Neurol. Psychiatry. *2*:137–148, 1939.
12. Boukobza, M., Guichard, J. P., Boissonet, M., et al.: Spinal epidural hematoma: Report of 11 cases and review of the literature. Neuroradiology *36*:456–459, 1994.
13. Brillman, J., and Howieson, J.: Transient midbrain syndromes as a complication of vertebral angiography. J. Neurol. *41*:71, 1974.
14. Brown, L. P., Bridwell, K. H., Holt, R. H., and Jennings, J.: Aortic erosions and lacerations associated with the Dunn anterior spinal instrumentation. Abstract presented at the 20th Annual Scoliosis Research Society, San Diego, CA, 1985.
15. Burrington, J. D., Brown, C., Wayne, E. R., and Odom, J.: Anterior approach to the thoracolumbar spine: Technical considerations Arch. Surg. *11*:456–463, 1976.
16. Cain, J. E., Jr., Major, M. R., Lauerman, W. C., et al.: The morbidity of heparin therapy after development of pulmonary embolus

in patients undergoing thoracolumbar or lumbar spinal fusion. Spine 20:1600–1603, 1995.

17. Capener, N.: The evolution of lateral richotomy. J. Bone Joint Surg. Br. 36:173–179, 1954.

18. Chan, D. P. K.: Pyogenic infections of the spine. In Evardez, C. M. (ed.): Surgery of the Musculoskeletal System. Vol. 2. New York, Churchill Livingstone, 1983, pp. 169–173.

19. Chou, S. N., and Seljeskog, E. L.: Alternative surgical approaches to the thoracic spine. Clin. Neurosurg. 20:306–321, 1973.

20. Chozick, B. A., Watson, P., and Greenblatt, S. H.: Internal Carotid Artery Thrombosis After Cervical Corpectomy. Vol. 19. Philadelphia, J. B. Lippincott Co., 1994, pp. 2230–2232.

21. Cloward, R. B.: The treatment of ruptured lumbar intervertebral disc by vertebral body fusion: Indications, operative techniques, and after care. Clin. Orthop. 193:5–15, 1985.

22. Cloward, R. B.: Spondylolisthesis: Treatment by laminectomy and posterior interbody fusion—review of 100 cases. Clin. Orthop. 154:74–82, 1981.

23. Cloward, R. B.: The treatment of ruptured lumbar intervertebral disc by vertebral body fusion. J. Neurol. 10:154–168, 1953.

24. Collis, J. S.: Total disc replacement: A modified posterior lumbar interbody fusion—report of 750 cases. Clin. Orthop. 193:64–67, 1985.

25. Cook, W. A.: Transthoracic vertebral surgery. Ann. Thorac. Surg. 12:54–65, 1970.

26. Cosgrove, G. R., and Theron, J.: Vertebral arteriovenous fistula following anterior cervical spine surgery: Report of two cases. J. Neurosurg. 66:297–299, 1987.

27. Crock, H. V.: Anterior and lumbar interbody fusion: Indications for its use and surgical technique. Clin. Orthop. 1985:157–163, 1982.

28. Denaro, V.: Surgical approaches. In Stenosis of Cervical Spine: Causes Diagnosis and Treatment. New York, Springer-Verlag, 1991, pp. 162–185.

29. DeSaussure, R. L.: Vascular injury coincidence to disc surgery. J. Neurol. 16:222–229, 1959.

30. DiChiro, G., Fried, L. C., and Doppman, J. L.: Experimental spinal cord angiography. Br. J. Radiol. 43:19–30, 1970.

31. Dommisse, G. F.: The blood supply of the spinal cord: A critical vascular zone in spinal surgery. J. Bone Joint Surg. Br. 56:222–235, 1974.

32. Dommisse, G. F., and Enslin, T. B.: Hodgson's circumferential osteotomy in the correction of spinal deformity. J. Bone Joint Surg. Br. 52:778, 1970.

33. Dwyer, A. F., and Schafer, M. F.: Anterior approaches to scoliosis: Surgical results in 51 cases. J. Bone Joint Surg. Br. 56:218–224, 1974.

34. Eder, L. I., Asassaro, L. I., and Spaccarelli, G.: Vertebral angiography as a cause of necrosis of the cervical spinal cord. Br. J. Radiol. 35:261–264, 1962.

35. Efsen, F.: Spinal cord lesions as a complication of abdominal aortography. Acta Radiol. 4:47–58, 1966.

36. Faciszewski, T., Winter, R. B., Lonstein, J. E., et al.: The surgical and medical complications in anterior spinal fusion surgery in the thoracic and lumbar spine in adults: A review of 1223 cases. Spine 20:1592–1599, 1995.

37. Feigleson, JJ., and Ravin, H. A.: Transverse myelitis following selective bronchial arteriography. Radiology 85:663–665, 1965.

38. Ferree, B. A., Stern, P. J., Jolson, R. S., et al.: Deep venous thrombosis after spinal surgery. Spine 18:315–319, 1993.

39. Ferree, B. A., and Wright, A. M.: Deep venous thrombosis following posterior lumbar spinal surgery. Spine 18:1079–1082, 1993.

40. Fidler, M. W.: Excision of prolapse of thoracic intervertebral disc: A transthoracic technique. J. Bone Joint Surg. Am. 66:518–522, 1984.

41. Fielding, J. W.: Complications of anterior cervical disk removal and fusion. Clin. Orthop. 284:10–13, 1992.

42. Flynn, J. C., and Hogue, M. A.: Anterior fusion of the lumbar spine. J. Bone Joint Surg. Am. 61:1143–1150, 1979.

43. Freebody, D., Bendal, R., and Taylor, R.: Anterior transperitoneal lumbar fusion. J. Bone Joint Surg. Br. 53:617–627, 1971.

44. Freeman, D. G.: Major vascular complications of lumbar disc surgery. West. J. Surg. Gynecol. Obstet. 69:175–177, 1961.

45. Gillilan, L. A.: The arterial blood supply of the human spinal cord. J. Comp. Neurol. 110:75–103, 1958.

46. Golfinos, J. G., Dickman, C. A., Zabramaski, J. M., et al.: Repair of vertebral artery injury during anterior cervical decompression. Spine 19:2552–2556, 1994.

47. Graham, A. W., Swank, M. L., Kinard, R. E., et al.: Posterior cervical arthrodesis and stabilization with a lateral mass plate. Spine 21:323–329, 1996.

48. Graham, J. J.: Complications of cervical spine surgery. Spine 14:1046–1050, 1989.

49. Gray, H.: The arteries and veins. In Goss, C. N. (ed.): Anatomy of a Human Body. Vols. 8, 9. Philadelphia, Lee & Febiger, 1973, pp. 561–716.

50. Hadley, L. E.: The co-vertebral articulations in cervical foramina encroachment. J. Bone Joint Surg. Am. 39:910–920, 1957.

51. Hardin, C. A.: Vertebral artery insufficiency produced by cervical osteophytic spurs. Arch. Surg. 90:629–633, 1965.

52. Harmon, P. H.: Anterior excision and vertebral body fusion operation for intervertebral disc syndromes of the lower lumbar spine. Clin. Orthop. 37:130–144, 1964.

53. Hodge, W. A., and DeWald, R. L.: Splenic injuries complicating the anterior thoracoabdominal surgical approach for scoliosis— a report of two cases. J. Bone Joint Surg. Am. 65:396–397, 1983.

54. Hodgson, A. R., Stock, F. E., and Fang, H. S. Y.: Anterior spinal fusion: The operative approach and pathologic findings in 412 patients with Pott's disease of the spine. Br. J. Surg. 48:172–178, 1960.

55. Hogan, E. L., and Ramanul, F. C. A.: Spinal cord infarction occurring during insertion of aortic graft. Neurology 16:67–74, 1976.

56. Hohf, R. P.: Arterial injuries occurring during orthopaedic operations. Clin. Orthop. 28:21–37, 1963.

57. Horschler, E. G.: Vascular complications of disc surgery. J. Bone Joint Surg. Am. 30:968–970, 1948.

58. Husni, E. A., Bell, H. S., and Storer, J.: Mechanical obstruction of the vertebral artery. JAMA 196:101–104, 1966.

59. Hutter, C. G.: Posterior intervertebral body fusion: A twenty-five year study. Clin. Orthop. 179:86–96, 1983.

60. Inoue, S., Watanabe, T., Hirose, A., et al.: Anterior discectomy and interbody fusion for lumbar disc disease. Clin. Orthop. 183:221–231, 1984.

61. Jarster, B. S., and Rich, N. M.: The challenge of the arteriovenous fistula formation following disc surgery: A collector review. J. Trauma 16:726–733, 1976.

62. Jenis, L. G., and LeClair, W. J.: Late vascular complications with anterior cervical diskectomy and fusion. Spine 19:1291–1293, 1994.

63. Keim, H. A., and Hilal, S. K.: Spinal angiography in scoliosis patients. J. Bone Joint Surg. Am. 53:904–912, 1971.

64. Killian, D. A., and Foster, J. H.: Spinal cord injury as a complication of contrast angiography. Surgery 59:969–981, 1966.

65. Kozak, J. A., Heilman, A. E., and O'Brien, J. P.: Anterior lumbar fusion options: Technique and graft materials. Clin. Orthop. 300:45–51, 1994.

66. Kraus, D. R., and Stauffer, E. S.: Spinal cord injury as a complication of elective anterior cervical fusion. Clin. Orthop. 112:55–61, 1975.

67. Lane, J. D., and Moore, E. S.: Transperitoneal approach to the intervertebral disc in the lumbar area. Ann. Surg. 127:537–551, 1948.

68. Lawton, M. T., Porter, R. W., Heiserman, J. E. et al.: Surgical management of spinal epidural hematoma: Relationship between surgical timing and neurological outcome. J. Neurosurg. 83:1–7, 1995.

69. Lazorthes, G., Gouaze, A., Zadeh, J. O., et al.: Arterial vascularization of the spinal cord: Recent studies of the anastomotic substitution pathways. J. Neurosurg. 35:253–262, 1971.

70. Leavens, M. E., and Bradford, F. K.: Ruptured intervertebral disc: Report of a case and defect in the anterior annulus fibrosus. J. Neurosurg. 10:544–546, 1953.

71. Lin, P. N.: Posterior Lumbar Interbody Fusion. Springfield, IL, Charles C Thomas, 1982, p. 154.

72. Lin, P. N., and Cautillira Joyce, N. F.: Posterior lumbar interbody fusion. Clin. Orthop. 180: 154–168, 1983.

73. Lindblum, K.: Intervertebral disc degeneration considered as a pressure atrophy. J. Bone Joint Surg. Am. *39:*933–945, 1957.

74. Linton, R. R. and White, P. D.: Arteriovenous fistula between the right common iliac artery and the inferior vena cava. Arch. Surg. *50:*6–13, 1945.

75. Livingston, M. C. P.: Spinal manipulation causing injury. Clin. Orthop. *81:*82–86, 1971.

76. Louis, R.: Fusion of the lumbar and sacral spine by internal fixation with screw plates. Clin. Orthop. *203:*18–33, 1986.

77. Louw, J. A., Mafoyane, N. A., Small, B., and Neser, C. P.: Occlusion of the vertebral artery in cervical spine dislocations. J. Bone Joint Surg. Br. *72:*679–681, 1990.

78. Lyness, S. S., and Simeone, F. A.: Vascular complications of upper cervical spine injuries. Orthop. Clin. North Am. *9:*1029–1038, 1978.

79. Mack, J. R.: Major vascular injuries incident to intervertebral disc surgery. Am. Surg. *22:*752–763, 1956.

80. Mack, J. R., Regan, J. J., McAfee, P. C., et al.: Video-assisted thoracic surgery for the anterior approach to the thoracic spine. Ann. Thorac. Surg. *59:*1100–1106, 1995.

81. Marsicano, J., Mirovsky, Y., Remer, S., et al.: Thrombotic occlusion of the left common iliac artery after an anterior retroperitoneal approach to the lumbar spine. Spine *19:*357–359, 1994.

82. Mayfield, F. H.: Complications of laminectomy. Clin. Neurol. *23:*435–439, 1975.

83. McAfee, P. C., Regan, J. R., Zdeblick, T., et al.: The incidence of complications in endoscopic anterior thoracolumbar spinal reconstructive surgery: A prospective multicenter study comprising the first 100 consecutive cases. Spine *20:*1624–1632, 1995.

84. Meyer, P. R.: Complications of treatment of fractures and dislocations of the dorsal lumbar spine. *In* Eppes, C. H. (ed.): Complications of Orthopedic Surgery. pp. 643–715.

85. Michele, A. A., and Krueger, F. J.: Surgical approach to the vertebral body. J. Bone Joint Surg. Am. *31:*873–878, 1949.

86. Micheli, L. J., and Hall, J. E.: Complications in management of adult spinal deformity and complications of orthopaedic surgery. *In* Eppes, C. H. (ed.): Complications of Orthopedic Surgery. pp. 1049–1051.

87. Moe, J. H.: Complications of scoliosis treatment. Clin. Orthop. *53:*21–30, 1967.

88. Moe, J. H.: The normal spine: Anatomy embryology and growth. *In* Moe, J. H., Winter, R. B., Bradford, P. S., and Lonstein, J. E. (eds.): Scoliosis and Other Deformities. Philadelphia, W. B. Saunders Co., 1978, pp. 25–39.

89. Moe, J. H., Purcell, G. A., and Bradford, D. S.: Zielke instrumentation (VDS) for the correction of spinal curvature: Analysis of results in 66 patients. Clin. Orthop. *180:*133–153, 1983.

90. Montorsi, W., and Ghiringhelli, C.: Genesis, diagnosis and treatment of vascular complications after intervertebral disc surgery. Int. Surg. *58:*233–235, 1973.

91. Moore, C. A., and Cohen, A.: Combined arterial, venous and ureteral injury complicating lumbar disc surgery. Am. J. Surg. *115:*574–577, 1968.

92. Moresch, F. P., and Sayre G. P.: Neurologic manifestations associated with dissecting aneurysm of the aorta. JAMA *144:*1141–1148, 1950.

93. Mouat, T. B.: The operative approach to the kidney of Bernard Fey. Br. J. Urol. *2:*126–132, 1939.

94. Nayak, U. K., Donald, P. J., and Stevens, D.: Internal carotid artery resection for invasion of malignant tumors. Arch. Otolaryngol. Head Neck Surg. *121:*1029–1033, 1995.

95. Nordestgaard, A. G., Bodily, K. C., Osborne, R. W., Jr., and Buttorff, J. D.: Major vascular injuries during laparoscopic procedures. Am. J. Surg. *169:*543–545, 1995.

96. Ortigliano, T. C., Al-Mefty, O., Leonetti, J. P., et al.: Vascular considerations and complications in cranial base surgery [see comments]. Neurosurgery *35:*351–362, 1994.

97. Ottolenghi, C. E.: Diagnosis of orthopaedic lesions by aspiration biopsy: Result of 1,061 punctures. J. Bone Joint Surg. Am. *37:*443–464, 1955.

98. Pfeifer, B. A., Friedberg, S. R., and Jewell, E. R.: Repair of injured vertebral artery in anterior cervical procedures. Spine *19:*1471–1474, 1994.

99. Phillips, D. G.: Surgical treatment of myelopathy and cervical spondylosis. J. Neurol. Neurosurg. Psychiatry *36:*879–884, 1973.

100. Prothero, S. R., Parkes, J. C., and Stinchfield, F. E.: The classic: Complications after low-back fusion in 1000 patients: A comparison of two series one decade apart. Clin. Orthop. *306:*5–11, 1994.

101. Riley, L. H.: Surgical approaches to the anterior structures of the cervical spine. Clin. Orthop. *91:*16–20, 1973.

102. Riseborough, E. J.: The anterior approach to the spine for the correction of deformity of the axial skeleton. Clin. Orthop. *93:*207–214, 1973.

103. Rizzoli, H.: Personal communication, 1985.

104. Robinson, R. A., and Southwick, W. O.: Surgical approaches to the cervical spine. Instr. Course Lect. *27:*299–330, 1960.

105. Sacks, S.: Anterior interbody fusion of the lumbar spine: Indications and results in 200 cases. Clin. Orthop. *44:*163–170, 1966.

106. Sacks, S.: Anterior interbody fusion of the lumbar spine. J. Bone Joint Surg. Am. *47:*211–223, 1965.

107. Schelhas, K. P., Latchaw, R. E., Wendling, L. R., and Gold, L. H. A.: Vertebral basilar injuries following cervical manipulation. JAMA *244:*1450–1453, 1980.

108. Schweighofer, F., Passler, J. M., Wildburger, R., and Hofer, H. P.: Interbody fusion of the lower cervical spine: A dangerous surgical method? Langenbecks Arch. Chir. *377:*295–299, 1992.

109. Scott, R. W., and Sancetta, S. M.: Dissecting aneurysm of the aorta with hemorrhagic infarction of the spinal cord and complete paraplegia. Am. Heart J. *38:*747–756, 1949.

110. Seeley, S. F., Hughes, C. W., and Jahnke, E. J.: Major vascular damage in lumbar disc operations. Surgery *35:*421–429, 1954.

111. Sen, C., Eisenberg, M., Casden, A. M., et al.: Management of the vertebral artery in excision of extradural tumors of the cervical spine. Neurosurgery *36:*106–115, 1995.

112. Shallat, R. F., and Klump, T. E.: Paraplegia following thoracolumbar sympathectomy. J. Neurol. *34:*569–571. 1971.

113. Sheehan, S., Bauer, R. B. and Myer, J. S.: Vertebral artery compression in cervical spondylosis. Neurology *10:*968–986, 1960.

114. Simeone, F. A., and Rashbaum, R.: Transthoracic disc excision. *In* Smecdt, H. H., and Sweet, W. H. (eds.): Operative Neurosurgery Techniques. Vol. 2. New York, Grune & Stratton, 1982, pp. 445–505.

115. Slover, W. P., and Kiley, R. F.: Cervical vertebral erosion caused by tortuous vertebral artery. Radiology *84:*112–114, 1965.

116. Smith, M. D., Emery, S. E., Dudley, A., et al.: Vertebral artery injury during anterior decompression of the cervical spine. J. Bone Joint Surg. Br. *75:*410–415, 1993.

117. Southland, S. R., Remedios, A. M., McKerrell, J. G., and Litwin, D.: Laparoscopic approaches to the lumbar vertebrae. Spine *20:*1620–1623, 1995.

118. Stambough, J. L., and Cheeks, M. L.: Central retinal artery occlusion: A complication of the prone position in spine surgery. J. Spinal Disord. *5:*363–365, 1992.

119. Stambough, J. L., and Rothman, R. H.: Indications for cervical spine surgery. *In* Wiesel, S. W., and Feffer, H. L. (eds.): Neck Pain. Charlottesville, VA, Michie Co., 1986, pp. 275–312.

120. Stambough, J. L., and Simeone, F. A.: Vascular complications in spine surgery. *In* Rothman and Simeone: The Spine. Philadelphia W. B. Saunders Co., 1992, pp. 1877–1885.

121. Stauffer, R. N., and Coventry, M. B.: Anterior interbody lumbar spine fusion. J. Bone Joint Surg. Am. *54:*756–768, 1972.

122. Stevens, W. R., Glazer, P. A., Rubery, P. T., and Bradford, D. S.: Ophthalmic complications after spinal surgery. (Abstract.) 30th annual SRS meeting, Asheville, NC, September 1995, p. 117.

123. Suh, H., and Alexander, L.: Vascular system of the human spinal cord. Arch. Neurol. Psych. *41:*659–677, 1939.

124. Tarlov, I. M.: The knee-chest position for lower spinal operations. J. Bone Joint Surg. Am. *49:*1193–1194, 1967.

125. Tew, J. M., and Mayfield F. H.: Complications of surgery of the anterior cervical spine. Clin. Neurosurg. *23:*424–434, 1975.

126. Tuohy, E. L., Boman, P. G., and Berdes, G. L.: Spinal cord ischemia in dissecting aortic aneurysm. Am. Heart J. *22:*305–313, 1941.

127. Verbiest, H.: A lateral approach to the cervical spine: Technique and indications. J. Neurosurg. *30:*191–203, 1967.

128. Wayne, S. J.: The tuck position for lumbar-disc surgery. J. Bone Joint Surg. Am. *49:*1195–1198, 1967.

129. West, J. L., and Anderson, L. D.: Incidence of deep vein thrombosis in major adult spinal surgery. Spine *17*(8 Suppl.):254–275, 1992.

130. Whitesides, T. E., and Kelly, R. P.: Lateral approach to the upper cervical spine for anterior fusion. South. Med. J. *59*:879–883, 1966.
131. Winter, R. B., Lonstein, J. E., Denis, F., et al.: Risks of paraplegia secondary to segmental vascular ligation: An analysis of 1,197 consecutive anterior operations. (Abstract.) 63rd annual AAOS meeting, Atlanta, GA, 1996, p. 215.
132. Winter, R. B., Moe, J. H., and Wang, J. F.: Congenital kyphosis: Its natural history and treatment as observed in a study of 130 patients. J. Bone Joint Surg. Am. *55*:223–256, 1973.
133. Young, P. H.: Complications of cervical spine microsurgery. *In* Dunsker, S. B. (ed.): Seminars in Neurological Surgery: Cervical Spondylosis. New York, Raven Press, 1980, pp. 185–189.
134. Zeidman, S. M., and Ducker, T. B.: Posterior cervical laminoforaminotomy for radiculopathy: Review of 172 cases. Neurosurgery *33*:356–362, 1993.
135. Zimmerman, H. B., and Farrel, W. J.: Cervical vertebral erosion caused by vertebral artery tortuosity. Am. J. Rheology *108*:767–770, 1970.

Neurologic Complications in Spine Surgery

Jeffery L. Stambough, M.D.

Frederick A. Simeone, M.D.

Neurologic injuries as a consequence of surgery fortunately are sporadic and rare.[7] These injuries can occur from direct insults, such as a laceration of the neural elements, or indirectly, such as an interruption of the blood supply to the spinal cord. The incidence of direct neural injury is dependent largely on the procedure performed, as well as the degree to which the procedure deals specifically with the neural elements.[82, 89] The incidence of indirect injury, such as disruption of the blood supply to the crucial neural elements, probably approaches one in every 2000 to 3000 cases involving cervical or thoracic spinal surgery.[69] Regardless of the cause, injury to the spinal cord or nerve roots may be transient or permanent. Once complete neural damage has occurred, the probability of recovery is limited or nonexistent. Consequently, the best and only effective management of most neural injuries is prevention.[2, 88]

Neurologic complications may be considered in several categories: (1) neurologic complications caused by delayed or protracted nonsurgical care, (2) neurologic complications related to patient positioning during surgery, (3) intraoperative neurologic injury, and (4) complications occurring postoperatively, some of which are specific to the type of spinal procedure or approach used. Neurologic complications are not always predictable but can be expected at a low rate if a significant number of spinal surgeries are performed.[41, 84, 86]

CERVICAL SPINE

Neurologic injury in the cervical spine may be prolonged or significant after appropriate surgical decompression or may result from an inappropriate delay in this surgical intervention. Diagnosing the extent of the patient's pathology is important. Consideration must be given to repeat neurodiagnostic imaging of the cervical spine in the event of progressive myelopathy postoperatively.[9] Syringomyelia has been shown to arise at a significant rate following surgery of the cervical spine, and the myelopathy will be more rapidly progressive after operations for arteriovenous malformation or intramedullary tumor than for those involving a herniated disc or spinal stenosis.[9] Magnetic resonance imaging (MRI) is the most sensitive test for diagnosing these complex clinical problems. An absolute indication for urgent spinal surgery is progressive neural deficit owing to spinal cord or nerve root compression.[50, 52]

Failure to recognize and respond to these cases in an urgent manner may prevent reversal of the existent neural damage, especially in cases involving the spinal cord. The magnitude and reversibility of any neural dysfunction caused by compression depend on the amount of force applied to the neural elements and the length of application of this force.[23, 53, 77] In general, the less force and the shorter the duration, the more likely the neural tissues are to fully recover. Furthermore, nerve roots tolerate this pressure better than the spinal cord in similar circumstances. The spinal nerve is more likely to recover than the intradural spinal nerve roots, because of the spinal nerve's protective perineurium and epineurium.[70] Weber[98] has confirmed clinically that the nerve root is much more forgiving to pressure.[87]

Trauma to the spinal cord or nerve roots during cervical spine surgery is not a common complication. Direct cervical nerve root laceration was reported in one of 650 cases of keyhole foraminotomy for cervical radiculopathy by Scoville.[81] Although cervical nerve root laceration is uncommon, nerve root dysfunction after decompressive procedures is not infrequent. The fifth cervical nerve root is particularly sensitive to these decompressive procedures, and the spinal cord is also exquisitely sensitive to manipulation. A case of severe, permanent paraparesis in a patient undergoing cervical laminectomy for severe cervical spinal stenosis due to spinal cord contusion is known to us. In general, the spinal cord is less forgiving to manipulation than either the cervical or the lumbar nerve roots. Direct neural injury is more likely in repeat operative cases in which excessive dissection of epidural scar tissues is necessary.[50] Direct intraoperative neural injury is best prevented, because no predictable or effective surgical management is known once injury has occurred. Complete and careful hemostasis coupled with magnification, adequate illumination, and visualization are essential ingredients in helping to avoid direct neural injury. Always working away from the neural element or parallel to the nerve roots also minimizes direct neural injuries. Excessive retraction should always be avoided. In general, the neural elements should not be retracted unless this is essential for adequate visualization. Spinal cord manipulation is to be strictly avoided. It is better and safer to widen the bony exposure than to produce excessive or overzealous retraction on the neural elements.[88] Intraoperative monitoring by evoked potentials when working intradurally with the spinal cord has become routine in many centers.[3, 24] Some controversy exists regarding the specificity and sensitivity of evoked potentials in cases involving direct spinal cord surgery, but not in other cervical spine surgical cases.[68]

Another source of possible cord injury is related to hyperextension of the neck during tracheal intuba-tion.[67] Hyperextension of the neck in a narcotized pa-tient may lead to acute cord compression, especially in the elderly stenotic cervical spine (Fig. 54–30A). Anes-thesia colleagues should be aware of the tolerable neck extension appropriate for the patient before induction, to avoid this devastating complication. This level of cervical extension should not be exceeded.[92] Alterna-tively, an awake intubation can be performed. This avoids reducing the canal diameter when the muscles of the neck relax after general anesthesia.[87] Patients with excessive degenerative changes in the lumbar spine with or without spondylolisthesis should be sus-pected of having similar changes in the cervical region, or vice versa. Lumbar spinal stenosis correlates very well with peripheral osteoarthritis, as well as with cervical degenerative disc disease.[28] A high index of

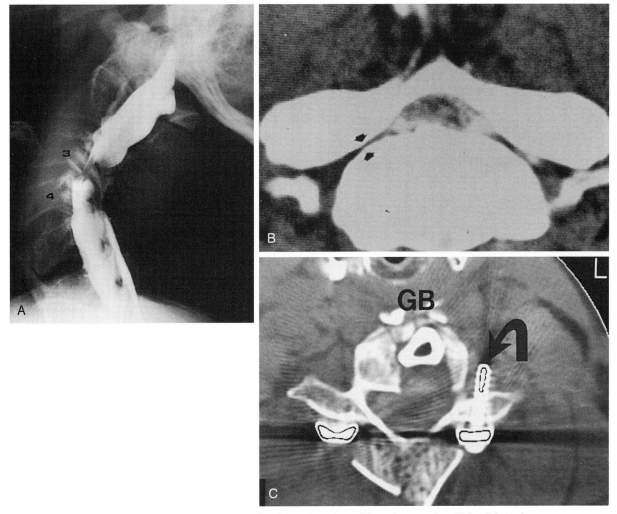

Figure 54–30. *A,* The stenotic cervical spine is made worse with neck extension. This oil-based myelogram demonstrates severe canal narrowing at C3–C4 in a patient with paraparesis following prone positioning for lumbar spine surgery. *B,* The stenotic cervical spinal canal illustrated by flattening of the cord, placing the cord or root (see arrows) at jeopardy with decompression (either anterior or posterior). Instruments should be directed away from the neural elements at all times. Specifically, spinal cord manipulation or retraction must be avoided. *C,* Malpositioned lateral mass screw at C6, producing severe C6 radiculopathy postoperatively (see arrow). The symptoms improved with screw removal and revision instrumentation.

suspicion is necessary, and careful positioning to avoid hyperextension of the spine is essential during surgical procedures involving the spine or other areas.

Cervical spinal procedures have neurologic complications that are procedure specific.[29, 76] The anterior approach for anterior cervical disc excision with or without fusion has a low, but definite, incidence of recurrent laryngeal nerve palsy and Horner's syndrome, estimated at 0.2 per cent in the series reported by Tew and Mayfield.[61, 92] Horner's syndrome occurred at a rate of 1.1 per cent in Bertalanffy and Eggert's series of 450 anterior approach cases.[13] Heeneman[43] reported an 11 per cent rate of postoperative voice changes in 85 cases; of these, three had permanent vocal cord paralysis. Intraoperative injury to the recurrent laryngeal nerve can be avoided by staying in fascial planes and avoiding sharp dissection. This nerve is less vulnerable on the left side of the neck because of its longer anatomic course and more protected position in the tracheoesophageal groove. The most likely cause of nerve injury is prolonged retraction against the trachea.[17, 39] Horner's syndrome and injury to the cervical sympathetic chain can be minimized by keeping the dissection medial to the longus colli muscles and by careful placement of the retractor blades under the medial edge of the muscles.

Rarely, transection of cranial nerves IX, X, XI, or XII may occur during an anterior approach when high in the neck, resulting in deficits involving phonation and swallowing.[100] These injuries can best be avoided with knowledge of the anatomy of the upper cervical area and by taking care to stay in the fascial planes during dissection. Assistance by an experienced head and neck surgeon should be considered if the spinal surgeon infrequently exposes the upper anterior cervical spine. The phrenic nerve, because of its lateral position on the longus colli, is rarely injured during anterior cervical spine surgery and is not usually at risk during routine anterior disc surgery, except when extensive exposure may be necessary.[4, 32] Avoiding the sympathetic chain as described earlier also indirectly protects against damage to the phrenic nerve.

When a fusion is performed with an anterior cervical discectomy, there is a potential risk of neural injury, especially if the posterior vertebral chondro-osseous bar is removed, allowing displacement of the cylindric bone graft posteriorly against the spinal cord (Fig. 54–30B).[1] Concussion of the cord, indicated by jerking of the limbs, may result in a postoperative increase in spastic paresis if residual osteophytes are driven against the spinal cord. A rare complication, sleep-induced apnea, has been reported in patients operated at the C3–C4 level.[32] Orthostatic hypotension, bradycardia, and cardiorespiratory instability are also features of this condition, which is secondary to damage to the descending respiratory pathway in the reticulospinal tract. Although usually self-limited, prompt recognition and treatment are necessary to prevent death.[92]

In those procedures that employ interbody fusion, such as the Cloward or Smith-Robinson techniques, there is a definite risk of extrusion of the bone graft postoperatively. In most series, posterior displacement occurs at a rate of approximately 2 per cent.[29, 61, 76, 92] If extrusion occurs in the immediate postoperative period, the patient will likely complain of dysphagia or pain in a radicular pattern. If the patient has these complaints, a lateral cervical spine radiograph is recommended to confirm graft location. If the graft is displaced, it is usually anteriorly, and proper steps for management can be initiated to avoid further neurologic complication or erosion into the esophagus.[69] Many grafts showing an abnormality (mild anterior extrusion or protrusion) on the postoperative radiograph can be managed without surgical replacement.[92]

In almost all series, the greatest incidence of complications of the anterior approach to the cervical spine is related to the harvesting of bone graft.[62] Although not life-threatening, these neurologic injuries can result in significant morbidity. Neurologic complications involving the bone graft harvest site, usually the iliac crest, have been reported to occur at a rate of 12 per cent.[102] Injury to the lateral femoral cutaneous, iliohypogastric, ilioinguinal, genital femoral, or cluneal nerves can result in painful syndromes. Injury to most of these nerves can be avoided by keeping the dissection superior and lateral to the anterior superior iliac spine when exposing the iliac crest. A parallel, rather than a transverse, incision also is helpful in avoiding painful neuroma formation.

The most catastrophic neurologic complication is that of spinal cord injury with resultant permanent quadriplegia or paraplegia. This may occur as a result of compression, traction, or laceration of the spinal cord. This neurologic complication is higher in stenotic, degenerative cases as compared with soft disc cases. Tew and Mayfield[92] reported a 0.2 per cent incidence of cord and neurologic injury in anterior cervical disc excision and fusion cases. Flynn reported a neurologic complication rate of 0.3 per cent in over 350 cases of anterior cervical disc excision and fusion.[35] The most common complication in the series of 450 cases of anterior disc excision reported by Bertalanffy and Eggert was worsening of pre-existing myelopathy, which occurred at a rate of 3.3 per cent.[13] Yonenobu and coworkers reported a rate of 5.5 per cent neurologic deterioration related to surgery in their series of 384 cases of cervical myelopathy operated on by anterior and posterior approaches.[101] In a review of 172 cases of radiculopathy treated by posterior cervical laminoforaminotomy, there was one instance of cord injury, resulting in a central cord syndrome that partially resolved after a few months.[41, 102]

In general, the neurologic complications associated with the posterior approach to the surgical management of acute disc herniation are few.[62] Graham, in his five-year review of complications related to cervical spine surgery, found the overall rate of neurologic injury to be higher when using the posterior approach than when operating anteriorly: 2.18 and 0.64 per cent, respectively.[39] The rate of cord injury was also higher with the posterior approach.[39] In addition, the cervical nerve roots are at risk of impingement from posterior mass screws used during posterior cervical spinal plating. Risks relate to the length of the screw and the direction of insertion, as well as the technique (Fig. 54–30C). Lateral angulation is preferable to lessen vertebral artery impairment, and superior angulation decreases the risk of nerve root impairment within the neuroforamina. If a nerve root irritation or deficit occurs, prompt removal is the preferred method of treatment.[39]

THORACOLUMBAR SPINE

Neurologic complications seen in anterior thoracic or thoracolumbar exposures and procedures are also rare. In these cases, vascular-related neurologic complications, such as disruption of the artery of Adamkiewicz resulting in delayed paraparesis or paraplegia, are also possible causes of neurologic complications.[22, 65] Faciszewski and associates described an overall 0.25 per cent neurologic complication rate.[31] This involved two nerve root injuries, for an incidence of 0.5 per cent. There were three Horner-Bernard syndromes in the high thoracic cases. The total high thoracic cases numbered 42, and there were three such syndromes noted, for an incidence of 7.2 per cent. The overall rate of lumbar plexus injuries out of 930 thoracolumbar cases was 0.01 per cent. Among 371 men operated on in the lower lumbar region, there were three cases of impotence, for an incidence of 0.8 per cent, and two cases of retrograde ejaculation, for an incidence of 0.6 per cent.

Attar and colleagues reported five cases of paraplegia following open thoracotomy for a variety of chest pathologies.[8] Intraoperative factors leading to neurologic deficits include bleeding at the costovertebral angle, migration of oxidized cellulose into the canal, thrombosis of the anterior thoracic spinal artery, epidural hematoma, epidural narcotic, and hypotension. The cervicothoracic junction represents a difficult area to access, expose, and operate on safely. Attar and colleagues reported 36 cases with neurologic complications, including pseudomeningocele, vocal cord paralysis, and Horner's syndrome.

Neurologic injury may be prolonged or significant after appropriate surgical decompression, or it can result from an inappropriate delay in this surgical intervention. Two absolute indications for urgent spinal surgery are known: (1) a progressive neural deficit owing to spinal cord compression, and (2) a progressive neurologic deficit involving a significant nerve root or roots (e.g., cauda equina syndrome).[50] Failure to recognize and respond to these cases in an urgent manner may result in failure to reverse the existent neural damage, especially in cases involving the spinal cord or cauda equina compression. In the lumbar spine, cauda equina compression is most often caused by massive disc rupture or postoperative epidural hematoma. The magnitude and reversibility of any neural dysfunction caused by compression depend on the amount of force applied to the neural elements and the length of application of this force.[23, 53, 77] In general, the

less force and the shorter the duration, the more likely the neural tissues are to fully recover. Weber has confirmed clinically that the nerve root is much more forgiving to pressure. Neurologic recovery in the 50 per cent of lumbar disc patients with neural deficits was generally good, with about 70 per cent of these patients improving, regardless of the type of treatment employed.[98] Severe sciatica and significant neural dysfunction were preselected for surgery in the series reported by Weber, however.[98] Hakelius has shown that neural recovery is better in patients operated on within three months of the onset of the neural deficit.[41] In general, progressive weakness in a major muscle such as the quadriceps or anterior tibialis should not be watched too long. Progressive weakness in muscles whose functional deficit is inconsequential to the patient, such as the extensor hallucis longus, can be observed for longer periods.

Once the diagnosis of lumbar cauda equina syndrome is established or suspected, surgical decompression is recommended on an urgent or emergent basis.[7, 16, 63] A recent report by Kostuik and others suggest that this surgery may be delayed for 24 to 48 hours without irreversible cauda equina damage.[50, 83] The incidence of cauda equina syndrome varies from 1 to 16 per cent in reported series, but most large series report incidences of less than 3 per cent. Motor and sensory dysfunction usually recover, but bowel and bladder function are particularly sensitive to prolonged or excessive compression. Loss of bowel and bladder function correlates poorly with other physical findings but is less likely to recover if perianal sensation is also lost (anocutaneous reflex; S1–S4). The classic tetrad of low back pain, bilateral sciatica, saddle anesthesia, and motor weakness in the lower extremities progressing to paraplegia with bowel and bladder incontinence is not frequently present, necessitating a high index of suspicion in all patients with symptomatic lumbar disc disease. Kostuik has documented that unilateral sciatica may be a predominant feature, further emphasizing the need to examine the patient for S1 through S4 dysfunction.

Intraoperative neurologic injury occurs by various methods but is an expected complication of spinal surgery. It occurs at a variable rate, depending on the exact type of procedure performed.[37, 68] Neural injury results from contusion, laceration, electrocauterization, or traction on the neural elements.[84] Spinal fixation with the use of transpedicular screws also risks direct neural injury, most commonly as the nerve root passes medial and inferior to the pedicle.[71] Other cases of mechanical compression from foreign objects have been reported.[84] Indirect neural injury resulting from inadvertent disruption of the blood supply to the spinal cord and nerve roots may also contribute to the etiology of intraoperative neural damage. This is most often seen in spinal surgery for scoliosis, where corrective distractive forces are applied to rather rigid spinal deformities during posterior spinal instrumentation.[54] Turker and colleagues reported two cases of thoracic paraplegia remote from the site of lumbar spine surgery.[93] Etiologies of this rare neurologic sequela were hypothesized to be spinal cord ischemia or infarction with spinal cord edema. Taylor and coworkers reported a case of delayed-onset paraplegia related to hypotension in an adult scoliosis case.[88] These changes were caused by hypovolemia and ischemia rather than embolization or direct trauma, and they were reversible. Spinal cord monitoring was helpful in the management of the case.

The risks of intraoperative neural injury start at the time of subperiosteal exposure of the posterior elements of the spine.[84] In this situation, care should be taken to avoid inadvertent canal penetration. Careful inspection of the preoperative radiographs for vertebral midline anomalies (e.g., spina bifida occulta), coupled with a careful subperiosteal dissection with a large periosteal elevator, diminishes the possibility of this complication. When this complication occurs, an immediate pool of clear cerebrospinal fluid is noted, heralding a tear in the dura mater. Injury to the lumbar nerve roots may occur without laceration per se. Bertrand described a syndrome related to incomplete lumbar nerve root injuries that he referred to as the "battered lumbar nerve root."[14] This clinical syndrome consists of preoperative sciatica that is treated by a lumbar laminectomy or laminotomy. Postoperatively, the patient notes partial relief of the leg pain with severe numbness in the distribution of the involved nerve. The leg pain reappears gradually, and the profound numbness persists. This constellation of symptoms strongly suggests intraoperative lumbar nerve root injury. Direct nerve root avulsion was reported in 0.4 per cent of cases reviewed by Tew and Mayfield.[57, 92]

Direct intraoperative neural injury is best prevented, because there is no effective surgical management once injury has occurred.[46] Complete and careful hemostasis coupled with magnification, good lighting, and visualization are essential ingredients to avoid direct neural injury. Also, always working away from the neural element and/or parallel to the nerve roots helps minimize direct neural injuries. Excessive retraction should be avoided.[45] In general, the neural elements should not be retracted unless this is essential for adequate visualization. It is better and safer to widen the bony exposure rather than to retract the neural elements excessively or overzealously. The use of cotton pledgets and gentle retraction that is intermittently released throughout the procedure also helps to minimize direct neural injury (Fig. 54–31). Always completely visualize and work laterally to the nerve root sleeve in the lumbar spine. Matsui and associates, studying the effects of lumbar nerve root retraction, correlated changes with the degree of (force) pressure and the length of that (force) pressure.[59] Lumbar nerve root blood flow is decreased by retraction. Concurrent electrophysiologic changes were also documented. These findings could be seen with retraction force as low as 70 g/cm².

Postoperative neurologic complications may persist from injuries occurring intraoperatively, or they may develop after a baseline normal postoperative neurologic examination. These latter problems tend to be reversible, but they must be promptly identified and

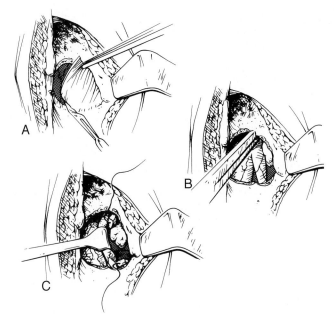

Figure 54–31. Safe technique of mobilization and retraction of a lumbar nerve root. After removing the ligamentum flavum *(A)*, the laminotomy is enlarged to clearly visualize the lateral border of the nerve root *(B)*. The nerve root is then mobilized and gently retracted medially and further protected with cotton pledgets superiorly and inferiorly along the lateral border of the nerve root. *(C)* (From Stambough, J. L.: Surgical technique for lumbar discectomy. Semin. Spine Surg. *1*:50, 1989.)

addressed. Cauda equina compression or direct nerve root compression resulting in cauda equina syndrome or radiculopathy, respectively, may develop after a successful operation owing to hematoma,[34, 75, 78] epidural abscess,[10–12, 33, 47, 48, 74, 95] malpositioning of an autogenous fat graft,[19, 72, 73] retained sponges,[90, 91] or failure to adequately relieve concomitant spinal stenosis.[5] Spinal cord or cauda equina ischemia caused by overdistraction or hypovolemia may develop in spinal deformity patients on a delayed basis.[93] Retroperitoneal fibrosis represents a late cause of neurologic deficits in anterior spinal procedures.[20] The incidence of this neurologic complication following lumbar spine surgery is approximately 0.2 per cent.[60] Neural traction injury and epidural scarring are generally the result of a limited exposure necessitating excessive manipulation of the lumbar neural elements (Fig. 54–32).[21] Clinical presentation is variable, but peroneal numbness, progressive motor loss, mild back and leg pain, and urinary retention requiring catheterization should alert one to the potential of this complication, even after an uneventful lumbar spinal surgery. The onset may be rapid or more insidious. CT scanning, MRI, and ultrasonography may be useful to confirm the suspected diagnosis.[53, 58] Once the diagnosis is established, the neural elements should be decompressed as soon as possible, preferably within 6 to 24 hours.

Dural tears or trauma that is unrecognized or inadequately repaired during surgery may result in the formation of a pseudomeningocele.[18, 40, 41, 43, 56, 80, 82] The

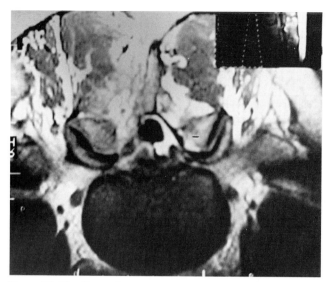

Figure 54–32. Excessive scarring about the right S1 nerve root following an L5–S1 discectomy. This man had burning dysesthetic pain involving the right S1 nerve root. Excessive manipulation and retraction of the nerve root were involved.

incidence is estimated to be between 0.07 and 2 per cent in lumbar spinal surgery cases.[41] This false sac may subsequently entrap, in a ball valve effect, either the spinal cord or the nerve roots, resulting in neurologic dysfunction and/or pain. Neural symptoms may also occur from the increased pressure within the pseudomeningocele sac. Lumbar pseudomeningoceles are much more common than cervical ones.[80] The onset of symptoms may be weeks to years after the surgical procedure and may present in a delayed and insidious fashion or as a sudden neurologic deficit with severe pain. The diagnosis is readily confirmed by CT scanning, MRI, or ultrasonography.[51] Once the diagnosis is established, surgical exploration and repair of the dural deficit are necessary to eliminate the patient's symp-

toms. Removal of the cyst wall per se is not necessary. The surgical outcome is generally good if this syndrome is promptly recognized and addressed.

Neurologic injury may occur as a result of anterior or posterior spinal instrumentation. Sublaminar wires in the cervical or thoracic spine may cause direct neurologic impairment during their passage or removal. Long-term effects are also suspected in animal models but have not been reported in humans. Hooks placed intralaminarly, supralaminarly, or into the facet can also cause direct neurologic injury. This is more likely along the concavity of the scoliotic curve, where the spinal cord is displaced owing to the chronic rotatory deformity. The authors are aware of one such case that only resolved partially. Anterior instrumentation that is now commonly employed in the cervical and thoracolumbar spine may impale the neural element if the screw is directed too far posteriorly (Fig. 54–33A). Thoracic and lumbar transpedicular screws also threaten the nerve root, especially as it passes medially or caudally around the corresponding pedicle (Fig. 54–33B). In large series of posterior transpedicular screw fixation, the incidence of direct or indirect neural injury is very low. This incidence can be reduced by (1) direct identification of the pedicle to nerve root anatomy intraoperatively (by open laminectomy or laminotomy); (2) careful identification of pedicle external landmarks—pars interarticularis, transverse process, and superior articular facet; and (3) the use of intraoperative biplanar image intensification or biplanar plane radiography. With attention to these details and principles, the incidence can be reduced to very low levels. Intraoperative electromyographic stimulation of the pedicle can also aid in identifying a violation of the pedicle cortical wall.

The incidence of neurologic injury caused by pedicle screw malpositioning varies in several large retrospective series from 0 to 6.5 per cent.[15, 30] These injuries include neurapraxia or irritation that clears with or without screw removal. Permanent nerve injury can

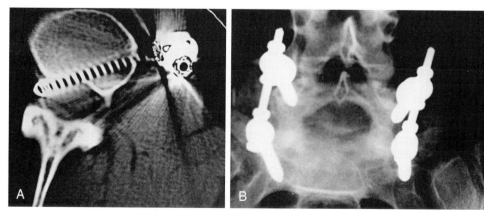

Figure 54–33. *A,* Malpositioned anterior vertebral body screw producing impingement of the dural sac and right L3 nerve root. Revision was required for persistent L3 radiculopathy. *B,* Malpositioned right L5 transpedicular screw producing right L5 radiculopathy. Removal and revision instrumentation was required. In both cases, the nerve root function recovered slowly.

occur as well, even with careful technique and radiographic guidance. In a large multiple-surgeon, multiple–implant system review of 617 pedicle screw cases, neurapraxia occurred in 15 cases (2.4 per cent) and permanent nerve root injury occurred in 14 cases (2.3 per cent). Overall, 32 cases (5.2 per cent) had unrecognized screw malpositioning, all without clinical significance. These as well as other types of complications were found to increase as the number of repeat surgeries increased.

Injury, partial or complete, to the fifth lumbar nerve root is frequent when reduction of high-grade spondylolisthesis is attempted. The incidence of fifth lumbar paraparesis varies from 20 to 65 per cent, depending on the series.[44, 82] Neurapraxia and axonotmesis can occur even if full reduction is not attempted or achieved. The fifth lumbar nerve root seems particularly vulnerable, probably because of chronic stretching and foraminal compromise. The authors have noted attenuation of this root in several cases in which the nerve root sleeve was only about one third the diameter of the adjacent S1 nerve root.

Neurologic impairment or injury has also been reported directly or indirectly in other clinical situations or associated with other therapeutic interventions. Eismont and Simeone reported a late case of paralysis caused by overgrowth of a bony fusion or possibly a pseudarthrosis within the fusion mass in a patient treated years earlier for scoliosis.[27] Direct neural injury can occur from transpedicular screw placement or from sublaminar wire passage.[38] It has also been noted in certain lumbar spine procedures that a certain incidence of reflex sympathetic dystrophy can be expected postoperatively.[40, 82]

Chemonucleolysis, which has fallen into disfavor in the United States, has a definite risk of transverse myelitis, thought to be caused by local reactions to the chymopapain enzyme.[25, 27, 53, 55] Based on early results, automated percutaneous discectomy does not seem to have the same risk of nerve root or spinal cord injury, because these patients are under local anesthesia and are fully awake to report any transient or symptomatic leg pain.[57] Direct neural injury occurred in about 6 per cent of cases in one series of percutaneous discectomies reported by Stern.[89] Neural injury in cases of posterior lumbar interbody fusions may result from graft displacement posteriorly, causing either nerve root or cauda equina compression.

PERIPHERAL NERVE

Peripheral nerve injuries can result from excessive pressure over vulnerable areas owing to improper positioning of patients during surgery (Fig. 54–34). These problems are best prevented by padding and inspecting suspicious areas during the surgical procedure. Spinal anesthesia for lumbar spine surgery also allows the patient to be awake during the surgical decompression so that the symptomatic problems can be identified and corrected immediately. These injuries may be the consequence of direct or prolonged pres-

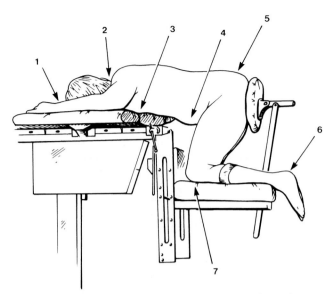

Figure 54–34. Kneeling position used during lumbar spine surgery. Care is taken to pad the ulnar nerves (1) and avoid hyperextension of the neck (2). The patient is in a three-point kneeling position (3, 7), and the abdomen is free, minimizing epidural venous congestion (4). The hip and knees are flexed, relaxing the formal and sciatic nerves. The back is horizontal (5), and antithrombotic stockings are worn (6). (From Stambough, J. L.: Surgical technique for lumbar discectomy. Semin. Spine Surg. 1:48, 1989.)

sure, excessive traction, or both. The ulnar nerve is the most frequently reported peripheral nerve to be injured as a consequence of positioning during surgery.[64, 66, 94] Other peripheral nerves reported injured as a consequence of malpositioning during surgery include the anterior interosseous nerve,[1] the radial nerve,[85] the lateral femoral cutaneous nerve, the median nerve,[77, 96] and the recurrent laryngeal nerve.[79] All these nerves are vulnerable to direct pressure as a result of their proximity to bone or cartilage or are particularly vulnerable to stretch by the fact that they cross a highly mobile joint (e.g., around the shoulder).[6, 99] Careful patient positioning for lumbar spine surgery may also help avoid these complications (see Fig. 54–30). Placing the patient in a kneeling position, allowing the abdomen to be free of pressure, minimizing compression on the retroperitoneal and epidural venous plexus, and allowing unimpeded respiratory exchange help decrease bleeding, facilitating better visualization and thereby lessening the possibility of direct neural injury as well.[26, 89, 95] Ford noted that flexion of the knees and hips also relaxes the sciatic and femoral nerves, lessening the possibility of injury due to retraction.[36] Nevertheless, this positioning does put the head and neck region, as well as the elbows and the knee areas, at some risk for direct pressure.[17] Prevention is the best management for these direct peripheral nerve injuries. Fortunately, most of these lesions recover postoperatively, unless the duration of compression has been excessive.

Spinal and epidural anesthesia may cause neurologic injuries either by direct neural damage or by the collection of an epidural mass effect from hematoma or abscess.[47, 49] The possibility of some vascular injury also exists. Serious and permanent paralysis is reported in less than 0.02 per cent of all cases of epidural and spinal anesthesia.[94] Patients on full anticoagulation, patients with elevated prothrombin time or activated partial thromboplastin time, or patients with disorders of platelet function should not have this type of anesthesia. Whether epinephrine can cause vasospasm and ischemia of the spinal arteries is still controversial. However, this has not been a significant clinical problem, and epinephrine is routinely utilized to increase the duration of spinal anesthesia. Overall, in our experience, this type of anesthesia has proved quite safe and predictable, with a very low complication rate.[48, 64]

CONCLUSION

Neurologic injuries as a consequence of spine surgery are rare. These injuries may result from a delay in surgical decompression, intraoperative neural injuries, neurologic problems related to positioning of the patient during surgery, or postoperative early or late complications. These complications are best prevented, because a definite treatment usually does not exist for these often irreversible lesions. Careful preoperative planning and surgical technique, concentrating on meticulous hemostasis, magnification, and adequate lighting and visualization, as well as well-applied surgical principles and knowledge of the anatomy, can help reduce the risk of neurologic complications in spine surgery.[88] The surgeon should always try to work away from the neural elements, especially the spinal cord, and minimize the retraction or direct manipulation of the nerve roots. Relative to the neural elements of the cervical or thoracolumbar spine, the adage "an ounce of prevention is worth a pound of cure" surely applies.

References

1. Albanese, S., Buterbaugh, G., Palmer, A., et al.: Incomplete anterior interosseous nerve palsy following spinal surgery: A report of two cases. Spine 11(10):1037–1038, 1986.
2. Albright, J., Flanigan, S., and Southwick W: Common complications of surgery of the cervical spine. Conn. Med. 32:725–733, 1968.
3. Aminoff, M. J.: Intraoperative monitoring by evoked potentials for spinal cord surgery: The cons. Electroencephalog. Clin. Neurophysiol. 73:378–380, 1989.
4. An, H. S., Vacarro, A., Cotler, J. M., and Lin, S.: Spinal disorders at the cervicothoracic junction. Spine 19(22):2557–2564, Nov. 15, 1994.
5. Anderson, J. T., and Bradley, W. E.: Neurogenic bladder dysfunction in protruded lumbar disc after laminectomy. Urology 8(1):94–100, 1976.
6. Anderson, J. M., Schady, W., and Markham, D. E.: An unusual cause of postoperative brachial plexus palsy. Br. J. Anesth. 72(5):605–607, 1994.
7. Armstrong, J. R.: The cause of unsatisfactory results from the operative treatment of lumbar disc lesions. J. Bone Joint Surg. 33B:31–35, 1951.
8. Attar, S., Hankins, J. R., Turney, S. Z., et al.: Paraplegia after thoracotomy: Report of five cases and review of the literature. Ann. Thorac. Surg. 59:1410–1415, 1995.
9. Avrahami, E., Tadmor, R., and Cohn, D. F.: Magnetic resonance imaging in patient with progressive myelopathy following spinal surgery. J. Neurol. Neurosurg. Psychiatry 52:176–181, 1989.
10. Baker, A. S., Ojemann, R. G., Swartz, M. N., and Richardson, E. P., Jr.: Spinal epidural abscess. N. Engl. J. Med. 293:463–468, 1975.
11. Bartel, A. D., Schiffer, J., Heilbronn, Y. D., and Yabel, M.: Anterior interbody fusion for cervical osteomyelitis. J. Neurol. Neurosurg. Psychiatry 35:133–136, 1972.
12. Benson, C., and Harris, A.: Acute neurologic infections. Med. Clin. North Am. 70:987–1011, 1986.
13. Bertalanffy, H., and Eggert, H. R.: Complications of anterior cervical discectomy without fusion in 450 consecutive patients. Acta Neurochir. 99:41–50, 1989.
14. Bertrand, G.: The battered root problem. Orthop. Clin. North Am. 6:305–310, 1975.
15. Blumenthal, S., and Gill, K.: Complications of the Wiltse pedicle screw fixation system. Adv. Orthop. Surg. 18:153–155, 1994.
16. Boccanera, L., and Laus, M.: Cauda equina syndrome following lumbar spinal stenosis surgery. Spine 12:712–715, 1987.
17. Bulger, R. F., Rejowski, J. E., and Beatty, R. A.: Vocal cord paralysis associated with anterior cervical fusion: Considerations for prevention and treatment. J. Neurosurg. 62:657–661, 1985.
18. Burres, K. P., and Conley, F. K.: Progressive neurological dysfunction secondary to postoperative cervical pseudo-meningocele in a C4 quadriplegic. J. Neurosurg. 48:289–291, 1978.
19. Cabezudo, J. M., Lopez, A., and Bacci, F.: Symptomatic root compression by a free fat transplant after hemilaminectomy: A case report. J. Neurosurg. 63:633–635, 1985.
20. Chan, F. L., and Chow, S. P.: Retroperitoneal fibrosis after anterior spinal fusion. Clin. Radiol. 34:331–335, 1983.
21. Choudhury, A., Taylor, J. C., and Whitaker, R.: Paraplegia complicating lumbar disc surgery. J. R. Coll. Surg. Edinb. 24:167–169, 1979.
22. Coselli, J. S.: Thoracoabdominal aortic aneurysms: Experience with 372 patients. J. Card. Surg. 9:638–647, 1994.
23. Dahlin, L. B., Rydevik, B., and McLean, W. G.: Changes in fast axonal transport during experimental nerve compression at low pressures. Exp. Neurol. 84:29–34, 1984.
24. Daube, J. R.: Intraoperative monitoring by evoked potentials for spinal cord surgery: The pros. Electroencephalogr. Clin. Neurophysiol. 73:374–377, 1989.
25. Eguro, H.: Transverse myelitis following chemonucleolysis. J. Bone Joint Surg. Am. 65:1328–1329, 1983.
26. Eie, N., Solgaard, T., and Kleppe, H.: The knee-elbow position in lumbar disc surgery: A review of complications. Spine 8:897–900, 1983.
27. Eismont, F. J., and Simeone, F. A.: Bone overgrowth (hypertrophy) as a cause of late paraparesis after scoliosis fusion: A case report. J. Bone Joint Surg. Am. 63:1016–1019, 1981.
28. Epstein, N. E., Epstein, J. A., and Carras, R.: Degenerative spondylolisthesis with an intact arch: A review of 60 cases with an analysis of clinical findings and the development of surgical management. Neurosurgery 13:555–561, 1983.
29. Esperson, J. O., Buhl, M., Eriksen, E. F., et al.: Treatment of cervical disc disease using Cloward's technique. 1. General results, effect of different operative methods and complications in 1106 patients. Acta Neurochir. (Wien) 70:97–114. 1984.
30. Esses, S. I., Sachs, B. L., and Dreyzin, V.: Complications associated with the technique of pedicle screw fixation: A selected survey of ABS members. Spine 18:2231–2239, 1993.
31. Faciszewzki, T., Winter, R. B., Lonstein, J. L., et al.: The surgical and medical perioperative complications of anterior spinal surgery in the thoracic and lumbar spine in adults: A review of 1223 cases. Spine 20:1512–1599, 1995.
32. Fielding, W. J.: Complications of anterior cervical disk removal and fusion. Clin. Orthop. 284:10–13, 1992.
33. Firsching, R., Frowien, R. A., and Nittner, K.: Acute spinal epidural empyema. Acta Neurochir. 74:68–71, 1985.
34. Flaschka, G.: Akutes, spinales epidural Hamatom bei Immunovasculitis. Neurochirurgia 25:174–176, 1982.
35. Flynn, T. B.: Neurologic complications of anterior interbody fusion. Spine 7:536–539, 1982.

36. Ford, L. T.: Position for lumbar disk surgery. Clin. Orthop. Rel. Res. 123:104, 1977.

37. Fujimaki, A., Crock, H. V., and Bedbrook, G. M.: The results of 150 anterior lumbar interbody fusion operations performed by two surgeons in Australia. Clin. Orthop. 165:164–167, 1982.

38. Goll, S. R., Balderston, R. A., Stambough, J. L., et al.: Depth of intraspinal wire penetration during the passage of sublaminar wires. Spine 13:503–509, 1988.

39. Graham, J. J.: Complications of cervical spine surgery. Spine 14:1046–1050, 1989.

40. Hadani, F. G., Knoler, N., Tadmor, R., et al.: Entrapped lumbar nerve root in pseudo-meningocele after laminectomy: Report of three cases. Neurosurgery 19:405–407, 1986.

41. Hakelius, A.: Prognosis in sciatica: A clinical follow up of surgical and nonsurgical treatment. Acta Orthop. Scand. Suppl. 129:1–78, 1970.

42. Hanakita, J., Kinuta, Y., and Suzuki, T.: Spinal cord compression due to postoperative cervical pseudomeningocele. Neurosurgery 17:317–319, 1985.

43. Heeneman, H.: Vocal cord paralysis following approaches to the anterior cervical spine. Laryngoscope 83:17–21, 1973.

44. Hu, S. S., Bradford, D. S., Transfeldt, E. E., and Cohen, M.: Reduction of high-grade spondylolisthesis using Edwards instrumentation. Spine 21:367–371, 1996.

45. Jayson, M. I.: The role of vascular damage and fibrosis in the pathogenesis of nerve root damage. Clin. Orthop. 279:40–48, 1992.

46. Jonsson, B., and Stromqvist, B.: Lumbar spine surgery in the elderly: Complications and surgical results. Spine 19:1431–1435, 1994.

47. Kalufman, D., Kaplan, J., and Litman, N.: Infectious agents in spinal epidural abscesses. Neurology 30:840–844, 1980.

48. Kannangara, D. W., Tanaka, T., and Thadepalli, H.: Spinal epidural abscess due to *Actinomyces israelii*. Neurology 31:202–204, 1981.

49. Katz, J., and Aidinis, S.: Current concepts review complications of spinal and epidural anesthesia. J. Bone Joint Surg. Am. 62:1219–1222, 1980.

50. Kostuik, J. P., Harrington, I., Alexander, D., et al.: Cauda equina syndrome and lumbar disc herniation. J. Bone Joint Surg. Am. 68:386–391, 1986.

51. Laffey, P. A., and Kricun, M. E.: Sonographic recognition of postoperative meningocele. AJR Am. J. Roentgenol. 143:177–178, 1984.

52. Larsson, E. M., Holtas, S., and Cronquist, S.: Emergency magnetic resonance examination of patients with spinal cord symptoms. Acta Radiol. 29:69–75, 1988.

53. Lundborg, G., Myers, R., and Powell, H.: Nerve compression injury and increased endoneural fluid pressure: A "miniature compartment syndrome." J. Neurol. Neurosurg. Psychiatry 46:1119–1124, 1983.

54. MacEwen, G. D., and Bunnell, W. P.: Acute neurological complications in treatment of scoliosis. J. Bone Joint Surg. Am. 57:404–408, 1975.

55. MacNab, I., McCulloch, J. A., Weinder, D. S., et al.: Chemonucleolysis. Can. J. Surg. 14:280–288, 1971.

56. Mariui, F., Corriero, G., Giamondo, A., et al.: Postoperative cervical pseudomeningocele. Neurochirurgia 31:29–31, 1988.

57. Maroon, J. C., and Onik, G.: Percutaneous automated discectomy: A new method for lumbar disc removal. J. Neurol. 66:143–146, 1987.

58. Masaryk, T. J., Modic, M. T., Geisinger, M. A., et al: Cervical myelopathy: A comparison of magnetic resonance and myelography. J. Comp. Assist. Tomog. 10(2):184–194, 1996.

59. Matsui, H., Kitagawa, H., Kawaguchi, T., and Tsuji H.: Physiologic changes of nerve root during posterior lumbar discectomy. Spine 20(6):654–659, Mar. 1995.

60. Mayfield, F.: Complications of laminectomy. Clin. Neurosurg. 23:435–439, 1975.

61. Mayfield, F. H.: Cervical spondylosis: A comparison of the anterior and posterior approaches. Clin. Neurosurg. 13:181–188, 1966.

62. McGuire, D. J.: Management of cervical disc disease. In Bridwell, K. H., and Dewald, R. L. (eds.): The Textbook of Spinal Surgery, Vol. 2 Philadelphia, J. B. Lippincott, 1991, pp. 749–770.

63. McLaren, A. C., and Bailey, S. T.: Cauda equina syndrome: A complication of lumbar discectomy. Clin. Orthop. Rel. Res. 204:143–149, 1986.

64. Meinecke, F. W.: Spinal cord lesions after diagnostic and therapeutic procedures. Paraplegia 17:284–293, 1979–1980.

65. Michel, F., Rubini, J., Grand, C., et al.: Neurological complications of surgery for spinal deformities. Rev. Chir. Orthop. Reparatrice Appar. Mot. 78:90–100, 1992.

66. Miller, R. G., and Camp, P. E.: Postoperative ulnar neuropathy. JAMA 242:1636–1639, 1979.

67. Newbery, J. M.: Paraplegia following general anesthesia. Anesthesia 32:78–79, 1977.

68. Nuwer, M. R., Dawson, E. G., Carlson, L. G., et al.: Somatosensory evoked potential spinal cord monitoring reduces neurologic deficits after scoliosis surgery: Results of a large multicenter survey. Electroencephalogr. Clin. Neurophysiol. 96:6–11, 1995.

69. Ogle, K., Palsingh, J., Hewitt, C., and Anderson, M.: Osteoptysis: A complication of cervical spine surgery. Br. J. Neurosurg. 6:607–609, 1992.

70. Parke, W. W., and Watanabe, R.: The intrinsic vasculature of the lumbosacral spinal nerve roots. Spine 10:508–515, 1985.

71. Pattee, G. A., Bohlman, H. H., and McAfee, P. C.: Compression of a sacral nerve as a complication of screw fixation of the sacroiliac joint: A case report. J. Bone Joint Surg. Am. 68:769–771, 1986.

72. Prusick, V. R., Lint, D. S., and Bruder, W. J.: Cauda equina syndrome as a complication of free epidural fat-grafting. J. Bone Joint Surg. Am. 70:1256–1258, 1988.

73. Quencer, R. M., Green, B. A., Montalvo, B. M., and Eismont, F. J.: Symptomatic spinal cord deformity secondary to a redundant intramedullary shunt catheter. Neuroradiology 27:176–180, 1985.

74. Ravicovitch, M., and Spallone, A.: Spinal epidural abscesses. Eur. Neurol. 21:347–357, 1982.

75. Reynolds, A. F., and Wilson, C. B.: Letters to the editor: Epidural bleeding in anterior discectomy. J. Neurosurg. 50:126–129, 1979.

76. Riley, L. H., Robinson, R. A., Johnson, K. A., and Walker, A. E.: The results of anterior interbody fusion of the cervical spine: Review of 93 consecutive cases. J. Neurosurg. 30:127–133, 1969.

77. Rydevik, B., and Lundborg, G.: Permeability of intraneural microvessels and perineurium following acute, gradual experimental nerve compression. Scand. J. Plast. Reconstr. Surg. 11:179–187, 1977.

78. Sang, H., and Wilson, C. B.: Postoperative epidural hematoma as a complication of anterior cervical discectomy. J. Neurosurg. 49:288–291, 1978.

79. Schmidt, C. R.: Peripheral nerve injuries with anesthesia: A review and report of three cases. Anesth. Analg. (Cleveland) 45:748–753, 1966.

80. Schumacher, H. W., Wassman, H., and Podlinski, C.: Pseudomeningocele of the lumbar spine. Surg. Neurol. 29:77–78, 1988.

81. Scoville, W. B.: Posterior keyhole laminotomy: Complication of cervical spondylosis. In Dunsker, S. B. (ed.): Seminars in Neurological Surgery: Cervical Spondylosis. New York, Raven Press, 1980, pp. 169–171.

82. Serena, S. H., Bradford, D. S., Transfeldt, E. E., and Cohen, M.: Reduction of high grade spondylolisthesis using Edwards instrumentation. Spine 21:367–371, 1996.

83. Sherman, J. E., Carr, J. B., and Delamarter, R. B. Cauda equina syndrome: Recovery following early or late decompression. AAOS Abstracts, 59th annual meeting, Washington, DC, February 20–25, 1992, p, 150.

84. Simmons, E. H., and Wilbur, R. G.: Complications of spinal surgery for discogenic disease and spondylolisthesis. In Epps, C. H. (ed.): Complications in Orthopaedic Surgery. Philadelphia, J. B. Lippincott, 1986, pp. 1181–1214.

85. Smith, R. B., Gramling, Z. W., and Volpitlo, P. P.: Problems related to the prone position for surgical operations. Anesthesia 22:189–193, 1961.

86. Spangfort, E. V.: The lumbar disc herniation. Acta. Orthop. Scand. Suppl. 142:1–95, 1972.

87. Stambough, J. L., and Rothman, R. H.: Indications for cervical spine surgery. *In* Wiesel, S. W., and Feffer, H. L. (eds.): Neck Pain. Charlottesville, VA, Michie Co., 1986, pp. 275–312.
88. Stambough, J. L., and Simeone, F. A.: Neurogenic complications in spine surgery. *In* Rothman and Simeone: The Spine. Philadelphia, W. B. Saunders Co., 1992, pp. 1885–1891.
89. Stern, M.: Early experience with percutaneous lateral diskectomy. Clin. Orthop. *238*:50–55, 1988.
90. Strand, C. L., King, R. L., and Echols, W. B.: Retained surgical sponge following laminectomy. JAMA *23*:1040, 1973.
91. Sutterlin, C., and Rechtine, G. R.: Using the Heffington frame in elective lumbar spinal surgery. Orthop. Rev. *17*:597–600, 1988.
92. Tew, J. M., Jr., and Mayfield, F. H.: Surgery of the anterior cervical spine: Prevention of complications. *In* Dunsker, S. B. (ed.): Seminars in Neurological Surgery: Cervical Spondylosis. New York, Raven Press, 1980, pp. 191–208.
93. Turker, R. J., Slack, C., and Regan, Q.: Thoracic paraplegia after lumbar spinal surgery. J. Spinal Disord. *8*:195–200, 1995.
94. Vandam, L.: Neurological sequelae of spinal and epidural anesthesia. Int. Anesth. Clin. *24*:231–255, 1986.
95. Verner, E. F., and Musher, D. M.: Spinal epidural abscess. Med. Clin. North Am. *69*:375–384, 1985.
96. Wadsworth, T. G., and Williams, J. R.: Cubital tunnel external compression syndrome. BMJ *1*:662–666, 1973.
97. Wayne, S. J.: A modification of the tuck position for lumbar spine surgery: A 15 year follow-up study. Clin. Orthop. Rel. Res. *184*:212–216, 1984.
98. Weber, H.: The effect of delayed disc surgery on muscular paresis. Acta Orthop. Scand. *46*:631–642, 1975.
99. West, C. G. H.: Bilateral brachial paresis following anterior decompression for cervical spondylosis. Spine *11*:176–178, 1986.
100. Wilkes, L. L.: Paraplegia from operating position and spinal stenosis in non-spinal surgery: A case report. Clin. Orthop. Rel. Res. *146*:148–149, 1980.
101. Yonenobu, K., Hosono, N., Asano, M., and Ono, K.: Neurologic complications of surgery for cervical compression myelopathy. Spine *16*:1277–1282, 1991.
102. Young, P. H.: Complications of cervical spine microsurgery. *In* Dunsker, S.B. (ed.): Seminars in Neurological Surgery: Cervical Spondylosis. New York, Raven Press, 1980, pp. 185–189.
103. Zeidman, S. M., and Ducker, T. B.: Posterior cervical laminoforaminotomy for radiculopathy: Review of 172 cases. Neurosurgery *33*:356–362, 1993.

Cerebrospinal Fluid Leaks: Etiology and Treatment

Gabrielle F. Morris, M.D.

Lawrence F. Marshall, M.D.

The most frequently encountered complication in spinal surgery is that of inadvertent dural entry. The increasing use of sophisticated instrumentation and a more aggressive approach to the repair of the thoracolumbar spine, particularly following severe injuries to the bony structures and the cord, mean that spine surgeons will increasingly encounter these leaks or inadvertently cause them. Dural tears that result in the leakage of cerebrospinal fluid (CSF) present a danger to the patient in several ways. First, if such leaks result in wound breakdown, the possibility of infection with meningitis is real. Second, the development of pseudomeningocele, occasionally with neural elements trapped within the pseudomeningocele, may produce intractable pain and, rarely, neurologic deficit. Finally, incapacitating headaches can occur if these fistulas go untreated. Fortunately, this complication can be reduced to a very rare occurrence by appropriate attention to meticulous surgical techniques. Even with the trend to a more aggressive approach in the repair of spinal column injuries and the increasing use of sophisticated instrumentation to treat degenerative disease, leaks should be relatively rare, particularly in patients undergoing their first procedure.

CLASSIFICATION

All classifications of CSF leaks are arbitrary, although logically they can be divided based on etiology. The two most common types are those that result from direct injury and those that occur because of an iatrogenic event. Further categorization, including description of the leakage location, the region along the spinal axis, and the relation within the spinal canal, is helpful in individual cases but does not contribute to our understanding of etiology or repair. Obviously, the extent of dural injury is also a factor, but it is relatively uncommon for dural injury to be so extensive that primary repair is not possible.

The progression of CSF leaks to true fistulas occurs only in the presence of breakdown of the overlying tissues. This is an important distinction, because infection, as a major risk of CSF leaks, becomes a factor only when one has a true fistula. Most leaks that are the result of trauma to the dura and often the cord are of no consequence unless the patient undergoes a surgical procedure that unroofs the bony coverings and ligamentous structures that, when combined with the clot that is often present, usually contain the leak. Perhaps the only exceptions are gunshot wounds, particularly those caused by large-bore missiles, in which a spontaneous fistula may develop, most often into the chest or dorsally in the upper back.

DIAGNOSIS

Clinical Findings

There is little diagnostic difficulty when clear fluid emanating from a wound is seen. Intraoperatively, close observation identifies such lesions where dural disruption allows free egress of CSF. As the thecal sac empties, there is a resultant decrease in local tissue pressure on the epidural veins. With this, rebleeding of previously adequately controlled areas may be seen and requires attention. One must also identify dural disruption that has not yet violated the arachnoid layer.

In most circumstances, a CSF leak, if one has a high index of suspicion, is not difficult to diagnose. Immediate causes for concern on physical examination include a visible and/or palpable subcutaneous fluid collection, severe headache exacerbated by upright posture, and signs or symptoms of infection. Known risk factors for poor wound healing must be considered, such as the patient's immune status, presence of diabetes, addiction to tobacco smoking, loss of integrity of overlying tissues, and history of radiation therapy in proximity. Whether instrumentation has been used and whether this is a reoperation are also important considerations. Certain traumatic injury patterns, especially those with extensive structural spinal damage, have higher associations with dural tears.

Radiographic Findings

Neurodiagnostic studies provide anatomic delineation of the extent of injury. Plain films identify injury. Computed tomography (CT) is best for bony detail, and magnetic resonance imaging (MRI) provides excellent soft tissue resolution. A combination of these studies is used in the initial patient evaluation and therapeutic planning. Some generalities can be gleaned. Most burst fractures at the thoracolumbar junction or in the lumbar spine do not have dural tears associated with them. However, if the degree of canal impingement exceeds 50 per cent, if there is an associated laminar fracture, and if a neurologic deficit is present, at least 70 per cent of such patients will have a dural tear.[2] It is usually located laterally at the nerve root exit or ventrally-dorsally. When a marked component of distraction as well as subluxation is present, associated dural tears are much more likely. Similarly, thoracolumbar junction and upper lumbar fractures with significant axial components, particularly lateral subluxation, have been associated with extensive dural tears. CSF leaks are unusual with cervical spine injuries. The primary leak a surgeon is likely to encounter is iatrogenic.

Occasionally, additional radiographic studies are needed. There are circumstances when the surgeon feels reasonably certain that there is no dural injury, yet the patient's complaints clearly raise that possibility. Here, MRI with interest directed to the soft tissues may be helpful in determining whether or not fluid is present in quantities in excess of that expected as postoperative changes. Water-soluble contrast media with high-quality fluoroscopy can be used to determine whether a leak is present and to further localize it.[15] The use of radionuclide myelography has also been suggested, but it has not gained widespread support.[8]

PREVENTION

The single best method to treat a CSF leak is to prevent its occurrence in the first place. Obviously, this is not possible if the patient's injury caused the leak. Con-

versely, all iatrogenic dural tears are potentially preventable. In general, dural injuries in patients who have not had previous surgery and in whom the spinal canal is anatomically intact are relatively rare. If they occur with any frequency, the surgeon must critically examine his or her technique.

Iatrogenic dural tears are frequently associated with reoperation; thus, greater caution must be exercised when working on these patients. Other factors that lead to a higher rate of iatrogenic dural entry include failure to attend to principles of modern surgery, inexperienced surgeons, and undue haste in carrying out the procedure.

Consistent and strict adherence to sound operative technique is required. This cannot be overemphasized. A conscientious surgeon attempts to minimize inadvertent dural tear with each intraoperative motion. Every bite with any rongeur involves two steps: first, identifying the structure to be excised under direct vision, and second ensuring that no dura mater comes between this and the instrument. The tearing of spinal ligaments with instruments that are not sharp or not properly placed should be avoided if possible. The introduction of the foot plate of the Kerrison rongeur should be perpendicular to the bone that is to be removed. Drills should be used in a medial to lateral direction so that if slippage occurs, it is less likely that the dura and the underlying spinal cord will be injured (Fig. 54–35).

Whenever possible, when operating within the canal, the dura and its underlying contents should be covered with cottonoids or other material to protect against inadvertent penetration. Of course, such materials should not be packed in where the canal is stenosed, but rather laid gently over the dura as bony removal is performed. In patients in whom the canal is especially tight, for example, in an elderly patient with lumbar stenosis, thinning of the bone laterally using a drill is helpful before using rongeurs, so that the risk of inadvertent dural entry during the removal of "thickened" bone can be reduced.

The frequency of lumbar laminectomy for disc disease in the United States makes opening of the ligamentum flavum during hemilaminotomy and discectomy the most frequent cause of inadvertent dural injury. In many patients, there is no need to remove the ligament overlying the thecal sac, because the protrusion is lateral. By carrying out a more lateral approach and not disturbing the ligamentum flavum over the thecal sac, the possibility of inadvertent dural entry can be reduced. Magnification, with enhanced lighting, is extremely helpful and also reduces the incidence of this complication. Adequate lateral traction as the ligament is being incised also reduces the risk of dural injury. The use of toothed forceps or a ligamentum flavum clamp permits this to be done without dural injury, assuming visualization of the ligamentum is unobstructed prior to grasping it. Tearing or ripping of ligaments using large Kerrison rongeurs should be avoided. As the ligament is being retracted laterally, a small cottonoid or dural elevator can be introduced to

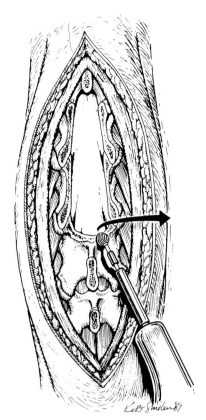

Figure 54–35.   The drill should always be used from medial to lateral.

separate the dura from the ligamentum flavum as the remaining ligament is removed.

Occasionally, the dura is torn somewhat more ventrally, and repair is difficult. Under such circumstances, adequate bony removal and complete exposure of the tear must be achieved to allow for successful closure, even though this results in the patient having a much larger procedure.

Reoperation for any indication puts patients at higher risk for dural injury and CSF leaks. Although meticulous technique must always be emphasized, it is in this patient group that careful preoperative planning and systematic surgical technique are essential to avoid tearing the scarred and often thinned dura. It is wise to begin the dissection in an area of normal tissue planes and then proceed toward the scarred region. In lumbar stenosis, beginning either proximal or distal to the previous operative site and working toward the hypertrophied facets is recommended. By dissecting the scar from the facets and then working medially, the lateral aspect of the canal can usually be identified. Under magnification along the gutter of the canal, the dura can gradually be freed so that the roots can be identified and the bony dissection continued. In general, trying to divide the scar in the midline and working laterally is technically quite difficult, but when the midline scar frees up easily, a groove director can be introduced and the scar divided. This facilitates access

to the roots for decompression. It is not necessary to remove the scar directly over the dorsal surface of the thecal sac, unless it is acting as a tether. The dissection should be gentle.

A less frequent cause of leaks in the lumbar spine is a failure to recognize spina bifida occulta preoperatively. It is important in this era of modern imaging that plain radiographs still be obtained in patients to identify this possibility preoperatively. A slip into the canal with a periosteal elevator or osteotome can produce extensive damage to the cauda equina that may be irreparable.

A by-product of the explosion of instrumentation techniques available for surgery in the thoracolumbar spine has been an increase in the frequency of iatrogenic CSF leaks. Because there is a small, but definitely increased risk with surgery using foreign materials, the possibility of inadvertent dural entry in these patients is potentially serious. Here again, the experience of the surgeon and strict adherence to basic surgical principles are the best way to minimize complications. Even in the best of hands, dural injury does occur, however. Recognition of the dural tear before wound closure, rather than after, is the most important determinant in reducing the risk of postoperative leak.

TREATMENT OF DURAL TEARS AND CSF FISTULAS

Primary Repair

Most dorsal CSF leaks occur as a result of iatrogenic injury, particularly when the canal or foramina are decompressed because of stenosis or when wires are passed for internal fixation beneath the lamina or through the spinous processes. Occasionally, the placement of hooks and/or pedicle screws, particularly in older patients, leads to dural injury, but these are often more lateral. The majority of dural tears can be identified under direct vision at operation and lend themselves to simple repair. Occasionally, supplemental techniques may be required. Only when conventional management fails should more invasive measures be pursued. The dural repair should attempt, if possible, to avoid compromise of the intraluminal diameter of the thecal sac and should result in immediate cessation of CSF leakage.

The first step in closure is complete exposure of the dural tear. It is imperative that the full extent of the dural rent be visible, including enough surrounding area for safe manipulation of the instruments in the repair process. The surgeon must ascertain whether there is only one area of dural injury. If not, full exposure of each is necessary. Magnification and adequate lighting are essential. The goal is apposition of dural edges free of tension, which requires meticulous placement of the sutures. A running locking stitch can achieve this. Attention must be paid to replacing the neural elements in their intrathecal location and avoiding their incorporation into the suture line. Leaks can often be closed with 6.0 cardiovascular suture such as Prolene. Some surgeons choose a 4.0-caliber suture, but it requires a much larger needle and is unsuitable when the dura is thinned, as in the elderly, or when the dural opening is very small. The recommended suture placement for dural closure is approximately 2 mm from each dural edge and 3 mm between stitches. Following completion of the dural closure, the surgeon should inspect the site of closure while the anesthesiologist carries out a Valsalva maneuver for the patient. If the leak persists, further steps are required, which can include the use of fibrin glue, further suture repair, or the placement of a small piece of Gelfoam over the area, which, when held gently for several minutes, often adheres to the dura and seals these very small residual leaks.

Once the best possible dural repair has been achieved, a multiple-layer, water-tight closure of the remaining tissues is essential. The fascia, which is by far the most important barrier, should be tightly closed without causing tissue necrosis. Interrupted sutures supplemented by running oversewing sutures are effective. Good approximation of subcutaneous tissue and the skin is also important. When a CSF leak has occurred, suturing the skin is preferable to stapling.

Surgeons historically have kept patients in the supine position following dural entry and repair to reduce the hydrostatic pressure on the suture line. More recently, however, we have ambulated patients after 24 hours of bed rest and have not observed an increase in the frequency of CSF leak. It is, of course, important to inspect the wound frequently to verify that it remains intact and dry and that there is no bulge.

Techniques for Reinforcement

Extensive, complex dural tears may not lend themselves to an anatomic tension-free primary repair. This can be seen in association with extensive anterior bony destruction, such as complex vertebral body fractures in the cervical and thoracic spine. The preservation of all local tissues, including lacerated fascia, for example, is extremely important when approaching such repairs. Often these materials can be used to assist in primary closure. The generation of local tissue flaps has often been extremely helpful in repairing these complex lateral dural injuries.

Patch grafting is an effective means of closing larger dural defects. Fascia from the paravertebral muscles is useful for this purpose. The patient's autologous graft can be relatively easily obtained. In general, the placement of initial anchoring stitches is helpful. A simple technique, with the initial stitch placed from the graft to the dura, as shown in Figure 54–36, is optimal.[5] After one side is secured, the graft can be trimmed to fit and should not be so redundant as to be floppy. Closure can then be completed, and the fascia tightly closed.

Occasionally, there are circumstances when the dural leak is small and cannot be visualized. This occurs under instrumentation or laterally along the proximal nerve root. Here, a bit of blood-soaked Gelfoam can be

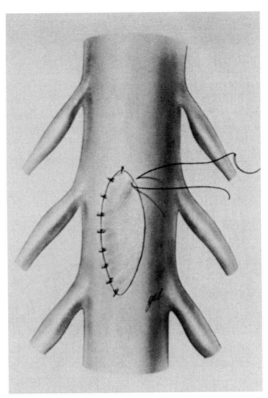

Figure 54–36. Dural repair using a fascia lata patch graft. Suture begins on the graft ends on the dura. (From Eismont, F. J., Wiesel, S. W., and Rothman, R. H.: Treatment of dural tears associated with spinal surgery. J. Bone Joint Surg. Am. *63*:1132–1136, 1991.)

applied and gently held for several minutes while it dries and adheres.

An alternative technique that is effective for small lateral leaks that cannot be sutured primarily is a lateral patch technique, as described by Mayfield and illustrated in Figure 54–37.[10] A small dorsal opening is made in the dura, and a transdural approach is then carried out to permit the placement of a suture from central to lateral. Attached to that suture is a small piece of fat or muscle that is then pulled from the outside in, thus producing a seal. Although a small durotomy is acceptable in the midline, it must not be so small that injury to the cord or the roots occurs when this technique is used.

Remember to check the final repair by performing a Valsalva maneuver, which often allows identification of points where continued leakage is occurring. These techniques must be applied to each site.

Fibrin Glue

The addition of fibrin glue to the armamentarium of the spine surgeon has been an advance in both the prevention and the treatment of CSF leaks. This substance, when properly formed and applied, results in an immediate barrier to the extradural egress of fluid. Additional benefit is derived during the healing pro-

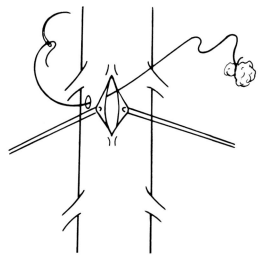

Figure 54–37. The lateral pull-through technique of Mayfield is shown for small lateral defects that are difficult to suture.

cess, when the presence of fibrin glue components incites an inflammatory response. The result is a tough, fibrous scar that overlies the dura and forms a watertight seal. No luminal compromise should occur. Indications for the use of fibrin glue as a sealant have been identified in a wide variety of surgical procedures. In complex spine surgery, fibrin glue is indicated when dural tears cannot be fully exposed anatomically, precluding adequate repair. It also has a role in reinforcing tenuous repairs, as well as providing an extra layer of protection in those patients in whom CSF leakage would be catastrophic.[6, 7, 12]

Fibrin glue is formed by equal volume mixtures of thrombin and cryoprecipitate solution, which is rich in clotting factors, especially fibrinogen. As these two liquids come into contact with each other, a biologic gel with strong adhesion properties is formed. The components must be kept separate until ready for application to the disrupted or freshly repaired dural surface. For the best result, certain details should be attended to. Cooling the individual components prior to mixing increases the repair strength of patched tissue defects.[14] Applying the solution as a spray may seal the dura better than the mixture method.[13] In contrast to common U.S. preparations, antifibrinolytic agents are added to the preparations in Europe. These agents include epsilon amino caproic acid, aprotinin, or similar compounds often used with calcium. Currently, there is no consensus that such agents are essential to the efficacy of fibrin glue.[1]

The major concern that has precluded the routine use of fibrin glue is the possibility of transmission of communicable diseases, specifically AIDS and hepatitis. The lack of literature reporting such problems suggests that current donor selection and serum testing protocols have reduced the risk of infectious transmission to a minimum. Previous problems with pooled-donor cryoprecipitate have been circumvented by the wide availability of single-donor cryoprecipitate.

Newer technologies also permit the generation of adequate fibrin glue from autologous donations. Although these methods may increase cost and require advance planning, they clearly eliminate the risk of infectious transmission.[3, 4]

Overall, fibrin glue provides spine surgeons with a biologic tissue sealant to help combat the problem of CSF leakage. Intuitively, the concept is logical. Many centers have reported the efficacy of this substance, but it is noted that at this time there is no adequately controlled clinical trial that conclusively confirms its benefit over standard meticulous microsurgical technique in dural repair. Fibrin glue is a good agent in addition to, but not instead of, adequate dural repair.

VENTRAL LEAKS FROM MISSILE INJURY

Almost all leaks into the chest or abdominal cavity are the result of missile injuries, which produce major vertebral body disruption with cord and dural destruction. The overwhelming majority of these patients have complete injuries. In contrast to surgical dictum in the past, such patients with complete injuries need not be routinely explored. These injuries are fundamentally different biomechanically from other traumatic injuries; usually, much of the ligamentous support of the spinal column is left intact, and unless multiple vertebral bodies and posterior elements are involved in the blast, operation for stabilization is usually not necessary. When multiple vertebral segments are involved with accompanying posterior element injury, a limited procedure done posteriorly to débride the wound is preferable, because large anterior and posterior operations are likely to make such dural leaks worse.

If ventral exploration is indicated in these patients, primary repair of the dura is difficult, unless there is extensive exposure. Here, the use of a fascia lata graft with fibrin glue is strongly recommended. In such patients, we place a distal lumbar drain, in an attempt to decompress the repair, for several days. This technique has been successful, and reoperation has been necessary in only one patient over the last decade.

LUMBAR MYELOMENINGOCELES

The increasing frequency of lumbar decompression for stenosis as the population ages appears to be leading to an increased incidence of lumbar pseudomyelomeningocele. These are more common than previously thought.[11] Although undoubtedly many small tears close spontaneously, others either continue to leak directly into the soft tissues until the skin breaks down or form a progressive meningocele. The former usually present with increasing headache, often quite severe, and a wound that has become progressively "swollen."

In contrast, in patients in whom a myelomeningocele develops, headache is less common, but they often have persistent sciatica, the complaint that led to their operation in the first place. Thus, a history of modest headache on standing, which is relieved by the recumbent position, and worsening persistence of sciatica in a patient operated on for degenerative disease of the lumbar spine suggests the possibility of pseudomeningocele. Such patients should be restudied. It is important to ask the radiologist to rule out the possibility of meningocele through the use of contrast myelography or MRI.

The patient should be reoperated on for primary closure of the dural leak, if at all possible. Usually this is relatively simple, because the leak can be easily recognized and the tear is small. On occasion, a larger, less easily reparable leak is identified, and here, techniques previously described (e.g., the lateral patch technique) are useful. Alternatively, fibrin glue can be applied and is likely to be successful. Although covering the site of dural injury with fat may be of some value, it is important not to pack the fat into the foramen, because this can exacerbate the underlying sciatica that the patient initially presented with.

CSF Diversion

For leaks that despite the surgeon's best efforts, cannot be primarily sutured or patched and are still leaking, a lumbar subarachnoid drain should be placed percutaneously at L3, L4, or L5. This allows CSF to be diverted via a low-resistance pathway.[9] The patient is placed on prophylactic antistaphylococcal antibiotics and kept on supine bed rest for 72 to 96 hours while continuous drainage into a sterile bag is performed. The drain is then clamped and the patient allowed to ambulate. The wound is inspected for an additional 24 to 48 hours. If it remains flat and dry, the drain is removed. If there is still a question of leak, drainage can be continued for a maximum of seven days. At that point, the risk of catheter-induced infection is likely to exceed the benefits of continued drainage, and the catheter should be removed. Lumbar catheter drainage is effective in most patients, with surgery reserved for those who fail.

CONTINUED CSF FISTULA IN THE FACE OF REPAIR

Occasionally, either because a leak is not recognized or because the primary repair is technically difficult or impossible, the patient has evidence of a CSF leak into the soft tissues or with early skin breakdown and fluid leak to the surface. Small leaks associated only with headache and a closed wound can be treated with strict bed rest and a pressure dressing. In most instances, if the wound is firmly healed, this can be done on an outpatient basis, and the patient can be re-examined at regular intervals.

CSF emanating from a wound is a relative emergency. If the surgeon is certain of the site of the leak, primary repair is often best. However, in the face of extensive metallic instrumentation, the risks of reopening the wound are increased, and here we prefer the use of a lumbar drain. Most leaks can be controlled and closed with lumbar diversion for four to seven days, but if the leak is brisk, this technique is not likely

to work. One must then weigh the risk of reoperation, particularly when instrumentation is in place, as compared with temporary lumboperitoneal or ventriculoperitoneal shunting. The placement of these shunting systems is a decision that should be made after thoroughly considering the alternatives. When there is no graft or instrumentation, re-exploration is clearly preferable if temporary external CSF diversion has not resulted in healing and sealing of the CSF leak. The surgeon must take into account the condition of the overlying tissues, the degree of the leak, and the patient's general medical status in making such a decision. Prolonged bed rest, especially in an older patient, is not without consequence, and this factor must also be considered. If prolonged bed rest is chosen as therapy, subcutaneous heparin should, in general, be administered to reduce the frequency of deep venous thrombosis and pulmonary emboli. In general, our preference is for reclosure, particularly if the leak is brisk.

SUMMARY

The basic principles and the treatment of CSF leaks have been described. Meticulous surgical technique will do much to reduce the frequency of this complication, but in some instances, because of the tremendous injuries that are now being operated on, leaks that appear impossible to close will be encountered. These will test the ingenuity and technical resources of the surgeon, but most should be possible to close primarily using a variety of suture techniques and fibrin glue.

References

1. Alving, B. M., Weinstein, M. J., Finlayson, J. S., et al.: Fibrin sealant: Summary of a conference on characteristics and clinical uses. Transfusion 35:783–790, 1995.
2. Cammisa, F. P., Eismont, F. J., and Green, B. A.: Dural laceration occurring with burst fractures and associated laminar fractures. J. Bone Joint Surg. Am. 71:1044–1051, 1989.
3. Cederholm-Williams, S. A.: Autologous fibrin sealants are not yet available. (Letter.) Lancet 344:336–337, 1994.
4. Cederholm-Williams, S. A.: Fibrin glue. (Letter.) BMJ 308:1570, 1994.
5. Eismont, F. J., Wiesel, S. W., and Rothman, R. H.: Treatment of dural tears associated with spinal surgery. J. Bone Joint Surg. Am. 63:1132–1136, 1991.
6. Gibble, J. W., and Ness P. M.: Fibrin glue: The perfect operative sealant? Transfusion 30:741–747, 1990.
7. Jane, J. A.: Neurosurgical applications of fibrin glue: Augmentation of dural closure in 134 patients. Neurosurgery 26:207–210, 1990.
8. Kadric, H., Driedger, A. A., and McInnes, W.: Persistent dural cerebral spinal fluid leaks shown by retrograde radionuclide myelography: A case report. J. Nucl. Med. 17:797–799, 1976.
9. Kitchel, S. H., Eismont, F. J., and Green B. A.: Closed subarachnoid drainage for management of cerebrospinal fluid leakage after an operation on the spine. J. Bone Joint Surg. Am. 71:984–987, 1989.
10. Mayfield, F. H., and Kurokawa, K.: Watertight closure of spinal dura mater: Technical note. J. Neurosurg. 43:639–640, 1975.
11. Miller, P. R., and Elder, F. W., Jr.: Meningocele pseudocysts (meningocele spurious) following laminectomy: Report of 10 cases. J. Bone Joint Surg. Am. 50:268–276, 1968.
12. Shaffrey, C. I., Spotnitz, W. D., Shaffrey, M. E., et al.: Neurosurgi-

cal applications of fibrin glue: Augmentation of dural closure in 134 patients. Neurosurgery *26*:207–210, 1990.

13. Terasaka, S., Sawamurra, Y., and Abe, H.: Sealing effect of fibrin glue spray on protection of cerebrospinal fluid leakage through the dura mater. No Shinkei Geka *22*:1015–1019, 1994.

14. Wiegand, D. A., Hartel, M. I., Quander, T., et al.: Assessment of cryoprecipitate-thrombin solution for dural repair. Head Neck *16*:569–573, 1994.

15. Wiesel, S. W.: Neurological complications in lumbar laminectomy: A standardized approach to the multiply operated lumbar spine. *In* Garfin, S. R. (ed.): Complications of Spine Surgery. Baltimore, Williams & Wilkins, 1989, pp. 65–74.

55

The Multiply Operated Low Back: An Algorithmic Approach

Sam W. Wiesel, M.D.

Scott D. Boden, M.D.

William C. Lauerman, M.D.

Unfortunately, low back surgery is not always successful. Patients who have undergone one or more back operations and continue to have significant discomfort are becoming an ever-increasing problem. It is estimated that 300,000 new laminectomies are performed each year in the United States alone and that 15 per cent of these patients will continue to be disabled.[44] The inherent complexity of these cases necessitates a method of problem solving that is precise, accurate, and cost efficient.

The best possible solution for recurrent symptoms after spine surgery is to prevent inappropriate surgery whenever possible.[18, 38] Proper surgical indications for the initial procedure should be strictly followed. Moreover, findings on diagnostic imaging studies must be precisely correlated with clinical signs and symptoms, owing to the high incidence of clinically false-positive myelograms, discograms, computed tomography (CT) scans, and magnetic resonance imaging (MRI) scans in asymptomatic individuals.[2, 20, 22, 49] The idea of "exploring" the low back when the necessary objective criteria are not met is no longer acceptable. In fact, even when there are objective findings but the patient is psychologically unstable or there are compensation-litigation factors, the outcome of low back surgery is uncertain.[40] Thus, the initial decision to operate is the most important one. Once recurrent pain arises after surgery, the potential for a solution is limited at best.

In the evaluation of recurrent symptoms following surgery, the problem confronting the physician is to distinguish the patient with a mechanical lesion from one with a nonmechanical condition. Mechanical lesions include recurrent herniated disc, spinal instability, and spinal stenosis. These three entities produce symptoms by causing direct pressure on the neural elements and may be amenable to surgical intervention. The nonmechanical entities consist of scar tissue (either arachnoiditis or epidural fibrosis), psychosocial instability, and systemic medical disease. These latter problems are not helped by any type of additional lumbar spine surgery.

The keystone for successful treatment is to obtain an accurate diagnosis. Despite the obviousness of this essential step, it often is not taken. Consequently, the rehabilitation of this patient group has been fraught with difficulty.

EVALUATION

When a multiply operated low back patient first arrives for evaluation, it is important to obtain all the vital information in an organized manner. Assessment of these patients must begin with the history, which can be quite involved. Many patients want to relate their entire story to the evaluating physician, and it is best to let them do so. However, there are three specific historic points that must be elucidated so that the proper decision-making process can be initiated.

The first is the number of previous lumbar spine operations the patient has undergone. It has been shown that with every subsequent operation, regardless of the diagnosis, the percentage of good results diminishes. Statistically, the second operation has a 50 per cent chance of success, and after two operations, patients are more likely to be made worse than better.[14, 45]

The second important historic point is the length of the pain-free interval after the previous operation. If the patient awoke from surgery with pain still present, it is likely that the nerve root was not properly decompressed, or that the wrong level was explored. If the pain-free interval was at least six months, the patient's recent pain may stem from a recurrent herniated disc at the same or a different level. If the pain-free interval was between one and six months and recurrent symptoms had a gradual onset, the diagnosis most often is some type of scar tissue, either arachnoiditis or epidural fibrosis.[14]

Finally, the patient's pain pattern must be carefully evaluated. If leg pain predominates, a herniated disc or spinal stenosis is most likely, although scar tissue is also a possibility. If back pain is the major component, instability, tumor, infection, and scar tissue are the major considerations. If there is both back and leg pain, spinal stenosis and/or scar tissue are the likely causes.

Physical examination is the next major step. The neurologic findings and existence of a tension sign, such as the sitting straight leg raising (SLR) test, must be noted. It is helpful to have the results of a dependable previous examination so that a comparison can be made between the preoperative and postoperative states. If the neurologic picture is unchanged from before the earlier surgery, and if the tension sign is negative, mechanical compression is unlikely. If, however, a new neurologic deficit has occurred since the last surgery or the tension sign is positive, pressure on the neural elements is possible. However, one must realize that epidural or perineural fibrosis can cause a positive tension sign; the tension sign is not pathognomonic for a mechanical lesion in these patients.

Roentgenographic studies are the last major component of the work-up. It is most helpful to have studies that were performed before the previous surgical procedure to compare the pre- and postoperative situations. Often, careful analysis may reveal that the initial operation was not warranted.

The plain radiographs must be evaluated for the extent and level of previous laminectomies and for any evidence of spinal stenosis. It should not be taken for granted that the correct level was decompressed; the laminectomy level on the plain radiograph must correspond to the level on the preoperative radiographic studies, to the level described in the operative report, and to the neurologic findings demonstrated by the patient. The standing (weight-bearing) lateral flexion-extension radiographs must be assessed for any evidence of abnormal motion (see "Lumbar Instability").

Metrizamide myelography is of limited value in the multiply operated back patient with chronic back pain.[18] This test can identify extradural compression but cannot distinguish between disc material and epidural scar.[8] The major use of myelography in these patients is for confirmation of arachnoiditis when the

diagnosis is otherwise uncertain. CT with metrizamide in the subarachnoid space is also a sensitive test for demonstrating the changes of arachnoiditis.[8]

CT is rarely used by itself for evaluating the multiply operated low back patient. It is generally employed, as stated earlier, following myelography. The size of the spinal canal, surgical deficits, and hypertrophied bony changes causing stenosis are well visualized.[41]

MRI is the most useful diagnostic tool to distinguish a recurrent residual disc herniation from epidural scar tissue.[21, 36] Intravenous contrast enhancement with gadolinium-diethylenetriaminepenta-acid/dimeglutamine (Gd-DTPA) will enhance (light up) scar tissue because it is vascular. A herniated disc is avascular and will not enhance after the injection of Gd-DTPA. However, it has been demonstrated that for the first six months after surgery, a gadolinium MRI may reveal pathologic changes, including persistent herniated disc material, despite the complete relief of symptoms.[1] There is an orderly progression of imaging changes during the first six months following lumbar surgery, which limits the interpretation of an MRI during this period. Thus, even in successfully decompressed patients, a residual mass effect on the neural elements may frequently simulate a recurrent or residual disc fragment. MRI scans during the initial six months after surgery, even when enhanced with gadolinium, must be interpreted with extreme caution.

Finally, the MRI is also a good screening tool for other types of processes that can cause low back pain and may be responsible for the continued symptoms after previous back surgery. These entities include metabolic abnormalities, infections, and tumors.

AN ALGORITHM FOR THE MULTIPLY OPERATED BACK

The primary goal of the evaluation of the multiply operated back patient is to arrive at a correct and specific diagnosis. The most common lesions accounting for failed back surgery syndrome include recurrent or persistent disc herniation (12 to 16 per cent), lateral (58 per cent) or central (7 to 14 per cent) stenosis, arachnoiditis (6 to 16 per cent), epidural fibrosis (6 to 8 per cent), and instability (less than 5 per cent).[7] To standardize and organize the physician's decision-making capabilities, a systematized approach to these patients has been developed in the form of an algorithm (Fig. 55–1). Its aim is to select the correct diagnostic category and proper treatment avenues for each patient.

The first step in the algorithm is to determine whether the patient's complaint has a nonorthopedic cause such as pancreatitis, diabetes, or an abdominal aneurysm. Thus, a thorough general medical examination should be routinely obtained. If this early examination reveals anything significant, it should be treated appropriately. In addition, if there is any indication of psychosocial instability, evidenced by alcoholism, drug dependence, depression, or compensation-litigation

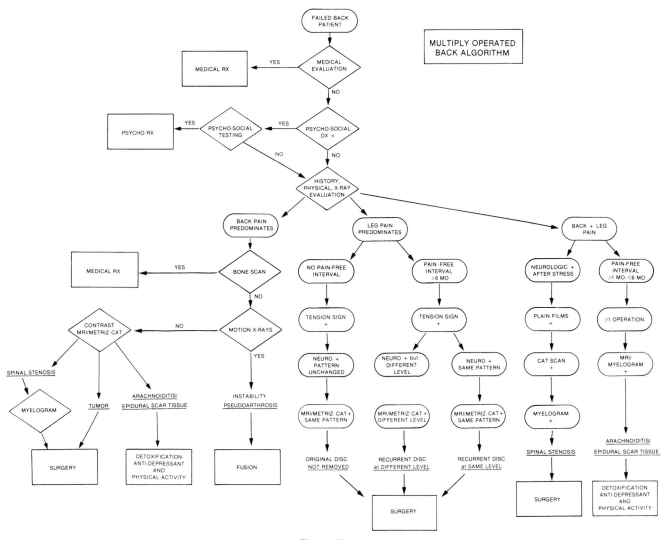

Figure 55–1.

involvement, a thorough psychiatric evaluation is necessary. It has been clearly demonstrated that patients with profound emotional disturbances and those involved with litigation do not derive any observable benefit from additional surgery.[46] Even if an orthopedic diagnosis is made, the psychosocial problem should be addressed first. In many cases, once a patient's underlying psychosocial problem has been treated successfully, the somatic back complaints and disability disappear.

Once the patients with medical and psychosocial problems have been identified, the physician is left with a group who have back and/or leg pain. The goal is then to separate patients with specific mechanical conditions from those whose symptoms are secondary to some form of scar tissue or inflammation. The former may benefit from additional surgery; the latter will not. It must be stressed that the incidence of surgically correctable problems is much lower than that of scar tissue.

HERNIATED INTERVERTEBRAL DISC

If the patient's pain is caused by a herniated disc, there are three possibilities. First, the disc that caused the original symptoms may not have been satisfactorily removed. This can happen if the wrong level was decompressed, if the laminectomy performed was not adequate to free the neural elements, or if a fragment of disc material was left behind. Such patients continue to have pain because of mechanical pressure on, and irritation of, the same nerve root that caused their initial symptoms. They complain predominantly of leg pain, and the neurologic findings, tension signs, and radiographic patterns remain unchanged from the preoperative state. The distinguishing feature is that they report no pain-free interval; they awake from the operation complaining of the same preoperative pain. Patients in this group can be aided by a technically correct laminectomy.

A second possibility is that there is a recurrent herniated intervertebral disc at the previously decompressed level. These patients complain of sciatica and have unchanged neurologic findings, tension signs, and radiographic studies. The distinguishing characteristic here is that their pain-free interval is greater than six months. Another operative procedure is indicated in these patients, provided that contrast-enhanced CT or MRI can demonstrate herniated disc material rather than just scar tissue.

Finally, a herniated disc may occur at a completely different level. Such patients generally have a pain-free interval longer than six months and suffer a sudden onset of recurrent pain. Sciatica predominates, and tension signs are positive. However, a neurologic deficit, if present, and the radiographic findings are noted at a different level from that in the original studies. A repeat operation for these patients is beneficial.

LUMBAR INSTABILITY

Lumbar instability is another condition that causes pain on a mechanical basis in the multiply operated back patient. Instability is an abnormal or excessive movement of one vertebra on another, causing pain. The cause may be the patient's intrinsic back disease or an excessively wide bilateral laminectomy.[22, 24] Pseudarthrosis resulting from a failed spinal fusion is included in this category, because the pain would be caused by the instability created at the failed fusion.

Patients with instability complain predominantly of back pain, and the physical examination may be negative. Sometimes the key to diagnosis of these patients is the weight-bearing lateral flexion-extension radiograph; however, it is often difficult to define precisely the anatomic origin of back pain in the presence of radiographic instability. Relative flexion–sagittal plane translation of more than 8 per cent of the anteroposterior diameter of the vertebral body, or a relative flexion–sagittal plane rotation of more than 9 degrees between adjacent segments, is the most commonly cited guideline for instability of the lumbar spine.[31, 45] At the lumbosacral junction, the criteria are slightly different: relative flexion translation of more than 6 per cent or rotation of more than 1 degree is significant. These criteria are based on maximal displacements on a single flexion or extension view; however, dynamic measurement of relative translation and rotation from flexion to extension may prove to be a more reliable indication of true instability.[3, 15]

Unfortunately, there is little information on why some patients with segmental instability develop back pain and others do not. If there is radiographic evidence of instability in symptomatic patients, spinal fusion (or repair of the pseudarthrosis) may be considered. Additional confirmatory evidence to determine the precise level of origin of the symptoms may be gathered from facet injections and discography; however, these tests have a substantial rate of false-positive results.[18]

SPINAL STENOSIS

Spinal stenosis in the multiply operated back patient can mechanically produce both back and leg pain. The etiology may be secondary to progression of the inherent degenerative spine disease, a previous inadequate decompression, or overgrowth of a previous posterior fusion. The physical examination is often inconclusive, although a neurologic deficit may occur after exercise; this phenomenon is termed a positive stress test with reproduction of the patient's symptoms.

The plain radiographs can be suggestive and may reveal facet degeneration, decreased interpedicular distance, decreased sagittal canal diameter, and disc degeneration. CT demonstrates bony encroachment on the neural elements; this is especially helpful in evaluating the lateral recesses and neural foramina. A metrizamide myelogram or MRI shows compression of the dural sac at the involved levels. It should be appreciated that spinal stenosis and scar tissue can coexist.[13] Good results can be expected from surgery in at least 70 per cent of properly selected patients; those with previous laminectomy and spinal fusion have less successful outcomes.[31] If there is definite evidence of bony compression, a laminectomy is indicated, but if substantial scar tissue is present, the degree of pain relief that the patient can anticipate is uncertain.

ARACHNOIDITIS, EPIDURAL SCAR TISSUE, AND DISCITIS

Scar tissue (arachnoiditis or epidural fibrosis) and discitis are nonmechanical causes of recurrent pain in the multiply operated back patient. Although the etiologies and specific locations of these lesions are different, they are discussed in the same section, because none of them improve significantly with additional surgical procedures.

Postoperative scar tissue formation can be divided into two main types on the basis of anatomic location. Scar tissue that occurs beneath the dura is commonly referred to as arachnoiditis. Scar tissue can also form extradurally, either directly on the cauda equina or around a nerve root.

Arachnoiditis is strictly defined as an inflammation of the pia-arachnoid membrane surrounding the spinal cord or cauda equina.[6] The condition may be present in varying degrees of severity, from mild thickening of the membranes to solid adhesions. In severe cases, the scarring may obliterate the subarachnoid space and block the flow of contrast agents.

This condition has been attributed to many causes; lumbar spine surgery and previous injections of contrast material seem to be the most frequent precipitating events.[34] Postoperative infection may also play a role in the pathogenesis. The exact mechanism by which arachnoiditis develops from these events is not clear.[9, 13]

There is no uniform clinical presentation for arachnoiditis. Statistically, the history reveals more than one previous operation and a pain-free interval of between one and six months. These patients often complain of back and leg pain. The physical examination is not conclusive; alterations in neurologic status may be on the basis of a previous operation. As mentioned earlier, myelography, CT, and MRI can be helpful in confirming the diagnosis.

At present, there is no effective treatment for arachnoiditis. Surgical intervention has not proved effective in eliminating the scar tissue or significantly reducing the pain. Along with much-needed encouragement, various nonoperative measures can be employed.[6, 9, 12, 17, 30, 32, 35, 38, 43] Epidural steroids, transcutaneous nerve stimulation, spinal cord stimulation, operant conditioning, bracing, and patient education have all been tried. None of these leads to a cure, but when used judiciously, they provide symptomatic relief for varying periods. Patients should be detoxified from all narcotics, placed on amitriptyline (Elavil), and encouraged to partake in as much physical activity as possible. Treating these patients is a real challenge, and the physician must be willing to devote time and patience to achieve optimal results.

Formation of scar tissue outside the dura on the cauda equina or directly on nerve roots is a relatively common occurrence.[28] This epidural scar tissue acts as a constrictive force about the neural elements and may cause postoperative pain. However, although most patients have some epidural scar tissue, only an unpredictable few become symptomatic.

Patients with epidural scarring may present with symptoms at any time, from several months to a year after surgery. They may complain of back pain, leg pain, or both. Commonly there are no new neurologic findings, but there may be a positive tension sign purely on the basis of scar formation around a nerve root. The condition is best differentiated from a recurrent herniated disc by means of a gadolinium-enhanced MRI.

Like arachnoiditis, there is no definitive treatment for epidural scar tissue. Prevention may be the best answer. Until recently, a free fat graft was commonly used as an interposition membrane to minimize epidural scar tissue after laminectomy.[26] However, routine use of free fat grafts is being reconsidered because of a possible increased risk of postoperative cauda equina syndrome. Once scar has formed, surgery is not successful, because scarring often re-forms in a greater quantity. The treatment program should be similar to that already described for arachnoiditis.

Discitis is an uncommon but debilitating complication of lumbar disc surgery. Its pathogenesis is postulated to be direct inoculation of the avascular disc space, but it is not completely understood.[10] The onset of symptoms is usually several weeks after surgery, and most patients complain of severe back pain. Physical examination sometimes reveals fever and a positive tension sign and occasionally a superficial abscess.

If discitis is suspected from the history and physical examination, the erythrocyte sedimentation rate (ESR), blood cultures, and plain radiographs should be obtained. Plain radiographs may demonstrate disc space narrowing and end plate erosion in the early stages. Contrast-enhanced CT or MRI should confirm the diagnosis.

Effective treatment of discitis has been a matter of controversy.[10] We recommend placing the patient on bed rest acutely, with immobilization of the lumbar spine in a brace or corset. If the patient experiences progressive pain after adequate immobilization or has constitutional symptoms, a needle aspiration should be performed. If a bacterial organism is identified, a six-week regimen of intravenous antibiotics is indicated. There is no need for open disc space biopsy, provided the patient responds to conservative therapy. With improvement of symptoms, the patient may ambulate as tolerated.

INSTRUMENTATION

Increasing numbers of patients with persistent pain have had instrumentation as part of their previous lumbar spine surgery. Although this complicates the approach to these patients in several ways, it is still essential to use a structured approach to their evaluation, with the goal of arriving at a specific diagnosis. Although there are several circumstances under which implant removal or revision or nonunion repair may be indicated, routine removal of pedicle screw instrumentation has not been reported to have a high rate of success in relieving back pain.[11]

Traditionally, the late finding of a broken Harrington rod was thought to indicate the presence of one or more pseudarthroses in the underlying fusion mass. Although pedicle screw instrumentation systems have several potential modes of failure, it should be noted that mechanical failure, particularly late screw breakage, does not routinely represent an indication for removal or revision. Screw breakage, typically at the shank–thread junction, was once quite common. Manufacturing changes have lessened the incidence of this occurrence, and it has also been demonstrated that a broken screw does not preclude the possibility of a solid arthrodesis.[47] Therefore, unless there are other objective indications for surgery, the presence of one or more broken screws does not routinely require reoperation. The most common mechanism of failure in most pedicle screw instrumentation systems is screw loosening at the bone–screw interface. This appears to be a relatively common finding on late radiographic follow-up, but no clear correlation between screw loosening and back pain has been reported. As noted earlier, pseudarthrosis may result in instability and persistent or recurrent back pain after a fusion. Dynamic flexion-extension radiographs demonstrating motion across the fused or instrumented segments are the most reliable means of confirming failure of fusion. Finally, the risk of late infection, occurring months or even years after otherwise successful surgery, should be considered in patients with these bulky implants. CT scanning, looking for a fluid collection around the implant, and aspiration of the wound should be considered when infection is a possibility.

Surgical Indications

Patients who have had pedicle screw instrumentation implanted are most appropriately evaluated using the algorithm for the multiply operated back. Before repeat surgery can be recommended, objective evidence of nerve root compression or instability should be documented. In addition to disc herniation or lateral spinal stenosis, nerve root compression can be caused by an aberrantly placed screw. In this situation, the patient commonly describes pain and paresthesias, occasionally with weakness, early in the postoperative period. In most cases, the symptoms are present prior to hospital discharge, but on occasion, the radicular symptoms do not manifest for weeks or even months after surgery. New radicular signs and symptoms following implantation of pedicle screws merit prompt radiographic evaluation to rule out the possibility of impingement by the implant. Thin-cut CT scanning of the lumbar spine, using bony windows, is capable of identifying most screws placed outside the pedicle. Nerve root compression can occur medial and lateral to the pedicle, as well as anterior to the sacral ala with impingement on the L5 root. It has been demonstrated that as many as 25 per cent of pedicle screws are imperfectly positioned, and a large majority of these do not cause symptoms. Therefore, close correlation between the patient's complaints and the CT findings is essential before deciding on repeat surgery. Once the diagnosis of symptomatic screw malposition has been made, screw removal is indicated.

Postoperative instability is a potential source of back pain in these patients and is evaluated as described earlier. A rigidly fixed pedicle screw implant provides temporary stability, but in the absence of bony fusion, loosening is likely to occur. Recurrent back pain after a pain-free interval is the most common history in a patient with a symptomatic pseudarthrosis following pedicle screw instrumentation and fusion. Plain radiographs may demonstrate loosening around the screws but are not accurate in assessing the integrity of the fusion mass.[29] Dynamic lateral radiography is the most reliable way to document painful instability in the presence of a pseudarthrosis, whether or not instrumentation has been used. Although no data exist at the present time that define the amount of motion that is clinically significant following lumbar spinal fusion or that clearly define which patients are likely to benefit from revision surgery, we believe that pseudarthrosis repair, in the absence of objective evidence of motion, has a low likelihood of relieving the patient's symptoms.

Implant removal, in the absence of objective evidence of nerve root compression or instability, is occasionally recommended. Because the bulk of the paraspinous musculature is adequate to provide soft tissue coverage in most patients, soft tissue problems like those seen with subcutaneous implants on long bones rarely occur. Routine exploration, therefore, has a limited role in addressing objective pathology. The results of routine implant removal confirm this limitation; in a recent review of patients undergoing removal of pedicle screw instrumentation, Davne and Myers reported that 32 per cent of patients improved significantly following implant removal when a solid fusion was discovered, and 35 per cent improved when a pseudarthrosis was demonstrated and revision of the fusion and instrumentation performed.[11]

SUMMARY

In conclusion, it should be stressed that the physician must take an organized approach to the evaluation of the multiply operated low back patient. In many cases, the origin of the problem is a faulty decision to perform the original surgical procedure. Further surgery on an exploratory basis is not warranted and will lead only to further disability. Another operative procedure is indicated only when there are objective physical findings confirmed by a diagnostic imaging study.

The etiology of each patient's complaint must be accurately localized and identified. In addition to orthopedic evaluation, the patient's psychosocial and general medical status must be thoroughly investigated. Once the spine is identified as the source of the symptoms, specific features should be sought in the clinical history, physical examination, and radiographic studies. The number of previous operations, the characteristics of the pain-free interval, and the predominance of leg pain or back pain are the major historic points. The most important aspects of the physical examination are the neurologic findings and the presence of a tension sign. Plain radiographs, motion films, CT, and MRI all have specific roles in the work-up. When all the information is integrated, the physician usually can distinguish patients with arachnoiditis, epidural scar, and discitis from those with mechanical conditions of the spine.

References

1. Boden, S. D., Davis, D. O., Dina, T. S., et al.: Contrast-enhanced MR imaging performed after successful lumbar disc surgery: Prospective study. Radiology 182:59–64, 1992.
2. Boden, S. D., Davis, D. O., Dina, T. S., et al.: Abnormal magnetic resonance scans of the lumbar spine in asymptomatic subjects: A prospective investigation. J. Bone Joint Surg. [Am.] 72:1178–1184, 1990.
3. Boden, S. D., and Wiesel, S. W.: Lumbosacral segmental motion in normal individuals: Have we been measuring instability properly? Spine 15:571–576, 1990.
4. Braun, I. F., Hoffman, J. C., Davis, P. C., et al.: Contrast enhancement in CT differentiation between recurrent disk herniation and post-operative scar: A prospective study. AJNR Am. J. Neuroradiol. 6:607–612, 1985.
5. Bundschuh, C. V., Modic, M. T., Ross, J. S., et al.: Epidural fibrosis and recurrent disk herniation in the lumbar spine: MR imaging assessment. AJR Am. J. Roentgenol. 150:923–932, 1988.
6. Burton, C. V.: Lumbosacral arachnoiditis. Spine 3:24–30, 1978.
7. Burton, C. V., Kirkaldy-Willis, W. H., Yong-Hing, K., and Heithoff, K. B.: Causes of failure of surgery on the lumbar spine. Clin. Orthop. 157:191–199, 1981.
8. Byrd, S. E., Cohn, M. L., Biggers, S. L., et al.: The radiographic evaluation of the symptomatic post-operative lumbar spine patient. Spine 10:652–661, 1985.
9. Coventry, M. B., and Stauffer, R. N.: The multiply operated back.

In American Academy of Orthopaedic Surgeons: Symposium on the Spine. St. Louis, C. V. Mosby Co., 1969, pp. 132–142.

10. Dall, B. E., Rowe, D. E., Odette, W. G., and Batts, D. H.: Postoperative discitis: Diagnosis and management. Clin. Orthop. *224*:138–148, 1987.

11. Davne, S. H., and Myers, D. L.: Results following removal or revision pedicle screw instrumentations. Orthop. Trans. *18*:257, 1994.

12. de la Porte, C., and Siegfried, J.: Lumbosacral spinal fibrosis (spinal arachnoiditis): Its diagnosis and management. Spine *8*:593–603, 1983.

13. Epstein, B. S.: The Spine. Philadelphia, Lea & Febiger, 1962.

14. Finnegan, W. J., Tenlin, J. M., Marvel, J. P., et al.: Results of surgical intervention in the symptomatic multiply-operated back patient. J. Bone Joint Surg. [Am.] *61*:1077–1082, 1979.

15. Friberg, O.: Lumbar instability: A dynamic approach by traction-compression radiography. Spine *12*:119–129, 1987.

16. Gabriel, K. R., and Crawford, A. H.: Magnetic resonance imaging in a child who had clinical signs of discitis. J. Bone Joint Surg. [Am.] *70*:938–941, 1988.

17. Ghormley, R. K.: The problem of multiple operations on the back. Instr. Course Lect. *14*:56, 1957.

18. Grubb, S. A., Lipscomb, H. J., and Gilford, W. B.: The relative value of lumbar roentgenograms, metrizamide myelography, and discography in the assessment of patients with chronic low-back syndrome. Spine *12*:282–286, 1987.

19. Hirsch, C.: Efficiency of surgery in low back disorders. J. Bone Joint Surg. [Am.] *47*:991–1004, 1965.

20. Hitselberger, W. E., and Witten, R. M.: Abnormal myelograms in asymptomatic patients. J. Neurosurg. *28*:204–206, 1968.

21. Hochhauser, L., Kieffer, S. A., Cacayorin, E. D., et al.: Recurrent postdiskectomy low back pain: MR-surgical correlation. AJNR Am. J. Neuroradiol. *9*:769–774, 1988.

22. Holt, E. P.: The question of lumbar discography. J. Bone Joint Surg. [Am.] *50*:720–726, 1968.

23. Hopp, E., and Tsou, P. M.: Postdecompression lumbar instability. Clin. Orthop. *227*:143–151, 1988.

24. Hueftle, M. G., Modic, M. T., Ross, J. S., et al.: Lumbar spine: Postoperative MR imaging with Gd-DTPA. Radiology *167*:817–824, 1988.

25. Johnsson, K. E., Willner, S., and Johnsson, K.: Postoperative instability after decompression for lumbar spinal stenosis. Spine *11*:107–110, 1986.

26. Lahde, S., and Puranen, J.: Disk space hypodensity in CT: The first radiological signs of postoperative diskitis. Eur. J. Radiol. *5*:190–192, 1985.

27. Langenskydd, A., and Kiviluoto, O.: Prevention of epidural scar formation after operations on the lumbar spine by means of free fat transplants. Clin. Orthop. *115*:92–95, 1976.

28. LaRocca, H., and MacNab, I.: The laminectomy membrane. J. Bone Joint Surg. [Br.] *56*:545–550, 1974.

29. Larsen, J. W., Rimoldi, R. L., Nelson, R. W., et al.: Identification of pseudoarthrosis in the presence of pedicle screw instrumentation. Presented at the sixty-first annual meeting of the American Academy of Orthopaedic Surgeons, New Orleans, LA, 1994.

30. Mooney, V.: Innovative approaches to chronic back disability. American Academy of Orthopaedic Surgeons Instructional Course Lecture, Dallas, TX, 1974.

31. Nasca, R. J.: Surgical management of lumbar spinal stenosis. Spine *12*:809–816, 1987.

32. Oudenhover, R. C.: The role of laminectomy, facet rhizotomy and epidural steroids. Spine *4*:145–147, 1979.

33. Posner, I., White, A. A., Edwards, E. T., and Hayes, W. C.: A biomechanical analysis of the clinical stability of the lumbar and lumbosacral spine. Spine *7*:374–389, 1982.

34. Quiles, M., Marchisello, P. J., and Tsairis, P.: Lumbar adhesive arachnoiditis: Etiologic and pathologic aspects. Spine *3*:45–50, 1978.

35. Rose, D. L.: The decompensated back. Arch. Phys. Med. Rehabil. *56*:51–58, 1975.

36. Ross, J. S., Masaryk, T. J., Modic, M. T., et al.: Lumbar spine: Postoperative assessment with surface-coil MR imaging. Radiology *164*:851–860, 1987.

37. Ross, J. S., Masaryk, T. J., Modic, M. T., et al.: MR imaging of lumbar arachnoiditis. AJNR Am. J. Neuroradiol. *8*:885–892, 1987.

38. Rothman, R. H.: Indications for lumbar fusion. Clin. Neurosurg. *71*:215–219, 1973.

39. Schubiger, O., and Valavanis, A.: CT differentiation between recurrent disc herniation and postoperative scar formation: The value of contrast enhancement. Neuroradiology *22*:251–254, 1982.

40. Spengler, D. M., and Freeman, D. W.: Patient selection for lumbar discectomy: An objective approach. Spine *4*:129–134, 1979.

41. Teplick, J. G., and Haskin, M. E.: CT of the postoperative lumbar spine. Radiol. Clin. North Am. *21*:395–420, 1983.

42. Teplick, J. G., and Haskin, M. E.: Intravenous contrast-enhanced CT of the postoperative lumbar spine, improved identification of recurrent disc herniation, scar, arachnoiditis, and diskitis. AJR Am. J. Roentgenol. *143*:845–855, 1984.

43. Tibodeau, A. A.: Management of the problem postoperative back. J. Bone Joint Surg. [Am.] *55*:1766, 1973.

44. Waddell, G.: Failures of disc surgery and repeat surgery. Acta Orthop. Belg. *53*:300–302, 1987.

45. Waddell, G., Kummel, E. G., Lotto, W. N., et al.: Failed lumbar disc surgery and repeat surgery following industrial injuries. J. Bone Joint Surg. [Am.] *61*:201–207, 1979.

46. Waring, E. M., Weisz, G. M., and Bailey, S. I.: Predictive factors in the treatment of low back pain by surgical intervention. Adv. Pain Res. Ther. *1*:939–942, 1979.

47. West, J. L., Bradford, D. S., and Ogilvie, J. W.: Results of spinal arthrodesis with pedicle-plate fixation. J. Bone Joint Surg. [Am.] *73*:1179–1195, 1991.

48. White, A. A., Panjabi, M. M., Posner, I., et al.: Spinal stability: Evaluation and treatment. Instr. Course Lect. *30*:457, 1981.

49. Wiesel, S. W., Bell, G. R., Feffer, H. L., et al.: A study of computer assisted tomography. Part I. The incidence of positive CAT scans in an asymptomatic group of patients. Spine *9*:549–551, 1984.

56

Redo Disc Surgery— Techniques and Results

Timothy A. Garvey, M.D.

Ensor E. Transfeldt, M.D.

"I shall return."

(Douglas MacArthur, March 11, 1942, leaving the Philippines)

The title of this chapter was a difficult one to select, as a "revision lumbar disc procedure" can encompass many different surgical procedures that have varied anatomic goals. We focus primarily on the patient who presents with persistent or recurrent dominant sciatica, for whom a revision lumbar nerve root decompression is being considered as a treatment option. A small percentage of patients truly have a recurrent ipsilateral herniated nucleus pulposus with resultant disabling leg pain, and they are candidates for a true "redo discectomy."[2–5, 10, 12, 19, 23, 25, 27, 45, 60, 64, 95, 100] However, it appears clear, from an abundant literature, that there are multiple pathoanatomic causes for the large number of patients seeking evaluation for potential revision lumbar surgery.[5, 10, 11, 13, 16, 19, 22, 23, 25, 27, 28, 32, 39, 45, 54, 60, 63, 64, 66, 82, 97, 100, 106, 111] It is imperative to recognize the importance of psychosocial factors in predicting the outcome of lumbar spine surgeries, be they initial or revision procedures.[6, 17, 22, 35, 45–49, 51, 68, 78, 79, 81, 89, 93–95, 106, 119]

Wiesel, Boden, and Lauerman presented their approach to the multiply operated low back pain patient in the preceding chapter. It is critical that we also address operative indications in relation to our approach, which allows rational surgical decision making to occur. The treating physician must use a consistent decision-making process. To us, this includes having a

base of knowledge of the pathophysiologic abnormalities of the lumbar spine, understanding the incidence of such findings in asymptomatic populations, and knowing the natural history of symptomatic patients with or without surgical intervention. The rational surgical decision-making process starts with the treating physician obtaining a pertinent medical history, performing an insightful physical examination, and interpreting imaging studies in the clinical context of the specific patient being evaluated. The past medical records are then studied. We prefer to review the records after taking the history and performing the physical examination, so as not to bias the evaluation. A psychosocial evaluation should be included to complete the assessment, and this important step is often overlooked by the initial surgeon. With a total assessment accomplished, the physician then counsels the patient regarding the known risk-benefit ratios for the operative and nonoperative options available for the specific diagnosis generated, as supported by peer-reviewed literature and a critical analysis of the clinical outcomes of the surgeon's own patients. The surgeon must then skillfully perform the technical aspects of the revision procedure. Finally, a postoperative physical and vocational rehabilitative program tailored to the needs of the patient is developed and implemented.

This chapter highlights and gives specific literature support for our approach to rational surgical decision making in revision lumbar spine surgery. We present a review of published clinical series reporting on redo disc surgery, as well as revision decompressions. We specifically detail our preferred techniques. Although much in current spine surgery is not practiced universally, a systematic, knowledgeable, literature-supported surgical decision-making process must be the standard. Although prospective randomized double-blinded studies are desirable (but often not practical in lumbar spine surgery), most of the present literature is of the retrospective or prospective nonrandomized type. However, we do gain useful information from this literature.

NATURAL HISTORY AND PATHOGENESIS

The magnitude of the social problem of low back pain is fairly well appreciated by most of those involved in the surgical care of such patients.[33, 35, 102, 106] Often-quoted figures indicate a lifetime prevalence of low back pain of 80 per cent, with a yearly incidence of 5 per cent.[24, 33, 35, 40, 41, 91] The estimate for surgical intervention in the form of laminectomies and discectomies is in the range of 200,000 to 300,000 such procedures a year in the United States.[33, 35, 63, 95] "Notwithstanding our earnest desire to ameliorate human suffering, the staggering economic consequences of lost productivity and direct medical costs makes assessment of each therapeutic intervention mandatory."[35] In properly selected patients, there is strong literature support for an approximate 85 to 95 per cent successful clinical outcome in individuals undergoing lumbar laminotomy and discectomy.[2, 24, 26, 34, 36, 41, 46, 51, 52, 91–95, 109, 117, 118] However, there also appears to be a significant population of patients—3 to 20 per cent of the surgical group—who present for repeat evaluation for a recurrent disc herniation and/or disabling postdiscectomy low back pain.[2, 5, 10–13, 16, 22, 23, 25, 27, 28, 32, 39, 41, 45, 54, 60, 63, 64, 66, 94,96, 97, 106, 111] If the initial operative indications are not well objectified, as has been suggested in published series analyzing failures of lumbar surgery, then the number of patients seeking re-evaluation will obviously continue to rise.[11, 13, 16, 27, 28, 63, 92, 97]

A critical factor is the natural history of the symptomatic individual. Most individuals with acute mechanical low back pain have resolution of their symptoms within the first three months—the vast majority within the first few weeks.[24, 32, 35, 40, 51, 52, 86, 91–93, 109] This occurs despite therapeutic interventions. Therefore, in assessing the success of a surgical procedure, one must analyze the clinical outcome in the context of the natural history of the untreated patient and the timing of that surgical intervention as it relates to resolution of the clinical symptoms.

In considering the natural history of the symptomatic patient with acute radiculopathy, Hakelius documented the long-term prognosis of sciatica in a retrospective review of 583 patients.[40] Of those patients who had severe unilateral sciatica, 93 per cent had a two-month period of rest and restriction of lumbar motion with a corset as their conservative management. The relief of symptoms with surgical intervention was statistically superior for the initial three months, as com-

pared with nonoperative management. At six months, the findings were not statistically different. Of interest, 526 patients were followed for an average of 7.3 years. At long-term follow-up, the nonoperative group complained of more low back pain (71 versus 48 per cent), greater residual sciatica (61 versus 44 per cent), more recurrence of sciatica pain flare-ups (20 versus 10 per cent), and greater lost work time. Nonetheless, Hakelius reported that only 19 per cent appeared to "need" surgical intervention by six months.[40]

Weber presented a controlled prospective study with 10 years of observation in those with lumbar disc herniations.[109] We encourage the reader to review the original work. The study randomized 126 patients with "uncertain indications" between operative and nonoperative care. Another group of 67 patients was felt to have a definite need for surgical decompression, and a third group of 87 patients was felt to have no indication for operative intervention. In the randomized group, four fifths of the nonoperative group who did well with nonoperative care had been identified by the three-month mark. It is of importance to note that of the 66 patients randomized to nonoperative care, 17 (26 per cent) did "require" surgery by 7.5 months. These patients were not reported as poor outcomes of nonoperative management; rather, they were carried out to long-term follow-up as a separate reporting group. Thus, although many state that the ultimate clinical outcome for operative and nonoperative care equilibrates at 10-year follow-up, if this group of 17 patients had been classified as unsatisfactory results of nonoperative management, then in addition to surgery having been statistically significantly superior at one-year follow-up for those with uncertain indications, it would have been statistically significantly superior at the four- and 10-year follow-up marks as well. Nonetheless, the stated conclusions of Weber's study are important: that operative management of lumbar disc herniations is statistically superior at one year, with less pronounced differences over the additional nine years of observation; that the natural history of radiculopathy due to disc pathology is more encouraging than anticipated; that patient education is important; that "back insufficiency" was the major complaint at final follow-up; and that there was little change between the 10- and four-year follow-up.

Saal and Saal emphasized that an aggressive rehabilitative approach can successfully treat those with lumbar radiculopathy secondary to a herniated lumbar intervertebral disc.[86] Important in understanding the applicability of this study is that the inclusion criteria required "a [computed tomography] CT scan demonstrating a herniated nucleus pulposus *without significant stenosis*." They felt that failure to respond to nonoperative management should suggest the presence of stenosis. This corroborates the report by Kornberg and Rechtine that those coming to surgical intervention for an L4–L5 disc herniation had congenitally smaller canals (i.e., stenosis) than an age- and sex-matched non–lumbar surgical group of patients.[61] Therefore, when considering the natural history of the patient with acute sciatica, the presence of bony lateral recess or foraminal stenosis may be a negative indicator, but typically this is appreciated only after the initial six to eight weeks of nonoperative management has failed to yield a good clinical outcome.

The natural history of the symptomatic patient with acute radiculopathy secondary to a lumbar herniated nucleus pulposus thus appears to be that a majority improve without surgical decompression. Those that do improve generally do so within the first two to three months. This leads to the suggested six to 12 weeks of nonoperative management that we and most authors utilize.[24, 25, 34, 35, 51, 52, 84, 91, 93, 95, 109] However, Hurme and Alaranta reported that better results could be achieved if surgery was done before two months' duration of disabling sciatica.[52] It appears that in addition to those with acute cauda equina syndrome or significant progressive radicular neurologic deficit, surgical decompression for patients with self-perceived disabling sciatica should be considered a conservative decision-making option.[24, 26, 34, 35, 40, 41, 51, 91, 94, 109, 120]

We know of no series that reports on the outcome of nonoperatively treated patients with the diagnosis of recurrent sciatica secondary to a recurrent herniated nucleus pulposus. The published series regarding recurrent lumbar disc herniations outline the clinical outcomes of surgical intervention. If a patient presents with a history and physical examination consistent with a recurrent herniation at another level in the lumbar spine or on the opposite side, we consider these patients to have a natural history similar to that of a patient with acute sciatica, as outlined earlier. For example, an individual who five years previously had a left S1 radiculopathy that resolved with an L5–S1 hemilaminotomy and discectomy now presents with the acute onset of low back pain and right leg pain radiating to the lateral calf. The patient is noted on examination to have a mildly weak extensor hallucis longus, with the presence of a positive straight leg raising sign and no evidence of a cauda equina syndrome. We would recommend that this individual be considered for treatment based on an algorithmic approach for the treatment of a suspected L5 radiculopathy, which is nonoperative management for a six- to eight-week period before considering surgical intervention. We would use our standard operative indications for a primary decompression. However, it is our experience, as well as that of others, that the patient with an ipsilateral same-level recurrent disc herniation does not have as favorable a natural history.[96] In fact, it appears that these individuals present with leg pain of greater intensity, and more often than not they require surgical intervention.

Pathophysiologically, the less favorable natural history for recurrent lumbar disc herniation likely has to do with the fact that the dura and affected nerve root are "tacked down," that is, scarred to the dorsolateral aspect of the annular end plate junction, and thus are less mobile. Therefore, for a given volume of herniated nucleus pulposus, such a patient may present with a greater intensity of leg pain and a more severe magni-

tude of neurologic deficits, as the nerve root has less mobility. In this group, we do not believe that the six- to eight-week period of nonoperative management is mandatory. Although we would typically start with nonoperative options, we would counsel the patient about this less favorable natural history. If the indication is disabling leg pain that interferes with the activities of daily living, we are not averse to considering surgical decompression before the six- to eight-week interval recommended in primary cases for those with suspected ipsilateral same-level recurrent herniated nucleus pulposus. Of course, a frank cauda equina syndrome or significant progressive neurologic deficit would make surgical treatment a more urgent consideration. This does not mean that an individual with recurrent ipsilateral same-level herniation cannot improve with a nonoperative program, only that it is less likely than in those with an initial presentation for herniated nucleus pulposus.

HISTORY AND PHYSICAL EXAMINATION

The initial evaluation of a patient who is a candidate for revision lumbar surgery includes several critical decisions.[38] These are whether (1) the pain is local, referred, or radicular; (2) the pain is mechanical or nonmechanical; (3) there is the presence or absence of significant neurologic dysfunction; and (4) there are significant psychosocial factors influencing the need for revision surgery. The history, as always, is most important and is supplemented by the physical examination. A review of available imaging studies with interpretation in the specific context of the clinical situation completes the initial evaluation.

We find a key question to be the percentage of pain that is back pain versus the percentage of pain that is buttocks and leg pain. Local pain is just that—pain in the lumbosacral area. Referred pain—pain felt away from the tissue of origin—is typically paralumbar and proximal buttocks. Radicular pain, true nerve pain, typically follows the dermatomal distribution and radiates into the calf and foot. If the patient's complaint is of dominant leg pain (i.e., greater than 50 per cent leg pain), the differential diagnosis of radiculopathy is focused on, and therapeutic options are directed toward this differential diagnosis. If the patient complains of 10 per cent leg pain and 90 per cent low back pain, it is relatively unimportant to know if there is a recurrent herniated nucleus pulposus, as treatment is pointed at mechanical low back pain and not nerve root compression. The physician must be alert to symptoms that suggest a nonmechanical source of pain, such as rest pain, night pain, lack of activity-related changes, and pain of atypical quality (e.g., colicky), and to constitutional symptoms. If nonmechanical pain is identified, a diagnostic work-up to exclude sources such as tumor, infection, renal colic, gastric ulcer, gynecologic abnormalities, and abdominal aortic aneurysm must be undertaken. Upon conclusion of documenting the history and reviewing a pain drawing and other self-rated disability scales, a critical decision is made, which should generally focus on whether the pain is recurrent or persistent radiculopathy with dominant buttocks and leg pain or dominant mechanical low back pain. Simplistically, if it is leg pain, think nerve root; if it is low back pain, think disc and joint pathology. Of course, many patients complain of 50 per cent low back pain and 50 per cent leg pain, and both issues must be considered.

The physical examination focuses on the neurologic examination of the lower extremities, the presence or absence of nerve root tension signs, and an evaluation for incongruency signs. Motor strength testing, sensory testing, and elicitation of deep tendon reflexes all look toward documenting an objective sign of radiculopathy. For example, acute recurrent posterior thigh and calf pain, diminution of the Achilles reflex, and decreased sensation on the plantar aspect of the foot suggest an S1 radicular problem.

The straight leg raising test and its variants are used to document nerve root tension by reproducing the presenting pain along the course of the affected nerve with a provocative physical examination maneuver.[24, 34, 35, 46, 51, 95] We recommend fully documenting the patient's response (e.g., leg pain reproduced at 45 degrees, or back pain occurring at 30 degrees), as opposed to recording a simple positive or negative response. Reproduction of back pain does not constitute a positive nerve root tension sign. A contralateral straight leg raising sign (pain reproduced in the affected leg by elevation of the unaffected leg) is thought to increase the likelihood of a disc herniation, often an extrusion, as the source of sciatica.[35, 96]

The nonorganic physical signs, as described by Waddell and colleagues, should be documented.[107] These incongruency signs are standardized physical maneuvers to detect *tenderness*, that is, nonanatomic or superficial; to *simulate* that a test is being done with axial loading or rotation; to *distract* and confirm physical findings, as with the supine versus the sitting straight leg raising test; to identify *regional* weakness or sensory changes; and to assess for *overreaction*. When three or more signs are present, formal psychologic evaluation is recommended. The presence of multiple nonorganic signs has a correlation with poor surgical outcome and should heighten the surgeon's awareness regarding treatment options.[107]

The psychosocial evaluation should be extended with the use of the Minnesota Multiphasic Personality Inventory (MMPI) or other similar index, especially in consideration of revision surgery.[22, 45-48, 52, 79, 93, 95] A formal psychologic evaluation is certainly indicated if the surgeon suspects that the psychosocial issues are negatively impacting the patient's perceived symptoms. It is probably a good idea to institute this formal psychosocial assessment on a routine basis in the management of revision surgical candidates, as some authors have suggested.[45-47, 79, 92, 93, 95, 119] We routinely use a pain drawing, a self-rated disability scale, a depression index, documentation of compensation or litigation status, and the documentation of nonorganic physical

signs as the psychosocial evaluation. One of us (T.A.G.) routinely uses the MMPI on all lumbar spine cases, and the other (E.E.T.) does so based on the initial screening. We make independent judgments as to the necessity for formal psychologic assessment based on these.

PSYCHOSOCIAL EVALUATION

The patient's psychosocial status is a critical decision-making element, and the psychosocial evaluation is important in making a total assessment of a patient being considered for a revision lumbar procedure. This sphere has often been overlooked in the past and likely contributed to failures of surgical management.

Spengler and coworkers[93, 95] and Herron and Turner[46] reported on objective rating systems in the selection of patients for elective discectomy. Twenty-five points on a 100-point objective rating system were attributed to "personality factors" or to the "psychosocial environment," of which the MMPI was the key objectifying test. Herron and associates noted that patients who were working preoperatively did significantly better than those not working and that the MMPI hypochondriasis (Hs) and hysteria (Hy) scales significantly related to the outcome.[46, 48] Spengler and coworkers noted that "the psychologic score was the best predictor of the outcome of treatment" and that "of seven patients who had herniation of a disc and a distinctly abnormal score on the MMPI, none had a good outcome."[95] Hurme and Alaranta additionally noted that "the social and psychologic factors influence the outcome more than the findings in the preoperative physical examination or the grade of the operative findings" in those undergoing initial decompression.[52]

The pain drawing is an inexpensive tool that can be used with all patients being evaluated for a lumbar spine problem. Whether an objective means of scoring pain drawings can differentiate between organic and nonorganic pathology or correlate with psychometric testing is at issue.[22, 49, 67, 68, 78, 81] Ransford and colleagues correlated a grading system using four penalty points: (1) unreal drawings with poor anatomic locations, (2) magnification or expansion (e.g., pain drawing with marks outside the body), (3) "I particularly hurt here" indication, and (4) "Look how bad I am" (i.e., a tendency toward total body pain). They concluded that 93 per cent of patients with poor psychometrics could be screened.[81] Parker and associates, more recently, could not differentiate between organic and nonorganic pain patterns, nor identify distressed patients with sufficient specificity and sensitivity, when studying the use of objective scoring systems for pain drawings.[78] Mann and colleagues reported that computer-graded patient pain drawings provide valid "initial impressions" of lumbar spine disorders.[68] It is in this light that we find the drawing useful. Whether or not pain drawings hold up to scientific scrutiny as to objectification, they appear to be an important part of the psychosocial evaluation in our perspective.

Interesting work in the psychosocial evaluation domain has been published recently regarding preinjury emotional trauma and childhood psychologic trauma. Schofferman and associates noted an 85 per cent likelihood of an unsuccessful surgical outcome when a patient had three of five serious childhood psychologic risk factors present.[89] These risk factors are (1) physical abuse, (2) sexual abuse, (3) alcohol or drug abuse in a primary caregiver, (4) abandonment, and (5) emotional neglect or abuse.[89] Blair and coworkers reported "a high rate of preinjury emotional trauma in patients with chronic back pain."[6] They noted that statistically more patients reported abandonment and emotional abuse than physical and sexual abuse.[6] Crauford and colleagues reported a significant excess of adverse life events in patients evaluated for back pain of "uncertain cause," and that these stressors (not psychiatric illness) that predated the onset of back pain were involved in the development of chronic back pain.[17]

IMAGING STUDIES

Although basic spinal radiographs are nonspecific and generally do not alter therapeutic decision making in acute low back pain, they are important in the potential revision surgical candidate.[32, 35, 42, 63] We use standing anteroposterior (AP) and lateral lumbosacral radiographs, combined with flexion-extension radiographs obtained in the lateral decubitus position.[8, 121] The AP radiograph is assessed for evidence of width and level of previous surgical decompression. The standing lateral radiograph provides evidence of loss of disc height, spondylolisthesis, spondylosis, and end plate irregularity. The standing film, in combination with the flexion-extension views, is used to check for instability. We use a dynamic translation in the anterior-posterior plane of greater than 8 per cent, contrasting the movement measured with the adjacent body width (i.e., body width = 50 mm and 4 mm of dynamic motion = 8 per cent), as constituting an abnormal measurement, as suggested by Boden and Wiesel.[8] We define abnormal dynamic angular motion as being greater than 12 degrees of angulation, as described by Wood and coworkers.[121] A previous controlled study at our institution in patients with spondylolisthesis documented the need for combining the lateral decubitus flexion-extension film series with a standing film to maximize the motion measurement.[121] Although objective lumbar instability is uncommon, it suggests the need for surgical arthrodesis if revision surgery is contemplated.

Advanced imaging, in the form of CT scanning and magnetic resonance imaging (MRI), both with and without contrast agents, has considerably increased our ability to understand potential surgical anatomy. However, it must be noted that a given scan can be interpreted only in the clinical context of a given patient.[35] Most are now well acquainted with the number of asymptomatic individuals who have significant anatomic abnormalities on imaging studies.[114, 122] Boden and colleagues documented that approximately 20 per cent of asymptomatic individuals younger than age 60

had a herniated nucleus pulposus on MRI.[7] Wiesel and associates showed that 30 to 35 per cent of asymptomatic individuals have CT scan abnormalities, again with younger patients having a herniated nucleus pulposus and older patients having lumbar stenosis.[114] We recently published a series reviewing asymptomatic individuals and documented that only one of three has a "normal" MRI of the thoracic spine.[122] It is therefore emphasized that the physician must treat the patient and not the MRI or CT scan.

The interpretation of a postoperative imaging study may be even more difficult than that of a preoperative study. A study ordered postoperatively is generally used to assess for compressive pathology, with the differentiation between recurrent herniated nucleus pulposus and perineural scarring being a critical one. Scans are scrutinized for the presence of lateral recess or foraminal stenosis. Most, if not all, patients who have had a previous lumbar decompression or discectomy of any variant will have morphologic abnormalities consistent with disc degeneration. Therefore, surgical decisions are not routinely based on interpretations of disc morphology alone. Additional studies, such as provocative discography, must be done if a surgical approach to mechanical low back pain is being considered.[15, 74, 85, 88, 108, 121] We focus on the interpretation of postoperative scans in assessing for lumbar radiculopathy.

The interpretation of postoperative scans is made even more difficult by knowledge of the natural history of asymptomatic postoperative individuals who have sequential scans performed. MRI studies have been followed in patients with clinically successful lumbar decompressions.[9, 21, 81, 82] Ross and colleagues followed 15 patients and noted that 69 per cent had mass effects in the acute postoperative period that were similar to the preoperative scan, although they did not correlate this with symptoms.[83, 84] Boden and coworkers followed a small series of patients with good clinical outcomes.[9] They also noted that about two thirds of scans showed a significant mass effect at the operative level. Importantly, they identified a rim enhancement pattern suggestive of a recurrent or residual disc fragment encompassed by perineural scar.[9] Deutsch and associates examined patients with "unequivocally successful" surgery for lumbar disc herniation and reported that 9 of 23 patients had near resolution of the disc herniation, 13 of 23 patients had persistent posterior contour deficits, and 4 of 23 patients had no appreciable change in the posterior disc margin.[20] Thus, posterior disc margin abnormalities and mass effects noted on postoperative MRI studies may be significant clinical findings, but they are also commonly encountered in studies of patients with successful disc surgery. Therefore, a complete clinical evaluation with correlation to the study is critical.

In the evaluation of a patient with recurrent radiculopathy, the postoperative MRI or CT scan is used to assess for nerve root compression. The differentiation of recurrent disc fragment from scar tissue is crucial, as surgery for neurolysis of fibrosis portends a poor outcome, but surgery for documented recurrent herniation or bony stenosis predicts a good outcome.[4, 13, 19, 23, 27, 28, 44, 54, 64, 102, 111] Simplistically, a recurrent fragment will have continuity with the parent disc, with scar tissue showing enhancement on gadopentetate dimeglumine (formerly called Gd-DTPA) early postinjection T1-weighted MRI scans; recurrent disc material remains unenhanced with the enhancement agent.[72, 81–83] Ross and coworkers reported a 96 per cent accuracy in differentiating scar from disc in 44 revision surgical cases.[83] Glicksten and Sussman reported a time dependency to perineural scar enhancement, with the greatest degree of enhancement occurring in the initial nine months after surgery, and less intense (even nonexistent) enhancement occurring with images made long after surgery.[38] Taneichi and colleagues presented interesting findings of intrathecal nerve root enhancement in 40 per cent of preoperative patients, suggesting pathologic radiculitis.[101] Unfortunately, 59 per cent of patients had postoperative enhancement, and 75 per cent of those who had preoperative enhancement and resolution of their symptoms with surgical decompression had continued enhancement in the early postoperative period. Late postoperative imaging was not done, so the usefulness of this finding in clinical situations remains to be seen.

Although we have focused on the use of MRI in postoperative lumbar spine evaluations, it should be noted that CT scanning with intravenous contrast has been reported to have an accuracy of 67 to 100 per cent in assessing for postoperative scar versus remnant or recurrent disc herniation.[71, 72, 112] Some have criticized the technique as being technically demanding and involving too large a load of IV contrast when compared with the information available from even unenhanced MRI.[72]

In studying the postoperative patient with recurrent radiculopathy, we are assessing for objective mechanical lesions. In addition to the presence of a recurrent or remnant disc herniation and/or dynamic instability, lumbar stenosis can cause neural compression and hence radicular symptoms. We previously reported on a series of 30 patients undergoing revision decompression with a diagnosis of lateral recess or foraminal stenosis as the cause of failure of their previous decompression.[19] Only 8 of those 30 patients had classic pseudoclaudicatory leg pain. Twenty-four of 30 patients (80 per cent) had self-perceived long-term relief of leg pain with revision decompression. Twenty-four of 30 patients had concurrent anatomic imaging compression and/or symptomatic relief with selective nerve root infiltration (i.e., a classic L5 dermatomal distribution with an L5–S1 foraminal narrowing, or greater than 50 per cent relief of leg pain with selective infiltration of the root to be decompressed if the pain was atypical or the compressive pathology was only marginal on the imaging studies), and of these 24, 21 (88 per cent) had good resolution of symptoms.

Terminology for and description of the anatomy of spinal stenosis vary in the literature. We prefer the term "lateral recess" and define this as the portion of the central canal that is medial to the pedicle and contained dorsally by the ascending medial articular process, as has been described by Heithoff as the "subarticular recess."[11, 42, 73] We prefer the term "foraminal stenosis" (as opposed to "lateral stenosis") for the anatomic area between the medial and lateral edge of the pedicle, where the root is often compressed by the annular end plate junction with a disc protrusion or uncal osteophyte formation.

Kent and colleagues criticized the available literature as lacking sufficient methodologic rigor to allow strong conclusions about the relative diagnostic accuracy of MRI versus CT scanning.[59] Modic and coworkers reported in a prospective blinded study that MRI and CT studies had similar prediction value compared with surgical findings, and that both had higher yields than myelography alone.[71] We agree with Kent and colleagues that what is most important is the patient's self-perceived clinical outcome based on specific selection inclusion criteria that lead to a specific operative procedure, and to what extent the imaging studies contribute to that selection process and hence to the prediction of outcome.

In this light, we, as well as Jonsson and Stromqvist and Akkerveeken, have reported on the relatively high predictive value of diagnostic nerve root infiltrations.[1, 19, 54] If there are marginal imaging study findings or an atypical pain pattern for a specific compressed neural lesion that is being considered for decompression, we recommend a diagnostic nerve root infiltration. If the patient has good resolution of the clinical pain symptoms in question, then the diagnostic infiltration appears to be a positive predictive factor for consideration of revision surgical decompression.

Although the clinical outcome based on the objective inclusion criteria for a surgical approach is clearly the most important concern, we should continue to study the basic pathophysiologic mechanisms for sciatica-type pain and low back pain. Mechanical compression is one of the factors that produce sciatica, and we surgeons focus on identifying anatomic compression, because we can address this with surgical decompression. This is especially reinforced when our patients awake with relief of their leg pain. Yet compression is only one factor in producing symptoms. The basic science literature shows us that in addition to mechanical deformation, chemical irritation, alteration of intraneural microcirculation, and neuropeptide level changes all likely play some part in pain generation.[77, 106] In a group of patients we surgically treated using local anesthesia, we anecdotally found similar results to the published results of Kuslich and associates as to the source of pain provocation in lumbar spine conditions.[62] They reported on tissue stimulation during operative decompression utilizing progressive local anesthesia in a consecutive series of 193 patients. Radicular leg pain was caused by stimulation of compressed inflamed nerve roots, and low back pain was most commonly generated by stimulation of the posterolateral annulus and posterior longitudinal ligament. This more current work reinforces the data of Hirsch and colleagues and Smyth and Wright.[50, 90]

At this point, we make note of our use of discography in the management of individuals being considered for lumbar fusion whose chief complaint is dominant mechanical low back pain. This is a distinctly different patient population from those with dominant leg pain, and there exists a whole surgical literature dealing with these patients. We have included some key references that support the option of arthrodesis as surgical treatment for mechanical low back pain, and many of these studies utilized discography in the selection of surgical candidates.[4, 12, 15, 39, 53, 65, 67, 74, 75, 87, 88, 97, 98, 100, 108, 113, 123, 125] One must realize that the dominant back pain population will yield a lower percentage of clinically successful outcomes in revision lumbar surgery and that, importantly, revision surgical decompression with the goal of relieving low back pain will most likely not accomplish that goal and will often make the symptoms worse.[28, 35, 58, 106] However, we strongly believe that a patient with chronic low back pain who has failed 12 to 18 months of nonoperative management, which includes a functional restoration–type approach; who has no obvious psychosocial contraindication; who has objective evidence of degeneration on MRI or CT scan; and who has concordant reproduction of pain on provocative discography has a surgical option available to him or her. Single-level pathology clearly has a higher rate of reported clinical success than multilevel pathology.[12, 15, 53, 65, 67, 75, 97, 113, 123] The charge to surgeons who believe that they are improving the quality of patients' lives with fusions will be to produce acceptable prospective clinical outcome studies to document this improvement. Our most recent five-year retrospective patient-perceived outcome study had 82 per cent of patients globally satisfied with their outcome for a posterolateral arthrodesis for a given diagnosis.[12] However, those with the diagnosis of postdiscectomy syndrome or degenerative disc disease did not report as great a percentage of success nor magnitude of relief of symptoms on a visual analog scale as did those with the diagnosis of spondylolysis or spondylolisthesis.

INDUSTRIAL LOW BACK PAIN AND LEG PAIN

Much work has been done in the industrial setting of patients with low back pain.[10, 22, 33, 90, 102, 115] Studies exist that document an inferior outcome for patients with compensation or litigation as a psychosocial risk factor.[4, 10, 41, 46, 52, 64, 106] Herron and Turner used the presence of these issues as 25 points of their 100-point scale for objective selection criteria for lumbar discectomy.[46] Bosacco and coworkers reported a dismal 74 per cent rate of permanent disability in patients undergoing laminectomy and discectomy in a Philadelphia city compensation clinic.[10] However, any modification of work status was considered unsatisfactory. The authors noted that an unrestricted disability plan was likely a significant factor in the patients' having unsuccessful

outcomes when stringent criteria for success are utilized. Wiesel and colleagues reported a 10-year prospective outcome study that used an algorithmic approach to unbiased monitoring of the injured worker.[116] They documented improved quality of care with a reduction in surgical cases and, importantly, improved clinical outcomes when surgery was performed, although the number of surgical cases was small. Similarly, Dzioba and Doxey documented an 82 per cent "prognosis success rate" when studying orthopedic and psychologic predictors of outcome of first-time lumbar surgery following an industrial injury.[22] The most significant predictive variables in Dzioba and Doxey's study were English proficiency, the nonorganic signs testing, the amount of back pain versus leg pain, the hypochondriasis scale of the MMPI, and the pain drawing.[22] So although the presence or absence of a compensation or litigation injury is an important psychosocial factor to document, it should not be viewed pejoratively and does not preclude good clinical surgical outcome in well-selected patients.

INDEX SURGICAL PROCEDURE

The main focus of this chapter is on the patient who has had previous disc surgery. This includes open standard laminotomy and discectomy, microdiscectomy with all its variants, percutaneous discectomy with all its variants, and a lesser number of patients having chemonucleolysis. It should be stressed that the initial decision to perform a procedure and the choice of a specific technique are more important than all these revision considerations. The key principle is to decompress the nerve root that is causing the radiculopathy. The removal of whatever combination of disc, ligament, or bone that is necessary must be done in a safe and efficient fashion. In properly selected patients, there should be an approximate 90 per cent chance of good clinical outcome as to resolution of leg pain.[24, 26, 34, 35, 40, 41, 46, 51, 80, 91–93, 95, 109, 117, 118, 124]

Chymopapain has fallen out of favor in the United States. Well-done prospective blinded studies have shown chemonucleolysis to be superior to placebo saline injection.[14, 30, 80, 82, 124] Approximately 70 per cent of injected patients have relief of leg pain, but it takes longer for that relief to occur in comparison to open decompression. The rare occurrence of anaphylaxis and neurologic complications was cited as a factor against chemonucleolysis by one recent reviewer, but another still believes chemonucleolysis to be a reasonable standard of treatment.[43, 70] There appears to be an increase in acute postinjection low back pain, as well as recurrent low back pain, in the chemonucleolysis group. This is intuitive as one considers the degeneration model by which chemonucleolysis destroys the nuclear compartment. We believe that there is a substantially greater number of patients with advanced disc degeneration and symptomatic low back pain among those who have had chemonucleolysis than among those who have had open discectomy. In patients undergoing chemonucleolysis, this increased risk of degeneration will likely result in more patients seeking evaluation for revision surgery, secondary to spondylitic narrowing of the lateral recess and foramen, as well as for mechanical low back pain at long-term follow-up, in addition to those who seek early surgical revision for failure to obtain relief of leg pain with the initial chemonucleolysis.

Percutaneous lumbar discectomy (PLD) has significantly increased in use in the last 10 years. Some surgeons find PLD to be a reasonable treatment option for those with acute sciatica that fails to improve with six to eight weeks of nonoperative management and in whom imaging studies reveal a contained disc herniation.[37] A PLD can be done manually, with or without an arthroscope; with a laser; or with an automated reciprocating device. The outcome for PLD seems to be similar to that for chymopapain, and conceptually, this makes sense, as both work from within the disc space. Gill favorably reviewed PLD and reported an approximate 75 per cent success rate, with a less than 1 per cent complication rate.[37] He stated, "The large number of patients, the large volume of literature, and the consistency of results reported in the literature support the conclusion that PLD may have efficacy in appropriately selected patients."[37] However, two controlled trials of APLD (automated PLD) have shown disappointing results. Revel and colleagues, in a prospective randomized multicenter trial of APLD versus chymopapain, showed only 37 per cent of patients having a good outcome with APLD, versus 60 per cent in the chymopapain group (which mimics the known chymopapain literature).[14, 82] Chatterjee and associates recently reported a controlled clinical trial comparing APLD and microdiscectomy in the treatment of contained lumbar disc herniations.[14] The study was halted, secondary to ethical concerns, when there was a high number of failures. Only 29 per cent of the APLD group, versus 90 per cent of the microdiscectomy group, had a satisfactory outcome. Chatterjee and associates concluded that APLD was ineffective in the treatment of contained lumbar disc herniations. In an economic companion study to the Chatterjee study, Stevenson and colleagues concluded that APLD was less cost-effective than microdiscectomy.[99] Finally, Kahanovitz and coworkers similarly concluded in a multicenter analysis of percutaneous discectomy that "this study clearly indicates that percutaneous discectomy does not appear to be as predictable or successful a treatment modality as surgical discectomy."[55] Thus, when multicenter and controlled trials are reviewed, it appears that extreme caution should be used in selecting a percutaneous discectomy option. We believe that PLD needs to prove itself in well-done prospective clinical series and that the technique lends itself to comparison with microdiscectomy or standard laminectomy and discectomy cases. Similarly to patients treated with chymopapain, we have seen post-APLD patients with inadequate initial decompression, foraminal stenosis, and dominant mechanical back pain, who are seeking a revision surgical option for their problem.

The potential controversy over microdiscectomy versus open discectomy is less an issue of substance than of technique. Whereas limiting the surgical dissection to minimize scar formation, and perhaps to decrease the length of stay, would favor microtechniques, the primary issue is really whether the surgeon accomplishes an adequate decompression of the nerve root in question. Treatment failure is more often related to poor patient selection and inadequate decompression than to perineural scarring or paraspinal muscle fibrosis. In comparisons of open discectomy versus microdiscectomy patients, it appears that the long-term outcomes are similar.[3, 24, 118] Future studies that compare open discectomy and microdiscectomy will favor the limited incision if decreased length of stay, decreased cost, and decreased postoperative morbidity are borne out, provided that the outcome remains the same and the clinical complications of inadequate decompression, dural laceration, and infection are not greater than has been suggested to date. We currently use a "microdiscectomy," which means a limited 2.5 to 3.0-cm incision, laminotomy and medial facetectomy as required, illumination with a headlight, and loop magnification ($\times 3.5$). Most patients are discharged within 24 to 36 hours of surgery.

Finally, as relates to simple fragment excision versus curettage of the disc space, we favor simple fragment excision. Spengler reported on limited discectomy and foraminotomy and noted an 83 per cent success rate, with 15 per cent of individuals having intermittent back or leg pain and 2 per cent having persistent symptoms, but no recurrent herniations were documented.[92] Balderston and colleagues compared simple fragment excision and disc space curettage, focusing on the reherniation rate.[2] They found no difference, with approximately 5 per cent of patients having reherniation at the same level, and 7 per cent having herniation at a new level, with an overall rate of recurrent herniated nucleus pulposus of 12 per cent. Because reoperation rates for the two techniques were similar, the authors recommended simple excision as a means to decrease the risk of retroperitoneal penetration and potential great vessel injury. In addition, we intuitively feel that once the goal of decompressing the nerve root has been accomplished, the intervertebral disc material should be left intact, if it is not a loose fragment, to continue to function as a biomechanical shock absorber.

SURGICAL SELECTION CRITERIA AND TECHNIQUE

As outlined, a comprehensive patient assessment is mandatory. A patient with a suspected new-level or opposite-side pathologic process, as determined by his or her clinical history and examination, is considered as if he or she had not had operative intervention. We generally use a six- to eight-week period of nonoperative management, and then order an MRI to assess for compressive pathology. If the symptoms indicate an ipsilateral same-level herniation, that timeline is typically shorter. Our operative indications include cauda equina syndrome, significant progression of neurologic deficit, and persistent patient-perceived disabling leg pain. These patients generally have dominant leg pain, a neurologic deficit that correlates to a root level, a positive tension sign, and concurrent anatomic imaging that objectifies the compressive pathology. We attempt to elucidate psychosocial contraindications. If there are atypical pain patterns or marginal imaging findings, we recommend a selective nerve root infiltration. Preoperatively, the patient has standing AP and lateral radiographs as well as lateral decubitus flexion-extension dynamic radiographs. We attempt to carefully inform the patient of the risks, benefits, and alternatives to the potential revision surgery being solicited.

We usually use general anesthesia, but we have done a fair number of cases using local anesthesia or local with epidural anesthesia. A Foley catheter is commonly used in a revision case and is removed immediately postoperatively if the length of the procedure was short. We generally use a four-poster frame with the abdomen free and the lumbosacral spine in extension. We believe that keeping the lumbosacral spine in extension, although making it somewhat more difficult to enter the interlaminar space, more closely mimics the upright posture and hence accentuates stenosis. This gives more of the feel of compression in the lateral recess and foramen. This stenosis is then addressed at the time of surgery. The abdomen is free in order to decrease abdominal pressure and thus minimize raised intravenous pressure on the epidural veins. We use extra gel pads on the posts for protection of the skin. The shoulders are flexed and abducted less than 90 degrees to decrease tension on the brachial plexus. The patient receives routine IV antibiotics preoperatively and for an additional 24 hours postoperatively. Intermittent compressive pneumatic stockings are used as a means of deep vein thrombosis (DVT) prophylaxis. Dura prep is routinely used after an alcohol wipe. A Betadine-impregnated Vi-drape is utilized.

When doing a microdiscectomy approach, we use a localizing radiograph with a metal marker on the skin to center the incision at the desired interlaminar level. We recommend having patience in obtaining the first radiograph, as palpation of landmarks alone can often lead one away from the desired location of the incision. The skin and subcutaneous tissue are infiltrated with a dilute lidocaine with epinephrine solution. We then sharply dissect the skin and subcutaneous tissue and again take a confirmatory localization radiograph with a large marker on the spinous process. We strongly recommend this confirmatory radiograph, as the complication of approaching the wrong level can be minimized. A careful study of the preoperative radiographs as well as the MRI or CT scan is made to ascertain if there is abnormal lumbar segmentation; then, intraoperative clinical correlation is done with the intraoperative film and preoperative film.

We use a combination of electrocautery and Cobb elevator dissection to subperiosteally dissect down the spinous process, out laterally on the lamina to the facet capsule. The capsule is protected. A McCulloch, Scoville, or similar self-retracting retractor is posi-

tioned. Anecdotally, we have noted an increased number of superficial wound problems with the use of a micro-Taylor retractor and have thus minimized its use. With the retractor set, the inner laminar space is exposed, revealing the inferior edge of the cephalad lamina and the superior edge of the caudad lamina, with the descending facet and its intact capsule (Fig. 56–1). We clear away excessive tissue and scar to the level of the laminar dorsal edge. Routinely, we use 3.5-loop magnification and a headlamp. If an operative scope is desired, it is now positioned. We emphasize the need to maintain meticulous hemostasis.

At this point, the canal is opened. We dissect with a sharp curet in a medial to lateral fashion to detach scar from the cephalad edge of the caudad lamina, coming laterally to the ascending medial facet (Fig. 56–2). Alternatively, we use a quarter-inch osteotome to perform a medical facetectomy of the descending medial facet (Fig. 56–3). The osteotome is positioned at a low trajectory, with the goal of removing minimal bone but exposing the whole ascending medial articular mass (Fig. 56–4). The straight curet, with its blunt edge medially facing the neural tissue and its sharp edge laterally opposed against the ascending medial facet, is used to detach the scar from the medial ascending articular mass and the laminar edge. A bony resection of lamina and ascending medial facet is then done with Kerrison rongeurs (Fig. 56–5). The key is to identify the lateral border of the traversing nerve root (Fig. 56–6). If difficulty in identifying the root is encountered, we recommend finding the medial pedicle and bluntly dissecting with a Penfield 4 retractor down the pedicle to the canal floor, where the lateral root border will be found.

At this stage, mobilization of the affected nerve root is performed. Forces are primarily in a cephalocaudad

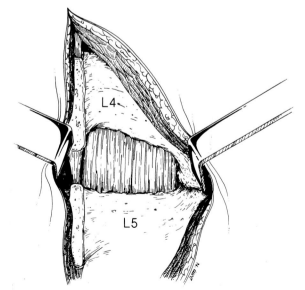

Figure 56–1. Representative view of exposed lamina above and lamina below, with a vertical scar between the L4 and L5 levels.

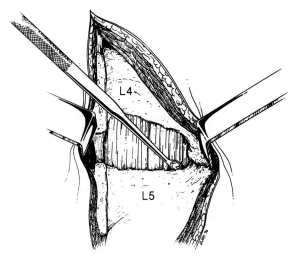

Figure 56–2. A sharp curet is used to detach the scar from the cephalad border of the caudad lamina with a medial to lateral motion, with the blunt edge of the curet toward the neural tissues.

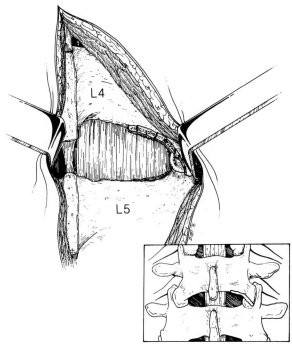

Figure 56–4. With the descending medial facet removed, the medial border of the ascending facet is visualized.

motion, paralleling the lateral border of the root. This minimizes the chance of traumatic damage to the root. We use a combination of blunt and sharp dissection, but our preference is for a Penfield 4 dissector or blunt nerve hook. Hemostasis at this point is critical and typically is the stumbling block for the inexperienced spine surgeon. We use bipolar electrocautery lateral

to the root and powdered Gelfoam mixed to a paste consistency with thrombin, which is gently compressed with a cottonoid against the dorsal floor of the bleeding spinal canal. The bony resection of lamina and facet continues until the entire lateral border of the root is

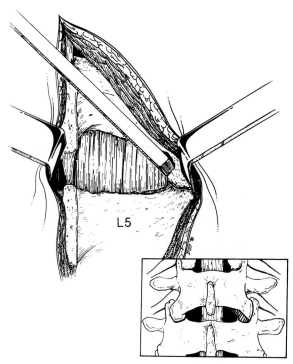

Figure 56–3. An osteotome is used to remove a small portion of the inferior descending medial facet. The inset figure shows the approximate portion of bone that is removed.

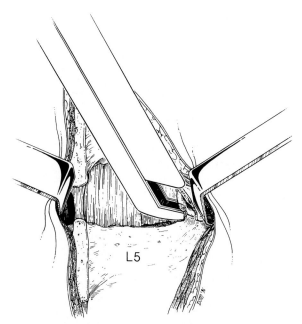

Figure 56–5. A Kerrison rongeur is used to resect a portion of the ascending medial facet. (This rongeur appears larger than would typically be used.)

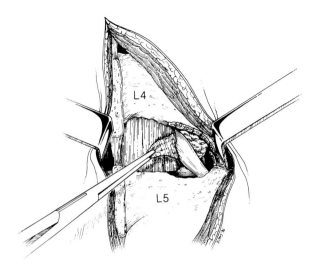

Figure 56–6. The exiting nerve root is being displaced medially by the recurrent disc herniation. The dorsal scar tissue is reflected medially. The key is to identify the lateral border of the nerve root in question.

visualized from its exit off the thecal sac to its departure into the lateral foramen. The root is gently mobilized medially over the disc fragment and protected with a root retractor. Any compressive disc material is then removed. We typically make a single vertical incision with a 15 blade if there is no obvious defect in the posterolateral annulus. We then use a pituitary rongeur to remove any loose fragments in the disc space. We routinely caution physicians in training not to place the tip of the pituitary rongeur into the disc space greater than 1.5 to 2 cm. The pituitary rongeur enters the space closed, is opened and advanced 1.5 to 2 cm, and then closed. It is used as a grasping, not a cutting, instrument. Upbiting or downbiting pituitary rongeurs may be used. We then palpate medially under the posterior annulus with a blunt Woodson dissector to ensure that there are no loose posterior fragments. This same instrument, or another blunt probe such as a Murphy ball, can be used to probe the root in the exiting foramen. At this point, the surgeon must be satisfied that the nerve root is mobilized and free of impingement from its exit off the thecal sac and is clear well into the distal foramen. Of course, preoperative planning should predict the expected pathology, and if any deviation occurs, intraoperative restudy of the anatomic imaging should be done. If concern about lack of pathologic compression exists, do not be embarrassed to take an additional radiograph with a marker in the disc space to confirm the level of decompression.

The previously described technique will adequately address central canal stenosis, a posterolateral herniated nucleus pulposus, and lateral recess stenosis. If foraminal stenosis is the primary pathology, then attention is focused there. The affected root can be traced distally and the dorsal roof of the foramen undercut with Kerrison rongeurs or angled curets. This traditional foraminotomy, however, has an increased risk of

causing an iatrogenic pars intra-articularis defect and subsequent instability. We prefer a "direct foraminotomy," by working caudad to the root in the foramen—that is, by approaching the L5 root from the L5–S1 interspace. From the opposite side of the table, we work at a low trajectory across the table and inferior and lateral to the root (Fig. 56–7). We resect some of the tip of the ascending facet with a Kerrison rongeur or osteotome. A curet is then rotated to resect the annular end plate junction, removing disc or osteophyte from the caudal aspect of the exiting nerve root. Hemostasis is again critical, and we use a combination of bipolar electrocautery, powdered Gelfoam with cottonoids, patience, and perseverance to maintain this hemostasis. In summary, we may combine dissection at the disc level (i.e., the L4–L5 interspace) to inspect the L5 root at the L4–L5 intervertebral disc and lateral recess, ensuring that it is free; then, if foraminal narrowing is suspected, we confirm the foraminal decompression from the L5–S1 interspace, viewing the undersurface of the L5 root in the L5–S1 intervertebral foramen.

If compression is far lateral in the foramen (i.e., a lateral disc herniation), we prefer an intertransverse approach. We expose the pars intra-articularis and transverse process at the pedicle above the root involved (i.e., the L4–L5 facet is the location of the L5 pedicle, the L5 transverse process, and the L5 root exiting below the L5 pedicle). The intertransverse membrane is detached from the caudal aspect of the transverse process with a similar technique to detaching scar or ligamentum flavum from the laminar edge. The dorsal root ganglion is identified exiting under the pars intra-articularis. The root is mobilized, and hemostasis is maintained with bipolar electrocautery. The disc fragment displacing the root is identified. The same technique of longitudinal dissection along the root coming back toward the canal, with similar hemostasis techniques, is utilized. The surgeon can now follow the root into the canal and ensure its mobil-

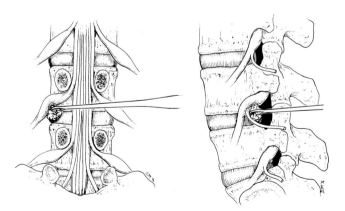

Figure 56–7. Removal of the osteophyte that is pushing up into the nerve root. This can be accomplished by working caudad to the nerve root at a low trajectory from across the table.

ity. An interlaminar approach as described previously is used if intracanal pathology is still suspected.

After having assured ourselves of adequate decompression, we then obtain final hemostasis in the canal. We irrigate copiously with antibiotic irrigation solution. A fat graft, thinned to 5 mm or less, is laid across the exposed neural tissue. If no fat is available, we place Gelfoam squares on the exposed neural tissues. The dorsal lumbar fascia is closed with a running suture. A drain is placed in the subcutaneous tissue. The skin is generally closed with a running subcuticular suture if the dermal edges are not compromised.

Postoperatively, we continue antibiotics for 24 hours. The patient typically receives a patient-controlled analgesia unit. We encourage walking immediately after surgery and try to minimize sitting for six to 12 weeks. The initial three months of rehabilitation focus on aerobic conditioning and light upper and lower extremity strengthening. We then start trunk strengthening. Throughout the preoperative and postoperative periods, the patient receives strong reinforcement regarding proper body posture and lifting mechanics.

SURGICAL RESULTS

It appears that first-time lumbar decompressions for those with acute persistent radiculopathy secondary to a herniated nucleus pulposus have a high rate of success.[2, 24, 26, 34, 41, 46, 51, 52, 91, 117, 118] Wisneski and Rothman documented with an algorithmic approach 90 to 95 per cent patient satisfaction, 90 to 95 per cent reduction of leg pain, and 80 to 85 per cent diminution of back pain in patients undergoing laminotomy and discectomy.[120] Hurme and Alaranta reported that 92 per cent of patients perceived themselves improved at the six-month follow-up.[52] Spengler and Freeman reported that 44 of 50 patients (88 per cent) had good results in a 1979 study evaluating an objective approach to selecting surgical candidates.[93] In 1990, Spengler and associates reported an additional experience with an objective method to select discectomy candidates.[95] Approximately 3 per cent of new patients screened were selected for primary lumbar discectomy. Of the 61 patients with sufficient data, 77 per cent had good results, 7 per cent fair results, and 16 per cent poor outcomes.

When Spengler reported on a limited discectomy technique in 1982, he reported 83 per cent good, 15 per cent fair, and 2 per cent poor results in 54 patients with no recurrent disc herniations.[92] Balderston and coworkers compared simple fragment excision and disc space curettage and reported overall good relief of leg pain, with a 12 per cent reherniation rate in both groups and no difference in the perceived clinical outcomes, other than that the curettage group reported greater back pain.[2] It appears from varied literature that the recurrence rate is approximately 5 to 10 per cent of patients, with 10 to 40 per cent of the recurrences being at the initially operated on level (Table 56–1).[2, 13, 16, 41, 91, 96, 111]

Herron and Turner, using an objective rating system, reported on 106 patients with 75 per cent good results,

Table 56–1. RECURRENCE RATE OF HERNIATED NUCLEUS PULPOSUS

Year	Author	Number of Patients	Reported Recurrence Rate (%)
1972	Spangfort[91]	2504	5.1
1978	Cauchoix et al.[13]	520	5.9 (12% at same level)
1980	Weir and Jacobs[111]	560	11.8
1989	Hanley and Shapiro[41]	87	7
1991	Balderston et al.[2]	83	12 (40% at same level)
1991	Connolly[16]	182	10
1994	Stambough[96]	111	4.5 (all at same level)

13 per cent fair results, and 12 per cent poor results.[46] Epstein and colleagues reported 97 per cent ultimate good to excellent results in 60 patients undergoing decompression of far lateral disc herniations and associated structural abnormalities, with 13 of 60 patients requiring second operative procedures before final assessment.[26]

Hanley and Shapiro looked at the development of low back pain after disc excision.[41] They reported on 120 primary discectomies, with 87 patients having comprehensive 24-month follow-up. Radiculopathy was relieved in 86 of 87 (99 per cent). However, 14 per cent of patients reported an operative failure secondary to disabling low back pain, and 7 per cent had recurrent disc herniations requiring operative revision procedures. An approximate 15 per cent incidence of chronic low back pain after disc excision appears to be a consistent finding in published series looking at this complaint.[23, 35, 41, 112] Weber, however, reported that at 10-year follow-up, none of his patients complained of greater than "some low back pain," whereas "considerable" pain had been reported at the four-year follow-up.[109]

When specifically looking at revision surgery, there is often a pessimistic attitude. However, it appears that if objective criteria are used to select surgical candidates, predictable results are achievable (Table 56–2).[1, 4, 5, 13, 16, 23, 25, 27, 28, 32, 39, 60, 63, 66, 96, 97, 111, 119] Conversely, authors analyzing failures of revision surgery point out an increased incidence of poor outcomes if surgery is performed without clear indications—that is, a specific anatomic lesion must be identified.[11, 27, 28, 64, 94, 102, 115] Surgery done to address scarring, or perineural fibrosis, generally portends a poor outcome.[3, 4, 23, 27, 28, 54, 64, 106] It is clear that both for the initial operative intervention and for any revision surgical intervention, a specific diagnosis with specified preoperative goals must be established.

Law and coworkers reported that only 28 per cent of 53 patients with reoperation after lumbar disc surgery had a successful outcome.[64] Waddell and colleagues reported that only 40 per cent of second operative procedures were successful, and less so thereafter, when surgery was "frequently undertaken without clear indications or evidence of correctable organic lesions."[106]

Table 56–2. RESULTS OF REVISION DISCECTOMY FOR RECURRENT HERNIATED NUCLEUS PULPOSUS

Year	Author	Number of Patients	Reported Outcome
1967	Epstein et al.[25]	47	81% good, 13% fair, 6% poor
1978	Law et al.[64]	53	28% successful
1978	Frymoyer et al.[32]	22	77% satisfied
1978	Cauchoix et al.[13]	9	5 good, 4 fair, 0 poor
1980	Weir and Jacobs[111]	102	46% complete relief, 47% partial relief, 7% no change
1989	Ebeling et al.[23]	92	22% excellent, 30% good, 29% fair, 19% unsuccessful (43% at same level)
1989	Hanley and Shapiro[41]	6	All good
1992	Kim and Michelsen[60]	15	13 satisfied
1993	Jonsson and Stromqvist[54]	19	16 excellent, 2 fair, 1 poor
1994	Stambough[96]	5	3 good, 2 fair
1994	Herron[45]	41	69% good, 26% fair, 7% poor (74% at same level)

When a specific diagnosis of lumbar radiculopathy is made, with an identifiable compressive lesion, repeat decompression appears to be a good option.[1, 4, 5, 13, 16, 23, 25, 27, 28, 32, 39, 60, 63, 66, 96, 97, 111, 119] Finnegan and associates noted that 80 per cent of outcomes were satisfactory in revision cases, particularly when mechanical compression or instability was objectively seen and when a pain-free interval followed the previous operation.[28] Ebeling and colleagues reported 81 per cent satisfactory outcomes (22 per cent excellent, 30 per cent good, and 29 per cent satisfactory) with a microsurgical reoperation following lumbar disc surgery.[23] Kim reviewed a series of revision surgical cases of Michelsen and reported an overall 66 per cent significant improvement in pain and function.[60] However, 13 of the 15 patients (86 per cent) whose intraoperative diagnosis was confirmed as recurrent herniated nucleus pulposus had a satisfactory result. Weir and Jacobs reported 44 per cent complete relief, 50 per cent partial relief, and 6 per cent no change in patients undergoing reoperation following lumbar discectomy, which was not significantly different from their reported results with first-time discectomy.[111] Herron recently reported on 46 patients with a diagnosis of recurrent herniated nucleus pulposus who had a repeat laminectomy and discectomy.[45] Of 41 patients with adequate follow-up, 69 per cent had good, 24 per cent fair, and 7 per cent poor results.

SPINAL STENOSIS

Taking a similar approach with the diagnosis of spinal stenosis yields a similar outlook for revision surgery. Verbeist described the morphology and long-term results of decompression for stenosis.[104, 105] He reported on 92 patients with long-term follow-up, of whom

approximately 93 per cent had relief of neurogenic claudication or sciatica, and 70 per cent had relief of lumbago. Katz and coworkers reported a 31 per cent rate of patient dissatisfaction in a retrospective series on decompressive laminectomies for lumbar stenosis.[57] A group led by Katz recently followed a prospective series of patients having similar procedures to document patient satisfaction at six-month follow-up.[58] Of 194 study patients, only 33 per cent stated that they were bothered more by leg pain than by back pain. In the dominant leg pain group, 69 per cent were satisfied and 15 per cent somewhat satisfied; among those with back pain predominating, only 49 per cent reported being very satisfied, with 27 per cent being somewhat satisfied.[58] Overall, 22 per cent of patients were dissatisfied. Dominant back pain, greater comorbidity, and poor preoperative functional status were significantly and independently associated with these results, and as expected, dominance of leg symptoms predicted a better outcome. Herno and colleagues reported on surgical results for lumbar spinal stenosis and compared those patients with previous back surgery to those without.[44] The outcome was good to excellent in 67 per cent of singly operated patients, versus 46 per cent of repeat surgical cases. They felt that there was a significant worsening effect of previous back surgery, even when a well-established diagnosis of stenosis by myelography was made.

Turner and associates reported an attempted meta-analysis of the literature on lumbar stenosis and noted no significant association between previous back surgery and outcome.[103] Nasca reported 83 per cent good results in those with revision surgery for stenosis,[73] whereas Herron and colleagues reported that previous unsuccessful surgery had a negative effect on the outcome of revision surgery for lumbar stenosis.[48]

Jonsson and Stromqvist recently published a prospective two-year evaluation of repeat lumbar nerve root decompressions in 93 consecutive patients.[54] A diagnosis of recurrent disc herniation in 19 patients, central spinal stenosis in 20 patients, lateral spinal stenosis in 19 patients, and periradicular fibrosis in 35 patients was confirmed surgically. At the two-year follow-up, of the 19 patients with recurrent herniated nucleus pulposus, there were 16 excellent, 2 fair, and 1 unchanged outcomes; of the 19 with central stenosis, there were 7 excellent, 7 fair, 4 unchanged, and 1 worse outcomes; of the 18 with lateral stenosis, there were 12 excellent, 4 fair, and 2 unchanged outcomes; and in the 35 with fibrosis, there were six excellent, 10 fair, 15 unchanged, and 4 worse outcomes. We recently reported on a subset of our revision cases of lumbar decompression for those with the diagnosis of foraminal or lateral recess stenosis.[19] Twenty-four of 30 patients (80 per cent) had long-term relief of symptoms. Twenty-four patients had a classic dermatomal distribution of pain, which was concordant with imaging study compression, or had symptomatic relief with a selective nerve root infiltration. Of this group, 21 (88 per cent) had relief of radiculopathy. Of interest, 15 of the patients had no relief with their original surgery, and 13 of these 15 had good relief despite no pain-free interval. This suggests a different forecast for those with the diagnosis of stenosis rather than recurrent or persistent herniated nucleus pulposus when there is no pain-free interval.

REVISION DECOMPRESSION WITH FUSION

The scope of this chapter does not allow a full discussion of the literature on arthrodesis. However, it should be noted that for many patients, both back and leg pain are important symptom complexes. When back pain accounts for 50 per cent or greater of the symptomatic complaint, we believe that a thoughtful consideration of lumbar fusion must be made. If objective lumbar instability is documented preoperatively at the revision level, or if iatrogenic instability is felt to be created at the time of the revision decompression, an arthrodesis should be considered.

The surgeon who performs revision decompression for the chief complaint of mechanical low back pain often contributes to the pool of those with failed back surgery syndrome, and we do not recommend this approach. We believe that there is reasonable literature support for consideration of a lumbar fusion for those with mechanical low back pain who have failed a prolonged course of nonoperative management, and the reader is referred to those sources.[12, 15, 39, 52, 53, 65–67, 74, 75, 97, 102, 108, 123] These reports have combined varied diagnoses with varied combinations of revision decompressions, posterior fusions, and anterior fusions, with or without instrumentation, and reported success rates generally from 55 to 80 per cent.[12, 15, 39, 52, 53, 65–67, 74, 75, 97, 102, 108, 123] We recently presented a five-year follow-up of those having posterolateral lumbar arthrodesis for the chief complaint of mechanical low back pain, broken down by diagnosis.[12] Overall, 82 per cent of patients were globally satisfied with their outcome. The worst group was those fused with the diagnosis of postlaminectomy syndrome. In this group, only 60 per cent of the patients reported greater than 50 per cent relief of symptoms at the five-year follow-up. This was for posterolateral arthrodesis alone, with no interbody fusion, and the group included some patients with adjacent segment degeneration who had recurrence of pain after a pain-free interval of one or two years.

SUMMARY

The treating physician for those being considered for revision lumbar surgical intervention has a clear charge to make a definitive, clinically correlated diagnosis and to define preoperatively clear anatomic pathology that is to be addressed with the revision surgery. Patients who have dominant lumbar radiculopathy, with demonstrable compressive pathology on imaging studies, have a good chance at resolution of their leg symptoms with repeat decompression. If the pathology is a new-level or opposite-side disc herniation, it should be addressed similarly to a first-time disc herniation. If the

patient has an ipsilateral same-level recurrent herniated nucleus pulposus, revision surgery may be technically more demanding, but should yield good clinical outcomes in approximately 80 per cent of patients. We believe that the natural history of those with ipsilateral same-level recurrent herniation is not as good as that of those with an initial herniated nucleus pulposus, and these patients often have leg pain worse than the original occurrence. Patients who have recurrent pseudoclaudicatory leg pain or radiculopathy secondary to lumbar stenosis generally do respond to revision decompression. Patients who have neurolysis for perineural scarring alone often do not have improvement of symptoms.

A lumbar fusion does not routinely have to be added to a revision decompression for dominant radiculopathy. If a patient has dominant mechanical low back pain, decompression alone does not appear to be a good surgical option, and arthrodesis should be considered.

The preoperative evaluation, which must include a psychosocial evaluation, that leads to the selection of the surgical candidate is as important as the exact technique of surgery to be done, if not more so.

Case 1

Patient R. G. had undergone previous surgery at the L5–S1 level with good resolution of leg pain. He presented with acute onset of left-sided L5 sciatica. The MRI shows degenerative change at the L5–S1 level, with previous scarring (Fig. 56–8). It shows what appears to be a new herniated nucleus pulposus at L4–L5 to the left affecting the L5 nerve root, with a high signal zone of intensity in the posterolateral annulus (Fig. 56–9). This patient would be treated as if this were

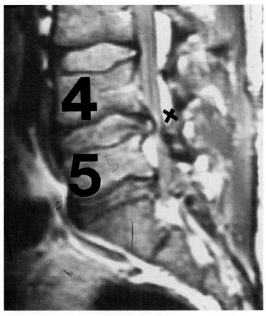

Figure 56–8.

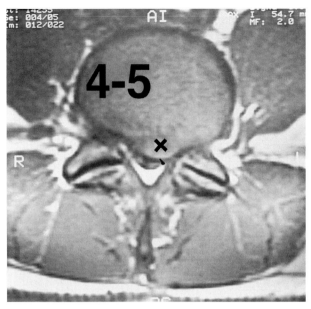

Figure 56–9.

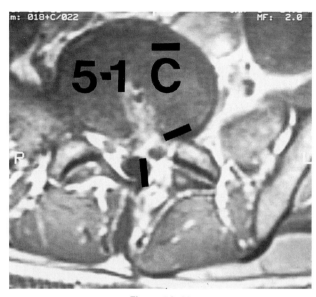

Figure 56–11.

a first-time occurrence, since it is a herniated nucleus pulposus at a new level. The MRI, with and without enhancing agent, shows the scar enhancement around the S1 nerve root at the previously operated on L5–S1 level (Figs. 56–10 and 56–11). This patient ultimately had surgery at the L4–L5 level, with good resolution of leg pain.

Case 2

D. T. represents a unique patient who demonstrates the natural history of recurrent herniated nucleus pulposus with multiple images. She was seen at a county hospital with a work-related injury. She had dominant left-sided leg pain, with a herniated nucleus pulposus at the L5–S1 level, as demonstrated in Figures 56–12 and 56–13. this demonstrates the displaced left s1 nerve root. She underwent surgery in April 1994, with complete resolution of leg pain.

This patient returned to work three months postoperatively doing home cleaning. She subsequently developed reoccurrence of leg pain in the same distribution. She was studied in July 1994 with an MRI that reveals what appears to be a recurrent herniated nucleus pulposus at the L5–S1 level. Sagittal MRIs

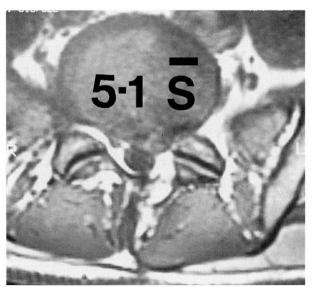

Figure 56–10.

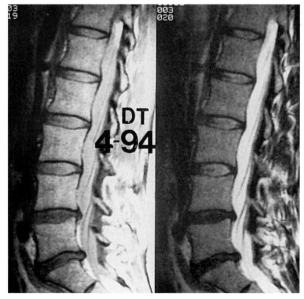

Figure 56–12.

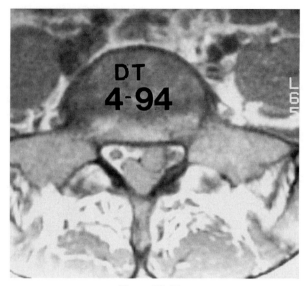

Figure 56–13.

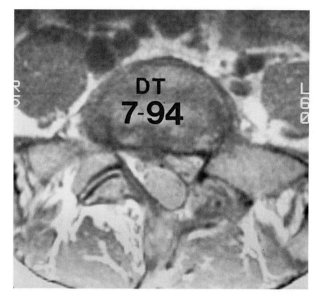

Figure 56–15.

show high signal of intensity inferior at the L5–S1 level. There appears to be a space-occupying lesion in the left L5–S1 region (Figs. 56–14 and 56–15). She was returned to surgery at the county hospital and awoke with left leg pain worse than she had experienced preoperatively.

The left leg pain persisted, and the patient had an additional MRI in September 1994. This was interpreted as showing small herniated nucleus pulposus at the right at L5–S1, with scar formation around the nerve root on the left, but no space-occupying lesion affecting the left S1 nerve root (Figs. 56–16 and 56–17). This was interpreted as persistent pain secondary to intraparenchymal damage to the left S1 nerve root.

Patient D. T. continued to be followed at the county hospital. She had continuing complaints of back pain and left leg pain. She began to develop symptoms of bladder dysfunction in February 1995. A subsequent MRI was ordered, which showed degenerative signal change at L4–L5 and L5–S1. It showed moderate scarring on the transverse images at the left L5–S1 level. There did not appear to be significant displacement of the S1 roots by the posterior annulus. Her symptoms continued to be left-side predominant (Figs. 56–18 through 56–20).

This patient subsequently was followed by the internal medicine department and had increasing

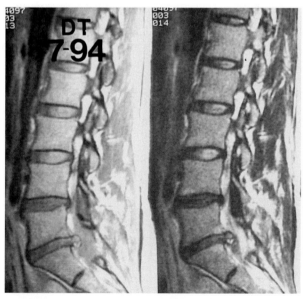

Figure 56–14.

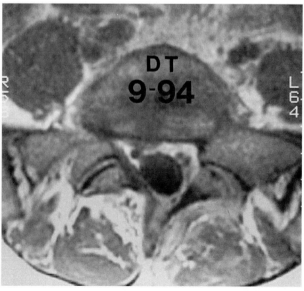

Figure 56–16.

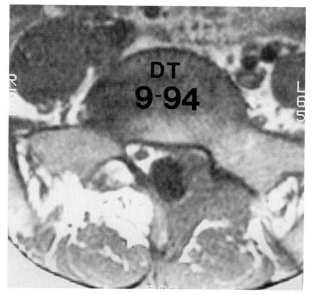

Figure 56–17.

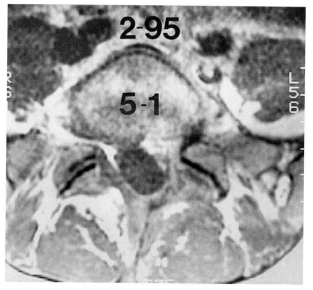

Figure 56–19.

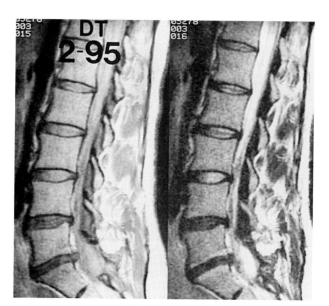

Figure 56–18.

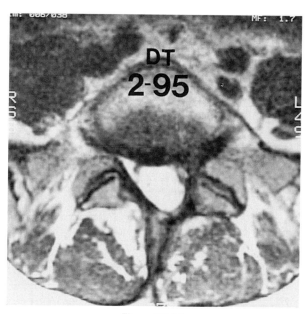

Figure 56–20.

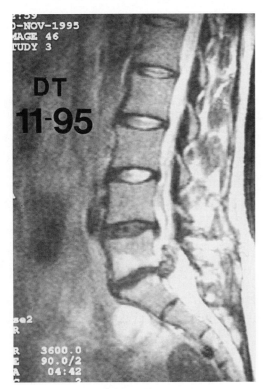

Figure 56–21.

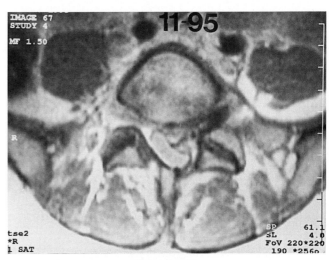

Figure 56–23.

complaints of bladder dysfunction. She was on a straight catheterization program and was wearing two fentanyl patches. A new MRI was obtained in November 1995, which showed a large extruded herniated nucleus pulposus at the L5–S1 level, with displacement of the thecal sac and compression of the S1 nerve root. She had complaints of back pain as well as left leg pain and urinary retention (Figs. 56–21 through 56–23).

She was subsequently referred to our center, where she had extensive preoperative evaluation. She was taken back to surgery for a revision decompression at the L5–S1 level, with instrumented arthrodesis from L4 through S1. At the three-month follow-up, she had significant improvement of leg pain. She continues with one fentanyl patch. She is no longer on an in-and-out catheterization program. The final outcome is pending.

This case represents an unusual history, with multiple MRIs in the same patient documenting the degenerative process with a recurrent herniated nucleus pulposus at the L5–S1 level.

References

1. Akkerveeken, P. F.: Pain patterns and diagnostic blocks. *In* Weinstein, J. N., and Wiesel, S. W. (eds.): The Lumbar Spine—ISSLS. Philadelphia, W. B. Saunders Co., 1990, pp. 107–132.
2. Balderston, R. A., Gilyard, G. G., Jones, A. M., et al.: The treatment of lumbar disc herniation: Simple fragment and excision versus disc space curettage. J. Spinal Disord. 4:22–25, 1991.
3. Barrios, C., Ahmed, M., Arrotegui, J., et al.: Microsurgery versus standard removal of the herniated lumbar disc: A 3 year comparison in 150 cases. Acta Orthop. Scand. *61*:399–403, 1990.
4. Bernard, T. N.: Repeat lumbar spine surgery. Spine *15*:2196–2200, 1993.
5. Biondi, J., and Greenberg, B. J.: Redecompression and fusion in failed back syndrome patients. J. Spinal Disord. 3:362–369, 1990.
6. Blair, J. A., Blair, R. S., and Rveckert, P.: Pre-injury emotional trauma and chronic back pain: An unexpected finding. Spine *19*:1144–1147, 1994.
7. Boden, S. D., Davis, D. O., Dina, T. S., et al.: Abnormal magnetic-resonance scan of the lumbar spine in asymptomatic subjects. J. Bone Joint Surg. Am. 72:403–408, 1990.
8. Boden, S. D., and Wiesel, S. W.: Lumbosacral segmental motion in normal individuals: Have we been measuring stability properly? Spine *15*:571–576, 1990.
9. Boden, S. D., Davis, D. O., Dina, T. S., et al.: Contrast-enhanced MR imaging performed after successful lumbar spine disk surgery: Prospective study. Radiology *182*:59–64, 1992.
10. Bosacco, S. J., Berman, A. T., Bosacco, D. N., et al.: Results of lumbar disk surgery in a city compensation population. Orthopedics *18*:351–355, 1995.

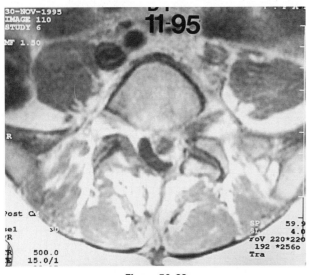

Figure 56–22.

11. Burton, C. V., Kirkaldy-Willis, W. H., Heithoff, K. B., et al.: Causes of failure of surgery in the lumbar spine. CORR 157:191–199, 1981.
12. Buttermann, G., Hunt, A. F., Garvey, T. A., et al.: Results of lumbar fusion related to diagnosis. Presented at North American Spine Society, Minneapolis, MN, 1994.
13. Cauchoix, J., Ficat, C., and Girard, B.: Repeat surgery after disc excision. Spine 3:256–259, 1978.
14. Chatterjee, S., Foy, P. M., and Findlay, G. F.: Report of a controlled clinical trial comparing automated percutaneous lumbar discectomy and microdiscectomy in the treatment of contained lumbar disc herniations. Spine 20:734–738, 1995.
15. Colhoun, E., McCall, I. W., Williams, L., et al.: Provocation discography as a guide to planning operations on the spine. J. Bone Joint Surg. Br. 70:267–271, 1988.
16. Connolly, E. S.: Surgery for recurrent lumbar disc herniation. In Proceedings of the Congress of Neurological Surgeons, Orlando, Florida, 1991: Clinical Neurosurgery. Baltimore, Williams & Wilkins, 1991, pp. 211–216.
17. Crauford, D. I., Creed, F., and Jayson, M. I.: Life events and psychological disturbance in patients with low-back pain. Spine 15:490–494, 1990.
18. Davis, G. W., Onik, G., and Helms, C.: Automated percutaneous discectomy. Spine 16:359–363, 1991.
19. Dekutoski, M. B., Garvey, T. A., Transfeldt, E. E., et al.: Residual lateral recess and foraminal stenosis: An etiology of failed lumbar surgery. Presented at annual meeting of Mid-America Orthopaedic Society, Hilton Head, SC, 1993.
20. Derby, R., Kine, G., Saal, J. A., et al.: Response to steroid and duration of radicular pain as predictors of surgical outcome. Spine 17:S176–S183, 1992.
21. Deutsch, A. L., Howand, M., Dawson, E. G., et al.: Lumbar spine following successful surgical discectomy: Magnetic resonance imaging features and implications. Spine 18:1054–1060, 1993.
22. Dzioba, R. D., and Doxey, N. C.: A prospective investigation into the orthopedic and psychological predictors of outcome of first lumbar surgery following industrial injury. Spine 9:614–623, 1984.
23. Ebeling, V., Kalbarcyk, H., and Reuben, H. J.: Microsurgical reoperation following lumbar disc surgery: Timing, surgical findings, and outcome in 92 patients. J. Neurosurg. 70:397–404, 1989.
24. Eismont, F. J., and Currier, B.: Current concepts review: Surgical management of lumbar intervertebral disc disease. J. Bone Joint Surg. Am. 71:1266–1271, 1989.
25. Epstein, J. A., Lavine, L. S., and Epstein, B. S.: Recurrent herniation of the lumbar intervertebral disc. Clin. Orthop. 52:169–178, 1967.
26. Epstein, N. E., Epstein, J. A., Carras, R., et al.: Far lateral lumbar disc herniation and associated structural abnormalities. Spine 15:534–539, 1990.
27. Fager, C. A., and Friedberg, S. R.: Analysis of failures and poor results of lumbar spine surgery. Spine 5:87–94, 1980.
28. Finnegan, W. J., Fenlin, J. M., Marvel, J. P., et al.: Result of surgical intervention in the symptomatic multiply operated back patient: Analysis of 67 cases followed three to seven years. J. Bone Joint Surg. Am. 61:1077–1082, 1979.
29. Fraser, R. D., Sawdhu, A., and Gogan, W. J.: Magnetic resonance imaging findings 10 years after treatment for lumbar disc herniation. Spine 20:710–714, 1995.
30. Friedman, W. A.: Percutaneous diskectomy: An alternative to chemonucleolysis? Neurosurgery 13:524–547, 1983.
31. Frymoyer, J. W., Hanley, E., Howe, J., et al.: Disc excision and spine fusion in the management of lumbar disc disease: A minimum ten year follow-up. Spine 3:1–6, 1978.
32. Frymoyer, J. W., Malteri, R. E., Hanley, E. N., et al.: Failed lumbar disc surgery requiring second operation: A long term follow-up study. Spine 3:7–11, 1978.
33. Frymoyer, J. W., and Cats-Baril, W. L.: An overview of the incidence and costs of low back pain. Orthop. Clin. North Am. 22:263–271, 1991.
34. Garfin, S. R., Glover, M., Booth, R. E., et al.: Laminectomy: A review of the Pennsylvania Hospital experience. J. Spinal Disord. 1:116–133, 1988.
35. Garvey, T. A.: Surgical decision making in lumbar disc herniations. Phys. Ther. Practice 1:10–19, 1992.
36. Garvey, T. A., and Wiesel, S. W.: Critical decisions in emergency medicine: Acute low-back pain. Critical Decisions in Emergency Medicine 5: Lesson 4, 1990.
37. Gill, K.: Percutaneous lumbar diskectomy. J. AAOS 1:33–40, 1993.
38. Glickstein, M. F., and Sussman, S. K.: Time-dependent scar enhancement in magnetic resonance imaging of the postoperative lumbar spine. Skeletal Radiol. 20:333–337, 1991.
39. Goldner, J. L., Urbaniak, J. R., and McCollom, D. E.: Anterior disc excision and interbody spinal fusion for chronic low back pain. Orthop. Clin. North Am. 2:543–568, 1971.
40. Hakelius, A.: Prognosis in sciatica: A clinical follow-up of surgical and non-surgical treatment. Acta Orthop. Scand. Suppl. 129:1–76, 1970.
41. Hanley, E. N., and Shapiro, D. E.: The development of low back pain after excision of a lumbar disc. J. Bone Joint Surg. Am. 71:719–721, 1989.
42. Heithoff, K. B.: Computed tomography and plain film diagnosis of the lumbar spine. In Weinstein, J. N., and Wiesel, S. W. (eds.): The Lumbar Spine—ISSLS. Philadelphia, W. B. Saunders Co., 1990, pp. 283–319.
43. Herkowitz, H. N.: Current status of percutaneous discectomy and chemonucleolysis. Orthop. Clin. North Am. 22:327–332, 1991.
44. Herno, A., Airaksinen, O., Saari, T., et al.: Surgical results of lumbar spinal stenosis: A comparison of patients with or without previous back surgery. Spine 20:964–969, 1995.
45. Herron, L.: Recurrent lumbar disc herniation: Results of repeat laminectomy and discectomy. J. Spinal Disord. 7:161–166, 1994.
46. Herron, L. D., and Turner, J.: Patient selection for lumbar laminectomy and discectomy with a revised objective rating system. Clin. Orthop. 199:145–152, 1985.
47. Herron, L. D., Turner, J., Clancy, S., et al.: The differential utility of the Minnesota Multiphasic Personality Inventory: A predictor of outcome in lumbar laminectomy for disc herniation versus spinal stenosis. Spine 11:847–850, 1986.
48. Herron, L., Turner, J., and Weiner, P.: A comparison of the Millon Clinical Multiaxial Inventory and the MMPI as predictors of successful treatment by lumbar laminectomy. CORR 203:232–238, 1986.
49. Hildebrandt, J., Frantz, C. E., Choroba-Mehnen, C., et al.: The use of pain drawings in screening for psychological involvement in complaints of low back pain. Spine 13:681–685, 1988.
50. Hirsch, C., Ingelmark, B. E., and Miller, M.: The anatomical basis for low back pain. Acta Orthop. Scand. 33:1–17, 1963.
51. Holmes, H. E., and Rothman, R. H.: The Pennsylvania Plan: An algorithm for the management of lumbar degenerative disc disease. Spine 4:156–162, 1979.
52. Hurme, M., and Alaranta, H.: Factors predicting the result of surgery for lumbar intervertebral disc herniation. Spine 12:933–938, 1987.
53. Jackson, R. K., Boston, D. A., and Edge, A. J.: Lateral mass fusion—a prospective study of a consecutive series with long term follow-up. Spine 10:828–832, 1985.
54. Jonsson, B., and Stromqvist, B.: Repeat decompression of lumbar nerve roots: A prospective 2 year evaluation. J. Bone Joint Surg. Br. 75:894–897, 1993.
55. Kahanovitz, N., Viola, K., Goldstein, T., et al.: A multicenter analysis of percutaneous discectomy. Spine 15:713–715, 1990.
56. Kambin, P., and Schaffer, J. L.: Percutaneous lumbar discectomy: Review of 100 patients and current practice. Clin. Orthop. 238:24–34, 1984.
57. Katz, J. N., Lipson, S. J., Larson, M. G., et al.: The outcome of decompressive laminectomy for degenerative lumbar stenosis. J. Bone Joint Surg. Am. 73:809–816, 1991.
58. Katz, J. N., Lipson, S. J., Brick, G. W., et al.: Clinical correlation of patient satisfaction after laminectomy for degenerative lumbar spinal stenosis. Spine 20:1155–1160, 1995.
59. Kent, D. L., Haynor, D. R., Larson, E. B., et al.: Diagnosis of lumbar spinal stenosis in adults: A metaanalysis of the accuracy of CT, MR, and myelography. AJR Am. J. Roentgenol. 158:1135–1144, 1992.

60. Kim, S. S., and Michelsen, C. B.: Revision surgery for failed lumbar back surgery syndrome. Spine 17:957–960, 1992.

61. Kornberg, M., and Rechtine, G. R.: Quantitative assessment of the fifth lumbar spinal canal by computed tomography in symptomatic L1–L5 disc disease. Spine 10:320–330, 1985.

62. Kuslich, S. P., Ulstrom, C. L., and Michael, C. J.: The tissue origin of low back pain and sciatica: A report of pain response to tissue stimulation during operations on the lumbar spine using local anesthesia. Orthop. Clin. North Am. 22:181–187, 1991.

63. LaRocca, H.: Failed lumbar surgery: Principles of management. In Weinstein, J. N., and Wiesel, S. W. (eds.): The Lumbar Spine—ISSLS. Philadelphia, W. B. Saunders Co., 1990, pp. 872–881.

64. Law, J. D., Lehman, R. A., and Kirsch, W. M.: Reoperation after lumbar intervertebral disc surgery. J. Neurosurg. 48:259–263, 1978.

65. Lee, C. K., Vessa, P., and Lee, J. K.: Chronic disabling low back pain syndrome caused by internal disc derangements. Spine 20:356–361, 1995.

66. Lehmann, T. R., and LaRocca, H. S.: Repeat lumbar surgery: A review of patients with failure from previous lumbar surgery treated by spinal canal exploration and lumbar spine fusion. Spine 6:615–619, 1981.

67. Lorenz, M., Zindrick, M., Schwaegler, P., et al.: A comparison of single-level fusions with and without hardware. Spine 16:S455–S458, 1991.

68. Mann, N. H., Brown, M. D., and Erger, I.: Statistical diagnosis of lumbar spine disorders using computerized patient pain drawings. Comput. Biol. Med. 21:383–397, 1991.

69. Margolis, R. B., Chibrall, J. T., and Tait, R. C.: Test-retest reliability of the pain drawing instrument. Pain 33:49–51, 1988.

70. McCulloch, J. A.: Alternatives to discectomy: Microsurgery and chemonucleolysis. Semin. Spine Surg. 6:243–255, 1994.

71. Modic, M. T., Masaryk, T., Boumphrey, F., et al.: Lumbar herniated disc disease and canal stenosis: Prospective evaluation by surface coil MR, CT and myelography. Neuroradiology 7:709–717, 1987.

72. Modic, M. T., and Ross, J. S.: Magnetic resonance imaging in the evaluation of low back pain. Orthop. Clin. North Am. 22:283–301, 1991.

73. Nasca, R. J.: Surgical management of lumbar spinal stenosis. Spine 12:809–816, 1987.

74. North American Spine Society: Position statement on discography. Spine 13:1343, 1988.

75. O'Beirne, J., O'Neill, D., Gallagher, J., et al.: Spinal fusion for back pain: A clinical and radiological review. J. Spinal Disord. 5:32–38, 1992.

76. Ohnmeiss, T., Vanharanta, H., and Guyer, R. D.: The association between pain drawings and computed tomographic/discographic pain responses. Spine 20:729–733, 1995.

77. Olmarker, K., and Rydevik, B.: Pathophysiology of sciatica. Orthop. Clin. North Am. 22:223–234, 1991.

78. Parker, H., Wood, D. L., and Main, C. J.: The use of the pain drawing as a screening measure to predict psychological distress in chronic low back pain. Spine 20:236–243, 1995.

79. Pheasant, H. C., Gilbert, D., Goldfarb, J., et al.: The MMPI as a predictor of outcome in low-back surgery. Spine 4:78–84, 1979.

80. Postacchini, F., Lami, R., and Massobrio, M.: Chemonucleolysis versus surgery in lumbar disc herniations: Correlation of the results to preoperative clinical pattern and size of the herniation. Spine 12:87–96, 1987.

81. Ransford, A. O., Cairns, D., and Mooney, V.: The pain drawing as an aid to the psychological evaluation of patients with low back pain. Spine 1:127–135, 1976.

82. Revel, M., Payan, C., Vallee, C., et al.: Automated percutaneous lumbar discectomy versus chemonucleolysis in the treatment of sciatica: A randomized multicenter trial. Spine 18:1–7, 1993.

83. Ross, J. S., Masaryk, T. J., Modic, M. T., et al.: Lumbar spine, postoperative assessment with surface-coil MR imaging. Radiology 164:851–860, 1987.

84. Ross, J. S., Masaryk, T. J., Schrader, M., et al.: MR imaging of the postoperative lumbar spine: Assessment with gadopentetate dimeglumine. AJR Am. J. Roentgenol. 155:867–872, 1990.

85. Ross, J. S., Modic, M. T., Masaryk, T. J., et al.: Assessment of extra-dural degenerative disease with Gd-DTPA enhanced MR imaging: Correlation with surgical and pathological findings. AJNR Am. J. Neuroradiol. 10:1243–1249, 1990.

86. Saal, J. A., and Saal, J. S.: Nonoperative treatment of herniated lumbar intervertebral disc with radiculopathy. Spine 14:431–437, 1989.

87. Schellhas, K. P.: Diskography. Spine, State of the Art Reviews 9:27–44, 1995.

88. Schellhas, K. P., Pollei, S. R., Gundry, C. R., et al.: Lumbar disc high intensity zone: Correlation of discography and MRI. Spine 2:79–86, 1996.

89. Schofferman, J., Anderson, D., Hines, R., et al.: Childhood psychological trauma correlates with unsuccessful lumbar spine surgery. Spine 17:S138–S144, 1992.

90. Smyth, M. J., and Wright, V.: Sciatica and the intervertebral disc: An experimental study. J. Bone Joint Surg. Am. 40:1401–1418, 1958.

91. Spangfort, E. V.: The lumbar disc herniation: A computer-aided analysis of 2,504 operations. Acta Orthop. Scand. Suppl. 142:1–95, 1972.

92. Spengler, D.: Lumbar discectomy results with limited excision and selective foraminectomy. Spine 7:604–607, 1982.

93. Spengler, D. M., and Freeman, C. W.: Patient selection for lumbar discectomy: An objective approach. Spine 4:129–134, 1979.

94. Spengler, D. M., Freeman, C., Westbrook, R., et al.: Low back pain following multiple lumbar spine procedures: Failure of initial selection? Spine 5:356–360, 1980.

95. Spengler, D. M., Ouellette, A. E., Battie, M., et al.: Elective discectomy for herniation of a lumbar disc. J. Bone Joint Surg. Am. 72:230–237, 1990.

96. Stambough, J. L.: Recurrent same-level, ipsilateral lumbar spine disc herniation. Orthop. Rev. 1994.

97. Stauffer, R. N., and Coventry, M. B.: A rational approach to failures of lumbar disc surgery: The orthopedist's approach. Orthop. Clin. North Am. 2:583–592, 1971.

98. Stauffer, R. N., and Coventry, M. B.: Posterolateral lumbar spine fusion. J. Bone Joint Surg. Am. 54:1195–1204, 1972.

99. Stevenson, R. C., McCabe, C. J., and Findlay, A. M.: An economic evaluation of a clinical trial to compare automated percutaneous lumbar discectomy with microdiscectomy in the treatment of contained lumbar disc herniations. Spine 20:739–742, 1995.

100. Stewart, G., and Sachs, B. L.: Patient outcomes after reoperation on the lumbar spine. J. Bone Joint Surg. Am. 78:706–711, 1996.

101. Taneichi, H., Abumi, K., Kaneda, K., et al.: Significance of Gd-DTPA-enhanced magnetic resonance imaging for lumbar disc herniations: The relationship between nerve root enhancement and clinical manifestations. J. Spinal Disord. 7:153–160, 1994.

102. Turner, J. A., Ersek, M., Herron, L., et al.: Patient outcomes after lumbar spinal fusions. JAMA 208:907–911, 1992.

103. Turner, J. A., Ersek, M., and Herron, L.: Surgery for lumbar spinal stenosis: Attempted meta-analysis of the literature. Spine 17:1–7, 1992.

104. Verbeist, H.: Pathomorphologic aspects of developmental lumbar stenosis. Orthop. Clin. North Am. 6:163–175, 1975.

105. Verbeist, H.: Lumbar spinal stenosis: Morphology, classification, and long term results. In Weinstein, J. N., and Wiesel, S. W. (eds.): The Lumbar Spine—ISSLS. Philadelphia, W. B. Saunders Co., 1990, pp. 546–589.

106. Waddell, G., Kummel, E. G., Lotto, W. N., et al.: Failed lumbar disc surgery and repeat surgery following industrial injuries. J. Bone Joint Surg. Am. 61:201–206, 1979.

107. Waddell, G., McCulloch, J. A., Kummel, E., et al.: Nonorganic physical signs in low-back pain. Spine 5:117–125, 1980.

108. Walsh, T. R., Weinstein, J. N., Spratt, K. F., et al.: Lumbar discography in normal subjects: A controlled, prospective study. J. Bone Joint Surg. Am. 72:1081–1088, 1990.

109. Weber, H.: Lumbar disc herniation: A controlled, prospective study with ten years of observation. Spine 8:131–140, 1983.

110. Weinstein, J.: Neurogenic and nonneurogenic pain and inflammatory mediators. Orthop. Clin. North Am. 22:235–246, 1991.

111. Weir, B. K., and Jacobs, G. A.: Reoperation rate following lumbar discectomy: An analysis of 662 lumbar discectomies. Spine 5:366–370, 1980.

112. Weiss, T., Treisch, J., Kazner, E., et al.: CT of the postoperative lumbar spine: The value of intravenous contrast. Neuroradiology 28:241–245, 1986.

113. West, J. L., Bradford, D. S., and Ogilvie, J. W.: Results of spinal arthrodesis with pedicle screw-plate fixation. J. Bone Joint Surg. Am. 73:1179–1184, 1991.

114. Wiesel, S. W., Tsourmas, N., Feffer, H. L., et al.: A study of computer-assisted tomography: The incidence of positive CAT scans in an asymptomatic group of patients. Spine 9:549–551, 1984.

115. Wiesel, S. W., Fefer, H. C., and Rothman, R. H.: Low back pain: Development and five year prospective application of a computerized quality-based diagnostic and treatment protocol. J. Spinal Disord. 1:50–58, 1988.

116. Wiesel, S. W., Boden, S. D., and Feffer, H. L.: A quality-based protocol for the management of musculoskeletal injuries: A ten year prospective outcome study. CORR 301:164–176, 1994.

117. Williams, R. W.: Microlumbar discectomy: A 12 year statistical review. Spine 11:851–852, 1986.

118. Wilson, D. H., and Harbaugh, R.: Lumbar discectomy: A comparative study of microsurgical and standard technique. In Hardy, R. (ed.): Lumbar Disc Disease. New York, Raven Press, 1982, pp. 147–156.

119. Wiltse, L. L.: Psychologic testing in predicting the success of low back surgery. Orthop. Clin. North Am. 6:317–318, 1975.

120. Wisneski, R. J., and Rothman, R. H.: Microdiscectomy techniques. Semin. Spine Surg. 1:54–59, 1989.

121. Wood, K. B., Popp, C. A., Transfeldt, E. E., et al.: Radiographic evaluation of instability in spondylolisthesis. Spine 19:1697–1703, 1994.

122. Wood, K. B., Garvey, T. A., Gundry, C., et al.: Magnetic resonance imaging of the thoracic spine: Evaluation of asymptomatic individuals. J. Bone Joint Surg. Am. 77:1631–1638, 1995.

123. Zdeblick, T. A.: A prospective randomized study of lumbar fusion. Spine 18:983–991, 1993.

124. Zeiger, H. E.: Comparison of chemonucleolysis and microsurgical discectomy for the treatment of herniated lumbar disc. Spine 12:796–799, 1987.

125. Zucherman, J., Derby, R., Hsu, K., et al.: Normal magnetic resonance imaging with abnormal discography. Spine 13:1355–1359, 1988.

Rehabilitation

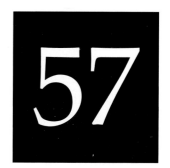

C H A P T E R

Workers' Compensation As It Affects the Spine

Compensation Low Back and Neck Pain

Scott D. Boden, M.D.

Sam W. Wiesel, M.D.

Low back pain has plagued health care systems dating back to at least the ancient Egyptians 5000 years ago.[95] Today, low back pain is one of the most common medical conditions in the Western world, afflicting up to 85 per cent of all persons at some time during their lives.[82] Although neck injuries occur in industry, the majority are caused by motor vehicle accidents. As a result, many neck injuries have both a compensation and a litigation component.[42, 54]

Low back pain and especially neck pain are illnesses of all people, not just workers. However, these problems pose special challenges in the industrial setting, and back pain has become the most common disabling musculoskeletal symptom in the Western workforce. Despite the magnitude of the problem, surprisingly little has been done to provide an organized approach to the management of low back or neck pain in industry. As a result, the potential for misuse and abuse of the workers' compensation system persists.[35]

In this chapter, the epidemiology and impact of compensation and the spine are outlined to establish a basis for the setting in which control strategies must function. Efforts at prevention as well as standardized evaluation and treatment programs are discussed, which may help reduce the impact of this ubiquitous problem.

PREVALENCE AND IMPACT OF INDUSTRIAL LOW BACK PAIN

The exact incidence and prevalence of low back pain in industry are unknown. It has been estimated that annually, 2 per cent of the United States' workforce incurs industrially related back injuries.[53] Several population studies in Sweden have demonstrated a prevalence of 60 to 80 per cent.[43] Rowe reviewed data from a large group of employees at the Eastman Kodak Company just before their retirement and found that at some time during their careers, 56 per cent of them had low back pain severe enough to require medical care.[74]

The impact of low back pain in the workplace is formidable. Kelsey and associates reported that back symptoms were the most common chronic condition resulting in decreased work capacity and reduced leisure-time activities for people below the age of 45 years.[48] Over a 10-year period in Sweden (1960–1971), back pain was responsible for 12.5 per cent of all sick days; of all available workdays, 1 per cent were lost each year because of back complaints (an average of 2.5 days for each working person yearly).[40] In Great Britain for 1969 to 1970, Benn and Wood found that 3.6 per cent of all workdays were lost because of low back pain.[6] In 1974, Wood and Badley reported that 1011 days per 1000 working persons were lost each year for the same reason.[94]

In the United States, based on estimates derived from the Bureau of Labor Statistics Annual Survey of Injuries and Illnesses, about 1 million workers suffered back injuries in 1980. Back injuries accounted for almost one out of every five injuries and illnesses in the workplace, although the frequency is variable, depending on the industry.[13] This 20 per cent ratio is similar to that reported in Great Britain and Canada.[2] Data from the National Health Survey indicate that in 1983, back impairment and intervertebral disc disorders were reported as chronic conditions by 8 million currently employed persons.[16] Only heart conditions and hypertension had a higher prevalence.

More recent data from the Department of Labor Injury and Illness Survey demonstrate that back injuries accounted for 23 per cent of all 1983 cases involving disability in the 18 states surveyed.[18] The majority of these disability cases (87 per cent) were sprains or strains, with 4 per cent dislocations and 2 per cent bruises or contusions. Although lumbosacral sprain is the most common diagnosis rendered in the compensation setting, herniated intervertebral discs, spinal stenosis, and spondylolisthesis are also seen. In addition, Rowe reported that inflammatory arthritis may be responsible for up to 20 per cent of "nonspecific" low back pain.[73]

Data from the records of the Liberty Mutual Insurance Company in 1989 indicate that low back pain cases represented 16 per cent of all claims but 33 per cent of all claims costs. The mean cost per case of low back pain was $8321. Medical costs represented 32 per cent of the total costs, and indemnity costs (payment for lost time) represented 66 per cent.[89] These data support the strategies that focus on minimizing lost time from work rather than purely minimizing the medical costs associated with low back pain episodes.

The financial impact of compensation low back pain is estimated to surpass $25 billion in annual expenditures by the end of the 1990s.[80] One study of a large industrial manufacturer found that claims related to back injuries constituted 19 per cent of all workers' compensation claims but were responsible for 41 per cent of the total injury costs.[82] Furthermore, it has been shown that the small percentage of claimants who receive permanent total or partial disability payments are responsible for a disproportionate amount of the total costs associated with back pain or injury. It is estimated that less than 10 per cent of back pain cases account for nearly 75 per cent of lost days, medical costs, and indemnity payments.[1] Careful evaluation of these cases will likely provide the greatest conservation of resources and increase in productivity.

RISK FACTORS FOR LOW BACK PAIN

It would be ideal if risk factors could be used to identify persons at high risk for low back pain or at risk for prolonged symptoms once injury occurs. Unfortunately, the complex epidemiology of this problem makes early identification and screening somewhat difficult. Although as many as 65 per cent of low back pain patients are unaware of any specific causative factor, several risk factors have been identified.[26, 73]

Low back pain typically begins in young adulthood, affecting the most productive years of life in an industrial worker. There is a rising prevalence with age until the fourth and fifth decades, after which there is a leveling off or decrease in prevalence.[73] Attacks of low back pain seem to be more common among those who have had back pain before. Buckle and colleagues found that among 68 patients, over 70 per cent reported at least one prior episode.[11] Rowe similarly noted that 85 per cent of low back pain patients had a history of intermittent episodes.[73]

Several studies have examined sex differences in the risk for low back injury.[3, 33] Women represent about 40 per cent of the working population but develop only 20 per cent of the industrial low back problems. This may be because women are typically employed in less physically demanding jobs. In a review of 31,000 employees of a manufacturer, Bigos and coworkers found that women had statistically fewer injuries than men but had an increased risk of becoming a high-cost injury claimant.[9] In occupations demanding strenuous physical efforts, Magora reported that women had a higher incidence of low back pain than men.[55] Other investigators report equal prevalence of back pain in men and women.[7]

Many investigators have examined the association between various radiographic abnormalities and the occurrence of back pain, usually concluding that no association exists.[30] Rowe reported that the prevalence of leg-length differences, increased lumbosacral angle, spondylolisthesis, transitional lumbosacral vertebrae, and spina bifida occulta among low back pain patients was not significantly different from that among a control group.[73] In a cohort study of 321 men, Frymoyer and associates found no correlation of back pain with transitional vertebrae, Schmorl's nodes, or the disc vacuum sign.[26] However, when there were traction spurs or disc space narrowing between the fourth and fifth lumbar vertebrae, an increased incidence of severe low back pain was evident.

At least two studies found low back pain to be more prevalent in cigarette smokers than in nonsmokers.[27, 79] It is not clear whether this association is a result of increased intradiscal pressure from chronic coughing and straining or if nicotine itself has a direct biochemical role in the pathophysiology of back injury.

Poor physical fitness may be a predisposing factor for back pain. Cady and colleagues, in a prospective study of firefighters, found that the least fit group of employees was 10 times more susceptible to developing back pain than the most fit group.[12]

One of the more well-studied risk factors for industrial low back pain is job type, but the data are inconsistent. The Bureau of Labor Statistics has identified construction and mining as the industries with the highest incidence of back injuries, followed closely by the trucking industry and the nursing profession.[49] Workers in government and finance were least likely to be affected. Accordingly, it has been hypothesized that the worker in heavy industry is most susceptible to back injury. Sairanen and coworkers, however, found no significant difference between lumberjacks and controls doing light work with regard to low back pain occurrence.[76] Nachemson has also maintained that there is not a high incidence among heavy laborers.[64] In a retrospective study of 2000 workers, Rowe found that 35 per cent of sedentary workers and 45 per cent of heavy handlers had visited physicians for low back pain within a 10-year period.[73] Eastrand's survey of Swedish workers suggested that the number of years spent doing heavy labor had a cumulative effect on predisposition to low back problems.[21]

Despite contradictory data, it seems likely that certain tasks in the workplace are important in the development of low back pain. Snook and associates found that handling tasks were responsible for 70 per cent of low back injuries, and Klein and colleagues reported similar findings.[49, 81] The weight of the object lifted has been implicated in lifting injuries. In a recent study, more than half the injured workers had lifted objects weighing at least 60 pounds.[17] The risk for low back pain is thought to be increased by prolonged sitting and exposure to vibration.[47] Less physically stressful but boring and repetitive jobs (assembly-line work) have also been linked to an increased incidence of back pain.[8]

Magora reported that workers who were not satisfied with their present occupation, place of employment, or social situation had a high incidence of low back pain.[56] This was also true of workers who felt that a high degree of responsibility and concentration was required of them. A correlation between back injuries and poor employee appraisal ratings by the supervisor has been demonstrated by Bigos and coworkers.[9] Frymoyer and associates showed an association between diminished spinal motion and specific abnormalities on formal psychologic testing in back pain patients.[28] Rossignol and colleagues showed that limitations in performing at work, limitations in activities of daily living, and a history of compensation (at any time) were the three indicators most likely to predict future work disability because of a low back problem.[72] It is difficult to determine whether unusual psychologic characteristics in the low back patient are primary problems or secondary to medical illness, however. Certainly it is clear that many job and workplace factors other than mechanical loading of the spine play a role in the development of industrial low back pain.

PREVENTION OF LOW BACK PAIN

In view of the elusive nature of the etiology of industrial low back pain, it is not surprising that attempts at prevention in industry have not met with great success. Previous efforts have focused on careful selection of workers, training in proper lifting techniques, and designing the job to fit the worker.

The goal of careful worker selection is to screen job applicants with the hope of identifying and bypassing those potential workers at increased risk for developing low back pain. The most commonly used screening tool is the pre-employment history and physical examination. Rowe, reviewing injuries at Kodak, found that only 10 per cent of workers who would subsequently develop low back problems could be identified from a pre-employment medical history and examination.[74] He found that the best predictor was a history

of back problems, but potential employees often do not volunteer such information.

Pre-employment lumbar spine radiographs have been advocated in the past.[60] Most recent investigations have shown that this procedure has little value.[62, 75] The American Occupational Medical Association has recommended that the lumbar spine roentgenographic examination not be used as a routine screening procedure for back problems but reserved as a diagnostic tool when there are appropriate clinical indications. Techniques such as biplanar radiography and new dynamic measurements of flexion-extension views may prove to be more sensitive indicators of early spine dysfunction.[10, 71] Further investigation with these methods will determine their role in the prediction of low back disorders.

Pre-employment strength testing is based on the premise that careful matching of the worker's strength to requirements of the job will help prevent low back injuries. The only strength testing method proved to be effective in industry is isometric simulation of the job, as advocated by Chaffin and coworkers.[14] In a series of studies, they found that a worker's likelihood of sustaining a back injury or musculoskeletal illness increased when job lifting requirements approached or exceeded the strength capacity demonstrated on an isometric simulation of the job.

Education and training on lifting methods have been allocated much time, effort, and expense. Despite endorsement from the National Safety Council, there is little evidence that such programs can reduce the incidence of low back problems.[95] Snook and colleagues found that back injuries were as common among workers who had participated in such instructional programs as among those who had not received training.[81]

Finally, it may be possible to alter the workplace and the job to better fit the abilities of the worker. The concept of matching the job to the worker, rather than the reverse, can be accomplished by defining workloads rather than selection of workers. Ergonomic redesign of the job, such as reducing the size of loads to allow them to be lifted between the legs or modifying the working methods involved, has been considered the most promising method for the prevention of low back injuries.[95]

FACTORS AFFECTING THE DURATION OF WORK LOSS

Once a low back pain episode has occurred, efforts must concentrate on returning the employee to work as soon as possible and identifying patients who will require permanent adjustments of their work duties. Although 90 per cent of patients return to work within six weeks of the onset of the back pain, the importance of early return to employment cannot be overemphasized. Longer delays in return are clearly associated with a decreased likelihood of ever returning to the workforce. McGill reported that workers with back complaints who are out of work over six months have only a 50 per cent possibility of ever returning to productive employment.[60] If they are off work over one year, this possibility drops to 25 per cent; if more than two years, it is almost zero. Accordingly, Frymoyer and Cats-Baril hypothesized that intensive rehabilitation early in the course of a disabling low back episode can prevent long-term disability and is cost effective.[25]

Although a multivariate model to predict disability from low back pain has not yet been developed, several factors have been shown to affect the duration of work absenteeism. First is the severity and type of injury. This may be difficult to evaluate, because the history provided by the patient may be consciously or unconsciously biased. Patients who have a potential for compensation typically identify the onset of a problem as acute rather than chronic. Most injuries, however, produce few objective physical findings.

Because objective findings are usually absent, other factors must be considered. Gallagher and associates concluded that psychologic factors rather than physical factors predict return to work among patients with low back pain.[29] Waddell and coworkers estimated that objective physical impairment accounts for only half the total disability that is also affected by psychologic reactions such as emotional distress.[87] Similar conclusions were reached by Deyo and Tsio-Wu, who found that low educational level and low income were strong correlates with work absenteeism.[19] In a study of 1483 patients, Hall and colleagues demonstrated that those discharged back to work with no restrictions were twice as likely to return to work successfully than those discharged with some restrictions based on reports of pain or unfounded fears of reinjury.[37] Parascandola found that information in a nursing history can predict extended lost time from low back problems.[69] That study found that individuals who live alone, do not actively participate in their treatment regimens, and/or have no family support systems are disabled significantly longer than those who live with others, actively participate in their medical care, and/or have support systems.

The role of compensation in the length of disability from low back pain is an issue that remains unresolved. Sander and Meyers found that patients injured on duty had a statistically significantly longer period of disability than those injured off duty.[77] Evaluation of the compensation patient may be complicated by malingering, conscious exaggeration and creation of symptoms, and subconscious amplification of the injury and symptoms. The conscious manipulator often arrives at the physician's office with extensive documentation and an above-average command of the medical jargon pertinent to his or her injury. These patients take a persistently defensive attitude, may be hostile, and may selectively withhold vital information. In contrast, documentation is less important to the subconscious exaggerator, whose defensive attitude is more transient; he or she rarely and only briefly expresses anger and does not knowingly withhold useful information. Hayes and associates studied the effect of financial compensation on responses to psychometric testing in 231 chronic low back pain patients and found signifi-

cantly higher inconsistency scores and nonorganic scores, suggesting that many psychometric test results are invalid for this group of patients.[39]

Sanderson and coworkers found that patients with compensation claims had greater disability as assessed by the Oswestry Score, but those claiming compensation and still working had significantly less disability than those claiming compensation who were unemployed.[78] This entitlement for workers in the United States stems from the Prussian paradigm as recounted by Nortin Hadler; however, the system is based on trying to relate physical impairment to disability—an impossible and imprecise task.[36] The federal government and the individual states have developed their own regulations, and compensation payments can amount to as much as 100 per cent of the worker's wage. Increased settlements for compensation claims and increases in the dollar value of compensation are highly associated with a subsequent increase in the number of claims made for alleged injury. Several investigations have concluded that a higher level of benefits prolonged the duration of back-related work loss.[88] The presence of compensation claims is also associated with a reduced rate of successful rehabilitation,[84] as well as less successful surgical results.[24, 25, 32, 50] There are studies that report successful multidisciplinary rehabilitation programs for patients with low back pain and workers' compensations claims.[20, 51]

Workers' compensation laws influence diagnostic evaluation, treatment, and recovery from injury.[88] Beals suggested that, paradoxically, financial compensation may discourage return to work, the appeal process may increase disability, an open claim may inhibit return to work, and recovering patients may be unable to return to work.[5] Although one study concluded that personal-injury litigants do not describe their pain as more severe than do nonlitigants,[61] other studies showed that if a lawyer becomes involved in the claim process, there is a greater probability of chronic pain and disability.[25, 34]

Health care providers also share responsibility for delaying return to work and escalating costs. Some physicians see the injured worker at unnecessarily frequent intervals. Others take advantage of the third-party fee-for-service payment system by liberally using their own radiography and physical therapy facilities, with questionable medical benefit to the patient. The result is a highly variable quality of health care and unnecessary expenditure of financial resources, both of which have served as the impetus for the development of standardized approaches to the diagnosis and treatment of industrial low back pain.

STANDARDIZED APPROACH TO THE DIAGNOSIS AND TREATMENT OF INDUSTRIAL LOW BACK PAIN

The vast majority of low back injuries are not serious, and most employees can return to work in a short time. However, employees return to work sooner and incur lower medical and compensation costs if an organized approach to evaluation, diagnosis, and treatment is used.[66, 91] There have been few standardized diagnostic or treatment protocols available in industry.

We recently evaluated the effect of such an organized approach in two industries. The study was prompted by a 1980 review of employee work loss at a public utility company that revealed that 45 per cent of all lost time was the result of back injuries.[4] In addition, the number of back operations performed on these employees was much higher than in a noncompensation setting.

Under a newly developed program, the clinical approach to every patient was standardized by using an algorithm for low back pain diagnosis and treatment. The algorithm was derived from information on previous patients with therapeutic successes as well as those who failed to respond. This protocol enabled the treating physician to make decisions based on well-delineated rules rather than on intuition or emotion. The monitoring physicians were unbiased, because they were not allowed to become involved in the patient's ongoing care. The algorithm has been modified to incorporate new data and technology since it was originally published.[91] We regard the use of a systematic and standardized approach as critical, even though we expect the pathways of the algorithm to evolve.

Two employee populations were studied with monitoring programs of differing intensity. "Passive" surveillance was used to follow back pain patients from the U.S. Postal Service, which employs 14,000 people in the Washington, DC, area. These patients were evaluated by one of the investigators (all orthopedic surgeons) after the initial episode of back pain. Computer forms were completed and, based on diagnostic data and impressions, a prediction was made regarding when the patient should return to work. This estimate was based in part on previous averages for specific diagnostic entities. The patient was seen again only if return to work was not achieved within five days of the predicted date or if surgical intervention was subsequently proposed by the treating physician. The study was conducted for one year (1982–1983) and resulted in a 41 per cent decrease in the number of low back pain patients, a 60 per cent decrease in days lost from work, and a 55 per cent decrease in compensation costs.

A second group of patients was "actively" followed. The Potomac Electric Power Company (PEPCO) employs 5380 workers, 75 per cent of whom are blue collar. Under the active monitoring program, PEPCO patients with back pain were seen weekly or biweekly by one of the investigators until their return to work. If there was any disagreement in management according to the algorithm between the monitoring orthopedic surgeon and the treating physician, the latter was contacted for discussion. If an acceptable agreement could not be reached, a third physician was consulted for an independent medical opinion.

PEPCO patients were followed in this fashion for 10 years (1981–1990). Using the standardized approach, there was an average 51 per cent decrease in the num-

ber of low back cases (from 59 a year before the study to 29 a year during the study years). There was also a 55 per cent decrease in days lost (from 3701 a year to 1684 a year). The average time lost per injury dropped by 40 per cent. The cost savings were dramatic: nearly $2.6 million was saved over the 10-year study (costs based on time lost from work; direct medical cost savings not included). The number of surgical procedures decreased from nine in the year before the study to an average of three per year over the study years. Perhaps more significant is that the surgical procedures performed under the algorithm criteria resulted in a much higher rate of successful patient return to work (90 vs. 56 per cent).[90]

Both the passive and the active surveillance systems produced important savings and reductions in work disability. Although many of the reductions were greater in the active system, such a program is more expensive. A cost-effectiveness study is needed to resolve this issue.

The cause of these large reductions with the standardized approach remains speculative. Workers may have realized that they were being closely observed by low back experts and that they would not get time off work without legitimate problems. Light duty was made available to recovering patients, and although there were no records concerning light-duty availability in prestudy years, this opportunity may have contributed to the savings. Finally, acceptance of the fact that surgical procedures would rarely return workers to very heavy duty and recognition that surgical indications were limited helped decrease the number of surgical procedures.

The employee response to this program has been enthusiastic. Our experience to date with this standardized approach to the diagnosis and treatment of low back pain has certainly accomplished the goals required of any health care system in industry: (1) early return to normal activity, (2) avoidance of unnecessary surgery, (3) efficient and precise use of diagnostic studies, and (4) a treatment format with affordable costs to society.

INCIDENCE OF NECK INJURIES

Various types of trauma can result in neck pain, but the most common cause is a hyperextension injury. The precise number of neck injuries is difficult to determine. It is estimated that over half a million cases of hyperextension occur each year.[70] These injuries represent 2.8 per cent of all occupants in police-reported automobile accidents. It is estimated that 85 per cent of all neck injuries result from motor vehicle accidents, and the majority involve rear-end collisions.[44, 45, 83]

LITIGATION IN ACUTE NECK INJURIES

The effect of litigation in acute neck injury has been the subject of several investigations. The typical accident leading to a hyperextension injury holds the striking vehicle at fault. In addition, the injured person rarely has an objective abnormality and appears to be a blameless victim incapacitated by subjective symptoms that are difficult to prove or disprove. In this setting, it is not surprising that more than half of the accident victims receive some type of settlement.[68]

Several studies have investigated the relationship between the presence or settlement of litigation and ultimate relief of symptoms. Gotten studied 100 patients whose whiplash injuries prompted them to sue; 88 per cent were asymptomatic after settlement.[31] Approximately 80 per cent of the patients who were satisfied with their settlements had no further symptoms, whereas only 25 per cent of those who were not satisfied with their settlements experienced complete relief. MacNab reported that 45 per cent of his study population (mostly hyperextension injuries) had persistent symptoms, even after settlement.[54] Although most reports maintain that litigation is a major negative influence on recovery from neck injuries, some studies have found no relationship between the presence or settlement of litigation and the ultimate relief of symptoms.[42, 67]

STANDARDIZED APPROACH TO THE DIAGNOSIS AND TREATMENT OF NECK PAIN IN INDUSTRY

Despite the prevalence of neck pain, industry has no standardized diagnostic and treatment protocols. Although most episodes of neck pain are self-limited, it has been shown that employees receive better care and return to work sooner if an organized approach to the evaluation and treatment of their neck problems is used.

A cervical spine algorithm has been developed and implemented in the same public utility company (PEPCO) as described earlier for the low back pain protocol.[92] Each injured employee was seen within one week of injury, and recovery was monitored using the algorithm. If a patient's clinical progress differed from that predicted by the algorithm, an independent medical examination was obtained.

The initial analysis indicated that 8 per cent of all time lost from work was caused by neck injuries. Results with the cervical spine algorithm were encouraging after the first year. Days lost from work and light-duty days because of neck injuries were reduced 65 per cent. The total number of acute neck accidents was 50 per cent less than during the previous (baseline) year. The number and type of automobile accidents reported were unchanged. Similar results were maintained during a 10-year follow-up period.[90]

The benefits of the standardized approach were similar to those for the low back pain algorithm. In comparing the two populations, neck cases were only 20 per cent as frequent as low back cases, but the amount of lost time and light-duty time per case were substantially higher for the neck patients.

IMPAIRMENT DETERMINATION

Despite successes in the diagnosis and management of low back and neck problems with these standardized approaches, some patients are unable to return to their preinjury level of function. Any physical injury that occurs in the work-related setting must be quantitated, especially if the patient is unable to return to his or her previous level of employment. For example, a laborer who undergoes back or neck surgery should not be expected to return to a position requiring heavy lifting. Such workers must be given a permanent partial impairment rating, a task that has had few satisfactory or accepted guidelines.

It is imperative to understand the distinction between physical impairment and physical disability. Physical impairment is an objective anatomic or pathologic dysfunction leading to loss of normal body ability.[86] Permanent impairment is an objective assessment of functional abnormality or loss after the acute injury phase and after maximal medical rehabilitation. Physical disability is a measure of reduced capacity to engage in gainful everyday activity as a result of some impairment.

Assessment of physical impairment is solely a medical responsibility.[85] However, the more subjective disability rating should be assigned by someone other than the treating physician. Disability rating is best calculated by administrative, vocational, or legal specialists from impairment ratings generated by the physician.[63]

A major problem for orthopedic surgeons is the paucity of useful guidelines to determine physical impairment ratings for the spine. One source is the American Medical Association's *Guide to the Evaluation of Permanent Impairment*.[22] The AMA *Guide* uses the concept of the "whole man," with each part of the body representing a part of the whole, based on functional use. In this system, the spine contributes a maximum of 90 per cent of the whole man (lumbar spine). The AMA *Guide* originally used loss of motion as the sole criterion for impairment and considered pain only when it could be substantiated by clinical findings. Measurement of spine motion, however, has a poor correlation with physical impairment, owing to large variations in normals as well as poorly reproducible measurement techniques.[15, 85] The third edition of the *Guide* replaced goniometer measurements with inclinometer readings, which may prove to be more reliable.[46, 59] The most recent fourth edition of the *Guide* de-emphasizes range of motion as the primary determinent of spinal impairment.[2a]

The other commonly cited source is the *Manual for Orthopaedic Surgeons in Evaluating Permanent Physical Impairment*, published by the American Academy of Orthopaedic Surgeons.[57] The AAOS *Manual* gives suggested impairment ratings for several diagnostic entities but relies heavily on subjective symptoms. Frequently, the patient with low back or neck pain has few or no objective clinical findings. The result is that many physicians take into consideration age, degree of pain, motivation, intelligence, education, and social factors and are actually rating disability rather than impairment.[33, 58]

The current smorgasbord of impairment guidelines and the vast spectrum of interpretations generate tremendous variation in ratings.[96] Clark and colleagues recently developed a new impairment schedule based on a comprehensive literature review and the collected opinions of a large number of back specialists.[15] Their goal was to develop a system that would give more consistent results by incorporating more objective data and less subjectivity. Preliminary results with a small number of cases have been favorable, but more extensive data are still awaited.

Perhaps one of the most workable guidelines available for evaluating the low back was described by Feffer.[23] This scheme uses a consensus of diagnosis-related impairment ratings compiled from a survey of members of the International Society for Study of the Lumbar Spine (ISSLS). The ISSLS ratings for a standardized set of diagnostic situations were then matched to the physical exertion requirements developed by the Social Security Administration. The result is a logical and integrated system of diagnosis-related low back evaluation guidelines (Table 57–1). A survey of members of the Cervical Spine Research Society has facilitated compilation of a similar database for neck injuries (Table 57–2).

In general, the physician should treat the back pain patient conservatively and wait up to six weeks for a response. The worker with an acute back strain should be able to return to work within two weeks; a heavy laborer may require three to four weeks of treatment. At the time of initial return to work, there should be some activity restrictions, such as the elimination of repeated bending, stooping, and twisting. Three weeks after return, these restrictions can be dropped, and most patients will have a complete recovery.

Treatment of the patient with an acute neck sprain, defined as a soft tissue injury of an otherwise normal neck, should permit return to normal activities within two to three weeks. The recovery period for hyperextension injuries from vehicle accidents depends on the severity of symptoms and the type of work to which

Table 57–1. WORK RESTRICTION CLASSIFICATION OF COMPENSABLE LOW BACK INJURIES

Work Category	Work Restriction	PPPI*	Relevant Diagnosis
Very Heavy	Occasional lifting in excess of 100 lbs Frequent lifting of 50 lbs or more	0%	Recovered acute back strain Herniated nucleus pulposus treated conservatively with complete recovery
Heavy	Occasional lifting of 100 lbs Frequent lifting of up to 50 lbs	0%	Healed acute traumatic spondylolisthesis Healed transverse process fracture
Medium	Occasional lifting of 50 lbs	<5%	Chronic back strain Degenerative lumbar intervertebral disc disease under reasonable control
	Frequent lifting of 25 lbs		Herniated nucleus pulposus treated by surgical discectomy and completely recovered Spondylolysis/spondylolisthesis under reasonable control Healed compression fracture with 10% residual loss of vertebral height
Light	Occasional lifting of no more than 20 lbs	10 to 15%	Degenerative lumbar intervertebral disc disease with chronic pain and restriction Herniated nucleus pulposus treated conservatively or operatively, but left with some discomfort, restriction, and neurologic deficit
	Frequent lifting of up to 10 lbs		Acute traumatic spondylolysis/spondylolisthesis, treated conservatively or operatively, but with residual discomfort and restriction Lumbar canal stenosis Moderately severe osteoarthritis accompanied by instability Healed compression fracture with 25 to 50% residual loss of vertebral height
Secondary	Occasional lifting of 10 lbs Frequent lifting of no more than lightweight articles and dockets	20 to 25%	Multiply operated back (failed back syndrome)

* PPPI, Permanent partial physical impairment.
Adapted from Social Security Administration Regulations.

Table 57–2. WORK RESTRICTION CLASSIFICATION OF COMPENSABLE NECK INJURIES

Work Category	Work Restriction	PPPI*	Relevant Diagnosis
Very Heavy	Occasional lifting of over 100 lbs Frequent lifting of 50 lbs or more Overhead work	0%	Neck strain with complete recovery Hyperextension injury with complete recovery
Heavy	Occasional lifting of 100 lbs Frequent lifting of up to 50 lbs Overhead work	0%	Herniated nucleus pulposus, treated conservatively, with complete recovery Pre-existing degenerative disease or cervical canal stenosis with secondary neck strain, with complete recovery
Medium	Occasional lifting of 50 lbs	5%	Chronic neck strain Degenerative cervical disc disease, under reasonable control
	Frequent lifting of 25 lbs		Herniated nucleus pulposus treated by surgical discectomy, with complete recovery Hyperextension injury with residual pain Healed odontoid/hangman's fracture treated nonoperatively
	Restricted overhead work		Pre-existing, radiologically evident degenerative disease with secondary hyperextension injury, with moderate pain and restriction
Light	Occasional lifting of no more than 20 lbs	10 to 15%	Degenerative cervical disc disease, with chronic pain and restriction Herniated nucleus pulposus treated conservatively or operatively, with residual discomfort, restriction, and neurologic deficit
	Frequent lifting of up to 10 lbs		Hyperextension injury with chronic pain and restriction Cervical canal stenosis Moderately severe osteoarthritis accompanied by instability
	No overhead work		Hangman's fracture treated with fusion Odontoid fracture treated with fusion Burst/compression fracture of lower cervical spine with no neurologic deficit, treated with external fixation or fusion
Sedentary	Occasional lifting of 10 lbs	25%	Multiply operated neck (constant pain) Pre-existing cervical stenosis with neck injury, treated by surgery, with patient subjectively and objectively worse

* PPPI, Permanent partial physical impairment.
Adapted from Social Security Administration Regulations.

the patient must return. Often, busy professional patients return to work after one week. Nonmanual laborers can usually return in two weeks. Patients employed in positions involving heavy manual labor may require three to four weeks of treatment. Generally, most patients are able to return to work by six weeks after injury and should be encouraged to do so, even if mild symptoms persist.

The majority of the small group of patients who remain symptomatic have continuing complaints without objective findings. In this case, if the physician believes the patient, a 5 to 10 per cent impairment rating is fair; otherwise, no impairment should be assigned. In either case, the physician should encourage early, gradual, biomechanically controlled return to activity and work for these patients with no objective findings.[65] If the patient will not cooperate, a more formal functional capacity evaluation may be war-

ranted to better define the capabilities and limitations of the worker and to assist in finding a more physically compatible job. The patient with a true radiculopathy should never be expected to return to very heavy work, nor should an operation be expected to qualify him or her for heavy work. After discectomy, impairment typically ranges from 10 per cent with an excellent operative result to 20 per cent if the patient has continued symptoms. An employee who is given a permanent partial impairment rating must have a restructuring of his or her work duties based on the new physical exertion restriction.

SUMMARY

The impact of compensation low back and neck pain on society has deemed it a significant health care problem. Specific risk factors have been implicated for spine problems in industry. Although many studies on risk factors are contradictory, it is evident that those who have had back pain in the past are likely to have it again. It is important to understand how the relationship of pain, impairment, and subsequent disability may be different in compensation patients. Accordingly, specially designed strategies for the standardized evaluation and treatment of lumbar and cervical spine pain in the industrial setting have proved to be effective at delivering quality care, decreasing the costs of medical treatment, and minimizing lost productivity. Prospective, randomized trials in the compensation setting are required to validate the reported results for multidisciplinary functional restoration programs.

References

1. Abenhaim, L., and Suissa, S.: Importance and economic burden of occupational back pain: A study of 2,500 cases representative of Quebec. J. Occup. Med. *29*:670–674, 1987.

2a. American Medical Association: Guides to the Evaluation of Permanent Impairment. 4th ed. Edited by T. C. Doege. Chicago, American Medical Association, 1993, pp. 94–138.

2. Akeson, W. H., and Murphy, R.: Editorial comments: Low back pain. Clin. Orthop. *129*:2–3, 1977.

3. Andersson, G. B. J.: Low back pain in industry: Epidemiological aspects. Scand. J. Rehabil. Med. *11*:163–168, 1979.

4. Bauer, W.: Scope of industrial low back pain. *In* Wiesel, S. W., Feffer, H., and Rothman, R. (eds.): Industrial Low Back Pain. Charlottesville, VA, Michie Co., 1985, pp. 1–35.

5. Beals, R. K.: Compensation and recovery from injury. West. J. Med. *140*:233–237, 1984.

6. Benn, R., and Wood, P.: Pain in the back. Rheumatol. Rehabil. *14*:121–128, 1975.

7. Bergenudd, H., and Nilsson, B.: Back pain in middle age; occupational workload and psychologic factors: An epidemiologic survey. Spine *13*:58–60, 1988.

8. Bigos, S. J., Spengler, D. M., Martin, N. A., et al.: Back injuries in industry: A retrospective study II. Injury factors. Spine *11*:246–251, 1986.

9. Bigos, S. J., Spengler, D. M., Martin, N. A., et al.: Back injuries in industry: A retrospective study III. Employee-related factors. Spine *11*:252–256, 1986.

10. Boden, S. D., and Wiesel, S. W.: Lumbosacral segmental motion in normal individuals—a dynamic measurement technique. *In* Transactions of the 35th Annual Meeting of the Orthopaedic Research Society, Las Vegas, 1988.

11. Buckle, P., Kember, P., Wood, A., et al.: Factors influencing occupational back pain in Bedfordshire. Spine *5*:254–258, 1980.

12. Cady, L., Bischoff, D., O'Connell, E., et al.: Strength and fitness and subsequent back injuries in firefighters. J. Occup. Med. *21*:269–272, 1979.

13. California, State of: Disabling Work Injuries Under Workers' Compensation Involving Back Strain per 1,000 Workers, by Industry, California 1979. San Francisco, Department of Industrial Relations, Division of Labor Statistics and Research, 1980.

14. Chaffin, D., Herin, G., and Keyserling, W.: Pre-employment strength testing: An updated position. J. Occup. Med. *20*:403–409, 1978.

15. Clark, W. L., Haldeman, S., Johnson, P., et al.: Back impairment and disability determination: Another attempt at objective, reliable rating. Spine *13*:332–341, 1988.

16. Department of Health and Human Services: Disability Days United States, 1983. Publication no. (PHS) 87-1586. Hyattsville, MD, National Center for Health Statistics, 1986.

17. Department of Labor, Bureau of Labor Statistics: Back Injuries Associated With Lifting. Bulletin 2144. August 1982.

18. Department of Labor, Bureau of Labor Statistics: Injury and Illness Data Available From 1983 Workers' Compensation Records. Announcement 86-1. March 1986.

19. Deyo, R. A., and Tsio-Wu, Y. J.: Functional disability due to back pain—a population-based study indicating the importance of socioeconomic factors. Arthritis Rheum. *30*:1247–1253, 1987.

20. Di Fabio, R. P., Mackey, G., and Holte, J. B.: Disability and functional status in patients with low back pain receiving workers' compensation: A descriptive study with implications for the efficacy of physical therapy. Phys. Ther. *75*:180–193, 1995.

21. Eastrand, N.: Medical, psychological, and social factors associated with back abnormalities and self reported back pain: A cross sectional study of male employees in a Swedish pulp and paper industry. Br. J. Ind. Med. *44*:327–336, 1987.

22. Engelberg, A. L.: Guide to the Evaluation of Permanent Impairment. 3rd ed. Chicago, American Medical Association, 1988, pp. 71–94.

23. Feffer, H. L.: Evaluation of the low back diagnosis related impairment rating. *In* Wiesel, S. W., Feffer, H. L., and Rothman, R. H. (eds.): Industrial Low Back Pain. Charlottesville, VA, Michie Co., 1985, pp. 642–665.

24. Franklin, G. M., Haug, J., Heyer, N. J., et al.: Outcome of lumbar fusion in Washington state workers' compensation. Spine *19*:1897–1904, 1994.

25. Frymoyer, J. W., and Cats-Baril, W.: Predictors of low back pain disability. Clin. Orthop. *221*:89–98, 1987.

26. Frymoyer, J. W., Newberg, A., Pope, M. H., et al.: Spine radiographs in patients with low-back pain. J. Bone Joint Surg. [Am.] *66*:1048–1055, 1984.

27. Frymoyer, J. W., Pope, M. H., Clements, J. H., et al.: Risk factors in low-back pain. J. Bone Joint Surg. [Am.] *65*:213–218, 1983.

28. Frymoyer, J. W., Rosen, J. C., Clements, J. H., et al.: Psychologic factors in low-back-pain disability. Clin. Orthop. *195*:178–184, 1985.

29. Gallagher, R. M., Rauh, V., Langelier, R., et al.: Psychological, but not physical, factors predict return to work in low back pain. Psychosom. Med. *48*:296, 1986.

30. Gibson, E. S.: The value of preplacement screening radiography of the low back. *In* Deyo, R. A. (ed.): Occupational Medicine: State of the Art Reviews. Vol. 3. Philadelphia, Hanley & Belfus, 1988, pp. 91–107.

31. Gotten, N.: Survey of one hundred cases of whiplash injury after settlement of litigation. JAMA *162*:856–857, 1956.

32. Greenough, C. G., Taylor, L. J., and Fraser, R. D.: Anterior lumbar fusion: Results, assessment techniques and prognostic factors. Eur. Spine J. *3*:225–230, 1994.

33. Greenwood, J. G.: Low-back impairment-rating practices of orthopaedic surgeons and neurosurgeons in West Virginia. Spine *10*:773–776, 1985.

34. Haddad, G. H.: Analysis of 2932 workers' compensation back injury cases—the impact on the cost to the system. Spine *12*:765–769, 1987.

35. Hadler, N. M.: Industrial rheumatology—the Australian and New Zealand experience with arm pain and backache in the workplace. Med. J. Aust. *144*:191–195, 1986.

36. Hadler, N. M.: The disabling backache: An international perspective. Spine *20*:640–649, 1995.

37. Hall, H., McIntosh, G., Melles, T., and Holowachuk, E.: Effect of discharge recommendations on outcome. Spine *19*:2033–2037, 1994.

38. Hansson, T., Bigos, S., Beecher, P., and Wortley, M.: The lumbar lordosis in acute and chronic low-back pain. Spine *10*:154–155, 1985.

39. Hayes, B., Solyom, C. A. E., Wing, P. C., and Berkowitz, J.: Use of psychometric measures and nonorganic signs testing in detecting nomogenic disorders in low back pain patients. Spine *18*:1254–1262, 1993.

40. Helander, E.: Back pain and work disability. Social Med. T. *50*:398–404, 1973 (Swedish).

41. Hirsch, C.: Etiology and pathogenesis of low back pain. Int. J. Med. Sci. *2*:362–370, 1966.

42. Hohl, M.: Soft tissue injuries of the neck in automobile accidents: Factors influencing prognosis. J. Bone Joint Surg. [Am.] *56*:1675–1682, 1974.

43. Hult, L.: Cervical, dorsal, and lumbar spine syndromes. Acta Orthop. Scand. Suppl. *17*:1–102, 1954.

44. Jackson, R.: The positive findings in alleged neck injuries. Am. J. Orthop. *6*:178–187, 1964.

45. Jackson, R.: Crashes cause most neck pain. Am. Med. News, December 5, 1966.

46. Keeley, J., Mayer, T. G., Cox, R., et al.: Quantification of lumbar function. Part 5: Reliability of range-of-motion measures in the sagittal plane and an in vivo torso rotation measurement technique. Spine 11:31–35, 1986.

47. Kelsey, J. L., and Golden, A. L.: Occupational and workplace factors associated with low back pain. In Deyo, R. A. (ed.): Occupational Medicine: State of the Art Reviews. Vol. 3. Philadelphia, Hanley & Belfus, 1988, pp. 7–16.

48. Kelsey, J. L., Pastides, H., and Bisbee, G.: Musculoskeletal Disorders: Their Frequency of Occurrence and Their Impact on the Population of the United States. New York, Neale Watson Academic Publications, 1978.

49. Klein, B. P., Jensen, R. C., and Sanderson, L. M.: Assessment of workers' compensation claims for back strains/sprains. J. Occup. Med. 26:443–448, 1984.

50. Knox, B. D., and Chapman, T. M.: Anterior lumbar interbody fusion for discogram concordant pain. J. Spinal Disord. 6:242–244, 1993.

51. Lanes, T. C., Gauron, E. F., Spratt, K. F., et al.: Long-term follow-up of patients with chronic back pain treated in a multidisciplinary rehabilitation program. Spine 20:801–806, 1995.

52. Laubach, L. L.: Comparative muscular strength of men and women: A review of the literature. Aviat. Space Environ. Med. 47:534–572, 1976.

53. Leavitt, S., Johnston, T., and Beyer, R.: The process of recovery: Patterns in industrial back injury. Part I. Cost and other quantitative measures of effort. Indust. Med. 40:7–14, 1971.

54. MacNab, I.: Acceleration injuries of the cervical spine. J. Bone Joint Surg. [Am.] 46:1797–1799, 1964.

55. Magora, A.: Investigation of the relation between low back pain and occupation: I. Age, sex, community, education and other factors. Indust. Med. Surg. 39:465–471, 1970.

56. Magora, A.: Investigation of the relation between low back pain and occupation: V. Psychological aspects. Scand. J. Rehabil. Med. 5:191–196, 1973.

57. Manual for Orthopaedic Surgeons in Evaluating Permanent Physical Impairment. Chicago, American Academy of Orthopaedic Surgeons, 1960, pp. 28–29.

58. Mayer, T. G.: Assessment of lumbar function. Clin. Orthop. 221:99–109, 1987.

59. Mayer, T. G., Tencer, A. F., Kristoferson, S., and Mooney, V.: Use of noninvasive techniques for quantification of spinal range-of-motion in normal subjects and chronic low-back dysfunction patients. Spine 9:588–595, 1984.

60. McGill, C. M.: Industrial back problems—a control program. J. Occup. Med. 10:174–178, 1968.

61. Mendelson, G.: Compensation, pain complaints, and psychological disturbance. Pain 20:169–177, 1984.

62. Montgomery, C.: Pre-employment back x-ray. J. Occup. Med. 18:495–498, 1976.

63. Mooney, V.: Impairment, disability, and handicap. Clin. Orthop. 221:14–25, 1987.

64. Nachemson, A.: Low back pain: Its etiology and treatment. Clin. Med. 78:18–24, 1971.

65. Nachemson, A.: Work for all—for those with low back pain as well. Clin. Orthop. 179:77–85, 1983.

66. National Safety Council: Accident Facts. Chicago, National Safety Council, 1978, p. 26.

67. Norris, S. H., Watt, I.: The prognosis of neck injuries resulting from rear end vehicle collisions. J. Bone Joint Surg. [Br.] 65:608–614, 1983.

68. O'Neill, B., Haddon, W., Kelley, A. N., and Sorenson, W.: Automobile head restraint—frequency of neck injury claims in relation to the presence of head restraint. Am. J. Public Health 62:399–406, 1972.

69. Parascandola, J. M.: A behavioral approach to determining the prognosis in patients with lumbosacral radiculopathy. Rehab. Nursing 18:314–317, 1993.

70. Partyka, S.: Whiplash and other inertial force neck injuries in traffic accidents. Paper for the Mathematical Analysis Division,

National Center for Statistics and Analysis, Washington, DC, December 1981.

71. Pearcy, M., Portek, I., and Shepherd, J.: Three-dimensional x-ray analysis of normal movement in the lumbar spine. Spine 9:294–297, 1984.

72. Rossignol, M., Lortie, M., and Ledoux, E.: Comparison of spinal health indicators in predicting spinal status in a 1-year longitudinal study. Spine 18:54–60, 1993.

73. Rowe, M. L.: Low back pain in industry—a position paper. J. Occup. Med. 11:161–169, 1969.

74. Rowe, M. L.: Low back disability in industry—undated position. J. Occup. Med. 13:476–478, 1971.

75. Rowe, M. L.: Are routine spine films on workers in industry cost or risk benefit effective? J. Occup. Med. 24:41–43, 1982.

76. Sairanen, E., Brushaber, L., and Kaskinen, M.: Felling work, low back pain, and osteoarthritis. Scand. J. Work Environ. Health 7:18–30, 1981.

77. Sander, R. A., and Meyers, J. E.: The relationship of disability to compensation status in railroad workers. Spine 11:141–143, 1986.

78. Sanderson, P. L., Todd, B. D., Holt, G. R., and Getty, C. J. M.: Compensation, work status, and disability in low back pain patients. Spine 20:554–556, 1995.

79. Sivensson, H., and Andersson, G.: Low back pain in 40 to 47 year old men, work history and environment factors. Spine 8:272–276, 1983.

80. Snook, S. H.: The costs of back pain in industry. In Deyo, R. A. (ed.): Occupational Medicine: State of the Art Reviews. Vol. 3. Philadelphia, Hanley & Belfus, 1988, pp. 1–5.

81. Snook, S. H., Campanelli, R. A., and Hart, J. W.: A study of three preventive approaches to low back injury. J. Occup. Med. 20:478–481, 1978.

82. Spengler, D. M., Bigos, S. J., Martin, N. A., et al.: Back injuries in industry: A retrospective study. I. Overview and cost analysis. Spine 11:241–245, 1986.

83. States, J. D., Korn, M. W., and Masengill, J. B.: The enigma of whiplash injuries. N. Y. State J. Med. 70:2971–2978, 1970.

84. Tollison, C. D.: Compensation status as a predictor of outcome in nonsurgically treated low back injury. South. Med. J. 86:1206–1209, 1993.

85. Waddell, G.: Clinical assessment of lumbar impairment. Clin. Orthop. 221:110–120, 1987.

86. Waddell, G., and Main, C. J.: Assessment of severity on low-back disorders. Spine 9:204–208, 1984.

87. Waddell, G., Main, C. J., Morris, E. W., et al.: Chronic low-back pain, psychologic distress, and illness behavior. Spine 9:209–213, 1984.

88. Walsh, N. E., and Dumitru, D.: The influence of compensation on recovery from low back pain. In Deyo, R. A. (ed.): Occupational Medicine: State of the Art Reviews. Vol. 3. Philadelphia, Hanley & Belfus, 1988, pp. 109–121.

89. Webster, B. S., and Snook, S. H.: The cost of 1989 workers' compensation low back pain claims. Spine 19:1111–1116, 1994.

90. Wiesel, S. W., Boden, S. D., and Feffer, H. L.: A quality-based protocol for the management of musculoskeletal injuries: A ten-year prospective outcome study. Clin. Orthop. 301:164–176, 1994.

91. Wiesel, S. W., Feffer, H. L., and Rothman, R. H.: Industrial low-back pain—a prospective evaluation of a standardized diagnostic and treatment protocol. Spine 9:199–203, 1984.

92. Wiesel, S. W., Feffer, H. L., and Rothman, R. H.: The development of a cervical spine algorithm and its prospective application to industrial patients. J. Occup. Med. 27:272–276, 1985.

93. Wiesel, S. W., Feffer, H. L., and Rothman, R. H.: Low back pain: Development and five-year prospective application of a computerized quality-based diagnostic and treatment protocol. J. Spinal Disord. 1:50–58, 1988.

94. Wood, P., and Badley, M.: Epidemiology of back pain. In Jeyson, M. (ed.): The Lumbar Spine and Back Pain. London, Pitman, 1980, pp. 29–33.

95. Yu, T. S., Roht, L. H., Wise, R. A., et al.: Low-back pain in industry—an old problem revisited. J. Occup. Med. 26:517–524, 1984.

96. Ziporyn, T.: Disability evaluation—a fledging science? JAMA 250:873–874, 879–880, 1983.

Management of the Workers' Compensation Patient With Low Back Pain

Dan M. Spengler, M.D.

Low back pain represents one of the major disabling symptoms that affect our society. Patients suffering from low back pain symptoms impose a significant financial burden, owing to the high cost of assessing and managing this condition. In addition, the symptom appears to be increasing in frequency, despite our advancing knowledge of its pathogenesis and management.

Low back pain affects approximately 80 per cent of Americans at some point in their lifetime.[2, 10] The symptom complex appears to be most prevalent in individuals during their prime productive period.[2, 10, 16] Approximately 2.4 million Americans are disabled because of low back pain, and nearly 9.1 million are significantly impaired.[8, 16] Frymoyer suggested that approximately 2 per cent of adult males in the United States will have some form of low back surgery during their lifetime.[8] Because of this high prevalence and the invasive treatment necessary for many people who suffer back symptoms, the costs are staggering. The cost to society for low back pain appears to be more than $20 billion per year.[1, 16, 17] This cost is even greater when one considers the adverse impact that this syndrome has on impaired and disabled workers. Costs associated with low back pain do not have a normal gaussian distribution.[16, 17] Studies consistently show that a small percentage of individuals account for a large percentage of total costs associated with this problem.[16, 17] A retrospective review of a large aircraft manufacturer in the Pacific Northwest revealed that 10 per cent of the workforce accounted for 80 per cent of the costs associated with back injury.[17] This skewed distribution of costs needs to be recognized, because it probably explains why well-intentioned concepts such as health promotion programs have not been financially effective. Moreover, these programs do not appear to have any significant impact on total health care costs.

Many studies have been published dealing with the problem of low back pain from a number of differing perspectives. Clearly, our knowledge of this problem has increased enormously over the past 20 years. In spite of this, Social Security disability awards for low back problems have increased 2700 per cent over a recent 20-year period. Precise explanations for this phenomenon remain elusive.

Because many episodes of low back pain are related to events that occur at work, a contentious, adversarial relationship often arises between the injured employee and the employer. Between 1974 and 1984, there was a twofold increase in the number of compensation claims brought to litigation.[9] The employee is often caught in a contest in which it is necessary to aggressively assert the relationship between the symptoms and the workplace.[9] Hadler clearly demonstrated that this adversarial situation retards wellness behavior.[9] Although employees who successfully litigate a compensation claim can initially be presented with a windfall of dollars,

the long-term outcome for such individuals appears to be grim. The initial expectations regarding the settlement are often overestimated. The settlement award dwindles appreciably after court costs and attorney's fees are deducted. The residual reward is typically dissipated within a short time. Moreover, the employee will have been labeled a compensation claimant, virtually eliminating future work. Many authors have reported a disintegrating quality of life for such individuals.

Physicians are also to blame for the prolongation of time lost from work in most industrial settings. Frequently, physicians do not clearly understand the nature of the task performed within the workplace, and they are placed in the position of serving as the patient's advocate. Instead of promptly evaluating the patient's complaints in a thorough and consistent manner, many physicians employ ineffective methods that result in increasing dependency needs on the part of the patient, which clearly retards prompt return to work.[5, 18] Thus, doctors are guilty of overtreating patients through ineffective methods and powerful medications.[18] In addition, many physicians routinely prescribe long periods of bed rest, which, though effective in the short term, are rarely of any value beyond four or five days.[7] Physiologic studies have demonstrated that an individual may lose up to 10 per cent of bone mass with only two weeks of bed rest.[4] Surgical intervention is likewise used to excess in the United States, where the incidence varies dramatically throughout the country, the highest rate per 100,000 being in the western United States.[8] Although many physicians and surgeons genuinely direct their efforts to assisting the patient with subjective symptoms, such good intentions often do more to prolong the symptom complex than more appropriate treatments that include behavior modification and reconditioning. More recent data suggest that many patients with low back symptoms may also be receiving inappropriate or suboptimal care. Support for this concept has been derived from studies that have shown rather dramatic regional variations in both the use of diagnostic studies and the treatment for patients who suffer from low back pain. The authors of these studies have suggested that these data are explained by a lack of consensus among doctors about what are appropriate assessment and treatment. In addition to the confusion among doctors, the back injury problem is further complicated by a system that creates incentives for the employee not to return to the workplace (disincentives). Lawyers are clearly part of the problem, as employees who engage attorneys for compensation-related issues seldom return to work. Costs also skyrocket when an attorney becomes involved.

Companies and management also bear responsibility for a portion of this problem, because a restrictive management style can threaten productive but temporarily injured workers. These workers resent the ha-

1783

rassment and the hurdles that are often put in their way. An example would be to refuse to provide temporary light duty to facilitate an employee's return to full duty. In addition, a confrontational style by a supervisor can do much to undermine trust and result in an adversarial encounter with an employee and his or her counsel.

Efforts to address low back pain are further impaired because of ignorance of the cause. A precise anatomic source of nociception cannot be recognized in over 80 per cent of patients who perceive low back symptoms.[13, 14] Several authors have suggested that the symptom of idiopathic low back pain probably does not represent a disease process at all but a short, self-limited, physiologic phenomenon.[13, 14]

Nevertheless, low back pain does indeed represent a symptom, not a diagnosis. A careful history and physical examination must be obtained for individuals who suffer from this symptom complex. In addition, a thorough assessment is necessary to exclude the multiple causes of low back pain, including neoplasia and referred pain. Nearly 2 per cent of patients who present to physicians with a complaint of chronic low back pain are shown to have metastatic or primary tumors. Another subset of patients presents with low back symptoms that reflect referred pain from disease processes such as dissecting aortic aneurysms or posterior perforating ulcers. Clearly, physicians who evaluate patients suffering from low back pain must be vigilant for these treatable entities. I believe that most physicians readily welcome new approaches to enhance the classification and treatment of patients with low back symptoms.

PATIENT EVALUATION

When evaluating a patient with low back complaints, the physician must be thorough to identify unusual causes for this common symptom. Patients who have aortic aneurysms, perforating ulcers, pyelonephritis, primary or metastatic tumors, and retroperitoneal lesions may all present with low back symptoms. The physician also needs to be aware of the unfortunate fact that some patients attempt to exacerbate their pain in an attempt to avoid returning to the workplace. Such patients can often be difficult to identify and to distinguish from patients with true pathologic processes. This places the physician in a difficult situation. All of us need to serve as advocates for our patients, but on occasion, we need to serve the best interests of our patients by directing them to return to the workplace. The goals for the physician who evaluates patients with compensation should be to provide a thorough evaluation, including a good history and a physical examination; return the patient to the workplace as soon as possible; recommend appropriate diagnostic evaluation when indicated; provide appropriate treatment and follow-up evaluation to optimize clinical outcome; and communicate with case managers to reinforce the plan. The recent publication by Bigos and colleagues, sponsored by the Agency for Health Care Policy and Research, provides an excellent reference for the management of acute low back pain problems in adults.[3] The essence of the algorithms presented in the document reflects my style of patient management for the last 20 years.

The history obtained from the patient should focus on the presenting complaint, onset, intensity, and pain distribution. In addition, the patient must be queried regarding "red flags" that could imply significant associated pathologic processes. Serious trauma, age, history of cancer, constitutional symptoms, risk factors for infection, and nighttime pain represent relevant areas that warrant further medical evaluation and diagnostic assessment. In workers' compensation patients, the specifics of any injury should be recorded. The existence of disincentives must also be addressed, including whether the patient has hired an attorney to deal with the compensation issues.

The physical examination should feature a general evaluation, including any significant pain behavior exhibited by the patient. Inappropriate physical findings, as reported by Waddell and coworkers, should be included in all assessments.[20] A complete back evaluation that includes range of motion with or without dysrhythmia, sciatic tension signs, and neurologic deficits and an evaluation of the abdomen and hips should be included. A pelvic examination is also indicated when evaluating a woman with elusive low back pain symptoms.

Following the history and physical examination, the physician must decide what additional diagnostic studies, if any, are indicated. If the patient has low back pain with or without sciatica, no studies are necessary initially, unless the examination reveals a significant red flag or neurologic deficit. Plain radiographs of the lumbar spine are unnecessary, as is magnetic resonance imaging (MRI). The patient should be advised as to the natural history of back pain (short duration, rapid improvement) and started on a symptom-control program. My preference is to recommend the use of ice massage to help with acute symptoms and to select a salicylate, acetaminophen, or nonsteroidal anti-inflammatory drug of choice. Rarely, a patient presents with pain and incapacitation of such magnitude that narcotics and/or hospital admission becomes necessary. Work modification may also be required for up to four weeks. At that time, the patient should be reassessed to evaluate improvement. If improvement is occurring, but at a slow pace, work modifications can be continued for up to a maximum of three months. I recommend a thorough evaluation if no improvement in symptoms is observed within 30 days and the patient has not been able to return to work in any capacity. Early identification of patients with problems is essential to optimize outcome and to prevent the patient from slipping into the category of "chronic pain." Activation of the patient following symptom resolution is essential. Appropriate aerobic activity and trunk strengthening (both extensors and flexors) improve the likelihood for resumption of full work activity.

If red flags are observed, the patient should undergo

appropriate laboratory evaluation and additional imaging studies to sort through the differential diagnosis. For example, a referral to a specialist in internal medicine, neurology, or vascular surgery may be warranted. Specifics of the referral are contingent on the physician's differential diagnosis. If a patient does not improve within 30 days and back symptoms with or without sciatica persist, a thorough evaluation is warranted. I perform plain radiographs without oblique films but with lateral flexion-extension views to look for evidence of segmental hypermobility or instability. In addition, I believe that MRI is useful to establish a diagnosis or to exclude a significant disc disorder. If a large disc herniation is identified, prompt surgical discectomy may be useful to relieve symptoms and to actually shorten the rehabilitation period in well-motivated individuals. Fortunately, most patients do not lapse into chronic pain behavior within this four-week time frame. If the MRI is normal, I continue activation and direct the worker back to the workplace over a two- to three-week period. For individuals who are engaged in heavy labor, transitional employment allows them to return to productivity more quickly and serves to restrict their lifting requirements on this temporary basis.

Psychologic problems, medication abuse, and the well-recognized disincentives that occur in the present workplace environment can all interfere with successful rehabilitation of the employee with a spinal disorder. I believe that the more promptly workplace disputes are resolved, the more rapidly the employee will be able to return to some form of productivity. Unfortunately, the current system can create an incredibly hostile environment, with finger-pointing by all. Legislative changes to create a system of incentives to return to work would represent a great improvement over the existing situation.

ASSESSMENT WITH A DYNAMOMETER

I continue to be pleased with the use of a three-axis dynamometer to quantify lumbar function. This device records motion, velocity, and torque simultaneously in three planes. Data are recorded on a computer software program. The dynamometer is useful for identifying patients who provide poor effort, quantifying trunk strength following recovery from either an injury or surgery, and documenting compliance with a rehabilitation program. Much has been written to highlight the negatives of these "costly" pieces of equipment. Nevertheless, I believe that such authors have not truly assessed the opportunities afforded by these devices, focusing instead on their initial cost. Our group has spent less than $500 per month on the B-200 dynamometer. When one considers the total cost outlays with respect to the problem of low back pain, I cannot be persuaded that this is excessive cost.

The B-200 dynamometer measures motion, velocity, and torque simultaneously in three planes. This information is stored for permanent record-keeping purposes on a floppy disc (Fig. 57–1). The pelvis and trunk are held by a snug-fitting, comfortable restraint system. Resistance to motion is constant and is tester determined.

The patient receives a consistent set of instructions regarding the lumbar spine evaluation protocol. He or she is placed in the machine, and the harnesses and stabilizers are fitted. The reproducible starting point is then determined, and the protocol is initiated. The patient is asked to flex and extend, laterally bend side to side, and rotate left to right without any resistance being applied. During these maneuvers, the patient begins to be less apprehensive about the testing and is reassured by the successful completion of these maneu-

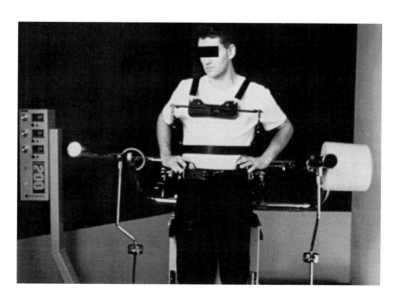

Figure 57–1. Multiaxis dynamometer.

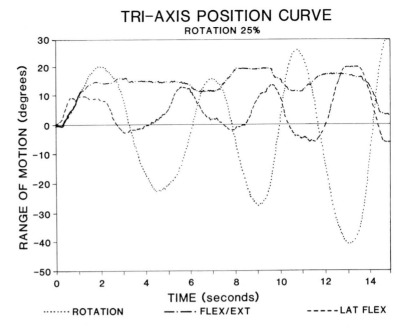

Figure 57–2. Output from a patient who has rotated to the right (positive numbers) and then rotated to the left (negative numbers). Note that both flexion and lateral bending occur simultaneously.

vers. After motion, all three axes are locked to determine isometric torques in each of the three planes. The patient is asked to exert a maximal resistance against a fixed object in the flexion-extension plane, lateral bending plane left and right, and rotation left and right. On the basis of the strengths exhibited during this portion of the testing, resistances are selected for dynamic testing. In general, these tests are performed at 25 and 50 per cent of isometric values. Once the isometric portion of the testing has been completed, motion, velocity, and torque are determined dynamically in each of the three axes at differing levels of resistance. In addition, the peak performances are inspected to ensure and verify consistency. At the completion of testing, data

are analyzed and compared with either a normative database or (preferably) previous data from the same individual. This approach can be used in employees who have had a baseline test before their employment.

One of the main strengths of dynamic multiaxis dynamometers is the ability to measure motion and torque in secondary axes as well as the primary axis.[9, 12] As seen in Figure 57–2, the patient is rotating to the right (positive numbers) and then to the left (negative numbers). There is also a significant element of lateral bending as well as flexion-extension. This is consistent with motion segment coupling, as reported by several investigators. Knowledge of these coupled motions becomes useful when classifying patients into the general

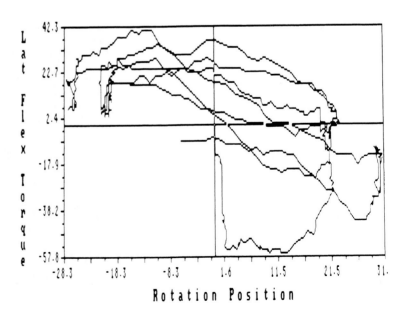

Figure 57–3. Lateral flexion torque (ordinate) versus rotation position (abscissa) in a patient with a known lumbar disc herniation. Note that the patient avoids rotation and lateral torque to the left lower quadrant of the illustration.

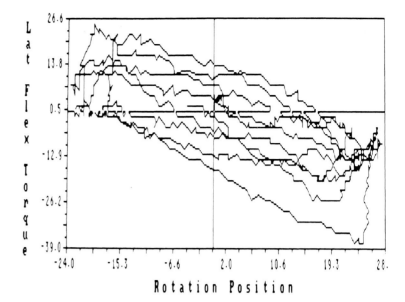

Figure 57–4. The patient in Figure 57–3 six weeks after successful lumbar discectomy. He no longer avoids rotation left with left lateral torque.

categories of normal, pathologic, and symptom amplifiers (Figs. 57–3 to 57–6).

Specific criteria that can be used to identify patients who are not cooperating fully or are amplifying symptoms are useful for the clinician who provides care to such patients. Inconsistencies are noted between the isometric and the dynamic portions of the test, as well as between trials for the same test (Fig. 57–7). For example, when dynamic torques in a particular motion plane exceed the isometric torques, a lack of effort explains the discrepancy. In addition, patients often exhibit more torque in a secondary axis than when asked to demonstrate torque in the primary axis (Fig. 57–8). Finally, feeble torque readings at extremely slow velocities also suggest symptom amplification (see Fig. 57–7).

To initially establish the value of a multiaxis dynamometer in sorting patients with various problems, we performed a study comparing known symptom amplifiers, patients with proved disc herniations, and a group of normal individuals with no history of any back or lower extremity problems. Table 57–3 lists the criteria for inclusion in each of the categories. During a standard multiaxis assessment of lumbar function, more than 200 variables are recorded; 13 of these accounted for 75 per cent of the variance in these groups. As can be seen from Figure 57–9, the computerized sort was most accurate in properly labeling normal patients with pathologic processes, and symptom amplifiers. In our initial review, only one mislabeling occurred. On reviewing this particular individual, a lumbar disc herniation was present, but the patient also

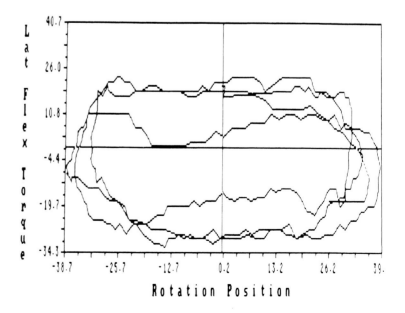

Figure 57–5. Lateral flexion torque versus rotation position in a 55-year-old man eight weeks after successful decompression for lateral recess stenosis. The situation is essentially normal except for decreased torque.

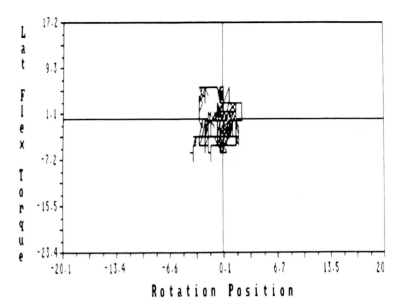

Figure 57-6. The patient in Figure 57-5 six weeks later, after hiring an attorney to assist him with job-related concerns. Note the feeble torques and unusual pattern, which indicates a clear lack of effort. A repeat MRI scan was normal. Four inappropriate physical findings as described by Waddell were noted on the physical examination.

exhibited signs of symptom amplification (positive Waddell's signs). Thus, the computer chose to classify this individual as an amplifier solely on the basis of the data from the dynamometer. If the entire clinical evaluation is performed, including history, physical examination, imaging studies, and dynamic assessment of lumbar function, a truly enhanced classification will result.

Multiaxis dynamometers appear to be useful for pre-employment assessments, injury management, comprehensive assessment, and rehabilitation. Pre-employment assessment of individuals in selected workplace activities provides baseline information for future refer-

ence should an individual sustain a back injury. Thus, if an employee suffers a back injury, recovers, and then considers returning to work, the pre-employment data are helpful in determining the percentage of recovery. Quantifying recovery allows the physician, the employee, and the employer to feel better about work release. The physician is reassured that the patient has recovered to preinjury status. The patient is much less anxious and undoubtedly will perform in a more effective manner. The employer realizes that the patient is qualified to return to work and that the risk of reinjury has been minimized.

Dynamometers are also useful in low back injury

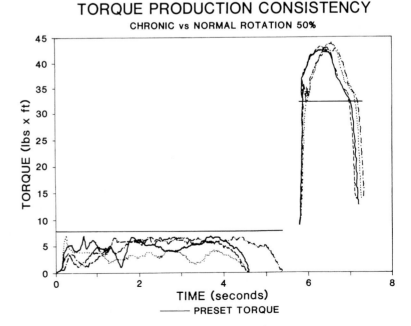

Figure 57-7. A patient demonstrating marked and feeble inconsistencies on the left compared with a very consistent performance by a different patient on the right.

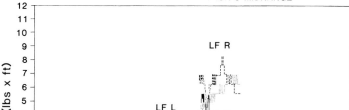

FLEX/EXT AXIS TORQUE PRODUCTION
FOR EACH MOVEMENT TASK'S MIDRANGE

Figure 57–8. A patient who had been unemployed for 18 months because of low back pain. No objective findings were observed; imaging studies were normal. Note that flexion torque during right and left lateral bending exceeded flexion torque when the patient was asked to flex, indicating a clear-cut lack of effort.

management. After an individual has recovered from an acute episode of symptoms, dynamic assessment of lumbar function can be performed and a specific strengthening program designed. Repeat assessments can be performed over time to provide visual feedback to the patient regarding progress. Because most individuals do not have pre-employment baseline data, normative databases exist for general comparison purposes. Thus, when an individual returns to normal, athletic and recreational activities and work become more comfortable.

Comprehensive assessment of individuals who have not recovered promptly or who have long-standing chronic symptoms is one of the best uses for dynamic assessment of lumbar function. Patients who have consistent abnormalities on dynamic assessment can be improved by subsequent rehabilitation efforts. Those

who demonstrate a dramatic lack of compliance or amplification of symptoms form a large subset of chronic patients who can be encouraged, but not coerced, to return to productivity. Impairment ratings also become easier with additional objective data. A big advantage of the multiaxis computerized dynamometer is the ability to determine an individual's effort. Thus, someone who exhibits decreased range of motion coupled with a dramatic decrease in effort is probably not cooperating with the test; thus, a high permanent impairment rating may not be appropriate.

Objective evaluation of lumbar function is also useful to provide feedback to highly motivated individuals during rehabilitation after injury and/or surgery. Repeat assessment in the dynamometer provides visual cues to improvement and positive feedback to individuals who continue working toward their objectives.

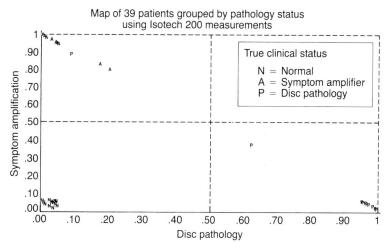

Figure 57–9. Classification that resulted after analysis of B-200 data from 39 subjects, which included normals (15), symptom amplifiers (14), and patients with known lumbar disc herniations (10). Only one patient was mislabeled as a symptom amplifier, but this patient showed clinical evidence of both a disc herniation and symptom amplification. (Courtesy of Dr. Charles F. Federspiel.)

Table 57–3. CRITERIA FOR CLINICAL CLASSIFICATION

Normal
  Young male
  Pre-employment assessment
  No history of back pain
Lumbar Disc Herniation
  Positive physical examination
    Sciatic tension signs
    Neural findings
Plus
  Positive imaging study
Symptom Amplifier
  Waddell's signs (three or more)
  MMPI (consistent with psychologic distress)
  Normal physical examination
  Normal imaging study

In summary, I believe that quantification of lumbar function represents a significant advance for the proper assessment and management of patients who suffer from low back and radicular symptoms, particularly in complex compensation patients. Further studies are indicated and will likely reaffirm the value of this new technology in our armamentarium.

References

1. Akeson, W. H., and Murphy, R. W.: Low back pain. Clin. Orthop. *129*:2–3, 1977.
2. Andersson, G. B. J., Svensson, H. O., and Oden, A.: The intensity of work recovery in low back pain. Spine *8*:880, 1983.
3. Bigos, S., Bowyer, O., Braen, G., et al.: Acute Low Back Problems in Adults. Clinical Practice Guideline No. 14. AHCPR Publication No. 95-0642. Rockville, MD, Agency for Health Care Policy and Research, Public Health Service, U.S. Department of Health and Human Services, December 1994.
4. Bortz, W.: The disuse syndrome. West. J. Med. *141*:691–694, 1984.
5. Deyo, R.: Conservative treatment for low back pain. JAMA *250*:1057–1062, 1983.
6. Deyo, R. A.: Non-operative treatment of low back disorders: Differentiating useful from useless therapy. *In* Frymoyer, J. W. (ed.): The Adult Spine: Principles and Practice. New York, Raven Press, 1991, pp. 1567–1580.
7. Deyo, R., Diehl, A., and Rosenthal, M.: How many days of bed rest for acute low back pain? N. Engl. J. Med. *315*:1064–1070, 1986.
8. Frymoyer, J.: Are we performing too much spinal surgery? Iowa Orthop. J. *9*:32–36, 1989.
9. Hadler, N. M.: Regional musculoskeletal diseases of the low back: Cumulative trauma versus single incident. Clin. Orthop. *221*:33–41, 1987.
10. Hult, L.: The Munkfors investigation. Acta Orthop. Scand. Suppl. 16, 1954.
11. Kelsey, J. L.: Idiopathic low back pain: Magnitude of the problem. *In* White, A. A., and Gordon, S. L. (eds.): American Academy of Orthopaedic Surgeons Symposium on Idiopathic Low Back Pain. St. Louis, C. V. Mosby Co., 1982, pp. 5–8.
12. McGill, S. M., and Norman, R. W.: Dynamically and statically determined low back moments during lifting. J. Biomech. *18*:877–885, 1985.
13. Nachemson, A.: Work for all. Clin. Orthop. *179*:77–85, 1983.
14. Nachemson, A.: Recent advances in the treatment of low back pain. Int. Orthop. *9*:1–10, 1985.
15. Parnianpour, M., Nordin, M., Kahanovitz, N., and Frankel, V.: Triaxial coupling of torque generation. Spine *13*:982–992, 1988.
16. Snook, S.: Low back pain in industry. *In* American Academy of Orthopaedic Surgeons Symposium on Idiopathic Low Back Pain. St. Louis, C. V. Mosby Co., 1982.
17. Spengler, D., Bigos, S., Martin, N., et al.: Back injuries in industry. Spine *11*:241–245, 1986.
18. Spitzer, W., LeBlanc, F., and Dupuis, M.: Quebec task force on spinal disorders. Spine *12* (Suppl. 75), 1987.
19. Turner, J. A., Ersek, M., Herron, L., et al.: Patient outcomes after lumbar spinal fusions. JAMA *268*:907–911, 1992.
20. Waddell, G., McCullough, J., Kummel, E., et al.: Nonorganic physical signs in low back pain. Spine *5*:117–125, 1980.
21. Wiesel, S., Feffer, H., and Rothman, R.: Industrial low back pain. Spine *9*:199–203, 1984.

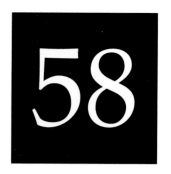

C H A P T E R

Spinal Functional Restoration: Tertiary Nonoperative Care

Tom G. Mayer, M.D.

Spinal rehabilitation has recently come to be recognized as a necessary part of the armamentarium for treating patients with painful spinal problems. Although the vast majority of such patients get well in a relatively short time without the need for extensive rehabilitative treatment, a small percentage of patients becomes severely disabled for long periods. For these patients, repeated passive therapy, manipulation, or surgical intervention has commonly been tried but has failed to relieve symptoms and overcome disability. These patients tend to produce the most significant cost to society in terms of medical care, disability payments, and loss of productivity. As such, they provoke a great deal of concern and interest. It is this difficult group of patients, failures of conservative care and/or surgery, for whom spinal functional restoration is intended.

No one has yet identified the unique structural pain generator in the chronic spinal disorder (CSD) patient. Description of such a site has eluded basic scientists, surgeons, internists, and psychologists and will probably continue to do so. The obvious reason for this is that pain is a subjective central experience of multifactorial origin. The source of the pain is deeply submerged and inaccessible to visual inspection (similar to headache and chronic abdominal pain), and the spine is subject to diverse influences, such as psychologic difficulties, social losses, and financial uncertainties. These secondary phenomena tend to be ignored by physicians and chiropractors, who have no mechanisms available to deal with these problems. As

a consequence, a critical part of our understanding of spinal disability is lost. Because interdisciplinary experience is not usually part of most physician training, lack of conceptualization and resolution in the area of chronic spinal disability is to be anticipated.

Concepts of nonoperative care, particularly for work injuries, are changing rapidly. In the past, the term "physical therapy" was loosely applied to any nonoperative management not specifically performed by physicians. A multitude of developments over the past two decades, however, has permitted the definition of several levels of care tied to the time since injury. *Primary care* refers to that provided during the acute phases of injury; it is usually intended for symptom control. This includes, but is not restricted to, the so-called passive modalities, including electrical stimulation, temperature modulation, or manual techniques. A variety of early assisted mobilization and educational programs are also included in this level. Treatment is customarily provided by a single therapist, with a limited number of treatments generally applied to a large number of patients entering the medical system.

Secondary care refers to therapy provided to a smaller number of patients not responding to initial primary treatment, whose more long-standing symptoms pass into the postacute or immediate postoperative period. In these cases, we now recognize that reactivation is the common need. Programs are generally adapted to provide appropriate exercise and education as the primary modalities, often assisted by additional passive modalities used for symptom control. In many cases, the secondary level of care lends itself to programmatic consolidation, particularly toward the end of the postacute period. Interdisciplinary consultation might be available for specialized situations but is not required on-site or in the majority of cases. The primary treaters in this phase are usually physical and occupational therapists, with physicians, psychologists, social workers, disability managers, and/or chiropractors (depending on the venue or community standards) available for consultation.

In the small number of patients who do not respond to secondary care (those whose pain becomes chronic) or who undergo complex surgical procedures, *tertiary care* is the final option. Tertiary care involves physician-directed, interdisciplinary team care, with all disciplines on-site and available to every patient. The Commission for Accreditation of Rehabilitation Facilities (CARF) pain management guidelines identify common standards of some tertiary care programs, although such treatment may be diverse and eclectic. The picture is further confused by the fact that not all "pain clinics" provide tertiary care, just as not all "work hardening" programs provide interdisciplinary consultative services needed to fulfill CARF definitions for this particular service. Specific programmatic terms are still in flux, but the concept of levels of care is becoming widely accepted. Thus, it is necessary to remain true to program definitions in terms of service provision if we are to achieve the goal of quality of care. It is with this in mind that a specific program—functional restoration, available at the Productive Rehabilitation Institute of Dallas for Ergonomics (PRIDE)—is discussed here as an example of tertiary care, mainly for work-related injury. The intent is to provide the reader with a direct understanding of the roles of each member of the interdisciplinary team within this particular type of tertiary care.[18, 39]

QUANTITATIVE EVALUATION OF PHYSICAL AND FUNCTIONAL CAPACITY

Although the so-called functional capacity evaluation (FCE) has become a popular term, highly variable methods are subsumed under this rubric. In fact, many of the developers of certification in this area teach opposing principles and criticize competitors as invalid. Few of the FCE methodologies use a quantitative approach, but instead use a qualitative, observational methodology that is traditional in physical therapy. Key principles of quantification using physics-based terminology are poorly understood by most therapists and physicians. In functional restoration, true quantification of function is required, because its absence would leave severely disabled and physically inhibited patients free to exercise without objective goals of improvement in "weak link" areas of injury. Greater understanding of accuracy, precision, and sources of error in any quantitative methodology is necessary.[38] In the PRIDE model of functional restoration, *physical capacity assessment* implies the assessment of the injured musculoskeletal weak link (lumbosacral, thoracic, or cervical spine region), generally involving assessment of mobility and strength around a given joint or region. The term *functional capacity assessment* implies measurement of whole-person performance in a task of daily living relevant to the injured body part (e.g., weight lifted, running speed, sitting tolerance time). The recent literature has focused both on pre– and post–functional restoration longitudinal studies of such measurements and on the development of specific normative databases.[4, 7, 28, 33–35, 40]

The reason for specific quantification techniques is the information required for the sports medicine approach. In the more than 40 years since DeLorme and Watkins,[8] we have learned much about the secondary physical changes attending disuse and immobilization that occur in the spine and extremities. Spontaneous healing or physician intervention can produce maximal recovery of disrupted soft tissues (ligaments, tendons, joint capsules, muscles, and discs) or osseous tissue. Quite often, in cases of severe injury, permanent tissue changes remain in the form of distorted bony structures or scar that has repaired soft tissue defects with a strong but less flexible and more easily injured fibrous tissue. In the musculoskeletal system, such changes may produce biomechanical derangements that prevent normal functioning through instability, stress risers, degenerative joint changes, and so forth. These problems are, at least to some extent, permanent derangements and can never be completely "fixed." Efforts of surgery, manipulation, and conservative care may be directed toward correcting or ameliorating these derangements to the greatest extent possible. This, however, is not the province of the rehabilitation physician.

Therapists in functional restoration are focused on the secondary changes brought about by the deconditioning syndrome. They assume that all activities that can be performed medically to correct the underlying structural deficit have been tried. In its wake, the structural deficit has left physical, deconditioning, and psychologic scars that need to be dealt with. These deficits can generally be overcome through exercise and education, through the patient's own active intervention. The goal of physical capacity assessment for this specialist is to identify these deficits.

Range of Motion Assessment

Trunk motion is a compound movement combining intersegmental and hip motion components. A patient with a completely fused spine can often bend forward to perform toe touches using hip motion alone. Although we are not yet able to measure intersegmental motion noninvasively, inclinometers may be used to separate the hip motion component from the lumbar spine motion component and derive valuable information.[20, 42] The basic information on inclinometry comes from British rheumatologists, and the system has been used, in one form or another, in Europe for more than 20 years.[25] As in all physical capacity measures, information obtained with range of motion techniques must be compared with a normative database, and an effort factor must be identified. For range of motion, the effort factor is the comparison between the hip motion component and the spine straight leg raising measurement.[29, 42] These measurements are isolated anatomic-physiologic physical capacity measurements, assessing the capabilities of a single functional unit of the body. These are ultimately compared with general functional or whole-body measurements, in which a synthetic task such as bending, climbing, or lifting is performed.

In the sagittal plane, the inclinometers, which are available in mechanical or computerized forms from various manufacturers, may be positioned at two points or moved from one point to another. Measurements are taken in both flexion and extension and checked through the effort factor of leg raising. A further effort factor is the reproducibility of the test within the same individual, looking to see whether the critical measurements are within 5 degrees or plus or minus 10 per cent on three consecutive test repetitions. There are many reasons for limitation of effort in any single test, so the effort factor is not primarily a test for malingering. Reduction of effort that impedes test validity may be produced by pain, fear of injury, physiologic perception of excess load, neuromuscular inhibition, or multiple psychologic factors of anxiety or depression, in addition to the rare cases of conscious effort to mislead the examiner.

In addition to sagittal movement of the spine, coronal movement can be assessed just as easily by simply rotating the inclinometer 90 degrees in the axial plane. Rotation may also be assessed where it is important, namely in the cervical and thoracic spine, through relatively simple techniques.[9] The smaller the range permitted in any given direction, the less reliable the test. However, if done in a standardized fashion with good effort, the techniques are highly reproducible.

The measurement techniques are used for several purposes. For assessment of function on a one-time basis, the technique can demonstrate the actual range of motion in the T12–S1 segment in the sagittal and coronal planes. In addition to assessing lumbar movement, the T1–T12 sagittal-torsional movement or the occiput–T1 cervical movement in all three planes can be assessed for rehabilitation or impairment evaluation purposes. Such tests can be performed multiple times to document progress.

Suboptimal effort may lead to more careful scrutiny of other components of the functional capacity test battery. However, even in the presence of poor effort, the determination of normal or abnormal motion can be made by comparing the spine and hip motion ratios. In the normally mobile lumbar spine, the sequence of forward bending generally involves spinal flexion considerably earlier than the hip flexion component, until the spine is "hanging on its ligaments." At this point, hip motion increases and further spine motion is constrained.[42] Even in the presence of suboptimal effort, if a normal spine-hip ratio exists, the clinician can usually conclude that normal spine mobility would have been present if the patient had provided sufficient effort. However, in the presence of an abnormal spine-hip ratio, with or without good effort, some actual limitation of spine mobility is likely to be present (postfusion ankylosis or postoperative or disuse scarring or stiffness).

The technique can also be used on multiple occasions to document progress through functional restoration training or as part of an impairment evaluation after maximal medical recovery has been reached. As part of the work capacity evaluation, this process is also important. Range of motion assessment is usually included as one part of the quantitative functional evaluation, a specific battery of physiologic tests for mobility, strength, endurance, and synthetic task performance.[4, 23, 29] There may be initial resistance to the use of this technique by clinicians, in that it is cumbersome and uses equipment not generally available at the present time. Among the devices that are available, the one in greatest use at PRIDE is the Cybex EDI-320 (Lumex, Ronkonkoma, NY), which is a single-head device whose computer calculates both simple and compound (spinal) joint measurements (Fig. 58–1). Another computerized device is made by MI Tech (Daytona Beach, FL), and mechanical devices are made by MedDesign

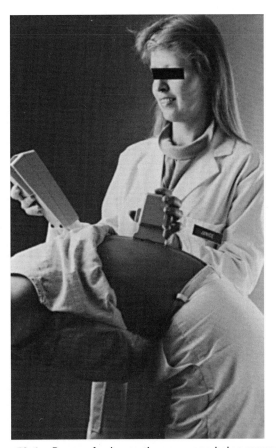

Figure 58–1. Range of spine motion: a person being measured with the Cybex EDI-320 for computerized inclinometric assessment of the cervical, thoracic, and lumbar spine regions.

(Liverpool, UK) and MIE (Leeds, UK). An inexpensive carpenter's level, available at most hardware stores, can also be used. With the mechanical devices, two inclinometers must be used simultaneously, and the calculations must be done by hand after measurements are taken. The advantages of versatility and internal calculation are provided by the computerized devices (at greater expense). Once mastered, both techniques are less time-consuming than obtaining a blood pressure, but the single-head devices require more care in anatomic placement than do dual inclinometer methods. Many medical specialists prefer to perform the tests themselves, but others have these measurements taken by assisting therapists, nurses, and technicians.

As in all other physiologic measurements, there is some variation in the normal population. Interestingly, our normative data show that mean true lumbar motion is almost the same in males and females, even though females tend to have greater hip and straight leg raising mobility components. Patient values are expressed as a "percent normal," as related to mean scores of the symptomatic subject population, normalized for such factors as age, gender, and body weight (when applicable).[28, 33, 34] The system allows the clinician to judge the significance of small variations from the anticipated value and, more importantly, to track the progress of the rehabilitation process from one examination to the next.

Isolated Trunk Strength Assessment

Several devices are commercially available for assessing isometric, isotonic, or isokinetic trunk strength in all planes of motion. Most involve some type of pelvic stabilization with application of force through a line projecting between the sternum and the scapulae, thus representing trunk strength as a torque (torsional force) around a pelvic fulcrum with a lever arm individualized to subject height. Cervical dynamic strength measurement devices have been seen in prototype form but are not currently available, leaving isometrics as the only alternative. Most of the devices are isokinetic: that is, they stabilize the variables of acceleration and velocity in order to provide torque as the primary independent variable. By limiting the number of independent variables, isokinetics tries to provide a more valid test by narrowing the normal distribution of values. Other devices may be purely isometric or isoinertial. Many laboratory model isometric testers using strain gauges have been used, but 1985 heralded the dawn of commercially available dynamic isokinetic trunk strength testing. Our experience has been primarily with the Cybex sagittal trunk extension-flexion (TEF) unit (Fig. 58–2), by the company that invented isokinetic dynamometers in the 1960s and has worked on prototype trunk strength testers since 1980. Other isokinetic devices include (not exclusively) the Lido Back (Loredan, Inc., Davis, CA), Kin-Com (Chattex, Chattanooga, TN), and Biodex (Biodex, Shirley, NY). Other devices are isometric (MedX, DeLand, FL) and isoinertial (Isotechnologies, Hillsboro, NC).

Results of normal subject testing have been compared with CSD patients, with and without prior surgery.[31–34, 41, 49] Substantial differences have been shown between these samples, and progressive improvements in trunk strength have been demonstrated during spinal rehabilitation of chronically disabled back pain patients.[4, 23, 36, 37] The intent of all the devices is to isolate the trunk strength component of the thoracolumbar functional unit by stabilizing above and below the area to be tested. This isolation through the vulnerable "weak link" portion of the vertebral biomechanical chain linking the shoulder girdle to the pelvis is intended to look at the critical area of strength and endurance, just as measuring quadriceps and hamstrings is of utmost importance to knee function. For any of the devices to be useful, one must be certain that the dynamometer gives an accurate and reproducible measure and that the protocol used conforms to that of the normative database. Moreover, such a database must be available, and the clinician must have a method for assessing effort in the patient to be tested.

Cardiovascular Fitness Assessment

The inactivity that leads to deconditioning in patients with spinal disorders also reduces cardiovascular fitness. The treadmill, bicycle, and upper body ergometry have long been used to measure the cardiovascular response to a measured workload. Significant deficits in aerobic capacity are frequently present in chronic and postoperative back pain patients, somewhat proportional to the duration of disability and the degree of inactivity. Because inactivity may also produce deconditioning of upper and lower extremity skeletal muscle, the ergometry test may be terminated because of extremity fatigue rather than lack of cardiovascular fitness. These alternatives can usually be distinguished by noting the heart rate achieved at the point of voluntary test termination, as well as by comparing the upper and lower body ergometric results. In most deconditioned patients, an exaggerated heart rate response to relatively low workloads is customarily the limiting factor of the test. Such testing leads to a determination of the extent to which aerobic capacity and/or lower and upper extremity strength training needs to be added to the functional restoration program.

Whole-Body Task Performance Assessment (Functional Capacity)

Whereas the preceding tests of mobility, strength, and endurance focus primarily on the injured isolated functional unit, measurements of task performance have more practical application. The body is certainly capable of functioning in the presence of spine rigidity, as in the case of a patient with a completely fused thoracolumbar spine. Using the spine as a rigid vertebral column may improve functional demands for substitution by other body structures, such as squatting and whole-body rotation to compensate for limitations in spine bending and twisting. Gait modifications may

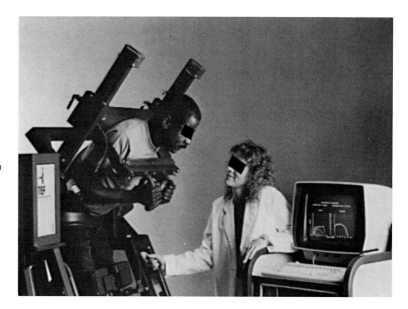

Figure 58–2. The Cybex TEF unit (trunk extension-flexion) for measuring sagittal torsion around an L5–S1 fulcrum isokinetically, or through multiposition isometrics. Also shown is computer graphics.

also be necessary to accommodate biomechanical losses to the "spinal engine" for locomotion.[15] Thus, functional task measurements help the clinician assess how the body performs as a whole rather than how the injured component is performing in isolation.

There is, however, a price to be paid for this "real world" information. Although we are interested in activities such as bending, lifting, and climbing, their measurement is difficult and imprecise. This leads to a wider distribution of normal values or, in other words, more uncertainty in identifying what is "normal." For this reason, a variety of methods for the measurement of lifting capacity might need to be used.

The classic measurement of whole-body activity involving the spine is that of lifting capacity. Because of its perceived importance as a mode of injury in industry, the ability to lift has become the measurement of greatest concern to those involved in ergonomic analysis and work capacity evaluations for functional limitations and job redesign. To give a full picture of lifting capacity, we must use several measures, including isometric,[6] isokinetic,[22] and isoinertial.[24, 26, 27, 30] The isometric testing measures are currently authorized for industrial use by National Institute of Occupational Safety and Health (NIOSH) guidelines. These tests are simple to perform and have a large industrial database to accompany them. Unfortunately, however, it appears that isometric and isokinetic measures can not be substituted for each other.[22] Isokinetic devices can usually be used for isometric measures, but they do not give the picture of a "real world" lift as an isoinertial test does. The complete lack of stabilization of independent variables in isoinertial tests, however, makes them imprecise, even though their outcomes are highly desirable. They are useful for screening purposes only. For the dynamic test, an effort factor in terms of curve reproducibility at intervals of one tenth of a second is used, whereas the progressive isoinertial lifting evalua-

tion (PILE) test uses a heart rate effort monitor. There is only limited correlation between isokinetic and isoinertial dynamic lifting measures. Similarly, there is only limited correlation between lifting capacity measures and trunk strength measures, because of the use of substitution in doing whole-body tasks. An anxious or fearful patient, particularly one who has been educated "never to lift anything heavier than a beer can," may show a paradoxic discrepancy in which lifting capacity measures are considerably lower than those anticipated on the basis of isolated trunk strength measures. Incomplete rehabilitation can be assessed by comparing the peak lifting force with the power generated at any given speed on an isokinetic test. The power indicates the area beneath the curve of the force versus velocity curve.

Positional and activity tolerance is another area of interest in functional task measurement directed toward return to productivity. Following spine injury, patients often cannot tolerate prolonged static positioning (sitting or standing) and often complain of inability to perform various tasks such as squatting, kneeling, walking, carrying, or climbing. A timed obstacle course requiring the use of multiple postures can be used to assess the patient's tolerance of daily living activities (Fig. 58–3). Observation of the patient through a testing or training session can give the therapist an idea of the patient's tolerance of various static postures. Because of the lack of corroborative tests, the latter measures are somewhat less objective than the multiple lift tests. As in the physical capacity assessment of the injured musculoskeletal joint or region, if the functional capacity assessment is to be quantitative rather than observational, there are two necessary conditions. First, normative data must be established to compare with data from injured workers.[22, 26, 30, 32, 35] Second, longitudinal studies must be provided demonstrating pre- and post-rehabilitation performance measures to document that

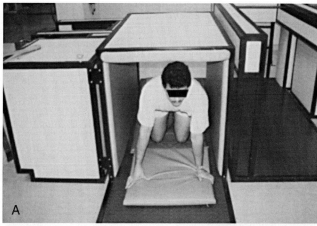

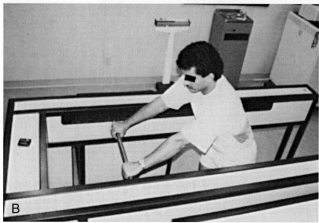

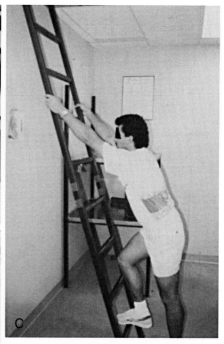

Figure 58–3. A timed obstacle course used at Productive Rehabilitation Institute for Dynamic Ergonomics (PRIDE) facilities for assessing whole body activity tolerance. *A,* Multiple components. *B,* Push-pull assessment. *C,* Climbing assessment.

differences are sufficiently large to allow tests of limited precision (i.e., with great human variability) to be used effectively as discriminating variables in a patient population.[7, 23]

In summary, quantification of physical function is a relatively new and important tool in assessing patients with chronic painful spinal disorders. Although the measures are in an early stage of development and standardization, experience with extremity rehabilitation suggests that these tests will, in time, become an important supplement to our sophisticated but expensive imaging devices. Quantification of physical functional capacity requires patient motivation, but because an effort factor can be identified with each physical capacity test, suboptimal effort can be recognized and used to validate the actual test scores.

PSYCHOLOGIC ASSESSMENT

Even though severe disability is what brings CSD patients to the attention of employers, attorneys, insurance companies, and vocational rehabilitation personnel, the patients enter the medical care system because of pain. Chronic pain is a complex and interactive psychophysiologic behavior pattern that cannot be broken down into distinct, independent physiologic and physical components. Thus, we are interested in as-

sessing the various psychosocial barriers to functional recovery that may impede patients in their rehabilitation programs. Rates of psychiatric illness (e.g., major depression, substance abuse, anxiety disorders, personality disorders, childhood trauma) that are much higher than the base rates for the U.S. population in general have been demonstrated for the CSD population at PRIDE and elsewhere.[13, 21, 46] The assessment generally breaks down into a number of tests that, when combined, can assist the clinician in identifying these barriers. They also demonstrate ways in which the health professional can work with the patient to overcome the barriers and return to productivity. At this time, no single comprehensive instrument has been developed specifically for chronic spinal pain. Thus, multiple tests are used for evaluation and to assist in the education and counseling of patients to guide them through functional restoration. These tests fall into a variety of categories.

Self-Report Tests

Self-report scores are totally subjective, in that they mirror only a patient's perception of pain, disability, and depression. As such, they have only limited value. However, in the last 15 years, a number of tests have been devised giving quantitative measures of self-reporting through various questionnaire formats that allow a number to be applied to the patient's level of perceived pain, discomfort, or disability. These instruments are simple to use and are repeated frequently during a course of rehabilitation to compare a patient's pain perception at different times. Many factors may increase pain, depression, and disability self-reporting (other than recurrence of injury), and the knowledge of such changes in any one individual is very useful. The large majority of chronic pain patients tend to be somatizing individuals (i.e., more pain sensitive and likely to exaggerate bodily responses compared with the general population). As such, their responses cannot be compared with a normative database; instead, an individual's response must be compared with that same individual's initial or baseline score obtained prior to treatment.

Quantified Pain Drawing

For more than a decade, quantified pain drawings have been used to give an assessment of pain location, severity, and subjective characteristics in a nonverbal communication by the patient.[45] An overlay over the pain drawing itself has been devised to give a numerical count of the trunk and extremity area covered, as well as whether the pain is limited within the bodily confines or is "outside the body." There is also a visual analog score to suggest whether the patient perceives the problem as more axial or extremity in origin and to gauge the severity of pain (Fig. 58–4). The overlay is on a transparent plastic sheet, permitting easy scoring by office personnel.[5]

Million Visual Analog Scale

This is a validated visual analog scale consisting of 15 questions and describing both pain and disability. Disability perception is a useful self-reporting tool.[43] Responses are expressed on a 10-cm line spanning the gamut from the minimum to the maximum possible severity on each item. In the original paper, high correlation was found between the subjective analog scores and the objective examination findings of the clinicians. Although this correlation may not be generally present in rehabilitation, it is a useful tool for documenting the patient's symptomatic improvement and the limitations on function that the pain imposes.

Beck Depression Inventory (BDI)

The BDI consists of 21 questions with a cumulative scoring system that looks at manifestations of depression including sleep disturbance, weight change, irritability, sexual dysfunction, and anhedonia. It was developed by Beck[3] as a means of assessing the cognitive components of depression. Depression, like anxiety, is a frequent concomitant of long-term back dysfunction and disability. Although it is unclear whether depression precedes or follows the onset of low back symptoms in the majority of cases, knowledge of its presence

can be quite helpful. Offering depressed patients pharmacologic treatment may encourage greater patient motivation and compliance, as well as reducing barriers to recovery. In fact, it appears that low-dose antidepressant medication may actually have a specific analgesic effect for chronic pain.[50]

Short Form 36

The Short Form 36 (SF-36) is a 36-item validated self-reporting test currently achieving wide acceptance as an outcome measure in many areas of medicine.[51] It has many advantages, including ease of comprehension, multiple dimensions of health status covered, and use in longitudinal studies of many diseases. Eight dimensions of physical and emotional functioning document self-perception of health status, with two global, comprehensive scores summarizing physical and mental health.

Psychologic Measures

A variety of more complex tests measure psychiatric and psychologic functioning, as well as personality factors. These tests have a scoring and interpretation system that is not immediately apparent to the subject taking the test. Many of these have been devised and "validated." Unfortunately, however, the usefulness of any particular test in the chronic spinal pain patient remains questionable, in spite of the hopes that have been raised over the past 30 years. The prediction of patient behavior is always risky.

Minnesota Multiphasic Personality Inventory (MMPI)

The MMPI is the "granddaddy" of all tests used in chronic pain patients and has been newly revised as the MMPI II. The main reason for its use appears to be that "everyone else uses it." By itself, it does not offer much help in choosing among treatment options. However, as part of a comprehensive evaluation using several other assessment tools, the MMPI can add valuable information.

Of the 10 major clinical scales by which the MMPI is classified, the hysteria, depression, and hypochondriasis scales are most frequently associated with chronic pain patients. Elevation of the hysteria and hypochondriasis scales with a normal depression scale provides a so-called Conversion V. This test profile was thought to be associated with pain that has a large psychologic component. However, it has been shown that, in reality, the Conversion V is a stress indicator and returns to a more normal profile after resolution of disability from whatever cause.[2] The test is more useful when a variety of personality profiles characteristic of patients with psychiatric or personality disorders is found, which may help in identifying techniques of counseling and therapy to be provided to these patients. For example, the McAndrews scale, initially standardized in an outpatient population of alcoholics, helps one recognize

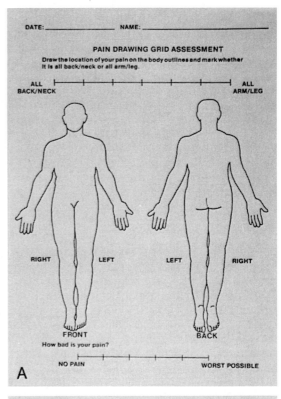

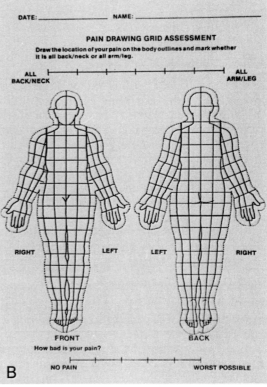

Figure 58–4. *A,* Quantified pain drawing filled out by the patient. *B,* Pain drawing with the transparent grid overlay. (From Mayer, T., and Gatchel, R.: Functional Restoration for Spinal Disorders: The Sports Medicine Approach. Philadelphia, Lea & Febiger, 1988, p. 190.)

patients with a drug-dependent personality type. The patient may not be actively abusing substances but has the personality tendency to fall into this mode of functioning under high levels of stress. Even reformed alcoholics generally show a substantial elevation on this scale.

Other Structured Evaluations

The SCID (Structured Clinical Interview for DSM-IV diagnosis) is a standard interview format specifically designed to provide a psychiatric diagnosis (if any) for the patient being assessed.[11] Because the rate of psychiatric illness is so high in chronically disabled patients—whether lifetime or secondary to the effects of disability—this test has become vital for the assessment of CSD patients. The Wechsler Adult Intelligence Scale (WAIS-R) is another important assessment tool.[52] Intelligence correlates well with the patient's ease of absorbing concepts involved in rehabilitation or with resistance to those concepts. The WAIS also correlates with prior education and skills, which are important for ultimate vocational reintegration. The Hamilton depression score is a clinician-administered assessment necessary to validate the self-reported BDI.[17] Major differences between clinical and subjective scores of depression can be important for identifying denial or extreme somatization.

The Clinical Interview

The interview is the most powerful clinical assessment tool available. It is difficult to standardize but is most important in looking at all the psychosocial and economic factors involved in continued disability and high pain report. Because of concern about specific problems, it can focus on such important areas as depression, personal and family medical history, patient and family substance abuse history, history of head injury or cognitive disorders, and signs of personality disorder. It also looks at past issues of finances, work (including job loss, job change, and job satisfaction), and pending litigation that may affect patient behavior as "secondary gain" disincentives to return to activity. Rehabilitation is ultimately a modification of patient behavior away from an unrealistic dependency on the medical system to "cure" the long-term pain source. Instead, the patient moves toward an independent approach to achieving the highest level of function possible and resuming a realistic level of productivity, given the severity of the permanent impairment that the patient has sustained. The process of this transition is discussed in the next section, but it can be facilitated only with an understanding of the psychologic impairments that are keeping the patient disabled, deconditioned, dependent, and drugged. Only if they can be identified by the medical professionals can they be dealt with in an appropriate manner.

THE FUNCTIONAL RESTORATION APPROACH TO REHABILITATION

Sports Medicine Concepts and Physical Training

The principles of sports medicine have come to be used not only for the rehabilitation of competitive athletes. Instead, they have been modified to emerge as a conceptual and methodologic framework for actively treating all individuals who wish to return to high levels of function. The component parts are shown in Table 58–1. Much of the initial work was done with extremity injury, but these concepts now involve the spine as well.

An injury can be seen either as a massive overload exogenously generated or as a cumulative trauma, termed degeneration, generated endogenously. Whatever the source of the musculoskeletal insult, the initial phases following overload are characterized by hemorrhage and edema. After several days, cellular infiltration and enzymatic degradation of necrotic tissues occur, with involvement of prostaglandins, bradykinins, and kallikreins. A proliferative phase follows, with its timing and duration related to the quality of the blood supply in the area and other systemic factors such as diabetes, cardiovascular and pulmonary disease, or cigarette smoking. Random deposition of collagen fibers takes place in the initial days of this phase. Subsequently, the collagen fibers align along lines of stress in a generalized form of Wolff's law called the law of mesothelial tissues. This basically states that tissue will align along lines of stress under conditions of both homeostasis and healing to produce the strongest, least adherent, and most efficient amounts of tissue. Clearly, a small amount of tissue injury with relatively good nutrition and low-grade stresses, such as might occur with a minor sprain or contusion, will proceed through this process quickly. Conversely, in the presence of extremely high stress, poor tissue nutrition (such as in large, avascular discs), and substantial injury, considerably delayed and poorer-quality healing can be anticipated. This is probably generally the case in the spine, just as it is in fractures of long bones. Finally, the injured area is left with a scar, visible or hidden, that has matured to fill the injured area but lacks the resilience, strength, and durability of the original tissue. If the scar is asymmetric in an axial structure, such as the

Table 58–1. COMPONENTS OF A FUNCTIONAL RESTORATION PROGRAM

Quantification of physical capacity
Quantification of psychosocial function
Reactivation for restoration of fitness
Reconditioning of the injured functional unit
Retraining in multiunit functional task performance
Work simulation
Multimodal disability management program
Vocational or societal reintegration
Formalized outcome tracking

spine, whether it is produced by injury, degeneration, or surgical trauma, one can anticipate severe disturbances of biomechanical performance in the critical spinal articulations as a secondary consequence of the healing process.

A particular characteristic of the injured individual is the tendency to splint and protect the injured area. This leads, in time, to delayed maturation of collagen,[1, 15] muscle atrophy,[44] adhesions and deficits in joint lubrication,[48] ligament atrophy,[1] and bone loss.[47] Subsequently, changes in endurance and aerobic fitness, called the deconditioning syndrome, progress, with declining physical capacity. Each pain episode increases patient fear, leading to more disuse, inactivity, and declining physical capacity.

The physiologic approach to the deconditioning syndrome involves exercise to address mobility, strength, endurance, cardiovascular fitness, and agility and coordination. The exercises must progress to involve simulation of customary physical activities to restore task-specific functions. Such exercises must be focused at the specific functional unit that has become deconditioned and ultimately be generalized to whole-body functions.

Strength can be restored after injury by a variety of means. Soon after injury, when continued immobilization may be necessary, isometric exercise may be the only type that the patient can perform. This involves exercising against fixed resistance without accompanying joint motion. These exercises may be done in a cast, splint, or brace, but the method has many drawbacks. First, it is the most fatiguing and least effective type of exercise.[19] There is a specificity of strength training to the length of the muscle fibers at the time of exercise, with rapid fall-off in training efficiency at different muscle fiber lengths. Additionally, there is limited translation of endurance and agility from isometric training to dynamic activities, although it can be used during the early rest phases to maintain muscle tone and produce relative resistance to atrophy. There is also some suggestion of the benefit of electrical muscle stimulation in combination with isometric exercise, but a higher injury potential may be associated with overvigorous contraction into a static pull.[16]

Dynamic muscle training, which has been shown to be the most efficient method of training, can also be used. It involves three basic modes: isotonic, isokinetic, and psychophysical (free weights).[10] Isotonic exercises are those in which the same force is applied throughout the dynamic range. The term is often inappropriately used for exercises in which a changing lever arm actually alters the applied torque. This type of exercise is most often associated with variable resistance devices, using a cam to equalize muscular demands throughout the dynamic range of motion.

Isokinetic devices require a sophisticated dynamometer that limits the speed to a preset value. In this mode, speed and acceleration are controlled, but the subject can produce essentially unlimited torque around a central axis, thereby eliminating the effect of acceleration on energy production. These devices can accommodate to force application, which provides injury protection, at least in the concentric (muscle shortening while contracting) type of contraction. Unlike variable resistance devices, however, high-speed training is possible for development of agility. Finally, isoinertial (psychophysical) strength training, using free weights, is limited to those postures in which weight can be attached to the body or held in the hands. The method is so termed because the subject self-selects the amount of weight that is acceptable. Although this is the closest to "real world" muscle loading, the maximal weight that can be handled is limited by the weakest portion of the dynamic range of motion and further compromised by limitations of the changing lever arm. However, if the exercise can be devised to simulate actual tasks or motions of the sport or work activity to which the patient is returning, this may be an effective training tool. Psychophysical and variable resistance lifting devices automatically produce both concentric and eccentric (muscle lengthening while contracting) contraction capability. This is more difficult and dangerous to accomplish in isokinetic devices, although computerized dynamometers are currently available to provide this type of training.

Secondary effects of a functional restoration program are also important. Physical training appears to have a specific beneficial effect on pain (possibly through increased synthesis of specialized neurotransmitters) and has been demonstrated to prevent scarring and adhesions while improving cartilage nutrition. Mobility appears to be the key, which can be done initially through passive and later through active means. Development of normal to supernormal strength and endurance in muscles acting around a joint may be beneficial in protecting a joint with cartilage damage or instability owing to ligamentous incompetence. This development of protective muscular mechanisms is particularly important when a complete return to normal joint architecture can no longer be anticipated.

Thus, the specific exercise interventions involve stretching exercises, strengthening exercises, and those designed to improve cardiovascular fitness, endurance, and agility. The application of these exercises is individualized, based on quantitative testing of function, and the exercise specificity and intensity change as repeated testing shows a more rapid clearing of some deficits than others. A variety of weight equipment is used in such a program (Fig. 58–5). A fitness maintenance program must be established to build on the gains made during the intensive, supervised program.

Psychosocial Interventions in Functional Restoration

The patient undergoing spinal rehabilitation is customarily one who has issues of prolonged disability, supplementing long-term pain. Traditional approaches have focused on pain management, which is intended to teach patients how to cope with pain and modify self-defeating behaviors. The essential flaw in this approach is the continued primary emphasis on the pa-

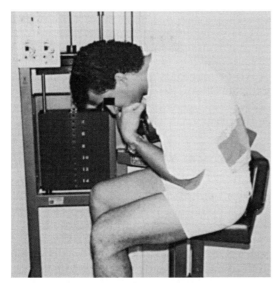

Figure 58–5. An abdominal weight machine used for trunk strengthening.

tient's self-reporting of pain, which is ultimately self-serving and unmeasurable. In functional restoration, the physician emphasizes the return to function and the setting of specific goals to achieve this return, recognizing that improved physical capacity, decreased stress and tension, and return of self-esteem and self-confidence will probably reduce the patient's pain perception. The rehabilitation process itself may be a tense, emotional, and physically painful "spring training" experience for the physically and psychologically deconditioned patient. As such, a variety of inspirational messages is necessary in the full half of the program devoted to education and counseling.

Individual and Group Counseling

A variety of defense mechanisms generally appears during sessions designed to overcome barriers to functional recovery. Emotional reactions and resistance to treatment must be discussed and overcome. Frustration regarding the pace of training inevitably occurs, making support during the difficult physical and psychologic tasks essential. This often takes place during one-on-one individual sessions. In groups, support is generally sought in a variety of ways. Patient groups can acknowledge difficulties with the process of rehabilitation, encourage the use of a "buddy system" with new patients, and encourage discussion of subjects such as psychologic testing, confidentiality, personal responsibility, and the work ethic. In addition, concerns about returning to work, litigation, fear of pain as a continued punishment, and medication and drug use are discussed. Finally, depression is recognized as part of the chronic pain problem. Reactions to treatment staff and the provision of honest feedback are strongly encouraged.

Behavioral Stress Management Training

Tension clearly accentuates the psychophysiologic experience of pain. Behavioral stress management is an important component of the treatment program. Biofeedback may be used to improve the patient's ability to relax physically and to gain better self-control over tense and painful muscles. The patient may also develop the ability to relax mentally by gaining control over unwanted thoughts and learning to self-direct his or her thinking. This is usually done in a cognitive-behavioral training program. Education in stress management is vital to teach patients the importance of proper breathing and to address their individual stress problems and accompanying symptoms. In group sessions, it is usually helpful to discuss the role of stress and relaxation in symptoms such as sleep disturbance, stiff joints, tight muscles, and emotional distress, so that patients integrate a response for relaxation when pain and tension increase.

Family Counseling

Families are an extremely important part of the disability process. They can encourage overprotectiveness and cocoon the patient, or they can act as instruments for recovery and return to independence. Involving spouses, parents, and children in treatment can be time-consuming but is usually a helpful part of the treatment process. During counseling for families, a variety of topics are discussed. Permission must be granted to family members to ignore illness behavior and be a potent force in attempts to modify it. Family members should participate in activities designed to encourage reactivation, including recreation, family exercises, walking in an interesting location, and so forth. Attempts to diffuse or redirect the anger of family members about a patient's own effort in his or her recovery should be encouraged, and fear of reinjury should be discussed realistically. There are clearly positive aspects of being disabled (e.g., more time at home with one's spouse), and the difficulties of giving these up with return to productivity must be covered. Finally, a full discussion of the negative impact of chronic spinal pain syndrome on families should be held. With family involvement, positive results can be anticipated. When family members work against the treatment team, a positive outcome is doubtful.

Functional Restoration Phases and Personnel

There are four phases associated with functional restoration treatment:

Phase I: Preprogram Stabilization

Phase I consists of one or two outpatient visits per week for two to four weeks prior to participating in the actual tertiary care program. The intent of this period is to establish initial mobility and tolerance of reasonable levels of activity, establish a home aerobics program, and reestablish a pattern of attendance and compliance with societal goals that previously characterized the patient's participation in work and recreation. Medication and substance abuse issues are dealt with prior to tertiary care, with detoxification and psychotropic drug stabilization performed as necessary. Antidepressant medications are commonly used, and major tranquilizers or anxiolytics may be necessary in certain cases. Narcotics, minor tranquilizers, and hypnotics are tapered, and anti-inflammatories may be used sparingly. Trust is established, and a pattern of home exercises commences, based on an initial quantitative functional evaluation and psychologic consultation. Compliance and attendance are carefully monitored as indicators of disability habituation.

Phase II: Intensive Tertiary Care Treatment

During this phase, a comprehensive multimodal disability management program is combined with a physical training program lasting up to eight hours a day. Strengthening exercises, aerobic fitness, and stretching are combined with work simulation and positional tolerance activities in the physical portion of the program. About half the day is spent in education, which includes group and individual counseling and classes on anatomy, physiology, assertiveness training, rational and emotive therapy, stress management, and quantitative test interpretation. The educational sessions are intended to fully inform the patient about the structural and functional issues that are critical to their recovery. Occupational counseling helps the patient focus on a work plan and return to productivity. Under ideal circumstances, such as at PRIDE in Texas, coordination with the State Vocational Rehabilitation Agency is facilitated, whenever necessary, immediately after medical rehabilitation. Even though vocational rehabilitation services are employed in only a minority of patients, their effectiveness is dramatically enhanced by receiving medically rehabilitated patients who are physically and mentally prepared for return to employment. The tertiary treatment plan is individualized, depending on the degree of utilization required, based on chronicity, physical testing, and psychosocial barriers. This intensive phase usually lasts two to four weeks (combining half days and full days), with limited psychologic intervention for those who can be functionally restored without it. Managed care agencies closely monitor utilization (which drives cost), usually necessitating justification of the individualized treatment plan.

Phase III: Work Transition

After completion of the intensive phase of the program, a period is often required to reintegrate the CSD employee into a work environment. Because the intensive tertiary care treatment includes work simulation, evaluation of permanent impairment, and preparation for closure of legal or administrative issues related to workers' compensation, the work transition phase is necessary only when the original job is not available, the patient is truly incapable of performing it, or vocational rehabilitation is problematic. This low utilization phase (two to four days over two to four weeks) involves further strengthening of the injured area, work simulation, and closure of occupational, legal, and administrative issues whenever necessary.

Phase IV: Outcome Tracking Phase

This important phase allows continued evaluation of the long-term effectiveness of the program, from both the patient's point of view and that of the staff. The patient is given the opportunity to consolidate gains and obtain feedback on maintenance of physical capacity goals by repeated quantitative functional evaluations performed at prescribed intervals. Telephone outcome tracking is performed at the first and second anniversaries of graduation by the staff, and assistance is offered whenever possible if new problems related to prior injury arise (Table 58–2). An effort is made during this phase to reinforce independence in the patient, so that visits are minimized to evaluations only, unless a new crisis requires a few "refresher sessions." An added benefit of a high rate of compliance in repeat testing and telephone tracking is the ability to perform one- and two-year follow-up studies such as have been performed at PRIDE.[12, 36, 37]

Staff and Duties

A supervising medical director guides the rehabilitation program and the treatment team. He or she must have a general background in sports medicine, musculoskeletal injury, psychoactive medications, disability management, and rehabilitation supervision. The medical director is usually assisted by a nurse "physician extender," who must be able to educate patients on medical matters, triage musculoskeletal problems, provide medication control, and communicate with outside agencies.

Physical therapists provide a vital service in working with the injured spinal segment or "weak link" functional unit. They supervise the progressive re-

Table 58–2. ONE-YEAR FOLLOW-UP OUTCOME GOALS FOR FUNCTIONAL RESTORATION

Outcome	Results
Return to work	>90%
Work retention (1 yr)	>80%
Posttreatment surgeries	<4%
Percentage unsettled claims	<15%
Spine-related medical visits (except for functional restoration or referring physician visits)	<5 visits/yr
Rate of recurrent injury claims (lost time) in patients returned to work	<2%/yr

sistive exercise and mobilization of this region. Occupational therapists tend to work more with whole-body work simulation, coordinating the injured segment with other body parts. Vocational counseling and assessment may be provided by vocational counselors working within an occupational department.

Psychologists have a dual role. They provide crisis intervention assistance through a cognitive-behavioral program, working with the rest of the team to deal with the barriers to functional recovery that characterize the patient's disabling spinal disorder. Using their assessment and personality knowledge, they provide valuable education and individual counseling for specific problems, as well as general classes in assertiveness training and stress management or coping methods. They also provide a staff support role through their assessment and interviewing skills by identifying teamwork barriers, their causes, and how to deal with them.

If these functions are performed well, they provide a complete rehabilitation program of proven efficacy and reasonable cost to patients with disabling CSDs. Such comprehensive tertiary rehabilitation is necessary for only the most chronic patients, those who have been refractory to all other forms of treatment. Other patients may be handled with simpler secondary care programs requiring considerably less supervision and fewer material resources. Hydrid secondary-tertiary approaches are available for injured workers on the cusp. For those who require functional restoration, the early application of rehabilitation is the surest way to resolve the patient's problem before the scourges of deconditioning, disability, depression, and drugs permanently alienate the patient from society.

References

1. Akeson, W., Amiel, D., and Woo, S.: Immobility effects on synovial joints: The pathomechanics of joint contracture. Biorheology *17*:95–100, 1980.
2. Barnett, J.: The Millon Behavioral Health Inventory and the Minnesota Multiphasic Personality Inventory compared as predictors of treatment outcome in a rehabilitation program for chronic low back pain. Ph.D. diss., Division of Psychology, University of Texas Southwestern Medical Center, 1986.
3. Beck, A.: Depression: Clinical, Experimental and Theoretical Aspects. New York, Harper & Row, 1967.
4. Brady, S., Mayer, T., and Gatchel, R.: Physical progress and residual impairment quantification after functional restoration. Part II: Isokinetic trunk strength. Spine *18*:395–400, 1994.
5. Capra, P., Mayer, T., and Gatchel, R.: Adding psychological scales to your back pain assessment. J. Musc. Med. *2*:41–52, 1985.
6. Chaffin, D.: Human strength capability and low-back pain. J. Occup. Med. *16*:248–254, 1974.
7. Curtis, L., Mayer, T., and Gatchel, R.: Physical progress and residual impairment after functional restoration. Part III: Isokinetic and isoinertial lifting capacity. Spine *18*:401–405, 1994.
8. DeLorme, T., and Watkins, A.: Progressive Resistance Exercise: Technic Medical Application. New York, Appleton-Century-Crofts, 1951.
9. Engelberg, A. (ed.): American Medical Association Guides to the Evaluation of Permanent Impairment. 3rd ed. Chicago, AMA Press, 1988.
10. Eriksson, E.: Sports injuries of knee ligaments: Their diagnosis, treatment, rehabilitation and prevention. Med. Sci. Sports *8*:133–144, 1976.
11. First, M. B., Spitzer, R. L., Gibbon, M., and Williams, J. B. W.: Structured Clinical Interview for DSM-IV Axis I Disorders. New York State Psychiatric Institute, Biometric Research Department, 1995.
12. Garcy, P., Mayer, T., and Gatchel, R.: Recurrent or new injury outcomes after return to work in chronic disabling spinal disorders: Tertiary prevention efficacy of functional restoration treatment. Spine (in press).
13. Gatchel, R., Polatin, P., Mayer, T., and Garcy, P.: Psychopathology and the rehabilitation of patients with chronic low back pain disability. Arch. Phys. Med. Rehabil. *75*:666–670, 1994.
14. Gelberman, R., Manske, P., Akeson, W., et al.: Kappa Delta Award paper: Flexor tendon repair. J. Orthop. Res. *4*:119–128, 1986.
15. Gracovetsky, S., and Farfan, H.: The optimum spine. Spine *11*:543–573, 1986.
16. Haggmark, T.: Comparison of isometric muscle training and electrical stimulation supplementing isometric muscle training in the recovery after major knee ligament surgery. Am. J. Sports Med. *7*:169–171, 1979.
17. Hamilton, M.: Anatomy scale for depression. J. Neurol. Neurosurg. Psychiatry *23*:56–62, 1960.
18. Hazard, R.: Spine update: Functional restoration. Spine *20*:2345–2348, 1995.
19. Hoshizaki, T., and Massey, B.: Relationships of muscular endurance among specific muscle groups for continuous and intermittent static contractions. Res. Q. Exerc. Sport *57*:229–235, 1986.
20. Keeley, J., Mayer, T., Cox, R., et al.: Quantification of lumbar function. Part 5: Reliability range of motion measures in the sagittal plane and in vivo torso rotation measurement technique. Spine *11*:31–35, 1986.
21. Kinney, R., Gatchel, R., Polatin, P., et al.: Prevalence of psychopathology in acute and chronic low back pain patients. J. Occup. Rehabil. *3*:95–103, 1993.
22. Kishino, N., Mayer, T., Gatchel, R., et al.: Quantification of lumbar function. Part 4: Isometric and isokinetic lifting simulation in normal subjects and low back dysfunction patients. Spine *10*:921–927, 1985.
23. Kohles, S., Barnes, D., Gatchel, R., and Mayer, T.: Improved physical performance outcomes following functional restoration treatment in patient with chronic low back pain: Early versus recent training results. Spine *15*:1321–1324, 1990.
24. Kroemer, K.: Human strength: Terminology, measurement and interpretation of data. Hum. Factors *12*:297–313, 1970.
25. Loebl, W.: Measurement of spinal posture and range in spinal movements. Ann. Phys. Med. *9*:103, 1967.
26. Mayer, T., Barnes, D., Kishino, N., et al.: Progressive isoinertial lifting evaluation. Part 1: A standardized protocol and normative database. Spine *13*:993–997, 1988.
27. Mayer, T., Barnes, D., Nichols, G., et al.: Progressive isoinertial lifting evaluation. Part 2: A comparison with isokinetic lifting in a disabled chronic low-back pain industrial population. Spine *13*:998–1002, 1988.
28. Mayer, T., Brady, S., Bovasso, E., et al.: Noninvasive measurement of cervical tri-planar motion in normal subjects. Spine *18*:2191–2195, 1993.
29. Mayer, T., and Gatchel, R.: Functional Restoration for Spinal Disorders: The Sports Medicine Approach. Philadelphia, Lea & Febiger, 1988.
30. Mayer, T., Gatchel, R., Barnes, D., et al.: Progressive isoinertial lifting evaluation: Erratum notice. Spine *15*:5, 1990.
31. Mayer, T., Gatchel, R., Betancur, J., and Bovasso, E.: Trunk muscle endurance measurement: Isometric contrasted to isokinetic testing in normal subjects. Spine *20*:920–927, 1995.
32. Mayer, T., Gatchel, R., Keeley, J., and Mayer, H.: Optimal spinal strength normalization factors among male railroad workers. Spine *18*:239–244, 1993.
33. Mayer, T., Gatchel, R., Keeley, J., et al.: A male incumbent worker industrial database. Part I: Lumbar spinal physical capacity. Spine *19*:755–761, 1994.
34. Mayer, T., Gatchel, R., Keeley, J., et al.: A male incumbent worker industrial database. Part II: Cervical spinal physical capacity. Spine *19*:762–764, 1994.
35. Mayer, T., Gatchel, R., Keeley, J., et al.: A male incumbent worker

industrial database. Part III: Lumbar/cervical functional testing. Spine 19:765–770, 1994.

36. Mayer, T., Gatchel, R., Kishino, N., et al.: Objective assessment of spine function following industrial injury: A prospective study with comparison group and one-year follow-up. 1985 Volvo Award in Clinical Sciences. Spine 10:482–493, 1985.

37. Mayer, T., Gatchel, R., Mayer, H., et al.: A prospective two-year study of functional restoration in industrial low back injury: An objective assessment procedure. JAMA 258:1763–1767, 1987.

38. Mayer, T., Kondrakse, G., Beals, S., and Gatchel, R.: Spinal range of motion: Accuracy and sources of error with inclinometric measurement. Spine (in press).

39. Mayer, T., Polatin, P., Smith, B., et al.: Contemporary concepts in spine care: Spine rehabilitation: Secondary and tertiary nonoperative care. Spine 18:2060–2066, 1995.

40. Mayer, T., Pope, P., Tabor, J., et al.: Physical progress and residual impairment quantification after functional restoration. Part I: Lumbar mobility. Spine 18:389–394, 1994.

41. Mayer, T., Smith, S., Keeley, J., and Mooney, V.: Quantification of lumbar function. Part 2: Sagittal plane trunk strength in chronic low back pain patients. Spine 10:765–772, 1985.

42. Mayer, T., Tencer, A., Kristoferson, S., and Mooney, V.: Use of noninvasive techniques for quantification of spinal range of motion in normal subjects and chronic low-back dysfunctional patients. Spine 9:588–595, 1984.

43. Million, R., Haavik, K., Jayson, M. I. V., et al.: Evaluation of low back pain and assessment of lumbar corsets with and without back supports. Ann. Rheum. Dis. 40:449–454, 1981.

44. Montgomery, J., and Steadman, J.: Rehabilitation of the injured knee. Clin. Sports Med. 4:333–343, 1985.

45. Mooney, V., Cairns, D., and Robertson, J.: A system for evaluating and treating chronic back disability. West. J. Med. 124:370–376, 1976.

46. Polatin, P., Kinney, R., Gatchel, R., et al.: Psychiatric illness and chronic low back pain: The mind and the spine—which goes first? Spine 18:66–71, 1993.

47. Ruben, C.: Osteoregulatory mechanisms—Kappa Delta Award. In Transactions of Annual Meeting, American Academy of Orthopedic Surgeons, New Orleans, 1985.

48. Salter, R., and Field, P.: The effects of continuous compression on living articular cartilage: An experimental study. J. Bone Joint Surg. [Br.] 43:376–386, 1961.

49. Smith, S., Mayer, T., Gatchel, R., and Becker, T.: Quantification of lumbar function. Part 1: Isometric and multispeed isokinetic trunk strength measures in sagittal and axial planes in normal subject patients. Spine 10:757–764, 1985.

50. Ward, N.: Tricyclic antidepressant for chronic low back pain: Mechanism of action and predictors of response. Spine 11:661–665, 1986.

51. Ware, J., and Sherbone, C.: The MOS 36-item short-form health survey (SF-36). Med. Care 30:473–483, 1992.

52. Wechsler, D.: Wechsler Adult Intelligence Scale—Revised. San Antonio, Psychological Corporation, 1981.

59

Chronic Pain Management

Nonsurgical Management of Chronic Back Pain

Mark S. Wallace, M.D.

Gordon Irving, M.D.

Joseph Dunn, M.D.

Tony Yaksh, Ph.D.

PHYSIOLOGY AND PHARMACOLOGY OF PAIN PROCESSING

Sensory Afferents

Peripheral nerves represent the initial pathway by which somatic and visceral stimuli gain access to the central nervous system. Mechanical, thermal, or chemical stimuli are able to generate afferent traffic in specific elements of this pathway, notably the small unmyelinated or lightly myelinated primary afferents. Table 59–1 summarizes the characteristics of these afferent components.

Under normal circumstances, small primary afferents display little or no spontaneous activity. Subpopulations of A-delta and C fibers are specifically activated by high-threshold mechanical and/or thermal stimuli, and the magnitude of their discharge increases as the stimulus intensity is increased. Because the firing frequency recorded from A-delta and C nociceptive fibers in the human correlates with subjective pain reports, it follows that the afferent traffic in these fibers contributes to generation of the pain state.

Aside from acute mechanical and thermal stimuli, local tissue injury yields (1) a persistent, spontaneous bursting activity in the primary afferent axons innervating the injured site, and (2) an exaggerated discharge in response to normally subthreshold and submaximal stimuli. The mechanisms of increased spontaneous activity and facilitated discharge have been widely considered and probably originate from

factors released into the periterminal milieu secondary to the injury.

As schematically indicated in Figure 59–1 after tissue injury, there is local cellular damage and an infiltration of inflammatory cells, which elaborate a variety of active products, including amines, kinins, lipidic acids, cytokines, and peptides. In addition, there is increased plasma extravasation secondary to damage to the local vasculature and an increase in capillary permeability at sites peripheral to the actual injury, mediated by the antidromic release of peptides from the peripheral terminal of the small afferent axon. These products are believed to contribute to the ongoing discharge and the persistent postinjury pain message (Table 59–2).

Afferent Neurotransmitters

Currently, excitatory amino acids such as glutamate and a number of peptides, including substance P (sP), vasoactive intestinal peptide (VIP), somatostatin, a VIP homologue (PHI), calcitonin gene related peptide (CGRP), bombesin, and related peptides, possess distinct nociceptive characteristics (Table 59–3). Most small primary afferents contain multiple transmitters, e.g., an excitatory amino acid and one or more peptides within the same terminal, and afferent depolarization releases these multiple pools of transmitters. Postsynaptically, excitatory amino acids produce a rapid, short-lasting depolarization. In contrast, peptides typically produce a delayed, long-lasting depolarization. Small

Table 59–1. CLASSIFICATION OF SENSORY AFFERENTS BY CONDUCTION VELOCITY, SIZE, AND EFFECTIVE STIMULUS

Fiber Class	Velocity	Effective Stimulus
A-beta (large myelinated) (12–20 μ diameter)	Group II (>40–50 msec)	Low-threshold mechanoreceptors Specialized nerve endings (Pacinian corpuscles)
A-delta (small myelinated) (1–4 μ diameter)	Group III (10–40 msec)	Low-threshold mechanical or thermal High-threshold mechanical or thermal Specialized nerve endings
C (small unmyelinated) (0.5–1.5 μ diameter)	Group IV (<2 msec)	High-threshold thermal, mechanical, or chemical Free nerve endings

The fiber class refers to an Erlanger-Gasser classification and is based on anatomic characteristics. Velocity groups are from the Lloyd-Hunt classification, defined on the basis of conduction velocity in muscle afferents.

primary afferents are sensitive to several neurotoxins, such as capsaicin, which stimulate and subsequently desensitize the terminal. The spinal terminals of small primary afferents are modulated by a variety of receptors (opiate, alpha-2 adrenoreceptor) that are found preterminally on the afferent. These receptors can inhibit the release of afferent neurotransmitters, leading to a block of C fiber transmission and analgesia.

Spinal Cord

The spinal cord is divided into several laminae characterized by a number of specific cell types and the specific afferent classes from which it receives excitatory input (Fig. 59–2).

Upon entering the spinal cord, the afferents collateralize, sending fibers rostrally and caudally up to several segments in the tract of Lissauer (small C fiber afferents) or into the dorsal columns (large afferents) and into the segment of entry. Upon penetrating into the parenchyma, the terminal fields also ramify rostrally and caudally for several millimeters.

Dorsal Horn Neurons

The second-order nociresponsive elements in the dorsal horn may be considered in several classes based on their response characteristics and their approximate anatomic location.

Cells may be classified as low threshold (i.e., driven by A-beta input), high threshold (i.e., driven by high-threshold A-delta or C fibers), or convergent (i.e., receiving input from A-beta/A-delta *and* C afferents). These latter cells are called wide dynamic range (WDR) neurons. Figure 59–3 presents schematically the firing pattern of a nociceptive-specific and a WDR dorsal horn neuron. In a broad sense, nociceptive-specific neurons provide an all-or-nothing signal, denoting the presence of a noxious stimulus; a WDR neuron possesses the ability to encode stimulus intensity by the frequency of its discharge.

In addition to the ability to encode stimulus intensity, WDR neurons display other properties that are useful in explaining certain properties of sensory encoding. Depending on the spinal level, a WDR neuron may be activated by stimulation of a variety of organ systems.

The same WDR neuron can be excited by cutaneous or deep (muscle and joint) input applied within the

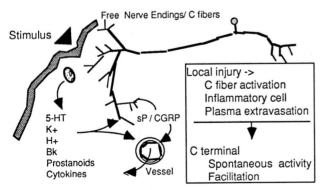

Figure 59–1. Primary afferent terminal. Local damaging stimulus leads to firing of the fine afferents and the local activation of inflammatory cells. Afferent fibers display antidromic release of neuromodulator peptides (sP/CGRP). Hormones, such as prostaglandins and cytokines, released from the inflammatory cells and plasma extravasation products result in additional stimulation and sensitization of the free nerve endings.

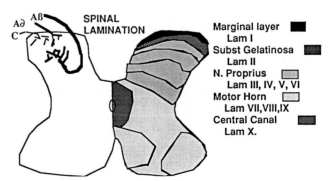

Figure 59–2. Schematic showing Rexed lamination (right) and the approximate organization of the afferents as they enter at the dorsal root entry zone and then penetrate into the dorsal horn to terminate in laminae I and II (A-delta/C) or penetrate more deeply to terminate as high as lamina III (A-beta).

Table 59–2. CLASSES OF AGENTS RELEASED BY TISSUE INJURY THAT INFLUENCE ACTIVITY AND SENSITIVITY OF SENSORY AFFERENTS

1. Amines
   Histamine (granules of mast cells, basophils, and platelets) and serotonin (mast cells and platelets) are released by a variety of stimuli, including mechanical trauma, heat, radiation, certain by-products of tissue damage, thrombin, collagen, and epinephrine, as well as members of the arachidonic acid cascade, leukotrienes, and prostanoids.
2. Kinin
   A variety of kinins, notably bradykinin, are released by physical trauma. Peptide is synthesized by a cascade that is triggered upon the activation of Factor XII by agents such as kallikrein and trypsin. Bradykinin acts by specific bradykinin receptors (B1/B2) to activate free nerve endings.
3. Lipidic acids
   Agents are synthesized by lipoxygenase or cyclooxygenase (prostanoids) upon the release of cell membrane–derived arachidonic acid secondary to the activation of phospholipase A_2. A number of prostanoids, including PGE_2, can directly activate C fibers. Others, such as PGI_2 and TXA_2, and several leukotrienes can markedly facilitate the excitability of C fibers. These effects are also mediated by specific membrane receptors.
4. Cytokines
   Cytokines such as the interleukins are formed as part of the inflammatory reaction involving macrophages and have been shown to exert powerful sensitizing effects on C fibers. Interleukins, such as IL-1, may sensitize C fibers via a prostaglandin intermediary.
5. Primary afferent peptides
   Calcitonin gene related peptide (CGRP) and substance P are found in and released from the peripheral terminals of C fibers and produce local cutaneous vasodilation, plasma extravasation, and sensitization in the region of skin innervated by the stimulated sensory nerve.
6. [H]/[K]
   Low pH activates the local axon reflex and results in the local release of CGRP, a potent vasodilator and modulator of plasma extravasation. A population of C nociceptors sensitve to noxious intensities of mechanical and thermal stimuli also respond in a stimulus-related fashion to solutions of increasing proton concentration injected into their receptive fields. These receptors develop a lower threshold and enhanced response to mechanical stimuli. Similar injections in humans induce a sustained graded pain and hyperalgesia.

dermatome that coincides with the segmental location of these cells. Thus, T1 and T5 root stimulation activates WDR neurons, which are also excited by coronary artery occlusion. In addition, these results likely account for the phenomenon of nocifensor tenderness, as revealed when the cutaneous receptor associated with an inflamed visceral organ is lightly percussed.

Repetitive stimulation of C but not A fibers produces a gradual increase in the frequency discharge of the WDR neuron until the neuron is in a state of virtually continuous discharge ("windup"). Under these conditions, the cell displays an enlarged receptive field and an increased response to a modestly aversive stimulus (e.g., hyperalgesia).

Ascending Spinal Tracts and Supraspinal Projections

Activity evoked in the spinal cord by high-threshold stimuli reaches supraspinal sites by several long and intersegmental tract systems that travel within the ventrolateral quadrant (Fig. 59–4). Pain that transverses a "crossed pathway" in that unilateral section of the ventrolateral quadrant yields a contralateral thermal/

Table 59–3. PUTATIVE NEUROTRANSMITTERS IN SMALL PRIMARY AFFERENTS

	Small DRG	Neuronal Excitation	Algesic Behavior*	Hyper-esthesia*
Peptides				
Substance P	+	Yes	+	+ +
CGRP	+	Yes	+	+
Somatostatin	+	Yes/no	+	0
Bombesin	+	Yes	+	+
Galanin	+	?	?	?
VIP	+	?	0	−
CCK	+/?	?	0	0
Excitatory Amino Acids				
Glutamate	+	+ + +	+ + +	+ + +
Aspartate	?	+ + +	+ + +	+ + +

DRG, dorsal root ganglion; ?, not known.
*Observed after spinal administration.
From Yaksh, T. L., and Malmberg, A. B.: Central pharmacology of nociceptive transmission. *In* Melzack, R., and Wall, P. (eds.): Textbook of Pain. 3rd ed. Churchill Livingstone, 1993, pp. 165–200.

mechanical analgesia in dermatomes below the spinal level of the section.

Spinothalamic Fibers

The cells of origin of this tract, the most extensively studied of the ventrolateral tract systems, are not limited to the dorsal gray, but are found throughout laminae I through VII and X of the spinal gray matter. Axons originating in the marginal layer and the neck of the nucleus proprius ascend predominantly in the contralateral ventral quadrant. Clinical experience suggests that the crossing may occur as much as several segments more rostrally. Thus, following cordotomy, the analgesic level may be several dermatomes caudal to the section. Although crossed fibers predominate, uncrossed fibers also represent an appreciable component of the spinothalamic population. Spinothalamic axons differentiate into a lateral and medial component in the posterior portion of the thalamus: the medial component passes through the internal medullary lamina to terminate in the nucleus parafascicularis and the intralaminar and paralaminar nuclei. The majority of fibers pass laterally through the external medullary lamina to terminate in small clusters scattered throughout the nucleus ventralis posterolateralis, the medial aspect of the posterior nuclear complex, and the intralaminar nuclei.

A significant proportion of the neurons projecting laterally in the thalamus (ventral posterior lateral complex) also project to the medial (central lateral nucleus or dorsal medial nucleus) portion. An additional popu-

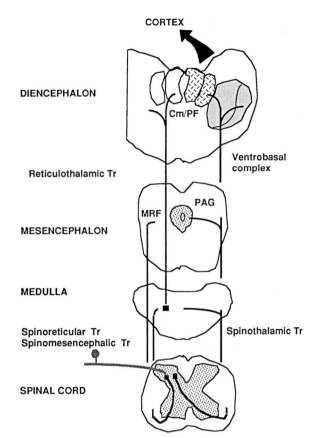

Figure 59–4. Schematic displaying organization of spinifugal systems through which nociceptive transmission is accomplished. Note that the diagram emphasizes crossed and uncrossed fibers, multisynaptic connections for the uncrossed fibers, collaterals into the medial medullary and mesencephalic core from all ascending afferents as they progress rostrally, and potential dual projection of STT fibers into the medial and lateral thalamus. STT, spinothalamic tract.

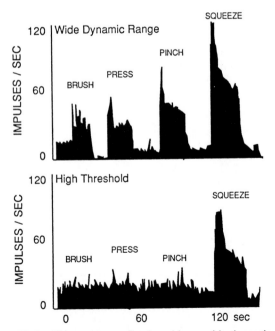

Figure 59–3. Firing pattern of a dorsal horn wide dynamic range (top) versus a high-threshold (bottom) spinothalamic neuron. Schematics present the neuronal response to graded intensities of mechanical stimulation applied to the receptive fields. (For examples of such cell activity, see works of Willis.)

lation projects solely to the medial nuclei. The importance of the ventrolateral tracts to pain is shown by the fact that ventrolateral tractotomies raise the threshold for visceral and somatic pain on the side contralateral to the lesion. The sensory level of the cordotomy indicates that the ascending tracts may travel rostrally several segments before crossing. Similarly, stimulation of the ventrolateral tracts in awake subjects undergoing percutaneous cordotomies results in reports of contralateral warmth and pain. Midline myelotomies that destroy fibers crossing the midline at the levels of the cut (as well as the cells in lamina X) produce bilateral pain deficits. These observations suggest that the relevant pathways for nociception are predominantly crossed. Although it is clear that spinal transmission of nociceptive information occurs in the ventrolateral funiculus, the relevance of other systems is suggested by (1) anomalous recovery of pain after 3 to 12 months, (2) persistence of contralateral pain sensations following a unilateral lesion, and (3) "breakthrough" of pain produced by afferent stimulation. Other systems may travel in the dorsal quadrant or within the central gray.

Supraspinal Systems

Certain supraspinal regions appear to participate in the processing of relevant pain information. The medullary reticular formation may present as a "relay station" for the rostral transmission of nociceptive information. Medullary reticular cell bodies are activated antidromically by stimulation in the thalamus; conversely, stimulation of the medullary reticular formation has been reported to activate thalamic neurons.

Units in the mesencephalic central gray and in the adjacent reticular formation are differentially responsive to innocuous and noxious cutaneous and electrical stimuli. Stimulation can evoke signs of intense discomfort in animals. In humans, autonomic responses are elicited, along with reports of dysphoria.

Cortex

The somatosensory areas (SI and SII) receive input indirectly from the three major spinal systems through which ascending sensory and noxious information may travel. Investigations have focused on the importance of the SII area in the reception and perception of pain information. Posterior SII receives input largely from the posterior thalamic complex. These neurons are polysensory, and a number of them respond to high-intensity mechanical stimuli. Discrete regions within the anterior cingulate gyrus of the cortex are activated by noxious, but not non-noxious, thermal stimuli.

Limbic System

The pain response has an overriding affective-motivational component that is as important to behavior as the initiating stimulus. A variety of lesion procedures in humans and animals have been shown to psychophysically dissociate the reported stimulus intensity from its affective component. Such disconnection syndromes are produced by prefrontal lobectomies, cingulotomies, and temporal lobe/amygdala lesions.

DYNAMIC COMPONENTS OF NOCICEPTIVE PROCESSING

The anatomic connectivity of the "pain pathway" does not provide insight into the dynamic nature of the processing of the afferent message, leading to a "pain state." Dynamic characteristics are essential in our understanding of the pain state generated after injury and inflammation and its management.

Peripheral mechanical and thermal stimuli evoke intensity-dependent increases in firing rates of small afferents, corresponding to the psychophysical report of pain sensation in humans and the vigor of the escape response in animals. Such stimuli also can induce a local tissue injury and the subsequent elaboration of active products. These products directly activate the local terminals of afferents (which are otherwise silent) and facilitate their discharge in response to otherwise submaximal stimuli. This then leads to an ongoing afferent barrage and the subsequent evolution of a state of facilitated processing, yielding hyperalgesia/hyperesthesia.

Acute Pain State: Transient Activation of High-Threshold Afferent Input

Afferent Organization of Acute Noxious Stimuli. Brief stimulation of small afferent fibers results in clearly defined pain behavior in humans and animals. This is believed to be mediated by the release of excitatory afferent transmitters and, consequently, the depolarization of projection neurons. There are proportional increases in the discharge rate as the intensity of the stimulus rises from innocuous to noxious, and there are corresponding parallels between the magnitude of the discharge of these projection neurons and the intensity of the pain sensation reported.

Modulation of Acute Afferent Evoked Excitation. Small afferent input is subject to modulation by a number of receptor systems within the spinal cord. In most cases, agonists for such receptors applied to the spinal cord reduce the magnitude of the response evoked by high-threshold afferent stimulation. In the case of agents such as those in the opioid class, considerable data emphasize that these agents diminish the magnitude of the response evoked and produce analgesia.

Many of these modulating substrates represent endogenous systems that are believed to function in the ongoing regulation of afferent processing. The best defined of these are the so-called bulbospinal aminergic pathways and the endogenous enkephalinergic systems that are believed to regulate afferent processing by a reflexly activated increase in spinal adrenergic, serotonergic, and opioid receptor activity, respectively. The direct spinal delivery of a number of agonists for these receptors has been shown to produce a powerful and selective inhibition for the processing of nociceptive input.

Post–Tissue Injury Pain State: Protracted Afferent Activation

Central Facilitation. WDR neurons in the dorsal horn display a stimulus-dependent response to the persistent activation of sensory C fibers. Repetitive stimulation of C (but not A) fibers results in a progressively facilitated discharge. This augmented response to a given stimulus is an important component of the pain message. Of equal importance is the fact that after such conditioning stimuli, low-threshold tactile stimulation also becomes increasingly effective in driving these neurons.

The role of afferent-evoked facilitation in the postinjury pain state cannot be minimized. After tissue injury, a local peripheral release of active factors is observed in the perineural space. Such active factors produce a prolonged activation of C fibers, which evoke a facili-

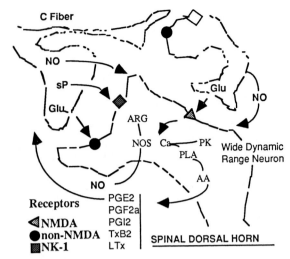

Figure 59–5. A schematic summary of the functional organization of elements in the dorsal horn discussed in the text that impact on the processing of afferent input. This organization reflects the response to acute stimulation, development of the hyperalgesic state induced by repetitive small afferent stimulation, and development of anomalous pain states secondary to large afferent stimulation.

tated state of processing in WDR neurons and lead to a facilitation of nociceptive processing.

Pharmacology of Central Facilitation. The pharmacology of central facilitation reflects more than the simple repetitive activation of an excitatory system (Fig. 59–5). The arrival of the first small afferent barrage appears to initiate the mechanisms leading to an augmented response to the peripheral stimulus. Blocking the initial input and/or preventing the augmentation is a goal for ongoing research. A number of classes of agents are known to influence the processing of this dorsal horn system, including opiates, non-*N*-methyl D-aspartate (NMDA) antagonists, neurokinin 1 (NK1) agonists, nonsteroidal anti-inflammation agents, and nitrous oxide.

Post–Nerve Injury Pain State

Low-intensity mechanical input, activating large low-threshold afferent axons, is not normally an aversive event. Following nerve injury, however, conditions such as causalgia or reflex sympathetic dystrophy may develop. In these states, aside from the spontaneous, sharp shooting pains that may evolve, light mechanical stimulation (touch) may be reported as exceedingly painful (allodynia). The pain state results from the activation of low-threshold mechanoreceptors (AB afferents), and the ability of light touch to evoke pain is evidence that the nerve injury has led to reorganization of central processing. Although the mechanism of this miscoding is poorly understood, certain sequelae of peripheral nerve injury appear relevant.

1. Persistent small afferent fiber activity originates

after an interval of days to weeks from the lesioned site (neuroma) and from the dorsal root ganglion (DRG) of the injured nerve.
2. Sprouting afferent terminals display a characteristic growth cone with transduction properties that were not possessed by the original axon, including mechanical and chemical sensitivity. Thus, these endings may be excited by a number of humoral factors, such as prostaglandins, catecholamines, and cytokines. Regenerating terminals have increased densities of various ion channels, notably those for sodium.
3. Following a peripheral sensory lesion, there is a hyperinnervation of the DRG cells by sympathetic terminals, and cross talk develops between A and C fibers.
4. Prominent morphologic changes have been identified in the spinal dorsal horn ipsilateral to the ligation. The mechanism of these changes is not clear, but the possibility of persistent changes secondary to the chronic afferent barrage or to a change in factors transported from the lesioned site seems likely.

An important class of neurons in the dorsal horn region are those interneurons that contain GABA and glycine. The spinal antagonism of GABA and glycine receptors yields a powerful facilitation of the response of WDR neurons to low thresholds; otherwise innocuous mechanical stimuli elicit prominent pain behavior in unanesthetized experimental animals following light touch.

PAIN-PRODUCING STRUCTURES IN THE SPINE (Table 59–4)

Zygapophysial Joint Pain

The facet joint has long been known to be a significant source of back pain. The facet joints are true diarthrodial joints with a rich nerve supply transmitting both nociception and mechanoreception.[261, 266] The synovial membrane of the facet joints is rich in free nerve endings associated with painful sensation.[78] In addition, morphologic studies on human[9, 18, 80, 101, 102, 109, 245] and animal[81] facet joints support the role of the facet joint in low back pain. These studies have demonstrated

Table 59–4. CRITERIA FOR DIAGNOSING FACET PAIN

Back pain associated with groin or thigh pain	30 points
Well-localized paraspinal tenderness	20 points
Reproduction of pain with extension-rotation	30 points
Corresponding radiographic changes	20 points
Pain below the knee	– 10 points

A score of 60 points or more indicates a very high probability of satisfactory response to facet joint injection.

From Helbig, T., and Lee, C. K.: The lumbar facet syndrome. Spine *13*:61–64, 1988.

neuropeptides and nerve endings in the facet joint capsule.

In spite of identification of pain fibers innervating the facet joints, many authors question the existence of true facet pain.[125, 216] Although it remains controversial, pathology within these joints appears to result in significant back pain. The exact pathophysiology of the facet that results in pain is unknown. However, Mooney and Robertson suggest three mechanisms of lumbar facet pain: (1) chronic synovial and/or capsular reaction to trauma, (2) spinal instability resulting in abnormal stresses on the facet joint, and (3) degenerative changes within the joints.[169]

Lumbar Facet Pain

Several investigators have demonstrated that painful lumbar facet joints refer pain into the low back, buttock, and upper posterior thigh.[136, 169, 170, 221] However, discogenic and myofascial pain can result in similiar pain referral patterns.[54, 84] Lumbar facet pain rarely produces true radicular pain into the extremity, but because of the close association of the facet joint with the nerve root, true radicular symptoms can occur with facet joint disease (e.g., synovial cysts, facet hypertrophy, or osteophytes).[25, 201, 223, 241, 253] Lumbar facet pain is worse in the morning and with inactivity and is aggravated by extension and lateral flexion of the spine to the diseased side. If lateral extension results in pain on the opposite side, soft tissue pain should be entertained.

Cervical Facet Pain

Cervical facet pain is a common etiology of neck pain, especially after whiplash injury.[7, 17] Painful cervical facets can refer pain unilaterally anywhere from the cranium to the lower border of the scapula.[73] Cervical facet pain may also result in autonomic dysfunction, resulting in dizziness, nausea, and blurred vision.[22] Typically, upper cervical facet pathology results in head pain, the middle cervical facets produce neck pain, and the lower facets produce lower neck and shoulder pain. There have been a few anecdotal reports of cervical facet pain radiating into the arm.[223, 241] Pain originating from the atlanto-occipital joint radiates mainly to the suboccipital region, although the pain may radiate anywhere from the vertex to C5.[73] Pathology of the C1–C2 facet may result in pain referred to the ipsilateral mastoid area, suboccipital area, or ear.[79, 106, 233]

Sacroiliac Joint

As with the facet joint, there has been controversy over the sacroiliac joint (SIJ) as a cause of low back pain. However, many clinicians believe that the potential for this joint to cause pain is underestimated.[21, 38, 39, 49, 59, 69, 95, 128, 144, 248] The largest study evaluating the incidence of SIJ pain revealed that SIJ pain and posterior joint syndromes were the most common referred-pain syndromes.[21] The SIJ is classified as a diarthrodial joint;

however, with age, the joint develops fibrous adhesions that restrict movement.[36, 124, 247] This restriction of movement decreases the joint's buffering capacity, which may lead to chronic pain. Like the facet joints, the SIJ is richly innervated with both free nerve endings and mechanoreceptors. The innervation has been extensively described and supports this joint as a pain-sensitive structure.[26, 32, 123] Most of the innervation of the SIJ is supplied dorsally, which results in the bulk of the innervation occurring in the dorsal segment of the joint.[107]

Pain from the SIJ is usually referred to the buttocks, groin, posterior thigh, and, occasionally, below the knee.[20, 47, 92, 93, 211] The pain is worsened with bending and prolonged sitting and improved with walking or standing.[20, 129] Neurologic examination is usually normal. Because of the anatomic location of the SIJ, this structure is difficult to examine, and many of the provocative tests can result in false-positives and intertester differences.[75, 188] However, there are several provocative tests that are reliable and easy to interpret.[21, 143]

Intervertebral Disc

The outer one third of the intervertebral disc (ID) is well innervated; however, there is controversy about whether it is a pain-producing structure.[24, 41, 43, 82, 254] There is little, if any, controversy over the role that a herniated disc plays in producing radicular pain; however, controversy arises over the role of isolated disc pathology without nerve compression as a cause of low back pain.[181] Nerve endings capable of transmitting pain impulses are abundant in the outer one third of the annulus fibrosus in both the cervical disc[26, 33, 110] and the lumbar disc.[108, 158, 267, 269] In addition, nerves within the ID contain neuropeptides that are involved in pain transmission.[250] Injuries in the annulus fibrosus may result in pain even though the external appearance of the disc remains normal and before nerve roots are affected.[30]

The referral pattern of pain originating solely from the disc is similar to that produced by facet joint pain.[84] Takahashi and colleagues suggest that disc pain is referred to the groin, because capsaicin applied to the rat lumbar ID caused extravasation in the groin skin.[237] Pain provocative maneuvers on physical examination to reproduce disc pain are nonspecific, and the diagnosis relies mainly on disc injections.[24] Moneta and coworkers analyzed 833 discograms and found that the outer annulus appears to be the origin of pain reproduction with this procedure.[168] The pain from diseased intervertebral discs may not arise directly from the disc but rather from other structures that develop abnormal stresses as a result of the diseased disc.[152] Other structures surrounding the disc are known to have pain fibers (e.g., facet joints, anterior and posterior longitudinal ligaments). However, Schwarzer and associates found that the combination of lumbar discogenic pain and lumbar zygapophyseal joint pain is uncommon.[214] This is in contrast to cervical pain, which seems to have a higher incidence of coexisting disc and facet pain.[28]

Ligaments of the Spine

There are many ligamentous structures in the spine that are innervated with free nerve endings. However, there is variability in the density of this innervation. Of all the ligamentous structures, the posterior longitudinal ligament appears to be the most heavily innervated with free nerve endings,[110, 185, 262] and the ligamentum flavum appears to be the least innervated.[198] Degenerative changes within these ligaments may result in sensitization of free nerve endings, leading to chronic pain. In addition, the close proximity of the anterior and posterior longitudinal ligaments to the discs makes the structures susceptible to exposure to the disc contents in the event of disc rupture. The disc contents may induce an inflammatory process in these ligaments, leading to pain.

Nerve Root

The nerve root is innervated by the sinuvertebral nerve, which branches from the segmental nerve and travels backward into the neural foramen. The arachnoidal covering of the nerve root is heavily innervated and can be a source of pain. Mechanical compression or irritation of these structures can lead to pain in the extremities that is associated with neurologic changes. The nerve root may be stimulated mechanically by disc herniation, osteophyte formation, foraminal narrowing owing to degenerative disc disease, or tumor invasion. In addition, it has been postulated that both the disc contents and the facet joint contents may induce an arachnoiditis; however, Haughton and colleagues showed this to be true only for the disc contents.[116]

DIAGNOSTIC AND THERAPEUTIC PROCEDURES FOR BACK PAIN

Zygapophyseal Joint Injections

History and Examination

Although careful history and examination may clinically implicate the zygapophyseal joint (Z-joint) as a cause of an individual's spinal pain, in the lumbar spine, there appear to be no specific pathognomonic clinical findings.[126] There is some correlation with older age, absence of leg pain, absence of exacerbation by cough, normal gait, absence of muscle spasm, and maximal pain on extension after forward flexion. Other studies have found no correlation between presenting pain in the groin, buttock, thigh, calf, or foot.[212] In one study there was no correlation between pain relief and pain provoked by passive extension and rotation movements.[126] No patients with central back pain responded to diagnostic blocks with Z-joints. Revel et al reported similar findings.[197]

In the cervical region, painful joints as defined by careful palpation have been shown to have a good correlation with Z-joint response to injections of local anesthetics.

Investigations

Although X-rays, computed tomography (CT) scans, and SPECT scans can identify abnormalities and arthritis of the Z-joints, some studies have shown little correlation with relief of pain following diagnostic injections in radiologically abnormal Z-joints.[61, 172, 203, 213] The validity of reports correlating CT findings and Z-joint pain has also been questioned by Schwarzer and coworkers.[218] They found marked interobserver variability in interpreting CT scans. Their conclusions were that CT has no value as a diagnostic test for lumbar Z-joint pain, and single-observer reporting of radiographic examination may be prone to significant error.

Prevalence

Schwarzer reported isolated lumbar Z-joint pain to have a prevalence of 15 per cent in chronic low back pain.[216] He used a double local anesthetic block technique, defining positive diagnosis when concordant pain relief followed the injection of a short-acting local anesthetic and, subsequently, on a different occasion, a longer-acting anesthetic gave a longer duration of pain relief. Other authors have reported prevalence rates ranging from 7.7 to 75 per cent.[46, 62, 83, 117, 150, 172, 197]

The prevalence of isolated cervical Z-joint–mediated pain in chronic neck pain may be at least 25 per cent.[7, 13, 28] If combined with provocative discography, Z-joint pain may contribute to the total pain in up to 64 per cent of subjects with nonradicular neck pain.[28] The incidence of thoracic Z-joint pain has not yet been reported in well-controlled studies.

Based on injection of either short-acting or long-acting local anesthetic into the joint or onto the medial branch of the dorsal primary ramus using placebo control, the incidence of false-positives has been as high as 38 per cent in the lumbar region and 30 per cent in the cervical region.[16, 213]

Technique

General Principles. Intra-articular Z-joint injections and injections of the medial branches of the dorsal primary rami should be done under fluoroscopy. Injections not using fluoroscopy have little, if any, diagnostic value.[13, 30, 61, 159] The medial branch block has been reported to have a similar specificity as intra-articular injection for diagnostic purposes.[13, 61] Light sedation may be given to obviate patient movement. However, if sedation is given, full recovery needs to occur before pain relief is quantified, even though the significance of concordant pain production has been doubted.[216] All blocks should be verified with contrast to confirm correct intra-articular placement and lack of intravenous or epidural spread, which would limit the diagnostic specificity of the injection.

The role of corticosteroids in any joint injectant has been questioned.[16, 46] These studies showed no long-term advantage of local anesthetic over local anesthetic combined with steroid or even saline. Dreyer and associates suggested that the role of corticosteroids intra-articularly may be to provide a window whereby the Z-joint can be mobilized.[71] They recommend that an intensive period of physical therapy or chiropractics be undertaken following intra-articular joint injections. Apart from anecdotal case descriptions, no controlled studies have been reported.

Despite the uncertainty of action, corticosteroid intra-articular Z-joint injections continue to be used. Open, uncontrolled studies of intra-articular cervical Z-joint injections have reported prolonged relief in 0 to 64 per cent of subjects.[121, 202]

Specific Principles. The patient is prone on the fluoroscopy table, and the C-arm is maneuvered obliquely until the joint line is clearly visualized. A 22- or 25-gauge spinal needle is introduced through the skin, directly in line with the direction of the fluoroscopy arm (gun barrel). The medial or lateral edge of the facet joint is touched, and the needle is carefully "walked off" into the joint (Fig. 59–6). Correct placement of the joint often causes a slight bend on the tip of the needle as it follows the direction of the joint. To confirm the intra-articular spread, 0.1 to 0.2 cc of contrast is injected (Fig. 59–7). Because the capsule may be

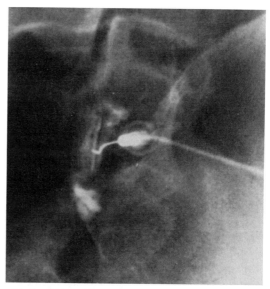

Figure 59–7. Oblique view showing correct needle placement for a lumbar intra-articular facet joint injection. Note the slight bend in the needle tip caused by entrance into the facet joint. Also, note the intra-articular spread of contrast dye inside the joint. (From Dreyfuss, P., Lagattuta, F., Kaplansky, B., and Heller, B.: Zygapophyseal joint injection techniques in the spinal axis. *In* Lennard, T. A. (ed.): Physiatric Procedures in Clinical Practice. Philadelphia, Hanley & Belfus, 1995, p. 223.)

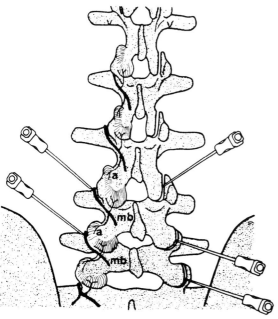

Figure 59–6. Illustration of the needle placement for a lumbar facet block. The left side illustrates the needle placement for a medial branch block, and the right illustrates the needle placement for an intra-articular facet joint injection. The medial branch of the dorsal ramus (mb) courses over the junction of the superior facet and transverse process. Each medial branch gives off an articular branch (a) above and below the joint it travels between. Thus, the L4–5 facet joint receives innervation from the L3 and L4 medial branches. (From Bogduk, N.: Back pain: Zygapophyseal blocks and epidural steroids. *In* Cousins, M., and Bridenbaugh, P. [eds.]: Neural Blockade in Clinical Anesthesia and Management of Pain. Philadelphia, J. B. Lippincott Co., 1988, p. 937.)

deficient in the superior or inferior recesses and dye may spread epidurally, it may be prudent to use a water-soluble dye for the facet arthrogram. (For further description, see reference 71.)

Thoracic Facet Injection. With the fluoroscopy unit in the anteroposterior (AP) position over the thoracic spine, a 22- or 25-gauge spinal needle is introduced at a level one lower than the Z-joint to be blocked. The needle is placed parallel to the spine, approximately 1 cm from the spinal process, and introduced onto the lamina just inferior to the joint to be blocked. While the bevel of the needle is turned downward, the needle is gently advanced along the lamina until it catches onto the coronally placed joint. Confirmation of intra-articular positioning can be made with a lateral view. This lateral view is often difficult to identify because of overlying ribs. Injection of 0.1 to 0.2 cc of contrast demonstrates the round discoid shape of the Z-joint on an AP appearance. Injectant containing local anesthetic with or without steroid in a volume of 0.7 cc can then be introduced. Concordant pain, if present, should be noted during the injection. (For further description, see reference 77.)

Cervical Z-Joint Injections. The approach can be either lateral or posterior (Fig. 59–8). If posterior, the C-arm needs to be positioned in a caudal-cephalad direction so the joints are clearly outlined. The needle has to pass through the muscles of the neck; thus, this approach tends to be more painful. The lateral approach positions the joints very close to the surface and is less painful. Introduction of a 22- or 25-gauge spinal needle is done with the needle first contacting the body of the joint and slowly walking off it into the joint itself. Verification of intra-articular spread is made with 0.1 cc of contrast (Fig. 59–9). The injectant volume should be less than 1 ml of local anesthetic with or without steroid. With the lateral approach, care must be taken regarding overenthusiastic placement of the needle. If the depth of needle insertion is uncertain, AP views can be taken to ensure that the needle does not go past the midline facetal line. For the first cervical occipital joint and the C1–C2 (atlantoaxial) joints, the reader is referred to reference 72.

Medial Branch Block. The best place to block the medial branch at the lumbar spine is at the junction of the superior facet and the transverse process (see Fig. 59–6). This is as it comes off the ventral nerve over the base of the transverse process below its level of origin. A 22-gauge needle is advanced until it hits the transverse process at the medial junction of the process and the base of the superior articular process. The injection should be done slowly over 20 seconds. Each joint is innervated by at least two medial branches. It is thus necessary to block two adjacent levels. To block the L4–L5 Z-joint, the L3 medial branch and the L4 medial branch need to be blocked as they go across the transverse process of L4 and L5, respectively. The L5 medial branch going to the L5–S1 Z-joint is blocked at the notch formed by the superior articular process of S1 and the ala of the sacrum. The L5–S1 joint also receives a small branch from the dorsal ramus of S1 as it emerges from the S1 posterior foramen. There is dis-

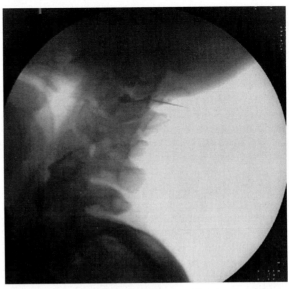

Figure 59–9. Intra-articular cervical facet joint using a lateral approach. Note the spread of contrast dye within the joint.

agreement about whether this nerve needs to be blocked to anesthetize the joint.[61] The cervical medial branch of the dorsal primary ramus position is well described and occurs in a consistent position.[13] With a lateral approach, the Z-joints of C3–C4, C4–C5, C5–C6, and C6–C7 are anesthetized by injecting 0.5 cc of local anesthetic onto the waist of the articular pillar of the same numbered vertebrae (see Fig. 59–8). The nerve is held against the waist by the tendons of the semispinalis capitus.[32] (For further descriptions, see references 13 and 72.)

Summary: Suggested Indications for Zygapophyseal (Facet) Joint Injections

1. Spinal pain of more than three weeks' duration with or without associated extremity pain.
2. Documented clinical findings, which may include the patient's pain being reproduced on moving the joint, especially in the cervical area.
3. Increased muscle tone over the joint.
4. Pain in a recognized joint referral zone.
5. Maximal site of tenderness over the joint area.
6. Failure of appropriate conservative therapy, which includes mobilization or manipulation of the joint by a physical therapist or chiropractor. Passive modalities such as heat, ultrasound, gentle massage, and exercise are not considered appropriate.

Sacroiliac Joint Injections

History and Examination

There appear to be no specific physical findings that accurately identify the SIJ as the source of pain. Injection of the SIJ in asymptomatic subjects caused a refer-

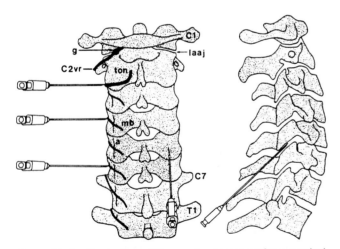

Figure 59–8. Illustration of the needle placement for a cervical facet block. The left side illustrates the needle placement for a medial branch block, and the right illustrates the needle placement for an intra-articular facet joint injection. The medial branch of the dorsal ramus (mb) courses around the waist of the articular pillar of the same numbered vertebra. Each medial branch gives off an articular branch (a) above and below the joint it travels between. Intra-articular injections can be achieved from a posterior approach, as shown here, or from a lateral approach. (From Bogduk, N.: Back pain: Zygapophyseal blocks and epidural steroids. *In* Cousins, M., and Bridenbaugh, P. [eds.]: Neural Blockade in Clinical Anesthesia and Management of Pain. Philadelphia, J. B. Lippincott Co., 1988, p. 937.)

ral zone in an area inferior to the ipsilateral posterior superior iliac spine.[92, 93] Schwarzer and colleagues, injecting the SIJ in patients with presumed SIJ dysfunction, reported that buttock, thigh, calf, or even foot pain referral patterns were present and did not distinguish SIJ-related pain from other pain generators.[211] Groin pain was the only pain referral pattern more commonly associated with a positive response to an SIJ block. There may be an increased risk of SIJ dysfunction in patients with a lumbar fusion or hip pathology.

On examination, the patient may have an antalgic gait, with the trunk shifted toward the normal side. Generally, the patient tends to sit with the painful side raised and often points to the posterior superior iliac spine as the place of greatest pain. Pain may be referred below the knee. The pain is often associated with ipsilateral paravertebral spasm and ipsilateral gluteus or piriformis spasm. Many clinical tests for SIJ dysfunction have been reported, but their accuracy has not been proved by fluoroscopically guided intra-articular injections of local anesthetic.[211]

Prevalence

Using fluoroscopically guided articular injections in 100 patients with low back pain, Aprill reported that the SIJ was the sole source of pain in 15 per cent.[4] It was part of the back pain syndrome in another 23 per cent. Schwarzer and colleagues, using a similar technique, reported a prevalence of SIJ-mediated pain in 13 to 30 per cent of the subjects tested.[211]

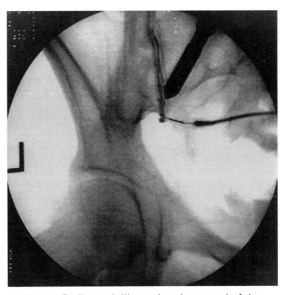

Figure 59–11. Radiograph illustrating the spread of the contrast dye injected into the sacroiliac joint. Note that the joint entry was achieved in the inferior aspect of the capsule.

Technique

General Technique. Many early reports of SIJ injections were nonfluoroscopically guided. The local anesthetic was usually injected, with steroid, blindly into the posterior ligamentous structures. The majority of the studies were noncontrolled, but still, approximately 60 per cent of these patients were reported to show at least some improvement.[118, 210] Two to four injections were usually made along the posterior SIJ line. Whether an intra-articular injection should be combined with postcapsular injections has not been investigated.

Specific Technique. The patient is prone on the fluoroscopy table, and either the fluoroscope or the patient is angled until the inferior part of the SIJ is clearly visualized. By shifting the C-arm obliquely, in some patients, the posterior aspect of the joint can be separated radiographically from the anterior aspect. The posterior aspect is seen as a more medial translucency (Fig. 59–10). A 25- or 22-gauge spinal needle is introduced through the skin onto the sacrum next to the posterior inferior joint capsule. The needle is walked off until it drops into the SIJ. A lateral view should confirm the needle placement inside the joint. Occasionally, the inferior joint is extremely narrow, and overenthusiastic advancement of the needle results in the needle being placed through the anterior capsule of the joint. Intra-articular placement of the needle is confirmed with 0.2 to 0.5 cc of contrast (Fig. 59–11). Concordant pain may be reproduced with the injection. On confirmation of the intra-articular spread of the contrast, local anesthetic with or without steroid can be introduced. The volume of the injectant should be no more than 3 ml. On occasion, attempting to inject

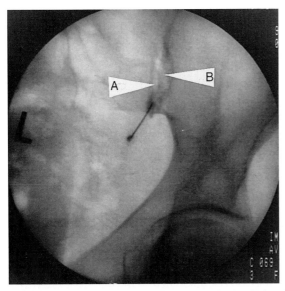

Figure 59–10. Sacroiliac joint injection. Note the medial and lateral translucencies. The medial translucency (A) is the posterior aspect of the sacroiliac joint and is the target for entering the joint. The lateral translucency (B) is the anterior aspect of the sacroiliac joint. Entry into the joint is usually achieved in the inferior aspect.

this volume is met with difficulty. This can usually be overcome by continuing to attempt to inject while turning the needle 90 degrees, because the bevel of the needle is presumably subarticular or abutting against the side wall of the joint. The SIJ injection is usually minimally painful and can be done without local sedation. (For a more detailed description, see reference 74.)

Therapy

If hypomobility of the SIJ is postulated as the cause of the patient's joint pain, injections of local anesthetic, with or without steroids, should logically be followed with manipulation and mobilization techniques, together with exercises and stretching.[74] Other therapies that may be of value in the acute phase of SIJ strain, such as occurs after trauma, include an SIJ belt, which must be worn tightly just above the greater trochanter, anti-inflammatories, and ice in the initial stage, followed by heat and gentle stretching exercises after 48 to 72 hours. Physical therapy or chiropractics should be used in subsequent stages to mobilize the often stiff SIJ. Mobilization or manipulation techniques may involve either end-of-range, low-amplitude, short-lever arm-thrust techniques or direct oscillation techniques, together with general muscle stretching techniques.[69, 137] Any leg length inequality of half an inch or more may be significant in prolonging the pain syndrome and should probably be corrected.[52] A home exercise program is important for general stretching and mobilization of the joint. Both postural and biomechanical education and correction may be necessary. An aerobic training program should also be included.

Prolotherapy is a technique that has been described to treat SIJ and low back pain.[138, 139, 180] A mixture of dextrose, glycerin, and phenol is combined with a local anesthetic and injected into the ligamentous posterior capsule. It is proposed that this causes collagen formation, with strengthening of proposed "weakened liga-

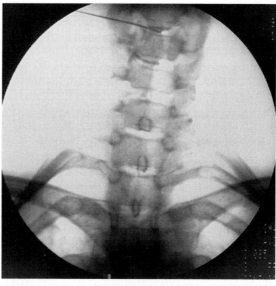

Figure 59–13. Anteroposterior radiograph showing correct needle placement for a cervical discography. The approach is right anterolateral to avoid entering the esophagus.

ments."[138, 139, 180] The injectant itself is neurolytic and may diminish pain not by stabilization but by denervation of the posterior capsule. Control studies on these techniques are still awaited.

Summary: Suggested Indications for SIJ Injection

1. Pain in the low back for more than six to eight weeks.
2. Maximal tenderness usually over the posterior superior iliac spine and ipsilateral buttock.
3. Failure of conservative therapy, including mobilization or manipulation and a home stretching program.
4. No neurologic deficit.

Therapeutic Procedures Based on Discography

Having demonstrated concordant pain with no extravasation of injectant into the epidural space, or when surgery is deemed to be difficult or hazardous for the patient, various therapeutic procedures have been proposed (Figs. 59–12 and 59–13).

Gray Ramus Communicantes Blockade/ Lumbar Sympathetic Block

The posterior aspect of the intervertebral disc and the posterior longitudinal ligament are innervated by the sinovertebral nerve (Fig. 59–14). This nerve innervates the disc at the level where it comes off the ventral root and one level higher.[26, 30, 158] The lateral aspect of the intervertebral disc is innervated by the gray rami communicantes, which come off the sympathetic lumbar

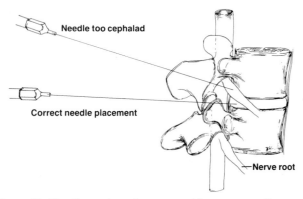

Needle too cephalad

Correct needle placement

Nerve root

Figure 59–12. Illustration of correct and incorrect needle placement for a lumbar discography. The needle should be directed immediately cephalad of the articular process to avoid the nerve root. (From Nordby, E. J.: Chemonucleolysis. *In* Frymoyer, J. W. [ed.]: The Adult Spine: Principles and Practice. New York, Raven Press, 1991, p. 1741.)

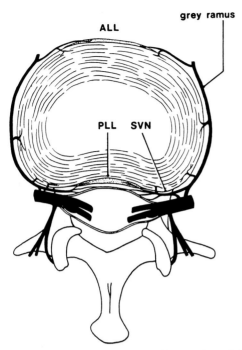

Figure 59–14. Illustration showing the innervation of the intervertebral discs, the anterior longitudinal ligament (ALL), and the posterior longitudinal ligament (PLL). The posterior aspect of the disc and the PLL are innervated by the sinuvertebral nerve (SVN). The lateral and anterior aspect of the disc is innervated by the gray rami communicantes, which comes off the sympathetic chain. (From Bogduk, N., and Twomey, L. T.: Clinical Anatomy of the Lumbar Spine. Edinburgh, Churchill Livingstone, 1991, p. 117.)

chain (Figs. 59–14 and 59–15). Bogduk suggests that although the gray rami communicantes send branches to the intervertebral discs, they may simply provide a route for nociceptive afferent fibers to return from the disc to the ventral root. There are numerous nerve endings of various types in the outer third of the annulus fibrosus that presumably have a nociceptive role.[158, 190] These nerve endings are densest on the lateral aspect of the disc, with fewer on the anterior aspect and slightly more on the posterior aspect. The rami communicantes also innervate the anterior longitudinal ligament.

The lumbar sympathetic trunks descend the lumbar region on either side of the ventrolateral border of the vertebrae.[200] White rami communicantes are distributed to the L1 and L2 ventral rami, and gray rami communicantes are distributed to every other ventral ramus.[26, 30] The number of the rami communicantes to each lumbar ventral root varies from one to three. In general, the rami run up the side of the vertebral body on the distal third of the vertebrae.

Technique of Blockade

The patient is prone on the fluoroscopy table. The vertebral body of the level to be blocked is identified. For the rami communicantes block, the needle is di-

rected to slip off the posterior third of the vertebral body just superior to the disc to be blocked. On the lateral view, the needle is placed at the junction of the superior third and distal third of the vertebra. Confirmation of the positioning is obtained with contrast, which should be seen to "hug" the side of the vertebral body. One to 2 cc of local anesthetic can be injected. There should be no somatic blockade.

Lumbar Sympathetic Blockade. The patient is placed in an oblique position, or the fluoroscopy C-arm is obliqued until the zygapophyseal joints are clearly visualized. The C-arm is then swung at a slightly caudal-cephalad projection to see more clearly into the transverse process. Using a "gun-barrel approach," in which the needle is directed in the axis of the fluoroscopy tube, the spinal needle is inserted some 5 cm from the midline onto the vertebral body. The needle is walked off the vertebral body until it lies just inferior when visualizing it in a lateral position (Fig. 59–16). On the AP projection, the needle should lie directly under the midzygapophyseal joint line (Fig. 59–17). Contrast should flow freely up and down the anterior of the vertebra in the loose areolar fat. There should be no spread in the psoas, as the sympathetic chain lies below the psoas muscle. The contrast often has an aerated appearance owing to the loose fat into which it is

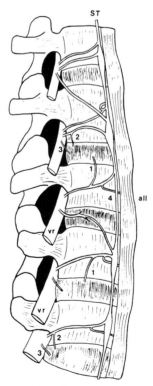

Figure 59–15. Lateral view illustrating the nerve supply to the intervertebral discs. Branches of the gray rami communicantes (1,2,4) supply the lateral and anterior aspect of the disc. The sinuvertebral nerve (3) supplies the posterior aspect of the disc. (From Bogduk, N., and Twomey, L. T.: Clinical Anatomy of the Lumbar Spine. Edinburgh, Churchill Livingstone, 1991, p. 117.)

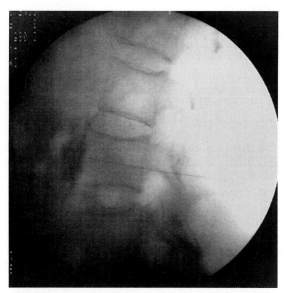

Figure 59–16. Lateral radiograph showing correct needle placement for a lumbar sympathetic block. The needle tip is located just anterior to the vertebral body, and the contrast dye should spread in a cephalad and caudad direction.

injected. Two to 5 cc of local anesthetic will block the sympathetic supply to this region.

If a ramus communicantes block, with or without a sympathetic block, significantly reduces the patient's pain, the procedure can be repeated using radiofrequency ablation, phenol, or a combination of both. With the use of phenol, care must be taken to ensure accurate placement, and small amounts should be used to avoid spillover onto the somatic nerves.[199, 226, 228]

Summary: Suggested Indications for Rami Communicantes/Lumbar Sympathetic Block

1. Chronic low back pain of more than six weeks' duration.
2. Back pain not associated with hard neurologic signs.
3. Back pain primarily unilateral and not responding to conservative therapy such as adequate bed rest, physical therapy, an exercise program, and medications.
4. X-ray confirmation of crushed vertebrae, e.g., from trauma or osteoporosis, with pain related to the dermatomal level of the disc innervation.

Epidural Steroid Injections

Rationale

Various substances are released by damage to the nucleus pulposus. One of the principal enzymes is phospholipase A_2. This enzyme can initiate the inflammatory cascade by the liberation of arachidonic acid, resulting in the formation of prostaglandins, leukotrienes, and peroxides. Corticosteroids act to inhibit the neuropeptide synthesis or action of phospholipase A_2.

They may also cause membrane stabilization of inflamed tissue and have anesthetic-like actions.[90, 132]

Technique

Epidural steroids may be injected by the caudal, lumbar, thoracic, or cervical route. There appears to be little consensus as to the volume of injectant or the dosages of steroids to be used. Theoretically, the injection of steroids via a transforaminal route onto the site of the inflamed nerve root and disc should result in a better clinical outcome. This still awaits clinical studies. Injecting the steroid with small amounts of local anesthetic via the transforaminal route also has the diagnostic advantage of identifying the level of the inflamed root.

If fluoroscopy is not used for the epidural injections, there is a significant failure rate. It has been reported that lumbar injections may fail to gain the epidural space in 17 to 30 per cent of patients.[22] Caudal injections have an even higher failure rate of 38 per cent. Even if the caudal space is entered, a large volume of injectant is required to reach the lumbar epidural space.

Side Effects and Complications

There appears to be little risk of serious complications associated with epidural steroids.[1] Spinal puncture in the lumbar epidural region has been reported to have an incidence as high as 5 per cent. The risk is of the steroid being injected into the subarachnoid space. Even without dural puncture, there is a 1 per cent risk of headaches with injection in the lumbar epidural region and approximately 5 per cent after caudal injec-

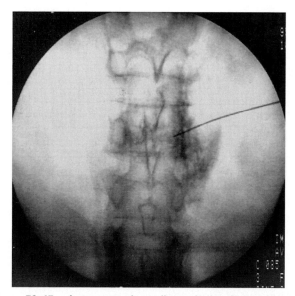

Figure 59–17. Anteroposterior radiograph showing correct needle placement for a lumbar sympathetic block. The needle tip is located directly caudad to the midzygapophyseal joint line. Contrast dye should spread in a cephalad and caudad direction.

tion. The incidence of headaches following cervical epidurals is extremely high. Hyperglycemia, fluid retention, arachnoiditis, epidural abscess, aseptic meningitis, and Cushing's syndrome have all been reported.[1] In his review of 64 series made up of nearly 7000 patients, Abram could not find any report of arachnoiditis as a complication of epidural steroid injection.[2] The pituitary adrenal axis is suppressed for several weeks after epidural injection.[42]

Indications

The indications are varied and often appear based on anecdotal case reports.

Results

White and colleagues found that epidural steroid injection responses decreased within three months.[252] Only 70 per cent of patients in their study still had pain relief at six months. A meta-analysis of the efficacy of epidural steroid injections in the treatment of low back syndromes concluded that perhaps 14 per cent of patients improved.[194] It is of note that the majority of studies did not use fluoroscopic control; thus, the beneficial results may have been falsely low.[251] The majority of beneficial reports were in patients with radicular sciatic pain with or without low back pain. Clinical improvement in these cases appeared to occur within a few days to a week, with improvement generally lasting no longer than several months.

The data on cervical epidural steroids are poor. Again, the patients with radiculopathy appeared to fare better than those with other presenting features.[85]

Summary: Suggested Indications for Epidural Steroid Injection

1. Spinal pain with associated extremity pain.
2. No more than one previous epidural steroid injection with documentation of relief lasting longer than seven days.
3. Failure of conservative therapy consisting of, but not limited to, appropriate bed rest, physical therapy, anti-inflammatory medications, or trigger point injections.
4. No "hard" neurologic deficits.

Differential Epidural/Spinal Block

The differential epidural was introduced as a technique to differentiate among somatic, sympathetic, and central (sometimes termed psychogenic) pain.[257] The theory was simple, in that it was proposed that low concentrations of local anesthetic would block the small sympathetic fibers first. Stronger concentrations would subsequently block the larger myelinated motor and nociceptive afferents.[96] A saline injection could be administered before the local anesthetic to try to counter any placebo effect. Unfortunately, this simplistic view of a relatively simple test has not stood up to examina-

tion. A number of studies have shown that although the preganglionic fibers of the sympathetic system are smaller than A-delta fibers, they are more resistant to a low concentration of local anesthetic.[19] Thus, the differentiation between sympathetic and somatic pain based on differing concentrations of local anesthetic is impossible. The technique, however, can still be used to differentiate between pain of somatic origin and central pain. It has been suggested that a subarachnoid block would be more effective than an epidural.[37] A microcatheter is inserted by a 25- or 26-gauge spinal needle into the subarachnoid space. Whether a catheter is inserted into the epidural or subarachnoid space, the following is injected:

1. First, 8 to 10 ml of saline solution is injected to control the placebo effect. If the patient reports marked pain reduction of more than 50 per cent, no further injections should be made until the pain relief has diminished. If after 30 to 60 minutes the patient still has significant pain relief, the procedure should be aborted.
2. If there is no pain relief or the pain relief is transitory, 2 per cent lidocaine is injected in increments to produce both a sensory and a motor block above the dermatomal level of the pain. Failure to block pain despite a dense motor and sensory block over the area indicates a central pain syndrome. If pain relief continues after the motor and sensory block has worn off, this may be due to sympathetic blockade. Unfortunately, because it is impossible to produce a pure sympathetic block or a pure block of the A-delta fibers as the dorsal horn is suffused with local anesthetic, it is unlikely that such a differential diagnosis between sympathetic and somatic can be made.

Another problem is that how the patient is questioned about his or her pain relief can contribute to difficulties in interpretation. If the differential technique is used, a stringent protocol of questions should be used to minimize bias.[100]

Summary: Suggested Indications for Differential Spinal/Epidural Block

1. Chronic low back pain with or without lower extremity pain of more than 12 weeks' duration.
2. Pain behavior or nonorganic signs that make differentiation of central pain from emotional exaggeration difficult.
3. In combination with an epidurogram, the differential block may suggest the potential for further therapy (e.g., adhesiolysis).

Prolotherapy

Prolotherapy (sclerotherapy) has been used for over 40 years.[112, 113] It is not a standard, generally used, or accepted mode of therapy, and it remains highly controversial. Its rationale is to strengthen weakened ligaments and supportive connective tissue around the lumbar spine. The connective tissue laxity allows segmental movement, which triggers nociceptive input from the densely innervated periosteum or periosteal attachment of tendons and ligaments. By injecting substances that cause collagen proliferation, it is hypothesized that this segmental movement will be decreased. Because most solutions used for prolotherapy are also neurotonic, this may explain their efficacy in decreasing back pain. Prolotherapy has been used for the treatment of trigger points in patients with fibromyalgia. In particular, it has been used at the musculotendinous junctions of recalcitrant trigger point–induced pain.[196]

Klein and coworkers injected a proliferant solution of glycerol, phenol, and dextrose in patients with low back pain. They showed a 60 per cent increase in collagen diameter at three months after six weekly proliferant injections. Two double-blind studies of the efficacy of dextrose, glycerol, and phenol injections in chronic low back pain patients have been reported.[138, 139, 180] These compared the injection of an anesthetic alone with the injection of anesthetic plus proliferant. At the six-month follow-up, statistically significant improvement in the range of motion, reduction in visual analogue pain score, and reduction in disability were seen in those patients who were treated with the proliferant solution. Some improvement was also seen in those patients injected with anesthetic alone.

Other proliferant solutions have been used. Recently, injections of growth factors into animal ligaments demonstrated growth enhancement. Human studies are still awaited.[146]

Any proliferant injections should be done by skilled practitioners. Further studies, especially with nonpainful solutions such as growth factors, are awaited with anticipation.

Summary: Suggested Indications for Prolotherapy

1. Central low back pain of more than three months' duration.
2. Failure of conservative therapy, i.e., active physical therapy, chiropractics, exercises, and appropriate medications.
3. No hard neurologic deficits.
4. A diagnostic local anesthetic injection into the interspinous and iliolumbar ligaments, if the pain is in the low back, significantly decreases the patient's pain.

Myofascial Trigger Points

Travell and Simons described a trigger point as a hyperexcitable spot, usually within a taut band of skeletal muscle or in the muscle's fascia. It is painful on compression and gives rise to a characteristic referred pain, tenderness, and autonomic phenomena. Palpation for trigger points may cause a twitch response in the muscle. The patient is often unaware of the trigger point, although he or she may spontaneously rub the area

because it is tight. As the examiner puts pressure over the point, the patient may wince or cry out and withdraw as a response to pain. This has been called the jump sign.[240]

The pressure required to cause pain over a trigger point can be measured by a pressure threshold meter or algometer.[87] This is a force gauge fitted with a 1 cm^2 rubber tip. The force required to produce pain can be measured at the trigger point. It should be 2 kg/cm^2 less than the force to produce pain at a comparable site in the muscle on the opposite side of the body. The algometer can be used to objectively quantify the trigger points and to follow the results of therapy.

Techniques of Injection

The trigger point, having been palpated with the muscle in a slightly stretched position, is affixed between two fingers. There are various methods of injecting trigger points that are well described.[88, 240] A needle with a syringe is inserted into the muscle until a hard band is felt and often after a twitch is seen. Then 0.1 to 0.2 cc of 0.25 per cent bupivacaine is injected into this band, and concordant pain in the trigger zone is looked for. The needle is then pulled out of the muscle and reinserted along the band, and another 0.1 to 0.2 cc is injected. This is done with several small injections up and down the band. Injection in small aliquots is also done across the band. The normal muscle has a softer feel than the presumed trigger point area. Importantly, after the trigger point has been injected, the patient is asked to do a range of movement exercises, such as flexion and extension, and is given a home exercise stretching program. Ideally, physical therapy with stretching should be done after the injection. Immediately after the injection, pressure should be applied, preferably with ice, for a few minutes to decrease any hematoma formation. No more than two areas should be injected, with three injections per area, for a maximum of six injections.

Local anesthetic is recommended for the injectant. There is no evidence that steroids add to the efficacy, and they may cause systemic problems and should probably be avoided. The type of local anesthetic, whether lidocaine, bupivacaine, or procaine, has not been evaluated in comparable studies. The purpose of the injectant is:

1. To chemically break up the taut band or trigger point.
2. To desensitize the tender point and allow an increased range of movement of the muscle and the joints to which the muscle is attached.
3. To decrease the soreness following the injection.

For low back pain, the quadratus lumborum is often extremely tender to palpation. These trigger points can be injected by placing the patient with the painful side uppermost. Palpation of the quadratus lumborum can isolate the trigger points, and these can be injected via a lateral insertion.[88]

Hopwood and Abram in 1994 reported a success

rate of 59.1 per cent in 193 patients who had trigger point injections.[120] They stated that the main causes of failure included lack of employment, prolonged duration of pain, and decreased social activity. There were no follow-up treatments given and no mention of patient education regarding perpetuating factors.

Trigger points can also be found in ligaments and capsules of joints. Injection of these areas as well as into scars can mechanically affect either the trigger points or the entrapped nerve tissue.

Summary: Suggested Indications for Trigger Point Injection

1. Documentation of abnormal local pressure sensitivity (tenderness). If an algometer is used, the pressure to cause pain should be at least 2 kg/cm^2 lower compared with the control side.
2. Reproduction of the patient's complaint when pressure is placed on the trigger point.
3. If previous injections have been given, pain relief should have lasted up to seven days.

PHARMACOLOGIC MANAGEMENT OF BACK PAIN

This section outlines one of several paradigms for a systematic approach to providing analgesic support for patients with chronic nonmalignant back pain. Traditionally, approaches to analgesia have been discussed as narcotic and nonnarcotic treatment. There are now enough mechanistic models to discuss a paradigm in terms of analgesics, antihyperalgesics, and analgesic adjuvants. This paradigm involves the characterization of pain, such as nerve ending (nociceptive) discomfort or abnormal nerve signaling (neuropathic). Further, it involves the initiation of dosing and subsequent titration according to the patient's individual pharmacologic responses and treatment goals. Paradigms that involve analgesic titration are subject to the following factors.

Pharmacology-Pharmacokinetics Versus Pharmacodynamics

Models of drug absorption, clearance, and end organ effect are used to predict the variability between the administration of a prescribed dose and the quality or intensity of drug effect. In the process of tracking a drug through the body, dosing errors or noncompliance changes the administered dose; once administered, variability in absorption, distribution in body compartments, binding in tissues, and elimination rate all alter the concentration at the site of drug effect (pharmacokinetics). As concentration of drug at the site of action builds, further variability occurs via drug-receptor interaction with changes in cellular physiology, pathology, genetic factors, other drugs, and tolerance (pharmacodynamics). Placebo effect—an unpredictable, unsustainable effect—and the functional state of an individual are other factors capable of altering the intensity of drug effect. Studies have revealed placebo response rates in chronic pain patients as high as 53 per cent.[45]

Tolerance

Tolerance is a poorly understood but essential piece of the conceptual framework for the adjustment and titration of drug dose to effect. Tolerance causes a decrease in drug effect that can be attributed to increases in clearance (pharmacokinetics), changes in drug-receptor interaction (pharmacodynamics), or depletion of neurotransmitters (tachyphylaxis). Cross-tolerance occurs frequently in central nervous system depressant drugs and is believed to be predominantly pharmacodynamically mediated.[127] An example of cross-tolerance would be the resistance to analgesics of a postoperative patient with a history of heavy alcohol abuse.

Psychoactive Substance Dependence

Psychologic dependence is an undisputed concern when providing long-term analgesic management. There are important distinctions between the physiologic and psychologic attributes of dependence.

Psychologic dependence or addiction is characterized as the continued craving for a drug to achieve a psychic effect. It is associated with aberrant drug-related behavior such as compulsive drug seeking, unsanctioned use or dose escalation of a drug, and its use despite harm to self or others.

Physiologic dependence, conversely, is associated with tolerance, withdrawal, and abstinence syndrome. Well-illustrated abstinence syndromes include the malignant hypertension after the sudden withdrawal of clonidine, severe flulike symptoms after the withdrawal of opiates, and delirium and/or seizures after the withdrawal of ethanol, sedatives, and muscle relaxants. Recognition of psychologic and physiologic dependence on analgesics, and thus the optimum management of these entities, necessitates a clear understanding of treatment goals and desired outcomes. These goals include contingency management for symptomatic painful episodes, around-the-clock procedures for blinded cocktails of analgesic medication, and weaning schedules for ineffective medications at risk of withdrawal.[91]

Toxic Effects

It is important for providers to familiarize themselves with the therapeutic window and the window of adverse reactions for any drug used in the therapeutic armamentarium. Toxicity must then be factored into the risk-benefit analysis of treatment goals—whether it be an allergic reaction; a dose-dependent adverse reaction, such as gastritis of nonsteroidal anti-inflammatories; or an idiosyncratic reaction, such as the dysrhythmias of the antihyperalgesic antiarrythmic agents.

TREATMENT GOALS AND DESIRED OUTCOMES

The exact etiology of the pain associated with back disorders can be elusive to even the most diagnostically skilled health care provider. Major categories of painful response can be recognized so that treatment goals and measurable outcomes can be employed to determine therapy. These categories, though partially overlapping, are classified as somatic or nociceptive, neuropathic, muscle spasm, visceral, and idiopathic.

Treatment of Postinjury States

Acute Injury. Acute back injury pain often results from a distinct site that involves somatic or nociceptive input. This initial pain is followed by hypersensitivity or secondary hyperalgesia. In turn, there is often reflex splinting and muscle spasm and sensitization of the nerve roots, either directly or by autonomic and/or spinal facilitation.

Use of this basic model provides a rationale for the administration of analgesics, antihyperalgesics, and adjuvants to treat the pain response process. Goals specific to this process include decreased painful input, decreased sensitization, and blunted autonomic output, so as to arrest or reverse inflammation and physiologic changes that may abnormally persist. Equally important goals that are not specific treatments are the use of the drugs for the augmentation of functional restoration or improvement with rehabilitation.

As medical treatment and impairment stabilize, pain as a sequela often limits treatment options to palliation. Often all other modalities fail, and patients with intractable back pain present with signs of severe deterioration in physical and role functioning. Whether opiate analgesics improve nonmalignant chronic pain such that discomfort intensity, duration, and frequency of aggravation are significantly reduced continues to generate intense debate.

Chronic Pain. A new willingness to critically examine the benefit of chronic opiate therapy for nonmalignant pain comes from the highly favorable outcomes demonstrated in the treatment of malignant pain. Long-term treatment provides adequate pain relief in 70 to 90 per cent of patients with chronic intractable cancer and is widely perceived to improve function and quality of life. This is coupled with observations that tolerance, physical dependence, and aberrant drug-related behaviors are not significant problems in the treatment of cancer pain.[186]

DRUG THERAPY FOR BACK PAIN

Opiates

Opium is derived from the unripe seed capsule of the poppy (*Papaver somniferum*), and its first reference can be found in Greece during the third century B.C. by the philosopher-botanist Theophrastus.[171]

Mechanism of Action

There are three sites of action for the opiate effects of analgesia: the supraspinal sites, the spinal sites, and the peripheral sites. Currently, three major classes of receptors are characterized: the mu-receptor resides across all three sites, the kappa-receptor is found chiefly along the spinal cord and peripheral C-fiber terminals, and the delta-receptors are located in the brain stem and spinal cord.

The mu- and delta-receptor increase potassium conductance, hyperpolarize the nerve, and decrease signal transmission and neurotransmitter release, thereby producing nociceptive analgesia. The kappa-receptor decreases calcium conductance and decreases neurotransmitter release at the peripheral nerve terminal, thus decreasing the hyperalgesia after injury.[234, 263–265]

Side Effects

The most common side effects of opioid therapy are respiratory depression, nausea and vomiting, constipation, and pruritus. Fortunately, the blood level of the opioid required to cause side effects is usually much higher than that required for analgesia. Also, these side effects are usually easily treated. Table 59–5 summarizes the treatment of opioid-induced side effects.

Respiratory depression is the most serious side effect but is rarely seen with the most common doses used in daily practice. It is produced by stimulation of the opiate receptors located in the brain stem. It is more likely to occur in opioid-naive patients and with very high doses. Also, pain stimulates respiration, which counteracts the respiratory depression caused by the opioid. Respiratory depression is rarely seen if one slowly titrates the opioid upward to achieve analgesic effect.

Table 59–5. MANAGEMENT OF OPIOID SIDE EFFECTS

Side Effect	Treatment
Respiratory depression	Dilute one ampule of naloxone (0.4 mg/cc) in 10 cc normosaline. Administer 1 cc (0.04 mg) every minute until respirations are >8/minute.
Nausea	Scopolamine patch every 72 hours. If above fails, add metoclopramide. If above fails, add ondansetron. If ondansetron fails, replace with prochlorperazine, trimethobenzamide, or hydroxyzine.
Constipation	Metamucil, 1 tbsp each A.M. Prune juice twice daily. Senokot-S, 2 tablets at bedtime. Encourage fluids. If no bowel movement in any 48-hour period: —Milk of Magnesia, 30 cc —Dulcolax, 10 mg at bedtime —Fleet Enema If patient is on antacids, choose Mylanta or Maalox.
Pruritus	Diphenhydramine

Nausea and vomiting are less serious side effects of the opioids but can be a great hindrance to their effective use. This side effect can usually be managed with the antinauseants targeted at the various supraspinal sites responsible for nausea and vomiting.

Constipation and pruritus are minor side effects of the opioids and are usually easily managed. Constipation results from the activation of the mu-receptor in the gastrointestinal tract. Prophylactic bowel maintenance is the most effective way to manage opioid-induced constipation, but mild laxatives may also be used. Pruritus results from activation of the mu-receptor in the spinal cord. It is more commonly seen with the intraspinal administration of opioids, which is discussed later.

Guidelines for Prescribing Opioids for Chronic Back Pain

The treatment of chronic benign back pain with opioids is somewhat controversial, but many chronic back pain patients can benefit from long-term opioid therapy. Opioids are not appropriate for all back pain syndromes. They are very effective in nociceptive pain (pain without coexisting nervous system pathology). Opioids, in general, are much less effective in neuropathic pain (pain secondary to nervous system pathology).[44] Many failed back syndrome patients suffer from neuropathic pain and may not respond as well to the opioids. This generalization does not apply to all patients, however; some patients with neuropathic pain respond to the opioids but usually require larger doses.

Opioid Monograms

Opioids are divided into agonists, agonists-antagonists, and antagonists. The agonists bind to one or more of the opiate receptors and activate them. The agonists-antagonists have agonist activity at one receptor and antagonist activity at another. The antagonists bind to the receptors without activation; therefore, they block agonist activity. The antagonists as well as the agonists-antagonists may induce withdrawal symptoms in opioid-dependent patients because of mu antagonism. Antagonists are frequently used to reverse life-threatening side effects of opioids such as respiratory depression from opioid overdose. Table 59–6 gives the equianalgesic doses for the most commonly used opioids.

Agonists

Morphine. Morphine sulfate is the reference standard for all opioids. Oral bioavailability is approximately one third the intravenous dose; therefore, when converting from intravenous to oral morphine, the dose must be tripled. The oral form comes in an immediate-release and a controlled-release preparation.

The immediate-release preparation has an onset of 15 to 20 minutes and a duration of three to four hours and therefore can be given every three to four hours. The controlled-release preparation has a slow onset but

Table 59–6. EQUIANALGESIC DOSES OF COMMONLY USED OPIOIDS

Drug	Equianalgesic Dose (mg)	
	IV	Oral
Morphine	10	30–60
Codeine	120	200
Fentanyl	0.1	—
Hydrocodone	—	30
Hydromorphone	1.5	7.5
Levorphanol	2	4
Meperidine	75	300
Methadone	10	10
Oxycodone	—	30
Oxymorphone	—	10
Propoxyphene	—	130
Butorphanol	2	—
Pentazocine	30	150

a prolonged duration of 8 to 12 hours. Controlled-release morphine is embedded in a wax base that slowly releases the morphine. The analgesia peaks in 90 to 120 minutes (compared with 30 to 90 minutes for the immediate-release preparation). The tablet cannot be broken, as this would release a large quantity of morphine. Controlled-release morphine should not be given more often than every eight hours. It is common to administer controlled-release morphine on a time-contingent basis (every 8 to 12 hours) and the immediate-release morphine on an as-needed basis for breakthrough pain (every three to four hours). This method allows for more stable blood levels of morphine without the peaks and valleys commonly seen with as-needed dosing. When treating back pain with chronic opioids, it is preferred that as-needed dosing with the short-acting opioids be avoided because of the risk of tolerance. Chronic opioid therapy is best accomplished with around-the-clock sustained-release methods.

Methadone. Methadone is slightly more potent than morphine. It is less likely to produce dependence because there is less euphoria and less sedation with methadone than with morphine. Oral bioavailability is almost 90 per cent; therefore, the intravenous and oral doses are almost equivalent. Methadone is poorly metabolized by the liver; therefore, it has an extremely long half-life. This makes the drug valuable in the prevention of withdrawal in drug addicts, because it requires only once-a-day dosing. However, the analgesia half-life is much shorter, and the drug must be administered every 6 to 12 hours for pain control. This dosing schedule makes it very popular for chronic opioid therapy. Methadone is also available in an elixir.

Meperidine. Meperidine is less potent than morphine but has a faster onset than morphine; therefore, the patient may experience more euphoria. Because of the metabolite normeperidine, which may induce seizures, it is not the opioid of choice. This effect of normeperidine may be significant at doses greater than 1 g per day or in patients with renal failure. In addition to analgesic effects, meperidine has atropine-like effects and local anesthetic effects. The atropine-like effects may lead to tachycardia. Also, meperidine has been known to induce a syndrome characterized by tachycardia, increased blood pressure, arrhythmias, and hyperthermia in patients taking monoamine oxidase inhibitors.

Hydromorphone. This opioid is six to eight times more potent than morphine. It is easily absorbed from the gastrointestinal tract and has fewer side effects than morphine. It has a fast onset and a short half-life; therefore, it requires frequent dosing (every two to three hours).

Codeine. Codeine is a weak opioid with less intense side effects. It has a higher oral bioavailability than morphine and a quicker onset; however, the duration is short. It is available only in acetaminophen-containing preparations and therefore is not intended for chronic use because of potential acetaminophen toxicity.

Hydrocodone. Hydrocodone has pharmacologic activity similar to that of codeine. It was previously used as an antitussive but is now a commonly used analgesic. It is available only in acetaminophen-containing preparations.

Oxycodone. Oxycodone is qualitatively similar to morphine in all respects. It is available in four preparations: oxycodone alone (immediate release), oxycodone with acetaminophen, oxycodone with aspirin, and a new sustained-release preparation.

Oxymorphone. This opioid is seven to 10 times more potent than morphine. It is a derivative of hydromorphone and comes in a 5-mg rectal suppository.

Levorphanol. Levorphanol is four times more potent than morphine. The incidence of nausea and vomiting and constipation is less than with other agents. The duration is somewhat longer than morphine.

Propoxyphene. Propoxyphene is a derivative of methadone. It is a less effective analgesic than codeine. Sixty mg is no more effective than 600 mg of aspirin, and 32 mg is no more effective than placebo. It has an alleged lower dependence potential, but this is disputed. Oral bioavailability is 50 per cent, and it has a large volume of distribution, which accounts for its long half-life of approximately 10 hours; however, its analgesic half-life is much shorter.

Fentanyl. Fentanyl is 100 times more potent than morphine. It is available in a transdermal patch only. A 25 to 50 mcg patch is equivalent to 30-mg sustained-release morphine every eight hours.

Agonists-Antagonists

Butorphanol. Butorphanol is a kappa and sigma agonist with weak mu antagonism. Because of the kappa agonism, significant sedation may result. There is 50 per cent less nausea and vomiting than with morphine, and other side effects are less common. This drug may also cause dysphoria. It is available in a nasal spray preparation. The success of this drug as a chronic analgesic has been limited and is not the opioid of choice.

Pentazocine. Pentazocine is a kappa and sigma agonist and mu antagonist. High doses may cause an increase in heart rate and blood pressure. There is a high incidence of psychomimetic effects (anxiety, dysphoria, nightmares, and hallucinations), which greatly limits the use of this drug.

Nonsteroidal Anti-Inflammatory Drugs (NSAIDs)

NSAIDs are a class of nonopioid analgesics that have anti-inflammatory, antipyretic, and analgesic properties. They are recommended for the relief of mild to moderate pain. If a strong inflammatory component is present, e.g., in acute back pain, the NSAIDs can be very effective. The use of NSAIDs for chronic back pain is limited because of the lack of an inflammatory component.

The mechanism of action of NSAIDs is through the inhibition of cyclooxygenase, thus preventing the production of prostaglandins.[89, 90] The breakdown of arachidonic acid by cyclooxygenase results in the production of prostaglandins, which sensitize free nerve endings to inflammatory products (bradykinin, histamine, substance P, and so forth).

Unfortunately, NSAIDs have side effects that greatly limit their use. These side effects are divided into gastrointestinal, hematologic, and renal. All are directly related to the inhibition of prostaglandin synthesis. As a group, the nonacetylated salicylates are less likely to cause these side effects.

Tramadol

Tramadol produces analgesia through two mechanisms. One relates to its weak affinity for the mu opioid receptor (about 6000-fold less than morphine, about 100-fold less than propoxyphene, and about the same as dextromethorphan, an antitussive found in cough syrup). Therefore, it is an extremely weak opioid agonist. Clinical trials suggest that the primary analgesic action of tramadol is through the nonopioid release or inhibition of neuronal reuptake of serotonin and norepinephrine. Thus, it has a similar action as seen with the antidepressants. Several lines of evidence suggest that the two mechanisms of action of tramadol combine synergistically to produce analgesia.

There are few side effects of tramadol. The most common is mild sedation. There is no abuse potential, although there have been isolated reports of addiction.

There is no withdrawal or tolerance seen with this drug.

Antidepressants

The antidepressants are commonly used in the treatment of back pain. The analgesic doses are lower than the antidepressant doses.[103] Whether the antidepressants actually treat underlying depression (which is known to exacerbate chronic pain) with a corresponding decrease in pain is unknown. However, it appears that these drugs have a direct analgesic effect on neuropathic pain conditions.[40] The antidepressants are most effective for diffuse, burning, and dysesthetic pain. Most patients can be managed at or below antidepressant doses. However, some patients may require antidepressant levels, in which case blood levels should be monitored.

The antidepressants inhibit the reuptake of norepinephrine and serotonin into the nerve terminals, which results in an increased concentration and duration of action of these neurotransmitters at the synapse. Both serotonergic and noradrenergic neurons in the brain stem project to and inhibit C-fiber input into the spinal cord. The antidepressants are thought to activate these descending inhibitory neurons. The opioids also activate these brain stem inhibitory neurons, and the antidepressants potentiate the action of the serotonin and norepinephrine released by the opioids.[86]

Unfortunately, the antidepressants have many side effects, including anticholinergic (dry mouth, constipation, urinary retention, sedation), antihistaminic (sedation), alpha-1 blockade (hypotension), and antidopaminergic (dystonia) effects. The sedation seen with these agents may be advantageous, as many chronic back pain patients suffer from a sleep disturbance.

The antidepressants are divided into three classes: tricyclics, serotonin specific reuptake inhibitors (SSRIs), and atypical antidepressants. The tricyclics are the oldest of the antidepressants, have the highest side effect profile, and have been clinically proved effective in neuropathic pain. They include amitriptyline, nortriptyline, imipramine, desipramine, doxepin, and amoxapine. The SSRIs are a new class of antidepressants that selectively inhibits the reuptake of serotonin. They do not seem to have as good an analgesic effect as the tricyclics. They are generally stimulating and, therefore, are given in the morning. It is not uncommon to administer an SSRI in the morning and a tricyclic at bedtime. The atypical antidepressants include trazodone, maprotiline, and venlafaxine. Trazodone is mildly sedating and is often used for sleep disturbances.

Because of the side effects of the antidepressants (especially the tricyclics), patient compliance may be poor. The most common cause of noncompliance with the tricyclics is starting at an initial dose that is too high. It is best to start at the smallest dose possible and gradually increase slowly over two to four weeks. The choice of the tricyclic depends on the patient. If the patient suffers from a sleep disturbance, a more sedating tricyclic (amitriptyline, doxepin, or imipramine) will be necessary. If there is no sleep disturbance, a less sedating tricyclic will be the drug of choice (nortriptyline, desipramine). Some patients may benefit from the stimulating effect of the SSRIs in the morning and the sedative effect of the tricyclics in the evening.

Therapeutic serum levels of the antidepressants that apply for depression do not apply for pain management; therefore, serum levels are not necessary. However, if the total dose is greater than 100 mg daily, serum levels may be necessary to avoid toxic levels.

Anticonvulsants

The anticonvulsant drugs have been demonstrated to be effective in pain syndromes with an intermittent lancinating quality.[236] The anticonvulsants used in back pain management include carbamazepine, gabapentin, phenytoin, valproic acid, and clonazepam. They are generally started at low doses and gradually increased until the emergence of toxicity or intolerable side effects. The "therapeutic" serum levels that apply for the treatment of epilepsy do not apply for pain management. Therefore, the drugs should be titrated to pain relief and side effects.

The mechanism of action of pain relief is unclear; however, the anticonvulsants appear to affect the peripheral nerves much the same way they affect the brain. Whereas the anticonvulsants suppress ectopic foci in the brain, thus preventing seizures, they also reduce the discharge from sites of ectopic foci in damaged peripheral nerves or dorsal horn cells thought to be responsible for intermittent lancinating pain. One mechanism of suppressing this abnormal activity is through sodium channel blockade.

Unlike the tricyclic antidepressants, the anticonvulsants are chemically unrelated and have different side effects. All the anticonvulsants, with the exception of gabapentin, may cause liver damage. Therefore, baseline liver function tests should be performed and monitored. Carbamazepine may cause aplastic anemia and the complete blood count should be monitored. Phenytoin may cause gingival hyperplasia. The most common side effects of gabapentin are sedation and ataxia, which usually subside with continued use. Gabapentin has no known systemic toxicities, nor have therapeutic blood levels been established. Doses as high as 3600 mg a day have been reported with no serious side effects.

Antiarrhythmics

Some of the antiarrhythmics have been shown to affect certain chronic pain syndromes. These drugs are useful in treating back pain with a lancinating quality. They are also effective in pain that has an allodynic or dysesthetic quality. Lidocaine is a potent analgesic that is available in intravenous form only. Intravenous lidocaine infusions are performed in pain clinics to determine the sensitivity of the pain to the sodium channel blockers.[238] The only two antiarrhythmics used orally for chronic pain are mexiletine and tocainide.

These drugs appear to act on ectopic foci in damaged nerves, much the same way as the anticonvulsants do. They suppress the abnormal activity in peripheral nerves through sodium channel blockade. The concentration required to suppress ectopic foci and abnormal activity is far below that required for frank nerve conduction blockade.

Side effects of the antiarrhythmics include nausea and vomiting, tremors and irritability, and seizures with high doses.

Alpha-1 Antagonists and Alpha-2 Agonists

The sympathetic nervous system (SNS) may be involved in chronic back pain with a neuropathic nature. This is especially true of chronic radicular symptoms with a burning dysesthetic pain in the extremity. Peripheral nerve terminals and dorsal root ganglion cells possess alpha receptors that may become active in neuropathic pain conditions.[165] The SNS releases norepinephrine, which stimulates these receptors and leads to pain. The alpha blockers block the action of norepinephrine on these receptors, and the alpha-2 agonists inhibit the release of norepinephrine from the postganglionic sympathetic nerve terminals. In this way, these agents produce a chemical sympathectomy.

Orthostatic hypotension is the most common side effect. As the body fluids shift to compensate for the change in vascular tone, this side effect usually disappears with time.

These drugs are well tolerated with few side effects. They must be titrated to blood pressure rather than pain relief. If unacceptable low blood pressure occurs before pain relief, these drugs must be discontinued.

Miscellaneous Drugs

Baclofen. Baclofen is a GABA-B agonist that has antispasmodic activity. It is most commonly used for spasms that result from spinal cord injury. It has been shown to be effective for pain with a lancinating or shooting quality. It also provides muscle relaxation. It is commonly used intrathecally in the management of spasticity of spinal origin.

Dantrolene. Dantrolene is a potent antispasmodic that dissociates the excitation-contraction coupling mechanism of skeletal muscle by interfering with the release of calcium from the sarcoplasmic reticulum. Fatal and nonfatal liver disorders may occur with dantrolene; therefore, this drug should be used in selected cases only.

Antihistamines. Because histamine can activate C fibers, it seems reasonable to administer an antihistamine to block this C-fiber activation. Hydroxyzine is the only antihistamine that has been proved to have intrinsic analgesic activity of its own. Hydroxyzine potentiates the effects of the opioids and is commonly administered with an opioid. Phenyltoloxamine and orphenadrine have also been used in pain management.

Skeletal Muscle Relaxants. The use of muscle relaxants is usually part of a therapeutic regimen; they are rarely given alone. In conjunction with the opioids, NSAIDs, and physical therapy, they can be quite effective in pain management. However, the long-term use of the skeletal muscle relaxants is controversial and is not recommended. The skeletal muscle relaxants are divided into the antispasmodics and the centrally acting muscle relaxants.

The centrally acting skeletal muscle relaxants include carisoprodol, chlorphenesin carbamate, chlorzoxazone, cyclobenzaprine hydrochloride, methocarbamol, and orphenadrine citrate. Many of these are available in combination with certain other drugs.

Sedatives, Hypnotics, and Tranquilizers. The use of these drugs in chronic back pain management is controversial. Despite this, their use in combination with opioids and antidepressants is not uncommon. It is still unclear whether these drugs have intrinsic analgesic activity. They should be reserved for selected cases.

Spinal Drug Delivery

Spinal infusions evolved from the work of Wall and Melzak in 1965. Demonstration of high opiod receptor density in the spinal cord provided a logical basis for spinal opiod use.[184]

In 1980, Matthews and Abrams reported that 2 to 4 mg morphine sulfate intrathecally provided 24 to 48 hours of analgesia.[160] Studies such as these led to high expectations that spinal opiates would become a rational alternative to systemic analgesics. However, these studies only sporadically discussed efficacy, side effects, and complications and intermittently observed variable results.

Abram's review of cancer and noncancer literature allowed a few generalizations to be made[1]:

1. There is a low mean opiate dose in all series that doubles every few months. Patients, particularly those in the terminal phase of disease, escalate their doses much more rapidly.
2. There is a tendency toward slower dose escalation with intrathecal administration. Epidural catheters may develop fibrosis, which causes pain on injection and tracks drug out of the epidural space.
3. Dose escalations are slower with infusions than with intermittent bolusing techniques. An accepted speculation is that bolus doses often provide higher receptor concentrations and may in turn accelerate tolerance mechanisms.
4. Neuropathic pain requires higher doses of opioid than does somatic pain. Visceral pain lies somewhere in between neuropathic and somatic requirements.
5. Pain with activity requires significantly more spinal or systemic drug than does pain at rest.

6. Higher systemic requirements predict higher spinal opioid requirements.
7. Chronic nonmalignant pain tends to be more resistant to management with spinal opiates. This may be related to psychosocial factors as opposed to biopsychologic issues, and therapy can last for many years in those nonterminal patients.

Complication reports in the literature are surprisingly rare. The most common complications for external access catheters are superficial catheter infection, catheter occlusion, and displacement. Epidural catheters can rarely expose patients to pain on injection, progressive decrement in efficacy, and subcutaneous leakage. Intrathecal systems may lead to the development of cerebrospinal fluid leaks (hygromas) or meningitis. This can be a major concern in diabetics or pancytopenic patients. Hematomas may occur in patients with coagulation abnormalities. Mechanical failures may occur but are fairly rare with current technology. Battery life is approximately three years. There have been reports of paradoxic hyperalgesia with high doses of intrathecal opiates, and this has been reproduced. Adverse reactions to spinal opiates are similar to those seen with systemic opiates but are more troublesome with opiate-naive patients. The most common side effects are nausea, pruritus, urinary retention, hypotension, and respiratory depression. These are treatable with low-dose naloxone (1 to 2 mcg per kg), which does not reverse the analgesic effect.

Safe ranges for converting systemic opiates to spinal opiates are usually 1 to 2 per cent of the daily systemic dose. Reasonable guidelines that have emerged from Oxford are as follows:

1. Oral to epidural morphine, divide the 24-hour dose by 10.
2. Subcutaneous to epidural morphine, divide the 24-hour dose by 5.
3. Epidural to intrathecal morphine, divide the 24-hour dose by 10.

Other drugs that are used for intrathecal delivery include baclofen and local anesthetics. Baclofen is approved for intrathecal delivery for the treatment of post–spinal cord injury spasticity. It may also be useful in chronic back pain with severe muscle spasms. It may also decrease the sharp shooting pain associated with nerve root injuries. The most common local anesthetics used for spinal delivery are bupivacaine and tetracaine. When delivering intrathecal local anesthetics, care must be taken not to cause motor weakness or sensory loss. These agents have been successfully used to treat chronic back pain without motor or sensory loss. Clonidine will soon be available for intrathecal delivery. It holds promise in treating pain that is sympathetically mediated.

NONPHARMACOLOGIC MANAGEMENT OF BACK PAIN

Spinal Cord Stimulation

The current use of electroanalgesia stems from the 1965 work on spinal gate control theory by Melzack and Wall.[258] Electric stimulation-induced analgesia is often separated into its anatomic target sites for discussion.

Although used for a variety of indications since its inception in 1967, the most common indication for spinal cord stimulation is chronic lumbar radiculopathy from multiple laminectomies. Outcomes have been traditionally hard to quantify, but those customarily measured, such as decrease in discomfort analogue, length of use of the device, and improvement in function and analgesic use, have demonstrated mixed effectiveness. Young in 1989 noted a 55 per cent initial improvement that dropped to 33 per cent beyond six months.[270] North and coworkers[176] and De La Porte and Van de Kelft[60] in 1993 noted long-term pain relief of approximately 50 per cent at mean intervals of seven and four years, respectively. This improvement in outcome over the last several years has been attributed to the evolution of programmable, multichannel electrodes and clinical selection.

Complications are divided into technical and medical problems. Technical problems with migration and malposition can cause reintervention rates as high as 55 per cent.[60] Infection is the major medical complication, with rates as high as 5 per cent.[60]

Selection of appropriate patients is achieved by screening based on medical indications, trial electrode placement, and psychologic readiness of the patient. Medical indication guidelines are useful and have evolved from a variety of sources. A representative example arises from the German Society for Neurosurgery. Its indications are as follows: failed back syndrome, incomplete plexus (cervical, brachial, lumbar) or peripheral nerve lesion, postamputation pain, sympathetic reflex dystrophy, and rest pain of vasular disease. Nonindications are complete tranverse lesions of the spinal cord, cancer, deafferentation pain in spinal root avulsion, and postherpetic neuralgia. Trial electrode placement determines whether stimulation paresthesias can adequately cover the painful region. Determination of psychologic readiness involves screening for untreated psychiatric illness or secondary gains. A history of drug abuse or addiction is a relative contraindication and should be addressed and treated separately from the pain issues.

Transcutaneous Electrical Nerve Stimulation (TENS)

There are more than 600 publications supporting the efficacy of TENS. Yet few individuals are offered TENS for back pain, despite a reported efficacy rate of up to 80 per cent in most acute low back pain problems and 50 per cent in less chronic problems.[222] The initial efficacy in chronic pain, unfortunately, tends to diminish over the course of a year.

The TENS equipment consists of a transistorized, battery-operated pulse generator designed to be worn on a belt or attached to the patient's clothing. The insulated leads connect the stimulator to the skin electrodes and are usually supple for patient comfort.

TENS Stimulation Variables

Pulse Frequency Width. Pulse frequency is adjustable on most units from 4 to 50 pulses per second, with some frequencies going up to 90 to 160 pulses per second. The most effective range appears to be between 50 and 100 pulses per second. The pulse width ranges from 9 to 350 milliseconds. The pulse width has a significant effect on the amount of stimulation actually received by the patient. When using a high amplitude, a low pulse width is usually used.

Waveform. Waveform differs among different commercial units. However, the waveform as measured by an oscilloscope may be grossly distorted by the time it reaches the nerve bundle.[122]

Intensity. Low-intensity impulses do not cause muscle twitch or contraction. They are applied at a high pulse rate (up to 100 pulses per second). The patient should barely perceive this stimulation. It is thought that this stimulation affects the larger myelinated afferents to excite the inhibitory cells in the dorsal horn. These act to diminish the nociceptive afferent input (closing the gate).

High-intensity impulses are applied to a tolerable level at approximately 10 pulses per second. If applied over any period of time, this becomes intolerable, and the high intensity must be modulated for patient comfort. It is thought that the high-intensity impulses work by releasing endorphins in the central nervous system. The effects can be antagonized by the injection of the opioid antagonist naloxone.[224]

Some patients may have no pain relief at one intensity but good pain relief at another intensity.[51]

Use in Acute Pain

The postoperative application of TENS may be one of its most beneficial uses. TENS is not effective enough to be the sole method of pain relief but can significantly reduce opioid requirements.[131] Care must be taken to remove all Betadine from the area by cleansing with alcohol before putting on the electrodes. The electrodes are placed on the skin on either side of the surgical scar. The electrode pads are changed on postoperative day two to avoid skin irritation. The patient is instructed on the use of TENS before surgery. In a controlled study of 100 patients undergoing lumbar back surgery, Jensen reported that 68 per cent of TENS patients felt that their pain was significantly reduced by the TENS.[131] Hospital stay was 1.74 days less in the TENS group. On average, the amount of pain medication received by the patients was decreased by almost half.

Use in Chronic Pain

It is difficult to predict who will respond to TENS for chronic pain. It is important that someone trained in

TENS application spend time with the patient initially, explain how it works, and try different electrode sites. A trial of TENS should be instituted with the patient trying different electrode placements and different stimulation patterns. If there is no improvement after a week, TENS will probably not be effective and it can be stopped. Johnson and colleagues in 1991 questioned almost 200 patients who had improvement of their pain with TENS.[133] They reported:

1. There was no significant relationship between response, diagnosis, or body area affected.
2. Patients usually applied the stimulation to create a strong but comfortable paresthesia within the painful area.
3. Almost half of the patients had their pain intensity reduced by more than 50 per cent. The onset of analgesia was within 30 minutes in over 75 per cent and within 60 minutes in over 95 per cent of the patients.
4. Pain relief lasted less than 30 minutes in 51 per cent of patients after turning off the TENS. It lasted more than one hour in 30 per cent and more than two hours in only 20 per cent.
5. Thirty per cent of patients used TENS more than seven hours a day. Seventy-five per cent used it on a daily basis.
6. Skin reactions to the electrodes, usually caused by drying out of the electrode jelly, occurred in 53 per cent of patients.

Contraindications and Side Effects

The main contraindications for TENS are its use over a pregnant uterus, over the carotid sinus in the neck, or in patients with demand-type pacemakers. Electrodes should not be placed over insensate or allodynic skin. The main side effect is from reaction to the electrodes or electrode jelly.

MANUAL THERAPY OF THE SPINE (MOBILIZATION AND MANIPULATION)

Manipulation of the spine has been used in therapy of spinal pain almost since the dawn of recorded medicine. Today, the manipulative therapist uses various methods of analysis when examining a patient with spinal pain.[106]

Testing Passive Intervertebral Joint Motion. The vertebral segment is passively moved through a range of movement around each major axis, and the end feel of the joint is ascertained. Passive movement may be rated on a 0 to 6 scale, with 0 being ankylosis, 3 being normal, and 6 unstable. Manual treatment ranges from no treatment if ankylosis is present to surgery if the segment is unstable. The more hypermobile the segment, the more likely it is that the treatment plan will be low-grade mobilization and stabilization exercises or external support.

Application of Specific Pressures on Bony Vertebral Processes.[157] The therapist presses on the spinous and transverse processes to ascertain the irritability of the segment. The grade of movement that produces irritability has been shown to be reliably reproduced by different examiners.[106, 157] Treatment is by mobilization of the joint up to and within the painful range.

Joint Position. Muscle spasm causes irritability within a segment. This may cause a compensatory scoliosis or antalgic deviation above or at the site of the problem. Treatment is usually on the basis of precise positional analysis, muscle energy techniques, or high-velocity thrust manipulations.

Mobilization

Mobilization describes passive joint movements in which repetitive, low-velocity movements within or at the limit of range of movement are given to the joint. The rationale is that these low-stress, small-amplitude movements cause effective synovial fluid distribution over and through articular cartilage and partial stretching of the ligamentous joint structures. These are considered necessary for efficient functioning and for repair of soft tissue structures.[95, 206, 243] The activation of mechanoreceptors in the capsule of the facet joint may also decrease pain by spinal gating mechanisms centrally.[106]

Manipulation

In manipulation, the joint, having been taken to the limit of range of movement, is subjected to a small-amplitude, high-velocity thrust. The joint is thus briefly taken beyond the restricted range of movement. Manipulation may be performed under anesthesia (MUA), but this is considered to involve a greater risk of tissue injury than manipulation when the patient is awake and cooperative. Comparison studies between MUA and awake manipulation have not been reported. The majority of studies on manipulation have been poorly done. Difabio identified 11 valid studies that demonstrated the efficacy of manipulation in the treatment of low back pain. He reported on three other valid studies, two for the cervical and one for the sacral region. The reported studies generally showed immediate and short-term symptomatic relief for low back pain in the manipulated group. Long-term differences between the manipulated and control groups were not significant. One of the cervical studies reported the manipulated group to be worse off than the control group.[68]

Techniques of manipulation vary considerably between different professions and even within the same profession. Many clinical trials are difficult to evaluate because of multiple techniques within the same study or poor descriptions of the techniques used, making replication of the study difficult. Difabio reported that rotational manipulation of the low back in the acute pain phase between 14 and 28 days after pain onset produced a significant improvement over a control

group.[68] This improvement, however, appears to disappear with time.[155] Manipulation of the spine in chronic pain often shows a small immediate improvement, but follow-up weeks later shows no difference between manipulated and control groups. This may emphasize the necessity of continuing an exercise program to maintain the health of a tissue that has had its range of movement improved. Koes and associates followed up patients for nonspecific chronic back and neck complaints for 12 months, comparing manipulation (on average, six sessions over nine weeks); physical therapy, which they described as heat, exercise, and massage (14 sessions over eight weeks); family physician treatment with medication and home exercises (no specific number of sessions reported); and placebo treatment consisting of detuned ultrasound (12 sessions over six weeks).[140] A total of 256 patients were assigned to one of the four groups. There was an 8 to 20 per cent dropout rate to follow-up at 12 weeks. There was a 15 to 26 per cent dropout rate to follow-up at 12 months. Their conclusions were that patients who had manipulative therapy fared slightly better than the physical therapy group and had fewer treatment sessions. Both groups did better than the physician/medication or placebo controls, although all groups showed improvement with time.[140] The fact that millions of people go to manipulative therapists every year for spinal pain has been cited as evidence that manipulation does work. Unfortunately, good controlled studies have yet to demonstrate this fact.

Whereas mobilization and lumbar spine manipulation appear to be relatively benign, there are recorded instances of mortality and morbidity associated with cervical manipulation. Herniation of a lumbar disc has been reported following manipulation, and damage has been reported following manipulation in patients with osteoporosis, fractures, or bony tumors.

Exercise

Manual therapy, whether by mobilization or manipulation of the spine, should always be combined with an exercise program. There are numerous studies showing the damaging effects of excessive rest on the spinal tissues. There are proponents of different exercise regimens based on extension[164] and flexion.[156] There is a rationale for both, and patients probably need both types of exercises. It must be remembered that whatever exercises are prescribed, they should be of relatively short duration and done more frequently than once a day. Patients must also be encouraged to get up and move around frequently during their daily routines. It has been suggested that sustained disc loading, such as occurs with poor posture and extended periods of sitting, is associated with disc degeneration and low back pain.[242, 243] Postural education and workplace ergonomics should be part of any back rehabilitation program. Several studies have shown that as lumbar function improves during an exercise regimen, the levels of back pain decline.[161, 242, 246] In patients with herniated lumbar discs, a vigorous exercise regimen has been shown to produce good or excellent outcomes when compared with nonexercising control groups.[205]

Summary: Suggested Indications for Manual Therapy

Mobilization

1. Pain in the cervical or lumbar region of more than six weeks' duration.

Manipulation

1. Acute low back pain of between two and four weeks' duration.
2. Acute or chronic thoracic pain.
3. Chronic low back or neck pain of more than six weeks' duration.
4. May be contraindicated in the elderly or in patients with osteoporosis or bone disease.

ACUPUNCTURE

Acupuncture is the stimulation of certain body points by needles. Many acupuncture points are situated on or very close to nerves or very close to major blood vessels, which are surrounded by their perivascular plexus of nervi vasorum. (The afferent impulses from the acupuncture needles probably travel via these nerves.) The acupuncture points themselves are areas of lowered skin impedance. This fact is used by many commercial acupuncture point finders, which indicate the lower resistance by a light or a noise. It has been suggested that these points are areas where there is a high concentration of acetylcholine, indicating increased sudomotor activity. The increased sweating in this small area would decrease resistance or increase conductance. Melzack and coworkers showed close correlation with so-called myofascial trigger points and acupuncture points,[166] and Liu and associates showed a correlation with motor points.[151] Stimulation of these points has been described as stimulating principally A-delta fibers, which may decrease nociceptive input from the C fibers. Classic Chinese acupuncture emphasizes points on so-called body meridians far away from the site of injury. Most Western practitioners, however, use sites in the segmental distribution of pain. Unfortunately, controlled studies comparing the two are not available.

Types of Acupuncture

There are many different traditions and styles of acupuncture, even within China. Acupuncturists from different schools recommend different points and needling techniques for the same patient. Although there is agreement on the site of classic acupuncture points, traditional acupuncturists may treat patients with similar conditions in different ways according to the patient's own unique constitution, lifestyle, and emotional state. The acupuncturist may assess signs such as the quality of the pulse, coloration of the tongue, the complexion, and the patient's smell. This information determines which points he or she will use. In contrast, the Western practitioner uses a formula type of treatment, usually using a small number of prescribed traditional acupuncture points. There are also acupuncturists who use the scalp, ear, or foot for treatment of chronic pain, including low back pain. Electrical acupuncture has been studied; it is usually applied at a rate between 4 and 10 Hz for 5 to 15 minutes. There are also hybrid techniques, such as electrical acupuncture[50] and Ryodoraku therapy.[179] These are derived from traditional acupuncture but are systematized using electrical methods of diagnosis and treatment. There are no control studies comparing the several techniques. One of the best results reported with acupuncture and low back pain was when a traditional acupuncturist was allowed to follow his clinical judgment and treatment was not limited to a specific formula.[55]

One major difficulty in assessing the efficacy of acupuncture in reported trials is the difficulty of having a control group. Most papers do not use control groups, or the control group may receive "sham acupuncture," where needles are placed in nonclassic acupuncture points, or "false acupuncture," where the needle is merely placed in the skin or even on top of the skin. TENS electrodes are placed over the area but not switched on.[148, 149] When controls have been used, it appears that acupuncture is more effective by some 20 to 35 per cent than placebo alone.

Gunn in 1980 described the use of dry needling of muscle motor points for chronic low back pain.[111] He placed the needle deep into the muscle belly at specified points that usually corresponded to tender or trigger points and stimulated the needle by rapidly moving it up and down (pecking). This pecking was often associated with a heavy feeling by the patient. This has been described by classic acupuncturists as *teh Ch'i*. This vague feeling of soreness, heaviness, pressure, numbness, fullness, or distention is possibly caused by excitation of various proprio- and mechanoreceptors. Gunn suggested that when *teh Ch'i* was elicited, the use of electrical acupuncture did not add anything to the results. Other authors have also suggested that unless *teh Ch'i* is described by the patient, the results of the acupuncture will be much poorer.

Most studies of acupuncture and low back pain have concentrated on short-term outcomes. Gunn followed patients for an average of 27.3 weeks.[111] Eighteen of 29 subjects who had failed conservative therapy and received needling of motor points had returned to their original or equivalent jobs, and 10 had returned to lighter employment. In the control group, which had conservative therapy alone, only four had returned to their original work, and 14 of 27 had returned to light employment. Nine were still disabled. Carlsson and Sjolund followed 211 patients who had acupuncture for chronic pain with a mean duration of 10.4 years.[48] Although the pain was not specifically back related, the results are of interest. The average number of treatments was 7.8. Follow-up continued for six months. In their experience, patients who had been classified as suffering from nociceptive pain (sensitive to opioids) responded the best to acupuncture, with some 48 per cent having initially good results. This decreased to 23.2 per cent after more than six months. The patients who were diagnosed as having neuropathic or psychologic pain had lower responses initially, and only 12 per cent (4 of 34) with neurogenic pain and more with psychogenic pain had improvement after more than six months. In an uncontrolled study of 20 patients with low back pain, 80 per cent improved initially, but only 15 per cent still had pain improvement after 12 months.[147] Lewith and colleagues reported on 151 patients, 70 per cent of whom had an immediate positive effect; 55 per cent were still better after three months.[149]

It is our experience that acupuncture should be only one modality in the treatment of low back pain. Acupuncture, whether done by needling into the trigger points and motor points as described by Cheng or by needling into the tender points as described by Baldry, has an effect not only on pain, which may be either dramatic or delayed, but also on muscle flexibility.[11, 51] It is our practice in patients with low back pain to place needles into the motor and trigger points to try to cause a feeling of *teh Ch'i*. If this feeling is achieved, pecking is used in the muscle surrounding this area, and the needle is left in situ for 10 to 15 minutes. Other painful areas of the low back are located, and these tender points have needles inserted subcutaneously for 30 seconds. The needle is subsequently removed as other tender points are found and the needle is inserted subcutaneously into them. Pressure over previously needled tender points usually elicits much less tenderness. With this technique of needling deep and superficial points, the muscles of the low back and buttocks are clinically much less tense following 15 to 20 minutes of therapy. This allows active stretching and range of movement exercises of the low back to be commenced. Like the treatment of trigger points as described by Travell and Simons,[240] acupuncture is useful in decreasing pain and relaxing the muscle to allow normal movement of the joint, but it is only part of the therapy. Stretching and range of motion exercises are the other important part. A significant number of individuals who are initially helped by acupuncture have an exacerbation of their pain one to two hours after the first treatment session. The patient must be warned of this exacerbation, or disillusionment with the treatment may occur.

Duration of Therapy

Members of the New York Society of Acupuncture for Physicians and Dentists suggest that an initial course of acupuncture therapy should consist of six treatments given initially biweekly and later, weekly.[145] If the patient does not improve at that point, therapy should be discontinued. The consensus was that approximately 50 per cent of patients who respond favorably to acupuncture do so within three treatments, and about 90 per cent within six treatments. The usual course of treatment in the literature appears to average seven sessions. Patients may not require further therapy for months or possibly years. However, it is our experience that many patients who have responded favorably to acupuncture return at some later time for further "top-up" treatments. These treatment sessions are usually fewer in number than the initial therapy and are usually as effective.

The needles should be stainless steel. Disposable round-bodied needles are available to obviate the risk of transmission of infection. The principal side effects are lightheadedness and syncope, which appear to occur in less than 1 per cent of patients. Hematoma formation is uncommon. There are only a few occasions when, using a 30-gauge needle, blood is seen on withdrawal of the needle. Pneumothorax has been reported following needle insertion of the upper trapezius into the apex of the upper lobe. There are few contraindications to acupuncture. Electrical acupuncture should not be used or should be used cautiously in patients with pacemakers. Patients with epilepsy should be recumbent during therapy, and vigorous needle stimulation should be avoided.

Summary: Suggested Indication for Acupuncture

1. Low back pain, especially associated with muscle spasms.

NEUROLYTIC TECHNIQUES FOR SPINE PAIN

Radiofrequency Lesioning

Specific techniques using a radiofrequency lesioner have been developed to treat pain emanating from certain structures in the spine that is resistant to conventional treatment. This technique has been successful in the treatment of pain arising from facet joints, nerve roots, and the annulus fibrosus. Because of the complexity of the innervation of the dura, the posterior longitudinal ligament, and the paraspinous musculature, it is not possible to use this technique to treat pain in these areas.

Basic Principles

Radiofrequency lesions are created by placing an insulated needle (electrode) with an uninsulated tip on neural tissue. An electric current is passed through the needle and dispersed through the uninsulated needle tip into the surrounding tissue. The tissue surrounding the needle tip creates an impedance to the current flow, which generates heat. The uninsulated needle tip absorbs the heat from the tissue, and an equilibrium is eventually reached between the needle tip and the surrounding tissue (equilibrium temperature). Because the current dissipates as it spreads away from the needle tip, the greatest current density is just around the needle tip; thus the hottest part of the lesion is in the tissue just adjacent to the needle tip. This results in heating and destruction of the tissue with smooth edges and a predictable distance around the electrode tip.[56]

To create an adequate lesion, it is important to hold the equilibrium for 30 to 60 seconds. The equilibrium temperature is established in approximately 60 seconds,[56] but cerebrospinal fluid or large blood vessels may convect the heat away and alter the equilibrium temperature, resulting in lesions with irregular borders. Modern needle electrodes are capable of accurately measuring temperature; therefore, one knows how long to hold the desired temperature. Tissue destruction occurs at 45°C; however, much higher temperatures are used to create a lesion (80 to 90°C). Temperatures above 90°C should not be used, because tissue boiling will occur.

Patient Selection

Because of the invasiveness of radiofrequency lesioning, it should not be a treatment of first choice. Only after conservative measures have failed should this technique be used. Before proceeding with any treatment plan for spinal pain, a diagnosis should be made as to the etiology of the pain. Unfortunately, the physical examination is frequently equivocal, and the definitive diagnosis is made with spinal diagnostic blocks.

The sequence of diagnostic blocks must proceed from ones with the lowest morbidity to ones with the most complications. Because radiating pain may result from mechanical low back pain, the source of this pain should be investigated first. The order of progression should be (1) facet blocks, (2) communicating ramus block at L4 and L5, and (3) sympathetic block at L4. If these blocks are negative, then radicular components of the pain can be investigated by blocking nerve roots segmentally.[228]

Radiofrequency Techniques for Spinal Pain

Facet Pain

The outcome of facet denervation is difficult to measure because of the subjectivity of the response criteria. Reports have suggested a success rate of 40 per cent in failed back patients and 80 per cent in patients who have not undergone surgery if one uses a 50 per cent reduction in pain as a successful outcome.[153, 220, 226, 228] In general, patients without previous back surgery seem to have a higher success rate than those with back surgery.

A few studies have demonstrated the value of prognostic blocks in predicting the success of radiofrequency facet denervation. North and associates showed that patients who reported at least a 50 per cent reduction in pain after a prognostic block had a 45 per cent chance of maintaining at least a 50 per cent reduction in pain long term (mean follow-up interval, 3.2 years)

after radiofrequency facet denervation.[175] Gallagher and coworkers demonstrated that radiofrequency facet joint denervation, when compared with placebo, is beneficial in patients who respond positively to periarticular injection with local anesthetic.[99]

Facet denervation is performed by lesioning the medial branch of the dorsal ramus as it crosses the medial edge of the transverse process. Because the facet joints receive innervation from two medial branches, the medial branch above and below the facet must be lesioned.

Disc Pain

The complex innervation of the discs precludes total denervation of this structure; however, if the pain is emanating from the anterolateral portion, gray rami or lumbar sympathetic lesions can effectively treat the pain.[228] This technique is performed by placing the lesion just anterior to the vertebral foramen where sensory fibers from the disc travel in the gray rami. Sensory fibers also traverse the sympathetic ganglion to reach the anterior portion of the disc.

The posterior portion of the disc is innervated by the sinuvertebral nerve, which branches from the segmental nerve and runs backward to supply the disc. It is not possible to lesion this nerve without damaging the segmental nerve root. Therefore, pain emanating from the posterior portion of the disc has not been accessible to radiofrequency lesioning. However, recently Sluijter and van Kleef described a technique in which the thermal electrode is placed into the posterior portion of the disc (Sluijter and van Kleef, unpublished observations). Because the annulus has a high impedance, heat is generated, which thermocoagulates nociceptors in the annulus. Although the risk of discitis is low with this procedure, the morbidity of discitis is high, and this lesion should be used as a last resort in severe cases.

Radicular Pain

Radicular pain that is unresponsive to epidural steroid injections or surgery may be effectively treated with radiofrequency lesioning. The technique involves a thermal lesion to a portion of the dorsal root ganglion. This procedure has been performed at the cervical, thoracic, lumbar, and sacral levels with good results.[174, 225] Care must be taken to preserve sensory and motor function, as there is a risk of deafferentation pain from this procedure.

The procedure is performed by placing the electrode into the appropriate lumbar foramen in the superior and dorsal quadrant of the foramina. At the thoracic level, a laminar osteotomy is required to enter the foramina and reach the dorsal root ganglion. This osteotomy can be performed percutaneously by drilling a hole in the lamina to create an entrance site for the electrode.

Epidural Adhesiolysis

This technique, first described by Racz, involves placing an epidural catheter into an area of scar tissue surrounding a nerve root that is causing significant pain and attempting adhesiolysis, or the breaking up of the scar tissue. Epidural scars are common following surgery and in themselves do not indicate a pain-producing mechanism. However, if the nerve roots that are surrounded by the scar tissue become clinically painful, which can be demonstrated by a selective local anesthetic nerve root block, adhesiolysis can be attempted. A firm spring guidewire-type catheter is introduced into the epidural space via the lumbar caudal or via first sacral foramen routes. Using a special needle (RK needle) or catheter introducer, the catheter is directed into the scar tissue surrounding the painful root, and 0.25 per cent bupivacaine plus hyaluronidase is injected into the site.[35, 191, 192] Following the onset of local anesthesia, hypertonic saline 10 per cent and steroid are injected in aliquots with water-soluble contrast in an attempt to open up the scar tissue around the root. It is important that the hypertonic injection not be done until it is demonstrated that the catheter is not placed subdurally or in the subarachnoid. Intrathecal injection of hypertonic saline may cause severe pain, muscle cramps, hypertension, cardiac arrhythmias, cerebral edema, cerebral infarction, and myelopathy.[134, 192, 207]

A second catheter has been used to approach the scar tissue both from above, via the lumbar epidural space, and from below, via the caudal space. Controlled studies comparing the two techniques have not been reported. Some physicians leave the catheter in and infuse the catheter for two days with hypertonic saline, hyaluronidase, and local anesthetic.[192] Again, before injection of the hypertonic saline, fluoroscopic verification of the catheter placement should be made with water-soluble contrast. After the third infusion of hypertonic saline, the catheters are removed. Other physicians do the procedure on an outpatient basis and repeat the catheter injection at weekly intervals for two visits. If there is a marked improvement after one or two injections, further treatments are postponed. At the 1993 World Congress, Arthur presented data on 100 patients drawn from a pool of 1500 patients, documenting that the addition of hyaluronidase reduced the failure rate measured at one month from 18 to 6 per cent.[8] Long-term outcomes for pain relief appear to be poor, however, with only a few patients having significant pain relief at 7 to 12 months. Similar poor long-term results were reported by Devulder and colleagues, but this study was criticized on technical grounds.[64, 191, 195]

Summary: Suggested Indications for Epidural Adhesiolysis

1. Low back pain with radiating nerve root pain, not amenable to surgical therapy.
2. Evidence by magnetic resonance imaging or epidurogram of scar tissue around the nerve root.
3. Diagnostic selective root block or differential epidural with local anesthetic significantly decreases or abolishes the pain.

References

1. Abram, S. E.: Advances in chronic pain management since gate control. Reg. Anesth. 18:66–81, 1993.
2. Abram, S. E., and O'Connor, T. C. Complications associated with epidural steroid injections. Reg. Anesth. 21:149, 1996.
3. Adams, M. A., and Hutton, W. C. The mechanical function of the lumbar apophyseal joints. Spine 8:327, 1983.
4. Aprill, C.: The role of anatomically specific injections into the sacroiliac joint. Presented at the First Interdisciplinary World Congress on Low Back Pain and Its Relation to the Sacroiliac Joint. San Diego, CA, November 5–6, 1992, pp. 373–380.
5. Aprill, C. N.: Diagnostic disc injection. In Frymoyer, J. W. (ed.): The Adult Spine: Principles and Practice. New York, Raven Press, 1991, p. 403.
6. Aprill, C., and Bodguk, N.: High intensity zone: A pathognomonic sign of painful lumbar disc on MRI. Br. J. Radiol. 65:361, 1992.
7. Aprill, C., and Bogduk, N.: The prevalence of cervical zygapophyseal joint pain: A first approximation. Spine 17:744–747, 1992.
8. Arthur, J., Racz, G. B., Heinrich, R., et al.: Epidural space: Identification of filling defects of lysis of adhesions in the treatment of chronic painful conditions. Abstracts, 7th World Congress on Pain, International Association for the Study of Pain, 1993, p. 557.
9. Ashton, I. K., Ashton, B. A., Gibson, S. J., et al.: Morphological basis for back pain: The demonstration of nerve fibers and neuropeptides in the lumbar facet joint capsule but not in the ligamentum flavum. J. Orthop. Res. 10:72, 1992.
10. Augustinsson, L. E., Carlsson, C. A., Holm, J., et al.: Epidural electrical stimulation in severe limb ischemia: Pain relief, increased blood flow, and a possible limb-saving effect. Ann. Surg. 201:104–110, 1985.
11. Baldry, P. E.: Acupuncture, Trigger Points and Musculoskeletal Pain. London, Churchill Livingstone, 1989.
12. Banks, A. R.: A rationale for prolotherapy. J. Orthop. Med. 13:54, 1991.
13. Barnsley, L., and Bogduk, N.: Medial branch blocks are specific for the diagnosis of cervical zygapophyseal joint pain. Reg. Anesth. 18:343, 1993.
14. Barnsley, L., Lord, S., and Bogduk, N.: Comparative local anesthetic blocks in the diagnosis of cervical zygapophyseal joint pain. Pain 55:99, 1993.
15. Barnsley, L., Lord, S., Wallis, B., et al.: False-positive rates of cervical zygapophyseal joint blocks. Crit. J. Pain 9:124, 1993.
16. Barnsley, L., Lord, S. M., Wallis, B. J., et al.: Lack of effect of intra-articular corticosteroids for chronic pain in the cervical zygapophyseal joints. N. Engl. J. Med. 330:1047, 1994.
17. Barnsley, L., Lord, S. M., Wallis, B. J., et al.: The prevalence of chronic cervical zygapophysial joint pain after whiplash. Spine 20:20–25, 1995.
18. Beaman, D. N., Graziano, G. P., Glover, R. A., et al.: Substance P innervation of lumbar spine facet joints. Spine 18:1044–1049, 1993.
19. Bengstsson, M., Losstrom, J. B., and Malmquist, L. A.: Skin conductant responses during spinal analgesia. Acta Anaesthesiol. Scand. 29:67, 1985.
20. Bernard, T. N., and Cassidy, J. D.: The sacroiliac joint syndrome—pathophysiology, diagnosis, and management. In Frymoyer, J. W. (ed.): The Adult Spine: Principles and Practice. New York, Raven Press, 1991, p. 2107.
21. Bernard, T. N., Jr., and Kirkaldy-Willis, W. H.: Recognizing specific characteristics of nonspecific low back pain. Clin. Orthop. 217:266–280, 1987.
22. Bogduk, N.: Back pain: Zygapophysial joint blocks and epidural steroids. In Cousins, M. J., and Bridenbaugh, O. (eds.): Neural Blockade in Clinical Anaesthesia and Pain Management. Philadelphia, J. B. Lippincott Co., 1990, pp. 935–954.
23. Bogduk, N.: The clinical anatomy of the cervical dorsal rami. Spine 7:317, 1983.
24. Bogduk, N.: Diskography. Am. Pain Soc. J. 3:149–154, 1994.
25. Bogduk, N.: Innervation and pain patterns of the cervical spine. In Grant, R. (ed.): Physical Therapy of the Cervical and Thoracic Spine. London, Churchill Livingstone, 1988, pp. 1–13.

26. Bodguk, N.: The innervation of the lumbar spine. Spine 8:286–293, 1983.
27. Bogduk, N.: The lumbar disc and low back pain. Neurosurg. Clin. North Am. 2:791–806, 1991.
28. Bogduk, N., and Aprill, C.: On the nature of neck pain, discography and cervical zygapophyseal joint blocks. Pain 54:213–217, 1993.
29. Bogduk, N., and Engel, R.: The menisci of the lumbar zygapophyseal joints: A review of their anatomy and clinical significance. Spine 9:454, 1984.
30. Bogduk, N., and Twomey, L. T.: Clinical Anatomy of the Lumbar Spine. 2nd ed. Melbourne, Churchill Livingstone, 1991.
31. Bogduk, N., Tynan, W., and Wilson, A. S.: The nerve supply to the human lumbar intervertebral discs. J. Anat. 132:39, 1992.
32. Bogduk, N., Wilson, A. S., and Tynan, W.: The human lumbar dorsal rami. J. Anat. 134:383–397, 1982.
33. Bogduk, N., Windsor, M., and Inglis, A.: The innervation of the cervical intervertebral discs. Spine 13:2–8, 1989.
34. Bonica, J. J.: Anatomic and physiologic basis of nociception and pain. In Bonica, J. J. (ed.): The Management of Pain. 2nd ed. Philadelphia, Lea & Febiger, 1990.
35. Borg, P. A., and Krijnen, H. J.: Hyaluronidase in the management of pain due to post-laminectomy scar tissue. Pain 58:273, 1994.
36. Bowen, V., and Cassidy, J. D.: Macroscopic and microscopic anatomy of the sacroiliac joint from embryonic life until the eighth decade. Spine 6:620–628, 1981.
37. Bowes, R. A., and Cousins, N. J.: Diagnostic neural blockade. In Cousins, M. J., and Bridenbaugh, P. O. (eds.): Neural Blockade in Clinical Anesthesia and Management of Pain. 2nd ed. Philadelphia, J. B. Lippincott Co., 1988, p. 885.
38. Broadhurst, N. A.: Sacroiliac dysfunction as a cause of low back pain. Aust. Fam. Physician 18:623–629, 1989.
39. Brockow, T.: Segmental functional disorders—a frequent cause of backache? Ther. Umsch. 51:403–409, 1994.
40. Bruera, E., and Ripamonti, C.: Adjuvants to opioid analgesics. In Patt, R. B. (ed.): Cancer Pain. 1st ed. Philadelphia, J. B. Lippincott Co., 1993, pp. 143–159.
41. Burchiel, K. J., Frank, E. H., and Keenen, T. L.: A plea for prospective studies on discography. APS J. 3:160–162, 1994.
42. Burn, J. M. B., and Langdon, L.: Duration of action of epidural methyl prednisolone: A study in patients with lumbosciatic syndrome. Am. J. Phys. Med. Rehabil. 53:29, 1974.
43. Campbell, J. N., and Belzberg, A. J.: Use of disk distention to diagnose pain of spinal origin. APS J. 3:157–159, 1994.
44. Campbell, J. N., Raja, S. N., Meyer, R. A., et al.: Myelinated afferents signal the hyperalgesia associated with nerve injury. Pain 32:89–94, 1988.
45. Capsaicin Study Group: Effect of treatment with topical capsaicin: Multicenter, double-blind, vehicle controlled study. Arch. Intern. Med. 15:159, 1992.
46. Carette, S., Marcoux, S., Truchon, R., et al.: A controlled trial of corticosteroid injections into the facet joints for chronic low back pain. N. Engl. J. Med. 325:1002, 1991.
47. Carey, I., Balague, F., and Waldburger, M.: Pseudo-sciatica of neoplastic origin: Apropos of an unusual case. Schweiz. Rundsch. Med. Prax. 84:197–199, 1995.
48. Carlsson, C. P. O., and Sjolund, B. H.: Acupuncture and subtypes of chronic pain: Assessment of long term results. Clin. J. Pain 10:290, 1994.
49. Cassidy, J. D.: The pathoanatomy and clinical significance of the sacroiliac joints. J. Manipulative Physiol. Ther. 15:41–42, 1992.
50. Chen, G. S., and Voll, R.: Twenty years of electro-acupuncture therapy using low frequency current pulses. Am. J. Acupunct. 3:291, 1975.
51. Cheng, R., and Pomeranz, B.: Electro-acupuncture analgesia could be mediated by at least two pain relieving mechanisms: Endorphins and non-endorphin systems. Life Sci. 25:1957, 1979.
52. Cibulka, M. T., and Koldunoff, R. N.: Leg length disparity and its effect on sacroiliac joint dysfunction. Clin. Management 6:10, 1986.
53. Clifford, J. R.: Lumbar discography: An outdated procedure. J. Neurosurg. 64:686, 1986.
54. Cloward, R.: Cervical diskography: A contribution of the etiology and mechanism of neck, shoulder and arm pain. Ann. Surg. 150:1052–1064, 1959.
55. Coan, R. M., Wong, G., and Coan, P. L.: The acupuncture treatment of neck pain: A randomized controlled study. Am. J. Chin. Med. 9:326, 1982.
56. Cosman, E. R., Nashold, B. S., and Bedenbaugh, P.: Stereotactic radiofrequency lesion making. Appl. Neurophys. 46:160–166, 1983.
57. Craig, A. D.: Supraspinal pathways and mechanisms relevant to central pain. In Casey, K. L. (ed.): Pain and Central Nervous Systems Disease: The Central Pain Syndromes. New York, Raven Press, 1991, pp. 157–170.
58. Crock, H. V.: Internal disc disruption: A challenge to disc prolapse 50 years on. Spine 11:650, 1986.
59. Daum, W. J.: The sacroiliac joint: An underappreciated pain generator. Am. J. Orthop. 24:475–478, 1995.
60. De La Porte, C., and Van de Kelft, E.: Spinal cord stimulation in failed back surgery syndrome. Pain 52:51–61, 1993.
61. Derby, R., Bogduk, N., and Schwarzer, A.: Precision percutaneous blocking procedure for localizing spinal pain. Part 1: The posterior lumbar compartment. Pain Digest 3:89, 1993.
62. Destouet, J. M., Gilula, L. A., Murphy, W. A., et al.: Lumbar facet joint injection: Indication, technique, clinical correlation and preliminary results. Radiology 145:321, 1982.
63. Devor, M.: Neuropathic pain and injured nerve: Peripheral mechanisms. Br. Med. Bull. 47:619–630, 1991.
64. Devulder, J., Bogaert, L., Castille, F., et al.: Relevance of epidurography and epidural adhesiolysis in chronic failed back surgery patients. Clin. J. Pain 11:147, 1995.
65. Deyo, R. H., Diehl, A. K., and Rosenthal, M.: How many days of bed rest for acute low back pain? N. Engl. J. Med. 315:1064, 1986.
66. Dickenson, A. H., and Sullivan, A. F.: Evidence for a role of the NMDA receptor in the frequency dependent potentiation of deep rat dorsal horn nociceptive neurones following C fibre stimulation. Neuropharmacology 26:1235–1238, 1987.
67. Dickenson, A. H., and Sullivan, A. F.: Peripheral origins and central modulation of subcutaneous formalin-induced activity of rat dorsal horn neurones. Neurosci. Lett. 83:207–211, 1987.
68. Difabio, R. P.: Efficacy of manual therapy. Phys. Ther. 72:853, 1992.
69. Don Tigny, R. L.: Anterior dysfunction of the sacroiliac joint as a major factor in the etiology of idiopathic low back pain syndrome. Phys. Ther. 70:250–265, 1990.
70. Don Tigny, R. L.: Function and pathomechanics of the sacroiliac joint: A review. Phys. Ther. 65:35, 1985.
71. Dreyer, S. J., Dreyfuss, P., and Cole, A. J.: Zygapophyseal (facet) joint injections: Intra-articular and medial branch block techniques. In Kraft, G. H., and Weinstein, B. M. (eds.): Physical Medicine and Rehabilitation Clinics of North America. Philadelphia, W. B. Saunders Co., 1995, p. 715.
72. Dreyfuss, P.: Atlanto-occipital and lateral atlanto-axial joint injection techniques. In Lennard, T. A. (ed.): Physiatric Procedures in Clinical Practice. Philadelphia, Hanley and Belfur, 1995, p. 227.
73. Dreyfuss, P., and Calodney, A.: Cervical facet pain. Pain Digest 3:197–201, 1993.
74. Dreyfuss, P., Cole, A. J., and Pauza, K.: Sacroiliac joint injection techniques. Phys. Med. Rehabil. Clin. North Am. 6:785, 1995.
75. Dreyfuss, P., Dryer, S., Griffin, J., et al.: Positive sacroiliac screening tests in asymptomatic adults. Spine 19:1138–1143, 1994.
76. Dreyfuss, P., Michaelsen, M., and Fletcher, D.: Atlanto-occipital and lateral atlanto-axial joint pain patterns: A study in five normal subjects. Spine 19:1125–1131, 1994.
77. Dreyfuss, P., Tibiletti, C., and Dreyer, S.: Thoracic zygapophyseal joint pain: A review and description of an intra-articular block technique. Pain Digest 4:44, 1994.
78. Edgar, M. A., and Ghadially, J. A.: Innervation of the lumbar spine. Clin. Orthop. 115:35–41, 1976.
79. Ehni, G., and Benner, B.: Occipital neuralgia and the C1–2 arthrosis syndrome. J. Neurosurg. 61:961–965, 1984.
80. Eisenstein, S. M., and Parry, C. R.: The lumbar facet arthrosis syndrome: Clinical presentation and articular surface changes. J. Bone Joint Surg. 69:3–7, 1987.

81. el-Bohy, A., Cavanaugh, J. M., Getchell, M. L., et al.: Localization of substance P and neurofilament immunoreactive fibers in the lumber facet joint capsule and supraspinous ligament of the rabbit. Brain Res. *460:*379–382, 1988.

82. Esses, S. I.: The diskography dilemma. APS J. *3:*155–156, 1994.

83. Fairbank, J. C. T., Park, W. M., McCall, I. W., et al.: Apophyseal injections of local anesthetic as a diagnostic aid in primary low back pain syndromes. Spine 6:596, 1981.

84. Feinstein, B.: Experiments of pain referred from deep somatic tissues. J. Bone Joint Surg. Am. *36:*981–997, 1954.

85. Ferrante, F. M., Wilson, S. P., Iacobo, C., et al.: Clinical classification as a predictor of therapeutic outcome after cervical epidural steroid injection. Spine *18:*730, 1990.

86. Fields, H. L.: Central nervous system mechanisms for control of pain transmission. *In* Fields, H. L. (ed.): Pain. New York, McGraw-Hill, 1987, pp. 99–131.

87. Fischer, A. A.: Documentation of myofascial trigger points. Arch. Phys. Med. Rehabil. *69:*286, 1988.

88. Fischer, A. A.: Local injections in pain management. *In* Kraft, G. H., and Weinstein, S. M. (eds.): Physical Medicine and Rehabilitation Clinics of North America. Philadelphia, W. B. Saunders Co., 1995, p. 851.

89. Flower, R. J., and Blackwell, G. J.: Anti-inflammatory steroids induced biosynthesis of a phospholipase A2 inhibitor which prevents prostaglandin generation. Nature *278:*456, 1979.

90. Flower, R. J., Mocada, S., and Vane, J. R.: Analgesic-antipyretics and anti-inflammatory agents; drugs employed in the treatment of gout. *In* Gilman, A. G., Rall, T. W., Nies, A. S., and Taylor, P. (eds.): The Pharmacologic Basis of Therapeutics. New York, Pergamon Press, 1985, pp. 674–715.

91. Fordyce, W. E.: Contingency management. *In* Bonica, J. J. (ed.): The Management of Pain. 2nd ed. Philadelphia, Lea & Febiger, 1990, p. 1707.

92. Fortin, J. D., Aprill, C. N., Ponthieux, B., and Pier, J.: Sacroiliac joint: Pain referral maps upon applying a new injection/arthrography techique. Part II: Clinical evaluation. Spine *19:*1483–1489, 1994.

93. Fortin, J. D., Dwyer, A. P., West, S., et al.: Sacroiliac joint: Pain referral maps upon applying a new injection/arthrography technique. Part I: Asymptomatic volunteers. Spine *19:*1475–1482, 1994.

94. Frank, A. M., and Trappe, A. E.: Are sacroiliac joint block and insertion tendinosis of the musculus erector trunici too rarely diagnosed as the etiology of failed back syndrome after intervertebral disk operation. Zentralbl. Neurochir. *5:*193–196, 1994.

95. Frank, C., Akeson, W. H., Woo, S. L.-Y., et al.: Physiology and therapeutic value of passive joint motion. Clin. Orthop. *185:*113, 1984.

96. Franz, D. N., and Perry, R. S.: Mechanisms for differential block among single myelinated and non-myelinated anions by procaine. J. Physiol. *236:*193, 1974.

97. Fraser, R. D.: Chymopapain for the treatment of intervertebral disc herniation: The final report of the double blinded study. Spine *9:*815, 1984.

98. Fraser, R. D., Osti, O. L., and Vernon-Roberts, B.: Iatrogenic discitis: The role of intravenous antibiotics in prevention and treatment, an experimental study. Spine *14:*1025, 1989.

99. Gallagher, J., Petriccione di Vadi, P. L., et al.: Radiofrequency facet joint denervation in the treatment of low back pain: A prospective controlled double-blind study to assess its efficacy. Pain Clinic *7:*193–198, 1994.

100. Ghia, J. N., Toomey, T. C., Maow, D. G., et al.: Toward an understanding of chronic pain mechanisms. The use of psychological tests and a refined differential spinal block. Anesthesiology 1979; 50:20.

101. Giles, L. G.: Pathoanatomic studies and clinical significance of lumbosacral zygapophyseal (facet) joints. J. Manipulative Physiol. Ther. *15:*36–40, 1992.

102. Giles, L. G., and Taylor, J. R.: Innervation of lumbar zygapophyseal joint synovial folds. Acta Orthop. Scand. *58:*43–46, 1987.

103. Glassman, A. H., Perel, J. M., Shostak, M., et al.: Clinical implications of imipramine plasma levels for depressive illness. Arch. Gen. Psychiatry *34:*197–204, 1977.

104. Goldthwaite, J. E.: The lumbosacral articulation: An explanation of many cases of lumbago, sciatica and paraplegia. Boston Med. Surg. J. *164:*365, 1911.

105. Greenman, P. E.: Principles of Manual Medicine. Baltimore, Williams & Wilkins, 1989, pp. 125–149.

106. Grieve, G. P.: Modern Manual Therapy: The Vertebral Column. 2nd ed. London, Churchill Livingstone, 1994.

107. Grob, K. R., Neuhuber, W. L., and Kissling, R. O.: Innervation of the sacroiliac joint of the human. Z. Rheumatol. *54:*117–122, 1995.

108. Groen, G., Baljet, B., and Drukker, J.: Nerves and nerve plexuses of the human vertebral column. Am. J. Anat. *188:*282, 1990.

109. Gronblad, M., Korkala, O., Konttinen, Y. T., et al.: Silver impregnation and immunohistochemical study of nerves in lumbar facet joint plical tissue. Spine *16:*34–38, 1991.

110. Gronblad, M., Weinstein, J. N., and Santavirta, S.: Immunohistochemical observations on spinal tissue innervation: A review of hypothetical mechanisms of back pain. Acta Orthop. Scand. *2:*614–622, 1991.

111. Gunn, C. C., Milbrandt, W. E., Little, A. S., et al.: Dry needling of muscle motor points for chronic lower back pain: A randomized clinical trial with long term follow up. Spine *5:*279, 1980.

112. Hackett, G. S.: Joint stabilization through induced ligament sclerosis. Ohio State Med. J. *49:*877, 1953.

113. Hackett, G. S.: Prolotherapy in whiplash and low back pain. Postgrad. Med. *27:*214, 1960.

114. Handwerker, H. O., and Reeh, P. W.: Nociceptors: Chemo pain and inflammation. Pain Res. Clin. Management *4:*59–70, 1991.

115. Hanesch, U., Heppelmann, B., Messlinger, K., Schmidt, R. F., et al.: Nociception in normal and arthic joints: Structural and functional aspects. *In* Willis, W. D. (ed.): Hyperalgesia and Allodynia. New York, Raven Press, 1992, pp. 81–106,

116. Haughton, V. M., Nguyen, C. M., and Ho, K. C.: The etiology of focal spinal arachnoiditis: An experimental study. Spine *18:*1193–1198, 1993.

117. Helbig, T., and Lee, C. K.: The lumbar facet syndrome. Spine *13:*61–64, 1988.

118. Hendrix, R. W., Lin, P. P., and Kane, B. J.: Simplified aspiration or injection technique for the sacroiliac joint. J. Bone Joint Surg. Am. *64:*1249, 1982.

119. Hijikata, S., Yamagishi, M., Nakayama, T., et al.: Percutaneous discectomy: A new treatment method for lumbar disc herniation. J. Toden Hospital *5:*5, 1975.

120. Hopwood, M. B., and Abram, S. E.: Factors associated with failure of trigger point injections. Clin. J. Pain *10:*227, 1994.

121. Hove, B., and Gyldensted, C.: Cervical analgesic facet joint arthrography. Neuroradiology 32:456, 1990.

122. Howson, D. C.: Peripheral neural excitability implications for transcutaneous electrical nerve stimulation. Phys. Ther. *12:*1467, 1978.

123. Ikeda, R.: Innervation of the sacroiliac joint: Macroscopical and histological studies. J. Nippon Medical School *58:*587–596, 1991.

124. Ishimine, T.: Histopathological study of the aging process in the human sacroiliac joint. J. Japanese Orthopaedic Assoc. *63:*1074–1084, 1989.

125. Jackson, R. P.: The facet syndrome. Myth or reality? Clin. Orthop. *279:*110–121, 1992.

126. Jackson, R. P., Jacobs, R. R., and Montesano, P. X.: Facet joint injection in low back pain: A prospective statistical study. Spine *13:*966, 1988.

127. Jaffe, H. J.: Drug addiction and drug abuse. *In* Gilman, A. G., Rall, T. W., Nies, A. S., and Taylor, P. (eds.): Goodman and Gilman's Pharmacological Basis of Therapeutics. 8th ed. New York, McGraw-Hill, 1990, pp. 522–574.

128. Jajic, I., and Jajic, Z.: The prevalence of osteoarthritis of the sacroiliac joints in an urban population. Clin. Rheum. *6:*39–41, 1987.

129. Jajic, Z., Jajic, I., Dubravica, M., et al.: Analysis of the location of pain related to sacroiliitis in ankylosing spondylitis. Reumatizam *41:*1–3, 1994.

130. Javid, M. J., Nordby, E. J., Ford, L. T., et al.: Safety and efficacy of chymopapain in herniated nucleus pulposus with sciatica: Results of a randomized double blind study. JAMA *249:*2489, 1983.

131. Jenson, J. E., Etheridge, G. L., and Hazelrigg, G.: Effectiveness

of transcutaneous neural stimulation in the treatment of pain. Sports Medicine 3:79–88, 1986.

132. Johansson, A., Hao, J., and Sjolund, B.: Local corticosteroid application blocks transmission in normal nociceptor C-fibers. Acta Anaesthesiol. Scand. 34:335, 1990.

133. Johnson, N. I., Ashton, C. H., and Thompson, J. W.: An in-depth study of long term users of transcutaneous electrical nerve stimulation (TENS): Indications for clinical use of TENS. Pain 44:221, 1991.

134. Kim, R. C., Porter, R. W., Choi, B. H., et al.: Myelopathy after intrathecal administration of hypertonic saline. Neurosurgery 22:942, 1988.

135. Kim, S. H., and Chung, J. M.: An experimental model for peripheral neuropathy produced by segmental spinal nerve ligation in the rat. Pain 50:355–363, 1992.

136. King, J. S., and Lagger, R.: Sciatica viewed as a referred pain syndrome. Surg. Neurol. 5:46–50, 1976.

137. Kirkaldy-Willis, W. H., and Cassidy, J. D.: Spinal manipulation in the treatment of low back pain. Can. Fam. Physician 31:535, 1985.

138. Klein, R. G., Bjorn, C. E., DeLong, B., et al.: A randomized, double blind trial of dextrose, glycerin, phenol injections for chronic low back pain. J. Spinal Disord. 6:23, 1993.

139. Klein, R. G., Dorman, T. A., and Johnson, C. E.: Proliferant injections for low back pain: Histological changes of injected ligaments and objective measurements of lumbar spine mobility before and after treatment. J. Neurol. Orthop. Med. Surg. 10:141, 1989.

140. Koes, B. W., Bouter, L. M., Mameren, H. V., et al.: Randomized clinical trial of manipulative therapy and physiotherapy for persistent back and neck complaints: Results of one year follow up. BMJ 304:601, 1992.

141. LaMotte, R., Shain, C., Simone, D., and Tsai, E. F.: Neurogenic hyperalgesia: Psychophysical studies of underlying mechanisms. J. Neurophysiol. 66:190–211, 1991.

142. Larson, S. J., Sances, A., Cusick, J. F., et al.: A comparison between anterior and posterior spinal implant systems. Surg. Neurol. 4:180–186, 1975.

143. Laslett, M., and William, M.: The reliability of selected pain provocation tests for sacroiliac joint pathology. Spine 19:1243–1249, 1994.

144. LeBlanc, K. E.: Sacroiliac sprain: An overlooked cause of back pain. Am. Fam. Physician 6:1459–1463, 1992.

145. Lee, M. H. M.: Acupuncture for pain control. In Mark, L. C. (ed.): Pain Control: Practical Aspects of Patient Care. New York, Masson Publishers, 1981.

146. Letson, A. K., and Dahners, L. E.: The effects of combinations of growth factors on ligament healing. Clin. Orthop. 308:207, 1994.

147. Leung, P. C.: Treatment of low back pain with acupuncture. Am. J. Chin. Med. 7:372, 1979.

148. Lewith, G. T., Field, J., and Machin, D.: Acupuncture compared with placebo in postherpetic pain. Pain 17:361, 1984.

149. Lewith, G. T., Turner, G., Machin, D., et al.: Effects of acupuncture on low back pain and sciatica. Am. J. Acupunct. 12:21, 1984.

150. Lippit, A. B.: The facet joint and its role in spinal pain: Management with facet joint injections. Spine 9:746, 1984.

151. Liu, Y. K., Varella, M., and Oswald, R.: The correspondence between some motor points and acupuncture loci. Am. J. Chin. Med. 3:347, 1977.

152. Loeser, J. D., Bigos, S. J., Fordyce, W. E., et al.: Low back pain. In Bonica, J. J. (ed.): The Management of Pain. Philadelphia, Lea & Febiger, 1990, pp. 1448–1483.

153. Lora, J., and Long, D.: So-called facet denervation in the management of intractable back pain. Spine 1:121–126, 1976.

154. Lysell, E.: Motion in the cervical spine. Acta Orthop. Scand. 123(Suppl.): 1, 1969.

155. MacDonald, R. S., and Bell, C. M. J.: An open controlled assessment of osteopathic manipulation in non-specific low back pain. Spine 15:364, 1990.

156. MacNab, I.: Backache. Baltimore, Williams & Wilkins, 1977.

157. Maitland, G. D.: Vertebral Manipulation. 5th ed. London, Butterworth's, 1986.

158. Malinsky, J.: The ontogenetic development of nerve terminations in the intravertebral discs of man. Acta Anat. 38:96–113, 1959.

159. Marks, R. C., and Houston, T.: Facet joint injection and facet nerve block: A randomized comparison in 86 patients. Pain 49:325, 1992.

160. Matthews, E. T., and Abrams, L. D.: Intrathecal morphine in open heart surgery. Lancet 1:543, 1980.

161. Mayer, T. G., Gathcel, R. J., Kishino, N., et al.: Objective assessment of spine function following industrial injury. Spine 10:482, 1985.

162. McCarron, R. F., Wimpee, M. W., Hudkins, P. G., et al.: The inflammatory effect of nucleus pulposus: A possible element in the pathogenesis of low-back pain. Spine 2:760–764, 1987.

163. McCulloch, J. A.: Chemonucleolysis: Experience with 2,000 cases. Clin. Orthop. Rel. Res. Jan.–Feb. (146):128–135, 1980.

164. McKenzie, R. A.: The Lumbar Spine. Waikanae, New Zealand, Spinal Publications, 1981.

165. McLachlan, E. M., Jang, W., Devor, M., and Michaelis, M.: Peripheral nerve injury triggers noradrenergic sprouting within dorsal root ganglia. Nature 363:543–546, 1993.

166. Melzack, R., Stillwell, D. M., and Fox, E. J.: Trigger points and acupuncture points for pain: Correlations and implications. Pain 3:3, 1977.

167. Mochida, J., Toh, E., Nishimura, K., et al.: Percutaneous nucleotomy in lumbar disc herniation: Patient selection and role in various treatments. Spine 18:2212, 1993.

168. Moneta, G. B., Videman, T., Kaivanto, K., et al.: Reported pain during lumbar discography as a function of annular ruptures and disc degeneration: A re-analysis of 833 discograms. Spine 19:1968–1974, 1994.

169. Mooney, V., and Robertson, J. A.: The facet syndrome. Clin. Orthop. 115:149–155, 1976.

170. Murley, A. H. G.: Facet joints and low-back pain. BMJ 2:125–126, 1978.

171. Murphy, M. R.: Opioids. In Barash, P. G., Cullen, P. F., and Stoelting, R. K. (eds.): Clinical Anesthesia. Philadelphia, J. B. Lippincott Co., 1989, p. 254.

172. Murtagh, F. R.: Computed tomography and fluoroscopy guided anesthesia instilled injection in facet syndrome. Spine 13:686, 1988.

173. Nachenson, A.: Editorial comment: Lumbar discography, where are we today? Spine 14:555, 1989.

174. Nash, T. P.: Clinical note percutaneous radiofrequency lesioning of dorsal root ganglia for intractable pain. Pain 24:67–78, 1986.

175. North, R. B., Han, M., Zahurak, M., et al.: Radiofrequency lumbar facet denervation: Analysis of prognostic actors. Pain 57:77–83, 1994.

176. North, R. B., Kidd, D. H., Zahurak, M., et al.: Spinal cord stimulation for chronic intractable pain: Experience over two decades. Neurosurgery 32:384–394, 1993.

177. Nwuga, V. C. B.: Relative therapeutic efficacy of vertebral manipulation and conventional treatment in back pain management. Am. J. Phys. Med. 61:273, 1983.

178. Ohba, S.: Morphological study of the sacroiliac joint of aged Japanese and macroscopic and microscopic observations on its articular surface. J. Japanese Orthopaedic Assoc. 59:675–689, 1985.

179. Okazaki, K.: Ryodoraku therapy for migraine headache. Am. J. Chin. Med. 3:61, 1975.

180. Ongley, M. J., Klein, R. G., Dorman, T. A., et al.: A new approach to the treatment of chronic low back pain. Lancet 2:143, 1987.

181. Paine, K. W. E., and Haung, P. W. H.: The lumbar disk syndrome. J. Neurosurg. 37:75–82, 1972.

182. Patsiaouras, T., Bulstrode, C., Cook, P., et al.: Percutaneous nucleotomy: An anatomical study of the risks of root injury. Spine 16:39, 1990.

183. Perry, S., and Heidrich, G.: Management of pain during debridement: A survey of US burn units. Pain 13:267–280, 1982.

184. Pert, C. B., and Snyder, S. H.: Opiate receptor: Demonstration in nervous tissue. Science 179:1011–1014, 1973.

185. Pionchon, H., Tommasi, M., Pialat, J., et al.: Study of the innervation of the spinal ligaments at the lumbar level. Bull. Assoc. Anat. 70:63–67, 1986.

186. Portenoy, R. K.: Opioid therapy for chronic nonmalignant pain: A review of the critical issues. J. Pain Symptom Manage. 11:203–217, 1996.

187. Porter, J., and Jick, H.: Addiction rare in patients treated with narcotics. N. Engl. J. Med. *312:*123, 1980.
188. Potter, N. A., and Rothstein, J. M.: Intertester reliability for selected clinical tests of the sacroiliac joint. Phys. Ther. *65:*1671–1675, 1985.
189. Privat, J. M.: Percutaneous nucleotomy-diskectomy techniques. Automated and manual techniques. Indications and results. Neurochirurgie *39:*116, 1993.
190. Rabischong, P., Louis, R., Vignaud, J., et al.: The intervertebral disc. Anat. Clin. *1:*55, 1978.
191. Racz, G. B., and Heavner, J.: Response to relevance of epidurography and epidural adhesiolysis in chronic failed back surgery patients. (Letter.) Clin. J. Pain *11:*151, 1995.
192. Racz, G., Heavner, J. E., Singleton, W., and Carline, N.: Hypertonic saline and corticosteroid injected epidurally for pain control. *In* Racz, G. B. (ed.): Techniques of Neurolysis. Austin, Kluwer, 1989, p. 73.
193. Raja, S. N., Meyer, R. A., and Campbell, J. N.: Peripheral mechanisms of somatic pain. Anesthesiology *68:*571–590, 1988.
194. Rapp, S. E., Haselkorn, J. K., Elam, J. K., et al.: Epidural steroid injection in the treatment of low back pain: A meta-analysis. Anesthesiology *81:*923, 1994.
195. Reed, K. L., and Will, K. G.: Letter. Clin. J. Pain *11:*154, 1995.
196. Reeves, K. D.: Treatment of consecutive severe fibromyalgia patients with prolotherapy. J. Orthop. Med. *16:*84, 1994.
197. Revel, M. E., Listrat, C. M., Chevalier, X. J., et al.: Facet joint block for low back pain: Identifying predictors of a good response. Arch. Phys. Med. Rehabil. *74:*824, 1992.
198. Rhalmi, S., Yahia, L. H., Newman, N., and Isler, M.: Immunohistochemical study of nerves in lumbar spine ligaments. Spine *18:*264–267, 1993.
199. Rocco, A. G.: Radiolumbar sympatholysis: The evolution of a technique for managing sympathetically maintained pain. Reg. Anesth. *20:*3, 1995.
200. Rocco, A. G., Palombi, D., and Raeke, D.: Anatomy of the lumbar sympathetic chain. Reg. Anesth. *20:*13, 1995.
201. Rothman, S. L., Glenn, W. V., and Kerber, C. W.: Postoperative fracture of lumbar articular facets: Occult cause of radiculopathy. AJR Am. J. Roentgenol. *145:*779–784, 1985.
202. Roy, D. F., Fleury, J., Fontaine, S. B., et al.: Clinical evaluation of cervical facet joint infiltration. J. Can. Assoc. Radiol. *36:*118, 1988.
203. Ryan, P. J., Divadi, L., Gibson, T., et al.: Facet joint injection with low back pain and increased facetal joint activity on bone scintigraphy with SPECT: A private study. Nucl. Med. Commun. *13:*401, 1992.
204. Saal, J. A., and Saal, J. S.: Non-operative treatment of herniated lumbar intervertebral disc with radiculopathy: An outcome study. Spine *14:*41, 1989.
205. Saal, J. S., Franson, R. C., Dobrow, R., et al.: High levels of inflammatory phospholipase A2 activity in lumbar disc herniations. Spine *15:*674–678, 1990.
206. Salter, R. B.: The biologic concept of continuous passive motion of synovial joints. Clin. Orthop. *242:*12, 1989.
207. Savitz, N. H., and Malis, L. I.: Intrathecal administration of hypertonic saline. Neurosurgery *23:*270, 1988.
208. Schellhas, K. P., Smith, M. D., Gundry, C. R., et al.: Cervical discogenic pain: Prospective correlation of magnetic resonance imaging and discography in asymptomatic subjects and pain sufferers. Spine *21:*300, 1996.
209. Schellhas, K. T., Pollei, S. R., Gundry, C. R., et al.: Lumbar disc high intensity zone: Correlation of MR and discography. Spine *21:*79, 1996.
210. Schuchmann, J. A., and Cannon, C. L.: Sacroiliac strain syndrome: Diagnosis and treatment. Tex. Med. *82:*33, 1986.
211. Schwarzer, A. C., Aprill, C. N., and Bodguk, N.: The sacroiliac joint in chronic low back pain. Spine *20:*31–37, 1995.
212. Schwarzer, A. C., Aprill, C. N., Derby, R., et al.: Clinical features of patients with pain stemming from the lumbar zygapophyseal joints: Is the lumbar facet syndrome a clinical entity? Spine *19:*1132–1137, 1994.
213. Schwarzer, A. C., Aprill, C. N., Derby, R., et al.: The false positive rate of single lumbar zygapophyseal joint blocks. Pain *58:*194, 1994.
214. Schwarzer, A. C., Aprill, C., Derby, R., et al.: The relative contributions of the disc and zygapophyseal joint in chronic low back pain. Spine *19:*801–806, 1994.
215. Schwarzer, A. C., Derby, R., Aprill, C. N., et al.: Pain from the lumbar zygapophysial joints: A test of two models. J. Spinal Disord. *7:*331–336, 1994.
216. Schwarzer, A. C., Derby, R., Aprill, C. N., et al.: The value of the provocation response in zygapophyseal joint injections. Clin. J. Pain *10:*309, 1994.
217. Schwarzer, A. C., Scott, A. M., Wang, S., et al.: The role of bone scintigraphy in chronic low back pain: Comparison of SPECT and planar images in zygapophyseal joint injection. Aust. N. Z. J. Med. *22:*185, 1992.
218. Schwarzer, A. C., Wang, S., Laurent, R., et al.: The ability of computed tomography to identify a painful zygapophyseal joint in patients with chronic low back pain. Spine *20:*907, 1995.
219. Schwetschenav, P. R., Ramirez, A., Johnston, J., et al.: Double blind evaluations of intradiscal chymopapain for herniated lumbar discs: Early results. J. Neurosurg. *45:*622, 1976.
220. Shealy, C. N.: Facet denervation in the management of back and sciatic pain. Clin. Orthop. *115:*157–164, 1976.
221. Shealy, C. N.: The role of the spinal facets in back and sciatic pain. Headache *14:*101–104, 1974.
222. Shealy, C. N., and Mauldin, C. C.: Modern medical electricity in the management of pain. Phys. Med. Rehabil. Clin. North Am. *4:*175, 1993; Clin. Podiatr. Med. Surg. *111:*161–173, 1994.
223. Shelkov, A.: Evaluation, diagnosis, and initial treatment of cervical disc disease. *In* Regan, J. (ed.): State of the Art Reviews: Cervical Spine Disease. Philadelphia, Hanley & Belfus, 1991, pp. 167–176.
224. Sjolund, B. H., and Eriksson, M. B. E.: The influence of naloxone on analgesia produced by peripheral conditioning stimulation. Brain Res. *173:*294, 1979.
225. Skubic, J. W., and Kostuik, J. P.: Thoracic pain syndromes and thoracic disc herniation. *In* Frymoyer, J. W. (ed.): The Adult Spine. New York, Raven Press, 1991, pp. 1443–1461.
226. Sluijter, M. E.: Percutaneous thermal lesions in the treatment of back and neck pain. Radionics Procedure Technique Series. Burlington, MA, Radionics, 1981.
227. Sluijter, M. E.: The RF disc lesion. *In* Radio-frequency Techniques in the Management of Chronic Pain. Sept. 9–10, 1995, Newport Beach, CA.
228. Sluijter, M. E.: The use of radiofrequency for pain relief in failed back patients. Int. Disabl. Studies *10:*1, 1988.
229. Sluijter, M. E., and Koetsveld-Baart, C. C.: Interruption of pain pathways in the treatment of cervical syndrome. Anaesthesia *35:*302–307, 1980.
230. Smith, L.: Enzyme dissolution of nucleus pulposus in humans. JAMA *187:*137, 1964.
231. Smith, L., Garvin, P. J., Jennings, R. B., et al.: Enzyme dissolution of the nucleus pulposus. Nature *198:*1311, 1963.
232. Smith Laboratories Inc., Northbrook, IL: Data from postmarketing surveillance, 1985.
233. Star, M. J., Curd, J. G., and Thorne, R. P.: Atlantoaxial lateral mass osteoarthritis: A frequently overlooked cause of severe occipitocervical pain. Spine *17S:*S71–76, 1992.
234. Stein, C.: Peripheral mechanisms of opioid analgesia. Anesth. Analg. *76:*182–191, 1993.
235. Stern, M. B.: Early experience with percutaneous lateral discectomy. Clin. Orthop. *238:*50, 1989.
236. Swerdlow, M., and Cundill, J. G.: Anticonvulsant drugs used in the treatment of lancinating pain: A comparison. Anaesthesia *6:*1129–1132, 1981.
237. Takahashi, Y., Nakajima, Y., Sakamoto, T., et al.: Capsaicin applied to rat lumbar intervertebral disc causes extravasation in the groin: A possible mechanism of referred pain of the intervertebral disc. Neurosci. Lett. *161:*1–3, 1993.
238. Tanelian, D. L., and MacIver, M. B.: Analgesic concentrations of lidocaine suppress tonic A-delta and C fiber discharges produced by acute injury. Anesthesiology *74:*934–936, 1991.
239. Torebjork, H., Lundberg, L., and LaMotte, R.: Central changes in processing of mechanoreceptive input in capsaicin-induced secondary hyperalgesia in humans. J. Physiol. *448:*765–780, 1992.

240. Travell, J. G., and Simons, D. G.: Myofascial Pain and Dysfunction. The Trigger Point Manual. Vols. 1 and 2. Baltimore, Williams & Wilkins, 1984, 1992.

241. Troot, P.: Manipulation therapy techniques in the management of some cervical syndromes. In Grant, R. (ed.): Physical Therapy of the Cervical and Thoracic Spine. London, Churchill Livingstone, 1988, pp. 219–242.

242. Twomey, L. T.: A rationale for the treatment of back pain and joint pain by manual therapy. Phys. Ther. 72:885, 1992.

243. Twomey, L. T., and Taylor, J. R.: Physical Therapy of the Low Back. 2nd ed. New York, Churchill Livingstone, 1994.

244. Van Haranta, H., Sachs, B. L., Spivey, M. A., et al.: The relationship of pain provocation to lumbar disc deterioration as seen by CT-discography. Spine 12:295, 1987.

245. Videman, T., Nurminen, M., and Troup, J. D.: 1990 Volvo Award in clinical sciences. Lumbar spinal pathology in cadaveric material in relation to history of back pain, occupation, and physical loading. Spine 15:728–740, 1990.

246. Waddell, G.: A new clinical model for the treatment of low back pain. Spine 12:632, 1987.

247. Walker, J. M.: Age-related differences in the human sacroiliac joint: A histological study; implications for therapy. J. Orthop. Sports Phys. Ther. 7:325–334, 1986.

248. Walker, J. M.: The sacroiliac joint: A critical review. Phys. Ther. 72:903–916, 1992.

249. Watts, C.: Complications of chemonucleolysis for lumbar disc disease. Neurosurgery 1:2, 1977.

250. Weinstein, J., Claverie, W., and Gibson, S.: The pain of discography. Spine 13:1344–1348, 1988.

251. Weinstein, S. M., Herring, S. A., and Derby, R.: Contemporary concepts in spine care: Epidural steroid injections. Spine 20:1842, 1995.

252. White, A. H., Derby, R., and Wynne, G.: Epidural injection for the diagnosis and treatment of low back pain. Spine 5:78, 1980.

253. Wilde, G. P., Szypryt, E. P., and Mulholland, R. C.: Unilateral lumbar facet joint hypertrophy causing nerve root irritation. Ann. R. Coll. Surg. Engl. 70:307–310, 1988.

254. Wilson, P. R.: Diskography is still investigational. APS J. 3:163–165, 1994.

255. Wilson, P. R.: Thoracic facet joint syndrome—a clinical entity? Pain Suppl. 4:S87, 1987.

256. Windsor, R. E., Falso, F. J. E., and Furman, M. B.: Therapeutic lumbar disc procedures. In Kraft, G. H., and Weinstein, S. M. (eds.): Physical Medicine and Rehabilitation Clinics of North America. Philadelphia, W. B. Saunders Co., 1995, p. 771.

257. Winnie, A. P., and Collins, V. S.: Differential neural blockade in pain syndrome of questionable etiology. Med. Clin. North Am. 52:123, 1968.

258. Wolf, C. J., and Thompson, J. W.: Stimulation-induced analgesia: Transcutaneous electrical nerve stimulation (TENS) and vibration. In Wall, P. D., and Melzack, R. (eds.): Textbook of Pain. 3rd ed. New York, Churchill Livingstone, 1994, pp. 884–896.

259. Woodward, J. L., and Weinstein, S. M.: Epidural injections for the diagnosis and management of axial and radicular pain syndromes. Phys. Med. Rehabil. Clin. North Am. 6:691, 1995.

260. Woolf, C. J., and Chong, M. S.: Preemptive analgesia—treating postoperative pain by preventing the establishment of central sensitization. Anesth. Analg. 77:362–379, 1993.

261. Wyke, B.: Articular neurology—a review. Physiotherapy 8:563–580, 1981.

262. Yahia, H., and Newman, N.: A light and electron microscopic study of spinal ligament innervation. Z. Mikroskopisch-Anatomische Forsch. 103:664–674, 1989.

263. Yaksh, T. L.: The spinal actions of opioids. Handbook Exp. Pharmacol. 104:53–89, 1993.

264. Yaksh, T. L., Al-Rohdhan, N. R. F., and Jensen, T. S.: Sites of action of opiates in production of analgesia. Prog. Brain Res. 77:371–394, 1988.

265. Yaksh, T. L., and Malmberg, A. B.: Central pharmacology of nociceptive transmission. In Melzack, R., and Wall, P. (eds.): Textbook of Pain. 3rd ed. New York, Churchill Livingstone, 1993, pp. 165–200.

266. Yamashita, T., Cavanaugh, J. M., el-Bohy, A. A., et al.: Mechanosensitive afferent units in the lumbar facet joint. J. Bone Joint Surg. 72:865–870, 1990.

267. Yamashita, T., Minaki, Y., Oota, I., et al.: Mechanosensitive afferent units in the lumbar intervertebral disc and adjacent muscle. Spine 18:2252–2256, 1993.

268. Yang, K. H., and King, A. I.: Mechanism of facet load transmission as a hypothesis for low back pain. Spine 9:557, 1984.

269. Yashizawa, H., O'Brien, J. P., Thomas-Smith, W., and Trumper, M.: The neuropathology of intervertebral discs removed for low-back pain. J. Pathol. 132:95–104, 1980.

270. Young, R. F.: Brain and spinal stimulation: How and to whom! Clin. Neurosurg. 35:422–447, 1989.

271. Young, R. F., and Rinaldi, P. C.: Brain stimulation for relief of chronic pain. In Wall, P. D., and Melzack, R. (eds.): Textbook of Pain. 3rd ed. New York, Churchill Livingstone, 1994, pp. 925–931.

272. Zuckerman, J., Derby, R., Shu, K., et al.: Normal magnetic resonance imaging with abnormal discography. Spine 13:1355, 1988.

Surgical Procedures for the Control of Chronic Pain

F. Todd Wetzel, M.D.

The results of surgical therapy for chronic benign pain syndromes involving the lumbar spine are generally poor.[153, 154, 176] Early neurosurgical experience with procedures such as cordotomy[28, 44, 45, 108, 120, 123, 151, 152] suggested that patients with neoplastic pain achieved satisfactory results more frequently than those whose pain was non-neoplastic in origin. Noordenbos and Wall[99] suggested that the longer life expectancy of chronic "benign" pain patients allowed neural plasticity to overcome surgical interruption. This was borne out in studies of cordotomy or dorsal rhizotomy,[1, 4, 15, 38, 82, 109, 111] in which the time to recurrence of a disabling pain syndrome appeared to be much less in patients with chronic benign pain. A distinct characteristic of refractory benign pain is that it appears to follow lesions of the nervous system. This is in contrast to malignant pain, which is thought to be nociceptive, i.e., resulting from chronic activation of nociceptors during such processes as malignant invasion of viscera or compression of nervous structures.

Thus, surgical intervention for chronic benign pain of lumbar origin is fraught with complications. The principles of such intervention can be clearly appreciated only if a basic understanding of neuropathologic mechanisms is attained.

MECHANISMS OF CHRONIC PAIN PRODUCTION

The immediate effect of injury is to activate receptors to cause firing in specific nerve fiber types. These include large myelinated A-beta fibers, small myelinated A-delta fibers, and small unmyelinated C fibers. The interaction of these afferents, through the substantia gelatinosa, forms the basis for the gate control theory of pain. The cell bodies of primary nociceptive neurons are located in the dorsal root ganglion, with afferent synapses in layer I or V. Layer I cells are nociceptor specific and somewhat less discriminatory. Layer V cells respond to many inputs, mainly repetitive nociceptive stimuli as well as nociceptive input. The primary nociceptive neurons synapse on rostrally projecting second-order neurons in the dorsal horn, the theoretic target of the "gate."[90] After postinjury discharge, the next normal event would be for the fibers to return to rest. In the face of persisting injury, however, repeated firings are provoked; some receptors become more sensitive to subsequent stimulation and can, in fact, fire without further stimulation.[78] This sensitization can arise from direct change in the structure of the nociceptor[12, 15, 17] or as a response to substances released in its milieu.[42, 63, 77, 126] As damaged tissue heals with scar formation, granulation tissue containing nerve sprouts and capillaries invades the area. This further changes the local environment and the properties of the nerve endings. Such changes have relevance in the healing of surgical wounds, such as those from laminectomy or spinal fusion; during healing, there may be significant pain problems generated by the wound itself.

The lumbar nerve root, subject to compression by a disc fragment or a stenotic foramen, as well as repetitive irritation by an unstable motion segment, is a likely candidate for nerve damage and all its ensuing consequences. Such roots are further subject to chemical irritation from the inflammatory process and to the edema and ischemia that result from compression. The end results of these pathologic processes are neural scar formation and demyelination.

The responses to nerve damage are complex and variable. Devor broadly classifies these into three groups. The first describes a state of sensitization of the nociceptor endings characterized by a reduced threshold for activation; in such a state, non-noxious stimuli may become capable of producing pain. Second, the nociceptive fibers themselves become a source of pain when they are activated at abnormal locations along their course; this is the phenomenon of ectopic electrogenesis. Third, pain could result from abnormal control processing of afferent impulses.[33] In the setting of chronic spinal pain syndromes, only the first two possibilities are germane.

Chemical[42, 77, 126] and mechanical[2, 51, 124] stimuli can invoke or modify repetitive discharge in the damaged nerve. Epinephrine and norepinephrine can both activate afferent fiber endings in neuromas; these responses are thought to be mediated by alpha-adrenergic receptors.[63, 131, 167] Experimental observation indicates that sympathetic system activity can produce abnormal sensation through neural transmitter release that stimulates afferent nerve sprouts possessing ectopic adrenergic chemosensitivity.[106, 167] The abnormal

sensations produced by these mechanisms may explain causalgia and other sympathetic dystrophies,[33, 155] along with the potential benefit of sympathectomy for such disorders.

The phenomenon of ectopic electrogenesis, which occurs in neuromas, can also develop in axons that have become demyelinated but remain in continuity. This issue relates directly to chronic low back and leg pain, in which a neuroma would not be expected to form, but in which demyelination of nerve roots is a known complication. Such demyelinated roots may exhibit either hypo- or hypersensitivity. Spontaneous discharge has been shown to occur at sites of peripheral demyelination.[55] These discharge patterns are similar to those found in neuromas.[33] Hence, nerves with regions of demyelination can behave just as neuromas do and demonstrate ectopic electrogenesis, which transfers nociceptor-like information into the central nervous system. Rhythmic firing, a characteristic of cell behavior not elicited until a certain threshold level of generation current is reached,[22] can be provoked in demyelinated regions by mechanical stimuli. This threshold characteristic is important, because Devor states that many injured nerves appear to be poised near the rhythmic firing threshold. Hence, brief or weakened stimuli can set off prolonged discharge that may persist beyond removal of the stimulus.[33] In experimental preparations, tetanic stimulation produces this so-called after-discharge, which is followed by a period of prolonged electrical silence.[81] It is evident that this could have implications in pain relief from spinal cord stimulation.

The dorsal root ganglion demonstrates mechanical sensitivity in its normal state and has such a high level of baseline excitability that some discharge occurs spontaneously[61]; after discharge occurs, stimulation is common. This baseline excitability is heightened after peripheral nerve injury. In this instance, the dorsal root ganglion contributes ectopic barrages above and beyond those generated by the region of peripheral injury.[165, 166] The state of excitability of the dorsal root ganglion is thus of clinical importance in root compromise.[55] In the chronically injured root, deafferentation in the form of ganglionectomy would, theoretically, remove this focus of irritability.

Damage to a peripheral nerve causes changes central to the lesion that may not be reversed by treating the original injury.[99] As noted earlier,[61, 166] these central changes include heightened sensitivity of the dorsal root ganglion to mechanical distortion and to neurotransmitters, such as epinephrine. Axons central to a nerve lesion also diminish their conduction velocity. Cells in the dorsal root ganglion may degenerate, with consequent degeneration of central axons. This leads to substantial loss of afferent fibers and produces deafferentation, which is another mechanism of pain. Additionally, the central terminals of C fibers change in response to peripheral nerve injury, and the result is a failure of feedback mechanisms that produce prolonged depolarization and inhibition. Peripheral nerve section is thus followed by a reduction in inhibition of afferent fibers.[165] As Wall has stated, the cord responds to diminished input (deafferentation) by diminishing inhibitions to the remaining input.[164] The spinal cord itself thus becomes a location for continuing provocation of pain through mechanisms of chronic afferent barrage accompanied by reduced inhibition. Not surprisingly, many central ablative procedures, such as cordotomy, have been proposed as treatments for chronic pain syndromes. However, the role of these more central procedures in the treatment of chronic spinal pain syndromes is limited.

Finally, the individual motion segment is richly innervated and is thus capable of generating postinjury pain in the absence of frank neural compression.[19, 93, 107, 114, 115, 169] This pain has, in the past, been somewhat blandly characterized as "mechanical" back pain, something of a misnomer. Many of the procedures discussed later are intended for the treatment of continued extremity pain caused by persistent neurogenic dysfunction; such procedures are not, in general, successful in dealing with disorders of the motion segment per se. Thus, entities such as posttraumatic lumbar strain, postdecompressive segmental instability, and persistent discogenic pain are not well served by deafferentation procedures. Additionally, reversible sources of neural compression producing continued sciatica, such as disc herniation, lateral recess, or central or foraminal stenosis, must be meticulously excluded before the consideration of any of these procedures. Indeed, the most effective way to deal with the "failed back" is to avoid creating it by judicious initial treatment and surgery as indicated. Wynn-Parry has noted a general belief among specialists that surgery for low back pain has been widely overprescribed in the past.[179] Indeed, this thought is underscored in the landmark study of Hakelius, in which he compared patients with sciatica who were treated conservatively with those who had been treated surgically with laminectomy and discectomy. Long-term functional results of the two groups were nearly identical.[50] As is the case with any surgical procedure, the key is meticulous patient selection. This is particularly true in chronic spinal pain syndromes, where the temptation to intervene in a rather desperate setting can be overwhelming for both patient and physician.

The surgery for chronic pain in this setting has revolved around two concepts: deafferentation, and enhancement of presynaptic inhibition. In the first case, the theoretic goal is diminution of the conduction of painful stimuli centrally by interrupting appropriate afferent pathways. Precise determination of these pathways can be difficult because of neuroplasticity and central mechanisms of continuing pain generation. In the second approach, enhancement of presynaptic inhibition, the goal is to achieve functional deafferentation by either chemical or physiologic means. Again, neuroplasticity complicates this approach.

Modulatory therapies that are germane to the concept of inhibition are nerve and cord stimulation and epidural implants. Destructive therapies are essentially deafferentation procedures: rhizotomy and ganglionec-

tomy. More central ablative procedures have no place in the current treatment of failed lumbar surgery syndromes. For example, the dorsal root entry zone (DREZ) lesion, produced by electrocoagulation, has been reported to yield a success rate of 54 to 82 per cent in brachial plexus avulsion[36, 46, 47, 156] and 50 per cent in neurogenic pain from spinal cord injury; however, in benign pain syndromes or arachnoiditis, dismal results have been reported.[96, 121, 122, 177] Cordotomy[145] has been extensively studied in cases of neoplastic pain and can be of major benefit in this instance.[28, 44, 108, 123] The procedure, in which the anterolateral pathways of the spinal cord are divided, thus interrupting pain and temperature transmission, has also been investigated in cases of lower cord or cauda equina injury. Porter and associates reported a 62 per cent rate of significant pain relief in follow-up ranging from eight to 20 years.[120] White and Sweet cited a 60 per cent rate of pain relief in patients with cord injuries and in four of seven with cauda equina damage.[176] The complications of this procedure are significant, however: urinary incontinence, sexual dysfunction, and leg weakness. Additionally, genitourinary dysfunction rates of 8 to 92 per cent have been reported.[44, 45, 120, 123, 176] Thus, cordotomy is not a reliable surgical procedure in the setting of the multiply operated lumbar spine and has never attained widespread acceptance or significant clinical reproducibility.

DEAFFERENTATION PROCEDURES

Little attention in the recent literature has been focused on the use of rhizotomy as a treatment for chronic backache and sciatica. It has, however, been widely investigated in other areas. As noted previously, results in tumor patients are generally superior to those achieved in chronic benign pain patients.[4, 133, 148, 157, 175, 178] In a comprehensive review, Barrash and Leavens analyzed dorsal rhizotomy for relief of tumor pain. Promising results of rhizotomy were noted in cases of central neoplasms, as well as neoplasms involving the breast, colon, head and neck, lung, and rectal and urogenital systems.[9] The problem of trigeminal neuralgia has been widely addressed as well. Van Loveren and associates reviewed their experience of 1000 patients with trigeminal neuralgia, comparing the techniques of percutaneous stereotactic rhizotomy and posterior fossa exploration. Of the 700 treated by percutaneous stereotactic rhizotomy, excellent or good results regarding pain relief were achieved in 125 patients treated with microsurgical vascular decompression or partial sensory rhizotomy.[161] These favorable results were corroborated by the report of Bederson and Wilson in 252 patients.[13] Additionally, glycerol rhizotomy for trigeminal neuralgia has been investigated.[5, 11, 14] In general, good or excellent results are reported in 70 to 72 per cent of the cases using this technique. Selective dorsal rhizotomy for spasticity in children with cerebral palsy, although controversial, has also been recommended. Cahan and associates and Kundi and associates emphasized the safety of the procedure, citing preservation of cortical

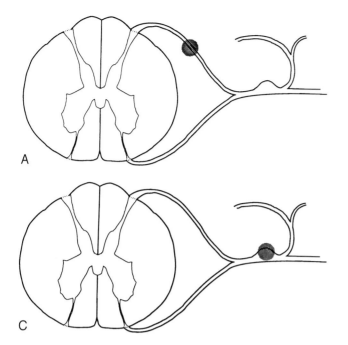

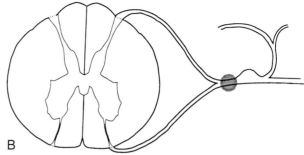

Figure 59–18. Rhizotomy and ganglionectomy. The shaded area represents the surgical lesion for (a) intradural rhizotomy, predominantly for use in cervical and thoracic areas; (b) extradural rhizotomy, predominantly used in the lumbosacral region; and (c) ganglionectomy. (From Wetzel, F. T.: Chronic benign cervical pain syndromes: Surgical considerations. Spine *17:* S367–S374, 1992.)

somatosensory evoked responses.[21, 68] Good results have also been reported by Arens and associates. In their series of 51 patients with spasticity, 42 demonstrated a marked reduction in motor tone and improved motor function after selective posterior rhizotomy. Sensory disturbances were minimal, and no evidence of spinal instability was demonstrated.[4] Similarly encouraging results have been reported by others.[40, 98, 111, 147] Intraspinal rhizotomy has been reported to diminish spasticity in patients with myelomeningocele as well.[86] Sacral rhizotomy in the treatment of hypertonic neurogenic bladder has also been investigated,[95, 128, 129, 157] as has control of spasticity resulting from posttraumatic paraplegia. Laitinen and associates reported the results of selective multilevel rhizotomies in a series of nine patients, all of whom showed good reduction of spasticity after the procedure.[69] Percutaneous radiofrequency rhizotomy resulted in improvement of spasticity in 24 of 25 patients in the series of Kadson and Lathi[59]; in Turnbull's series, percutaneous rhizotomy improved lower extremity spasm in paraparetic patients who were not hospitalized.[158]

Taken in concert with the results presented for the disorders reviewed earlier, the outcome of rhizotomy for chronic lumbar pain syndromes is particularly grim. In the case of chronic pain patients, preservation of function is essential, and the surgeon does not have the latitude to interrupt multiple roots, as is the case in many of the situations reviewed earlier. Additionally, the precise interpretation of pain reduction, which is necessarily subjective, complicates the evaluation of results of rhizotomy or ganglionectomy for chronic benign pain.

RHIZOTOMY AND GANGLIONECTOMY

Sectioning of the spinal nerves or excision of dorsal root ganglia can be accomplished at multiple levels.

Rhizotomy may be performed by intradural section of the dorsal root, extradural section of the dorsal root, or extradural section of the mixed root (Fig. 59–18). Additionally, the median branch of the posterior primary ramus may be interrupted, although this is usually by a percutaneous technique such as cryoablation or radiofrequency ablation (Fig. 59–19).

As Dubuisson[38] pointed out, intradural root section in the subarachnoid space is more frequently performed at cervical and thoracic levels where the cord segments are adjacent. The anatomic arrangement of the lumbosacral region—the cauda equina—in which nerve roots exit far caudal to the cord makes this more problematic. It is thus preferable to identify the dorsal roots near the intervertebral foramen of interest.

Sensory rhizotomy for the relief of chronic pain was first carried out by Abbe in 1888 but had been nearly abandoned by 1925 because of the relatively high failure rate and the subsequent interest in cordotomy.[1, 178]

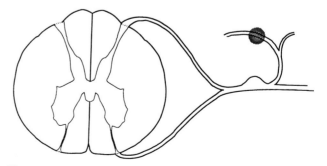

Figure 59–19. Facet rhizotomy. The shaded area represents the surgical lesion created. (From Wetzel, F. T.: Chronic benign cervical pain syndromes: Surgical considerations. Spine *17:* S367–S374, 1992.)

Rhizotomy may be performed at this level to include selective sensory fibers, or it may take the form of a complete rhizotomy. Characteristically, both ablative procedures are performed proximal to the ganglion.

The goal of rhizotomy or ganglionectomy is denervation of the area in which pain is felt without compromising spinal cord functions. It has frequently been assumed that root section should remove pain that is peripheral and circumscribed, because the afferent territory of a few adjacent nerves presumably completely delineates the pain for that region.[29, 38] Long-term results of rhizotomy fail to support this, however. In addition, results of selective sensory rhizotomy may be compromised because of the presence of denervation hypersensitivity, intersegmental cross-linking,[109] and overlapping dermatomes.[39, 43, 52, 139] Also, the Bell-Magendie law, maintaining that efferent motor impulses travel in anterior nerve roots and afferent sensory impulses travel in posterior roots, has been challenged by the discovery of unmyelinated axons in the ventral roots.[24, 150] Intraoperative stimulation of these roots has been shown to provoke pain.[48] If these ventral afferents comprise a significant portion of the ventral root, dorsal sensory rhizotomy may be providing insufficient deafferentation to interrupt pertinent sensory pathways. Thus, there are many possible mechanisms to explain the failure of rhizotomy to alleviate chronic extremity pain.

One of the central problems in planning surgery for persistent limb pain is the precise delineation of the involved roots. Many authors have attempted to select patients on the basis of their response to individual nerve root sheath blockade, as guided by electrophysiologic evidence of chronic radiculopathy and neurologic examination. Onofrio and Campa reported their results in 286 patients who underwent rhizotomy. Fifty-eight patients underwent lumbar rhizotomies—45 at S1, and 13 at L5. Only six of the 45 patients undergoing S1 rhizotomies were believed to have long-term pain relief; three of 13 patients who underwent lumbar rhizotomies had clinically successful results. These results were obtained despite consideration of dermatomal overlap and the use of selective nerve root blockade to plan the surgery.[109] Loeser reported the results of complete rhizotomy in 45 patients with chronic pain syndromes of various etiologies. Sixteen of the patients had undergone previous lumbar disc surgery. His initial success rate of 75 per cent at three months declined to 14 per cent at long-term follow-up of up to 10 years. Arachnoiditis, in the setting of failed disc surgery, seemed to be correlated with poor results, and preoperative nerve root blocks provided little diagnostic or prognostic information. Loeser offered several reasons for these results, including incomplete root sectioning, inadequate numbers of roots divided, and a higher threshold of fibers in adjacent nerves, which may begin to produce chronic pain syndromes after the effects of local anesthetics from root blocks have worn off. He also speculated that central alterations may be important.[82] Additionally, the utility of "diagnostic" nerve root blocks must be questioned. The selective root

sheath injection appears to be nonspecific in not only a dermatomal sense but in a central and peripheral sense as well: several authors have reported on the ability of distal blocks to produce temporary relief.[60, 173, 180] Jain believed that selective extradural sensory rhizotomy was not successful in the setting of arachnoiditis,[57] and several authors have reported poor results after rhizotomy for failed lumbar surgery.[15, 16, 117, 173]

In a compendium of results from multiple sources,[1] Dubuisson noted a 74 per cent rate of immediate success following rhizotomy at L4, L5, and S1, which dropped to 33 per cent three months after surgery.[16, 38, 57, 82, 109, 148] These results are corroborated by the reports of others.[15, 16, 117, 173] White, in reviewing a series of sensory rhizotomies for 10 patients with failed lumbar surgery, noted 80 per cent good to excellent results; however, follow-up was variable, ranging from four months to 11 years, and no specifics were available in a temporal sense. He did, however, agree that there was little pain relief when arachnoiditis was present.[175] Wetzel and colleagues reported poor outcomes (14 per cent success) in patients undergoing selective sensory rhizotomy at a mean follow-up of two years. All patients had undergone previous unsuccessful lumbar surgery.[174]

Thus, it is difficult to recommend rhizotomy for the treatment of chronic benign lower extremity pain. Seemingly, the most reliable indication for rhizotomy is pain caused by deafferentation itself. This is addressed by the report of Tasker and associates[155] in a retrospective review of 168 patients. The quality of the patients' pain was divided into two groups: spontaneous and hyperpathic. The latter implies pain production induced by normally non-noxious stimulation within adjacent areas of increased somatosensory thresholds. Overall, the pain in this group was nearly always causalgic or dysesthetic in quality and was associated with sensory loss. This was dramatically ameliorated by intravenous sodium thiopental, but not by morphine, and was usually relieved by proximal local anesthetic blockade. Various deafferentation procedures, including rhizotomy, neurectomy, and cordectomy and cordotomy, were reviewed, and each of these ablative procedures failed to relieve most patients of deafferentation pain. Hyperpathia, which occurred in incompletely deafferented areas, however, was partially relieved by surgical completion of the deafferentation, although the authors noted that pain may persist at the periphery of the sensory loss. Additional studies are required to assess this completely, but at the current time, the only reasonable recommendation for rhizotomy in benign pain syndromes is completion of a prior sensory rhizotomy in certain patients with deafferentation pain and hyperpathia.

Sectioning of the dorsal root ganglion has been shown to provide the best results in terms of pain relief when performed for benign truncal neuralgias.[112] The results of ganglionectomy (see Fig. 59–18c) at the caudal lumbar roots in cases of failed lumbar surgery are as disappointing as those reported for rhizotomy.[57, 82, 103, 109, 112] At this time, it is impossible to differentiate meaningfully between rhizotomy and ganglionectomy as distinct therapeutic tools in this setting.

Technique

The patient is placed in a prone position under general anesthesia, and hemilaminectomy and partial facetectomy are used to expose the involved root. The root sheath is clearly identified and opened longitudinally for 8 to 10 mm proximal to the dorsal root ganglia. The dural septum, which separates dorsal and ventral roots, is identified, and a small nerve hook is passed between root filaments. Osgood and associates[112] noted that several distinct root fascicles are usually present. With electrocautery at a low setting, electrical stimulation is used to distinguish between motor and sensory fibers. As Bertrand has noted, however, caution must be used in relying on this test exclusively, because chronically damaged roots may exhibit a higher threshold for motor excitation response than normal.[16] Thus, a wake-up test may be required. When appropriate sensory fibers are identified, they can be sectioned with electrocautery or a microsurgery blade.

FACET RHIZOTOMY

Facet denervation is not nerve root surgery in the same sense that open rhizotomy is; rather, the theory behind this procedure involves destruction of the median branch of the posterior primary afferent nerve that supplies the facet joint (see Fig. 59–19). As demonstrated by Pedersen and associates,[115] the median branch of the posterior primary ramus descends through a notch at the base of the transverse process and is covered by a ligament at the anteroinferior border of the facet joint at this level. This ligament is a continuation of the intertransverse membrane, and it is here that several small twigs are given off to the facet joint. These twigs then enter the facet joint capsule. Each posterior primary ramus supplies at least two facet joints, and each facet joint receives innervation from at least two spinal levels. Clinical features of facet joint syndrome have been well described by Mooney and Robertson.[93]

Rees is generally credited with performing the first facet rhizotomies. These were done percutaneously with a knife and reportedly resulted in immediate relief of symptoms in 998 of the 1000 patients who had facet pain in concert with the "intervertebral disc syndrome."[125] Shealy performed the procedure in North America but had an unusually high frequency of wound hematomas. This led to the adoption of a radiofrequency probe. Shealy reported a 90 per cent success rate in previously nonoperated patients.[135] That pain relief was achieved by the interruption of afferent impulses generated as a result of pathology within the facet joint has been suggested by the anecdotal reports of many authors who have noted immediate relief of pain in patients undergoing lumbar fusion.

Candidates for facet rhizotomy are those patients with back pain caused by facet dysfunction who have

failed to respond to conservative therapy. Sluijter drew an important distinction between posterior and anterior mechanical pain.[143] Posterior mechanical pain, resulting from irritation of the medial branch of the posterior primary ramus, is different in character and nondermatomal. Facet tenderness may be noted, and, as a rule, the neurologic examination is negative. Anterior mechanical pain from irritation of structures anterior to the transverse processes is mediated by nociceptive afferent transmission by the recurrent nerve of Luschka. This type of pain is unresponsive to diagnostic maneuvers involving blockage of the facet and the median branch of the posterior primary ramus.[143] The key diagnostic maneuver to establish this is the facet block. This involves percutaneous insertion of a needle into the joint, under fluoroscopic guidance, followed by joint injection with Xylocaine combined with steroids or contrast agents.[32, 93, 94] Patients in whom this procedure yields temporary relief are considered candidates for facet rhizotomy.[143] The diagnostic value of facet joint injections must, however, be rigorously scrutinized. Moran and associates noted that in only nine of 54 patients in whom facet syndrome was suspected was the diagnosis confirmed by facet joint arthrography. The authors noted extravasation into the epidural space after rupture of the capsule; clearly, introduction of steroid or local anesthetic into this space would confound the results.[94]

In the series of Shealy, a satisfactory clinical result was noted in 79 per cent of patients who had undergone no previous surgery. In patients who had undergone previous laminectomy, this number fell to 41 per cent, and in those who had undergone previous fusion, to 27 per cent.[135] Of the 82 patients of McCulloch, followed from six to 20 months after facet rhizotomy, 50 per cent had satisfactory results. This fell to 33 per cent in those receiving workers' compensation, and increased to 64 per cent in the group not on compensation. Interestingly, in this group, three required repeat surgery.[85] Schaerer reported on 71 patients who underwent lumbar facet rhizotomy. There were five distinct subgroups in his review: (1) lumbar facet disease without disc involvement (discography negative), (2) lumbar facet involvement with disc involvement (discography positive), (3) lumbar facet disease with discopathy and root signs, (4) facet signs with osteoarthritis, and (5) postlaminectomy pain. At a mean follow-up of 13.7 months, patients were evaluated using a pain profile. Thirty-five of 71 were believed to have satisfactory results. The highest percentage of success was in the author's first group—those who had a "pure" facet syndrome (seven of 15 patients). No attempt was made to determine statistically significant differences in outcome between these groups.[132] Florez and associates reported a series of 30 patients, achieving satisfactory results in 76 per cent. Twenty-six of the patients were followed for three to nine months. The best results were noted in patients without previous operations and those with shorter duration of symptoms.[41] Oudenhoven reported 377 patients with "pseudoradicular" pain in whom a lumbar facet syndrome was diagnosed by facet blocks. At a mean follow-up of 26 months, 83 per cent were judged to be clinical successes. The author noted that a unilateral facet rhizotomy did not control pain, and reported that 22 per cent of patients who were judged to be clinical successes noted some return of symptoms 18 to 24 months postoperatively.[113] None of the authors reported any significant complications with the procedure. Lord and coworkers reported on 19 patients who underwent cervical percutaneous neurotomy for neck pain of at least three months' duration following motor vehicle accidents. They found that results varied by level. Of the 10 patients who underwent C2–C3 rhizotomy, three obtained greater than six months of pain relief, and one was pain-free at four months follow-up; the remaining six had return of symptoms over three weeks. Of the 10 who underwent more caudal neurotomies, seven obtained "clinically useful" pain relief. The authors noted that C2–C3 results may have been compromised by technical failure, including the relatively large diameter of the nerves and their variable course.[84]

After a thorough review of the literature, one is tempted to recommend this procedure after diagnosis of facet syndrome with facet arthrography and blocks. Although the low morbidity and mortality rates associated with the procedure may seem to justify such a conclusion, it should be remembered that with the exception of the report of Oudenhoven,[113] no long-term follow-up studies support any lasting benefit from this procedure. It is nonetheless attractive to consider the procedure in any patient in whom the appropriate diagnostic modalities have yielded the specific diagnosis of facet syndrome.

Technique

The procedure for this is well described.[85, 143] It is recommended that it be performed in the operating room or radiology department. Local anesthetic is adequate; the patient should be in the supine position for cervical rhizotomy or the prone position for thoracic and lumbar rhizotomy. Image intensification is required. Fourteen-gauge needles are placed unilaterally in the region of the appropriate facet(s) and nerves. A 5-mm bare-tipped probe is then positioned in the area of the facet and the 14-gauge needle is partially withdrawn, leaving only the probe in the space between the superior facet and the transverse process immediately adjacent to the superior facet. The depth of the probe is controlled by lateral image intensification. A stimulation frequency of 100 Hz and from 0.1 to approximately 3 V is used to localize the tip away from the anterior ramus, as noted by the absence of paraesthesia in the ipsilateral extremity. Once the depth is appropriate—adjacent to the posterior primary ramus—and stimulation reproduces a pain pattern familiar to the patient, the lesioning is performed. A temperature-controlled lesion is produced by setting the controls at 25 V and 100 mA for approximately 60 seconds, at 80°C. During the final 20 seconds, the amperage is slowly increased to the point where the milliamperage starts to diminish

and voltage rises. This takes the temperature to approximately 90°C. After this, the probe is withdrawn, the wound dressed, and the patient mobilized.

SYMPATHECTOMY

Sympathetic dystrophy represents a constellation of disorders of sympathetic nerve functions that accentuate or perpetuate chronic pain. Historically, Lankford[70] divided sympathetic dystrophy into two types, based on the type of injury. A minor causalgia is associated with an injury to a sensory nerve, and a major causalgia with injury to a mixed nerve. Traumatic dystrophy is also subdivided into two types: minor dystrophy caused by a limited musculoskeletal injury, such as a sprain, or major dystrophy secondary to a major skeletal injury, such as a fracture. Recently, Stanton-Hicks and colleagues[146] presented a revised taxonomic classification for reflex sympathetic dystrophy (RSD), regrouping the subtypes into a single entity—complex regional pain syndrome (CRPS). The diagnosis of CRPS requires regional pain and sensory changes following the index injury, coupled with skin color changes, temperature changes, abnormal sudomotor response, and edema. CRPS Type I occurs without a specific nervous lesion and corresponds to RSD or traumatic dystrophy; Type II refers to a discrete nervous lesion, equivalent to the former definition of causalgia. Obviously, many features of chronic spinal pain syndrome may fall into these various categories.

Given the multiplicity of complaints in patients with chronic extremity pain and the anatomic relationship of the sympathetic chain to the mixed lumbar root, the coexistence of autonomic dysfunction in the setting of chronic lumbar pain and radiculopathy is plausible. Patients with a pattern of persistent limb distress after spinal surgery may have signs and symptoms suggestive of sympathetic dysfunction. These include vasomotor changes, alterations in skin temperature, and joint stiffness.

The anatomic constancy of the sympathetic trunk, with respect to the outer annulus, has been well demonstrated by Bogduk and associates.[19] Pain fibers traveling lateral to the vertebral column in the sympathetic trunk may be prone to irritation owing to injury to the motion segment. Likewise, tears of the annulus fibrosus have been thought to be capable of producing a cold, painful limb on the ipsilateral side,[107] and Hodgson described a pattern of intractable lower extremity pain, associated with diminished temperature, in patients with failed lumbar surgery.[53]

Despite defined clinical findings, the precise histopathology of sympathetic irritation in the setting of failed lumbar surgery has not been well characterized. Hodgson noted large pools of blood and dilated veins without evidence of inflammatory reaction in ganglia harvested from patients after anterior interbody fusion.[53] In contrast, others have noticed a marked inflammatory reaction of the prevertebral tissues with hyperemia in the ganglia.

Sympathectomy has been investigated in the treat-

ment of limb distress of other causes, most notably vascular disease. Norman and House[100] reported the results of lumbar sympathectomy for peripheral vascular disease in 153 patients. Five years after sympathectomy, 67 per cent of the patients who experienced claudication and 54 per cent of those who experienced rest pain had avoided further surgery. The authors concluded that sympathectomy was a valuable adjunct in the treatment of these disorders. Van Driel and associates also reported favorable results from sympathectomy in 66 patients who had suffered from lower limb ischemia.[160] Jones also noted a beneficial effect of digital sympathectomy in treating ischemia of the hand in systemic disease.[58]

In the setting of persistent neurogenic dysfunction, however, the results of sympathectomy have been far less predictable. A central problem remains in establishing the diagnosis. The most reproducible standard by which the diagnosis of autonomic dysfunction is made is thought to be response to sympathetic blockage.[3, 60, 169, 170] Thermography has come to represent an additional diagnostic technique for detecting skin surface temperature changes associated with autonomic dysfunction.[116, 119, 172, 173] Even with the use of both modalities, however, doubts have been raised regarding the validity of patient selection in chronic lumbar pain syndromes.[172, 173]

Mockus and associates reported a series of 34 patients who underwent lumbar sympathectomy. In 13 of these, the precipitating incident responsible for the autonomic dysfunction was lumbar disc surgery. Overall, they reported good results, with only one patient failing to obtain satisfactory relief.[92] In the author's experience with a series of 17 patients in whom sympathectomy was performed, the results were not as promising, with only four patients maintaining satisfactory pain relief at a mean follow-up of 18 months. In this group, the patients' response to block was not as significant in predicting response to surgery as was their initial thermographic diagnosis.[172, 173] Before the formulation of any definitive statement, however, more investigation into this area is required. Thus, at the present time, lumbar sympathectomy cannot be recommended with any strong conviction in the setting of chronic benign lumbar pain syndromes.

Technique

The patient is positioned in the lateral decubitus position with the appropriate side up. A standard retroperitoneal approach is used, with a short transverse flank incision spreading each of the three layers of the anterior abdominal muscles, inferior to the level of the kidneys. This may be modified by a long, oblique incision from the twelfth rib to the lower abdomen, permitting access to bodies of all the lumbar vertebrae. The lateral and inferior fibers of the latissimus dorsi and serratus posterior lie over the twelfth rib and may be partially transected. The distal half of the twelfth rib may be resected subperiosteally as well. The external oblique muscle is split in line with its fibers. The inter-

nal oblique and transverse abdominis are cut across their fiber in the same direction as the skin incision. Deep to the transversus is the peritoneum, and posterior to this is the renal fascia. The renal fascia and the retroperitoneal fat must be dissected en bloc and taken anteriorly. The major dissection is posterior to the kidney, between Gerota's fascia and the quadratus lumborum and psoas.

The lumbar veins and arteries are anterior to the vertebral bodies, and mobilization is facilitated with ligation of some of the segmental vessels. The sympathetic chain can then be plainly seen on the lateral aspect of the lumbar vertebra, with the most caudal ganglion usually at the L4 level. These ganglia should be dissected free from the underlying tissue, clipped, and removed. The wound is then closed in layers, with or without drainage as required.

STIMULATION THERAPY

Epidural and Intraspinal Implants

Selective nerve root blockade or epidural blockade has been successfully used in many intraoperative and postoperative situations.[56, 87, 171, 181] Likewise, implanted epidural narcotic reservoirs have been used in the treatment of intractable spinal and limb pain in a variety of neoplastic conditions.[26, 27, 31, 37, 49, 110, 130] Downing and associates reported 23 patients with cancer pain refractory to other methods of pain control. Excellent response rates to implanted reservoirs were noted, with minimal complications.[37] Sjogren and associates reported on 48 cancer patients receiving long-term treatment with epidural opioid catheters. The overall effect was "satisfactory." Twenty-nine patients were able to be stabilized on epidural opioid treatment, and of these, 21 were judged to be clinical successes. Somewhat ominously, however, a tendency toward better relief of non-neurogenic pain was noted.[142] The largest series reported to date is that of Liew and Hui.[79] In their 252 patients, good to excellent pain relief was obtained in 85 per cent. For patients who survived more than three months, the daily morphine requirement increased progressively from 3.5 to 19.5 mg per day. The authors noted that features of drug tolerance developed, but not drug addiction.

The use of implantable narcotic reservoirs in patients with chronic benign pain syndromes is less well studied. Several encouraging reports have appeared in the literature, however. In 1985, Auld and associates reported the results of intraspinal narcotic analgesia in 43 patients with chronic benign pain syndromes. Thirty-two of the 43 had continuous delivery systems, and 65 per cent reported good to excellent relief of pain in a follow-up longer than two years. The authors noted neither serious side effects nor evidence of addiction.[6] In an attempt to eliminate the bulkier continuous infusion system, Auld and associates investigated the effects of intraspinal narcotic analgesic on 20 patients using a smaller system consisting of an epidural catheter and subcutaneous reservoir. After an appropriate epidural trial, the catheters were inserted. Acceptable pain relief was obtained in 14 patients. The authors believed that the results of this system were comparable with those obtained using a continuous delivery system and speculated that bolus injections saturated pain receptors as completely as continuous infusion.[7]

It appears that the implantation of an indwelling narcotic reservoir is a promising technique that should be considered in the management of chronic limb distress; however, several notes of caution must be sounded. As previously noted, neuroplasticity in the setting of chronic benign pain tends to diminish the results of ablative therapies over time. Conceivably, this may also apply to pharmacotherapy. Additionally, the observations of Liew and Hui,[79] noting progressively increasing narcotic requirements in neoplastic patients, must be viewed with some alarm. Keeping these cautions in mind, the following recommendation can be made. An appropriate patient is one who is chronically disabled, not a surgical candidate, not appropriate for behavioral operant therapy, and psychologically sound. Whether a trial of electrical stimulation (see later) should precede consideration of an intraspinal implant is a matter of debate; additionally, it appears to be the case that certain types of pain (e.g., nociceptive predominant) may be relatively stimulator-resistant and are treated more effectively by intrathecal narcotics. After a careful discussion of the potential risks and benefits, a trail of epidural blockade may be recommended. If this provides relief, consideration can be given to an epidural or intraspinal narcotic implant.

Technique

An epidural block of 0.5 to 1.0 mg of morphine mixed with saline is injected through a 22-gauge spinal needle. The degree and duration of pain relief are then noted in relation to side effects. Occasionally, an indwelling catheter of several days' duration may be required.

If a satisfactory response to the block is noted, an epidural or intrathecal catheter is placed subcutaneously through the T12–L1 or L1–L2 interlaminar space and brought through a subcutaneous tunnel to the flank. The tunnel is then taken anteriorly, where a pocket is created for the reservoir. The procedure can be done under local anesthesia.

SPINAL CORD STIMULATION

In 1965, Melzack and Wall, in proposing the gate control theory of pain, ushered in a new era of thinking regarding chronic pain programs.[90] This theory seemed to specify that low-threshold, primary, afferent fibers might be electrically activated peripherally, the result being central suppression of nociceptive influences. Several authors[149, 168] applied this idea to the treatment of pain in the distribution of a peripheral nerve, with encouraging results. Subsequently, Shealy and associates[136, 137] suggested stimulation of the dorsal columns of the spinal cord to control chronic, intractable lower

extremity pain. This seemed physiologically correct, because the dorsal column fibers represent direct extensions of large-diameter primary afferent fibers running centrally. Thus, their stimulation should allow pain control over a wide region of the body. There are numerous reports in the literature addressing this.[52, 64, 97] The initial concept revolved around stimulation of the dorsal columns. However, as Larson and associates[71] demonstrated, ventral electrode placements can be as effective. Thus, active pathways are difficult to determine, and the physiological basis of pain relief from spinal cord stimulation is uncertain. Whether electrical stimulation activates specific axons, inhibiting central transmission, or blocks transmissions in nociceptive fibers is unknown at the current time. Additionally, the mechanism by which spinal cord stimulation achieves the desired effect may not be limited to electrical depolarization of certain fiber populations. The work of Bashbaum and Fields[10] has characterized a descending modulatory pathway; this lends credence to theories recommending the electrical and pharmacologic stimulation of *descending* pathways for the treatment of chronic pain. In this descending pathway, fibers from the midbrain and hypothalamus synapse in the dorsal pons and rostroventral medulla. Efferent, inhibitory impulses travel via the dorsolateral funiculus to synapses in the dorsal horn. These projections may functionally inhibit the target cells that give rise to the spinothalamic tract. The release of neuromediators in the dorsal horn has been documented in animal models. Linderoth and coworkers, in a cat model, noted increased levels of substance P–like immunoreactivity in microdialysate from the dorsal horn after spinal cord stimulation. Release of serotonin was also noted, but no effects on extracelluar levels of amino acids were detected. The authors speculate that serotonin release may be relevant for pain, based on the existence of descending neurons in the dorsolateral funiculus that store both substance P and serotonin, and have a putative role in pain inhibition.[80]

Initially, it was assumed that most of the effects of stimulation were attributed directly to stimulation of the dorsal columns. It has, however, become clear that application of an electrical field to the dorsal epidural space may activate a larger number of neural structures. It is likely that paresthesias are elicited from intraspinal neural structures both inside and outside the cord. Barolat and colleagues[8] noted that paresthesias ipsilateral to stimulating electrodes were perceived as tingling sensations; they believed that this reflected stimulation of large afferent myelinated fibers and most likely involved the dorsal columns, dorsal roots, dorsal root entry zone, and dorsal horn. Thus it is proposed that the older term "dorsal column stimulation" be abandoned in favor of the term "spinal cord stimulation."

Clinically, the results of stimulation have improved over time. Krainick and Thoden summarized the results of 726 patients in a European study group. Of the 726 patients available for evaluation of early results, 38 per cent reported pain relief greater than 50 per cent.

Of the 468 available for late follow-up, only 22.5 per cent reported any lasting pain relief.[64] These figures, however, represent the results of dorsal column stimulator implantation for syndromes of various etiologies. Husson and associates reported good preliminary results in their 20 patients, who were suffering from radicular pain secondary to arachnoidepiduritis or postoperative pain. They based their selection criteria on a pain relief level of at least 50 per cent after a month of transcutaneous stimulation.[56] Wester, in reporting on a series of 35 patients, 30 of whom were selected for implants, noted that 15 months postoperatively, 43.5 per cent used the stimulator regularly. He noted an increase in the amount of pain relief among patients with failed lumbar surgery syndromes and arachnoiditis.[171] Young, in his series of 51 patients who underwent stimulator implantation, reported much less satisfactory results. Twenty-five of these patients had undergone previous lumbar surgery, and in all patients pain had been present for at least 24 months. Thirty-seven patients underwent open laminectomy for implantation, 11 had electrodes placed percutaneously, and three, after an initial trial of percutaneous implantation, required open laminectomy. The author noted no major complications but stated that minor complications (e.g., paresthesia not in the desired location, infection, cerebrospinal fluid leak, lead migration, and breakage) required an additional 33 procedures. At a mean follow-up of 38 months, his results were disappointing. In the immediate postoperative period, 47 per cent had significant relief, but no functional improvement (e.g., return to work) was noted in any patient. Young thus raised the question whether a spinal cord stimulator is an effective treatment for chronic benign pain.[181]

Overall, with increased technical support, clinical experience, and the use of multichannel programmable devices, results have improved. Pain relief ranging from 0 to 85 per cent has been reported.[8, 18, 20, 23, 30, 31, 34, 54, 65–67, 72–76, 88, 89, 91, 101, 102, 104, 105, 118, 127, 134, 138, 140, 141, 159, 162, 163] All these studies, however, suffer from the same flaws: retrospective study design, variable definitions of criteria for success, and outcome comparisons independent of pain etiology. As the techniques and selection criteria improve, an overall trend in the literature is apparent, with increased maintenance of pain relief over time. Regarding efficacy in benign pain syndromes, the work of North and coworkers appears to be illustrative.[105] Successful outcomes, defined as 50 per cent or greater pain relief, have been realized in 50 to 53 per cent of patients with follow-up as long as 20 years.

Recent work by North and coworkers bears special mention.[104] In this prospective randomized study, spinal cord stimulation was compared with reoperation (laminectomy) for "failed back surgery syndrome." Fifty-one patients were randomized into stimulation and reoperation groups, with cross-over permitted. Failure of stimulation was defined as cross-over into the surgical group from the stimulator group, and failure of reparation was defined as cross-over into the stimulator group. Results for the first 27 patients reach-

ing the six-month cross-over point showed a statistically significant (p = .018) advantage for spinal cord stimulation compared with reoperation. Additionally, in a group of patients who opted for reparation, followed outside the study, 42 per cent crossed over to spinal cord stimulation at six-month follow-up.[104]

The selection criteria for patients who may be candidates for spinal cord stimulation are of paramount importance. Krainick and associates[65] performed an initial trial with an electrode inserted into the arachnoid space using a small cannula. Stimulation was performed above the segmental level of pain for 30 minutes. In 73 patients, 28 obtained more than 50 per cent pain relief. The value of a trial stimulation was also addressed by Neilson and associates.[97] In 96 of 221 patients who underwent a percutaneous trial, the stimulation was found to provide insufficient pain relief. Surprisingly, 28 of these 96 underwent permanent spinal cord stimulator implantation and, not surprisingly, failed to obtain *any* relief from the procedure.

Use of spinal cord stimulation to treat benign lumbar pain syndromes remains controversial. The most rigorous set of guidelines espoused for patient selection and technique are those of Krainick and associates[64, 65]: use of multiple electrodes, open epidural placement, localization of electrodes above the pain segments, absence of secondary gain, and localized rather than diffuse pain. These guidelines represent the ideal candidates for spinal cord stimulation. With the use of multiple electrodes to treat more complex pain syndromes,[72, 101] the open laminotomy or laminectomy approach is becoming less common; fluoroscopically guided percutaneous insertion has proved to be the preferred approach for insertion (see Fig. 59–20).

Technique

There are several methods by which spinal cord stimulator implantation can be performed. These include percutaneous threading of the electrodes into the epidural space, epidural electrode insertion through an open laminotomy, or creation of an intradural pouch. The latter is not clinically useful.

For most procedures, the patient is taken to the operating room and positioned prone. If the procedure is to be done percutaneously, local anesthesia with intravenous sedation is used. If an open laminotomy is preferred, the epidural space is directly visualized and the lead inserted. It is recommended that, for chronic lumbar pain syndromes, leads be inserted in the T12–L1 interlaminar space and traverse at least three levels cranially. This must be done under fluoroscopic control. The intradural pouch, well described by Burton,[20] also requires an open laminotomy.

Once the catheter is threaded, an unscrubbed assistant is given the lead to verify extension and efficacy of placement and to arrive at baseline parameters of stimulus intensity and frequency. After this, the lead is anchored in the fascia with a suture. A temporary lead extension is then tunneled and externalized for a trial. If a trial is done on the table and is successful, the

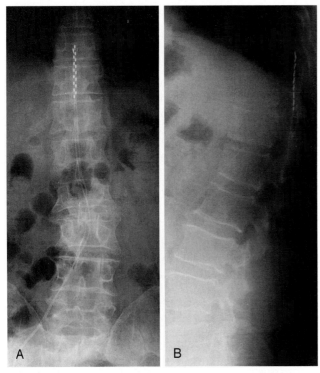

Figure 59–20. *A,* Note the symmetry around the midline and the thoracic placement. *B,* Spinal cord stimulation, with multiple electrodes placed via a percutaneous epidural approach. These electrodes are in the optimal area for control of six to seven dermatomes involving the low back and lower extremities.

lead and pulse generator are implanted permanently. A subcutaneous pouch and tunnel are created, and the lead is connected to the power source. The wounds are closed in a routine manner, and compressive dressings are applied.

SUMMARY

As can be appreciated in the previous discussion, the results of surgery for chronic lumbar pain syndromes are far from satisfactory. In ablative therapy, the results of rhizotomy and ganglionectomy are singly disappointing and can be recommended only when completion of the rhizotomy would result in alleviation of peripheral hyperpathia. Likewise, sympathectomy in the setting of chronic limb distress is unpredictable. The stimulatory therapies seem to offer much more promise, with additional work required to determine the proper role of implantable narcotic reservoirs. The spinal cord stimulator appears to be useful in carefully selected patients. Overall, however, these disappointing results further underscore the need to emphasize careful preoperative planning before any lumbar surgery, with the objective of creating fewer chronic benign pain syndromes.

References

1. Abbe, R.: Intradural section of the spinal nerves for neuralgia. Boston Med. Surg. J. *135*:329–335, 1889.

2. Adriansen, H., Gybels, J., Handwerker, H. O., and VanHees, J.: Nociceptor discharges and sensations due to prolonged noxious mechanical stimulation—a paradox. Hum. Neurobiol. *3*:53–58, 1984.
3. Amadio, P. C.: Pain dysfunction syndrome. J. Bone Joint Surg. Am. *70*:944, 1988.
4. Arens, L. J., Peacock, W. J., and Peter, J.: Selective posterior rhizotomy: A long-term study. Childs Nerv. Syst. *5*:148–152, 1982.
5. Arias, M. J.: Percutaneous retrogasserian glycerol rhizotomy for trigeminal neuralgia: A prospective study of 100 cases. J. Neurosurg. *65*:32–36, 1986.
6. Auld, A. W., Maki-Jolkela, A., and Murdoch, D. W.: Intraspinal narcotic analgesia in the treatment of chronic pain. Spine *10*:778–781, 1985.
7. Auld, A. W., Murdoch, D. W., and O'Laughlin, K. A.: Intraspinal narcotic analgesic pain management in the failed laminectomy syndrome. Spine *12*:953–955, 1987.
8. Barolat, G., Massaro, F., He, J., et al.: Mapping of sensory responses to epidural stimulation of the intraspinal neural structures in man. J. Neurosurg. *78*:223–239, 1993.
9. Barrash, J. M., and Leavens, M. E.: Dorsal rhizotomy for the relief of intractable pain of malignant tumor origin. J. Neurosurg. *38*:755–757, 1973.
10. Bashbaum, A. I., and Fields, H. L.: Endogenous pain control mechanisms: Review and hypothesis. Ann. Neurol. *4*:451–462, 1978.
11. Beck, D. W., Olson, J. J., and Urig, E. J.: Percutaneous retrogasserian glycerol rhizotomy for treatment of trigeminal neuralgia. J. Neurosurg. *65*:28–31, 1986.
12. Beck, P. W., Handwerker, H. O., and Zimmerman, M.: Nervous outflow from the cat's foot during noxious radiant heat stimulation. Brain Res. *67*:373–386, 1974.
13. Bederson, J. B., and Wilson, C. B.: Evaluation of microvascular decompression and partial sensory rhizotomy in 252 cases of trigeminal neuralgia. J. Neurosurg. *71*:359–367, 1989.
14. Bennett, M. H., and Lunsford, L. D.: Percutaneous retrogasserian glycerol rhizotomy for tic douloureux. Part 2. Results and implications of trigeminal evoked potential studies. Neurosurgery *14*:431–435, 1984.
15. Bernard, T. N., Broussard, T. S., Dwyer, A. P., and LaRocca, S. H.: Extradural sensory rhizotomy in the management of chronic lumbar spondylosis with radiculopathy. Orthop. Trans. *11*:23, 1987.
16. Bertrand, G.: The battered root problem. Orthop. Clin. North Am. *6*:305–310, 1975.
17. Besson, P., and Pere, E. R.: Response of cutaneous sensory units with unmyelinated fibers to noxious stimuli. J. Neurophysiol. *32*:1025–1043, 1969.
18. Blume, H., Richardson, R., and Rojas, C.: Epidural nerve stimulation of the lower spinal cord and cauda equina for the relief of intractable pain in failed low back surgery. Appl. Neurophysiol. *45*:456–460, 1982.
19. Bogduk, N., Tynan, W., and Wilson, A. S.: The nerve supply to the human lumbar intervertebral disc. J. Anat. *132*:39, 1981.
20. Burton, C.: Instrumentation for dorsal column stimulator implantation. Surg. Neurol. *2*:39–40, 1974.
21. Cahan, L. D., Kundi, M. S., McPherson, D., et al.: Electrophysiologic studies in selective dorsal rhizotomy for spasticity in children in cerebral palsy. Appl. Neurophysiol. *50*:459–463, 1987.
22. Calvin, W. H.: Generation of spike trains in CNS neurons. Brain Res. *84*:1–22, 1975.
23. Clark, K.: Electrical stimulation of the nervous system for control of pain: University of Texas Southwestern Medical School experience. Surg. Neurol. *4*:164–166, 1975.
24. Coggeshall, R. E.: Afferent fibers in the ventral root. Neurosurgery *4*:443–448, 1979.
25. Coombs, D. W., Saunders, R. L., Gaynor, M., and Pagean, M. G.: Epidural narcotic infusion reservoir: Implantation and efficacy. Anesthesiology *56*:469, 1982.
26. Coombs, D. W., Saunders, R. L., and Pagean, M. G.: Continuous intraspinal narcotic analgesia: Technical aspects of an implantable infusion system. Reg. Anesth. *7*:110, 1982.
27. Cosendy, B. A., Dupasquier, G., Buchser, E., and Chapuis, G.:

Epidural administration of morphine by a completely implantable device. Helv. Chir. Acta *56:*125, 1986.

28. Cowie, R. A., and Hitchcock, E. R.: The late results of anterolateral cordotomy for pain relief. Acta Neurosurg. *64:*39–50, 1982.

29. Davis, L., and Pollock, L. J.: The peripheral pathway for painful sensation. Arch. Neurol. Psychiatry *24:*883–898, 1930.

30. De La Porte, C., and Siegfried, J.: Lumbosacral spinal fibrosis (spinal arachnoiditis): Its diagnosis and treatment by spinal cord stimulation. Spine *8:*593–603, 1983.

31. De La Porte, C., and Van de Kelft, E.: Spinal cord stimulation in failed back surgery syndrome. Pain *52:*55–61, 1993.

32. Destouet, J. M., Giula, L. A., Murphy, W. A., and Monsees, B.: Lumbar facet joint injection: Indication, technique, clinical correlation and preliminary rehabilitation. Radiology *145:*321–345, 1982.

33. Devor, M.: Nerve pathophysiology and mechanisms of pain in causalgia. J. Auton. Nerv. Syst. *7:*371–384, 1983.

34. Devulder, J., De Colvenaer, I., Rolly, G., et al.: Spinal cord stimulation in chronic pain therapy. Clin. J. Pain *6:*51–56, 1990.

35. Devulder, J., Vermeulen, H., De Colvenaer, L., et al.: Spinal cord stimulation in chronic pain: Evaluation of results, complications, and technical considerations in sixty-nine patients. Clin. J. Pain *7:*21–28, 1991.

36. Dieckmann, G., and Veras, G.: Plexus avulsion pain (neurogenic pain): High frequency coagulation of the dorsal root entry zone in patients with deafferentation pain. Acta Neurosurg. *33*(Suppl.):445–450, 1984.

37. Downing, J. E., Busch, E. H., and Stedman, P. M.: Epidural morphine delivered by a percutaneous epidural catheter for outpatient treatment of cancer pain. Anesth. Analg. *67:*1159, 1988.

38. Dubuisson, D.: Root surgery. *In* Wall, P. D., and Melzack, R. (eds.): Textbook of Pain. 2nd ed. New York, Churchill Livingstone, 1989, pp. 784–794.

39. Dykes, R. W., and Terzis, J. K.: Spinal nerve distributions in the upper limb: The organization of the dermatome and afferent myotome. Philos. Trans. R. Soc. Lond. (Biol.) *293:*509–554, 1981.

40. Fassano, V. A., Broggi, G., and Zeme, S.: Intraoperative electrical stimulation for functional posterior rhizotomy. Scand. J. Rehabil. Med. Suppl. *17:*149–154, 1988.

41. Florez, G., Eiras, J., and Ucar, S.: Percutaneous rhizotomy of the articular nerve of Luschka for low back and sciatic pain. Acta Neurochir. Suppl. *24:*67–71, 1977.

42. Fock, S., and Mense, S.: Excitatory effects of 5-hydroxytryptamine, histamine and potassium ions of muscular group IV afferent units: A comparison with bradykinin. Brain Res. *105:*459–469, 1976.

43. Foerster, O.: The dermatomes in man. Brain *56:*1–39, 1933.

44. Frankel, S. A., and Prokop, J. D.: The value of cordotomy for the relief of pain. N. Engl. J. Med. *264:*971–974, 1961.

45. French, L. A.: High cervical tractotomy: Techniques and results. Clin. Neurosurg. *21:*239–245, 1974.

46. Friedman, A. H., and Bullitt, E.: Dorsal root entry zone lesions in the treatment of pain following brachial plexus avulsion, spinal cord injury, and herpes zoster. Appl. Neurophysiol. *51:*164–169, 1988.

47. Friedman, A. H., Nashold, B. R., and Bronec, P. R.: Dorsal root entry zone lesions for the treatment of brachial plexus avulsion injuries: A follow-up study. Neurosurgery *22:*369–377, 1988.

48. Frykholm, R., Hyde, J., Norlen, G., and Skogluna, C. R.: On pain sensations produced by stimulation of ventral roots in man. Acta Physiol. Scand. Suppl. *106:*457–469, 1953.

49. Greenberg, H., Ensminger, W., Tarin, J., and Doan, K.: Benefit from and tolerance to continuous intrathecal infusion of morphine for intractable cancer pain. Clin. Res. *30:*417A, 1982.

50. Hakelius, A.: Prognosis in sciatica. Acta Orthop. Scand. Suppl. *129:*1076, 1970.

51. Handwerker, H. O., Anton, F., and Rees, P. W.: Discharge patterns of afferent cutaneous nerve fibers from the rat's tail during prolonged noxious mechanical stimulation. Exp. Brain Res. *65:*493–504, 1987.

52. Head, H.: On disturbances of sensation with especial reference to the pain of nerve disease. Brain *16:*1–133, 1893.

53. Hodgson, A. R.: Mechanisms of spinal pain. *In* Wall, P. D., and

Melzack, R. (eds.): Textbook of Pain. 2nd ed. New York, Churchill Livingstone, 1989, p. 245.

54. Hoppenstein, R.: Electrical stimulation of the ventral and dorsal columns of the spinal cord for relief of chronic intractable pain: Preliminary report. Surg. Neurol. *4:*187–194, 1975.

55. Howe, J. F., Loeser, J. D., and Calvin, W. H.: Mechanosensitivity of dorsal root ganglia and chronically injured axons: A physiological basis for the radicular pain of nerve root compression. Pain *3:*25–41, 1977.

56. Husson, J. L., Meadeb, J., Eudier, F., and Maase, A.: Treatment of chronic pain of the musculoskeletal system by epidural stimulation. J. Chir. (Paris) *125:*522–524, 1988.

57. Jain, K. K.: Nerve root scarring and arachnoiditis as a complication of lumbar intervertebral disc surgery: Surgical treatment. Neurochirurgia *17:*185–192, 1974.

58. Jones, N. F.: Ischemia of the hand in systemic disease: The potential role of microsurgical revascularization and digital sympathectomy. Clin. Plast. Surg. *16:*547–556, 1989.

59. Kadson, D. L., and Lathi, E. S.: A prospective study of radiofrequency rhizotomy in the treatment of post-traumatic spasticity. Neurosurgery *15:*526–529, 1984.

60. Kibler, R. F., and Nathan, P. W.: Relief of pain and paraesthesia by nerve block distal to a lesion. J. Neurol. Neurosurg. Psychiatry *23:*91–98, 1960.

61. Kirk, E. J.: Impulses in dorsal spinal nerve rootlets in cats and rabbits arising from dorsal root ganglia isolated from the periphery. J. Comp. Neurol. *2:*165–176, 1974.

62. Koeze, T. H. E., Williams, A. C. de C., and Reiman, S.: Spinal cord stimulation and the relief of chronic pain. J. Neurol. Neurosurg. Psychiatry *50:*1424–1429, 1987.

63. Korenman, E. M. D., and Devor, M.: Ectopic adrenergic sensitivity in damaged peripheral nerve axons in rats. Exp. Neurol. *72:*63–81, 1981.

64. Krainick, J. U., and Thoden, U.: Spinal cord stimulation. *In* Wall, P. H., and Melzack, R. (eds.): Textbook of Pain. 2nd ed. New York, Churchill Livingstone, 1989, p. 924.

65. Krainick, J. U., Toden, U., and Reichert, T.: Spinal cord stimulation in post amputation pain. Surg. Neurol. *4:*167–170, 1975.

66. Kumar, K., Nath, R., and Wyant, G. M.: Treatment of chronic pain by epidural spinal cord stimulation: A 10-year experience. J. Neurosurg. *75:*402–407, 1991.

67. Kumar, K., Wyant, G. M., and Ekong, C. E. U.: Epidural spinal cord stimulation for relief of chronic pain. Pain Clinic *1:* 91–99, 1986.

68. Kundi, M., Cahan, L., and Starr, A.: Somatosensory-evoked potentials in cerebral palsy after partial dorsal root rhizotomy. Arch. Neurol. *46:*524–527, 1989.

69. Laitinen, L. V., Nilsson, S., and Fugl-Meyer, A. R.: Selective posterior rhizotomy for treatment of spasticity. J. Neurosurg. *58:*895–899, 1983.

70. Lankford, L. L.: Reflex sympathetic dystrophy. *In* Hunter, J. M. (ed.): Rehabilitation of the Hand. 2nd ed. St. Louis, C. V. Mosby Co., 1989, pp. 509–532.

71. Larson, S. J., Sances, A., Jr., Cusick, J. F., et al.: A comparison between anterior and posterior spinal implant systems. Surg. Neurol. *4:*180–186, 1975.

72. Law, J. D.: A new method for targeting a spinal stimulator. Appl. Neurophysiol. *58:*437–438, 1987.

73. Law, J. D.: Targeting a spinal stimulator to treat the "failed back surgery syndrome." Appl. Neurophysiol. *58:*437–438, 1982.

74. Leclercq, T. A., and Russo, E.: La stimulation epiduralale dan le traitement des douleurs chroniques. Neurochirurgie *27:* 125–128, 1981.

75. LeDoux, M. S., and Landford, K. H.: Spinal cord stimulation for the failed back syndrome. Spine *18:*191–194, 1993.

76. LeRoy, P. L.: Stimulation of the spinal neuraxis by biocompatible electrical current in the human. Appl. Neurophysiol. *44:*187–193, 1981.

77. Levine, J. D., Gooding, J., Donatoni, P., et al.: The role of polymorphonuclear leukocytes in hyperalgesia. J. Neurosci. *5:*3025–3029, 1985.

78. Lewis, T.: Experiments related to cutaneous hyperalgesia and its spread through somatic fibers. Clin. Sci. *2:*373–423, 1935.

79. Liew, E., and Hui, Y.: A preliminary study of long-term epidural

morphine for cancer pain via a subcutaneously implanted reservoir. Ma Tsui Hsuech Tsa Chi 27:5–12, 1989.

80. Linderoth, B., Gazellus, B., Franck, J., and Brodin, E.: Release of neuromediators in cat dorsal horn by dorsal column stimulation: Studies using microdialysis. Pain Suppl. 5:228, 1990.

81. Linsey, S. J. W., and Devor, M.: After discharge and interactions among fibers in damaged peripheral nerve in the rat. Brain Res. 415:122–136, 1987.

82. Loeser, J. D.: Dorsal rhizotomy for the relief of chronic pain. J. Neurosurg. 36:745–750, 1972.

83. Long, D. M., Erickson, D., Campbell, J., and North, R.: Electrical stimulation of the spinal cord and peripheral nerves for pain control: A 10-year experience. Appl. Neurophysiol. 44:207–217, 1981.

84. Lord, S. M., Barnsley, L., and Bogduk, N.: Percutaneous radiofrequency neurotomy in the treatment of cervical zygoapophyseal joint pain. Neurosurgery 36:732–739, 1995.

85. McCulloch, D. W.: Percutaneous radiofrequency lumbar rhizolysis (rhizotomy). Appl. Neurophysiol. 39:87–96, 1976.

86. McLaughlin, T. P., Banta, J. V., Gahm, N. H., and Raycroft, J. F.: Intraspinal rhizotomy and distal cordectomy in patients with myelomeningocele. J. Bone Joint Surg. Am. 68:88–94, 1986.

87. Meglio, M., Cioni, B., Prezioso, A., and Talamonti, G.: Spinal cord stimulation in the treatment of post-therapeutic pain. Acta Neurochir. Suppl. (Wien) 46:65–66, 1989.

88. Meglio, M., Cioni, B., and Rossi, G. F.: Spinal cord stimulation in management of chronic pain: A nine year experience. J. Neurosurg. 70:519–524, 1989.

89. Meilman, P. W., Leibrock, L. G., and Leong, F. T. L.: Outcome of implanted spinal cord stimulation in the treatment of chronic pain: Arachnoiditis versus single nerve root injury and mononeuropathy. Clin. J. Pain 5:189–193, 1989.

90. Melzack, R., and Wall, P. D.: Pain mechanisms: A new theory. Science 150:971–979, 1965.

91. Mittal, B., Thomas, D. G. T., Walton, P., and Calder, I.: Dorsal column stimulation (DCS) in chronic pain: Report of 31 cases. Ann. R. Coll. Surg. Engl. 69:104–109, 1987.

92. Mockus, M. G., Rutherford, R. B., Rosales, C., and Peach, W. H.: Sympathectomy for causalgia: Patient selection and long-term results. Arch. Surg. 122:688, 1987.

93. Mooney, V., and Robertson, J.: The facet syndrome. Clin. Orthop. 115:149–156, 1976.

94. Moran, R., O'Connell, P., and Walsh, M. G.: The diagnostic value of facet joint injection. Spine 13:1402–1410, 1987.

95. Mulcahy, J. J., and Young, A. B.: Percutaneous radiofrequency sacral rhizotomy in the treatment of the hyporeflexic bladder. J. Urol. 120:557–558, 1978.

96. Nashold, B. S., and Ostdahl, R. H.: Dorsal root entry zone lesions for pain relief. J. Neurosurg. 51:59–69, 1979.

97. Neilson, K. D., Adams, J. E., and Hosobuchi, Y.: Experience with dorsal column stimulation for relief of chronic intractable pain. Surg. Neurol. 4:148–154, 1975.

98. Neville, B. G.: Selective dorsal rhizotomy for spastic cerebral palsy. Dev. Med. Child Neurol. 30:395–398, 1988.

99. Noordenbos, W., and Wall, P. D.: Implications of the failure of nerve resection and graft to cure chronic pain produced by nerve diseases. J. Neurol. Neurosurg. Psychiatry 44:1068–1073, 1981.

100. Norman, P. E., and House, A. K.: The early use of lumbar sympathectomy in peripheral vascular disease. J. Cardiovasc. Surg. (Torino) 29:717–722, 1988.

101. North, R. B., Ewend, M. G., Lawton, M. T., and Piantadosi, S.: Spinal cord stimulation of chronic, intractable pain: Superiority of "multi-channel" devices. Pain 44:119–130, 1991.

102. North, R. B., Ewend, M. G., Lawton, M. T., et al.: Failed back surgery syndrome: 5-year follow-up after spinal cord stimulator implantation. Neurosurgery 28:692–699, 1991.

103. North, R. B., Kidd, D. H., Campbell, J. N., and Long, D. M.: Dorsal root ganglionectomy for failed back surgery syndrome: A five year follow-up study. J. Neurosurg. 74:236–242, 1991.

104. North, R. B., Kidd, D. H., Lee, M. S., and Piantadosi, S.: A prospective, randomized study of spinal cord stimulation versus reoperation for failed back surgery syndrome: Initial results. Stereotact. Funct. Neurosurg. 62:2067–2072, 1994.

105. North, R. B., Kidd, D. H., Zahurak, M., et al.: Spinal cord stimulation for chronic intractable pain: Experience over two decades. Neurosurgery 32:384–395, 1993.

106. Nunn, D., Gregg, J., Ambrose, W., and Hanker, J.: Histochemical study of autonomic fiber sprouting in traumatic neuromata. J. Dent. Res. 61:258, 1982.

107. O'Brien, J. P.: Mechanisms of spinal pain. In Wall, P. D., and Melzack, R. (eds.): Textbook of Pain. 2nd ed. New York, Churchill Livingstone, 1989, p. 244.

108. O'Connell, J. E.: Anterolateral cordotomy for intractable pain in carcinoma of the rectum. Proc. R. Soc. Med. 62:1223–1225, 1969.

109. Onofrio, B., and Campa, H.: Evaluation of rhizotomy. J. Neurosurg. 36:751–755, 1972.

110. Onofrio, B., Yaksh, T., and Arnold, D.: Continuous low-dose intrathecal morphine administration in treatment of chronic pain of malignant origin. Mayo Clin. Proc. 45:516, 1981.

111. Oppenheim, W. L.: Selective posterior rhizotomy for spastic cerebral palsy: A review. Clin. Orthop. 253:20–29, 1990.

112. Osgood, C. P., Dujorney, M., Faille, R., and Abassy, M.: Microsurgical ganglionectomy for chronic pain syndromes. J. Neurosurg. 45:113–118, 1976.

113. Oudenhoven, R. C.: The role of laminectomy, facet rhizotomy, and epidural steroids. Spine 4:145–147, 1979.

114. Pallie, W.: The intersegmental anastomoses of posterior spinal rootlets and their significance. J. Neurosurg. 16:188–195, 1959.

115. Pedersen, H. E., Blunck, C. F. J., and Gardner, E.: Anatomy of lumbosacral posterior rami and meningeal branches of spinal nerves. J. Bone Joint Surg. Am. 38:377, 1956.

116. Perelman, R. B., Adler, D., and Humphreys, M.: Reflex sympathetic dystrophy: Electronic thermography as an aid in diagnosis. Orthop. Rev. 16:561, 1987.

117. Phillips, F. M., Wetzel, F. T., Bernard, T. N., et al.: Extradural sensory rhizotomy in the management of chronic radiculopathy after failed lumbar surgery. Orthop. Trans. 19:361, 1995.

118. Pineda, A.: Dorsal column stimulation and its prospects. Surg. Neurol. 4:157–163, 1975.

119. Pochaczevsky, R.: Thermography in post-traumatic pain. Am. J. Sports Med. 15:243, 1982.

120. Porter, R. W., Hohmann, G. W., Bors, E., and French, J. D.: Cordotomy for pain following cauda equina injury. Arch. Surg. 92:765–770, 1986.

121. Powers, S. K., Adams, J. E., Edwards, M. S. B., et al.: Pain relief from dorsal root entry zone lesion made with argon and carbon dioxide microsurgical lasers. J. Neurosurg. 61:841–847, 1984.

122. Powers, S. K., Barbaro, N. M., and Levy, R. M.: Pain control with laster produced dorsal root entry zone lesions. Appl. Neurophysiol. 51:243–254, 1988.

123. Rashkind, R.: Analytical review of open cordotomy. Int. Surg. 51:226–231, 1969.

124. Reeh, P. W., Bayer, J., Kocher, L., and Handwerker, H. O.: Sensitization of nociceptive cutaneous fibers from the rat tail by noxious mechanical stimulation. Exp. Brain Res. 65:505–572, 1987.

125. Rees, W. E. S.: Multiple bilateral subcutaneous rhizolysis of segmental nerves in the treatment of the intervertebral disc syndrome. Ann. Gen. Pract. 16:126, 1971.

126. Richardson, B. P., and Engel, G.: The pharmacology and function of 5HT3 receptors. Trends Neurosci. 9:424, 1986.

127. Richardson, R. R., Siqueira, E. B., and Cerullo, L. J.: Spinal epidural neurostimulation for treatment of acute and chronic intractable pain: Initial and long term results. Neurosurgery 5:344–348, 1979.

128. Rockswold, G. L., Bradly, W. E., and Chou, S. N.: Differential sacral rhizotomy in the treatment of neurologenic bladder dysfuncion: Preliminary report of six cases. J. Neurosurg. 38:748–754, 1973.

129. Rockswold, G. L., Chou, S. N., and Bradly, W. E.: Re-evaluation of differential sacral rhizotomy for neurological bladder disease. J. Neurosurg. 48:773–778, 1978.

130. St. Marie, B.: Administration of intraspinal analgesia in the home care setting. J. Intra. Nurs. 12:164, 1989.

131. Scadding, J. W.: Development of ongoing activity, mechanosensitivity and adrenalin sensitivity in severed peripheral nerve axons. Exp. Neurol. 73:345–364, 1981.

132. Schaerer, J. P.: Radiofrequency facet rhizotomy in the treatment of chronic neck and low back pain. Int. Surg. *63*:53–59, 1978.

133. Scoville, W. B.: Extradural spinal sensory rhizotomy. J. Neurosurg. *25*:94–95, 1966.

134. Shealy, C. N.: Dorsal column stimulation: Optimization of application. Surg. Neurol. *4*:142–145, 1975.

135. Shealy, C. N.: Percutaneous radiofrequency denervation of spinal facets: Treatment for chronic back pain and sciatica. J. Neurosurg. *43*:448, 1975.

136. Shealy, C. N., Mortimer, J. T., and Hagfor, N. R.: Dorsal column electroanalgesia. J. Neurosurg. *32*:560–564, 1970.

137. Shealy, C. N., Mortimer, J. T., and Resturek, J. B.: Electrical inhibition of pain by stimulation of the dorsal column: Preliminary clinical report. Anesth. Analg. *46*:489–491, 1967.

138. Shelden, C. H., Paul, F., Jacques, D. B., and Pudenz, R. H.: Electrical stimulation of the nervous system. Surg. Neurol. *4*:127–132, 1975.

139. Sherrington, C. S.: Experiments in the examination of the peripheral distribution of the fibers of the posterior roots of some spinal nerves. Philos. Trans. R. Soc. Lond. (Biol.) *190*:45–186, 1898.

140. Siegfried, J., and Lazorthes, Y.: Long-term follow-up for dorsal cord stimulation for chronic pain syndrome after multiple lumbar operations. Appl. Neurophysiol. *45*:201–204, 1982.

141. Simpson, B. A.: Spinal cord stimulation in 60 cases of intractable pain. J. Neurol. Neurosurg. Psychiatr. *54*:196–199, 1991.

142. Sjogren, P., Banning, A. R., and Henriken, H.: High dose epidural opioid treatment of malignant pain. Ugeskr. Laeger *151*:25–28, 1989.

143. Sluijter, M. E.: Percutaneous facet denervation and partial posterior rhizotomy. Acta Anaesthesiol. Belg. *1*:63–69, 1981.

144. Spiegelmann, R., and Friedman, W.: Spinal cord stimulation: A contemporary series. Neurosurgery *28*:65–71, 1991.

145. Spiller, W. G., and Martin, E.: The treatment of persistent pain of organic origin in the lower part of the body by division of the anterolateral column of the spinal cord. JAMA *58*:1489–1490, 1912.

146. Stanton-Hicks, M., Janig, W., Hassenbusch, S., et al.: Reflex sympathetic dystrophy: Changing concepts and taxonomy. Pain *63*:127–133, 1995.

147. Storrs, B. B., and Nishide, T.: Use of the H reflex recovery curve in selective posterior rhizotomy. Pediatr. Neurosci. *14*:120–123, 1988.

148. Strait, T. A., and Hunter, S. E.: Intraspinal extradural sensory rhizotomy in patients with failure of lumbar disc surgery. J. Neurosurg. *54*:193–196, 1981.

149. Sweet, W. H., and Wepsic, J. G.: Treatment of chronic pain by stimulation of fibers of primary afferent nerves. Trans. Am. Neurol. Assoc. *93*:103–107, 1968.

150. Sykes, M. T., and Coggeshall, R. E.: Unmyelinated fibers in the human L4 and L5 ventral roots. Brain Res. *63*:490–495, 1973.

151. Tasker, R. R.: Percutaneous cordotomy—the lateral high cervical technique. *In* Schmidek, H. H., and Sweet, W. H. (eds.): Operative Neurosurgical Techniques: Indications, Methods, and Results. New York, Grune & Stratton, 1982, pp. 1137–1153.

152. Tasker, R. R.: Percutaneous cordotomy—the lateral high cervical technique. *In* Schmidek, H. H., and Sweet, W. H. (eds.): Operative Neurosurgical Techniques: Indications, Methods, and Results. New York, Grune & Stratton, 1988, pp. 1191–1205.

153. Tasker, R. R., and Dostrovsky, J. O.: Deafferentation and central pain. *In* Wall, P. D., and Melzack, R. (eds.): Textbook of Pain. 2nd ed. New York, Churchill Livingstone, 1989, pp. 154–186.

154. Tasker, R. R., Gervasio, T. C., DeCarvahlo, T. C., and Dolan, E. J.: Intractable pain of spinal cord origin: Clinical features and implications for surgery. J. Neurosurg. *77*:373–378, 1992.

155. Tasker, R. R., Organ, L. W., and Hawrylyshyn, P.: Deafferentation and causalgia. *In* Bonica, J. J. (ed.): Pain. New York, Raven Press, 1980, pp. 305–329.

156. Thomas, D. E. T., and Sheehy, J.: Dorsal root entry zone coagulation (Nashold's procedure) in brachial plexus avulsion. J. Neurol. Neurosurg. Psychiatry *45*:949, 1982.

157. Toczek, S. K., McCullough, D. C., Gargour, G. W., et al.: Selective

158. Turnbull, I. M.: Percutaneous lumbar rhizotomy for spasms in paraplegia. Paraplegia *21*:131–136, 1983.

159. Urban, B. J., and Nashold, B. S.: Percutaneous epidural stimulation of the spinal cord for relief of pain: Long term results. J. Neurosurg. *48*:323–328, 1978.

160. van Driel, R., van Bockel, J. H., and van Schilfgaarde, R.: Lumbar sympathectomy for severe lower limb ischemia: Results and analysis of factors influencing the outcome. J. Cardiovasc. Surg. (Torino) *79*:310–314, 1988.

161. van Loveren, H., Tew, J. M., Jr., Keller, J. T., and Nurre, M. A.: A ten-year experience in the treatment of trigeminal neuralgia: Comparison of percutaneous stereotaxic rhizotomy and posterior fossa exploration. J. Neurosurg. *57*:757–764, 1982.

162. Vogel, H. P., Heppner, B., Humbs, N., et al.: Long-term effects of spinal cord stimulation in chronic pain syndromes. J. Neurol. *233*:16–18, 1986.

163. Waisbrod, H., and Gerbershagen, H. U.: Spinal cord stimulation in patients with a battered root syndrome. Arch. Orthop. Trauma. Surg. *104*:62–64, 1985.

164. Wall, P. D.: Introduction. *In* Wall, P. D., and Melzack, R. (eds.): Textbook of Pain. 2nd ed. New York, Churchill Livingstone, 1989, p. 13.

165. Wall, P. D., and Devor, M.: The effect of peripheral nerve injury on dorsal root potentials and on transmission of afferent signals into the spinal cord. Brain Res. *209*:95–111, 1981.

166. Wall, P. D., and Devor, M.: Sensory afferent impulses originate from the dorsal root ganglia as well as from the periphery in normal and nerve injured rats. Pain *17*:321–339, 1983.

167. Wall, P. D., and Gutnick, M.: Ongoing activity in peripheral nerves: The physiology and pharmacology of impulses originating from a nerve. Exp. Neurol. *45*:576–589, 1974.

168. Wall, P. D., and Sweet, W. H.: Temporary ablation of pain in man. Science *155*:108–109, 1967.

169. Walsh, J. A., Glynn, C. J., Cousiss, M. I., and Basidow, R. W.: Blood flow, sympathetic activity and pain relief following lumbar sympathetic blockade or surgical sympathectomy. Anesth. Int. Care *13*:18, 1985.

170. Wang, J. K., Johnson, K. A., and Istrup, C. M.: Sympathetic blocks for reflex sympathetic dystrophy. Pain *23*:13, 1985.

171. Wester, K.: Dorsal column stimulation in pain treatment. Acta Neurol. Scand. *75*:151–155, 1987.

172. Wetzel, F. T., LaRocca, S. H., and Adinolfi, M.: The role of sympathectomy in treatment of chronic limb distress following failed lumbar surgery: A preliminary report. Clin. Ther. *1*:71–76, 1989.

173. Wetzel, F. T., LaRocca, S. H., and Adinolfi, M.: The treatment of chronic extremity pain in failed lumbar surgery: The role of lumbar sympathectomy. Spine *17*:1462–1468, 1992.

174. Wetzel, F. T., Phillips, F., Bernard, T. N., et al.: Extradural sensory rhizotomy in the management of chronic lumbar radiculopathy: A minimum two year follow-up study. Spine *22*:2283–2292, 1997.

175. White, J. C.: Posterior rhizotomy: A possible substitute for cordotomy in otherwise intractable neuralgia of the trunk and extremities of nonmalignant origin. Clin. Neurosurg. *13*:20–41, 1965.

176. White, J. C., and Sweet, W. H.: Pain and the Neurosurgeon: A 40-Year Experience. Springfield, IL, Charles C Thomas, 1969.

177. Wiegand, H., and Winkelmuller, W.: Behandlung des Deafferentierungsschmerzes durch Hoch-frequenzlasion der Hinterwurzeleintrittszone. Deutsch. Med. Wochenschr. *110*:216–220, 1985.

178. Wilkins, R. H.: Neurosurgical Classics. New York, Johnson Reprint Corp., 1968, pp. 504–515.

179. Wynn-Parry, C. B.: The failed back. *In* Wall, P. D., and Melzack, R. (eds.): Textbook of Pain. 2nd ed. New York, Churchill Livingstone, 1989, pp. 341–354.

180. Xavier, A. V., McDanal, J., and Kissin, I.: Relief of sciatic radicular pain by sciatic nerve block. Anesth. Analg. *67*:1177–1180, 1988.

181. Young, R. R.: Evaluation of dorsal column stimulation in the treatment of chronic pain. Neurosurgery *3*:373–379, 1978.

sacral rootlet rhizotomy for hypertonic neurogenic bladder. J. Neurosurg. *42*:567–574, 1975.

Index

Page numbers in *italics* refer to illustrations; numbers followed by t indicate tables.

Paralysis (*Continued*)
  ascending, in cervical cord injury, 977, *978, 979,* 980
  in idiopathic scoliosis, intraoperative, 363, 369
    postoperative, 363, 369
  in tuberculosis, 1246
    pathogenesis of, 1236
  in vertebral osteomyelitis, pathogenesis of, 1211, *1212–1215*
  predisposing factors for, 1211, 1229
Paraneoplastic myelopathies, 1424–1425
Paraplegia. See also *Neurologic complications; Paralysis; Spinal cord injury.*
  after open thoracotomy, 1727
  birth injury, 419
  degenerative sacroiliac changes in, anky-losing spondylitis vs., 436, *437*
  due to cervical spine surgery, 1726
  due to vascular complications, 1715
  hereditary spastic, 1427
  postoperative, remote from surgical site, 1728
Parapophyses, 29, *34, 35*
Parasitic myelopathy, 1420
Paraspinal muscles, denervation of, after surgery, 693
Paraspinous abscess, in vertebral osteomyelitis, 1210, *1212–1215*
Parastremmatic dysplasia, 313–314
Parathyroid hormone, in calcium homeostasis, 1266
Paravertebral abscess, in tuberculosis, drainage of, 1241
Paraxial mesoderm, 4
Paroxysmal torticollis of infancy, benign, 264
Pars interarticularis, 30–31, *30, 31*
  defects in, in pediatric patient, 197–198, *200–202*
    magnetic resonance imaging of, 196
    repair of, for spondylolisthesis, 856
  fracture of, in pediatric patient, 198, 424–425
  in spondylolisthesis, 839
Pars laminalis, 30, *30.* See also *Lamina(e).*
Pars pedicularis, 30, *30.* See also *Pedicle(s).*
Patch grafting, for dural tear, 1736, *1736*
Patellar tendon reflex, in lumbar radiculopathy, 632
Patient positioning, for lumbar spine surgery, vascular complications and, 1719–1720
  for posterior spinal surgery, complications related to, 1695
  peripheral nerve injury and, 1730–1731, *1730*
Peak plate, 536
Pediatric patients, 185–425
  back pain in, 187–220. See also *Back pain, pediatric.*
  cervical laminectomy in, kyphosis after, 1687–1688
    prevention of, 1689
  cervical spine mobility in, normal varia-tions in, 228, *229,* 251
  congenital anomalies in. See also specific anomalies.
    of cervical spine, 221–264
    of spinal cord, 267–302
  disc calcification in, 219, 585
  disc herniation in, lumbar, 203–205, *204, 205*
    microsurgery for, 710
  discitis in, 210–211, 317–322
  epidural abscess in, treatment of, 1234–1235

Pediatric patients (*Continued*)
  halo skeletal fixator application in, *1120,* 1122–1123
  inflammatory rheumatic disorders in, 218–219
  intraspinal infection in, 1377–1378
  kyphosis in, 405–414
  limb pain in, differential diagnosis of, 211t
  metabolic disorders in, 311–313. See also specific disorders.
  osteomyelitis in, 212
    clinical presentation of, 1211, *1216,* 1218
    prognosis in, 1229
  psychosomatic pain in, 219–220
  roentgenographic examination of cervical spine in, 904
  Scheuermann's disease in, 207–208, *208*
  scoliosis in, 209–210, 325–369. See also *Scoliosis.*
  skeletal dysplasias in, 303–311. See also specific disorders.
  slipped vertebral apophysis in, 206–207, *206*
  spinal trauma in, cervical, mechanisms of, 891–892
    lumbar, 417–425
    thoracic, 417–425
  spondylolisthesis in, 197–199, *199,* 199t, *200*
    symptoms of, 841–842
  spondylolysis in, 197–199, 200–202
  tuberculosis in, clinical presentation of, 1237
    kyphotic deformity due to, 1245–1246
  tumors in, of bone, 212–215, 1189–1190, 1189t
    of spinal cord, 216–218, *217*
Pedicle(s), 29–30, *30*
  fracture or sclerosis of, spondylolisthesis and, 846
  of axis, fracture of, 926–927, *926*
  of lumbar vertebrae, *34, 35*
  of thoracic vertebrae, *34, 35*
  width of, 1655, *1655*
Pedicle screw fixation, 1700
  anatomic considerations in, 1569–1570, *1569, 1570*
  complications of, *1696, 1697, 1699,* 1701–1702
  failure of, 1745–1746
  for lumbar disc disease, 666, 667
  for lumbar trauma, 1026–1029, *1028–1031*
  for spondylolisthesis, 870
  for thoracolumbar fracture, 1040
    complications of, 1044
  history of, 1643–1644, *1645*
  in vitro testing of systems for, 1051–1052, *1051–1054*
  indications and contraindications for, *1654*
  neurologic injury due to, 1729–1730, *1729*
  regulatory status of, 1644
  techniques for, 1654–1655, *1655, 1656*
Pelvic fracture, sacral fracture with, 893, 894
Pelvic splanchnic nerve, *1562,* 1565
Pelvic torsion test, in sacroiliac joint dysfunction, 772
Penicillin, for actinomycosis, 1247
  for spinal syphilis, 1420
Pennsylvania Plan Algorithm, for low back pain evaluation, 615–616, *616*
Pentazocine, 1823t, 1824
Peptic ulcer, in ankylosing spondylitis, 1351
Percutaneous discectomy. See under *Discectomy.*
Perichondrial zone blastema, 5, *6, 7*

Perichordal discs, 5–7, *6,* 13
Perichordal tube, 5
Perineural cyst, sciatica due to, 100, *100*
Perineurium, of spinal nerve, 84, *85*
Peripachymeningitis. See *Epidural abscess.*
Peritoneal perforation, with iliac crest harvest, 548, 1598, *1598*
Pernicious anemia, myelopathy due to, 1424
Peroneal nerve, common, injury to, with fibular graft harvest, 1599
  deep, injury to, with fibular graft harvest, *1592,* 1599
  entrapment of, *90,* 92
Peroneal neuropathy, diabetic, lumbar radiculopathy vs., 632, *632*
Peroneal vessels, injury to, with fibular graft harvest, *1592,* 1599
Pharyngeal approach to cervical spine, 1496–1498, *1498*
  for odontoid resection in ankylosing spon-dylitis, 1305–1307, *1307*
Pharyngeal artery, ascending, 53, *54,* 55–56
Pharyngeal nerve, 1482
Pharyngovertebral veins, 61
  hematogenous spread of infection and, 1210
Phencyclidine, for spinal cord injury, animal studies of, 1156
Phenoxybenzamine (Dibenzyline), for hypertensive crisis, after spinal cord injury, 994
Phenytoin, for chronic pain, 1825
  surgical complications with, 374
Philadelphia collar, *1099,* 1102–1103, *1105*
  applications for, 1110, *1111*
  cost of, 1116t
Phosphate homeostasis, 1265
Phospholipase A$_2$, activation of, in spinal cord injury, 1151, 1152
  in nucleus pulposus, inflammatory re-sponse to disc herniation and, 657–658
Phospholipase C, activation of, in spinal cord injury, 1151
Phosphoribosylpyrophosphate synthetase, excessive activity of, in gout, 448–449
Photodensitometry, radiographic, bone density assessment using, 1273
Phrenic nerve, *1467, 1481, 1482, 1483,* 1546–1547
  injury to, in cervical spine surgery, 545, 1512, 1726
Phrenic nerve stimulator, after spinal cord injury, 1136
Physeal plate, in immature spine, 418
  injury to, in immature spine, healing po-tential of, 423, *423*
Physical capacity assessment, in spinal functional restoration, 1792–1794, *1793, 1795*
Physical therapy. See also *Exercise; Manipulation.*
  for cervical disc disease, 493–494
  for lumbar disc disease, 643
  for sacroiliac pain, 1816
  levels of care in, 1791–1792
  with trigger point injection, 1820
Physiologic load, 1080
Pilonidal sinus, 296
Pin headrest, three-point, for intraoperative stabilization of cervical spine, 1495, *1496, 1497*
Piriformis syndrome, *90,* 91–92
Piroxicam, for back pain, in lumbar disc disease, 638